QM

24

D1577164

WITHDRAWN
FROM STOCK
QMUL LIBRARY

WN 17
4wk→
KEA
2001
(ORA)

D1577164

Atlas of NORMAL ROENTGEN VARIANTS THAT MAY SIMULATE DISEASE

Other Books by Theodore E. Keats

An Atlas of Normal Developmental Roentgen Anatomy
SECOND EDITION, with Thomas A. Smith

Emergency Radiology
SECOND EDITION

Atlas of Roentgenographic Measurement
SEVENTH EDITION

Radiology of Musculoskeletal Stress Injury
SECOND EDITION

Atlas of NORMAL ROENTGEN VARIANTS THAT MAY SIMULATE DISEASE

SEVENTH EDITION

Theodore E. Keats, M.D.

Professor of Radiology
Department of Radiology
University of Virginia Health System
Charlottesville, Virginia

Mark W. Anderson, M.D.

Associate Professor of Radiology
Department of Radiology
University of Virginia Health System
Charlottesville, Virginia

Mosby, Inc.
A Harcourt Health Sciences Company
St. Louis   London   Philadelphia   Sydney   Toronto

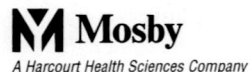
Mosby
A Harcourt Health Sciences Company

Acquisitions Editor: Janice M. Gaillard
Manuscript Editor: Jeffrey L. Scheib
Production Manager: Natalie Ware
Illustration Specialist: Peg Shaw
Book Designer: Marie Gardocky-Clifton

Copyright © 2001, 1996, 1992, 1988, 1984, 1979, 1973 by Mosby, Inc.

All rights reserved. No part of this publication may be reproduced or transmitted in any form or by any means, electronic or mechanical, including photocopy, recording, or any information storage and retrieval system, without permission in writing from the publisher.

Permission to photocopy or reproduce solely for internal or personal use is permitted for libraries or other users registered with the Copyright Clearance Center, provided that the base fee of $4.00 per chapter plus $.10 per page is paid directly to the Copyright Clearance Center, 222 Rosewood Drive, Danvers, Massachusetts 01923. This consent does not extend to other kinds of copying, such as copying for general distribution, for advertising or promotional purposes, for creating new collected works, or for resale.

Mosby, Inc.
A Harcourt Health Sciences Company
11830 Westline Industrial Drive
St. Louis, Missouri 63146

Printed in the United States of America.

Library of Congress Cataloging-in-Publication Data

Keats, Theodore E. (Theodore Eliot)

Altas of normal roentgen variants that may simulate disease / Theodore E. Keats, Mark W. Anderson.—7th ed.

p.   cm.

Includes index.

ISBN 0–323–01322–8

1. Radiography, Medical—Atlases.   2. Diagnostic errors—Atlases.   I. Anderson, Mark   II. Title.

RC78.2.K42 2001
616.07′572—dc21   00–051974

00 01 02 03 04 GW/KPT 9 8 7 6 5 4 3 2 1

To Dr. John F. Holt—
teacher, friend, and
the source of inspiration for this work

Foreword

My interest in anatomic variants dates back to World War II when, as a young 4-F Instructor in Radiology, it was my duty to intercept residents' film-reading queries on the way to "The Chief," hoping to save precious moments for our one and only professor, who was swamped with countless administrative problems in those days of severe manpower shortage. Eventually I kept score and discovered that, during one three-month period, the questions brought up by residents and fellow staff members regarding anatomic and physiologic variants outnumbered those concerning pathologic entities by three to one. Admittedly, a few of the aberrations that we initially thought to be variants eventually proved to be pathologic in nature, but the converse was true far more often, so I am reasonably certain that this ratio is at least as high today as it was thirty years ago.

When Caffey's classic text, *Pediatric X-Ray Diagnosis*, appeared in 1945 with its novel emphasis on anatomic variations, my interest in the subject was spurred again. In ensuing conversations and correspondence, Dr. Caffey repeatedly emphasized the great need for a comprehensive text on variants and artifacts encompassing both children and adults. He urged me to undertake the project alone, while generously offering his own collection of pediatric variants for my use in any way I saw fit. Subsequent informal discussions, lectures, and instruction courses at national meetings on my part clearly supported Caffey's convictions. Preliminary plans for the book were formulated and the gathering of additional material was begun.

Despite encouragement and support from all sides, this project did not reach fruition. There are a number of reasons why this was so, but one in particular stands out. As the collection of variants progressed in the form of films, negatives, photographic prints, and countless notations in books and on cards, it became first a steamroller and then an avalanche, resulting in eventual disorganization and utter frustration. No cutoff point ever came clearly into view, and the book became unaffectionately known as "The Monster." It was with a feeling of great relief that I happily relinquished any claims I had on the book to the eager and able hands of Ted Keats, former resident and longtime close friend, who had been quietly assembling his own collection of variants over the years.

Keats has neatly and effectively sidestepped my dilemma in several ways. Rather than trying to present all possible variants of the paranasal sinuses, the sella turcica, or the small intestine (just to cite three of many possible examples), he has wisely included only those that truly simulate recognizable disease entities. In so doing he has avoided the impossible and, more important, has brought the subject into practical perspective and has spared the reader much irrelevant trivia. His use of the atlas format in dealing with this material is also to be commended. The old argument that an atlas automatically precludes true scholarly achievement is just not valid in many aspects of diagnostic roentgenology and is nicely refuted by this particular volume. The carefully selected roentgenograms that have been so meticulously reproduced herein speak for themselves in a most eloquent manner.

Congratulations, Ted, on a job well done.

JOHN F. HOLT
Co-Director, Division of Pediatric Radiology (Retired)
C. S. Mott Children's Hospital
University of Michigan Medical Center
Ann Arbor, Michigan

Preface to the SEVENTH EDITION

The scientist who collects and catalogs and the child who wanders barefoot through the woods are equally awestruck by the sheer profusion of creatures that populate this planet.
PAUL BRAND and PHILIP YANCEY

The above quotation states perfectly my awe of the infinite variety with which nature has provided us. Despite my 28 years of gathering normal roentgen anatomic variants, scarcely a day or a week goes by without my finding some variation that I have not recognized previously. Fortunately, most of these are sufficiently obvious that they do not arouse any concern of pathology. Nevertheless, I have still managed to accumulate a large number that do raise suspicion, and these constitute the new additions to this seventh edition.

In order to keep the size of the book manageable, I have seriously considered which entities I could reasonably eliminate. I have removed the variants demonstrated by bronchography, since this technique has disappeared, but there is little else that is not still applicable. I am a bit saddened to note that interpretation of conventional radiography of the skull is rapidly becoming a lost art because of the advent of CT. Perhaps this section might be removed or limited in future editions, but at present I have retained it, since in some less technically sophisticated societies it is still a first line of investigation.

With this edition I am introducing my friend and colleague, Dr. Mark W. Anderson, associate professor of Radiology here at the University of Virginia, as co-author. Dr. Anderson is an accomplished musculoskeletal radiologist who will help carry on this work. His expertise in CT and MRI will enhance future editions with improved explanatory supplemental studies. Dr. Anderson and I serve as emergency radiologists in our department, and the material from this source will also provide us with additional bone and soft tissue variants for future inclusion.

Once again, I wish to express my thanks to the many radiologists in the United States and abroad who have submitted cases for my review. Their interest and gracious permission to include their material in the book is much appreciated.

Again, I owe special recognition to my secretary, Patricia West Steele, for many years of loyalty and dedication, and to my wife, Patt, for her long interest in and support of this work.

THEODORE E. KEATS

Preface to the SIXTH EDITION

The return from your work must be the satisfaction which that work brings you and the world's need of that work. With this, life is heaven, or as near heaven as you can get.
WILLIAM EDWARD BURGHARDT DU BOIS (1958)

For the most part, the stimulus for my continued interest in the field of normal variation comes from the many physicians who have personally communicated their appreciation for the help they have received from this atlas. These comments were offered by a wide spectrum of radiologists ranging from residents toiling in emergency settings to senior radiologists who have found a variant that has clarified a clinical problem.

However, I have concerns that the volume of material that I continue to present may become so large that it may be difficult to contain it in a single volume. Considering the wide range of experience of my audience, it is a difficult decision to eliminate some entries because of their simplicity and others due to their rarity. To alleviate this problem in part I have omitted the section on cholecystography since this technique has virtually disappeared from current clinical practice. Other changes included in this edition are a wide range of new variations that may be troublesome, better examples of previously documented entities, and the addition of MRI images, which help to explain the nature of some of the variations. In the future, I hope to provide more MRI correlations.

I would be remiss in not pointing out that some of the normal skeletal variations presented may be productive of clinical symptoms. These variants represent areas of relative structural weakness and when stressed may become symptomatic. Some of these are described by Dr. Jack Lawson* in a recent publication.

I wish to again express my appreciation to the many physicians the world over who have sent me material for inclusion in the book and who have offered suggestions for improvement of the presentation. The warm reception of this work by the readership has been most gratifying in the satisfaction I have gained from this effort and in finding enthusiasm for its continuance.

I owe special recognition to my secretary, Patricia West, for years of loyalty and dedication; and to my wife, Patt, for her long interest in and support of my work.

THEODORE E. KEATS

---

*Lawson P: Clinically significant radiologic variants of the skeleton. *Am J Roentgenol* 163:249, 1994.

Preface to the FIFTH EDITION

Say not "This is the truth" but "So it seems to me to be as I now see the things I think I see."

Inscription above a doorway at the German Naval Officers School in Kiel, quoted by John McPhee in *Rising From the Plains*

The many expressions of acceptance of this work have been most gratifying and have provided me with the stimulus to continue to collect and explain many of the normal phenomena that we see in our everyday work.

As I have collected normal roentgen variants over the years, I have heard the repeated criticism that the material is unproven, and in many cases the comment is true. Exploration of findings that are unrelated to symptomatology is not a usual undertaking. The quote above states the situation exactly. The inclusion of what I present is often based largely on the fact that the findings are incidental and asymptomatic, or have been seen repeatedly in other patients in a similar clinical setting. In the first edition, I stated that all entries are subject to further scrutiny and exclusion if necessary. I am delighted to state that over the years only a few have failed to survive the test of time.

In this edition I have included more CT images and some MR examinations to establish the developmental nature of some of the new entries. Unfortunately, not many incidental findings are subjected to these kinds of examinations, and only time will permit further documentation.

Mother Nature is inexhaustible in the infinite variety of human development she provides. Since this edition has gone to press, I have collected a great number of new variants for subsequent publications. The task is endless, but it is a labor of love.

I would like to express my appreciation to the many physicians who have sent me material and have graciously granted permission to publish these images. I would like to particularly acknowledge the invaluable expertise of Dr. Evan A. Lennon of Sydney, Australia, for his careful proofreading of the manuscript. Thanks are also due to my secretary, Patricia West; my editorial assistant, Carol Chowdhry, Ph.D.; and my wife, Patt, for her encouragement in this work.

THEODORE E. KEATS

Preface to the FOURTH EDITION

To study the phenomena of disease without books is to sail an unchartered sea, while to study books without patients is not to go to sea at all.

SIR WILLIAM OSLER

The publication of this fourth edition reflects the gratifying response of the medical profession to the earlier editions. I have been particularly rewarded by the comments of many radiologists who have indicated that the illustration of these many normal variants has been of great help in their clinical work and in convincing their clinical colleagues of the innocent nature of these findings. I have compiled most of the new entries during the course of my day's work when I can examine and question patients and try to document the nature of the radiographic findings.

Most of the entities in the last edition have stood the test of time. I have removed the illustration of what I believed to be the nutrient foramen of the tibia since I became aware of the typical appearance of the posterior tibial runners' stress fracture.

This illustration has been replaced with a correct version. I have added a great deal of new material on the cervical spine. I find this portion of the skeleton extremely difficult to interpret and full of pitfalls for the unwary radiologist, not only because of its anatomic structure, but also as a result of faulty positioning and projection.

The reader will also find some important new material concerning relationships of joints, particularly in the wrist and the acromioclavicular joint, that violate accepted criteria.

I wish to express my appreciation to the many physicians who have permitted me to publish material sent for consultation. I wish to express special appreciation to Dr. Christian Cimmino, of Fredericksburg, Virginia, for his many contributions and his invaluable assistance in unraveling many anatomic riddles. Thanks are also due my secretary, Patricia West; my editorial assistant, Carol Chowdhry; and my wife, Patt, for making my task easier.

THEODORE E. KEATS

Preface to the FIRST EDITION

Things are seldom what they seem. Skim milk masquerades
as cream.
GILBERT & SULLIVAN'S *H. M. S. Pinafore*

The problem of normal variation is a lifelong one for the radiologist, and the mark of his experience is often his ability to recognize a wide range of these entities. Cataloging and describing normal variants demonstrated by roentgenology is of more than academic interest, for recognition of the abnormal first requires full knowledge of the normal. Variation is inseparably related to the study of normal anatomy. In addition, the error of overdiagnosis of a normal variation as evidence of pathology may be more serious than omission and may lead to needless and harmful therapy.

When one studies the field of normal variation in detail, he is apt to be overwhelmed by the seemingly infinite variety nature has provided. A detailed study of all of these would be a valuable, but limitless, undertaking. Of more significance are those variations that may simulate disease in the radiograph. It is these variations that form the substance of this initial effort. Those that are shown here represent problems in diagnosis based on my personal experience, on that of my associates as well as on that of successive generations of residents in training. An interest in the subject of normal variations seems to induce spontaneous generation of additional entities so that, at the time of this writing, there appears to be no end in sight, but it is necessary to make a start. It is anticipated that subsequent editions will add additional troublesome variants as well as correct or amplify those herein as new information is obtained.

The distinction between a normal anatomic variation and a congenital anomaly is an arbitrary one. I have tried to avoid inclusion of anomalies of development, which are obvious in themselves and often productive of signs and symptoms, but rather have tried to concentrate on those alterations that are essentially incidental findings and significant only in their potential for misinterpretation.

The proof of the validity of the material presented is largely subjective, based on personal experience and on the published work of others. It consists largely of having seen the entity many times and of being secure in the knowledge that time has proved the innocence of the lesions. In other cases, follow-up studies indicated that the lesion in question represents a phase of growth that is eliminated by maturation. Still other variants were detected in examination of the side opposite that in question when a radiograph was made for purposes of comparison. Further experience may prove some of these concepts incorrect; all are, therefore, considered subject to future modification or elimination.

This book is arranged in atlas form with the concept that a photographic reproduction of a normal variant is far superior to a text description. The illustrative material, therefore, is emphasized and the text minimal and concise. References are included where the subject is still considered controversial or where documentation is thought necessary. The interested reader is referred to the works *Pediatric X-Ray Diagnosis* by John Caffey and Dr. Alban Kohler's *Borderlands of the Normal and Early Pathologic in Skeletal Roentgenology*. These books represent pioneer efforts in the field of Skeletal Roentgen variants. This atlas confines itself to roentgen variants seen in conventional roentgenology with no attempt to include those encountered in the specialized fields of angiocardiography, neuroradiology, or the other radiologic specialties. The latter will provide a fruitful source for future study.

Included are a number of normal entities that simulate pathology by virtue of growth, or projection, or both. These are not anatomic variations in the true sense, but since they introduce a similar problem, they are included as well.

The atlas is arranged by anatomic areas. However, certain specific entities are repeated in more than one section, so the reader searching for a variant may encounter it not only in the anatomic area of its origin, but also in the anatomic section of the lesion it simulates. It is hoped this repetitive arrangement will facilitate recognition, particularly for the less experienced observer.

Special acknowledgment is due to Dr. John F. Holt, Professor of Radiology at the University of Michigan, who, as my teacher, first interested me in the subject of normal variation. Throughout his professional career, he has been a student of the subject and has graciously contributed his collection of variants for inclusion in this work. He has also generously contributed time and constructive criticism during the development of this atlas. Without his inspiration and help this work could not have been accomplished.

I wish to express my appreciation also to the many unnamed physicians who have contributed to this collection and, in particular, to Drs. Christian Cimmino and Donald Kenneweg of Fredericksburg, Virginia, and Drs. William R. Newman and Clinton L. Rogers of Cumberland, Maryland, for many valuable cases. My thanks, too, to Miss Anne Russell, R.B.P., of the Section of Medical Photography at the University of Virginia, for her invaluable help in the preparation of the illustrations and to my secretary, Miss Ann Rutledge, for her patience and aid in manuscript preparation.

THEODORE E. KEATS

Contents

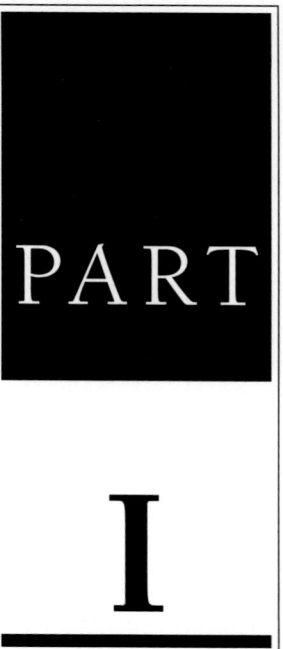

PART

I

The Bones

CHAPTER

1

The Skull

The Calvaria

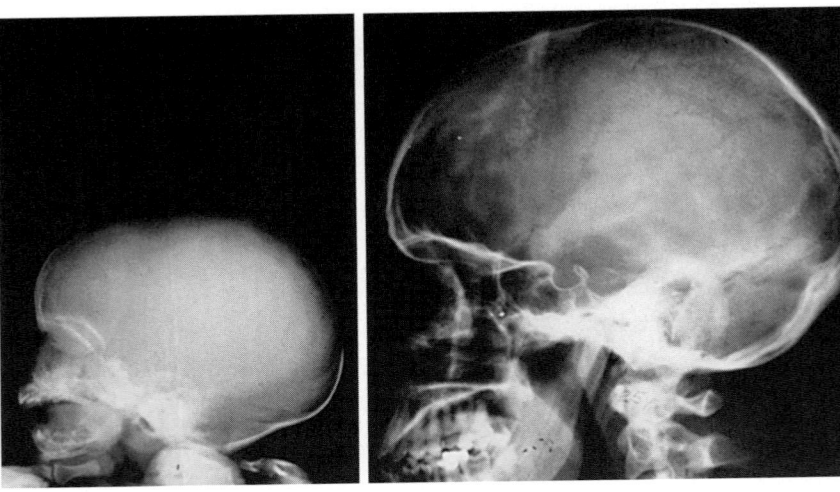

Figure 1–1. The relative proportions of the cranial vault size to face size in the infant differ strikingly from those of the adult and may suggest a disproportionate increase in vault size in the infant if adult standards are applied. At birth the head-to-face ratio is approximately 4:1. In adults this ratio is 3:2. (Ref: Watson EH, Lowrey GH: *Growth and development of children*, 5th ed. St. Louis, Mosby, 1967.) (From Keats TE: Pediatric radiology: Some potentially misleading variations from the adult. *VA Med* 96:630, 1966.)

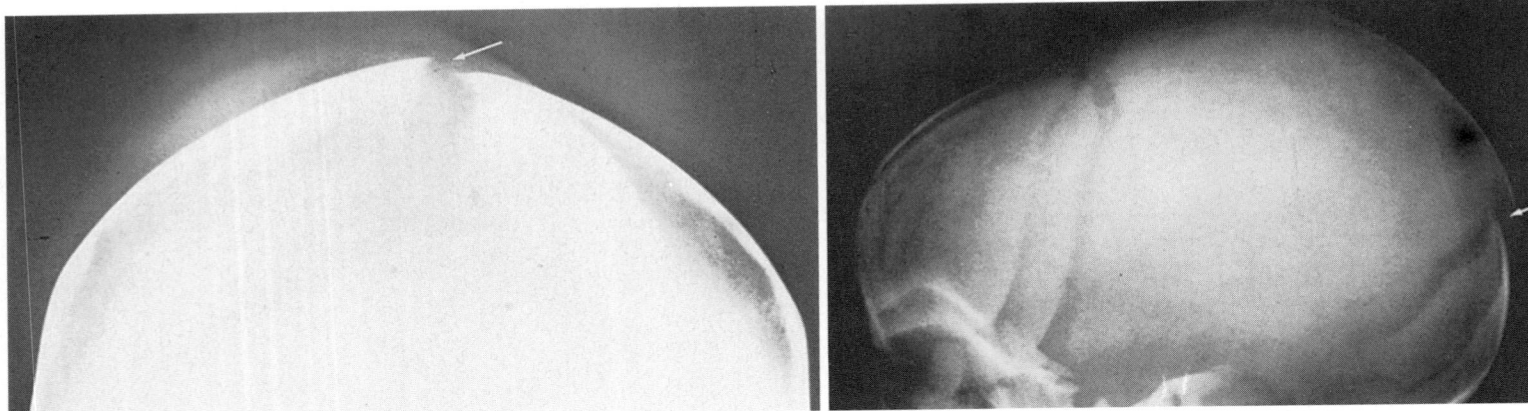

Figure 1–2. Overlapping sutures in a neonate secondary to molding of labor.

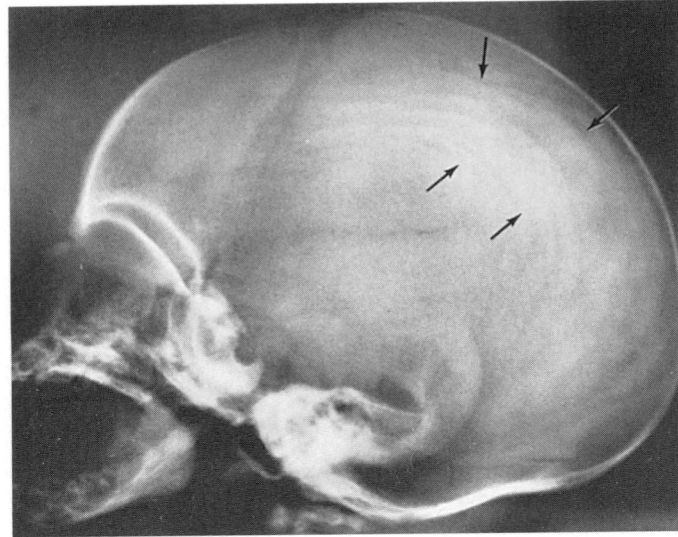

Figure 1–3. Scalp folds in a neonate, producing an unusual appearance in the parietal region.

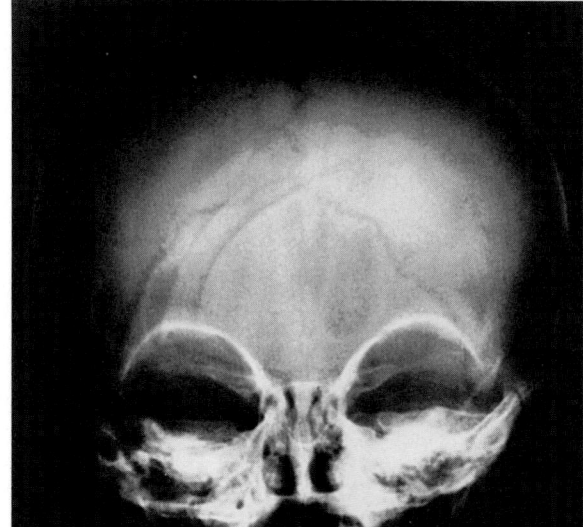

Figure 1–4. Occipital skin folds.

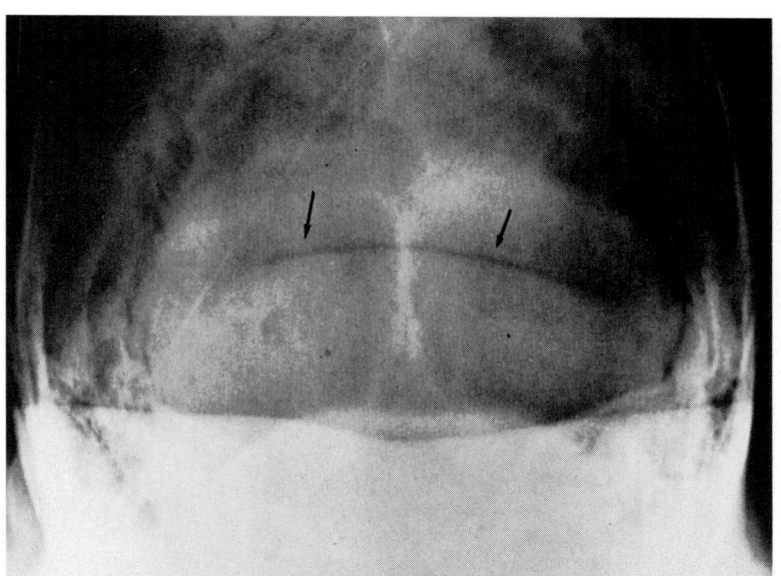

Figure 1–5. Scalp fold in the occipital region, which could be mistaken for a fracture.

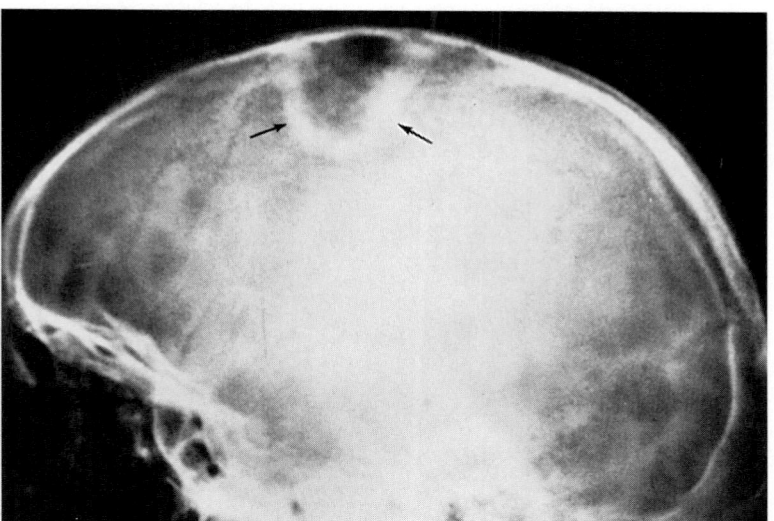

Figure 1–6. Hair braids producing an unusual shadow at the vertex of skull.

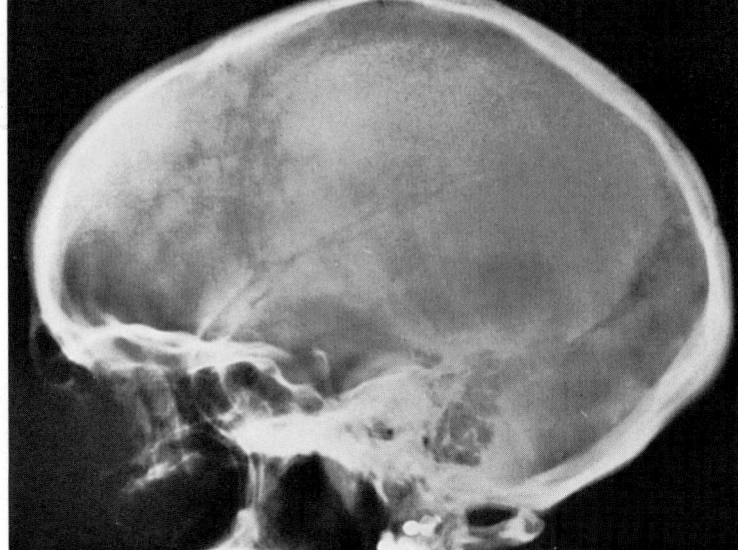

Figure 1–7. Striations over the parietal area caused by hair.

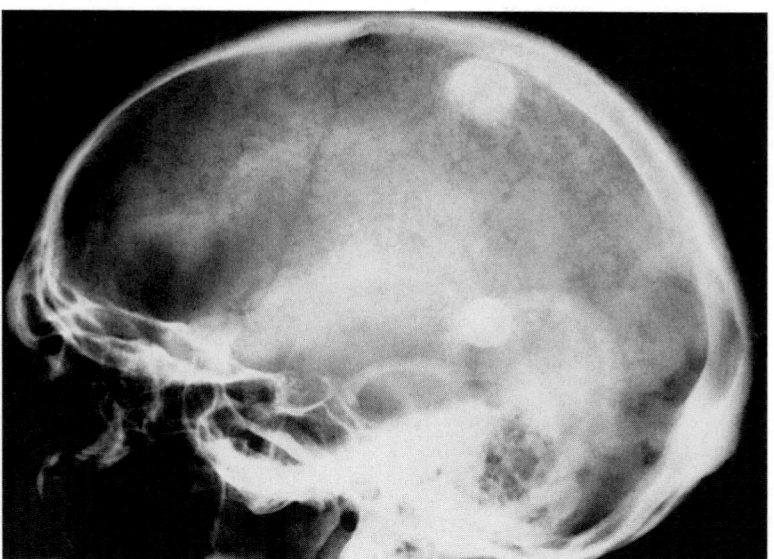

Figure 1–8. Hair braids with surrounding elastic bands, simulating sclerotic lesions.

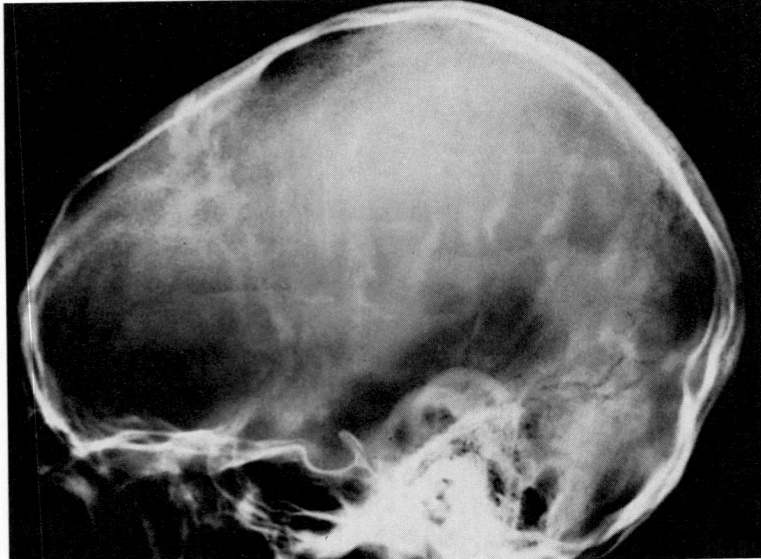

Figure 1–9. Multiple small hair braids ("corn rows"), producing unusual shadows in the frontal and parietal areas.

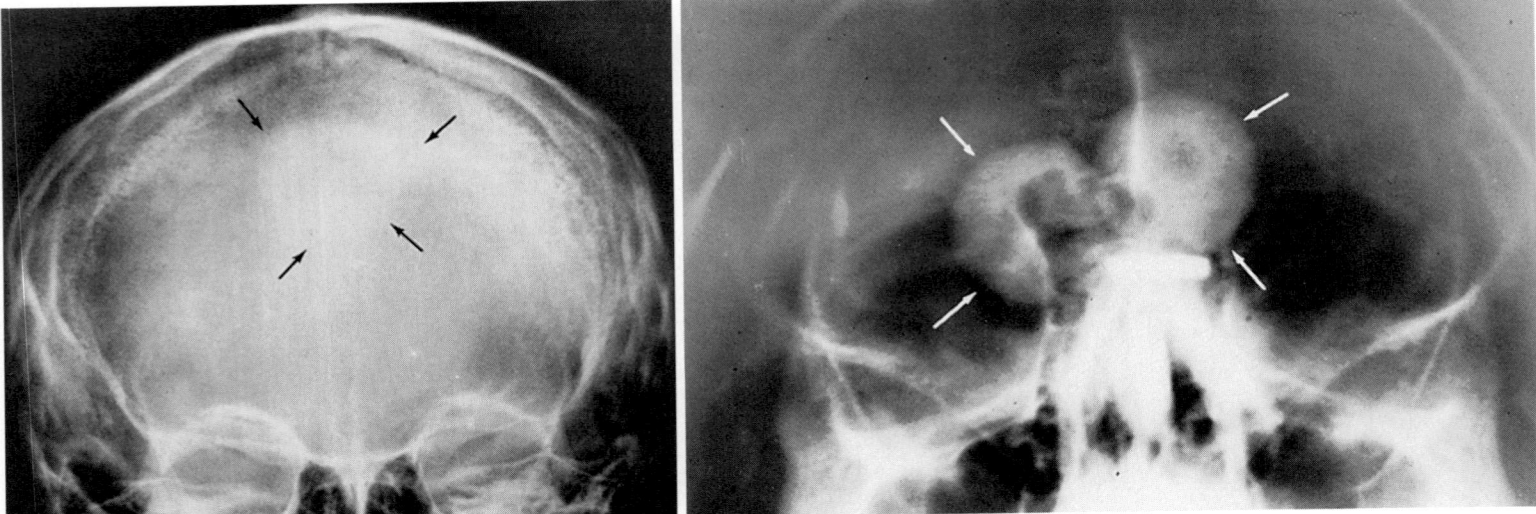

Figure 1–10. Hair arrangements—in these two cases a ponytail—may produce unusual shadows.

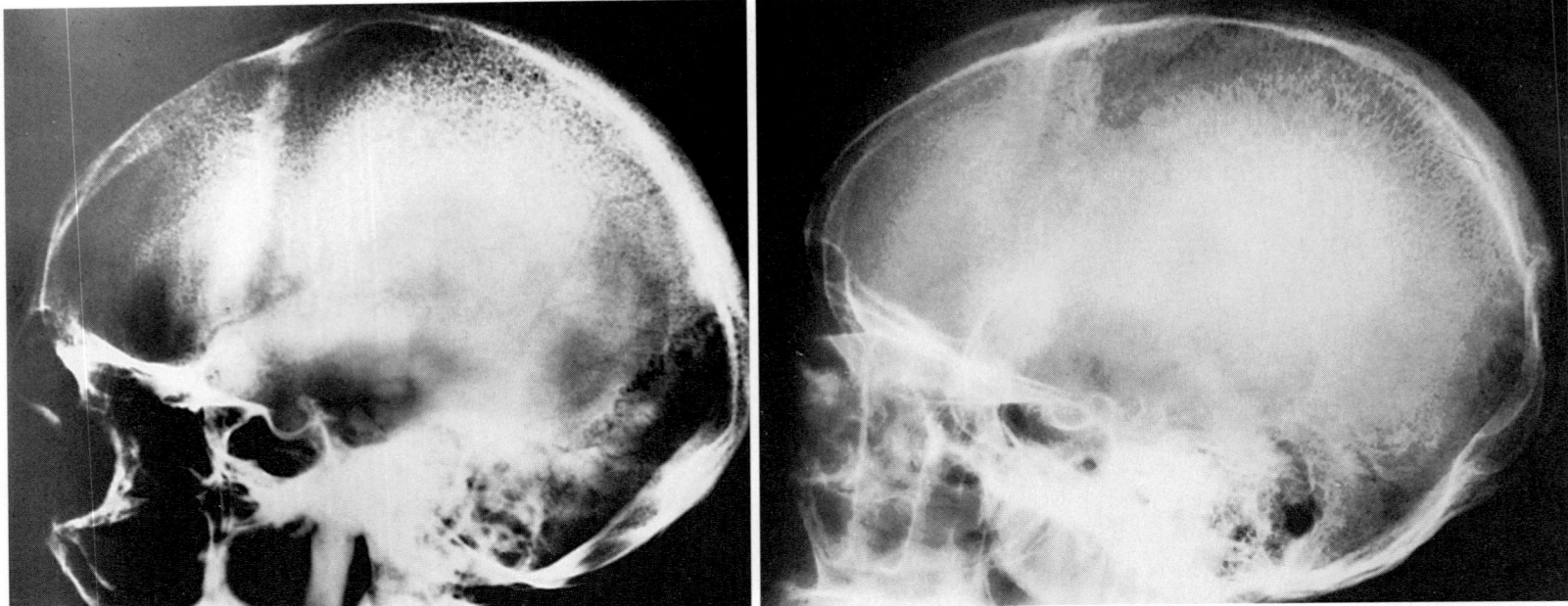

Figure 1–11. Two examples of prominent but normal diploic pattern of the calvaria.

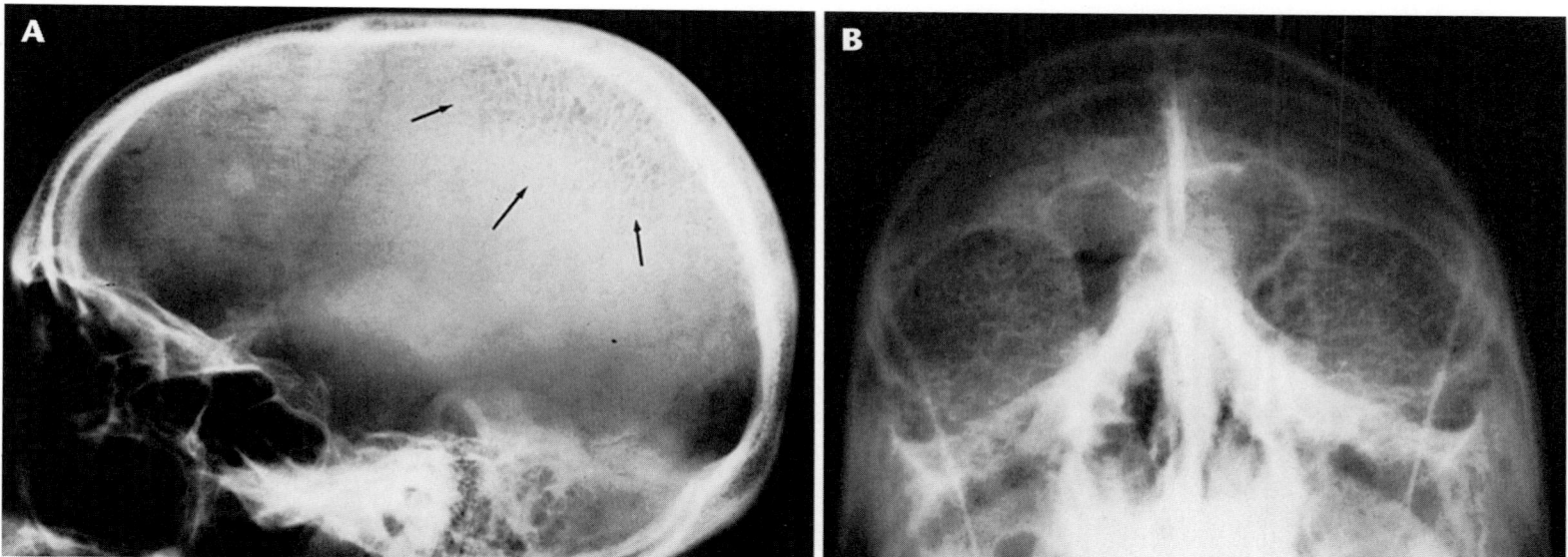

Figure 1–12. Localized prominent diploic pattern in the parietal bone **(A)** produces a striking appearance in Waters' projection **(B)**.

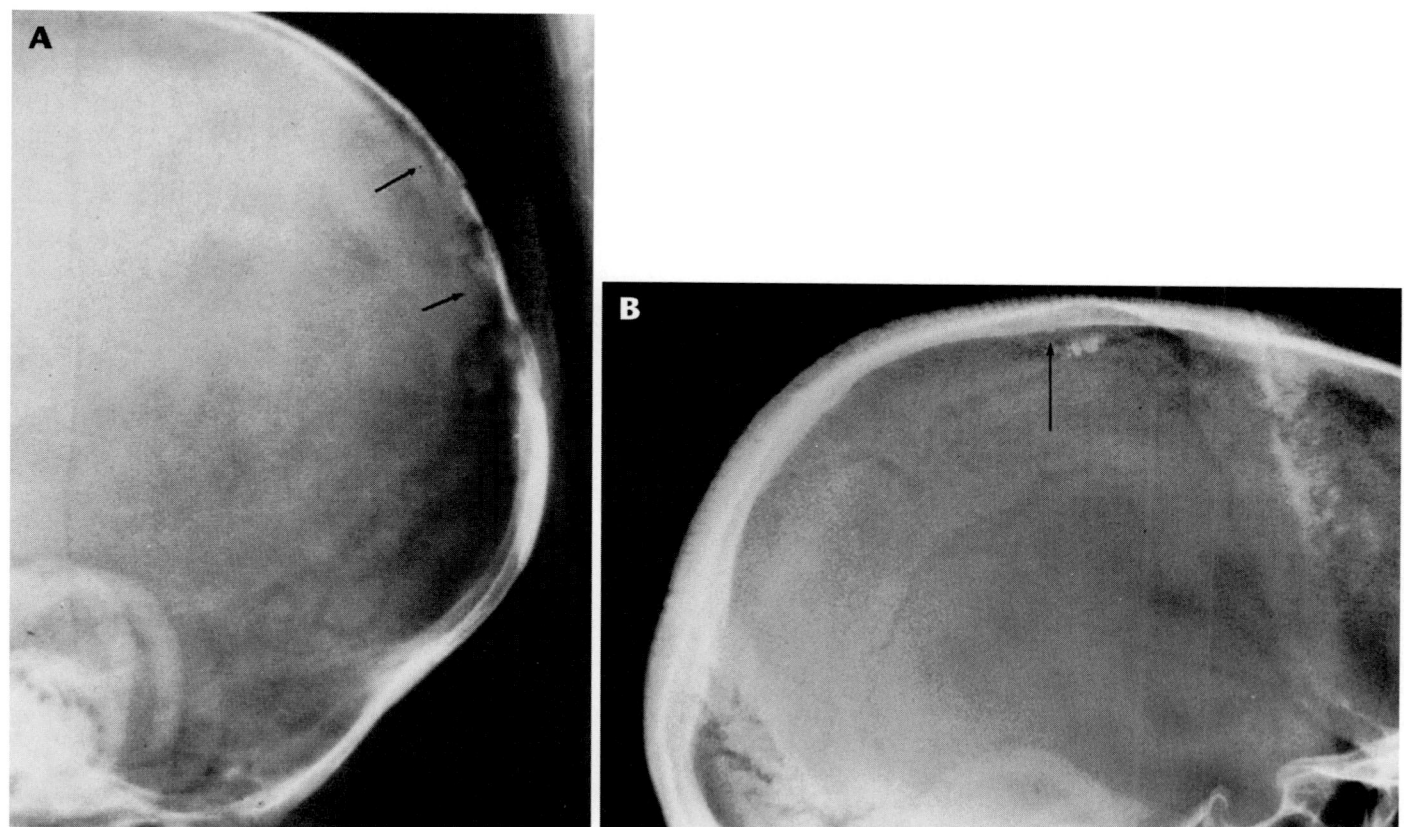

Figure 1–13. Irregularities and striations in the vertex of the parietal bone caused by the serrations of the sagittal suture. **A,** Neonate; **B,** 19-year-old man. (Ref: Sawar M et al: Nature of vertex striations on lateral skull radiographs. *Radiology* 146:90, 1983.)

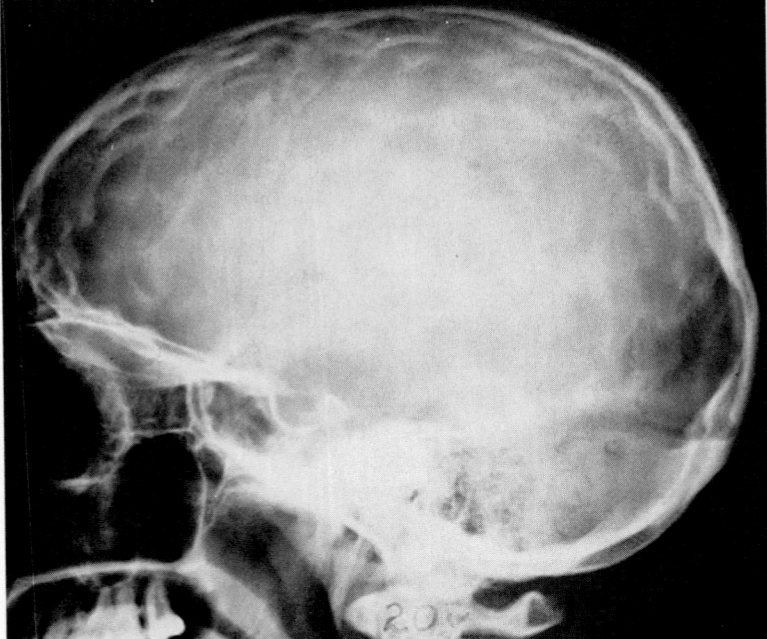

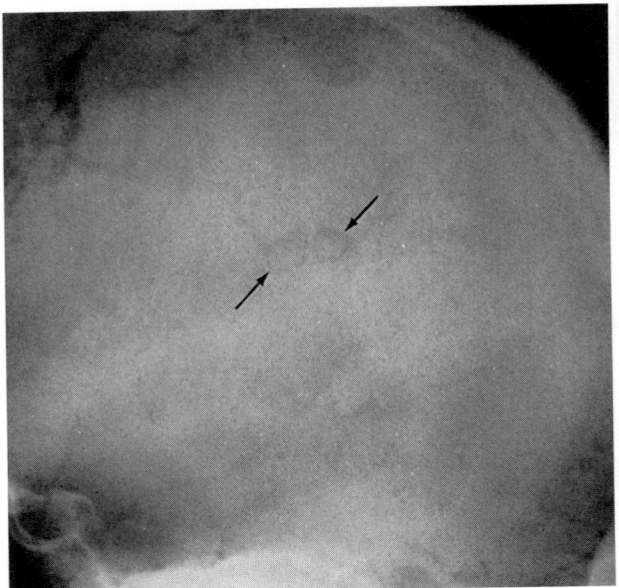

Figure 1–15. Vascular channels in the parietal bone, simulating button sequestra.

Figure 1–14. Prominent digital markings. The prominence of calvarial digital markings varies widely, particularly between the fourth and tenth years. They do not in themselves necessarily reflect increased intracranial pressure. (Ref: Macaulay D: Digital markings in the radiographs of children. *Br J Radiol* 24:637, 1951.) It should be noted that infants may occasionally be born without neurologic disease but having lacunar skulls, which resolve spontaneously. (Ref: Taylor B, Barnat HB, Seibert JJ: Neonatal lacunar skull without neurologic disease. *South Med J* 75:875, 1982.)

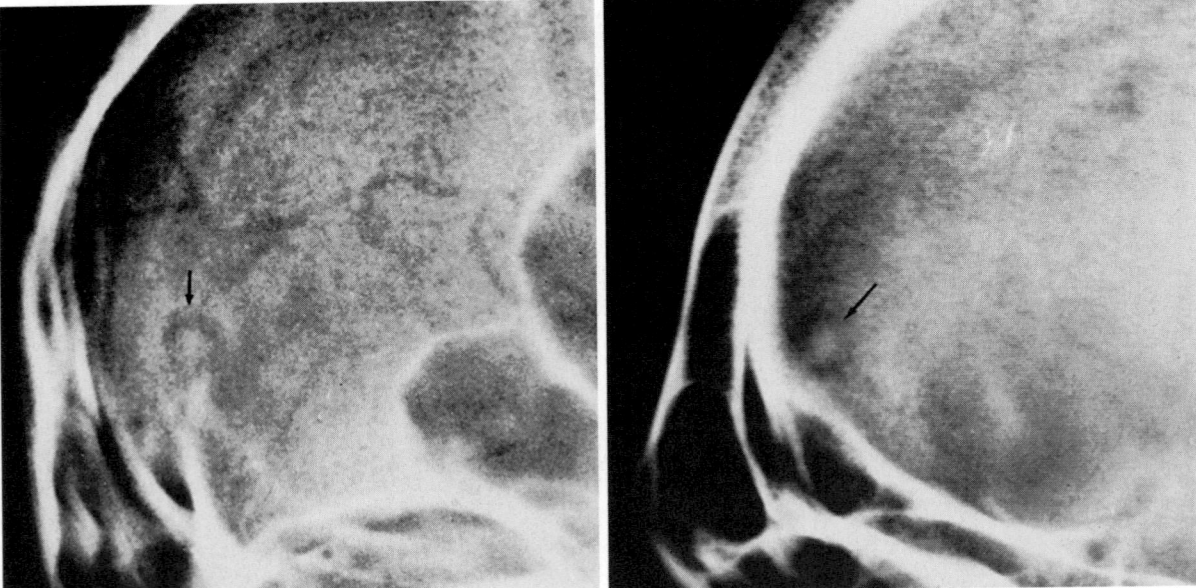

Figure 1–16. Vascular channels in the frontal bone, simulating button sequestra.

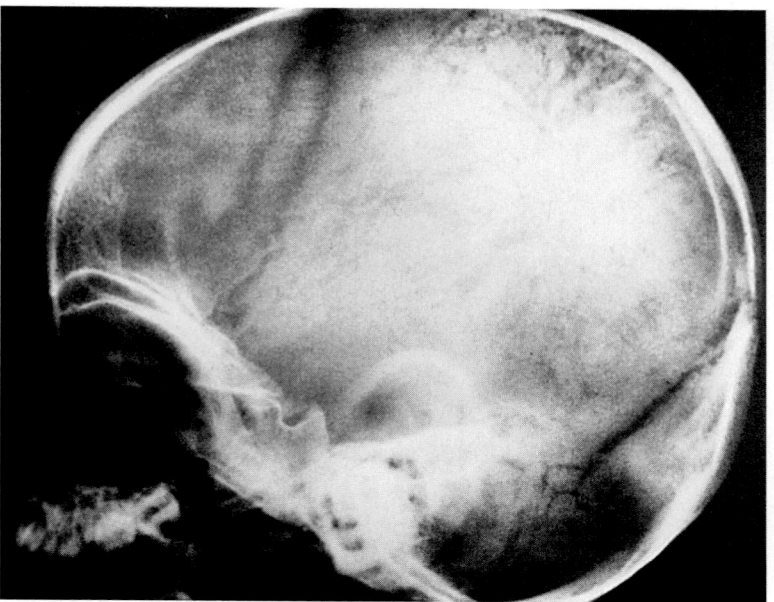

Figure 1–17. Prominent diploic vascular pattern in a child.

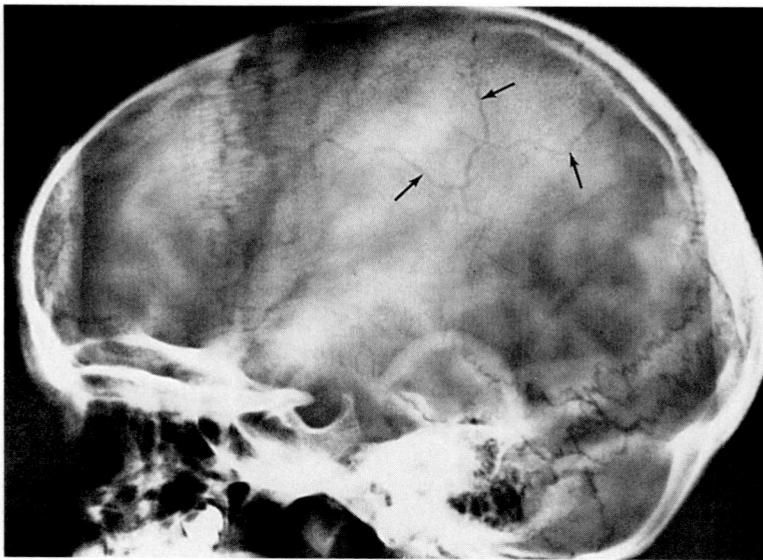

Figure 1–18. Unusual calvarial vascular pattern, simulating fractures.

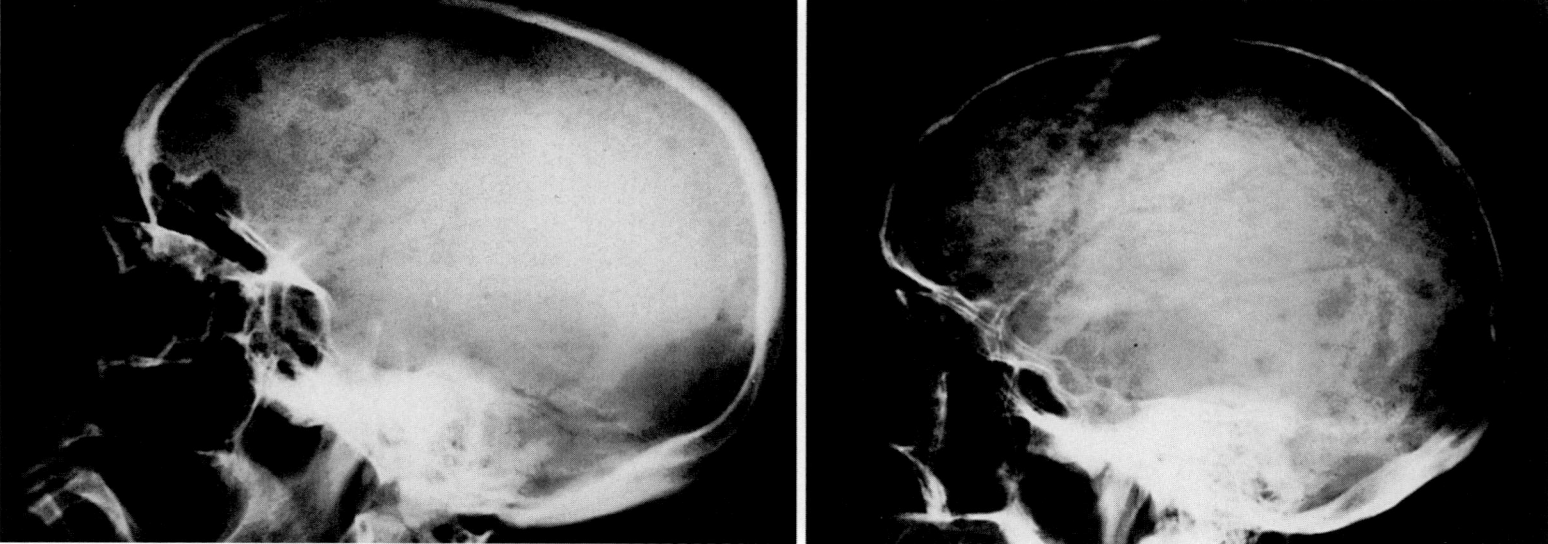

Figure 1–19. Two examples of multiple diploic venous lakes, which may simulate metastatic neoplasm. Both patients showed no change on long-term follow-up examination.

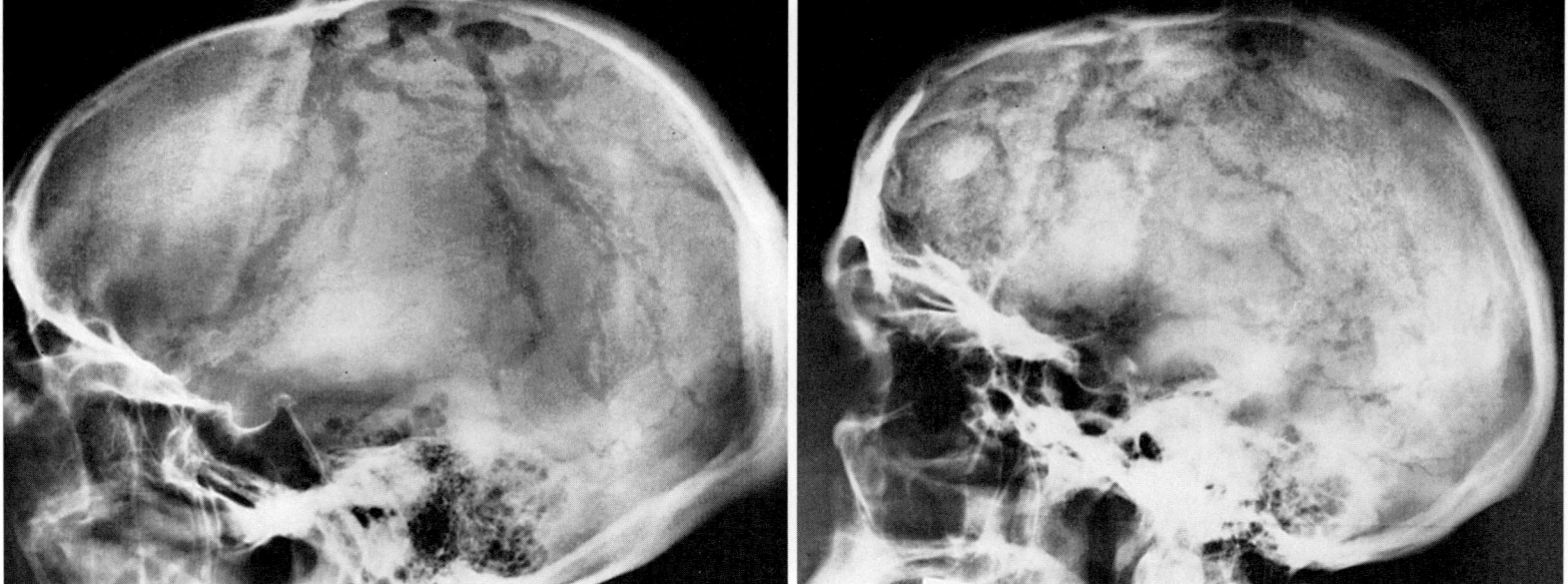

Figure 1–20. Two examples of prominent but normal diploic vascular patterns.

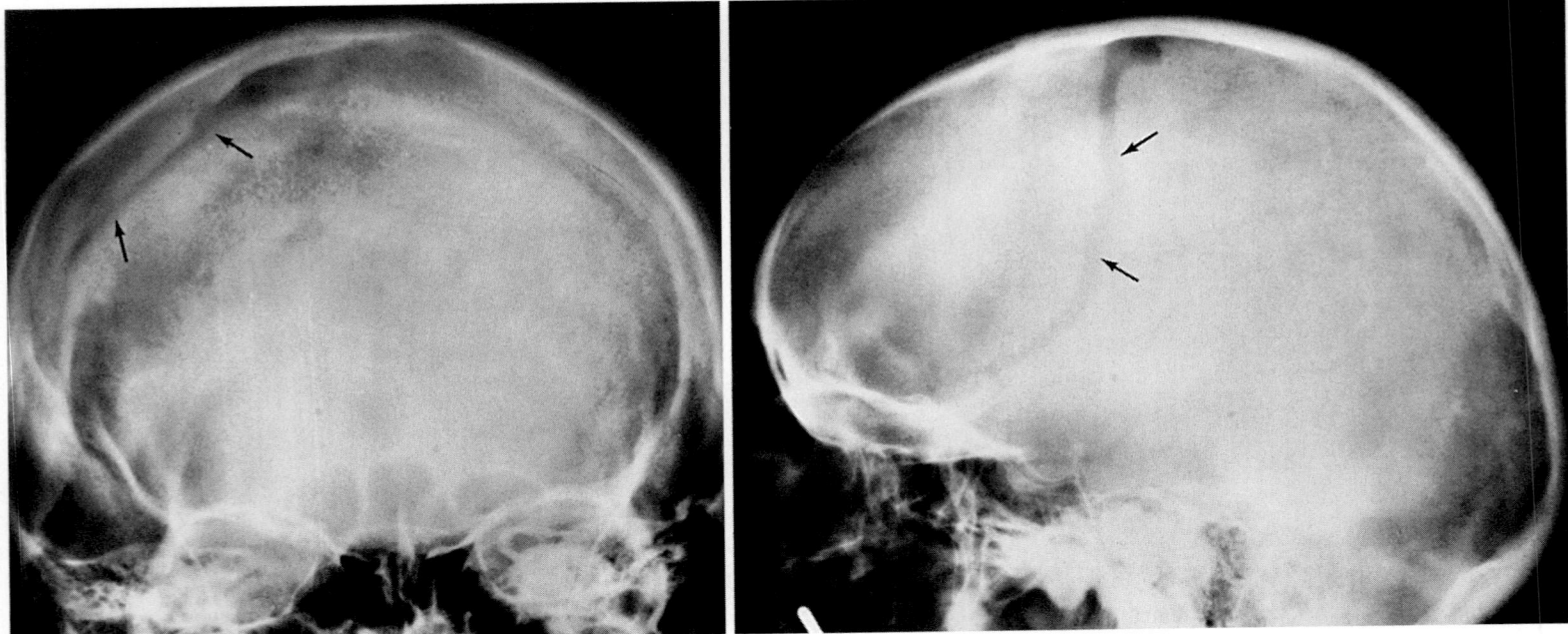

Figure 1–21. A prominent but normal groove for the sphenoparietal venous sinus.

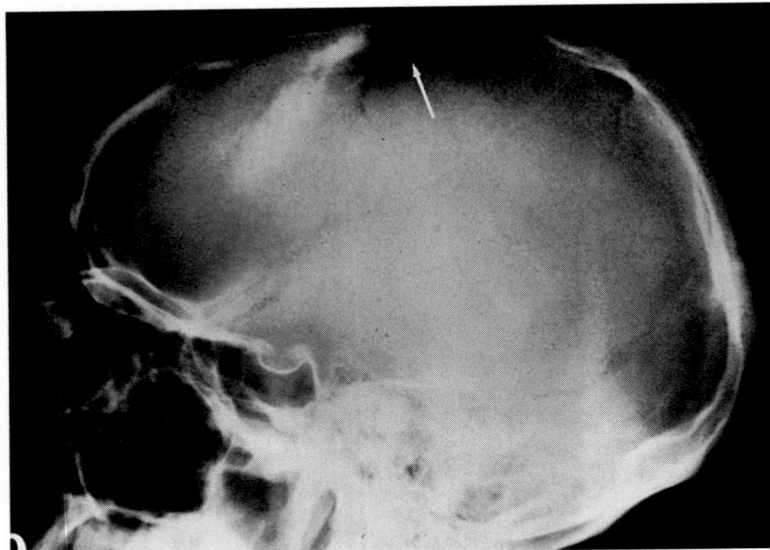

Figure 1–22. Prominent venous vascular groove at the vertex of the skull.

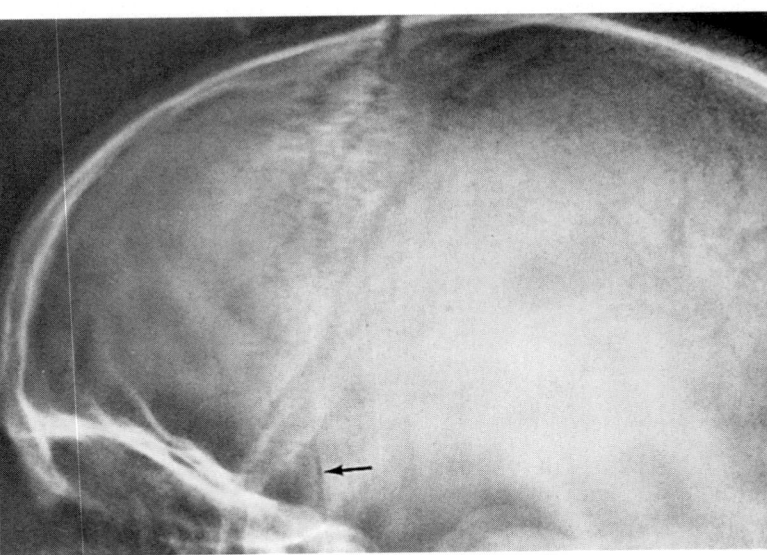

Figure 1–23. Vascular groove (sphenoparietal sinus), simulating fracture.

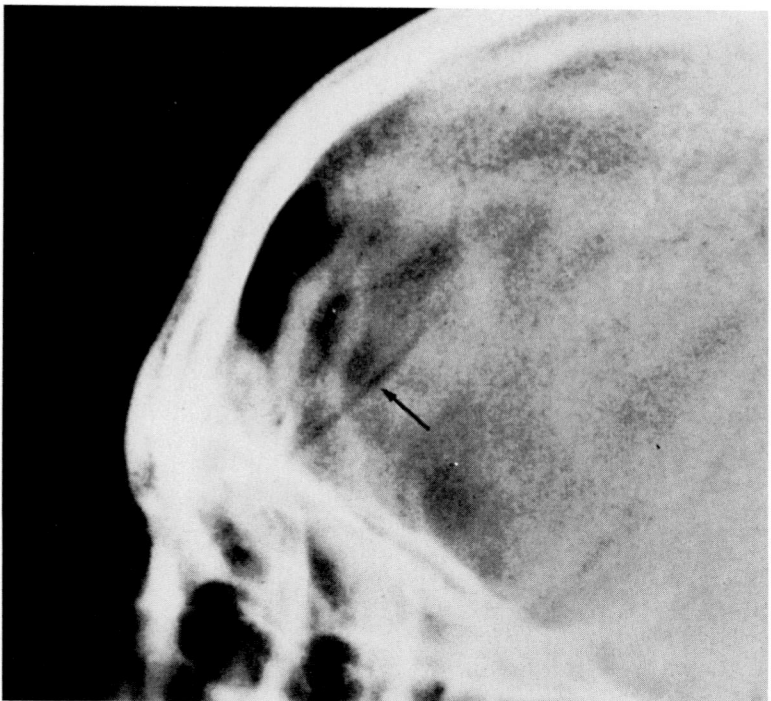

Figure 1–24. Venous vascular groove in the frontal bone, which may be mistaken for fracture.

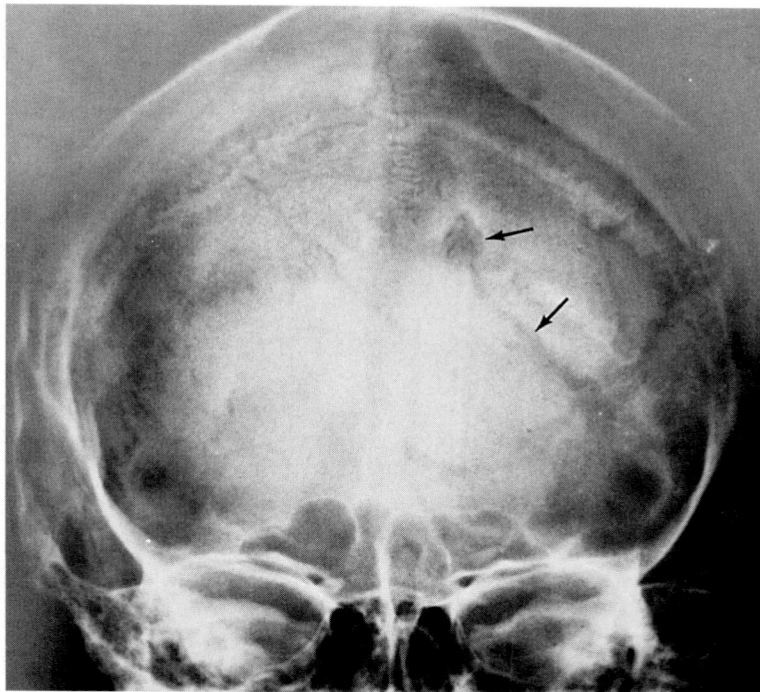

Figure 1–25. Lucent depression of a pacchionian granulation with a large draining vein.

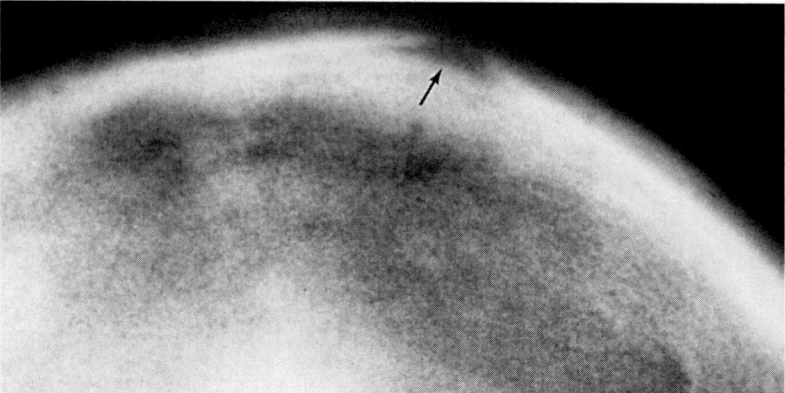

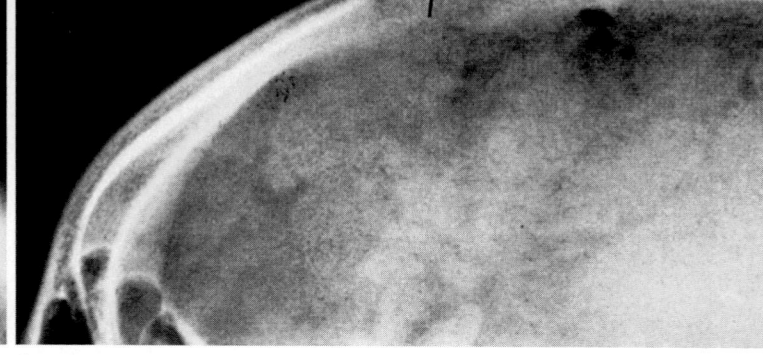

Figure 1–26. A rather poorly defined pacchionian depression, simulating a destructive lesion, particularly in the lateral projection. (Ref: Branan R, Wilson CB: Arachnoid granulations simulating osteolytic lesions of the calvarium. *Am J Roentgenol* 127:523, 1976.)

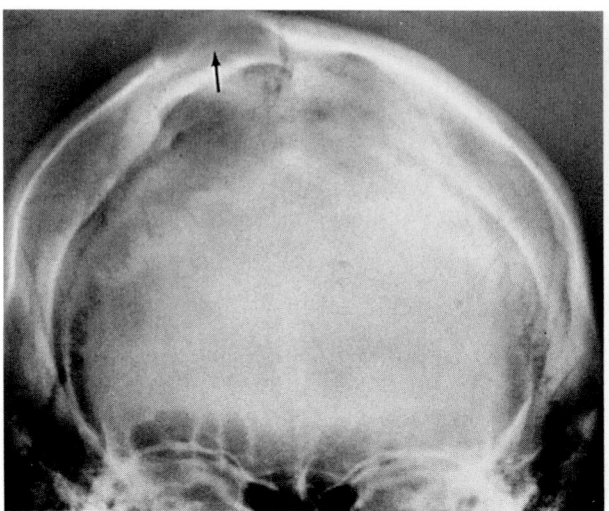

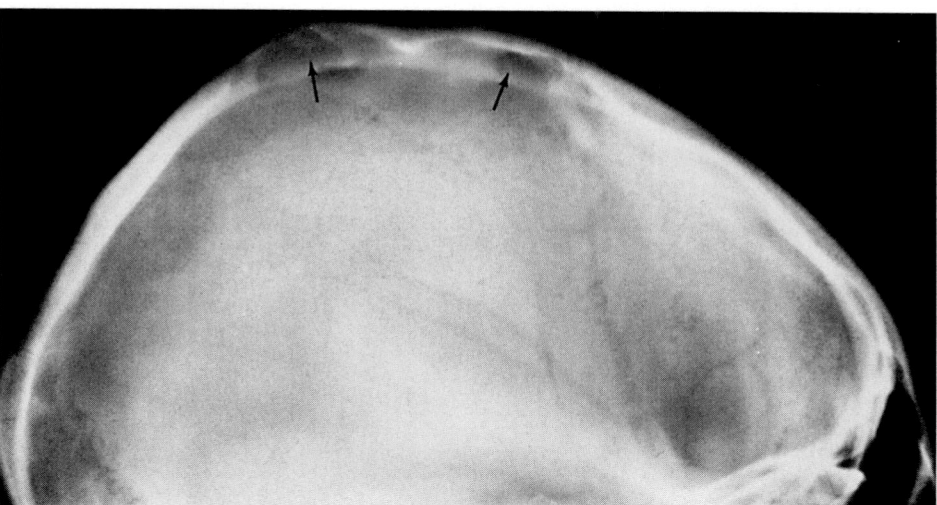

Figure 1–27. Deep but typical pacchionian depressions. The external table of the calvaria is bowed, and the internal table is apparently absent. Failure to appreciate these features may lead to an erroneous diagnosis of erosion of the inner table of the skull.

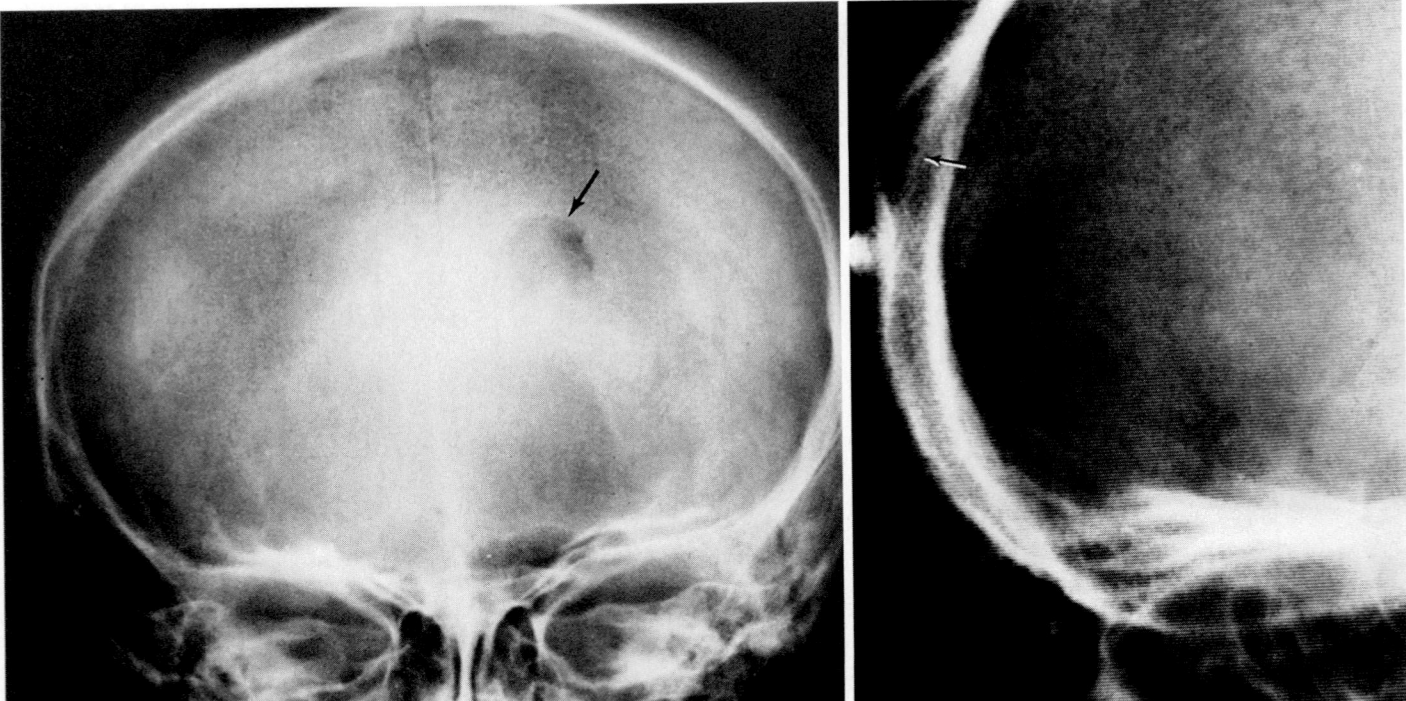

Figure 1–28. Typical pacchionian depression in the frontal bone. In the frontal view this lucency is often mistaken for a destructive lesion.

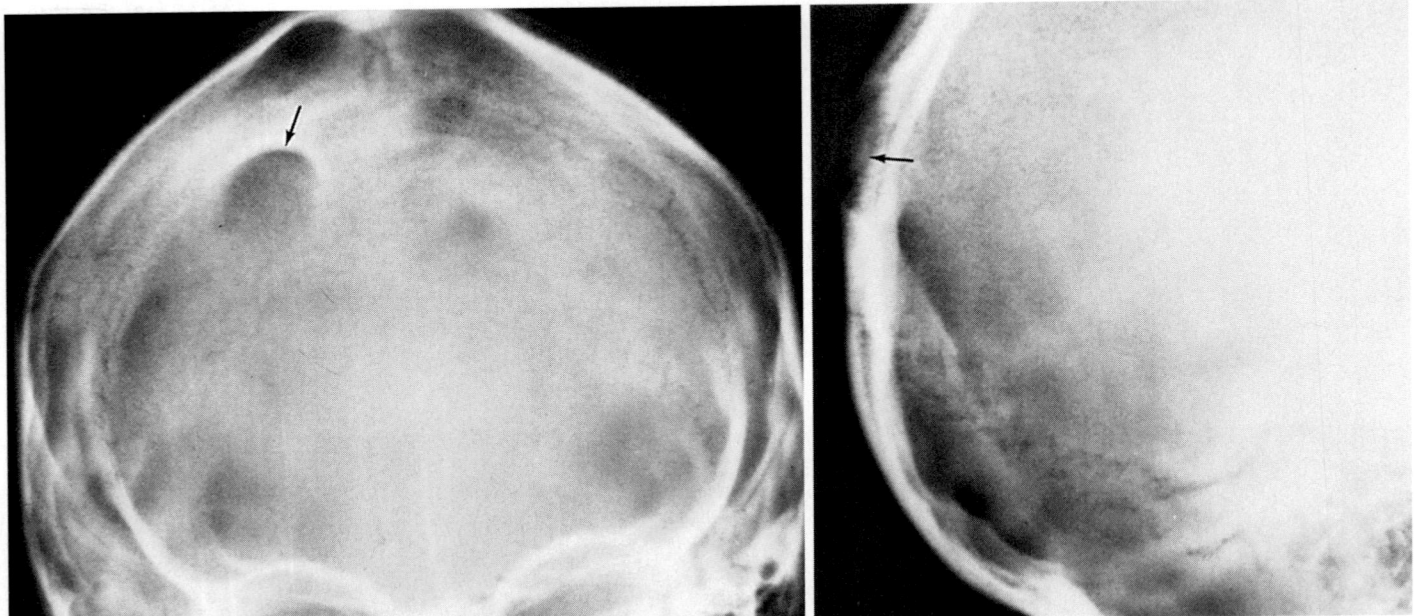

Figure 1–29. Pacchionian depressions in the occipital bone, an unusual location for this normal entity.

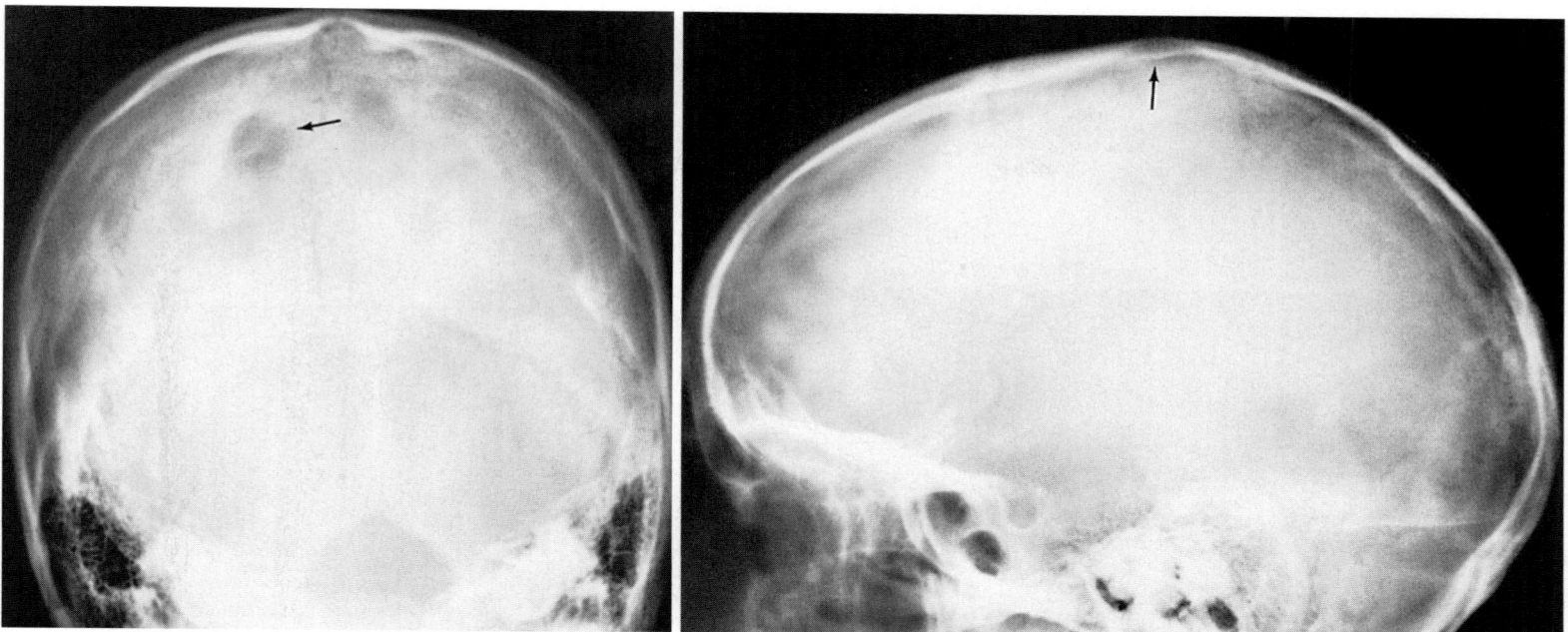

Figure 1–30. Pacchionian depression with a central area of density. This appearance is often mistaken for a significant lesion such as an eosinophilic granuloma. (Ref: Branan R, Wilson CB: Arachnoid granulations simulating osteolytic lesions of the calvarium. *Am J Roentgenol* 127:523, 1976.)

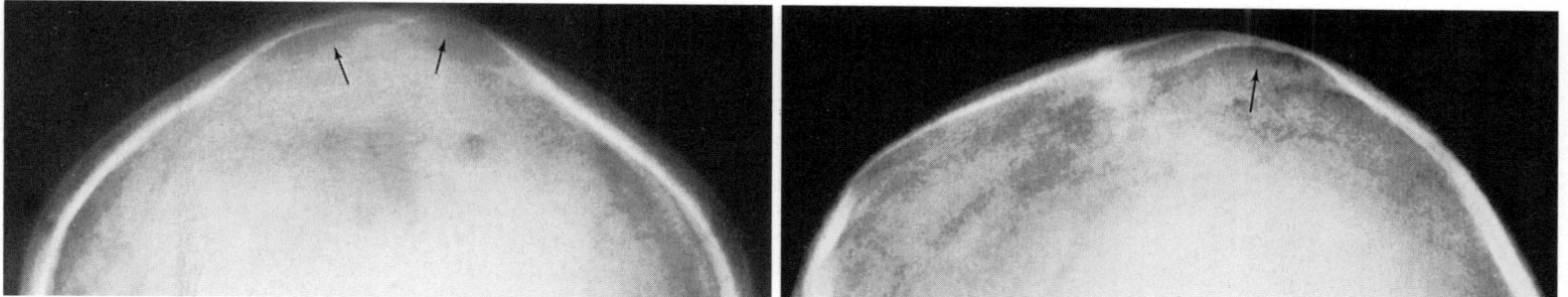

Figure 1–31. Large pacchionian granulations of the vertex of the skull, lending an unusual configuration to the vertex.

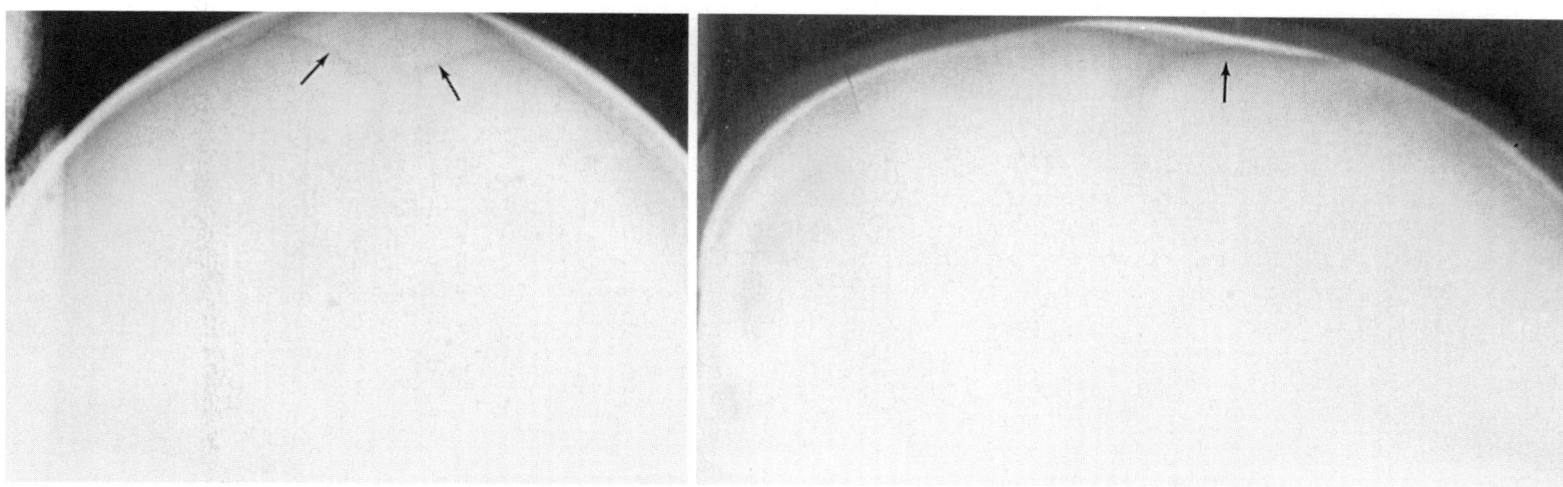

Figure 1–32. Anterior fontanel bone.

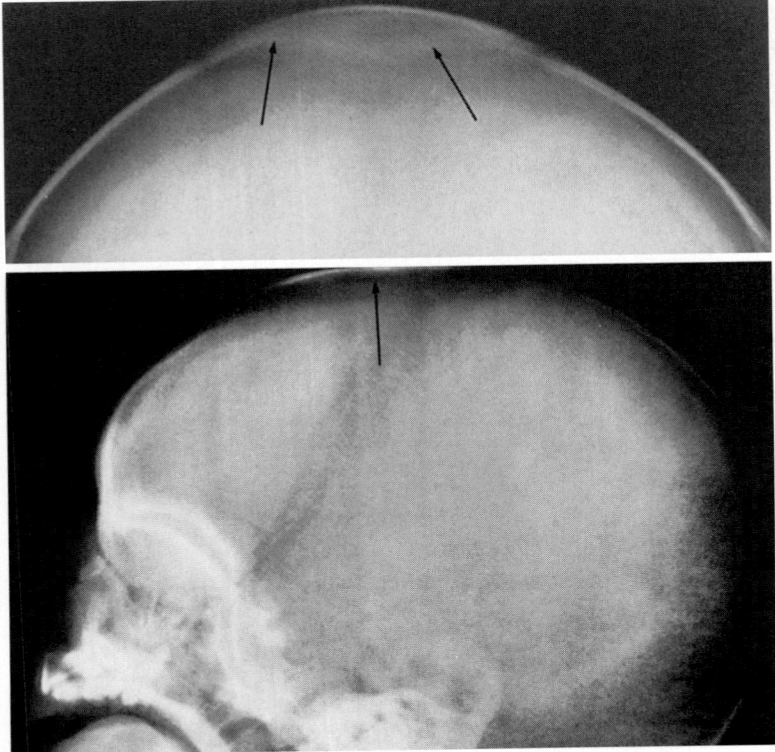

Figure 1–33. Huge anterior fontanel bone in a 1-month-old child.

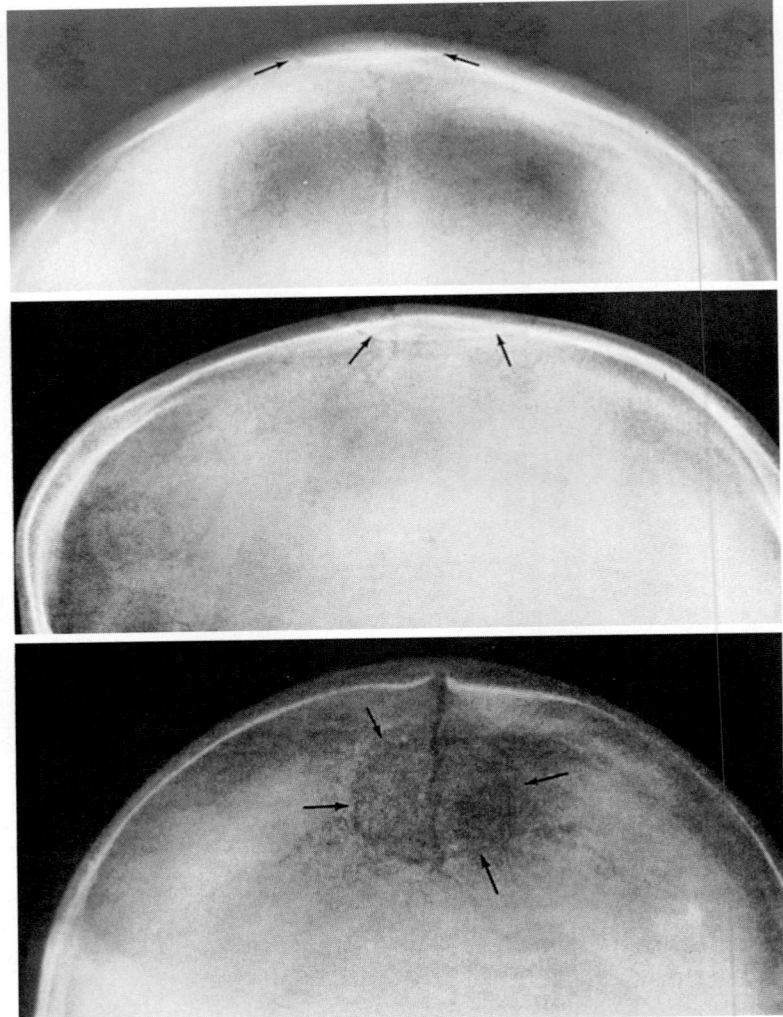

Figure 1–34. Fusing anterior fontanel bone in a 3-year-old boy. This appearance may be confused with a depressed fracture in the lateral projection. (Ref: Girdany BR, Blank E: Anterior fontanel bones. *Am J Roentgenol* 95:148, 1965.)

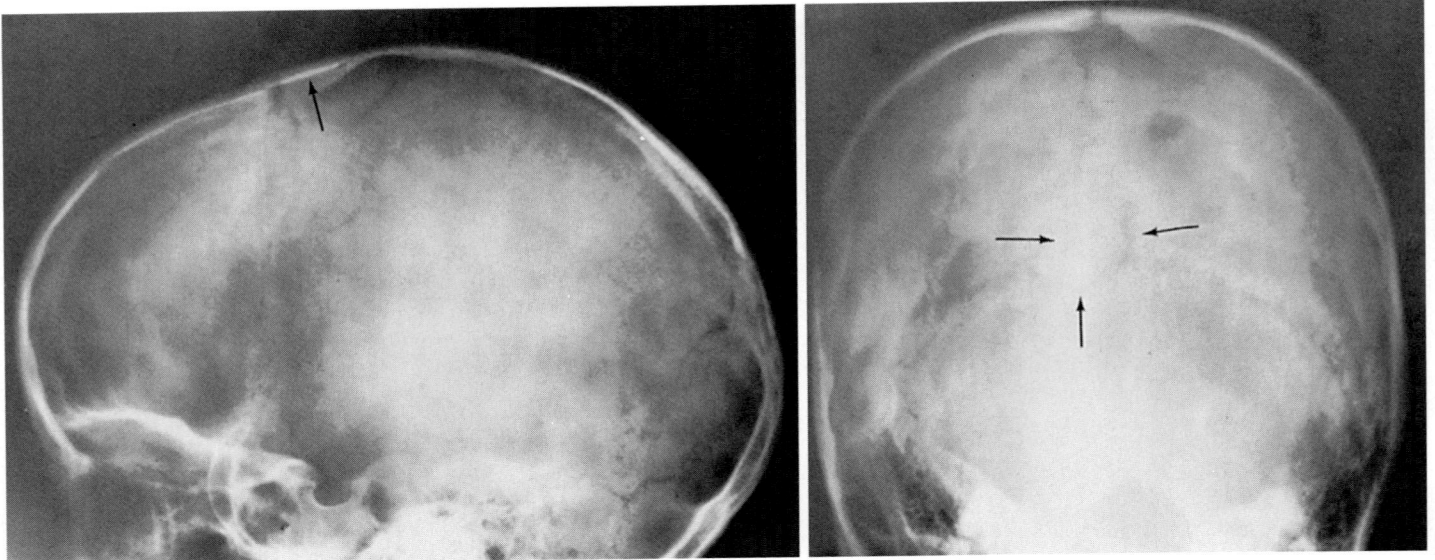

Figure 1–35. Anterior fontanel bone in a 5-year-old boy. Note its characteristic appearance in Towne's projection.

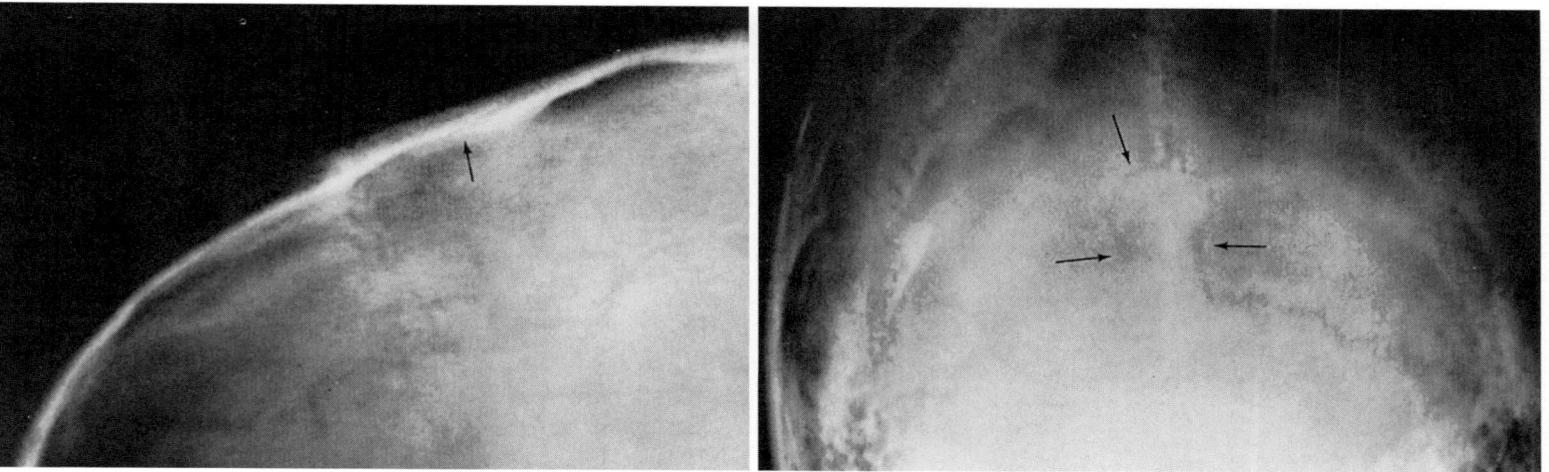

Figure 1–36. Closing anterior fontanel bone in an 11-year-old boy.

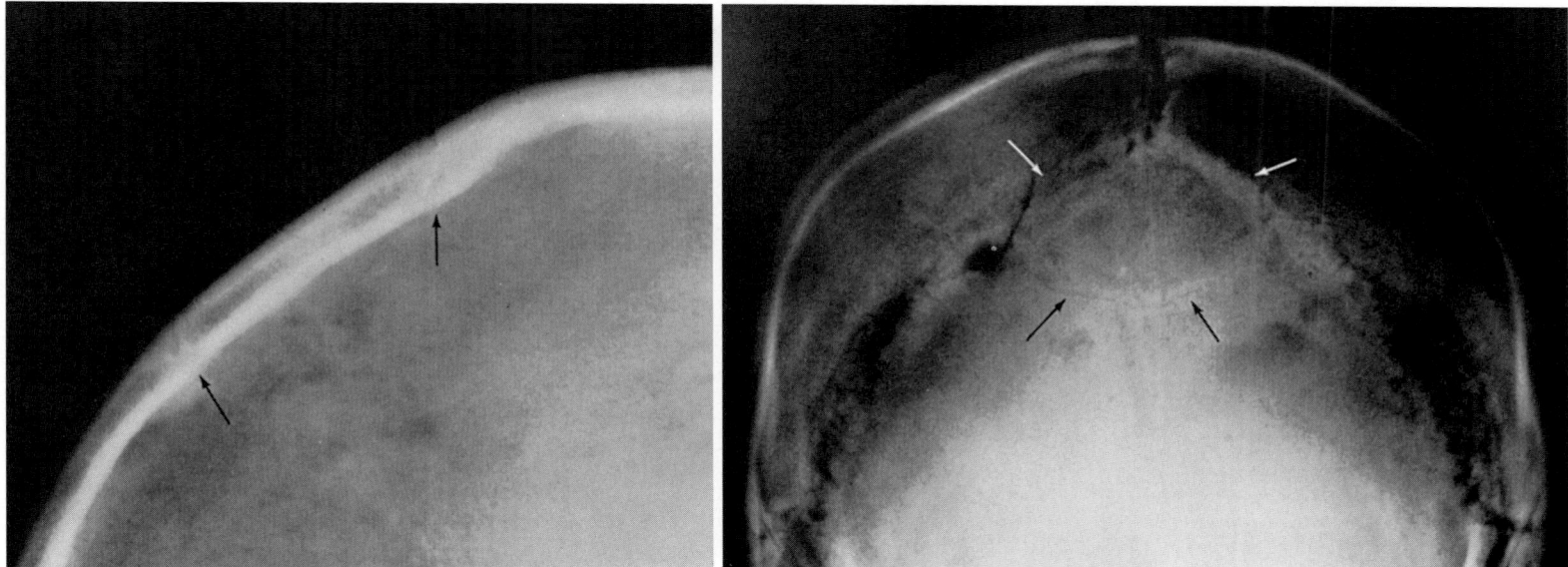

Figure 1–37. Remnants of the anterior fontanel bone in a 50-year-old man.

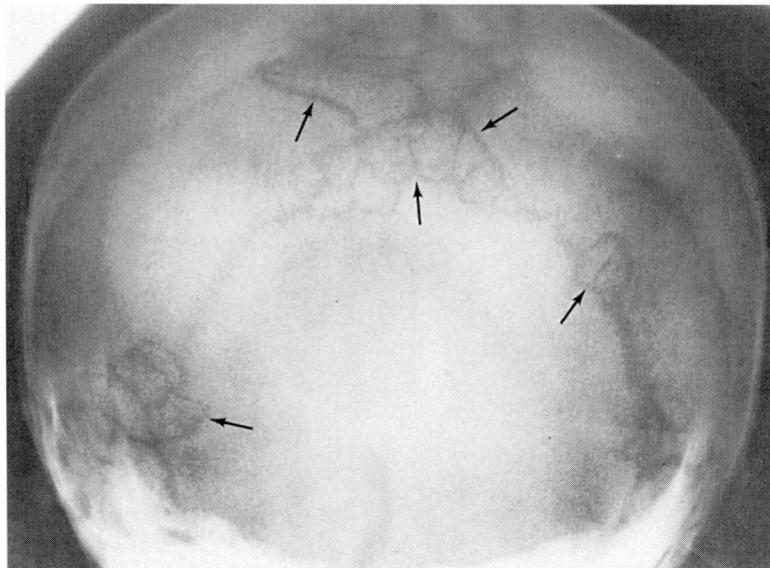

Figure 1–38. Wormian (sutural) bones in a 7-year-old child. These may be seen as a normal variant as well as in osteogenesis imperfecta and cleidocranial dysostosis.

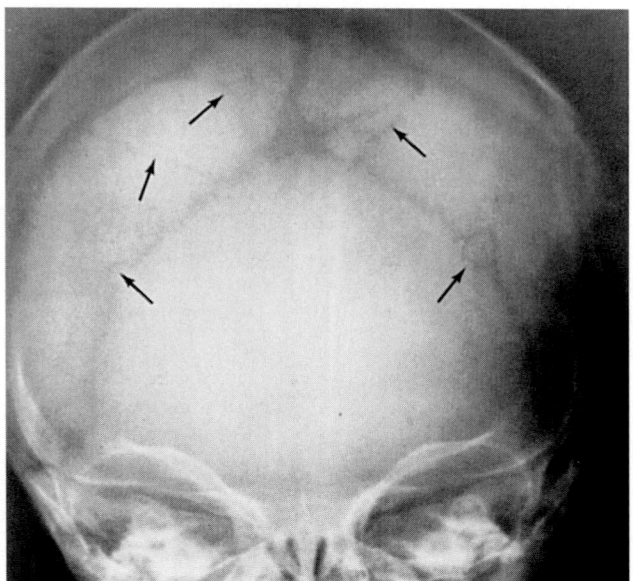

Figure 1–39. Wormian bones in a 9-year-old boy.

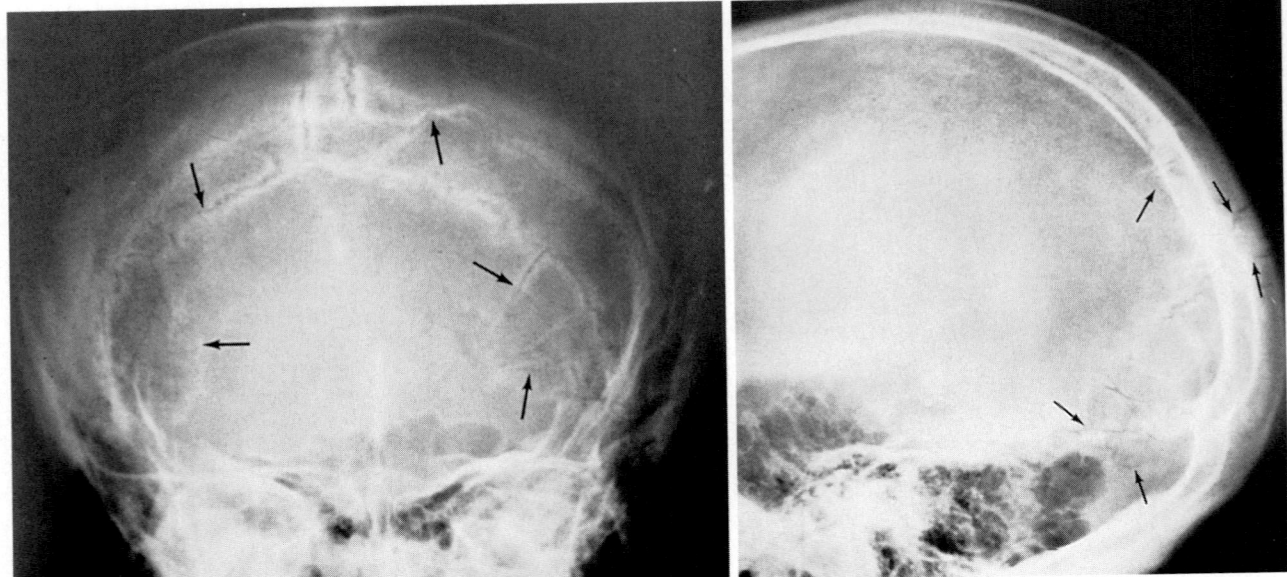

Figure 1–40. Wormian bones in a 19-year-old man.

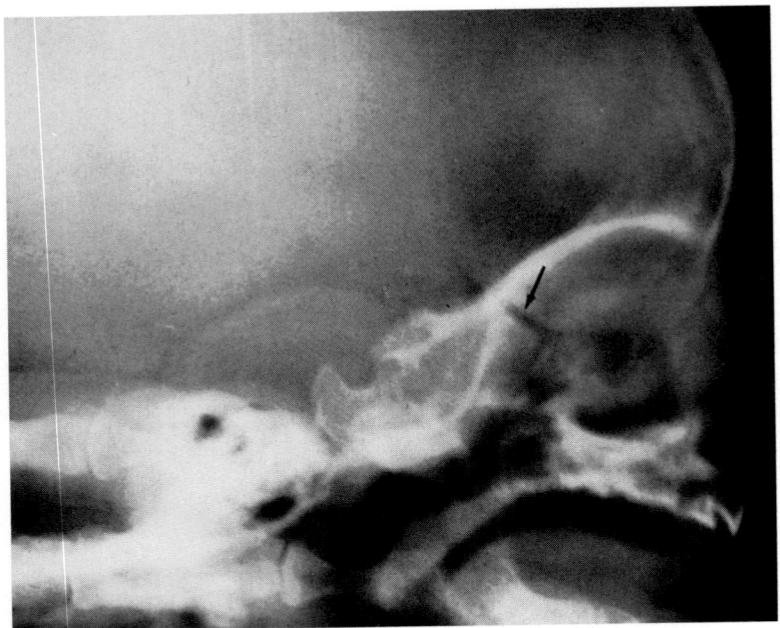

Figure 1–41. The zygomaticofrontal suture in a neonate.

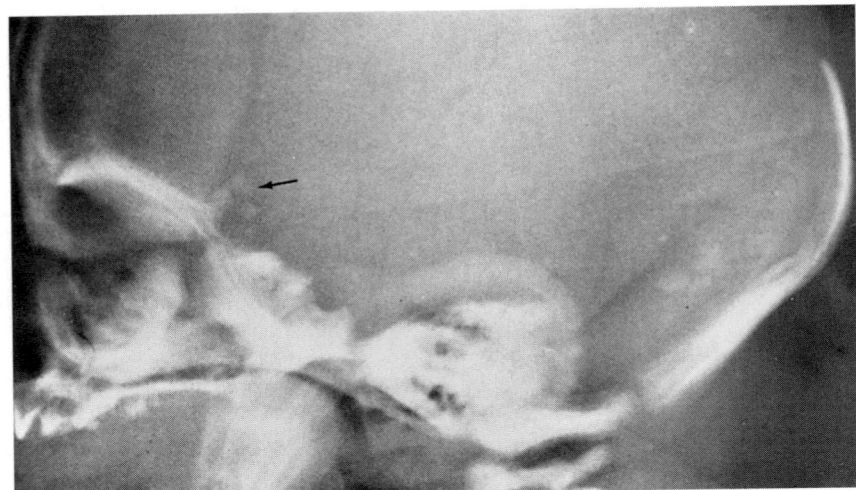

Figure 1–42. Wormian bones at the base of the coronal suture in a newborn (epiteric bones).

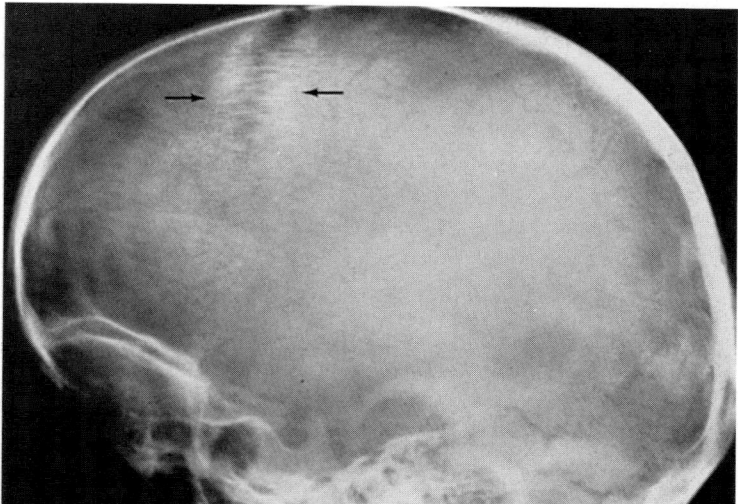

Figure 1–43. Simulated spread of the coronal sutures in a 4-year-old boy. Sutural prominence is extremely variable, particularly from ages 4 to 8, and should not be mistaken for evidence of increased intracranial pressure. Such early perisutural sclerosis accentuates the prominence of the sutures.

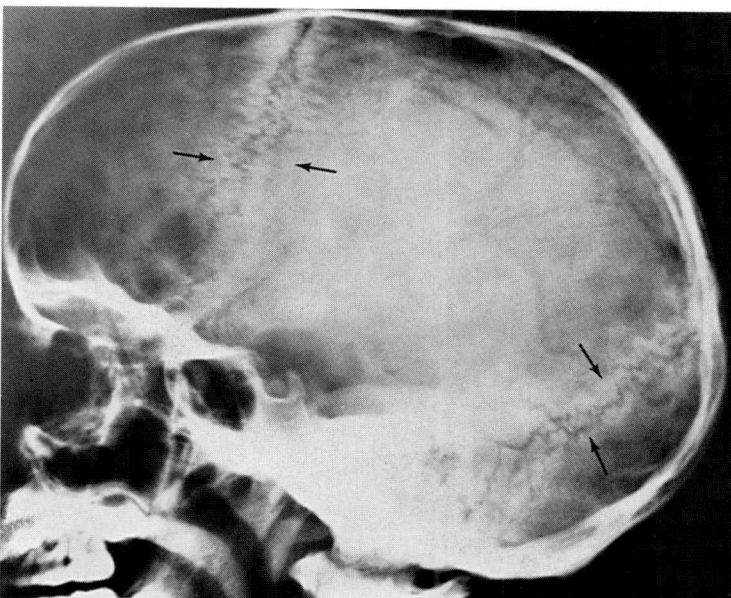

Figure 1–44. Simulated spread sutures in an 8-year-old boy.

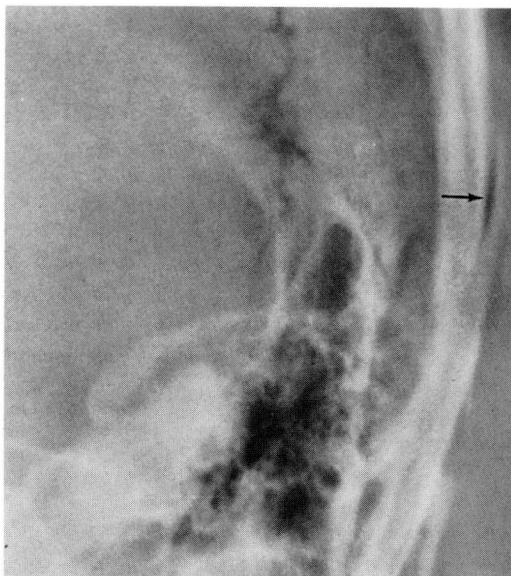

Figure 1–45. Normal squamosal suture projected tangentially, simulating a fracture.

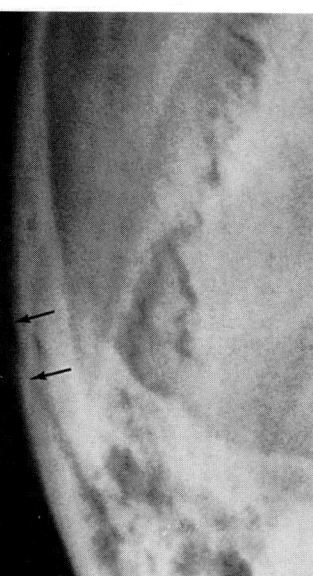

Figure 1–46. Tangential projection of the squamosal suture, producing a less obvious simulated fracture.

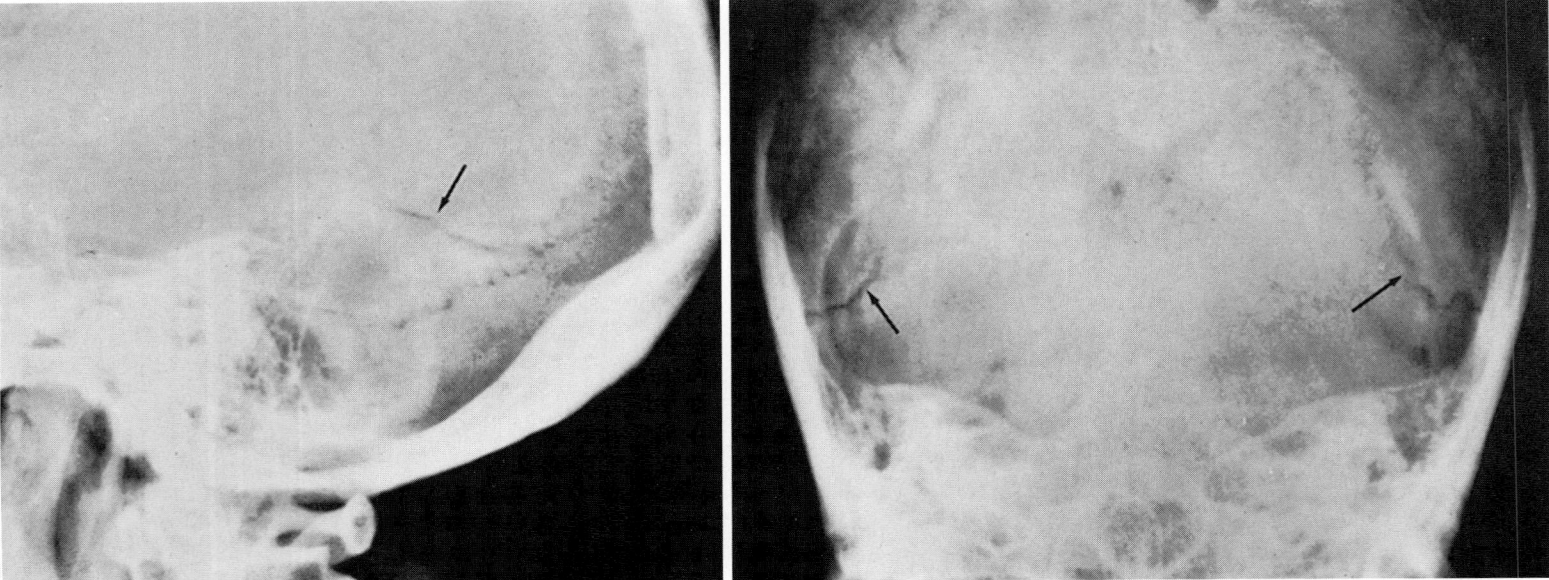

Figure 1–47. The posterior portion of the squamosal suture, which may simulate a fracture, particularly in the lateral projection.

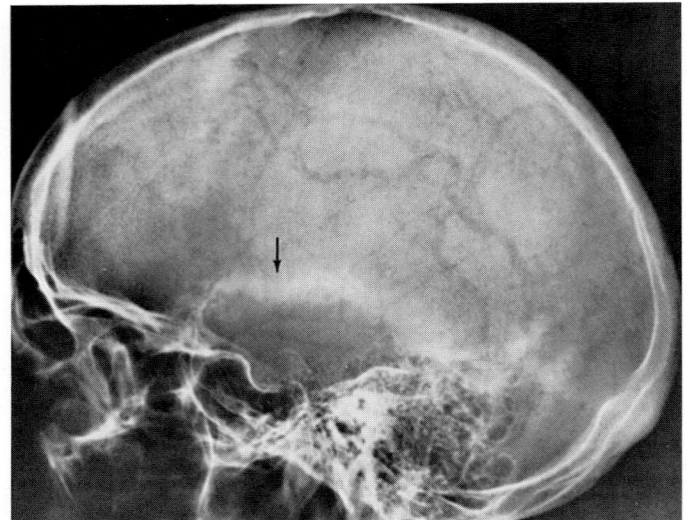

Figure 1–48. Normal sutural sclerosis of the squamosal suture.

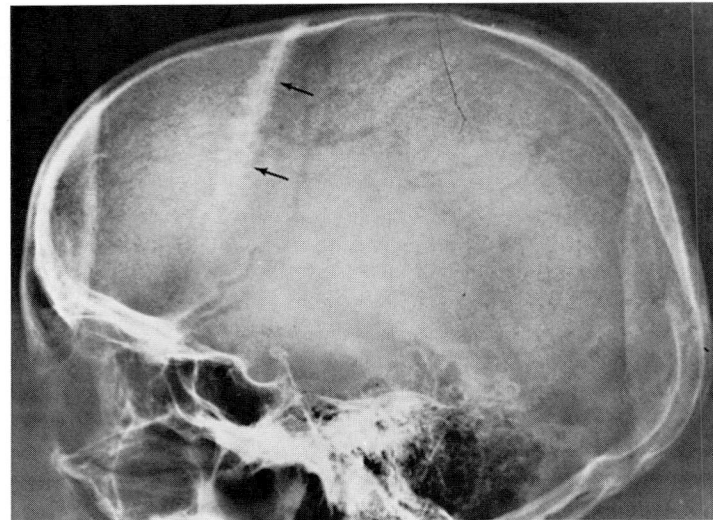

Figure 1–49. Normal sutural sclerosis of the coronal suture.

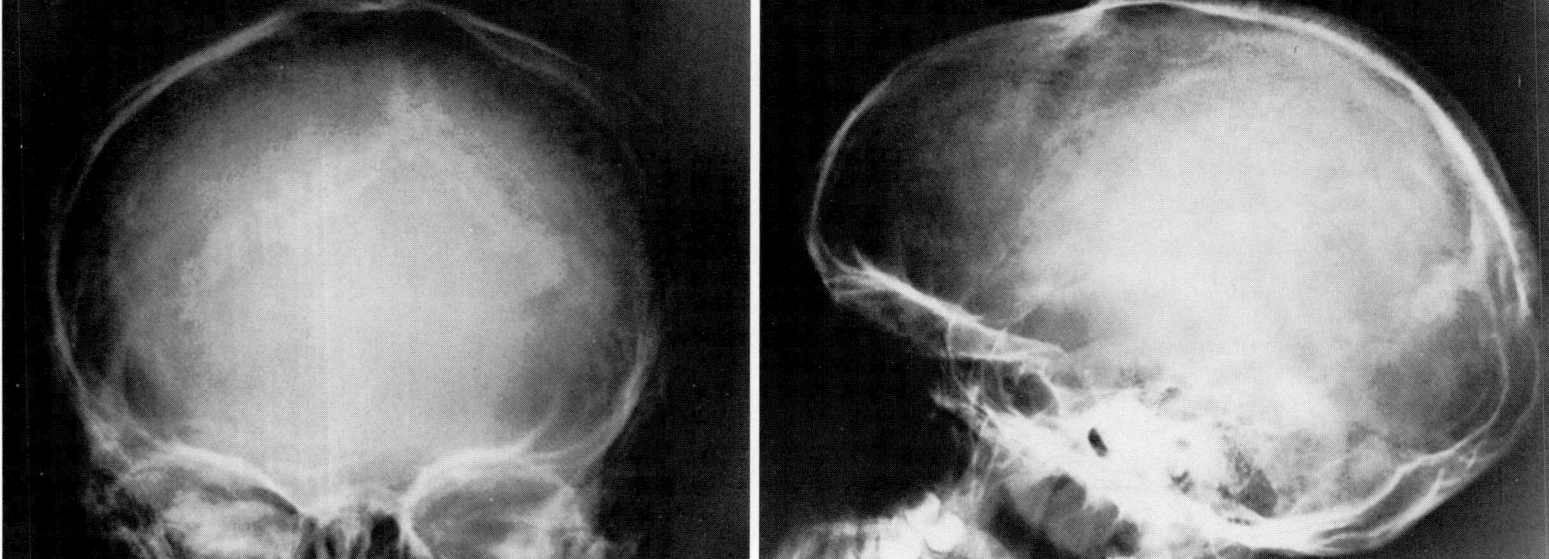

Figure 1–50. Early sutural sclerosis in a 12-year-old boy.

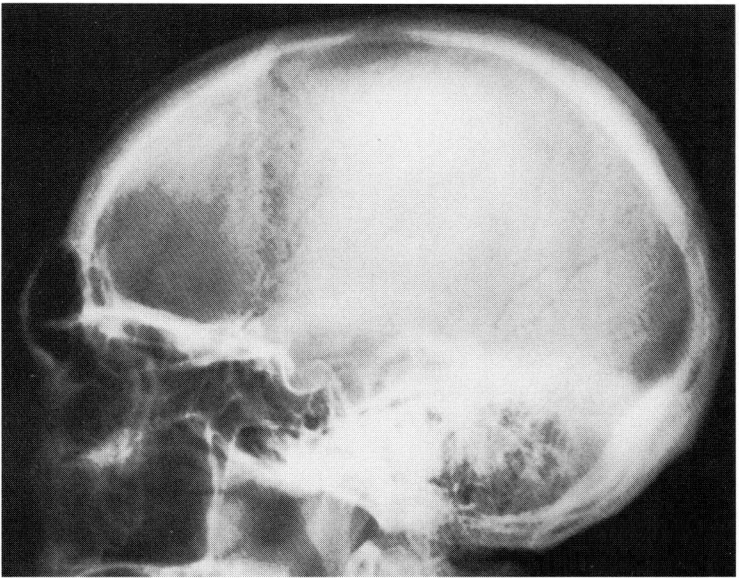

Figure 1–51. Thick but normal calvaria in a 30-year-old man.

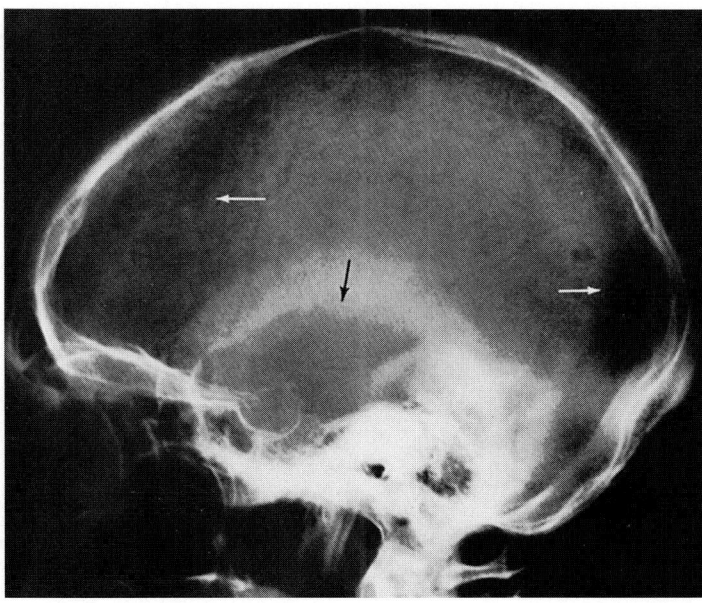

Figure 1–52. Normal frontal, temporal, and occipital lucencies seen in the aging calvaria.

Figure 1–53. Striking occipital radiolucency in a 32-year-old woman. These localized normal radiolucencies should not be mistaken for osteoporosis circumscripta of Paget's disease.

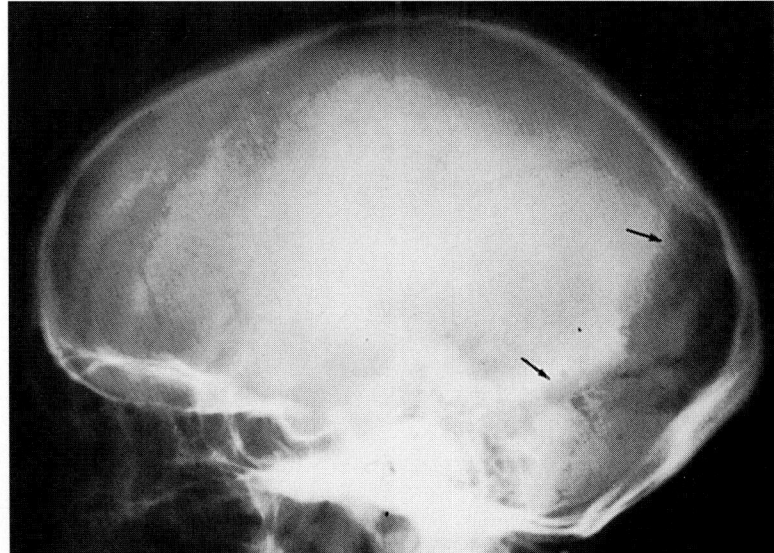

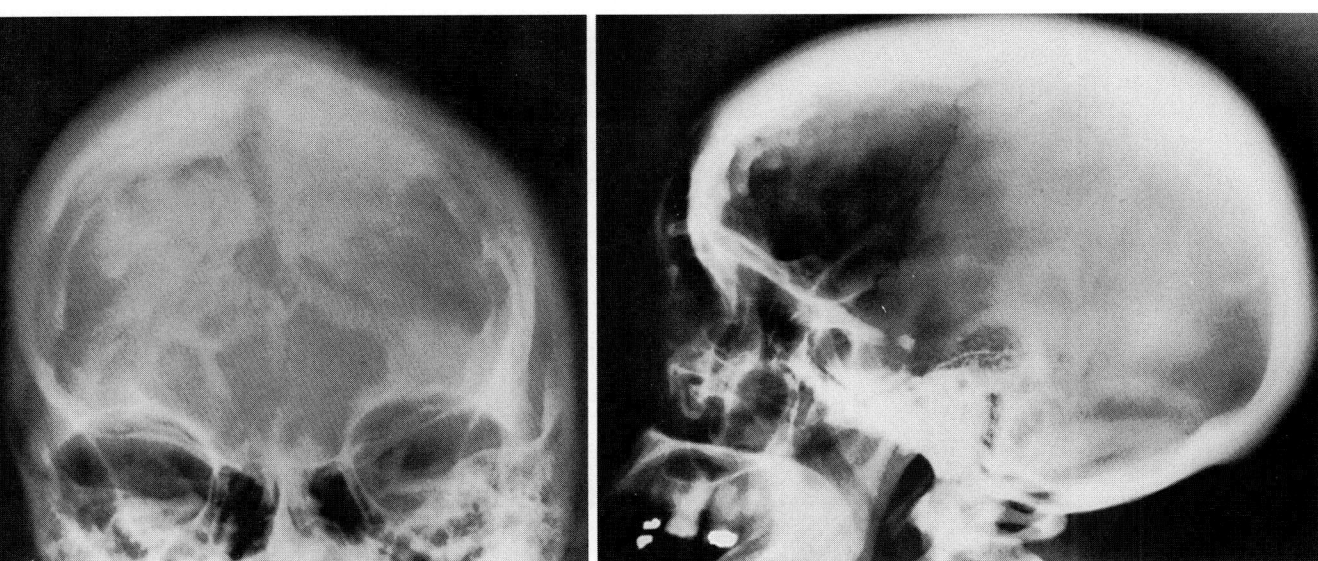

Figure 1–54. Generalized and frontal benign cranial hyperostosis in a 38-year-old woman.

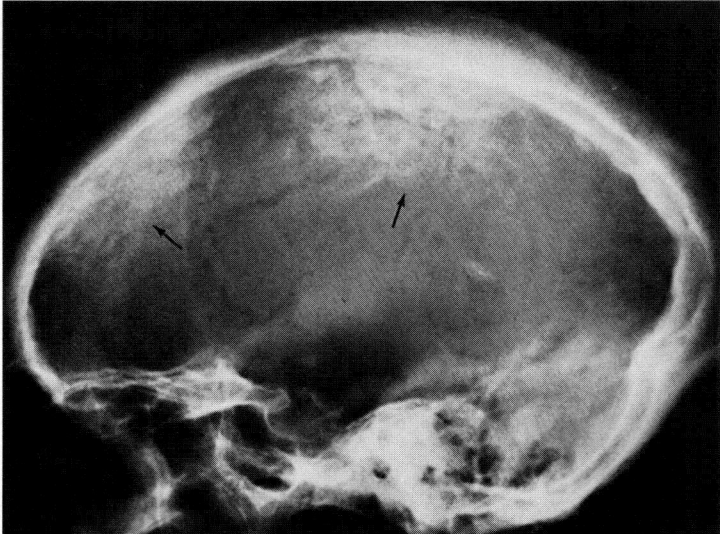

Figure 1–55. Benign cranial hyperostosis in a 65-year-old woman. Diffuse thickening of the calvaria is present as well as localized internal hyperostosis of the frontal and parietal bones.

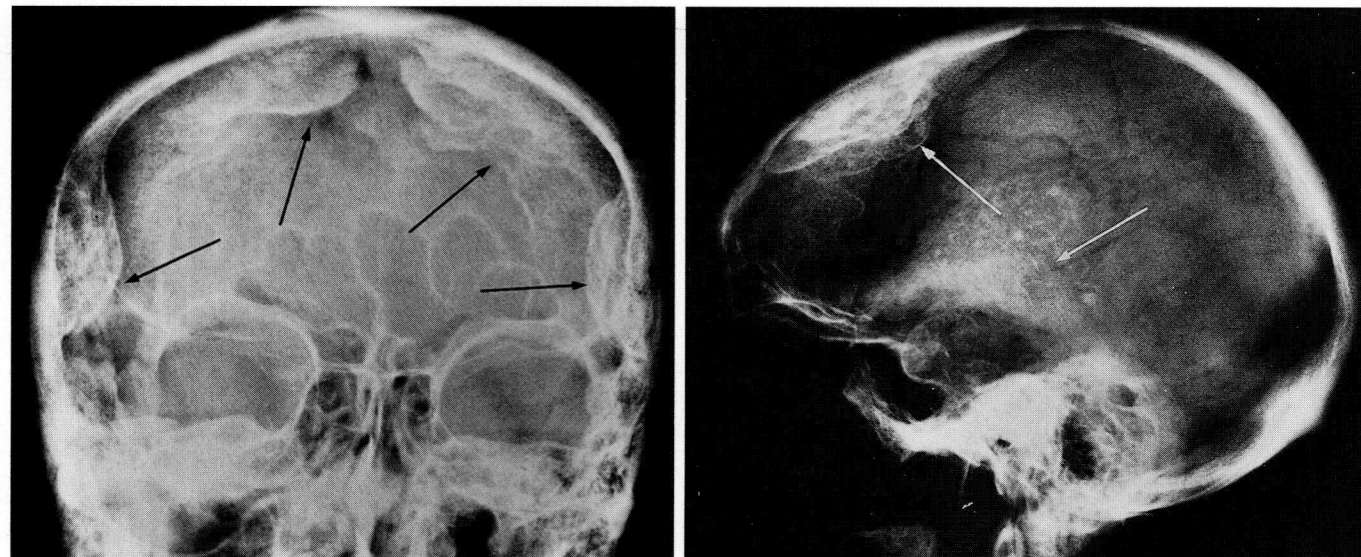

Figure 1–56. Frontal and temporal benign cranial hyperostosis in an 81-year-old woman.

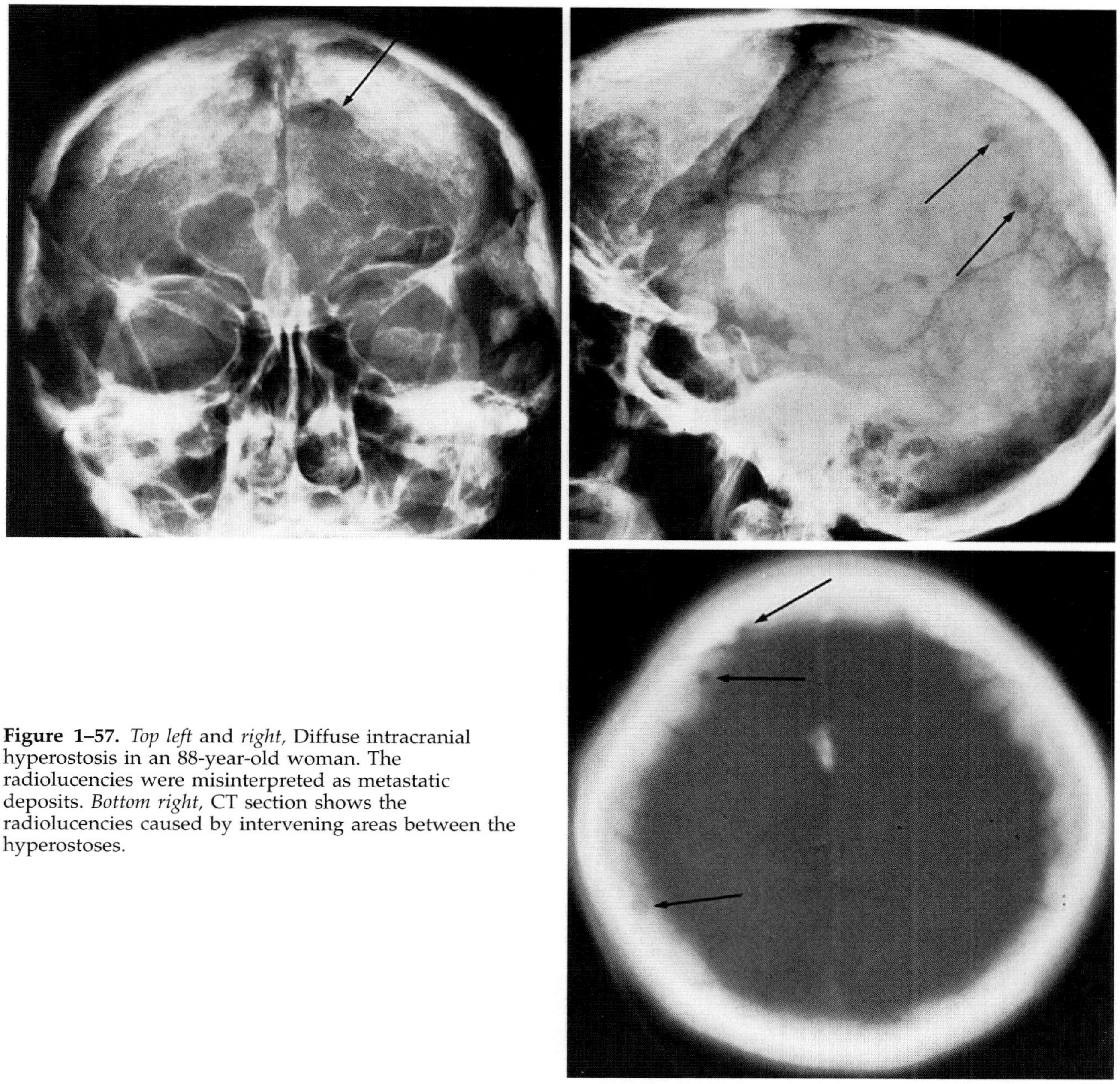

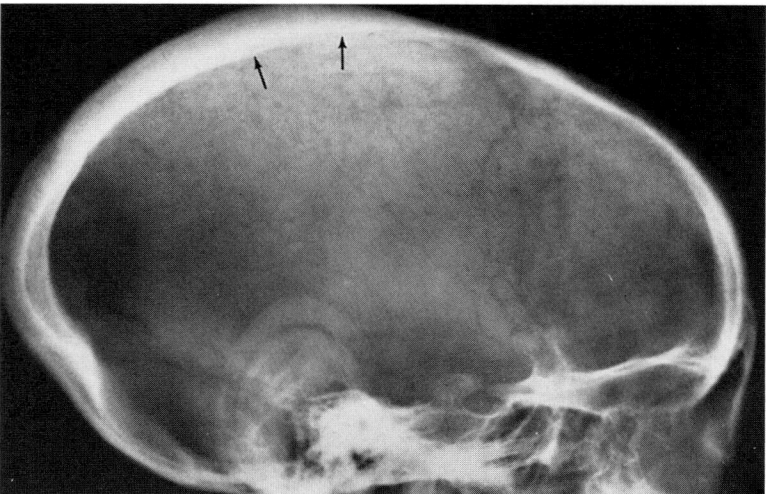

Figure 1–57. *Top left* and *right,* Diffuse intracranial hyperostosis in an 88-year-old woman. The radiolucencies were misinterpreted as metastatic deposits. *Bottom right,* CT section shows the radiolucencies caused by intervening areas between the hyperostoses.

Figure 1–58. Localized thickening of the parietal bone, a normal variation.

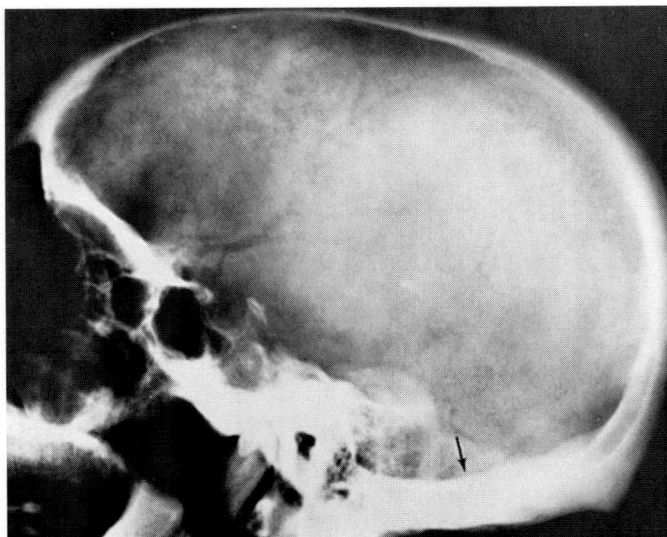

Figure 1–59. Localized thickening of the occipital bone, a normal variation.

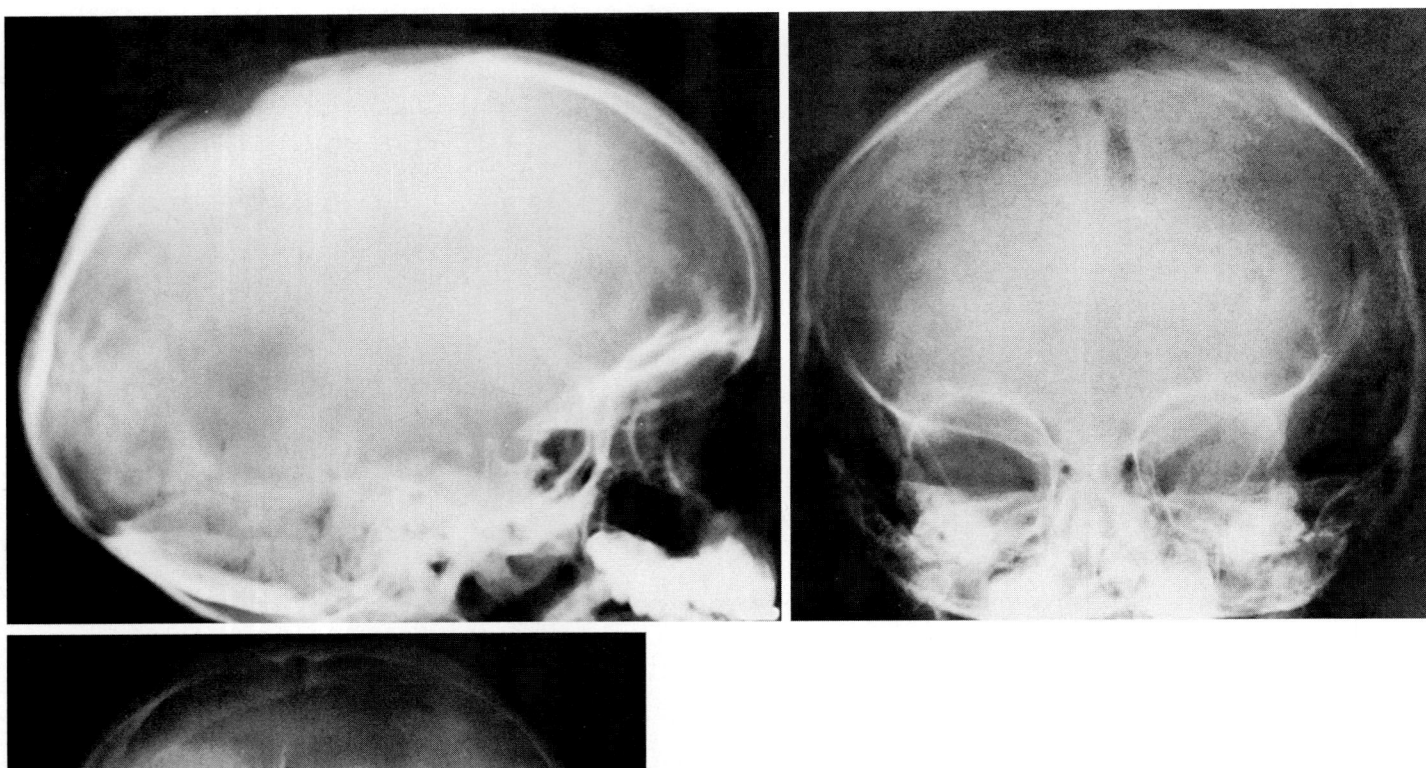

Figure 1–60. Cranium bifidum occultum. Incomplete closure of the midline of the skull in a 7-year-old boy, not to be mistaken for a destructive process. Such closure defects may be unassociated with bone dysplasia (see Figs. 1–99 to 1–102). (Ref: Inoue Y et al: Cranium bifidum occultum. *Neuroradiology* 25:217, 1983.)

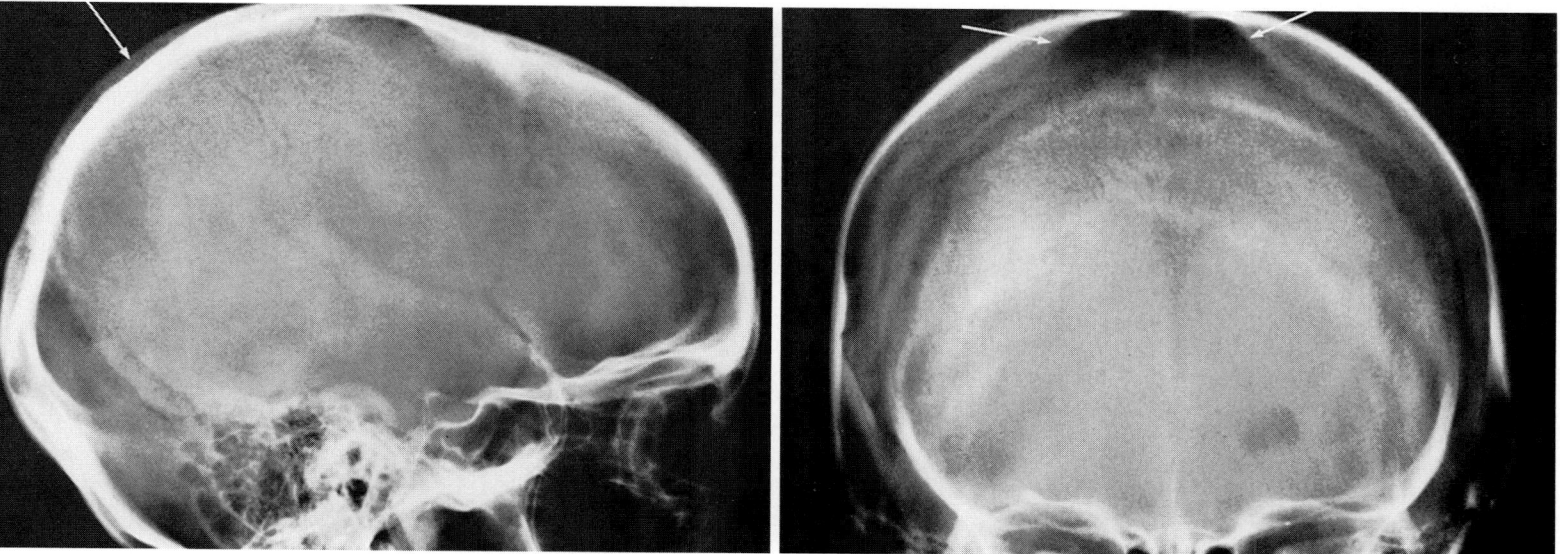

Figure 1–61. Localized palpable thinning of the outer table of the skull in an asymptomatic 21-year-old woman. This probably represents an incomplete form of cranium bifidum occultum (see Fig. 1–60).

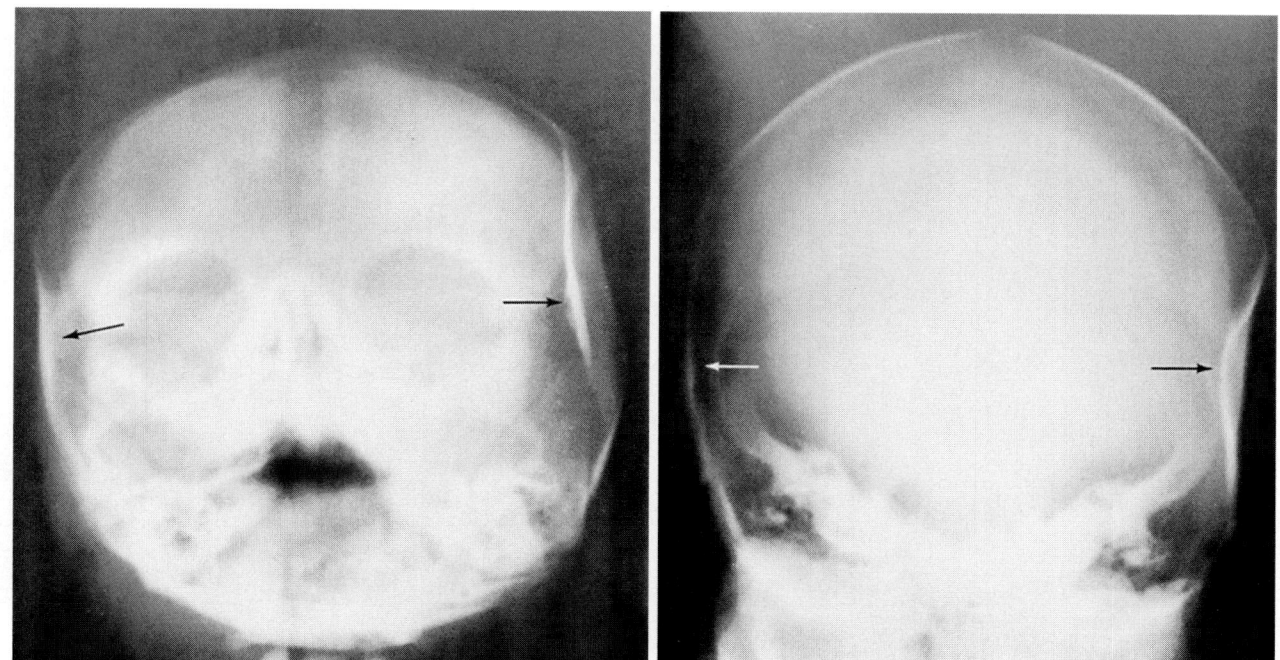

Figure 1–62. Congenital depressions of the calvaria caused by faulty fetal packing. Such depressions manifest at birth and, when not associated with edema or hemorrhage of the overlying soft tissues, are usually due to faulty position with long-standing pressure from the fetal feet or maternal sacral promontory. (Ref: Caffey J: *Pediatric x-ray diagnosis,* 8th ed. St. Louis, Mosby 1985; Eisenberg D, Kirchner SG, Perrin EC: Neonatal skull depressions unassociated with birth trauma. *Am J Roentgenol* 143:1063, 1984.)

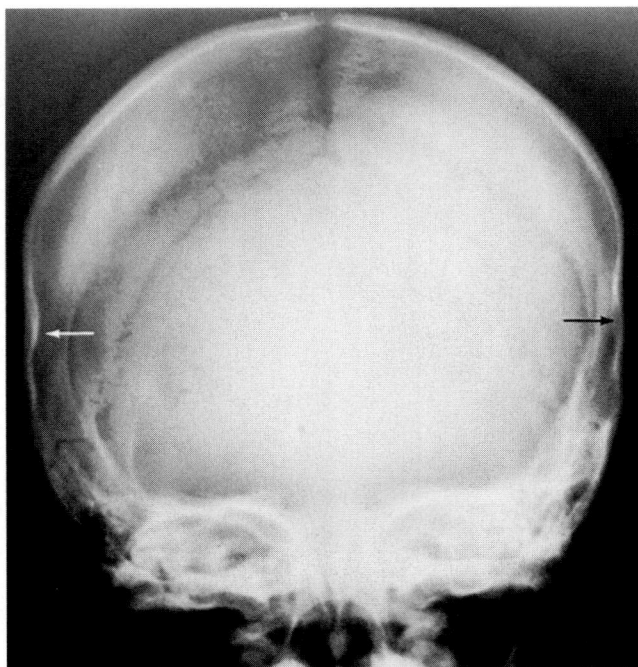

Figure 1–63. Slight calvarial depressions in an 18-month-old child, probably representing residuals of faulty fetal packing. These depressions usually regress spontaneously without treatment.

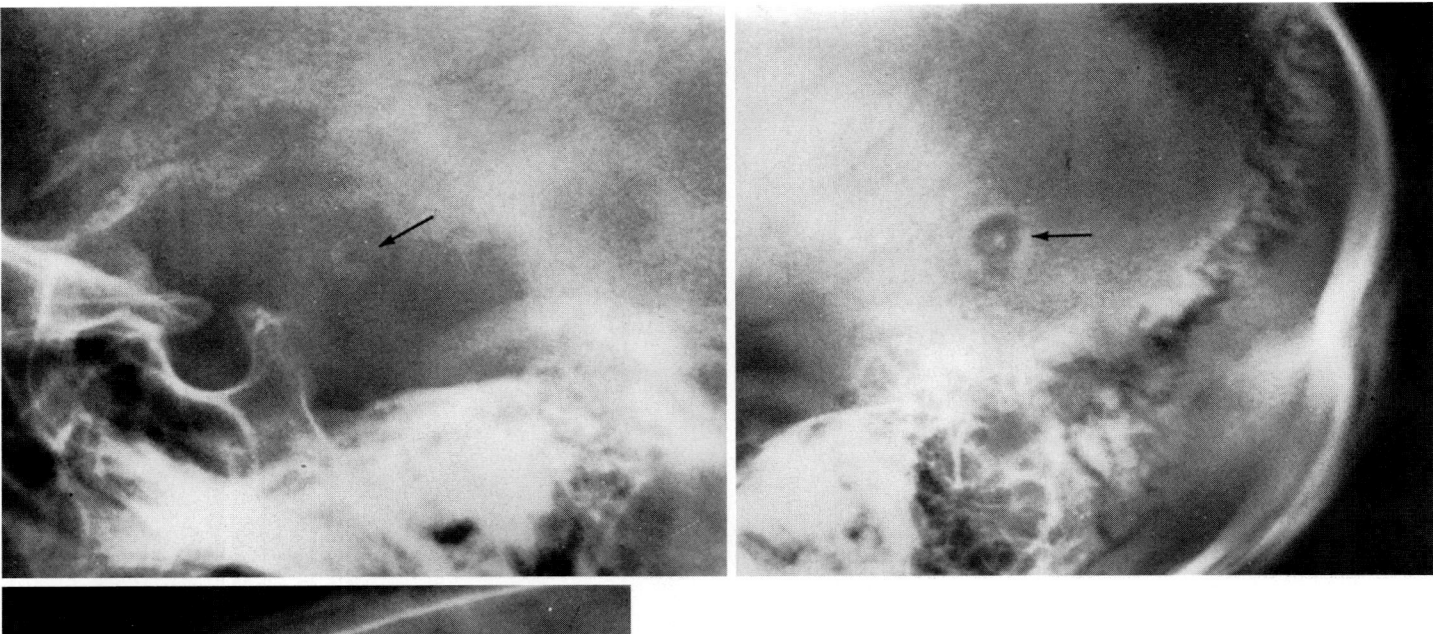

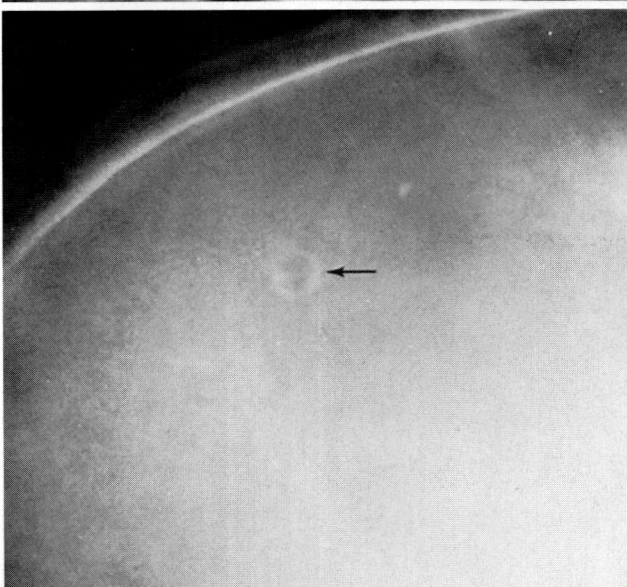

Figure 1–64. Three examples of "doughnut lesions." These are not clinically significant and may be seen in any part of the calvaria, including juvenile skulls. They may or may not contain a central area of sclerosis. (Ref: Keats TE, Holt JF: The calvarial "doughnut lesion": A previously undescribed entity. *Am J Roentgenol* 105:314, 1969.)

Physiologic Intracranial Calcifications

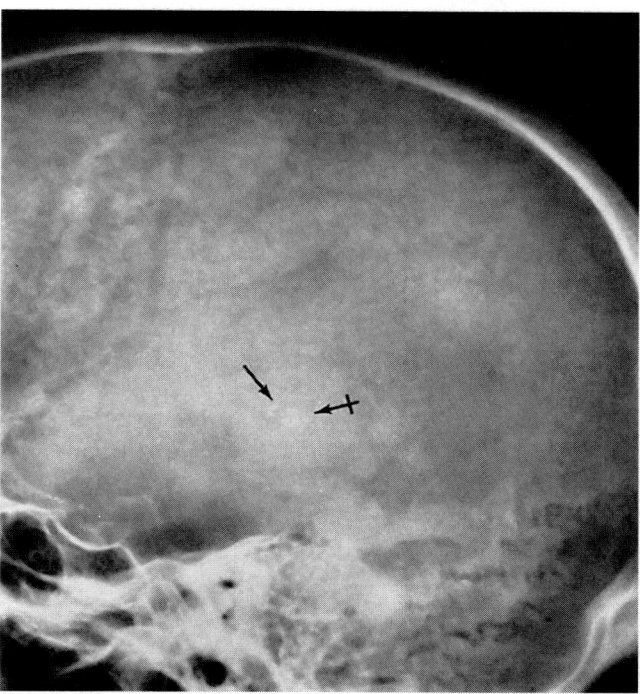

Figure 1–65. The habenular commissure (←) and the pineal gland (⟷).

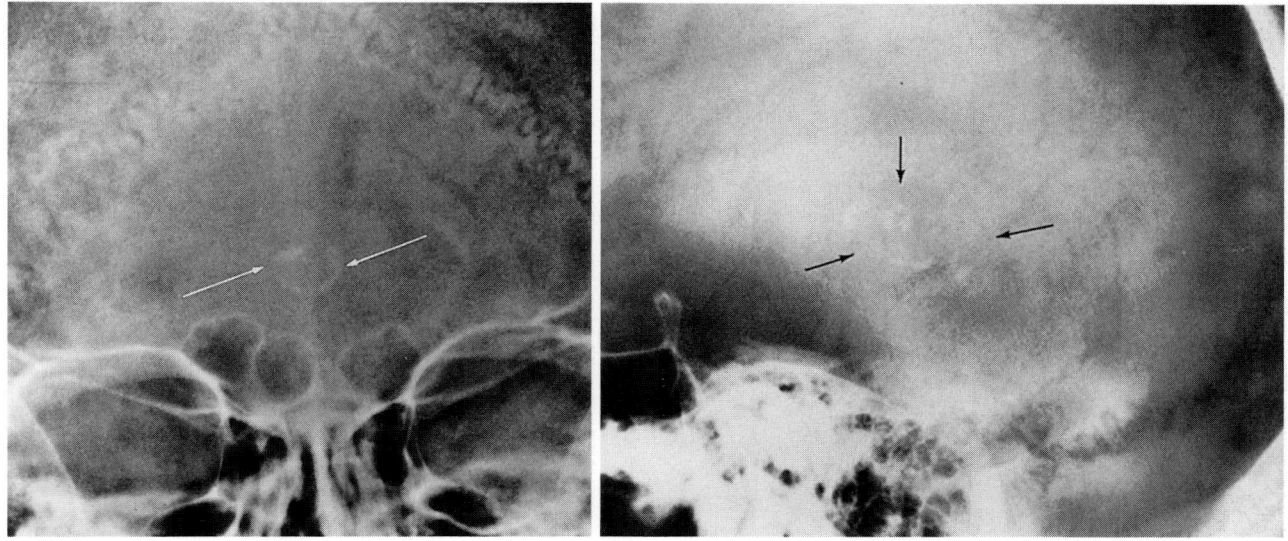

Figure 1–66. Large cystic pineal gland in a 60-year-old man. This finding in itself is of no clinical significance.

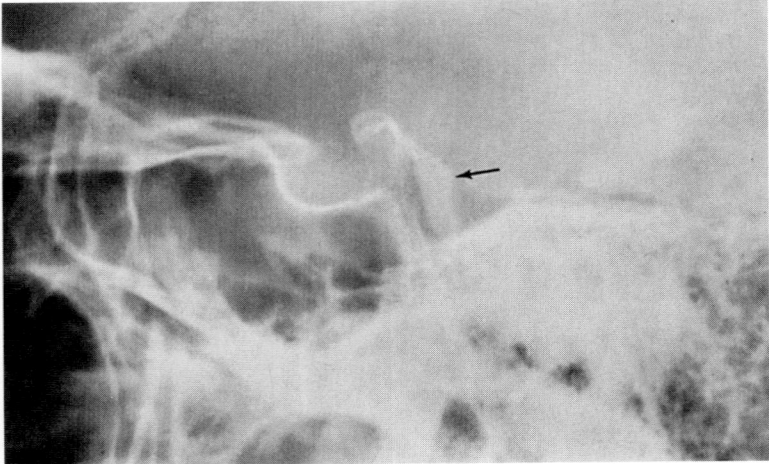

Figure 1–67. Petroclinoid ligament with heavy calcification.

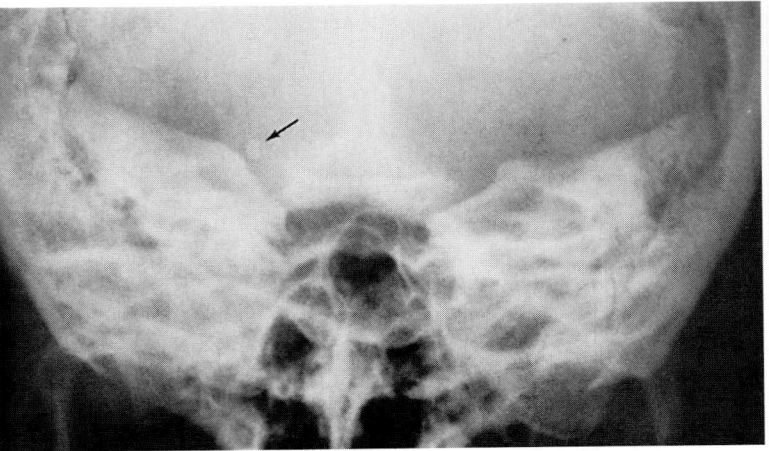

Figure 1–68. Petroclinoid calcification in the half-axial projection.

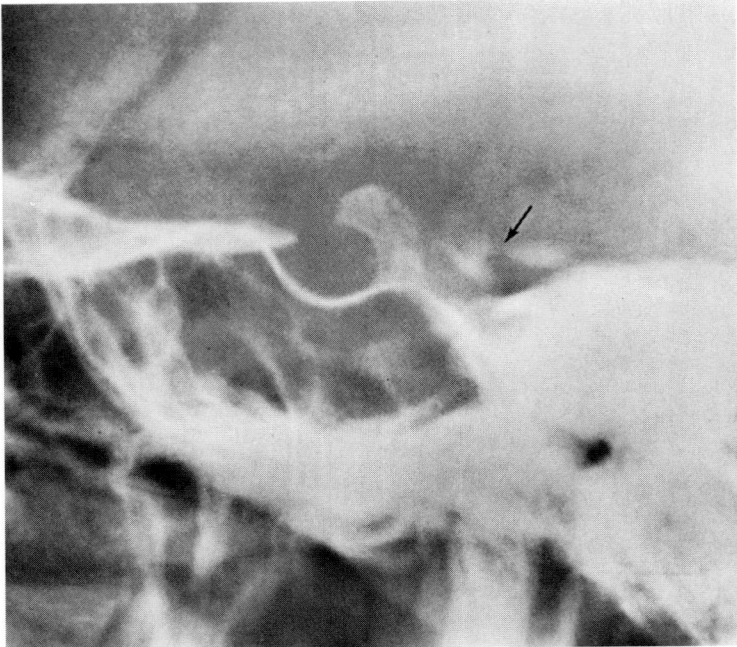

Figure 1–69. Petroclinoid ligament with irregular calcification.

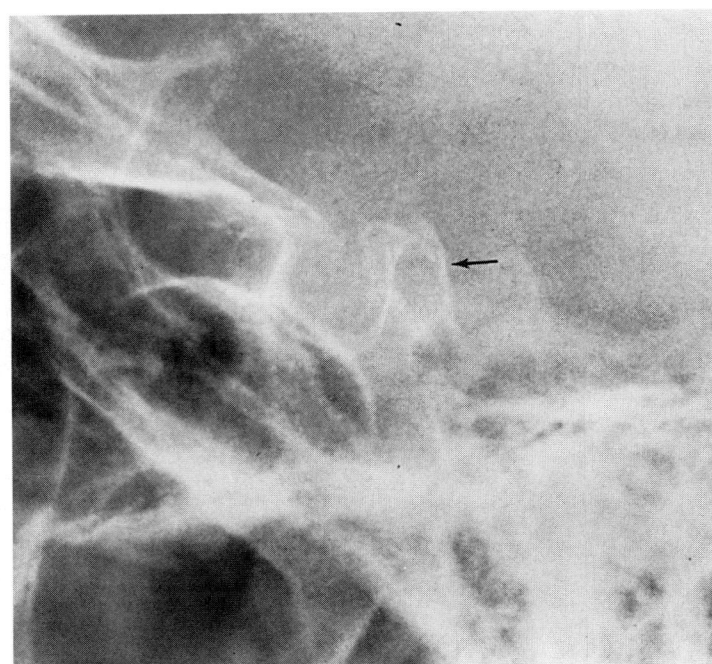

Figure 1–70. Petroclinoid ligament with an unusual pattern of calcification.

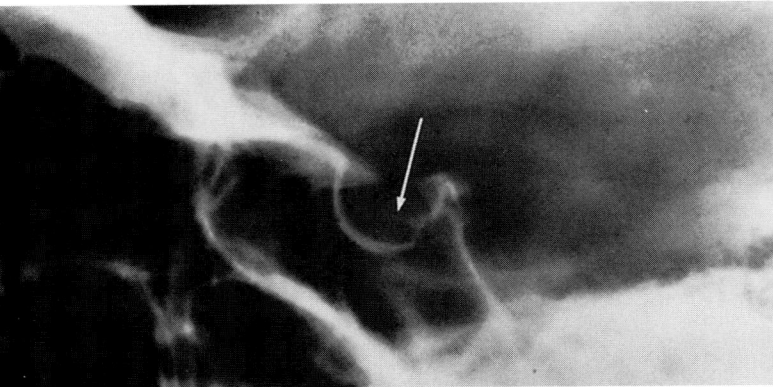

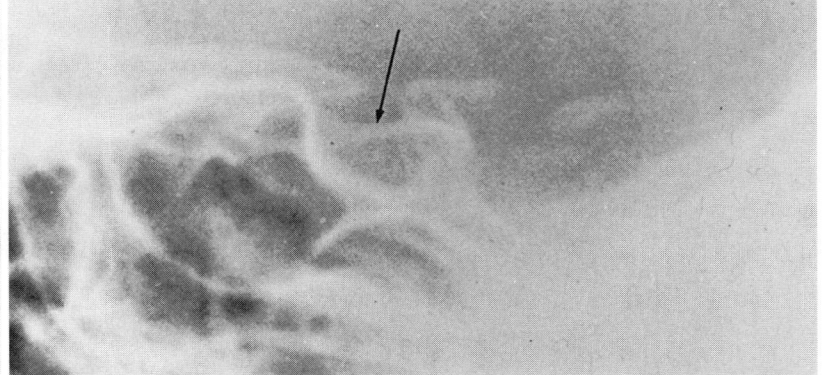

Figure 1–71. Two examples of calcification between the middle and posterior clinoid processes.

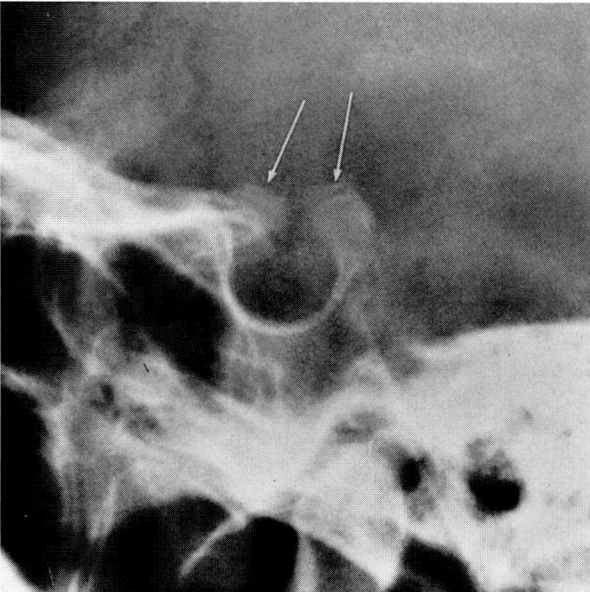

Figure 1–72. Unusual dural calcifications above anterior and posterior clinoid processes.

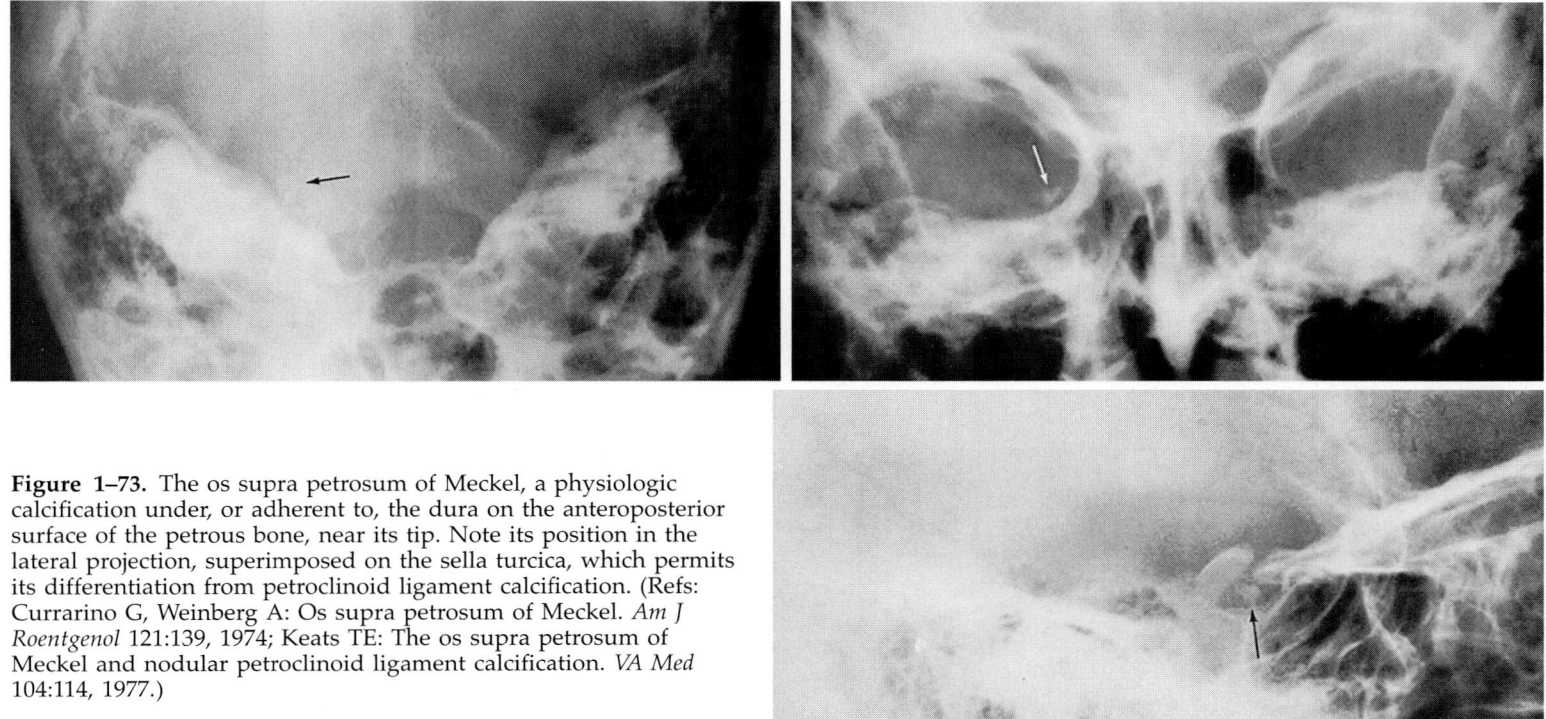

Figure 1–73. The os supra petrosum of Meckel, a physiologic calcification under, or adherent to, the dura on the anteroposterior surface of the petrous bone, near its tip. Note its position in the lateral projection, superimposed on the sella turcica, which permits its differentiation from petroclinoid ligament calcification. (Refs: Currarino G, Weinberg A: Os supra petrosum of Meckel. *Am J Roentgenol* 121:139, 1974; Keats TE: The os supra petrosum of Meckel and nodular petroclinoid ligament calcification. *VA Med* 104:114, 1977.)

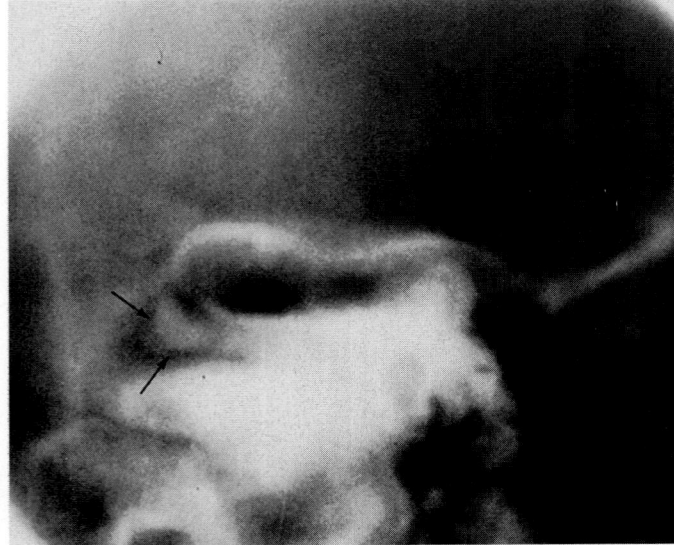

Figure 1–74. The os supra petrosum of Meckel, seen by polytomography.

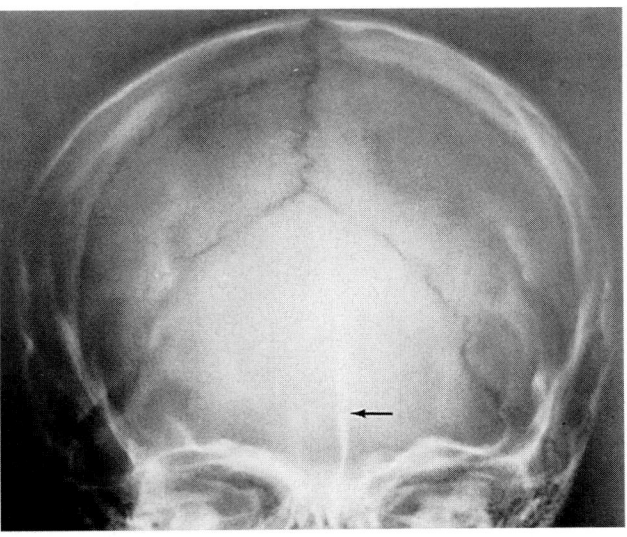

Figure 1–75. Prominent frontal crest on the internal surface of the frontal bone, simulating calcification of the falx cerebri in a healthy 4-year-old boy.

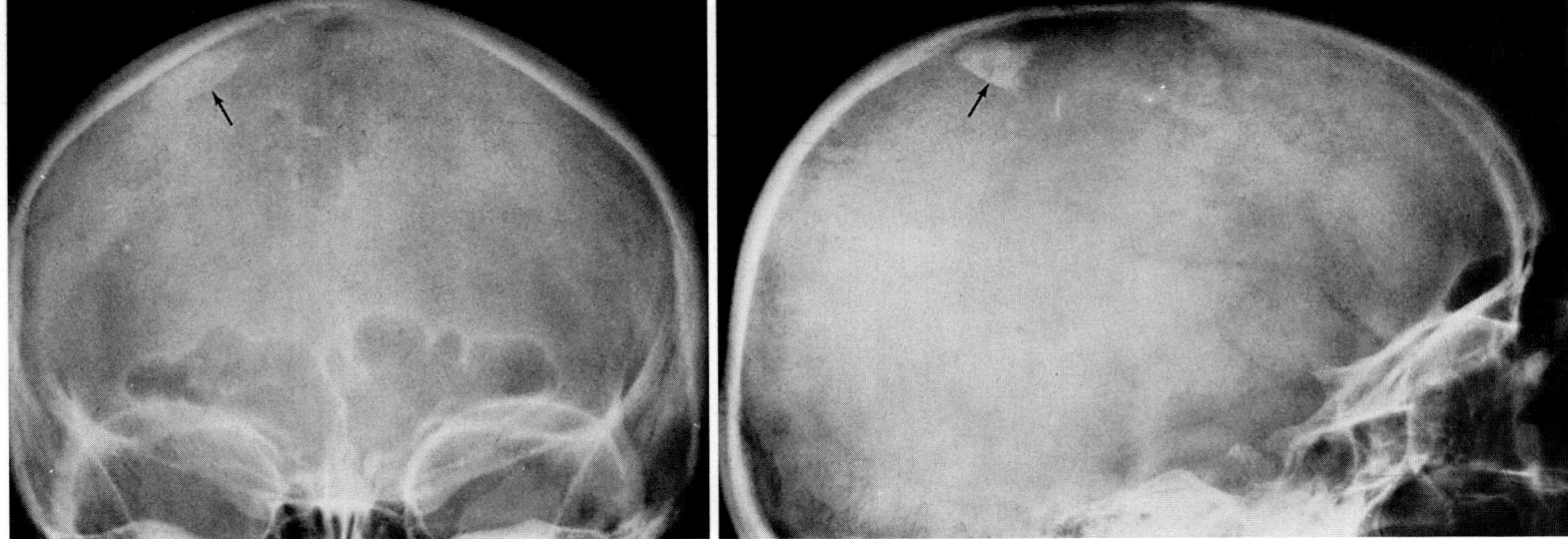

Figure 1–76. Localized focal dural calcification in the parietal area.

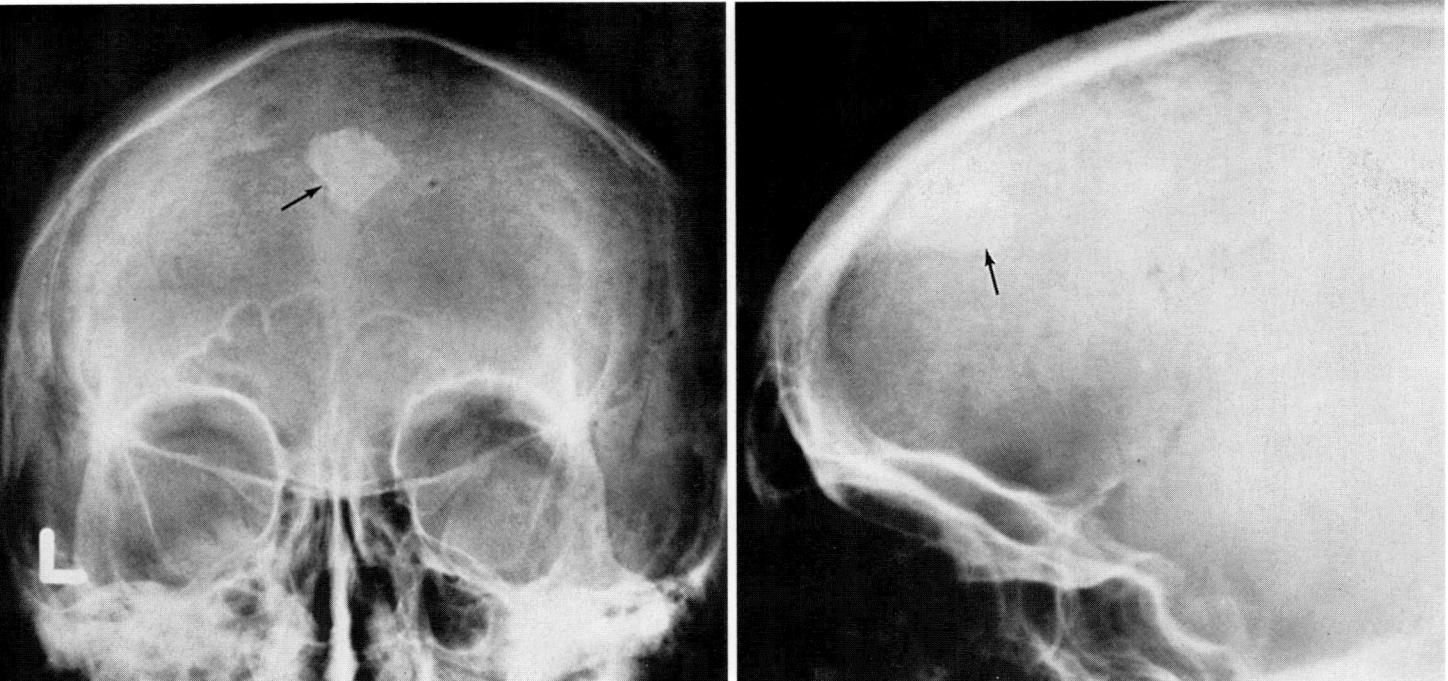

Figure 1–77. Localized focal dural calcification in the frontal area.

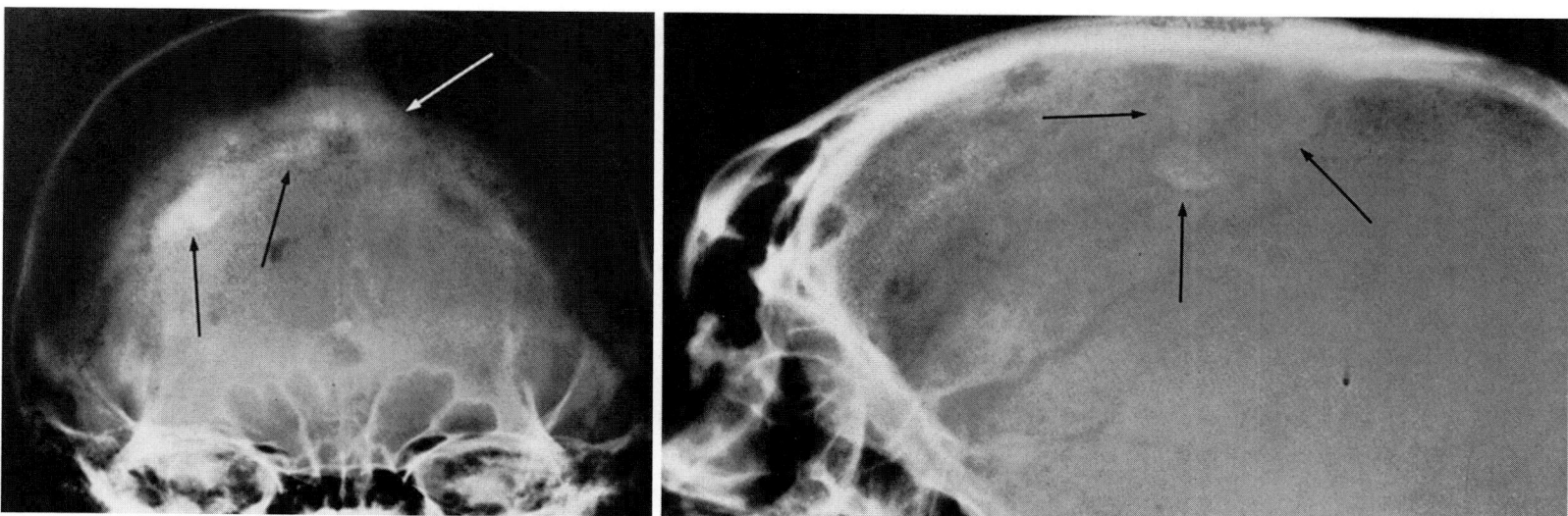

Figure 1–78. Multiple focal areas of dural calcification in a 71-year-old man.

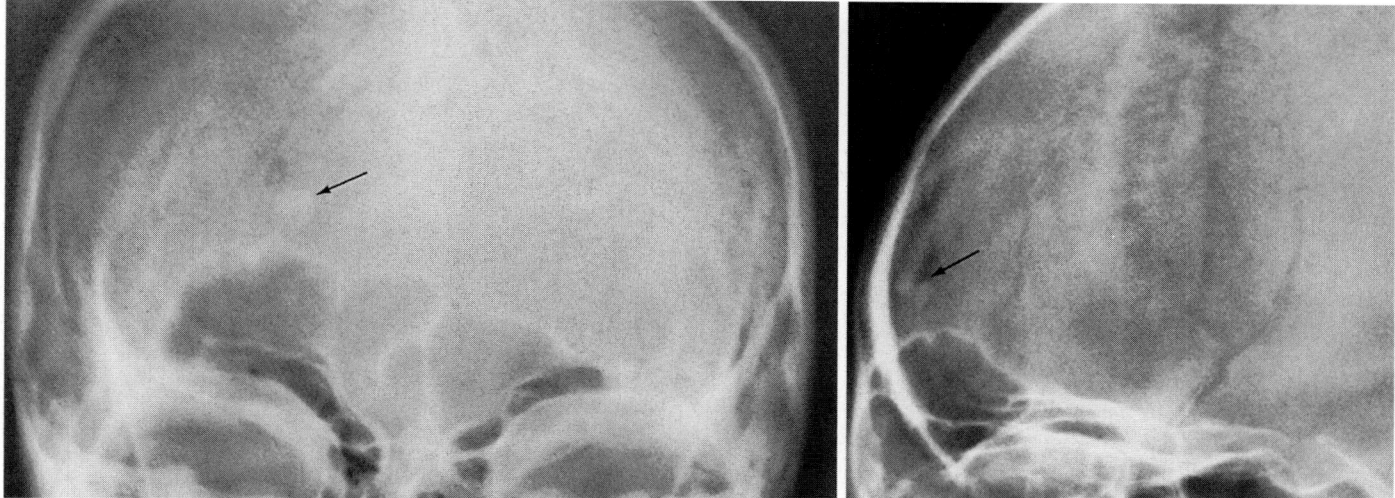

Figure 1–79. Small localized focal dural calcification in the frontal area.

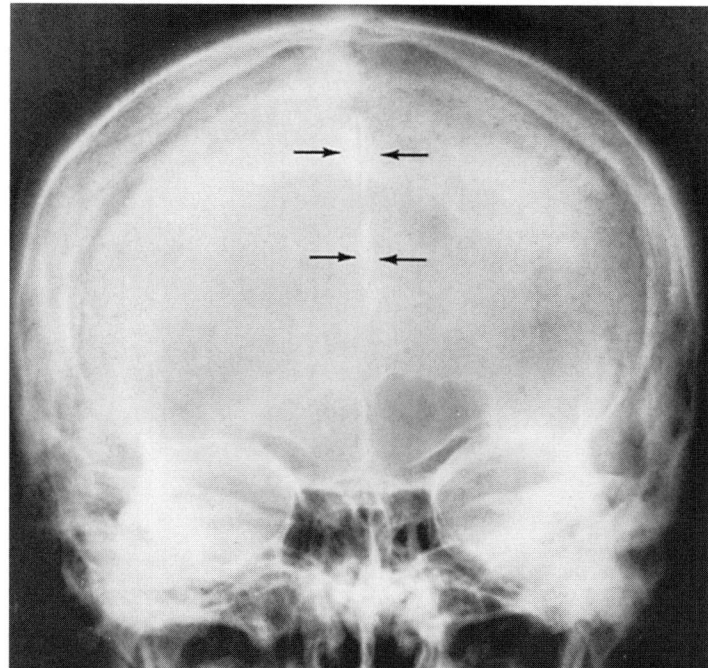

Figure 1–80. Calcification of the falx cerebri.

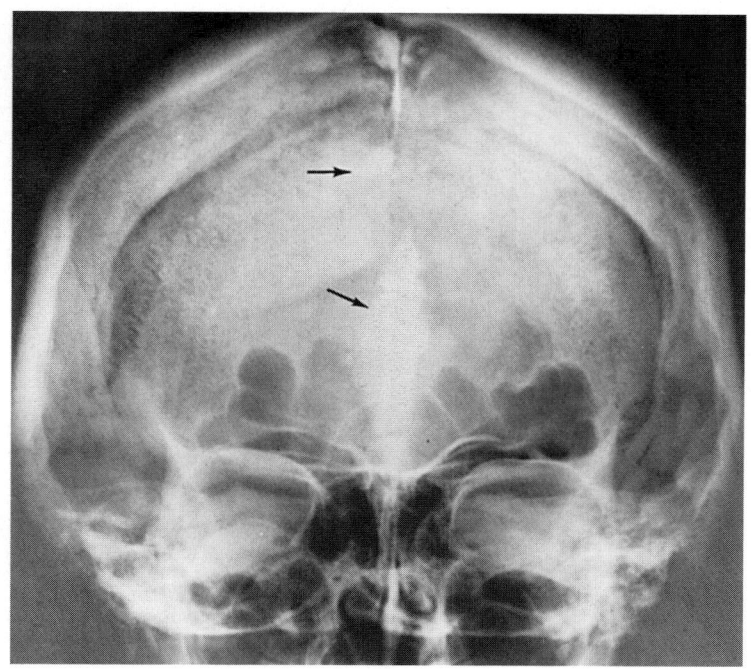

Figure 1–81. Heavy calcification of the falx cerebri.

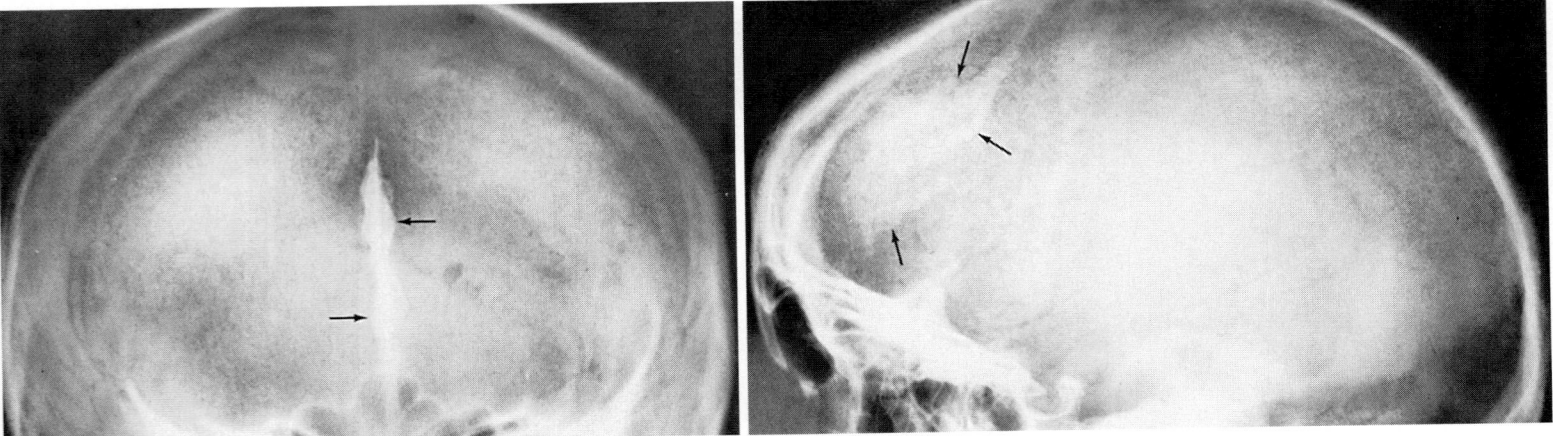

Figure 1–82. Heavy calcification in the falx cerebri in frontal and lateral projections.

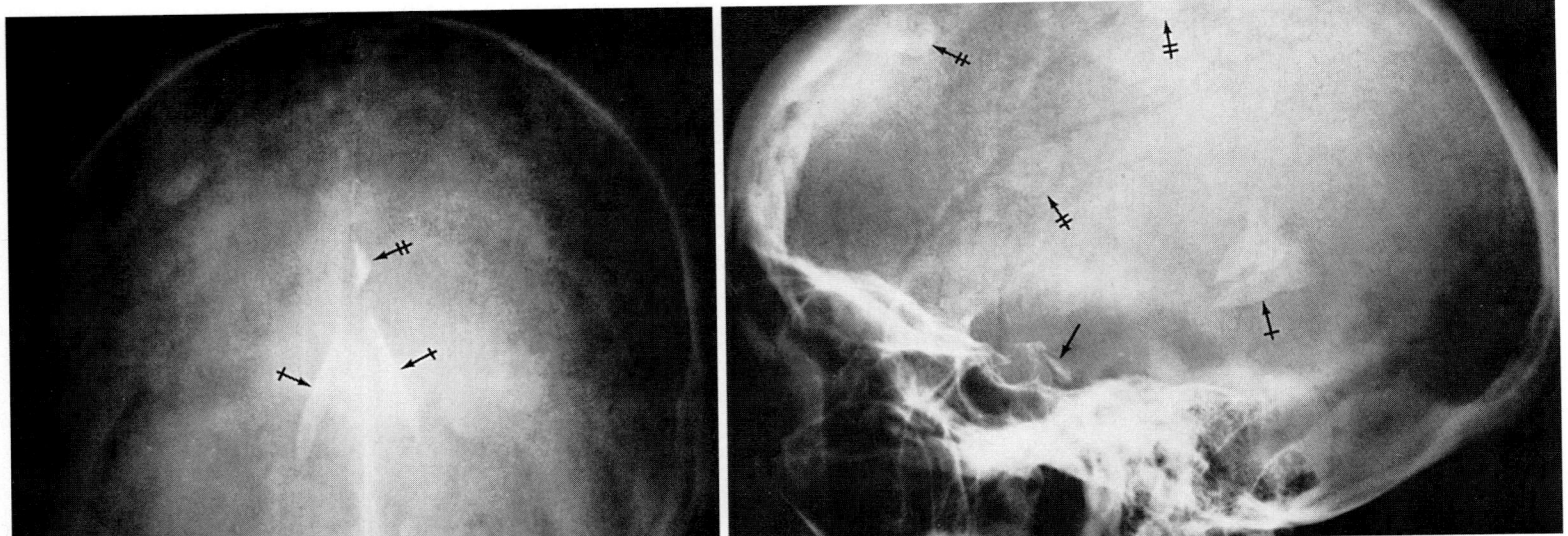

Figure 1–83. Three types of physiologic calcification. Demonstrated are petroclinoid ligament (←), heavy calcification of the tentorium cerebelli (↔), and falx cerebri (⇤).

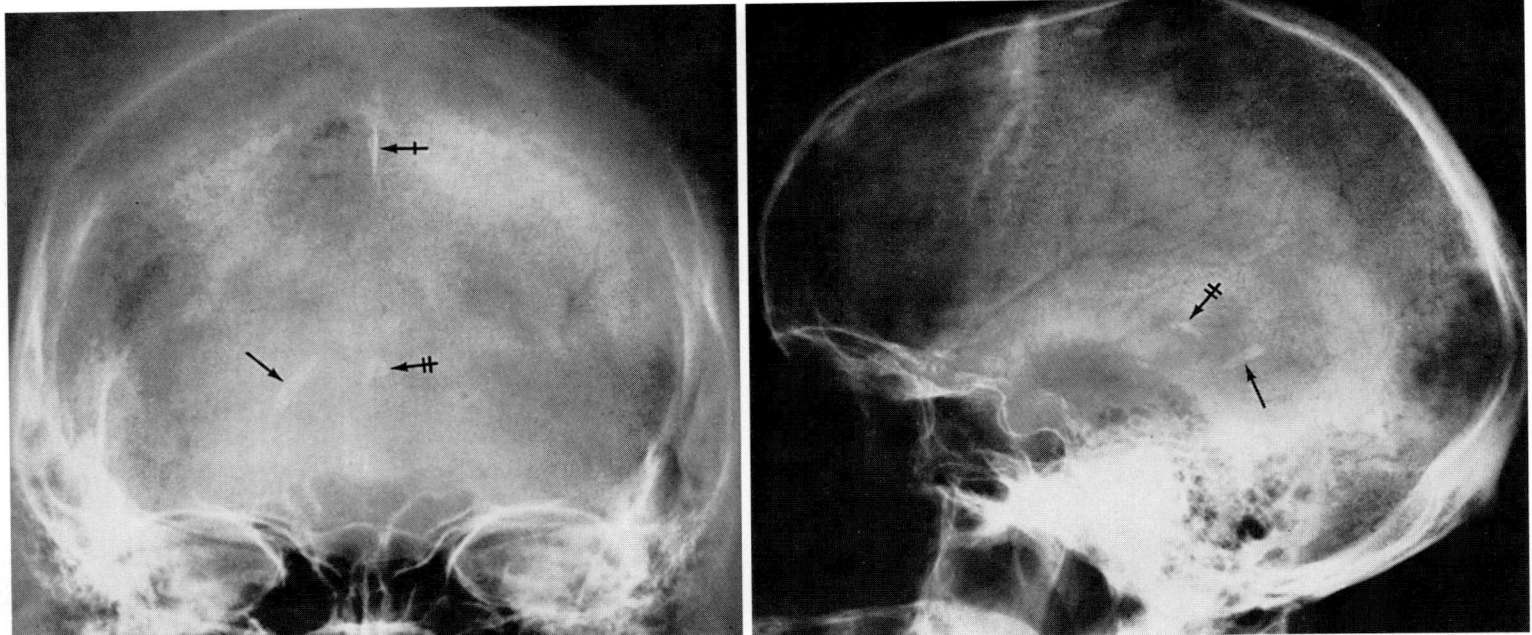

Figure 1–84. Minor calcification of the tentorium cerebelli (←). Calcification is also present in the falx (↔) and the pineal gland (⇤). (Ref: Saldino RM, De Chiro G: Tentorial calcification. Radiology 111:207, 1974.)

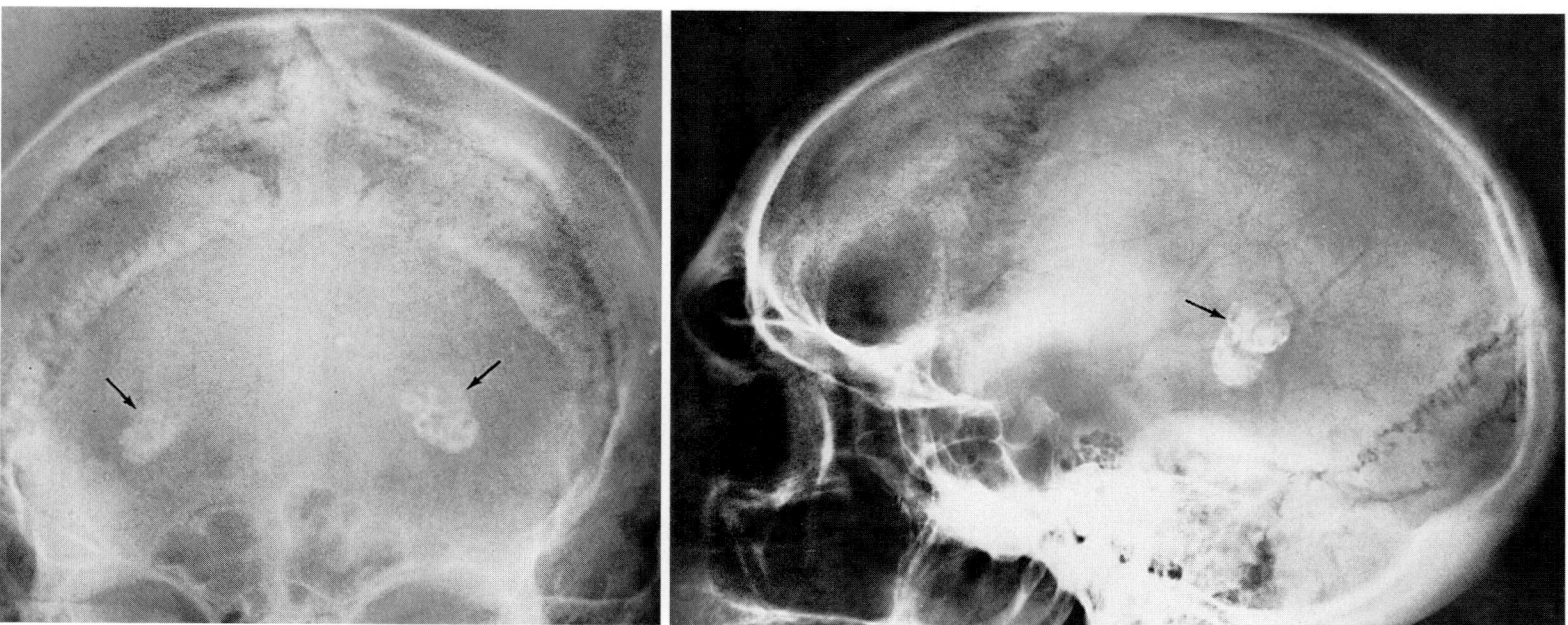

Figure 1–85. Calcification in the glomus of the choroid plexus of each lateral ventricle.

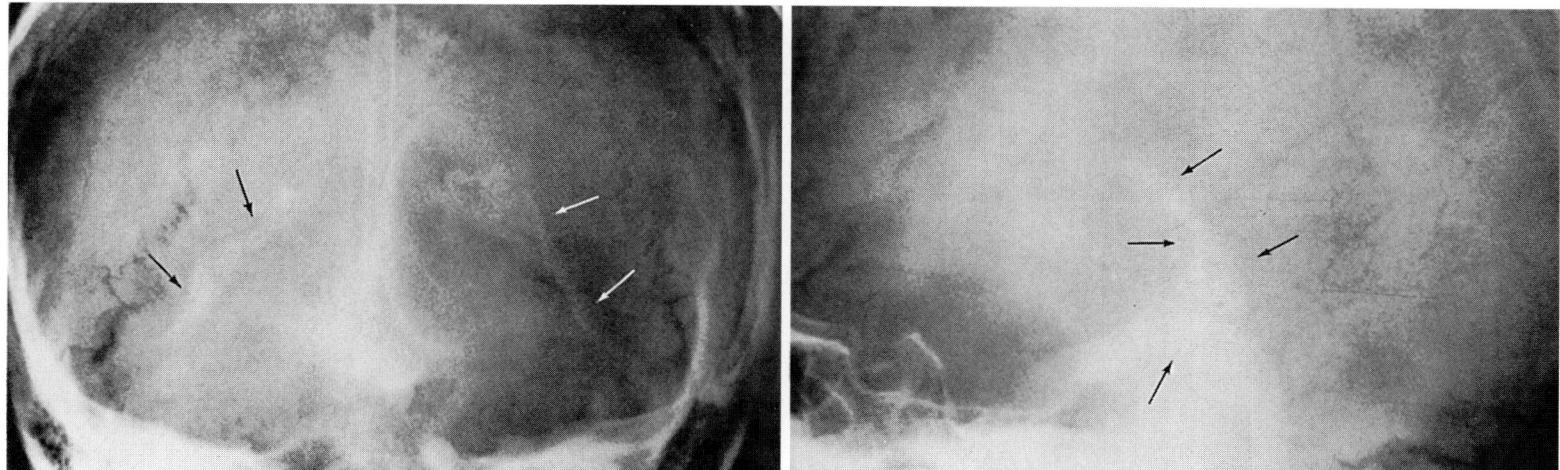

Figure 1–86. Calcification in the glomus of the choroid plexus (boomerang configuration).

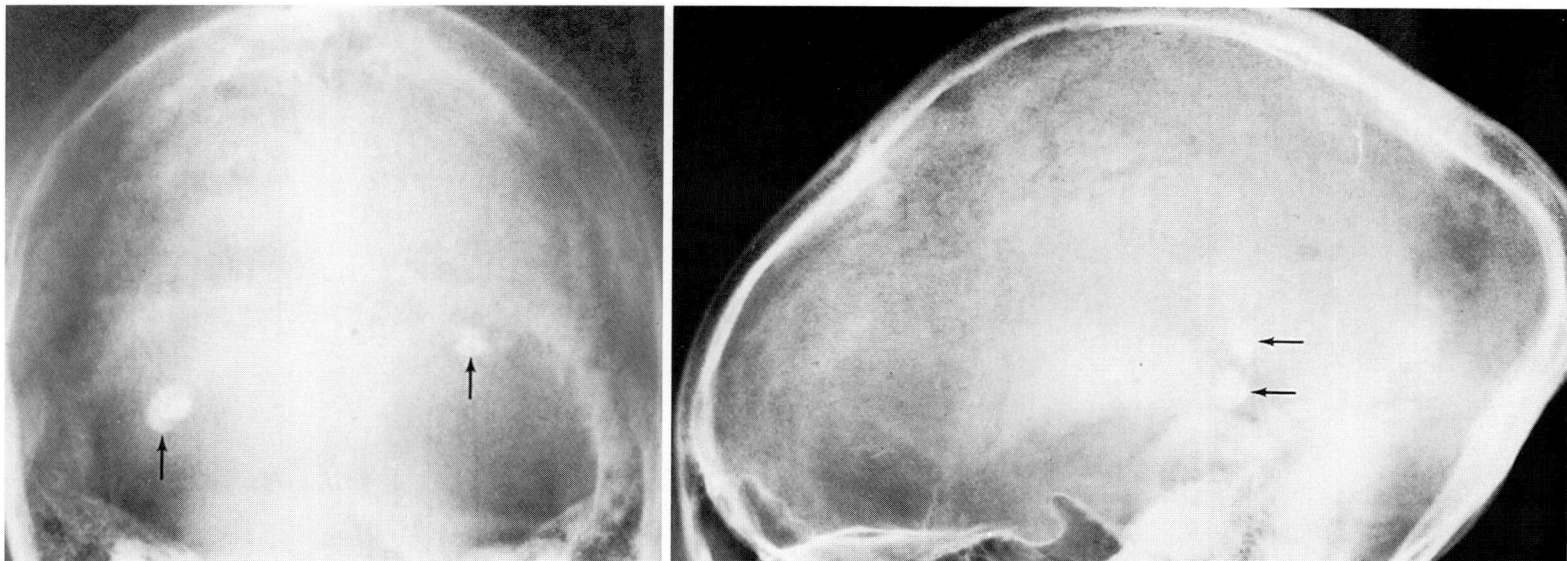

Figure 1–87. Normal asymmetry of the calcified glomera of the choroid plexus. These cannot be reliably used for evidence of intracranial abnormality.

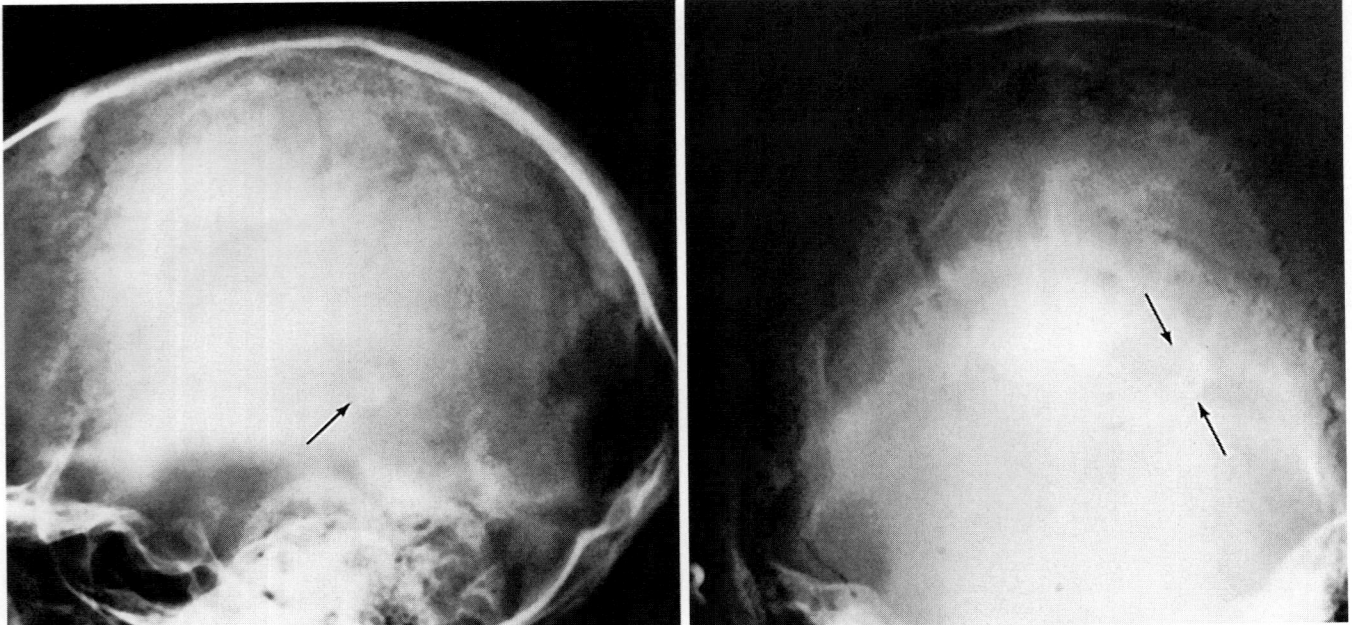

Figure 1–88. Unilateral calcification of the glomus of the choroid plexus.

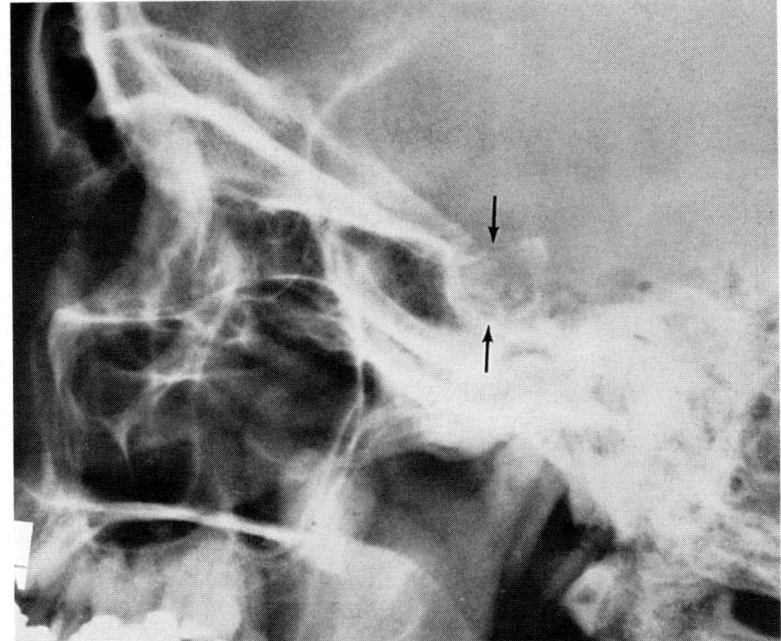

Figure 1–89. Calcification of the internal carotid arteries.

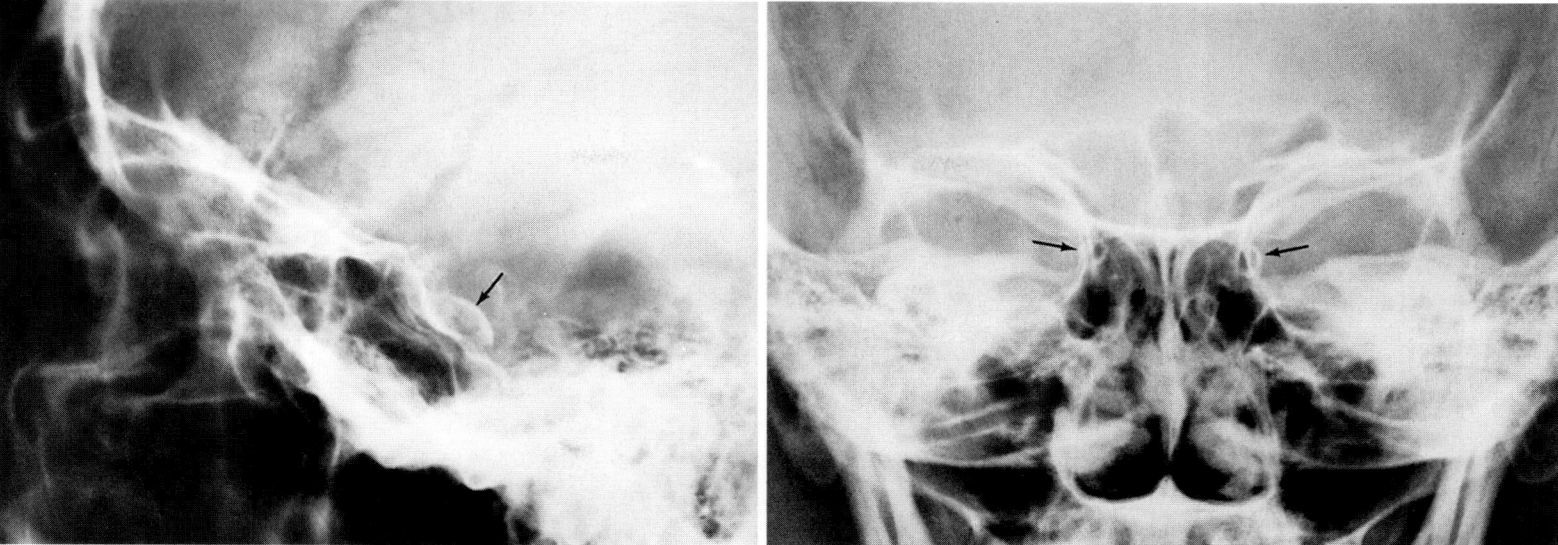

Figure 1–90. Calcification of the internal carotid arteries with very dense calcification in the lateral projection.

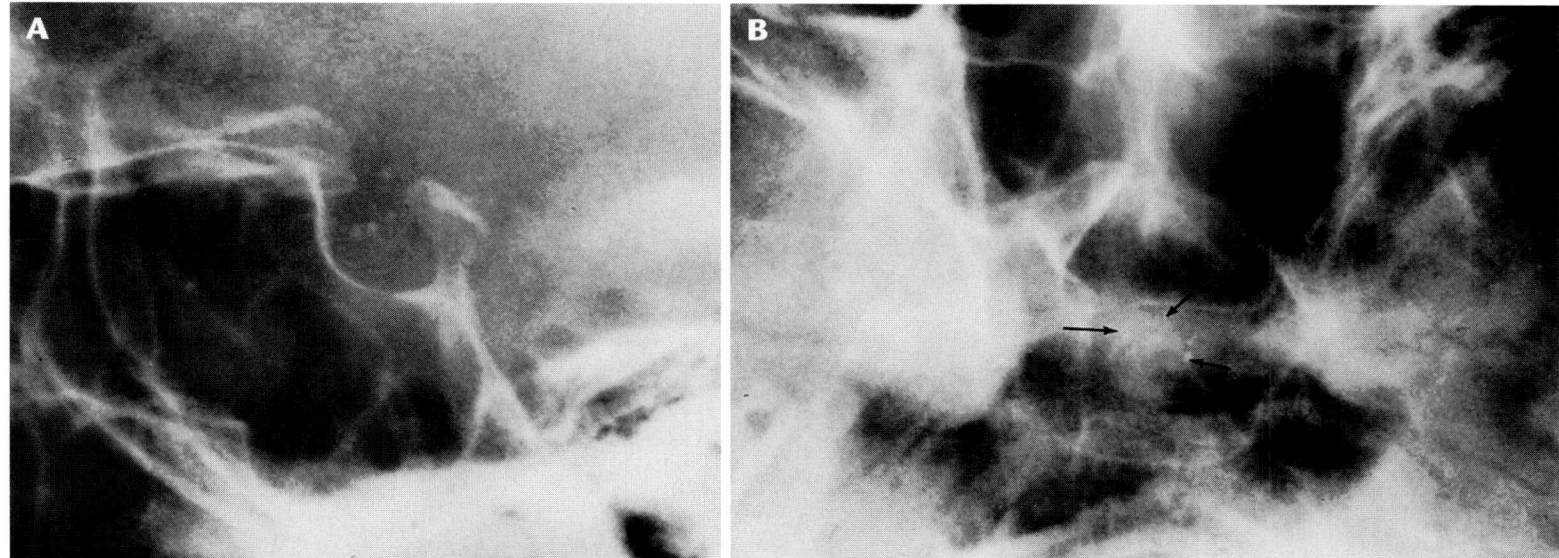

Figure 1–91. Pituitary stones seen in lateral **(A)** and basal **(B)** projections in a 46-year-old man. These may be seen in asymptomatic patients as well as in those with hypopituitarism. (Ref: Taylor HC et al: Pituitary stones and associated hypopituitarism. *JAMA* 242:751, 1974.)

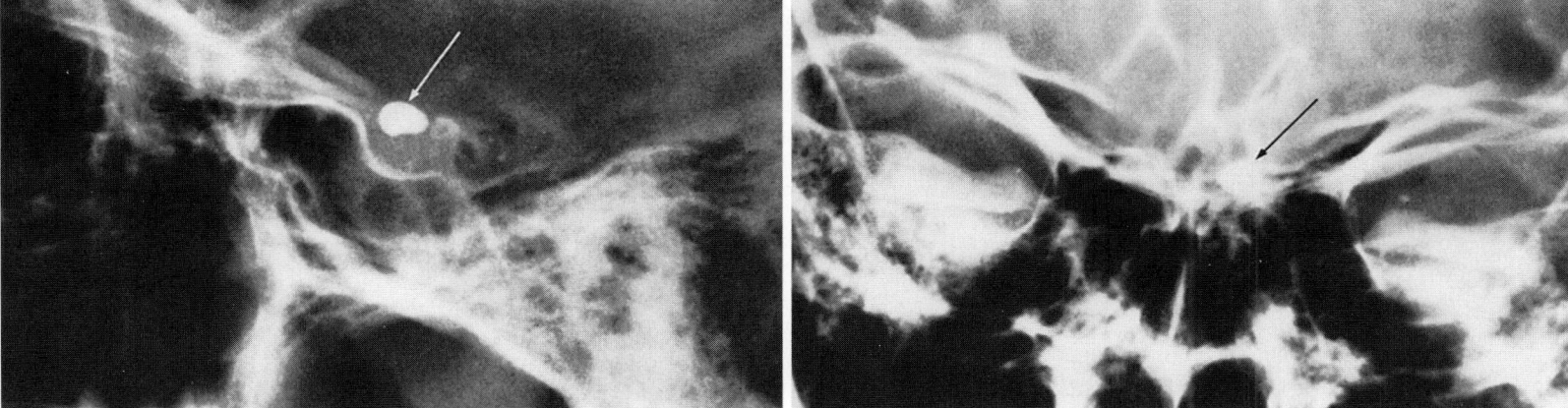

Figure 1–92. Large pituitary stone in a 20-year-old woman.

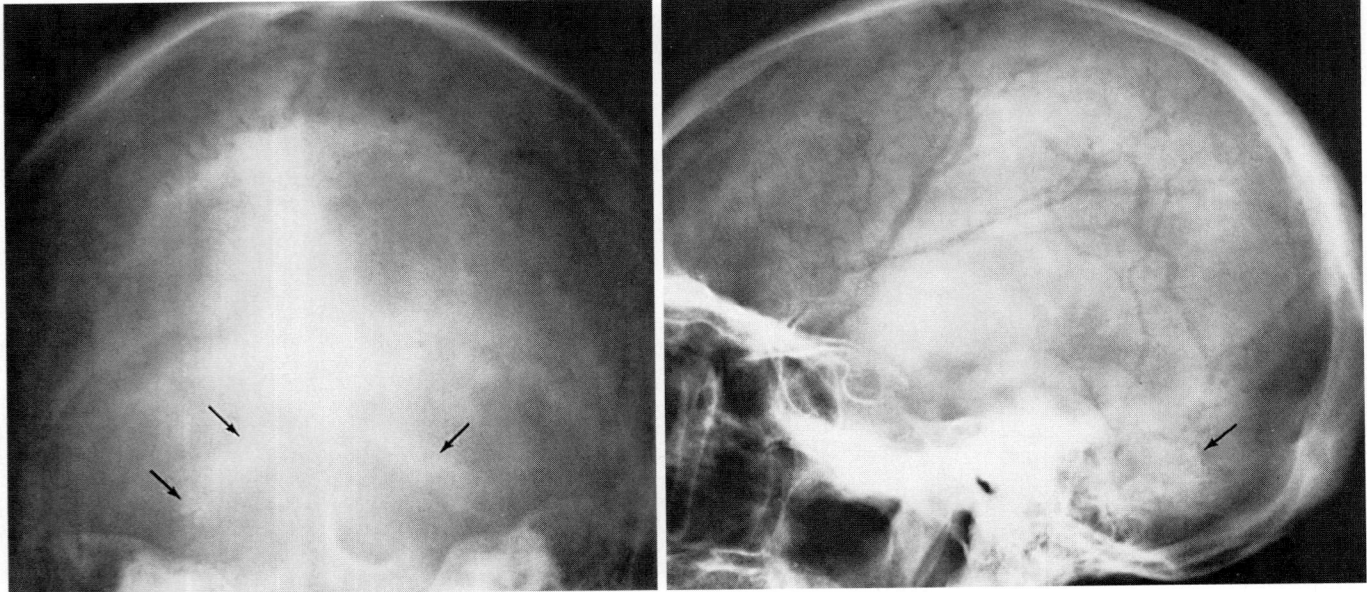

Figure 1–93. Calcification in the dentate nucleus of the cerebellum. This form of calcification is not necessarily of clinical significance and may be physiologic.

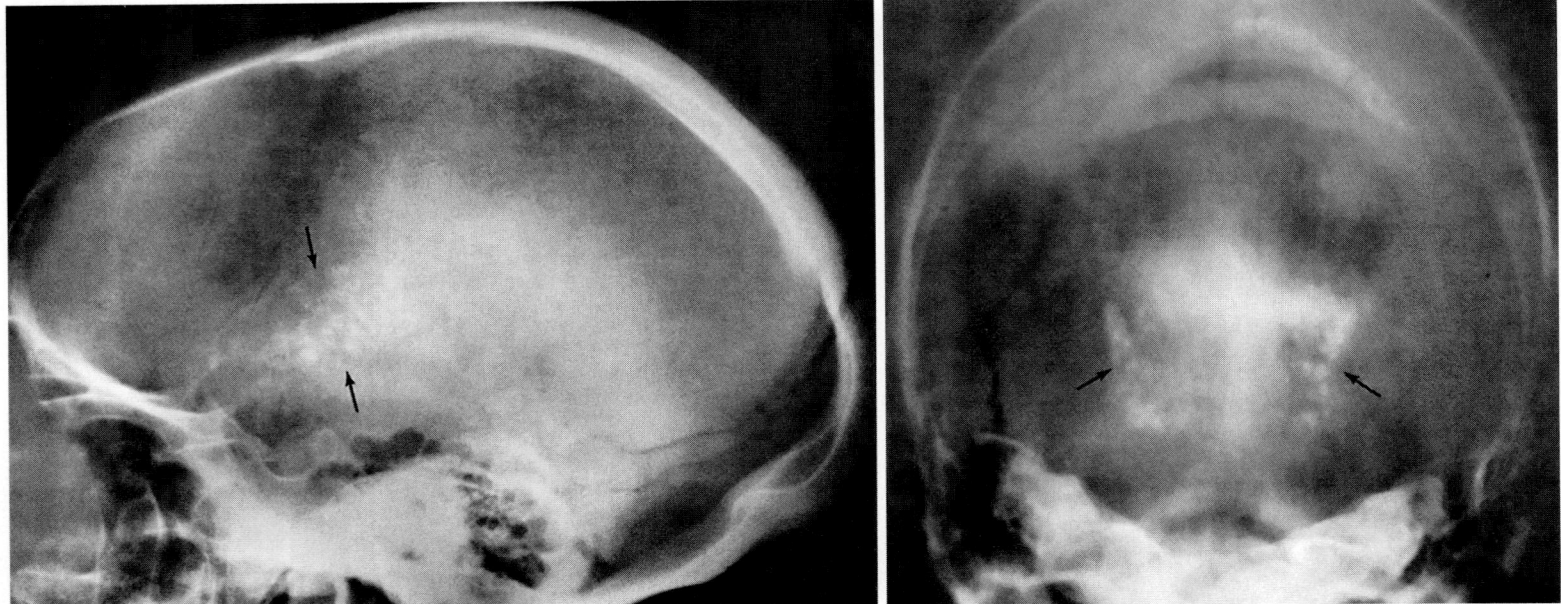

Figure 1–94. Idiopathic calcification of the basal ganglia may be familial and unassociated with other disease.

The Frontal Bone

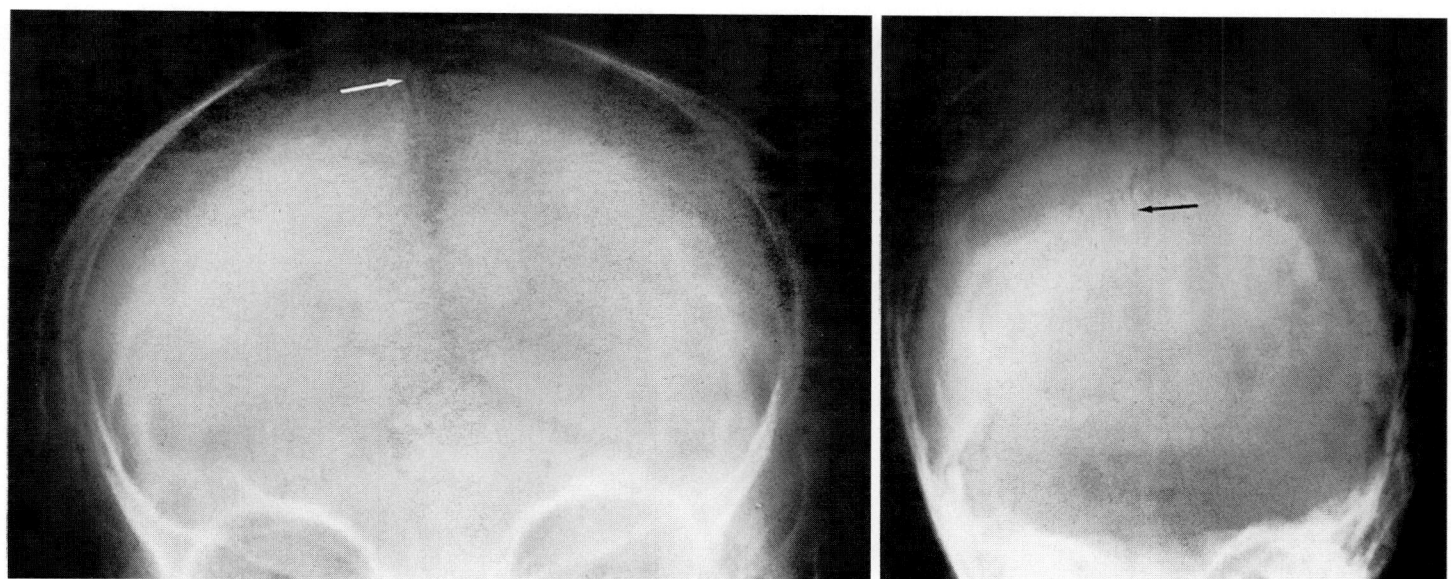

Figure 1–95. Closing metopic suture mistaken for a fracture in a 1½-year-old boy. Closure occurs last in the cephalic end of the suture.

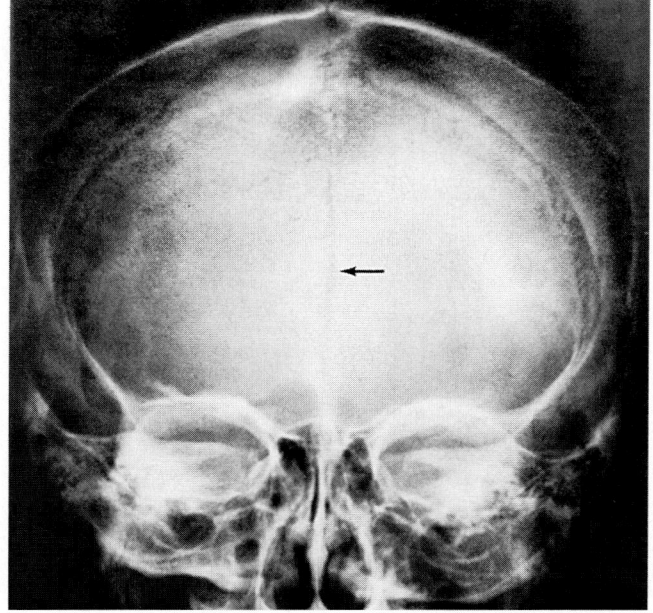

Figure 1–96. Persistent metopic suture in a young adult. This suture may persist throughout life and may be mistaken for a fracture.

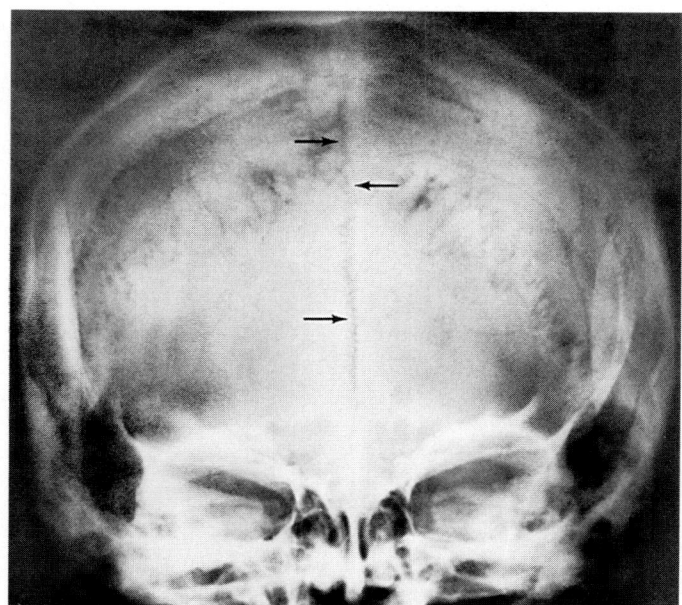

Figure 1–97. Persistent metopic suture, showing unusual serrations. The straight line is in the inner table, the serrated in the outer.

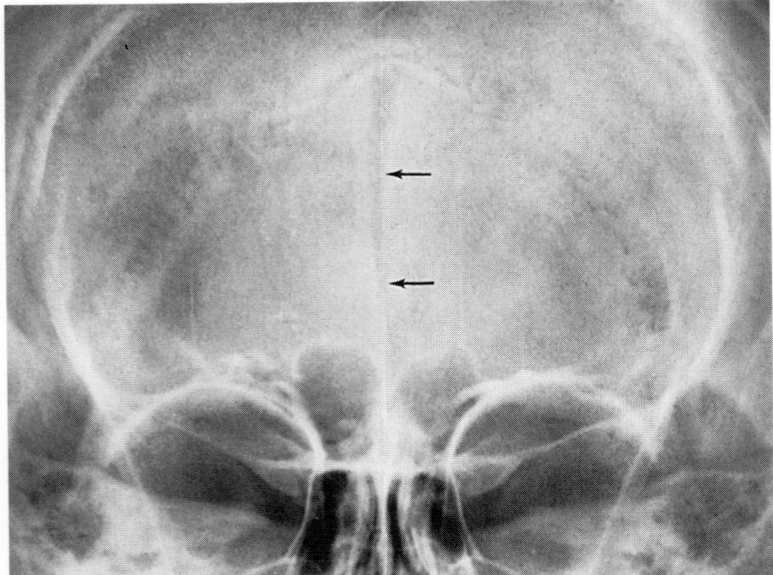

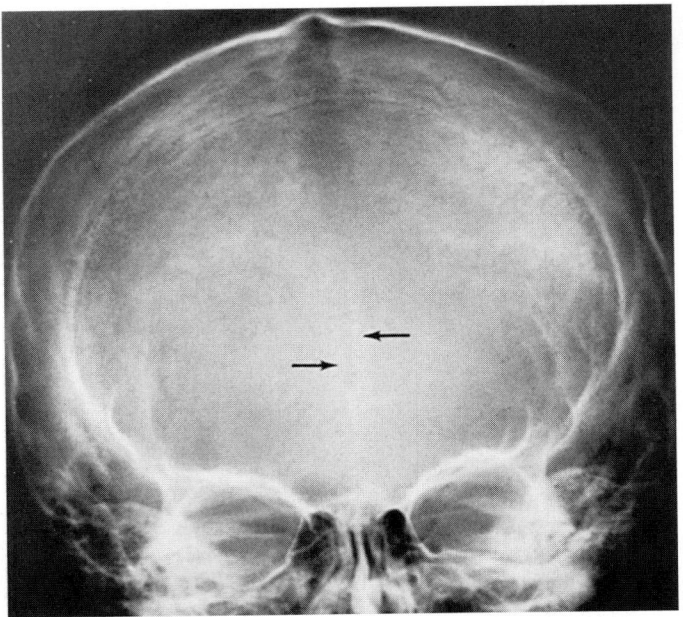

Figure 1–98. Groove for the sagittal suture projected through the frontal bone, simulating a metopic suture.

Figure 1–99. Unfused areas in the midline of the frontal bone (cranium bifidum occultum) in a 15-year-old child.

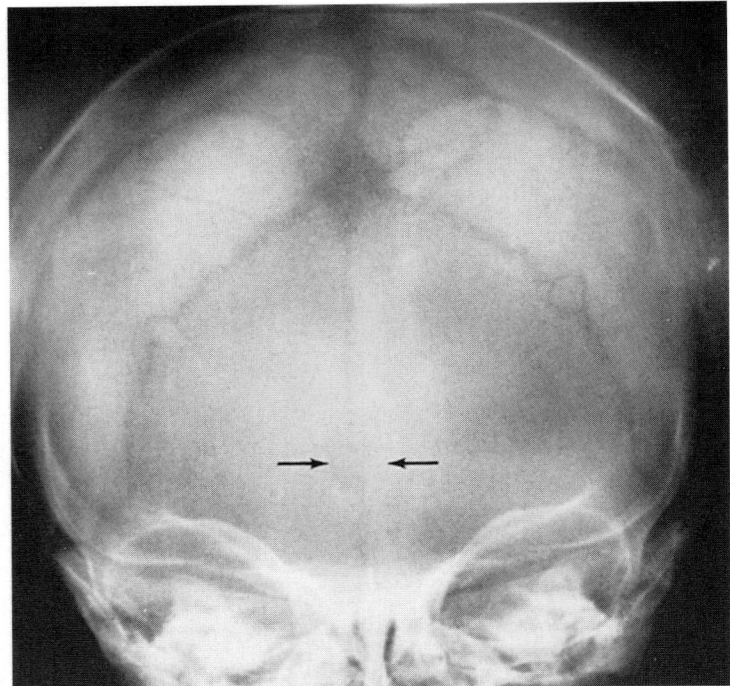

Figure 1–100. Cranium bifidum occultum in a 9-month-old girl.

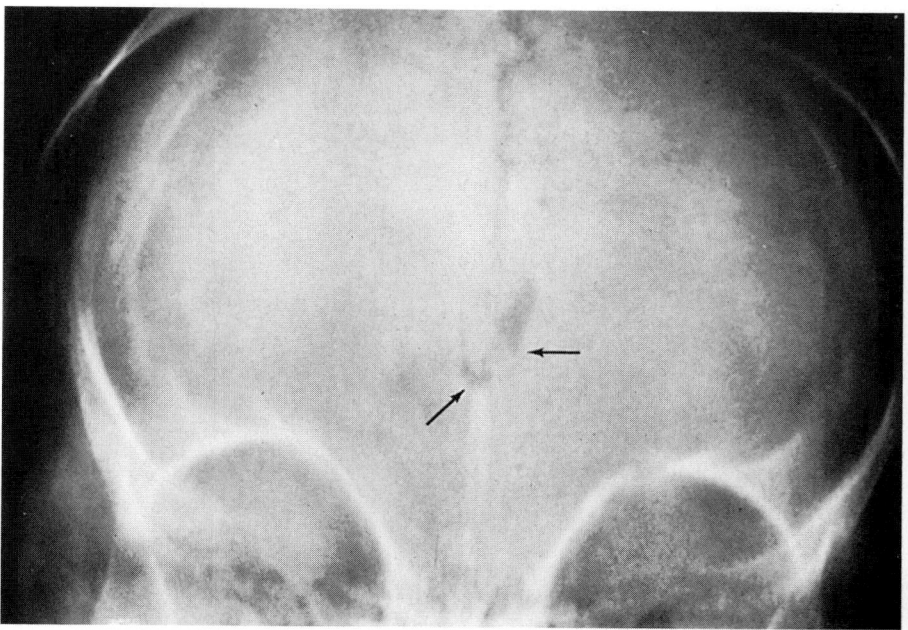

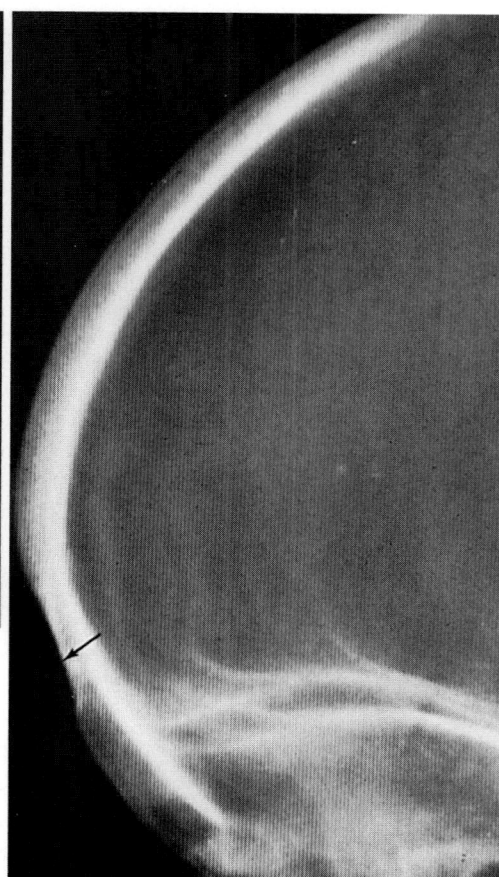

Figure 1–101. Cranium bifidum occultum in a 14-month-old boy.

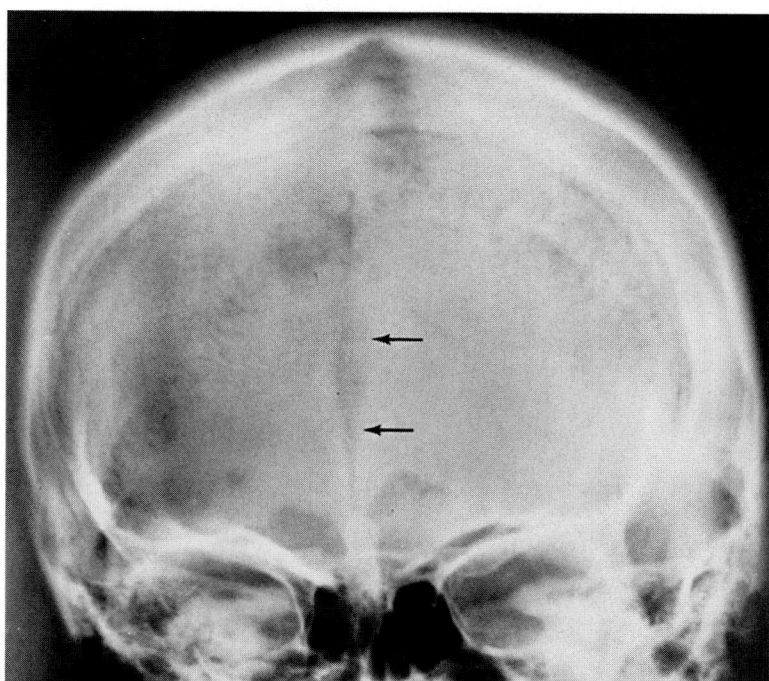

Figure 1–102. Cranium bifidum occultum in a 28-year-old woman.

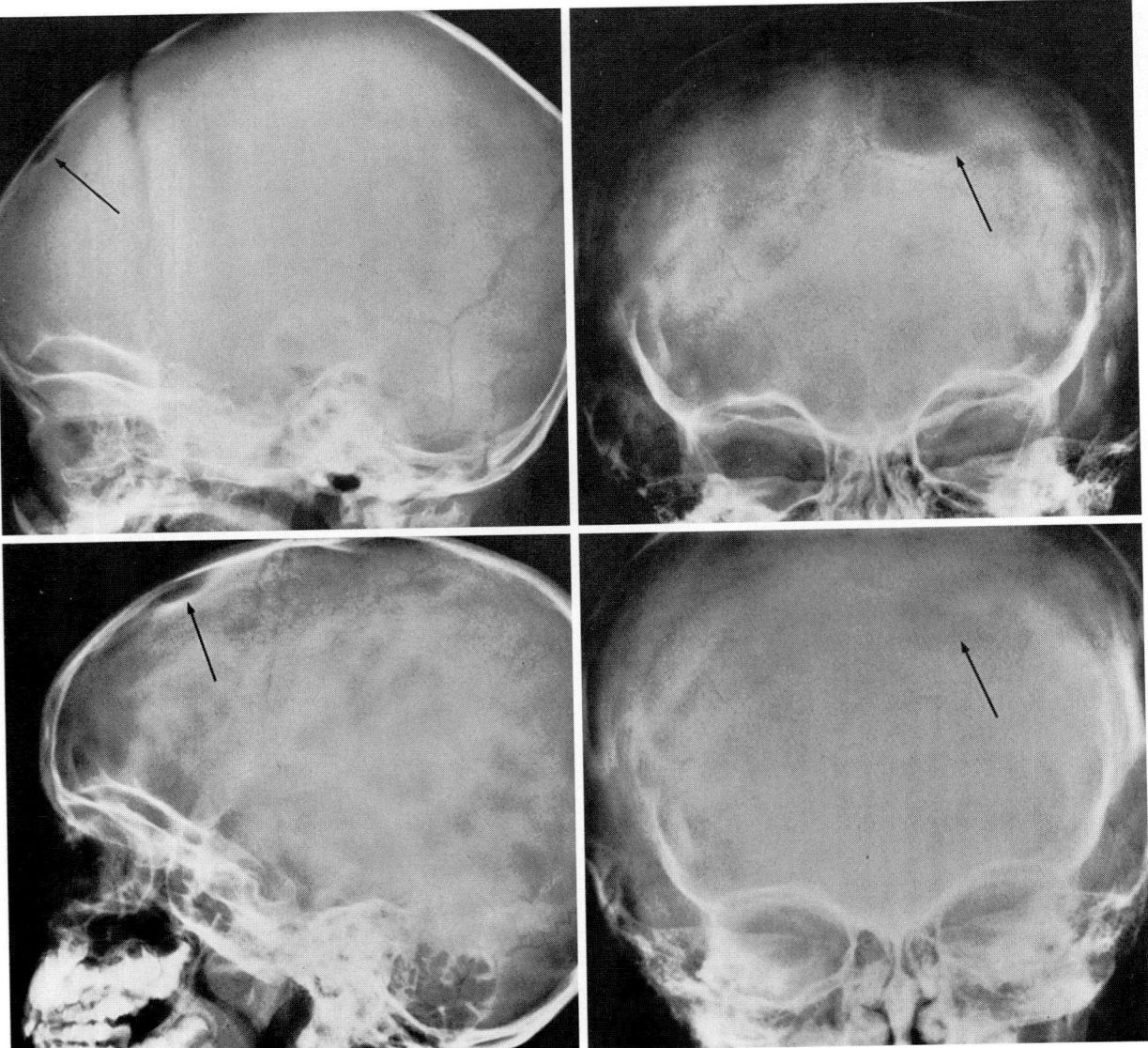

Figure 1–103. *Top,* Asymptomatic palpable developmental fossa in the frontal bone in an 8-month-old child. *Bottom,* At 5 years of age fossa is still present, essentially unchanged.

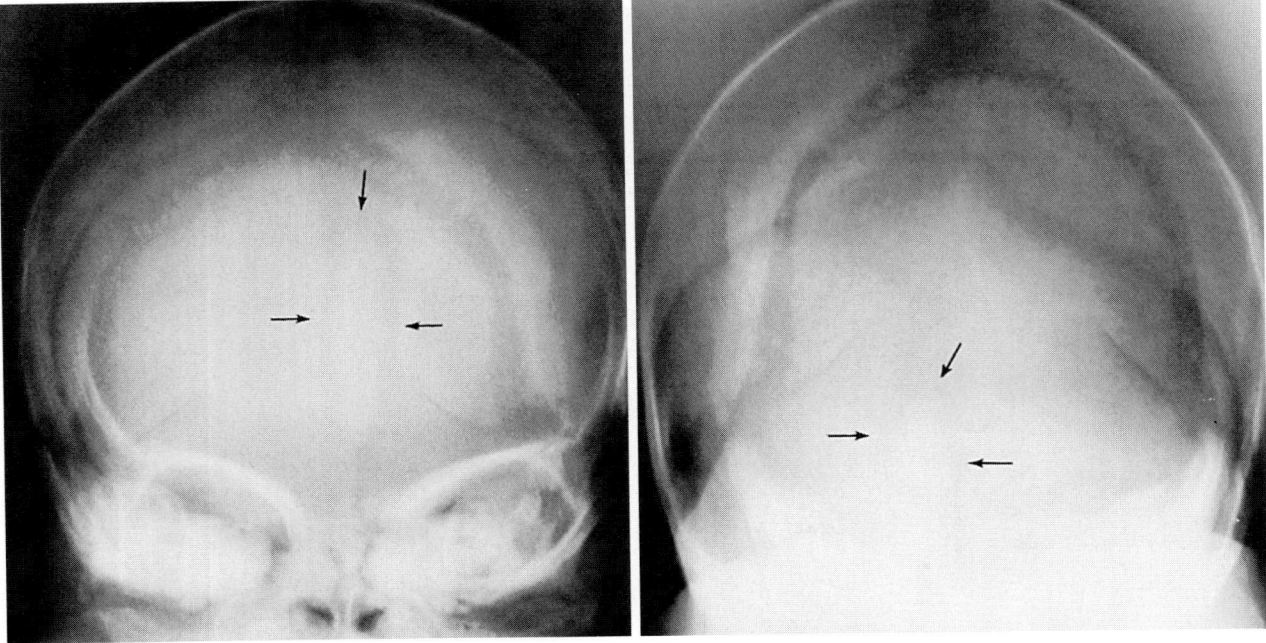

Figure 1–104. Midline frontal accessory bone in an 11-month-old boy.

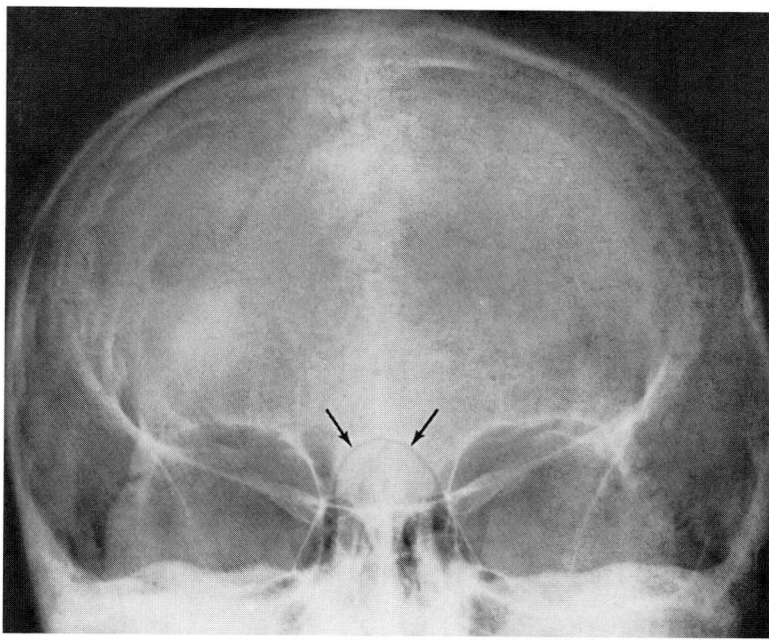

Figure 1–105. Prominent nasofrontal suture, not to be mistaken for a fracture. This suture may persist into adult life.

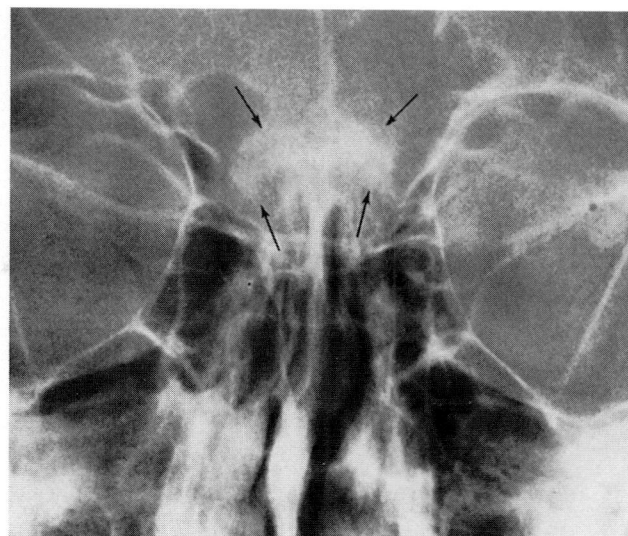

Figure 1–106. Sclerosis of the nasofrontal suture, which might be mistaken for a meningioma of the anterior fossa.

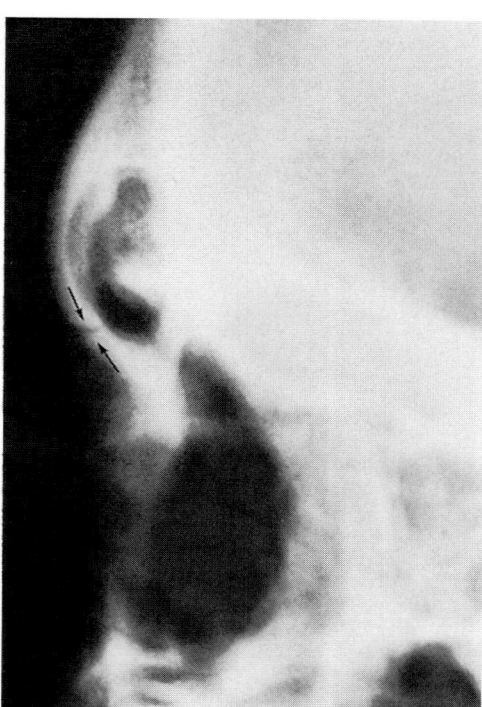

Figure 1–107. The nasofrontal suture in lateral projection.

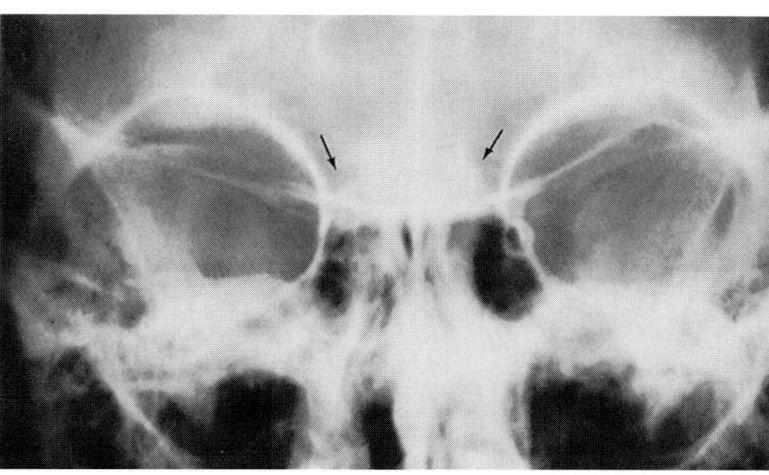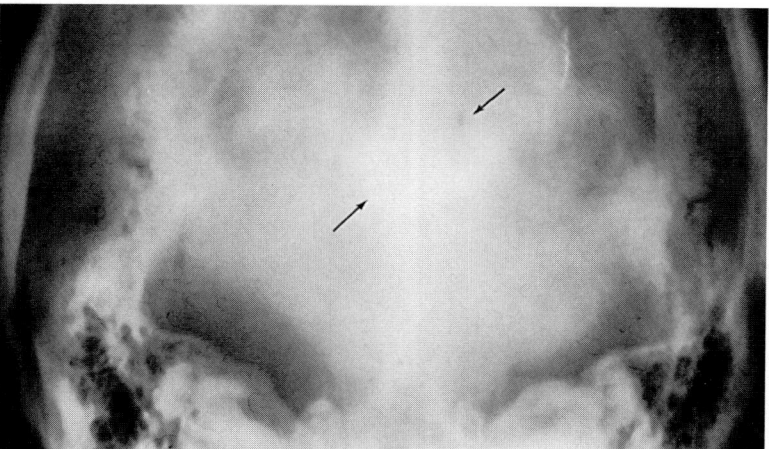

Figure 1–108. Large external occipital protuberance projected through frontal bone, simulating meningioma of the anterior fossa.

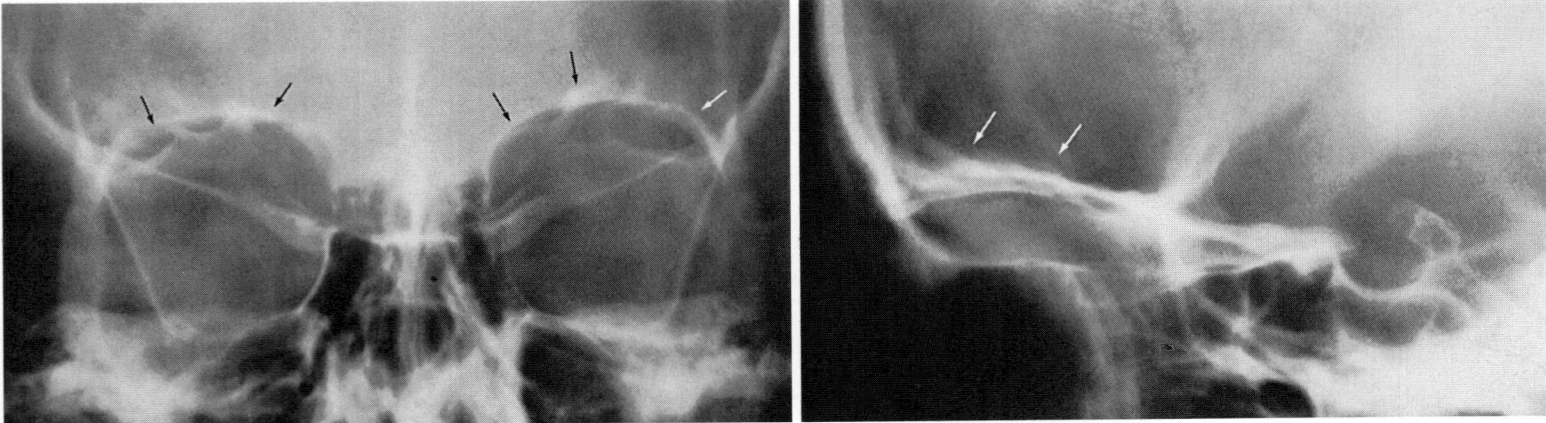

Figure 1–109. Unusual scalloped appearance of the floor of the anterior fossa.

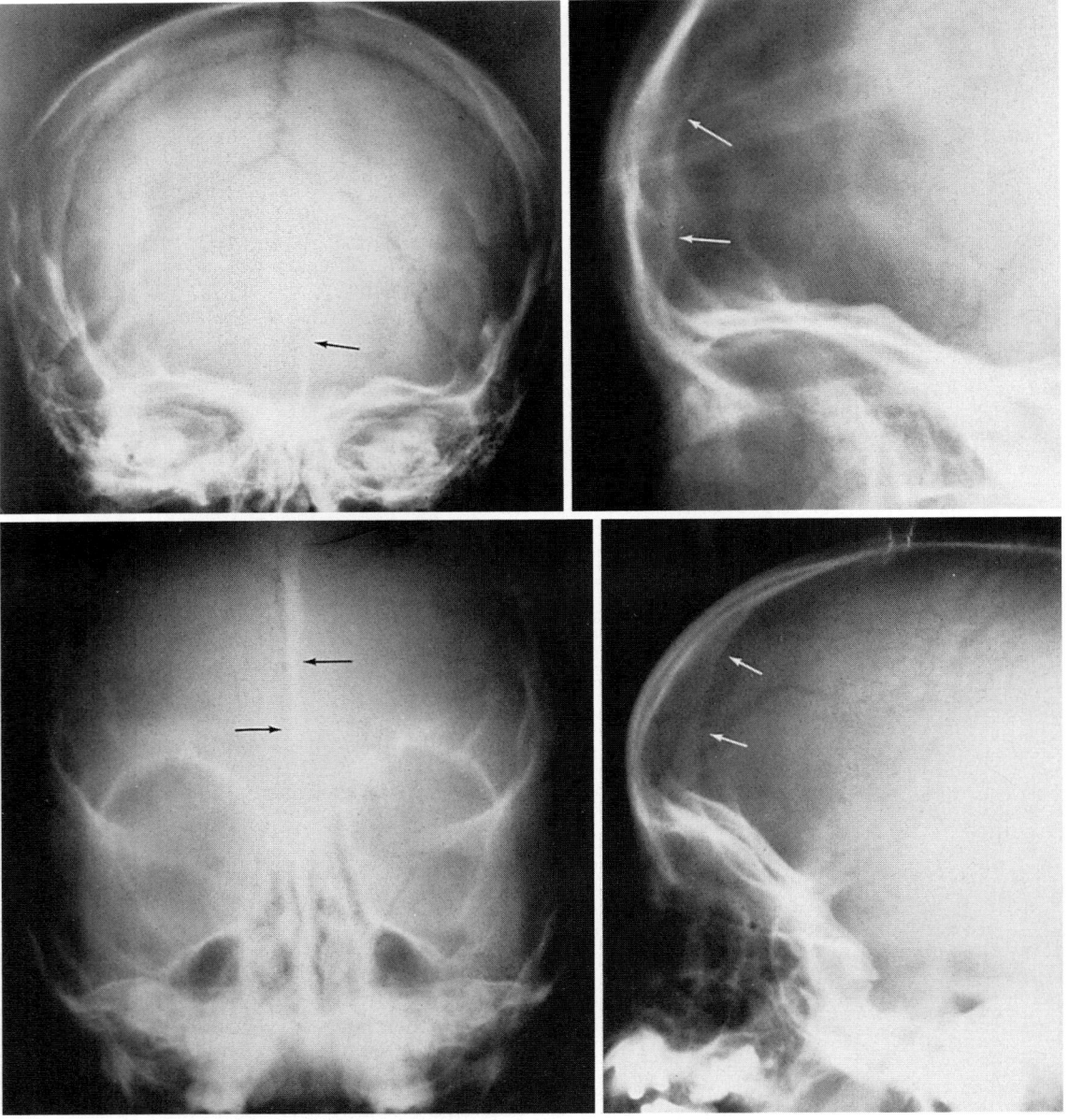

Figure 1–110. Two examples of prominent frontal crests in children, simulating falx calcification.

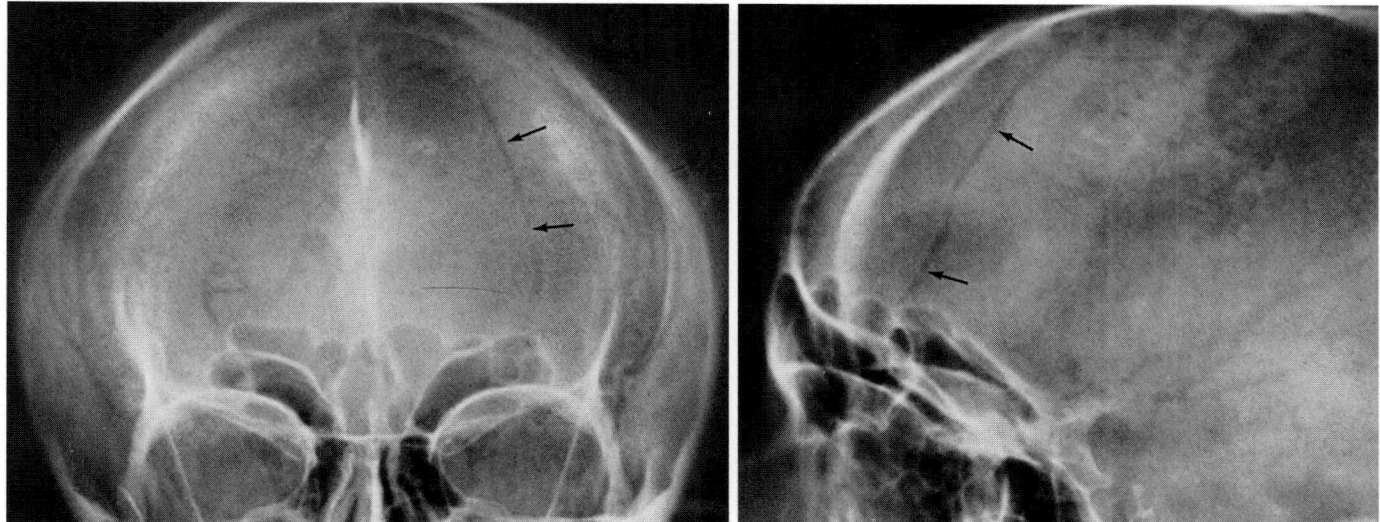

Figure 1–111. Vascular channel simulating a skull fracture. (Ref: Schunk H, Maruyama Y: Two vascular grooves of the external table of the skull which simulate fractures. *Acta Radiol* 54:186, 1960.)

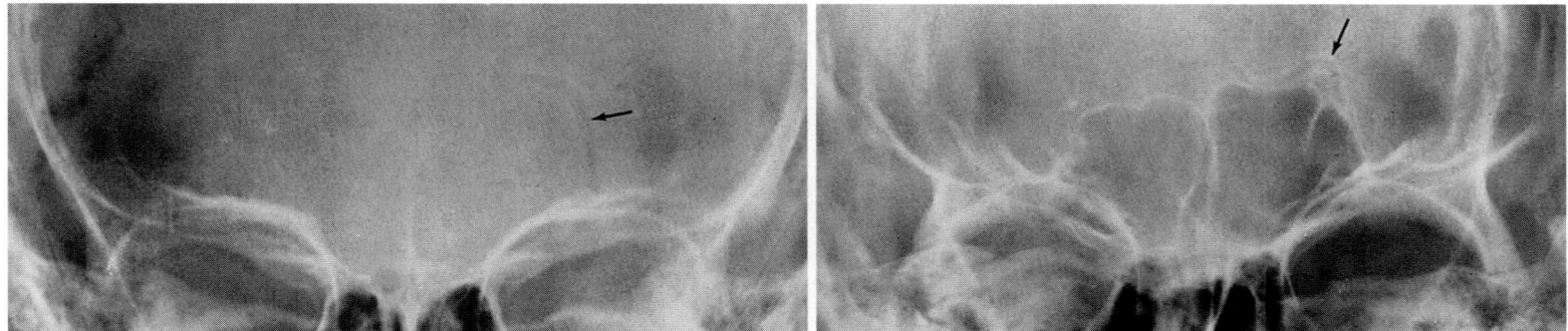

Figure 1–112. Unilateral serpentine vascular channels in the frontal bone.

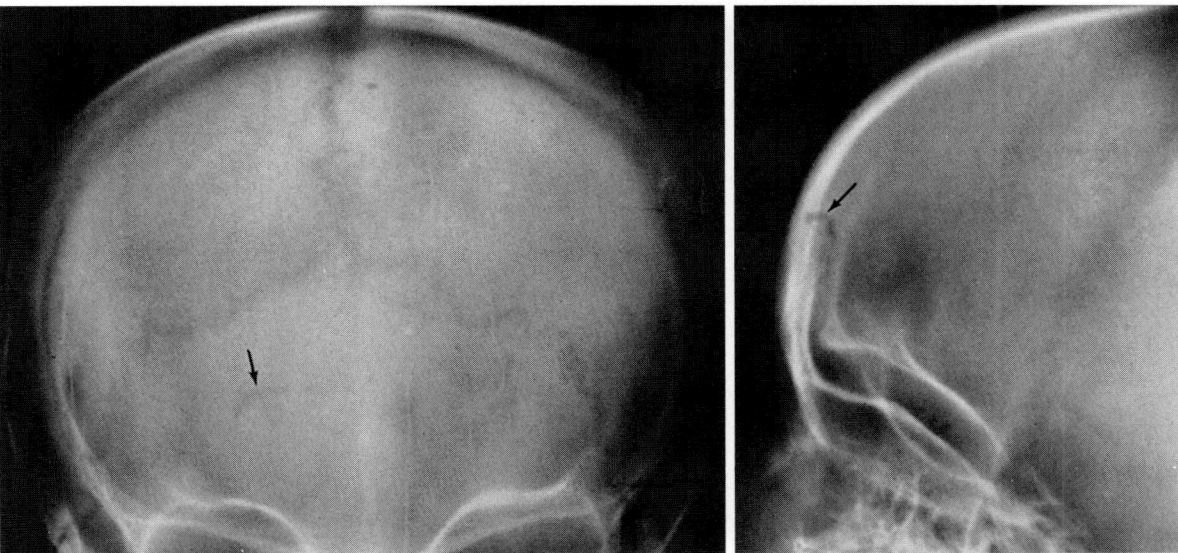

Figure 1–113. Vascular groove simulating a fracture in a 1-year-old boy.

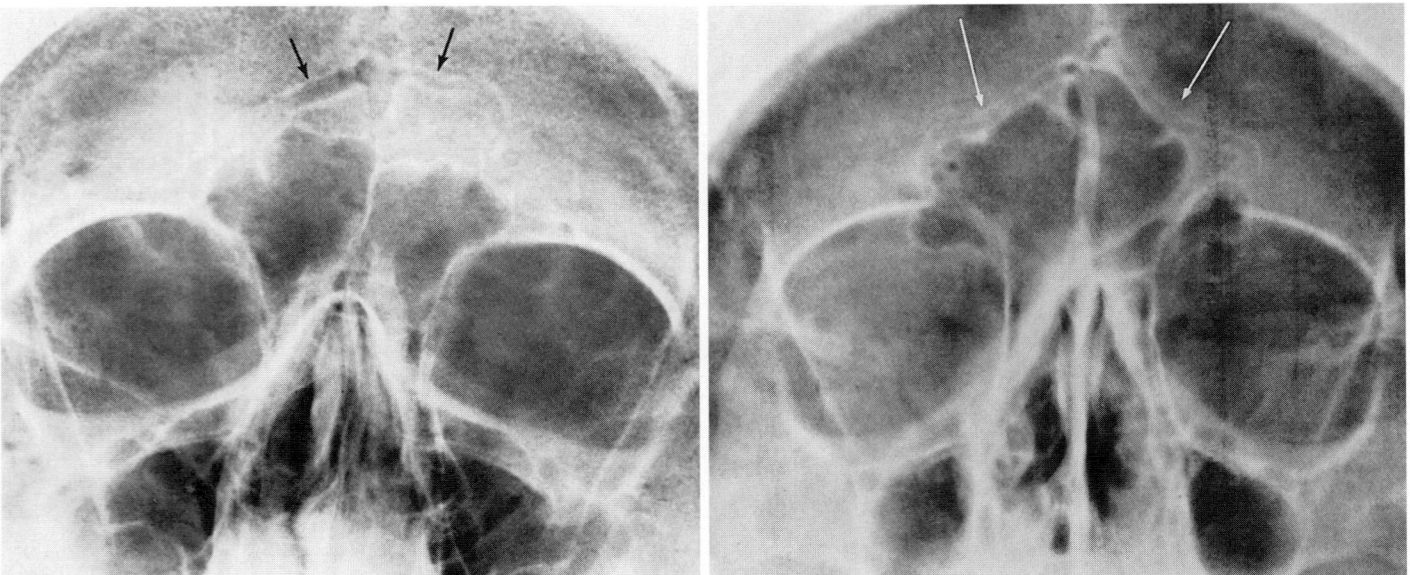

Figure 1–114. Vascular channels above the frontal sinuses.

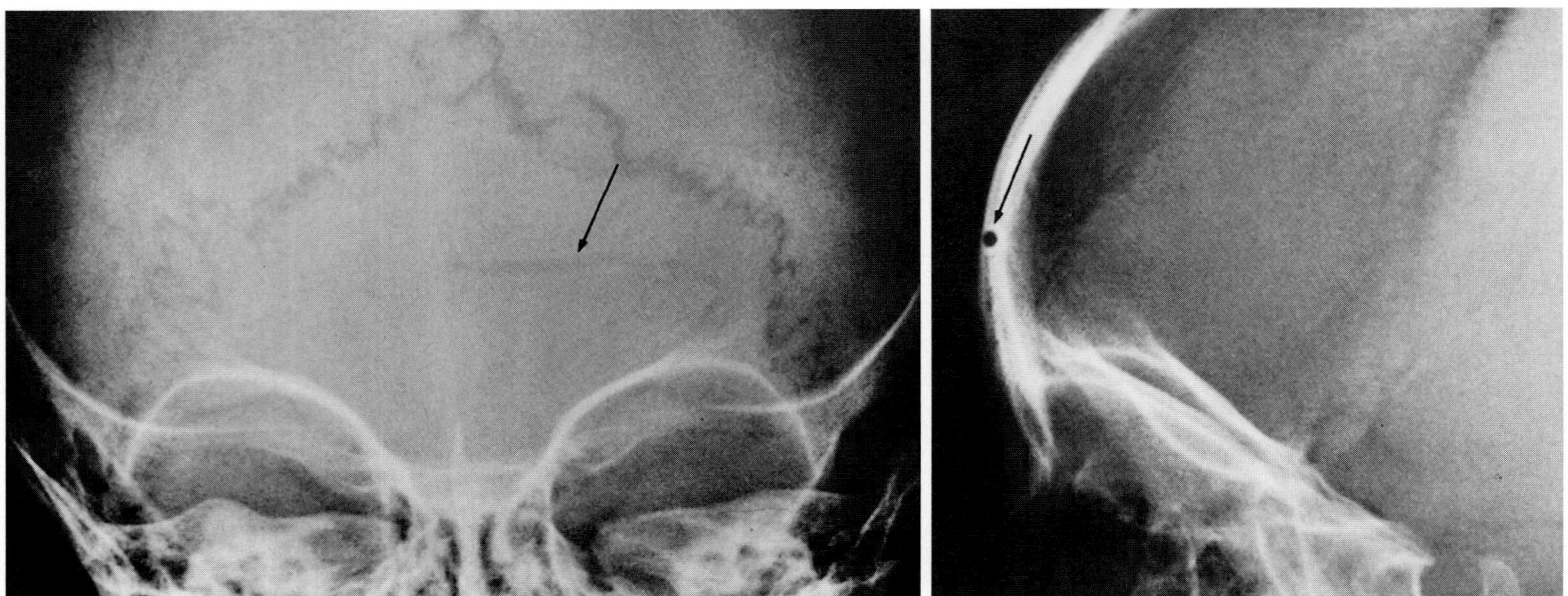

Figure 1–115. Vascular channel of the frontal bone, unusually well seen in lateral projection. (Courtesy of Dr. Wa'el M.A. Al-Bassam.)

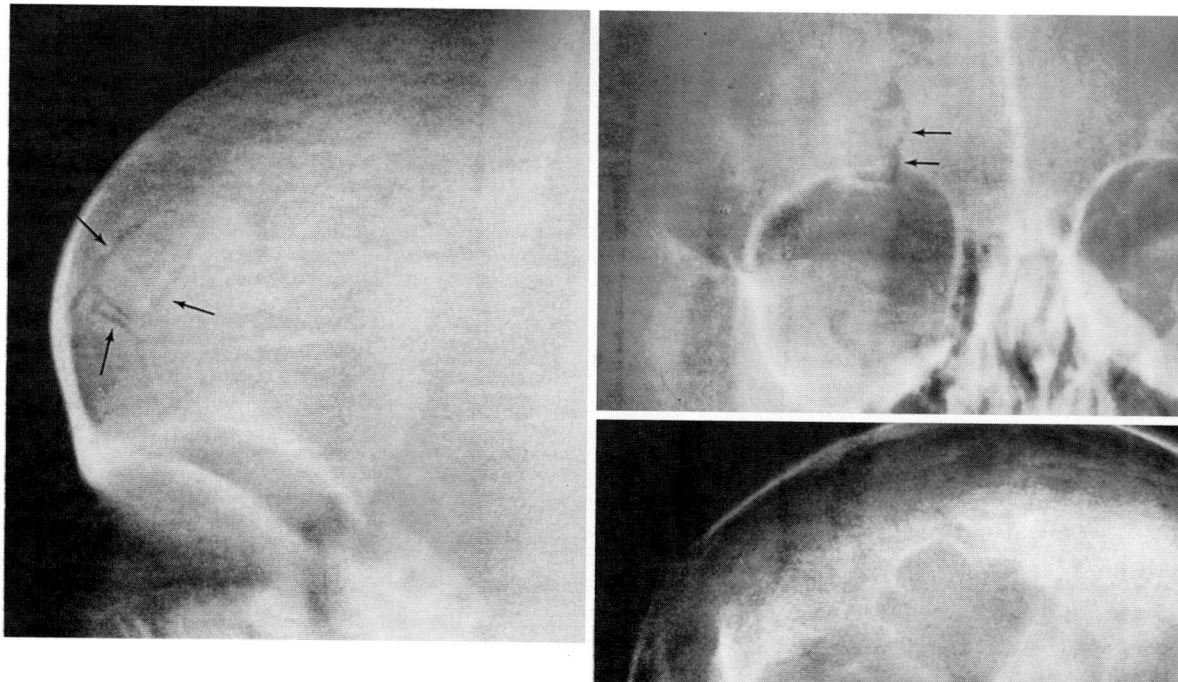

Figure 1–116. Three additional examples of frontal bone vascular grooves, which might be mistaken for fractures.

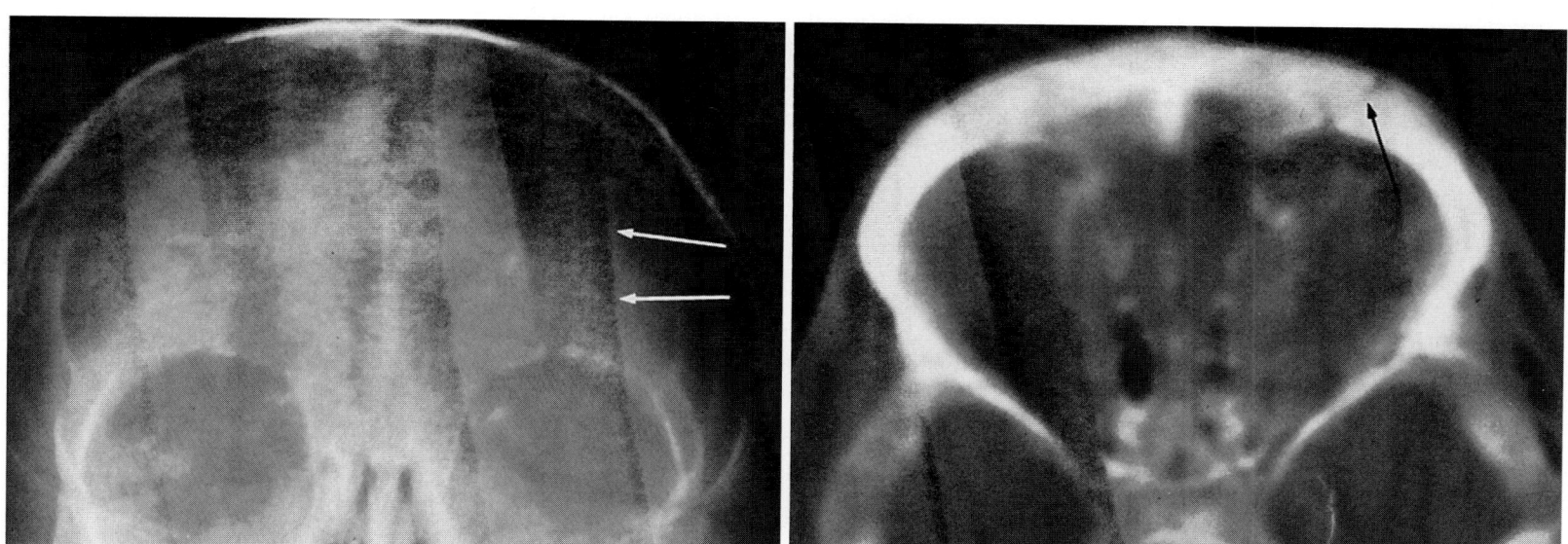

Figure 1–117. Vascular groove in the frontal bone mistaken for a fracture. *Left,* Plain film. *Right,* CT.

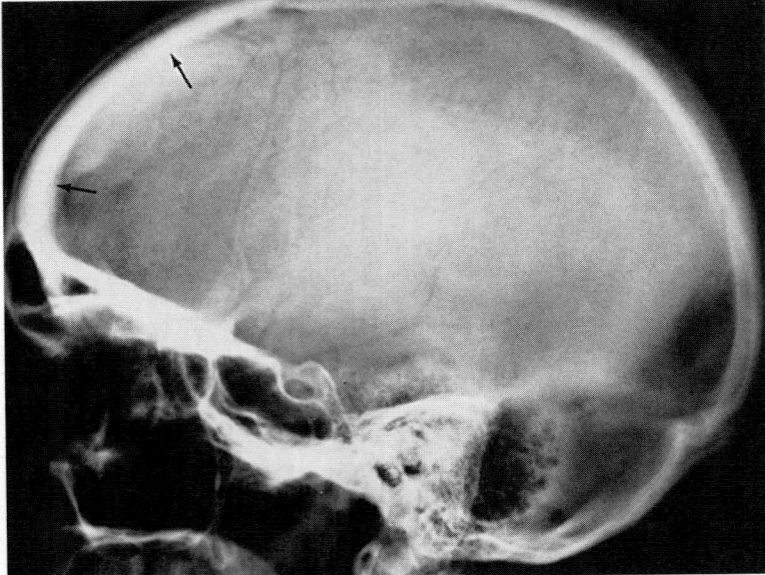

Figure 1–118. Focal thickening of the inner table of the frontal bone.

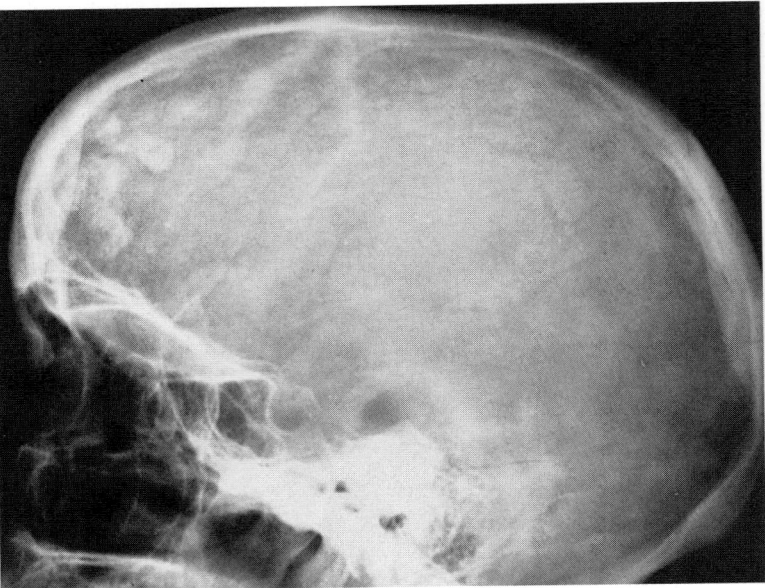

Figure 1–119. Nodular benign hyperostosis frontalis interna.

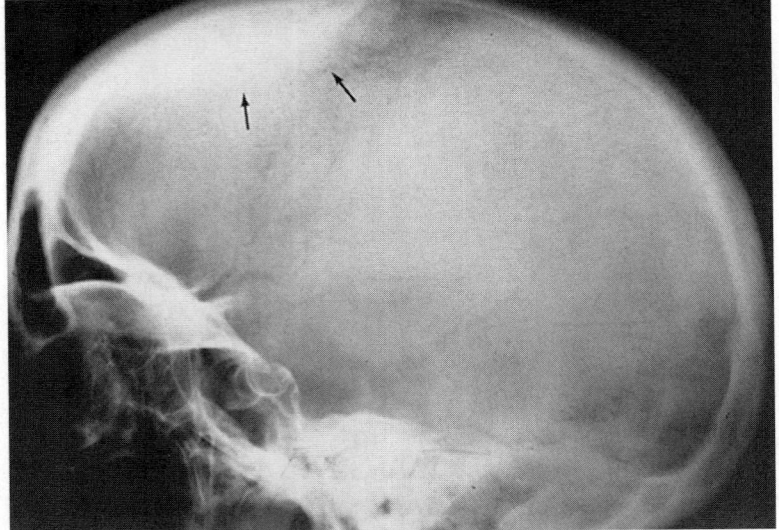

Figure 1–120. Nebular hyperostosis frontalis interna.

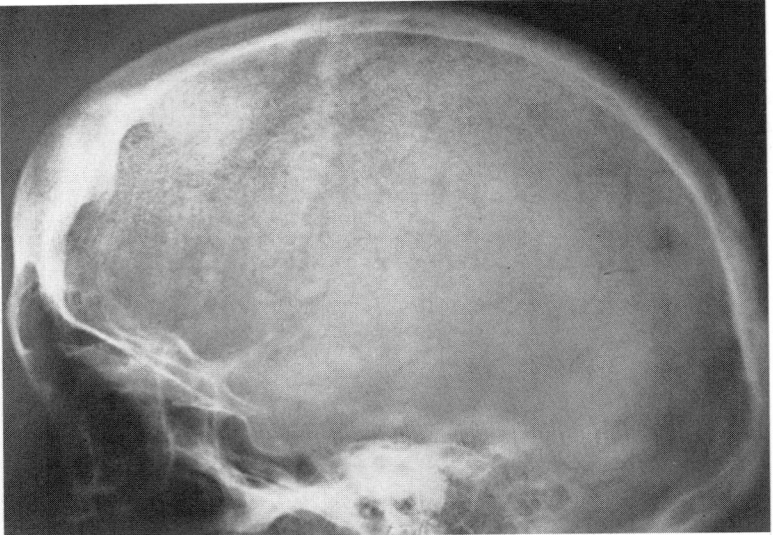

Figure 1–121. Diffuse benign hyperostosis of the frontal bone.

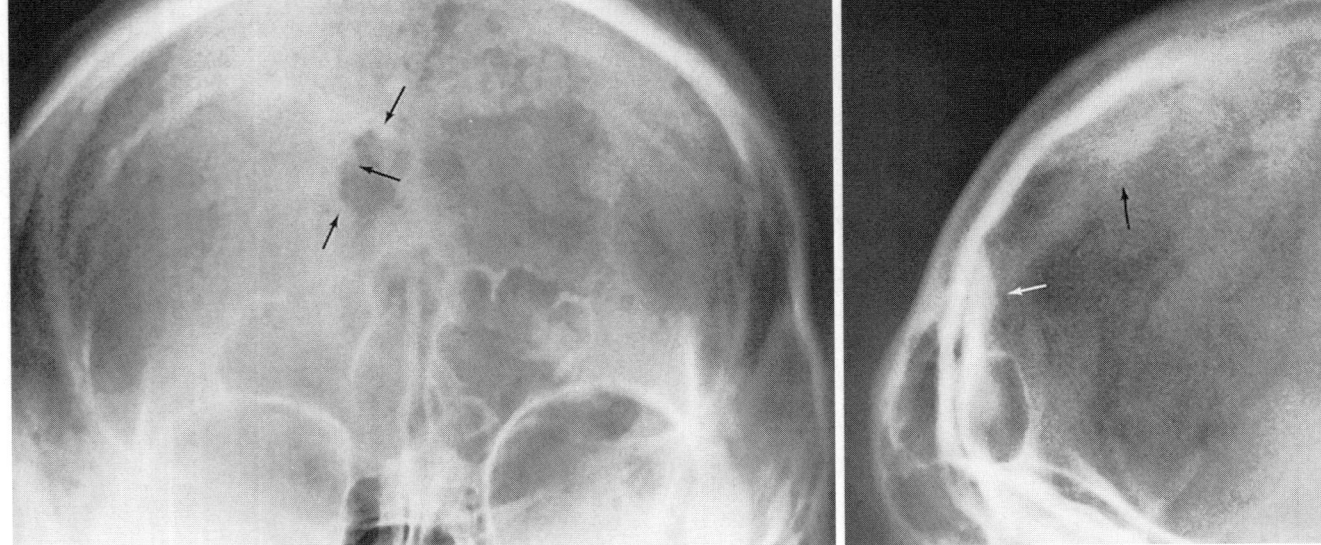

Figure 1–122. Asymmetric localized hyperostosis frontalis interna in a 20-year-old woman.

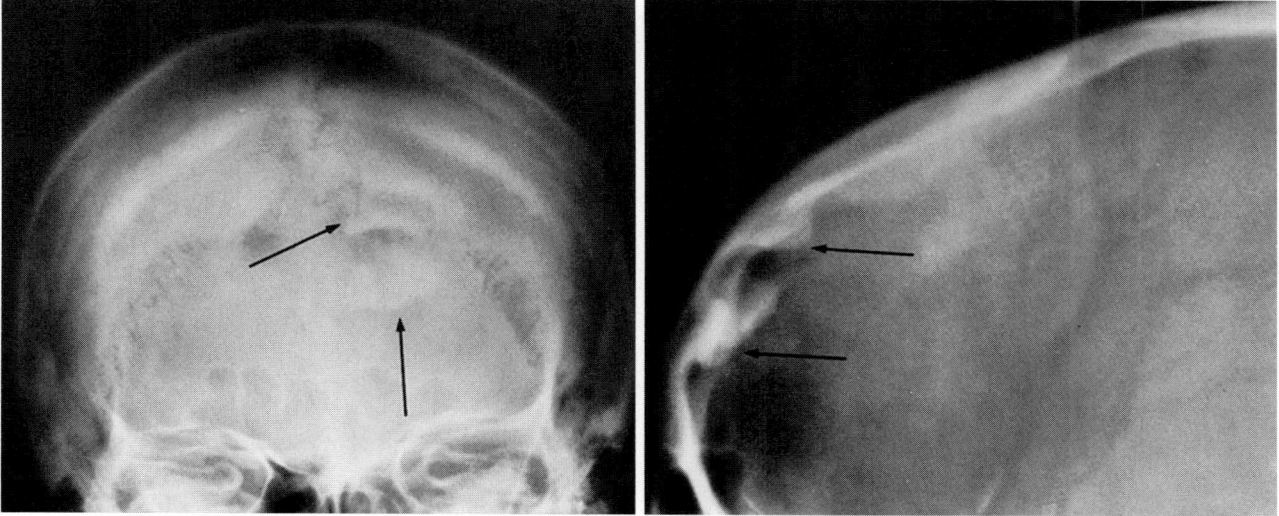

Figure 1–123. Asymmetric unilateral hyperostosis frontalis interna in a 28-year-old woman.

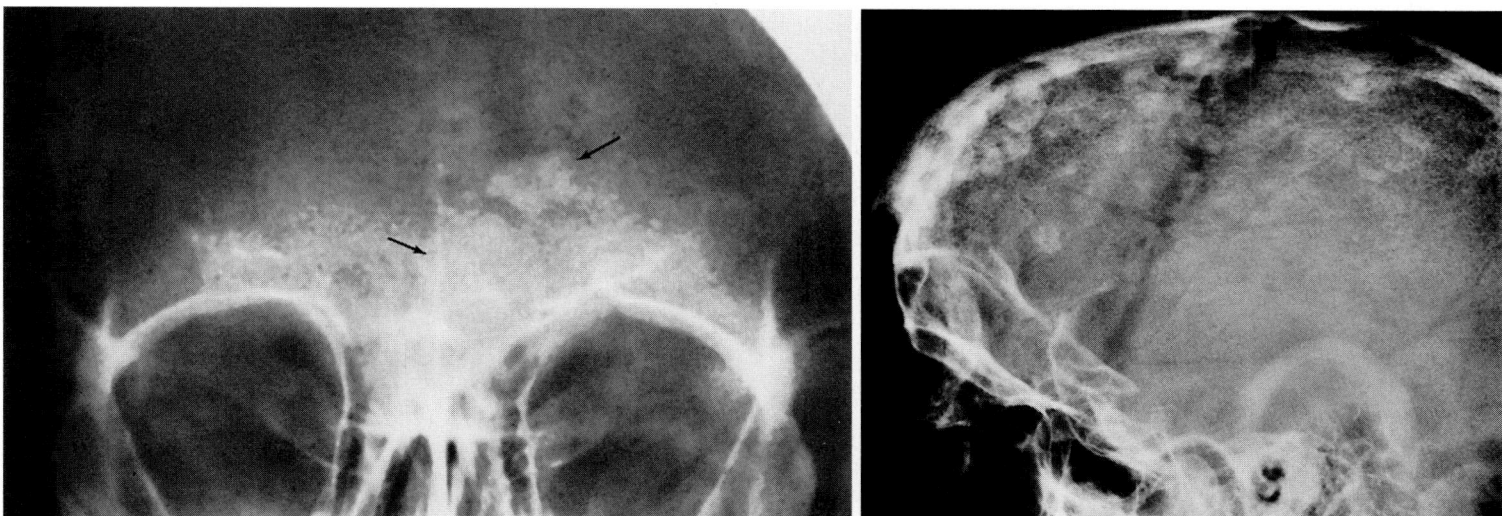

Figure 1–124. A, B. Early asymmetric hyperostosis frontalis interna in a 35-year-old man. This entity is much less common in males.

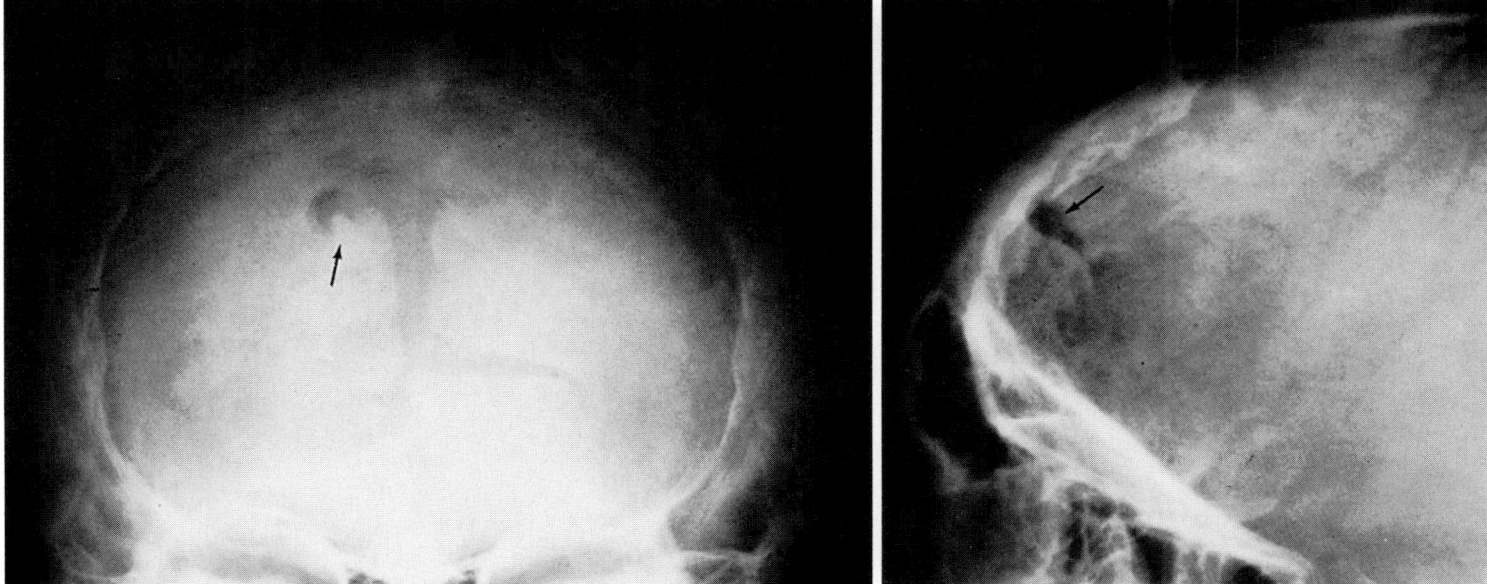

Figure 1–125. Hyperostosis frontalis interna with a simulated sequestrum.

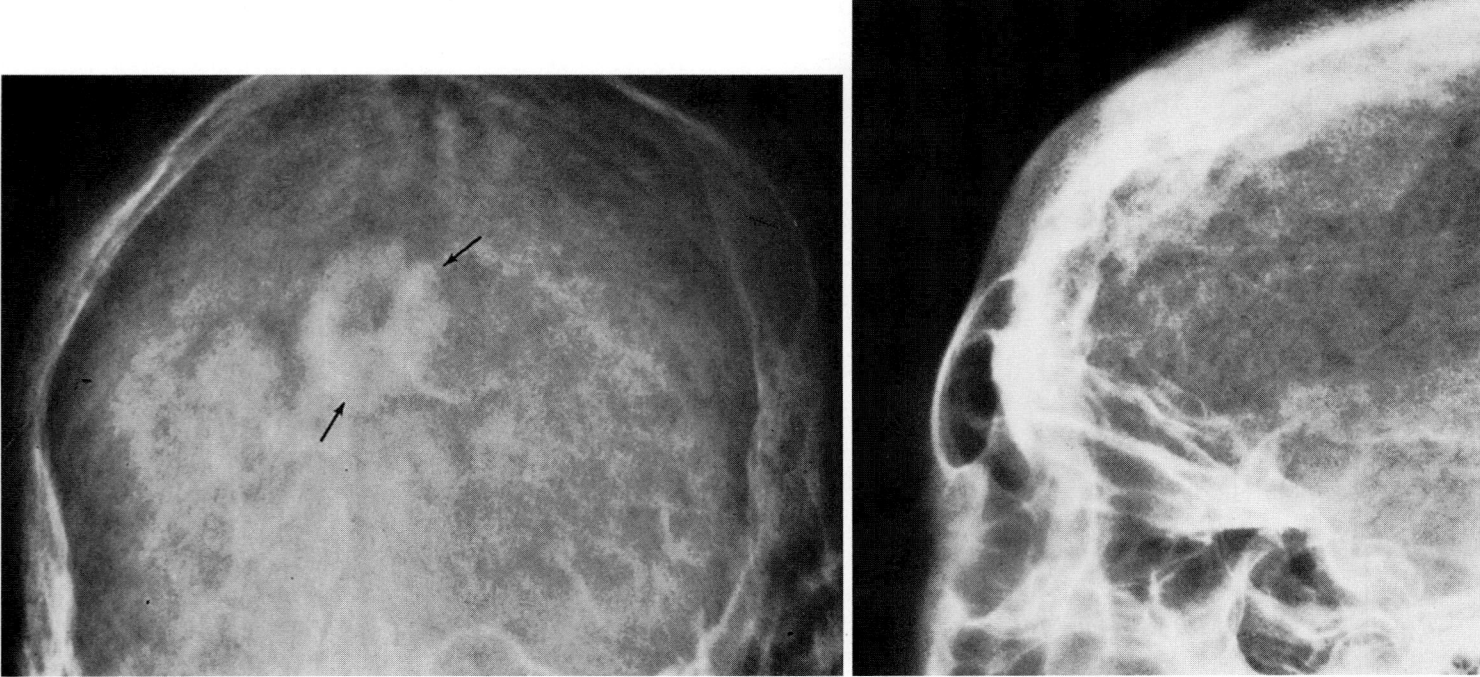

Figure 1–126. Hyperostosis frontalis interna with a simulated doughnut lesion.

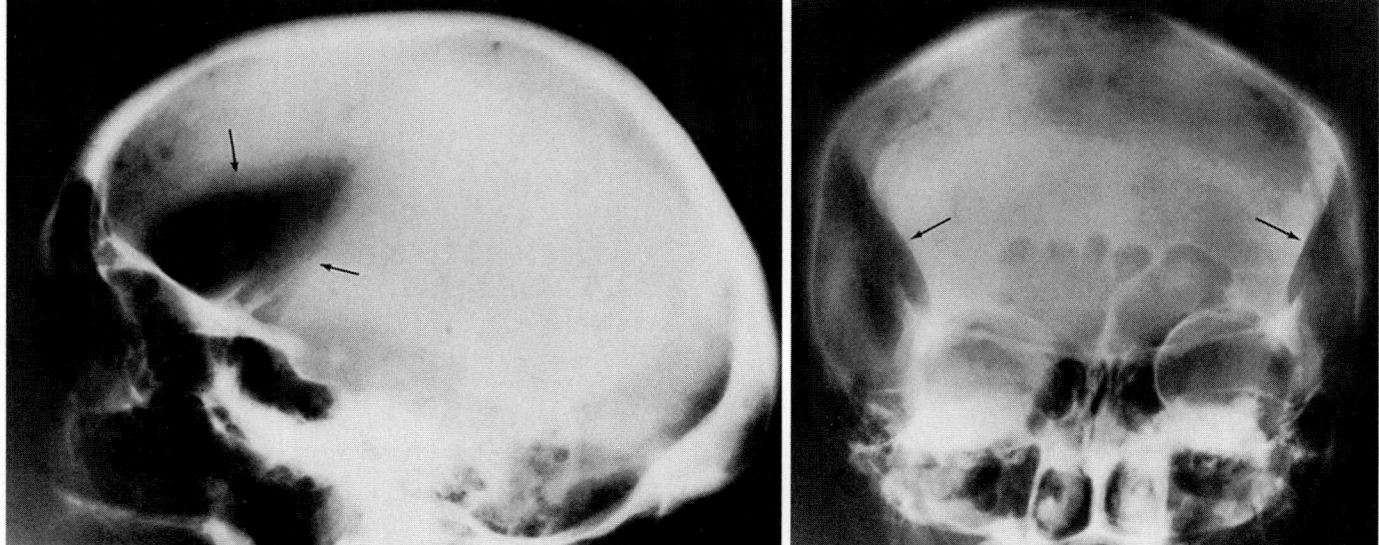

Figure 1–127. Localized frontal calvarial osteoporotic thinning in an 84-year-old woman.

The Parietal Bone

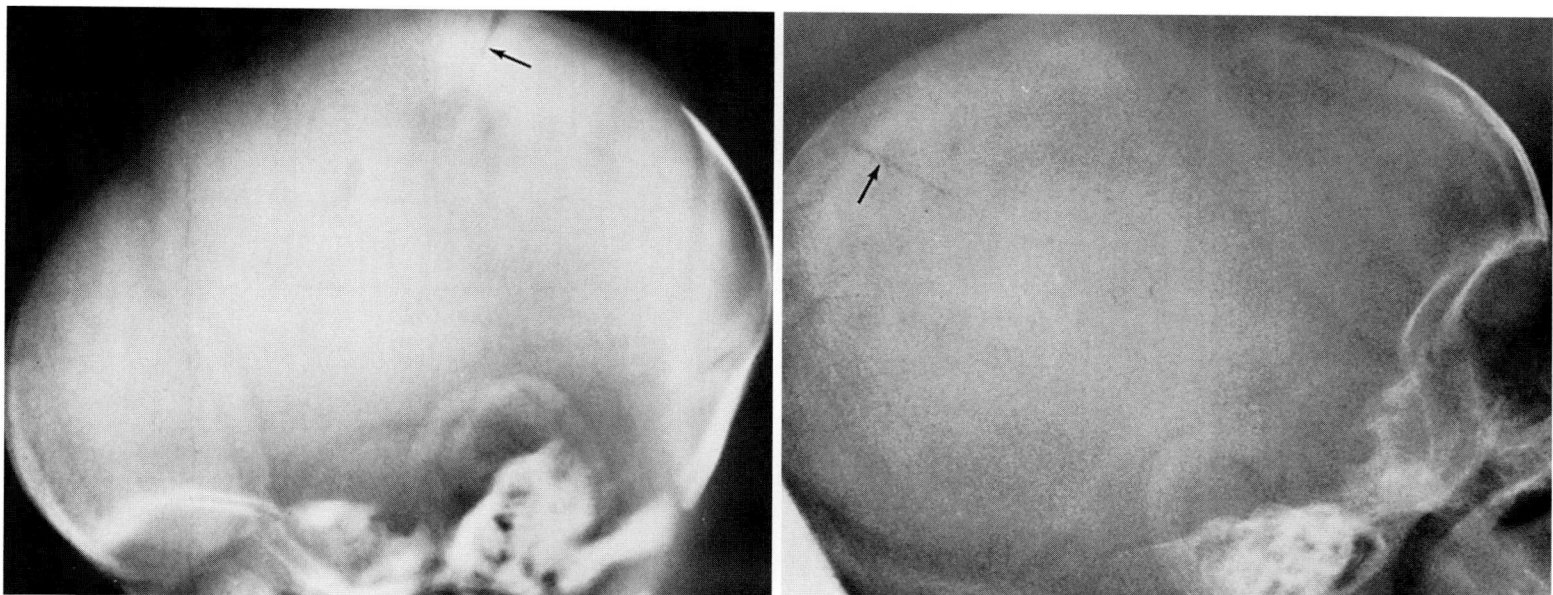

Figure 1–128. Two neonates showing parietal fissures caused by persistent strips of membranous bone matrix. These fissures disappear as the child matures and are often mistaken for fractures.

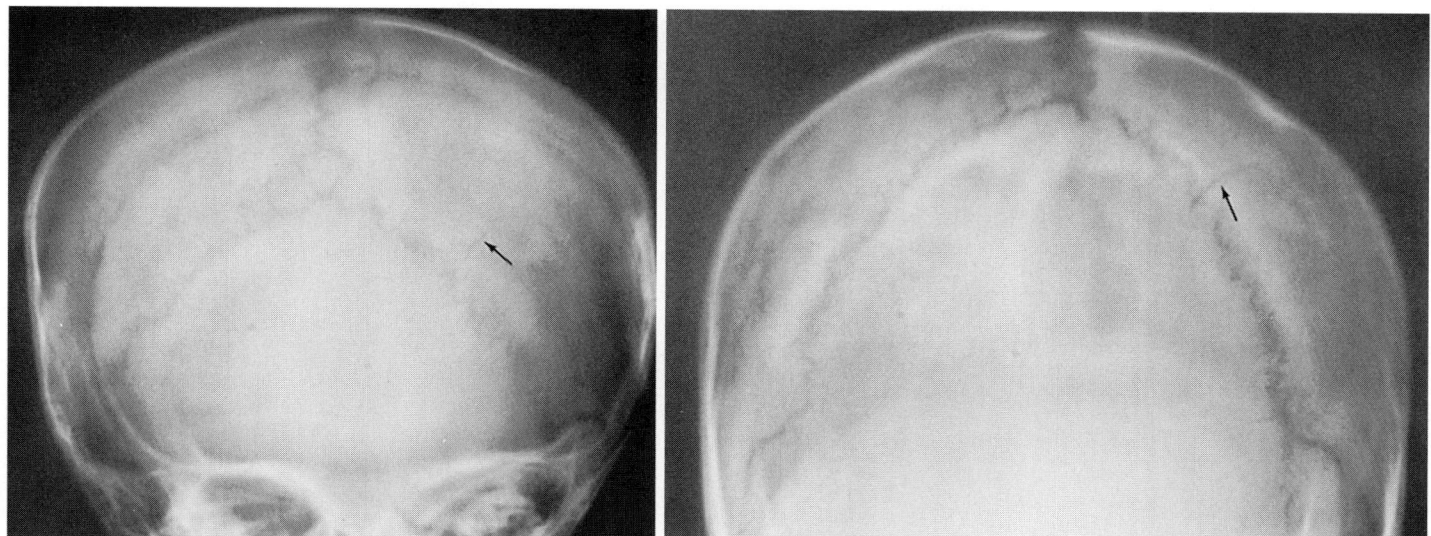

Figure 1–129. Persistence of parietal fissure in a 1-year-old child, simulating a fracture.

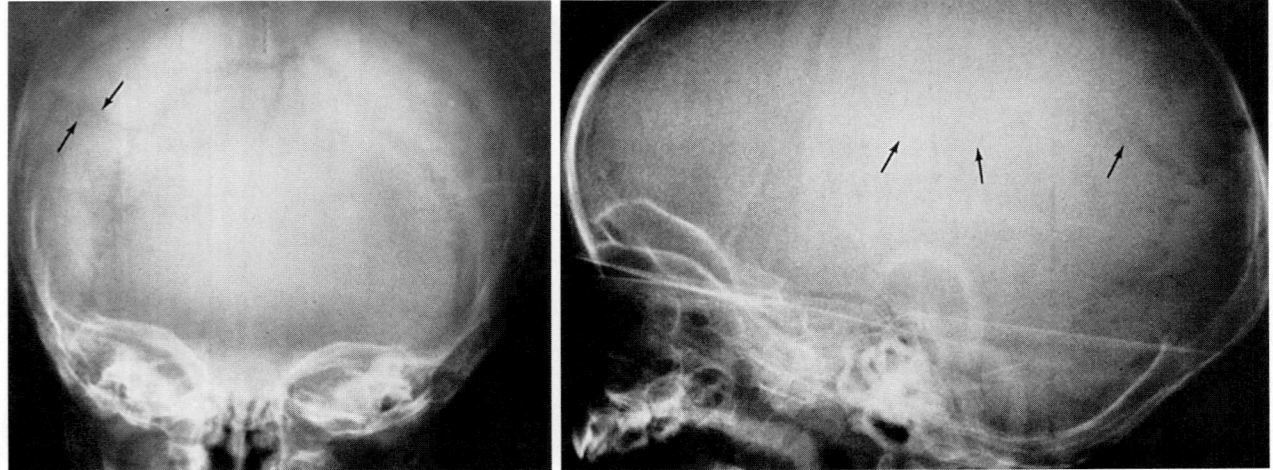

Figure 1–130. Unilateral intraparietal suture, which divides the parietal bone into an upper and lower segment. This suture may also occur bilaterally and extends from the coronal suture to the lambdoid suture. (Ref: Shapiro R: Anomalous parietal sutures and the bipartite parietal bone. *Am J Roentgenol* 115:569, 1972.)

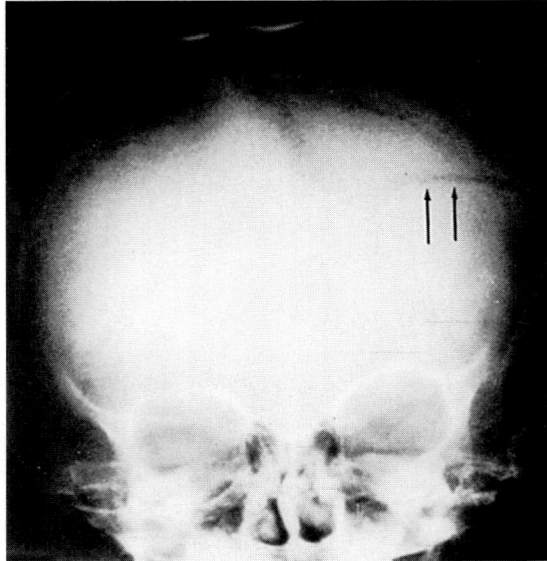

Figure 1–131. Unilateral intraparietal suture. When this suture is unilateral, the skull may be asymmetric, with the side harboring the intraparietal suture being larger than the opposite side, as in this case.

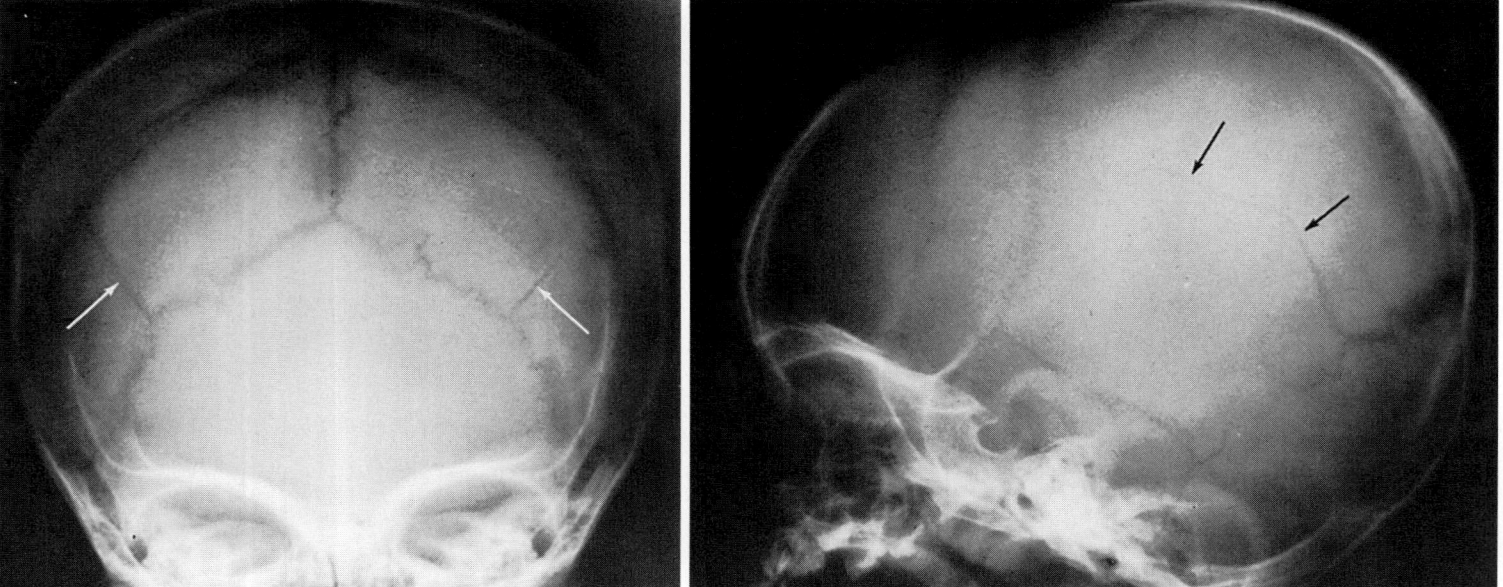

Figure 1–132. Bilateral subsagittal sutures in a 1-year-old child.

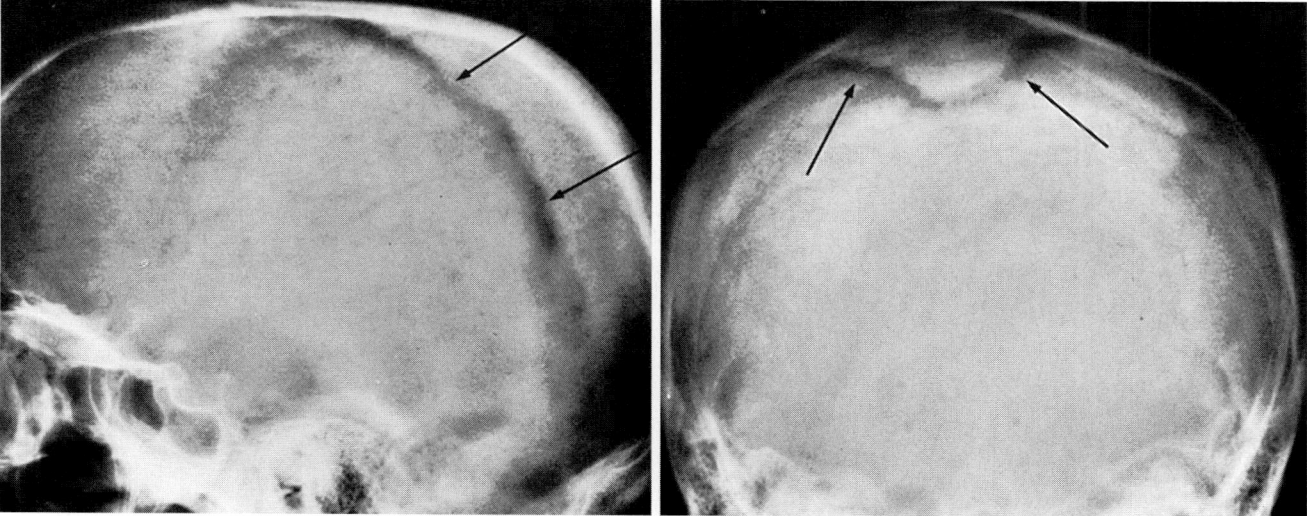

Figure 1–133. Unusual lucencies in the parietal bones crossing the midline, apparently representing a sagittal intrasutural bone, an incidental finding in an adult woman.

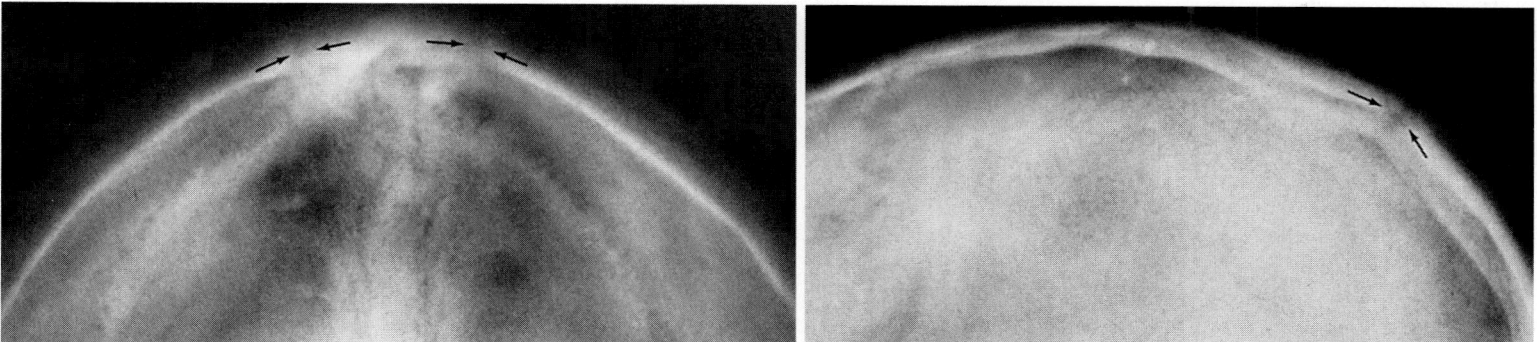

Figure 1–134. Normal parietal foramina, which transmit the emissary veins of Santorini.

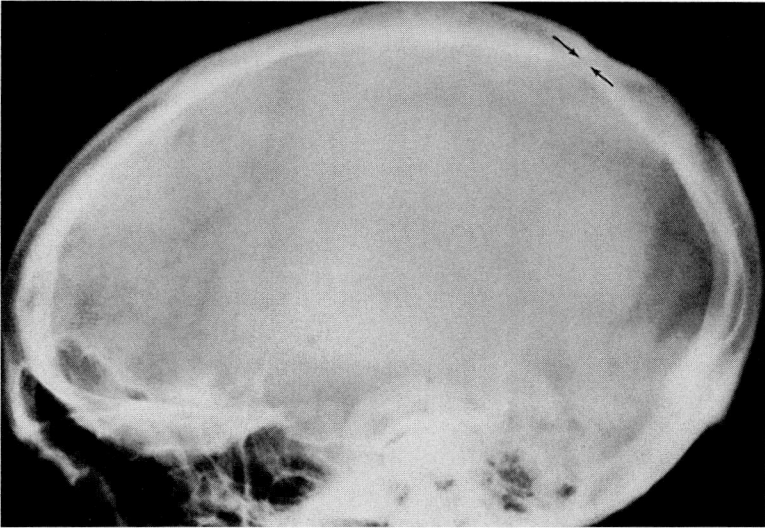

Figure 1–135. Parietal emissary vascular channel. Note the depression in the outer table at its point of exit.

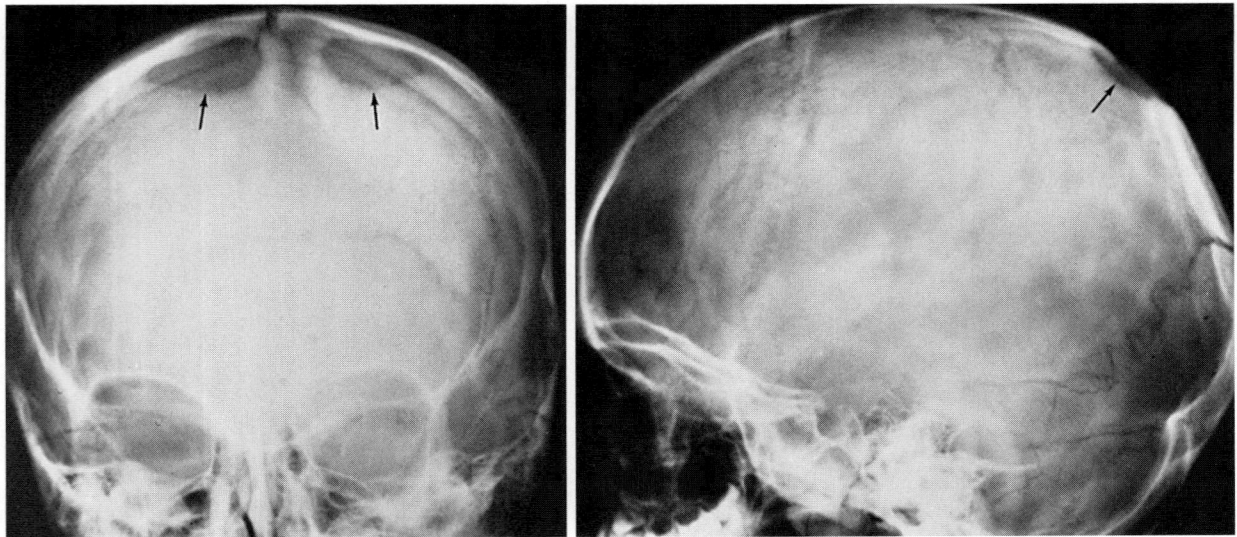

Figure 1–136. Parietal foramina. These congenital defects vary in size, but they are consistent in location and are often symmetric. They are not significant except in the differential diagnosis of cranial defects, including burr holes.

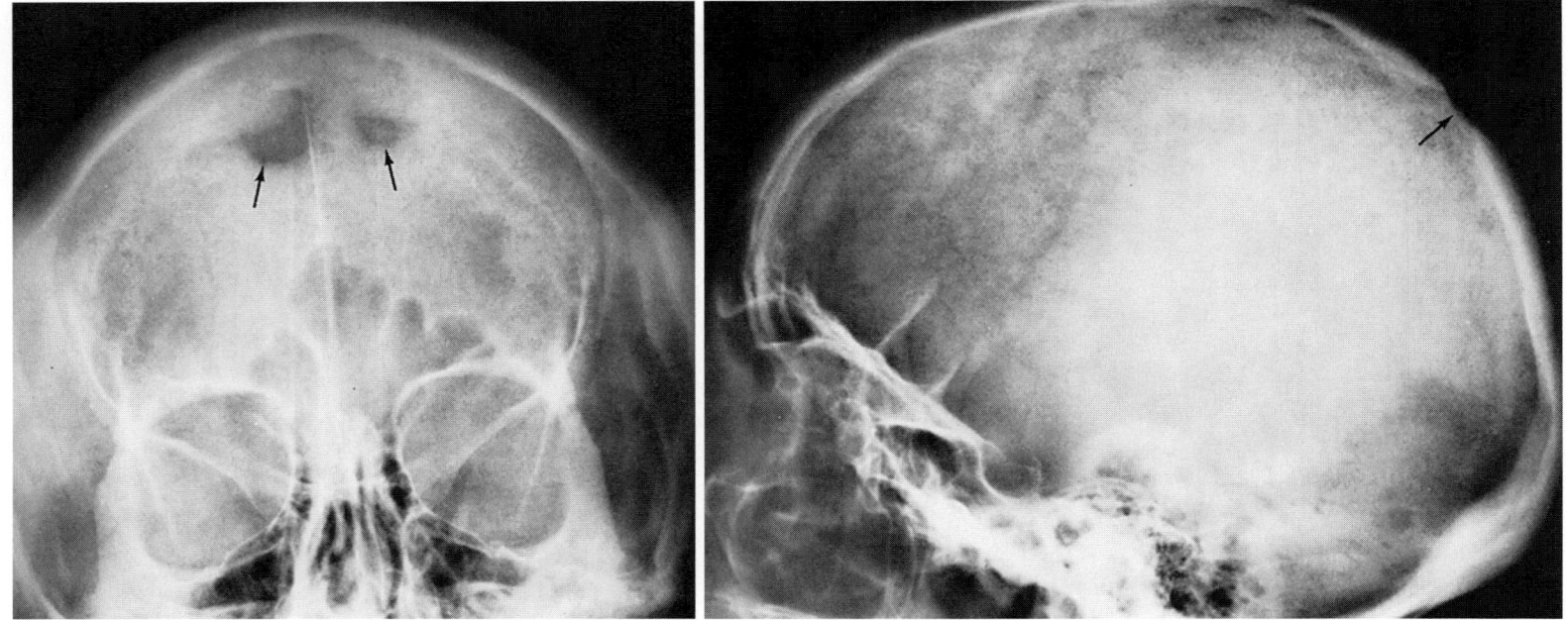

Figure 1–137. Parietal foramina showing some asymmetry.

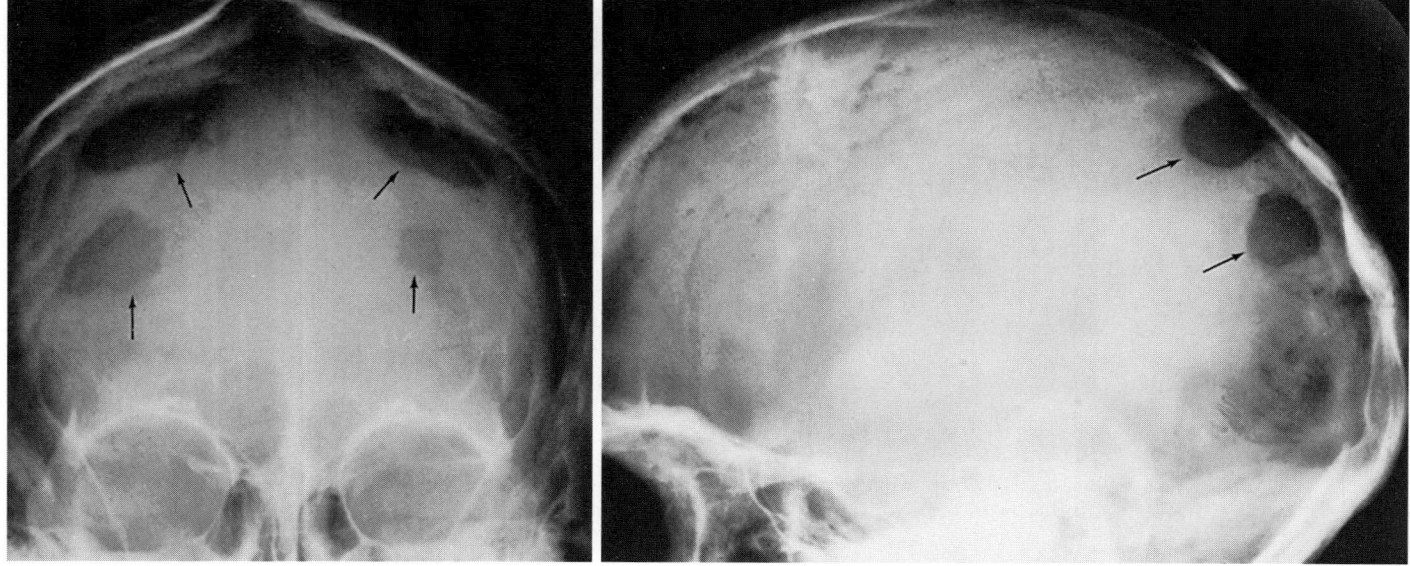

Figure 1–138. Paired parietal foramina, an unusual variant.

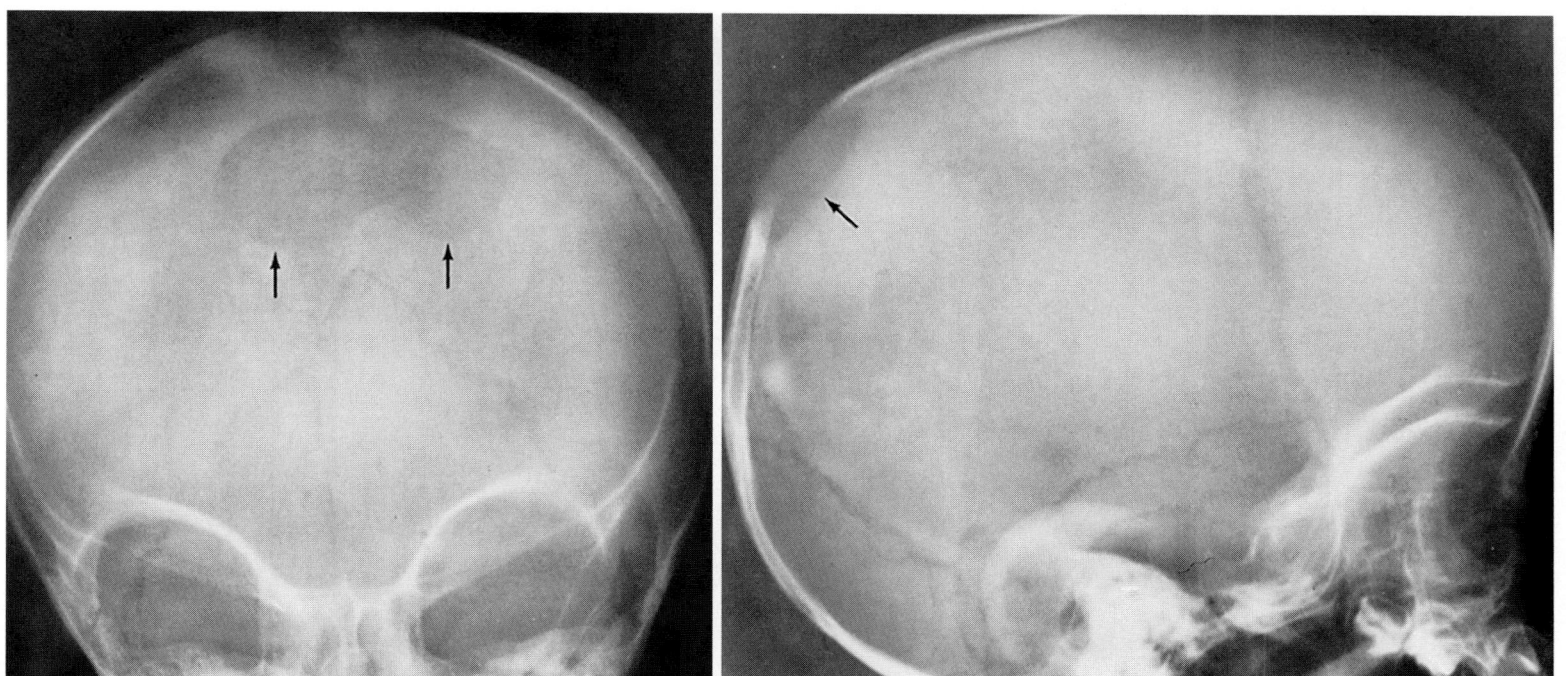

Figure 1–139. Parietal foramina in a 15-month-old child without central dividing strip.

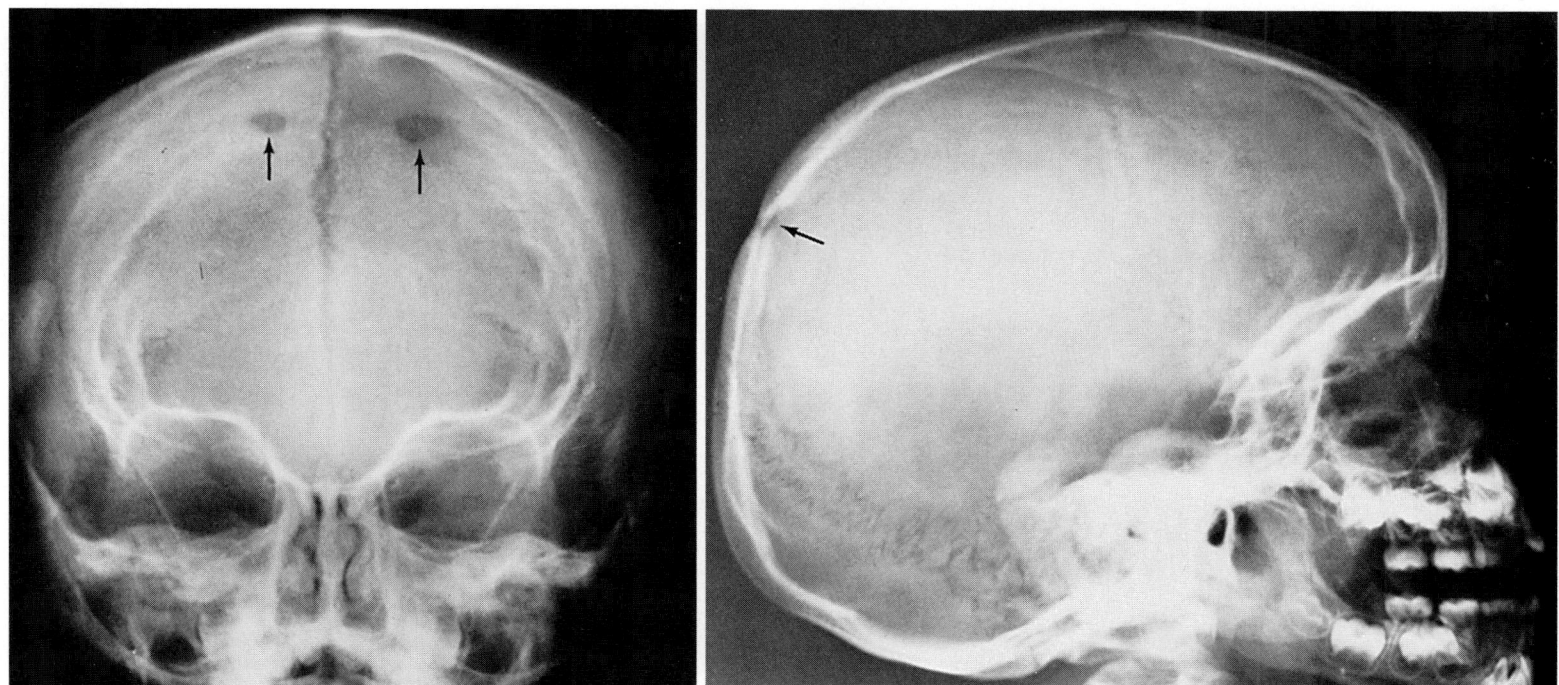

Figure 1–140. Asymmetric and irregular parietal foramina.

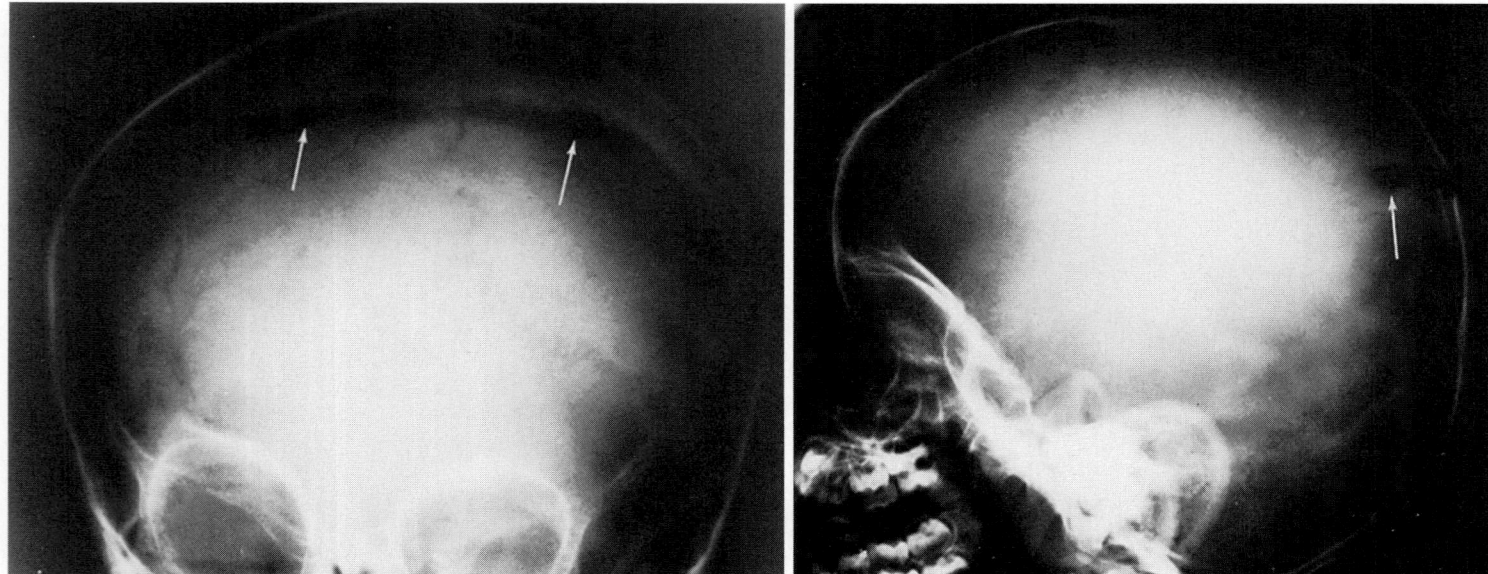

Figure 1–141. Unusual parietal foramina.

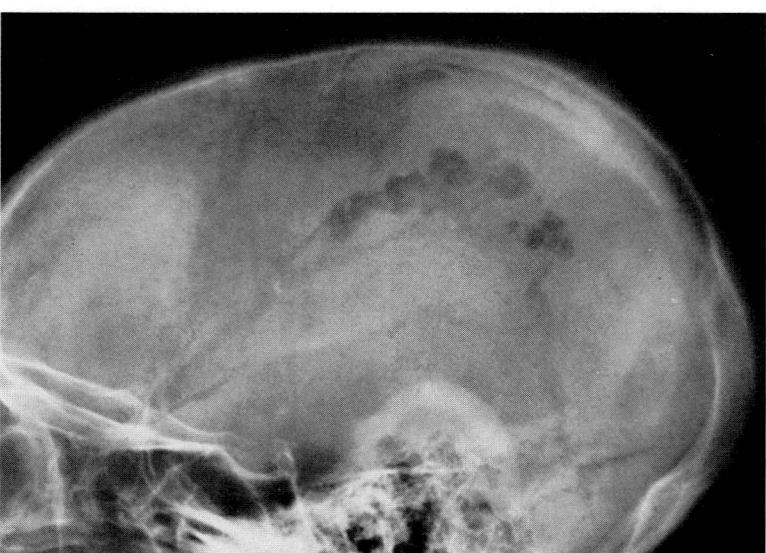

Figure 1–142. Unusual venous vascular markings in parietal bone. This area frequently shows a striking vascular pattern.

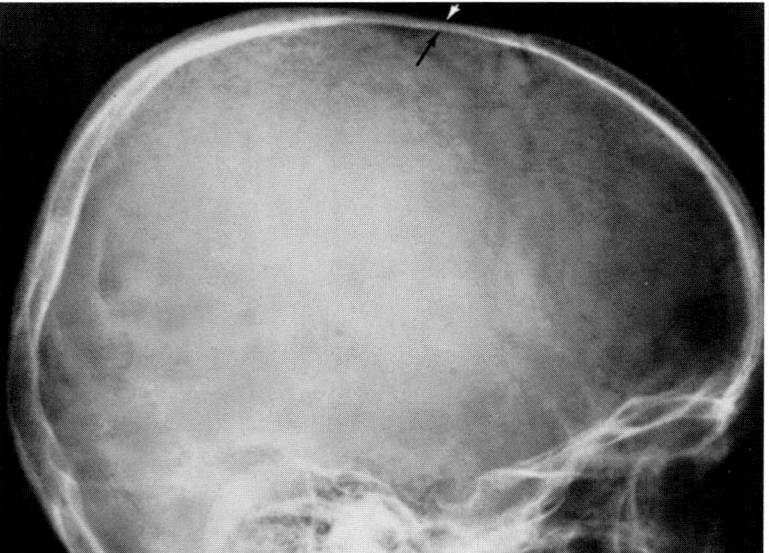

Figure 1–143. Localized area of thinning of the external table at the site of the anterior fontanel. This should not be mistaken for erosion of the outer table.

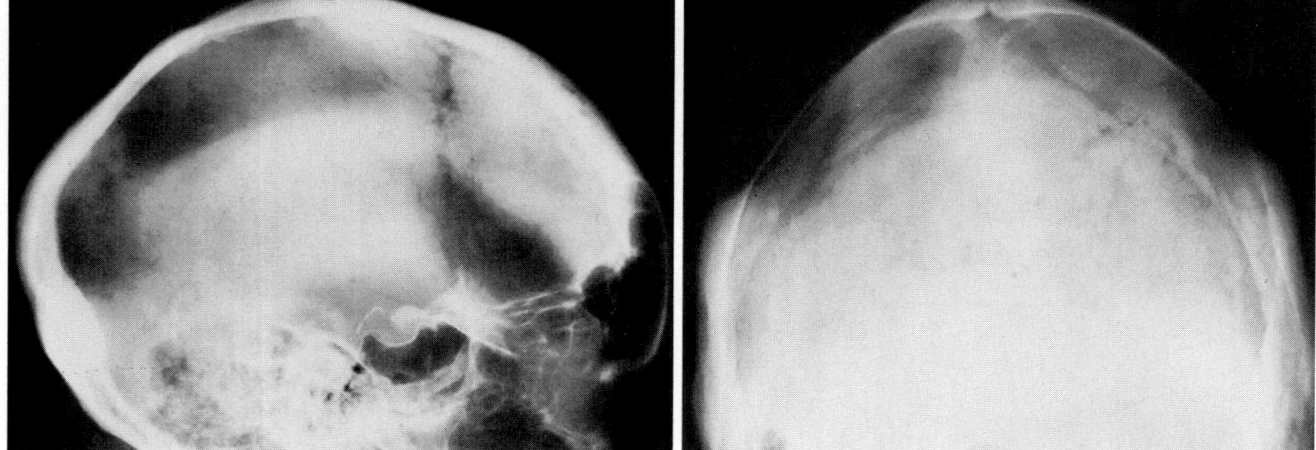

Figure 1–144. Parietal thinning, a manifestation of postmenopausal osteoporosis. The outer table is lost, with characteristic preservation of the inner table. Note also similar localized thinning of the frontal bone in the lateral projection. (Ref: Steinbach HL, Obata WG: The significance of thinning of the parietal bones. *Am J Roentgenol* 78:39, 1957.) Parietal thinning may rarely be unilateral. (Ref: Wilson AK: Thinness of parietal bones. *Am J Roentgenol* 58:724, 1947.)

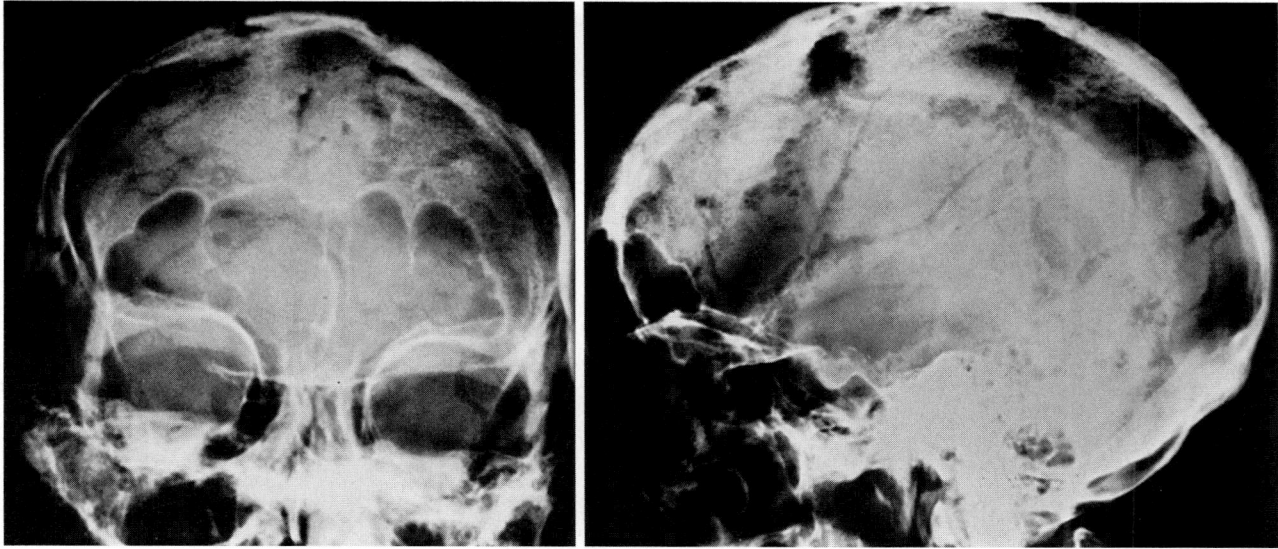

Figure 1–145. Combined parietal thinning and venous lakes and grooves in a 56-year-old woman.

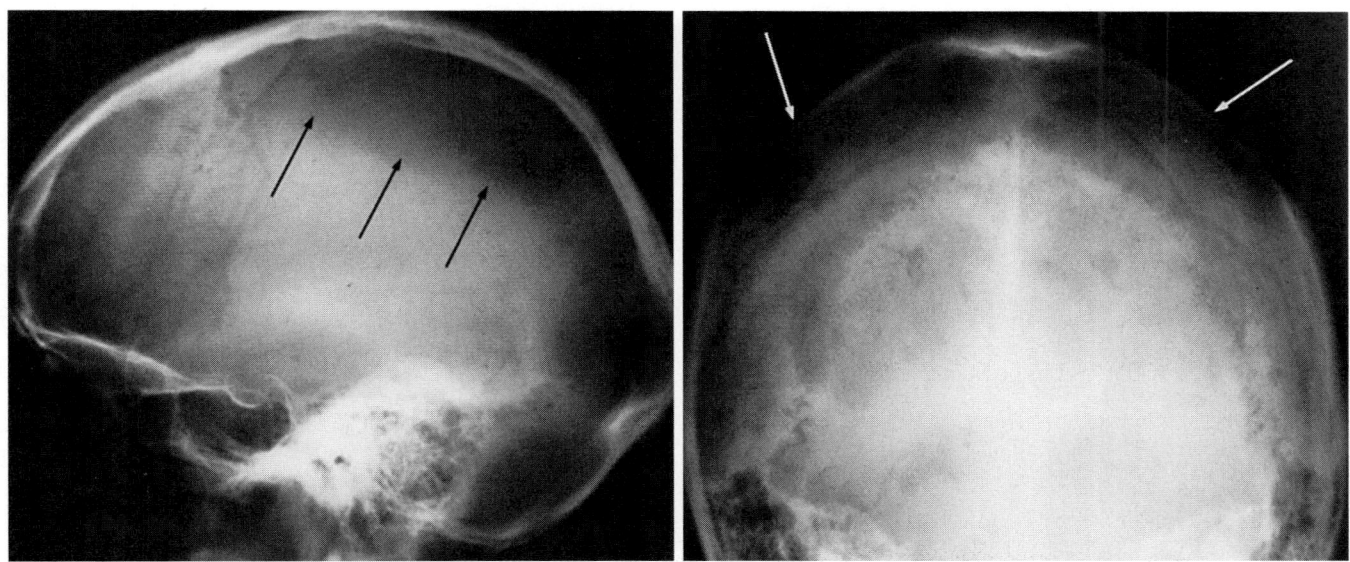

Figure 1–146. An 82-year-old man with parietal thinning. This entity is much less common in males.

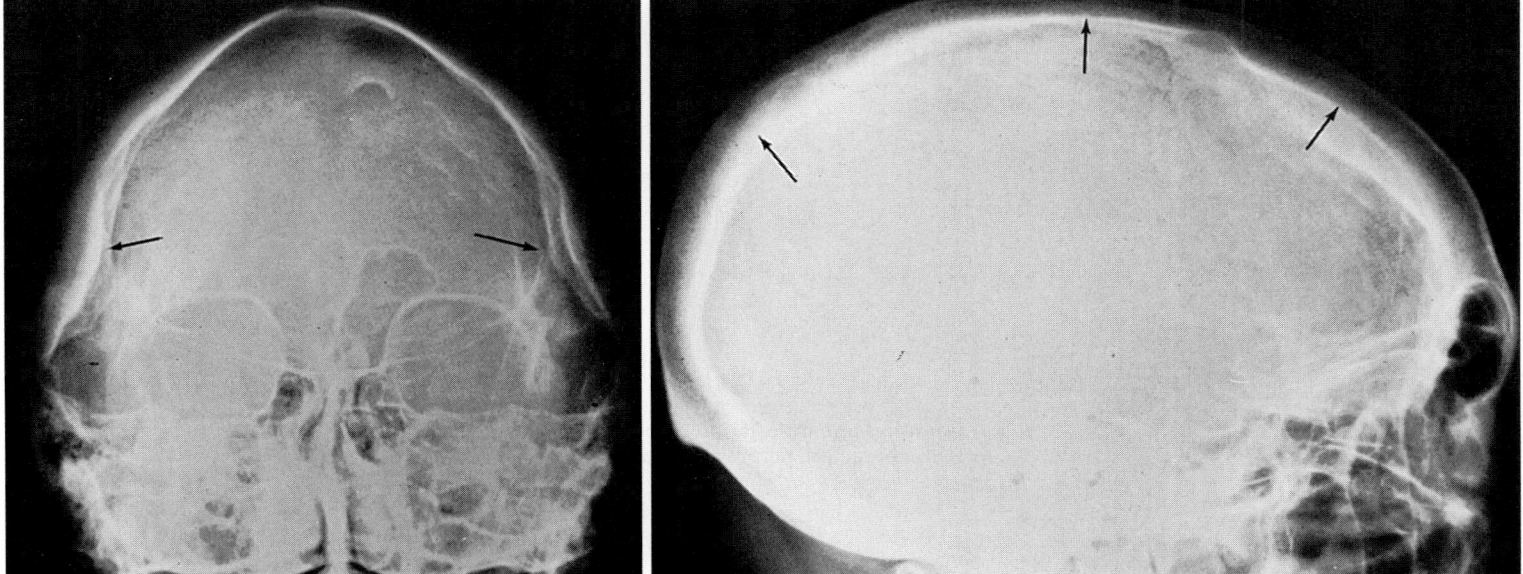

Figure 1–147. Hyperostosis generalisata and parietalis.

The Occipital Bone

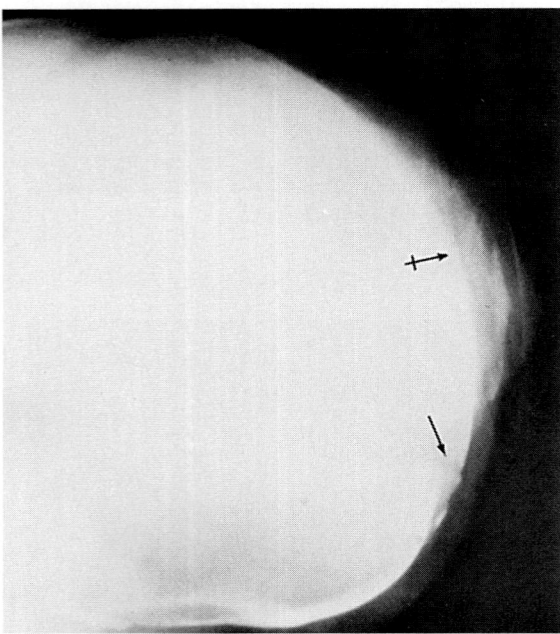

Figure 1–148. Apparent malalignment of the parietal and occipital bones caused by molding of labor, not to be mistaken for fracture (→). A cephalohematoma is present (↔).

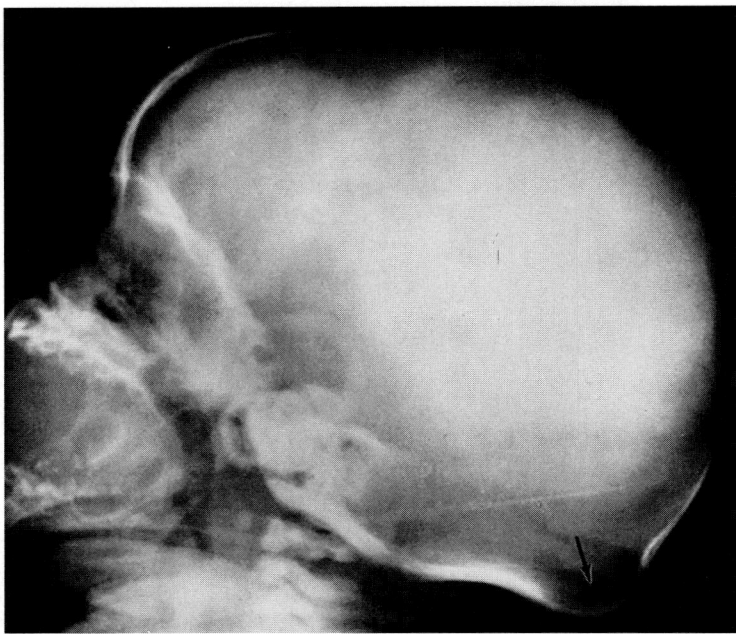

Figure 1–149. Unusual occipital configuration in the newborn is due to the molding of labor.

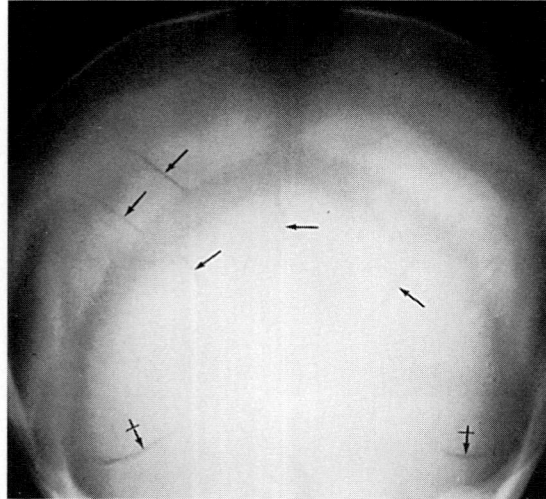

Figure 1–150. Occipital and parietal fissures caused by persistent strips of membranous bone, a common finding in infants that may simulate fracture. The mendosal sutures are evident (↔).

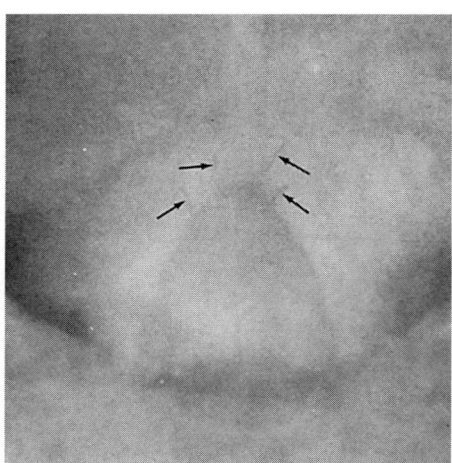

Figure 1–151. Fissures in an infant around foramen magnum similar to those of Fig. 1–150.

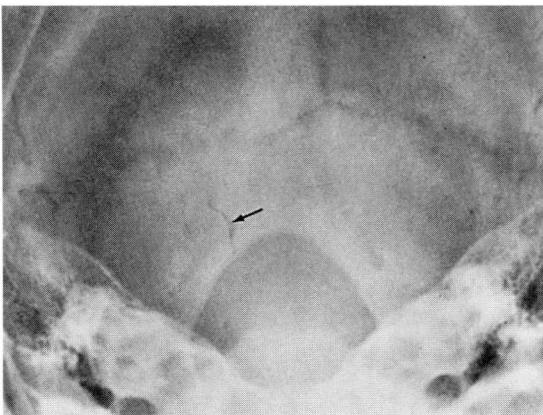

Figure 1–152. Persistent membranous fissures simulating a fracture in an adolescent girl.

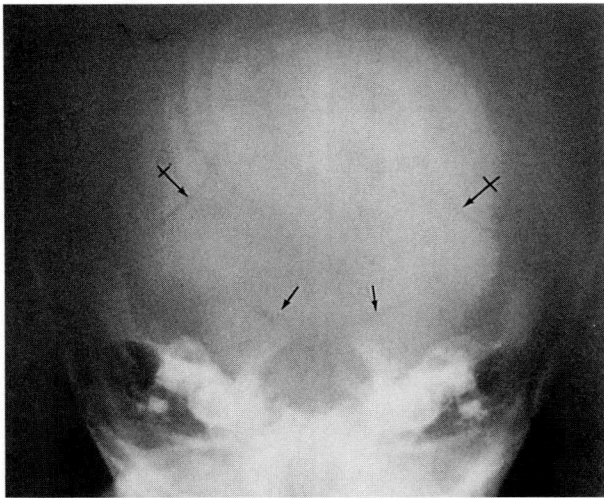

Figure 1–153. The synchondroses between the supraoccipital and exoccipital portions of the occipital bone in a 6-week-old child (→). The mendosal sutures are also seen (↦).

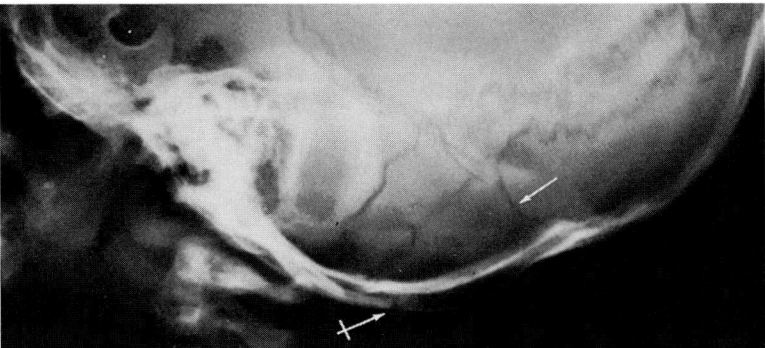

Figure 1–154. The mendosal suture (→) and synchondrosis between the supraoccipital and exoccipital portions of the occipital bone (↦) in lateral projection in a 1-month-old child.

Figure 1–155. Accessory ossicle of the supraoccipital bone (Kerckring's ossicle) in a normal infant. (Ref: Caffey J: On accessory ossicles of supraoccipital bone; some newly recognized roentgen features of normal infantile skull. *Am J Roentgenol* 70:401, 1953.)

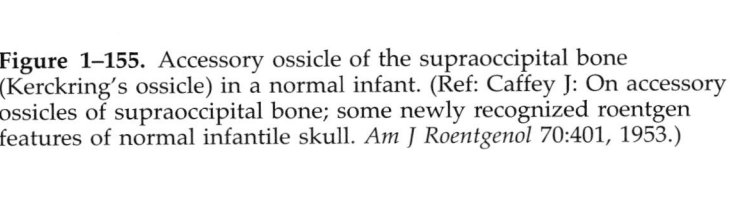

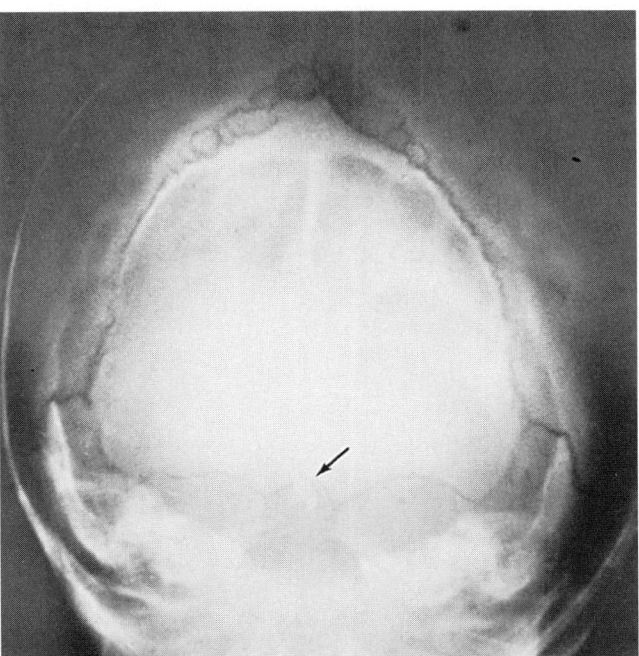

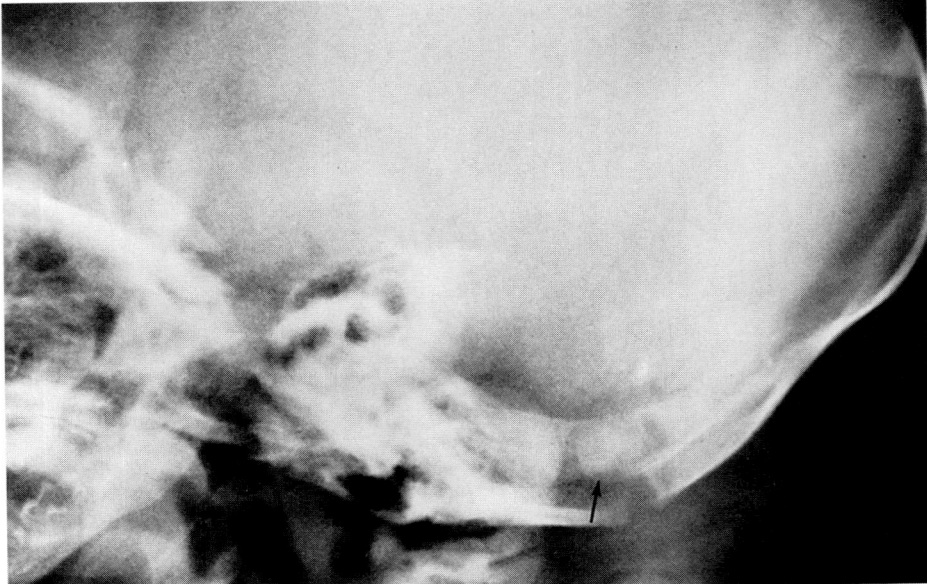

Figure 1–156. Appearance of the accessory supraoccipital ossicle in the lateral projection.

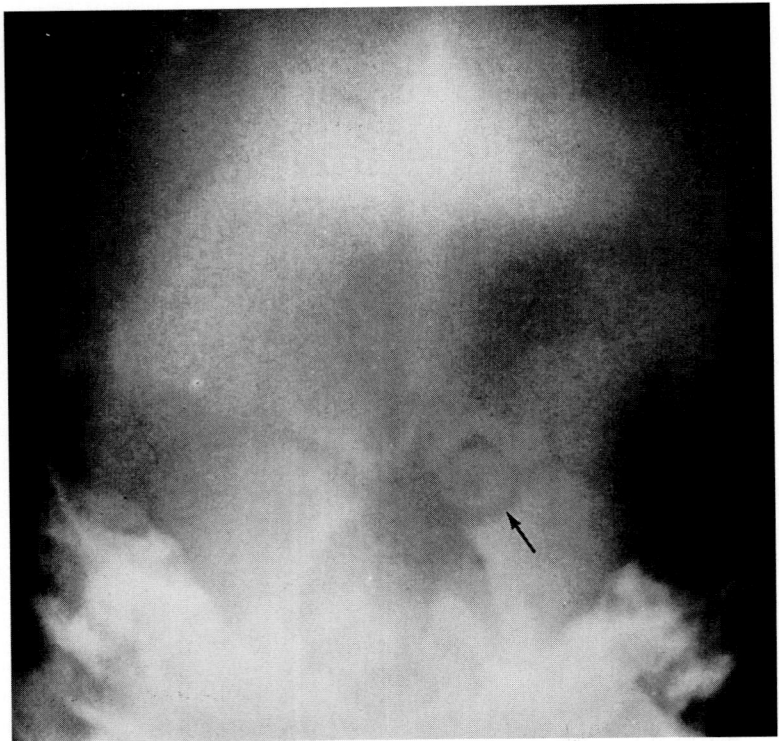

Figure 1–157. Unilateral ossicle of the supraoccipital bone.

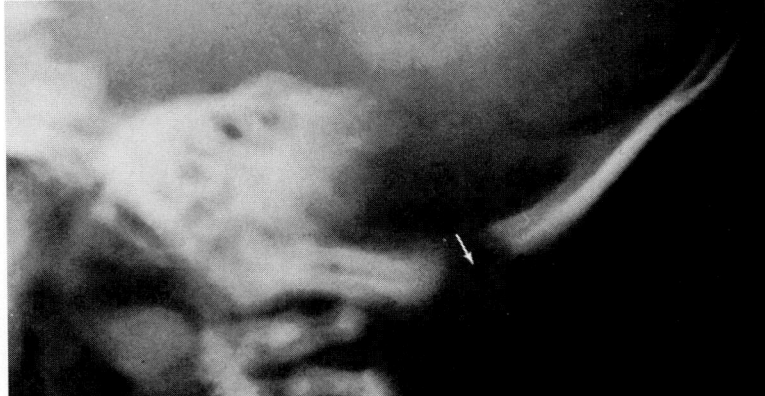

Figure 1–158. Occipital ossicle in the lateral projection.

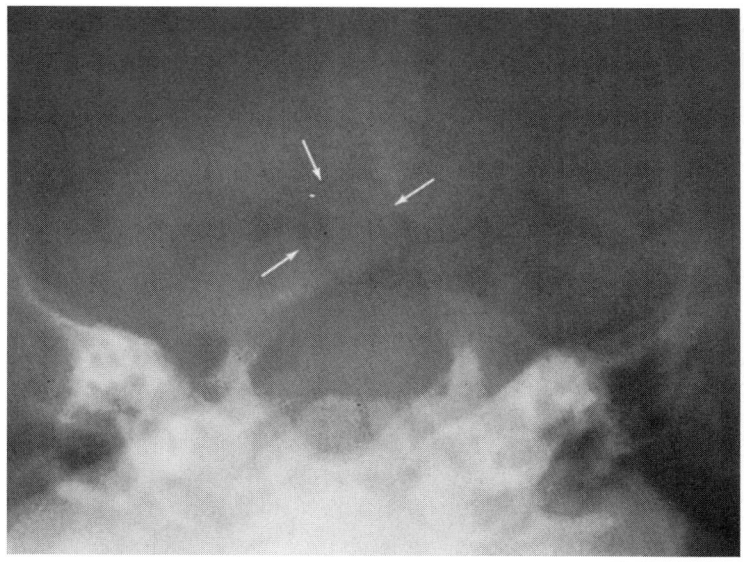

Figure 1–159. Irregular midline occipital ossicle in a 6-month-old girl.

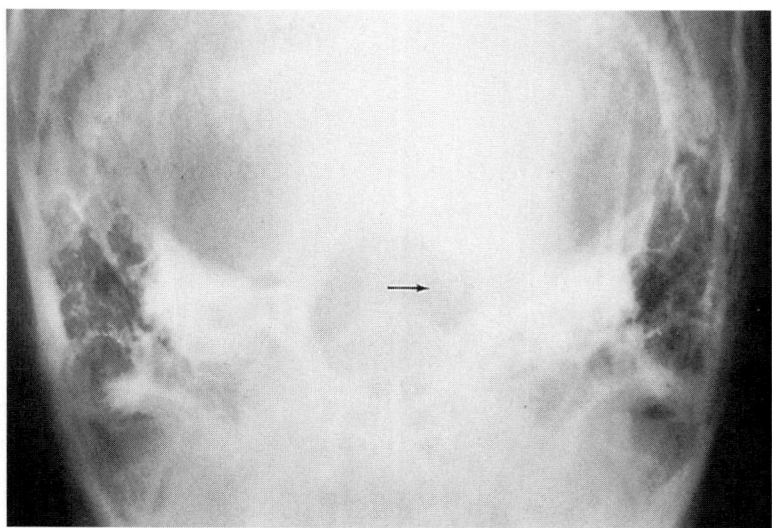

Figure 1–160. Persistence of an occipital ossicle in a 22-year-old man.

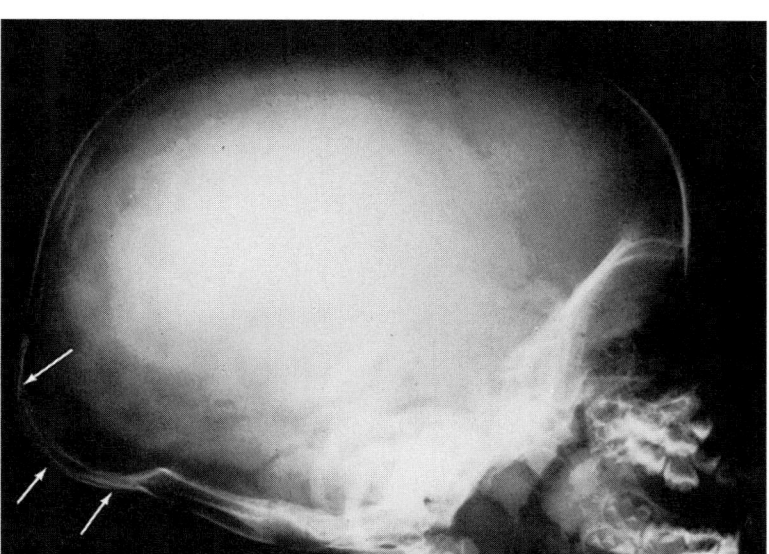

Figure 1–161. Bathrocephaly in a 1-year-old child.

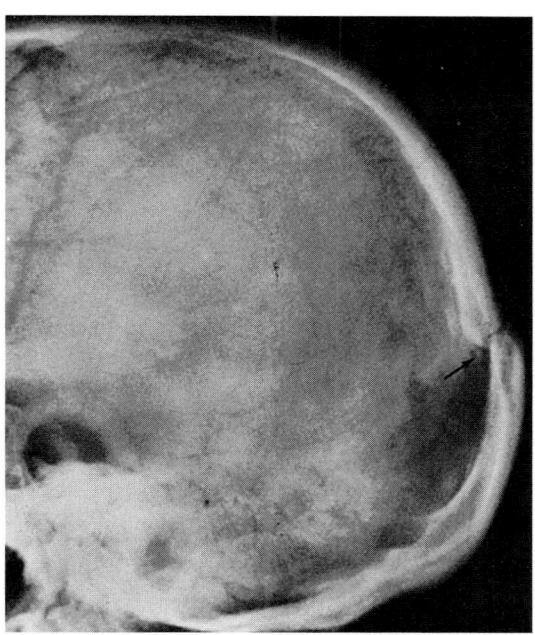

Figure 1–162. Bathrocephaly in an adult, which may be confused with a fracture.

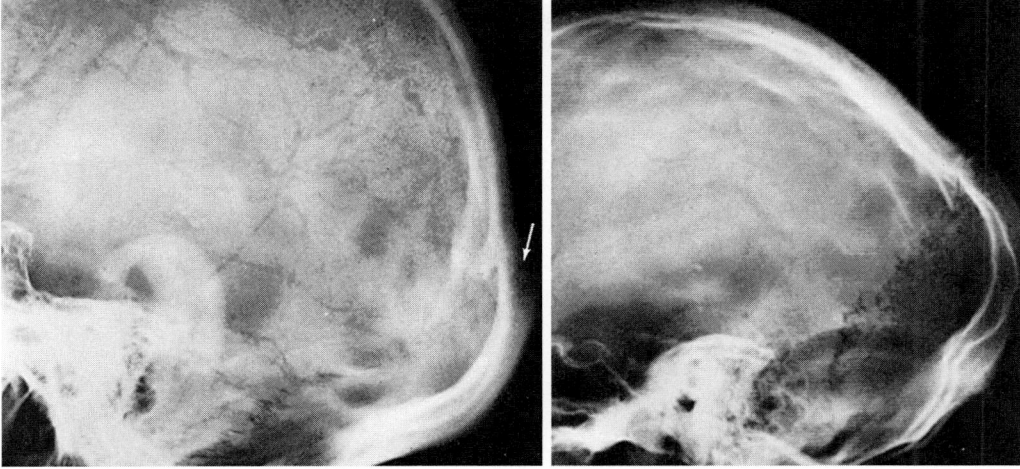

Figure 1–163. Bathrocephalic occiputs in adults.

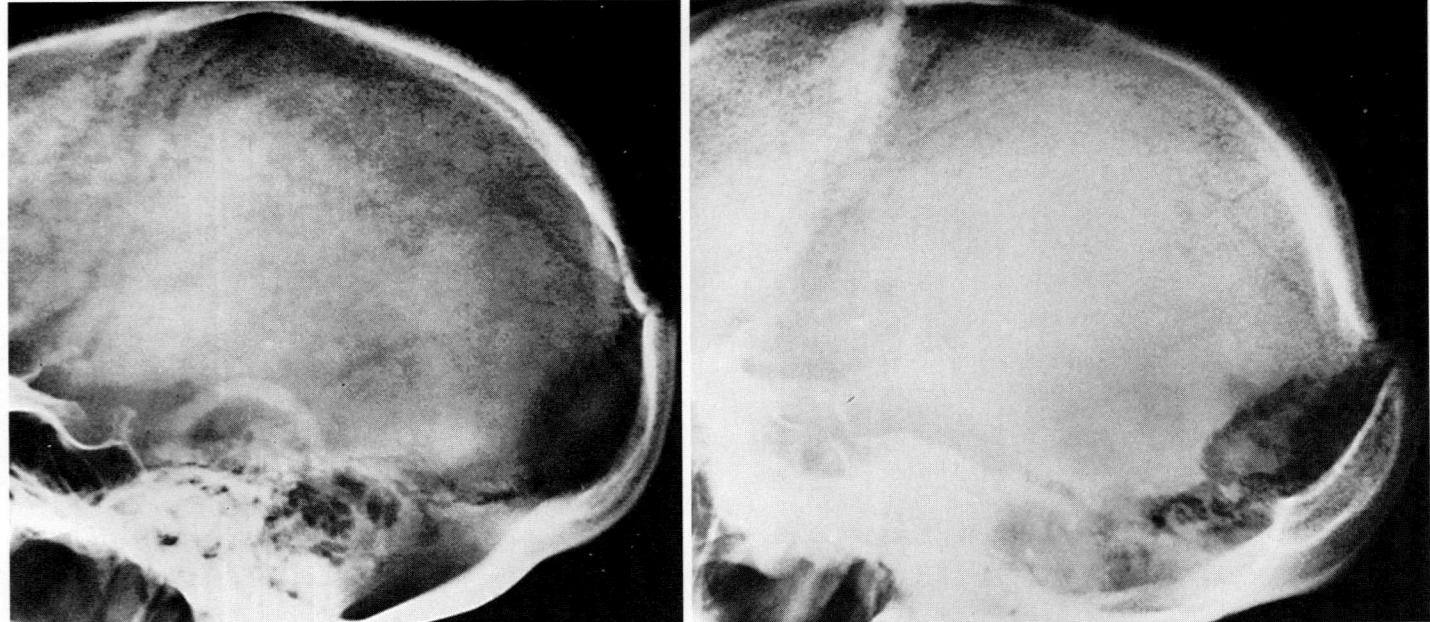

Figure 1–164. Bathrocephalic occiputs in adults.

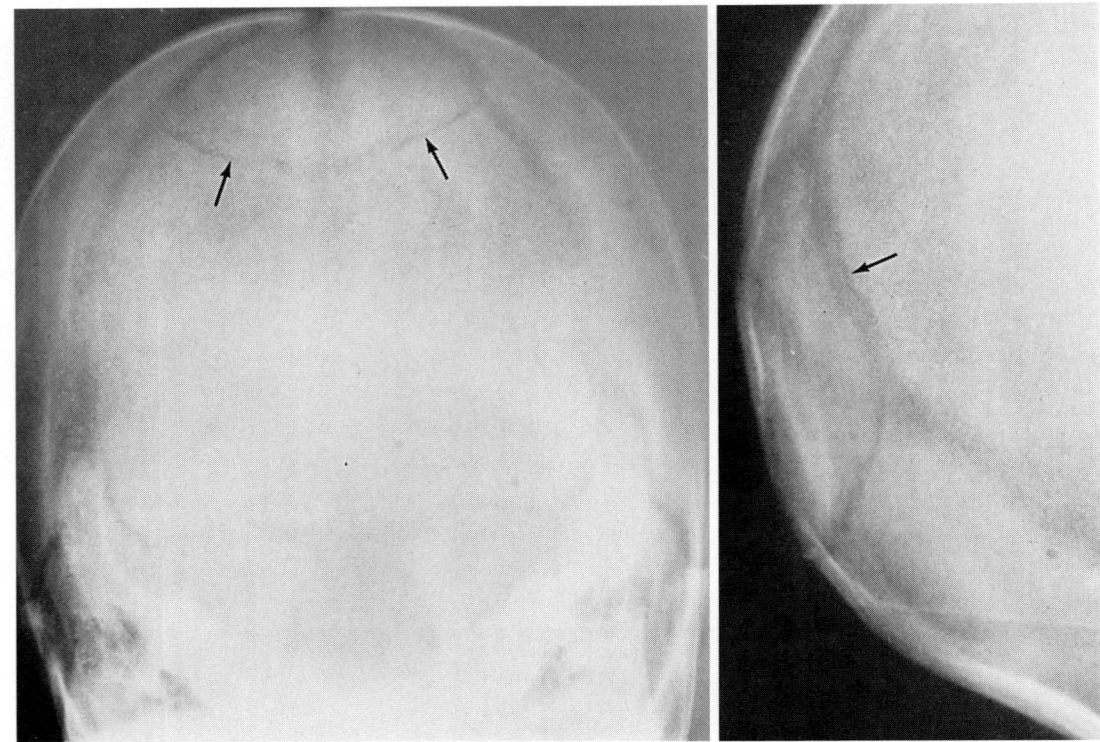

Figure 1–165. Normal large interparietal bone in a 3-month-old child in frontal and lateral projections.

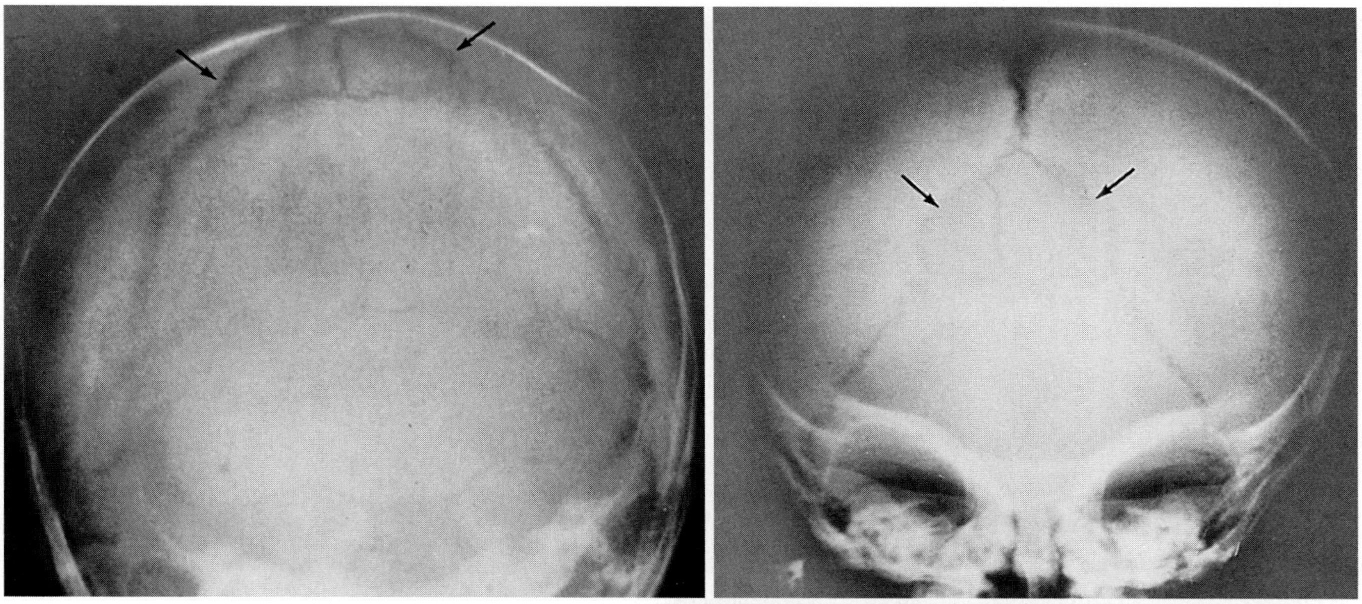

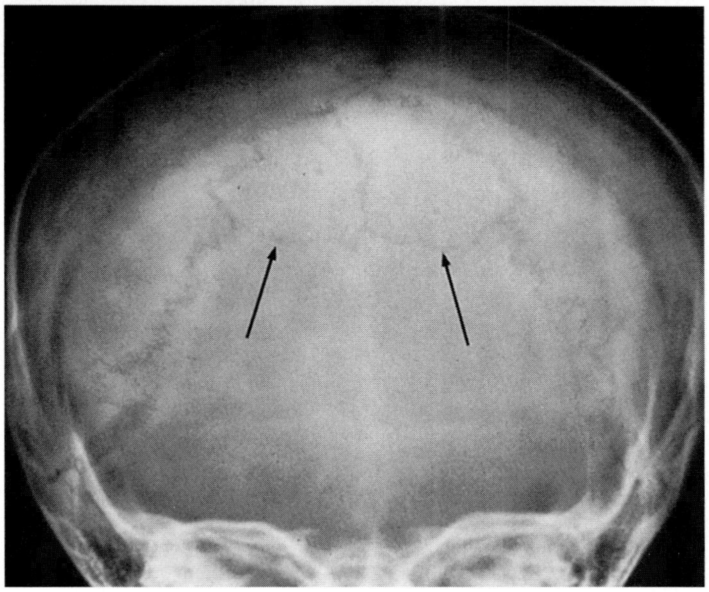

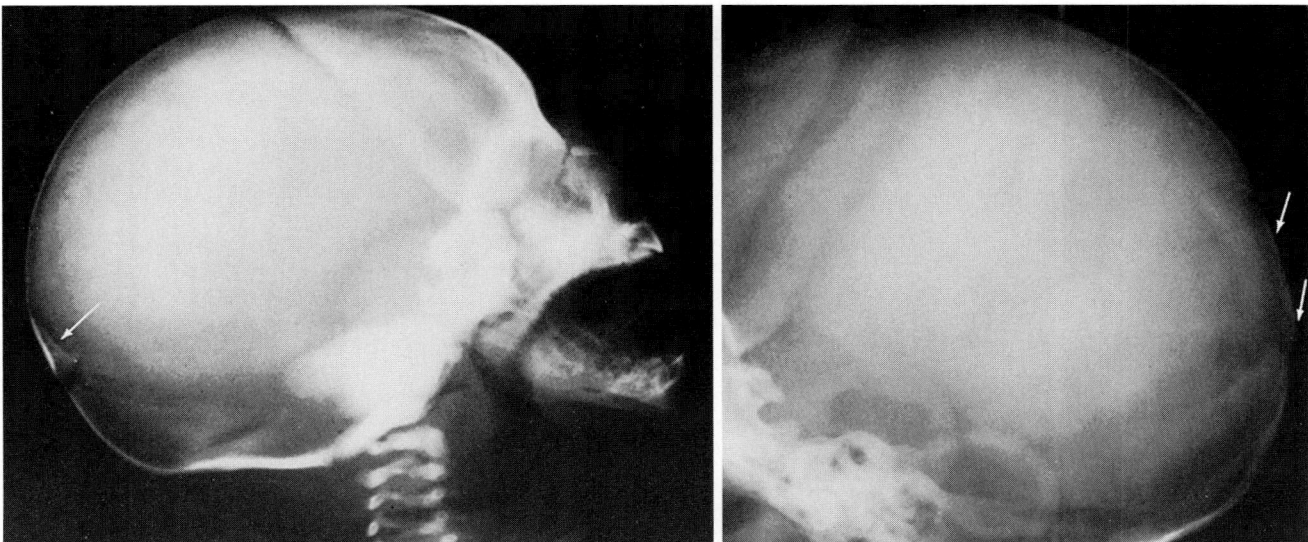

Figure 1–166. Three examples of bifid interparietal bones (Inca bone). This should not be mistaken for a fracture. (Ref: Shapiro R, Robinson F: The os incae. *Am J Roentgenol* 127:469, 1976.)

Figure 1–167. Two examples of how Inca bones may simulate fractures in the lateral projection.

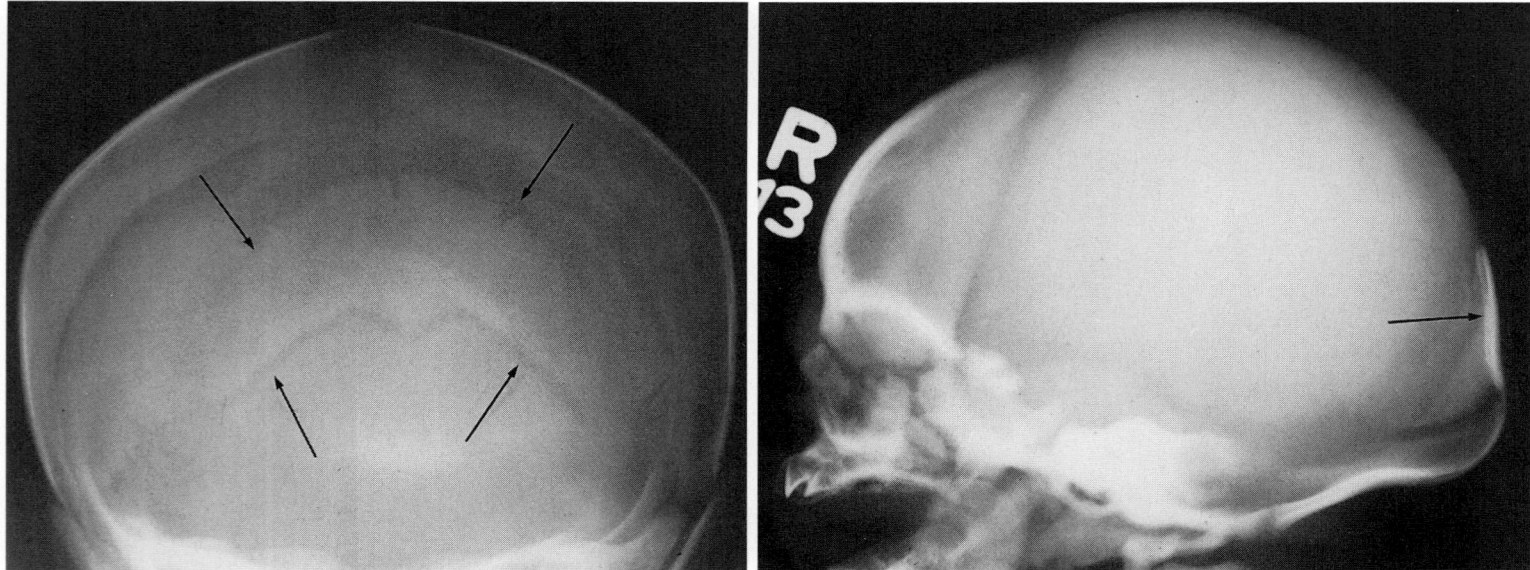

Figure 1–168. M-shaped Inca bone and occipital molding (breech head). This abnormal head shape is identified as a positive deformation associated with breech intrauterine position. It resolves during infancy with no residual impairment in most cases. (Ref: Haberkern CM, Smith DW, Jones KL: The "breech head" and its relevance. *Am J Dis Child* 133:154, 1979.)

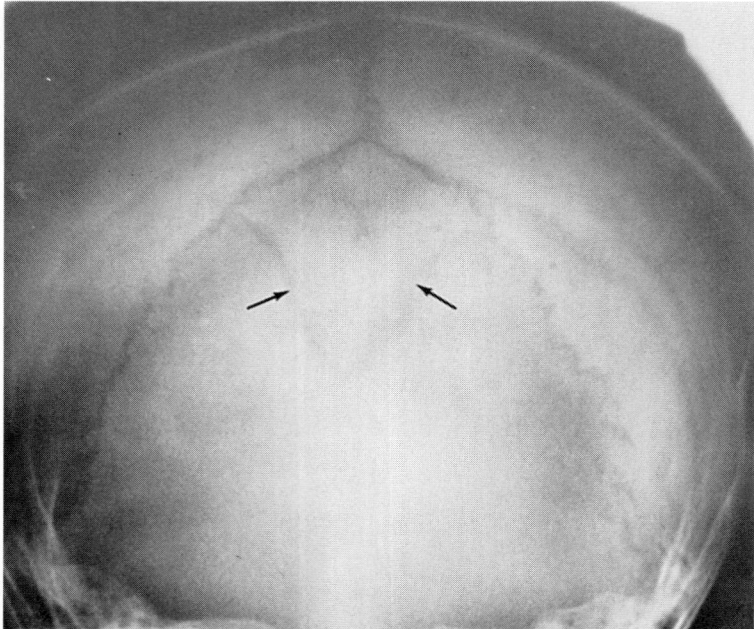

Figure 1–169. Cone-shaped interparietal bone.

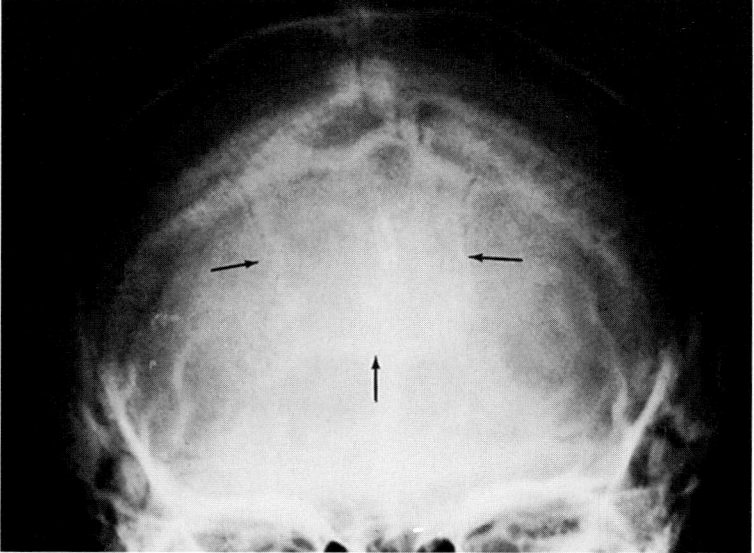

Figure 1–170. Rectangular interparietal bone in an adult.

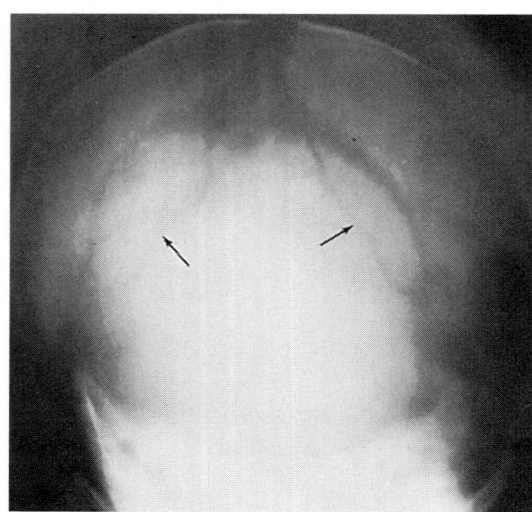

Figure 1–171. Paired, laterally placed interparietal bones.

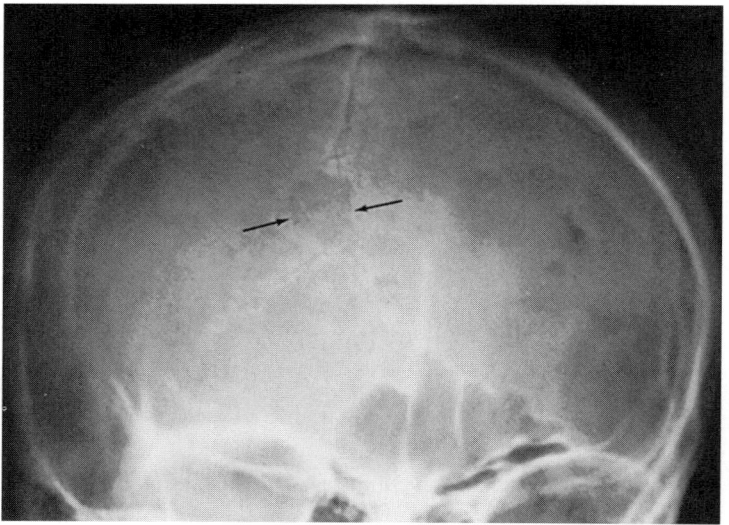

Figure 1–172. Small interparietal bone that has persisted into adult life.

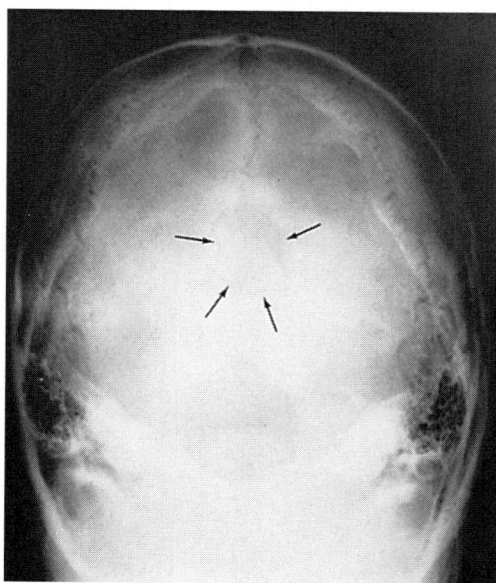

Figure 1–173. Anterior fontanel bone seen in the occipital projection in a 14-year-old.

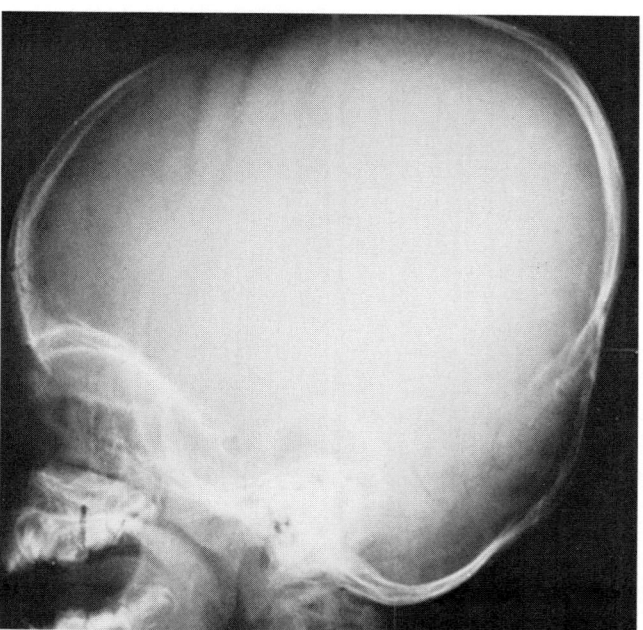

Figure 1–174. Occipital flattening caused by postural pressure, not to be confused with changes of craniostenosis.

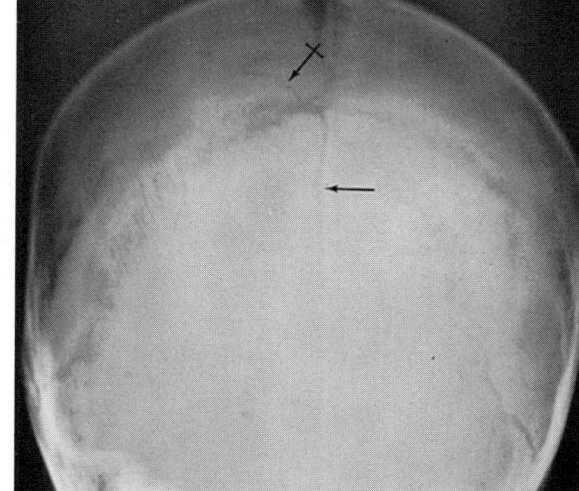

Figure 1–175. The superior median fissure of the occipital bone in a 21-month-old child, which should not be mistaken for a fracture. Note also persistence of a strip of membranous bone simulating a fracture (↦).

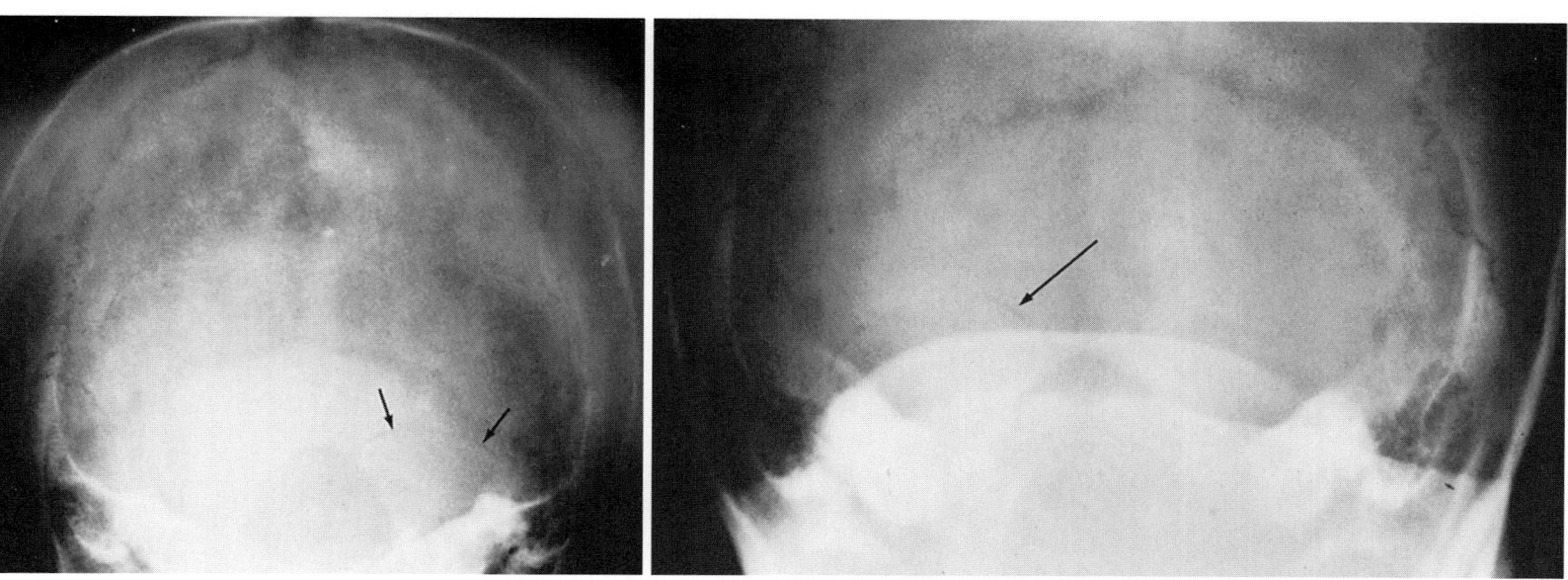

Figure 1–176. Examples of asymmetric closure of the synchondrosis between the supraoccipital and exoccipital portions of the occipital bone. *Left*, 15-month-old infant. *Right*, 12-month-old infant. The open suture may be mistaken for a fracture.

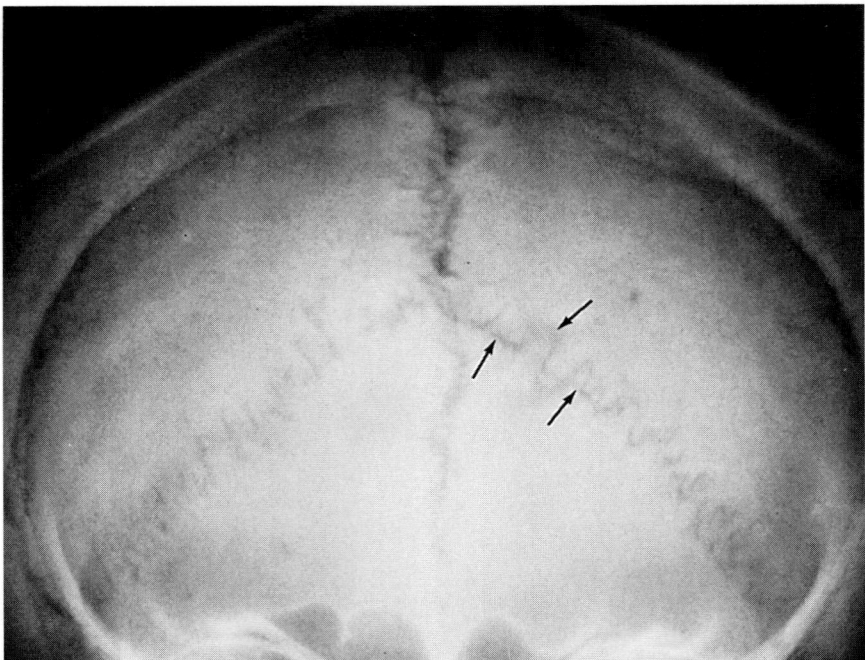

Figure 1–177. Visualization of the inner and outer aspects of the lambdoidal suture, suggesting diastatic fracture.

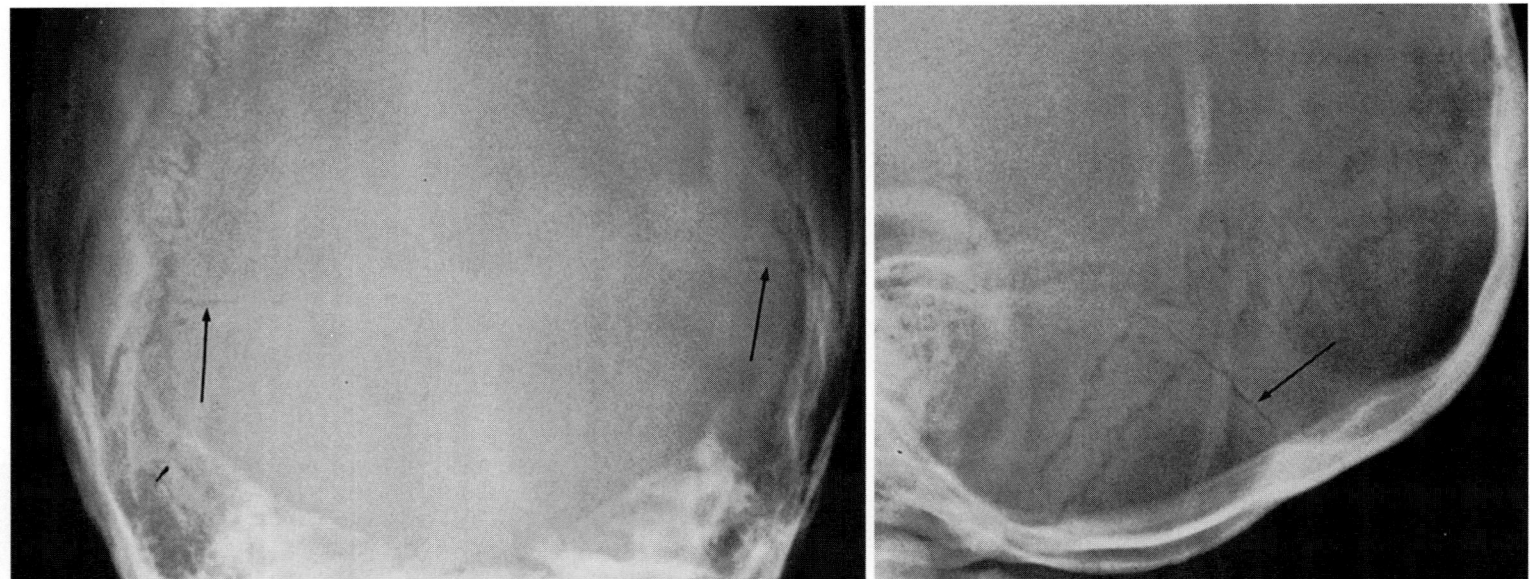

Figure 1–178. Persistent mendosal sutures in a 17-year-old boy.

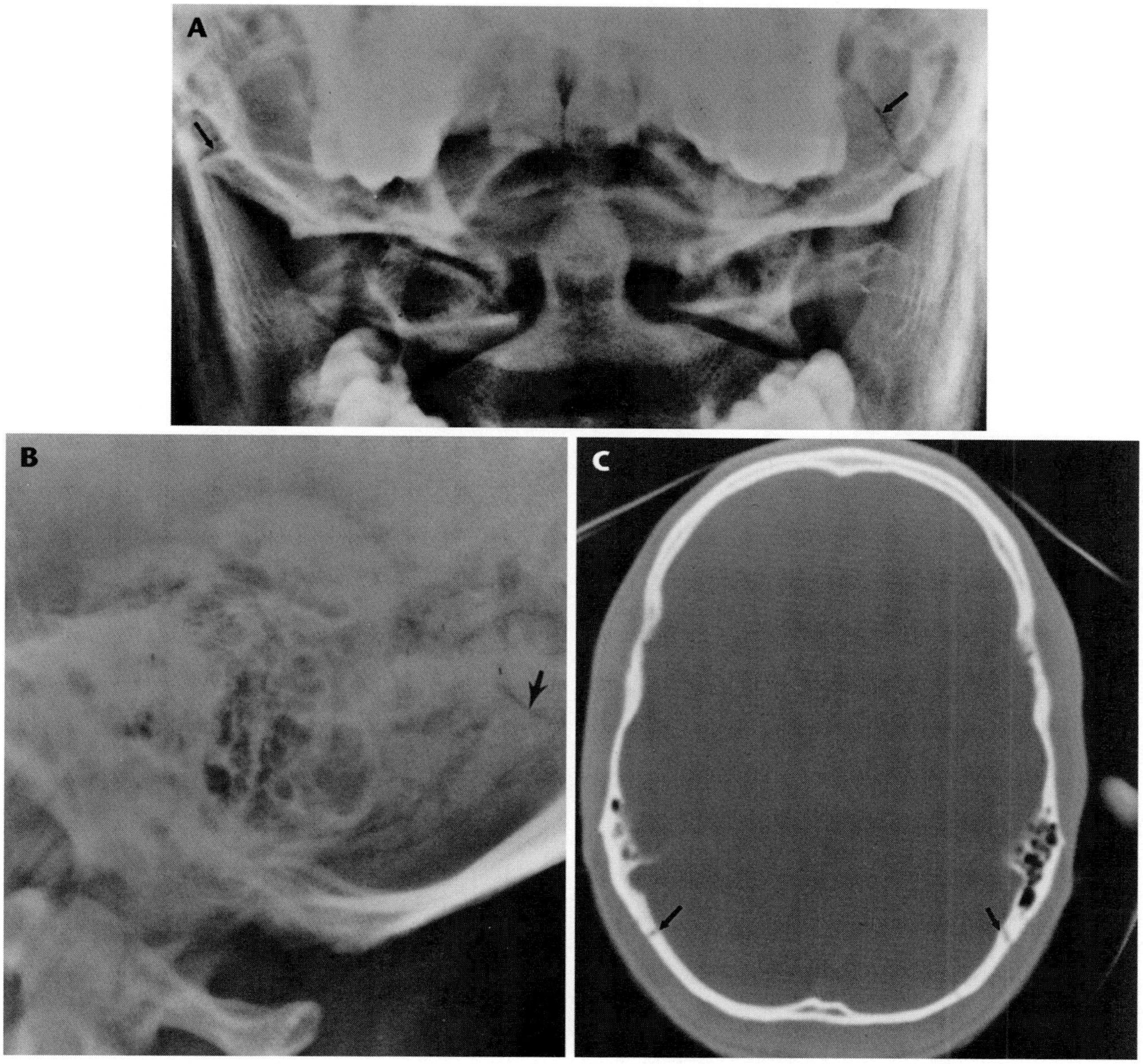

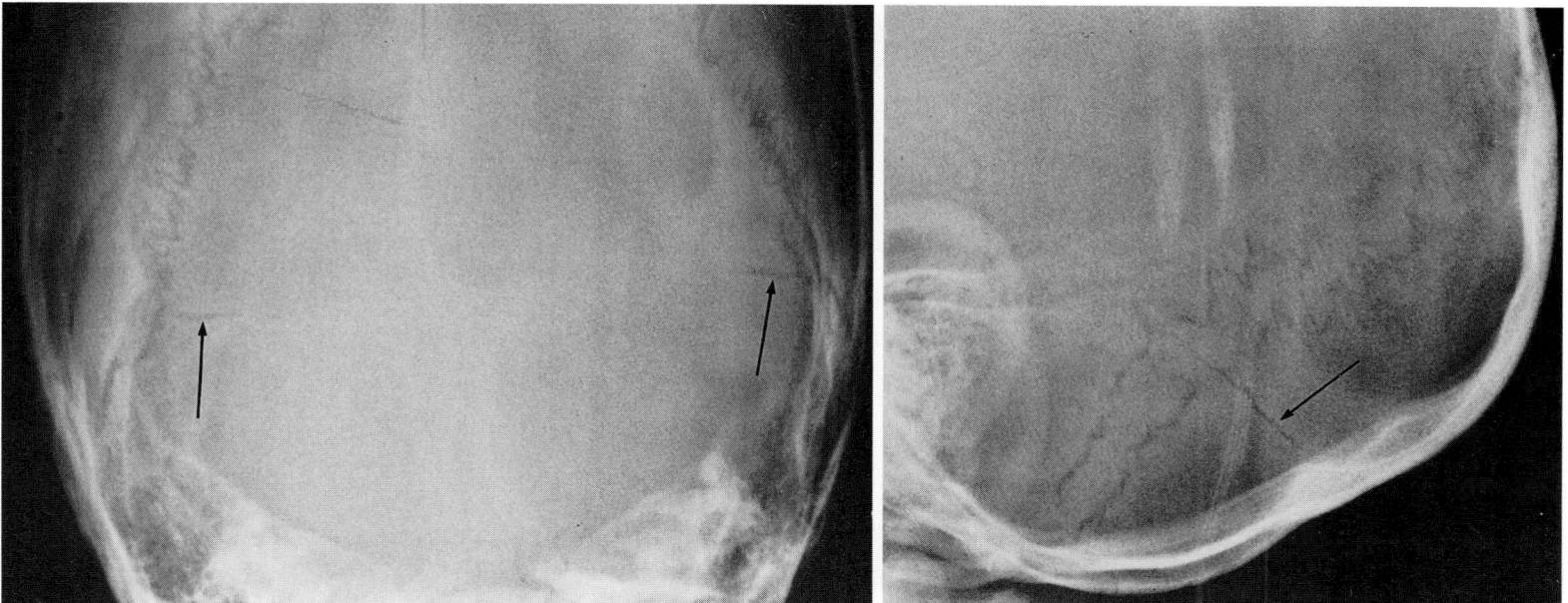

Figure 1–179. Persistent mendosal sutures in a 25-year-old man. **A**, Open-mouth odontoid view. **B**, Lateral projection. **C**, CT.

Figure 1–180. Mendosal suture in a 29-month-old child, mistaken for a fracture.

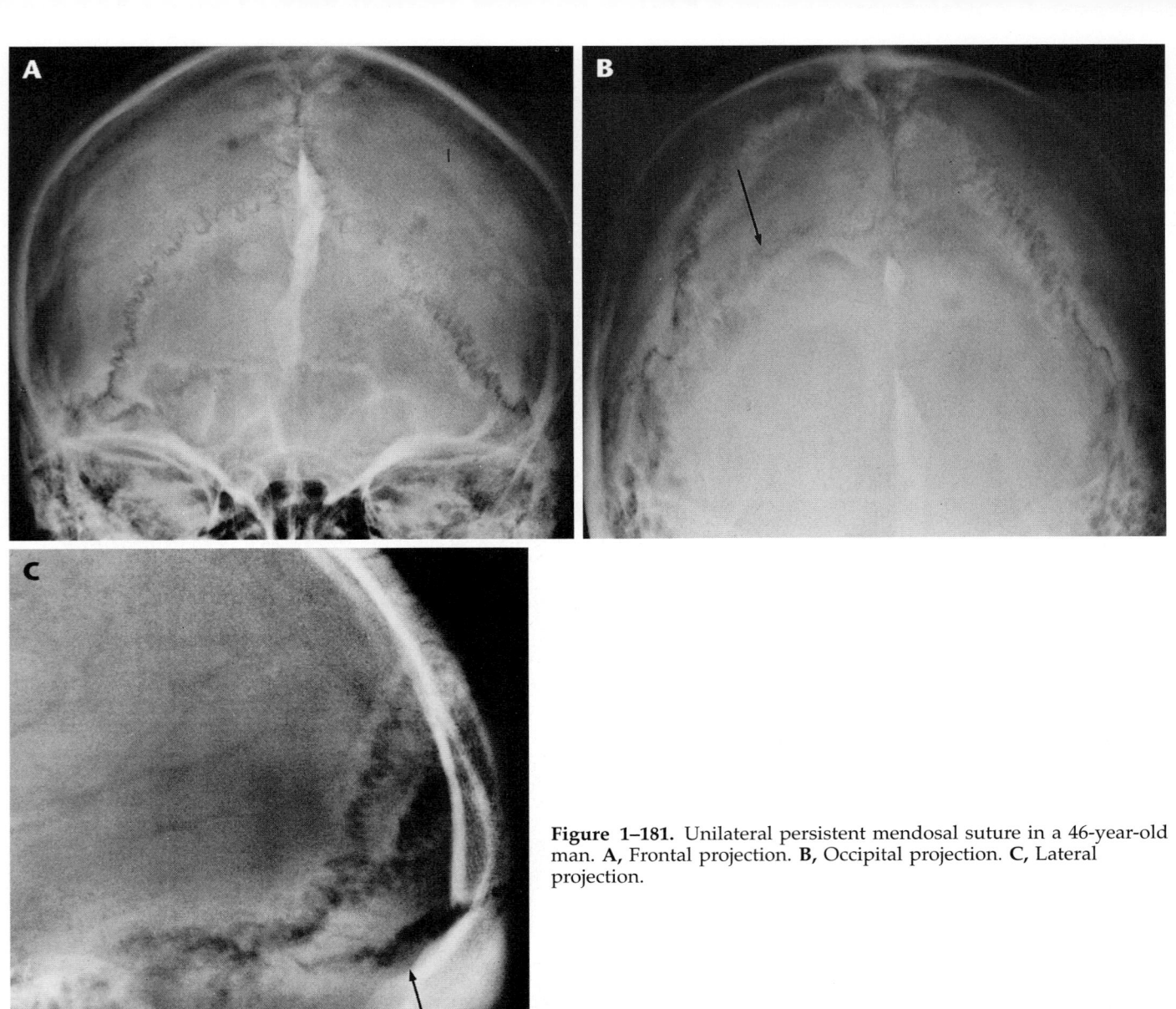

Figure 1–181. Unilateral persistent mendosal suture in a 46-year-old man. **A,** Frontal projection. **B,** Occipital projection. **C,** Lateral projection.

Figure 1–182. PA and AP projections showing an anomalous occipital suture, probably a remnant of the mendosal suture.

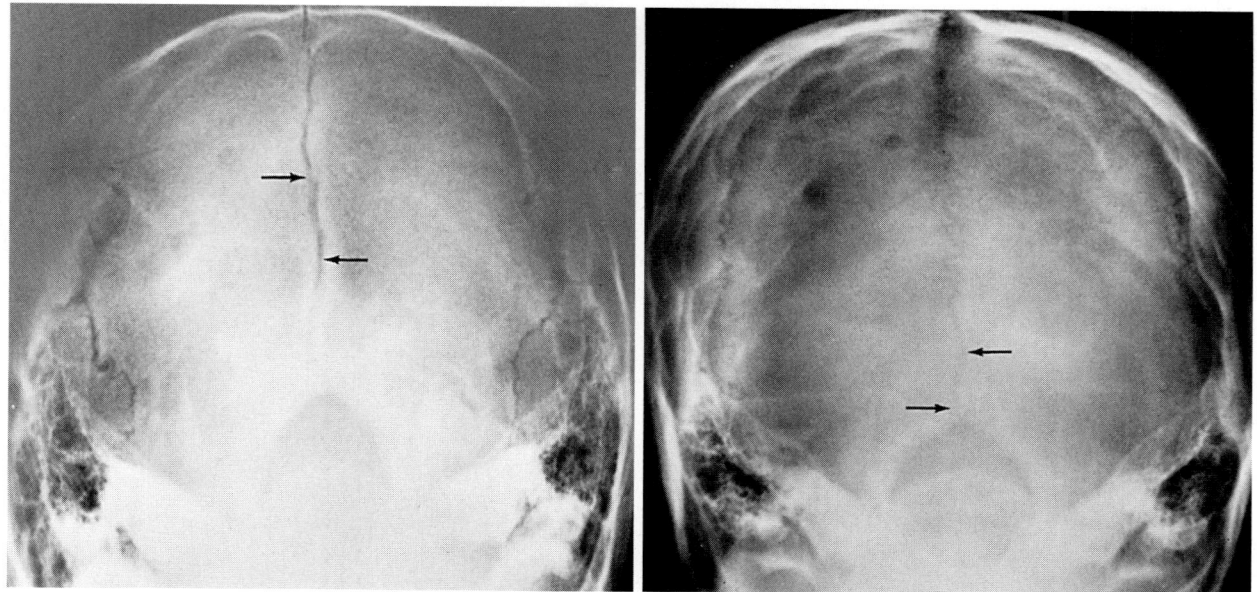

Figure 1–183. Anomalous midline occipital suture (cerebellar synchondrosis). This is also a common site of fractures in small children, and so the diagnosis of an anomalous suture should be made with caution. *Left,* Adult with sutural sclerosis evident. *Right,* Child with no history of trauma. (Ref: Franken EA Jr: The midline occipital fissure: Diagnosis of fracture versus anatomic variant. *Radiology* 93:1043, 1969.)

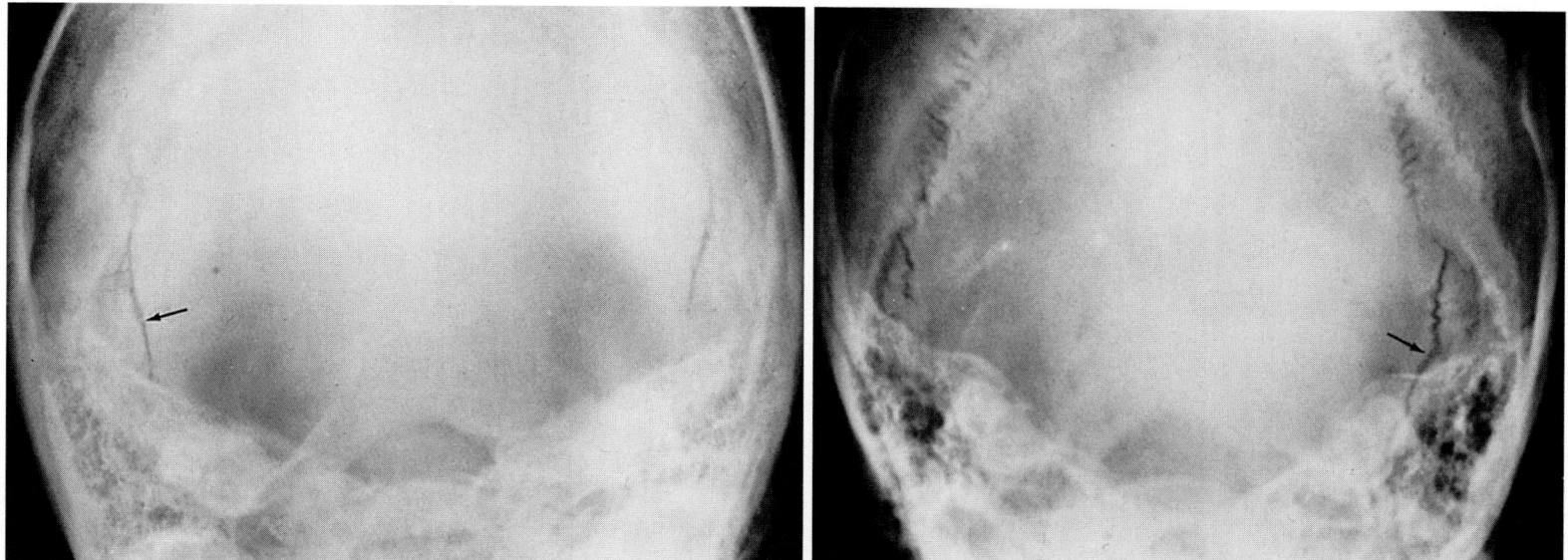

Figure 1–184. Two examples of asymmetric prominence of one occipitomastoid suture, suggesting fracture.

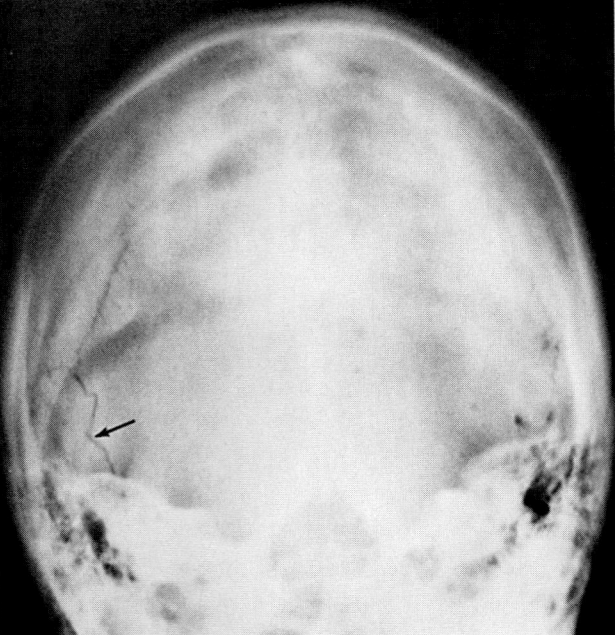

Figure 1–185. Striking example of asymmetric prominence of one occipitomastoid suture, suggesting fracture, accentuated by slight rotation.

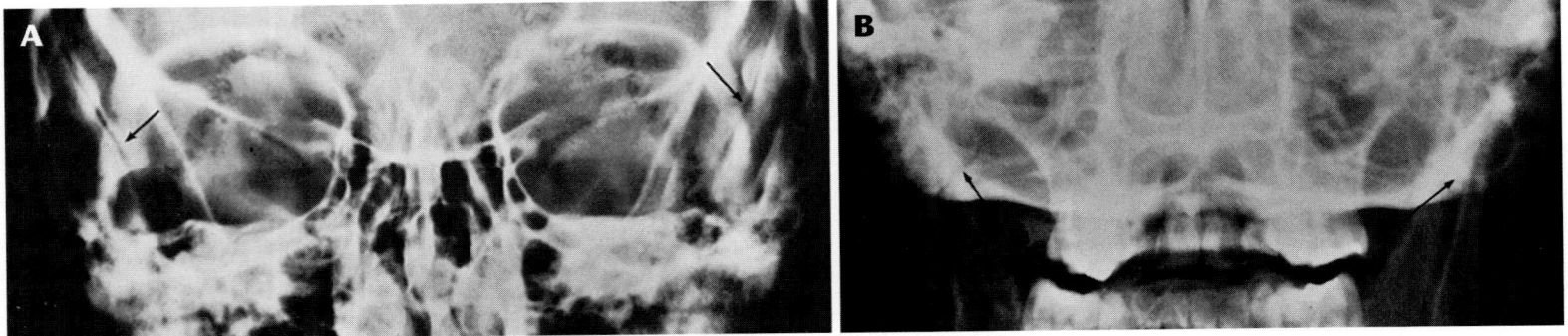

Figure 1–186. Occipitomastoid sutures in frontal projections.

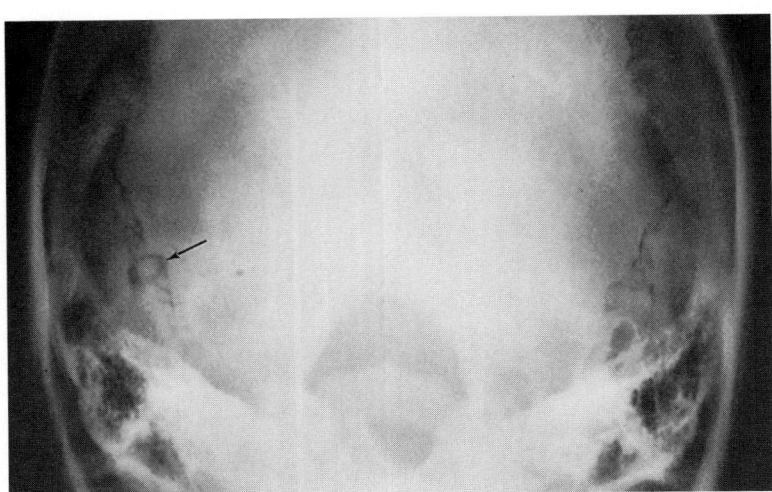

Figure 1–187. Sutural bone in the occipitomastoid suture.

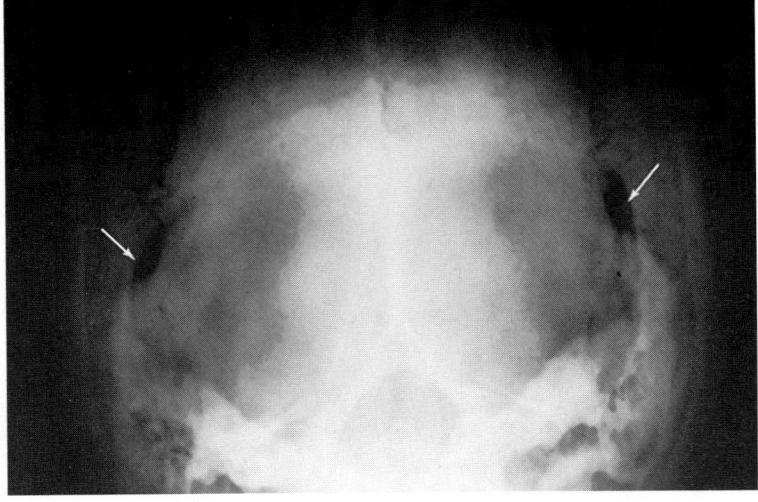

Figure 1–188. Defects in the lambdoid suture, presumably representing persistent mastoid fontanels. The patient did not have neurofibromatosis.

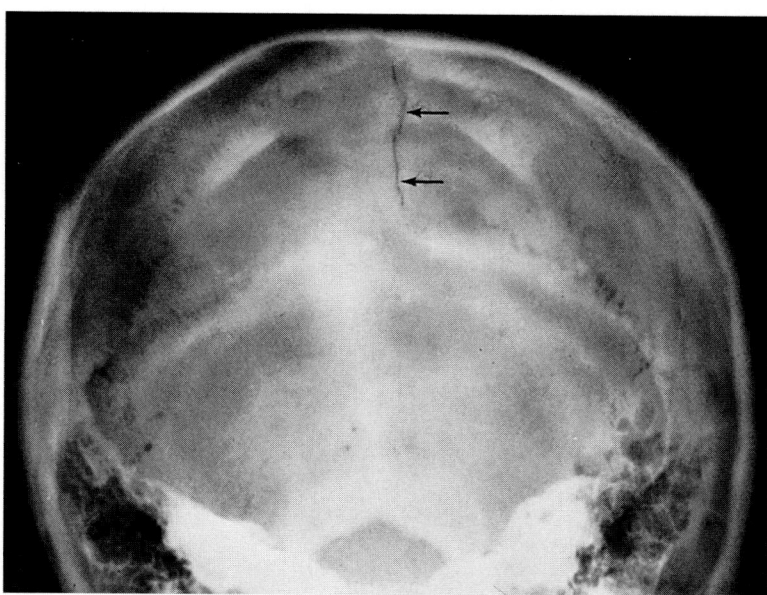

Figure 1–189. A portion of the sagittal suture seen through the occipital bone, simulating a fracture.

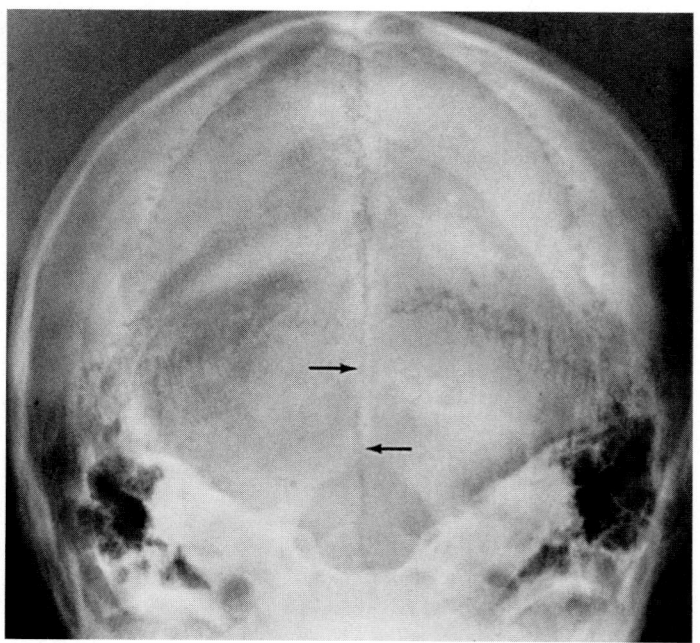

Figure 1–190. The metopic suture may be seen in Towne's projection and confused with a fracture. Note its continuation across the outline of the foramen magnum.

Figure 1–191. Metopic suture, simulating occipital fracture in a 22-month-old child. Note the lack of sutural serrations.

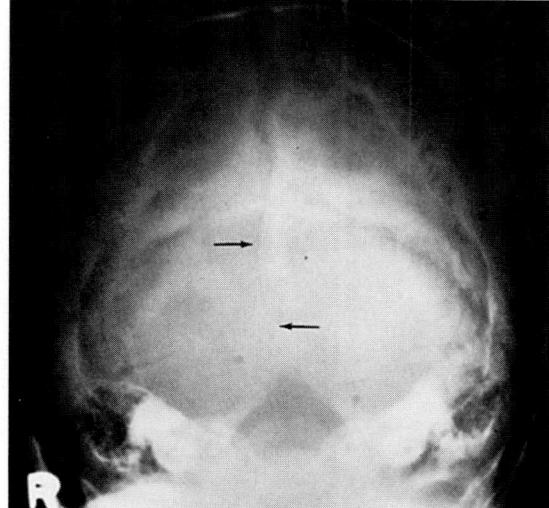

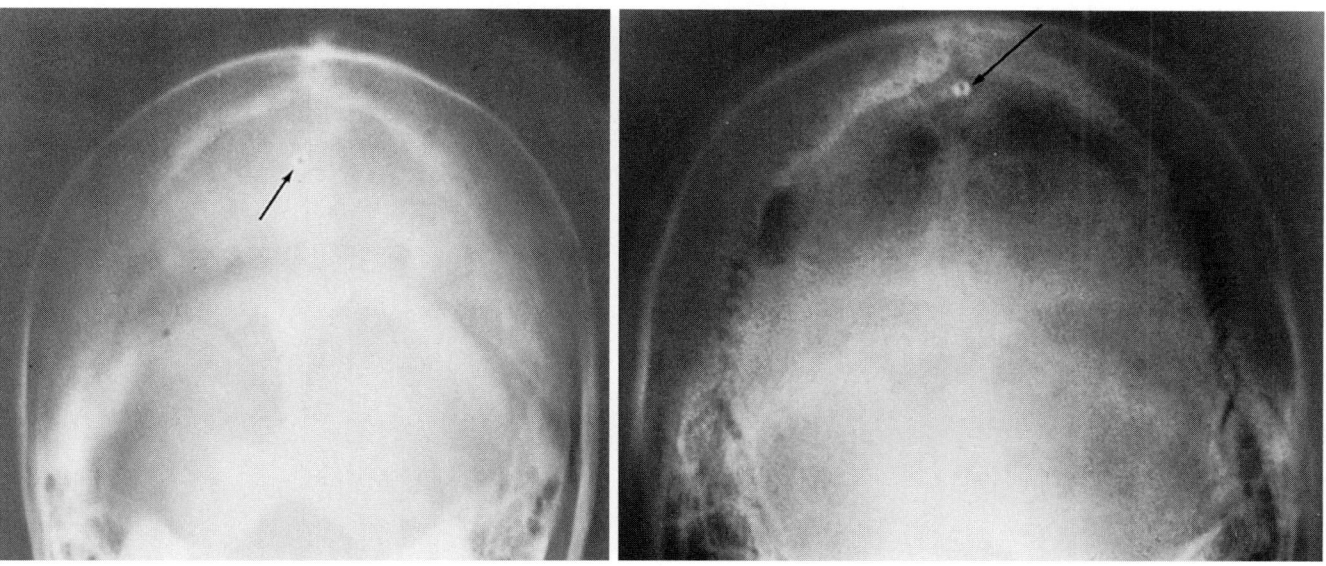

Figure 1–192. Examples of occipital emissary channels.

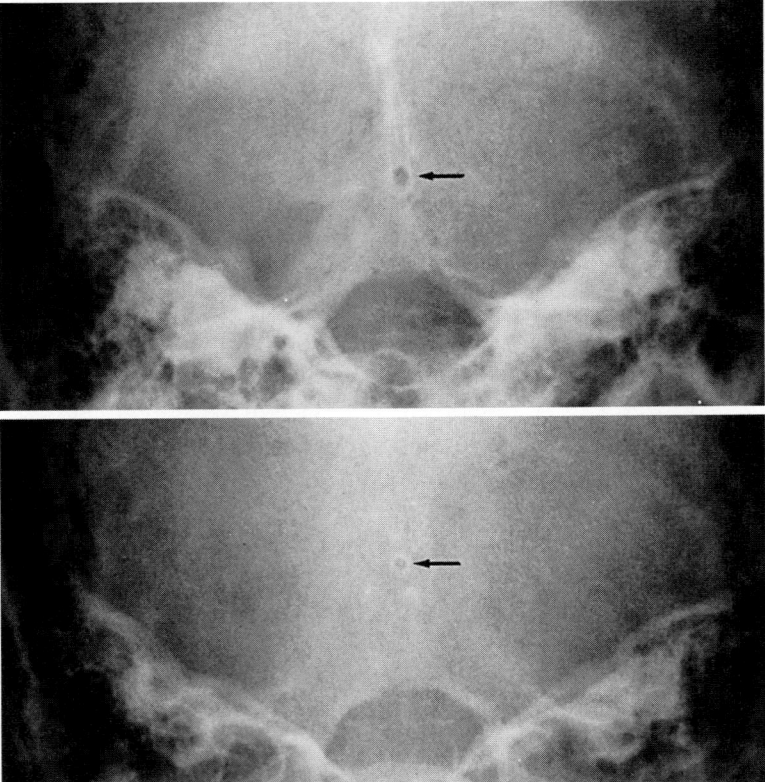

Figure 1–193. Two examples of the foramen for the occipital emissary vein, the inioendineal canal. This is a midline structure in contrast to the venous lakes, which are seen on both sides of the midline. (Ref: O'Rahilly R: Anomalous occipital apertures. *Arch Pathol* 53:509, 1952.)

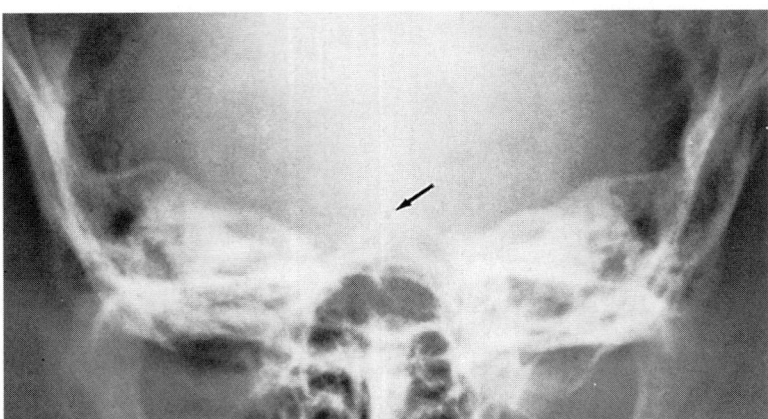

Figure 1–194. An unusual occipital emissary vein immediately above the foramen magnum.

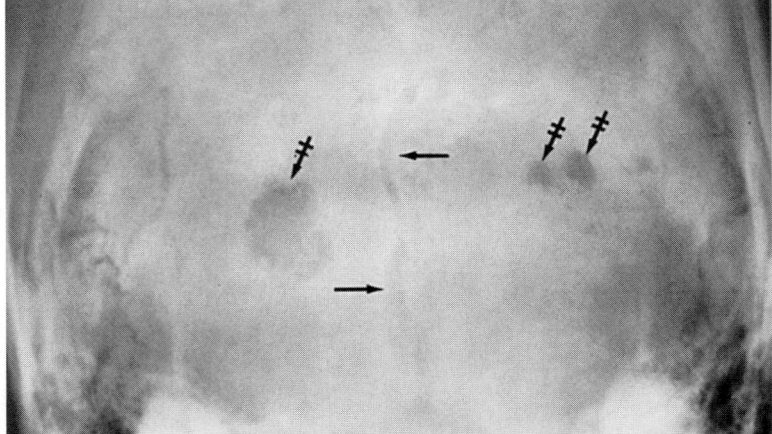

Figure 1–195. Midline vascular channel (←). Occipital venous lakes are also present (⇇).

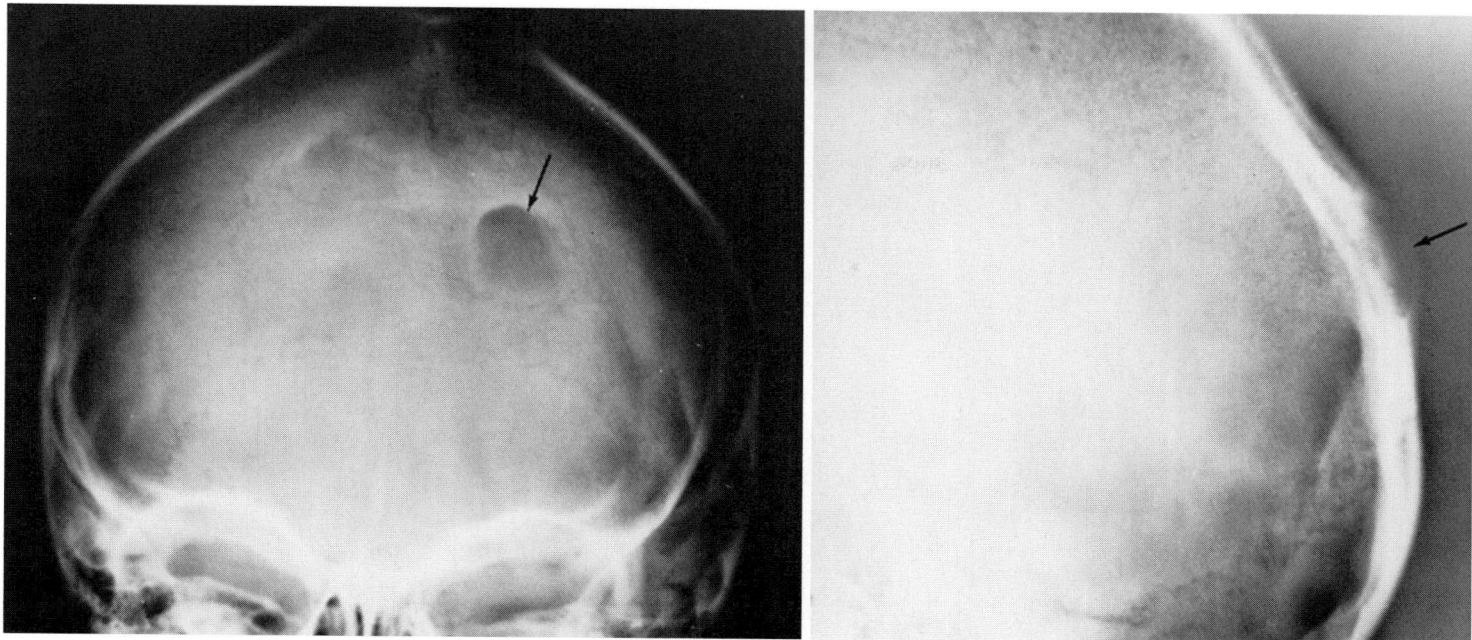

Figure 1–196. Occipital pacchionian impression.

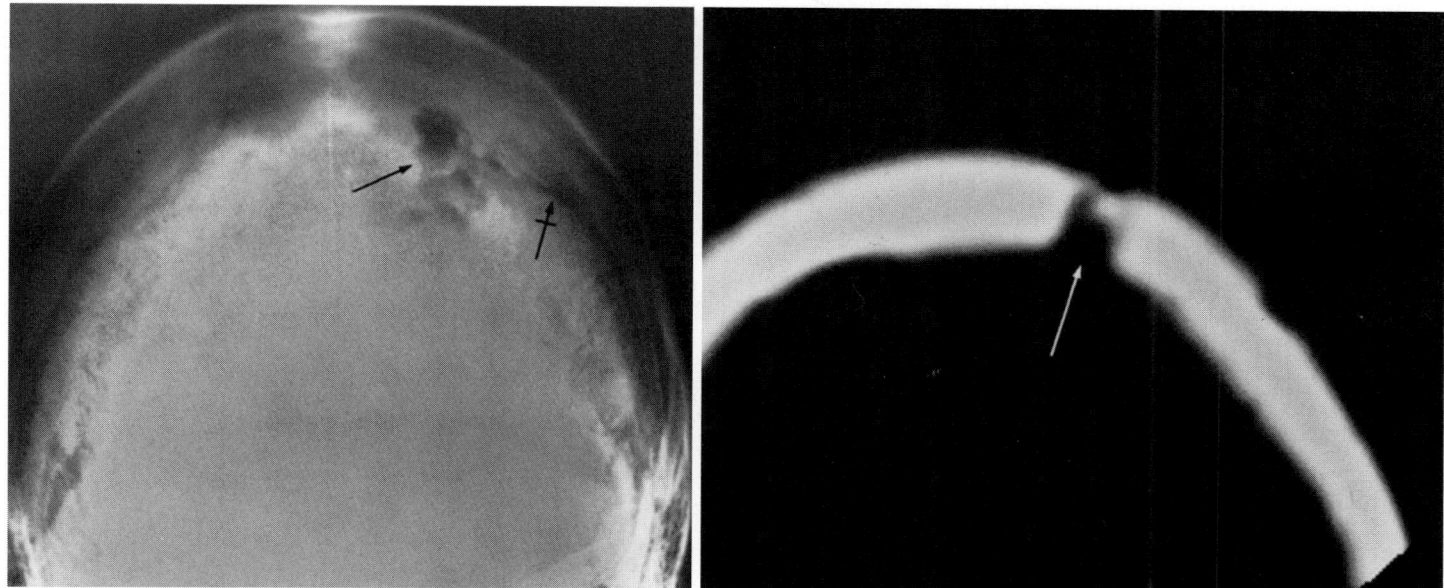

Figure 1–197. *Left,* Occipital pacchionian impression (←). Note the draining vein (↞). *Right,* CT confirmation. (Ref: Skully RD, Mark EJ, McNeely BV: Case 42-1984: Pacchionian granulation. *N Engl J Med* 322:1036, 1984.)

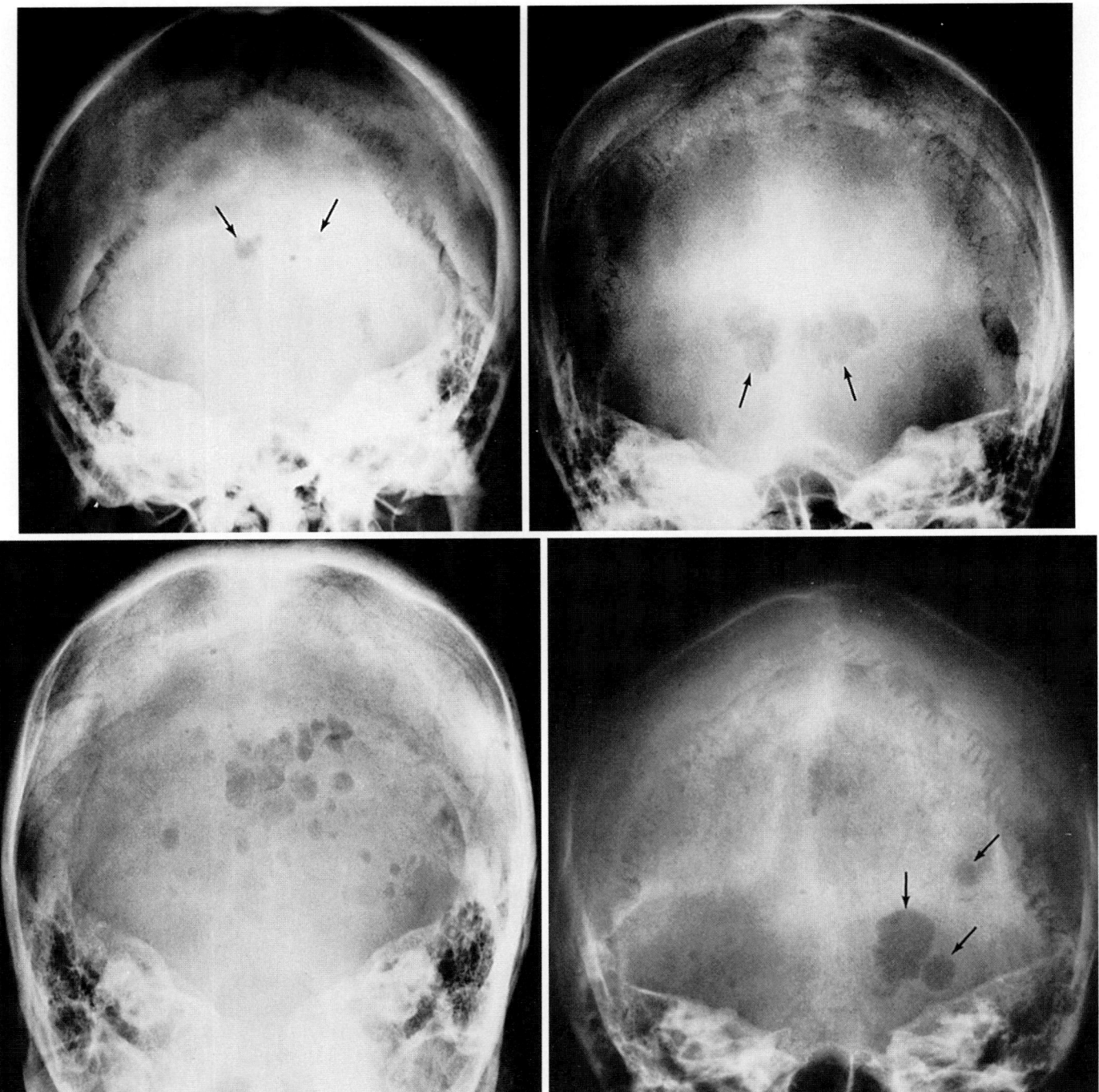

Figure 1–198. Occipital venous lakes. These structures vary widely in number and appearance. They are usually seen near the midline of the occipital bone, most commonly in older individuals. These lakes lie in the diploic space and are of no clinical significance. (From Keats TE: Four normal anatomic variations of importance to radiologists. *Am J Roentgenol* 78:89, 1957.) There is evidence that identical occipital radiolucencies may be the product of ectopic neural tissue. These are without clinical significance. (Ref: Goldring S et al: Ectopic neural tissue of the occipital bone. *J Neurosurg* 21:479, 1964.)

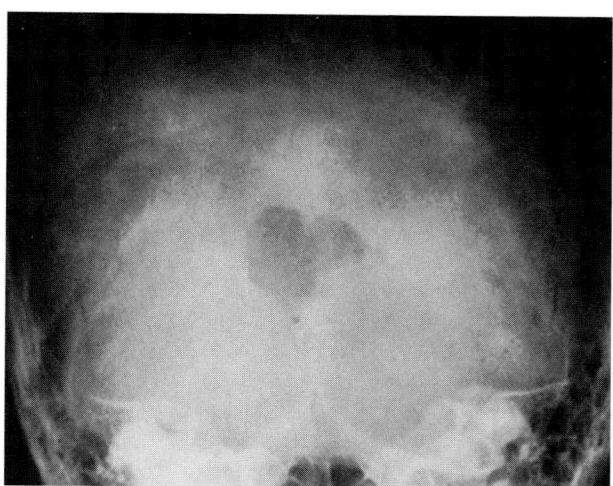

Figure 1–199. Large midline occipital venous lake.

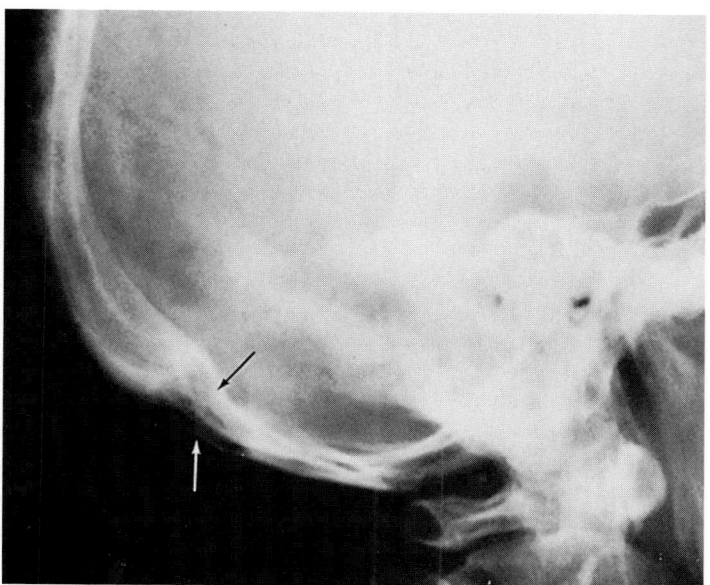

Figure 1–200. Venous lakes may often be seen in the diploic space in the lateral projection.

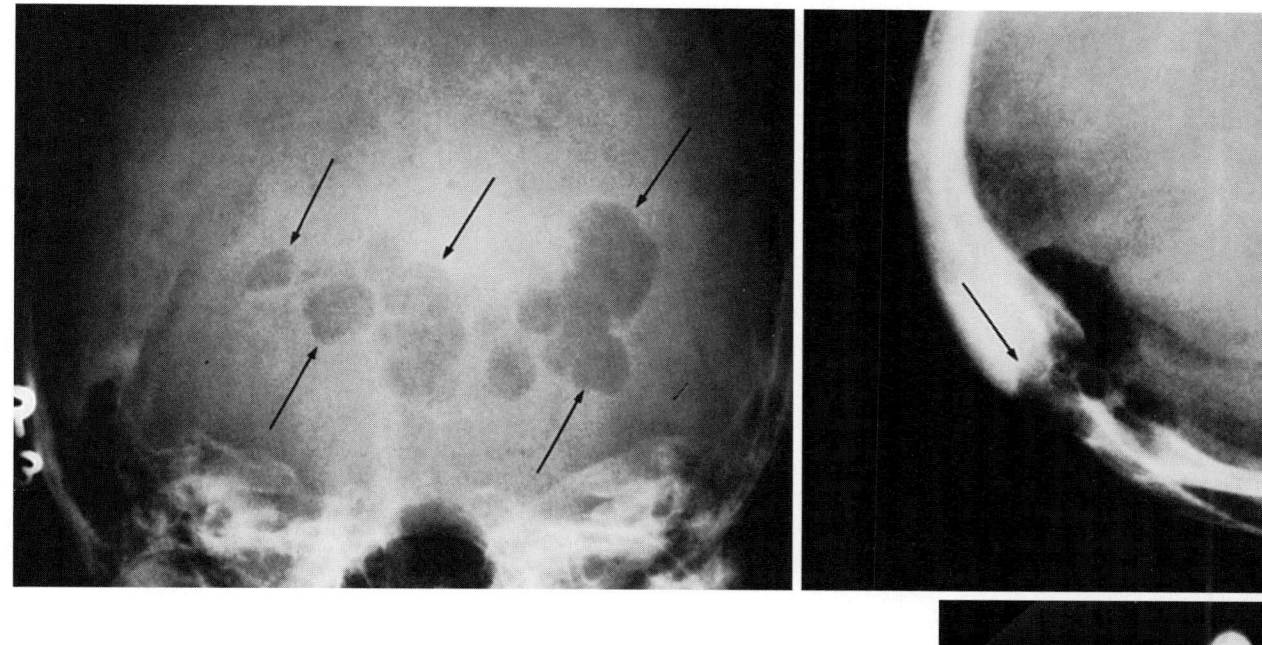

Figure 1–201. Similar occipital radiolucencies with CT demonstration.

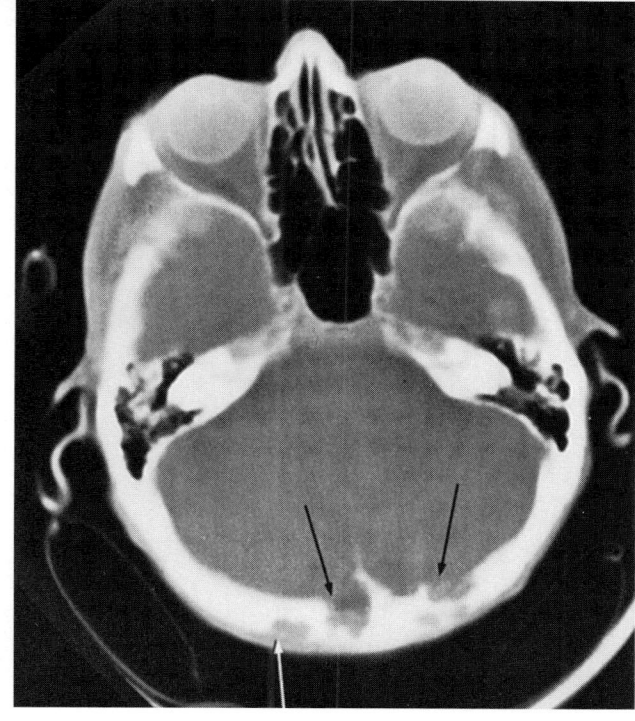

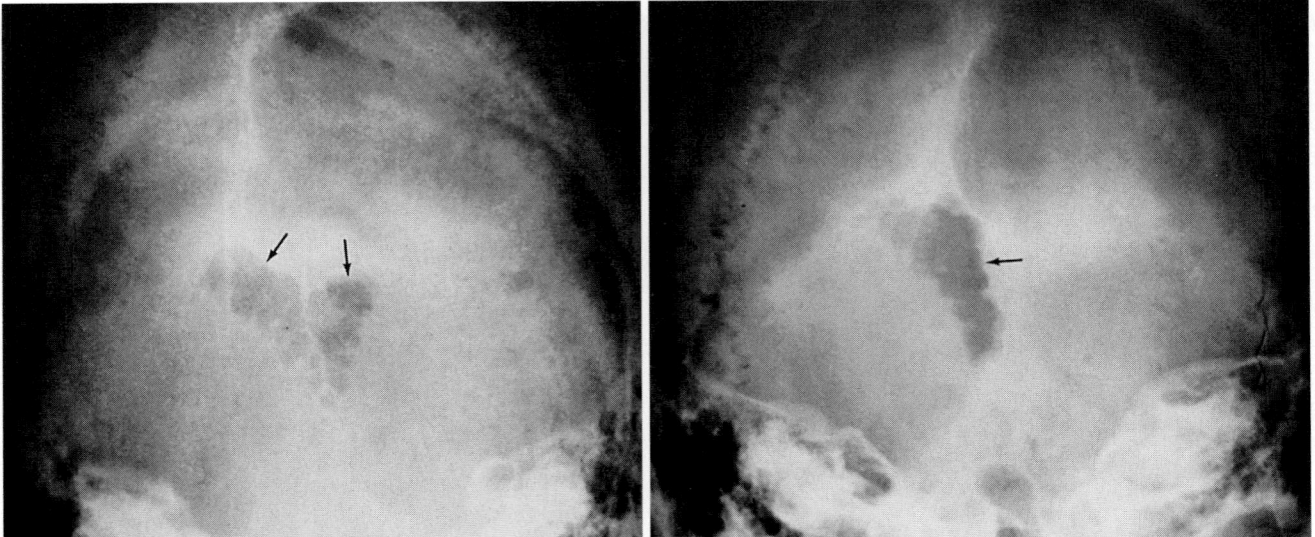

Figure 1–202. Other variations of occipital venous lakes.

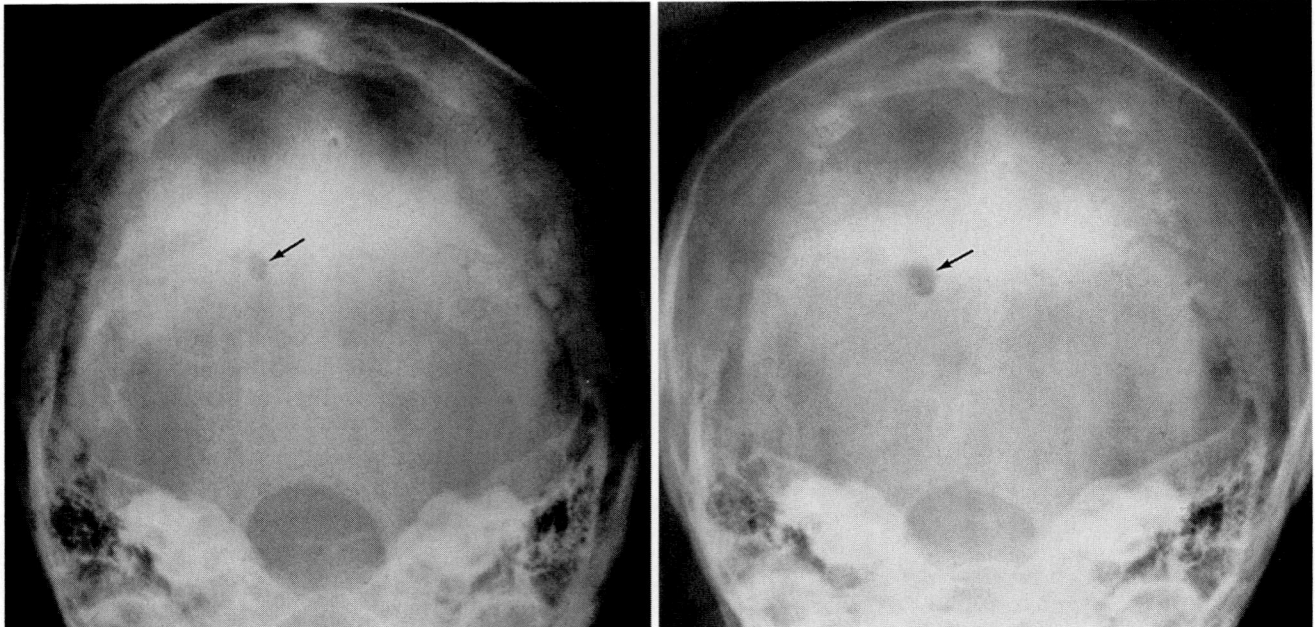

Figure 1–203. Development of occipital venous lake. The film on the right was exposed 16 years after the film on the left.

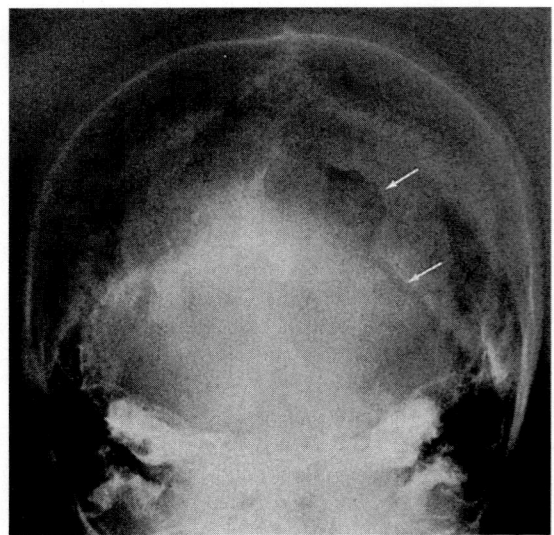

Figure 1–204. Occipital venous lake with a prominent draining venous channel.

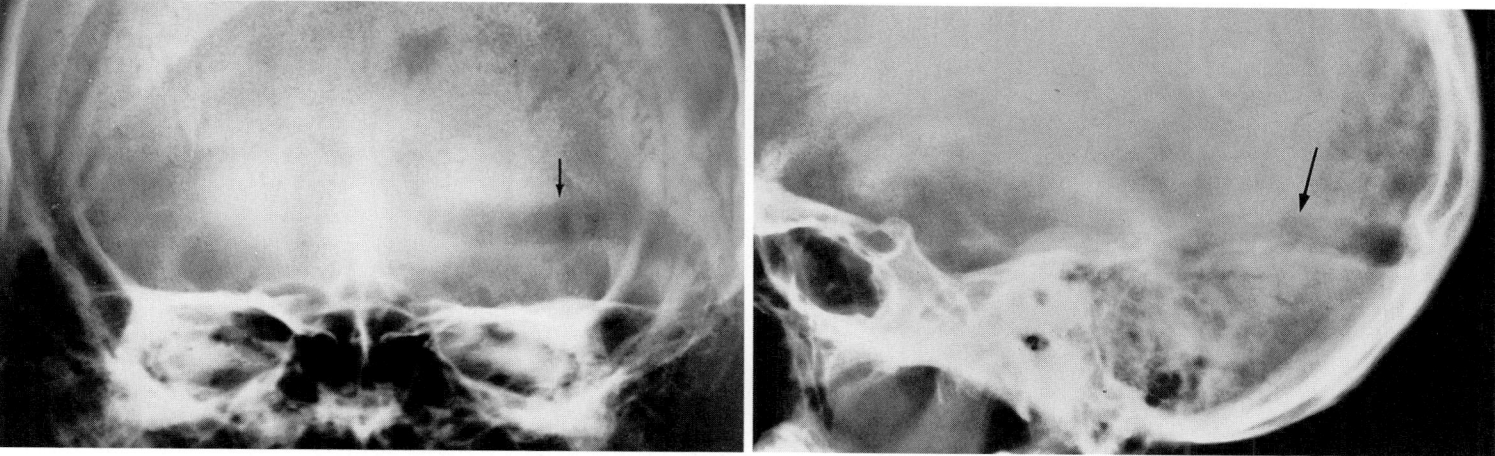

Figure 1–205. Normal unilateral prominence of the groove for the transverse venous sinus.

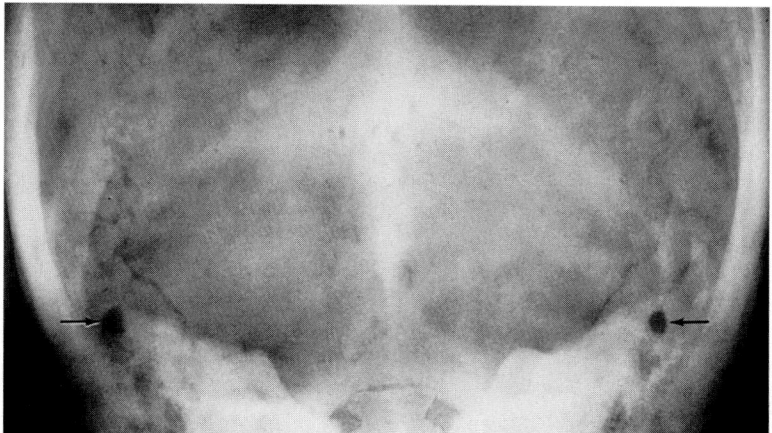

Figure 1–206. The transverse sinuses seen on end, evidenced as lucencies in the mastoids.

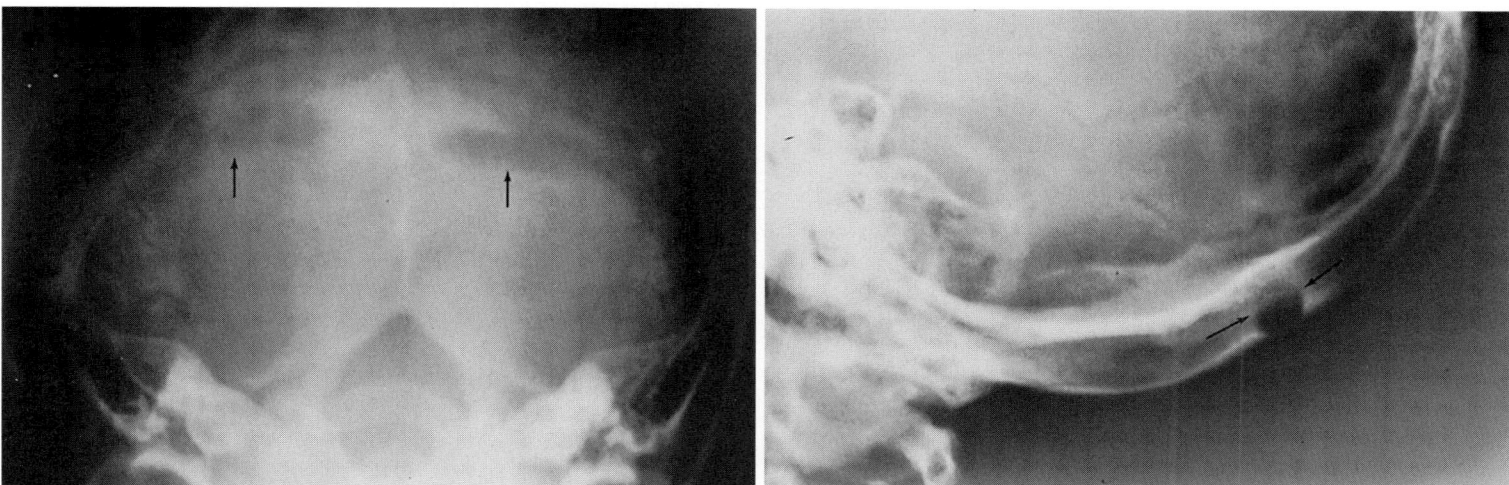

Figure 1–207. Prominent transverse venous sinuses, producing striking radiolucency in the lateral projection.

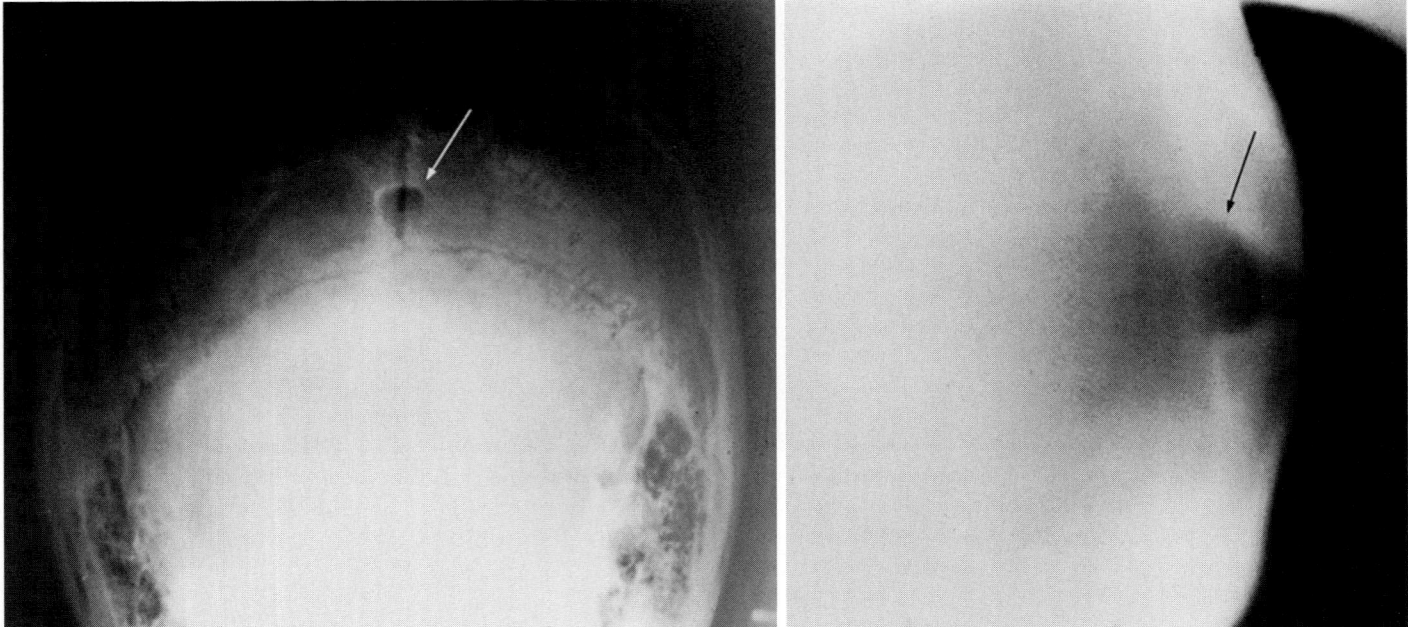

Figure 1–208. Occipital midline radiolucency, probably representing a closure defect. There were no associated clinical findings.

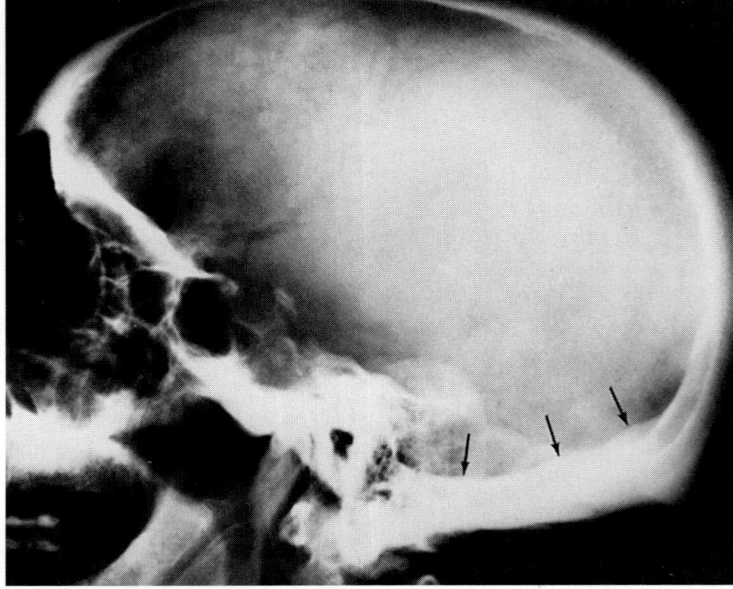

Figure 1–209. Localized thickening of the occipital bone, a normal variant.

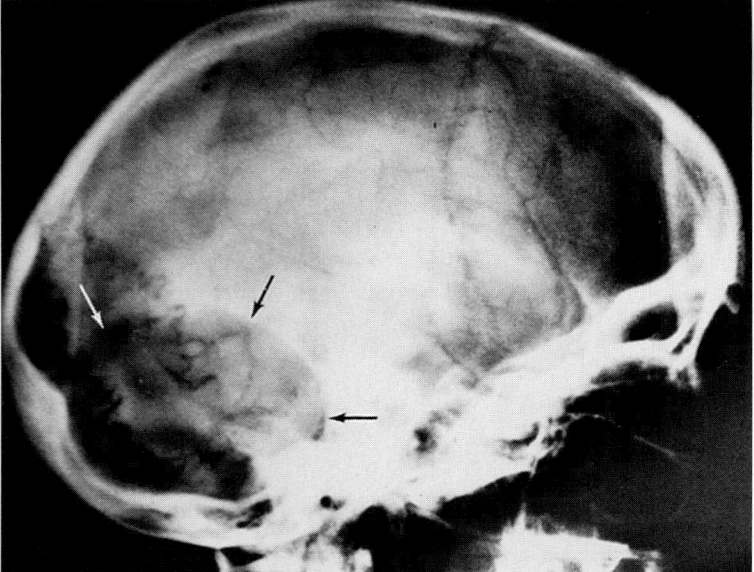

Figure 1–210. Striking appearance of the occipital region produced by venous sinuses and normal lucency of the occipital bones.

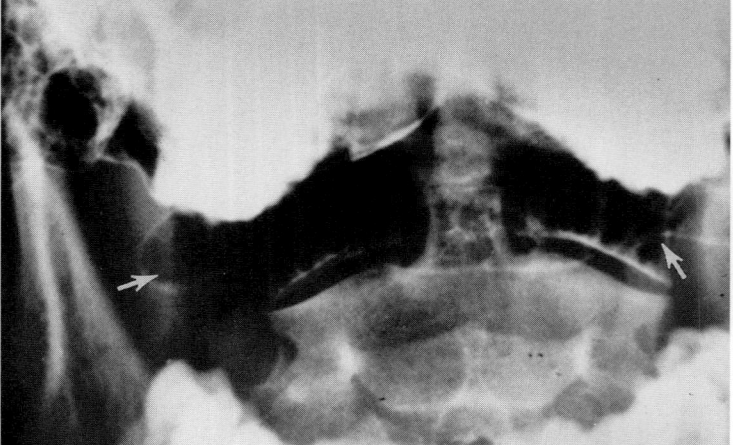

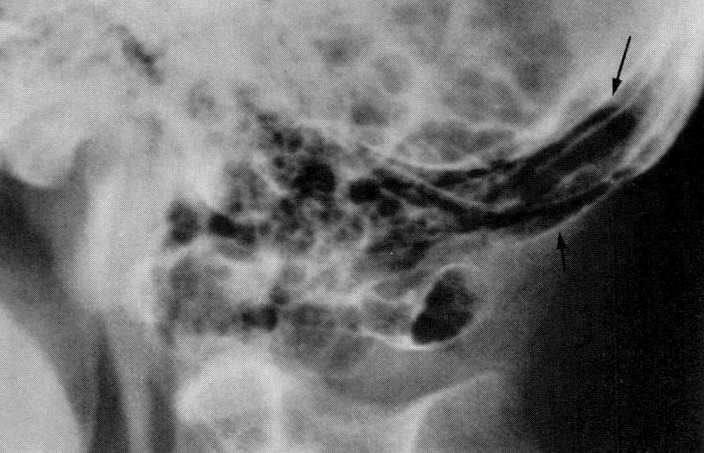

Figure 1–211. Pneumatization of the occipital bone as an extension from the mastoids.

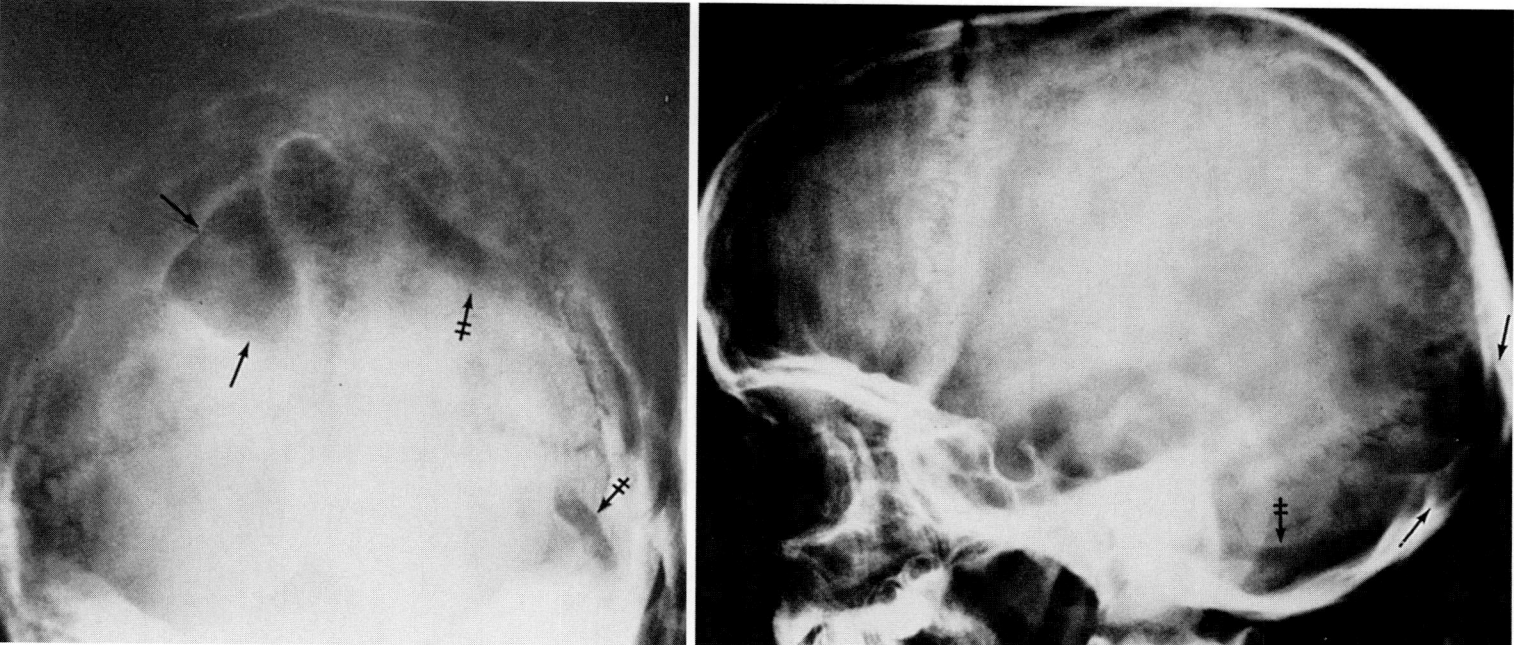

Figure 1–212. The occipital bone may have a variety of symmetric and asymmetric areas of thinning near the midline, which may simulate erosion of the inner table. Some of them relate to the configuration of the transverse venous sinuses. It is important that the innocence of these variants be recognized. The crossed arrows (⇥) indicate the venous sinuses.

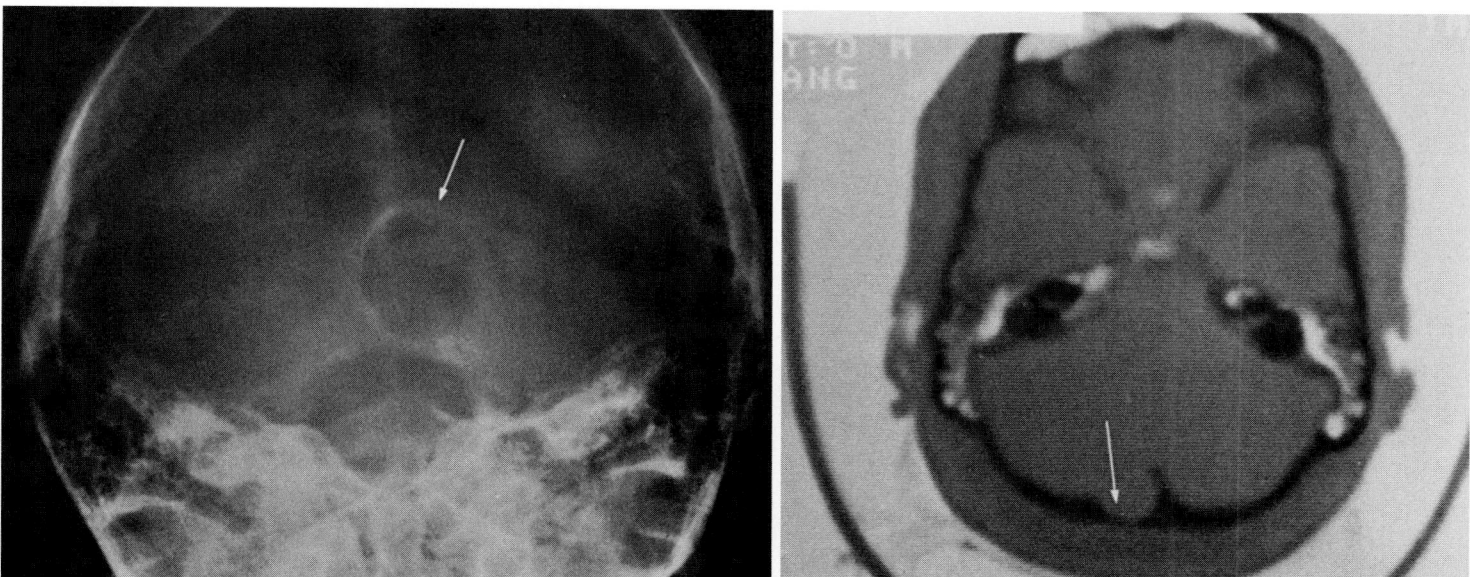

Figure 1–213. Developmental thinning of the occipital bone **(A)** proved by CT. The defect contains normal brain tissue **(B)**. (From Haden MA, Keats TE: The anatomic basis for localized occipital thinning: A normal anatomic variant. *Skeletal Radiol* 8:221, 1982.)

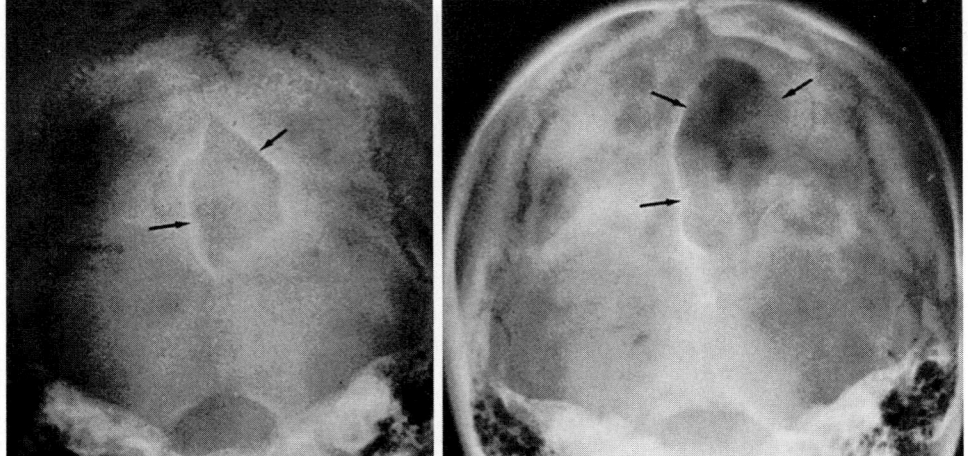

Figure 1–214. Additional examples of occipital thinning. Note similarity to changes of erosion of inner table.

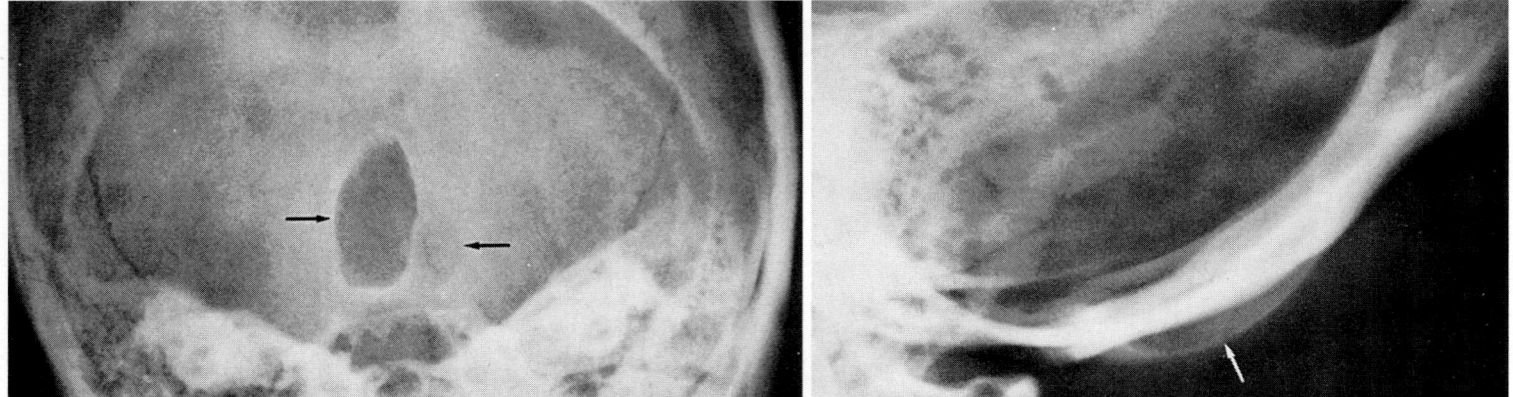

Figure 1–215. Asymmetric occipital thinning below the torcula in a 28-year-old woman.

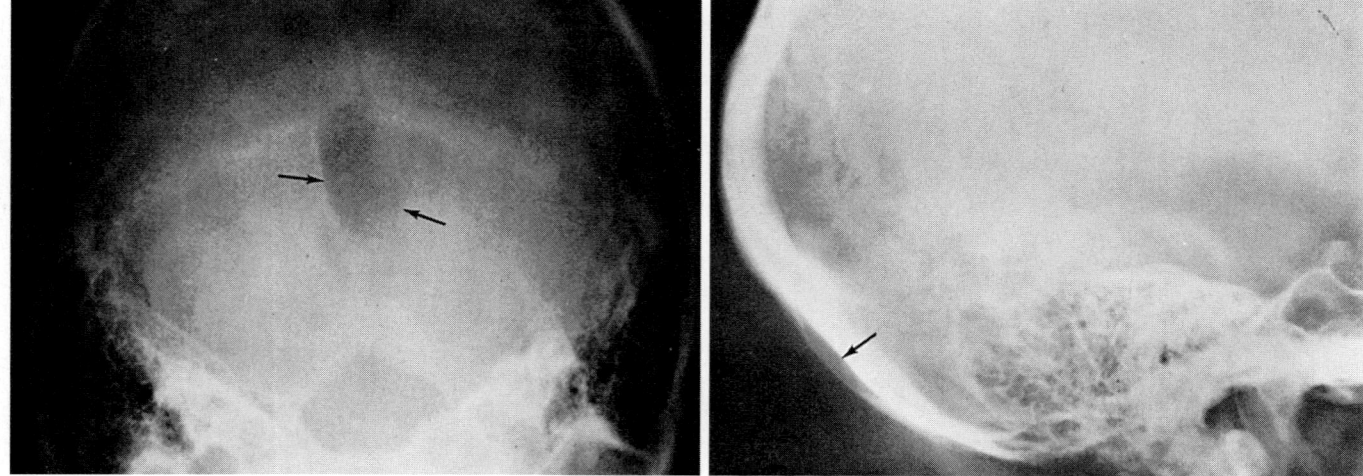

Figure 1–216. Occipital thinning near the midline.

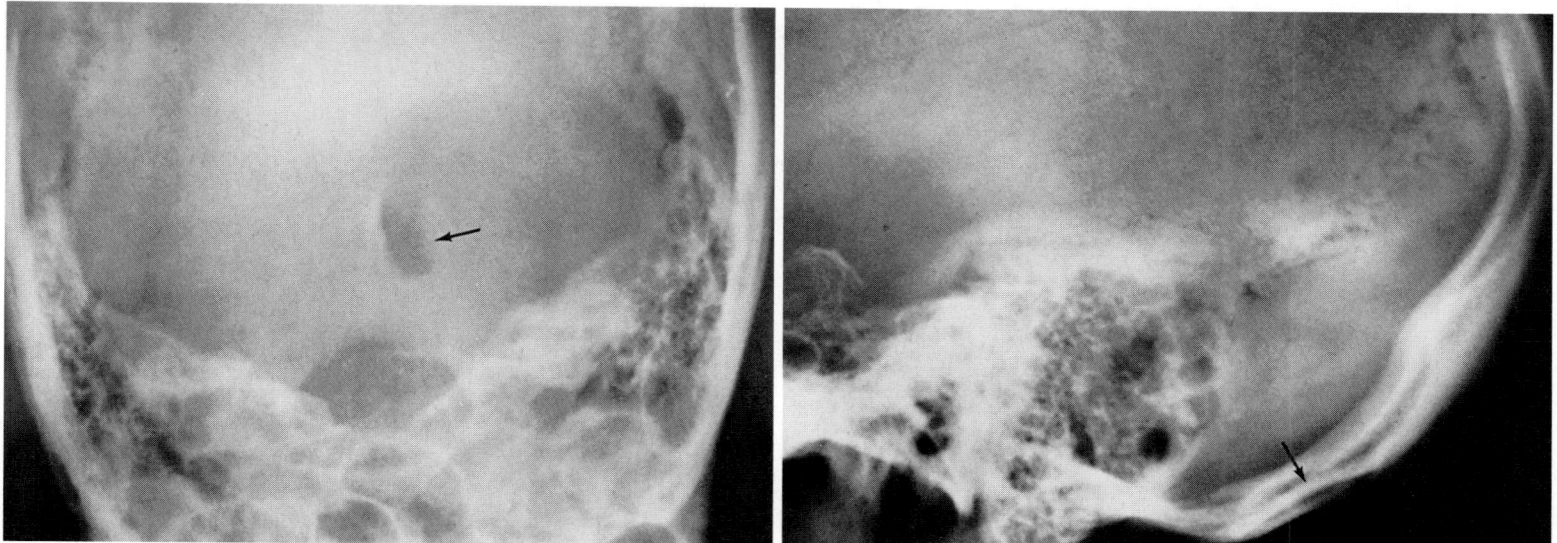

Figure 1–217. Small discrete area of occipital thinning.

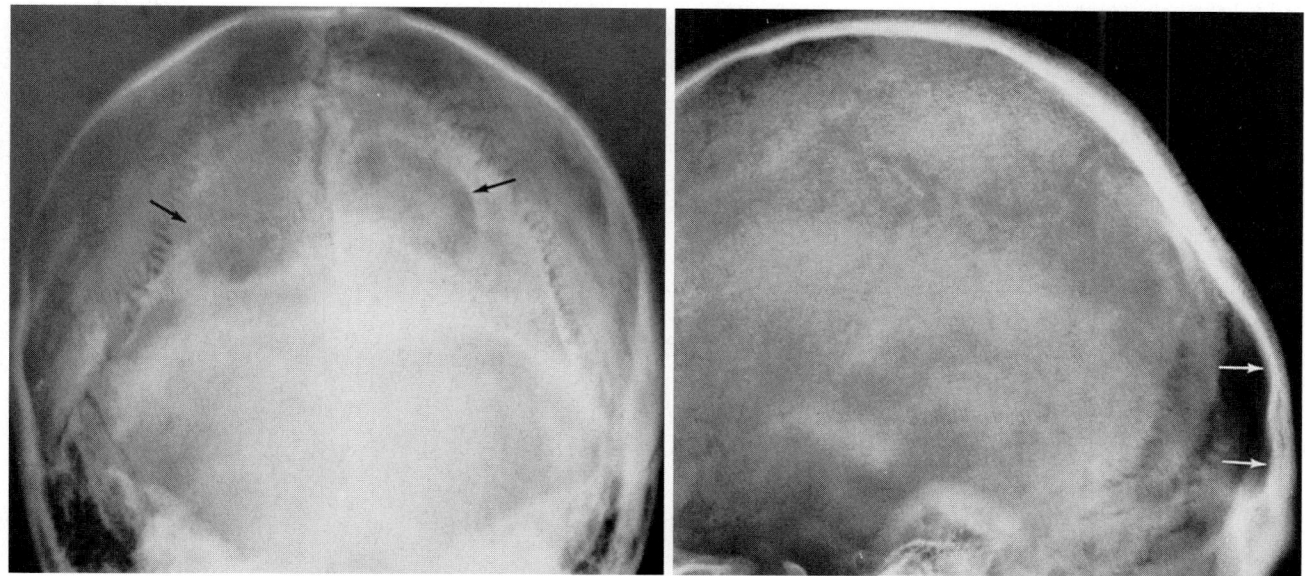

Figure 1–218. Symmetric occipital thinning above the torcula in a 26-year-old woman. It has been suggested that the lucencies in this location may coincide with the occipital poles, best observed in patients with thin cranial vaults. (Ref: Newton TH, Potts DG: *Radiology of the skull and brain,* vol. 1. St. Louis, Mosby, 1971.)

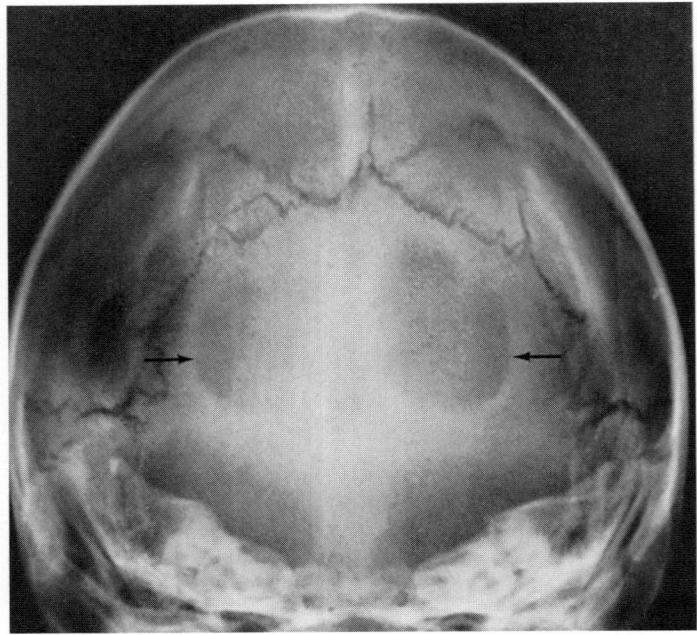

Figure 1–219. Symmetric areas of occipital thinning, simulating a pneumoencephalogram.

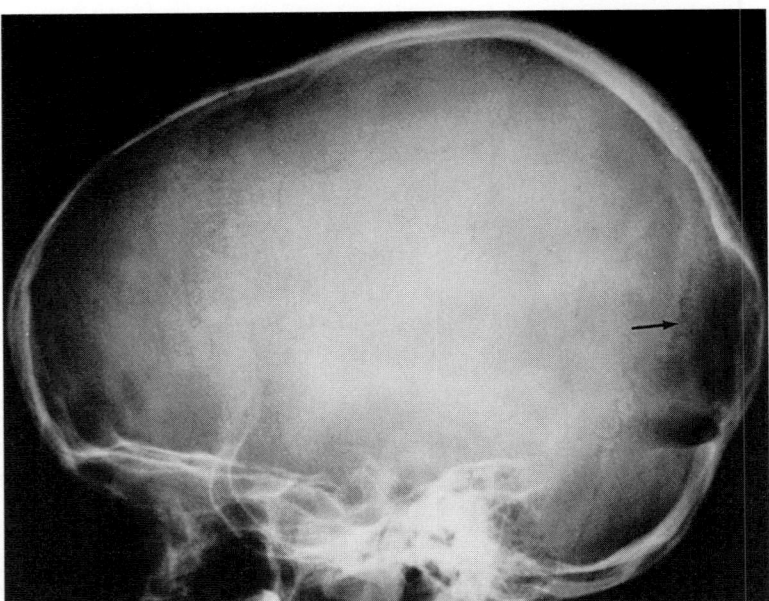

Figure 1–220. Occipital thinning seen in lateral projection above the transverse sinuses. Note the apparent loss of the inner table of the calvaria.

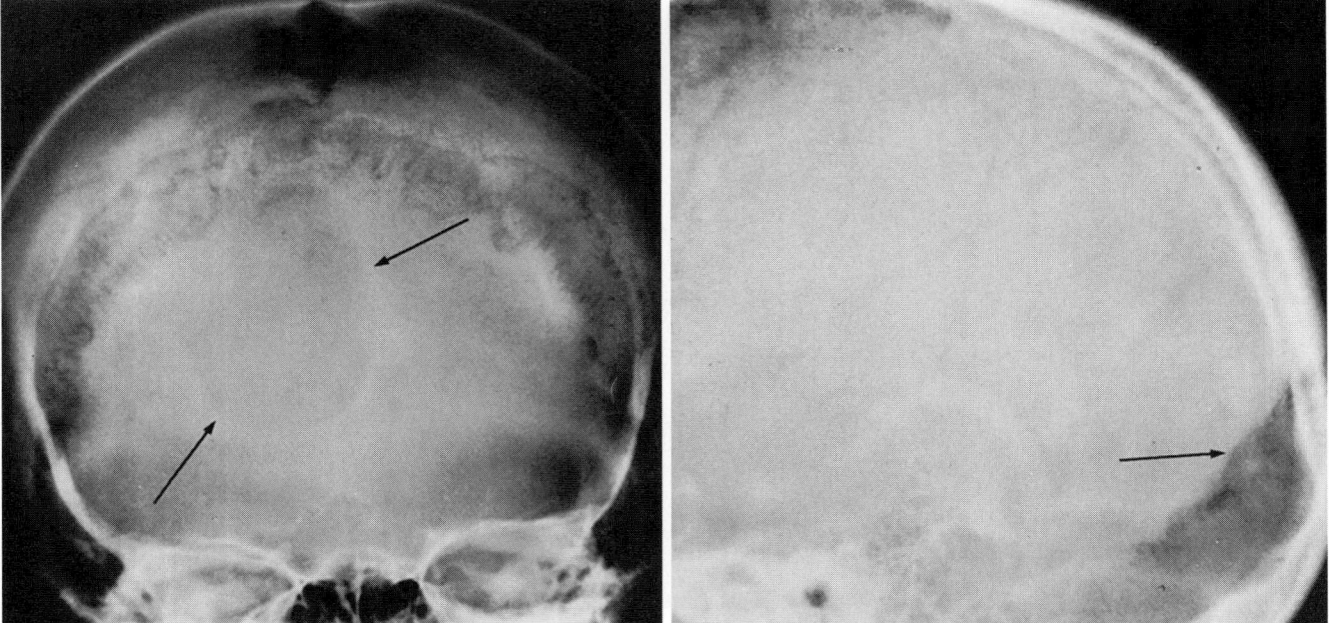

Figure 1–221. Large asymmetric occipital thinning in a 43-year-old woman.

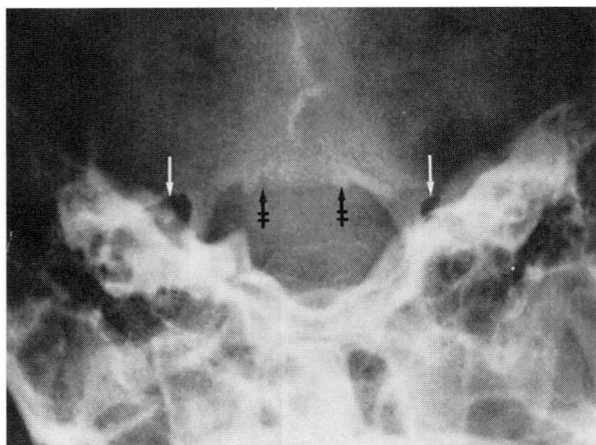

Figure 1–222. Normal asymmetry of the condyloid canals (←). A small ossicle is present in the right canal. Note also the normal irregularity of the posterior margin of the foramen magnum (⇥). (Ref: Gathier JC, Bruyn GW: The so-called condyloid foramen in the half-axial view. *Am J Roentgenol* 107:515, 1969.)

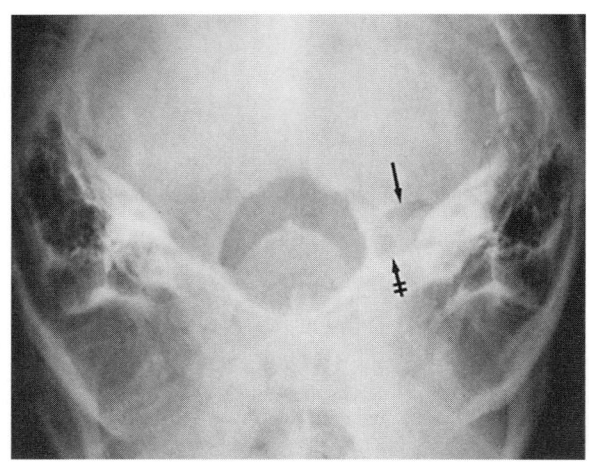

Figure 1–223. Asymmetric condyloid fossae with a large fossa on the patient's left (←). The condyloid canal is seen within the fossa (⇥).

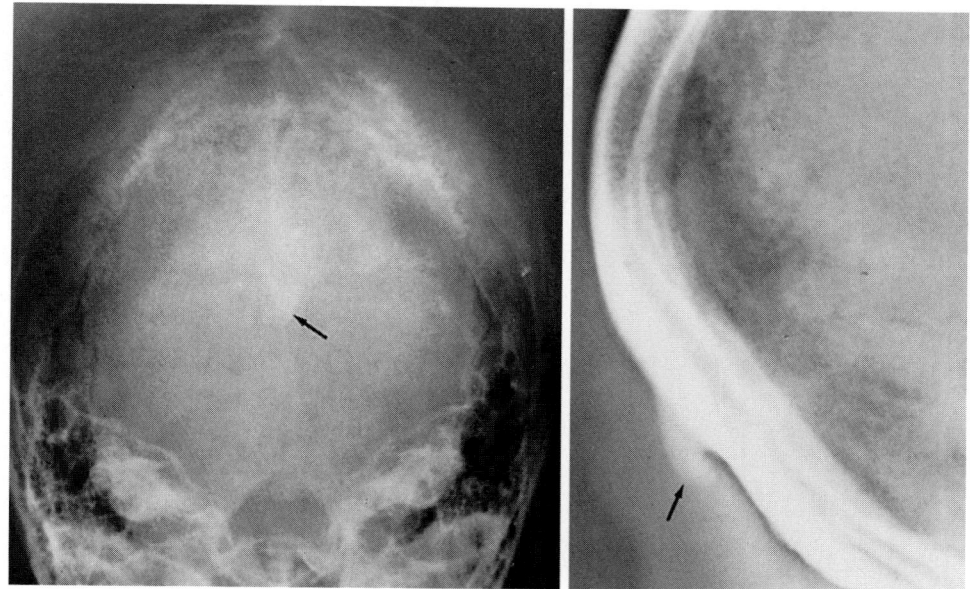

Figure 1–224. Prominent external occipital protuberance producing a midline density in the half-axial projection.

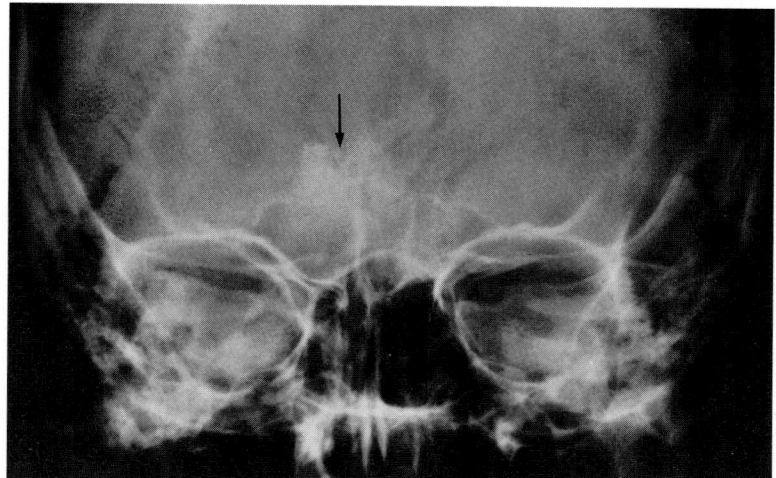

Figure 1–225. The external occipital protuberance producing a vague density superimposed on the frontal sinus.

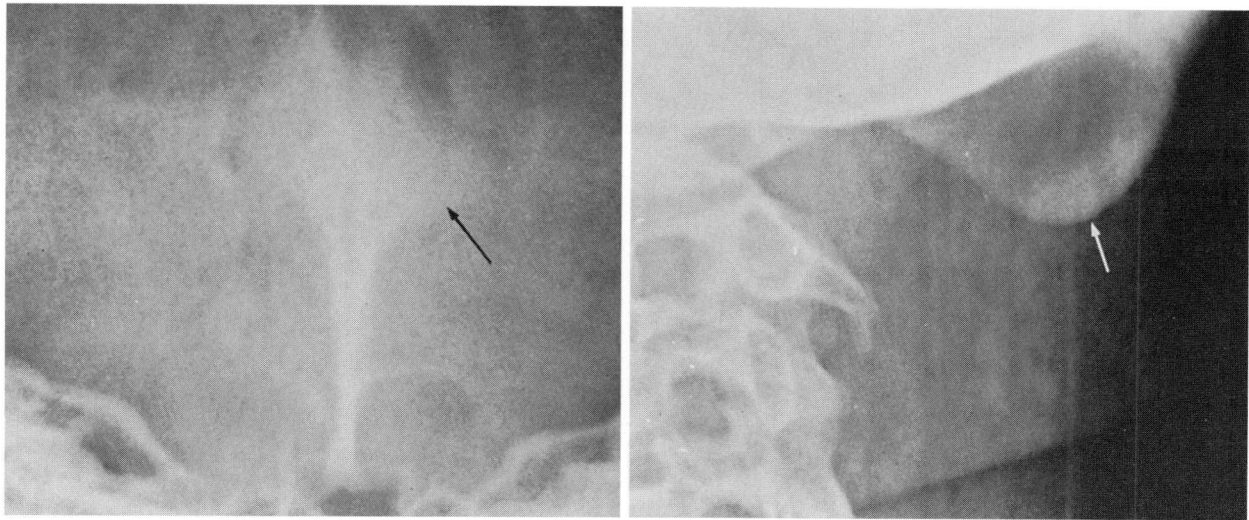

Figure 1–226. Huge external occipital protuberance.

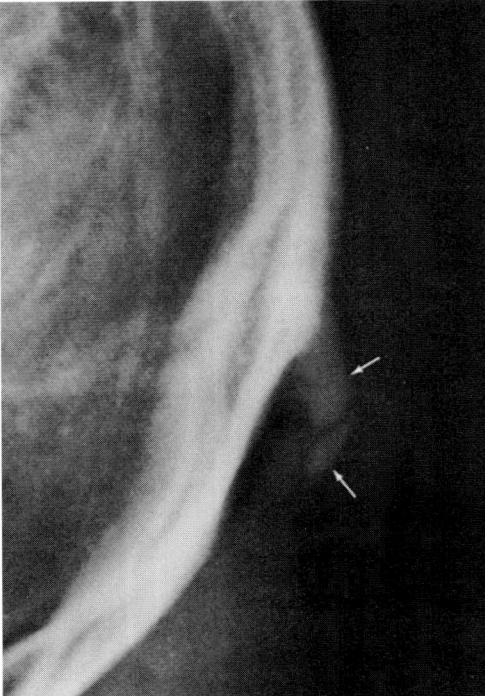

Figure 1–227. Prominent external occipital protuberance with adjacent calcification in the ligamentum nuchae.

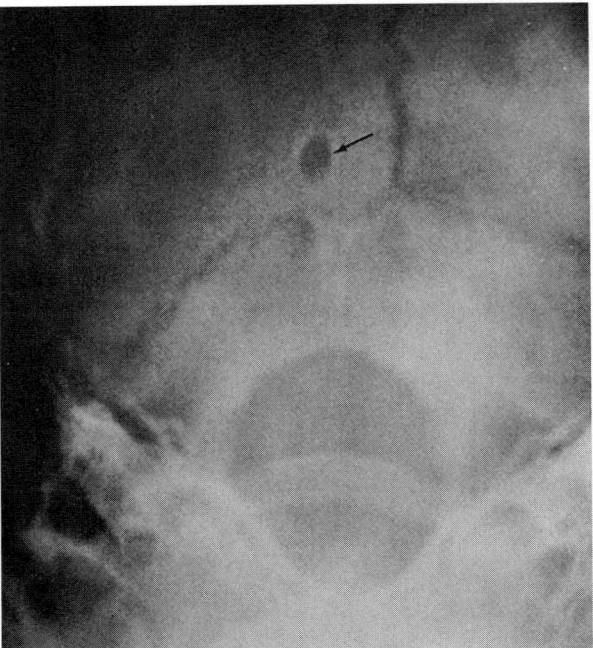

Figure 1–228. Radiolucency produced by the base of the external occipital protuberance.

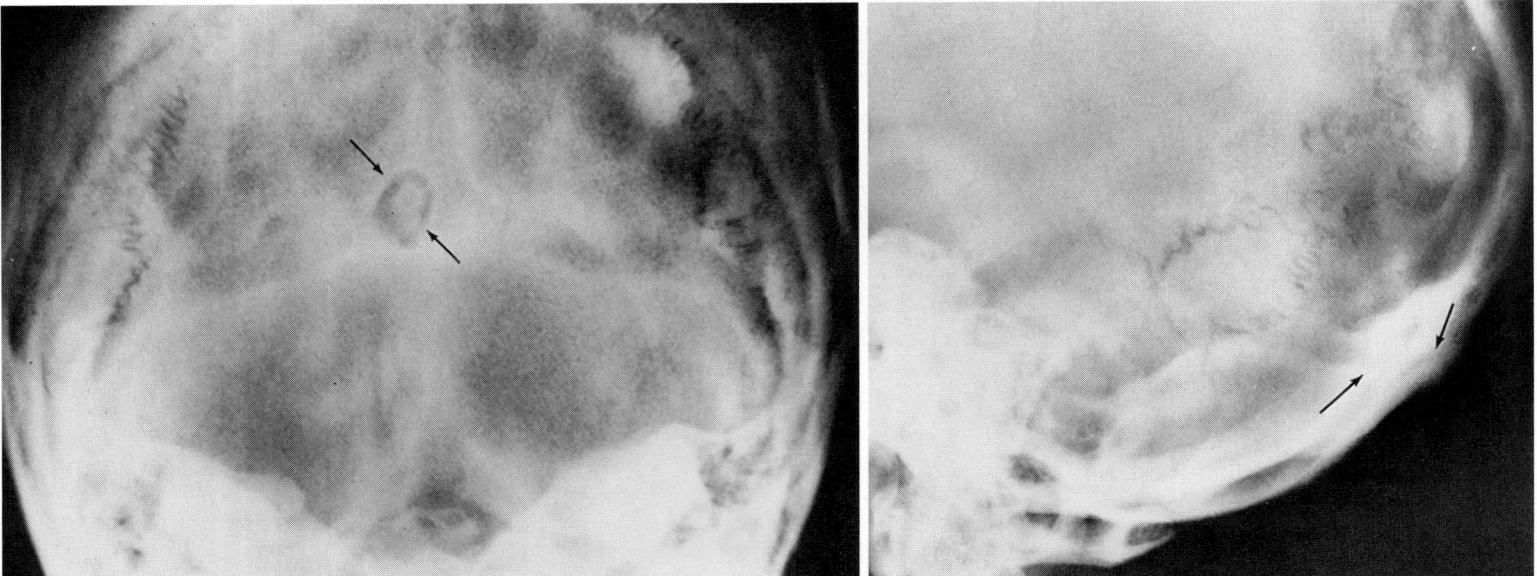

Figure 1–229. Unusual appearance produced by superimposition of external occipital protuberance and confluence of the venous sinuses.

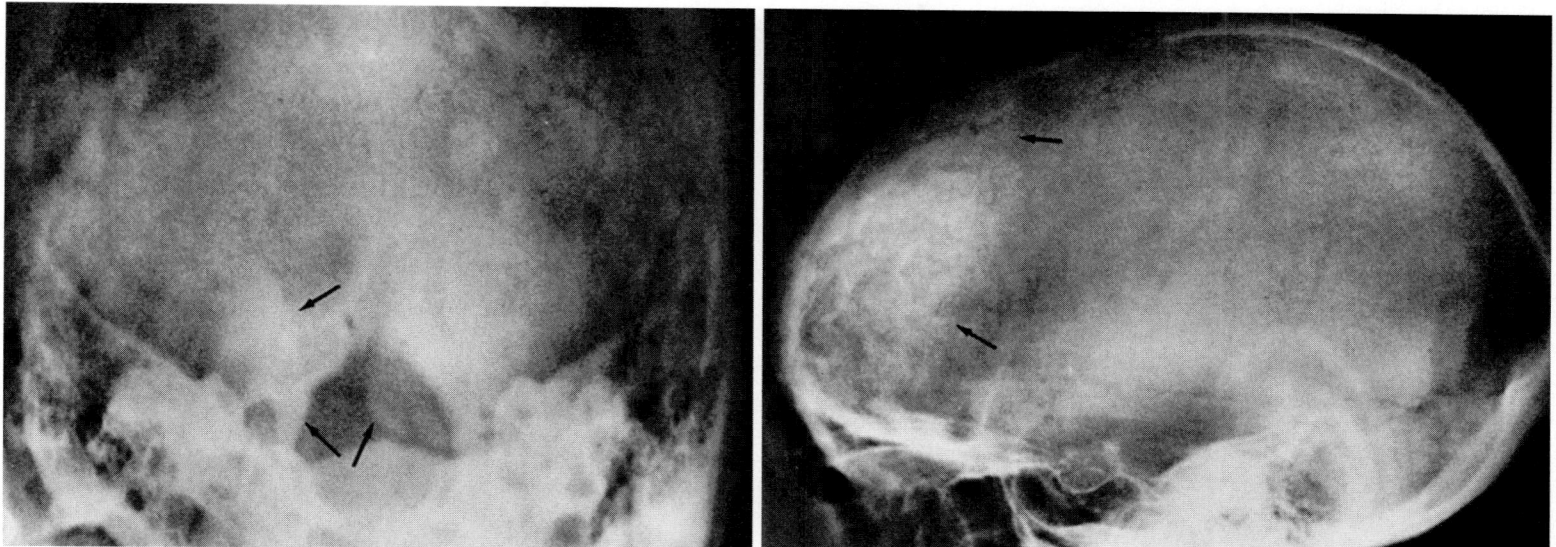

Figure 1–230. Simulated abnormality of foramen magnum, produced by superimposed projection of benign hyperostosis of the internal surface of the frontal bone.

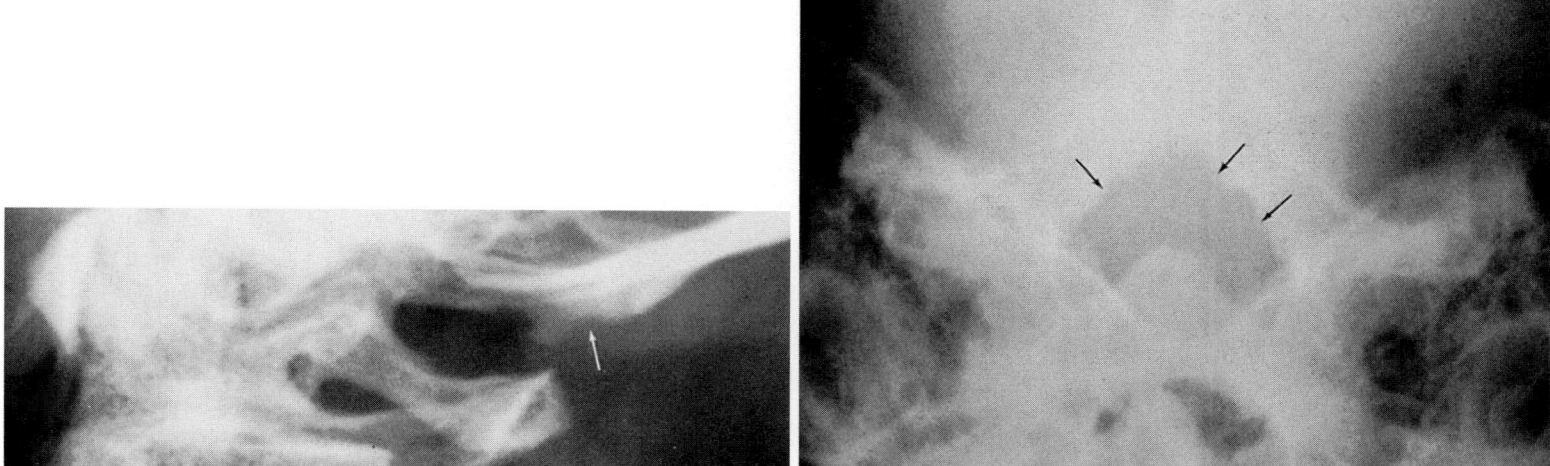

Figure 1–231. Two examples of normal irregularities of the margins of the foramen magnum.

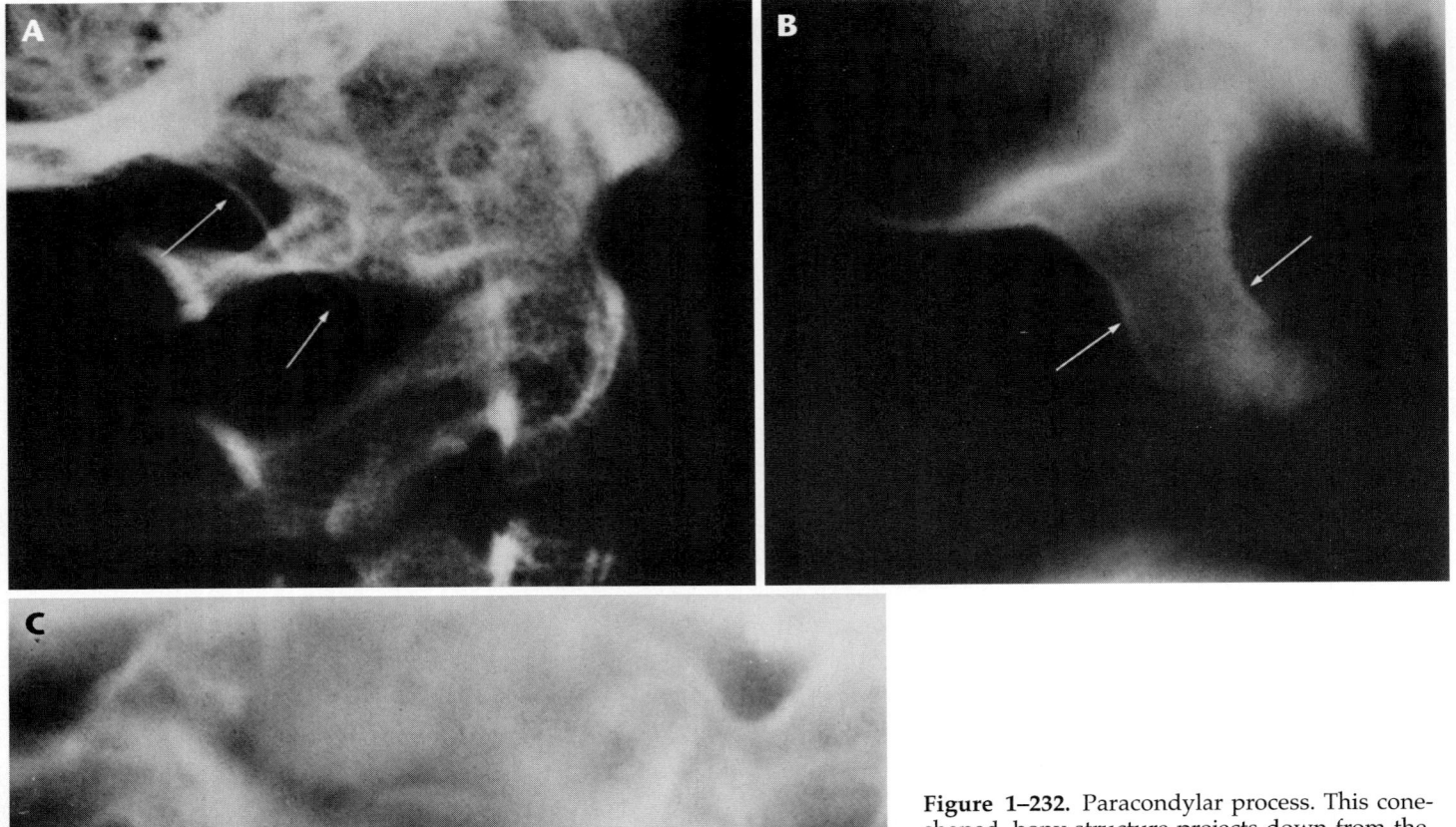

Figure 1–232. Paracondylar process. This cone-shaped, bony structure projects down from the lateral aspect of the occipital condyle toward the transverse process of C1. It may be unilateral or bilateral. **A,** Lateral projection. **B** and **C,** Tomograms. (Ref: Shapiro R, Robinson F: Anomalies of the craniovertebral border. *Am J Roentgenol* 127:281, 1976.)

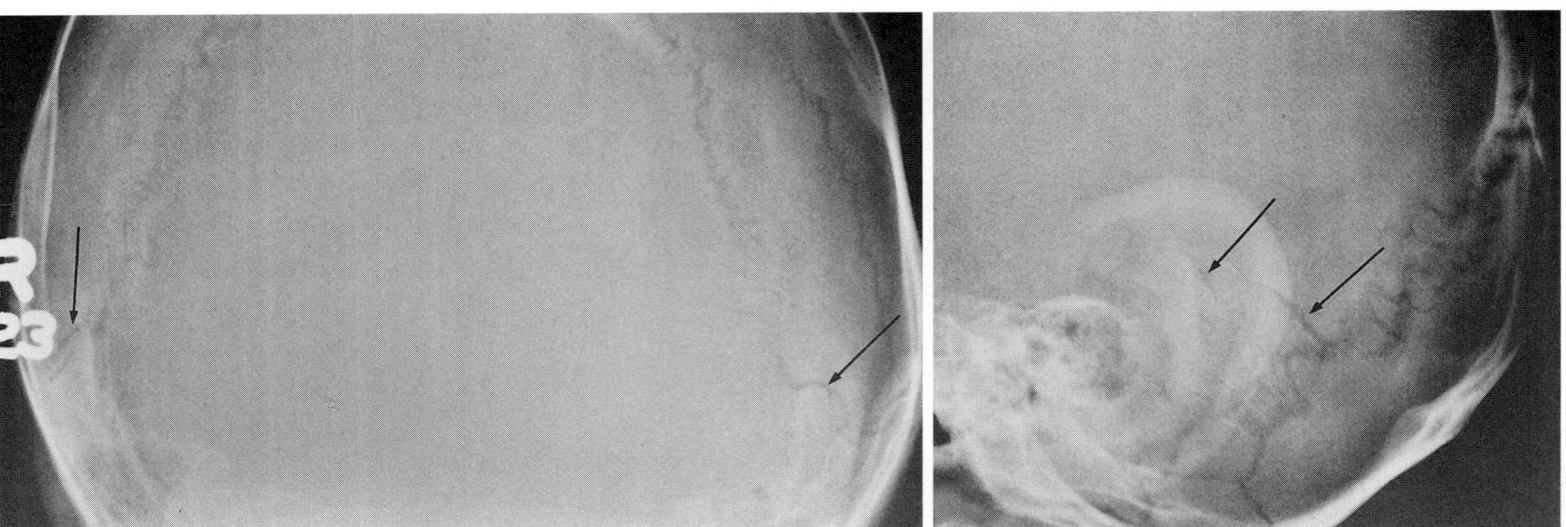

Figure 1–233. Squamoparietal suture in an 8-month-old should not be mistaken for a fracture (see Fig. 1–47).

The Temporal Bone

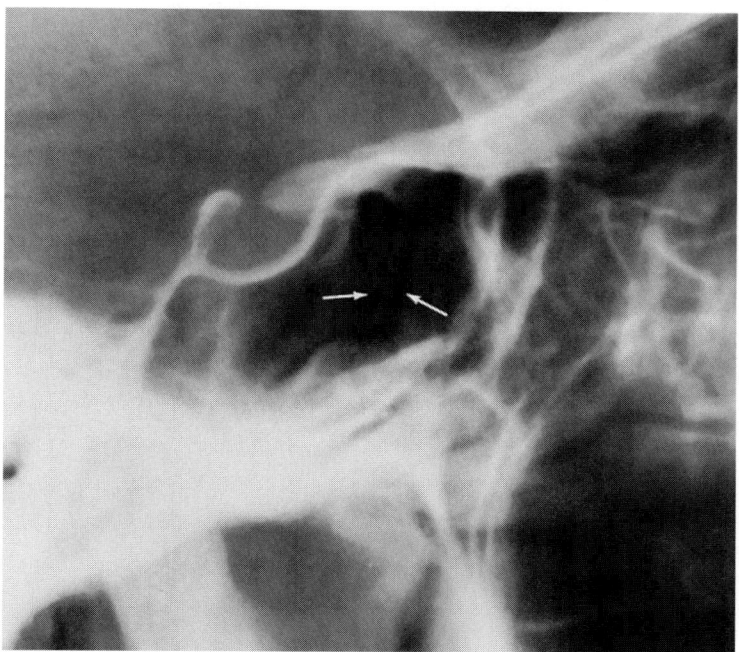

Figure 1–234. Vascular grooves in the temporal bone seen through the sphenoid sinus, simulating fractures.

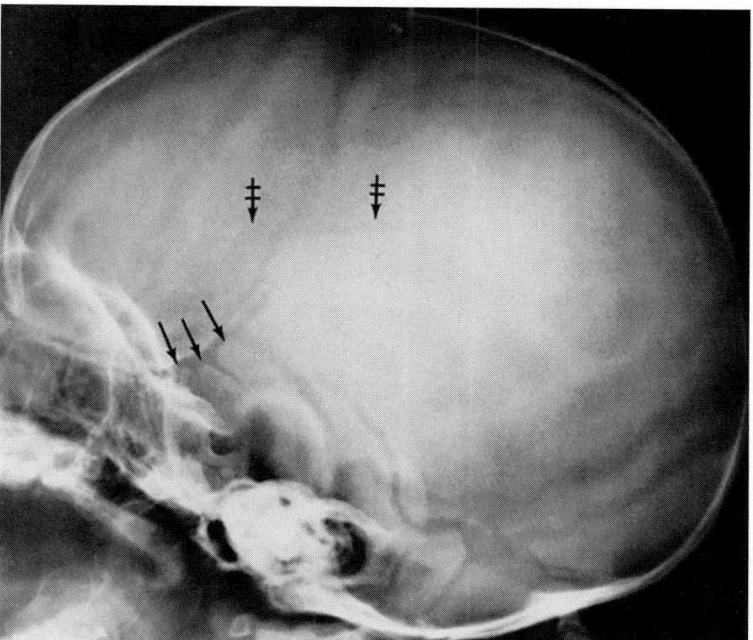

Figure 1–235. Skull of a 3-month-old infant, showing wormian bones in the anterior end of the squamosal suture (←). Note also the vascular groove in the parietal bone that simulates fracture (↔). The skull is rotated on its vertical axis, and the groove is projected across the coronal sutures.

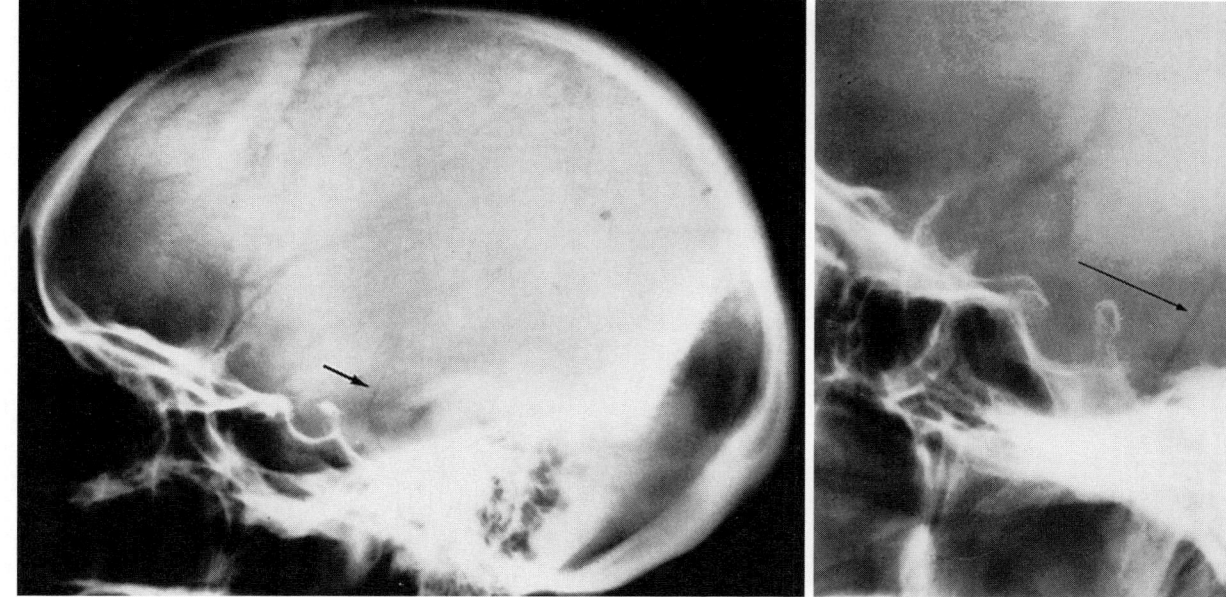

Figure 1–236. Two examples of grooves for the middle temporal artery, simulating fractures. (Ref: Schunk H, Maruyama Y: Two vascular grooves of the external table of the skull that simulate fractures. *Acta Radiol* 54:186, 1960.)

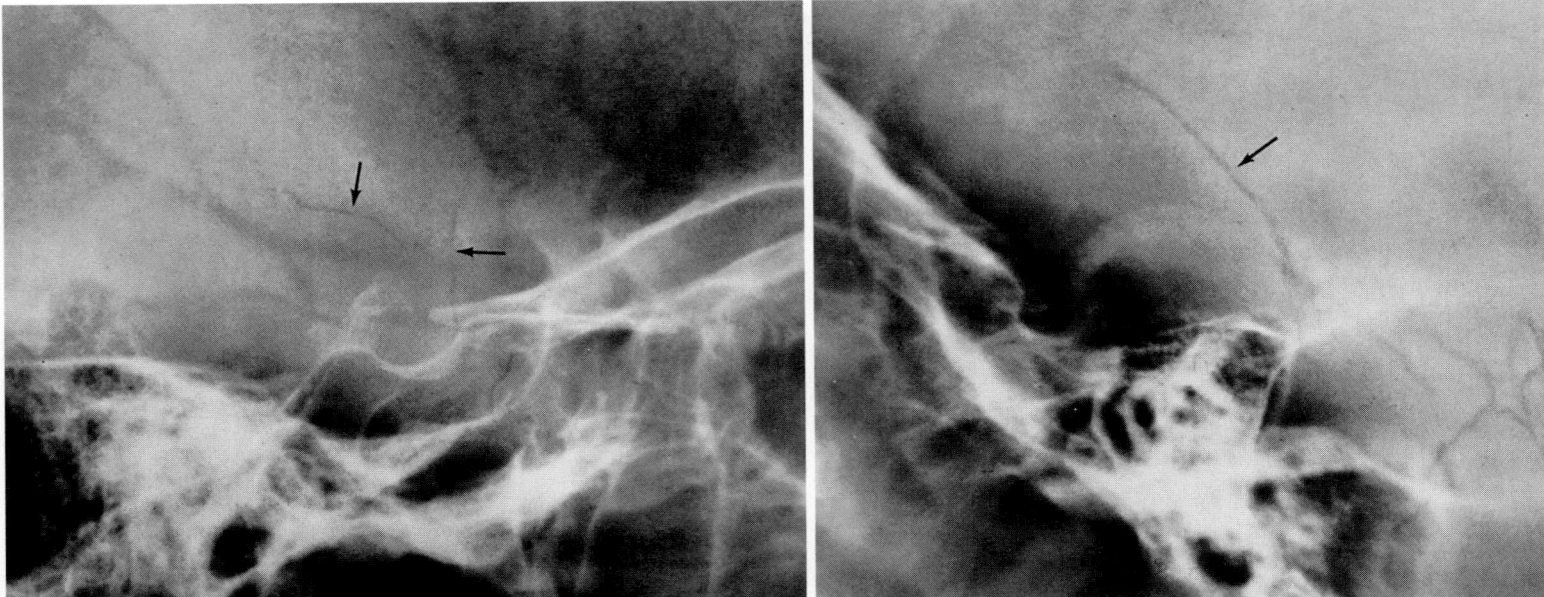

Figure 1–237. Two examples of vascular grooves in the temporal bone, simulating fractures. (Ref: Allen WE et al: Pitfalls in the evaluation of skull trauma. *Radiol Clin North Am* 11:479, 1973.)

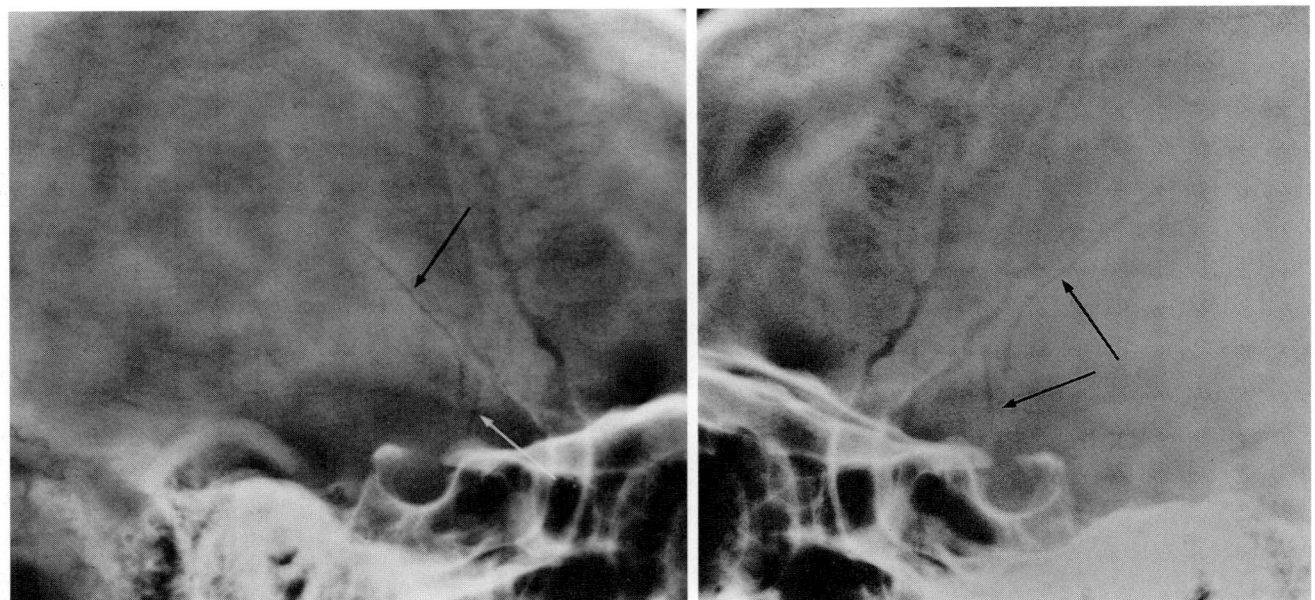

Figure 1–238. Additional examples of vascular grooves that may be mistaken for fractures.

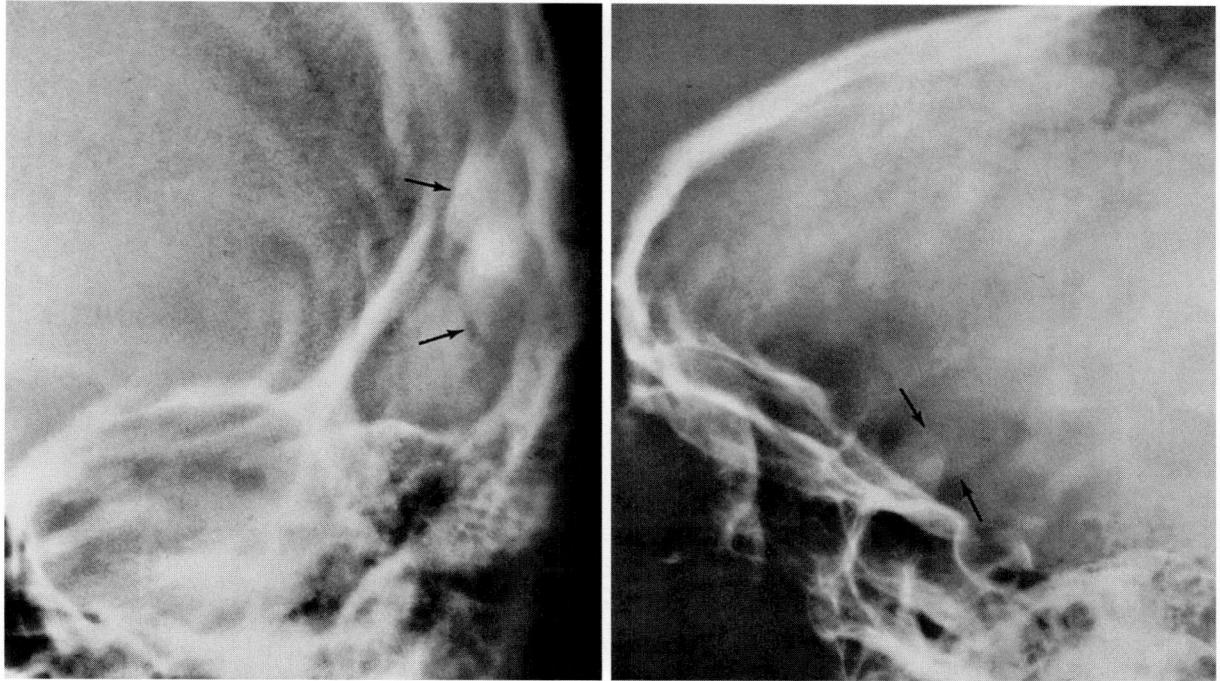

Figure 1–239. Convolutional impressions. The scalloping of the inner table of the middle cranial fossa is normal in adults. (Ref: Lane B: Erosions of the skull. *Radiol Clin North Am* 12:257, 1974.)

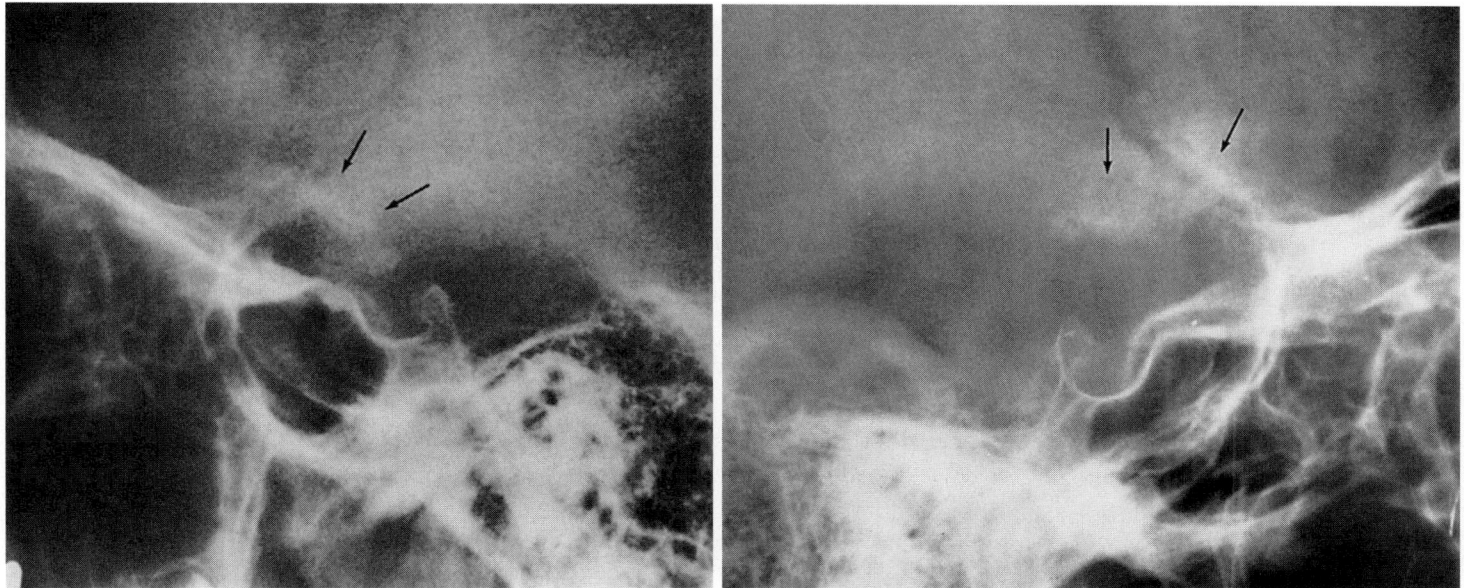

Figure 1–240. Two examples of temporal sutural sclerosis, simulating suprasellar calcification.

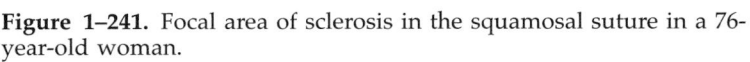

Figure 1–241. Focal area of sclerosis in the squamosal suture in a 76-year-old woman.

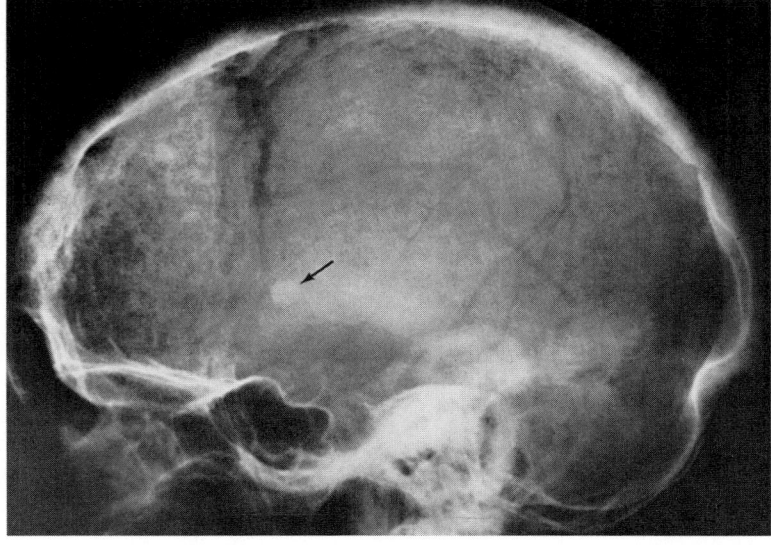

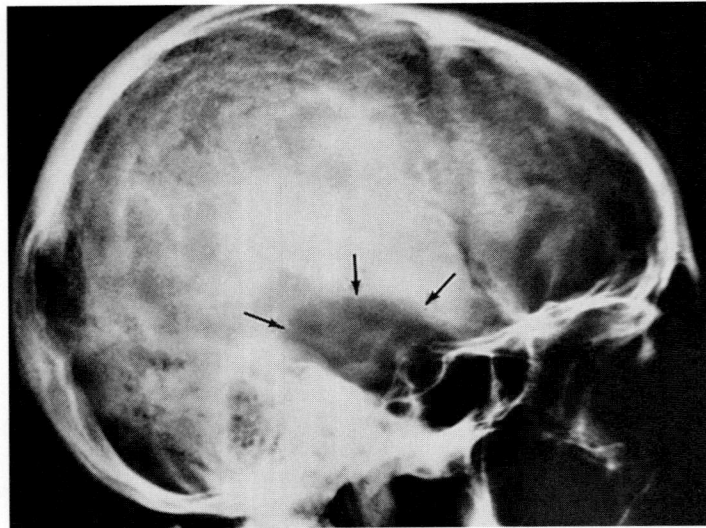

Figure 1–242. Exaggeration of the normal lucency of the squamosal portion of the temporal bone.

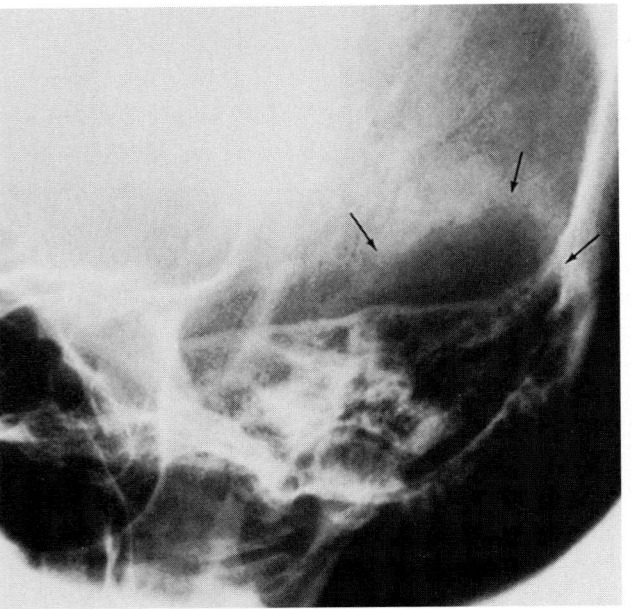

Figure 1–243. Temporal thinning in Stenvers' projection, simulating destruction of the calvaria.

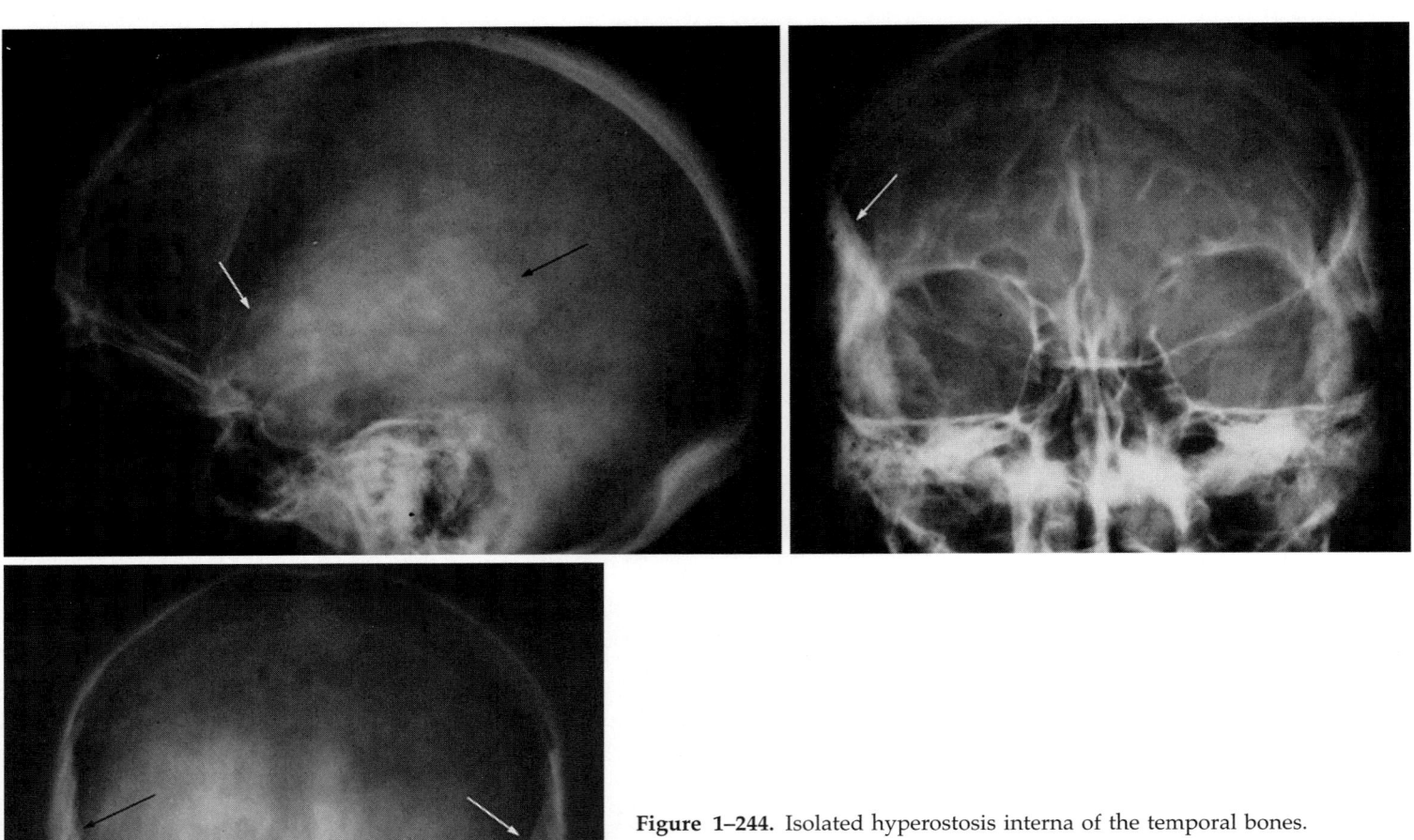

Figure 1–244. Isolated hyperostosis interna of the temporal bones.

The Mastoid

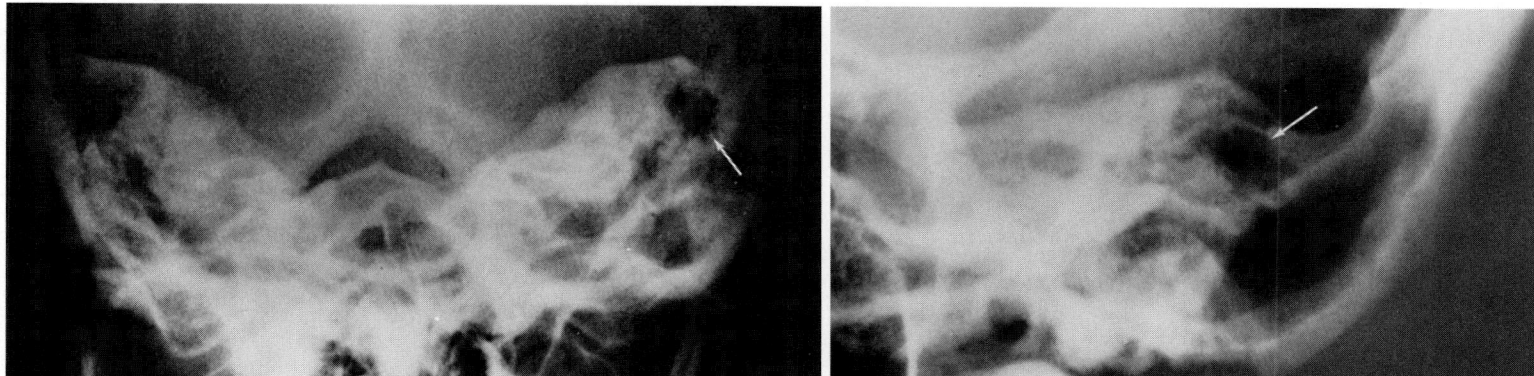

Figure 1–245. Large antrum, simulating a destructive lesion.

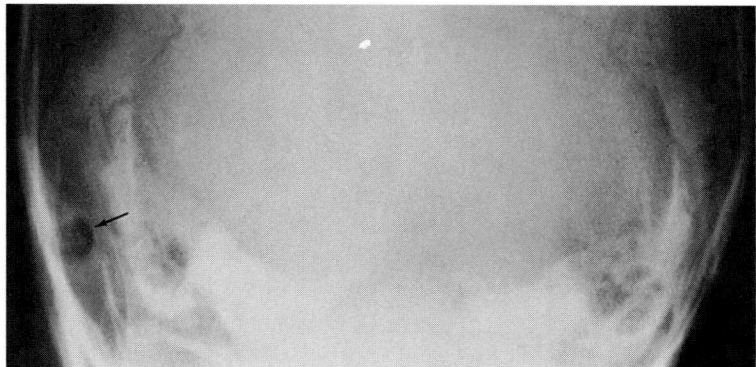

Figure 1–246. Air in the external auditory canal, seen as discrete radiolucency.

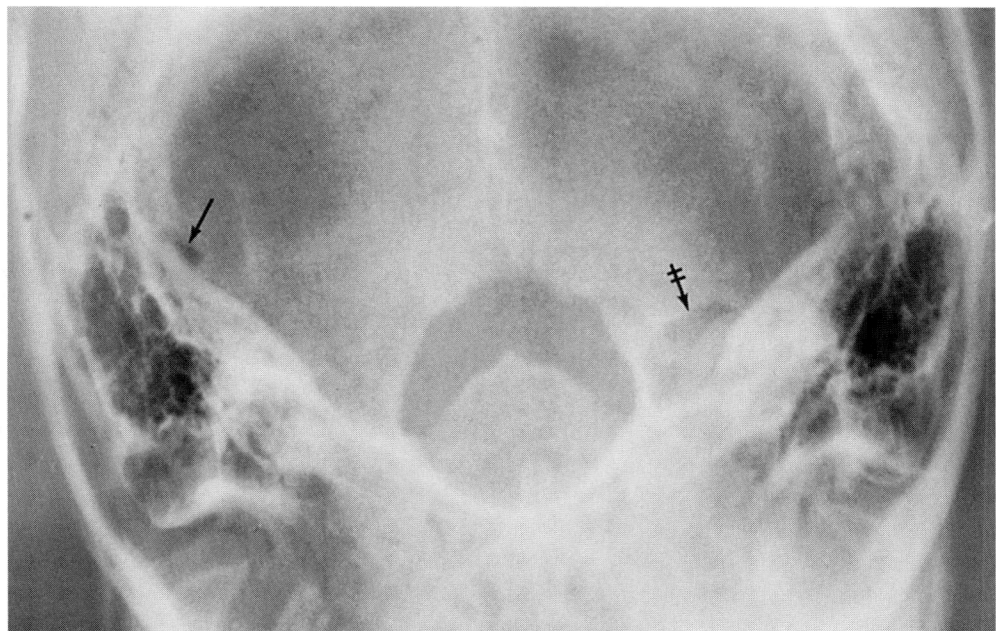

Figure 1–247. Mastoid emissary vein seen unilaterally in Towne's projection (←). Note the prominent condyloid fossa on the opposite side (⟵).

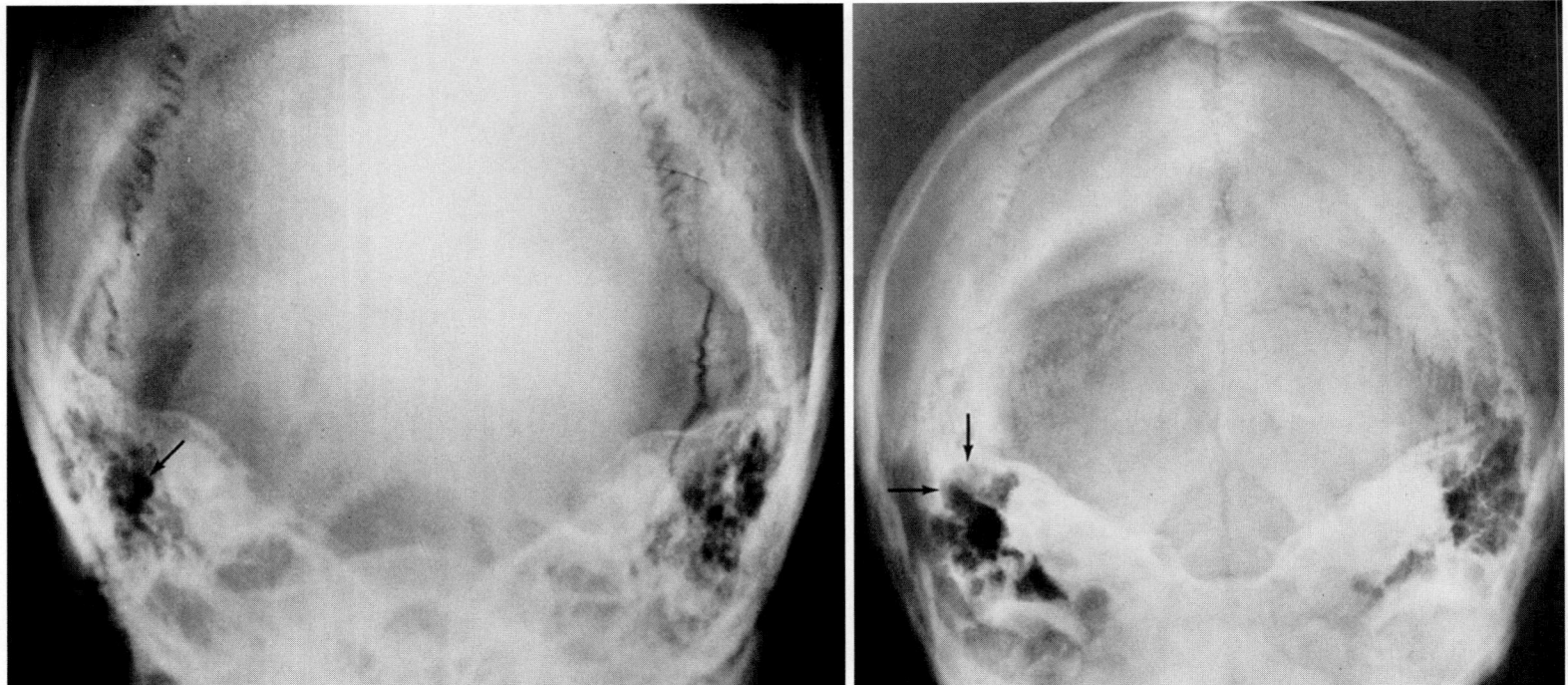

Figure 1–248. Large mastoid antra, which might be mistaken for cholesteatomas. (Ref: Tillitt R et al: The large mastoid antrum. *Radiology* 94:619, 1970.)

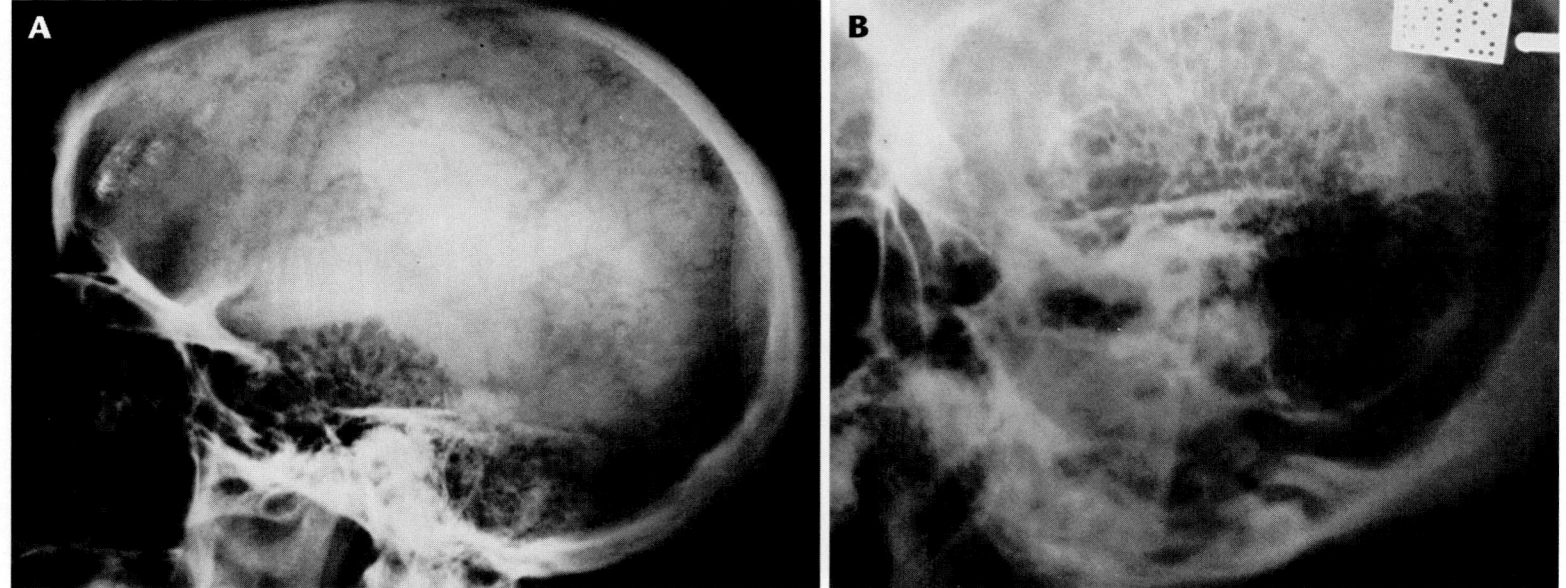

Figure 1–249. A, An example of unusually marked pneumatization of the mastoids. **B,** A detailed view of the mastoid air cells.

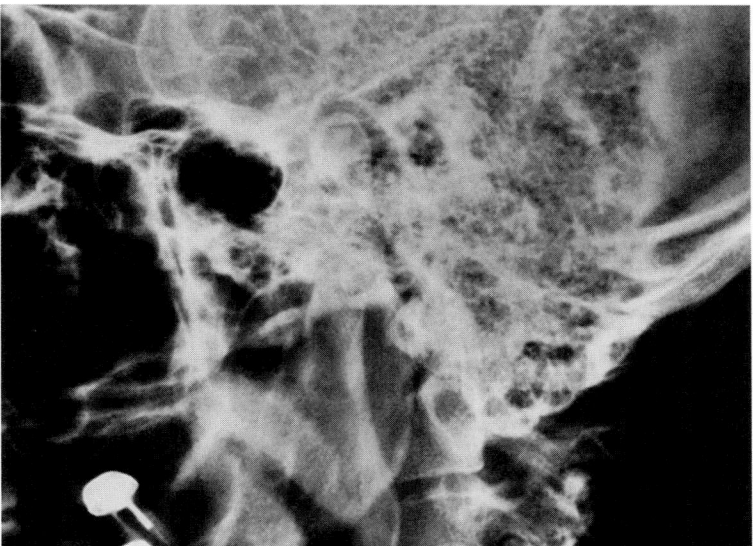

Figure 1–250. Extremely marked pneumatization of the mastoid.

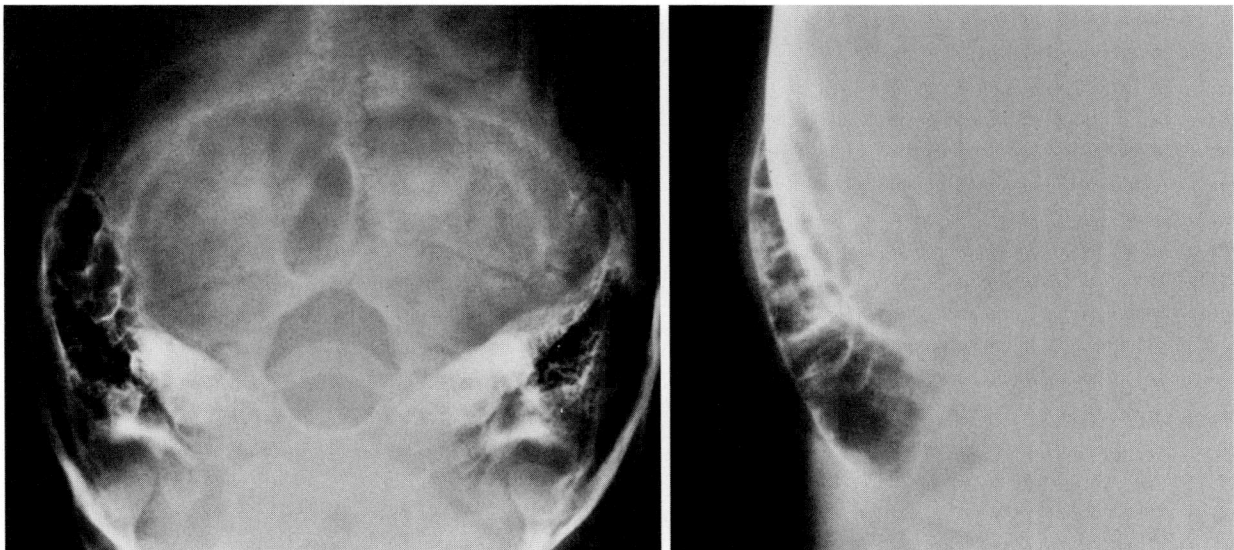

Figure 1–251. *Left,* A symmetric development of the mastoids in a 5-year-old child, with marked overdevelopment in the patient's right side. Note lucency in the midline of the occipital bone, which represents a normal variant. *Right,* A detailed view of the right mastoid.

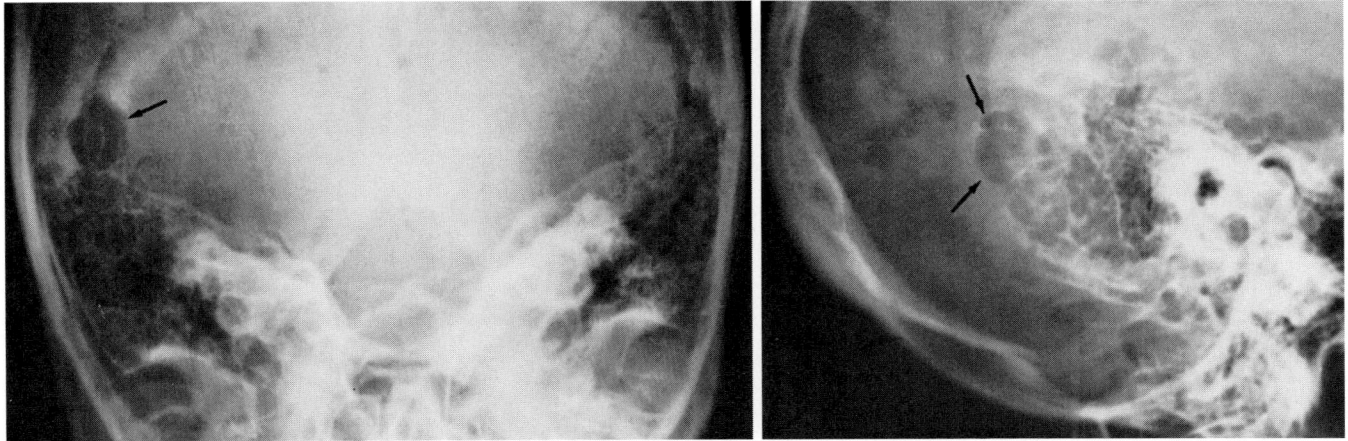

Figure 1–252. Large asymmetric mastoid air cell, which might be mistaken for an area of bone destruction.

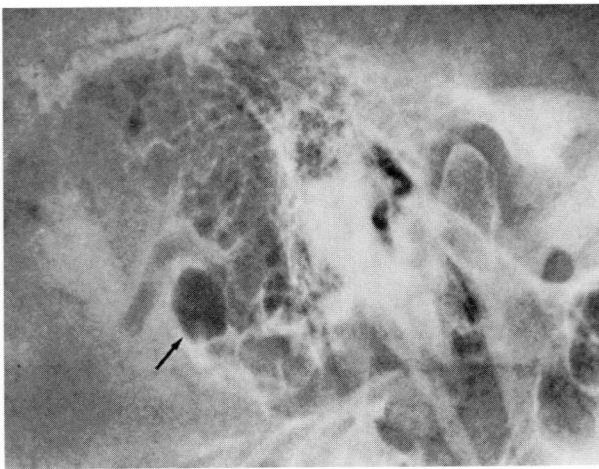

Figure 1–253. Large mastoid air cell below the emissary vein, simulating an area of bone destruction.

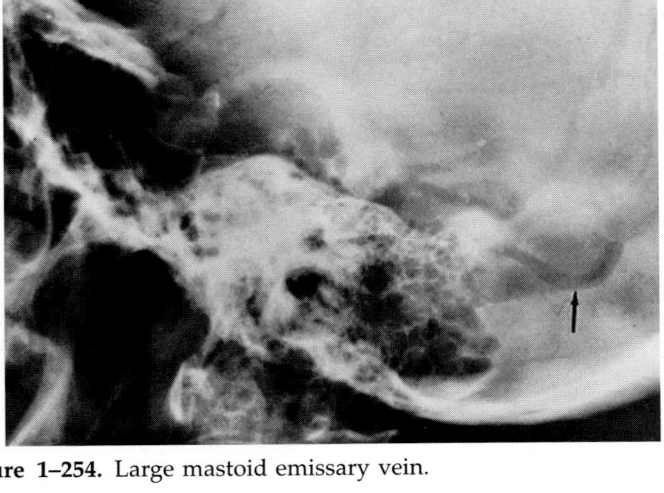

Figure 1–254. Large mastoid emissary vein.

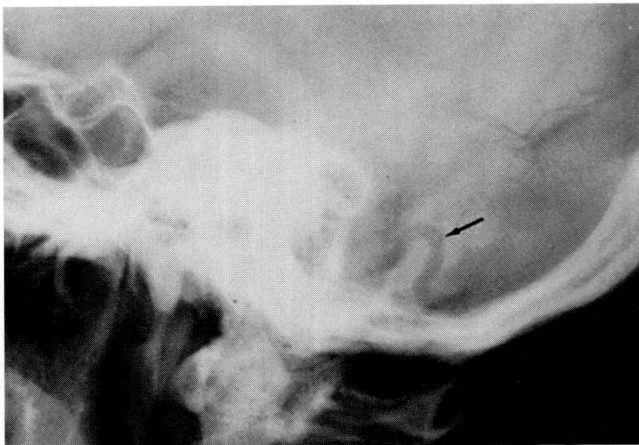

Figure 1–255. Large mastoid emissary vein.

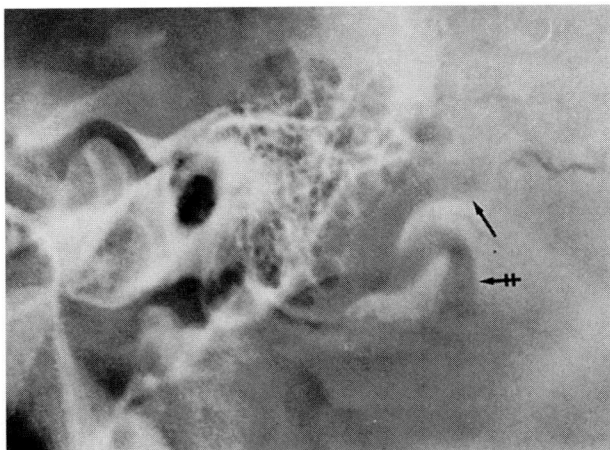

Figure 1–256. Sigmoid sinus (←) and mastoid emissary vein (⇇).

The Petrous Pyramid

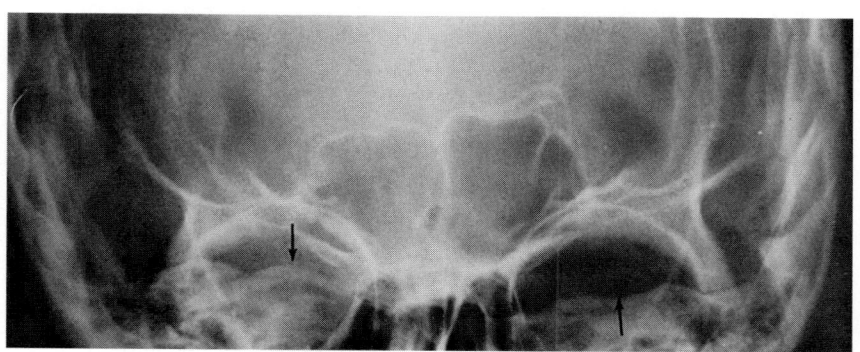

Figure 1–257. Normal asymmetry in height of the petrous ridges. This entity may be associated occasionally with trigeminal neuralgia. (Ref: Obrador S et al: Trigeminal neuralgia secondary to asymmetry of the petrous bone. *J Neurosurg* 33:596, 1970.)

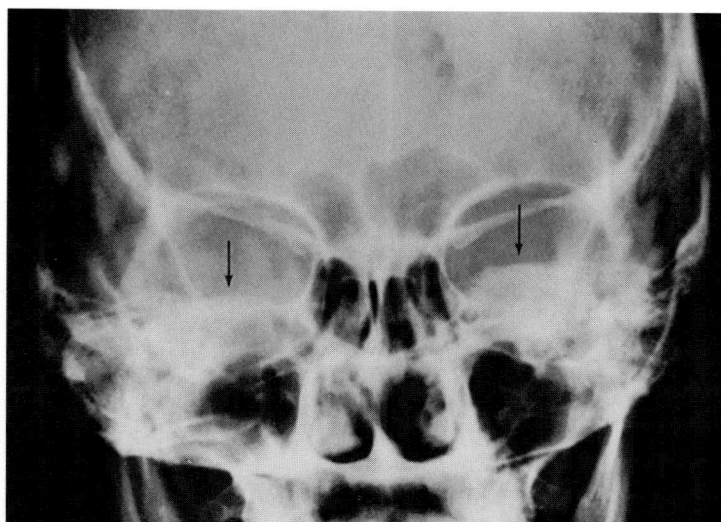

Figure 1–258. Two examples of normal asymmetry in height and configuration of the petrous ridges.

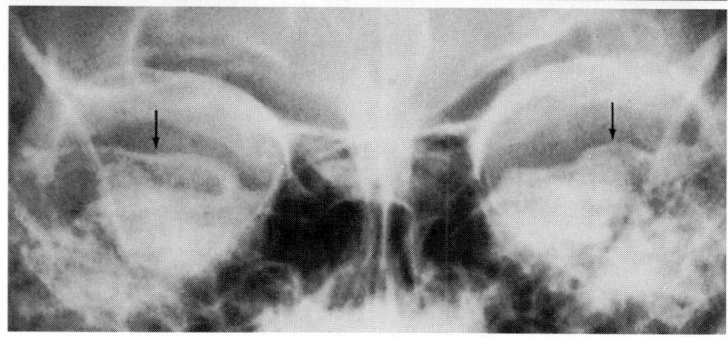

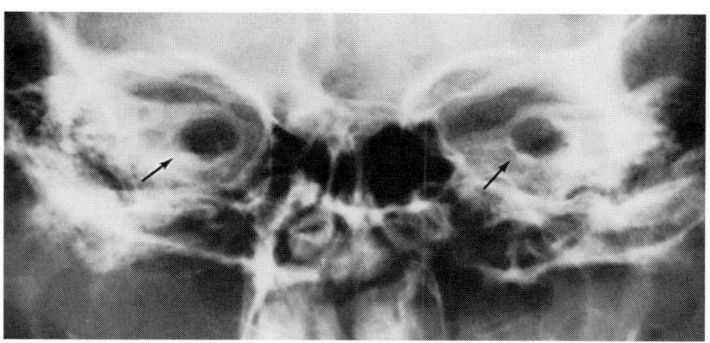

Figure 1–259. Large mastoid air cells at the petrous tips, simulating the changes of acoustic neuroma. (Ref: Dubois PJ, Roub LW: Giant air cell of petrous apex. *Radiology* 129:103, 1978.)

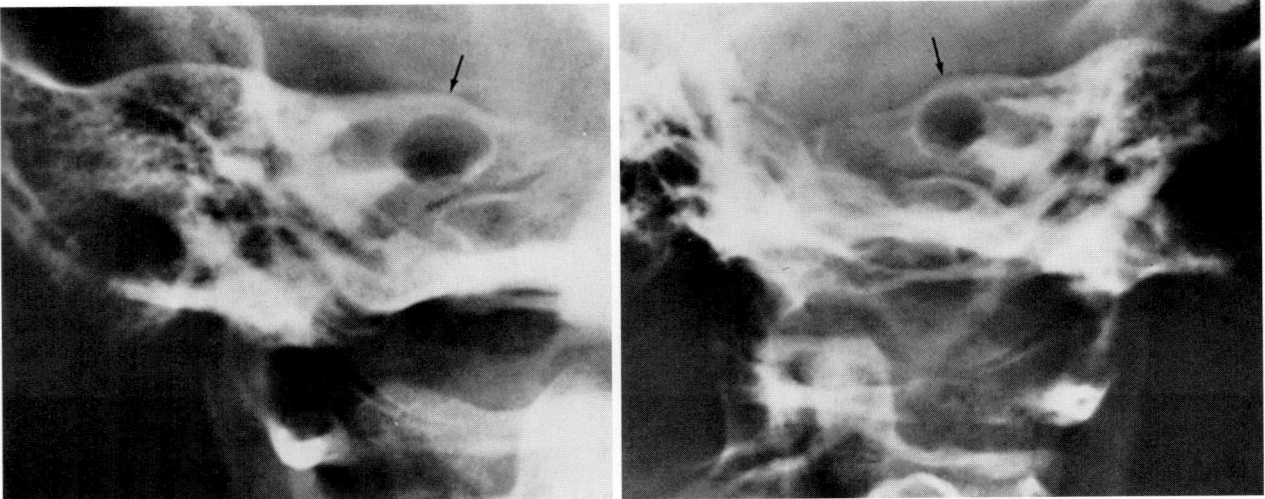

Figure 1–260. Stenvers' projection of the petrous tips of the case illustrated in the preceding figure.

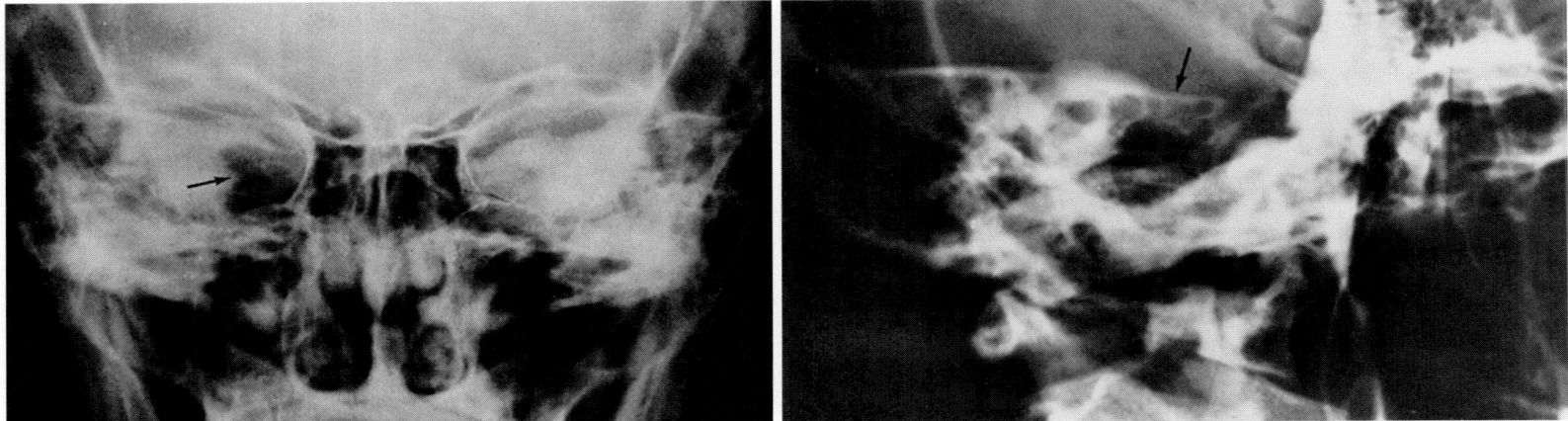

Figure 1–261. Pneumatization of one petrous tip simulating enlargement of the internal auditory meatus.

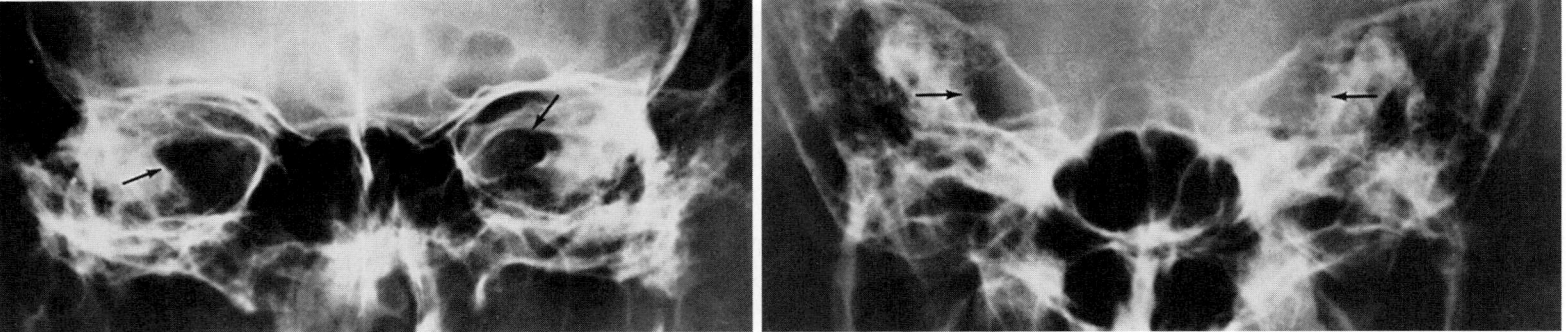

Figure 1–262. Apparent destruction of the petrous tips caused by pneumatization.

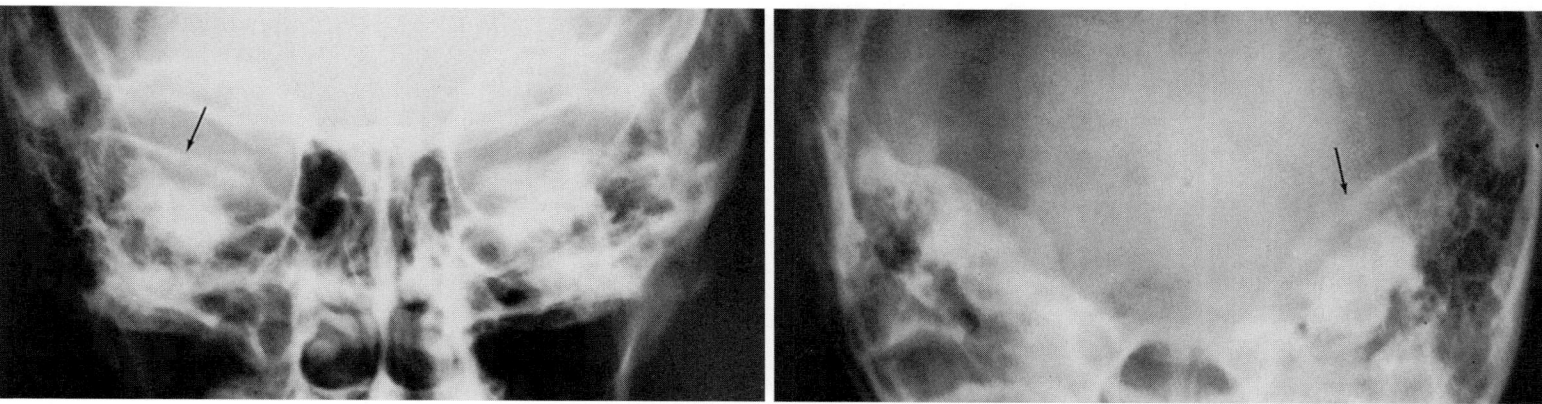

Figure 1–263. Asymmetric pneumatization of the petrous ridges.

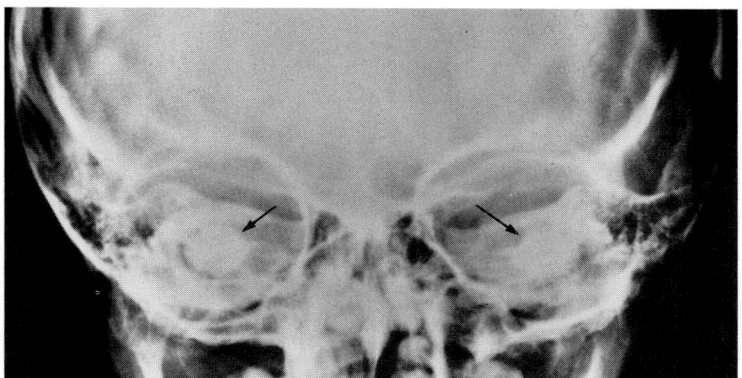

Figure 1–264. Unusual cochlear densities in a patient without symptoms referrable to the inner ear.

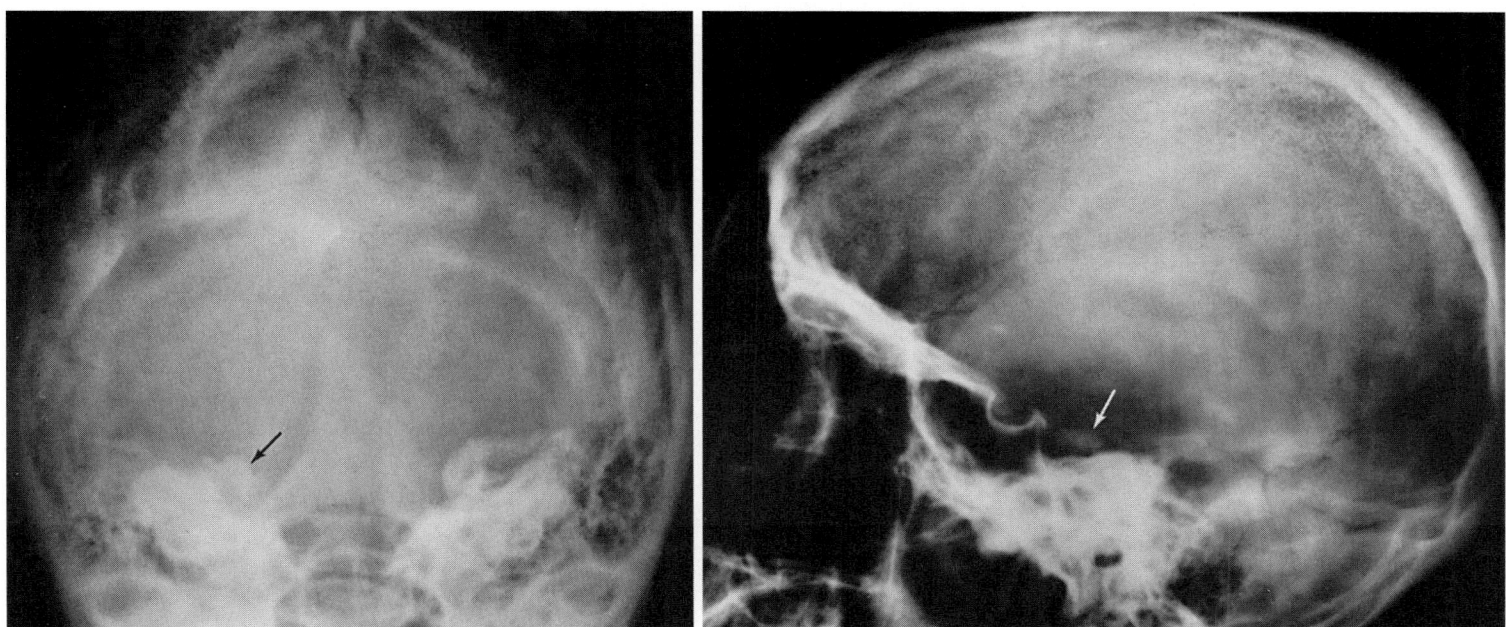

Figure 1–265. Dense nodular form of calcification of the petroclinoid ligament, simulating asymmetric development of one petrous bone, with the dense portion seen in the lateral projection.

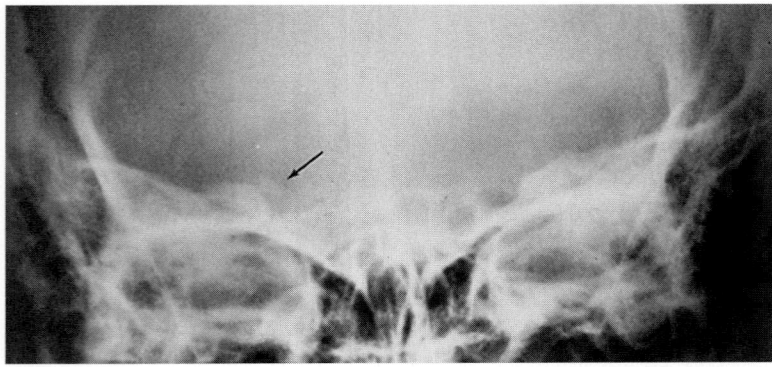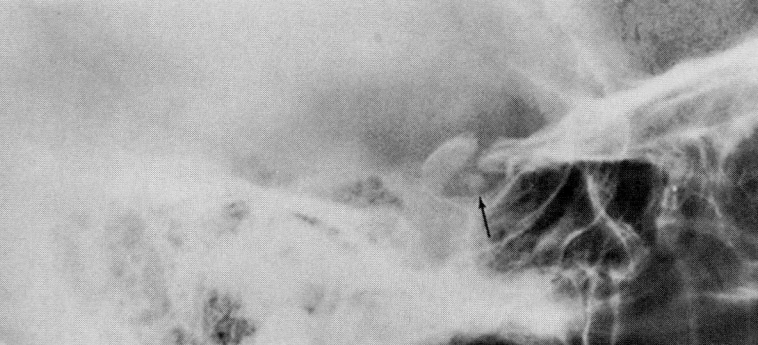

Figure 1–266. The os supra petrosum of Meckel (see Fig. 1–73).

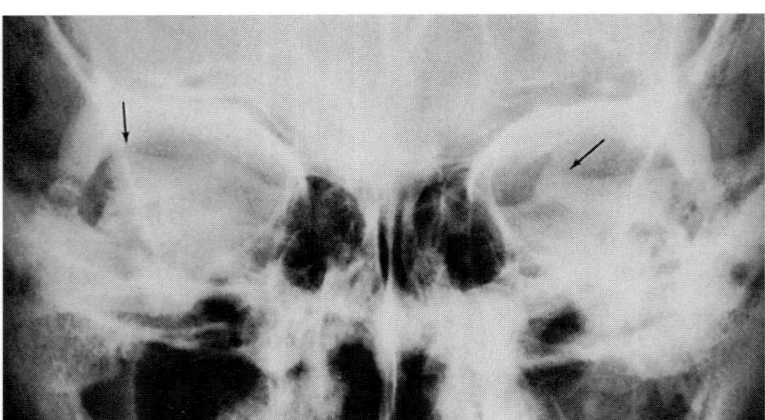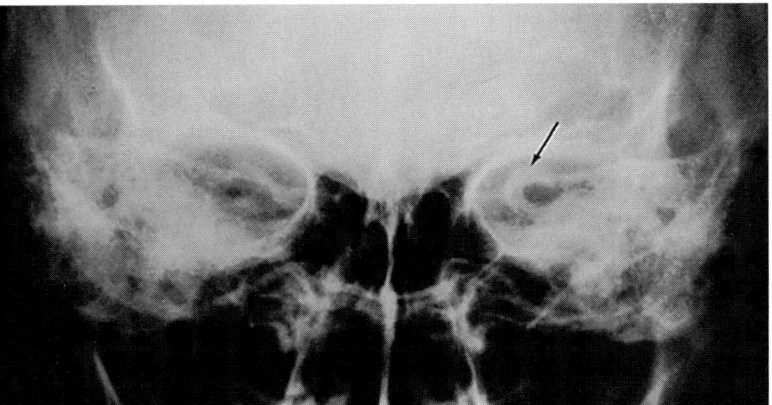

Figure 1–267. *Left,* Small, rounded bony knob on the superior margin of the petrous bones. This finding is usually unilateral but may be bilateral, as in this case. (Ref: Shapiro R: An interesting normal variant of the temporal bone. *Radiology* 128:354, 1978.) *Right,* Bony, ring-like configuration of the petrous tip.

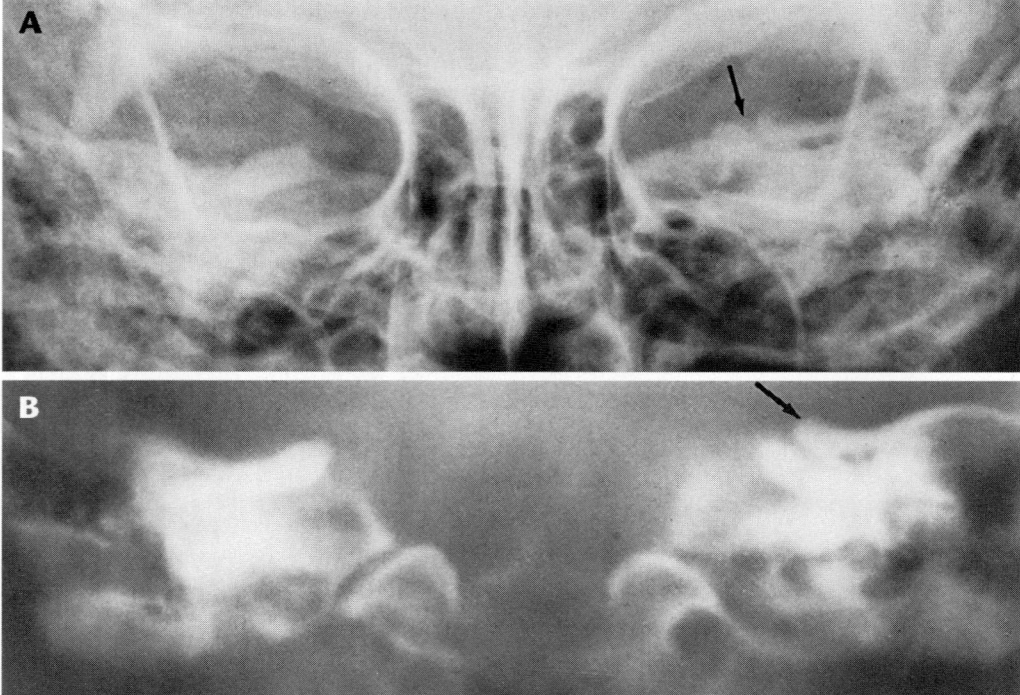

Figure 1–268. Variation in development of the petrous ridges, producing an anomalous "foramen" on one side. **A,** Plain film. **B,** Tomography.

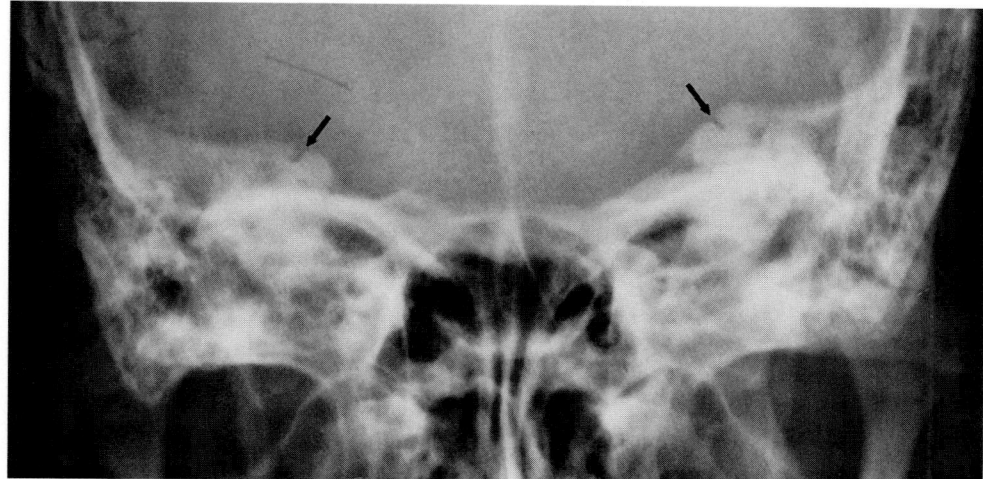

Figure 1–269. The same phenomenon as in preceding figure seen bilaterally.

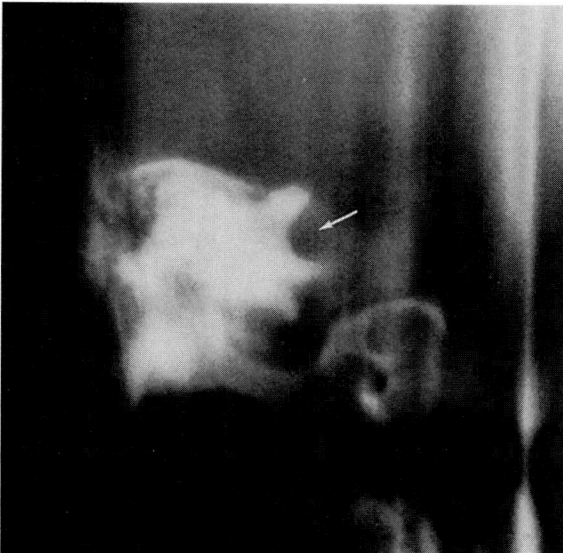

Figure 1–270. "Fish-mouth" internal auditory meatus by tomography, one of the normal variations in configuration.

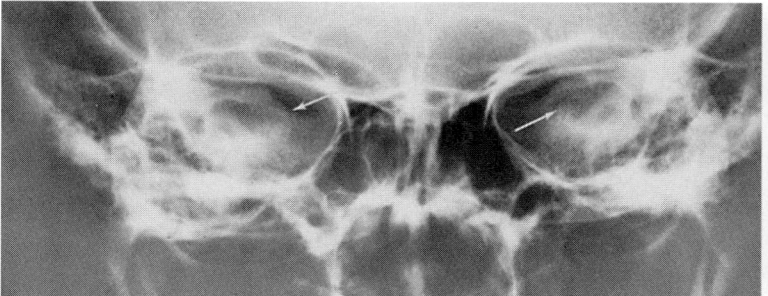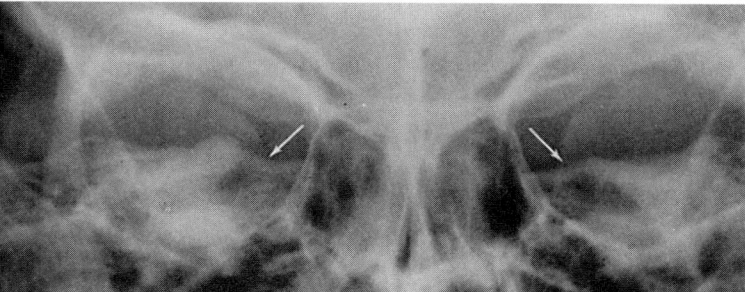

Figure 1–271. Two examples of normal asymmetry of the configuration of the internal auditory canals. (Ref: Fraser RA, Carter BL: Unilateral dilatation of the internal auditory canal. *Neuroradiology* 9:227, 1975.)

The Sphenoid Bone

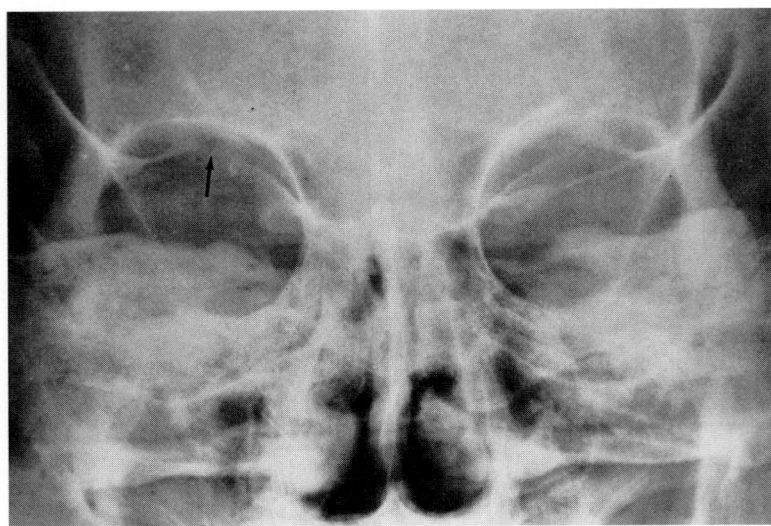

Figure 1–272. Normal asymmetry of the lesser wings of the sphenoid. Note the arching of the wing on the right.

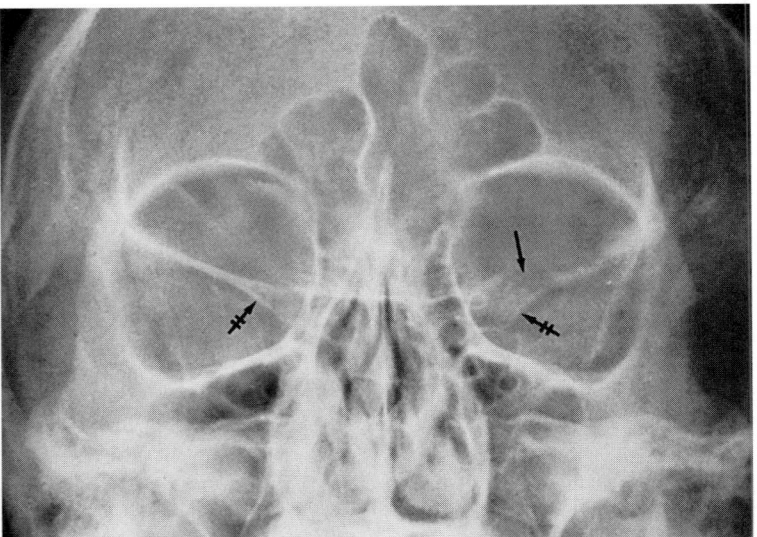

Figure 1–273. Asymmetry of the lesser wings of the sphenoid in a normal individual, simulating bone destruction of the left (←). Note also the normal asymmetry of the superior orbital fissures (↤). (Ref: Shapiro R, Robinson F: Alterations of the sphenoidal fissure produced by local and systemic processes. *Am J Roentgenol* 101:814, 1967.)

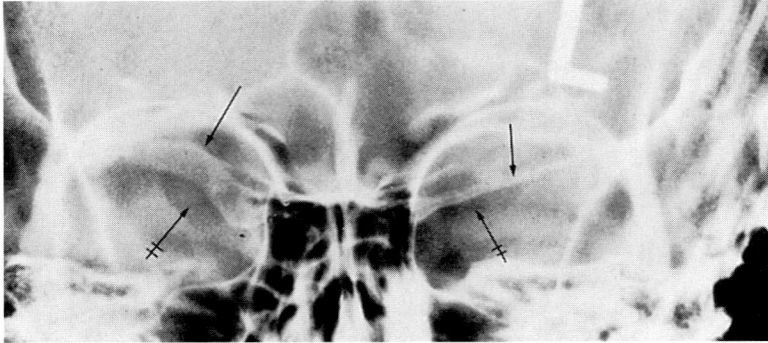

Figure 1–274. Asymmetry of the lesser wings of the sphenoid (←) and superior orbital fissures (↤).

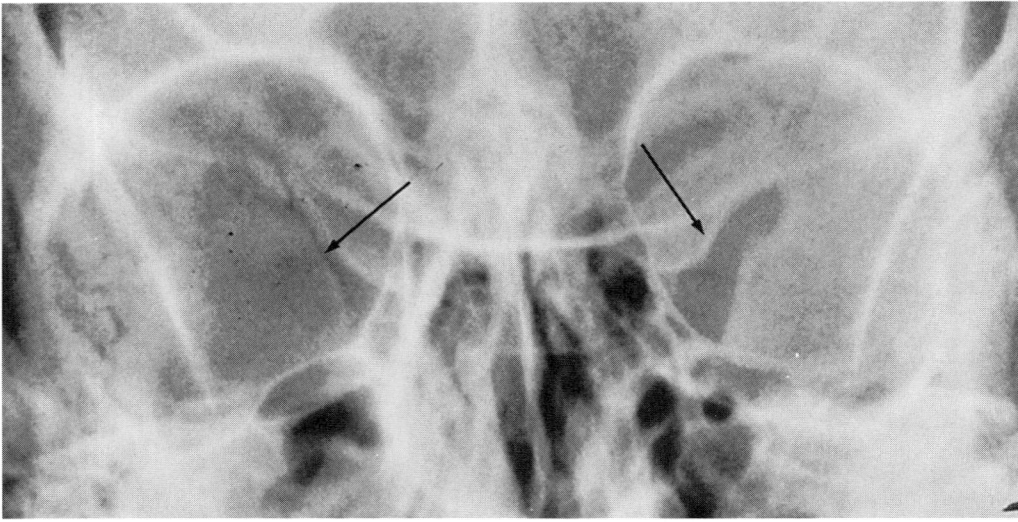

Figure 1–275. Marked asymmetry of the superior orbital fissures.

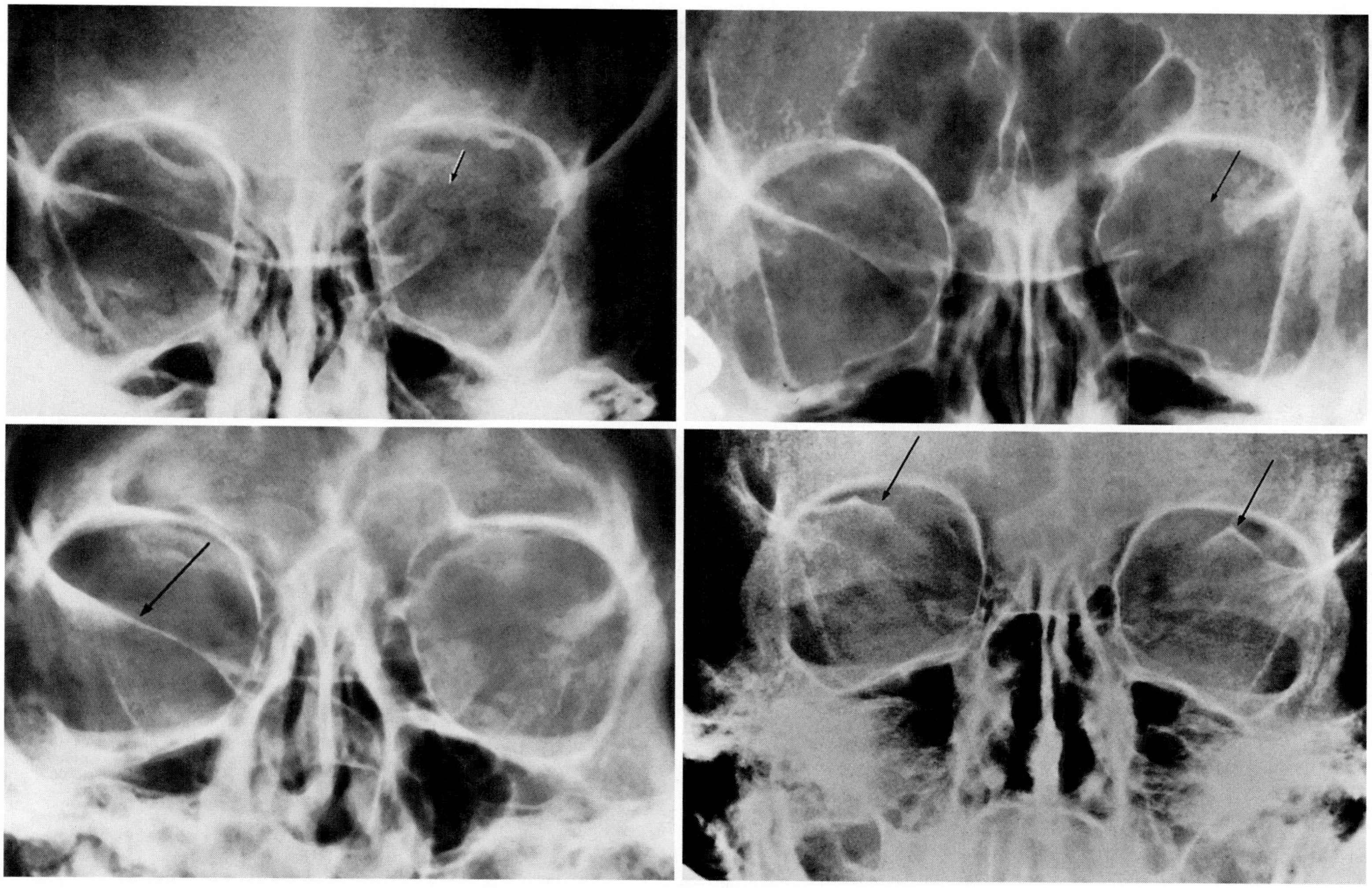

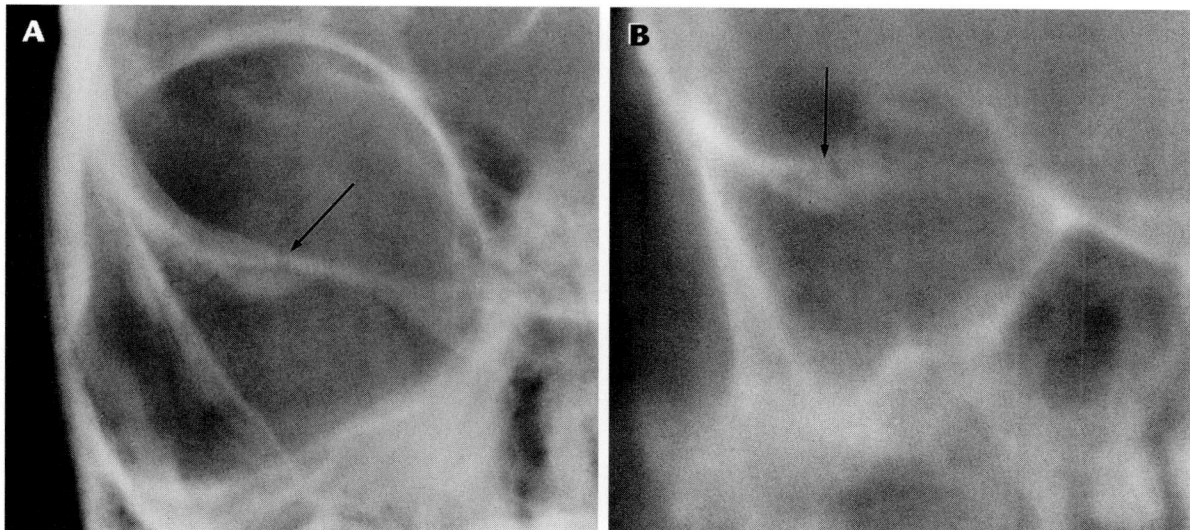

Figure 1–276. Four additional examples of normal variation and asymmetry of the lesser wings of the sphenoid.

Figure 1–277. Simulated fracture of the lesser wing of the sphenoid by anatomic variation not present on opposite side. **A,** Plain film. **B,** Tomography.

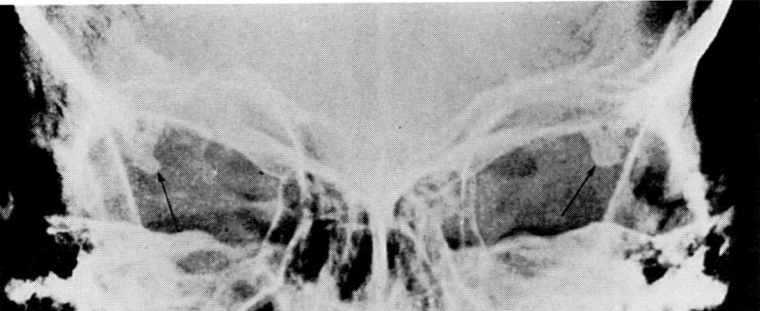

Figure 1–278. Developmental spurs from the lesser wings of the sphenoid.

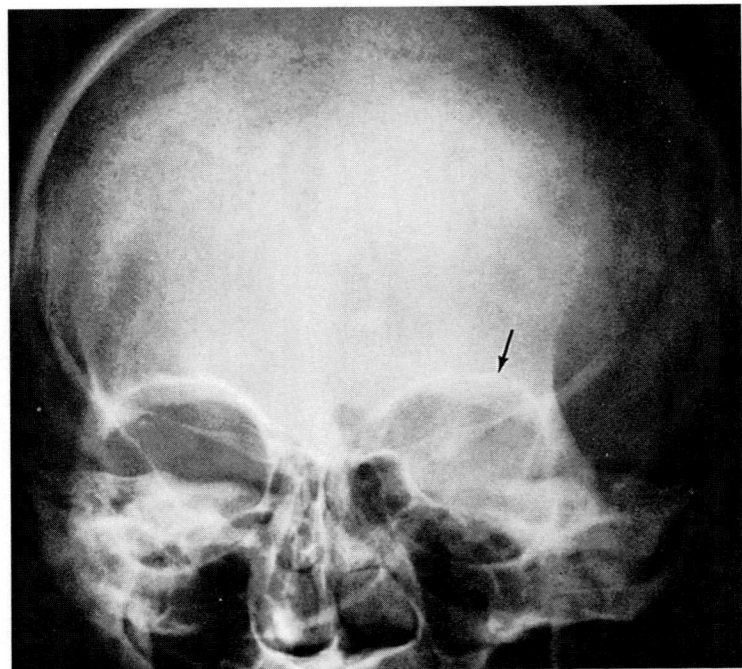

Figure 1–279. Slight rotation of the head and the superimposition of a prominent external occipital protuberance, appearing on the right, simulating the changes of a sphenoid wing meningioma.

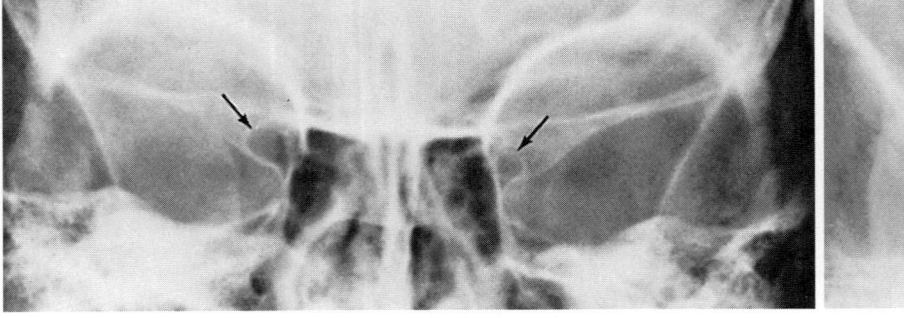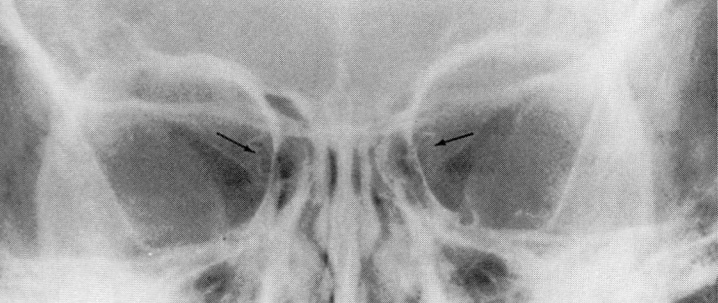

Figure 1–280. Two examples of pneumatization of the anterior clinoid processes, simulating enlargement of the optic foramina.

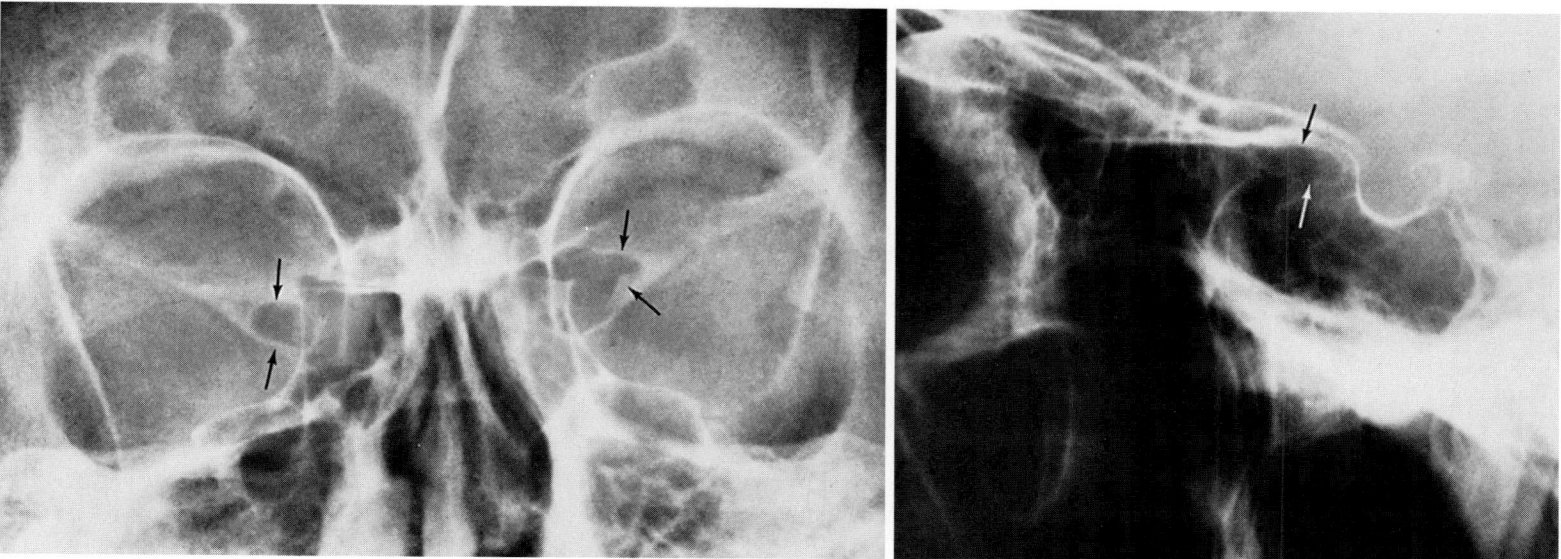

Figure 1–281. Asymmetric pneumatization of the anterior clinoid processes, simulating abnormality of the optic canals.

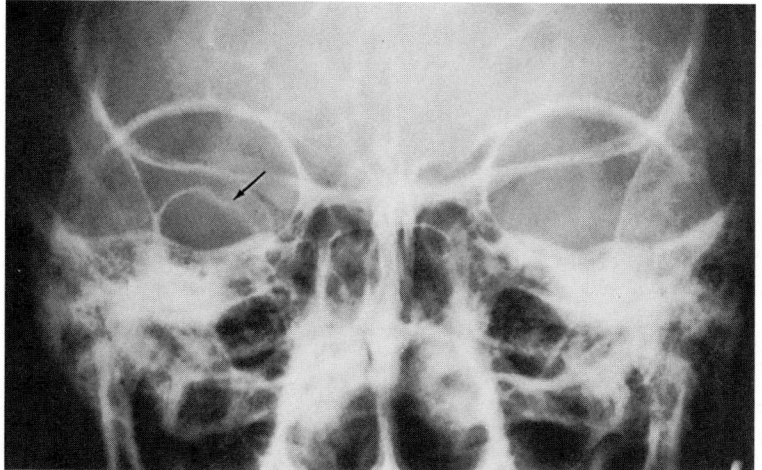

Figure 1–282. Lateral extension of sphenoidal sinus air cell into the greater wing of the sphenoid, simulating a destructive lesion.

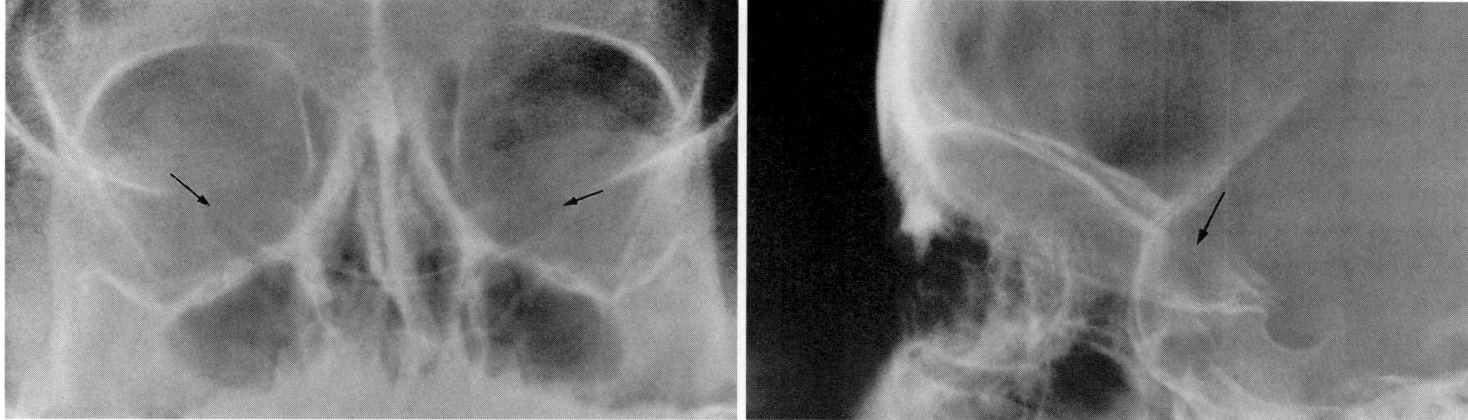

Figure 1–283. Pneumatization of the sphenoid sinus extending into the greater wings of the sphenoid, producing apparent defects in the floor of the anterior fossa in the lateral projection.

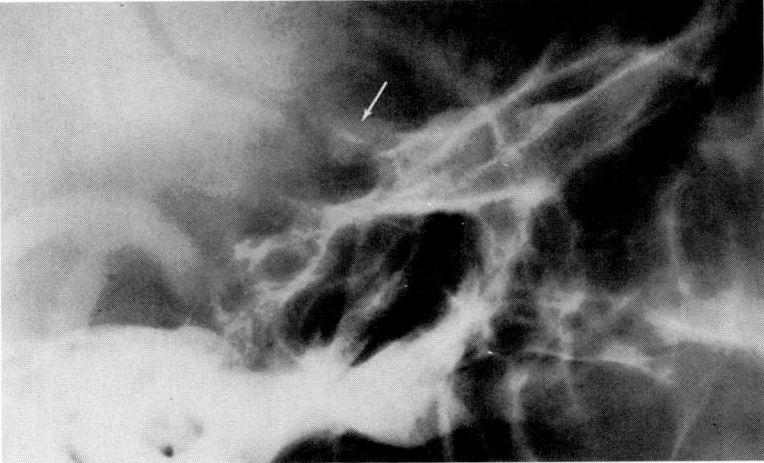

Figure 1–284. Lateral strut of the lesser wings of the sphenoid, simulating changes of a meningioma.

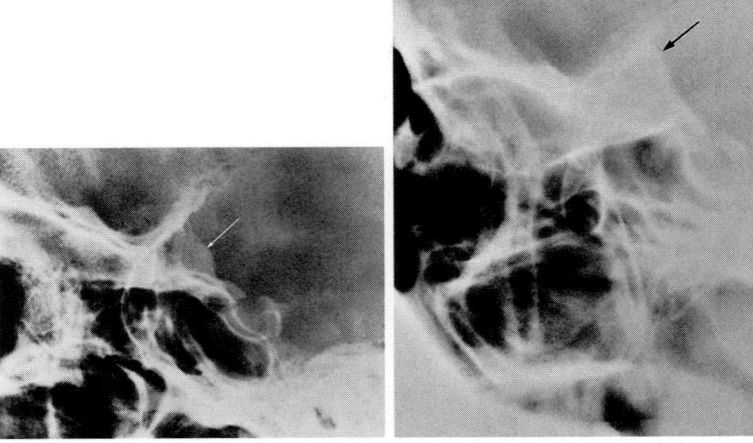

Figure 1–285. Two examples of the pterion, which may simulate a meningioma of the planum sphenoidale.

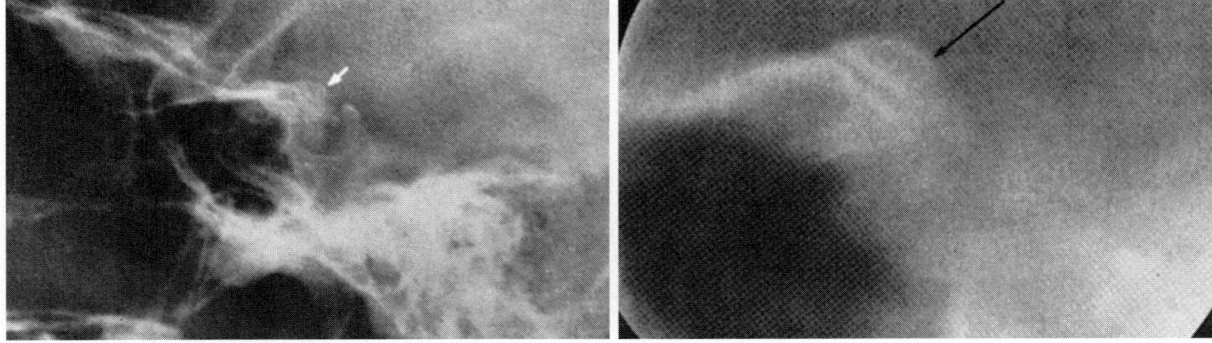

Figure 1–286. Nonunited ossification center of the presphenoid bone, which might be mistaken for evidence of a meningioma. *Left,* Separate well-corticated ossicle *(arrow)* posterior and superior to the anterior clinoid. *Right,* lateral tomogram showing separate center at the anterior clinoid process. The anterior clinoids are superior and the inferior clinoids are inferior. (From Ratner LM, Quencer RM: Nonunited ossification center of the presphenoid bone: Pseudomeningioma. *Am J Roentgenol* 143:503, 1983.)

The Base of the Skull

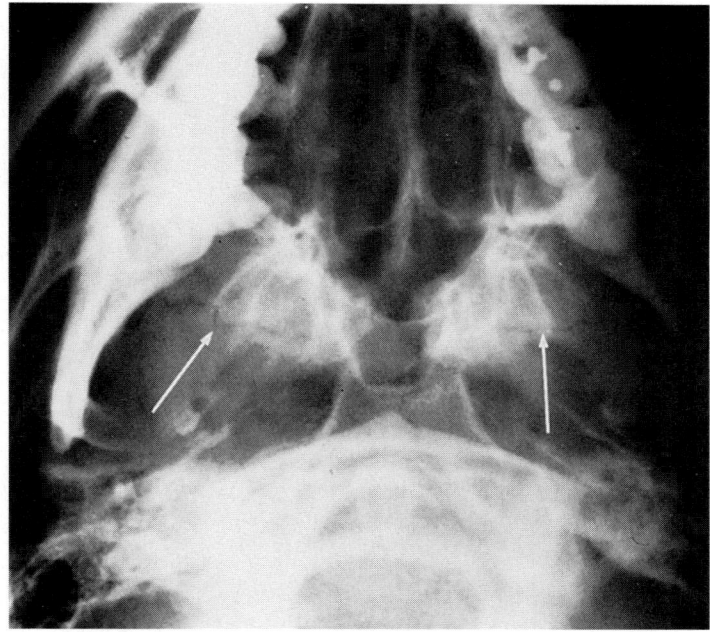

Figure 1–287. Coronal suture seen in the base view, simulating a fracture.

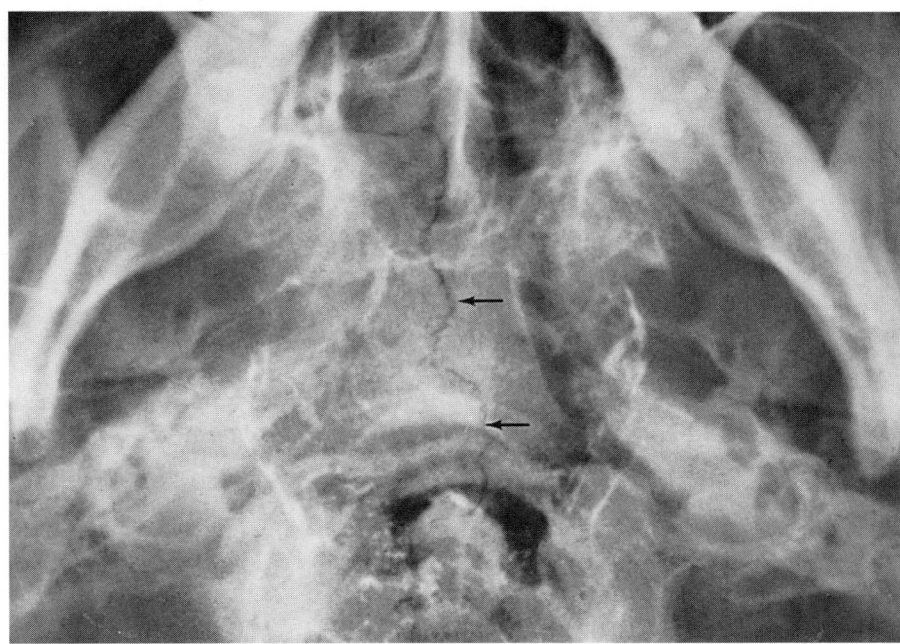

Figure 1–288. The sagittal suture, seen in the base view, simulating a fracture.

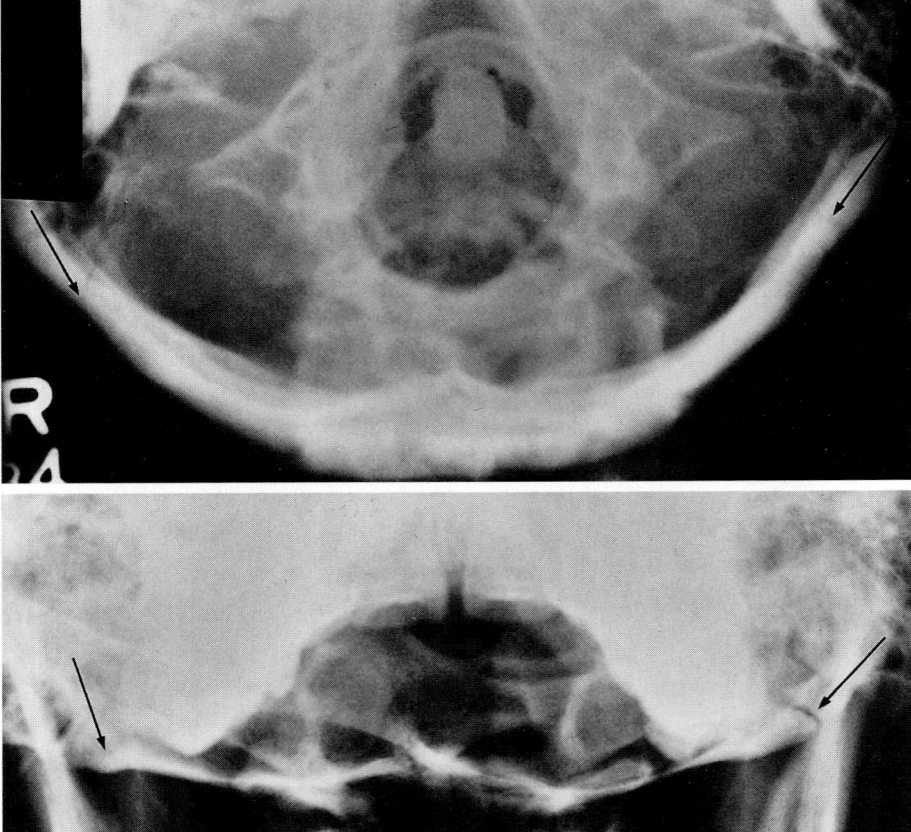

Figure 1–289. Occipitomastoid sutures in the basal views of the skull.

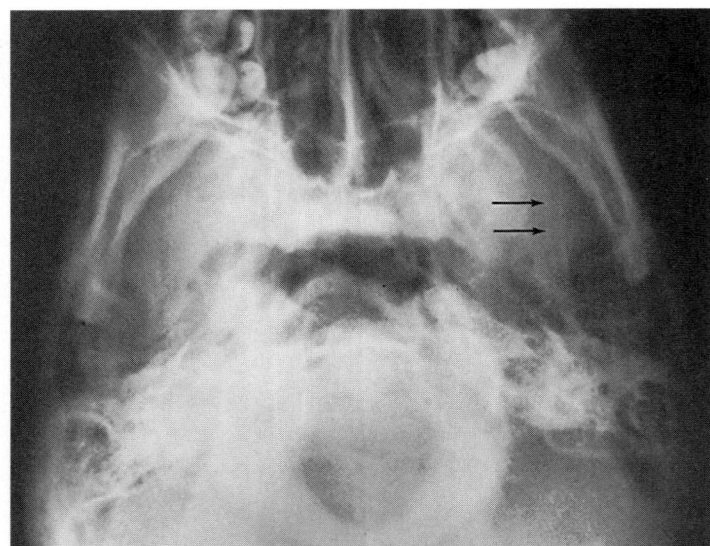

Figure 1–290. Squamosal suture in the base view.

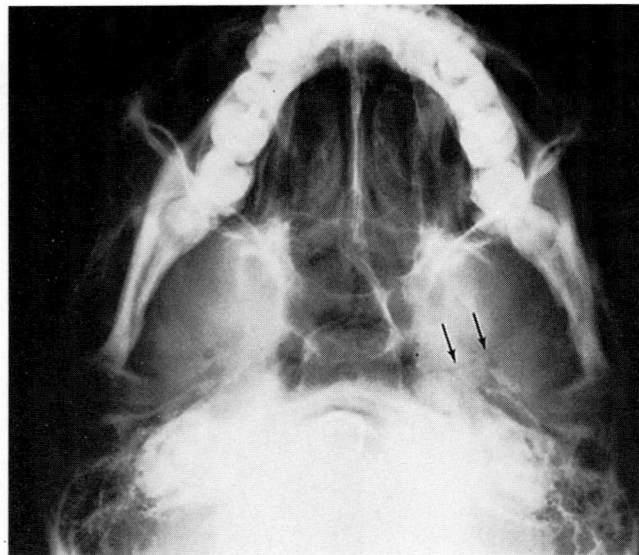

Figure 1–291. Vascular groove in the vertex of the skull, simulating a basal skull fracture.

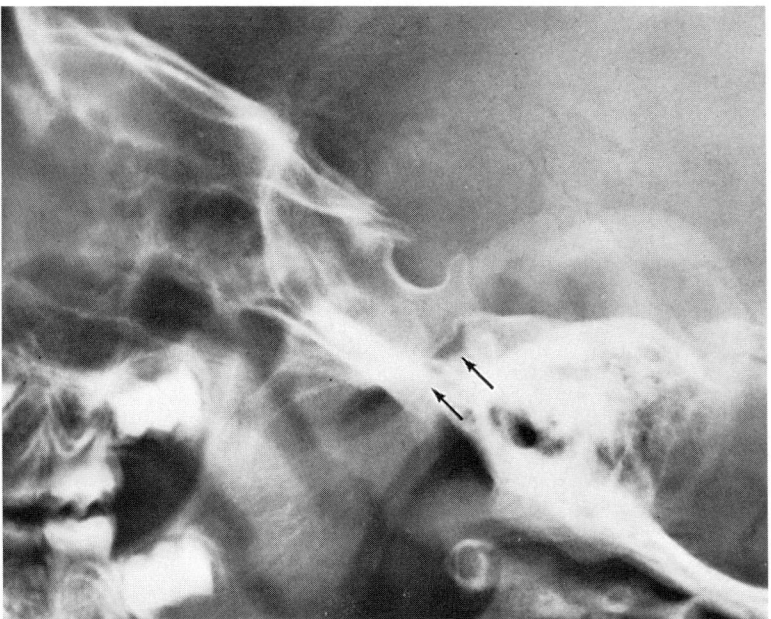

Figure 1–292. Synchondrosis between the basisphenoid and basiocciput in a 2-year-old boy. This suture normally closes near puberty but may persist until 20 years of age. It is at times mistaken for a fracture.

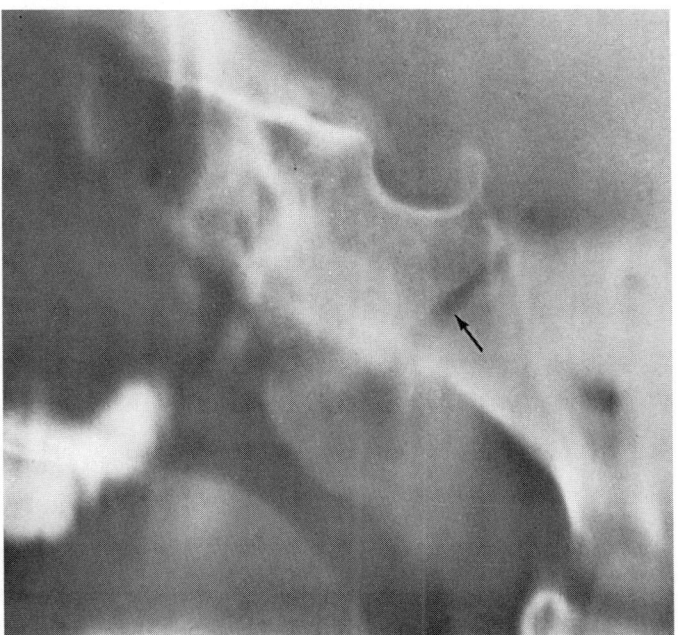

Figure 1–293. Basisphenoid-basiocciput synchondrosis in a 5-year-old girl, shown by tomography.

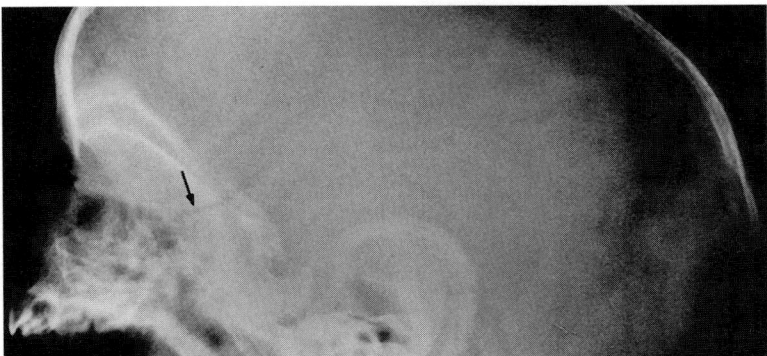

Figure 1–294. Sphenofrontal suture in a 3-month-old child.

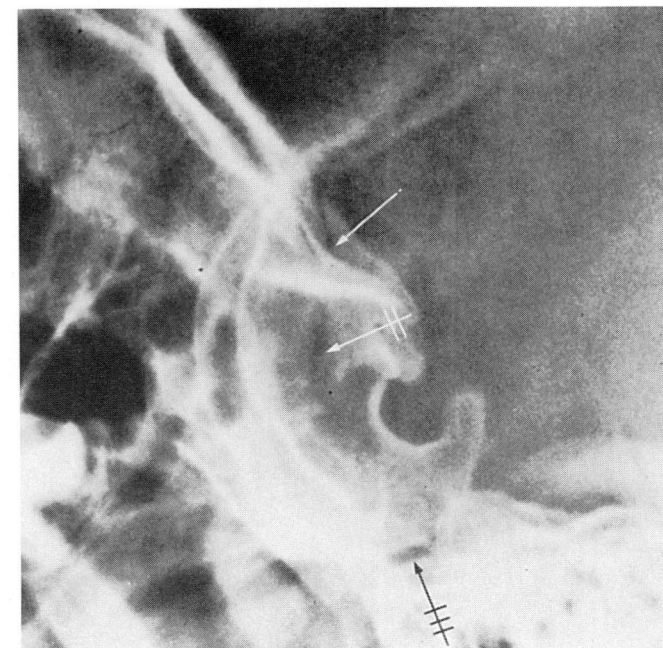

Figure 1–295. Sphenofrontal suture (←) and the sphenotemporal sutures (⇇) in an 18-month-old child. Note also the basisphenoid-basiocciput synchondrosis (⇚).

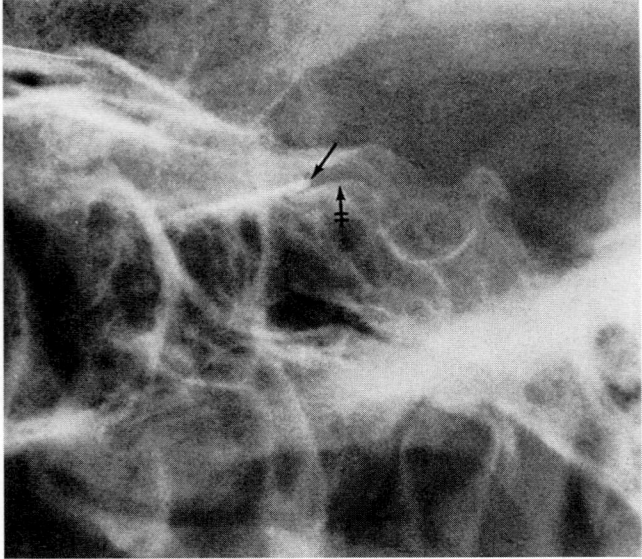

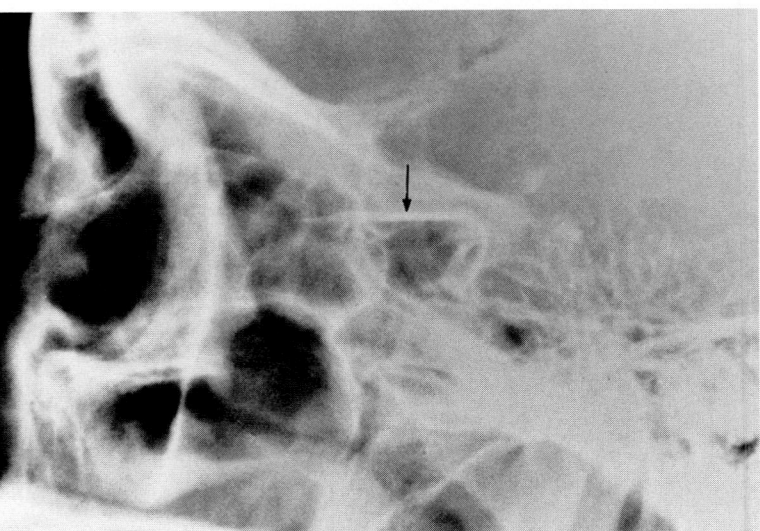

Figure 1–297. Normal planum sphenoidale for comparison with the preceding figure.

Figure 1–296. Unfused planum sphenoidale (←), simulating a fracture. This is a developmental variation. In fractures, the anterior fragment of the planum is depressed, as compared with this variation, in which the planum is superior to the chiasmatic sulcus (↔). (Ref: Smith TR, Kier EL: The unfused planum sphenoidale: Differentiation from fracture. *Radiology* 98:305, 1971.)

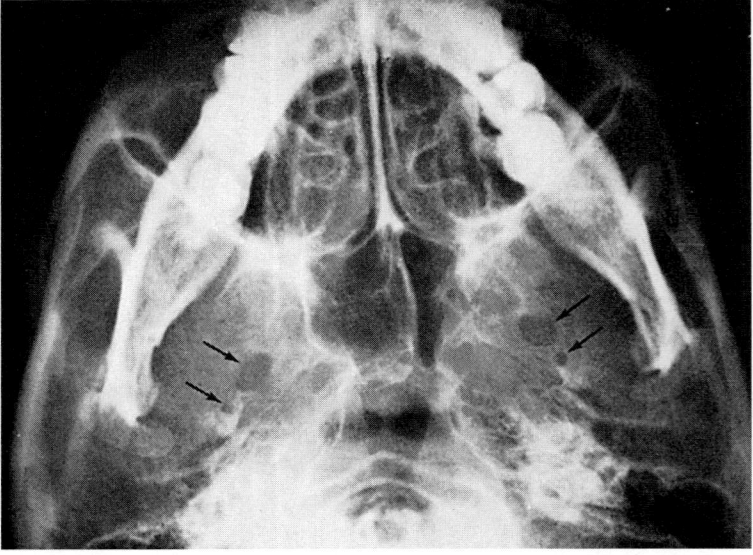

Figure 1–298. Normal asymmetry of the basal foramina. (Ref: Shapiro R, Robinson F: The foramina of the middle fossa: A phylogenetic, anatomic and pathologic study. *Am J Roentgenol* 101:779, 1967.)

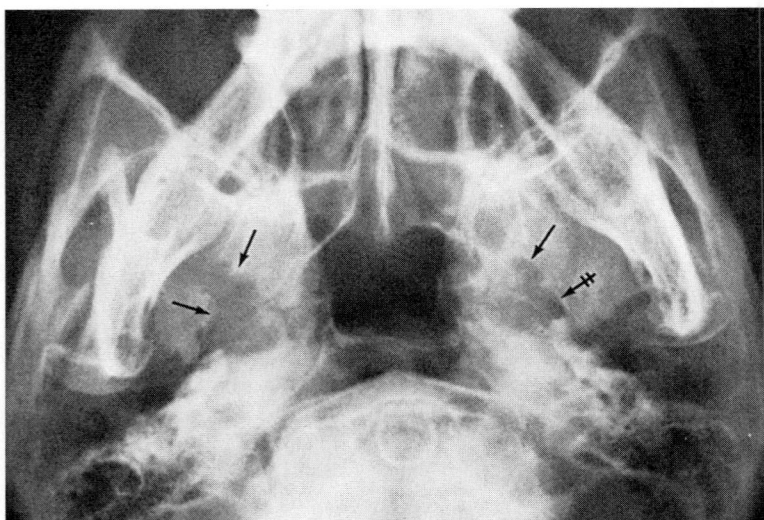

Figure 1–299. An example of striking asymmetry of the basal foramina. The foramen ovale (*upper arrows*) and the foramen spinosum (*lower arrows*) are confluent on the patient's right side, simulating destruction of the base of the skull. (Ref: Newton TH, Potts DG: *Radiology of the skull and brain,* vol. 1. St. Louis, Mosby, 1971.)

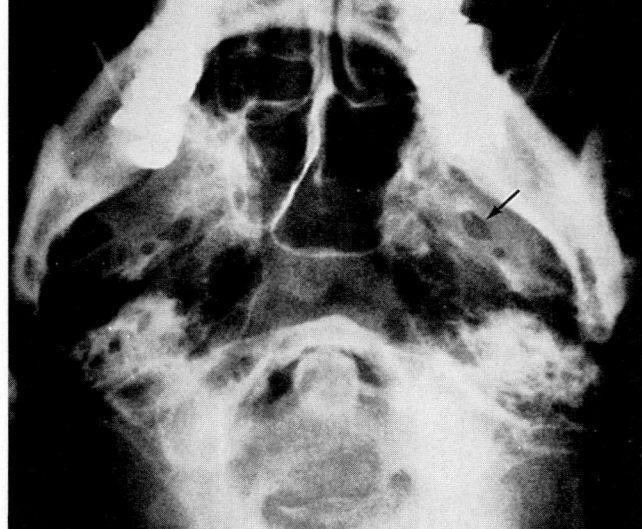

Figure 1–300. Foramen ovale with a petroalar bar. (Ref: Newton TH, Potts DG: *Radiology of the skull and brain,* vol. 1. St. Louis, Mosby, 1971.)

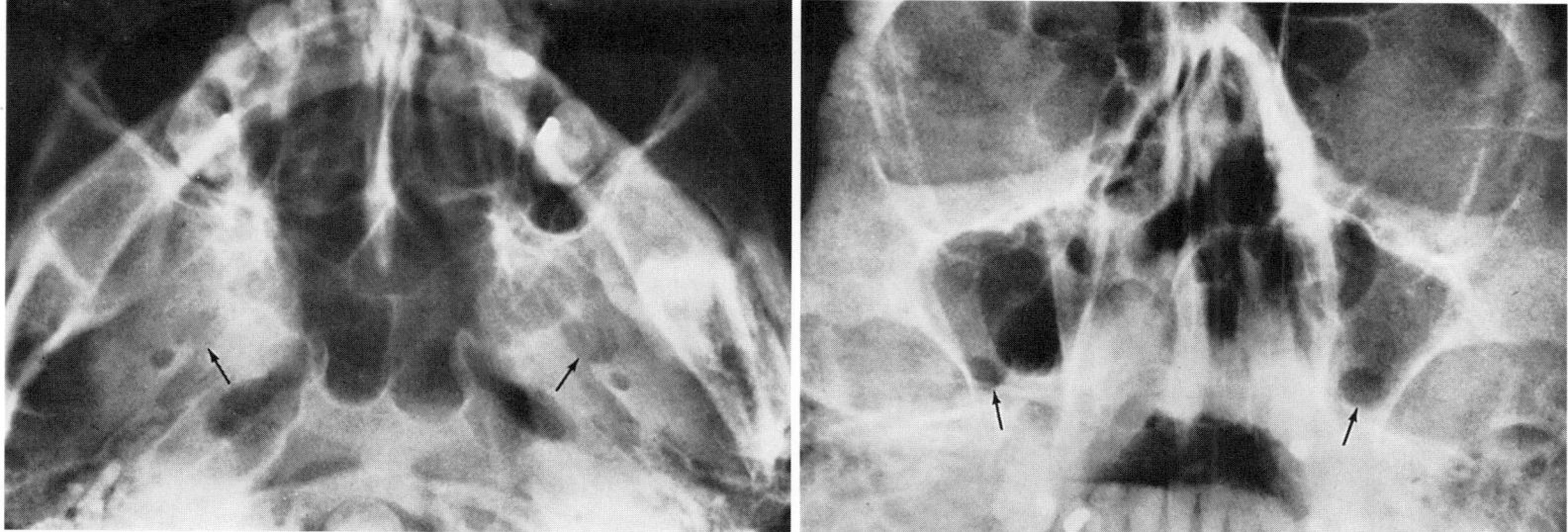

Figure 1–301. Normal asymmetry of the foramina ovale, also seen in Waters' projection on the right.

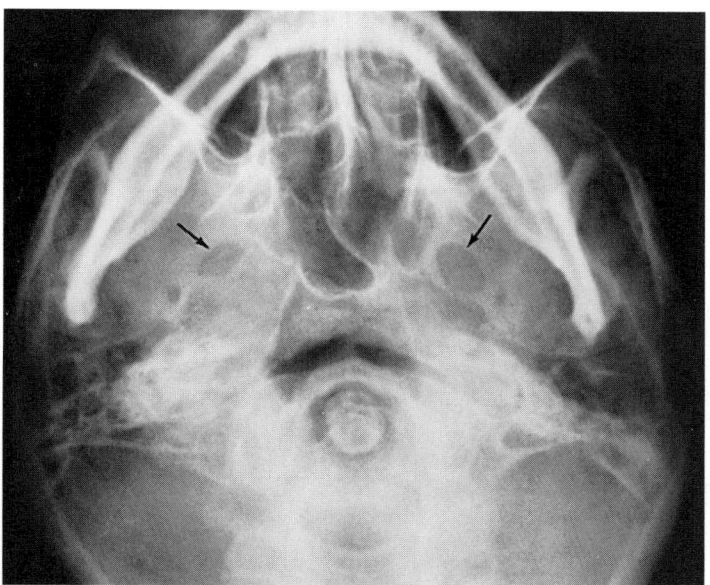

Figure 1–302. Marked asymmetric development of the foramina ovale.

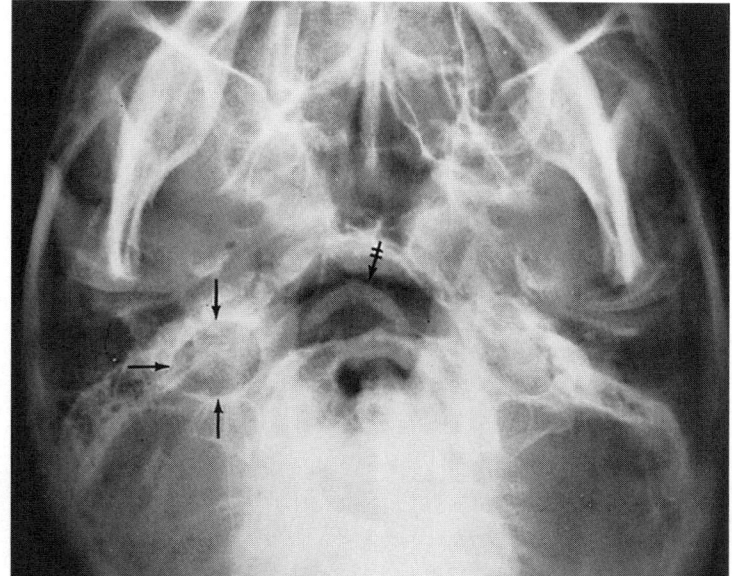

Figure 1–303. Very large jugular foramina with striking prominence on the right (←). Note the unusual shadow in the nasopharynx caused by the epiglottis (↔).

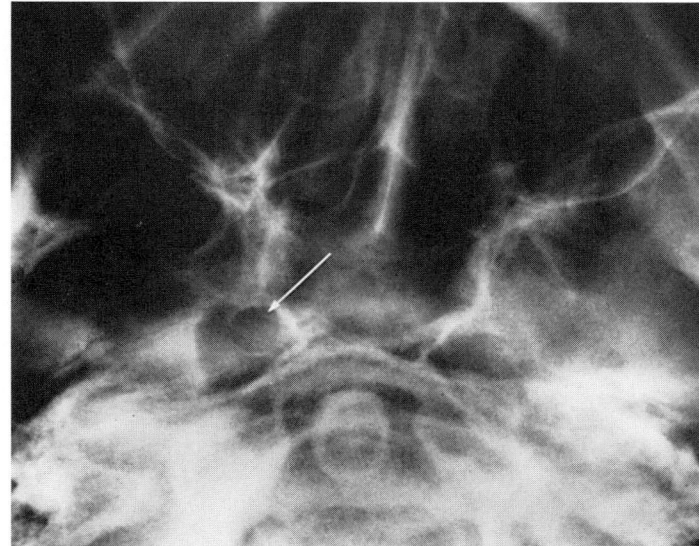

Figure 1–304. Large carotid foramen seen unilaterally.

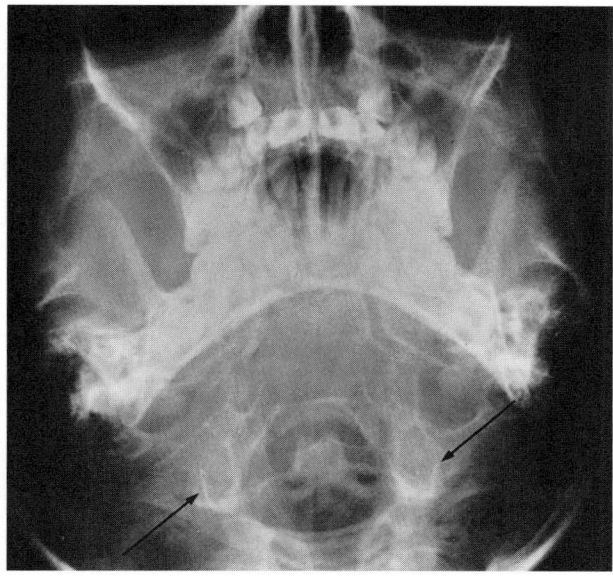

Figure 1–305. Simulated fossae produced by the rectus capitis muscle attachments.

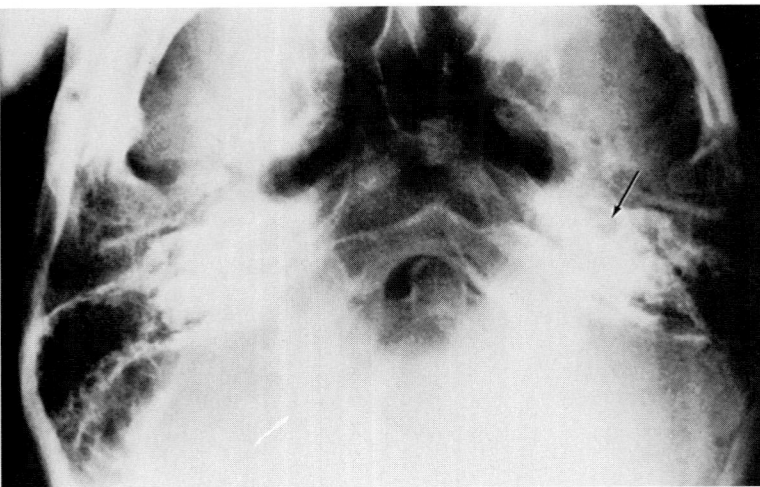

Figure 1–306. Foramen ovale with a pterygospinous bar. (Ref: Newton TH, Potts DG: *Radiology of the skull and brain,* vol. 1. St. Louis, Mosby, 1971.)

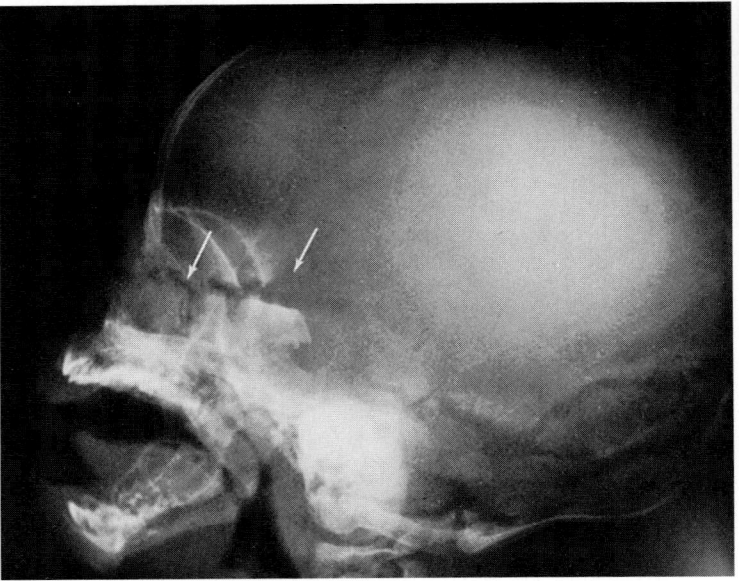

Figure 1–307. Junction of the frontal and ethmoid bones in a 3-month-old child might be mistaken for a fracture.

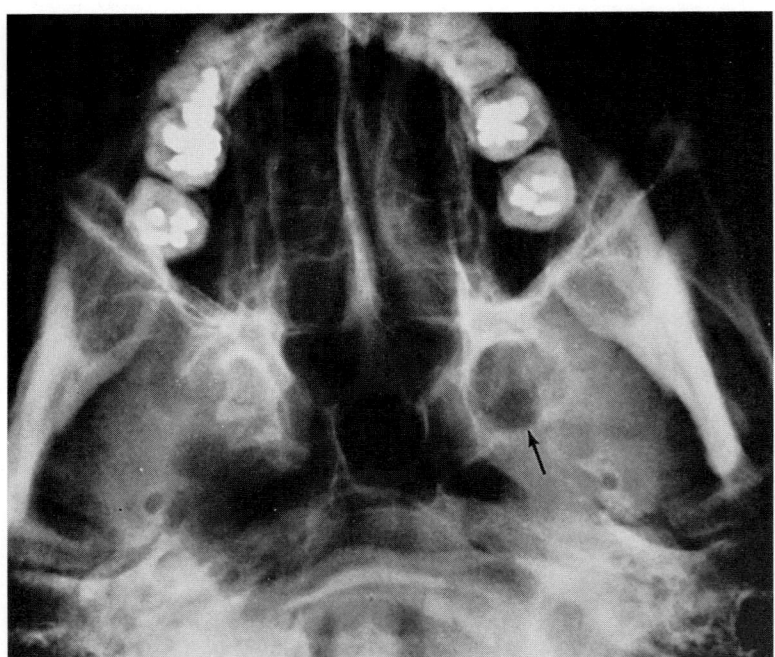

Figure 1–308. Large sphenoidal air cell, simulating an enlarged basal foramen.

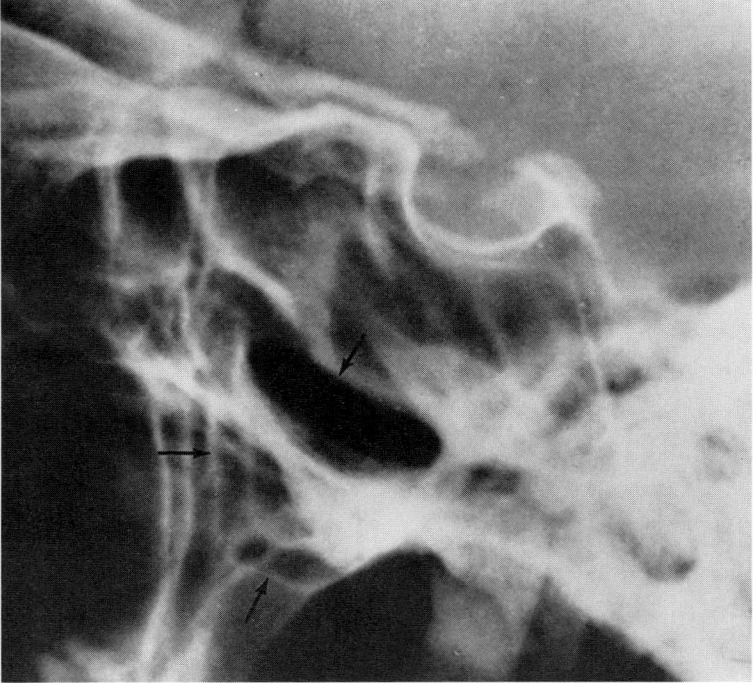

Figure 1–309. Pneumatization of the pterygoid bones producing unusual radiolucency in the base of the skull.

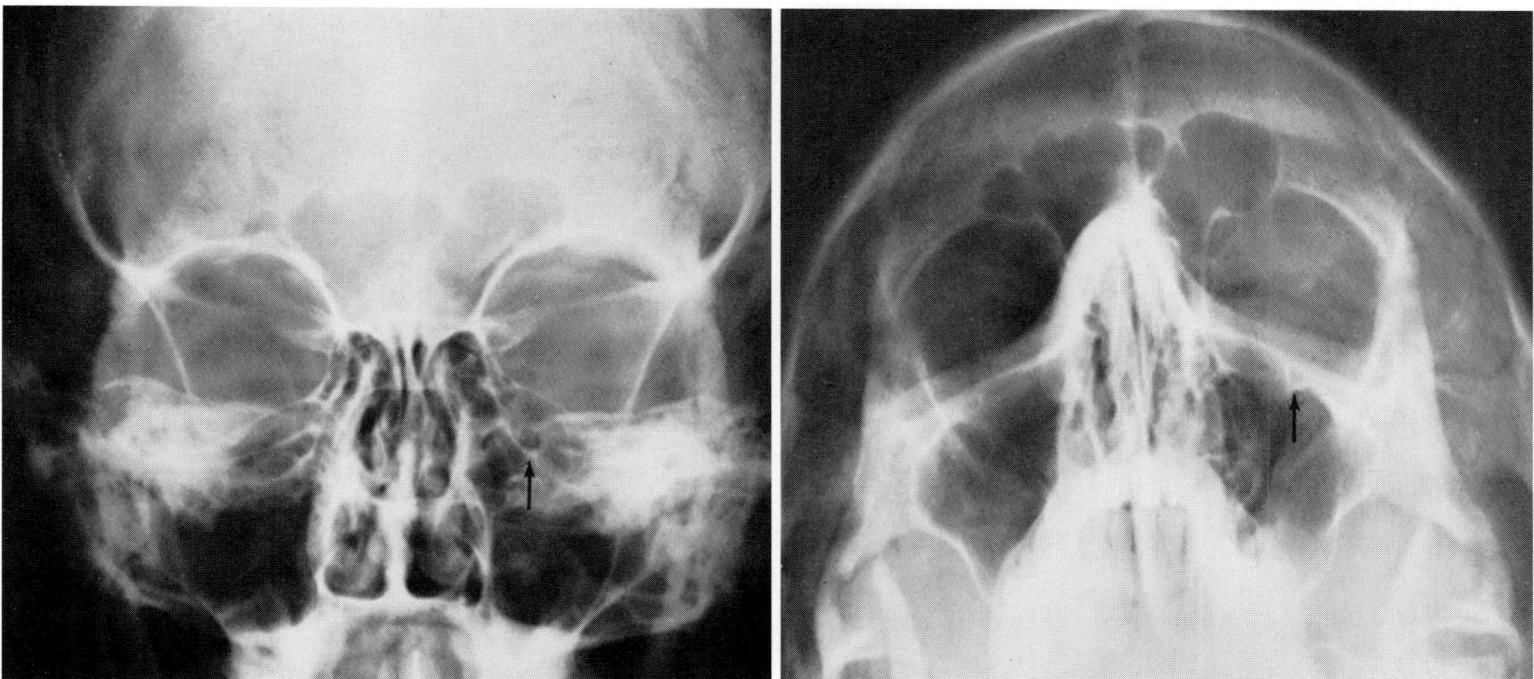

Figure 1–310. Normal asymmetry of foramina rotunda seen in Caldwell's projection *(left)* and asymmetry of the infraorbital foramina seen in Waters' projection *(right)*.

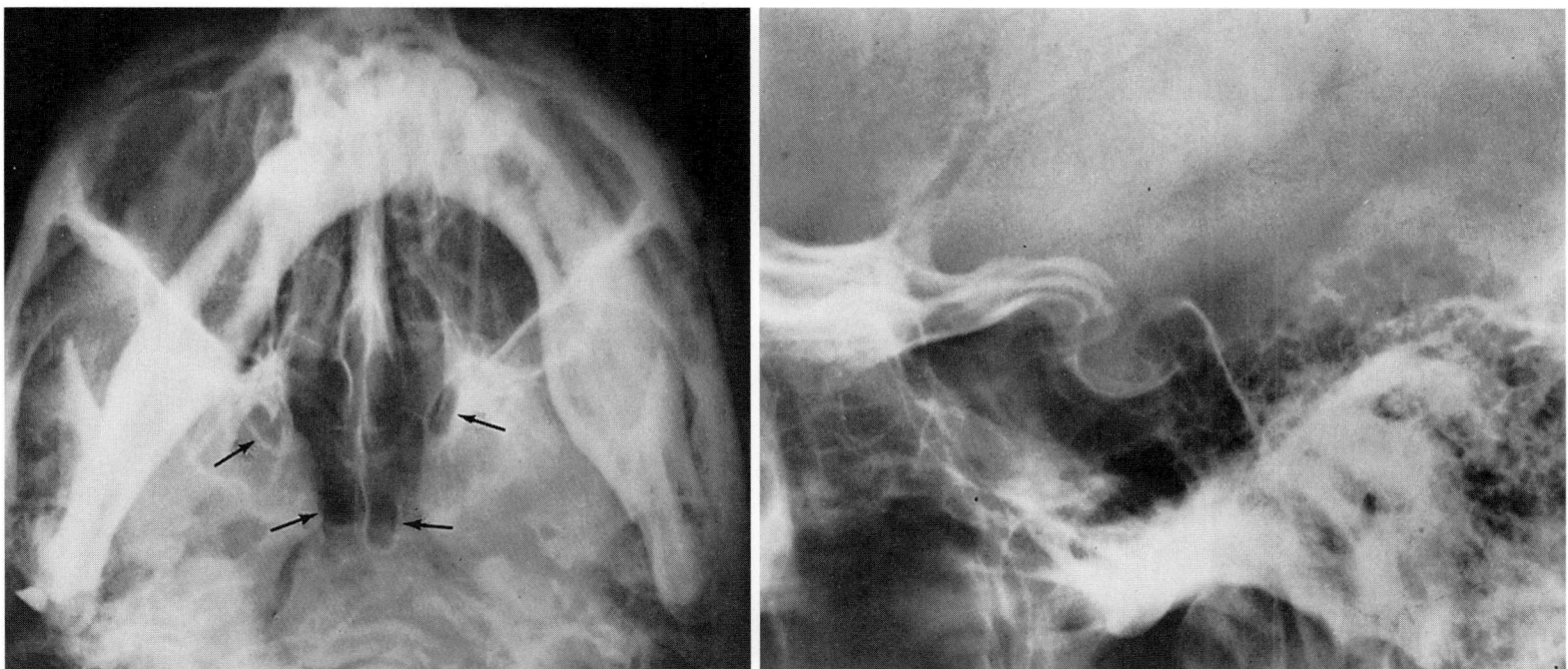

Figure 1–311. Pneumatization of the clinoid processes may produce spurious foramen-like shadows in the basal view.

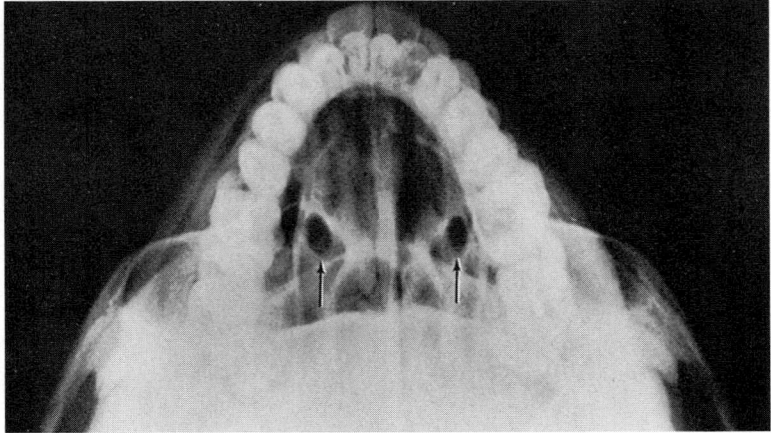

Figure 1–312. Nasolacrimal canals.

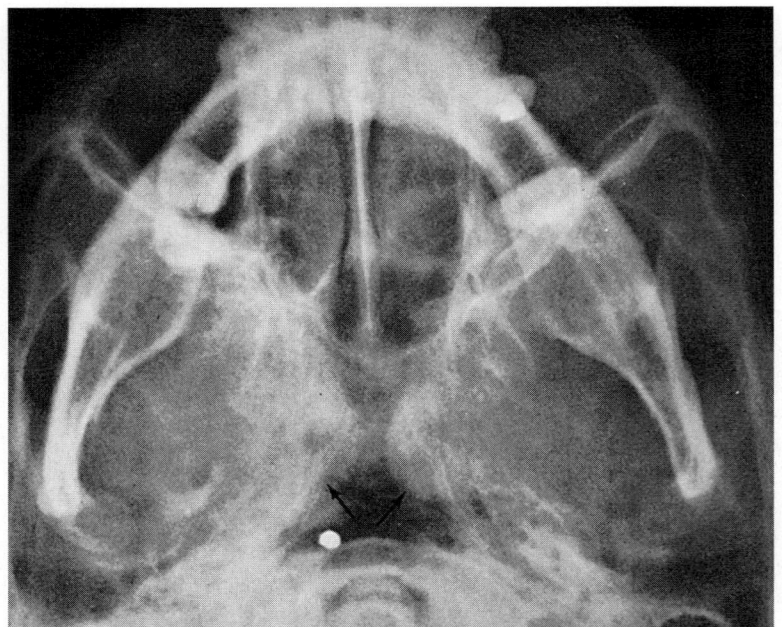

Figure 1–313. Soft tissue masses seen in the nasopharyngeal air shadow, representing large pharyngeal tonsils.

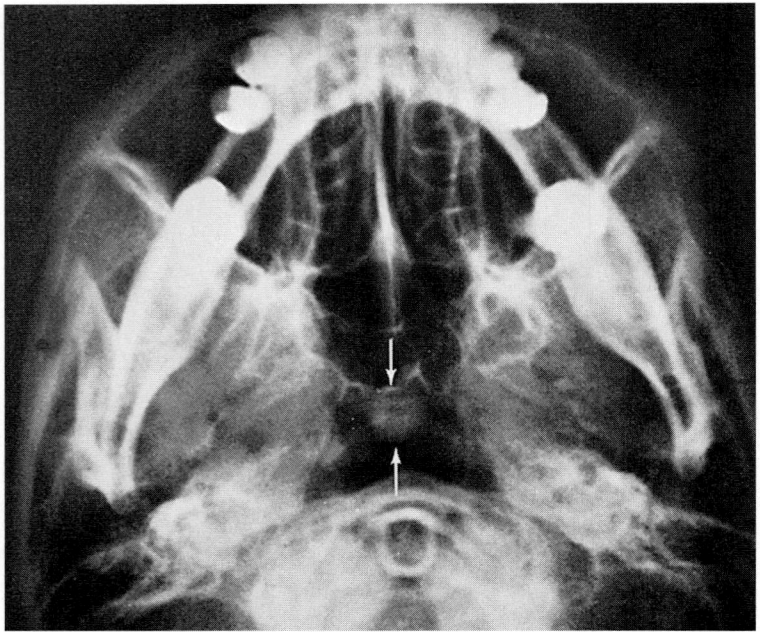

Figure 1–314. Uvula seen in the nasopharyngeal air shadow.

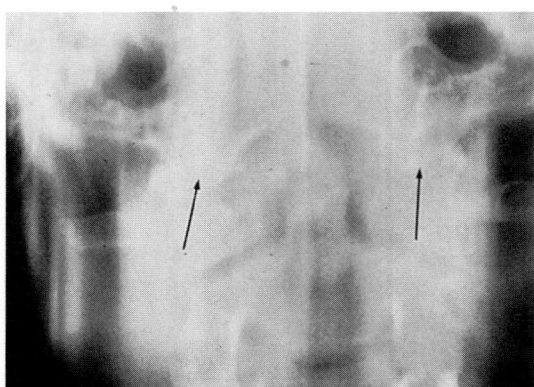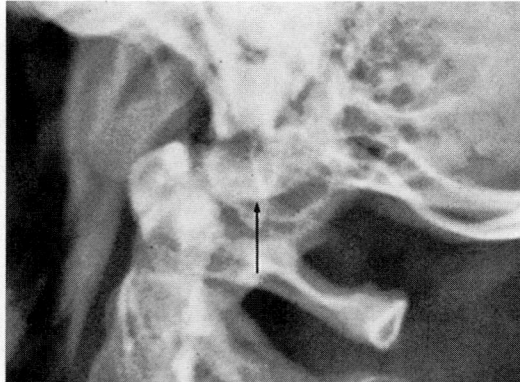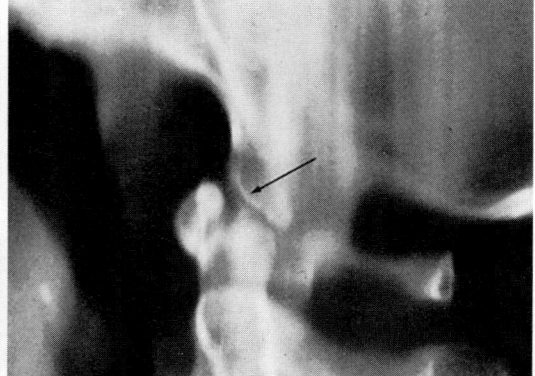

Figure 1–315. Large occipital condyles. *Left,* AP projection. *Center,* Lateral projection. *Right,* Tomogram.

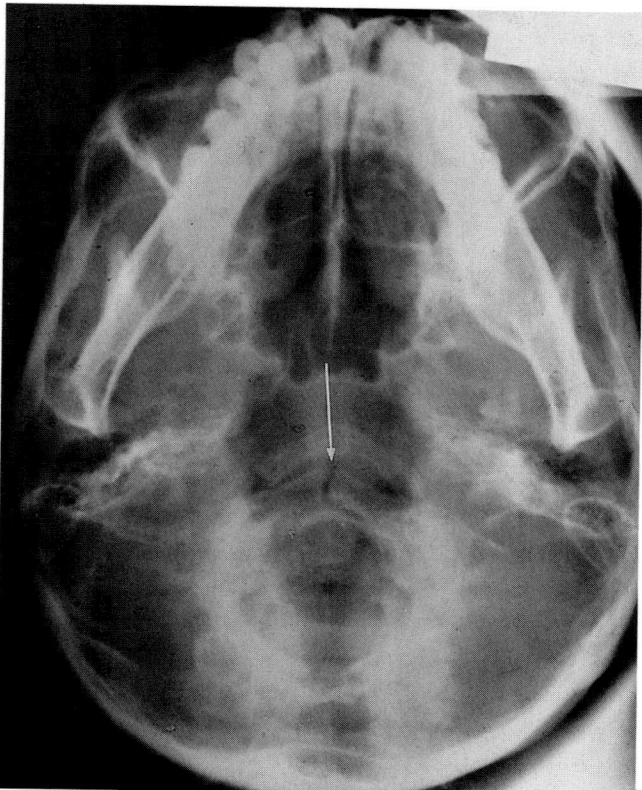

Figure 1–316. Unfused anterior arch of C1 vertebra in a basal view of the skull.

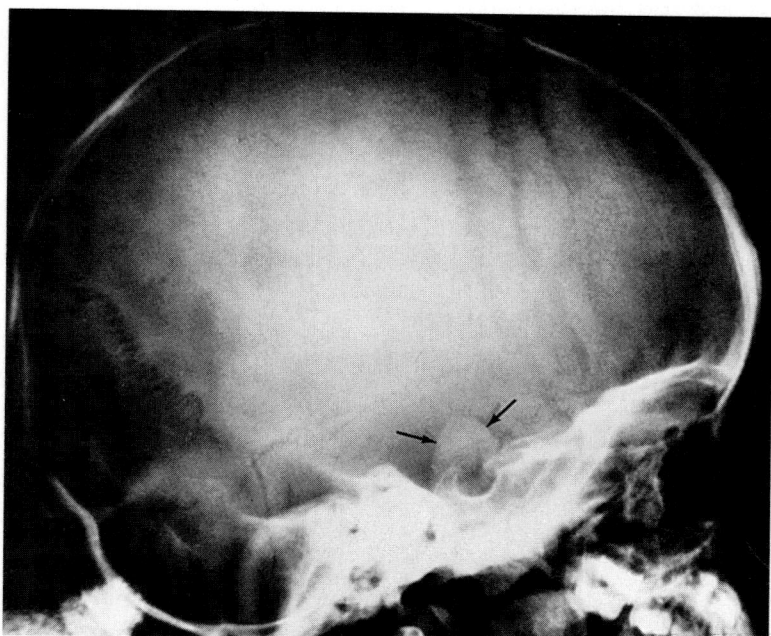

Figure 1–317. Shadow of the folded ear, simulating suprasellar calcification.

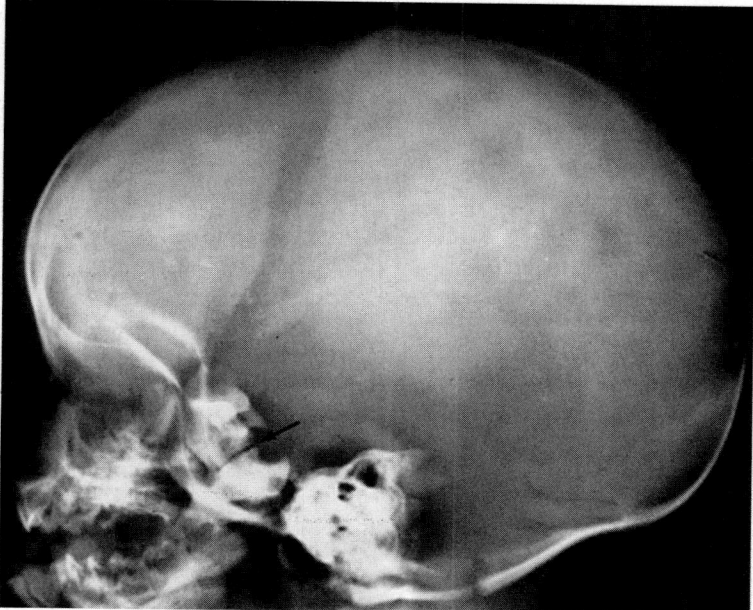

Figure 1–318. Intersphenoidal synchondrosis in a newborn. This entity should not be mistaken for a fracture, a persistent basipharyngeal canal, or the spheno-occipital synchondrosis. It has no pathologic significance and usually disappears by 3 years of age. (Ref: Shopfner CE et al: The intersphenoid synchondrosis. *Am J Roentgenol* 104:184, 1968.)

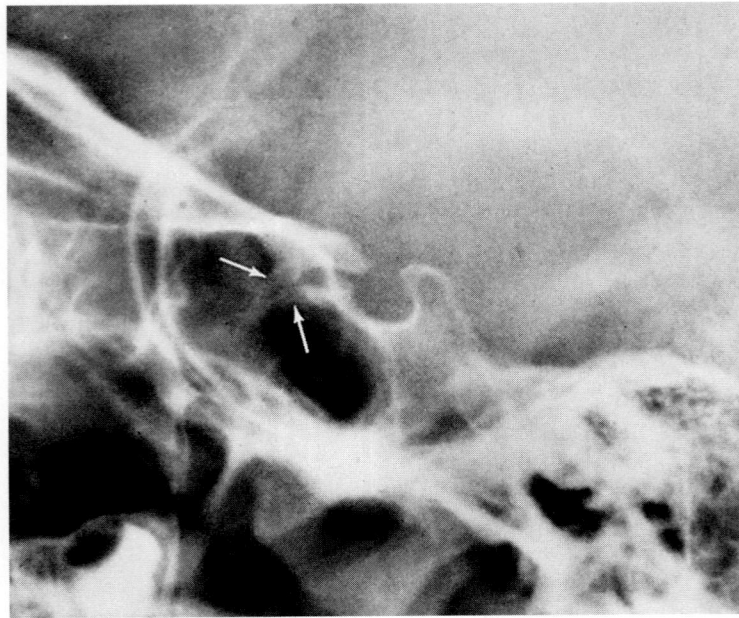

Figure 1–319. Partially obliterated intersphenoidal synchondrosis in a 2-year-old child.

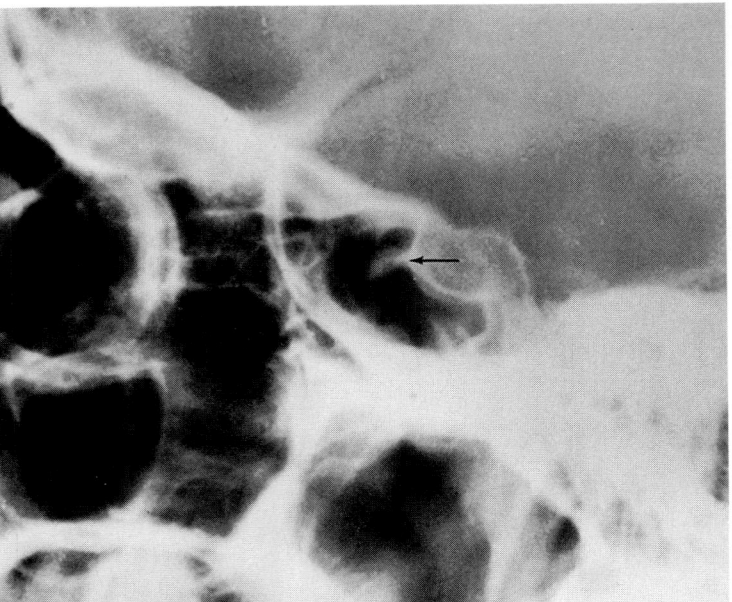

Figure 1–320. Obliterated intersphenoidal synchondrosis in an adult.

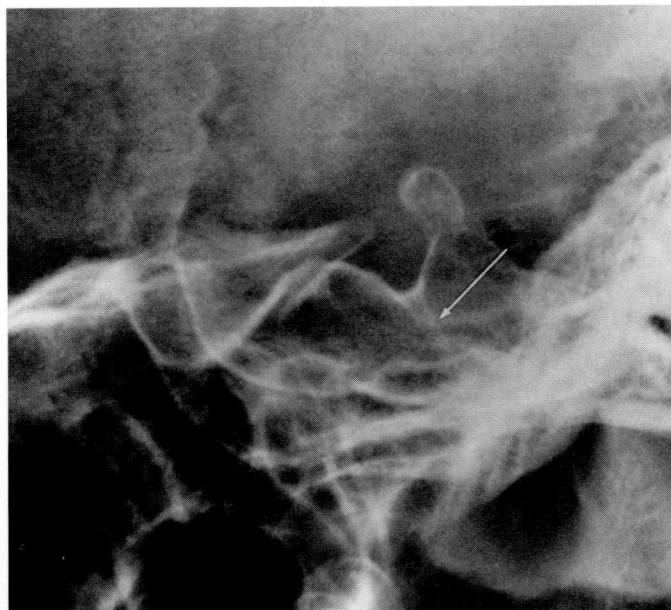

Figure 1–321. Basipharyngeal canal in a 10-year-old boy.

The Sella Turcica

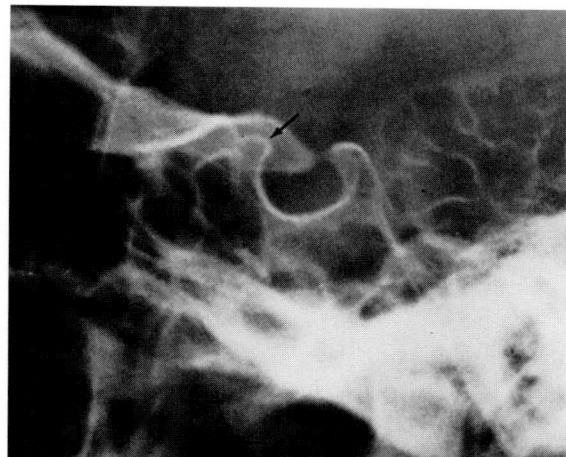

Figure 1–322. Large normal tuberculum sellae.

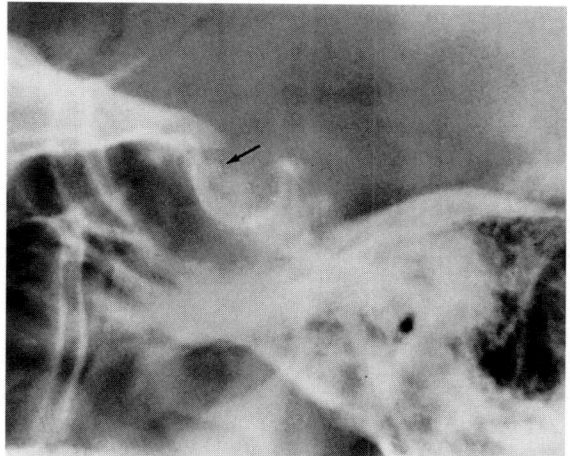

Figure 1–323. Well-defined middle clinoid process.

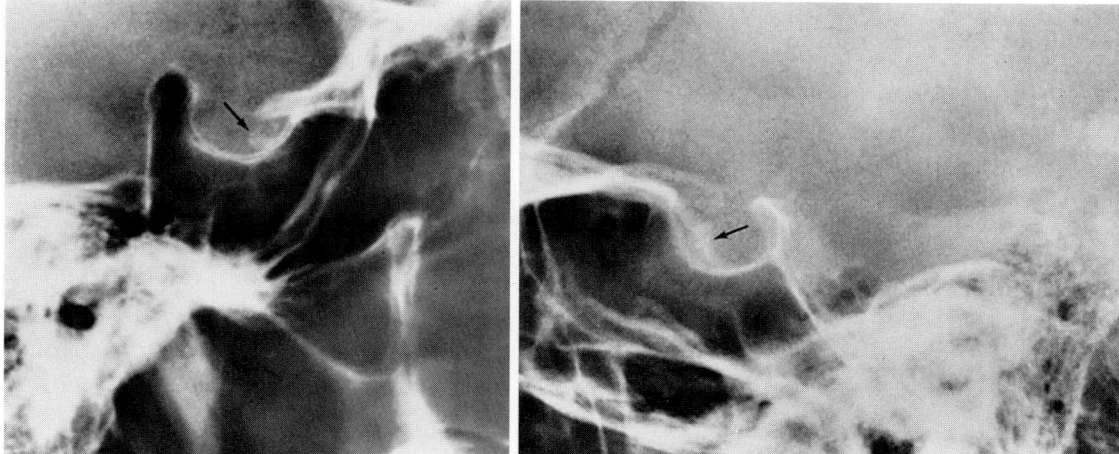

Figure 1–324. Additional examples of prominent middle clinoid processes.

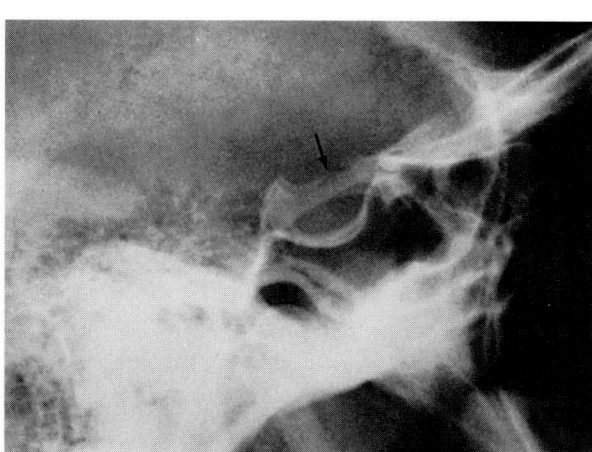

Figure 1–325. Bridging of the sella caused by calcification of the interclinoid ligaments.

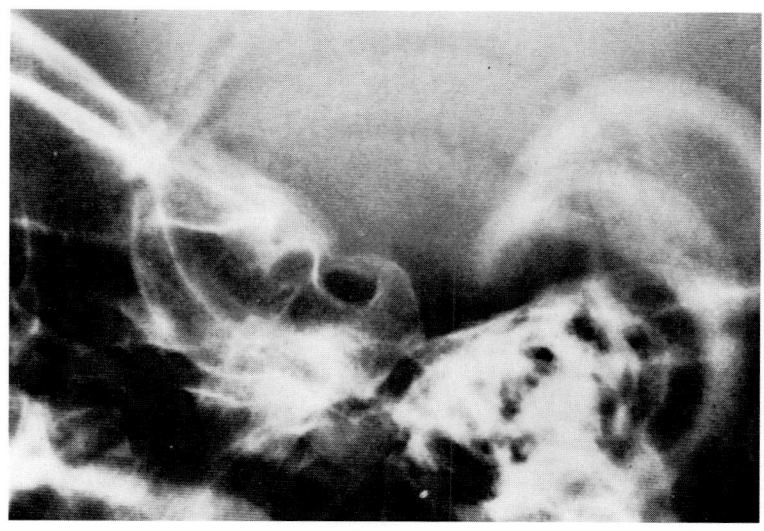

Figure 1–326. Bridging of the sella in a 5½-month-old child.

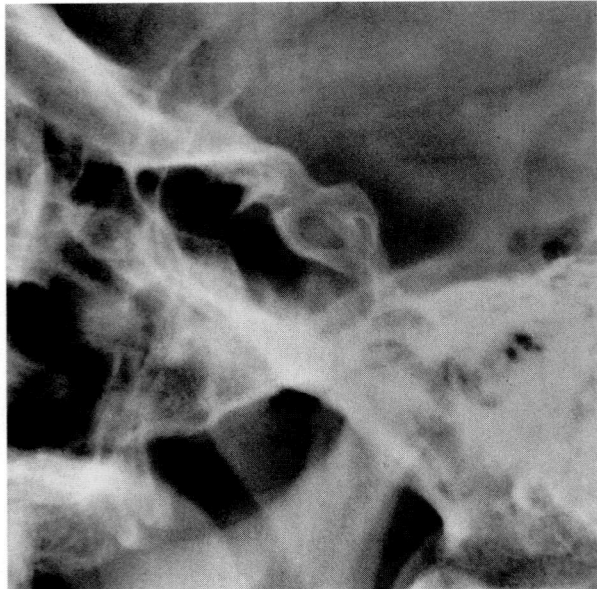

Figure 1–327. Heavy bridging of the sella turcica.

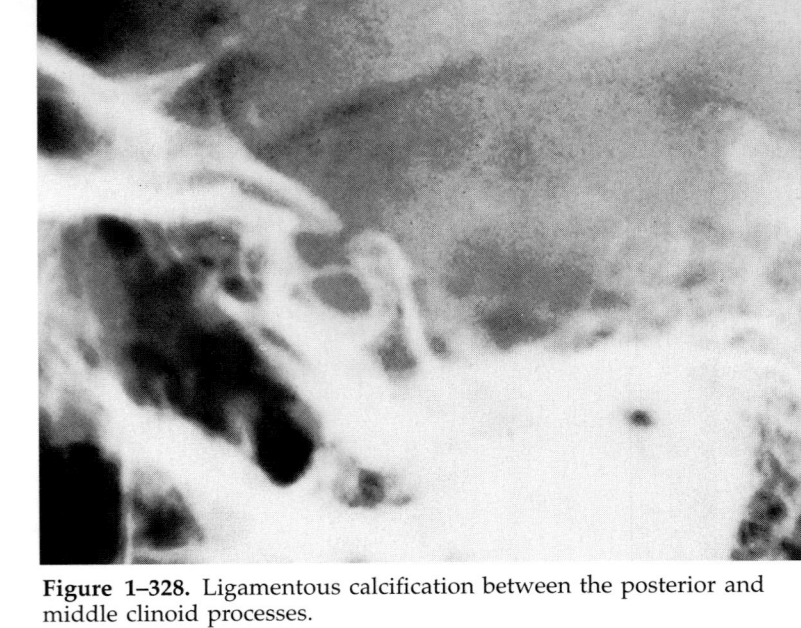

Figure 1–328. Ligamentous calcification between the posterior and middle clinoid processes.

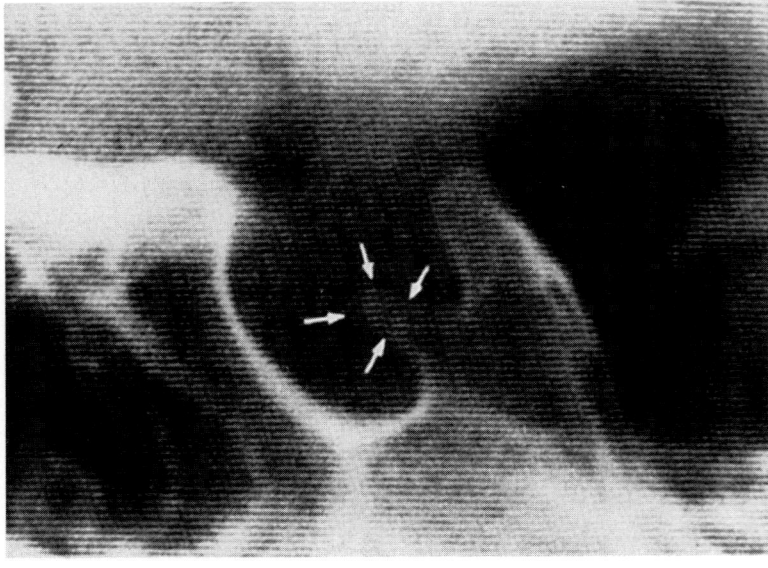

Figure 1–329. Sellar spine, an anatomic variant of no clinical significance. (From: Dietemann JL et al: Anatomy and radiology of the sellar spine. *Neuroradiology* 21:5, 1981.)

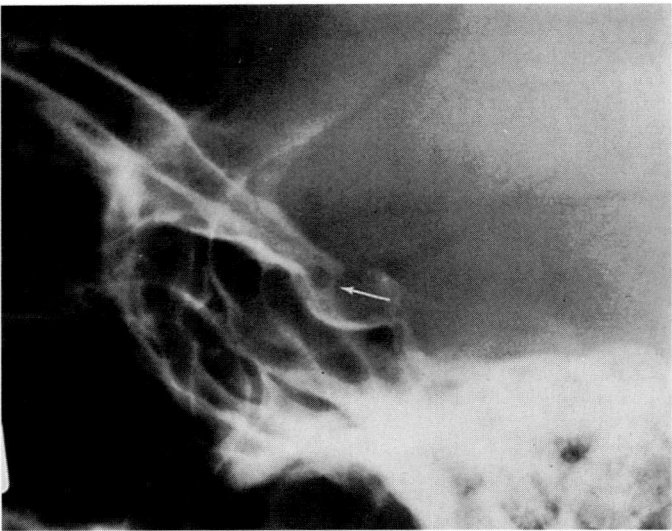

Figure 1–330. Bridging between the anterior and middle clinoid processes.

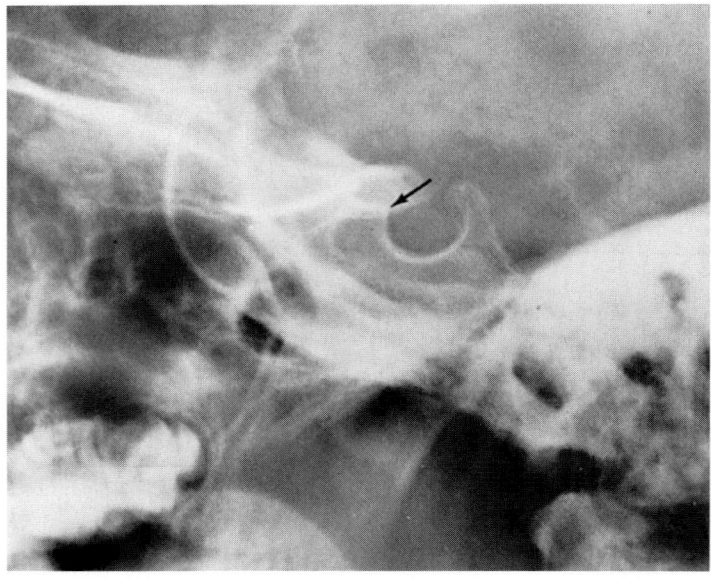

Figure 1–331. Well-defined tuberculum sellae.

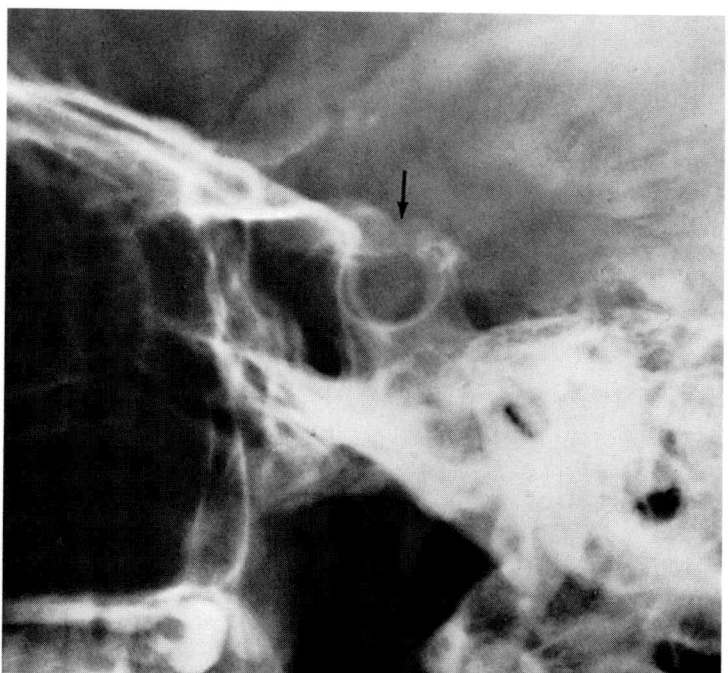

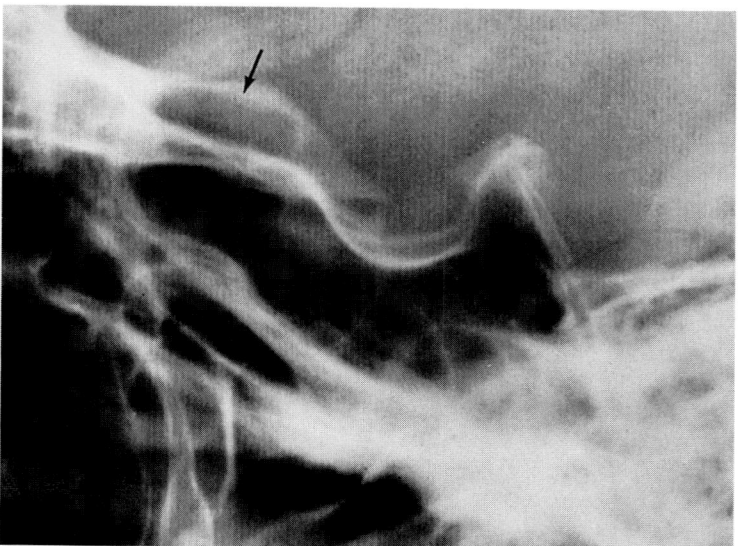

Figure 1–333. Pneumatization of the planum sphenoidale, producing an unusual appearance.

Figure 1–332. Very large clinoid processes, producing apparent bridging of the sella.

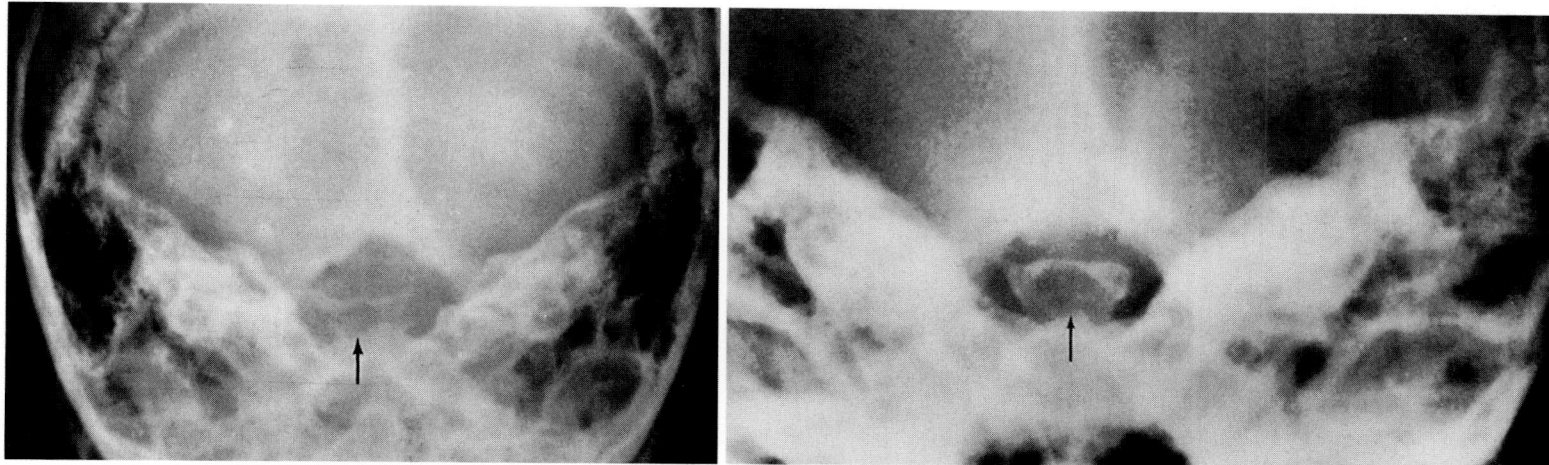

Figure 1–334. Two examples of the radiolucency of a thin dorsum sellae, simulating a destructive process.

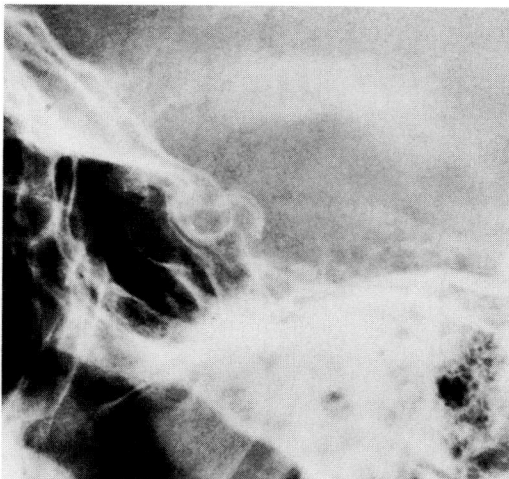

Figure 1–335. Mushroom configuration of the posterior clinoid processes.

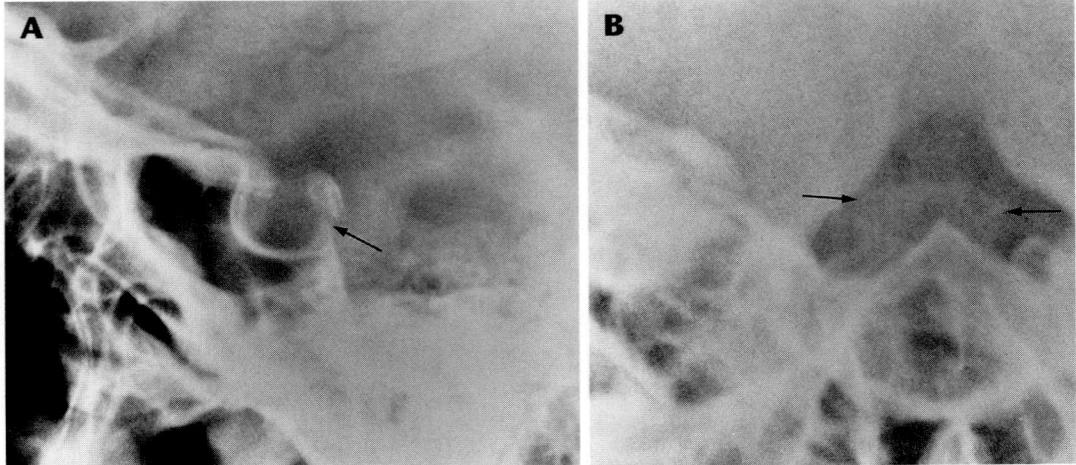

Figure 1–336. A, B, Apparent cleft in the posterior clinoids secondary to lateral extensions of the dorsum sellae (*arrows* in **B**).

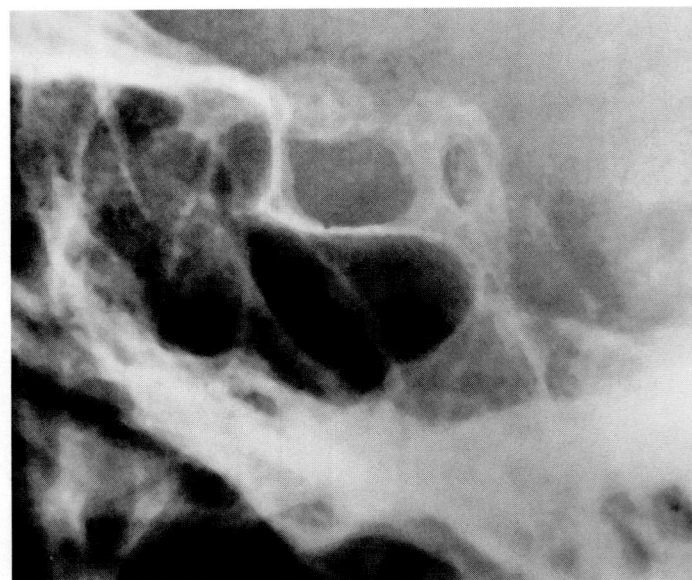

Figure 1–337. Unusual appearance of the dorsum sellae caused by heavy calcification of the petroclinoid ligament.

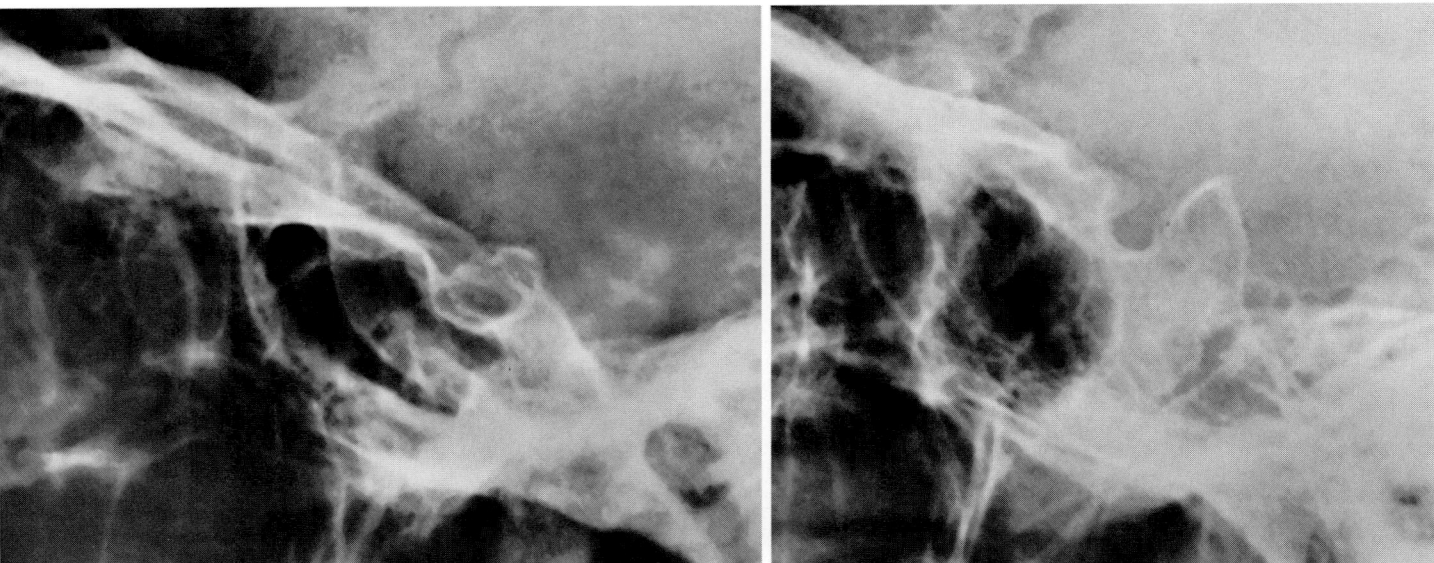

Figure 1–338. Normal variations in the shape of the sella turcica. Tiny sellae may normally be seen. (Ref: Swanson HA, Du Boulay G: Borderline variants of the normal pituitary fossa. *Br J Radiol* 48:366, 1975.)

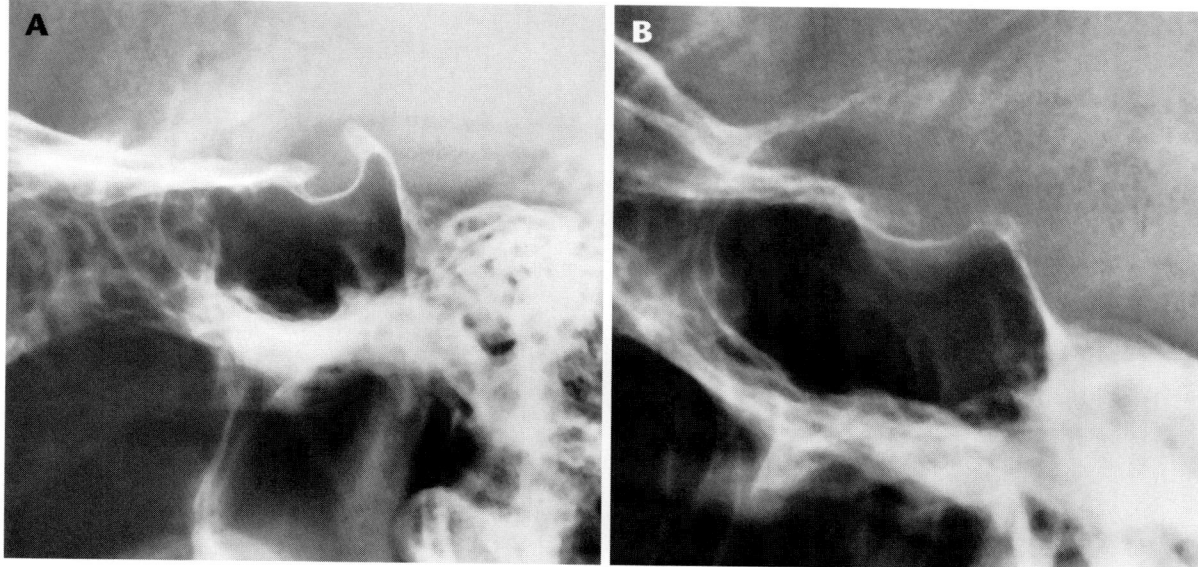

Figure 1–339. Normal variations in the shape of the sella turcica. **A,** The small sella. **B,** The shallow sella.

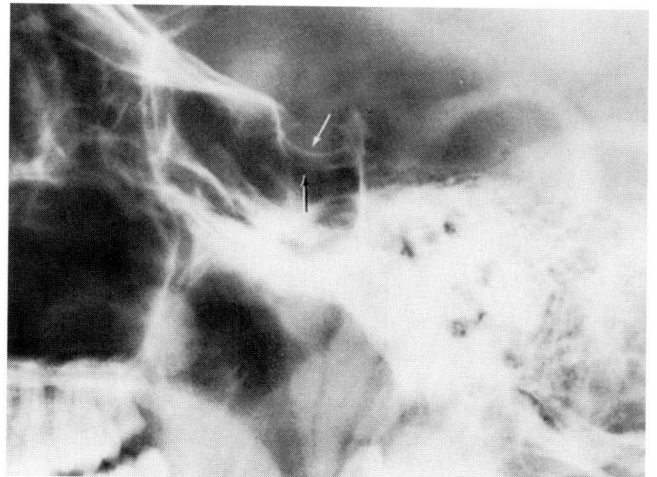

Figure 1–340. Double floor of the sella, produced by filming in less than true lateral projection.

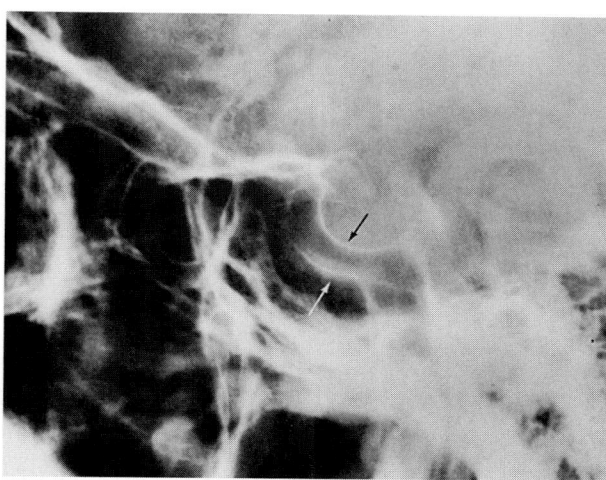

Figure 1–341. Double floor of the sella, simulated by the carotid groove.

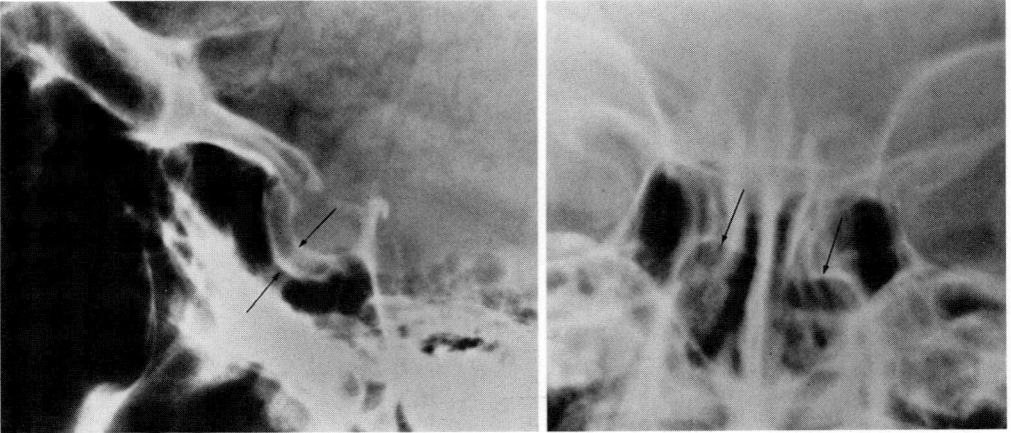

Figure 1–342. Double floor of the sella due to inclination of the sella. (Ref: Tenner MS, Weitzman I Jr: Pitfalls in the diagnosis of erosive changes in the expanding lesions of the pituitary fossa. *Radiology* 137:393, 1980.)

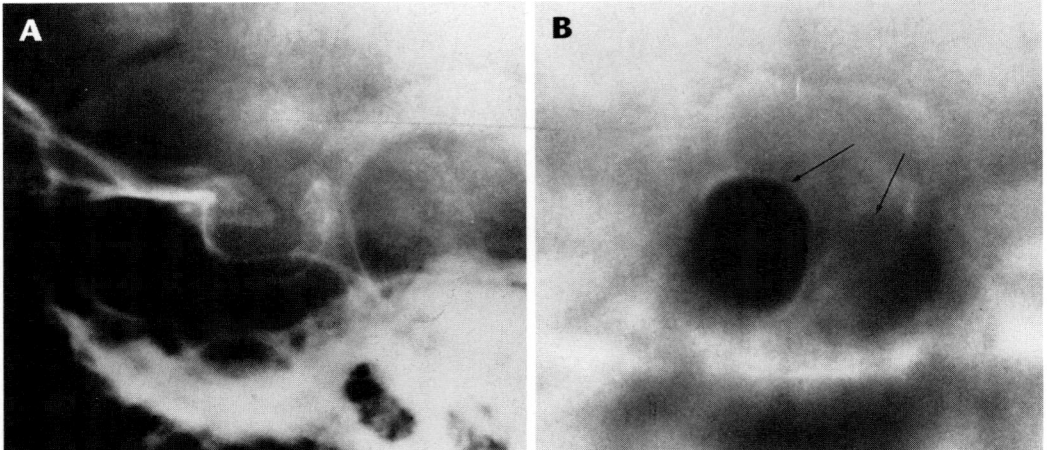

Figure 1–343. Double floor of the sella due to unequal sphenoid sinus development. **A,** Lateral projection. **B,** AP tomogram. (Ref: Bruneton JN et al: Normal variants of the sella turcica. *Radiology* 131:99, 1979.)

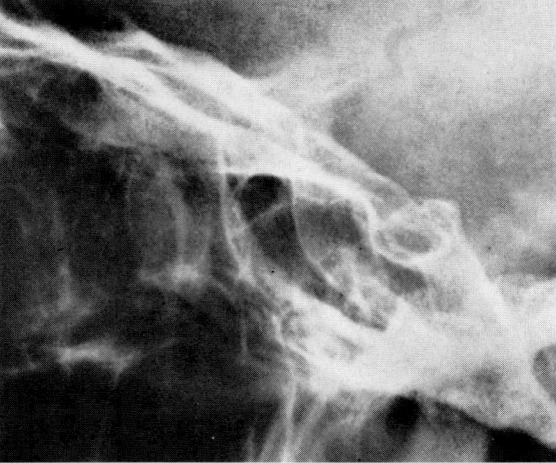

Figure 1–344. Normal variation of the sella turcica. Note the small bridged sella.

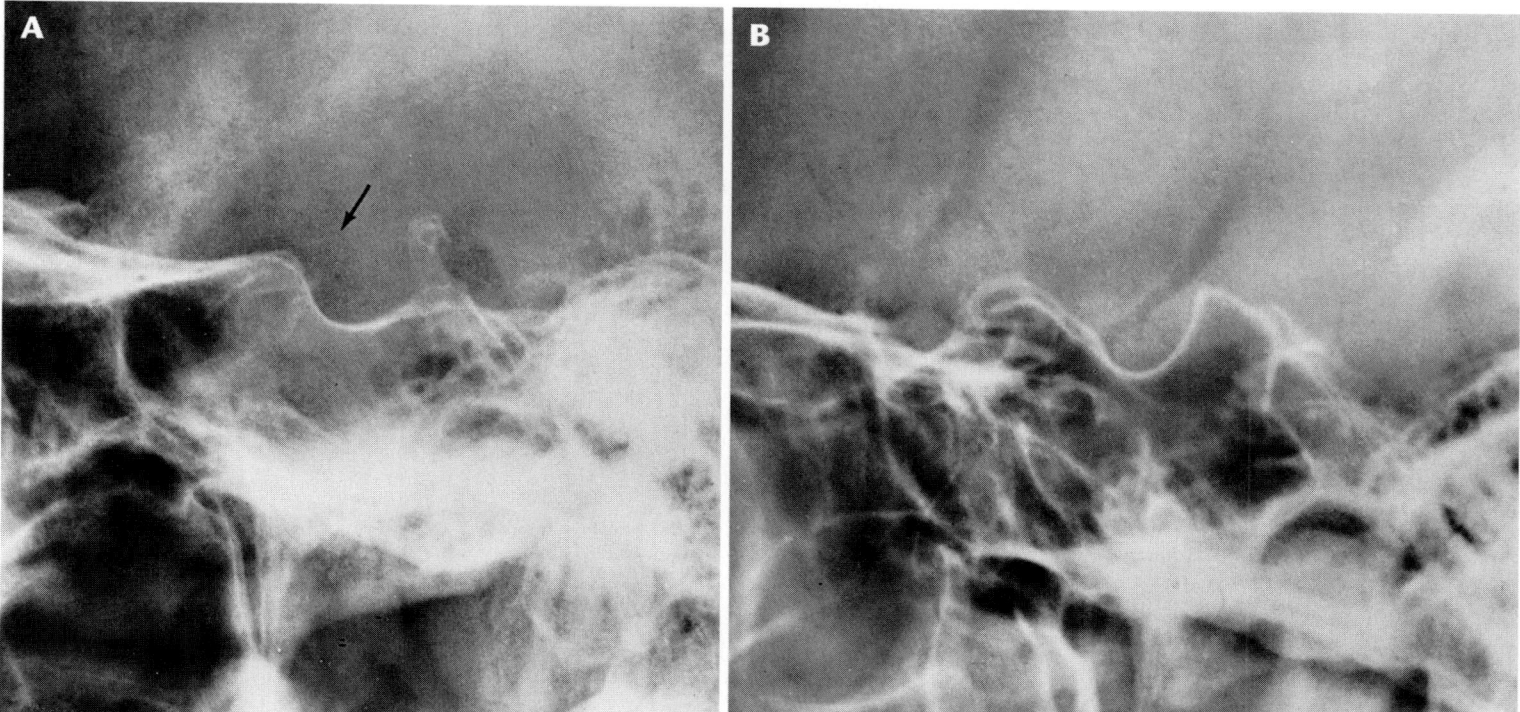

Figure 1–345. Normal variations of the sella turcica. **A,** Hidden anterior clinoid processes caused by pneumatization. **B,** Extensive pneumatization of the clinoid processes and dorsum sellae.

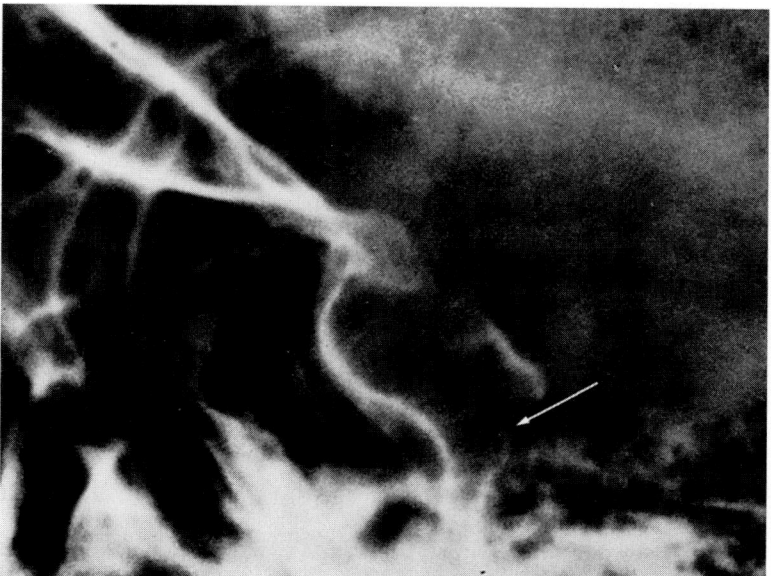

Figure 1–346. Extensive pneumatization of the dorsum sellae, simulating erosion.

CHAPTER 2

The Facial Bones

The Orbits

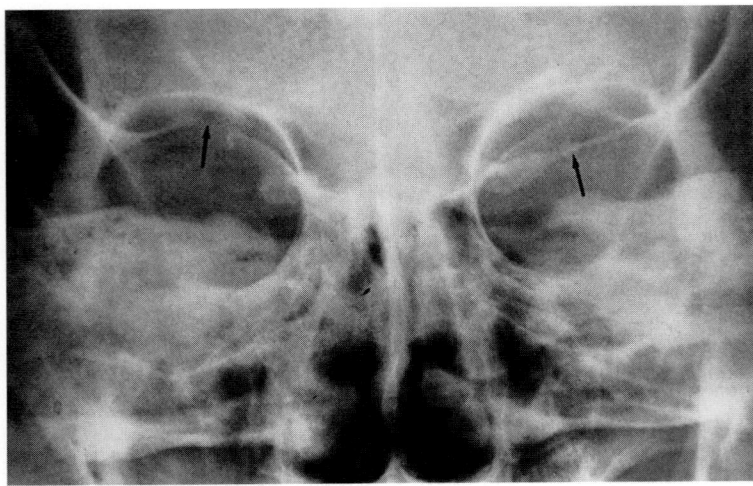

Figure 2–1. Normal asymmetry of the lesser wings of the sphenoid.

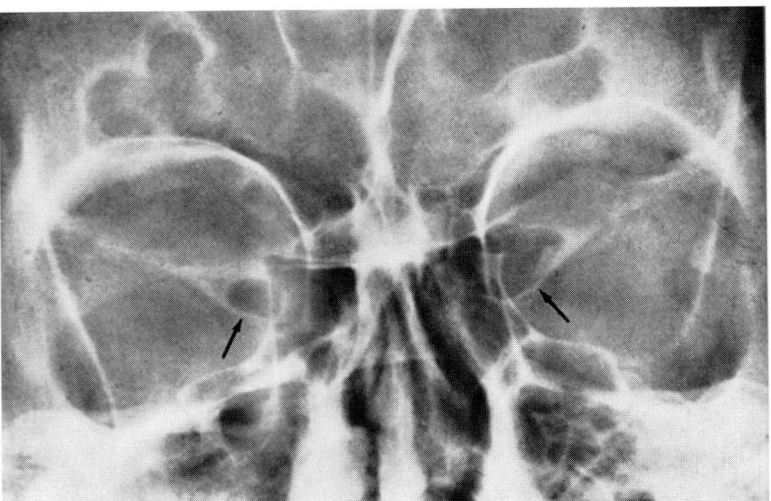

Figure 2–2. Pneumatization of the anterior clinoid processes, simulating enlargement of the optic canals.

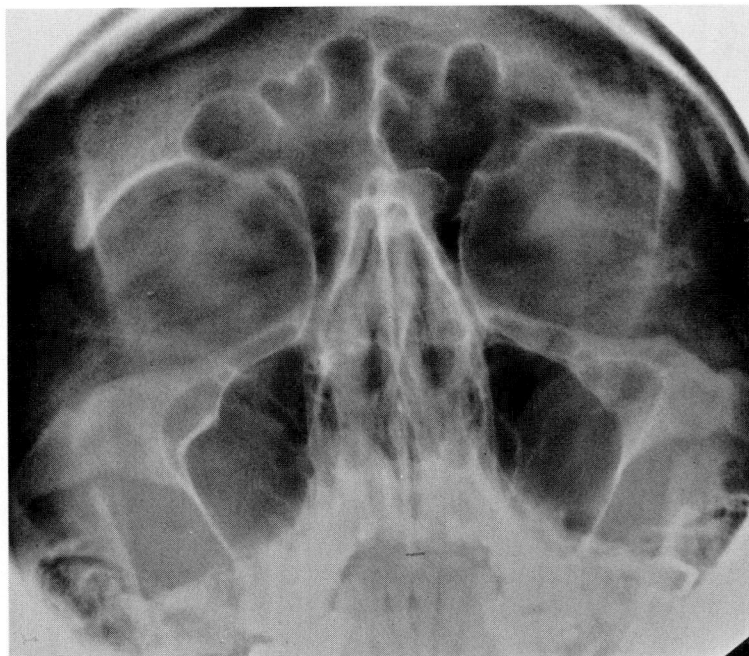

Figure 2–3. Bilateral congenital absence of the orbital processes of the zygoma.

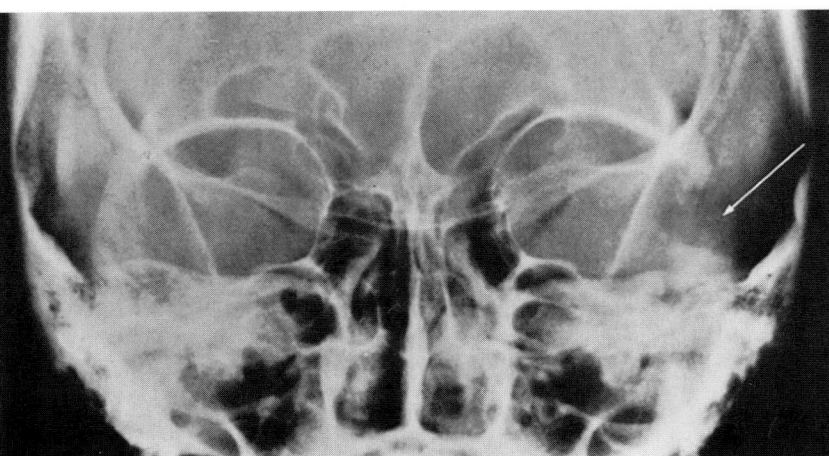

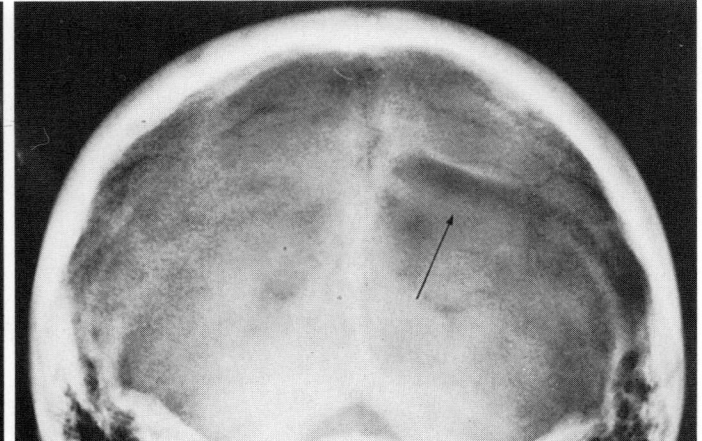

Figure 2–4. Simulated destruction of the lateral wall of the orbit, resulting from through-projection of the transverse venous sinus.

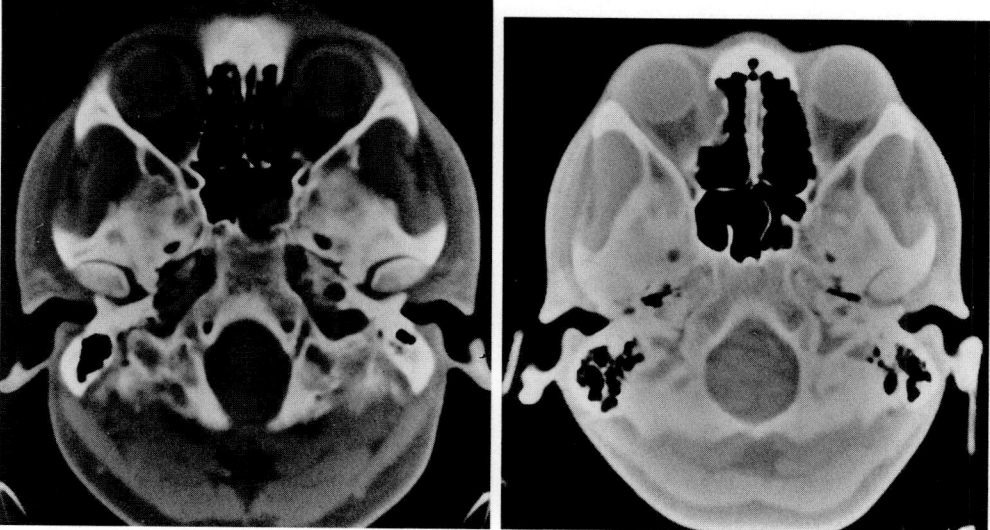

Figure 2–5. Two examples of absence of the medial walls of the orbits, a finding of no clinical significance.

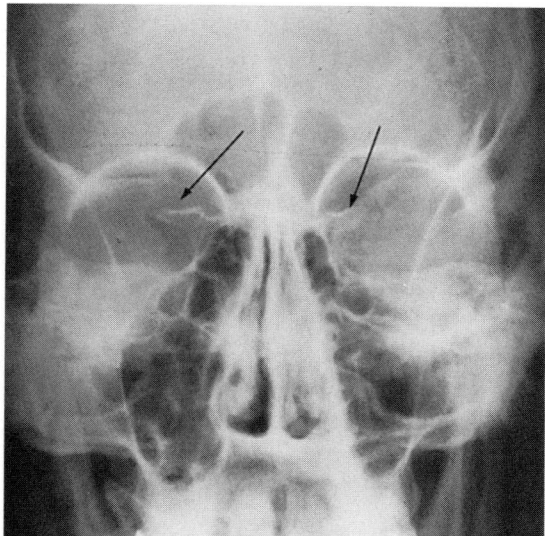

Figure 2–6. The anterior clinoid processes superimposed on the superior orbital fissures.

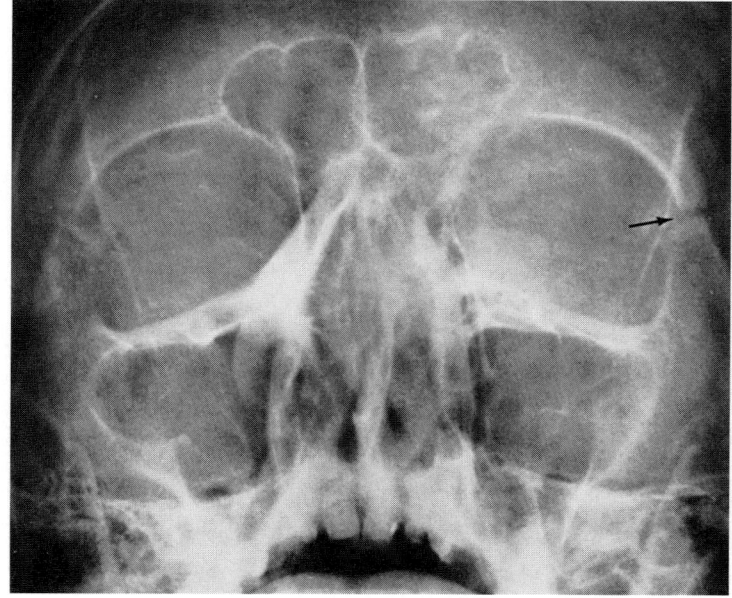

Figure 2–7. Simulated fracture through zygomaticofrontal suture, produced by a slight rotation of the head.

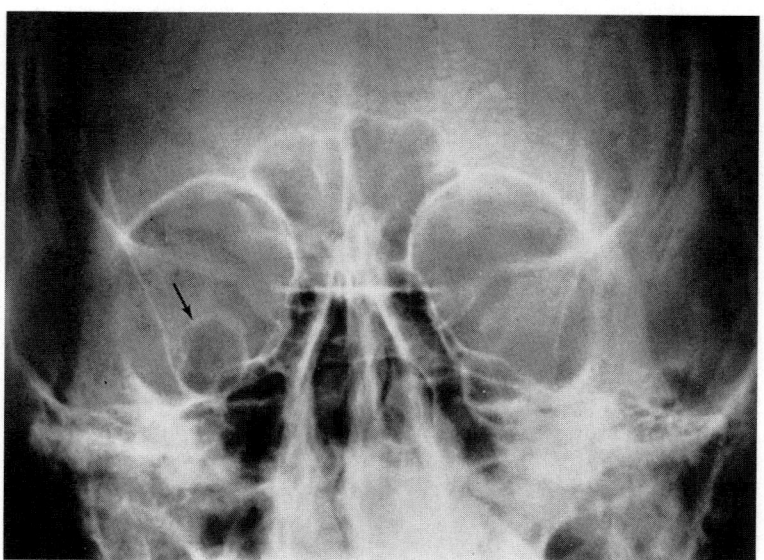

Figure 2–8. Unusual appearance produced by extension of a sphenoidal air cell into the greater wing of the sphenoid.

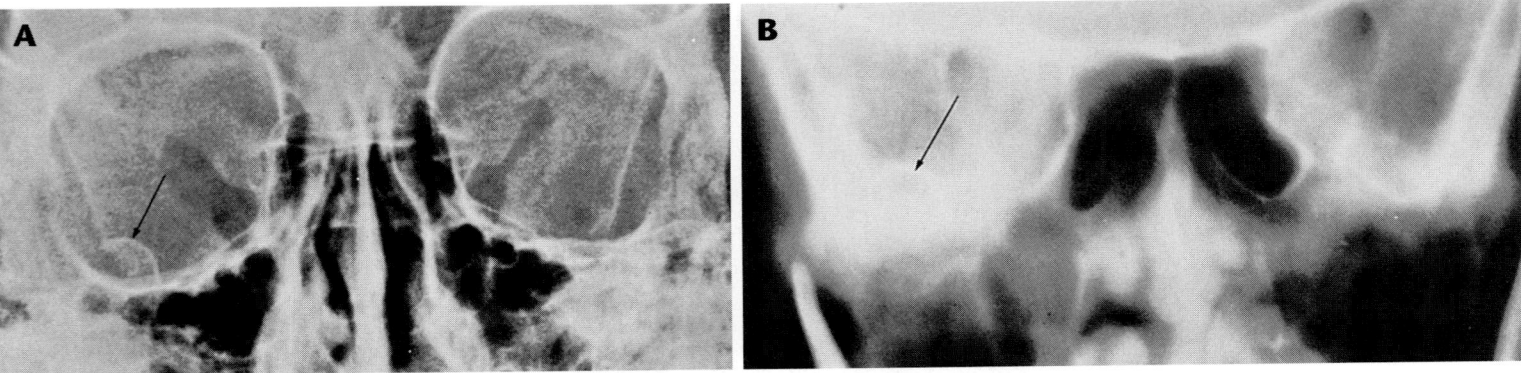

Figure 2–9. Ethmoid air cell, simulating trauma in a patient with facial trauma.
A, Plain film. **B,** Tomogram.

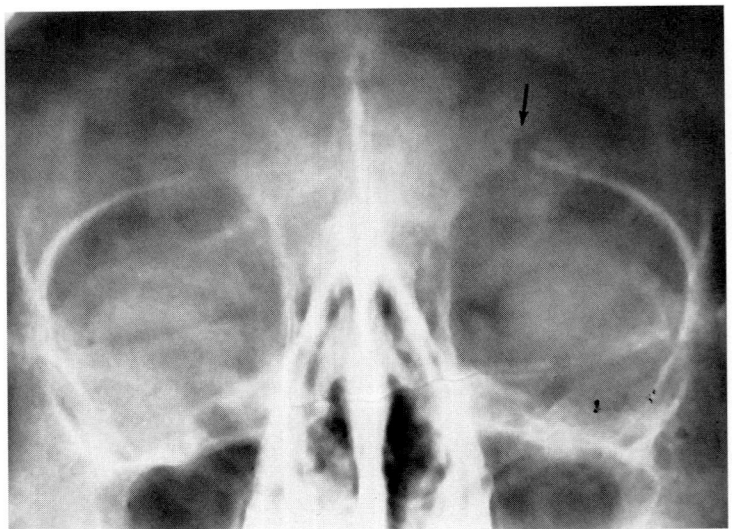

Figure 2–10. Asymmetric supraorbital foramina. This may be confused with a localized destruction of the orbital rim.

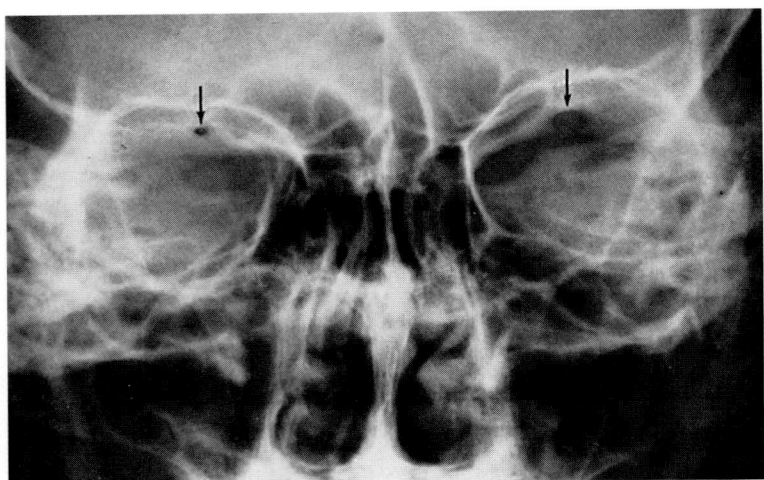

Figure 2–11. Asymmetric supraorbital foramina.

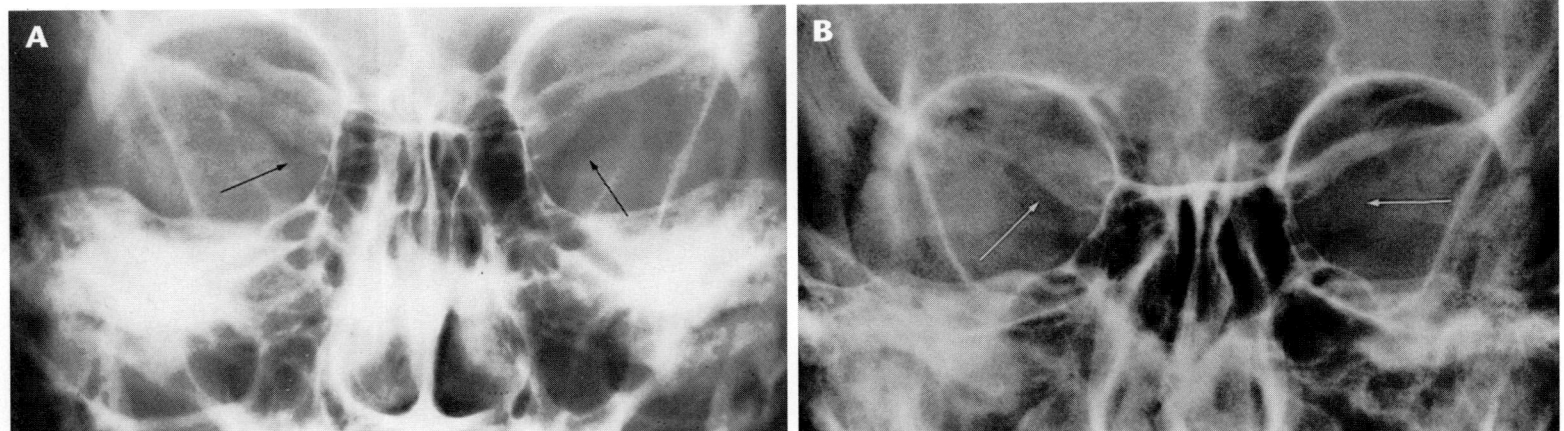

Figure 2–12. A, B, Two examples of normal asymmetry of the superior orbital fissures.

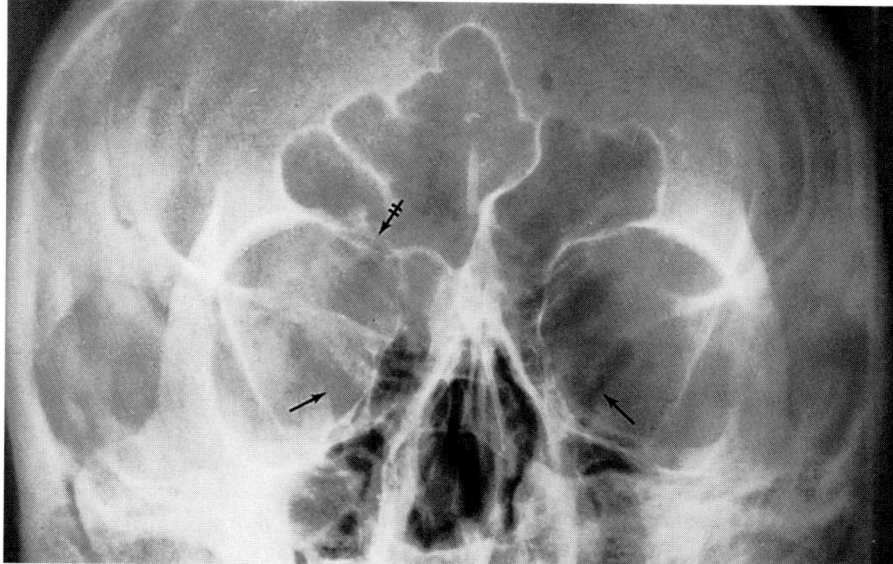

Figure 2–13. Normal asymmetry of the superior orbital fissures (←). Note also the asymmetric density of the sphenoidal wings and the apparent loss of the superior medial aspect of the right orbital rim (⇻).

Figure 2–14. Factitial increased density of the left orbit caused by a slight rotation of the head and a prominent superimposed external occipital protuberance.

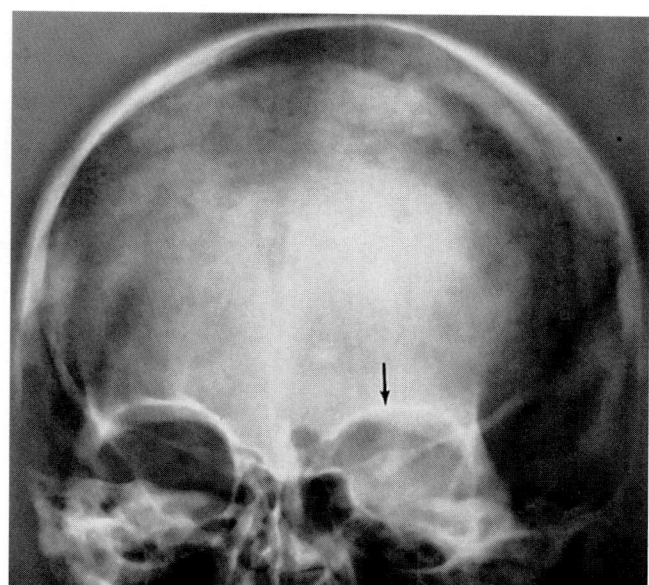

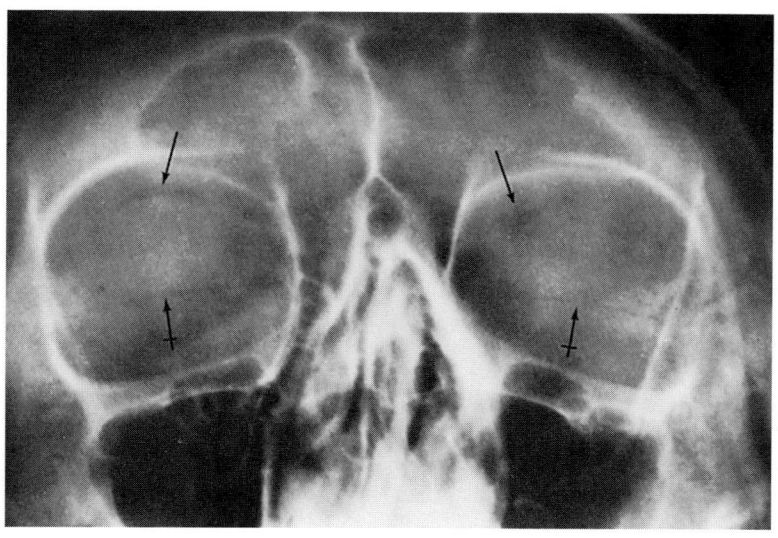

Figure 2–15. Periglobal fat, simulating air in the orbits (→). Note also the shadow of the closed eyelids (↦).

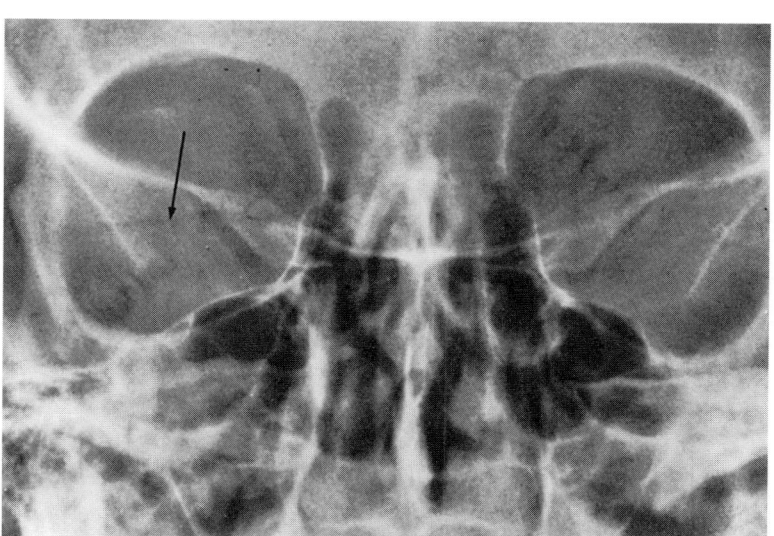

Figure 2–16. The shadow of the eyelid seen unilaterally.

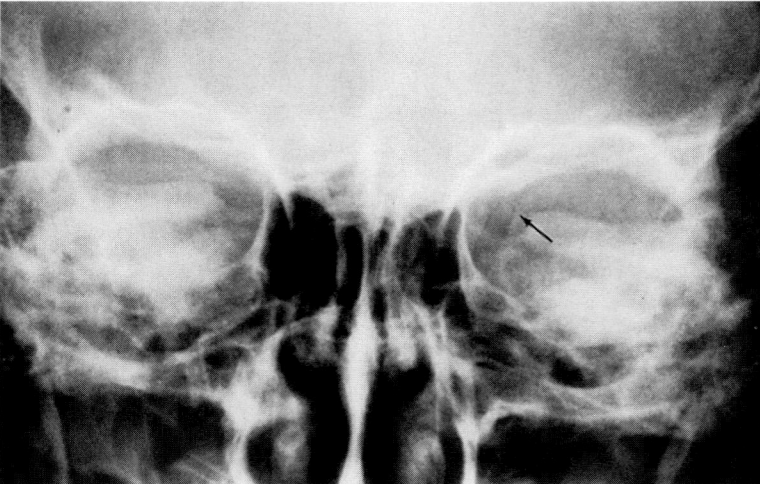

Figure 2–17. The edge of the superior orbital fissure, not to be mistaken for calcification in the globe.

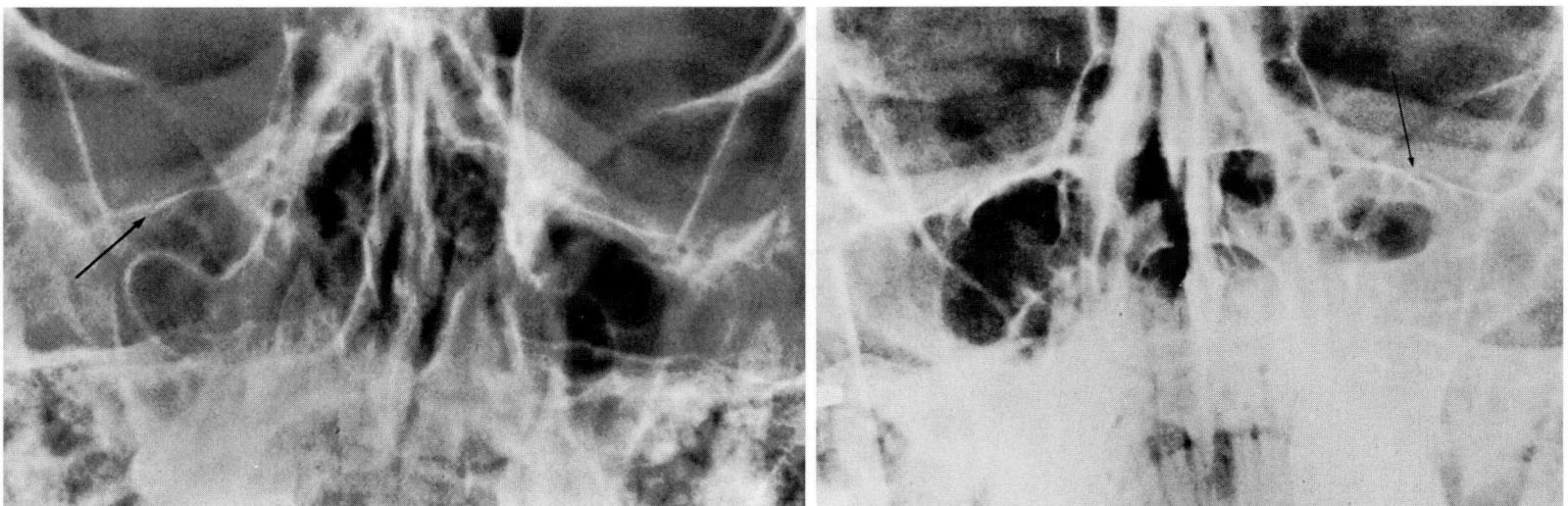

Figure 2–18. Two examples of the infraorbital groove, simulating a fracture of the floor of the orbit. The patient on the right has sinusitis.

The Paranasal Sinuses

The Maxillary Sinuses

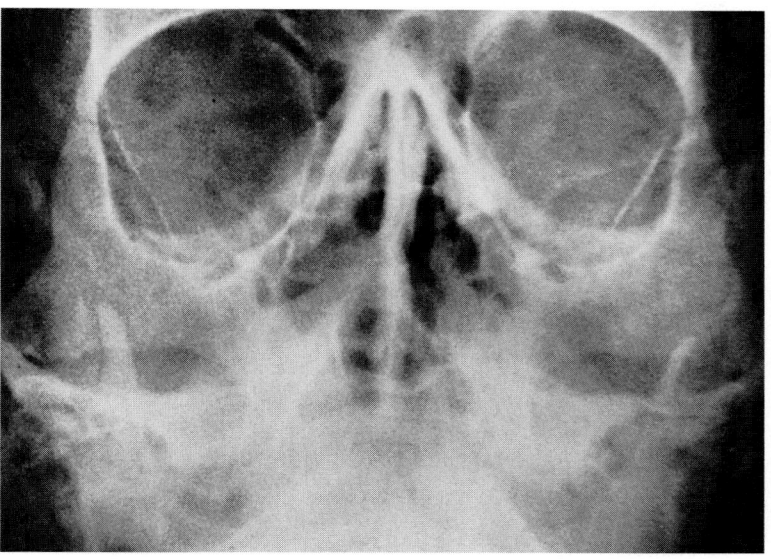

Figure 2–19. Hypoplasia of both antra, simulating sinus disease.

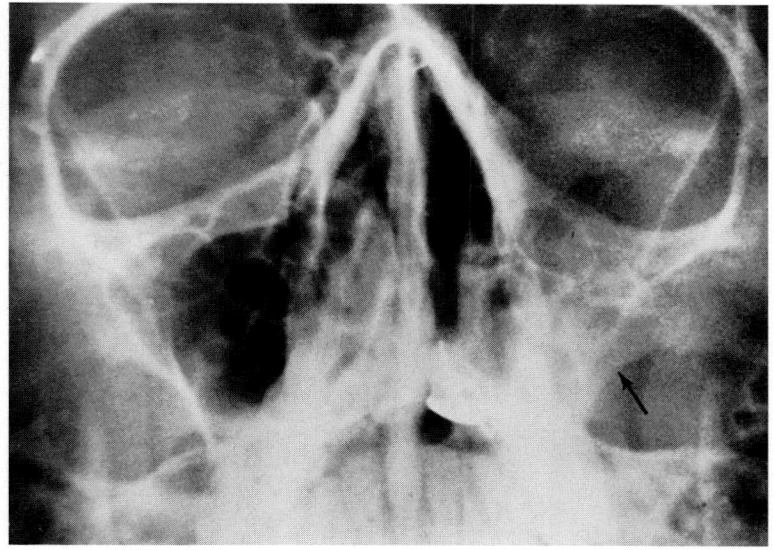

Figure 2–20. Hypoplasia of the maxillary antrum, simulating sinus disease.

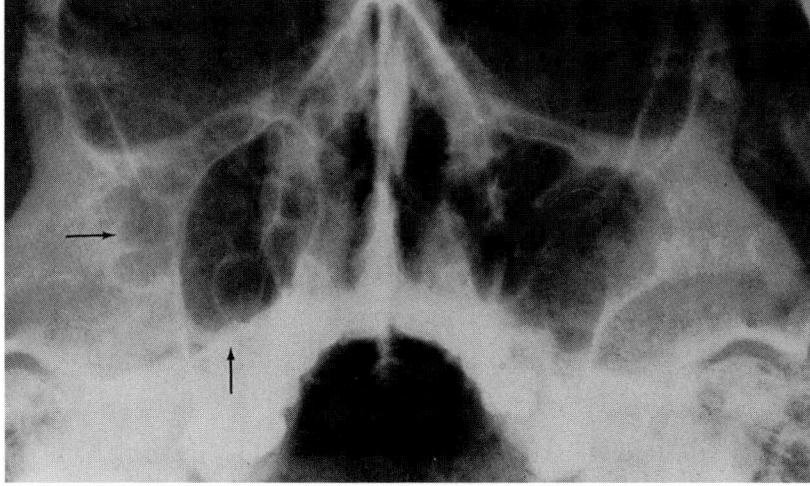
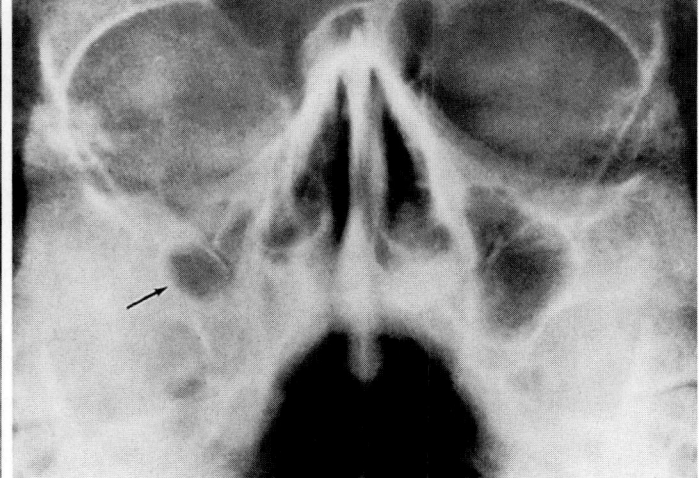

Figure 2–21. Two examples of unilateral hypoplasia of the maxillary antrum. This condition may be associated with asymmetry of the superior orbital fissures. (Ref: Bassiouny A et al: Maxillary sinus hypoplasia and superior orbital fissure asymmetry. *Laryngoscope* 92:441, 1982.)

Figure 2–22. Hypoplasia of the maxillary antrum. Note enlargement of the orbit on the same side, a finding that frequently accompanies hypoplasia of the antrum. (Ref: Bierny JP, Dryden R: Orbital enlargement secondary to paranasal sinus hypoplasia. *Am J Roentgenol* 128:850, 1977.)

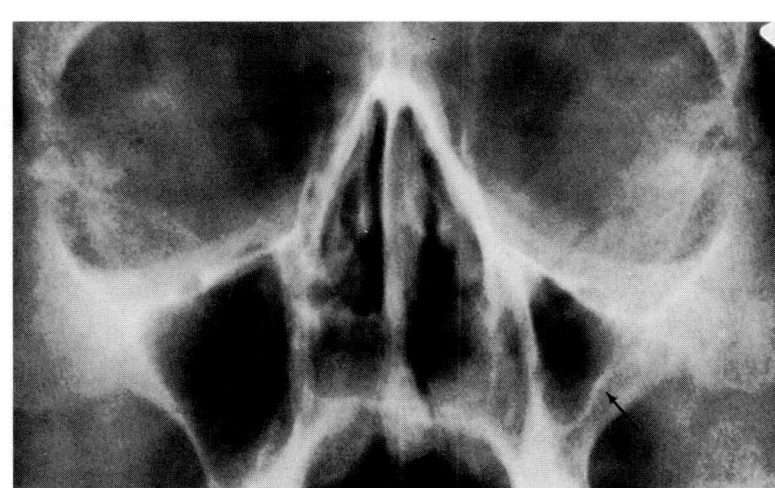

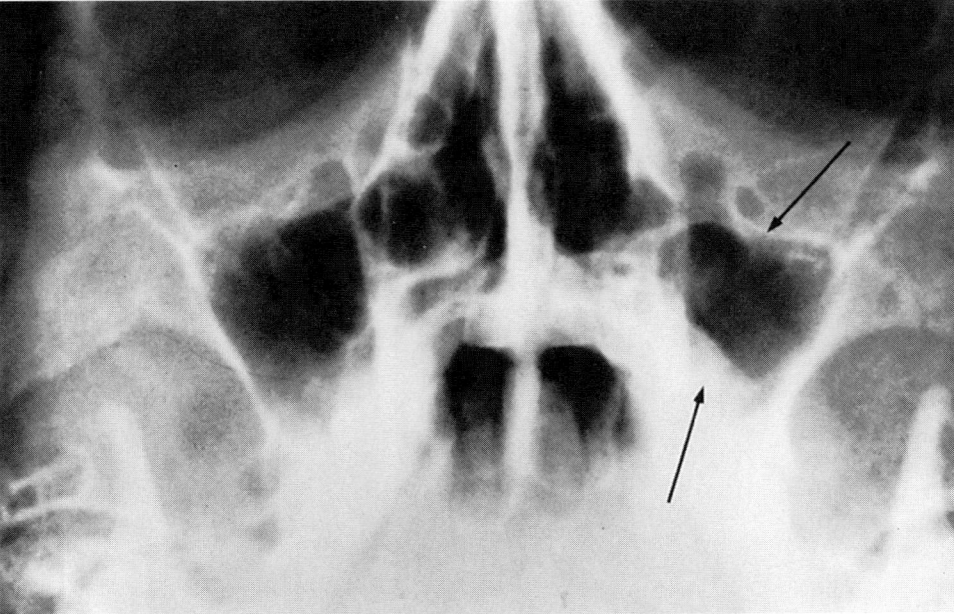

Figure 2–23. Hypoplasia of the left maxillary antrum.

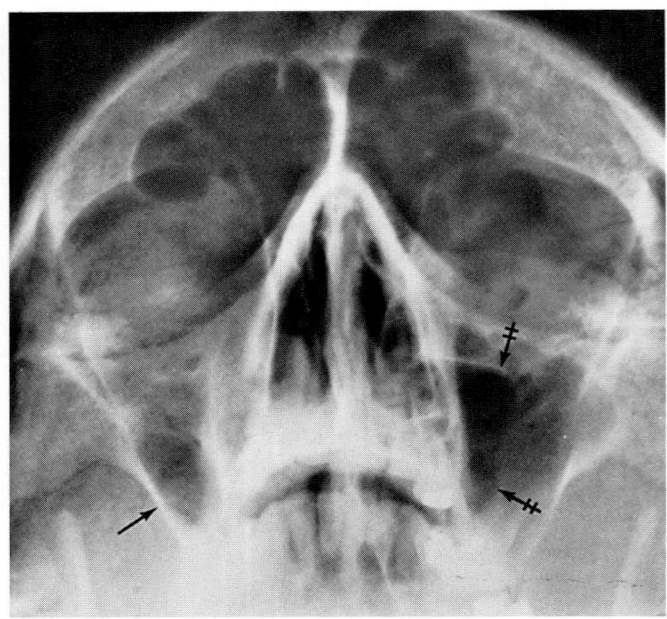

Figure 2–24. Hypoplasia of the antrum on the right (←). Note also the lateral extension of the left sphenoid sinus, producing an apparent loculation of the antrum (⇥).

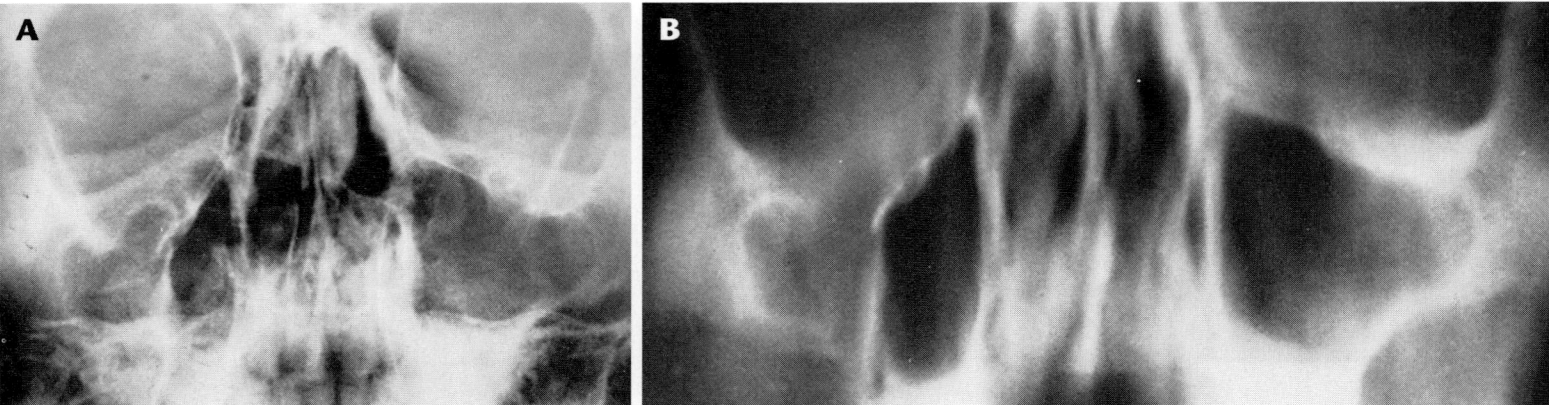

Figure 2–25. Unusual development of the maxillary antra. **A,** Plain film. The left antrum is huge and extends far laterally. The right antrum contains at least two loculi, the medial one being deeper and more lucent than the lateral. **B,** Tomogram.

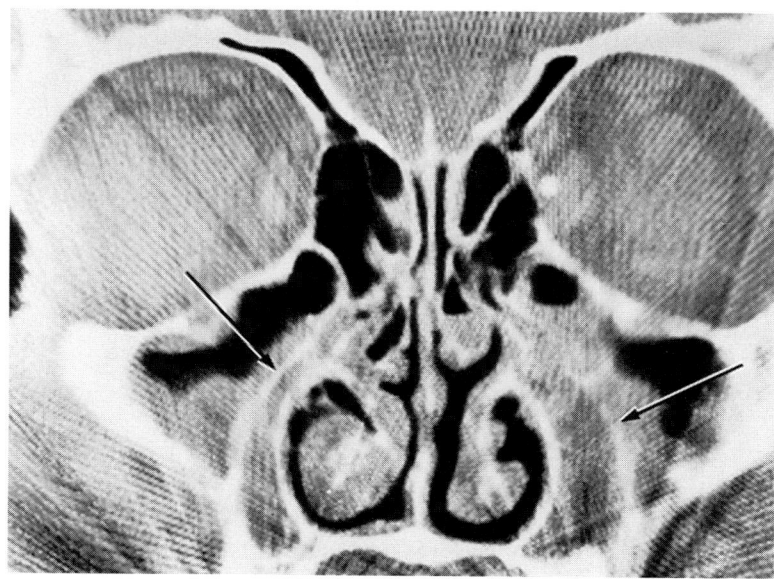

Figure 2–26. Compartmented antra in a patient with sinusitis.

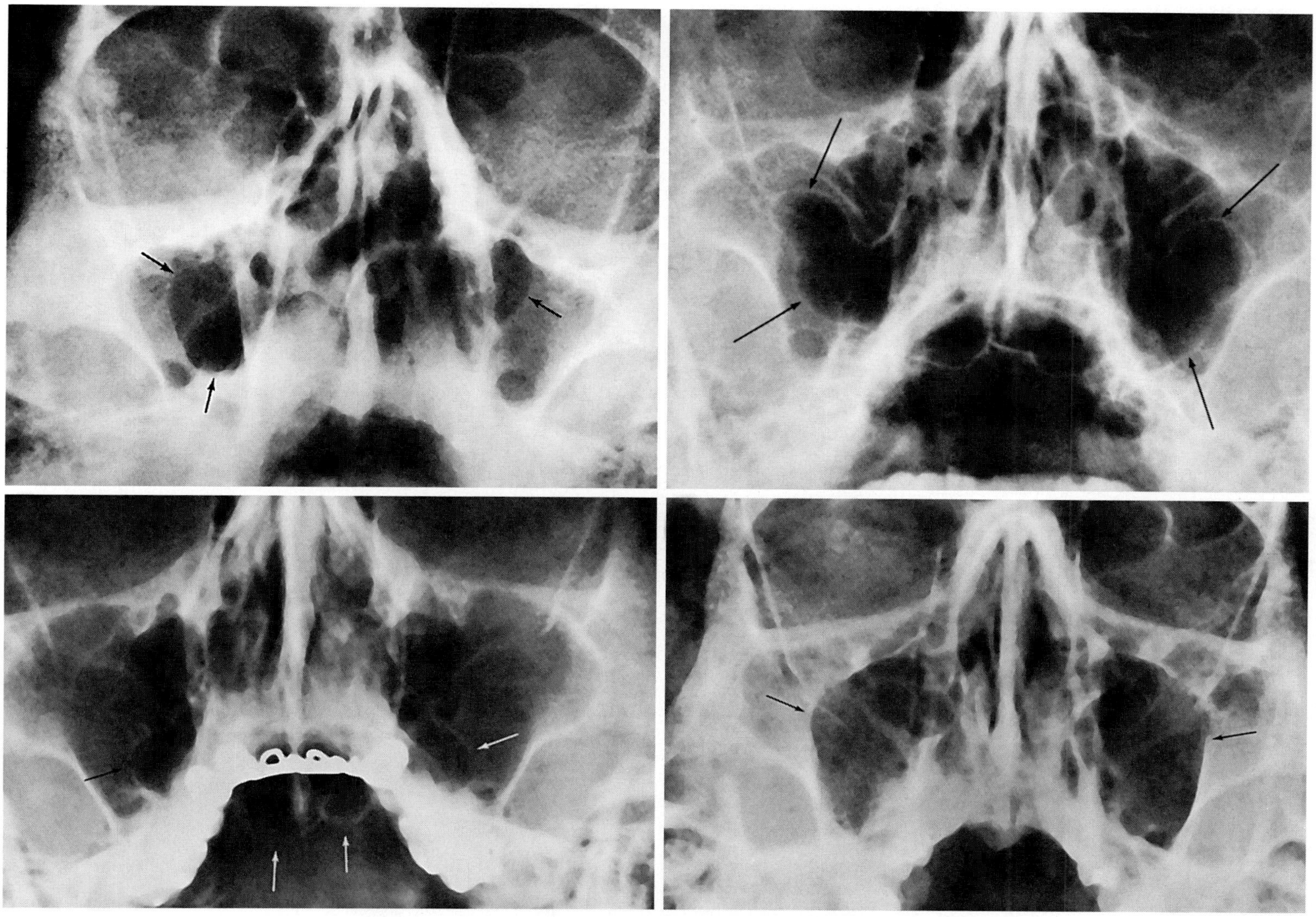

Figure 2–27. Four examples of apparent loculation of the antra, produced by lateral extension of sphenoidal sinus air cells.

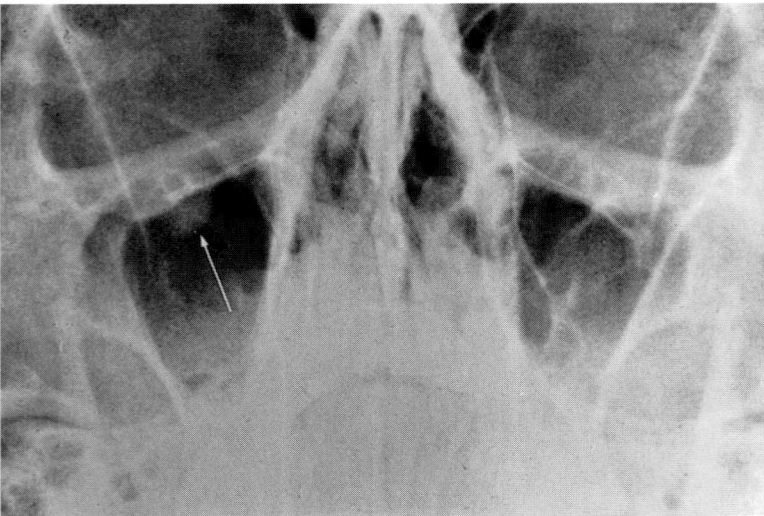

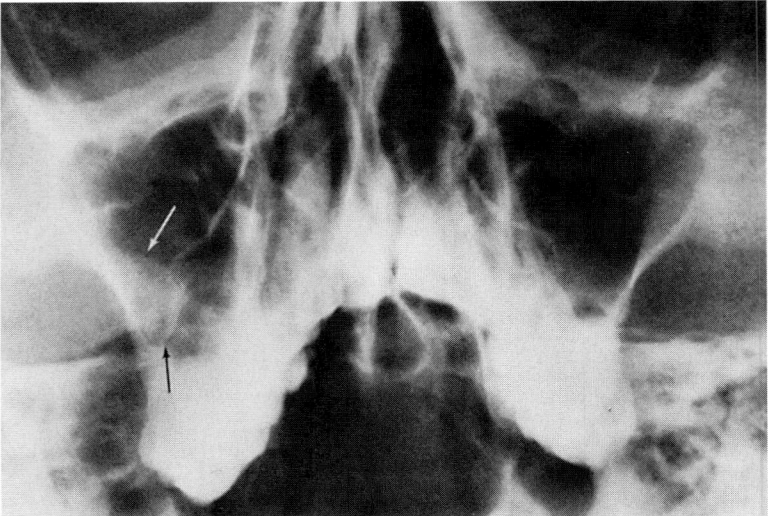

Figure 2–28. Localized bony excrescence in roof of antrum probably caused by incomplete aeration around the infraorbital canal and foramen.

Figure 2–29. Localized bony thickening of the lateral wall of the maxillary antrum.

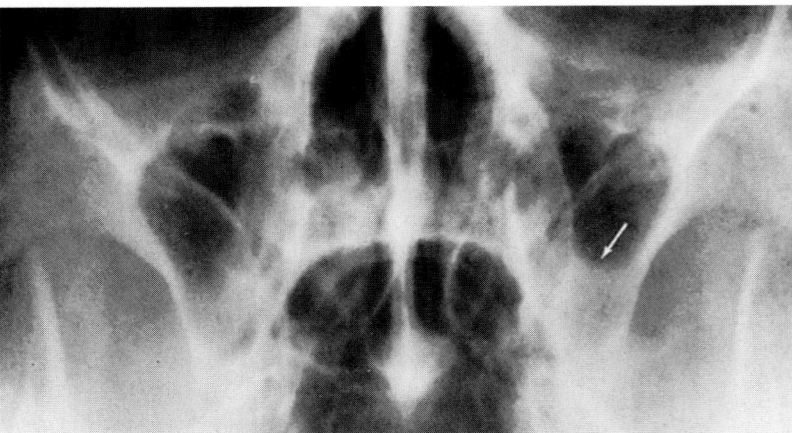

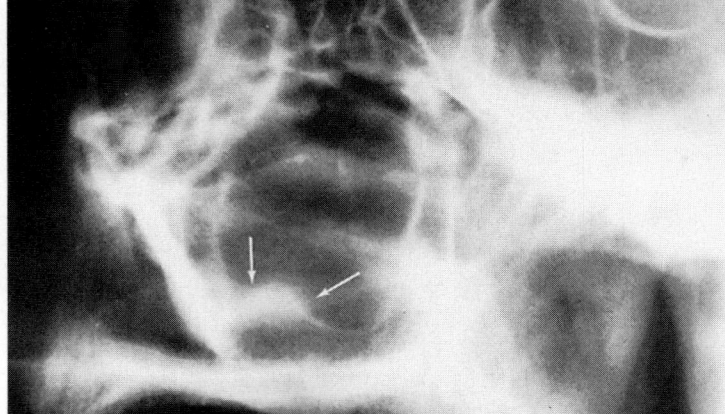

Figure 2–30. Localized bony excrescence in the floor of the maxillary antrum.

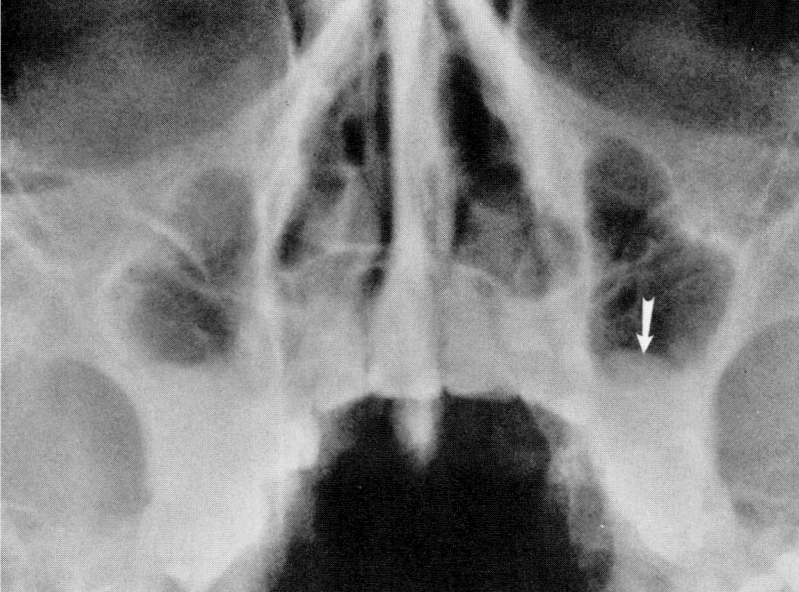

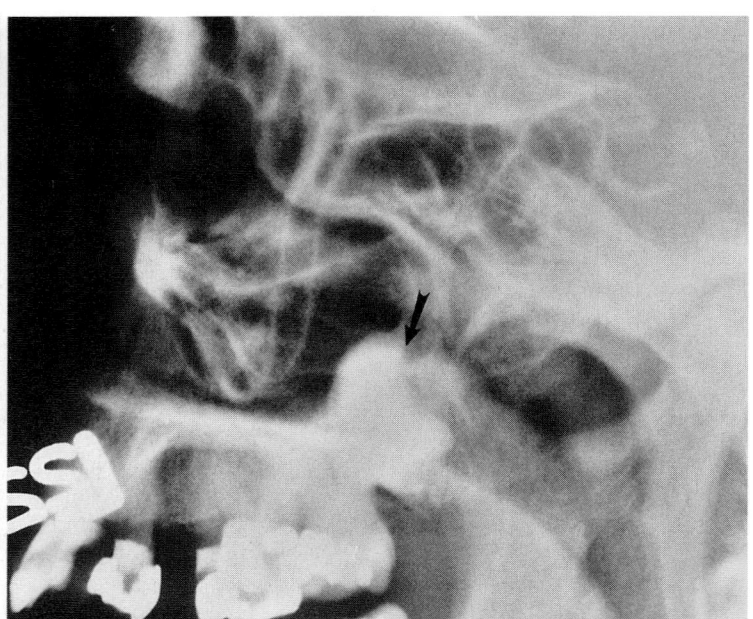

Figure 2–31. Impacted third maxillary molar producing a convex density in the floor of the maxillary antrum.

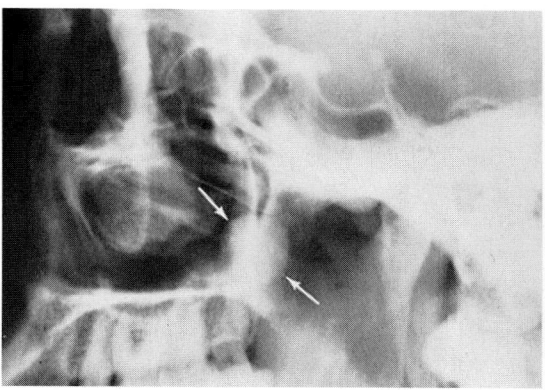
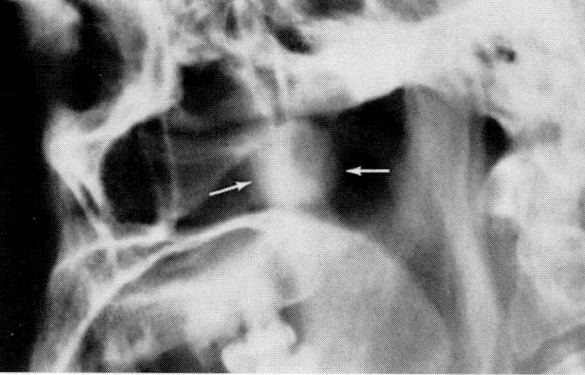

Figure 2–32. Two examples of simulated tumor of the antrum, produced by superimposition of the turbinates on the coronoid process of the mandible. (Ref: Sistrom CL, Keats TE, Johnson CM III: The anatomic basis of the pseudotumor of the nasal cavity. *Am J Roentgenol* 147:782, 1986.)

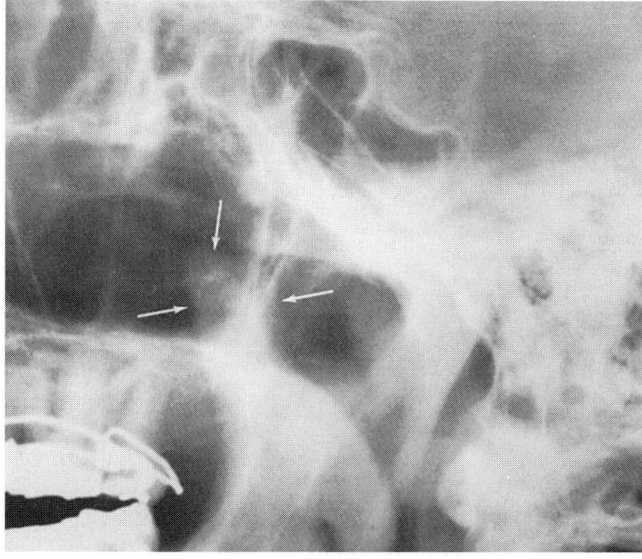

Figure 2–33. The coronoid process of the mandible, illustrating the mechanism of production of the pseudotumor shown in the preceding figure.

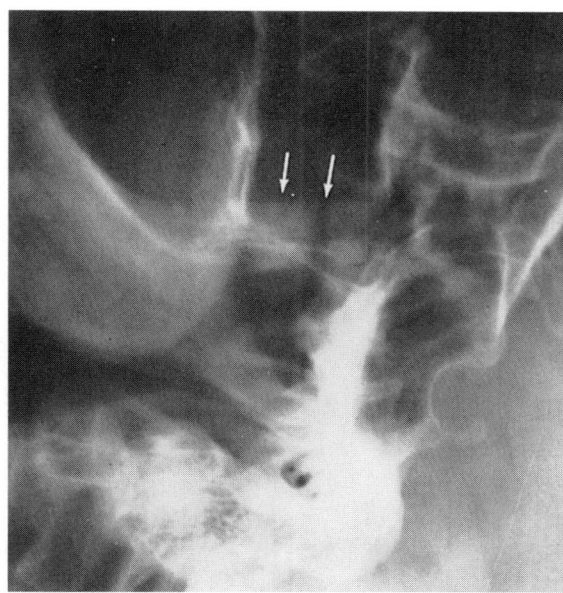

Figure 2–34. The coronoid process of the mandible in the brow-up projection, simulating an air-fluid level in the maxillary antrum.

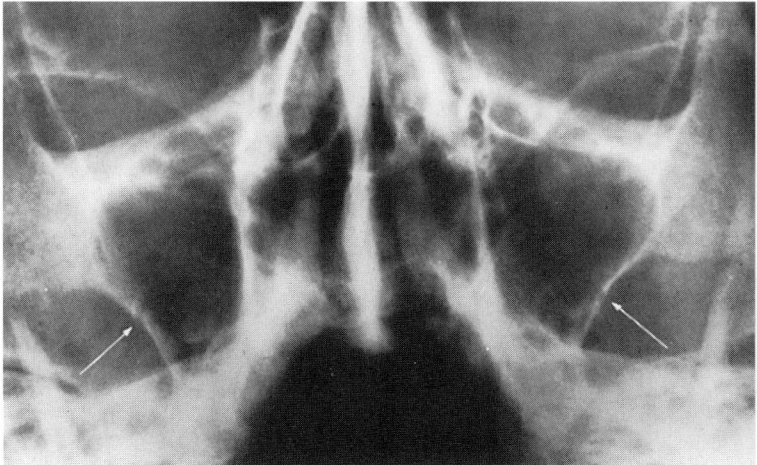
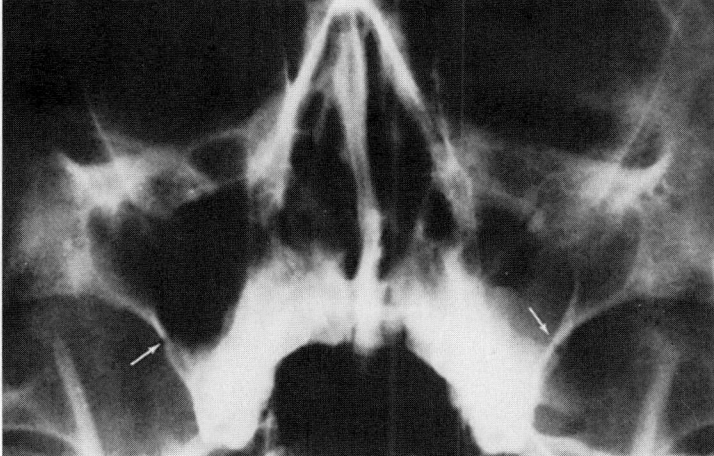

Figure 2–35. Simulated fractures of the lateral wall of the maxillary antrum, produced by the posterior superior alveolar canal. (Ref: Chuang VP, Vines FS: Roentgenology of the posterior superior alveolar foramina and canals. *Am J Roentgenol* 118:426, 1973.)

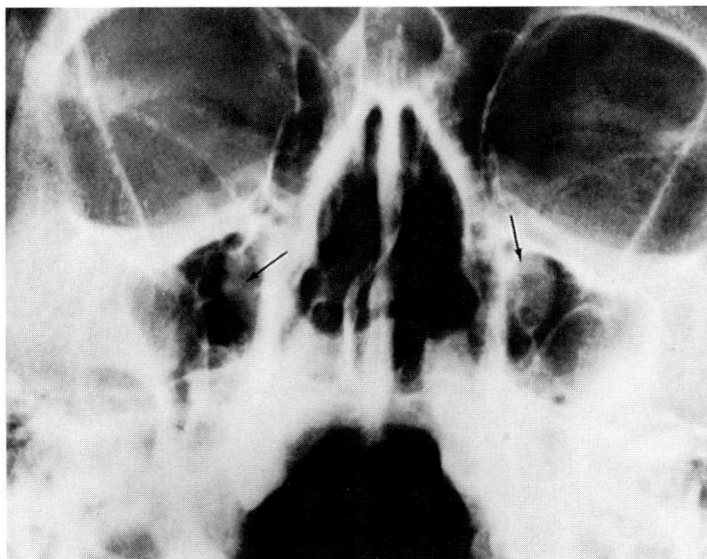

Figure 2–36. The nares superimposed on the antra, simulating polyps.

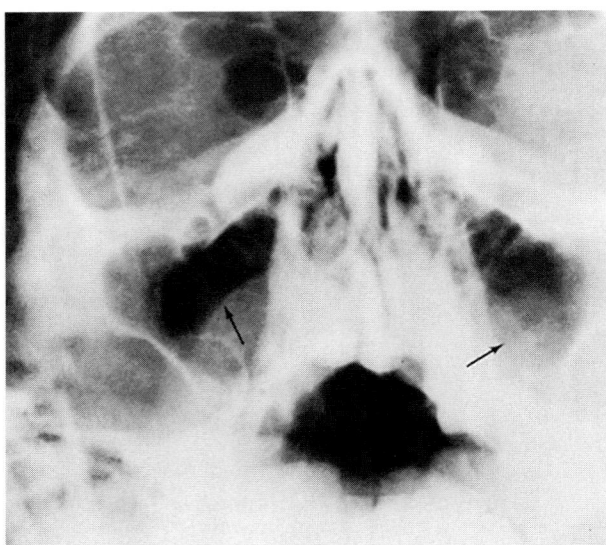

Figure 2–37. The upper lip superimposed on the antra, simulating retention cysts.

The Frontal Sinuses

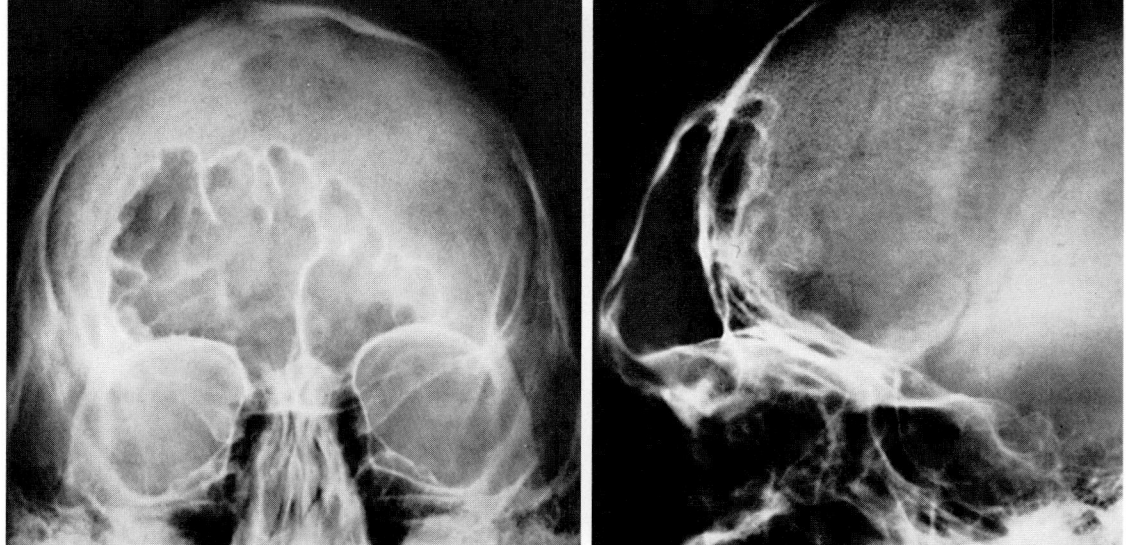

Figure 2–38. Overdevelopment of the frontal sinuses without associated disease.

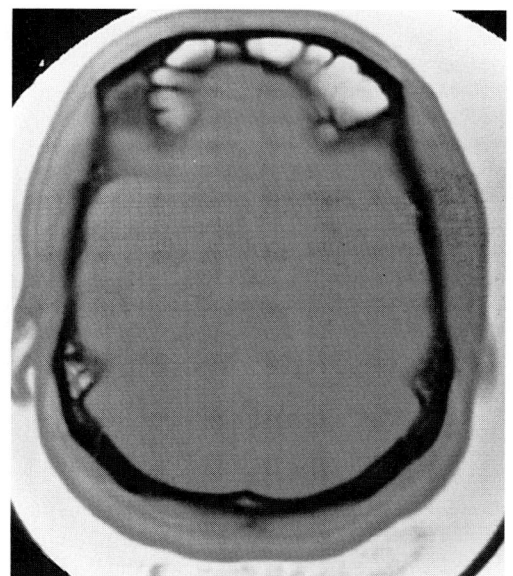

Figure 2–39. Marked pneumatization of the frontal bone by CT.

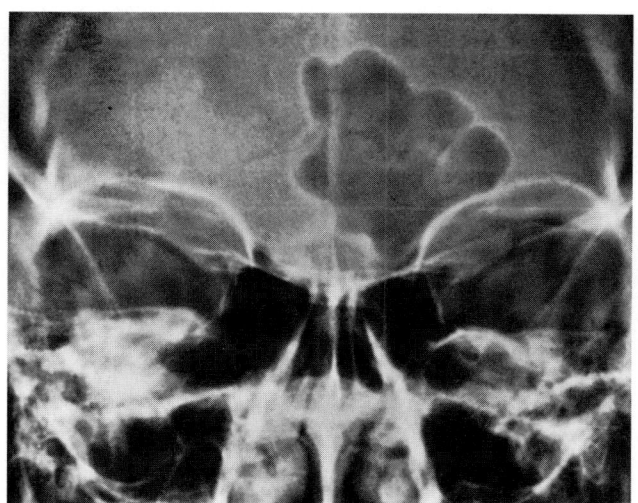

Figure 2–40. Unilateral development of the frontal sinuses.

Figure 2–41. Unusual variation in pneumatization of the frontal sinus with an anomalous air cell, simulating an intradiploic epidermoid.

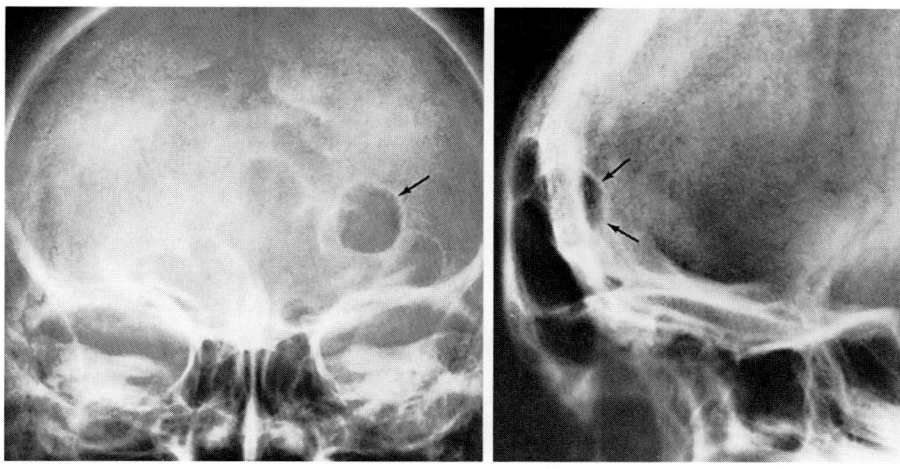

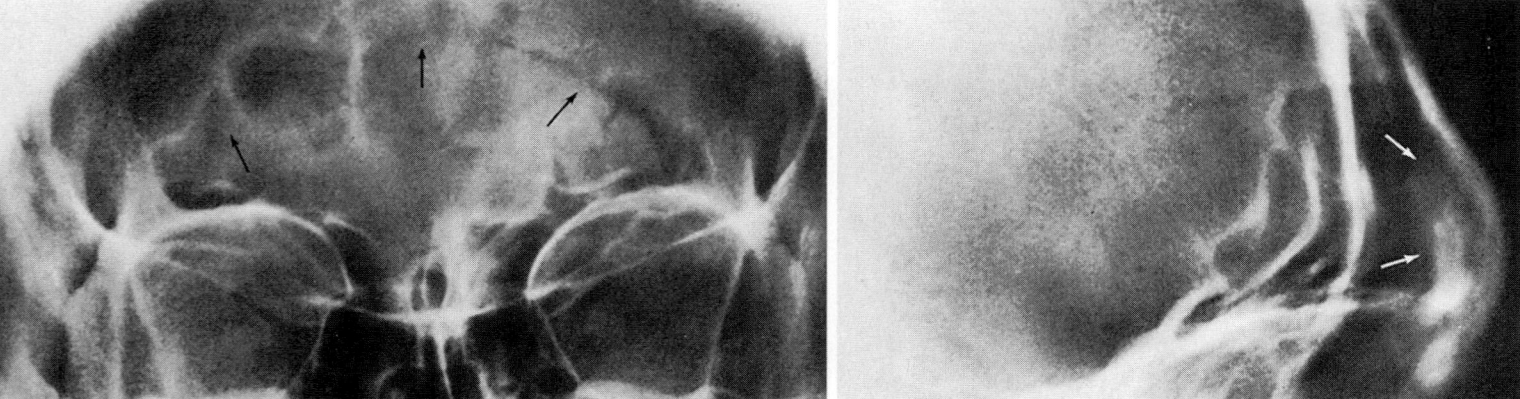

Figure 2–42. Incomplete pneumatization of the anterior wall of the frontal sinus, producing a mass effect in the sinus.

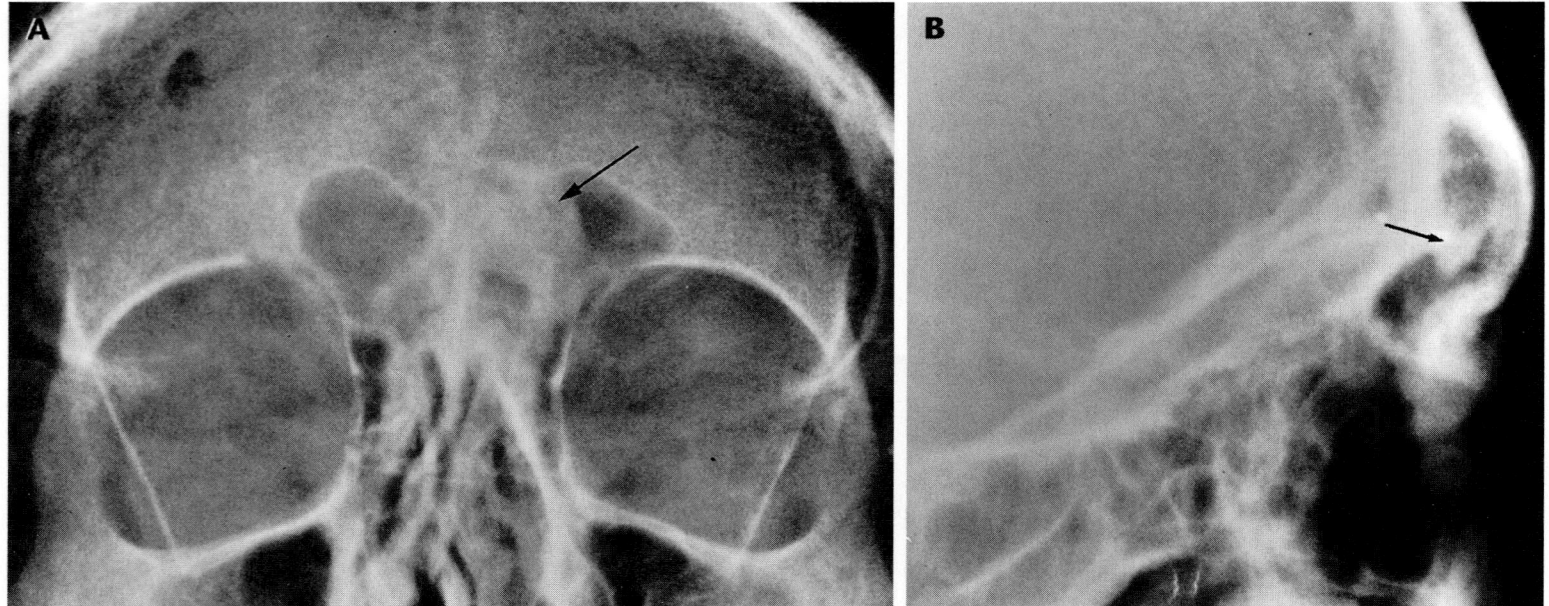

Figure 2–43. A, B, Incomplete aeration of the left frontal sinus simulating clouding of sinusitis.

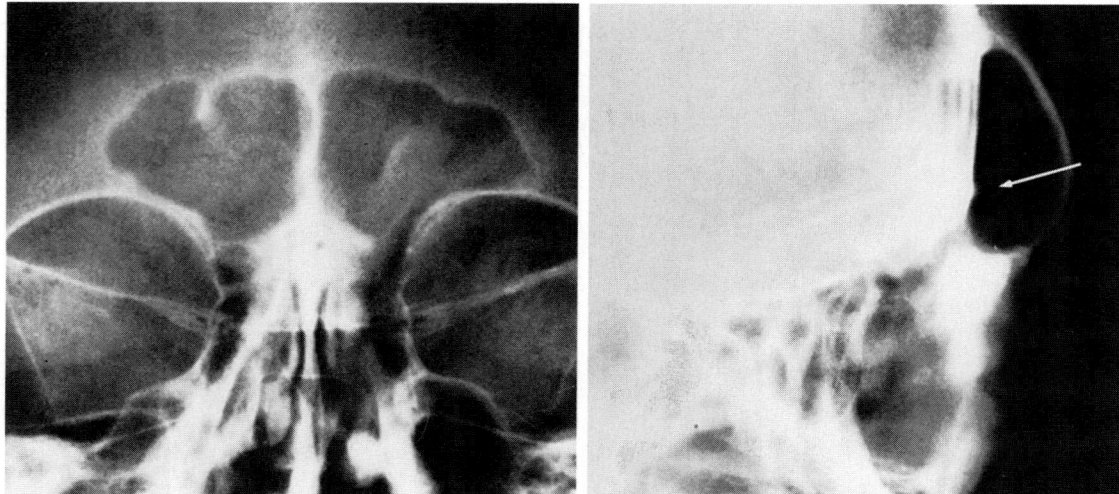

Figure 2–44. Incomplete aeration of the frontal sinus, producing shadowing of the frontal sinuses. Osseous shadows are evident in the lateral projection (*arrow*).

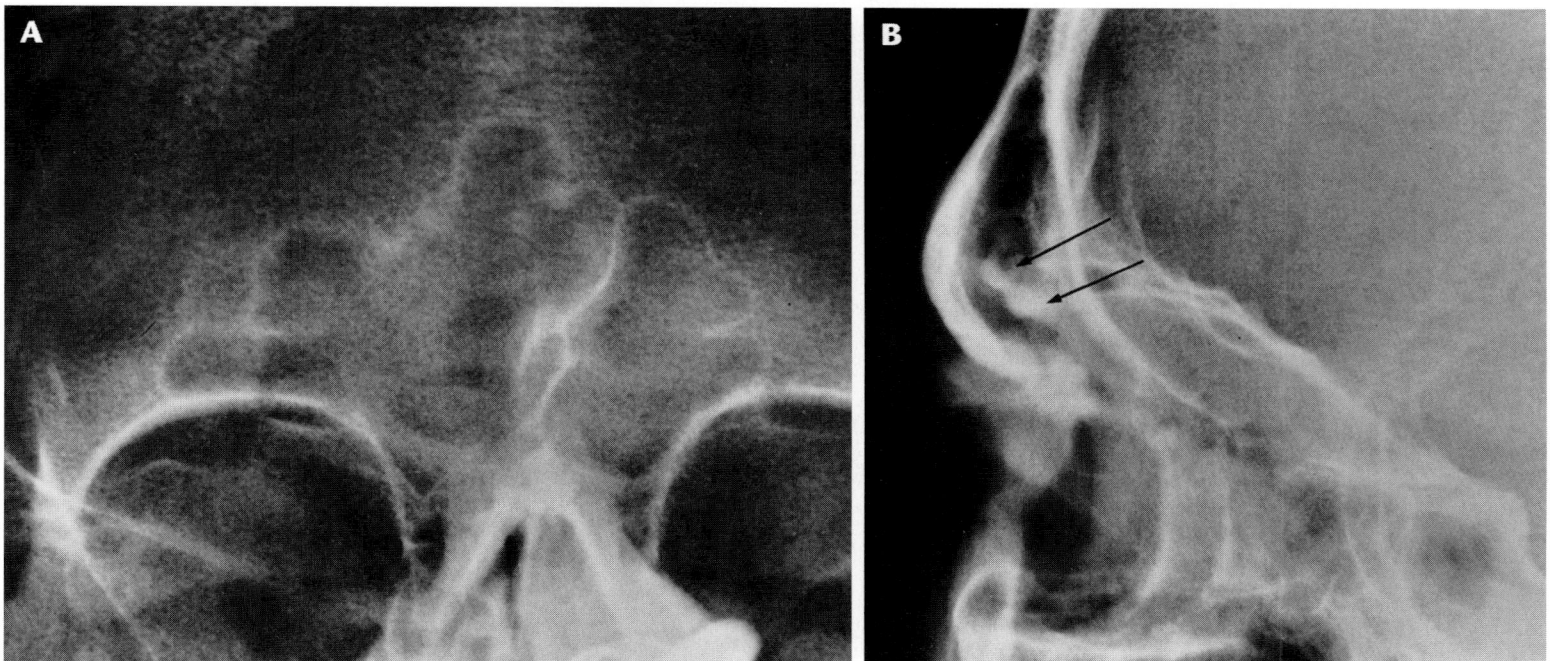

Figure 2–45. A, B, Uneven aeration of the frontal sinuses caused by irregularity of the posterior wall.

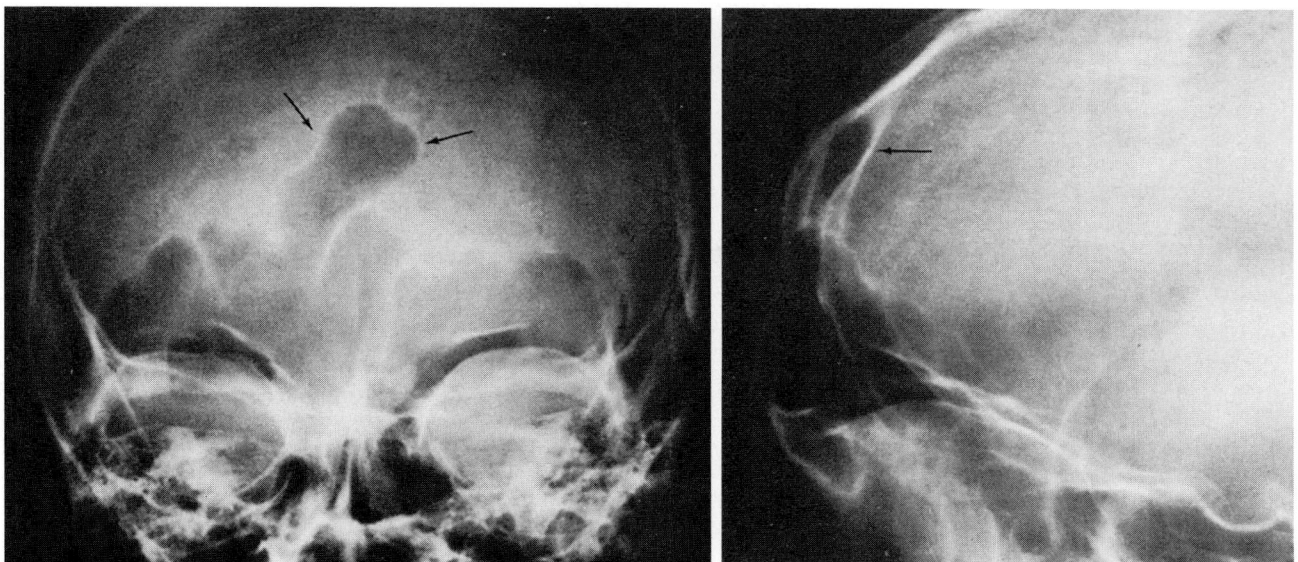

Figure 2–46. Marked cephalad extension of the frontal sinus.

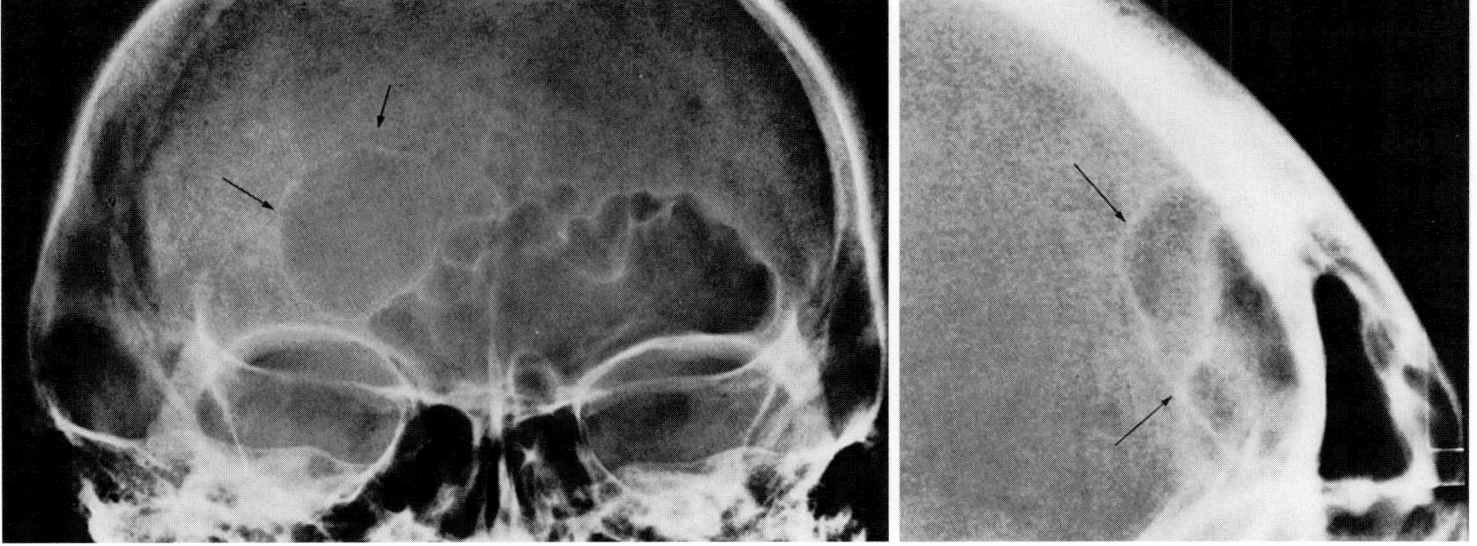

Figure 2–47. Large lateral locule of the frontal sinus.

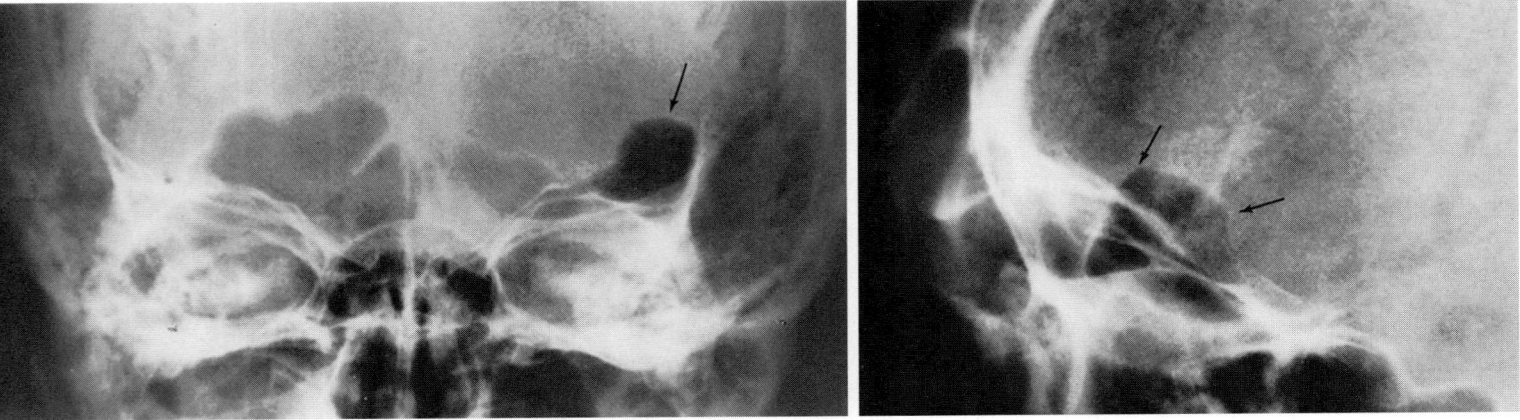

Figure 2–48. Marked lateral extension of the frontal sinus.

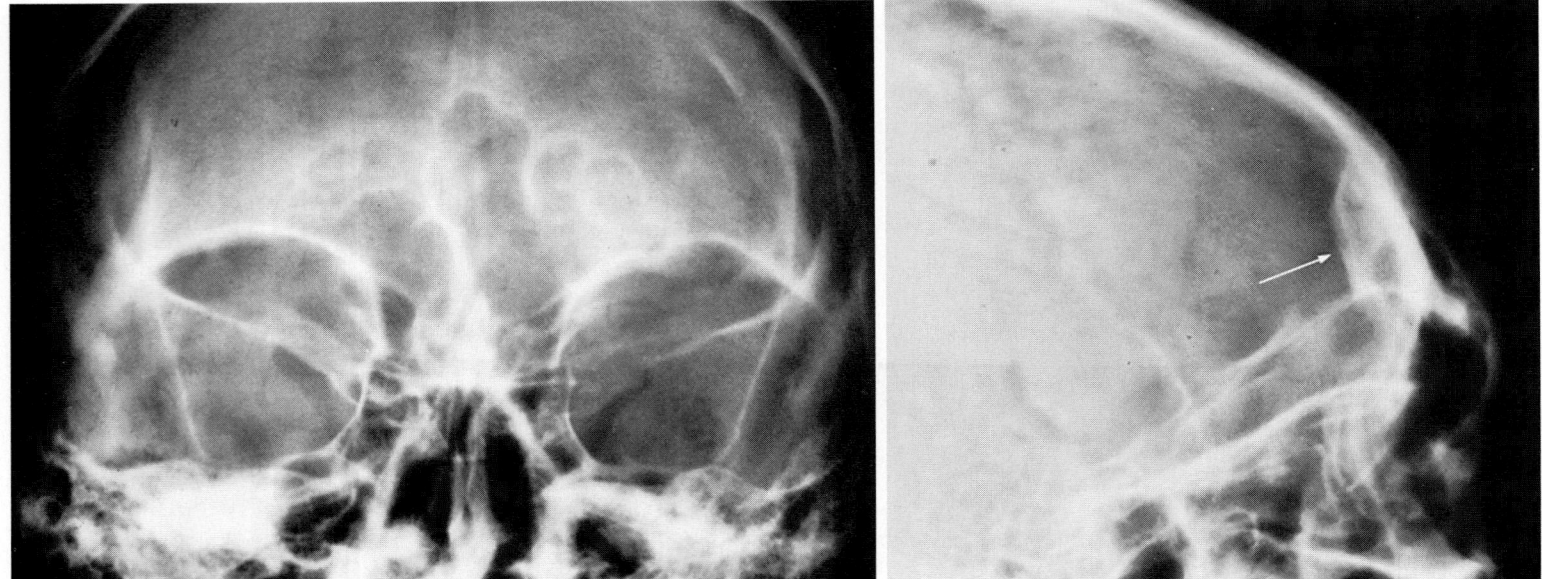

Figure 2–49. Marked posterior extension of the frontal sinuses.

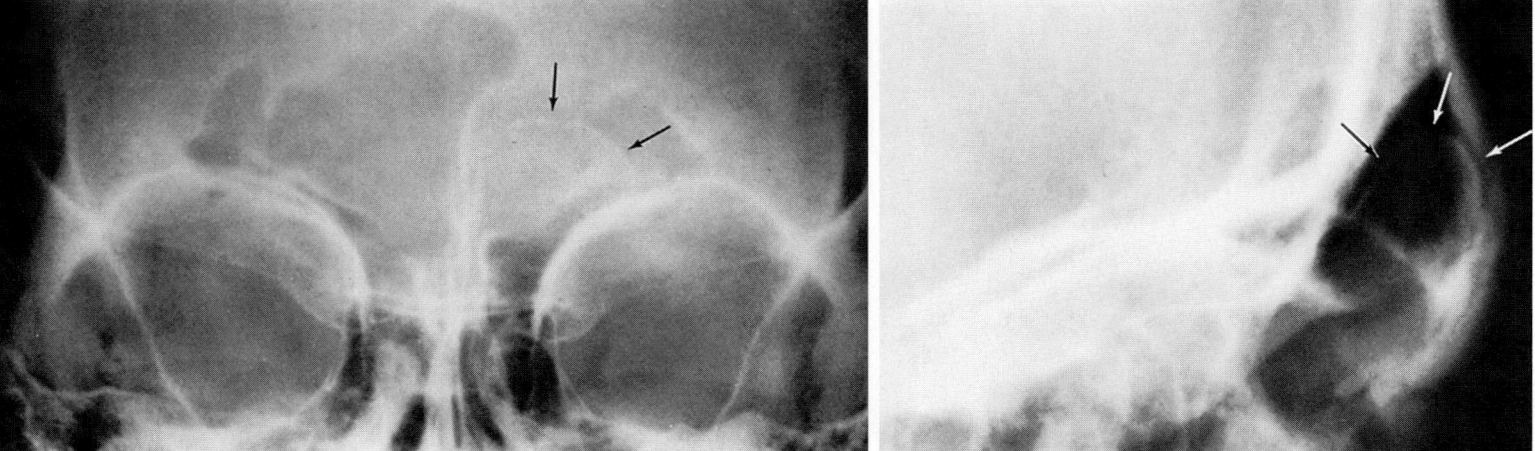

Figure 2–50. Discrete cellule within the frontal sinus, probably arising from an ethmoidal air cell.

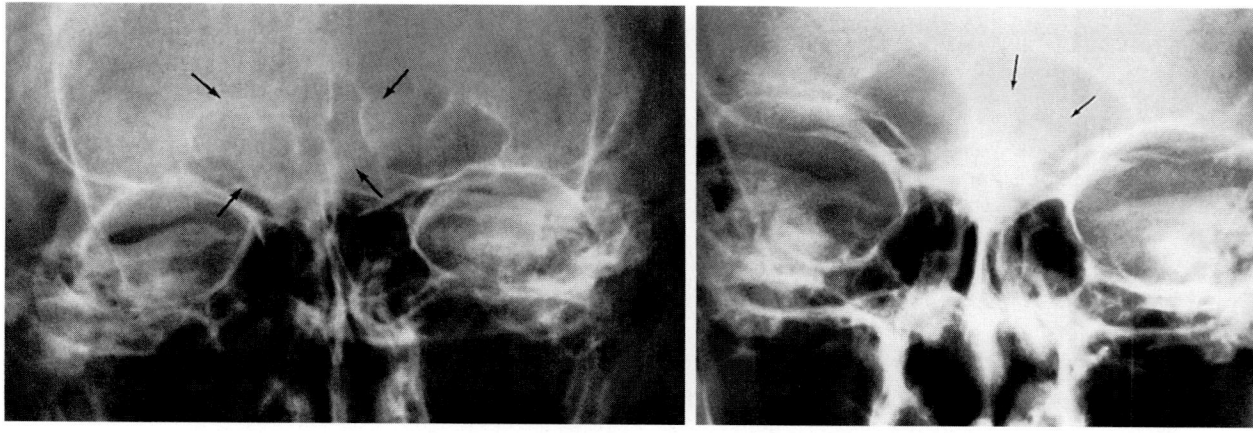

Figure 2–51. Two examples of factitial clouding of the frontal sinus, produced by superimposition of a large external occipital protuberance.

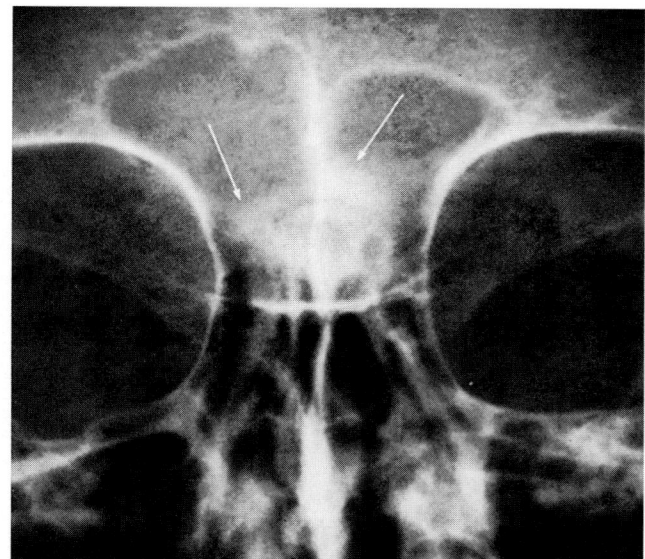

Figure 2–52. Sclerosis of the nasofrontal suture.

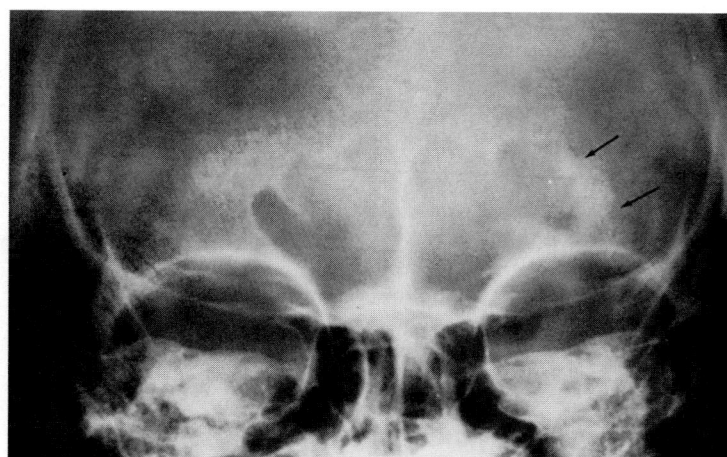

Figure 2–53. A sclerotic lambdoidal suture superimposed on the edge of the frontal sinus, mistaken for osteomyelitis.

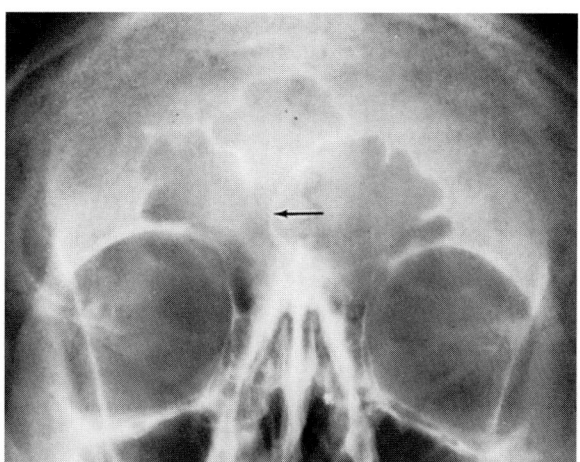

Figure 2–54. Bowed central septum of the frontal sinus.

The Ethmoid Bone and Ethmoidal Sinuses

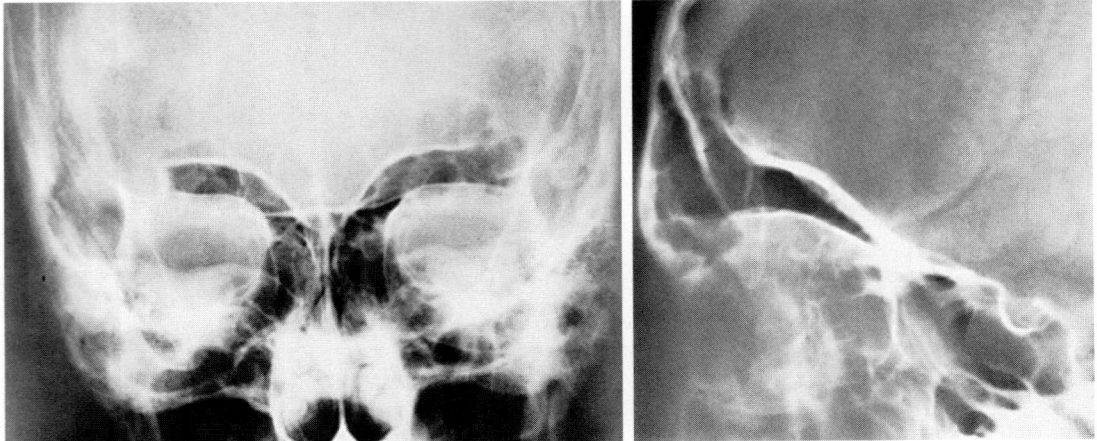

Figure 2–55. Remarkable overdevelopment of the ethmoidal air cells with extension into the floor of the anterior fossa.

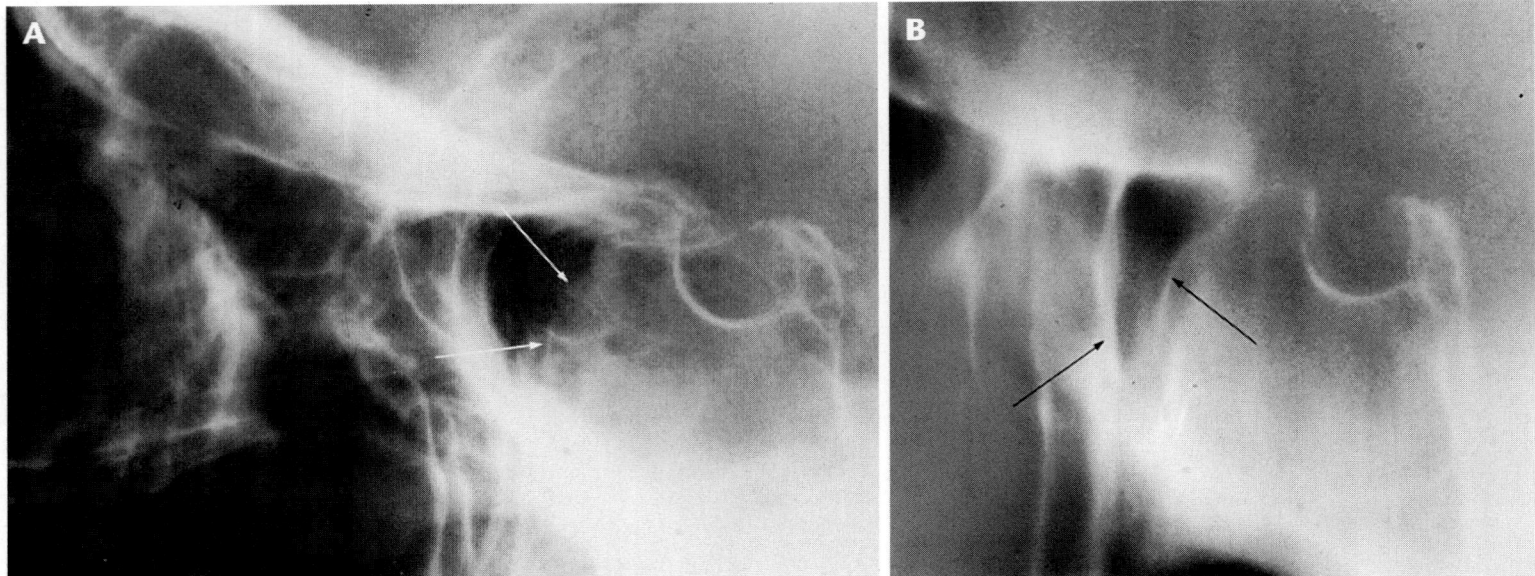

Figure 2–56. Ethmoidal cell extending into a nonaerated sphenoid sinus, resulting in a mass effect in the sphenoid sinus. **A,** Plain film, **B,** tomogram.

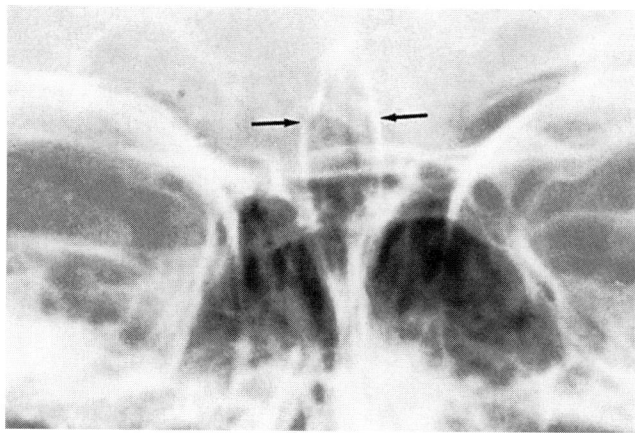

Figure 2–57. Marked pneumatization of the crista galli.

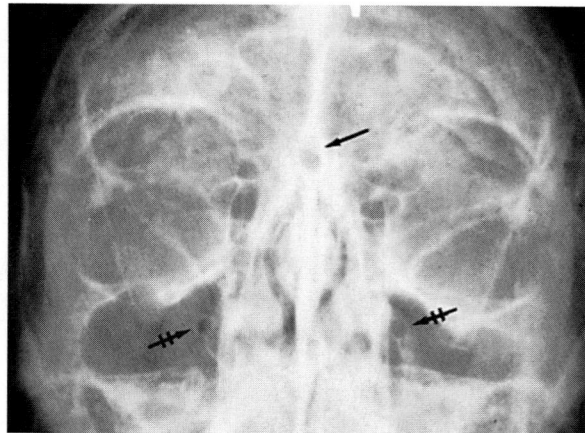

Figure 2–58. Less marked pneumatization of the crista galli (←). The arrows below (←╫) indicate the foramina rotunda.

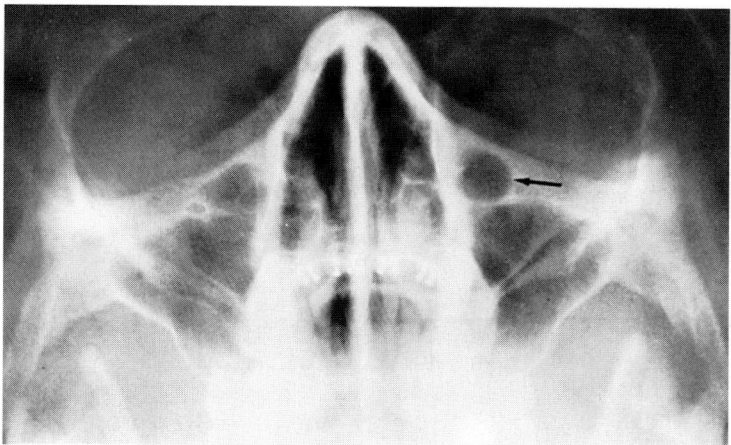

Figure 2–59. An anomalous ethmoidal air cell in the floor of the orbit.

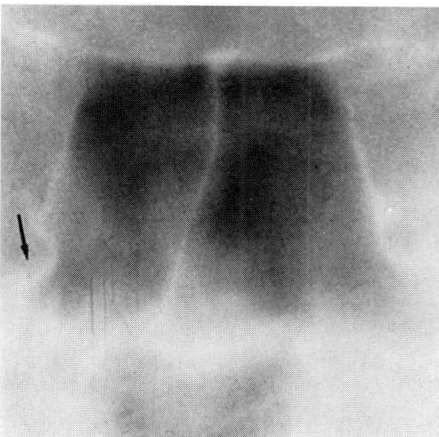

Figure 2–60. Tomogram of the ethmoidal region, showing asymmetric development of the foramina rotunda with poor definition of the lateral aspect of one of the foramina.

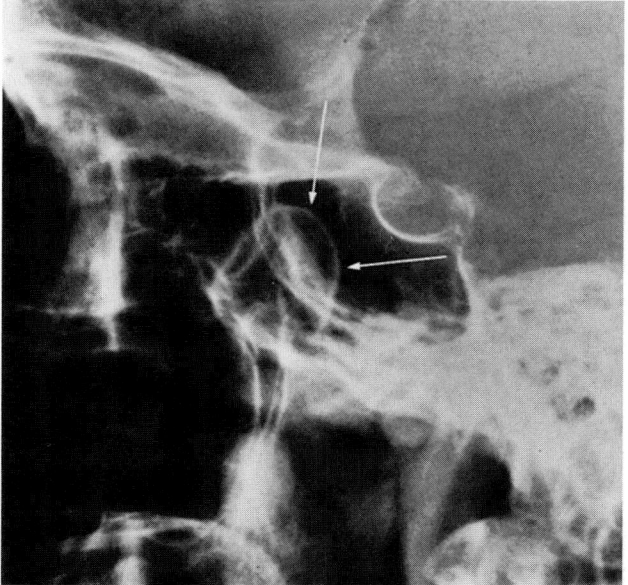

Figure 2–61. Ethmoidal cell extending into the sphenoid sinus.

The Sphenoidal Sinuses

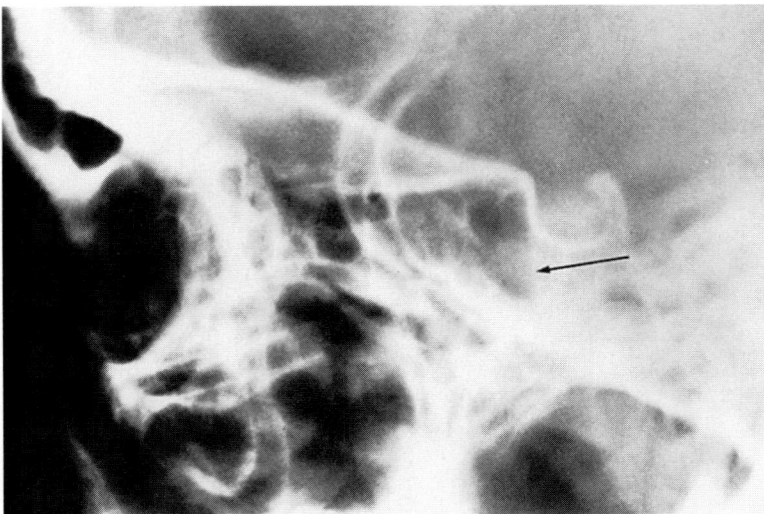

Figure 2–62. Apparent air-fluid level in the sphenoid sinus produced by incomplete aeration. The film was made upright but not brow-up.

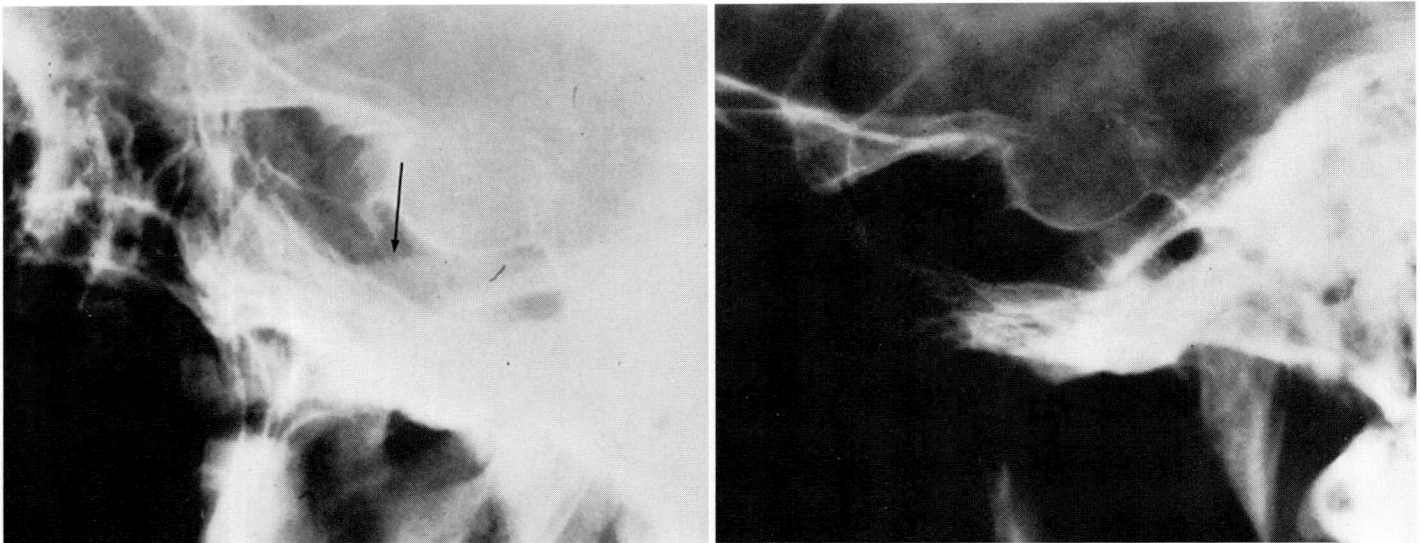

Figure 2–63. *Left,* Simulated air-fluid level in the sphenoid sinus produced by the zygomatic arch. *Right,* heavier exposure shows bony detail to better advantage. (Ref: Swenson WE: Zygomatic arch simulating an air-fluid level in the sphenoid sinus. *Br J Radiol* 61:518, 1988.)

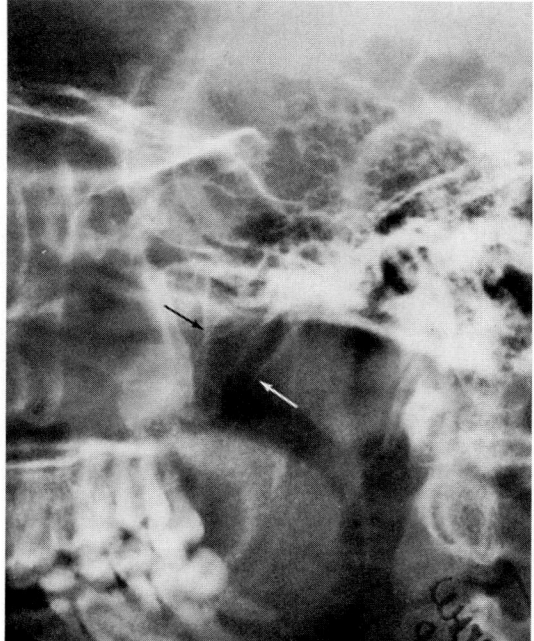

Figure 2–64. Pneumatization of the pterygoid plates.

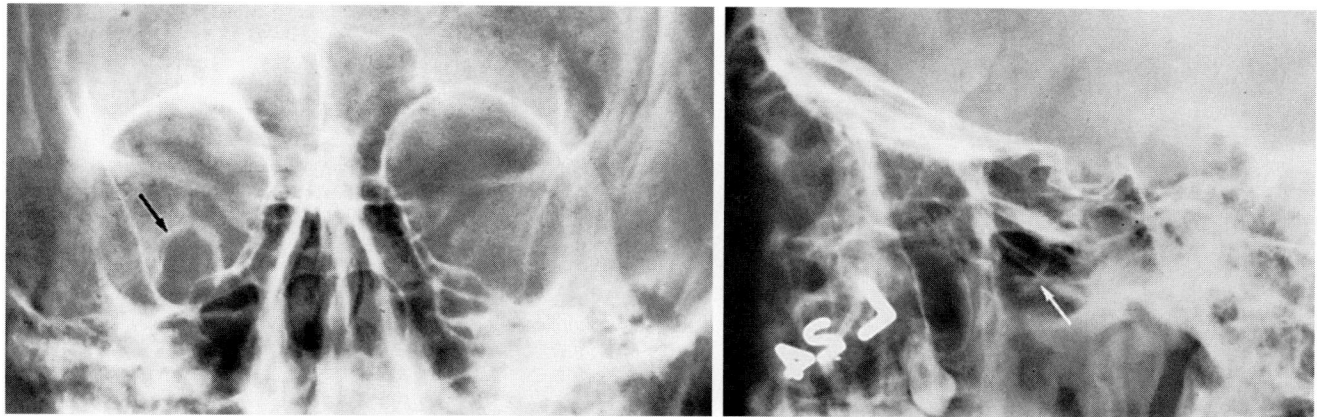

Figure 2–65. Unusual appearance produced by extension of a sphenoidal air cell into the greater wing of the sphenoid. (Ref: Yune HY et al: Normal variations and lesions of the sphenoid sinus. *Am J Roentgenol* 124:129, 1975.)

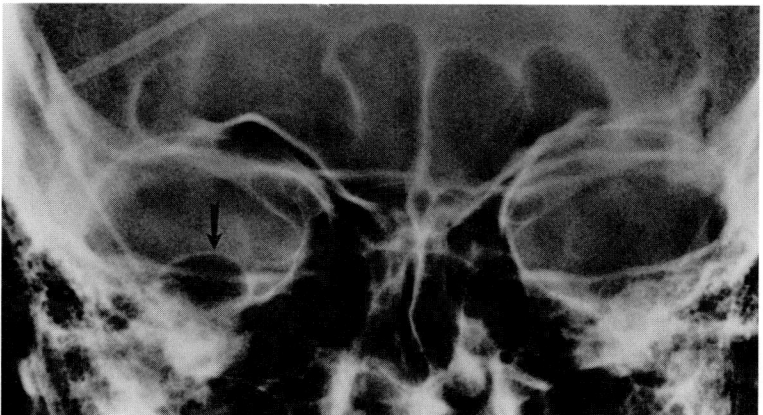

Figure 2–66. Another example of sphenoidal air cell in the greater wing of the sphenoid.

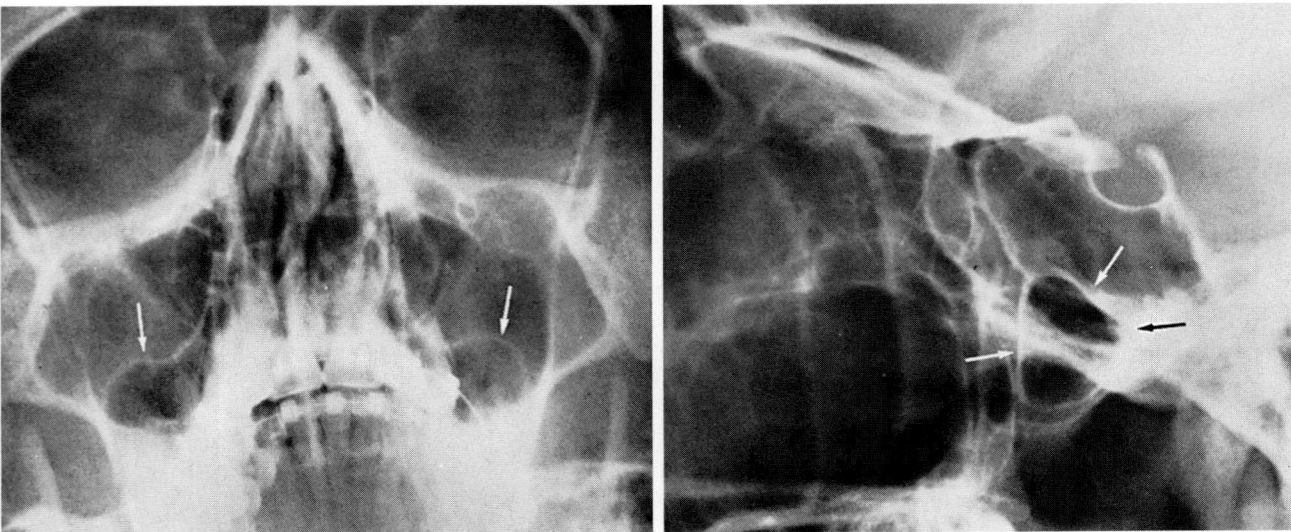

Figure 2–67. Marked lateral and inferior extensions of the sphenoid sinuses.

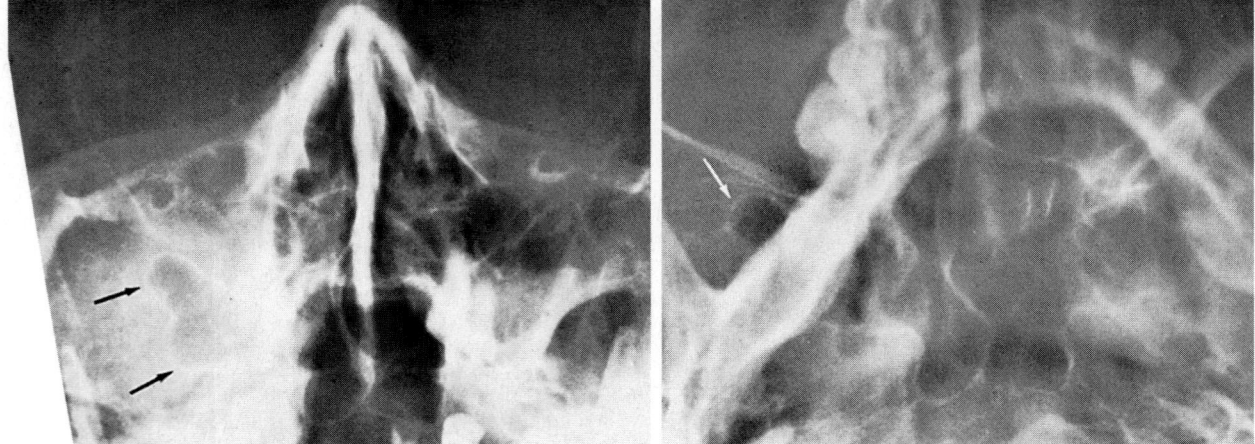

Figure 2–68. Unusually marked lateral extension of the sphenoid sinuses. (Ref: Kattan KR, Potter GY: Lateral extension of sphenoid sinuses. *Med Radiogr Photogr* 59:9, 1983.)

The Zygomatic Arch

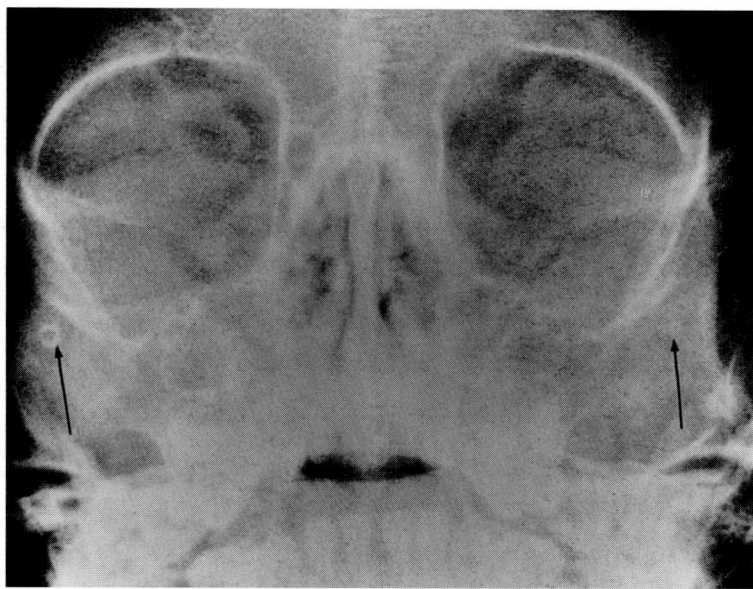

Figure 2–69. The zygomaticotemporal foramen (Hyrtl's foramen). (Ref: Yanagisawa E, Smith HW: Normal radiographic anatomy of the paranasal sinuses. *Otolaryngol Clin North Am* 6:434, 1973.)

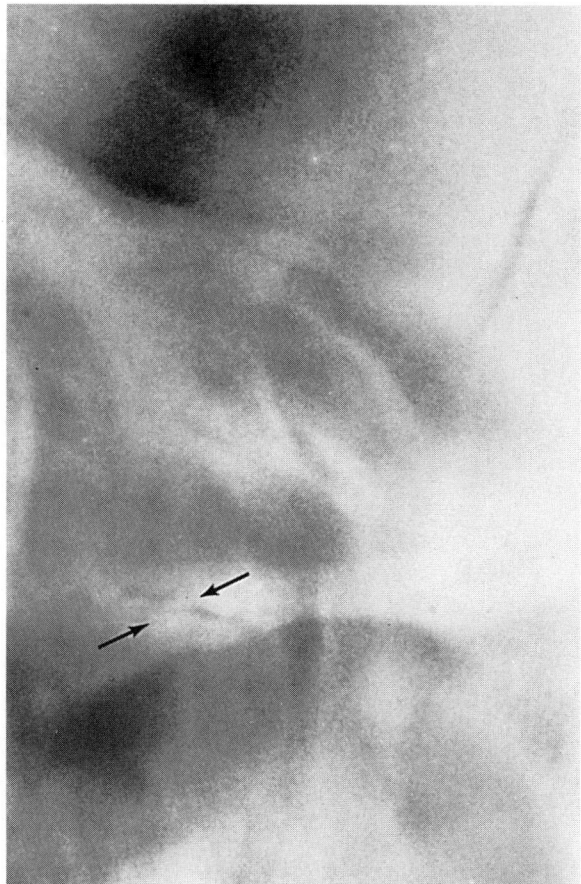

Figure 2–70. Tomogram of the zygomatic arch showing the suture between the zygomatic bone and the zygomatic process of the temporal bone. This suture may be confused with a fracture line.

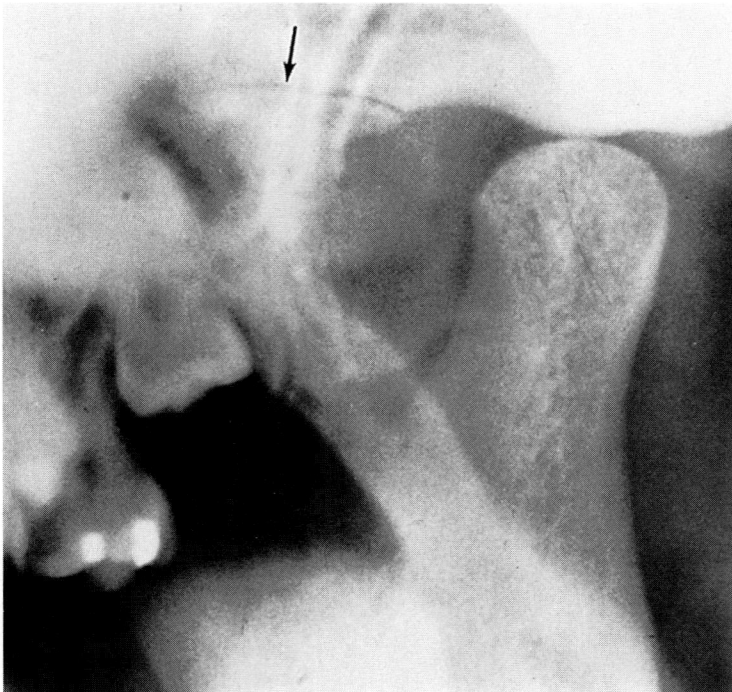

Figure 2–71. The suture between the zygomatic bone and the zygomatic process of the temporal bone seen in oblique projection, simulating a fracture.

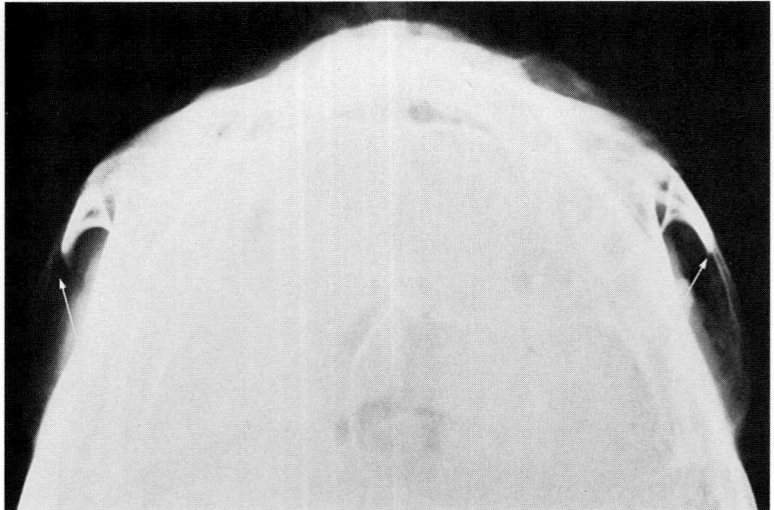

Figure 2–72. Simulated fracture of the zygomatic arch, produced by overlapping shadows of the base and arch of the bone.

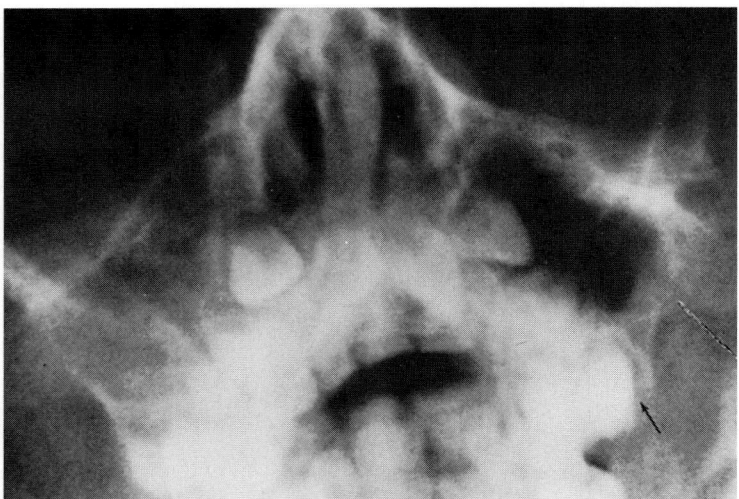

Figure 2–73. The zygomaxillary suture in a 6-year-old boy, simulating a fracture.

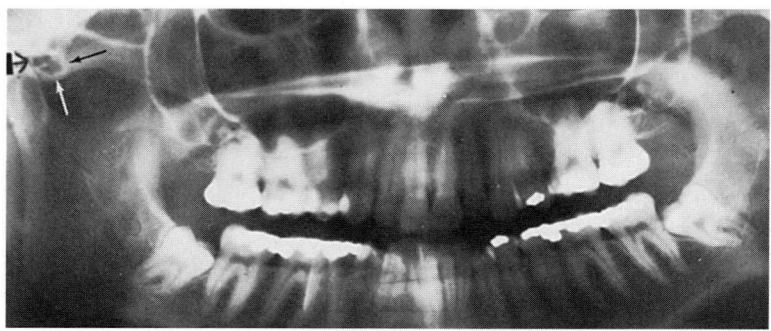

Figure 2–74. Air cell in the zygomatic arch.

The Mandible

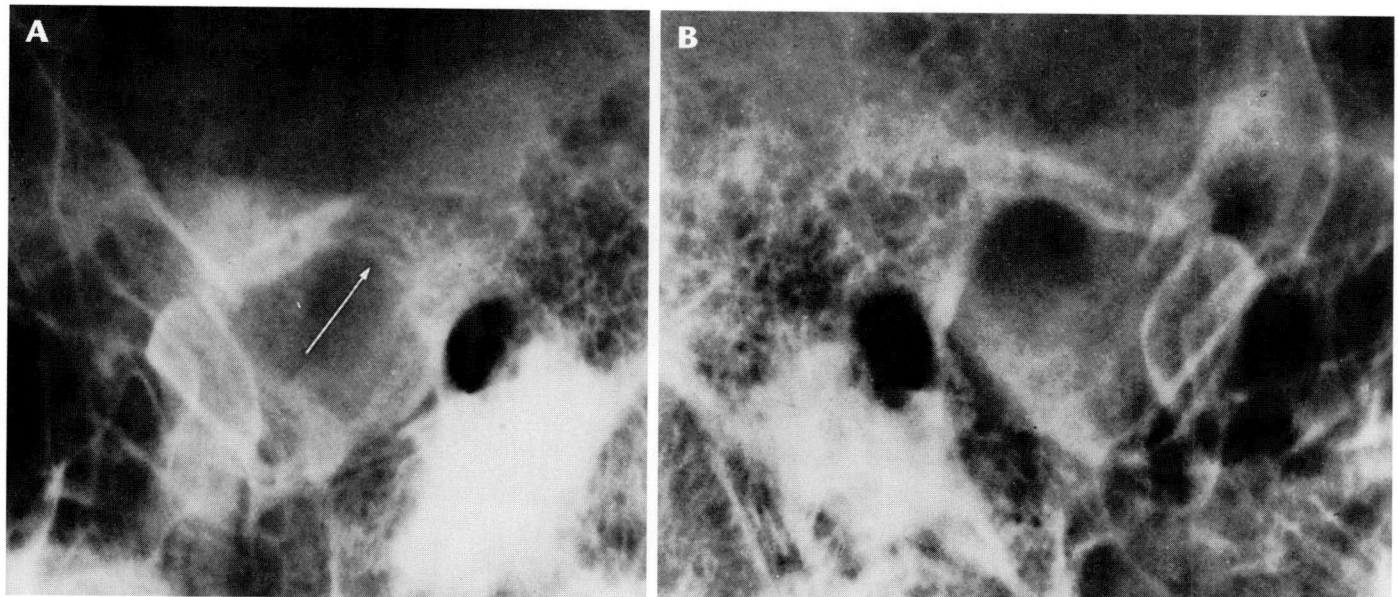

Figure 2–75. Pneumatization of the condylar fossa (**A**), which might be mistaken for arthritic change. Compare with opposite side (**B**).

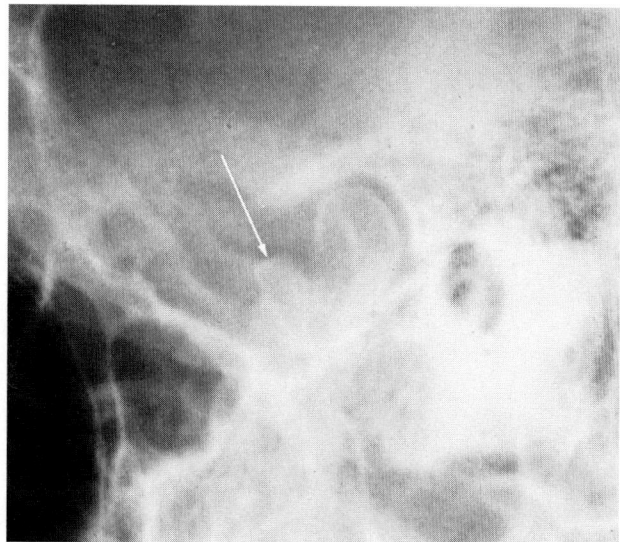

Figure 2–76. Spurlike insertion of the temporomandibular ligament.

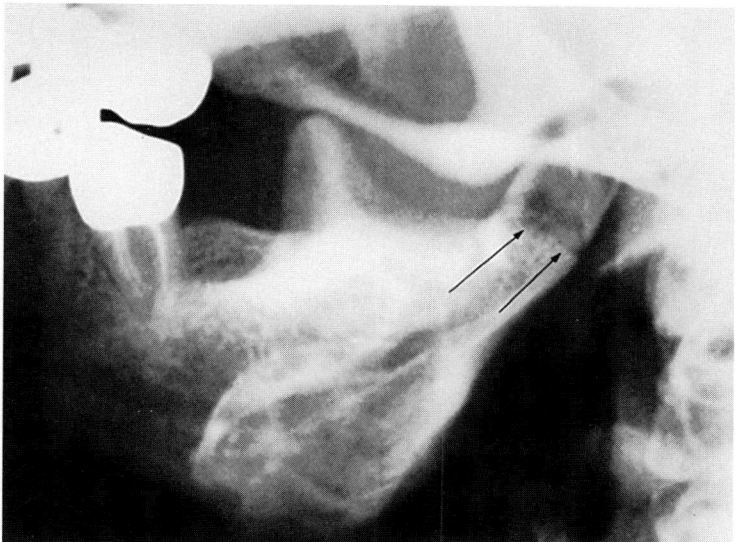

Figure 2–77. Overlapping shadow of the tongue, simulating fracture of the condyle of the mandible. (Courtesy of Dr. Rahmat O. Kashef.)

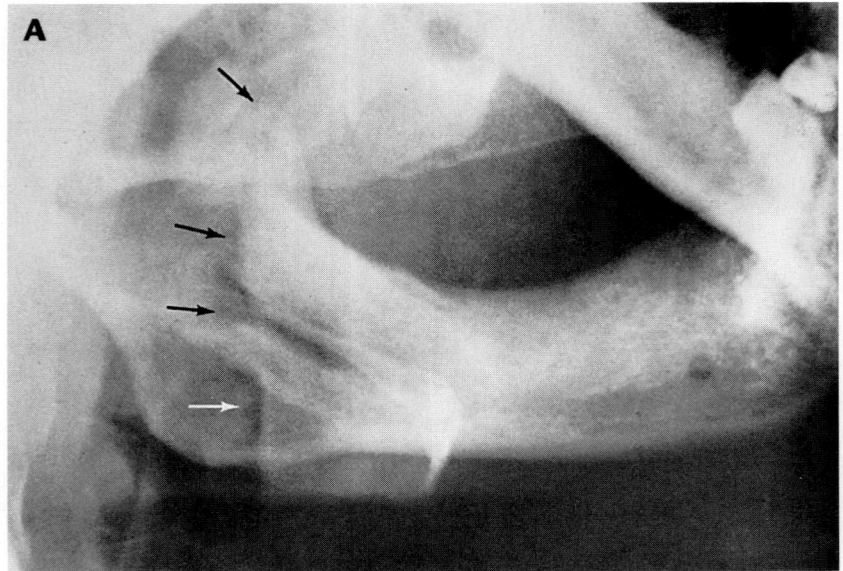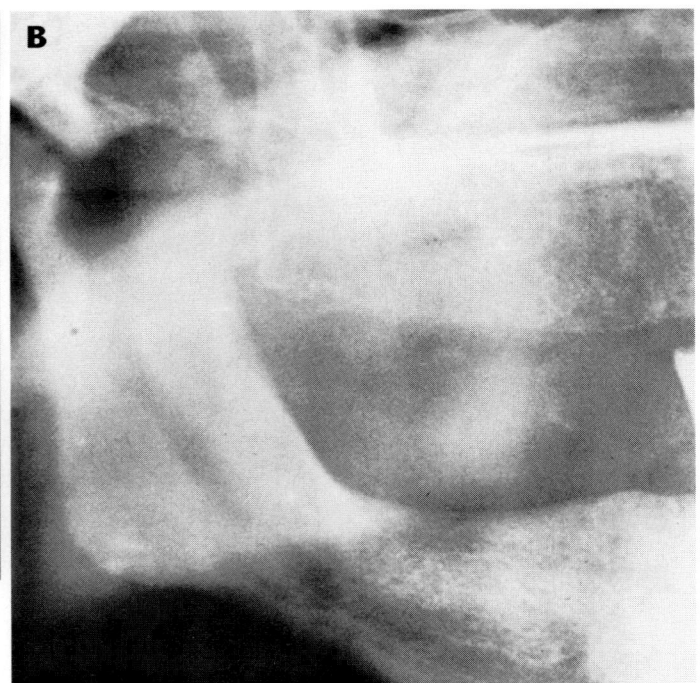

Figure 2–78. A, Pharyngeal air shadow over the base of the tongue superimposed on the mandible simulates a fracture. **B,** Panorex film made at same session shows that no fracture is present.

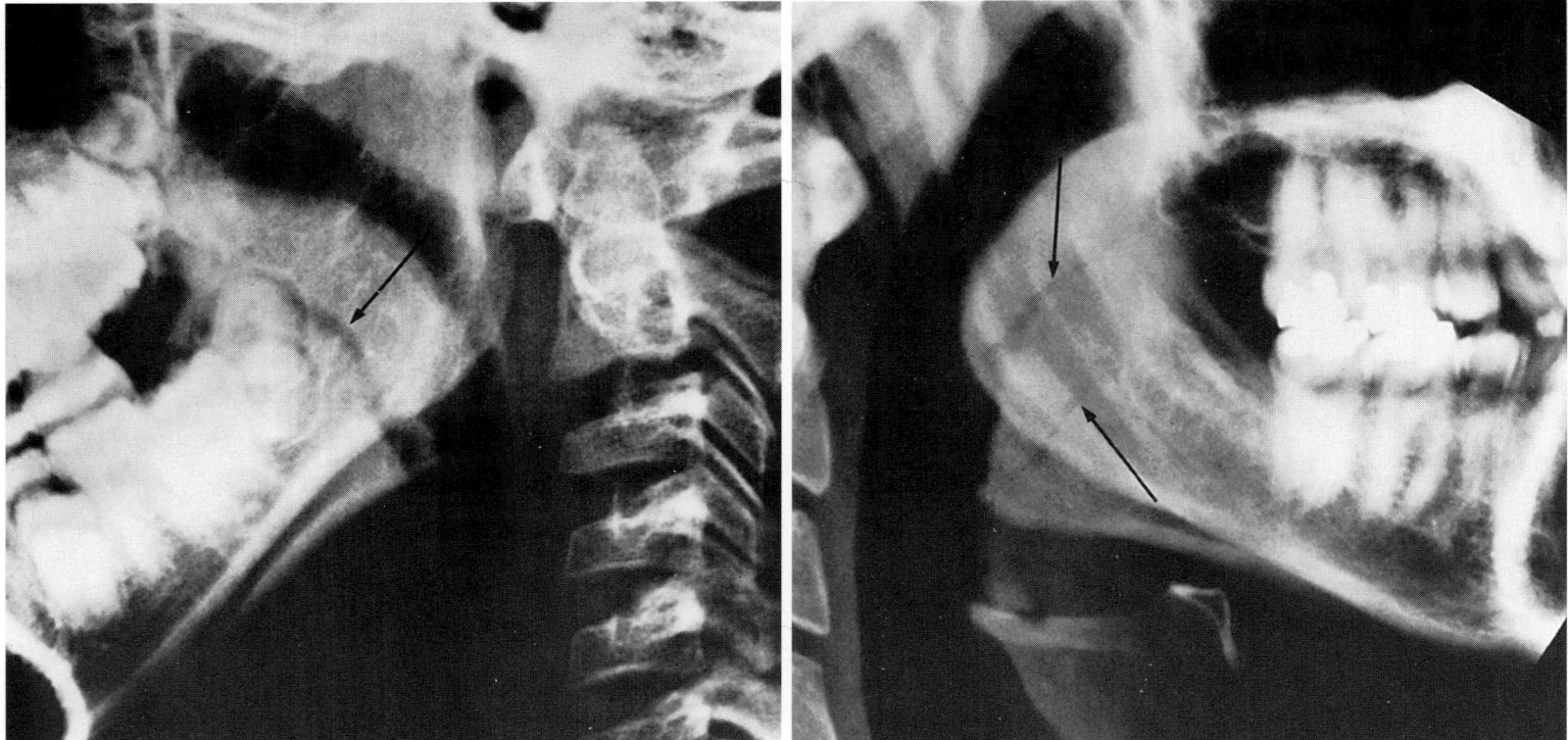

Figure 2–79. Two examples of how the pharyngeal air shadows may simulate a fracture of the mandible.

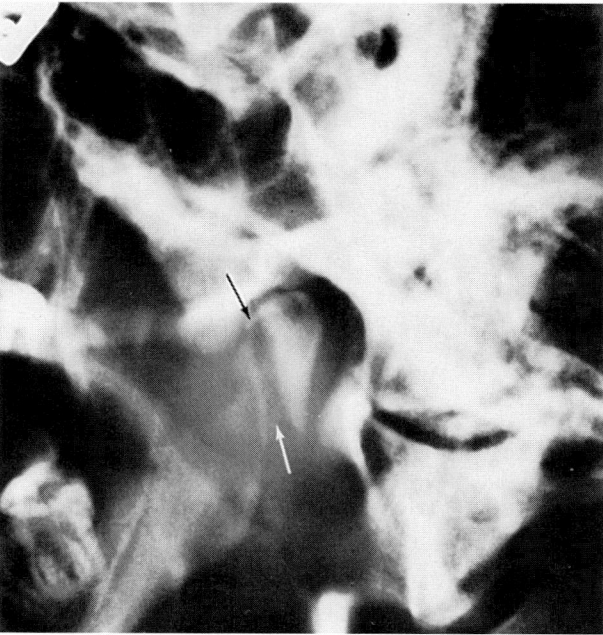

Figure 2–80. Superimposition of the airway, producing an apparent fracture of the mandibular condyle.

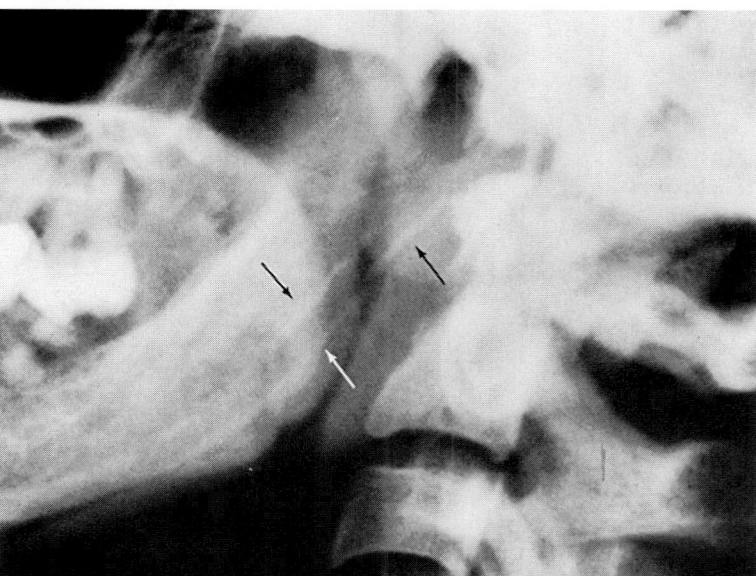

Figure 2–81. The mandibular canal, simulating calcification in soft tissues.

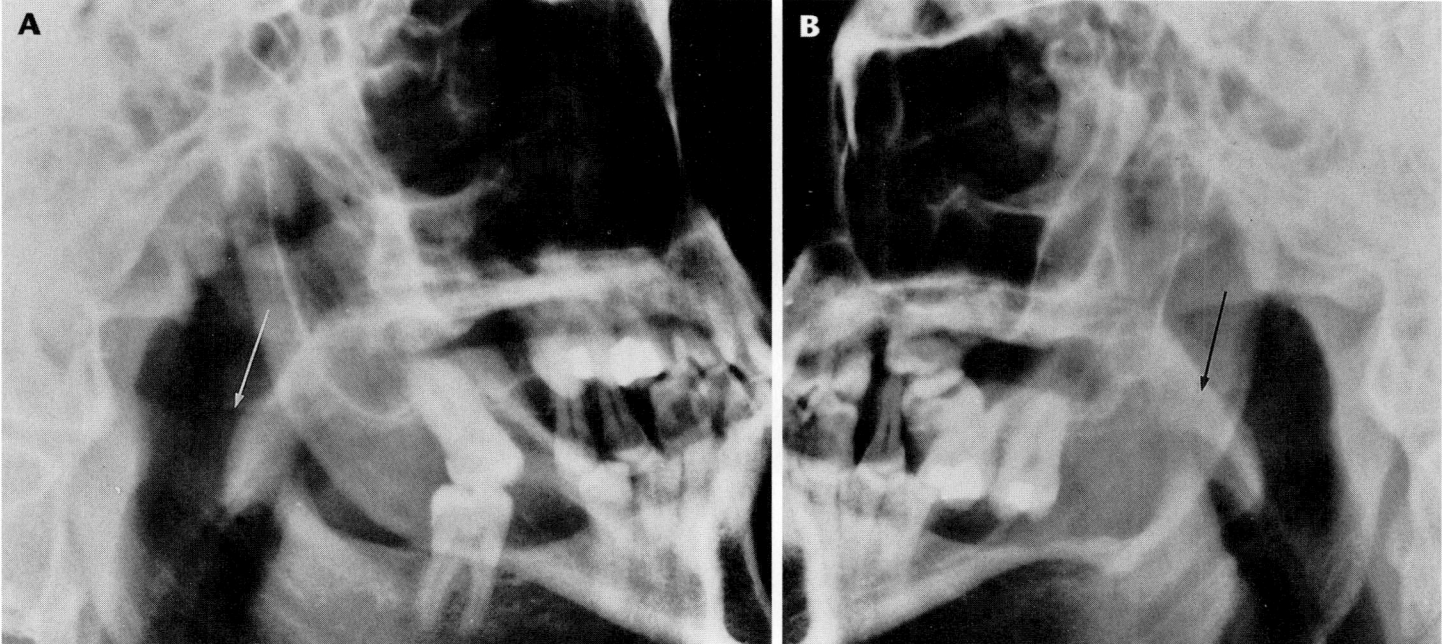

Figure 2–82. Simulated fractures of the coronoid processes produced by superimposition of the lateral pterygoid plates.

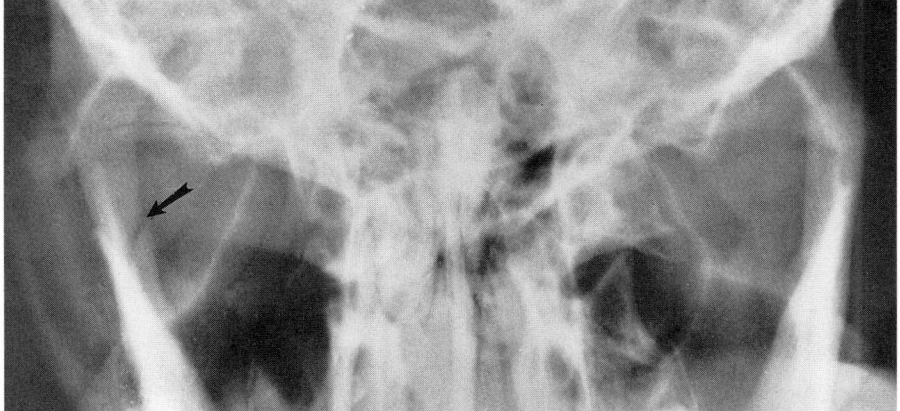

Figure 2–83. Simulated fracture of the ascending ramus of the mandible caused by overlapping of the coronoid process.

145

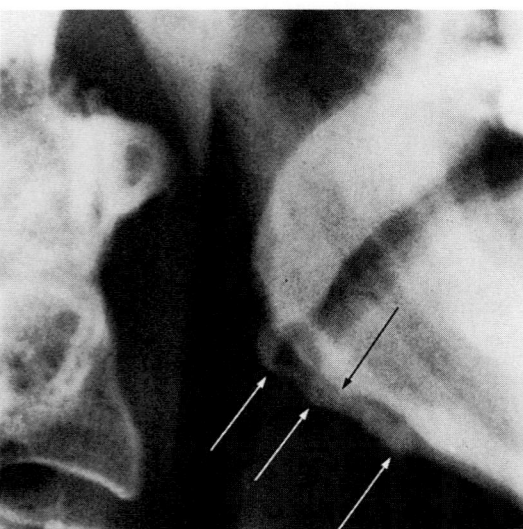

Figure 2–84. Irregularity of the mandibular angles caused by the insertion of the masseter muscles.

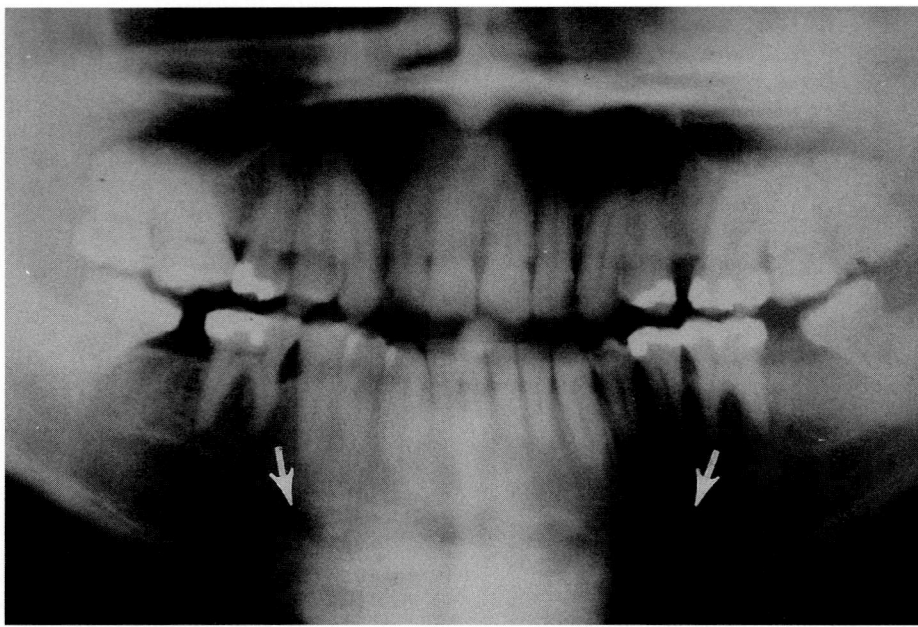

Figure 2–85. Prominent submandibular fossae, which should not be mistaken for area of bone destruction.

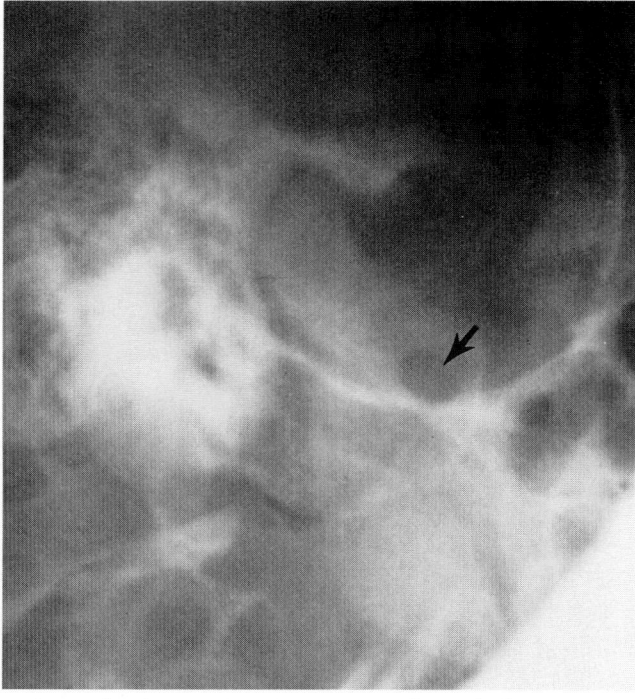

Figure 2–86. The foramen ovale projected through the ascending ramus of the mandible.

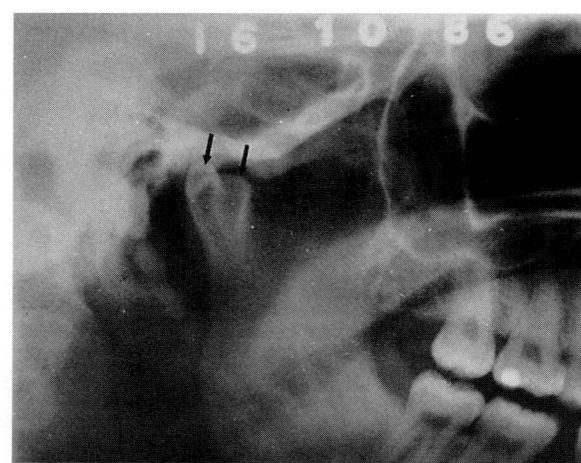

Figure 2–87. Bifid mandibular condyle. (From Loh FC et al: Bifid mandibular condyle. *Oral Surg Oral Med Oral Path* 69:24, 1990. By permission of the publisher.)

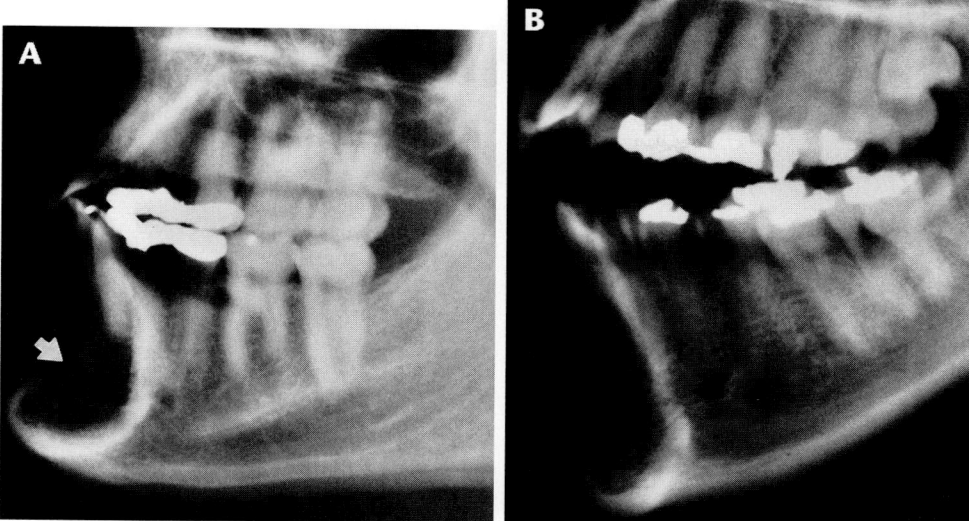

Figure 2–88. A, Simulated destructive lesion of the mandible produced by rotation at time of filming. **B,** Improved positioning corrects apparent lesion.

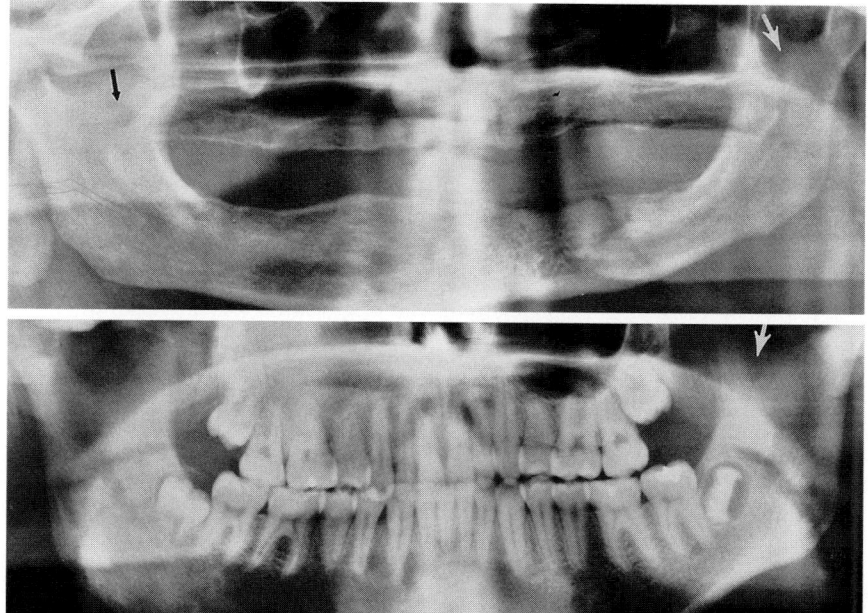

Figure 2–89. Lucencies in the ascending ramus of the mandible caused by fossae (Ref: Honig JF: Anatomical correlation of alveolar subsemilunar translucence on the ascending ramus of the mandible. *Electromedica* 59:58, 1991.)

Figure 2–90. Prominent mandibular angles simulating exostoses.

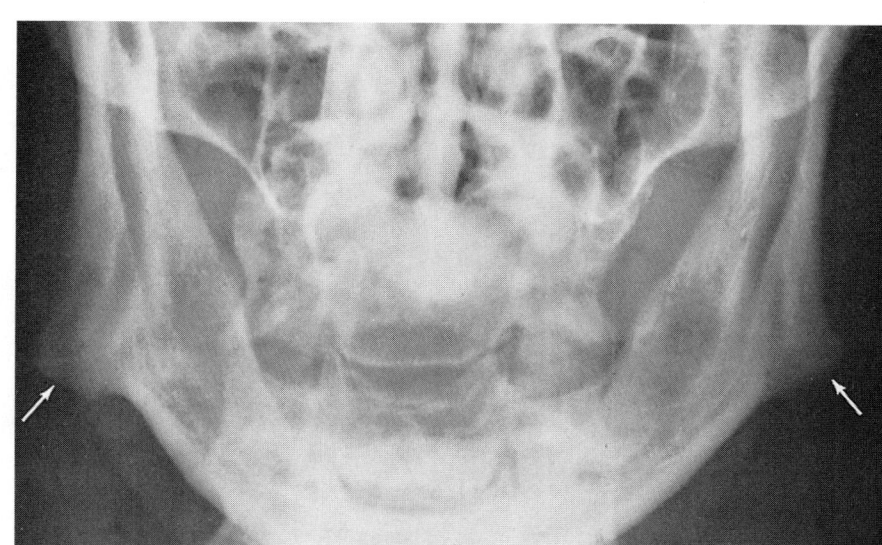

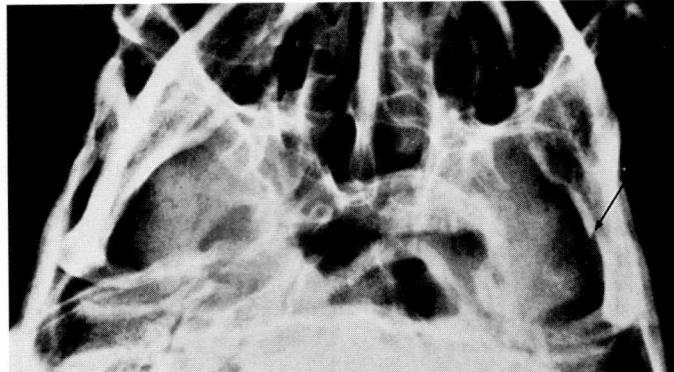

Figure 2–91. Entry point of the mandibular nerve simulating fracture of the mandible.

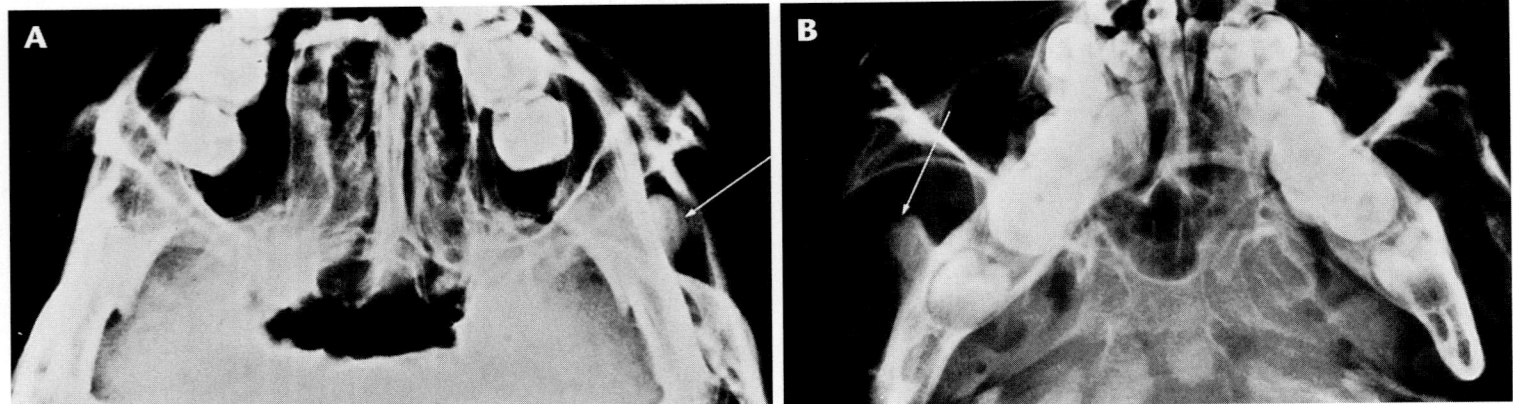

Figure 2–92. A, Coronoid process of the mandible mistaken for an osteoma.
B, Basal view in another patient illustrates the origin of the density seen in **A.**

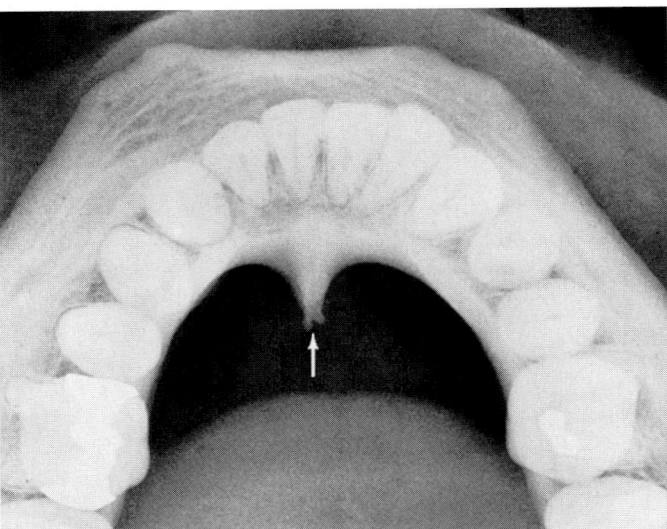

Figure 2–93. Very large geniohyoid tubercle.

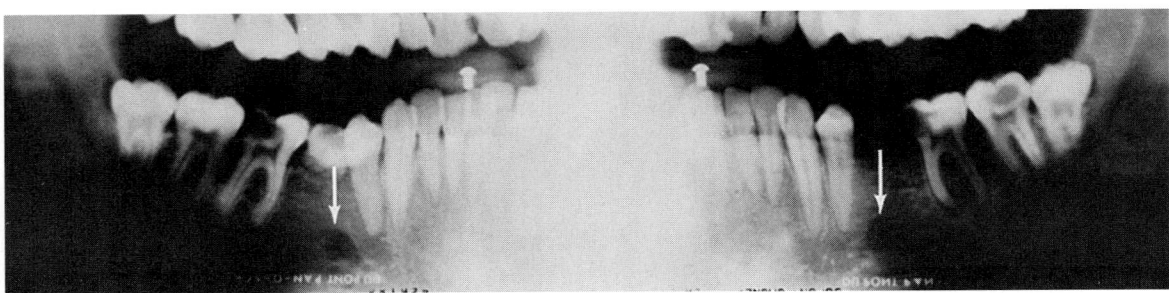

Figure 2–94. The normal mental foramina.

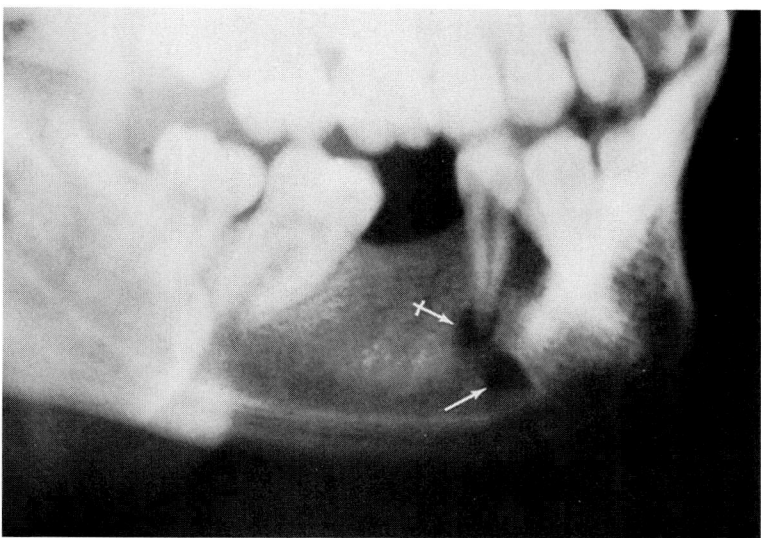

Figure 2–95. The mental foramen (→). Note how it can be mistaken for an apical abscess (↦).

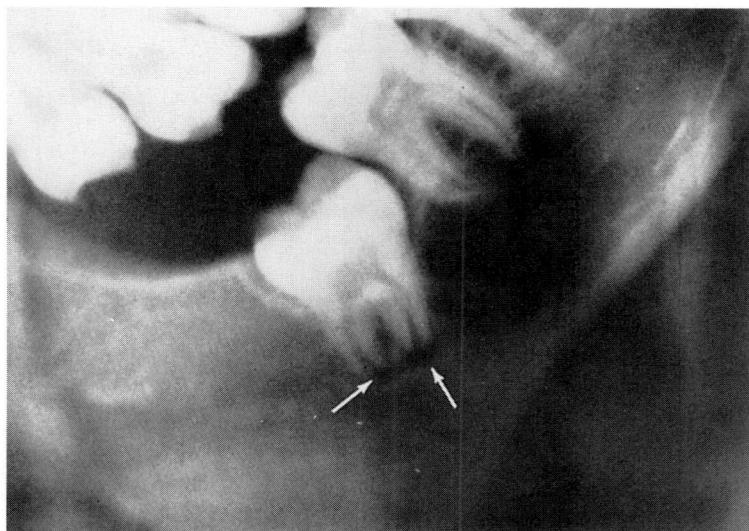

Figure 2–96. The dental crypt of a partially erupted molar should not be mistaken for an apical abscess.

Figure 2–97. Crypts for the third molars in a 9-year-old child, which should not be mistaken for dental cysts.

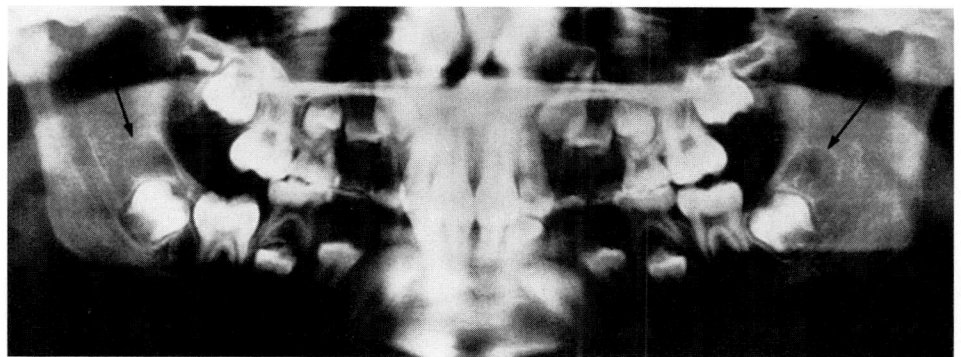

Figure 2–98. Prominent mandibular canals.

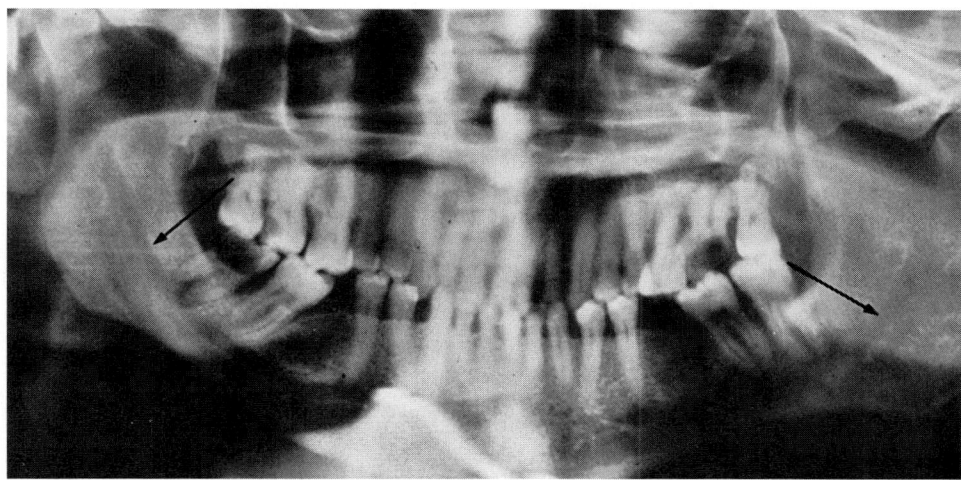

Figure 2–99. The earlobes visualized by Panorex radiography.

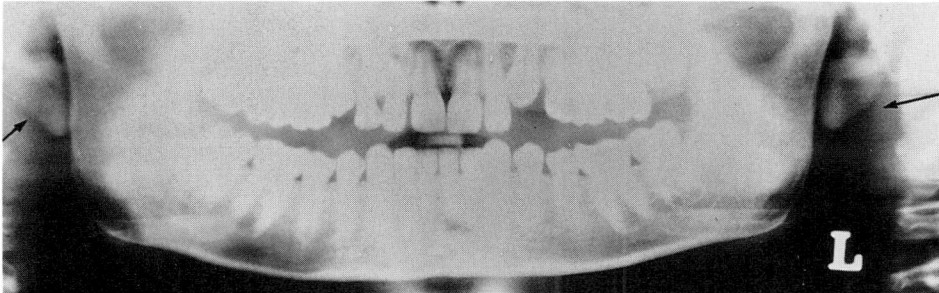

The Nose

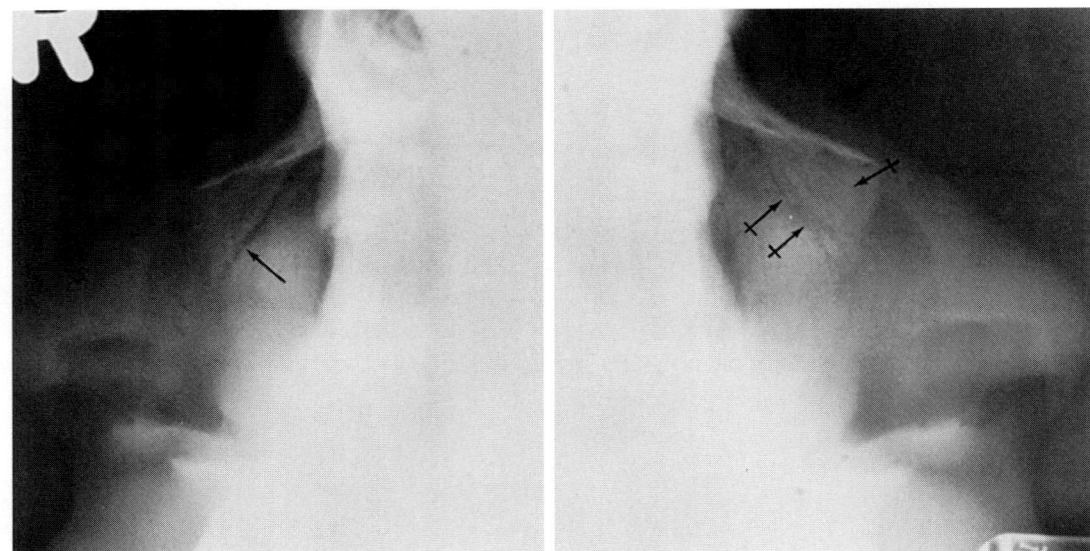

Figure 2–100. The normal nasal bone. Note the nasomaxillary suture (→) and the grooves for the nasociliary nerves (↦). No grooves should cross the nasal bridge. (Ref: de Lacey GJ et al: The radiology of nasal injuries: Problems of interpretation and clinical relevance. *Br J Radiol* 50:412, 1977.)

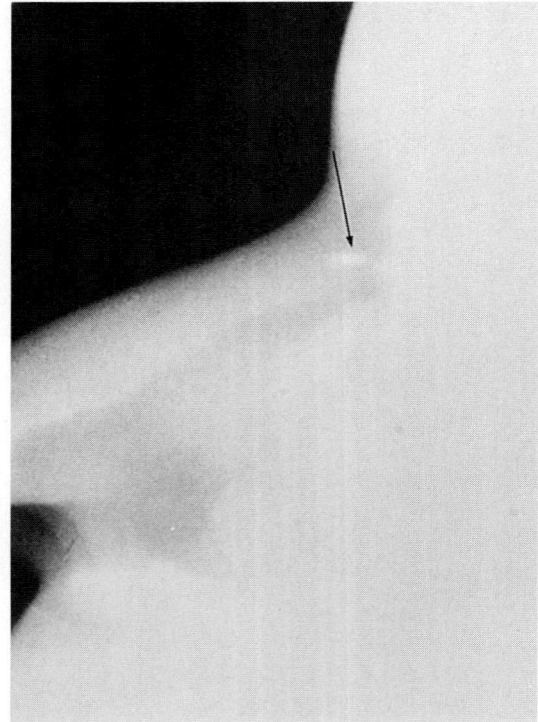

Figure 2–101. Hypoplasia of the nasal bone.

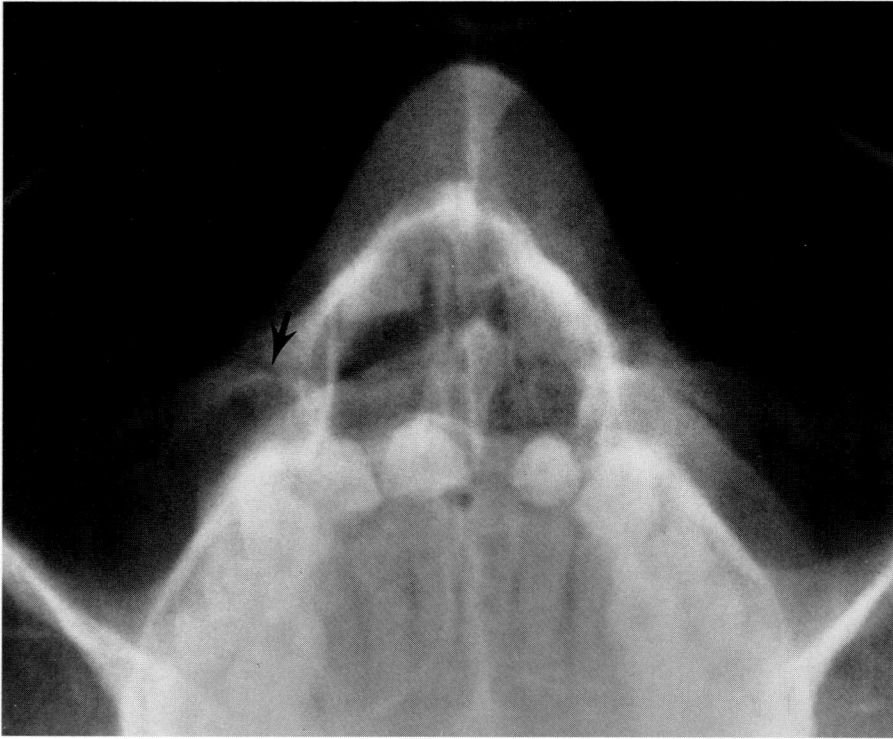

Figure 2–102. Simulated fracture of the nasal bone produced by the shadow of the superimposed coronal suture in an exaggerated Waters' projection. (Ref: Emberton P, Finlay DB: Letter to the Editor. *Clin Radiol* 43:217, 1991.)

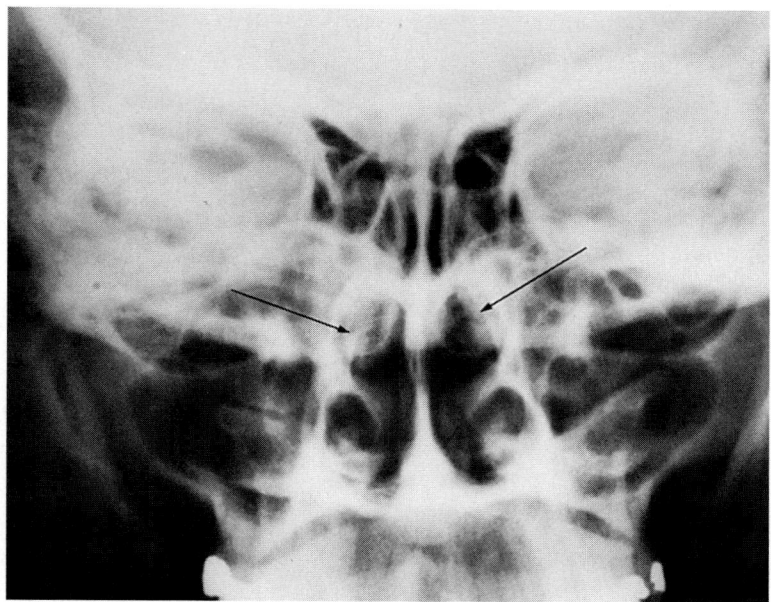

Figure 2–103. Pneumatized middle turbinates (concha bullosa).

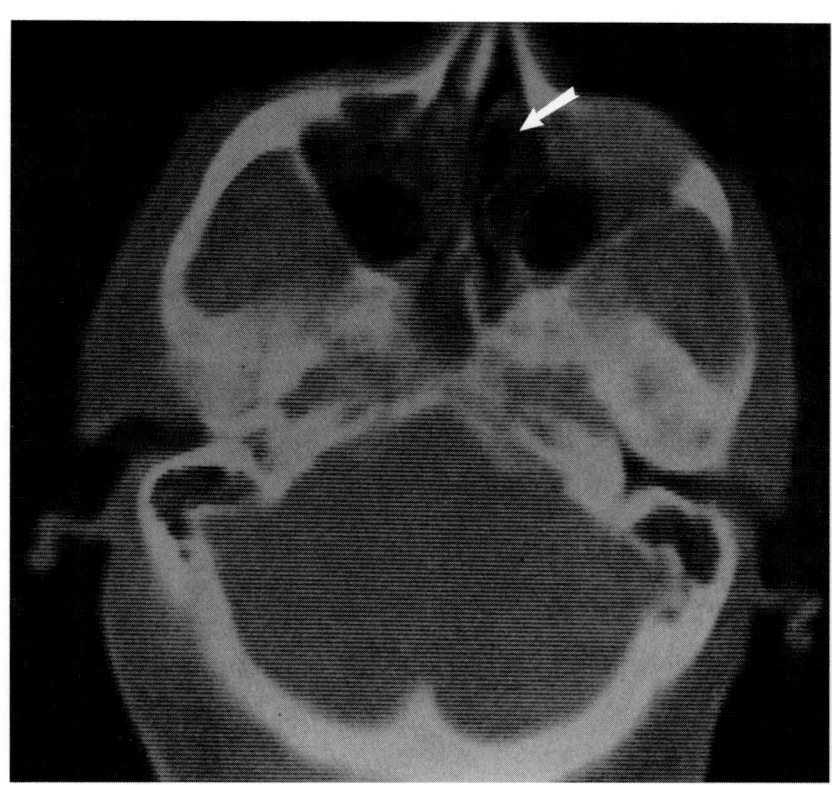

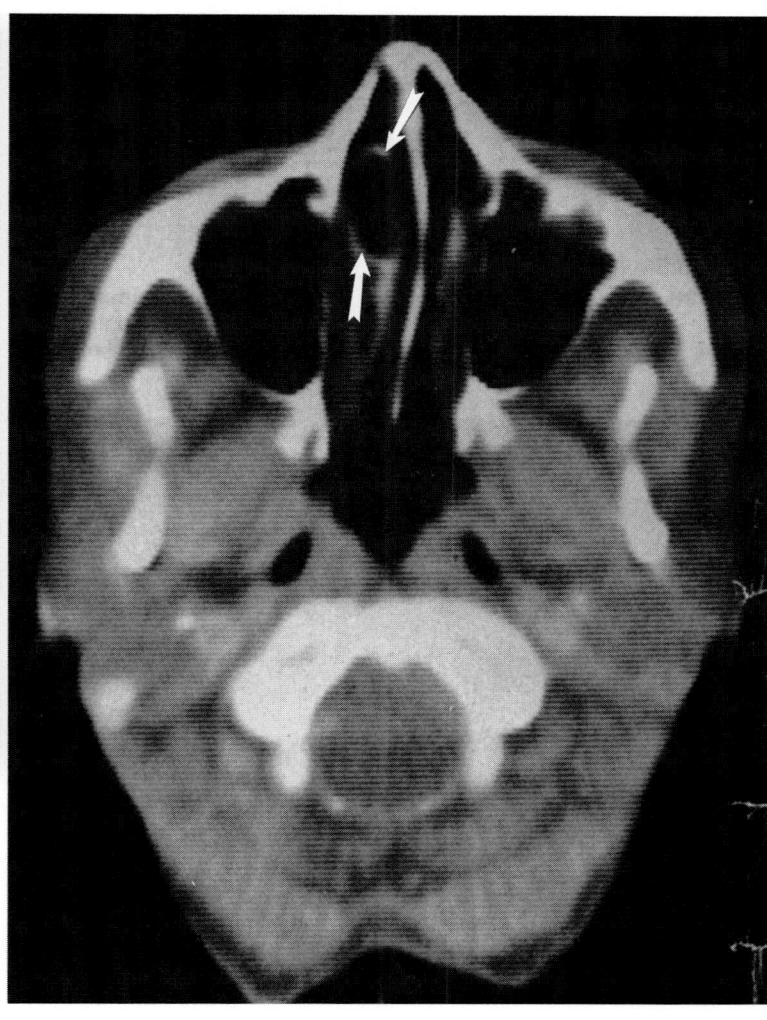

Figure 2–104. Concha bullosa by CT.

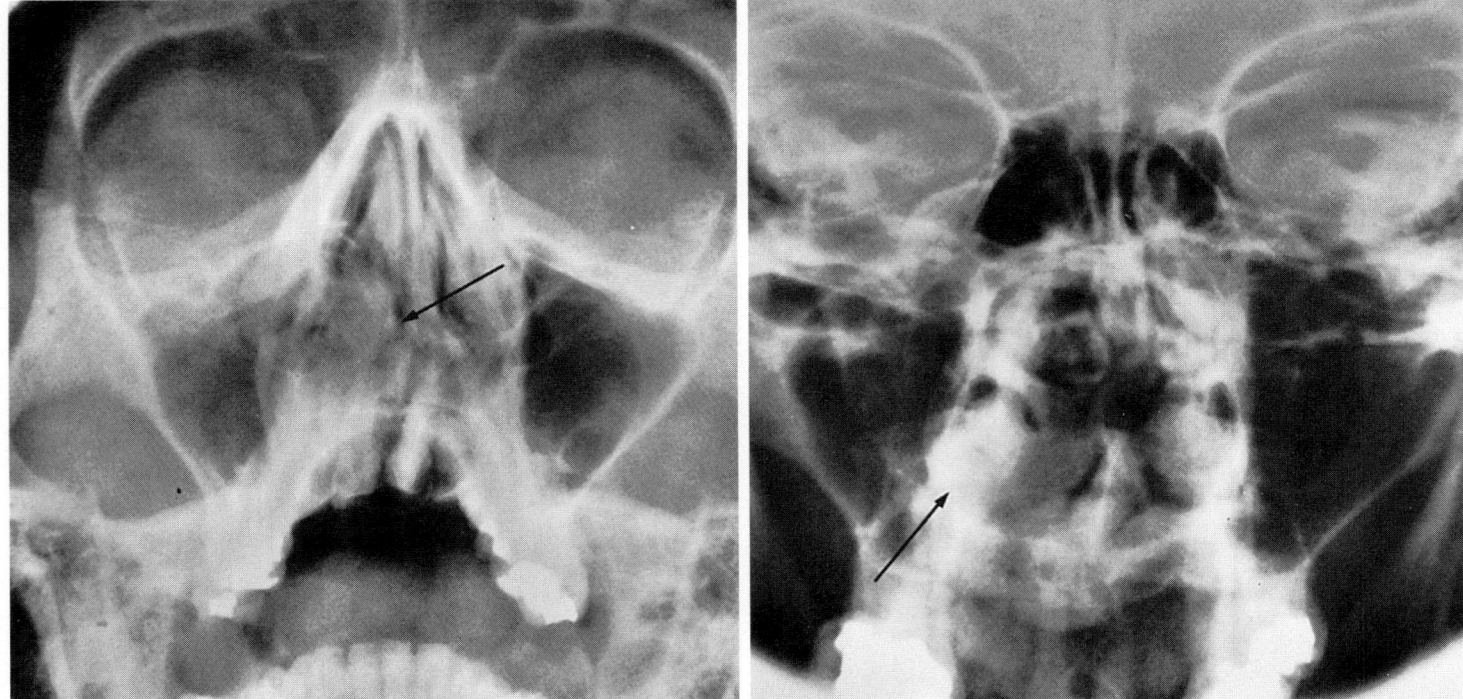

Figure 2–105. *Left,* Waters' projection suggesting a mass in the nasal passage produced by a large inferior turbinate. *Right,* The nature of the mass effect is evident in Caldwell's projection.

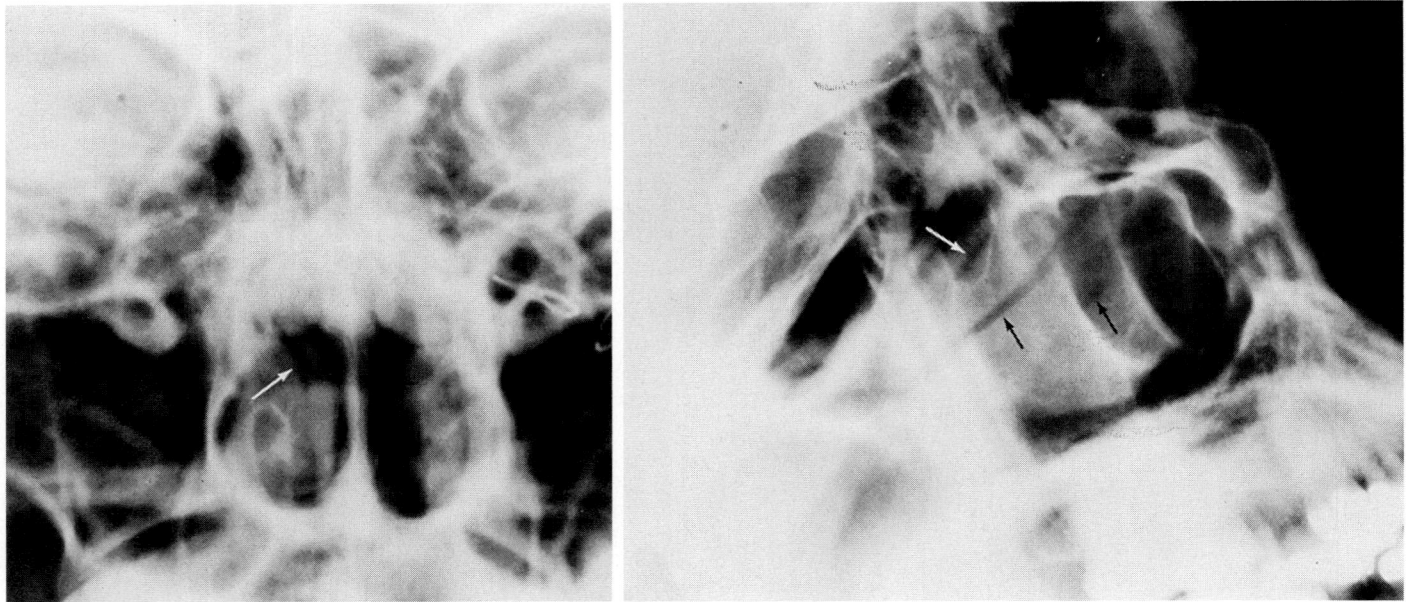

Figure 2–106. Turbinate air stripes.

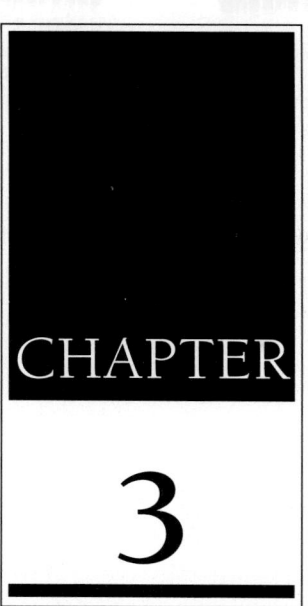

CHAPTER 3

The Spine

The Cervical Spine

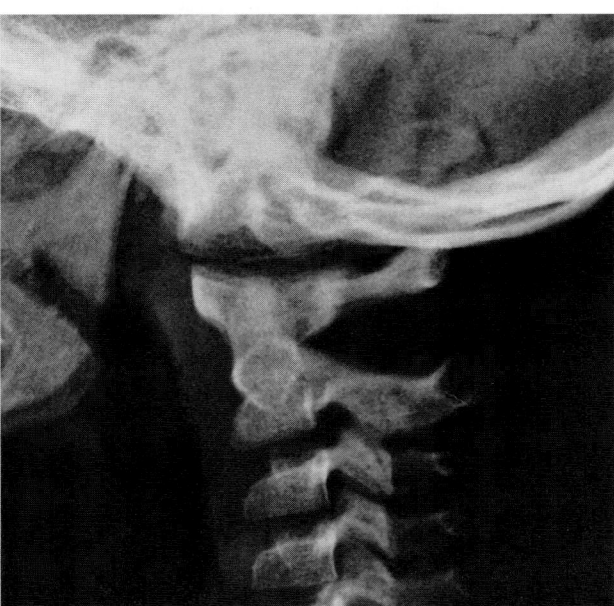

Figure 3–1. Note the remarkable apparent separation of the base of the skull and cervical spine in this 4-year-old child, not to be mistaken for craniovertebral separation. This appearance is most often seen in children younger than this age.

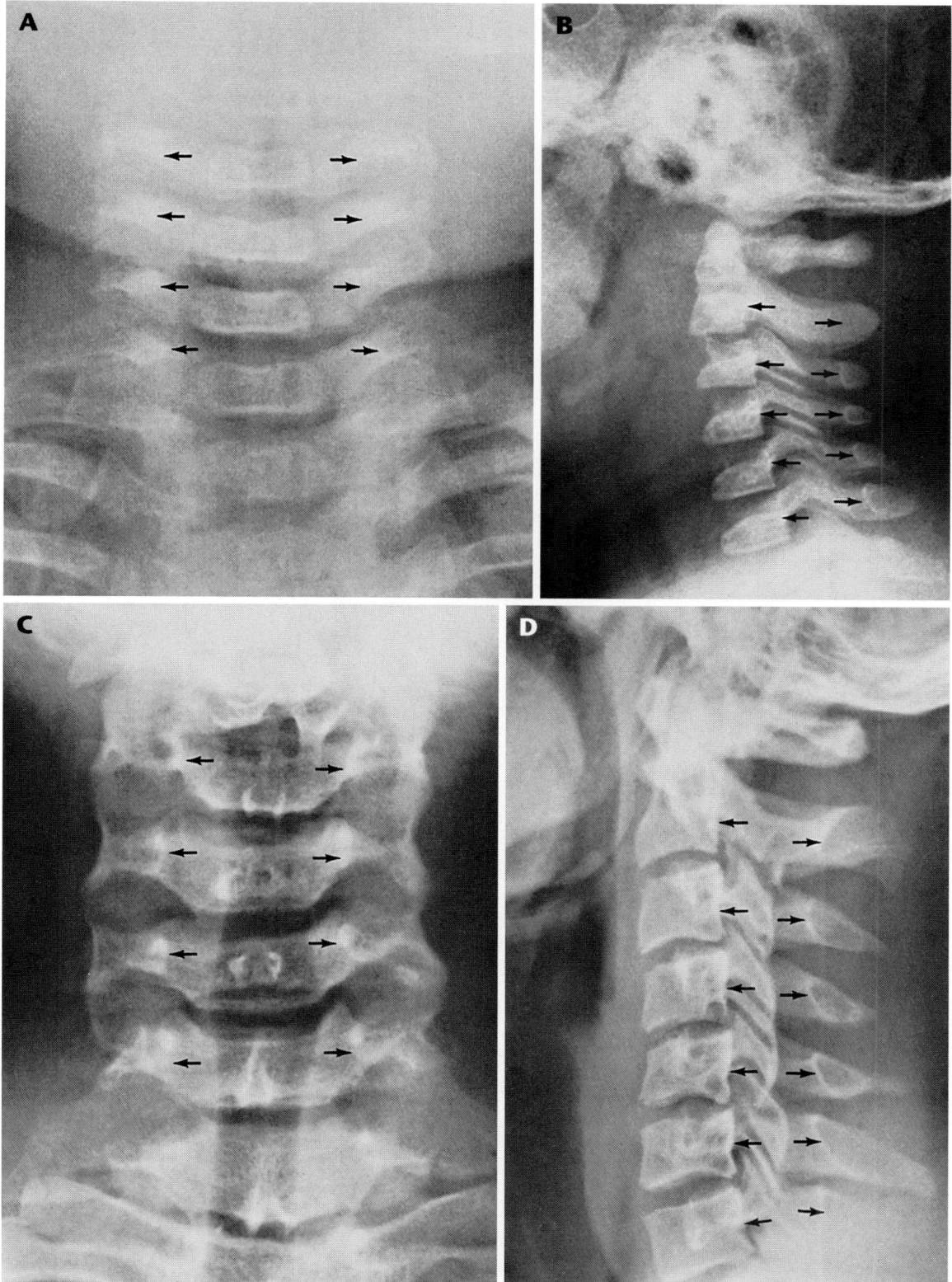

Figure 3–2. The neural canal in the infant is proportionately larger than in the adult. This difference is often overlooked in the infant and may be misinterpreted as a manifestation of pathologic expansion of the spinal canal. **A** and **B**, 4-month-old infant. **C** and **D**, 18-year-old man.

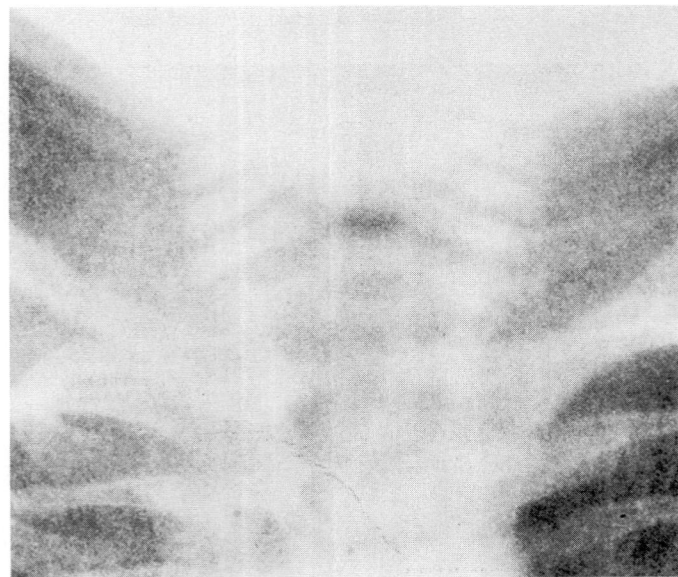

Figure 3–3. Apparent enlargement of the cervical spinal canal in a neonate as a result of flexion of the head at the time of filming and lordotic projection.

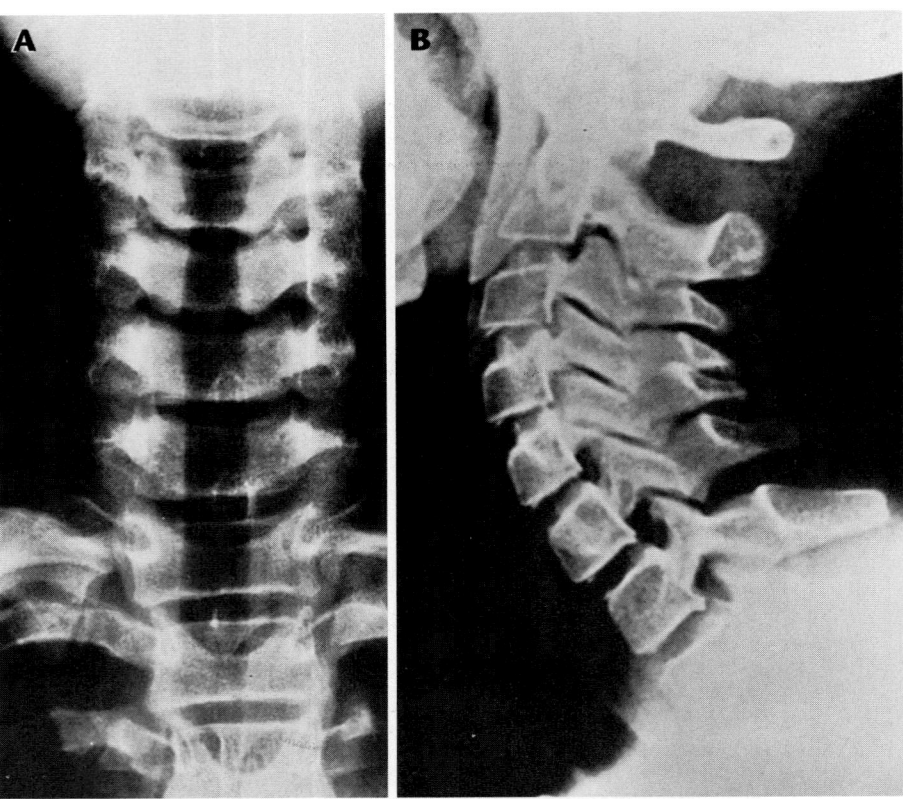

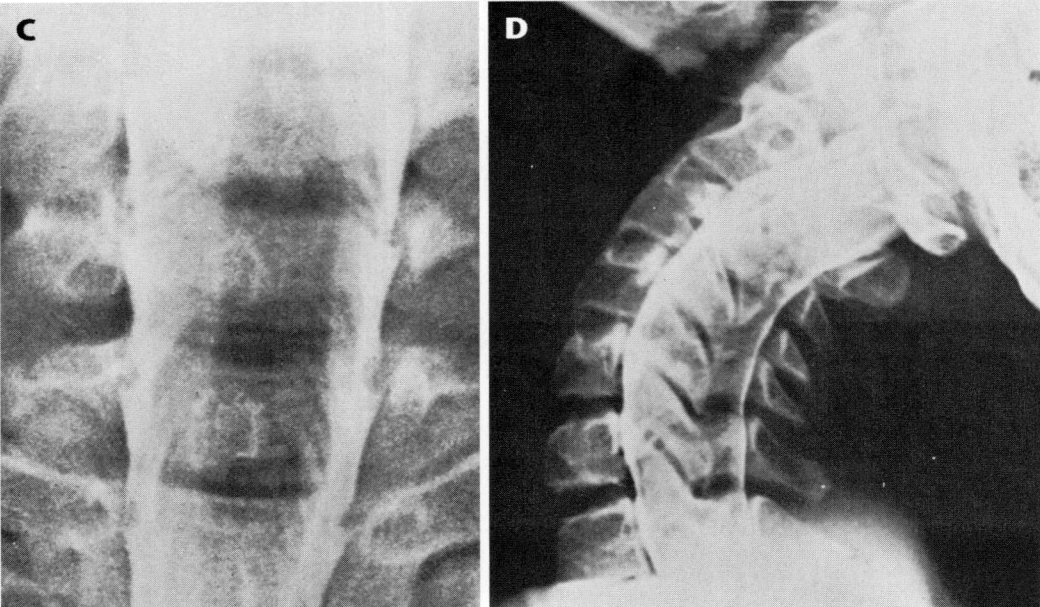

Figure 3–4. Enlargement of the cervical canal with no evidence of cervical cord lesions in normal children. **A** and **B,** Plain films showing marked enlargement of cervical canal. **C** and **D,** Myelograms showing large dural sac with normal cord. The same phenomenon may also be seen in the thoracic spine. (Ref: Yousefzadeh DK et al: Normal sagittal diameter and variation in the pediatric cervical spine. *Radiology* 144:319, 1982.)

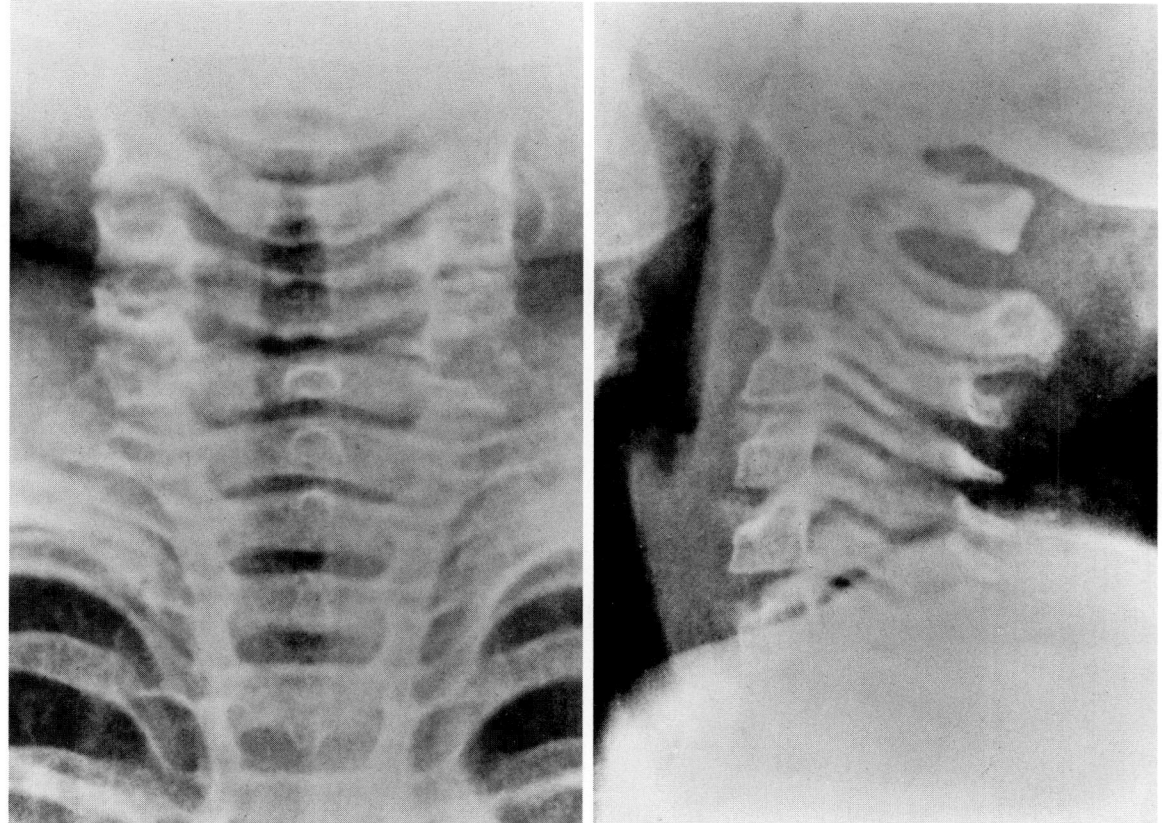

Figure 3–5. Large cervical canal in a healthy 4½-year-old girl.

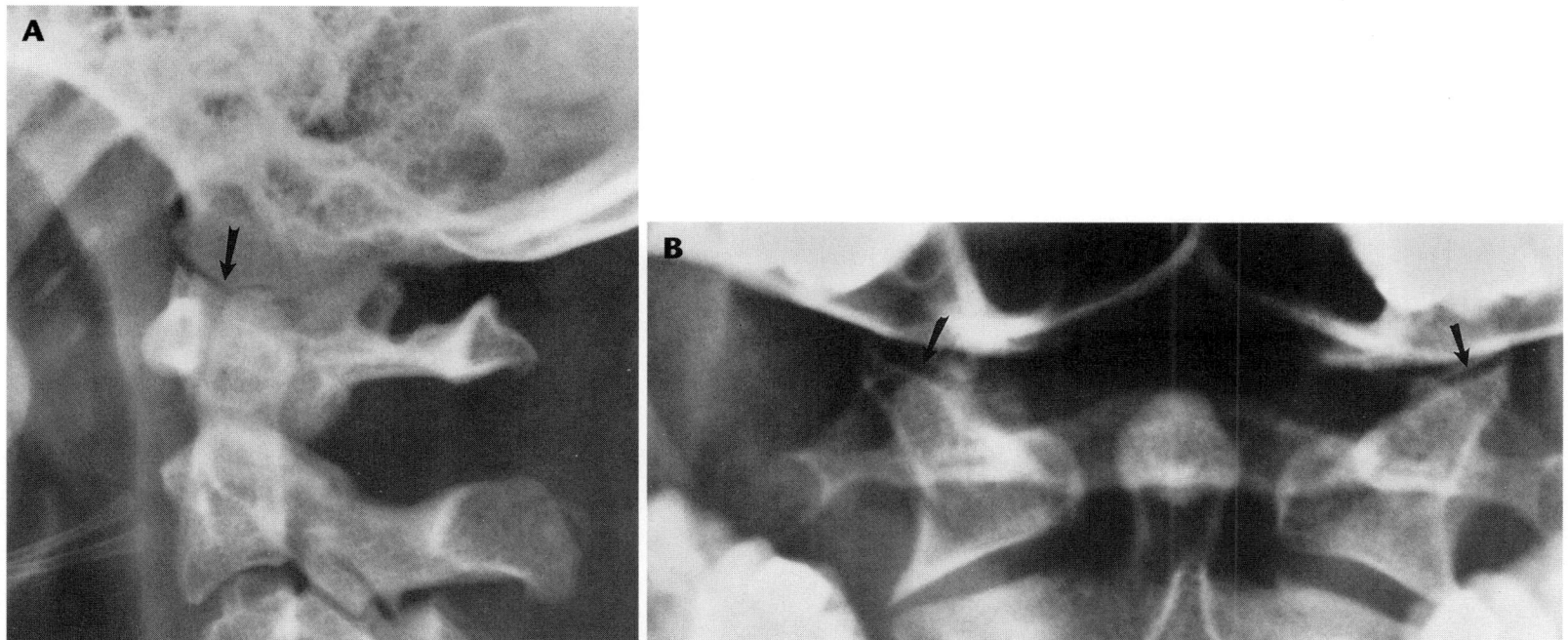

Figure 3–6. A, Prominent occipital condyles. **B,** The articulation between the occipital condyles and the lateral masses of C1.

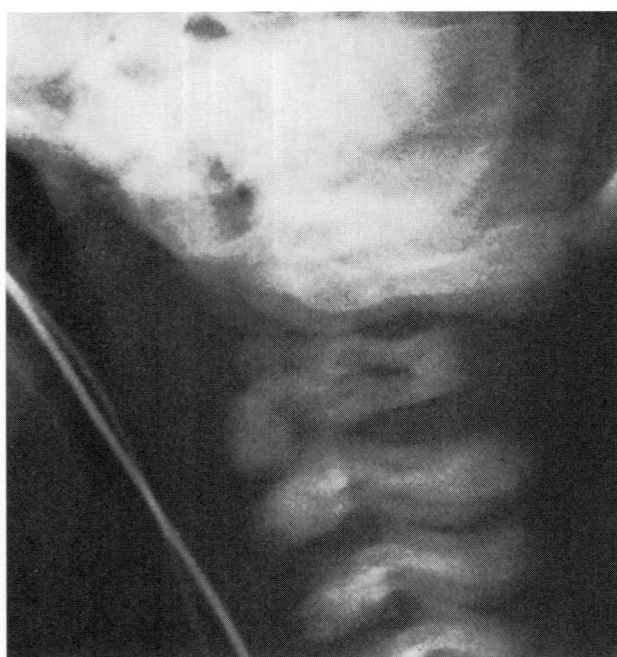

Figure 3–7. Absence of ossification in the anterior arch of C1 in a neonate. This is the normal situation in many neonates. (Ref: Dedick AP, Caffey J: Roentgen findings in the skull and chest in 1030 newborn infants. *Radiology* 61:13, 1953.)

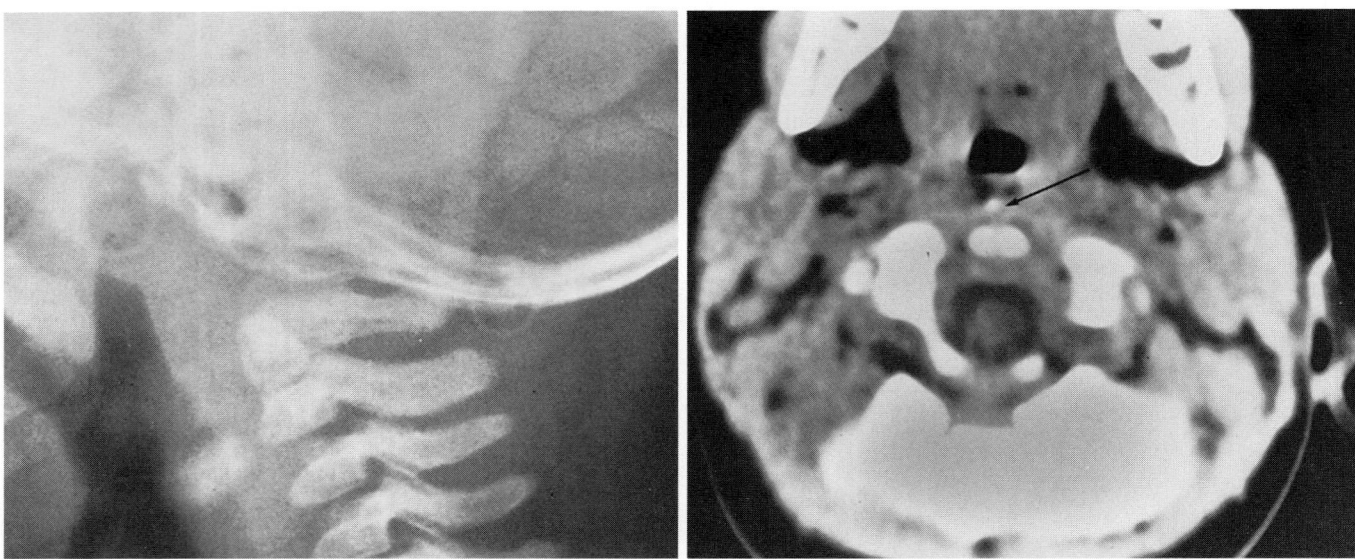

Figure 3–8. *Left,* Apparent absence of the anterior arch of C1 in a 29-month-old child. Ordinarily this should be evident by 12 months of age. *Right,* CT shows a small ossific nucleus for the anterior arch.

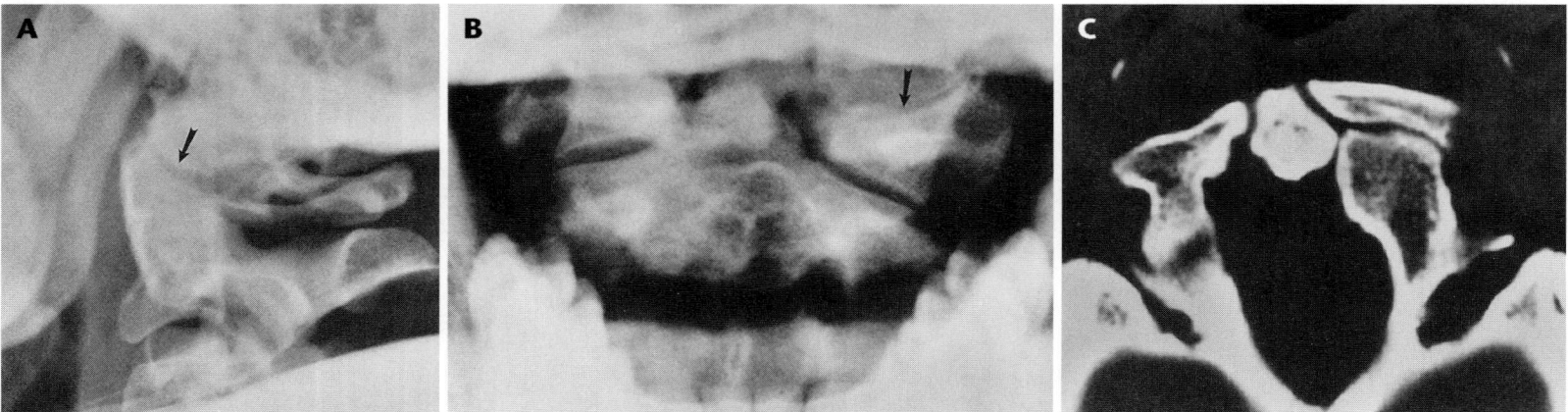

Figure 3–9. Absence of the anterior arch of C1. The left lateral condyle is huge *(arrow)*; the right is hypoplastic. **A,** Lateral; **B,** AP tomogram; **C,** CT.

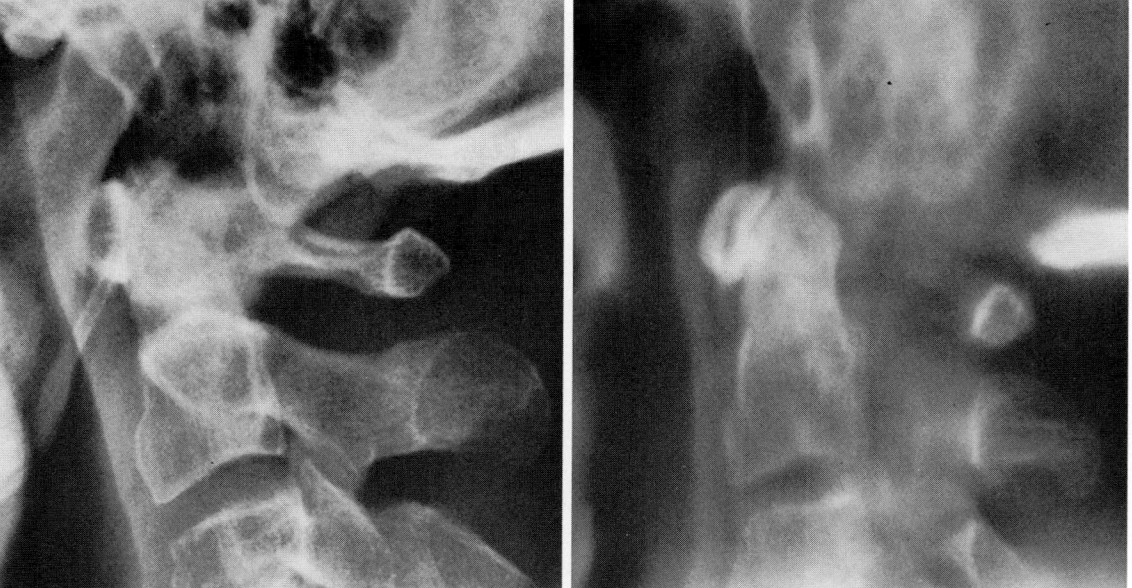

Figure 3–10. Simulated craniovertebral dislocation resulting from a slight tilting of the head at the time of filming. *Right,* Tomogram shows normal relationships of C1 to base of skull.

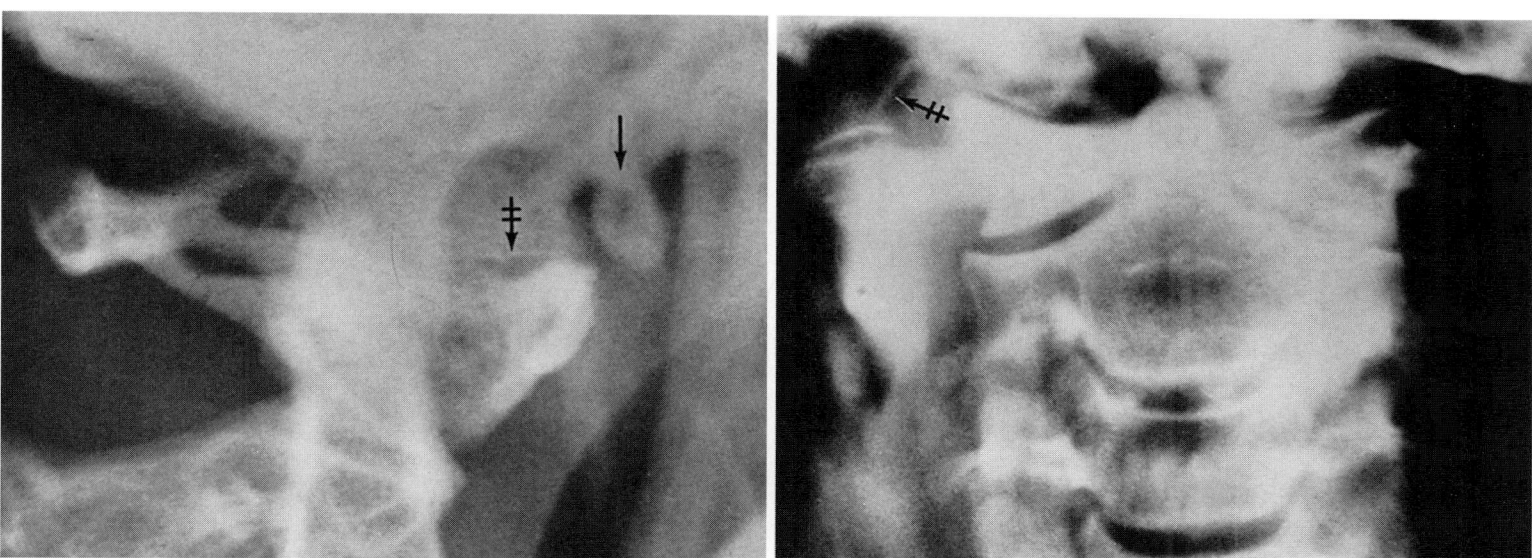

Figure 3–11. Occipital vertebra; the third condyle (←). A unilateral paracondylar process is present, which articulates with the transverse process of the atlas (⇇). (Ref: Lombardi G: The occipital vertebra. *Am J Roentgenol* 86:260, 1961.)

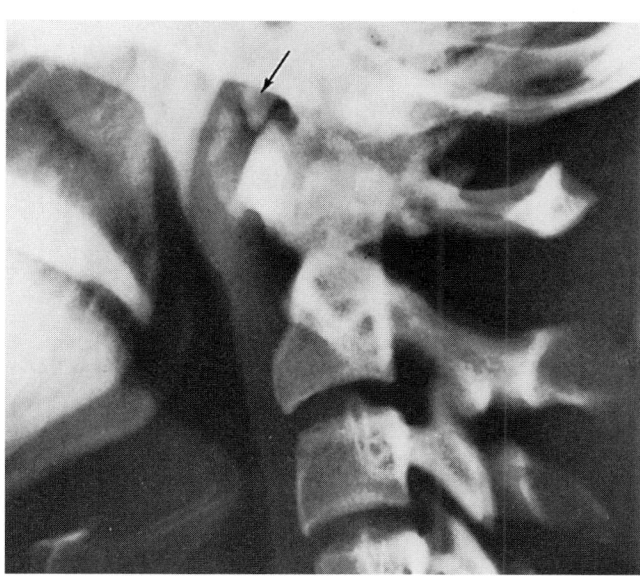

Figure 3–12. A smaller third occipital condyle.

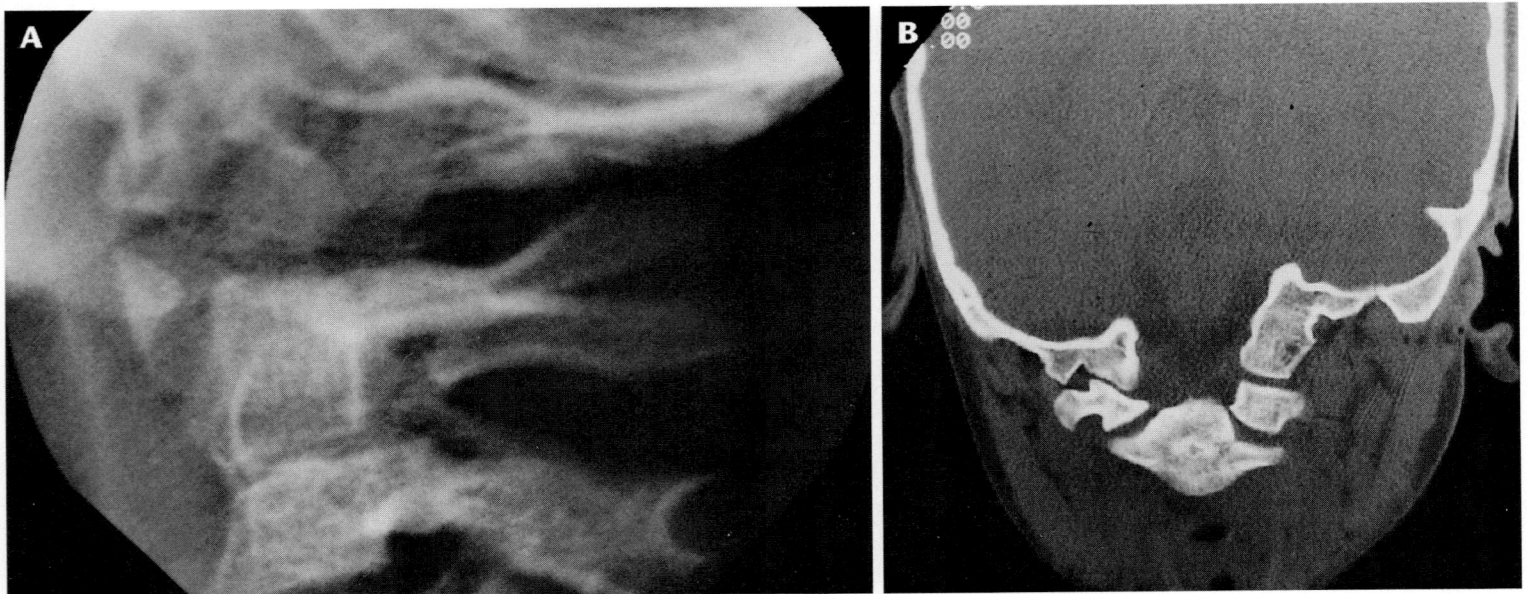

Figure 3–13. Assimilation of the left hemi-proatlas or occipital vertebra.
A, Lateral projection. **B,** Coronal CT.

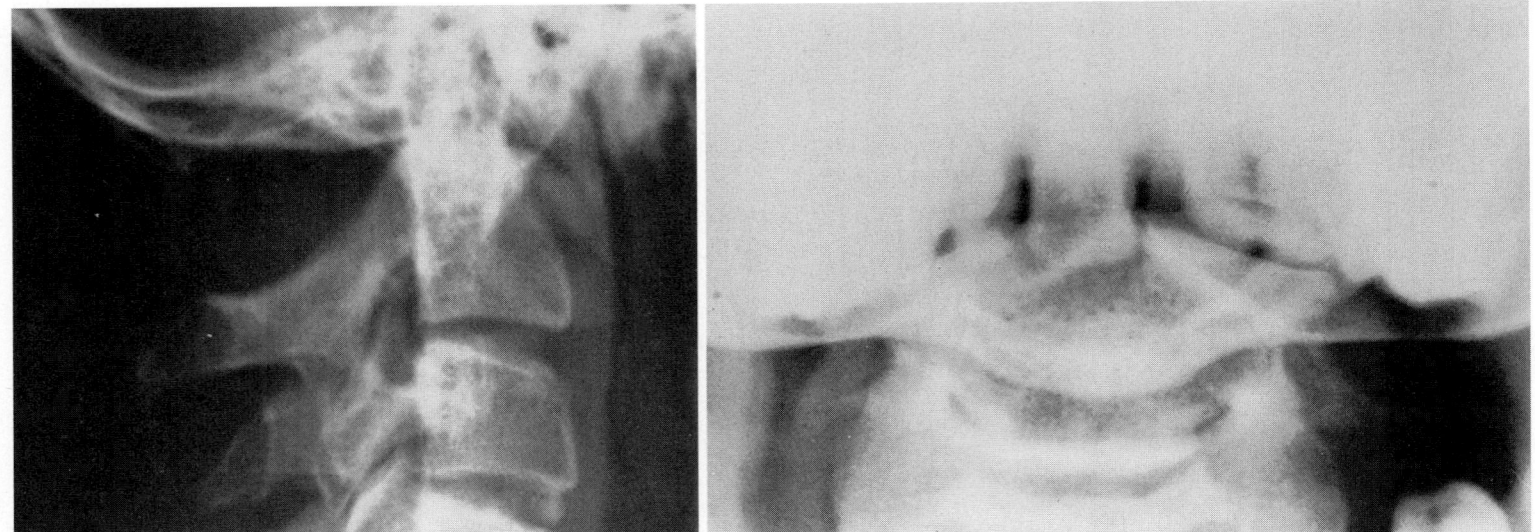

Figure 3–14. Complete incorporation of C1 into the base of the skull (assimilation of the atlas).

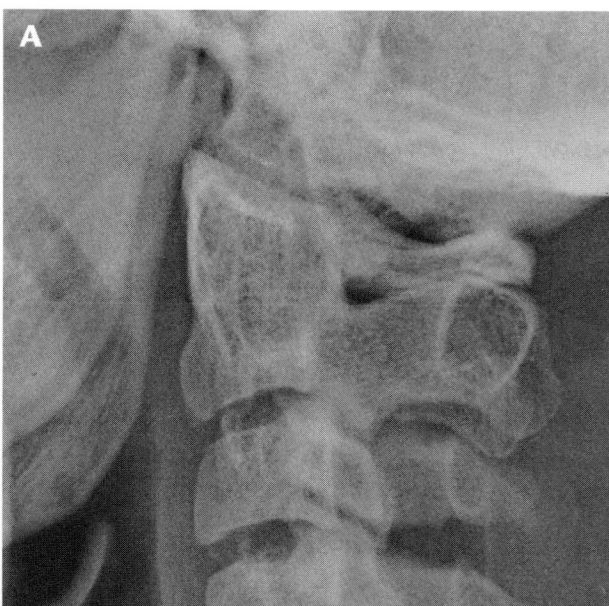

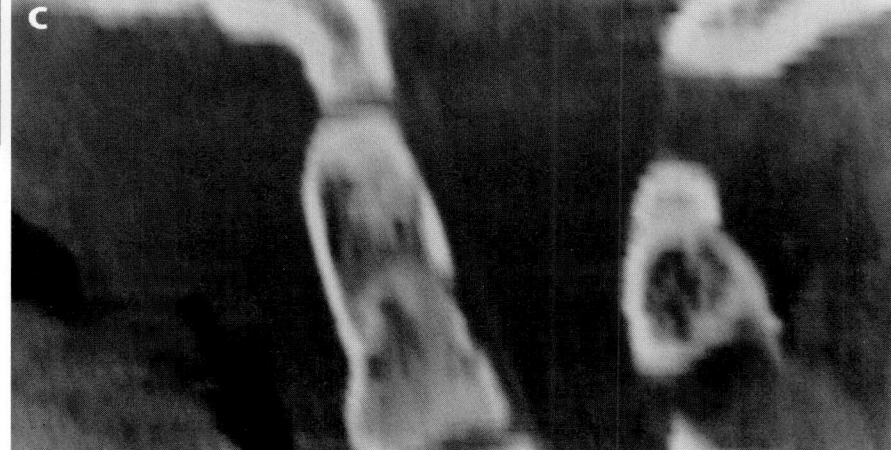

Figure 3–15. Partial incorporation of C1 into the base of the skull. Note the incomplete segmention of C1–C2 as well. **A,** Plain Film. **B** and **C,** CT sections.

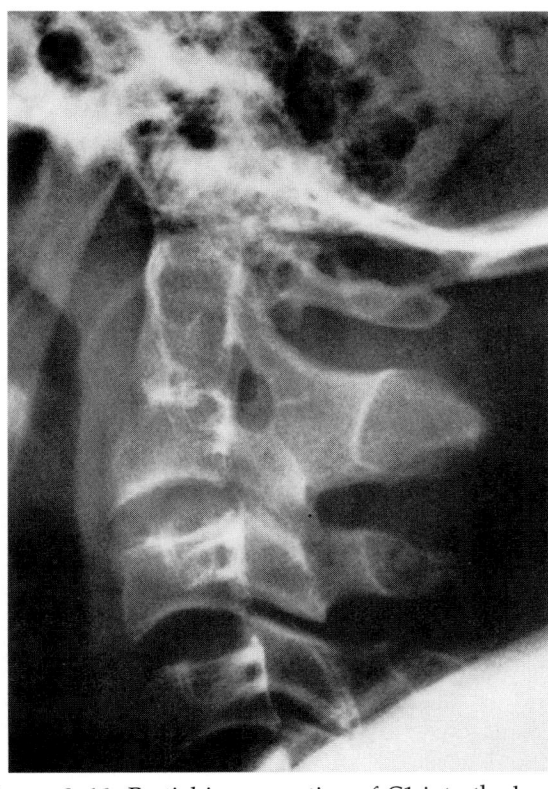

Figure 3–16. Partial incorporation of C1 into the base of the skull to a lesser degree than that pictured in Figure 3–15. Note also the similar incomplete segmentation of C2–C3.

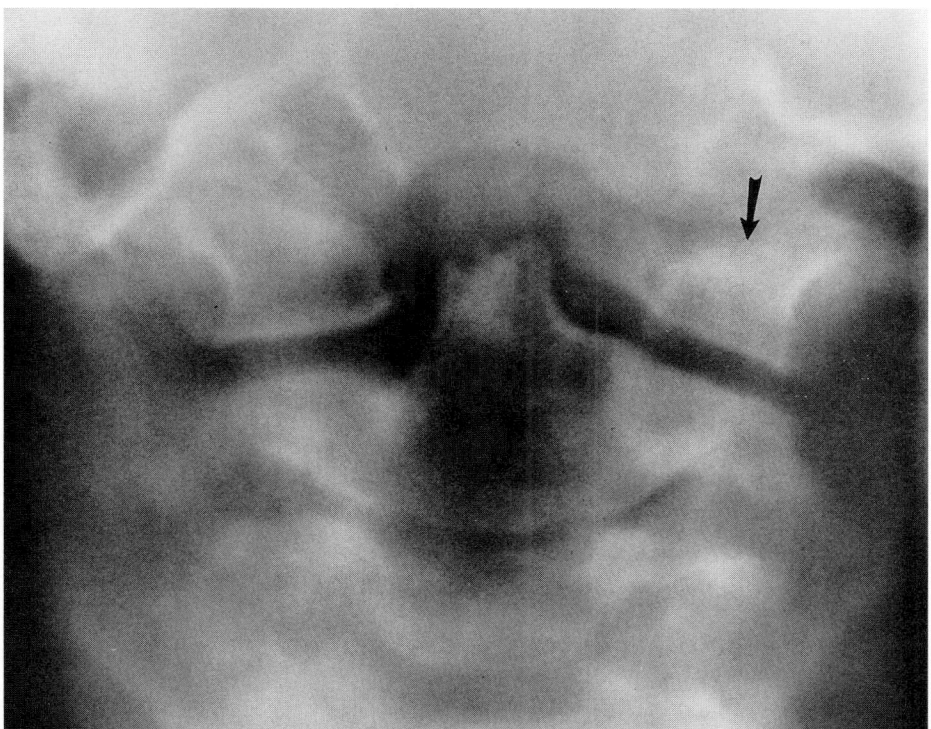

Figure 3–17. Partial assimilation of the left lateral mass of C1 at the base of the skull. Note the asymmetry of the lateral masses of C1 that accompanies this variation.

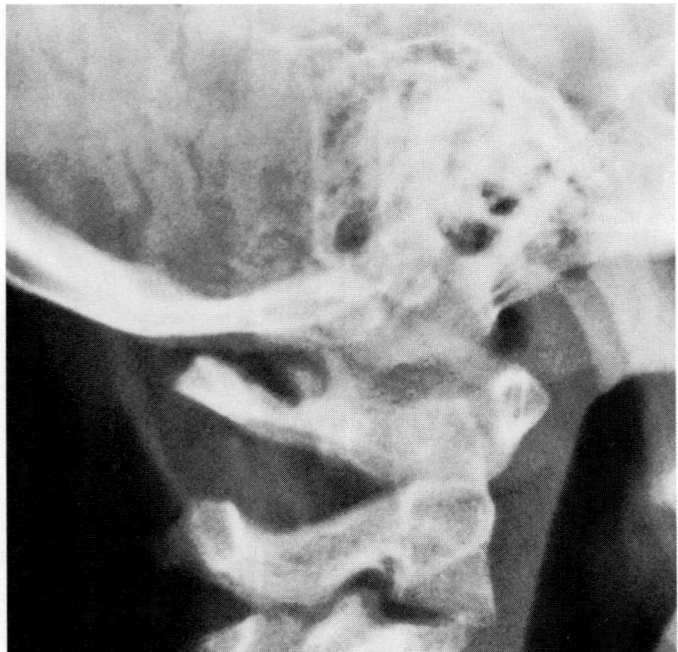

Figure 3–18. Uptilted neural arch of C1.

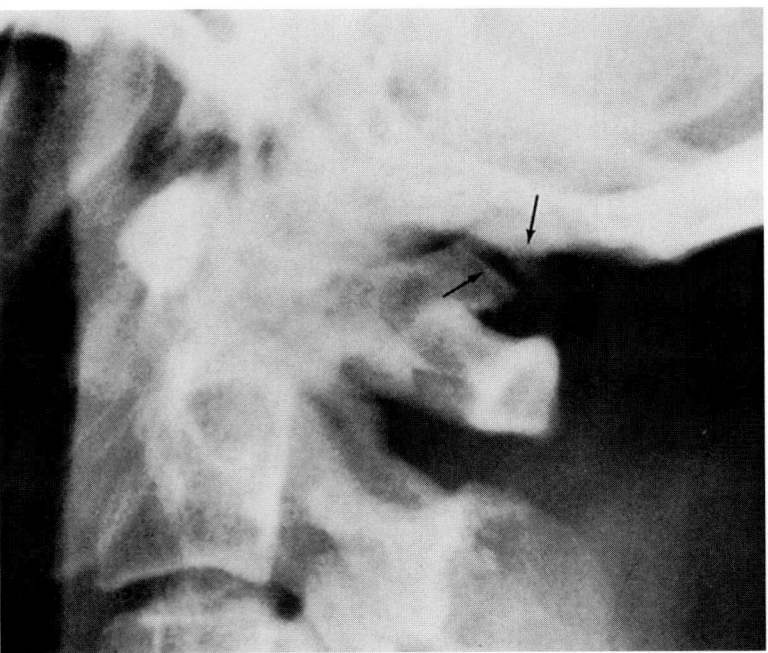

Figure 3–19. Anomalous articulation between the posterior arch of C1 and the base of the skull.

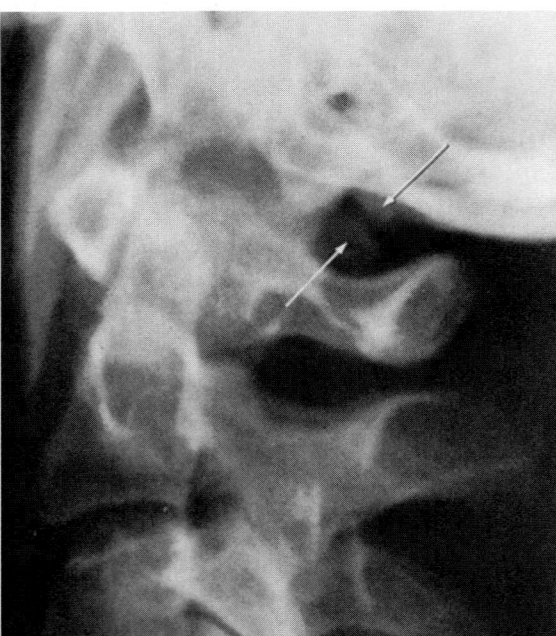

Figure 3–20. A second example of anomalous articulation between the posterior arch of C1 and the base of the skull.

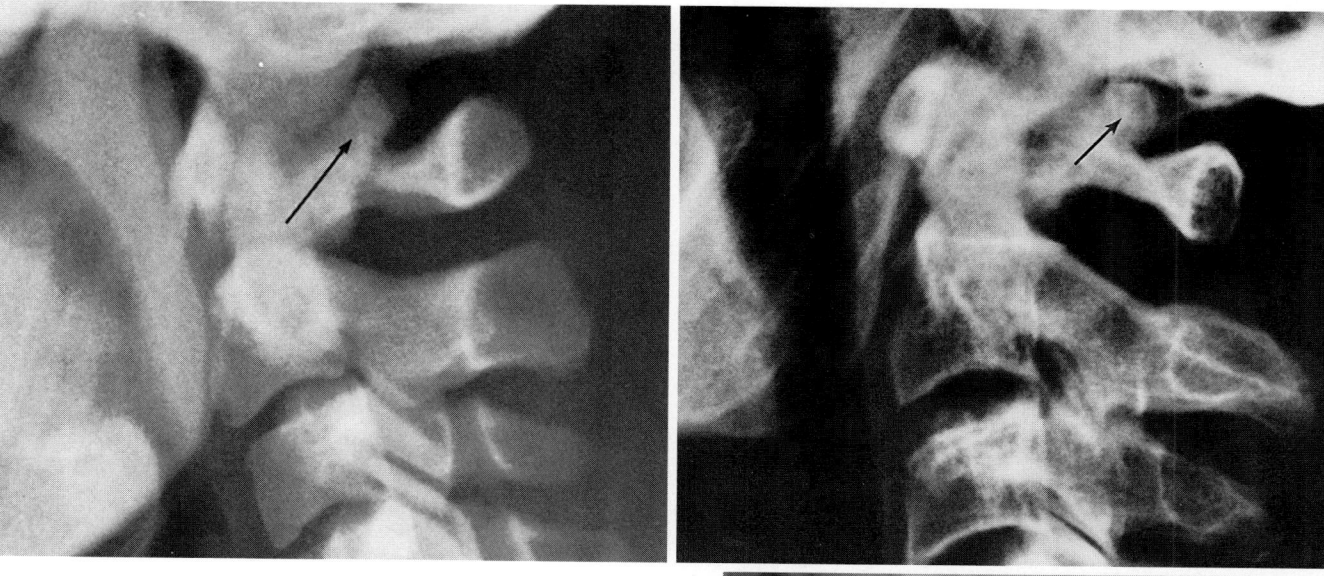

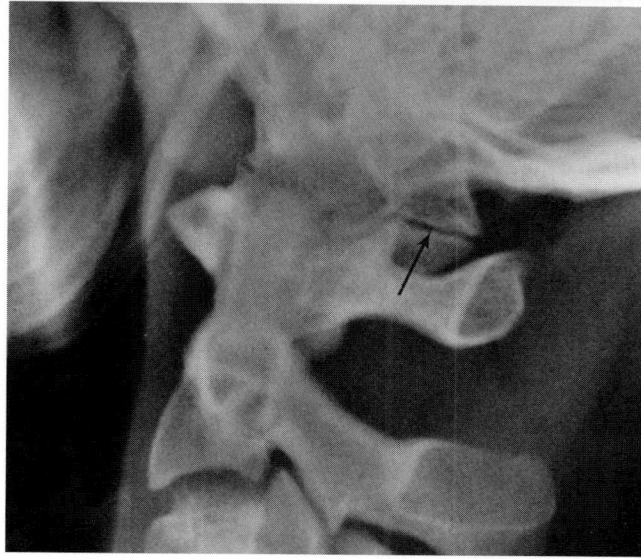

Figure 3–21. Three examples of anomalous articulation between the posterior arch of C1 and the base of the skull.

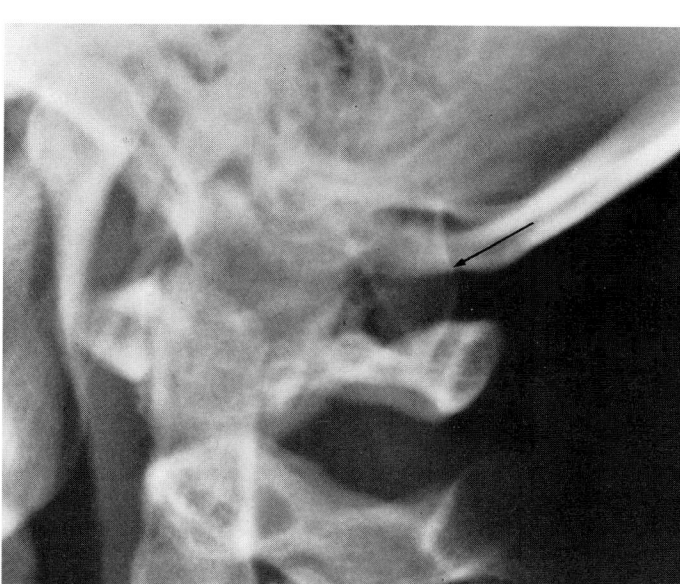

Figure 3–22. Paracondylar process arising from the occipital bone.

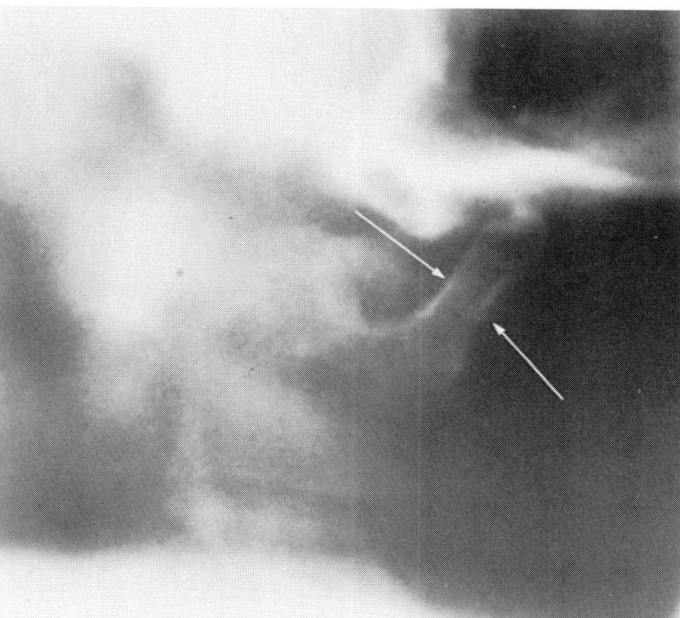

Figure 3–23. Epitransverse process arises from the transverse process of the atlas and projects cranially toward the occipital condyle. It is a mirror image of the paracondylar process. The epitransverse process may be unilateral or bilateral and may coexist with the paracondylar process. (Ref: Shapiro R, Robinson F: Anomalies of the craniovertebral border. *Am J Roentgenol* 127:281, 1976.)

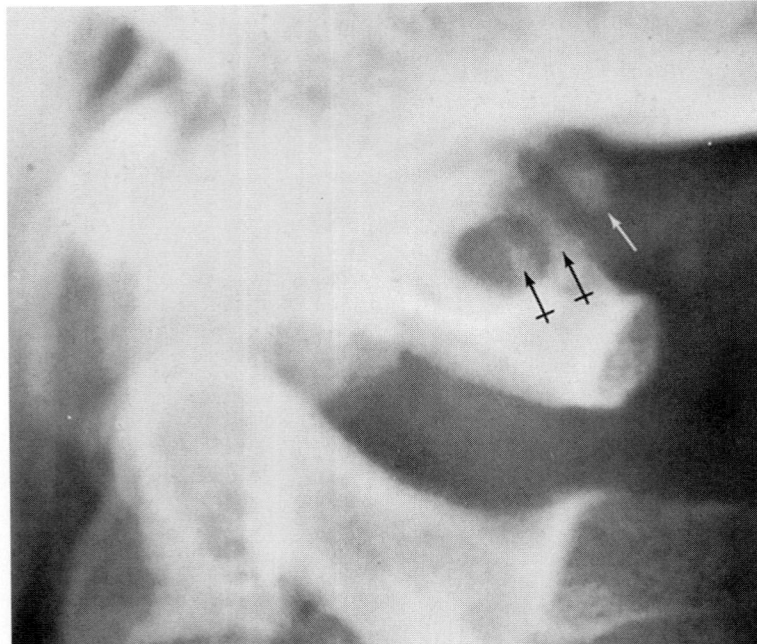

Figure 3–24. Bony spur arising from the base of the skull, simulating a neural arch (→). Note the arcuate foramina for the vertebral arteries (↦).

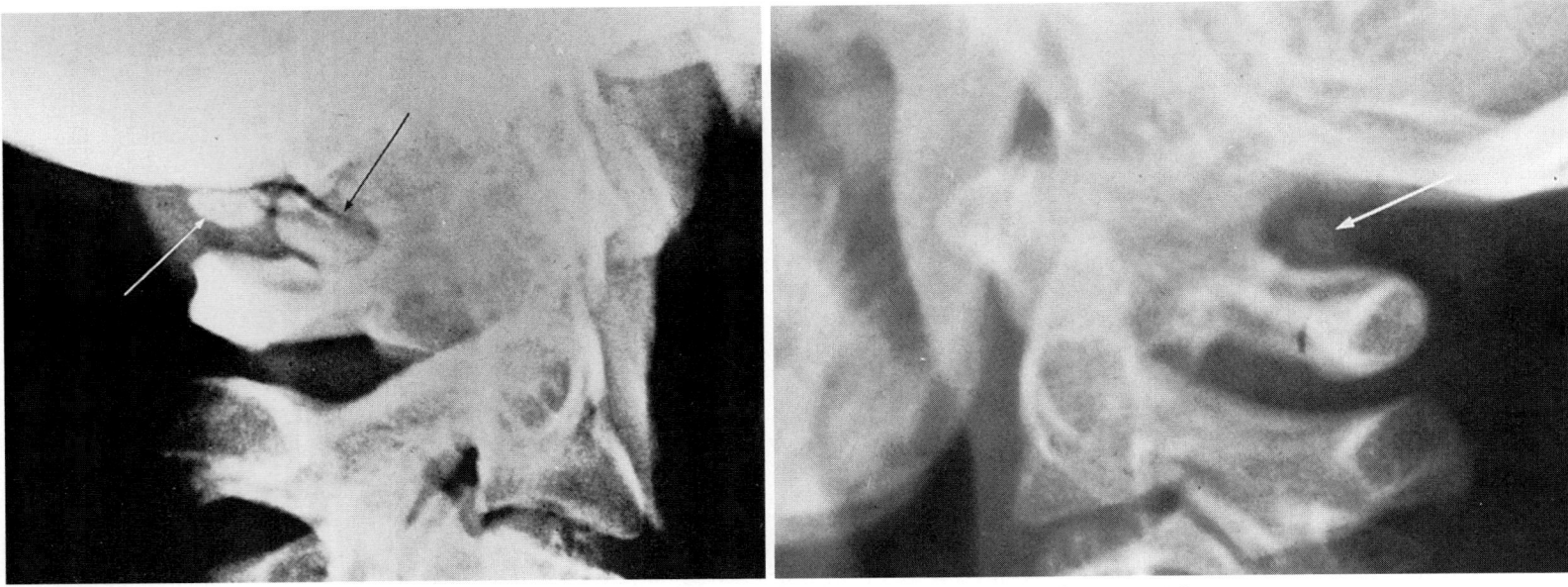

Figure 3–25. Two examples of accessory bony elements between the base of the skull and the neural arch of C1.

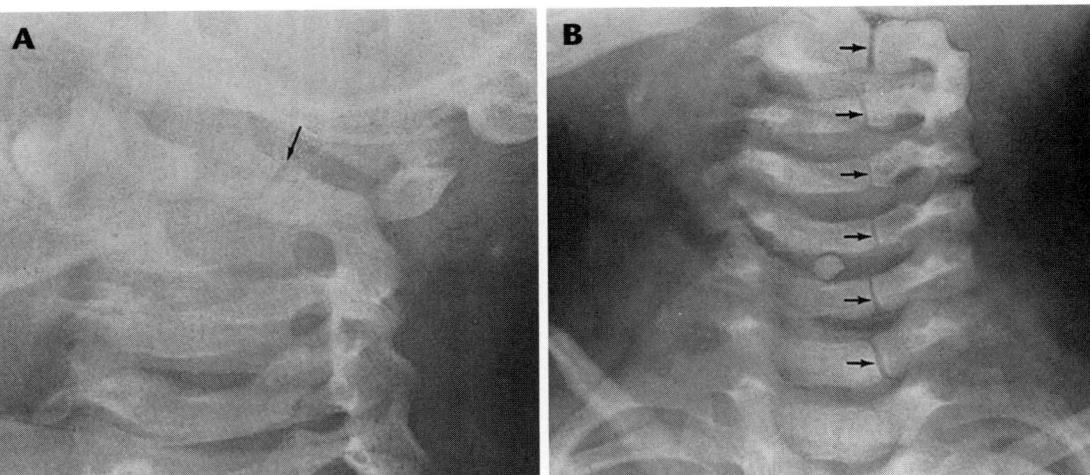

Figure 3–26. A, Normal cleft in the neural arch of the axis in a 1-year-old child. **B,** Normal clefts in the neural arches of all the cervical vertebrae in an 11-month-old child. These neurocentral synchondroses may persist until 3 to 6 years of age and may persist unilaterally for several months after the other side has closed. (Ref: Swischuk LE et al: The dens-arch synchondroses vs. the hangman's fracture. *Pediatr Radiol* 8:100, 1979.)

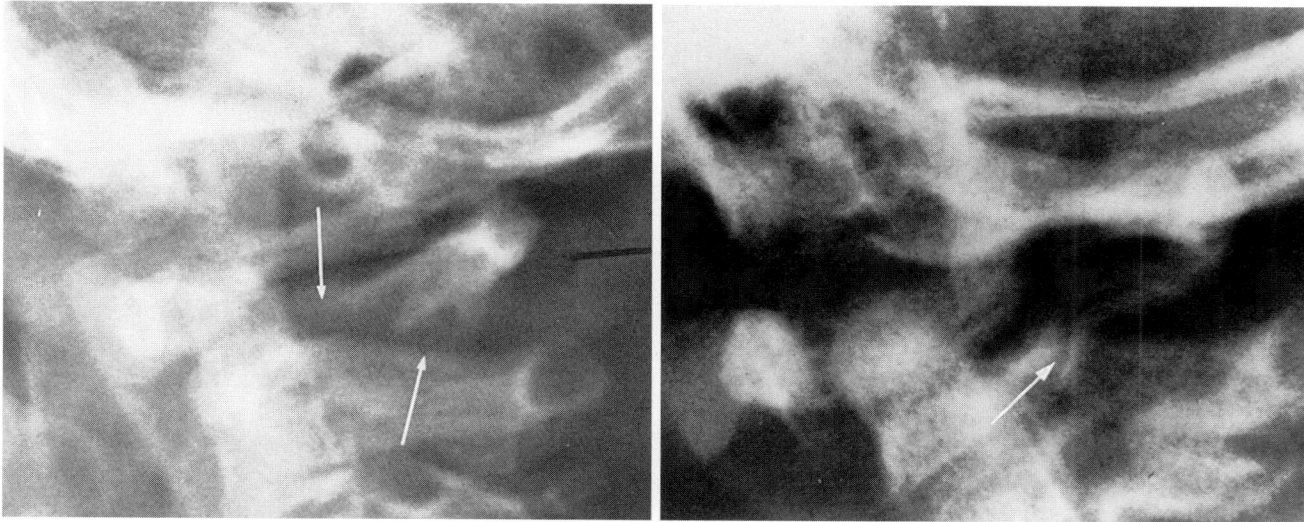

Figure 3–27. Incomplete closure of the neural arch of C1 in a 2-year-old child. These normally close at 3 to 6 years of age.

Figure 3–28. Complete absence of the posterior neural arch of C1. (Ref: Dalinka MK et al: Congenital absence of the posterior arch of the atlas. *Radiology* 103:581, 1972.)

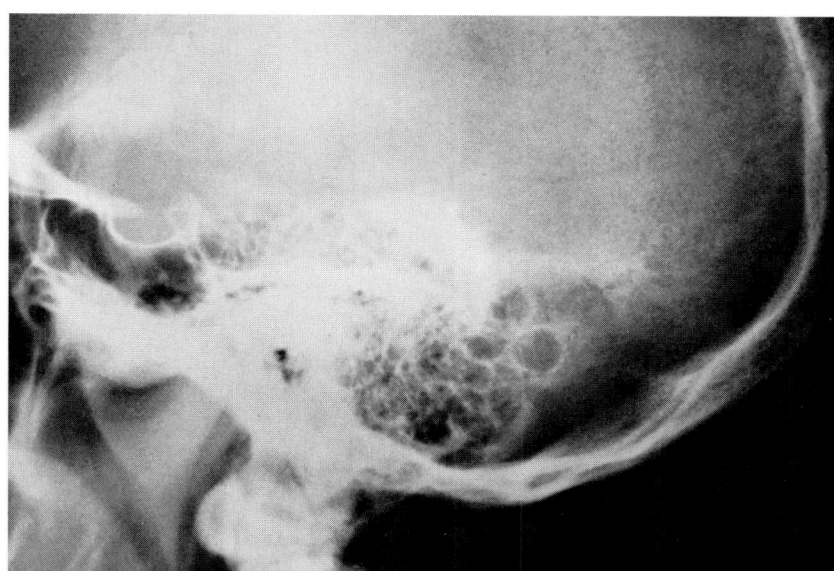

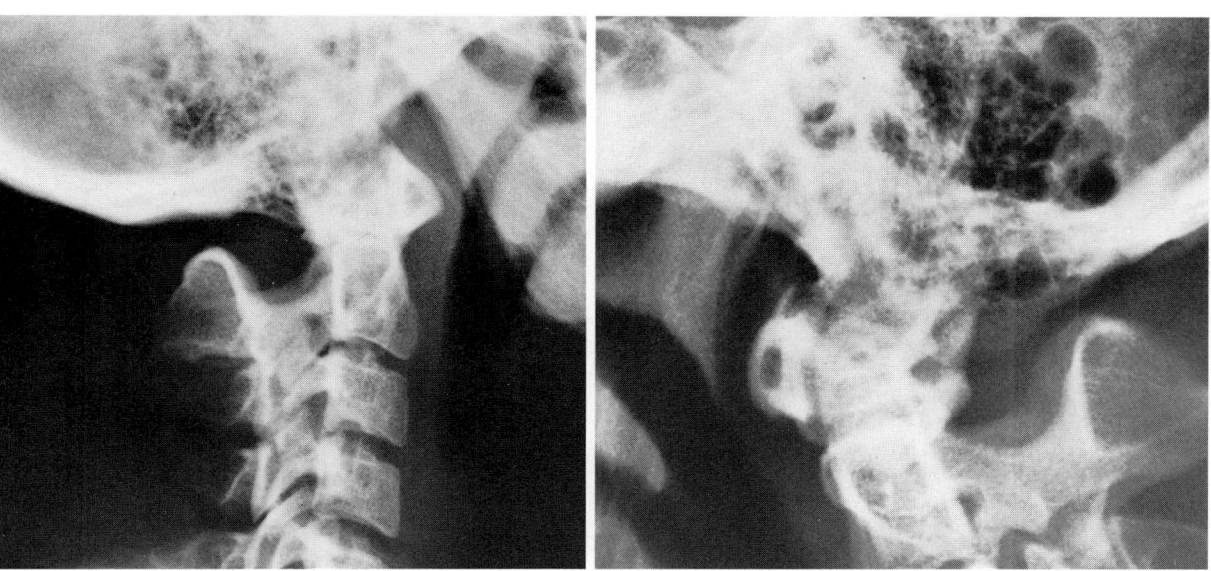

Figure 3–29. Two examples of absence of the posterior arch of C1. Note the marked overgrowth of the spinous process of C2.

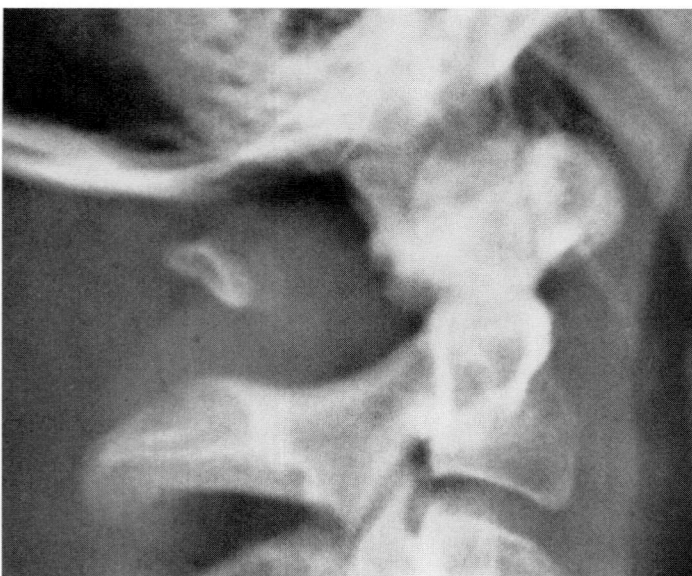

Figure 3–30. Absence of the laminae of C1. (Ref: Logan WW, Stuard ID: Absent posterior arch of the atlas. *Am J Roentgenol* 118:431, 1973.) This entity is not necessarily innocent and may be associated with instability. (Ref: Schultze P, Bourman R: Absence of the posterior arch of the atlas. *Am J Roentgenol* 134:178, 1982.)

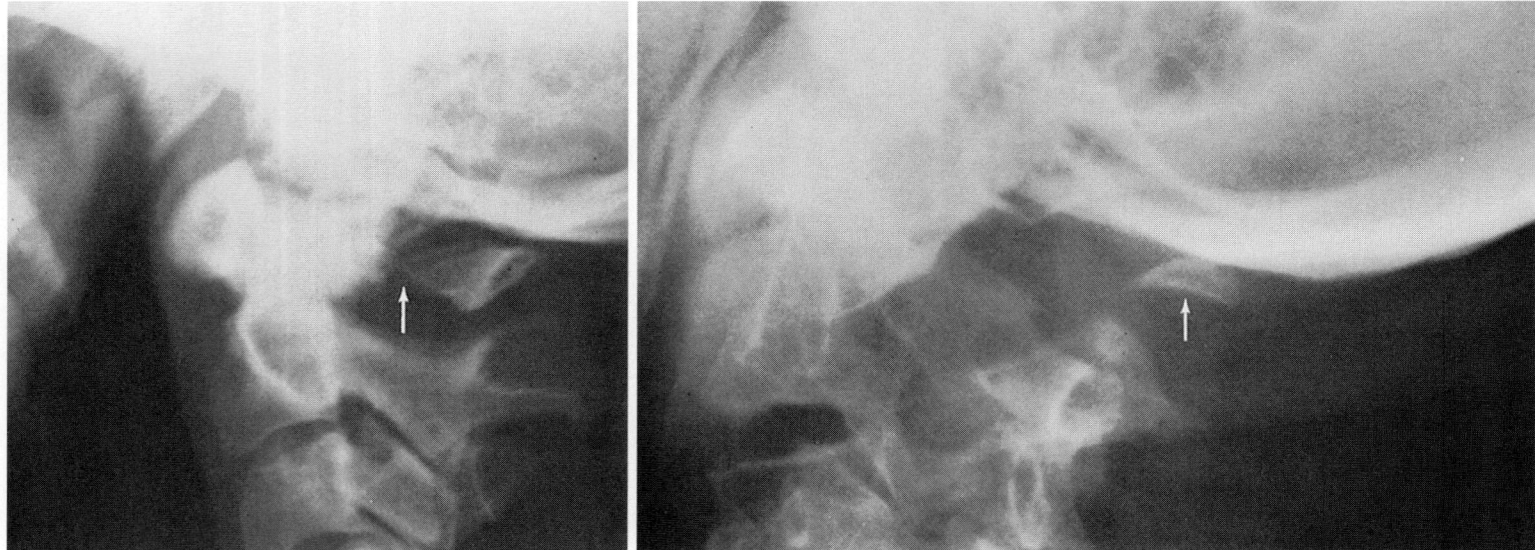

Figure 3–31. Two examples of incomplete formation of the posterior neural arch of C1.

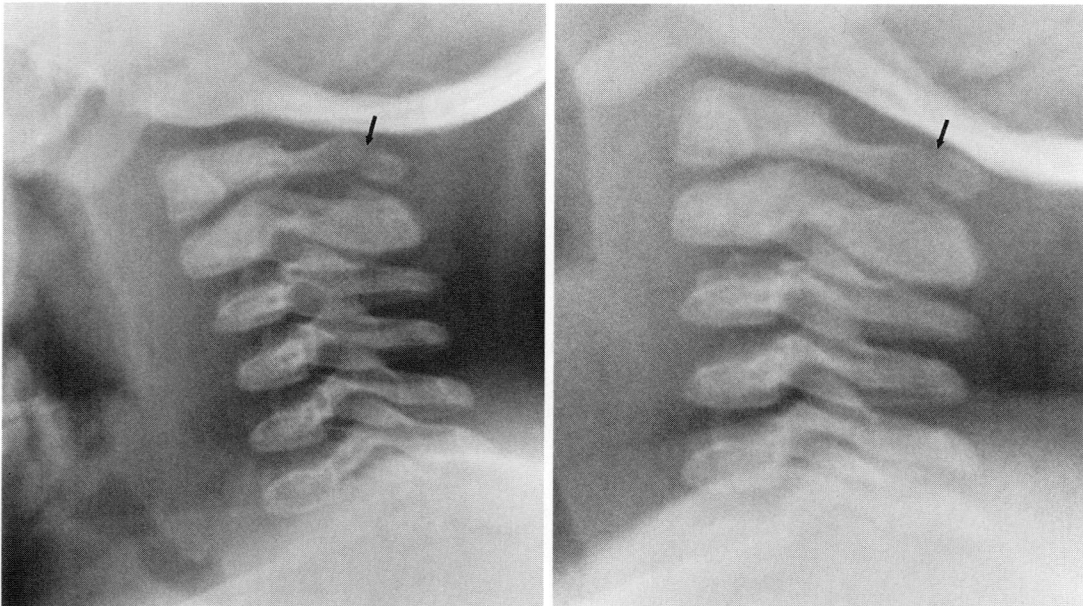

Figure 3–32. Two examples of incomplete development of the neural arch of C1 in infants.

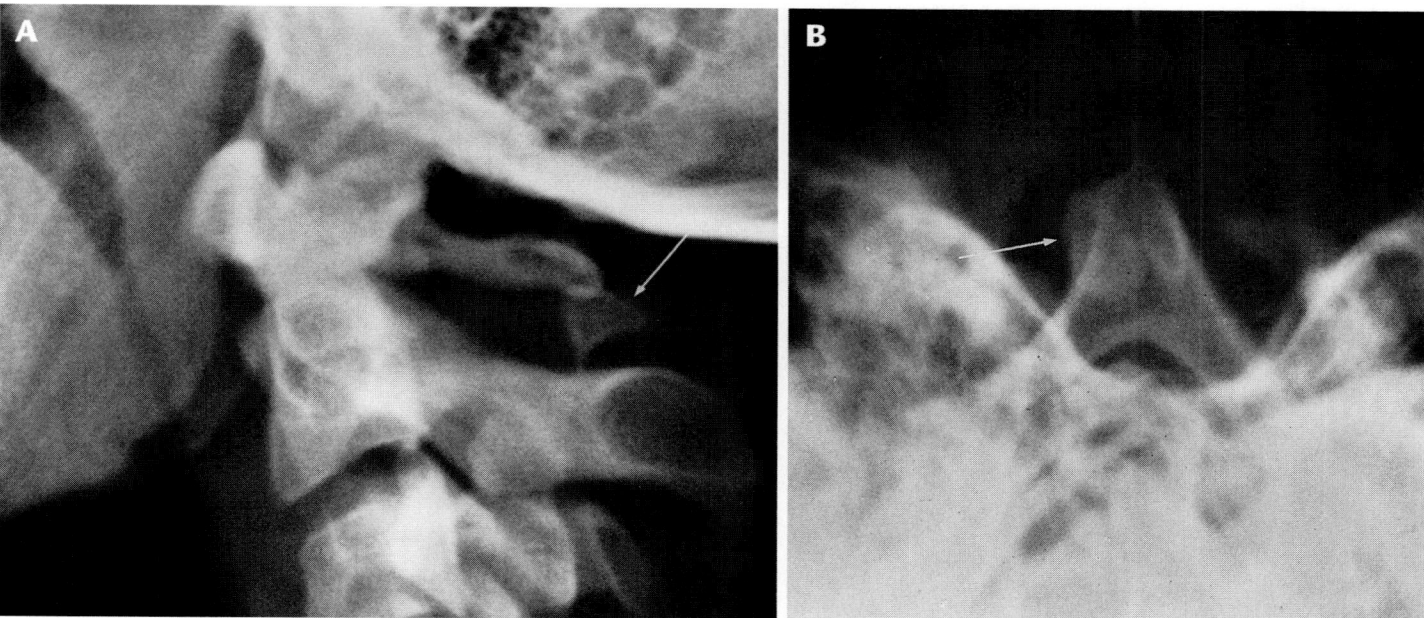

Figure 3–33. Incomplete formation of the neural arch of C1 with fragment seen in lateral projection **(A)** and in Towne's projection **(B)**.

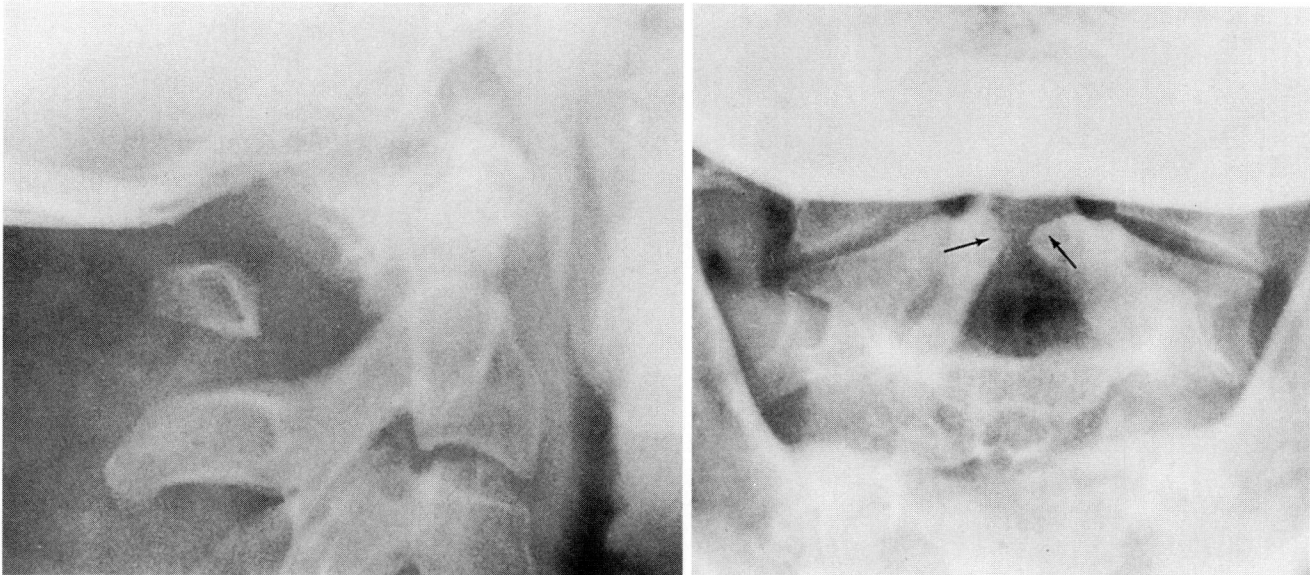

Figure 3–34. Incomplete formation of the posterior arch of C1 with spina bifida occulta seen in the frontal projection (→).

Figure 3–35. Unilateral incomplete neural arch of C1.

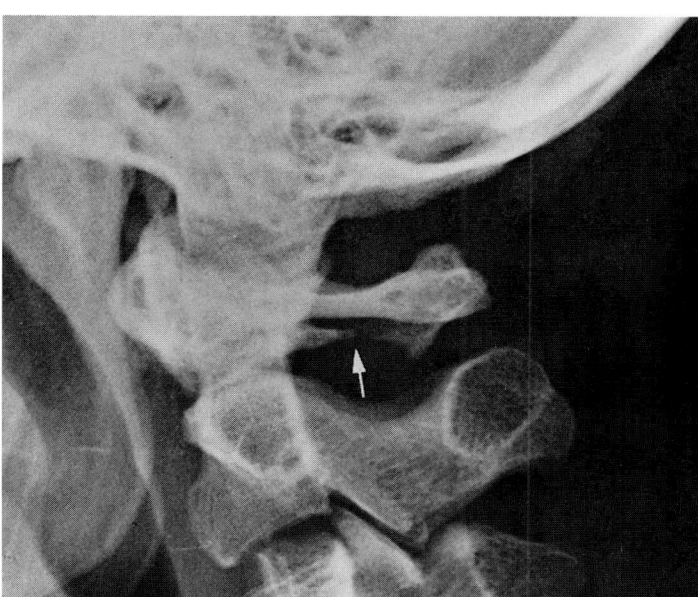

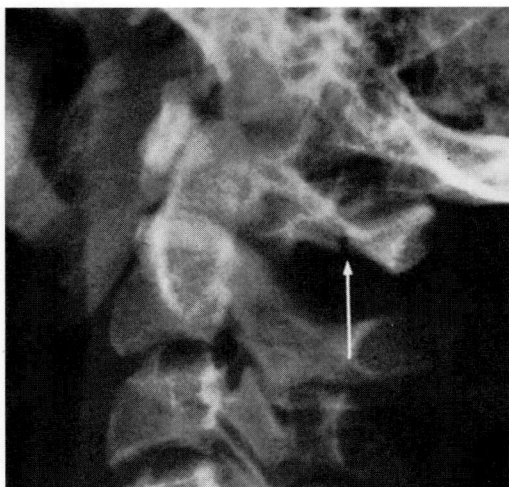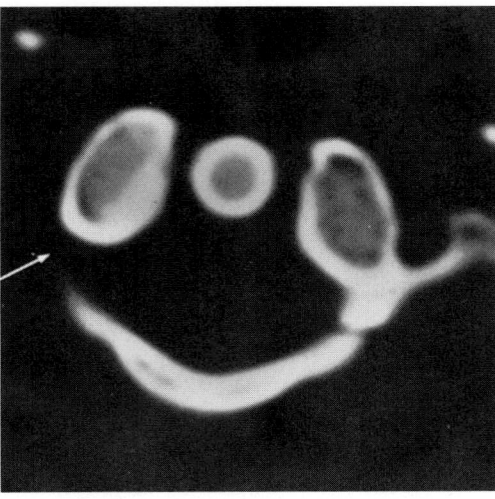

Figure 3–36. *Left,* Incomplete development of the neural arch of C1, simulating a fracture. *Right,* CT shows partial formation on the right side of the neural arch.

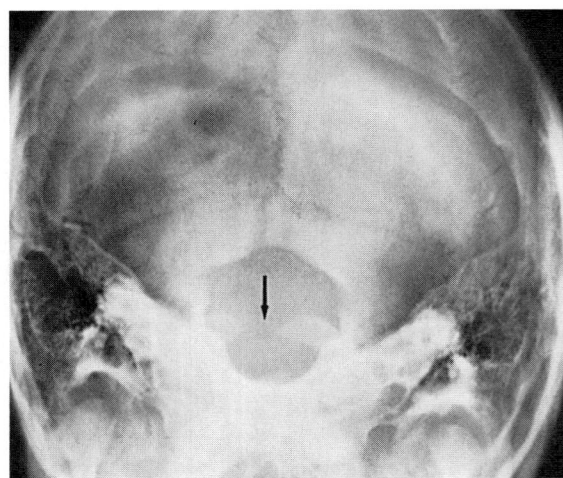

Figure 3–37. Failure of fusion of the posterior portion of the neural arch of C1 in an 8-year-old boy.

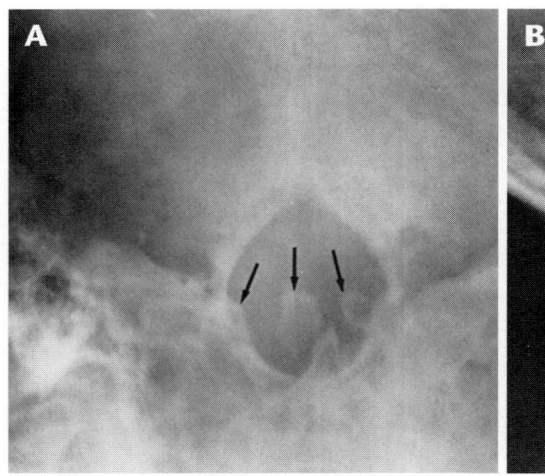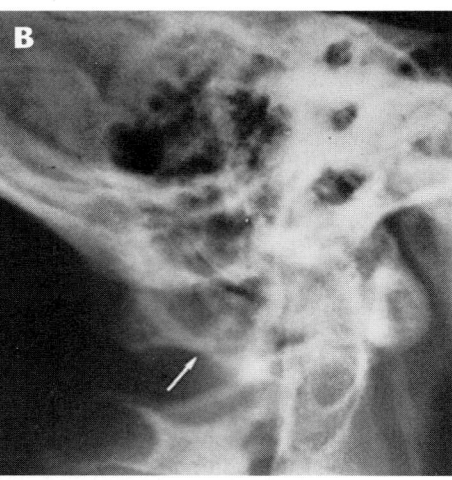

Figure 3–38. A, B, Incomplete formation of the neural arch of C1, seen best in the occipital view **(A).**

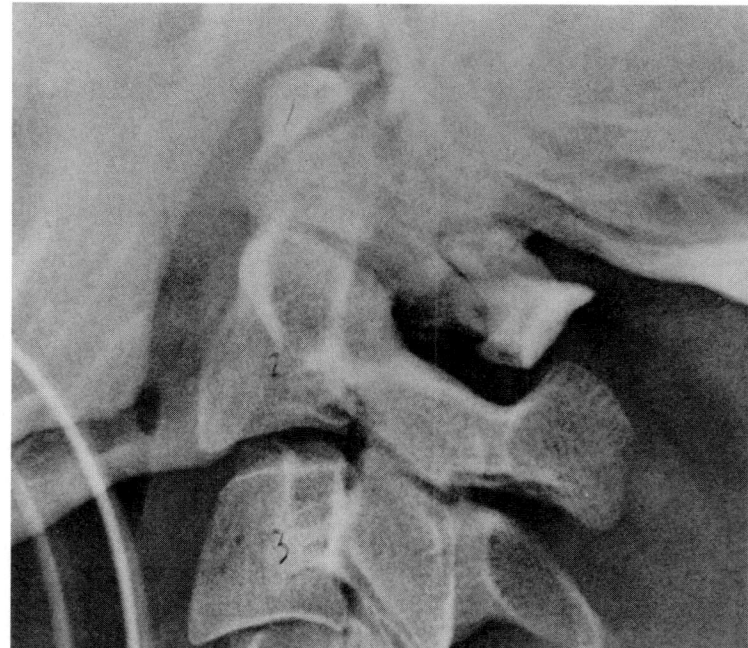

Figure 3–39. Incomplete development of the neural arch of C1 simulating a fracture. Proved by CT.

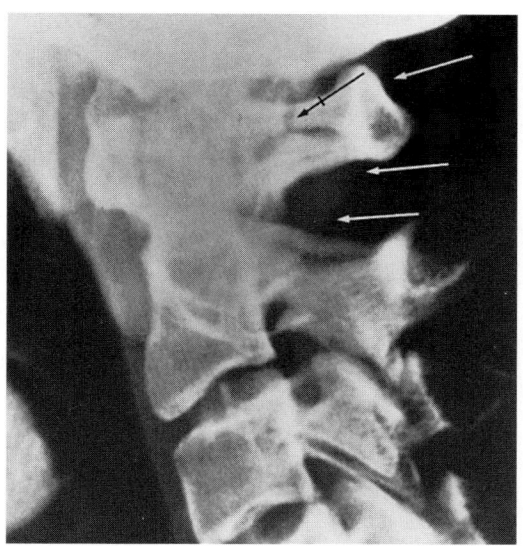

Figure 3–40. Air in the pinna (←) simulating a fracture of the neural arch of C1 (↔).

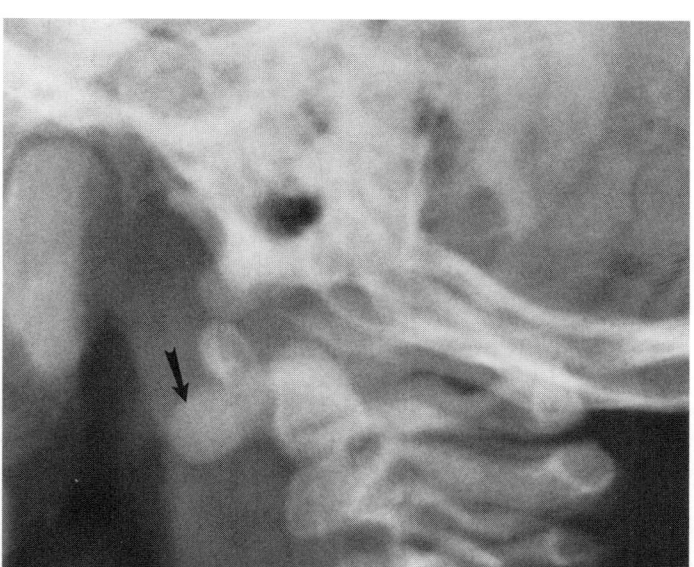

Figure 3–41. The lobe of the ear superimposed on the anterior arch of C1.

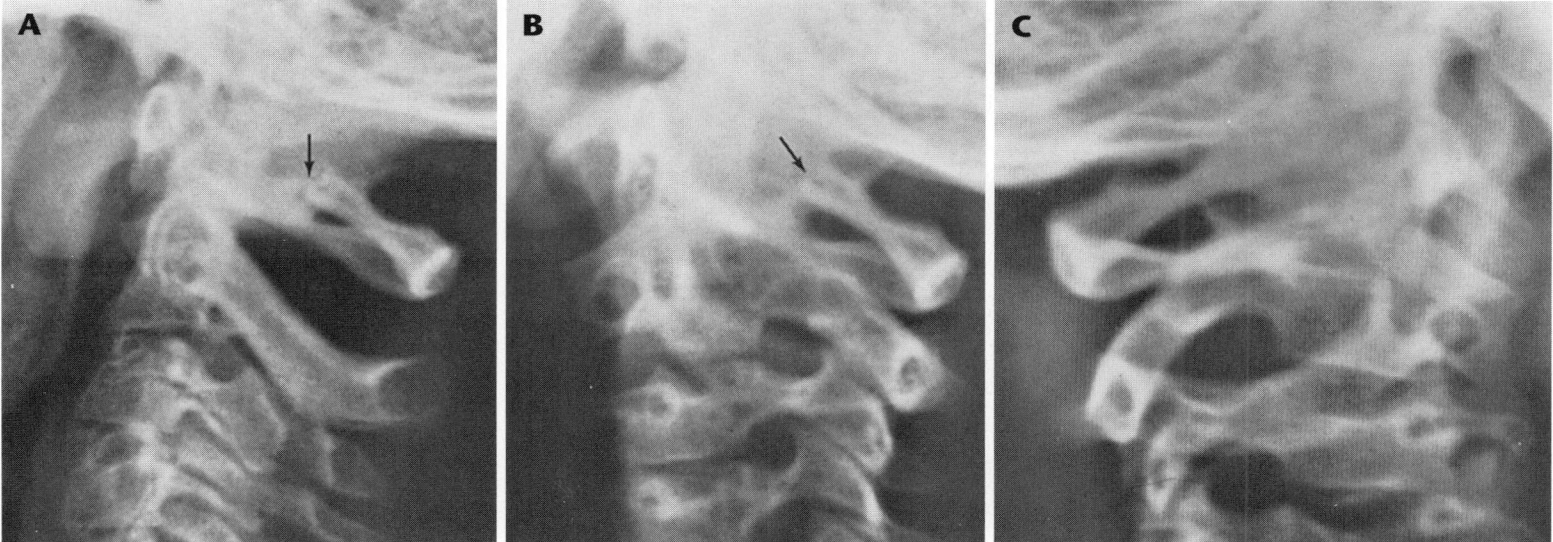

Figure 3–42. Unilateral absence of a portion of the neural arch of C1. **A,** Defect seen in lateral projection. **B,** Defect seen in oblique projection. **C,** Normal side of comparison. (Ref: Karasick S, Karasick D, Wechsler RJ: Unilateral spondylolysis of the cervical spine. *Skeletal Radiol* 9:259, 1983.)

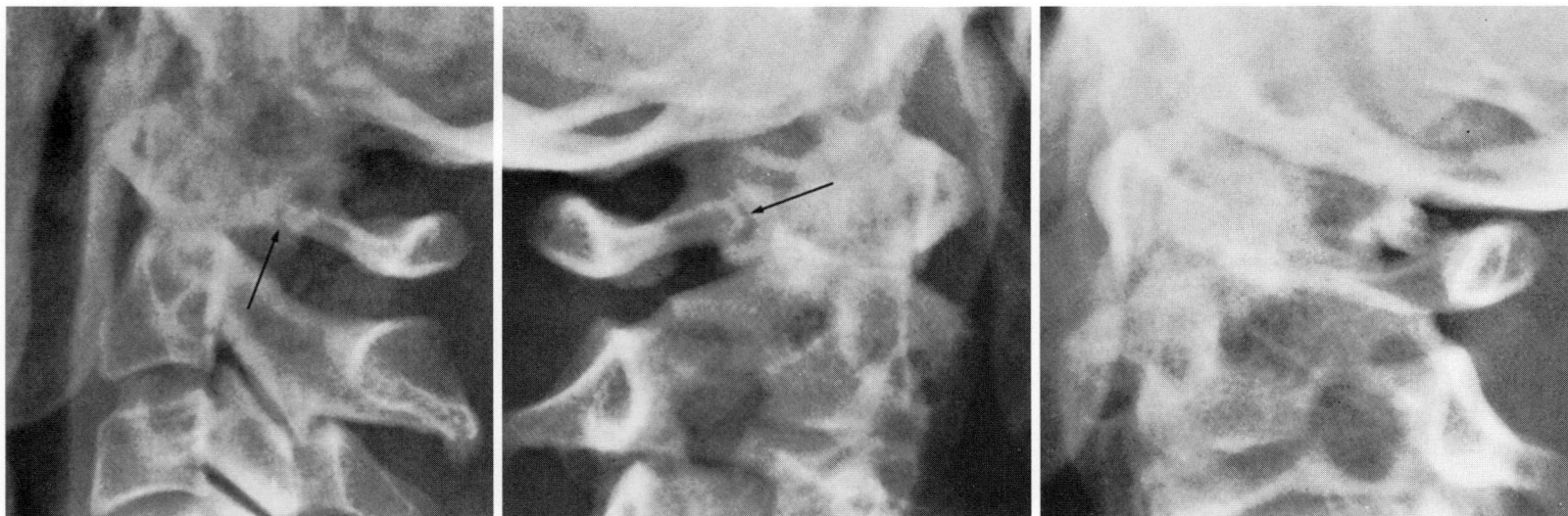

Figure 3–43. Unilateral spondylolysis of C1 with sclerosis at the site of the lysis, best seen in the center figure (←).

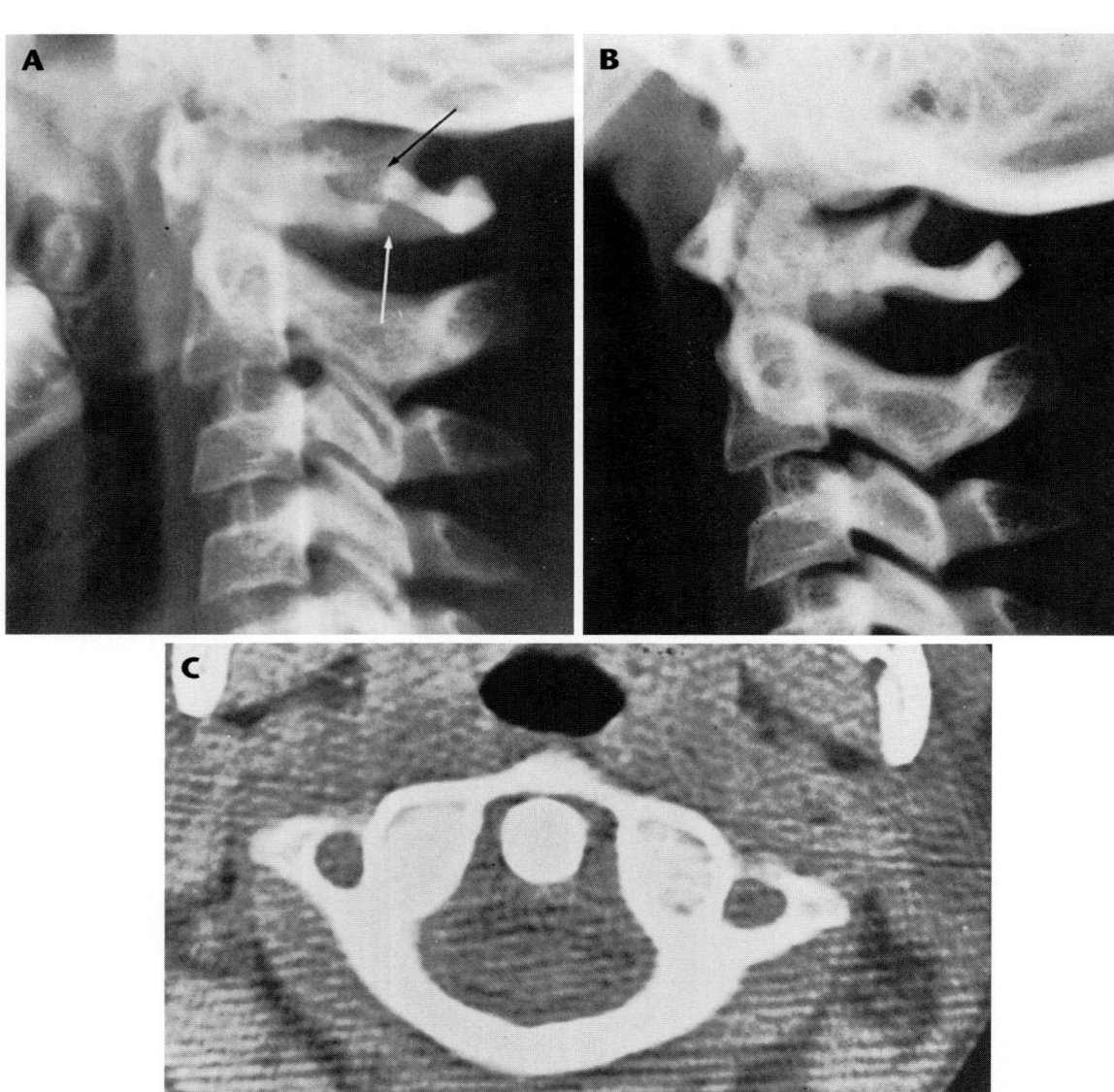

Figure 3–44. An appearance similar to that in Figure 3–43 may be produced by faulty positioning. **A,** Apparent defects in neural arch of C1 in off-lateral projection. **B,** Defects not seen in true lateral projection. **C,** CT shows the neural arch to be intact.

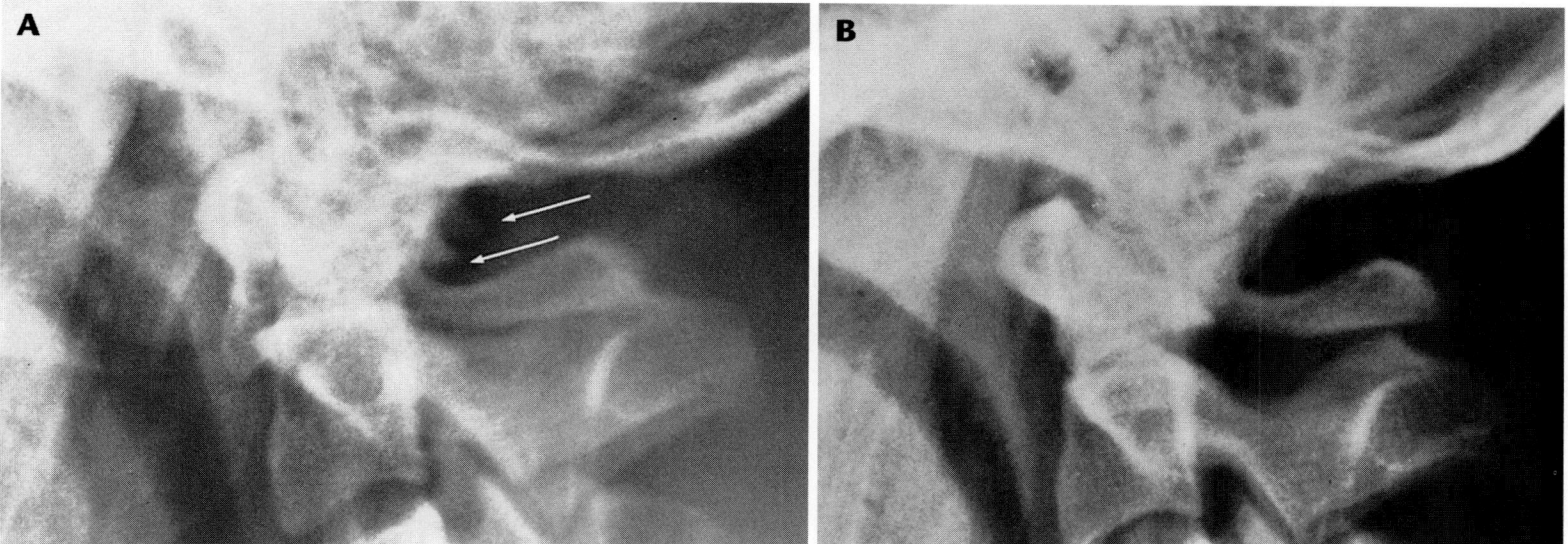

Figure 3–45. Spondylolysis of C1 seen in off-lateral projection **(A)** but not in true lateral projection **(B)**.

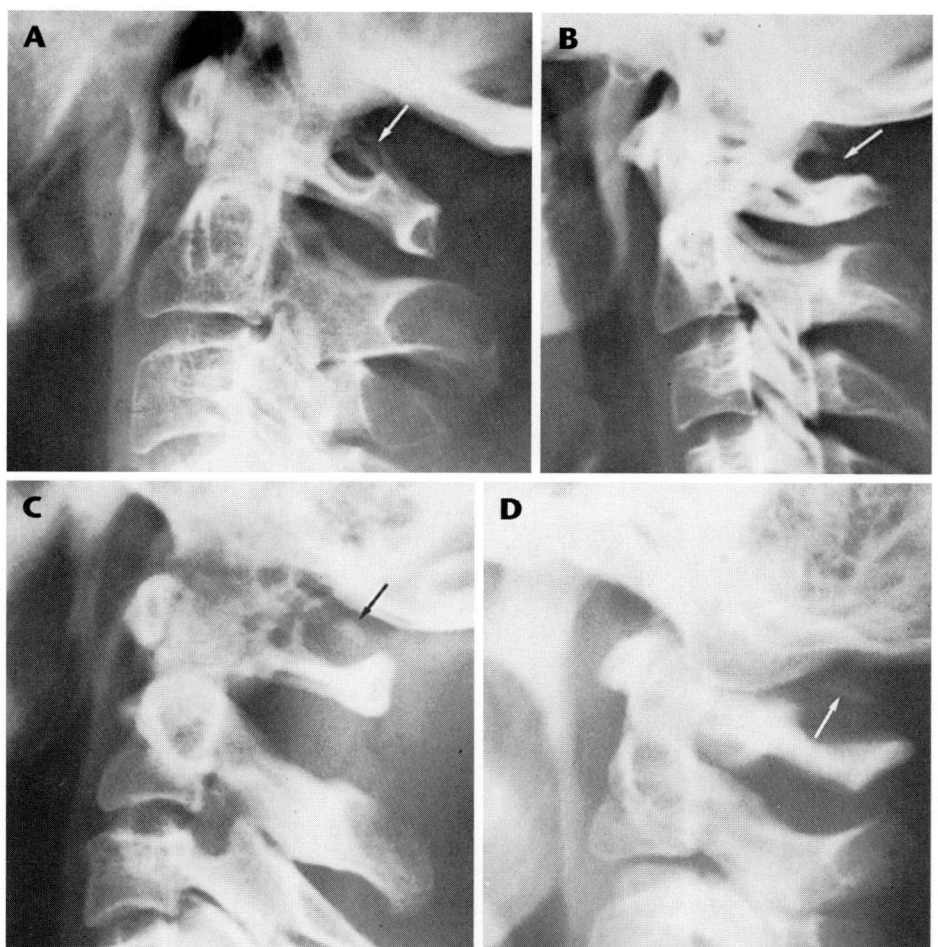

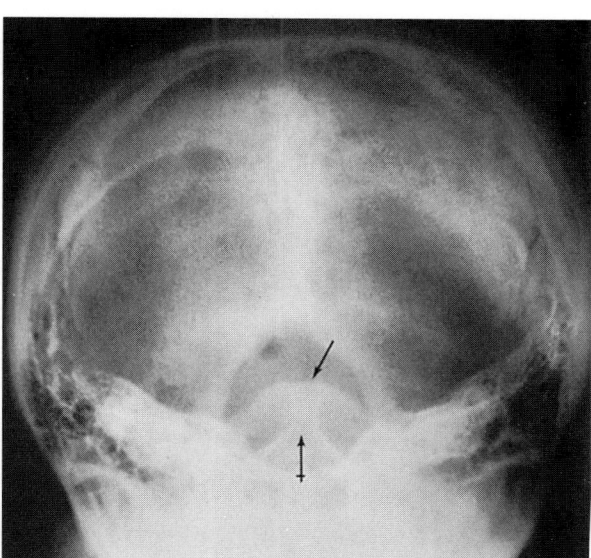

Figure 3–47. The posterior arches of C1 (→) and C2 (↠) seen in the steep Towne's projection.

Figure 3–46. The arcuate foramina formed by calcification of the oblique atlantooccipital ligaments. The vertebral arteries pass through these foramina. **A,** complete foramen. **B,** Incomplete foramen. **C** and **D,** Calcification in the oblique atlantooccipital ligaments forming incomplete arcuate foramina.

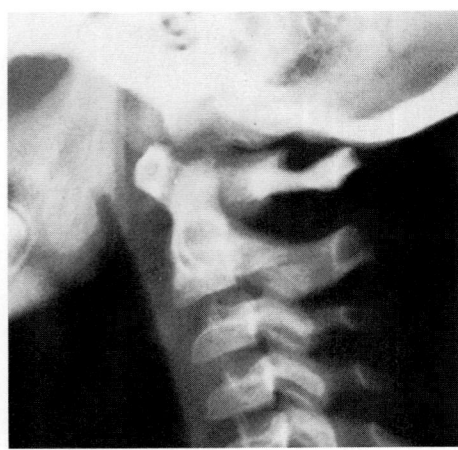 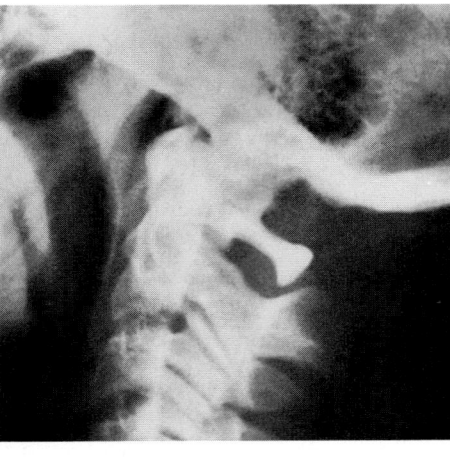

Figure 3–48. Normal exaggerated density of the posterior elements of C1 in a 7-year-old girl *(left)* and a 15-year-old girl *(right)*.

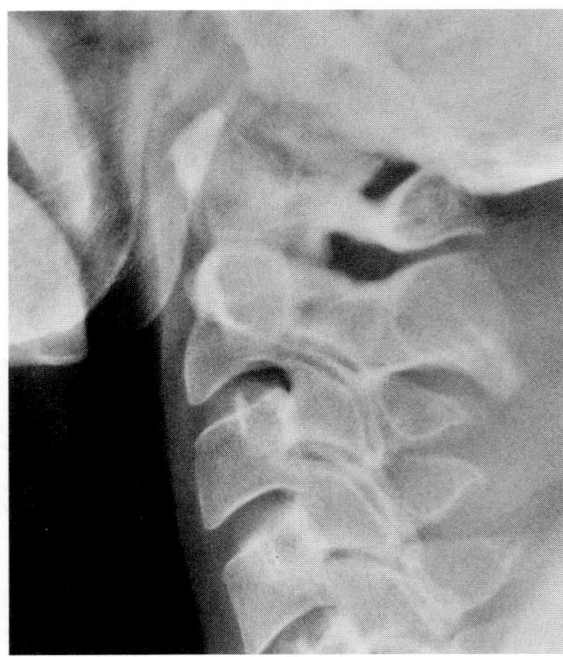

Figure 3–49. Sclerotic neural arch of C1 in an adult.

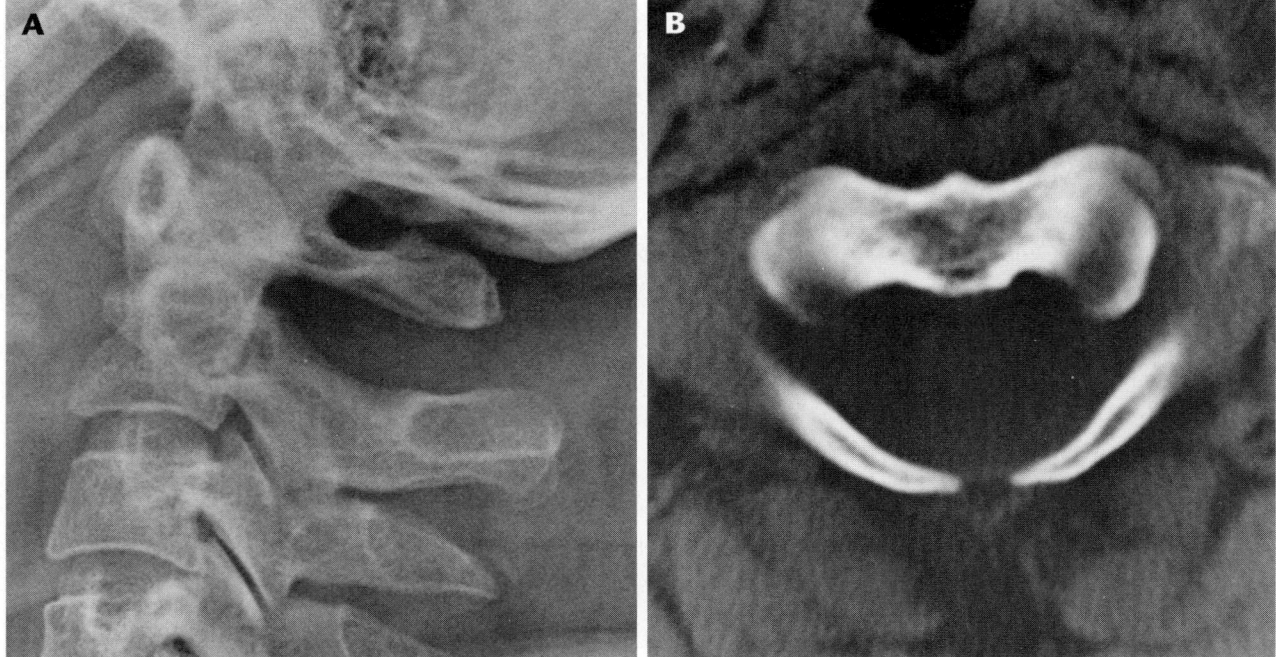

Figure 3–50. Absence of the spinolaminar line at C1 secondary to spina bifida occulta. **A,** Lateral projection. **B,** CT.

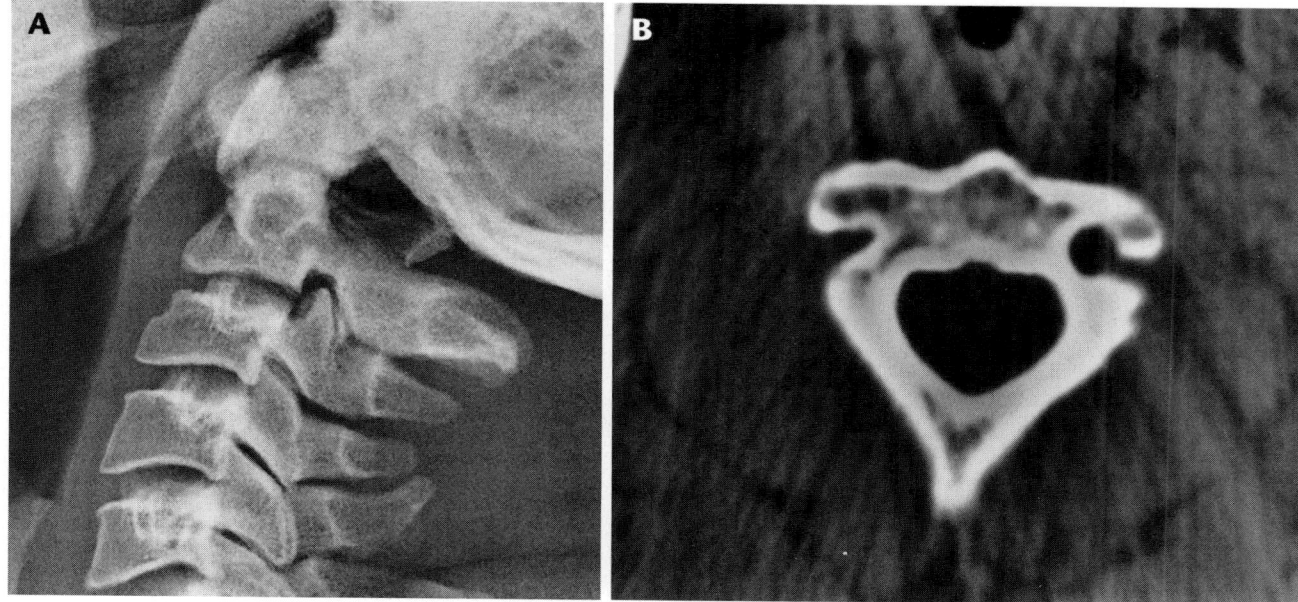

Figure 3–51. Failure of the spinolaminal line at C2, probably related to the large size of the neural arch. **A,** Lateral projection. **B,** CT.

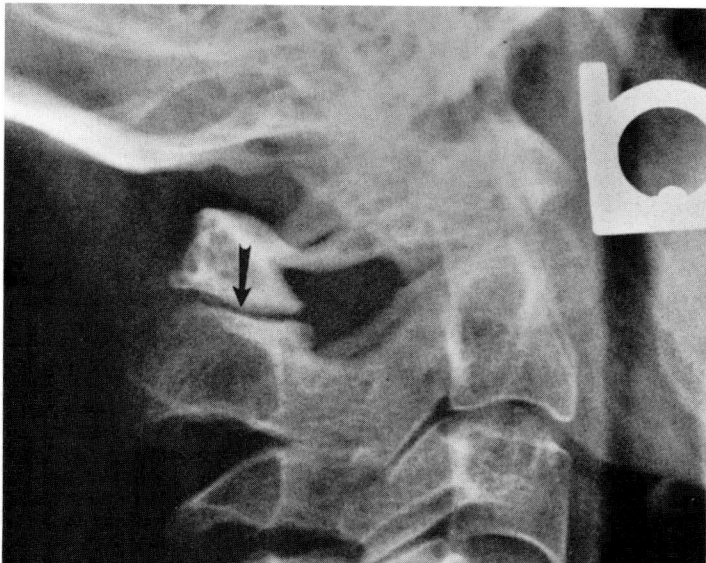

Figure 3–52. Anomalous articulation between the spinous processes of C1 and C2.

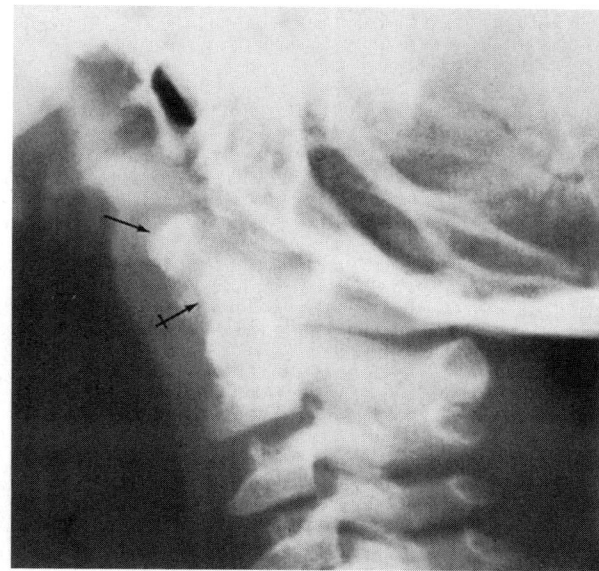

Figure 3–53. Normal position of the anterior process of C1 (→), with relationship to the odontoid (↦) when head is in extension. This may be mistaken for a posttraumatic event.

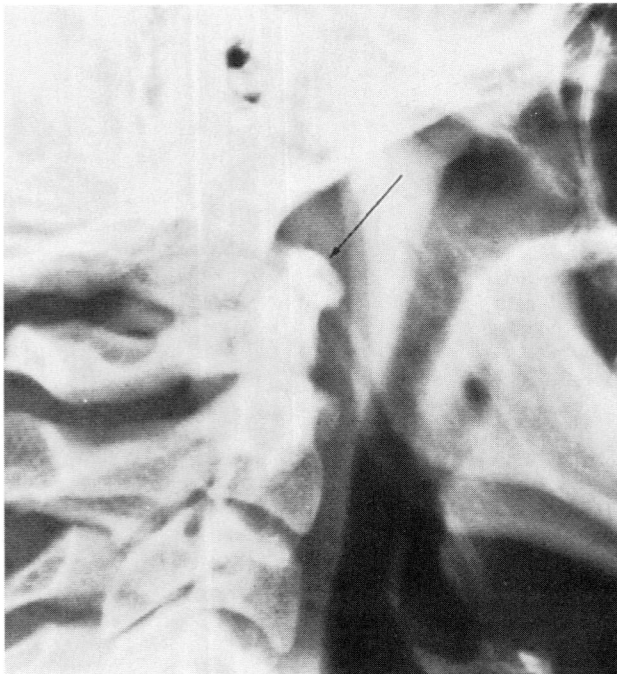

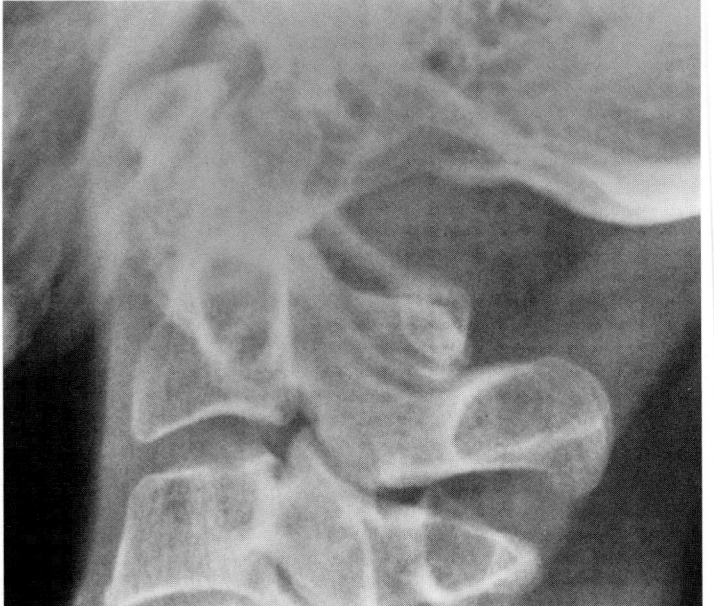

Figure 3–55. Tipped axis of C1 with high position of the anterior arch and low position of the neural arch.

Figure 3–54. High position of the anterior arch of C1 may be seen in normal individuals, even with the head in neutral position.

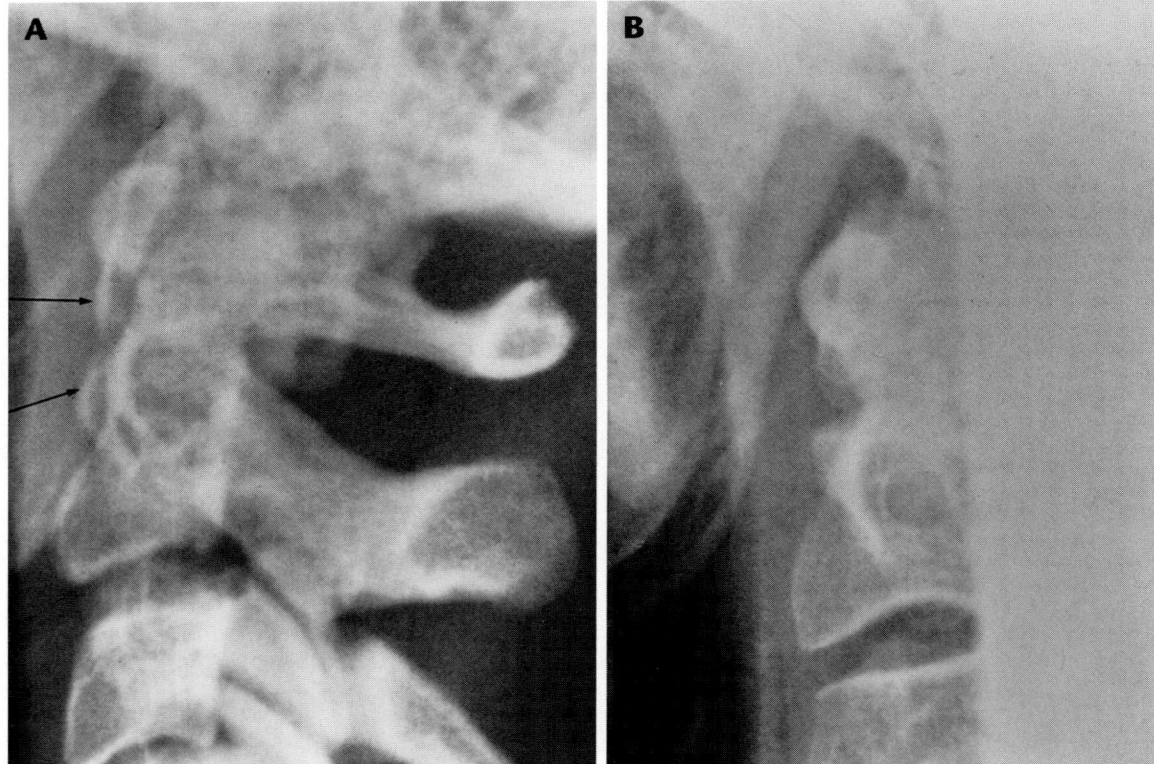

Figure 3–56. A, Double contours of the anterior aspects of C1 and C2 as a result of rotation. **B,** Normal appearance with proper positioning.

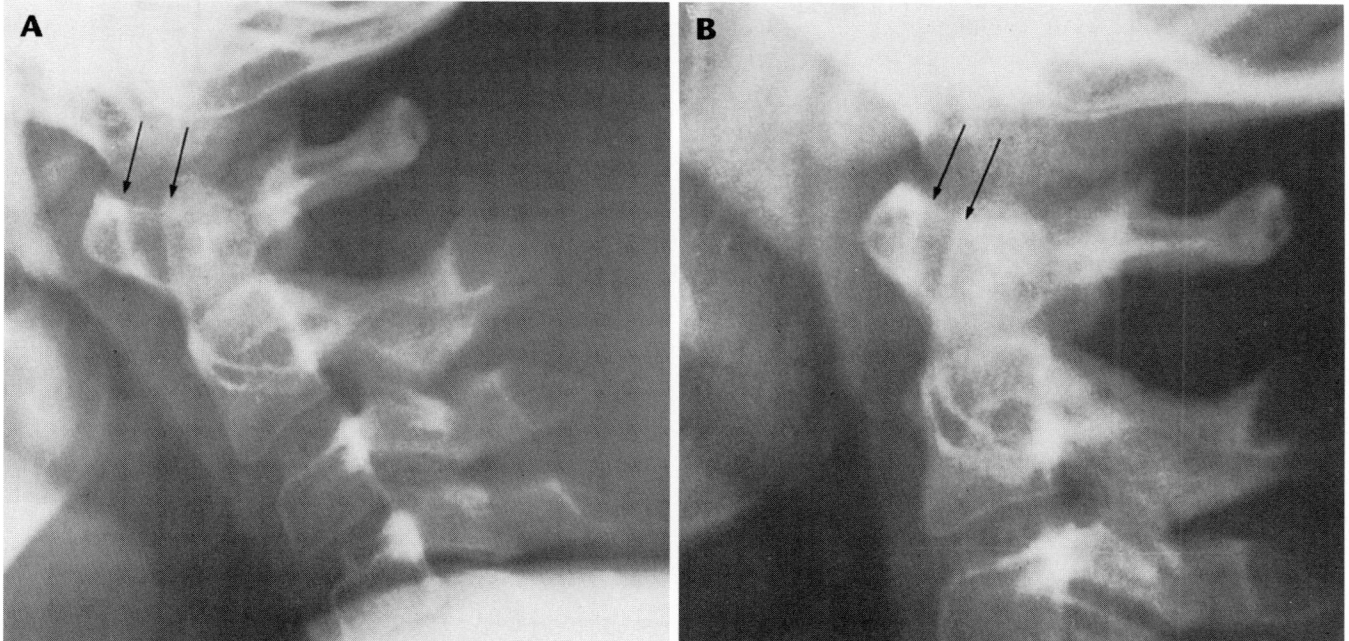

Figure 3–57. The dens–C1 interval normally increases with the head in flexion, particularly in children. **A,** Flexion; **B,** Neutral position. (Ref: Locke GR, Gardner JI, Van Epps EF: Atlas-dens interval in children. *Am J Roentgenol* 97:135 1966.) The V-shaped predens space is a normal variation and does not necessarily indicate damage to the transverse ligament. (Ref: Bohrer SP, Klein A, Martin W III: V shaped predens space. *Skeletal Radiol* 14:111, 1985.)

Figure 3–58. The dens–C1 interval may change in flexion and extension in this 10-year-old boy. This interval tends to remain fixed in adults. Note the shift of the posterior laminar line as well. (Ref: Swischuk LE: The cervical spine in childhood. *Curr Probl Diagn Radiol* 13:98, 1987.)

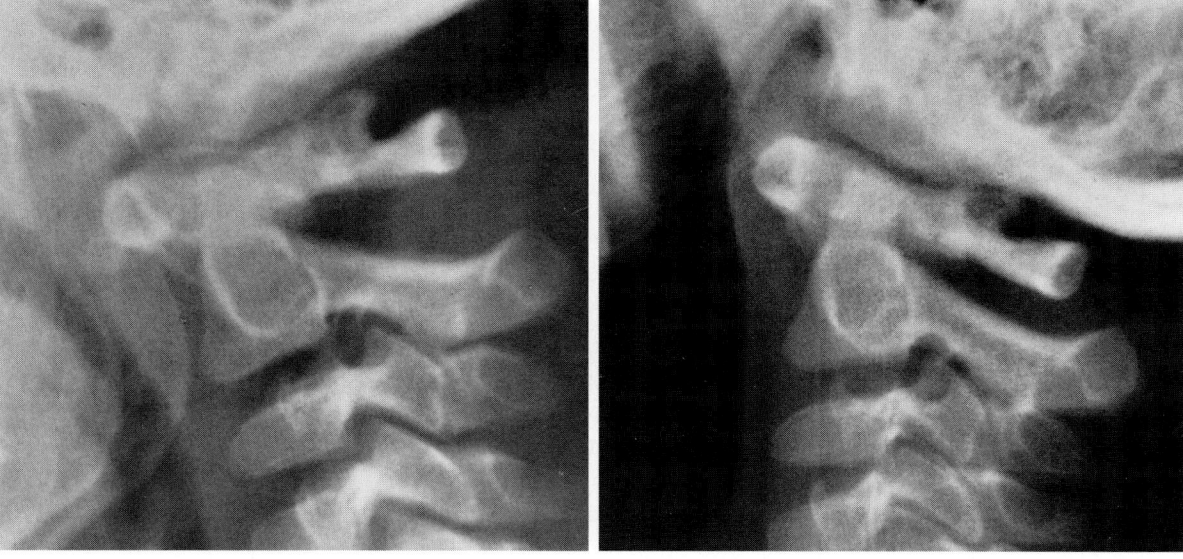

Figure 3–59. Accessory ossicle posterior to C1, articulating with the neural arch of C1.

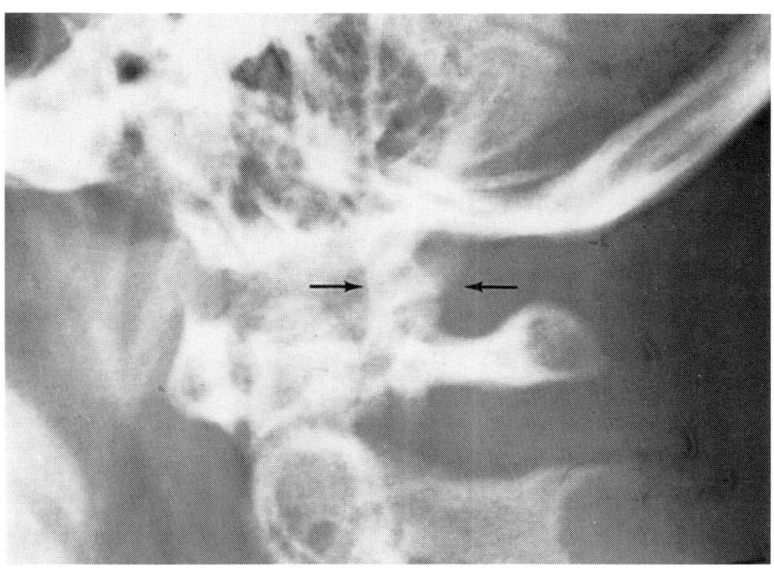

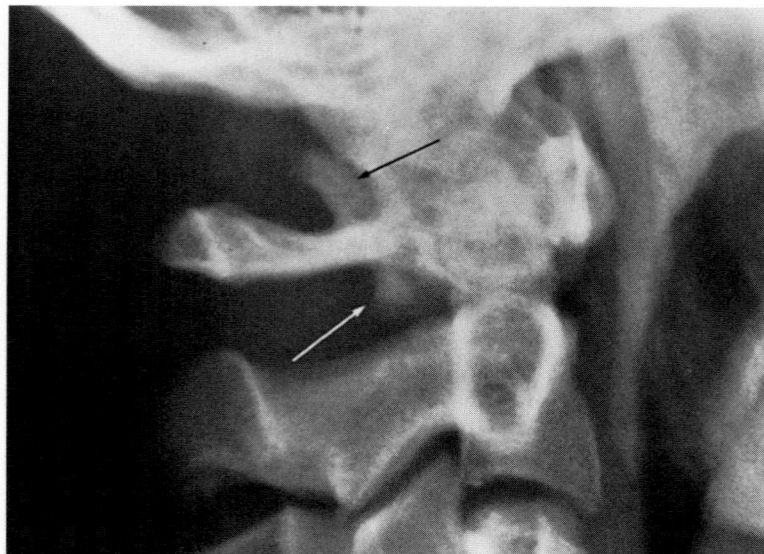

Figure 3–60. Osseous processes above and below the posterior arch of C1.

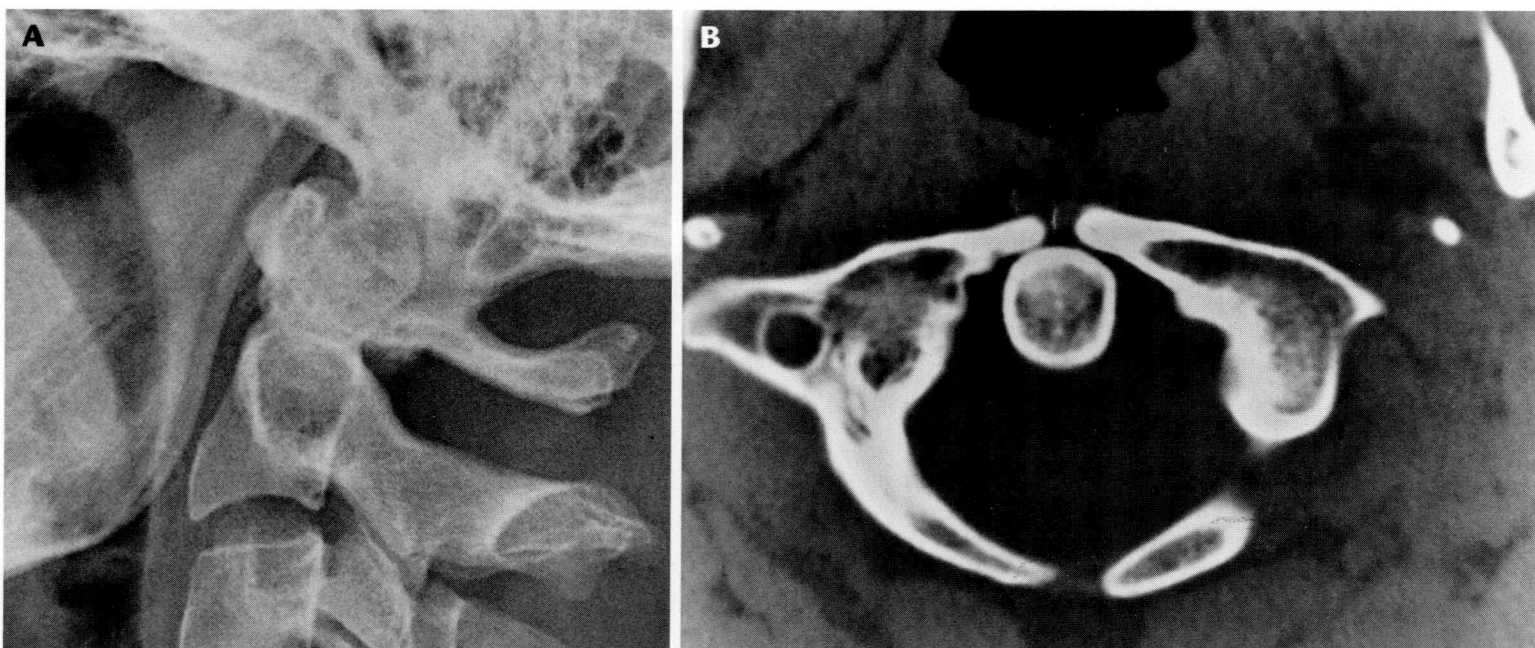

Figure 3–61. Unusual appearance of the anterior arch of C1 secondary to closure defects in the anterior and posterior neural arches.

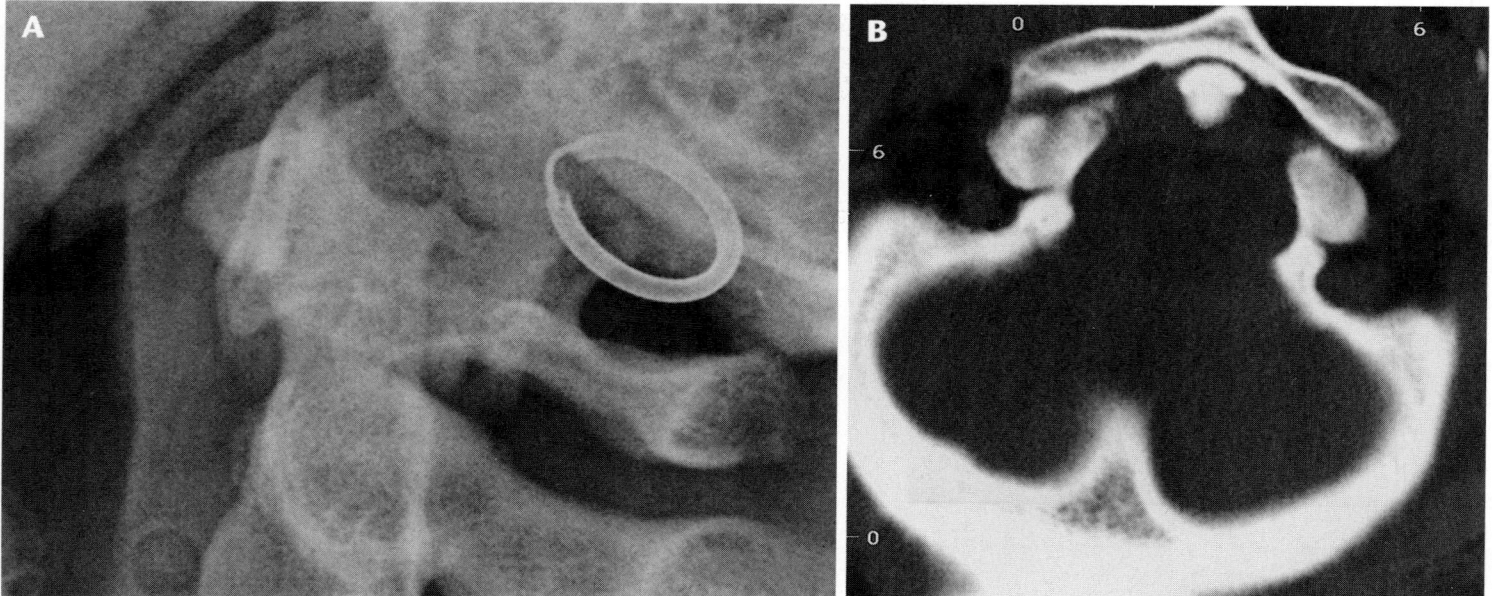

Figure 3–62. Unusual contour of the anterior arch of C1 with a spur-like configuration and double contour. **A,** Lateral projection. **B,** CT.

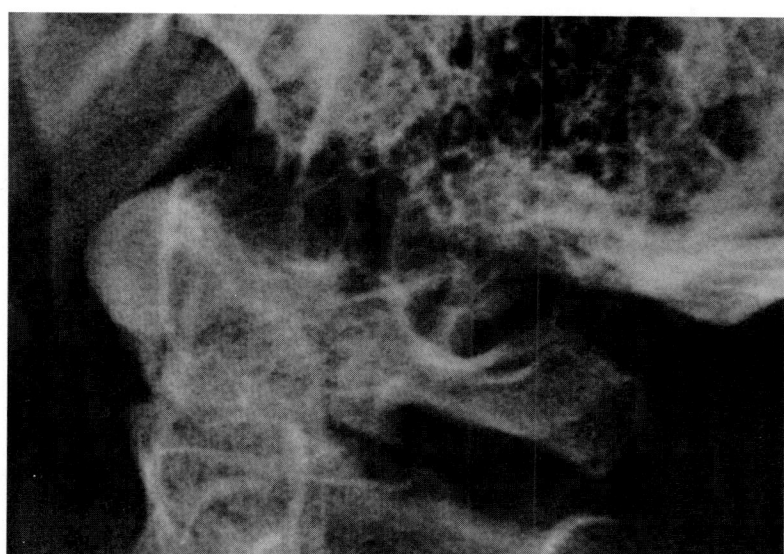

Figure 3–63. Huge anterior arch of C1 in the absence of other anomalies.

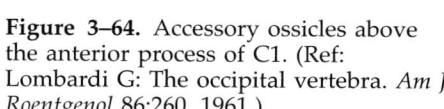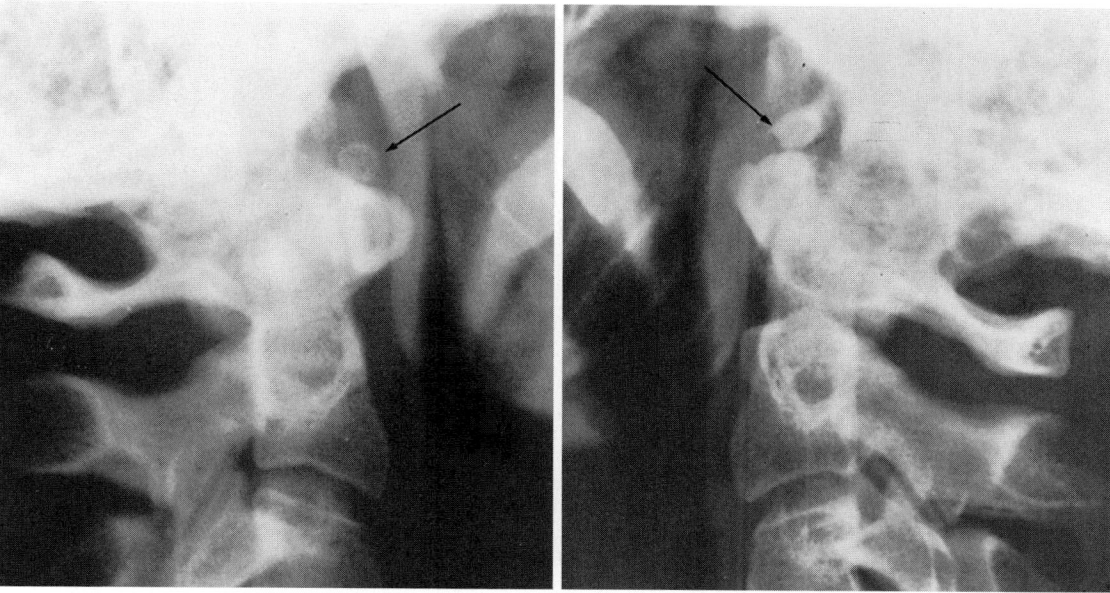

Figure 3–64. Accessory ossicles above the anterior process of C1. (Ref: Lombardi G: The occipital vertebra. *Am J Roentgenol* 86:260, 1961.)

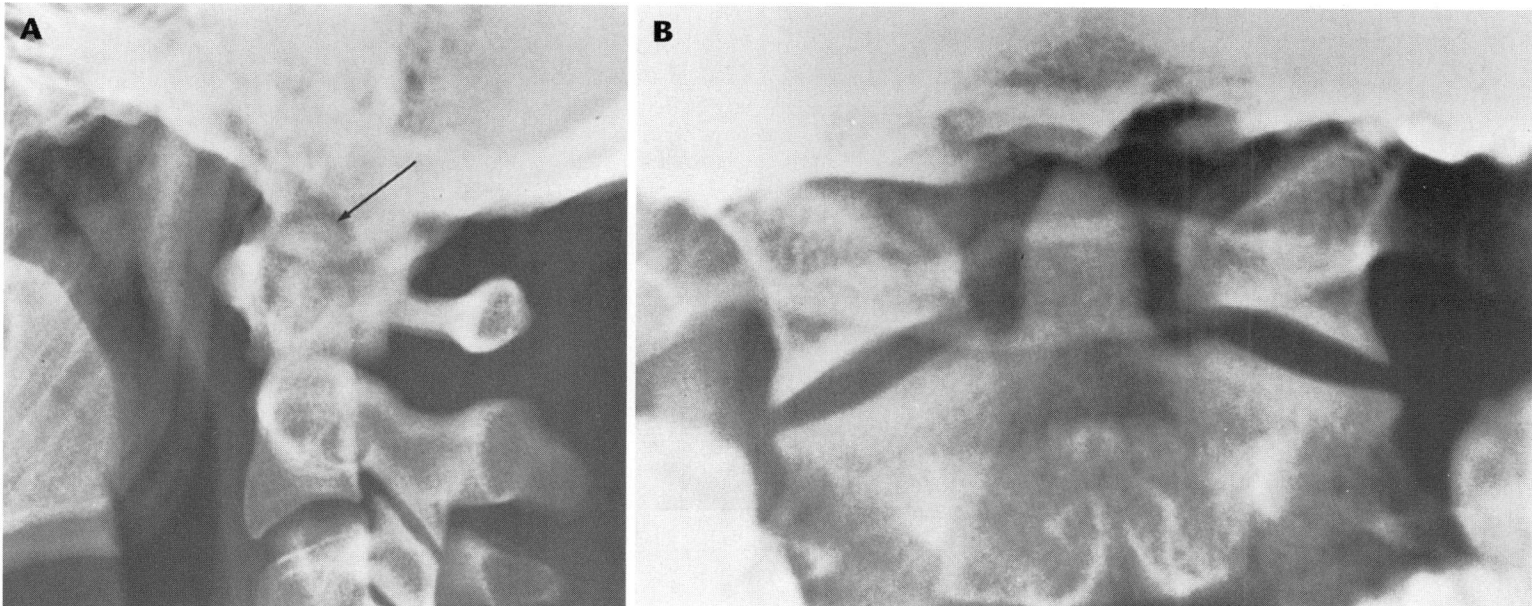

Figure 3–65. A, Simulated ossicle at the tip of the odontoid joint produced by the mastoid tip. **B,** Ossicle not seen in AP projection.

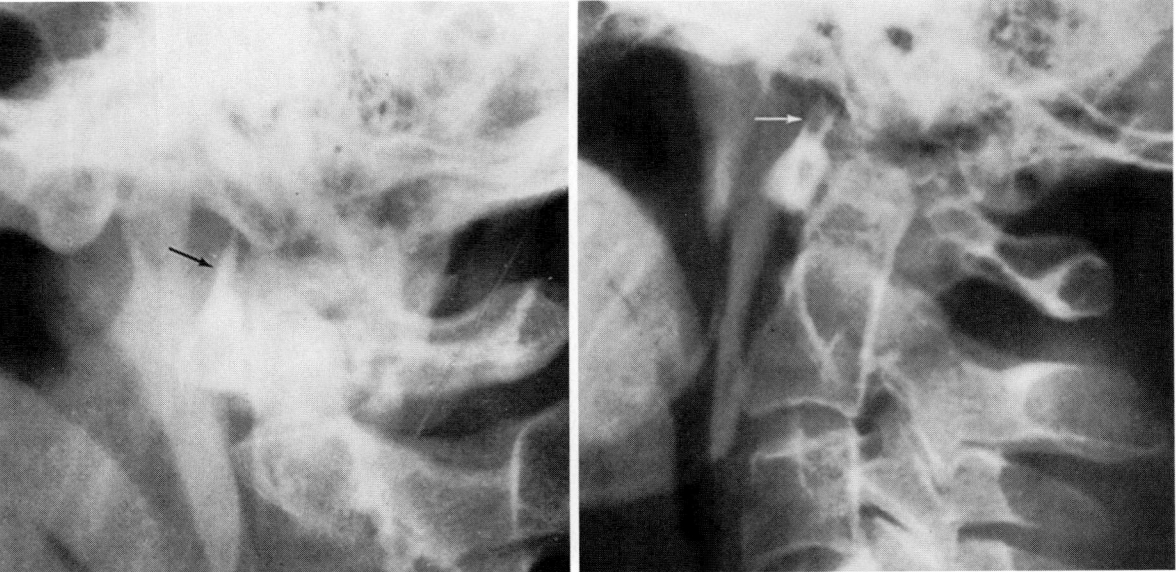

Figure 3–66. Examples of calcification of the anterior longitudinal ligament above the anterior process of C1.

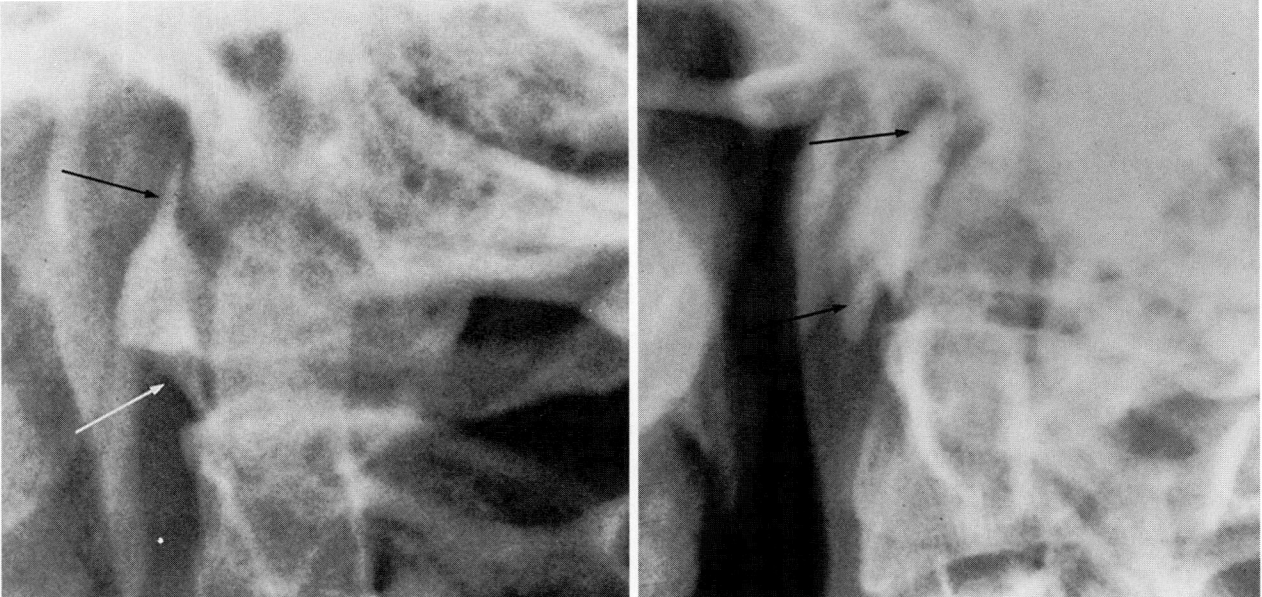

Figure 3–67. Calcification of the anterior longitudinal ligament above and below the anterior process of C1. *Left,* 14-year-old boy; *right,* 44-year-old man. In older individuals, these kinds of changes may be associated with degenerative arthritis of the atlanto-odontoid joint. (Ref: Genez BM et al: CT findings of degenerative arthritis of the atlantoodontoid joint. *Am J Roentgenol* 154:315, 1990.)

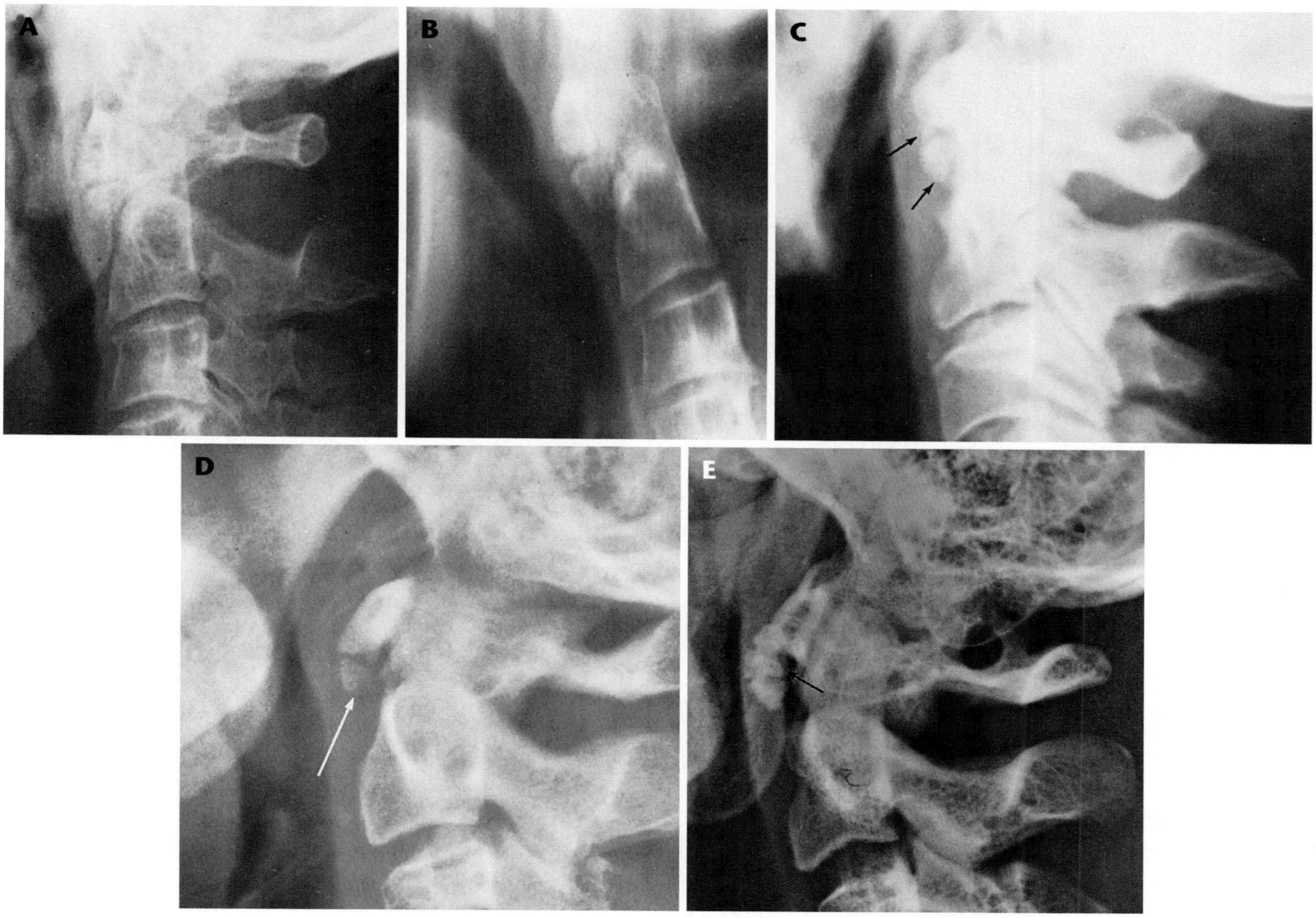

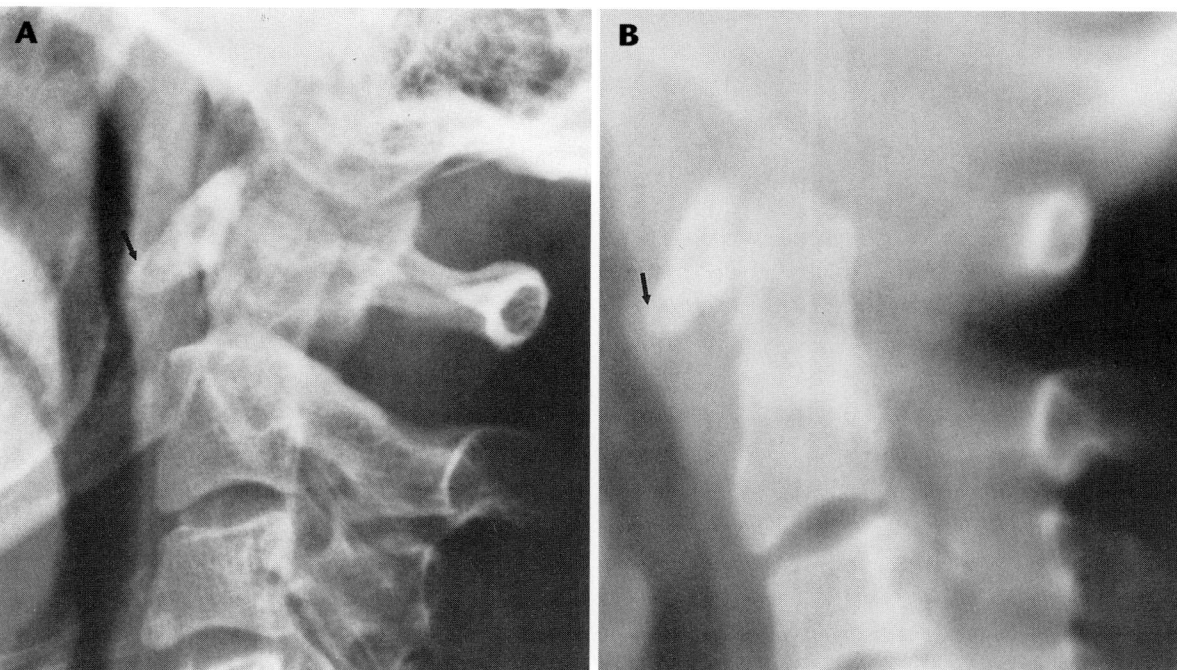

Figure 3–68. Five examples of the variable appearance of the accessory ossicle of the anterior arch of the atlas. The tomogram in **B** indicates an articulation with the inferior aspect of the anterior arch of C1. This articulation may be confused with a fracture. The ossicle should not be confused with calcific tendinitis of the longus colli muscle. (Ref: Haun C: Retropharyngeal tendinitis. *Am J Roentgenol* 130:1137, 1978.) (From Keats TE: Inferior accessory ossicle of the anterior arch of the atlas. *Am J Roentgenol* 101:834, 1967.)

Figure 3–69. An unusual ossicle of the anterior arch of C1. Note the displacement of the retropharyngeal soft tissues. **A,** Lateral projection. **B,** Tomogram.

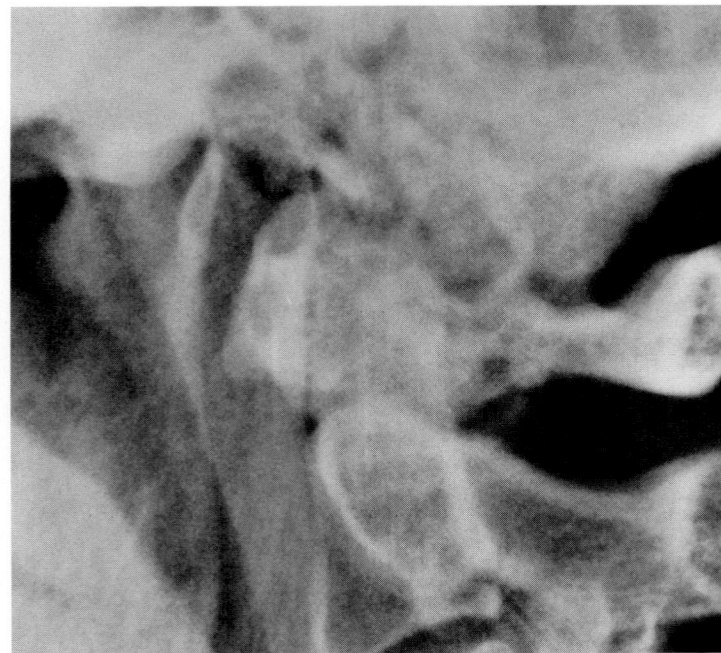

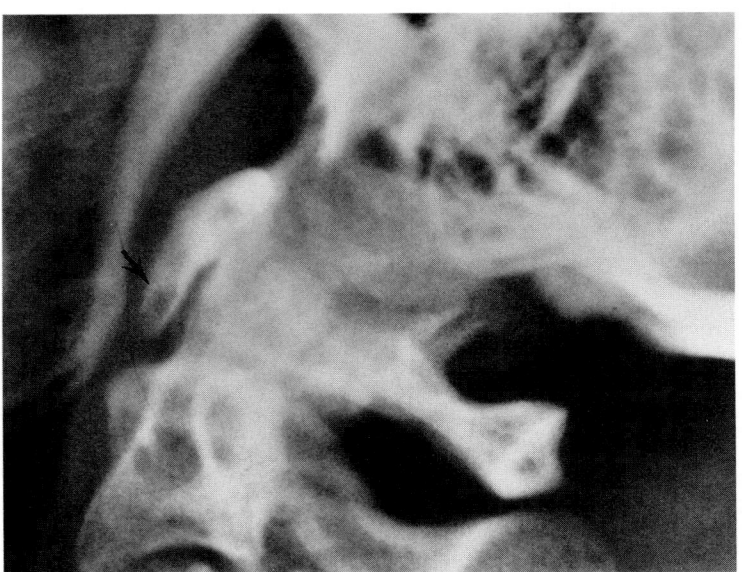

Figure 3–71. Huge ossicle fused to the anterior arch of C1.

Figure 3–70. Fused ossicle above the anterior arch of C1.

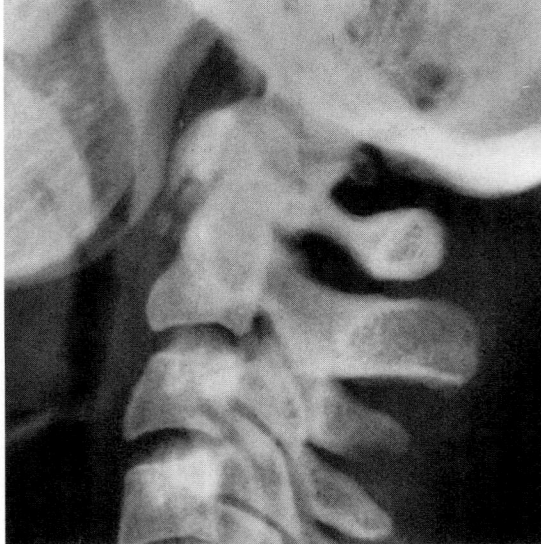

Figure 3–72. Constellation of ossicles and ligamentous calcification below the anterior arch of C1 in a 35-year-old woman.

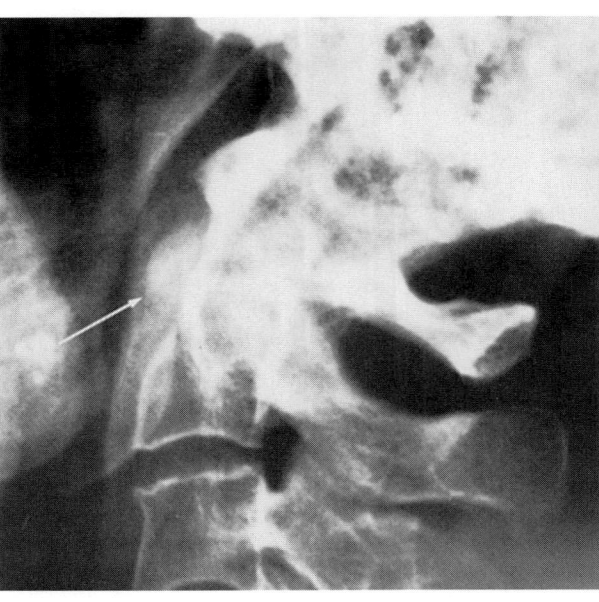

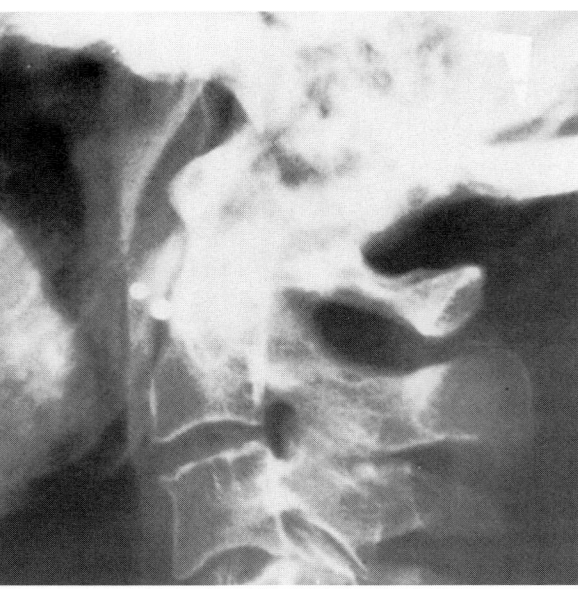

Figure 3–73. *Left,* Ear lobe simulating calcific tendinitis of the longus colli muscle. *Right,* The ear lobes identified with metallic markers to confirm the nature of the shadow seen in the left figure.

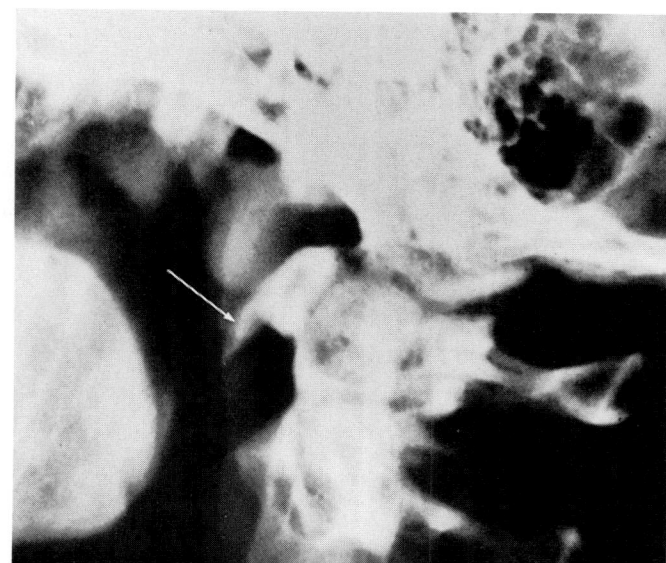

Figure 3–74. Probable calcification in the anterior longitudinal ligament below the anterior arch of C1. Compare with Figure 3–66.

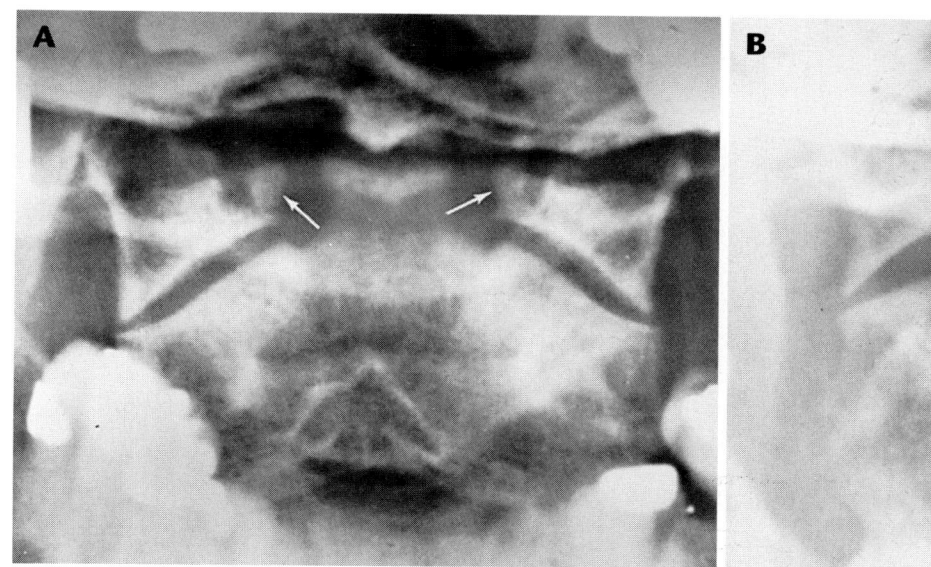

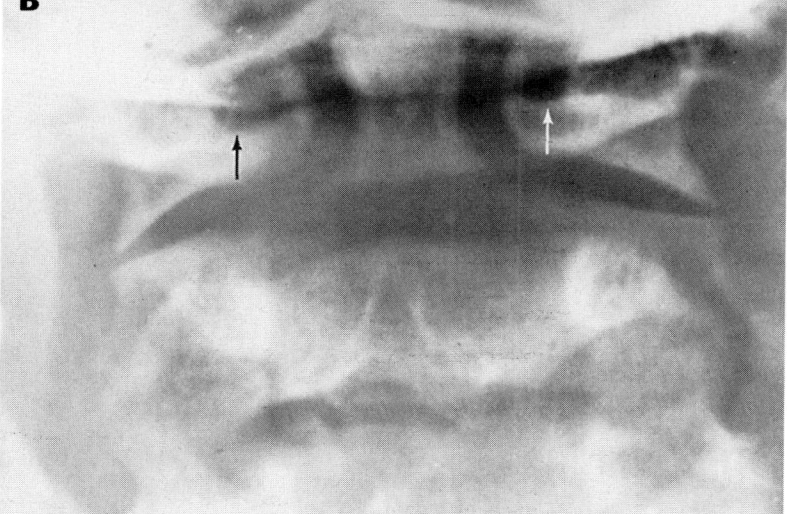

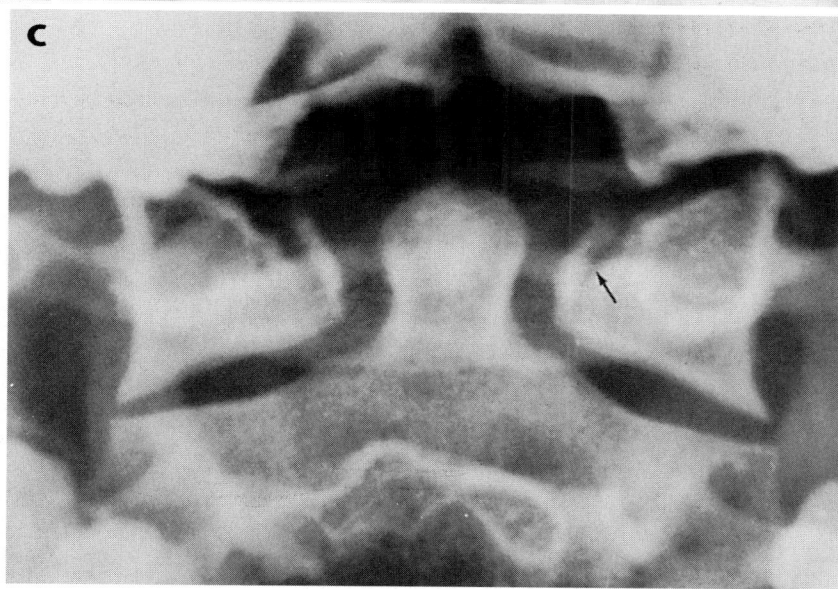

Figure 3–75. Normal variations in the appearance of the lateral masses of C1. **A,** Spurlike configurations of the medial borders. **B,** Foramenlike configuration of the medial borders. **C,** Pseudofracture. These variants should not be mistaken for manifestations of trauma. (Ref: Meghrouni V, Jacobson G: The pseudonotch of the atlas, *Radiology* 72:260, 1959.)

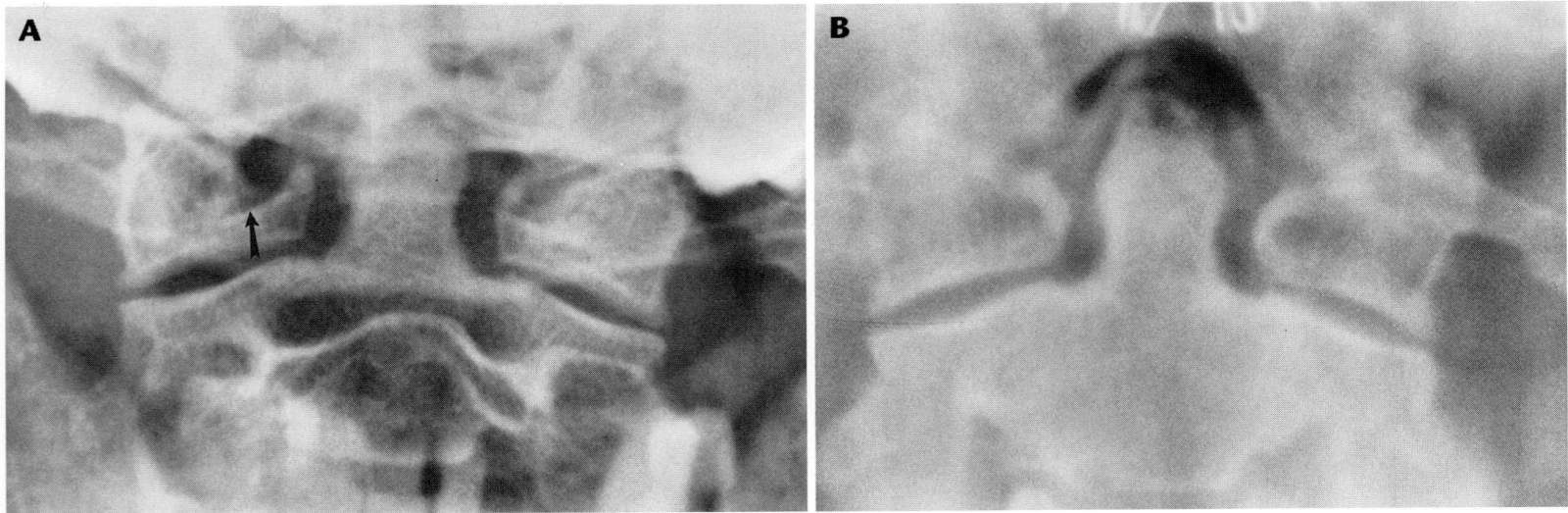

Figure 3–76. A, Shadow of the airway simulating a fracture of the lateral mass C1. **B,** Tomogram shows no fracture.

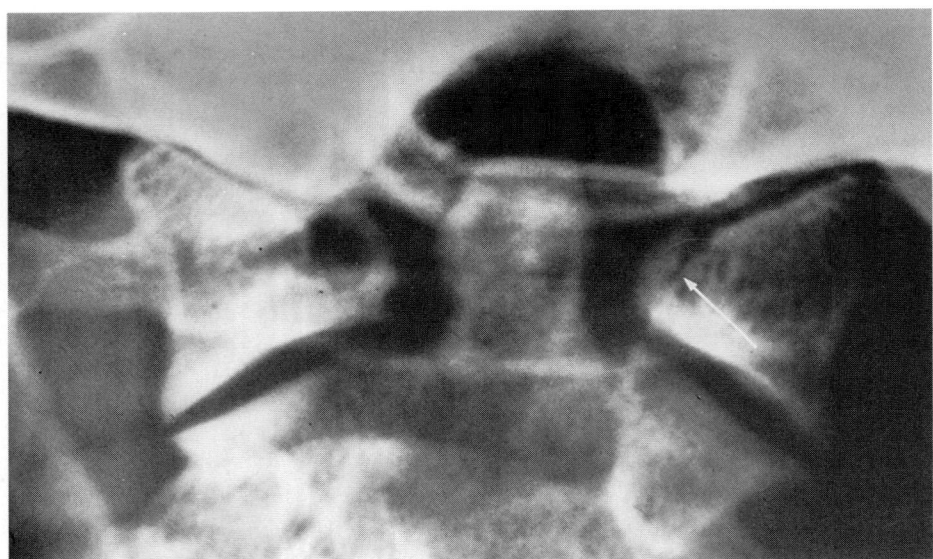

Figure 3–77. Pseudonotch of the atlas mistaken for a fracture. These notches form the attachment site of the transverse ligament.

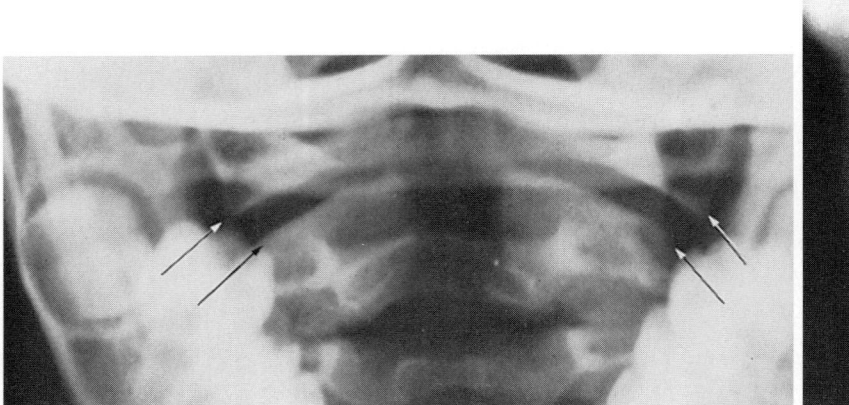

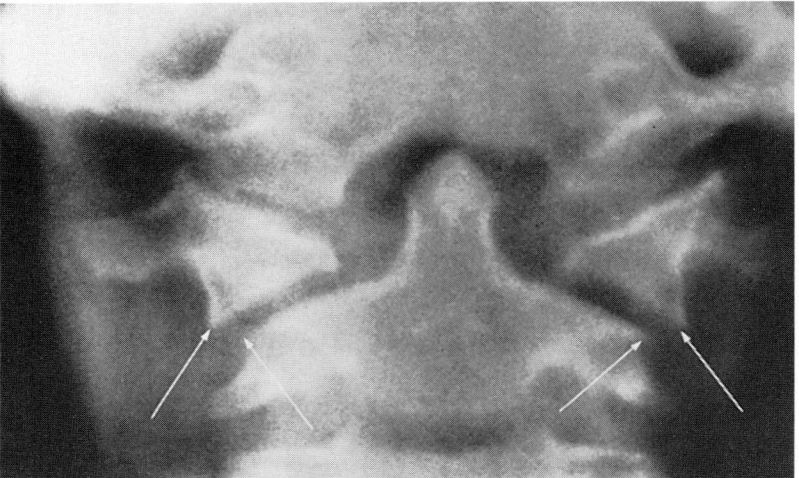

Figure 3–78. Two examples of developmental bilateral offsets of the lateral masses of C1 and C2 in children. This appearance in an adult would be presumptive evidence of a fracture of the neural arch of C1. This entity is believed to be secondary to a disparity of growth of the atlas and axis vertebrae in children and is most commonly seen in children approximately 4 years old. (Ref: Suss RA, Zimmerman RD, Leeds NE: Pseudospread of the atlas: False sign of Jefferson fracture in children. *Am J Roentgenol* 140:1079, 1983.)

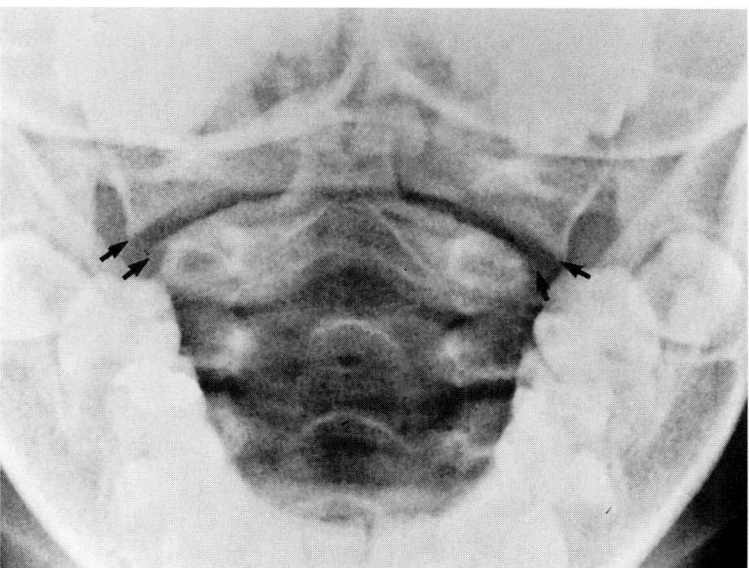

Figure 3–79. Developmental bilateral offset of the lateral masses of C1 on C2 may persist in older children as well, as seen in this 6-year-old.

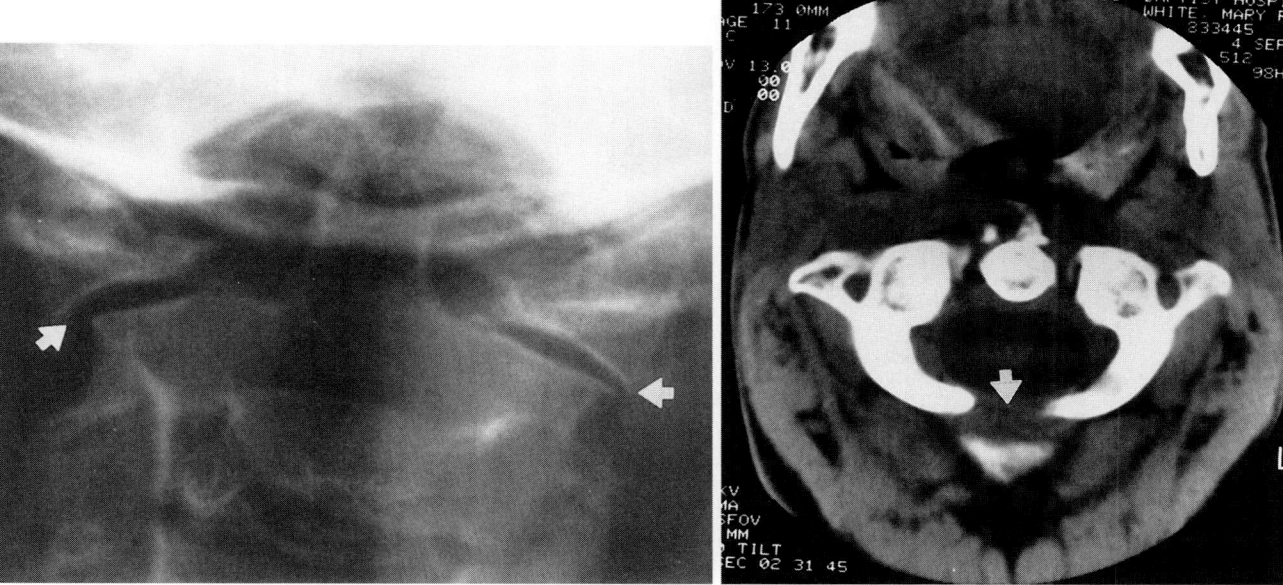

Figure 3–80. Offsets of C1 and C2, which may simulate Jefferson's burst fracture, may be seen in patients with incomplete neural arches. This patient has a spina bifida occulta of C1 posteriorly. (Ref: Rossitch JC and Bohrer SP: Case of the month. *Appl Radiology* 20:56, 1991.)

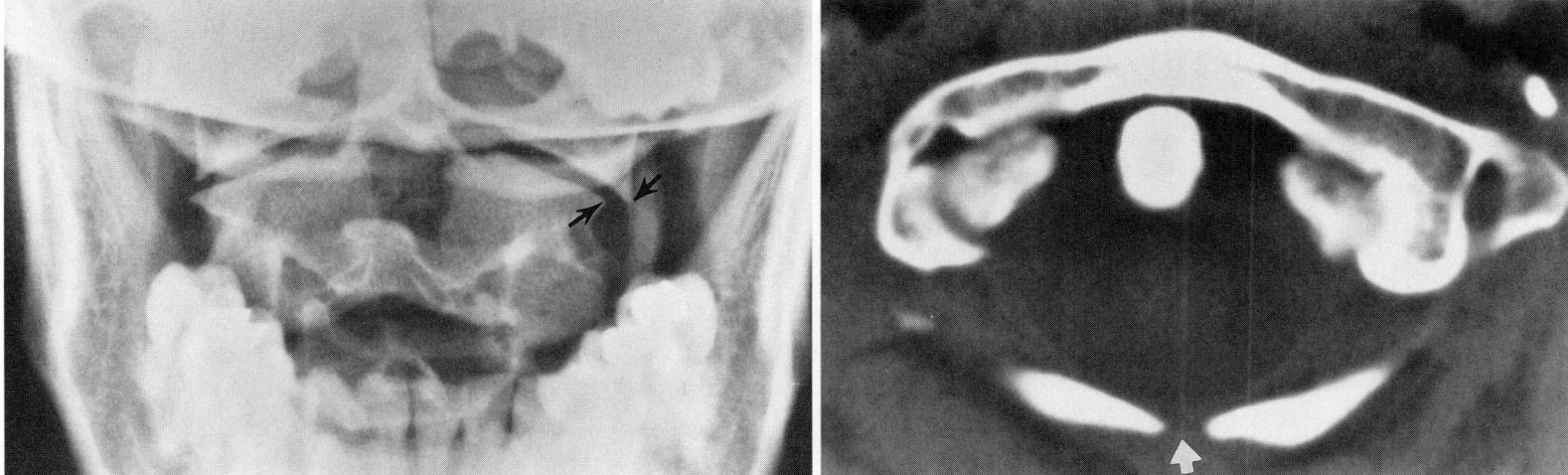

Figure 3–81. Unilateral offset of the left lateral mass C1 is associated with spina bifida occulta of the neural arch of C1.

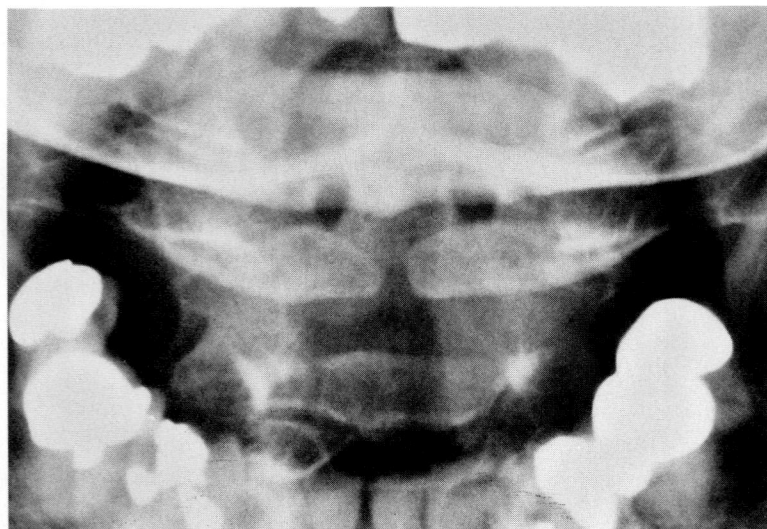

Figure 3–82. Spina bifida occulta of C1 seen in the open-mouth view of the odontoid process.

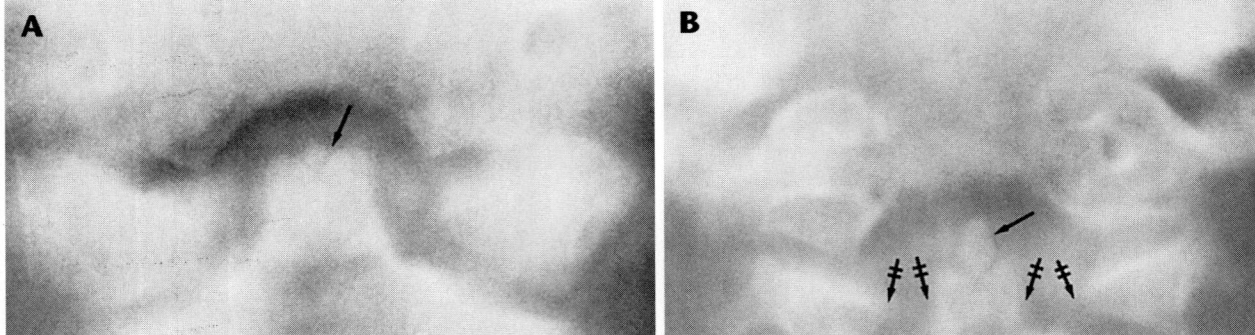

Figure 3–83. Normal ossification centers for the tip of the odontoid process. This center appears at age 2 and fuses at age 12. **A,** 5-year-old boy. **B,** 7-year-old boy. Minor variations in the width of the interval between the odontoid process and the lateral masses, as shown in **B,** are due to rotation of the head at the time of filming and should not be mistaken for evidence of trauma (⇥). (Ref: Wortzman G, DeWar FP: Rotary fixation of the atlantoaxial joint: rotational atlantoaxial subluxation. *Radiology* 90:479, 1968.)

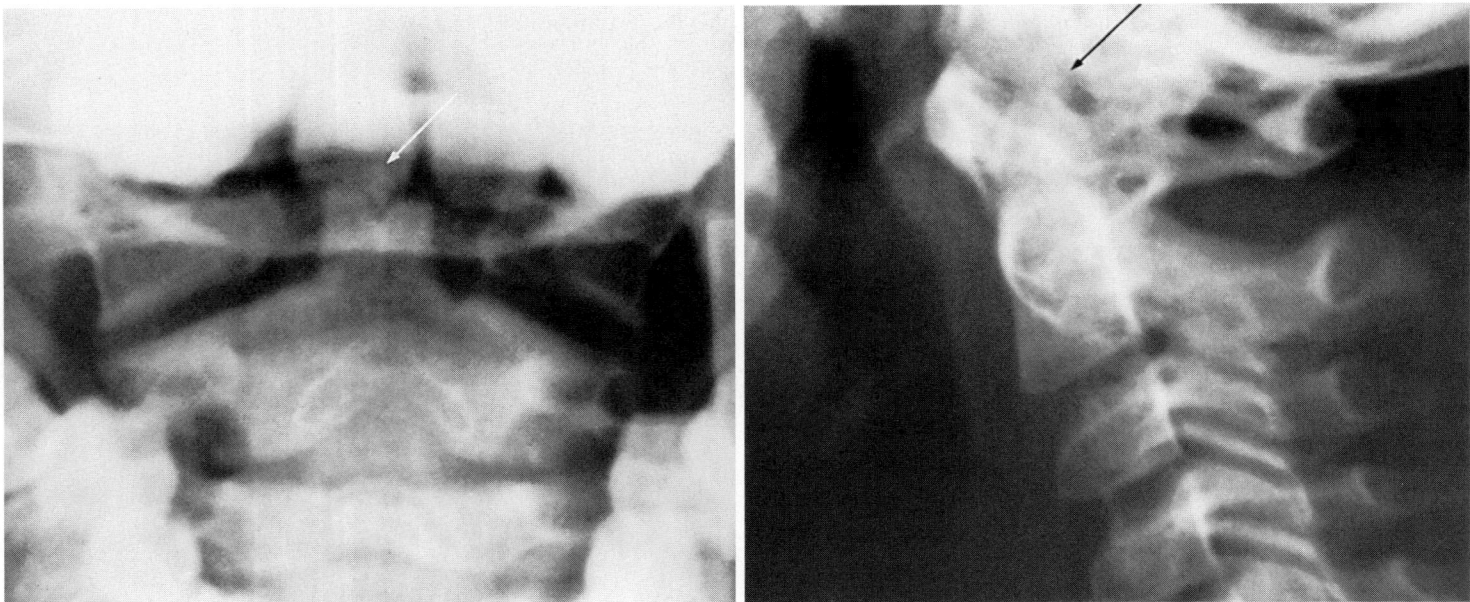

Figure 3–84. Ossification of the tip of the odontoid process (os terminale) in frontal and lateral projections in a 9-year-old boy.

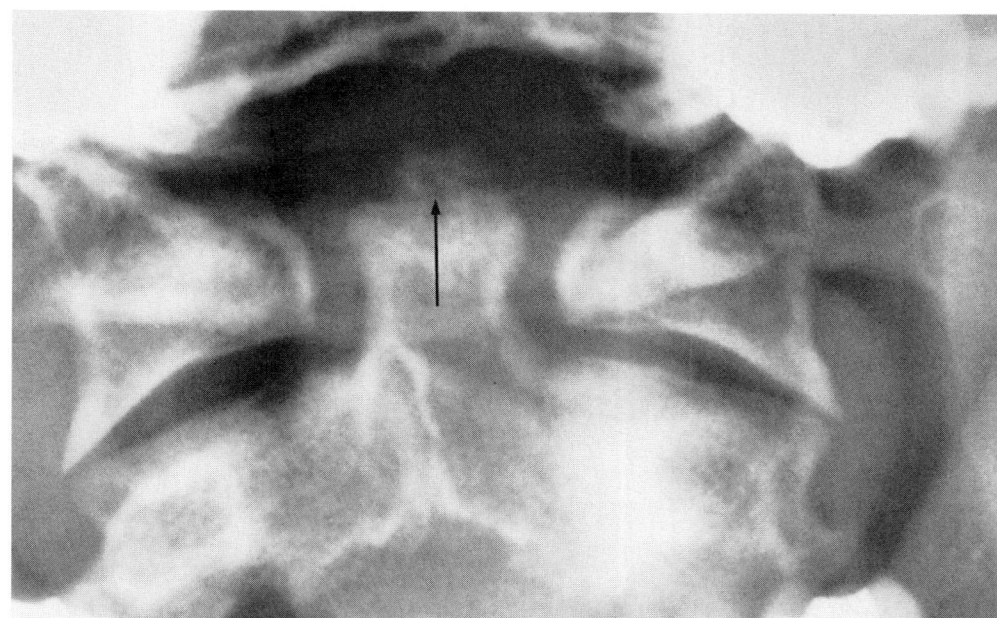

Figure 3–85. Mach effect produced by the shadow of the tongue, simulating an ununited ossification center of the tip of the odontoid process.

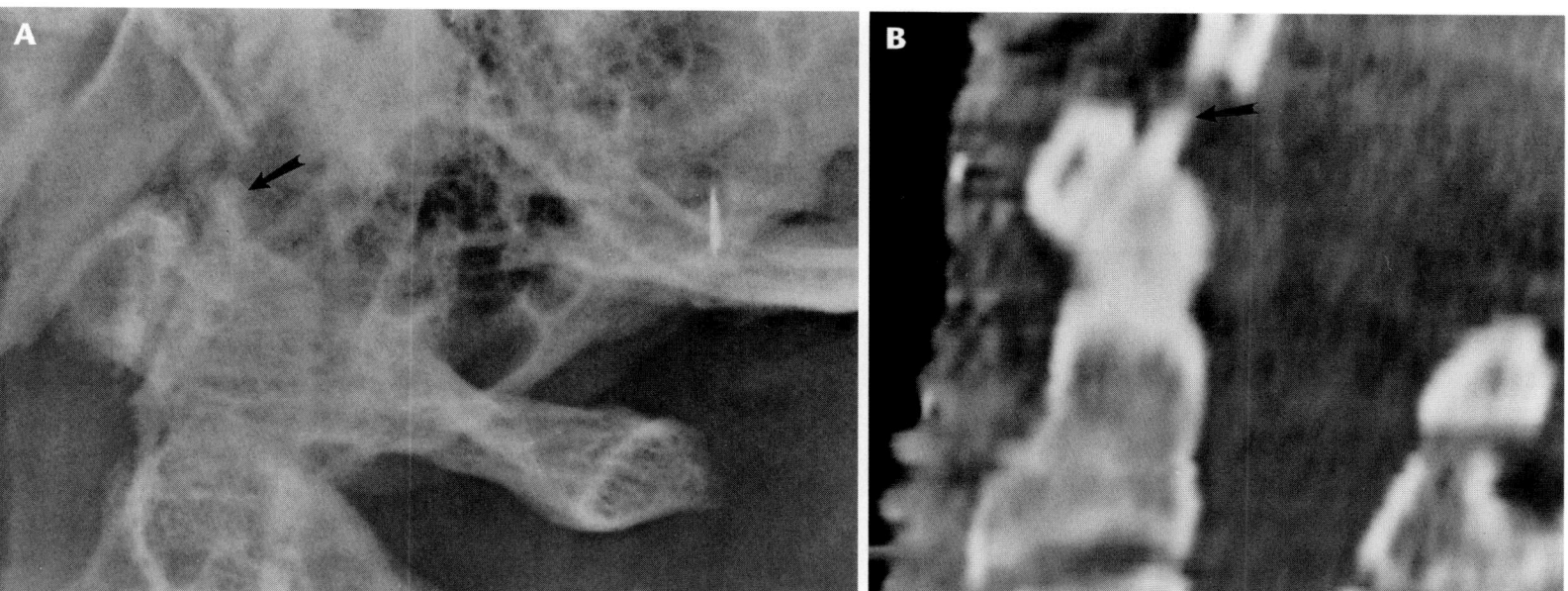

Figure 3–86. Calcification of the apical ligament of the odontoid. **A,** Lateral projection. **B,** Reformatted CT.

Figure 3–87. The midline cleft in the odontoid is usually closed at birth. It has persisted in this 4-year-old boy. (Ref: Ogden JA: Radiology of postnatal skeletal development. XII. 2nd cervical vertebra. *Skeletal Radiol* 12:169, 1984.)

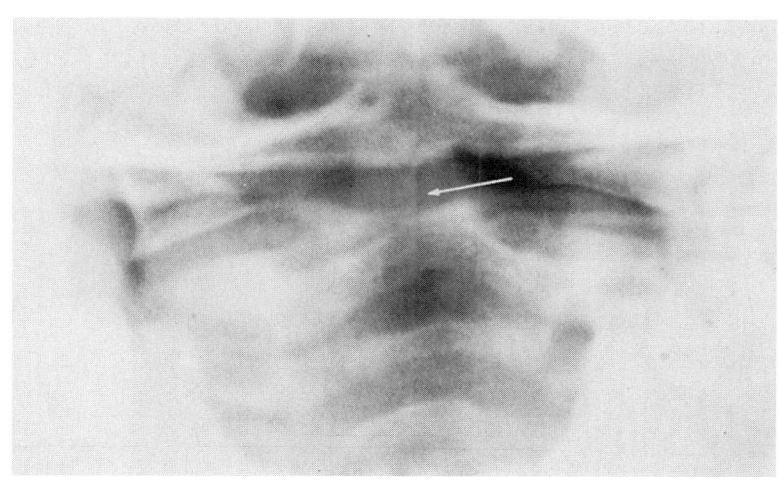

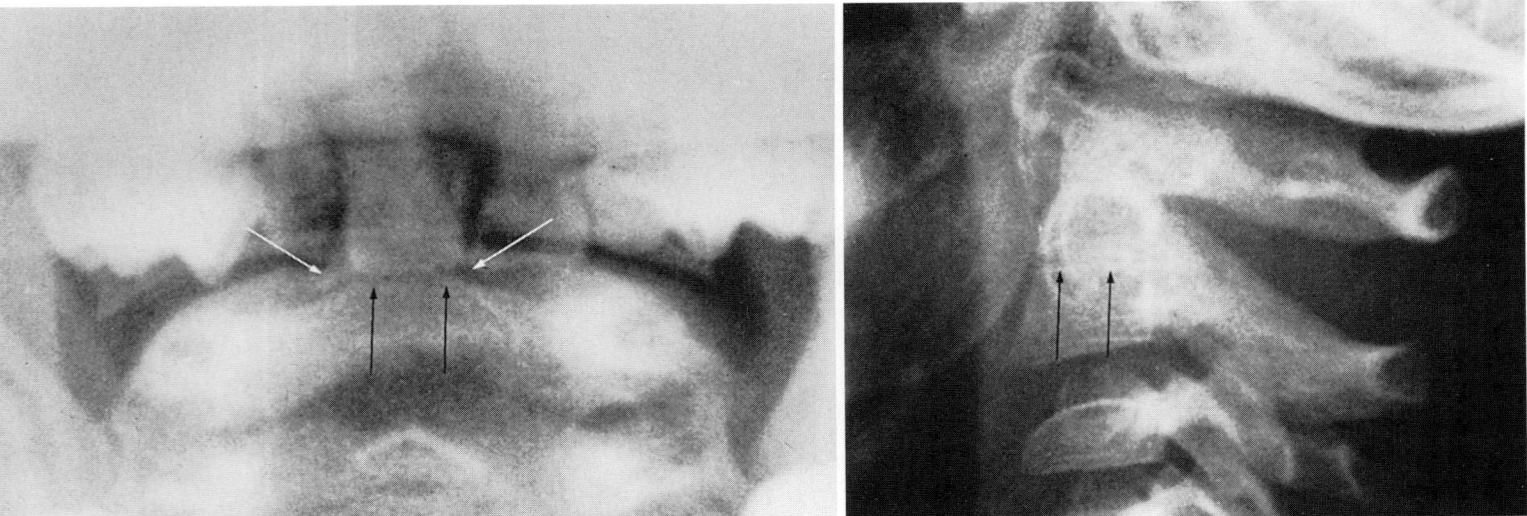

Figure 3–88. Normal synchondrosis of the base of the odontoid process in a child.

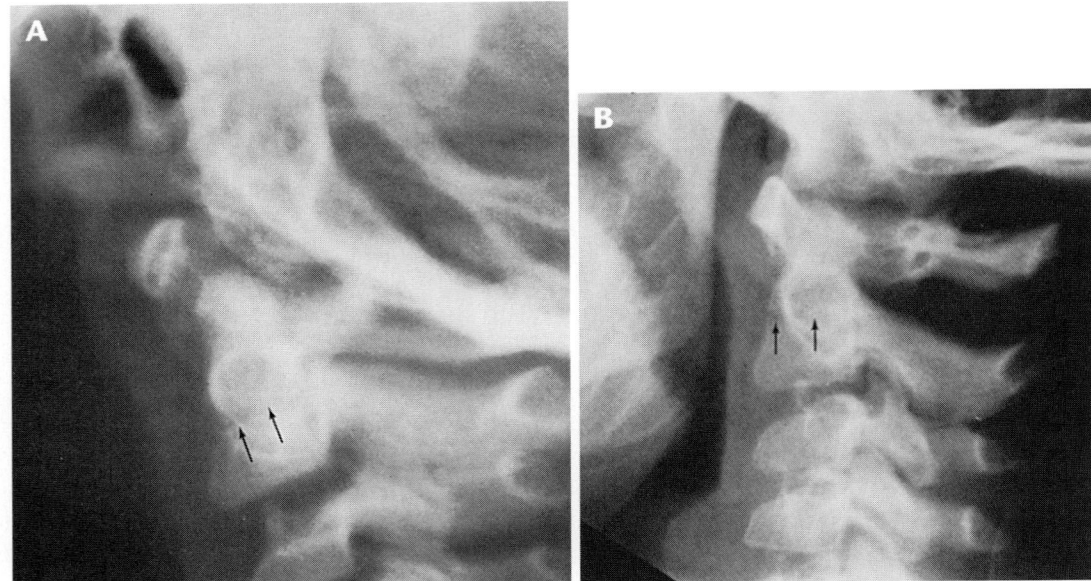

Figure 3–89. Synchondrosis at the base of the odontoid process may be mistaken for a fracture in children. The junction usually closes by age 7. **A,** 2-year-old child. **B,** 3-year-old child.

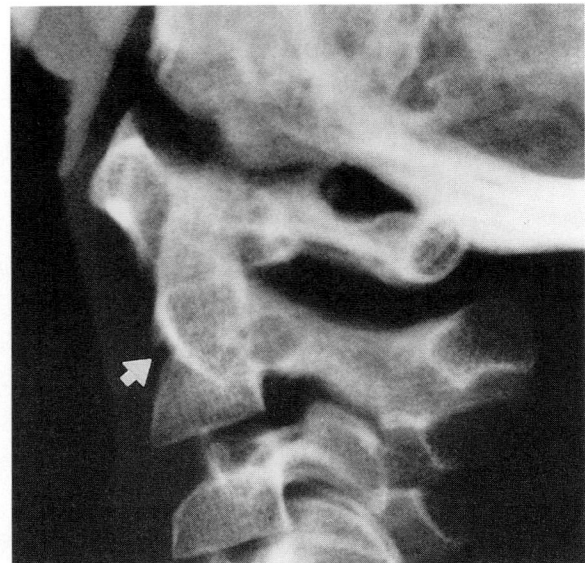

Figure 3–90. Persistence of a portion of the odontoid synchondrosis in a 9-year-old boy.

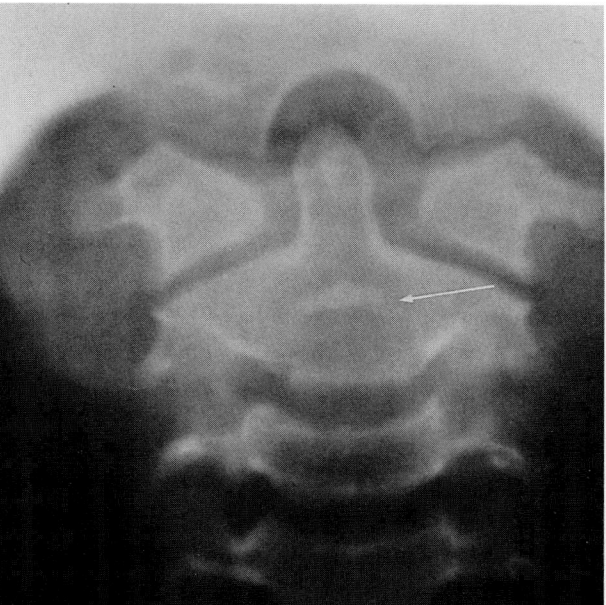
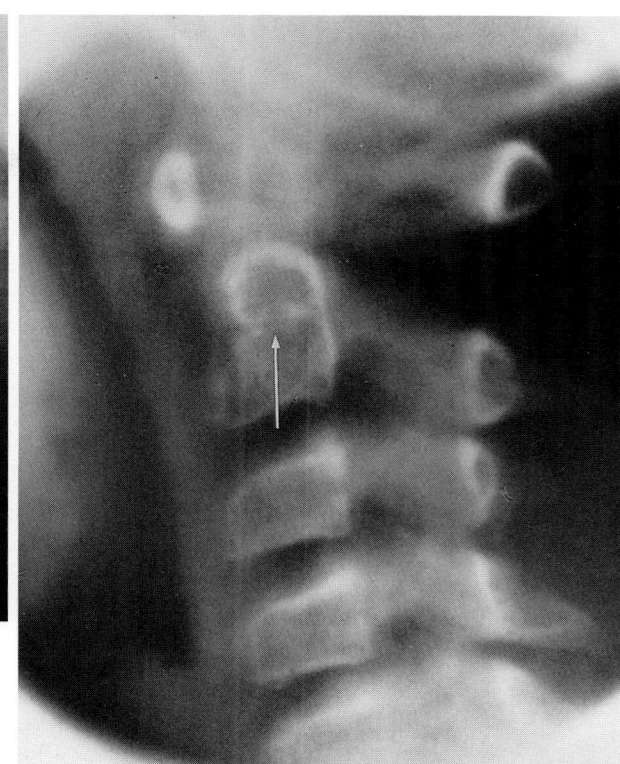

Figure 3–91. Persistence of a portion of the odontoid synchondrosis in a 13-year-old boy.

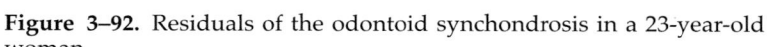
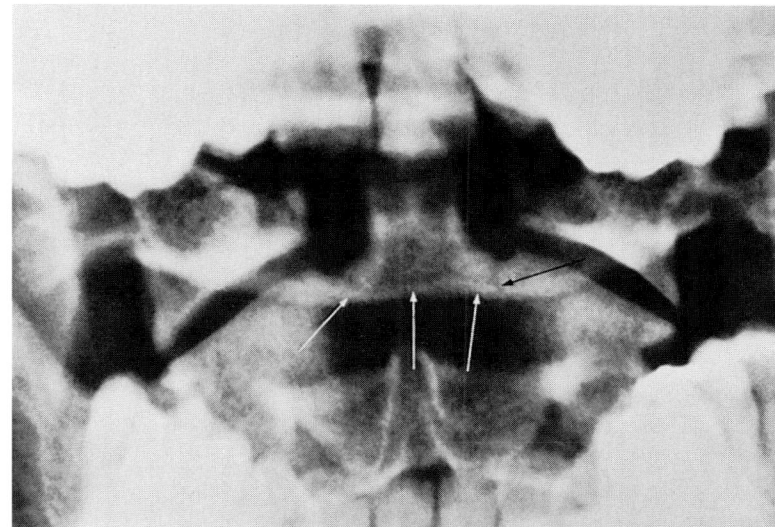

Figure 3–92. Residuals of the odontoid synchondrosis in a 23-year-old woman.

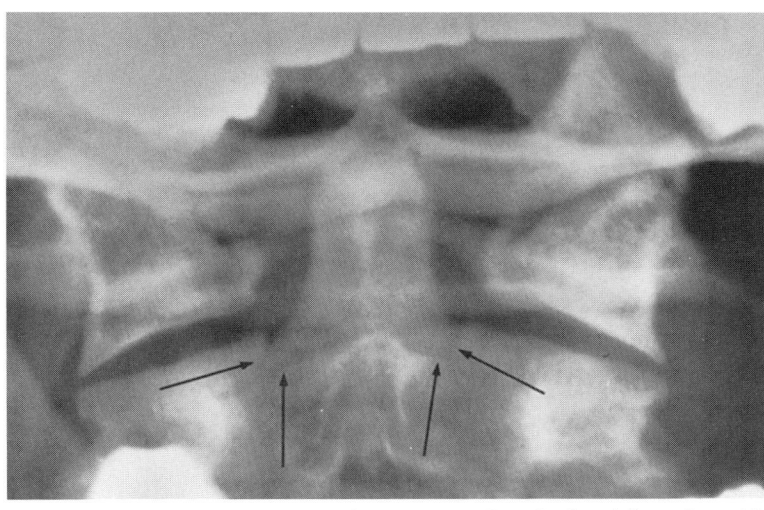
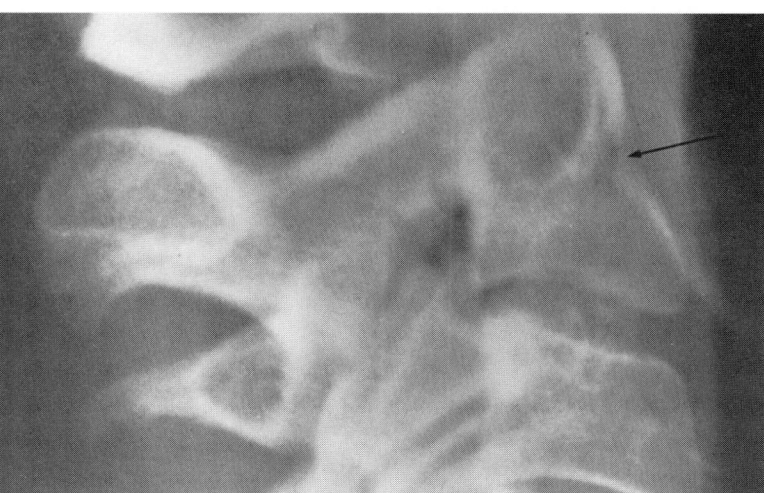

Figure 3–93. Residuals of the odontoid synchondrosis in a 28-year-old woman.

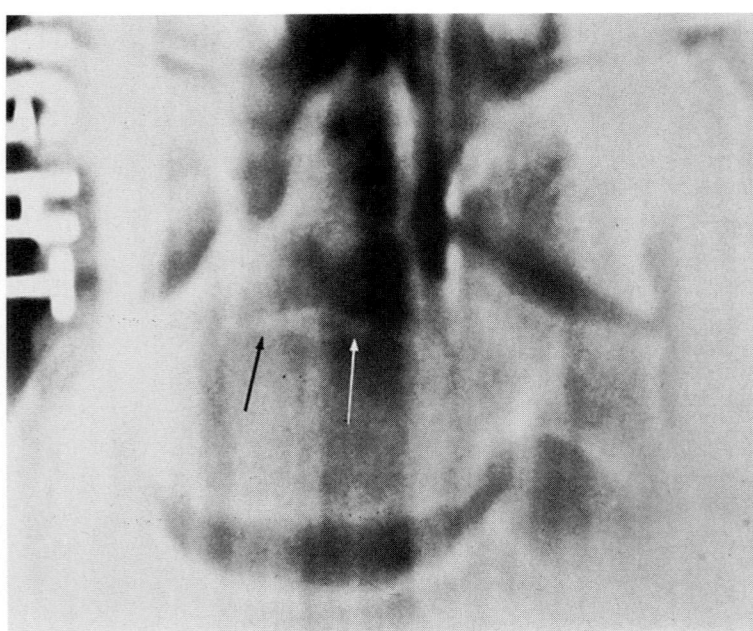

Figure 3–94. Sclerosis of the odontoid synchondrosis and asymmetry of the odontoid process.

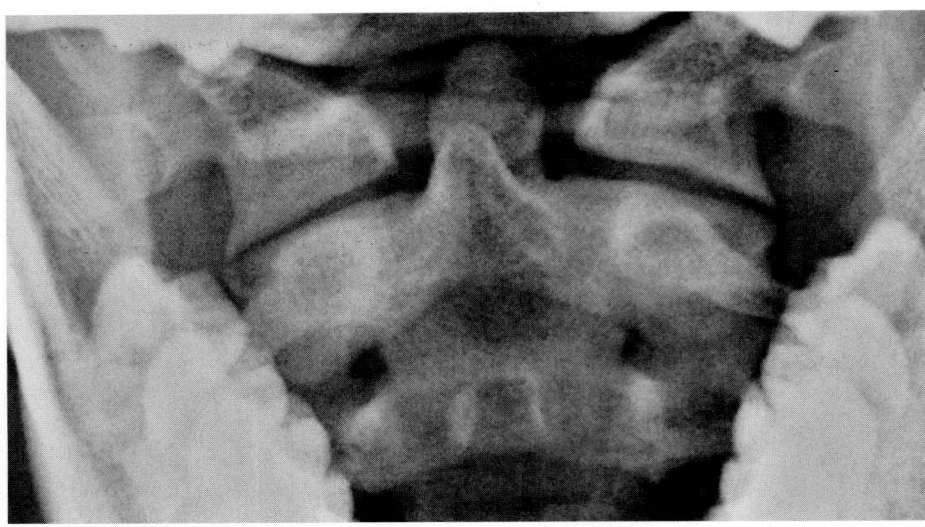

Figure 3–95. "Double odontoid" produced by superimposition of the neural arch of C2.

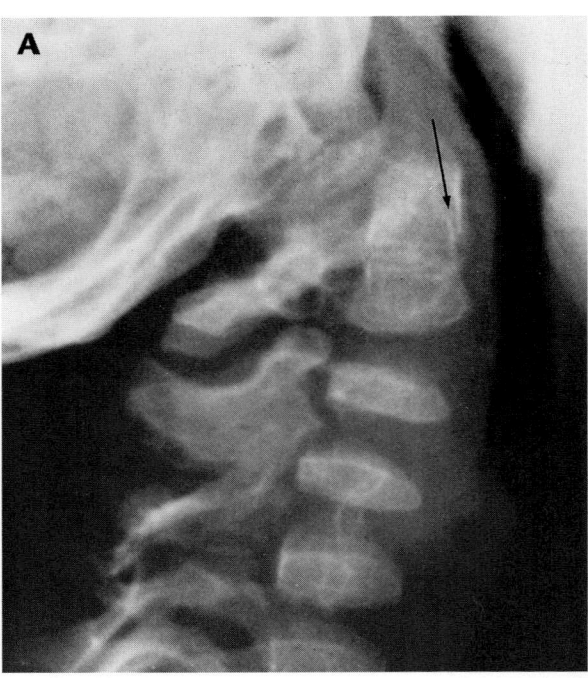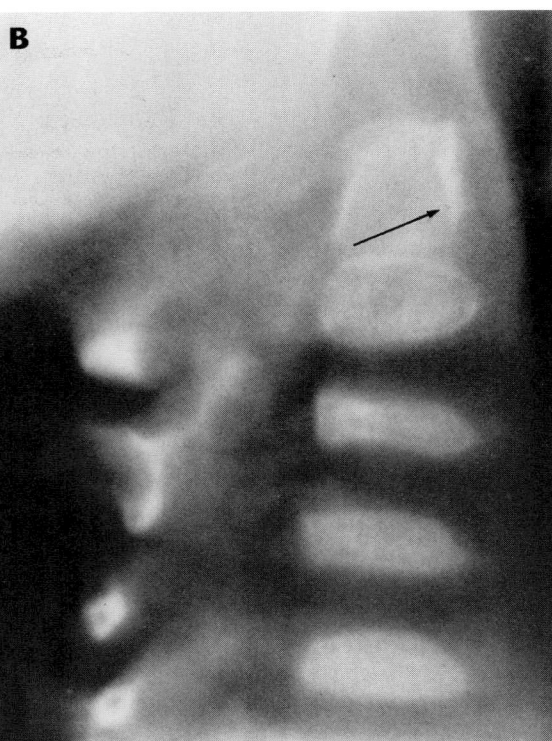

Figure 3–96. Fusion of the anterior arch of C1 to the odontoid process in a 3-year-old boy. **A,** Plain film. **B,** Tomogram. (Ref: Olbrantz K, Bohrer SP: Fusion of the anterior arch of the atlas to dens. *Skeletal Radiol* 12:21, 1984.)

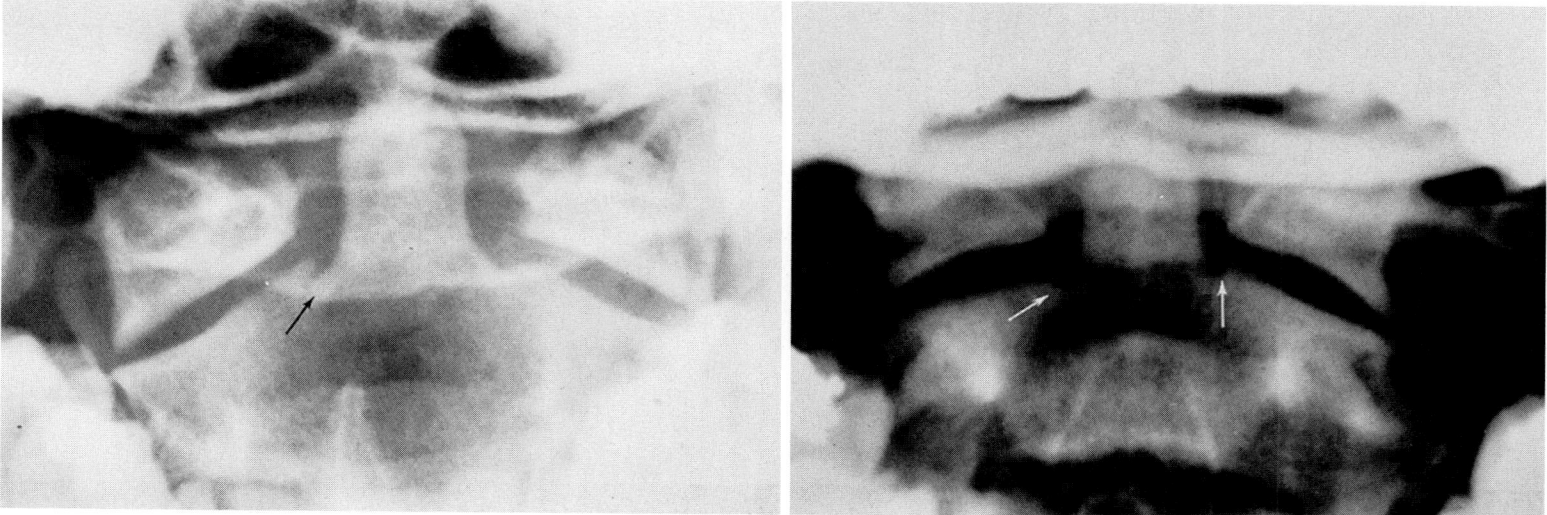

Figure 3–97. Normal developmental clefts at the base of the odontoid process, remnants of the synchondrosis.

Figure 3–98. Congenital absence of the odontoid process and posterior arch of C1 detected as an incidental finding. Note characteristic overdevelopment of the anterior arch of C1, seen in congenital absence of the odontoid process and in failure of union of the odontoid process. (Ref: Swischuk LE et al. The os terminale–os odontoideum complex. *Emergency Radiology* 4:72, 1997.)

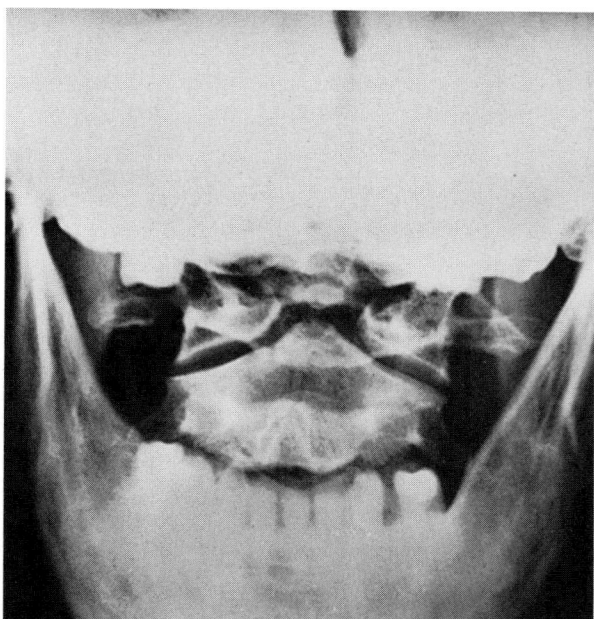
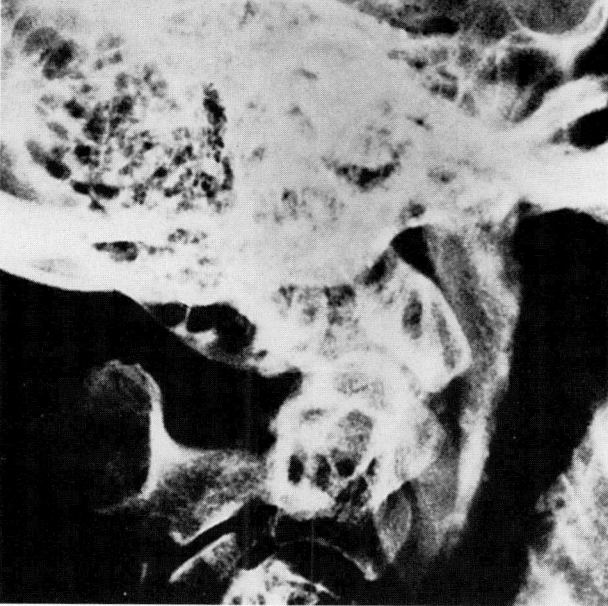

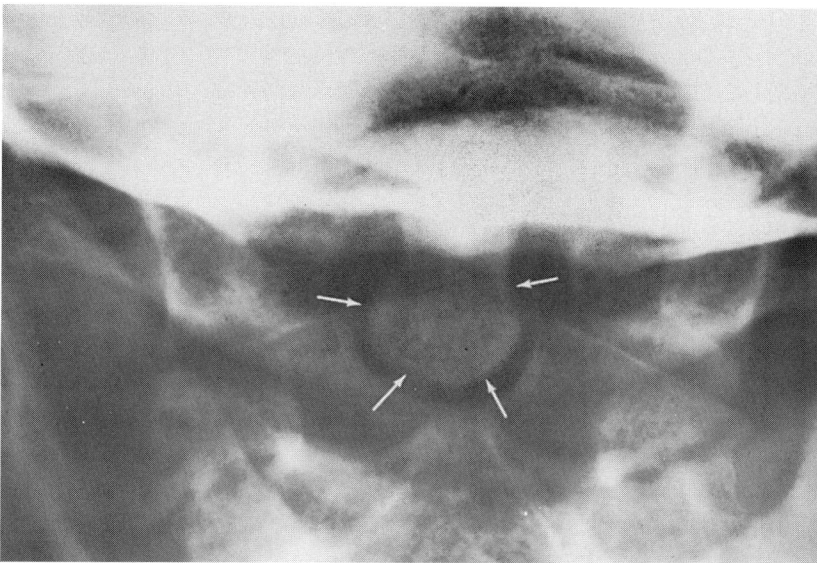
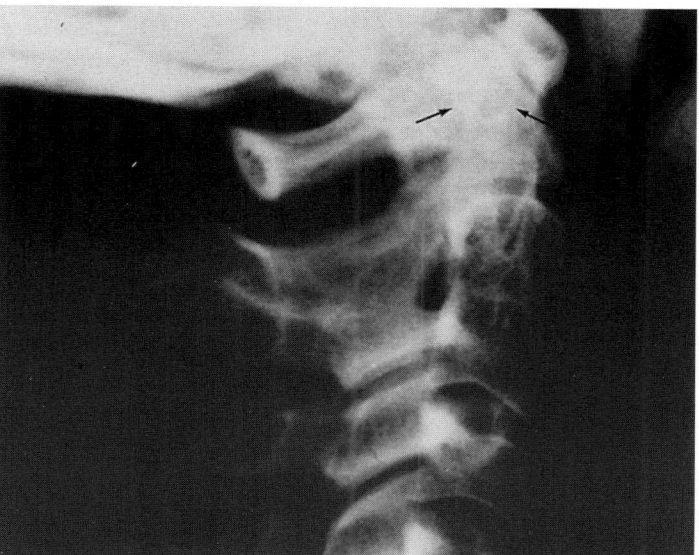

Figure 3–99. Failure of union of the odontoid process with a separate os odontoideum (→). Note also the failure of segmentation of C2. Os odontoideum is often difficult to differentiate from an old odontoid fracture. It is potentially dangerous if excessive motion is present. (Refs: Roback DL: Topics in radiology. *JAMA* 245:963, 1981; Dawson LG, Smith L: Atlantoaxial subluxation in children due to vertebral anomalies. *J Bone Joint Surg* 61A:582, 1979.)

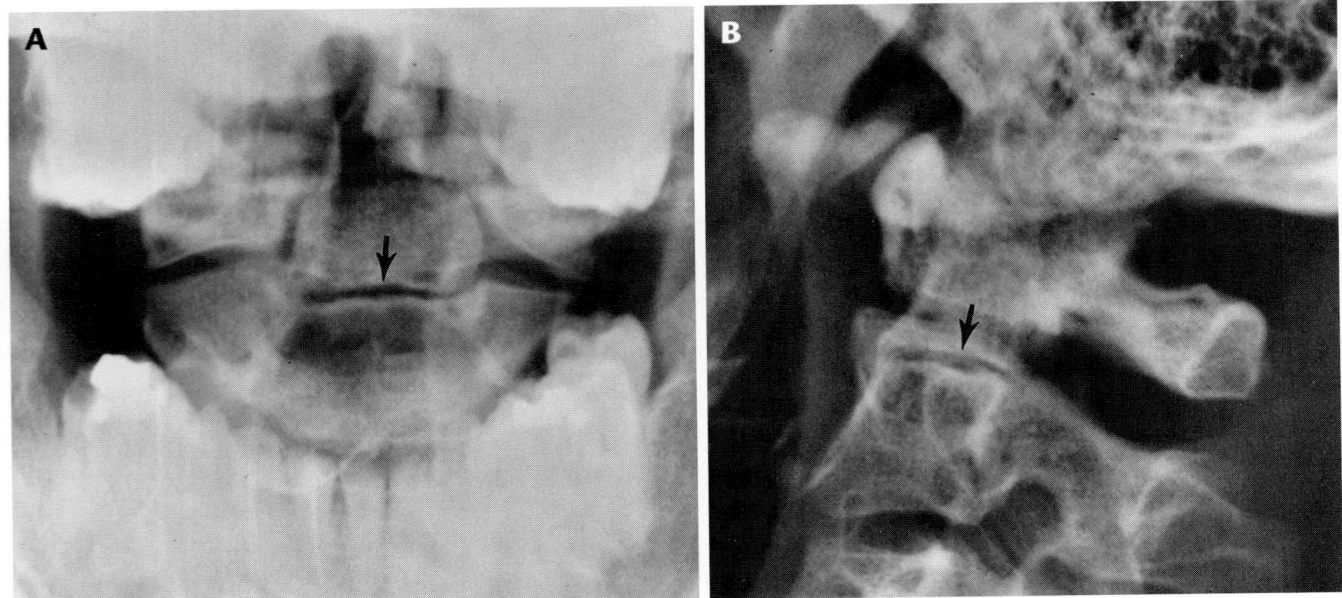

Figure 3–100. A, B, Os odontoideum resting in the original synchondrosis.
This case and the case in Figure 3–99 indicate that some os odontoidea are
developmental in origin and not secondary to trauma.

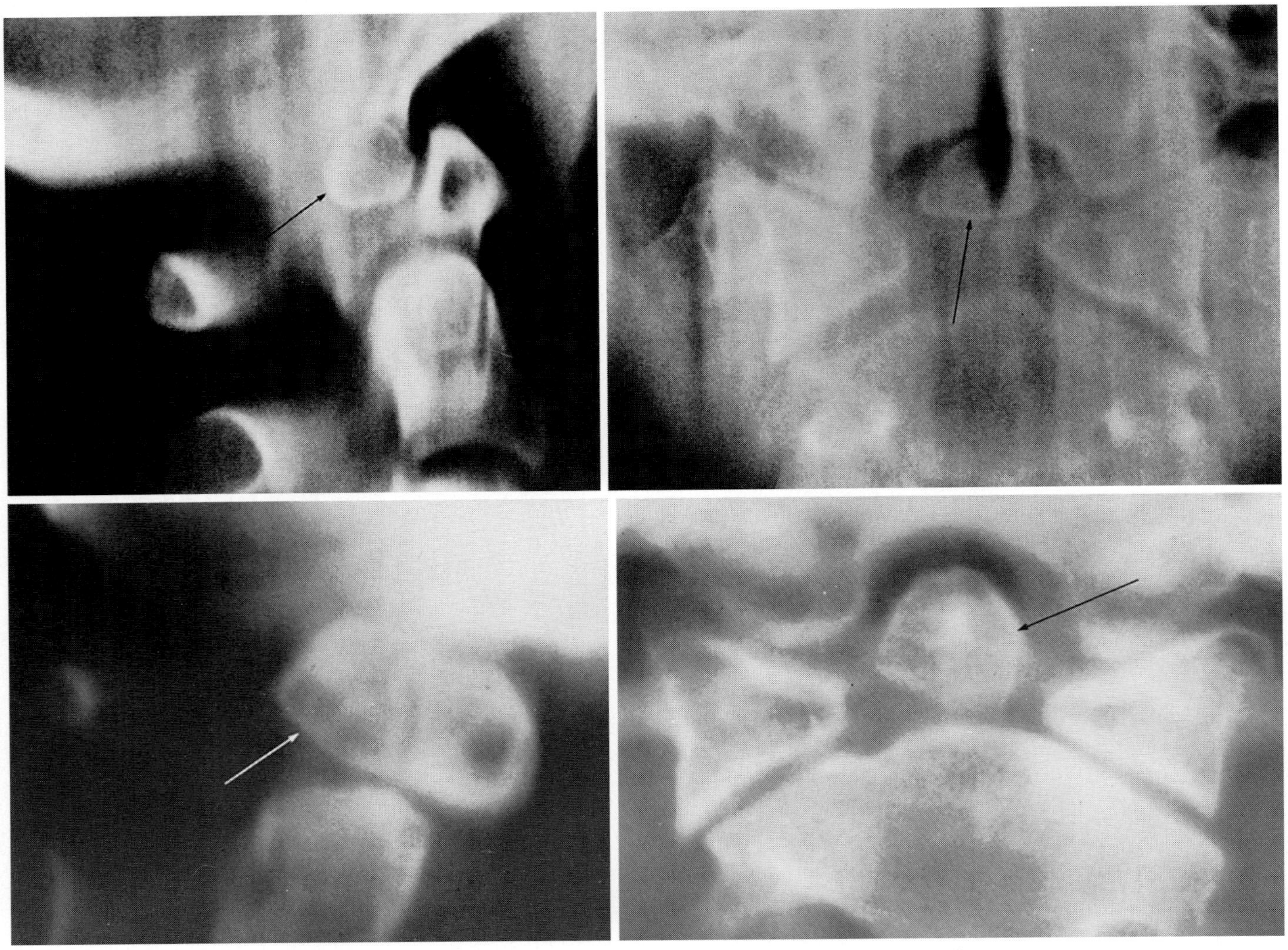

Figure 3–101. Two additional examples (two views each) of os odontoideum.
Note the overgrowth of the anterior arch of C1. The hypertrophy of the anterior
arch is a useful sign in differentiating os odontoideum from acute dens fracture.
(Ref: Holt RG et al: Hypertrophy of C1 anterior arch: Useful sign to distinguish os
odontoideum from acute dens fracture. *Radiology* 173:207, 1989.)

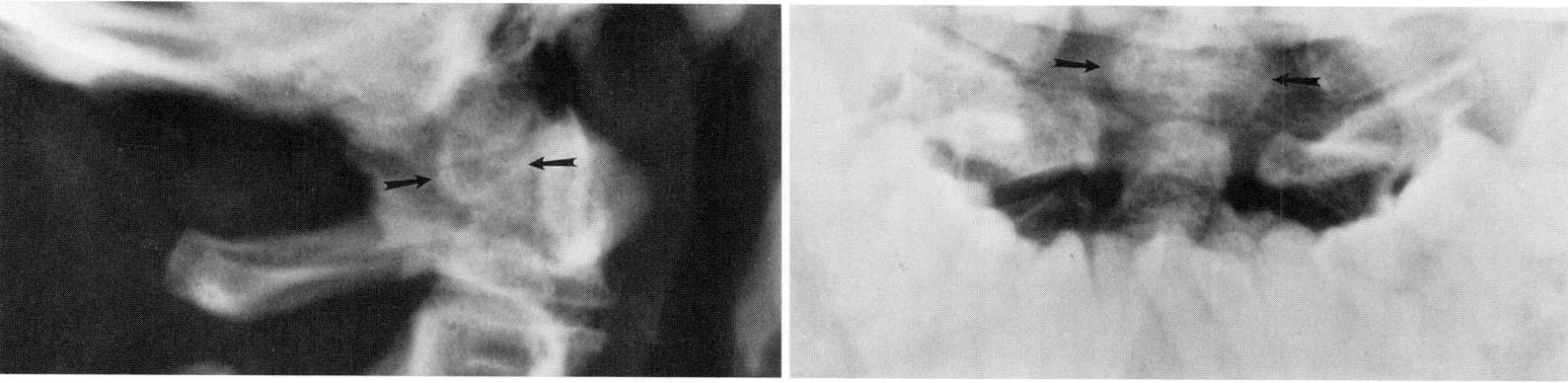

Figure 3–102. Huge os odontoideum. Note also the hypertrophy of the anterior arch of C1.

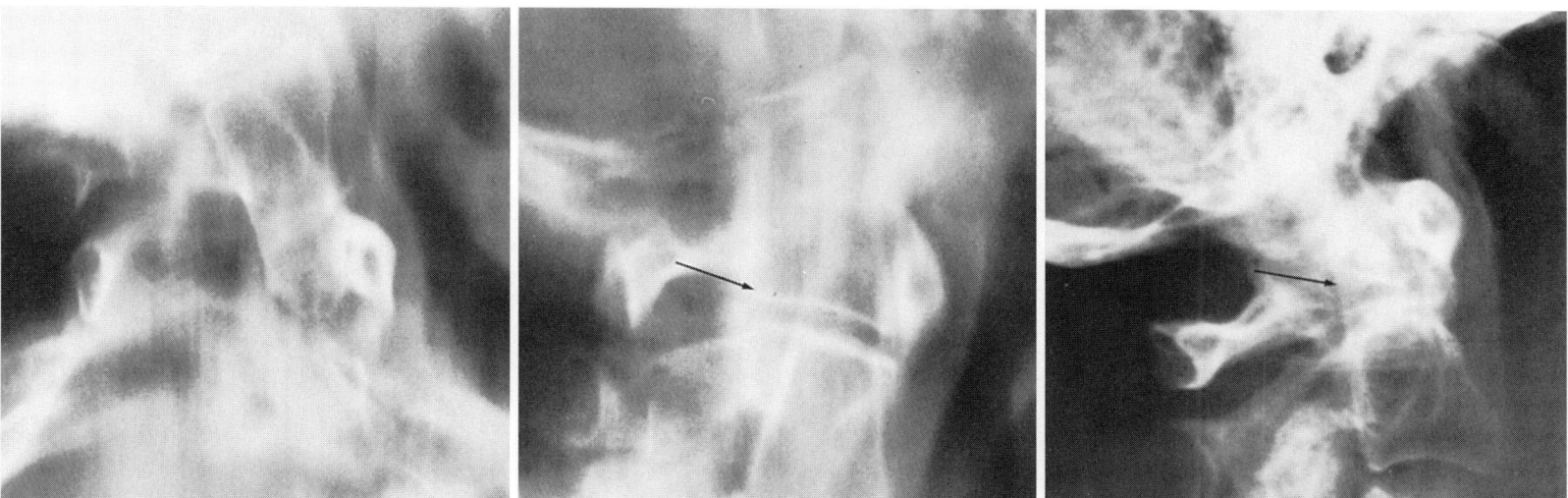

Figure 3–103. *Left,* Simulated os odontoideum produced by the lateral masses of C1. *Center,* Tomogram shows the lateral mass that produces the apparent discontinuity of the odontoid. *Right,* Tomogram shows no os odontoideum.

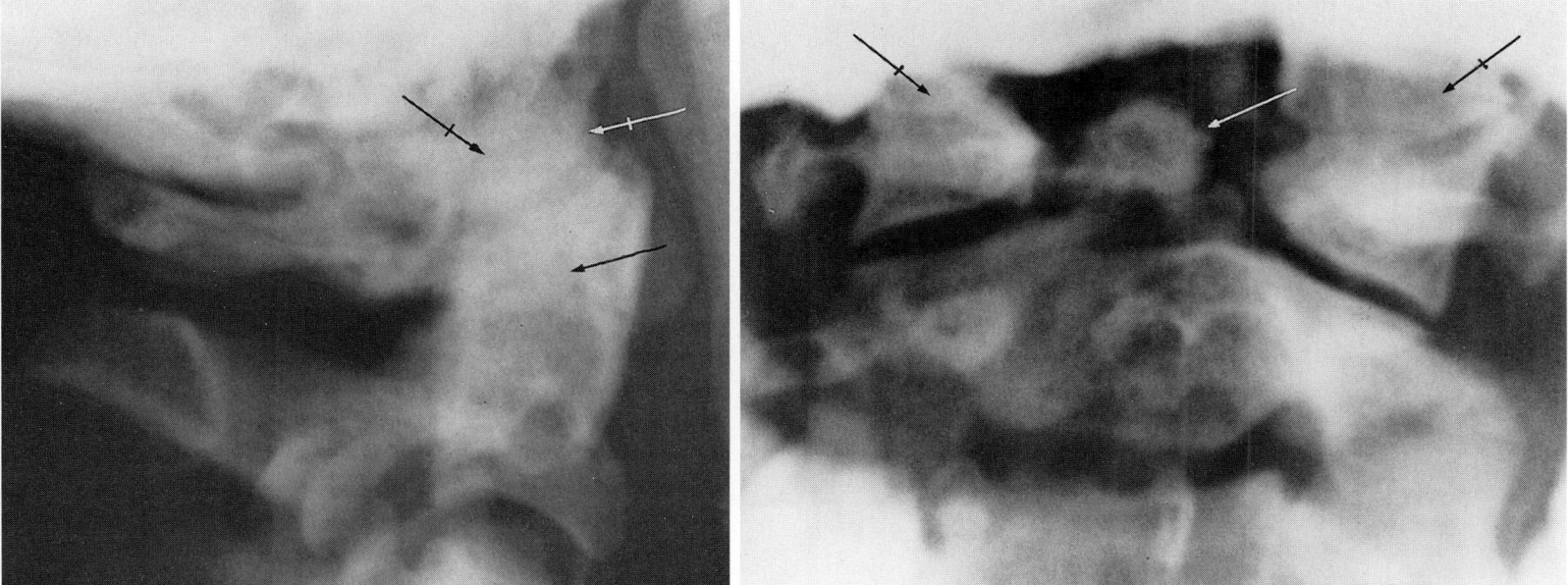

Figure 3–104. Odontoid hypoplasia (←) with large occipital condyles (↔). (Ref: McManners T: Odontoid hypoplasia. *Br J Radiol* 56:907, 1983.)

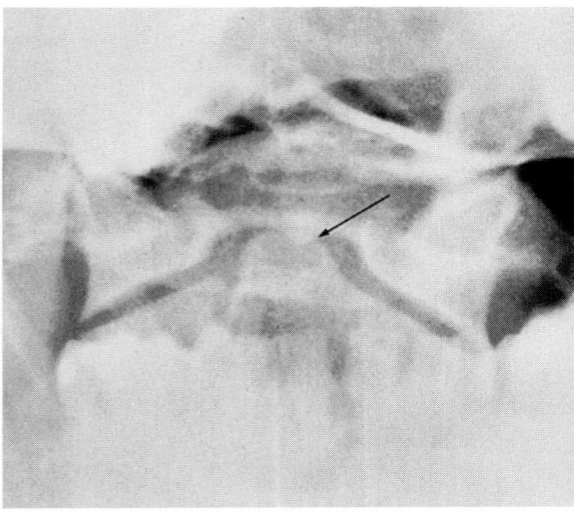
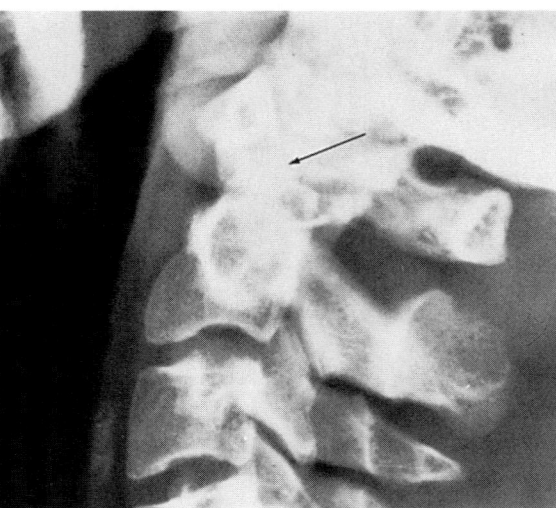

Figure 3–105. Odontoid hypoplasia. This entity may be associated with C1–C2 instability.

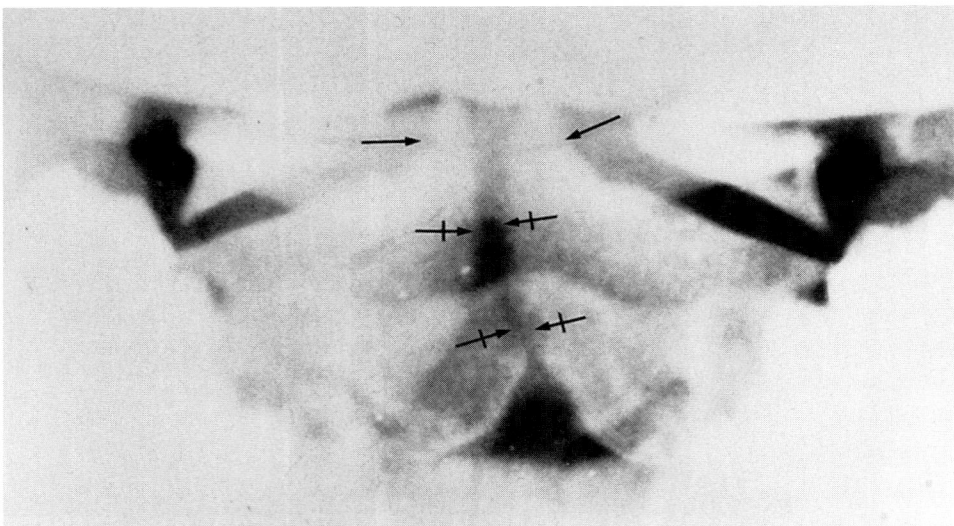

Figure 3–106. Hypoplastic odontoid (←). There is a spina bifida occulta of C2 and C3 producing an apparent cleft in the odontoid process (↔).

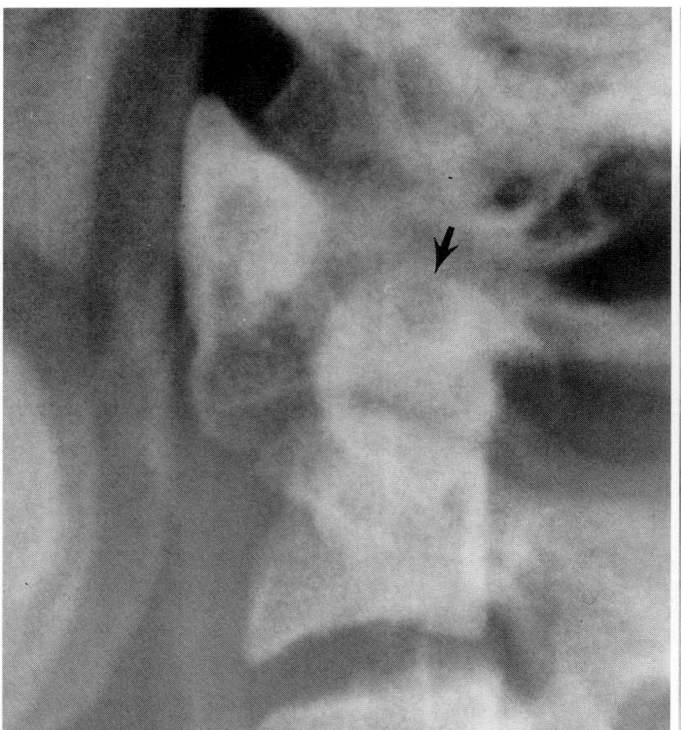
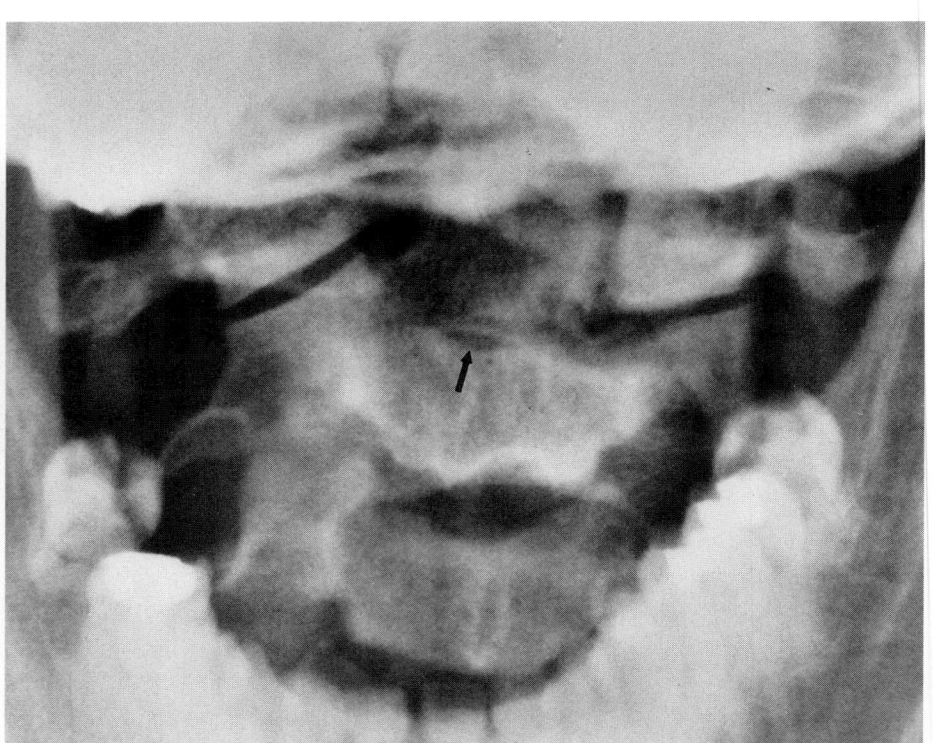

Figure 3–107. Hypoplastic odontoid process with inclination to the left and asymmetry of the lateral masses. Note the remnant of the synchondrosis at the base (*arrow*).

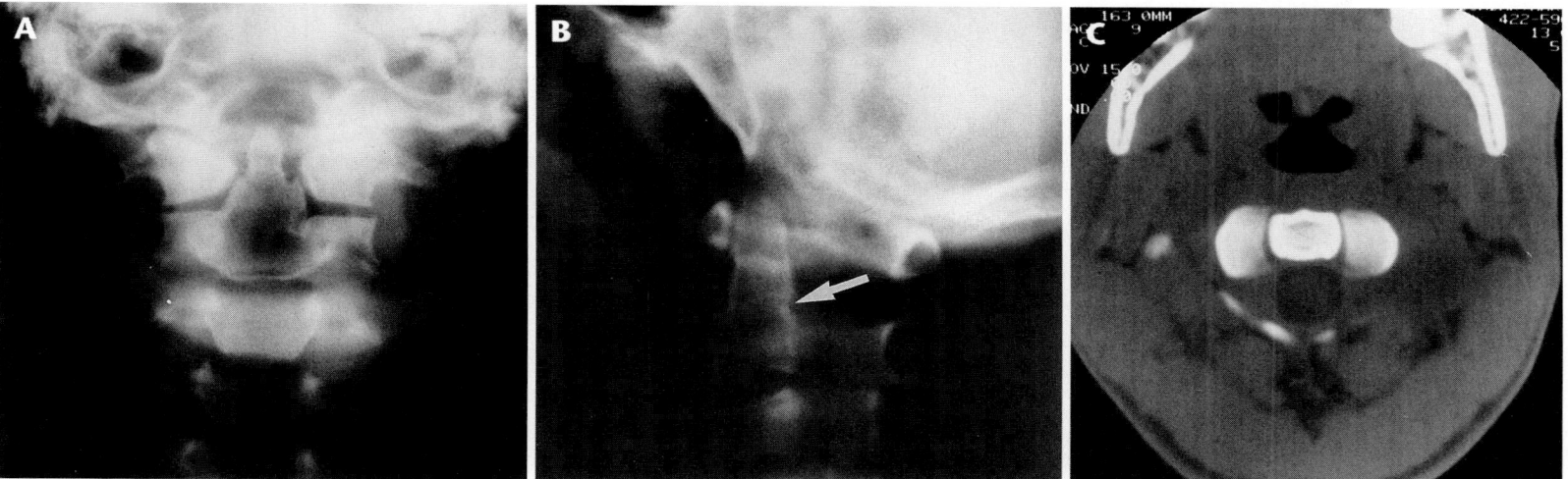

Figure 3–108. Persistent infantile odontoid process in an 18-year-old man. This variation produces the broad base of the odontoid process in **A,** the simulated fracture in **B,** and the broad-based odontoid process in **C. A** and **B,** Tomograms; **C,** CT. The asymmetrics of the base of the odontoid illustrated in the following six figures are products of this type of development. (Ref: McClellan R et al: Persistent infantile odontoid process: A variant of abnormal atlantoaxial segmentation. *Am J Roentgenol* 158:1305, 1992.)

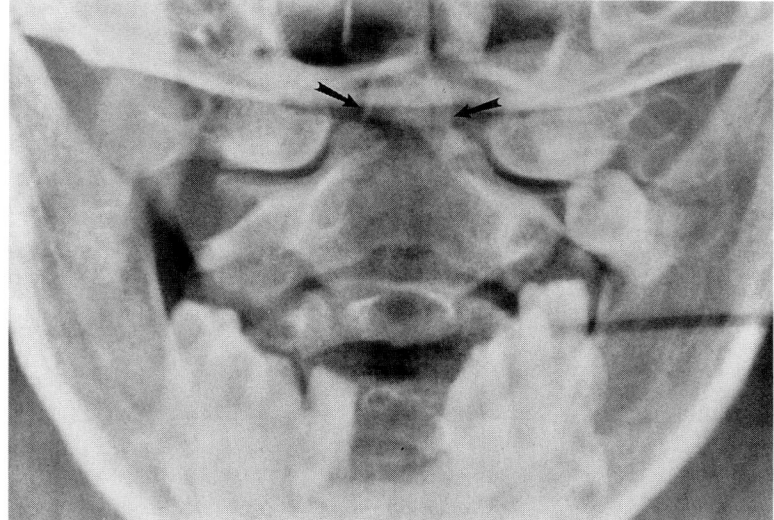

Figure 3–109. An additional example of persistent infantile odontoid process.

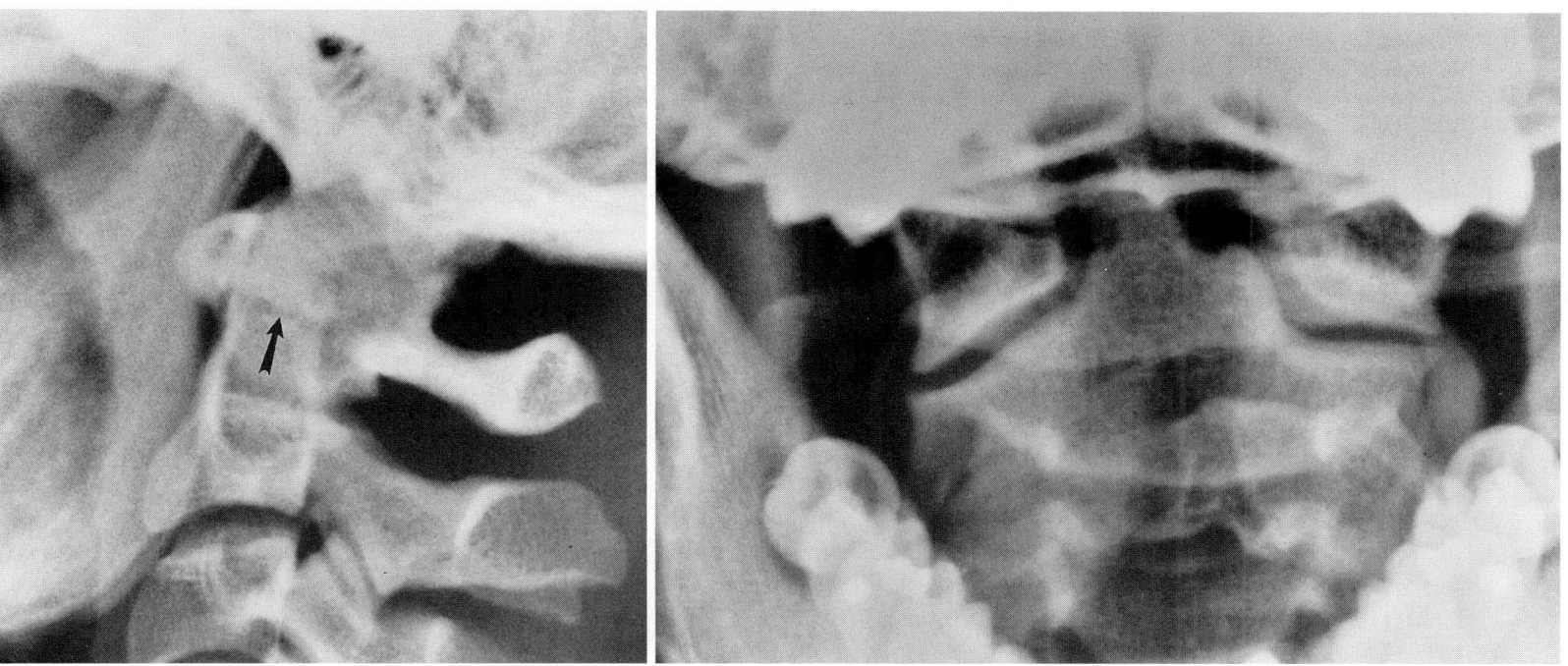

Figure 3–110. Simulated fracture of the odontoid resulting from persistent infantile odontoid process.

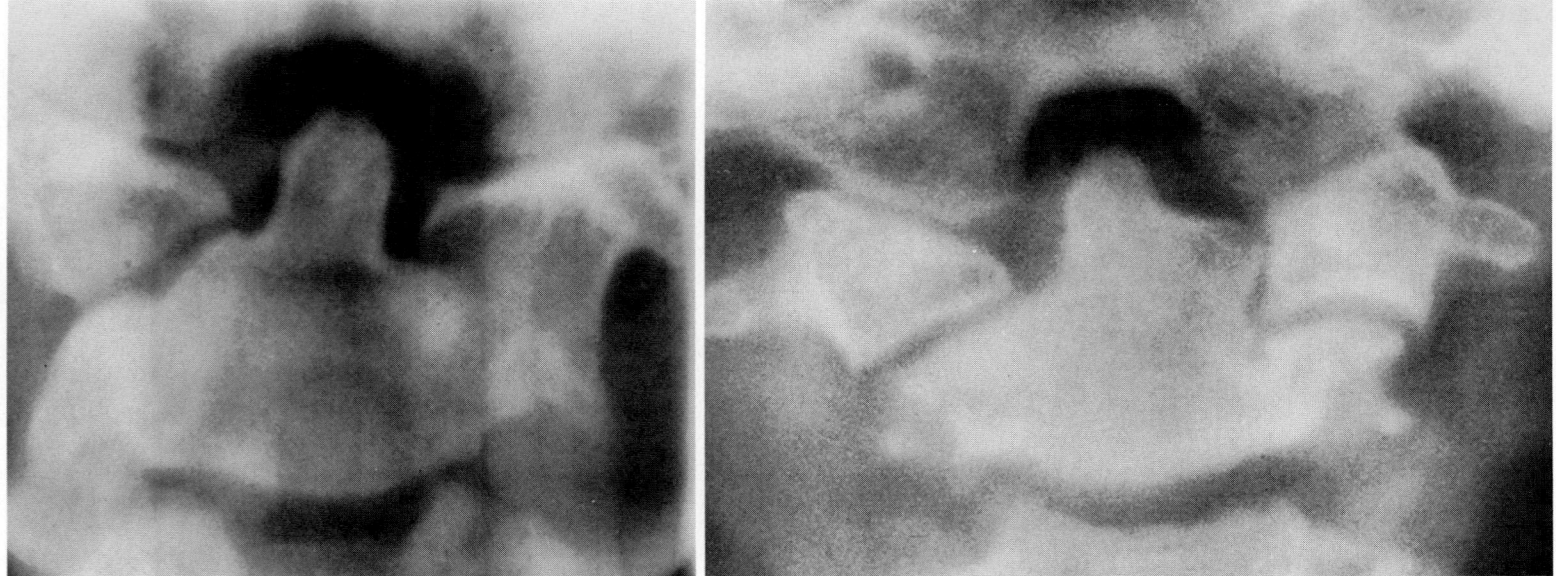

Figure 3–111. Two examples of anomalous development of base of the odontoid process. Note the corresponding deformity of the lateral masses of C1.

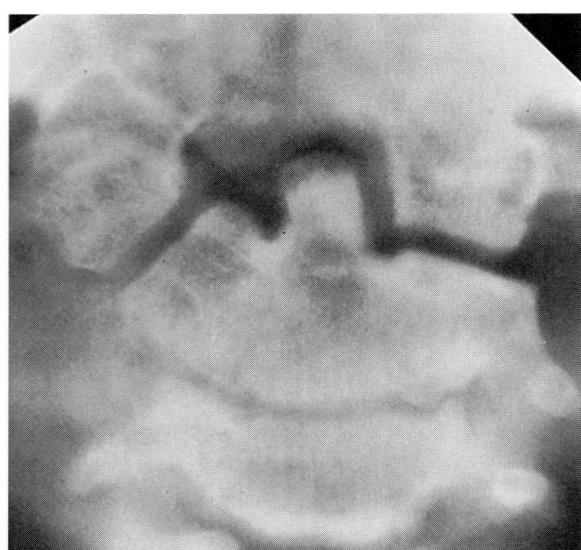

Figure 3–112. Asymmetric development of the occipital condyles and the lateral masses of C2 as well as the odontoid process. There is also incomplete segmentation of C2 and C3.

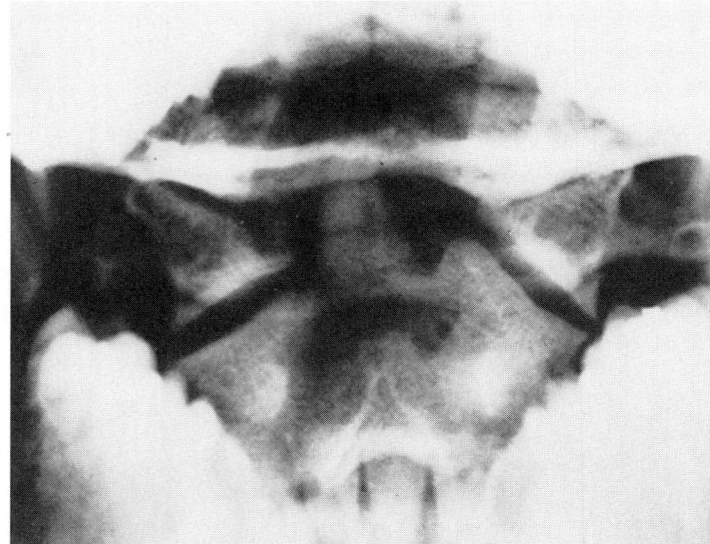

Figure 3–113. Asymmetry of development of the lateral masses of C2 with lateral deviation of the odontoid process.

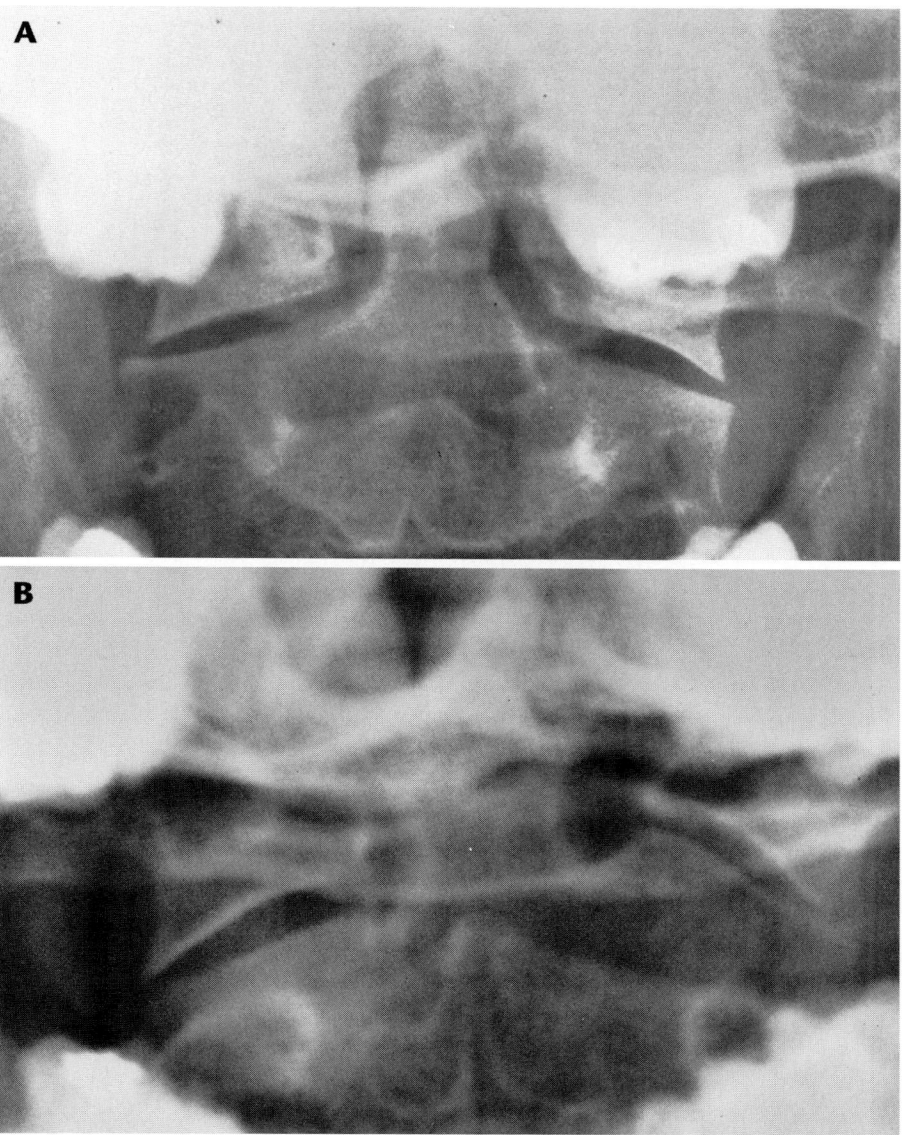

Figure 3–114. A, B, Two examples of asymmetry of the lateral masses of C1 and C2.

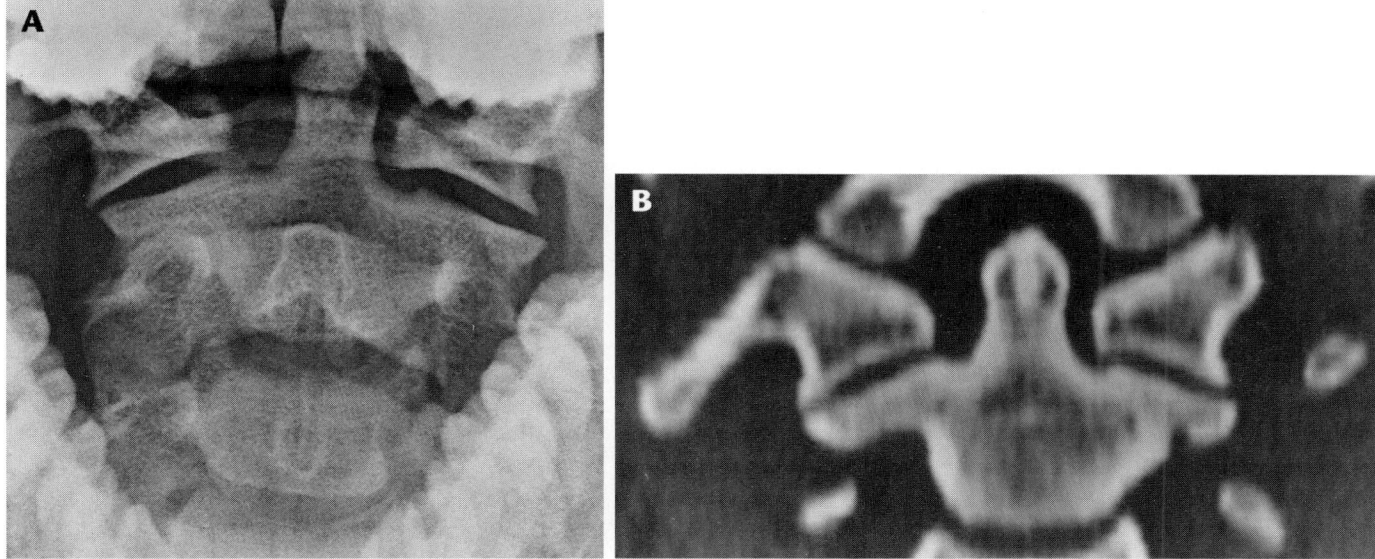

Figure 3–115. A, B, Asymmetry of the odontoid and lateral masses of C2 in the absence of rotation secondary to asymmetrical development of the articular planes of C2.

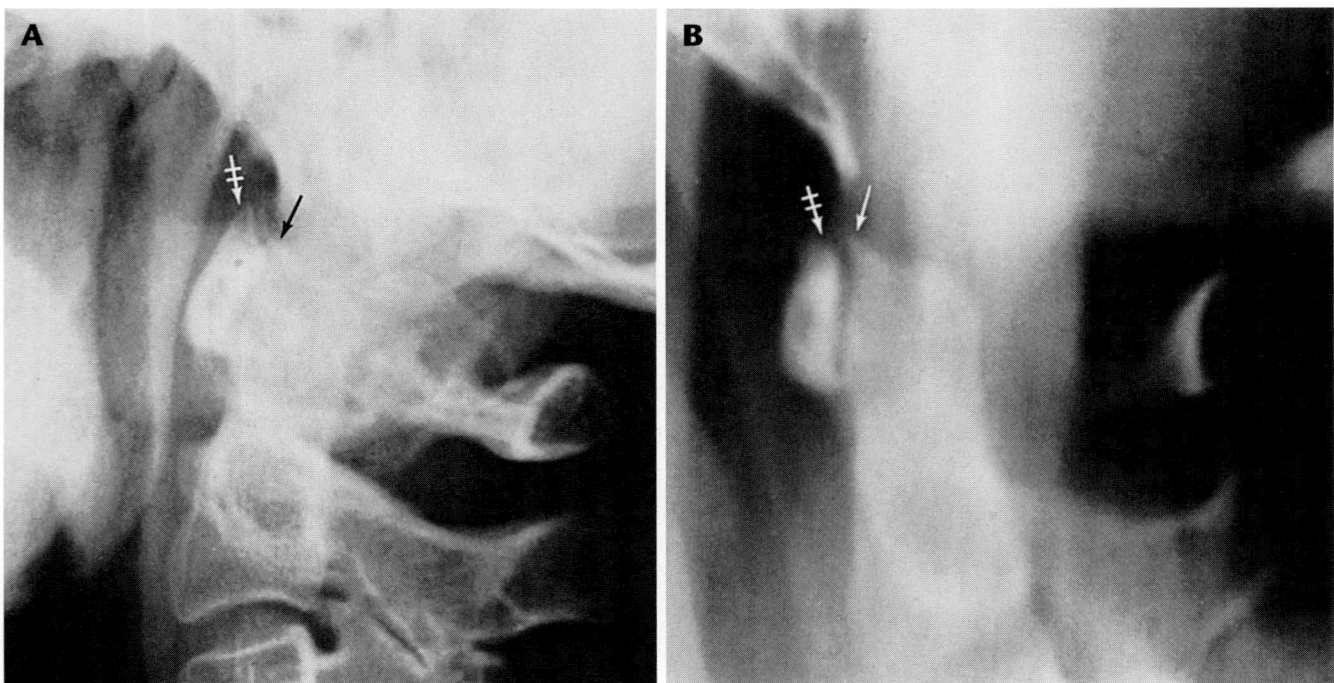

Figure 3–116. Unusual pointed anterior aspect of the odontoid process, not to be confused with the product of bony erosion (←). **A,** Plain film. **B,** Tomogram. Note also the spurlike extension from the superior aspect of the anterior arch of C1 (⇜).

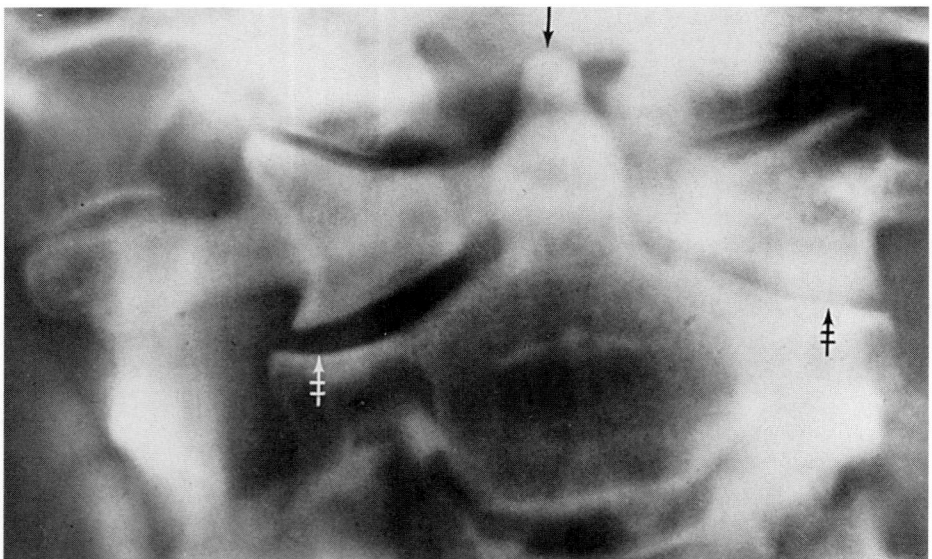

Figure 3–117. Unusual configuration of the tip of the odontoid process (←). Note also the normal asymmetry of the Luschka joints as a result of the positioning of the head (⇜).

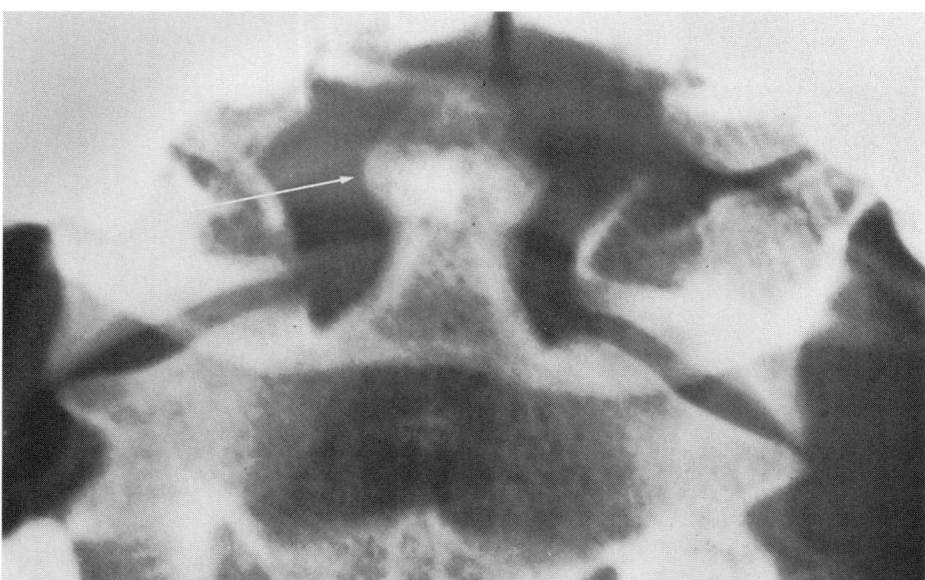

Figure 3–118. Turbinal configuration of tip of the odontoid process.

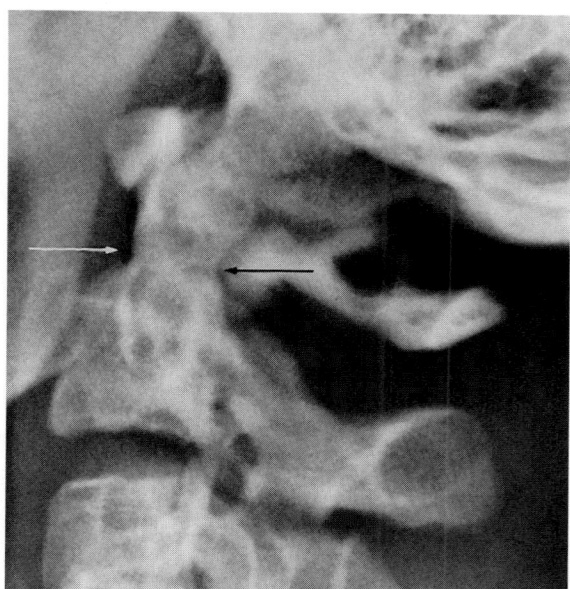

Figure 3–119. Marked "waist" in the midodontoid process.

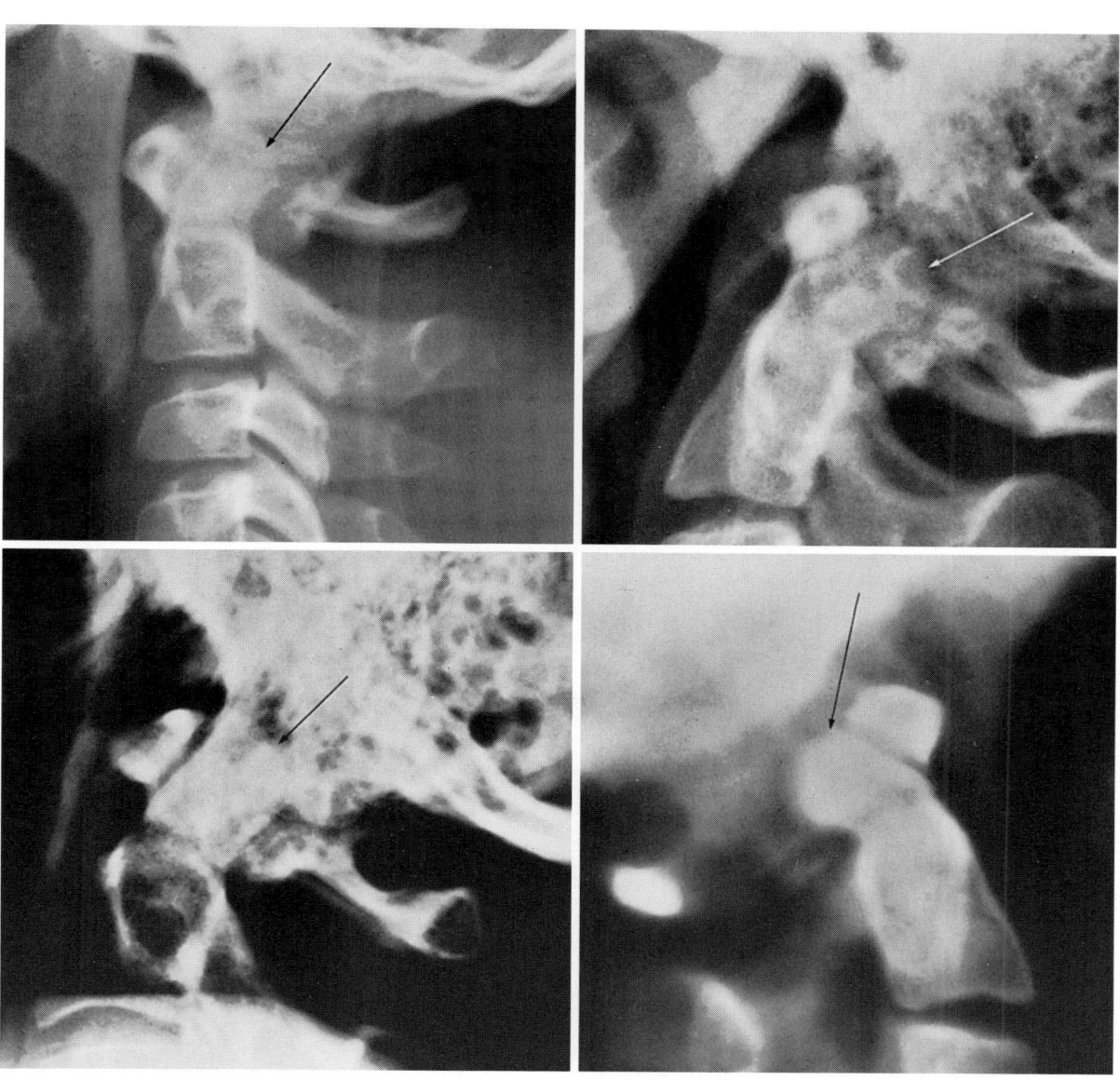

Figure 3–120. Four examples of posterior inclination of the odontoid process that should not be confused with fracture. Note characteristic high position of the anterior arch of C1. (Ref: Swischuk LE et al: The posterior tilted dens: Normal variation simulating fracture. *Pediatr Radiol* 8:27, 1979.)

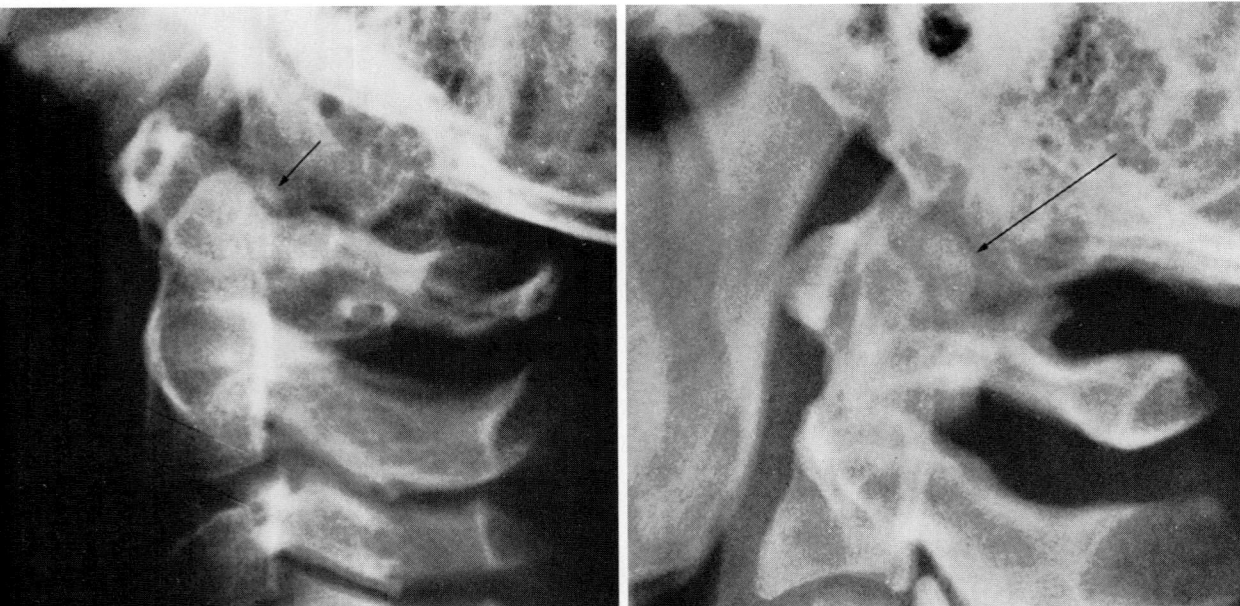

Figure 3–121. Two examples of ossicles around the tip of the odontoid process.

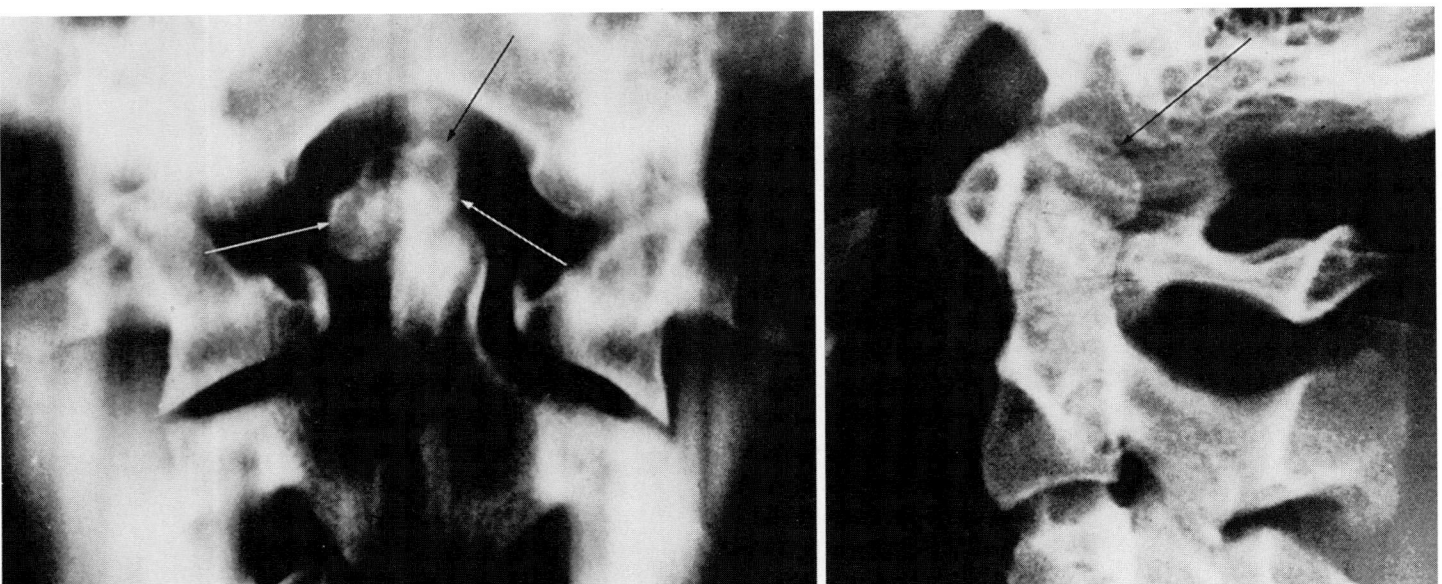

Figure 3–122. Large ossicle at the tip of the odontoid process.

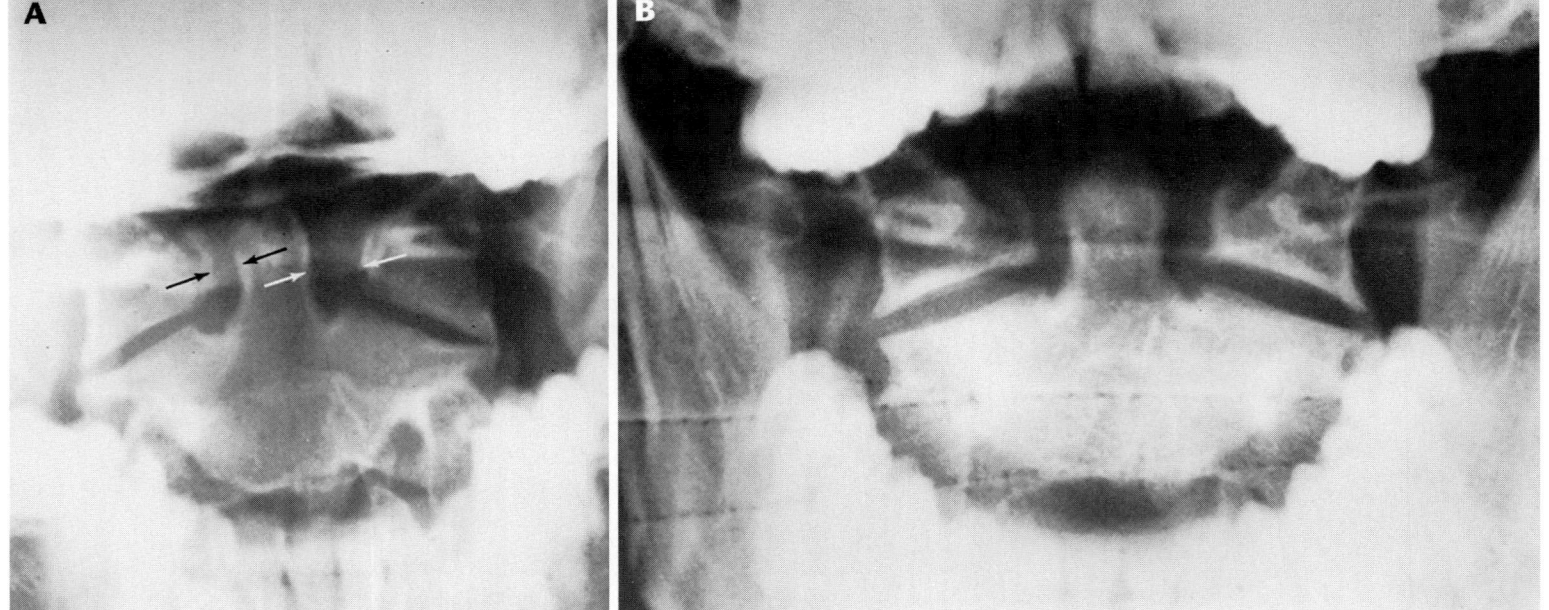

Figure 3–123. A, Normal asymmetry of the intervals between the odontoid process and the lateral masses of C1, produced by rotation of the head. **B,** Same patient with head in neutral position.

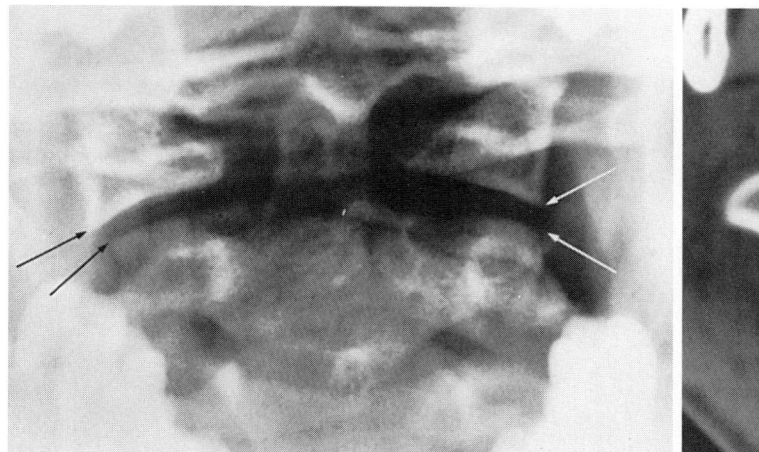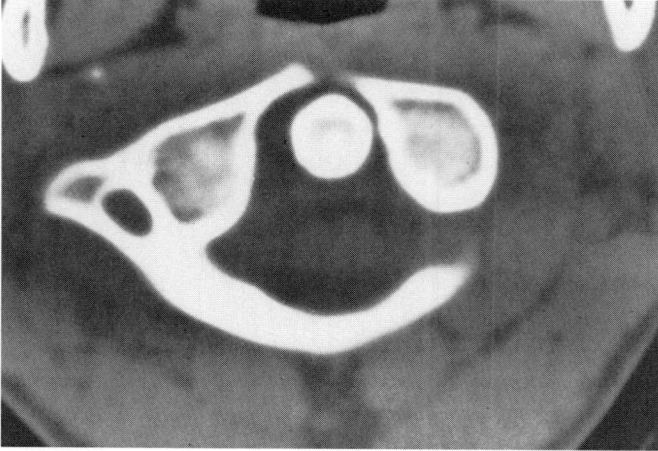

Figure 3–124. *Left,* The effect of the head tilting to the right. The atlas has glided to the patient's right side. The space between the left lateral mass and the dens has decreased, while that on the right has widened. The lateral margins of the lateral atlantoaxial joint spaces are asymmetric *(arrows)*. The spinous processes are deviated to the left. *Right,* CT shows the corresponding asymmetry of the spaces between the lateral masses of C1 and the dens. (Ref: Harris JH; Edeiken-Monroe B: *The radiology of acute cervical spine trauma,* 2nd ed. Baltimore, Williams & Wilkins, 1987, p. 19.)

Figure 3–125. Altered relationships between the lateral masses of C1 and the odontoid process, resulting from combined rotation and tilting of the head.

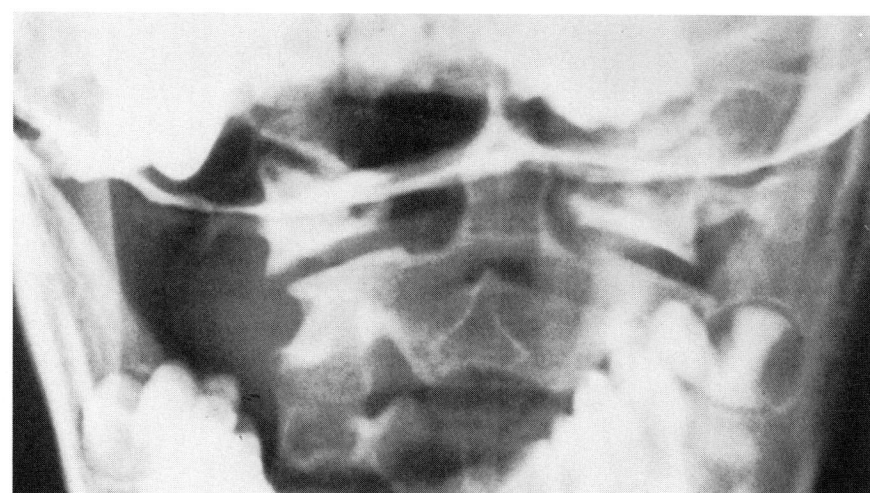

Figure 3–126. Rotation of the head producing an unusual elongated appearance of the lateral mass of C2 *(arrow).*

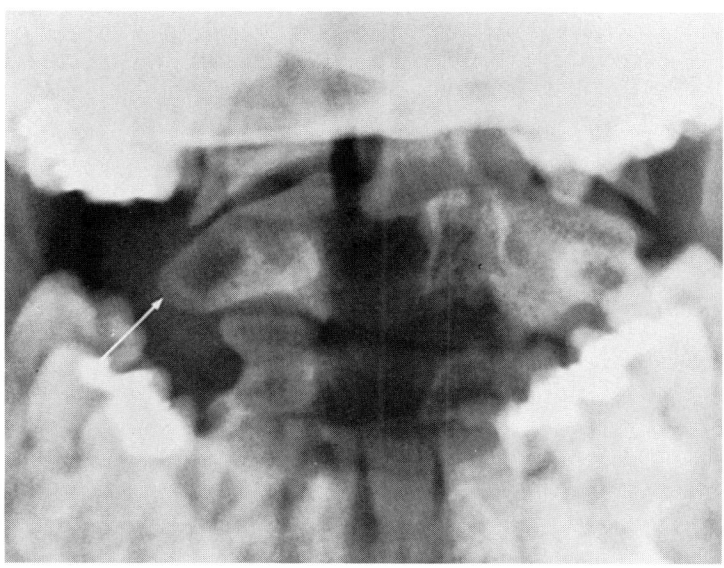

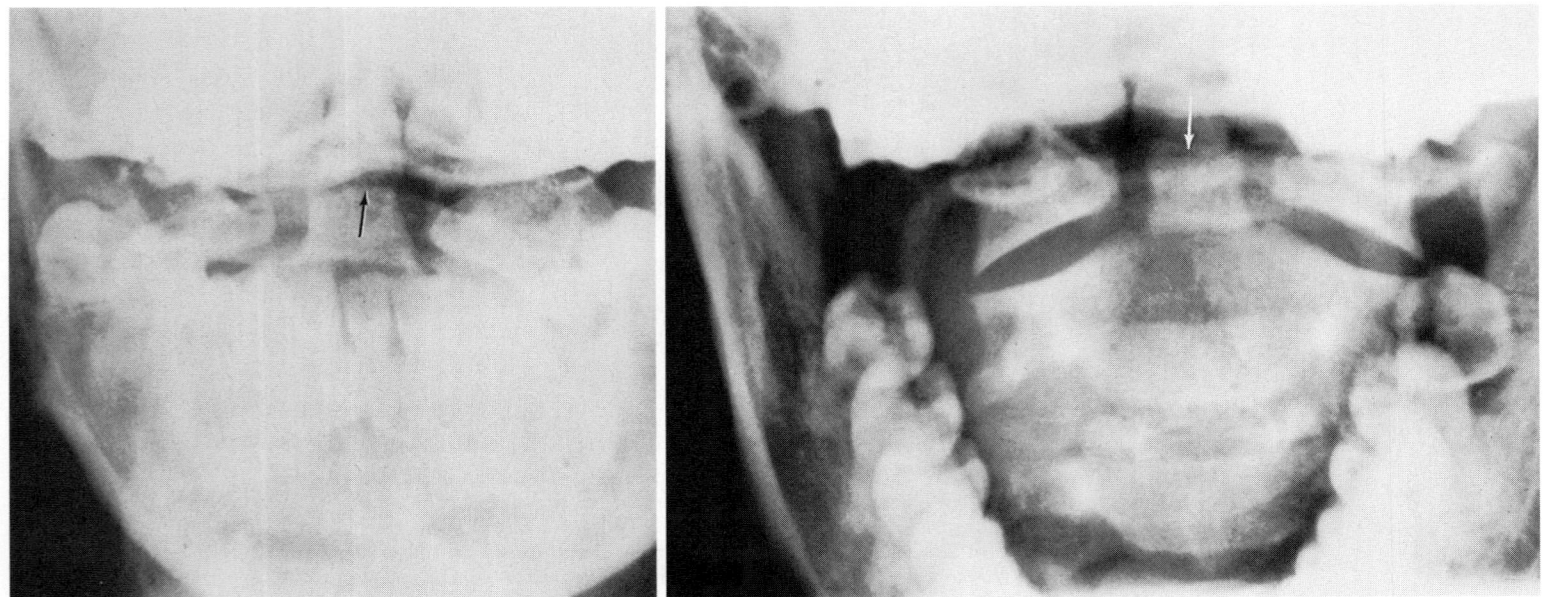

Figure 3–127. Pseudofractures of the odontoid process, produced by overlapping shadows of the central maxillary incisors.

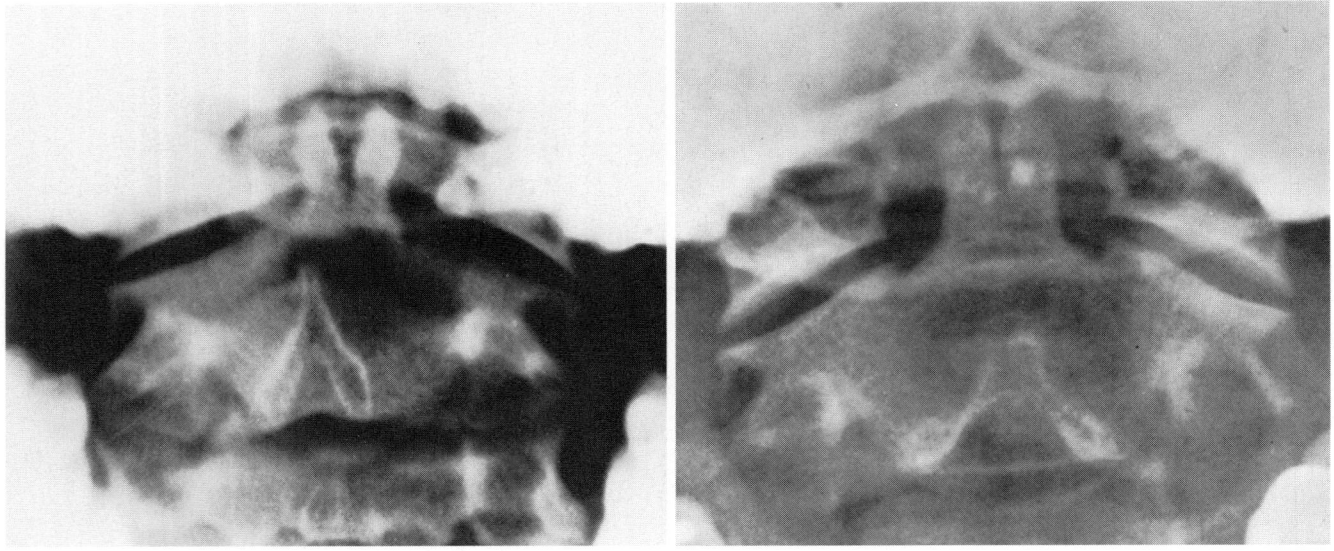

Figure 3–128. Two examples of the lucency between the maxillary central incisors superimposed on the odontoid process, simulating a split odontoid.

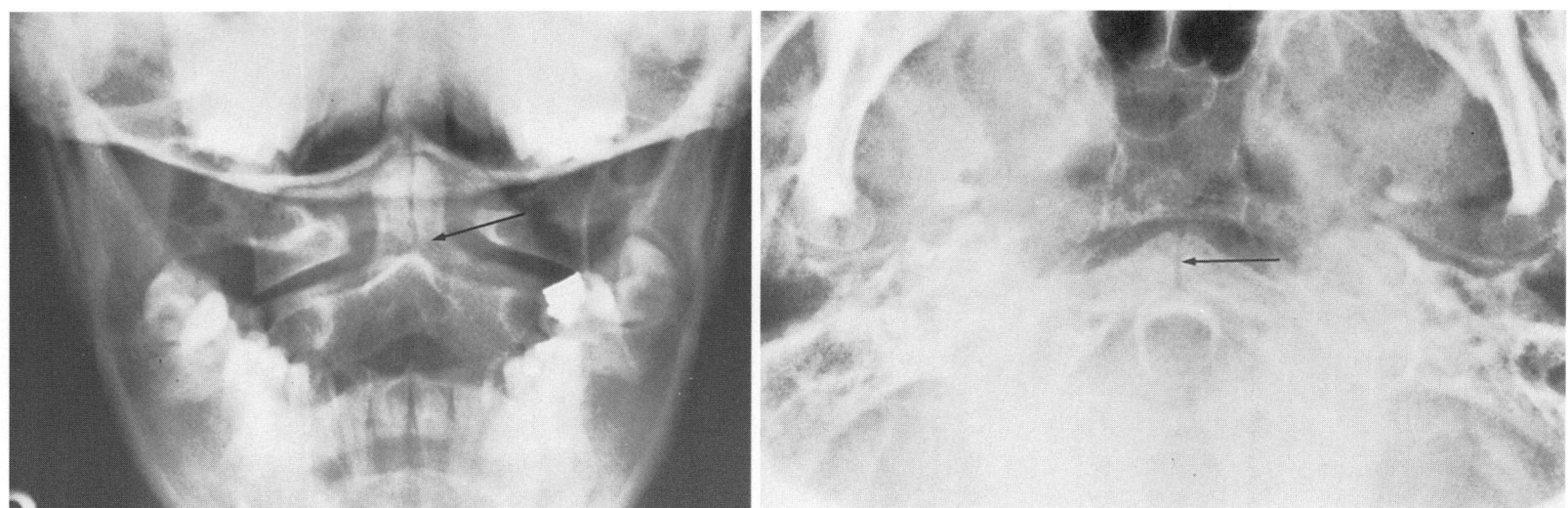

Figure 3–129. Simulated cleft in the odontoid process, produced by midline closure defect in the anterior arch of the atlas.

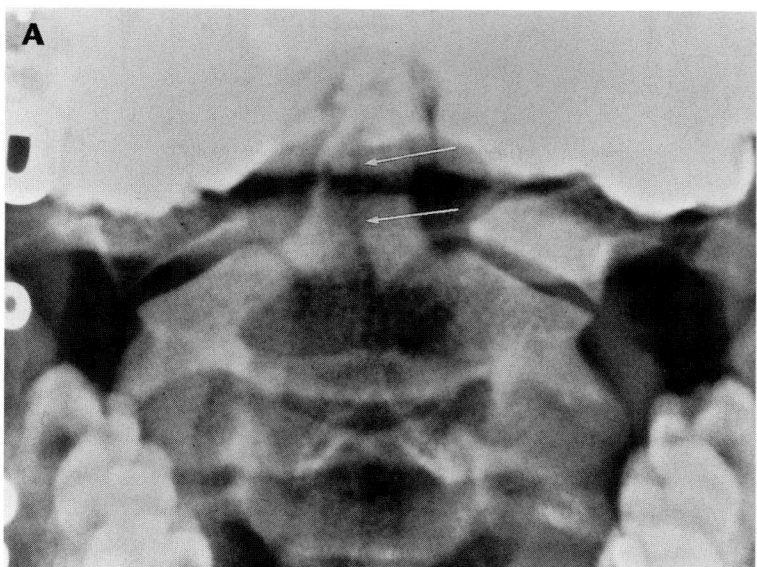

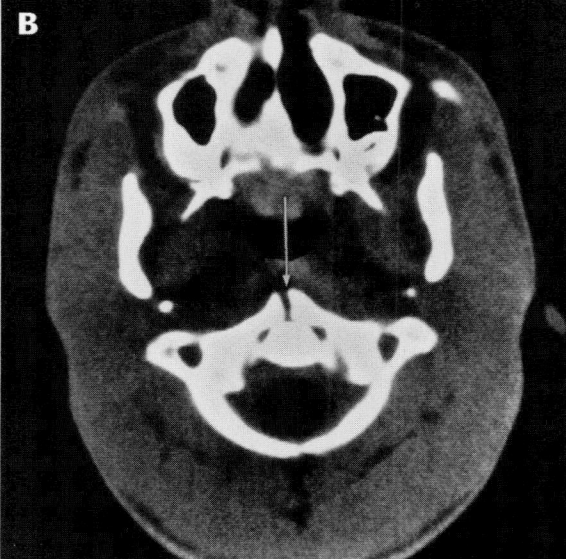

Figure 3–130. Closure defect in the anterior arch of C1, producing an apparent fracture of the odontoid process. **A,** Open-mouth view of the odontoid process. **B,** CT. (Ref: Chalmers AG: Spondyloschisis of the anterior arch of the atlas. *Br J Radiol* 58:761, 1985.) Closure defects may be present in the anterior and posterior arches in the same patient, resulting in a bipartite atlas vertebra. (Ref: Saifuddin A, Renwick, GH: Case of the month: A pain in the neck. *Br J Radiol* 66:379, 1993.) The bipartite atlas may also demonstrate hypertrophy of the anterior arch. (Ref: Walker J Biggs I: Bipartite atlas and hypertrophy of its anterior arch. *Acta Radiol* 36:152, 1995.)

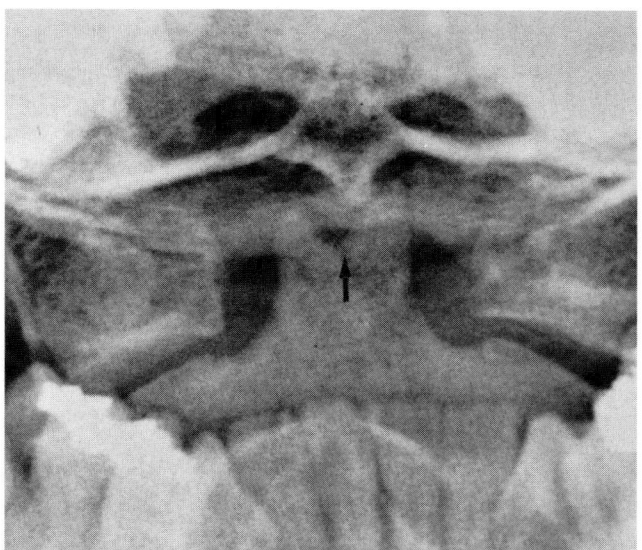

Figure 3–131. Deep median sulcus of the tongue superimposed on the odontoid simulating a vertical fracture of the odontoid.

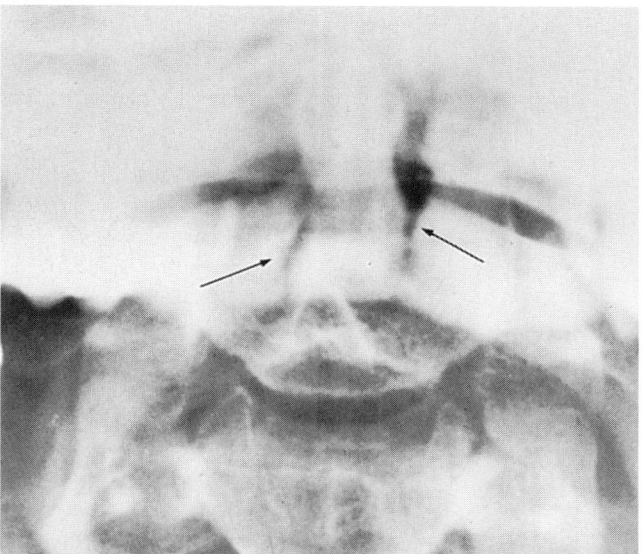

Figure 3–132. Pseudofracture of the body of C2, produced by overlapping shadows of the teeth.

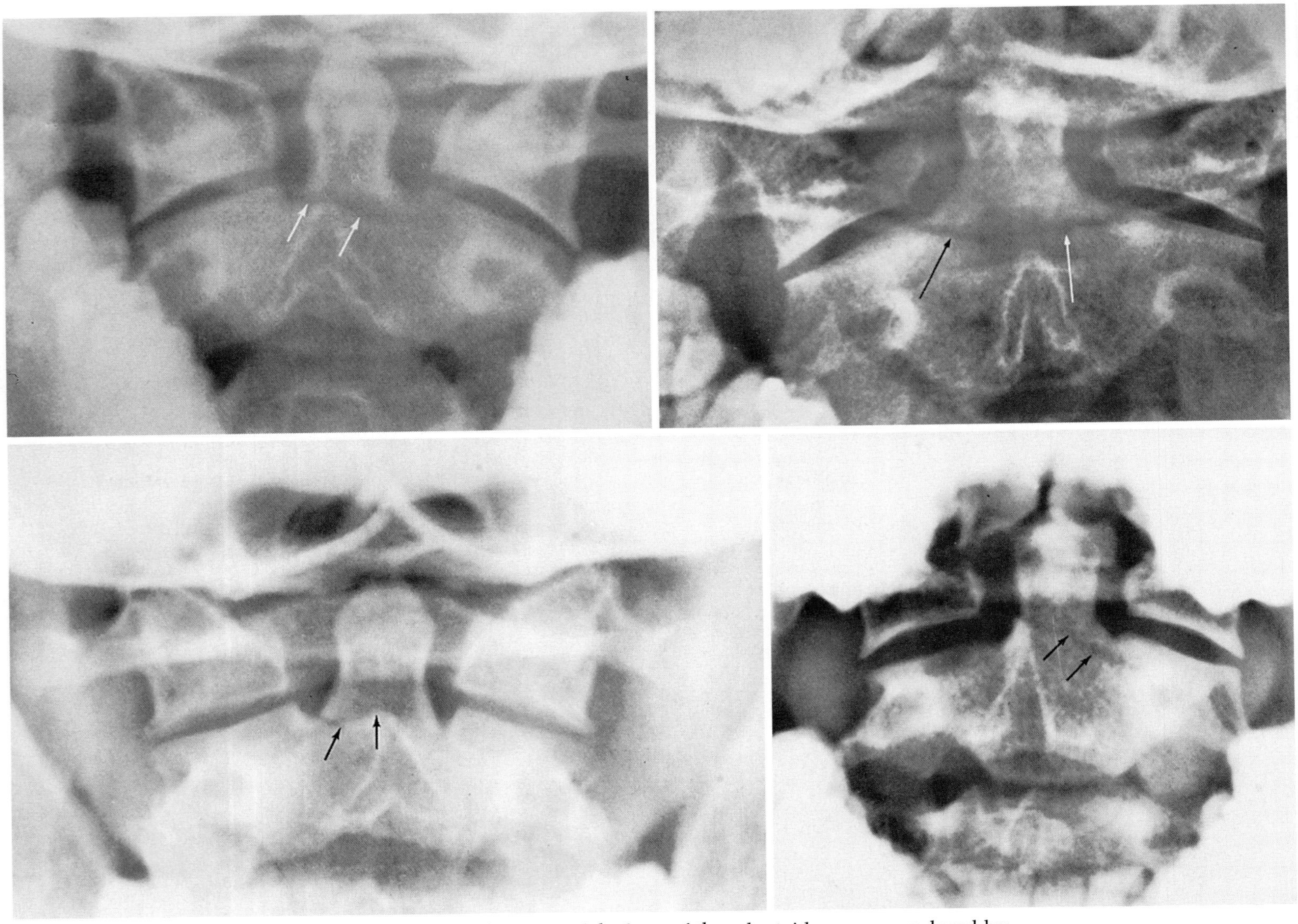

Figure 3–133. Pseudofractures of the base of the odontoid process, produced by the Mach effect from overlapping shadows of the posterior arch of C1, the tongue, or the occiput. Each was proved a pseudofracture by tomography. (Ref: Daffner RH: Pseudofracture of the dens: Mach bands. *Am J Roentgenol* 128:607, 1977.)

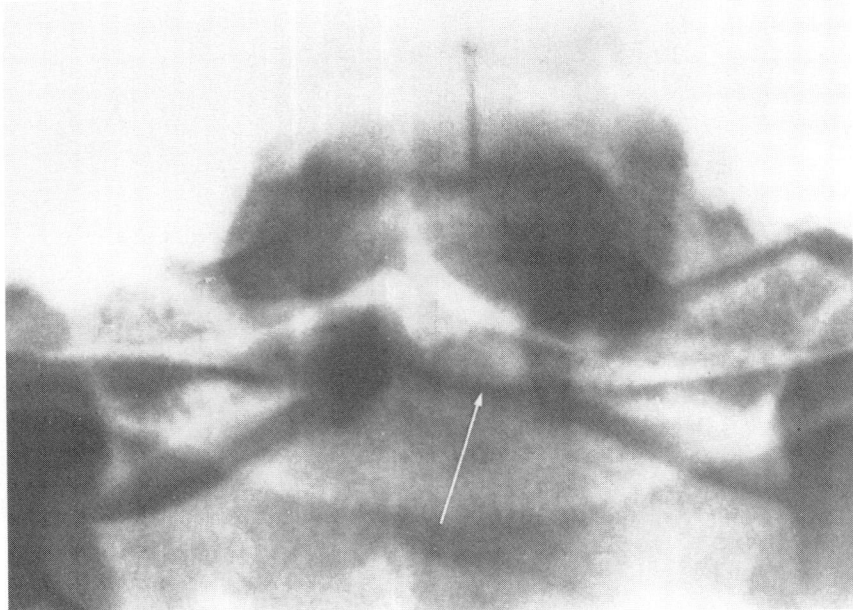

Figure 3–134. Pseudofracture of the odontoid process, produced by overlapping of the base of skull.

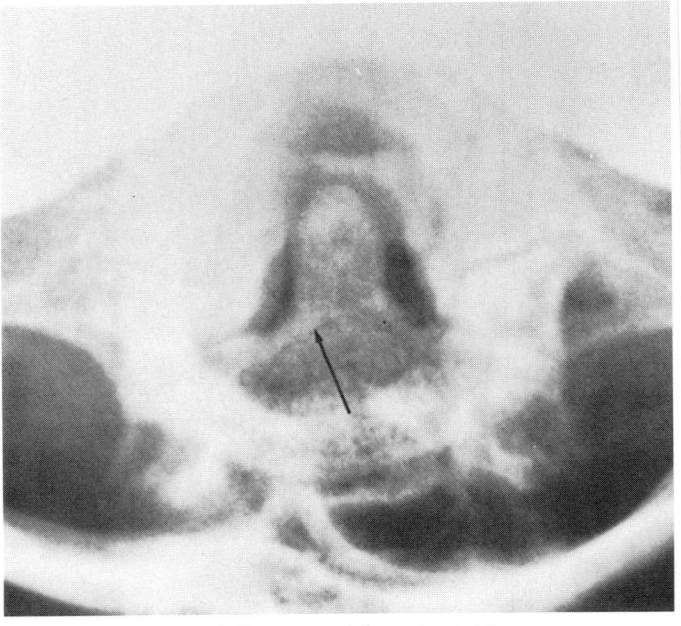

Figure 3–135. Pseudofracture of the odontoid process, produced by a vascular groove in the skull.

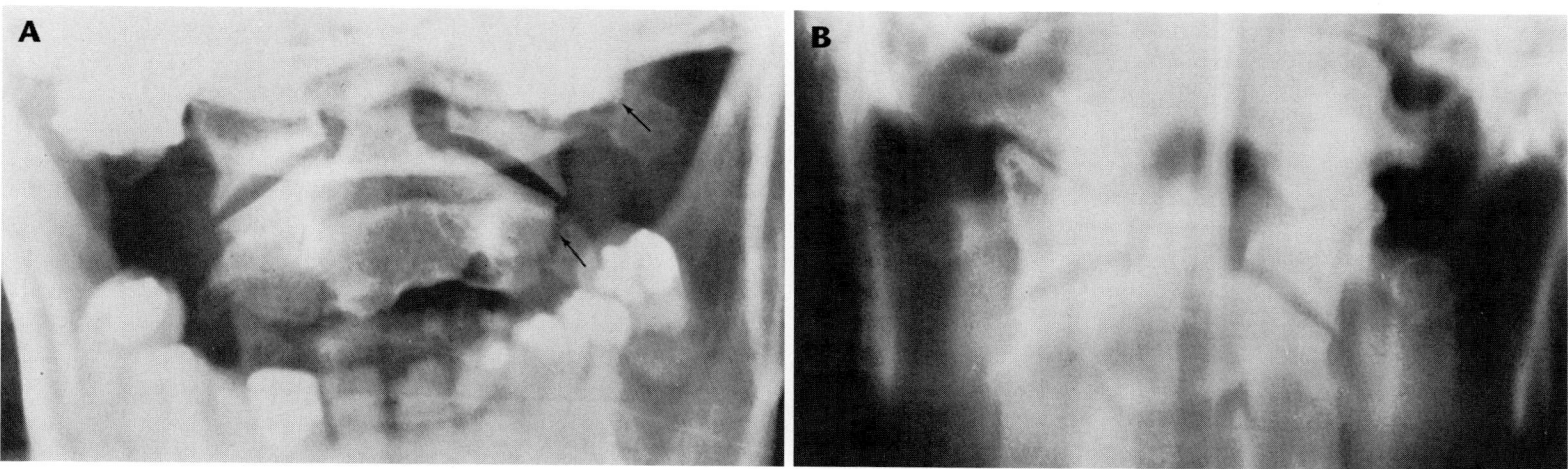

Figure 3–136. A, Pseudofractures of the transverse processes of C1 and C2, produced by Mach bands, probably overlapping the shadow of the anterior tonsillar pillar. **B,** Tomography shows no evidence of a fracture.

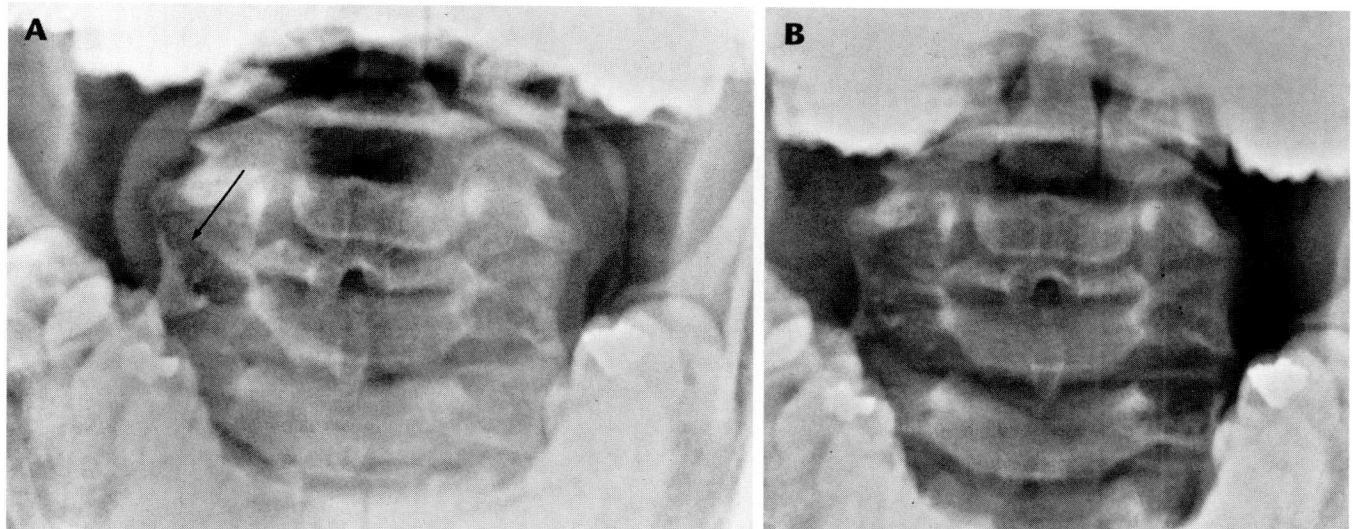

Figure 3–137. A, Mach effect from shadows of the lips, producing a simulated fracture. **B,** Reexamination shows no evidence of fracture.

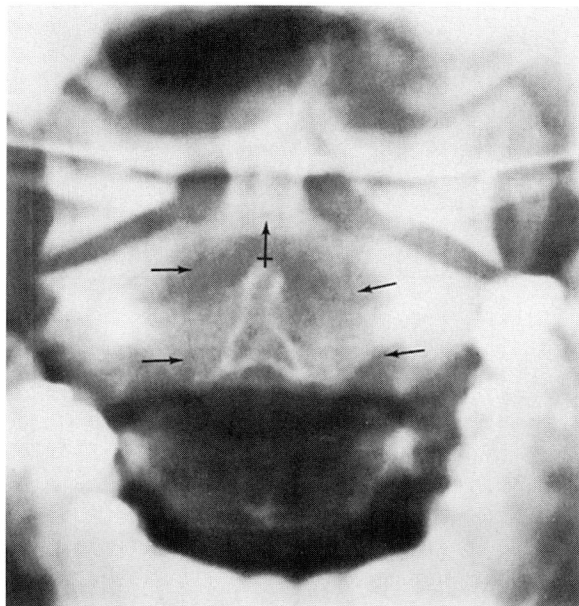

Figure 3–138. Remnants of the synchondroses of the primary ossification centers of C2 (→). Note also the pseudofracture of the base of the odontoid process (↦).

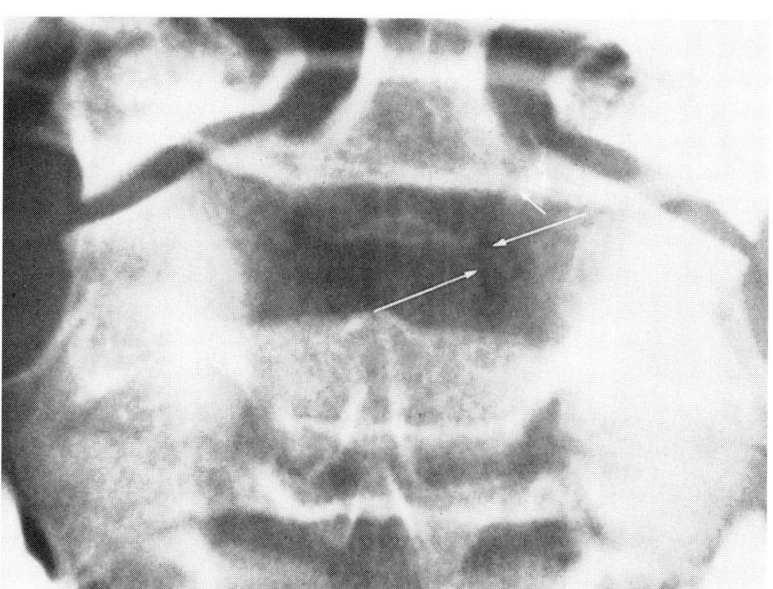

Figure 3–139. Pseudofracture of the body of C2, produced by overlapping pharyngeal soft tissue shadows.

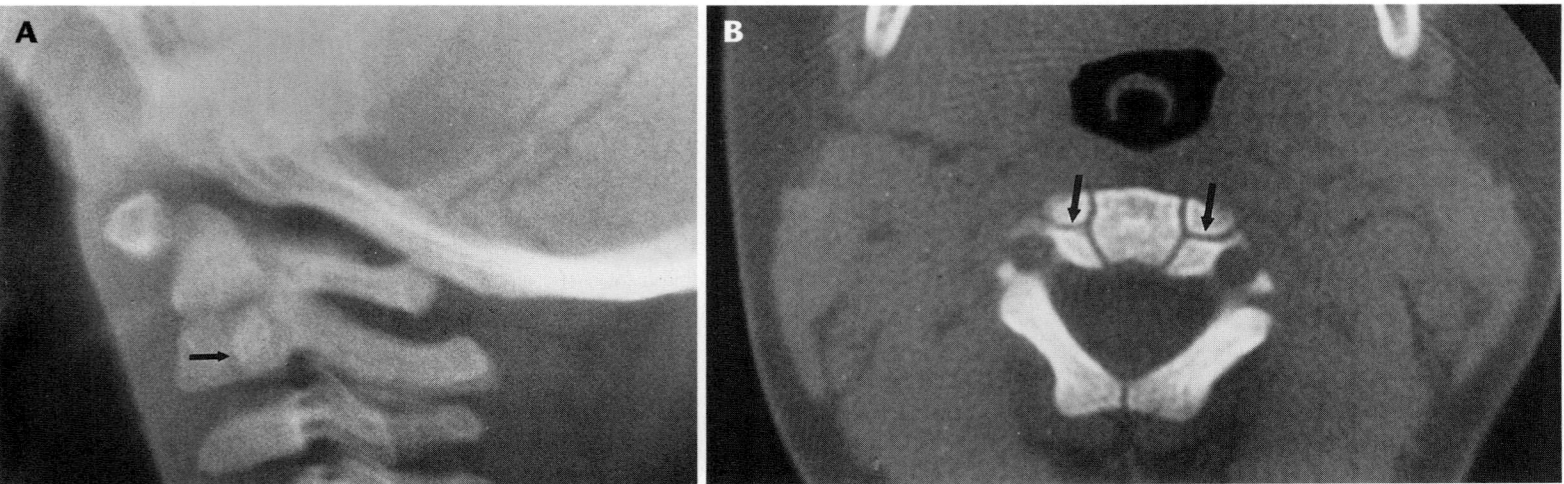

Figure 3–140. Coronal cleft of C2 in a 7-month-old infant, a transient developmental variant. **A,** lateral. **B,** CT.

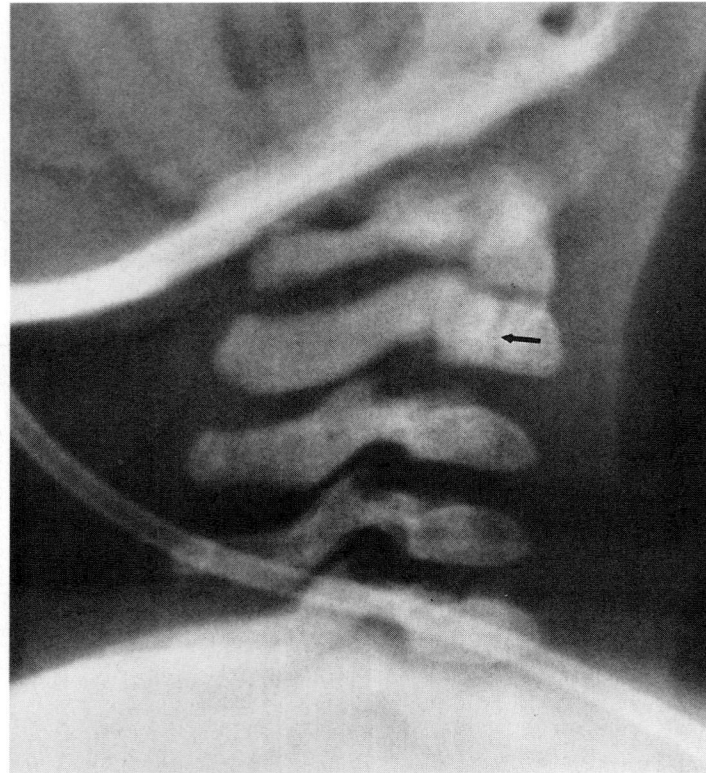

Figure 3–141. Additional example of coronal clefting of C2 in a 6-month-old infant.

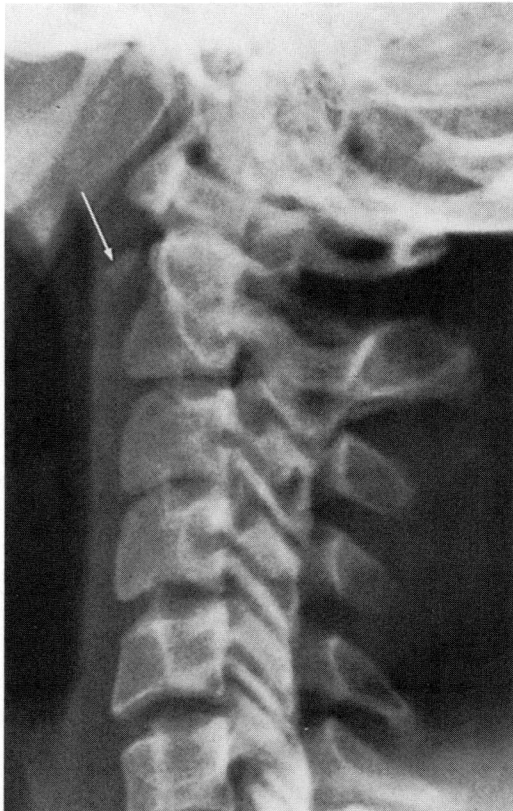

Figure 3–142. Osseous density representing the lateral mass of C2 thrown into relief by rotation and tilting of the head.

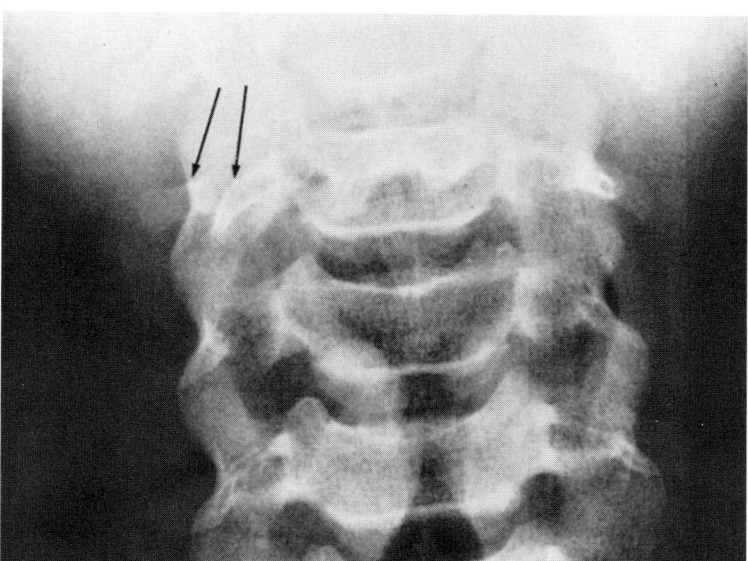

Figure 3–143. Persistent apophysis for the transverse process of C2. (Ref: Kohler A, Zimmer EA: *Borderlands of normal and early pathologic findings in skeletal radiography,* 4th ed. New York, Thieme, 1993, p. 451.)

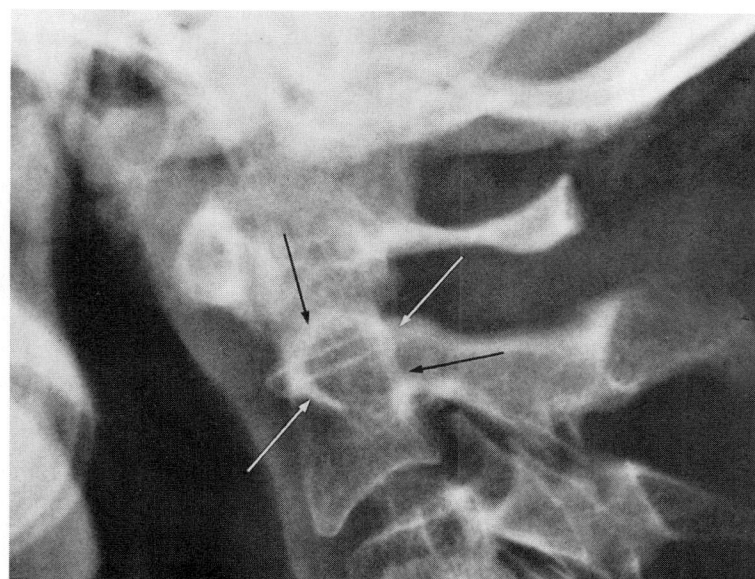

Figure 3–144. The C2 "target" composite shadow is a projectional variant not formed by a single anatomic structure. (Ref: Nicolet V et al: C-2 "target" composite shadow. *AJNR Am J Neuroradiol* 5:33, 1984.) Disruption of the ring shadow is a good indication of a low type (type III) odontoid fracture. (Ref: Harris JH et al: Low (type III) odontoid fracture: A new radiographic sign. *Radiology* 153:353, 1984.)

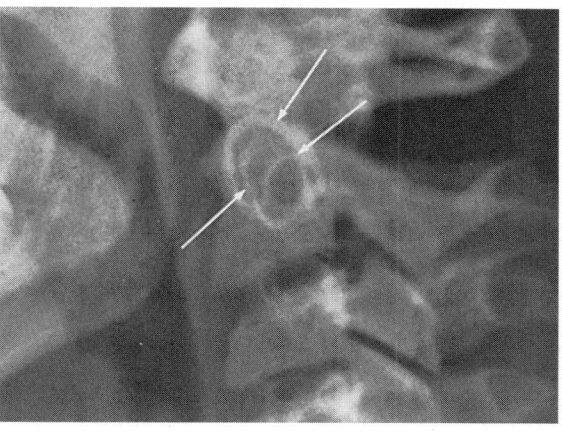

Figure 3–145. In the younger patient the C2 target shadow may appear as several rings, as shown in this 13-year-old boy.

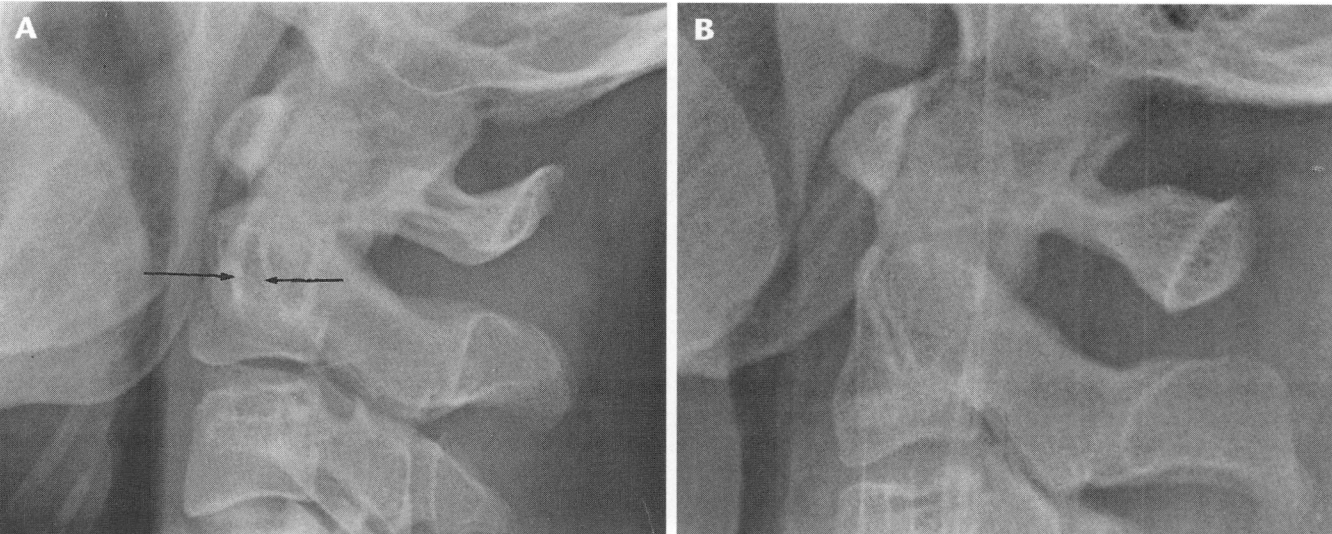

Figure 3–146. A, Duplication of the ring shadows of C2 caused by obliquity *(arrows).* **B,** True lateral projection reduces the appearance.

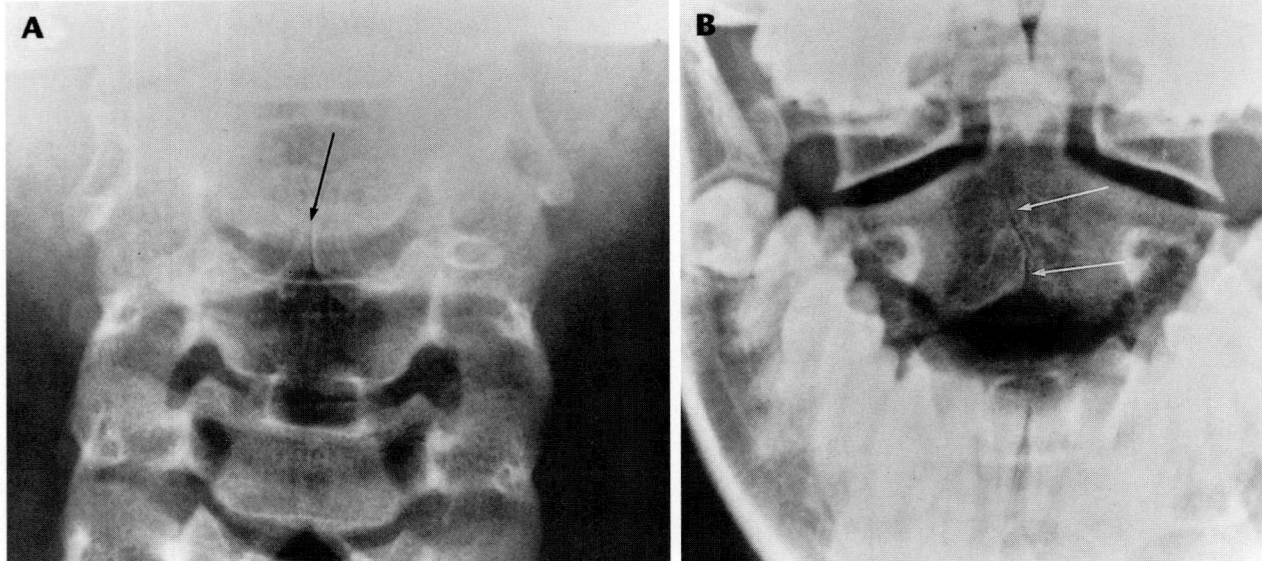

Figure 3–147. A, B, Spina bifida C2, simulating a fracture.

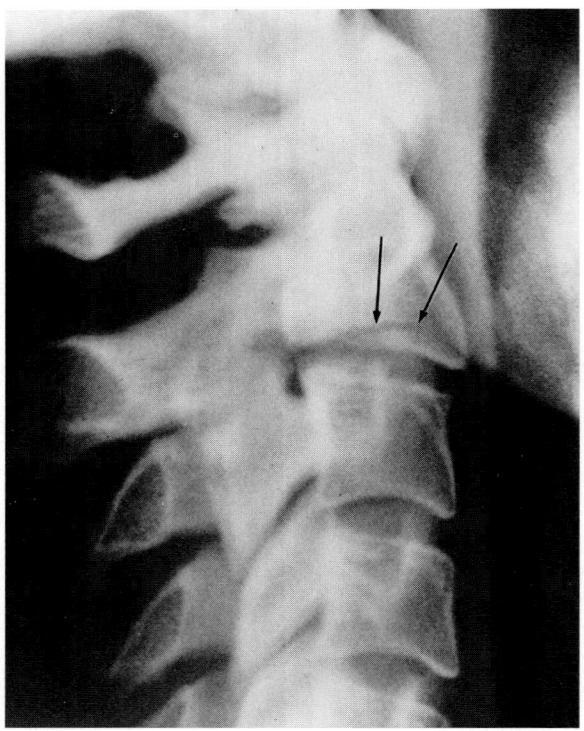

Figure 3–148. Pseudofracture of C2 produced by overlapping of large uncinate processes. (Ref: Daffner R: Pseudofracture of the cervical vertebral body. *Skeletal Radiol* 15:295, 1986.)

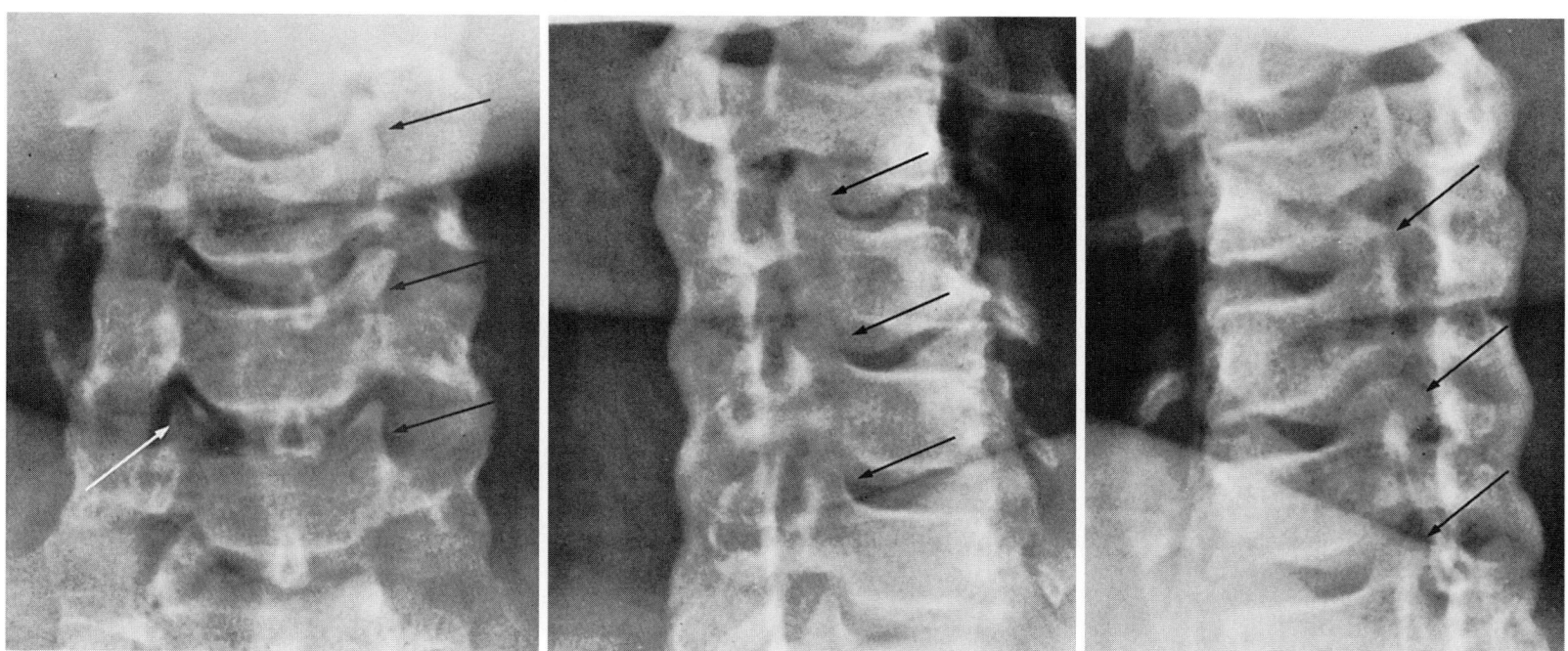

Figure 3–149. Very large uncovertebral processes in a 33-year-old woman.

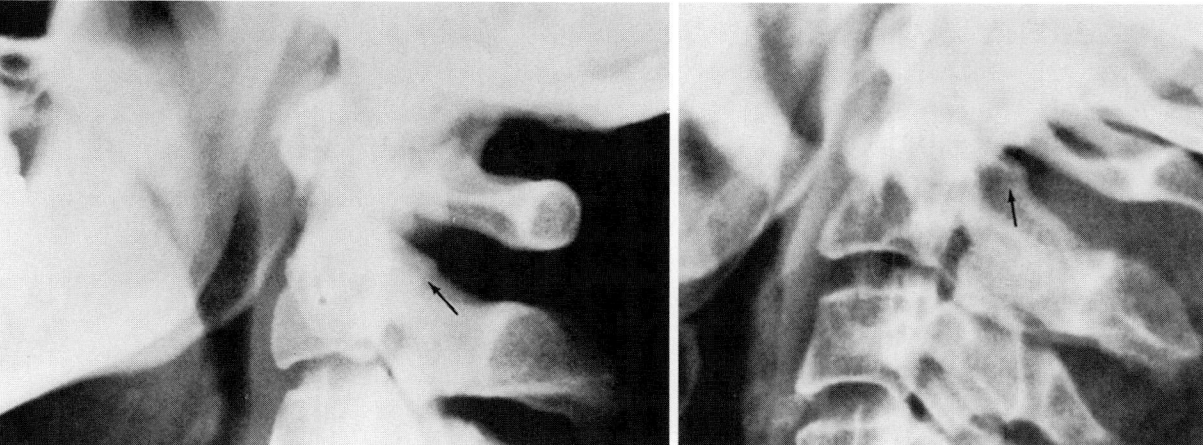

Figure 3–150. Normal contour alterations in the neural arch of C2 can produce pseudofractures.

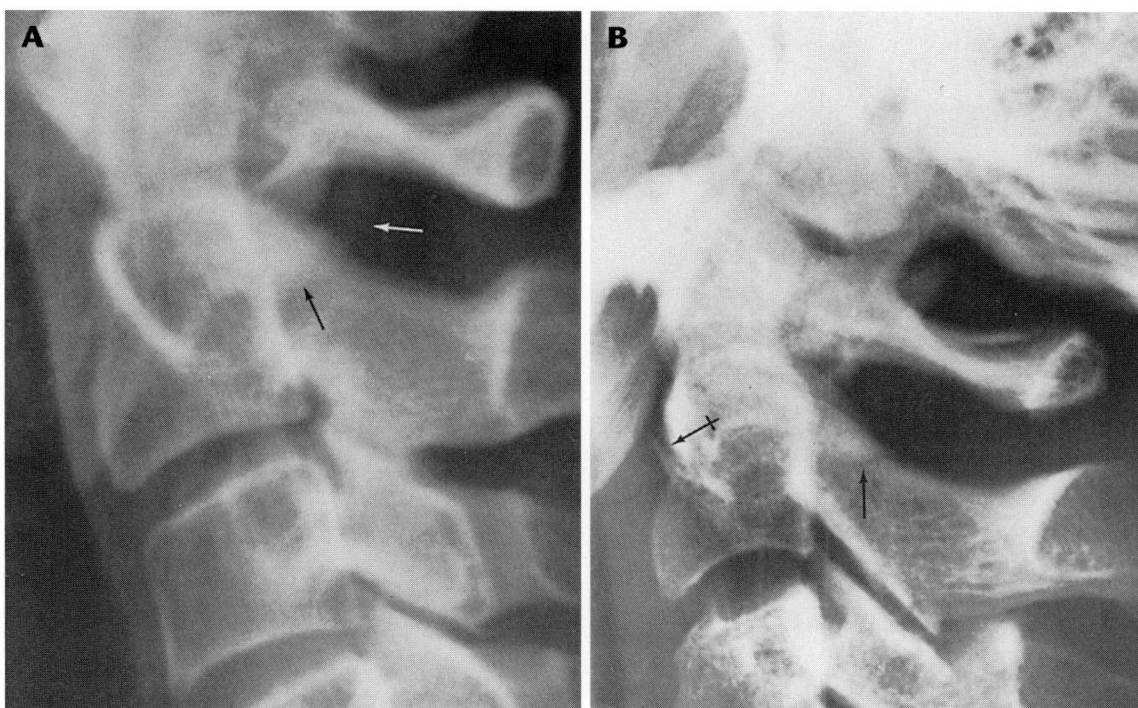

Figure 3–151. The superimposed lobe of the ear may produce shadows similar to those shown in Figure 3–150 and can simulate a fracture (→). Note in **B** the cleft in the anterior aspect of the vertebral body, which is probably a remnant of the synchondrosis for the odontoid process (↠).

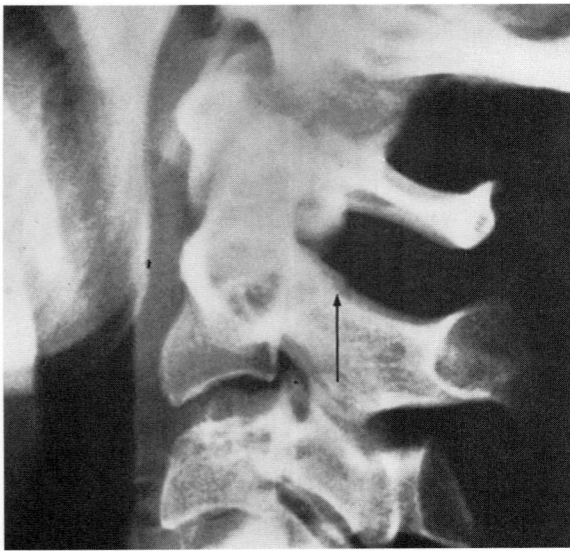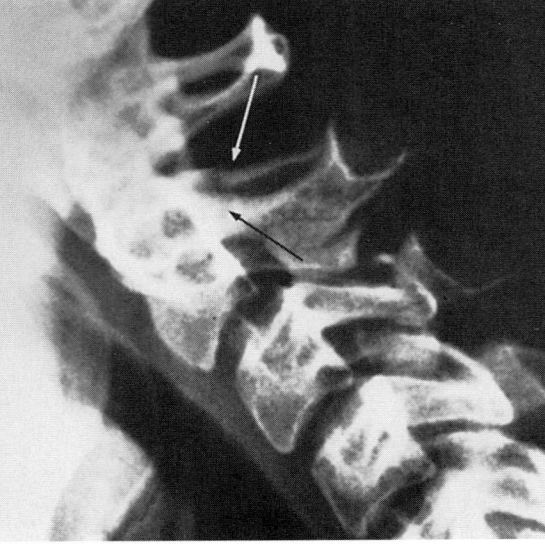

Figure 3–152. *Left,* Many patients exhibit a shallow groove at the superior aspect of the neural arch of C2 (←) that could be mistaken for a hangman's fracture: *Right,* in flexion these grooves are seen bilaterally. The physiologic subluxation of C2 on C3 reinforces the impression of a hangman's fracture.

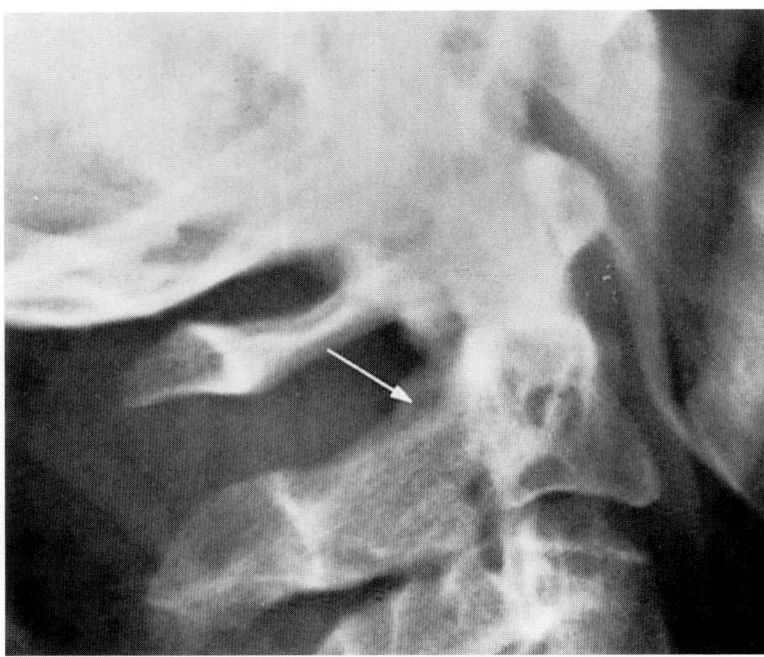

Figure 3–153. Additional example of the groove of the neural arch of C2 that can be mistaken for a fracture.

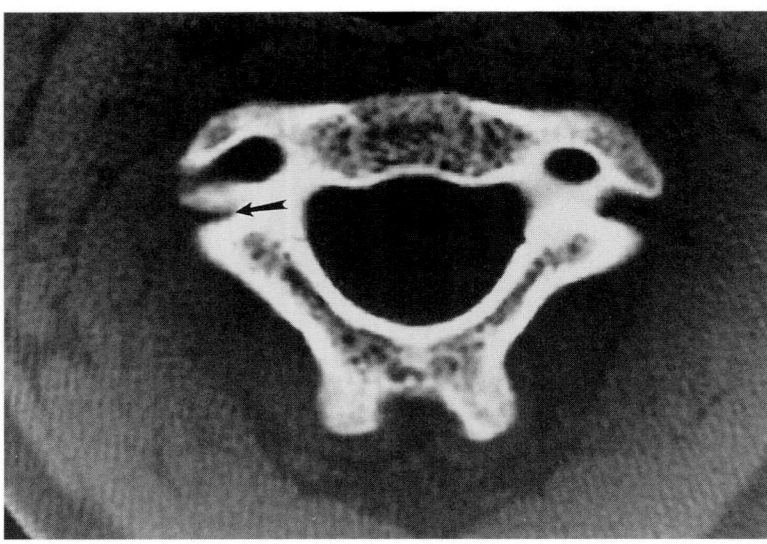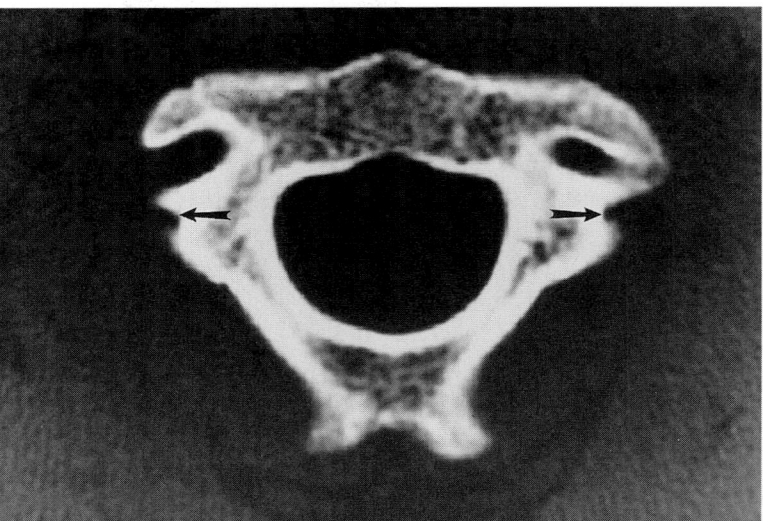

Figure 3–154. The grooves illustrated in the preceding figure can also be demonstrated by CT.

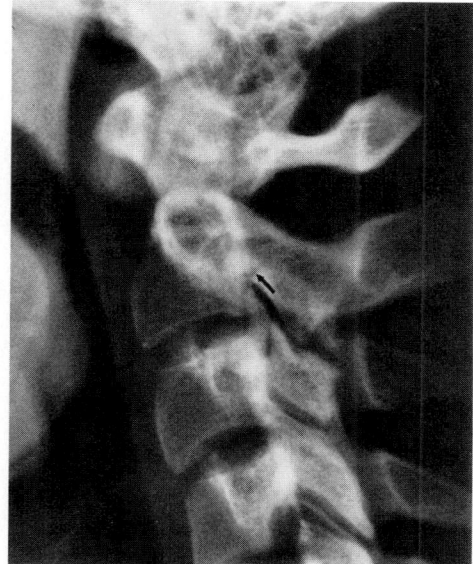

Figure 3–155. Cleft or groove simulating a fracture of C2.

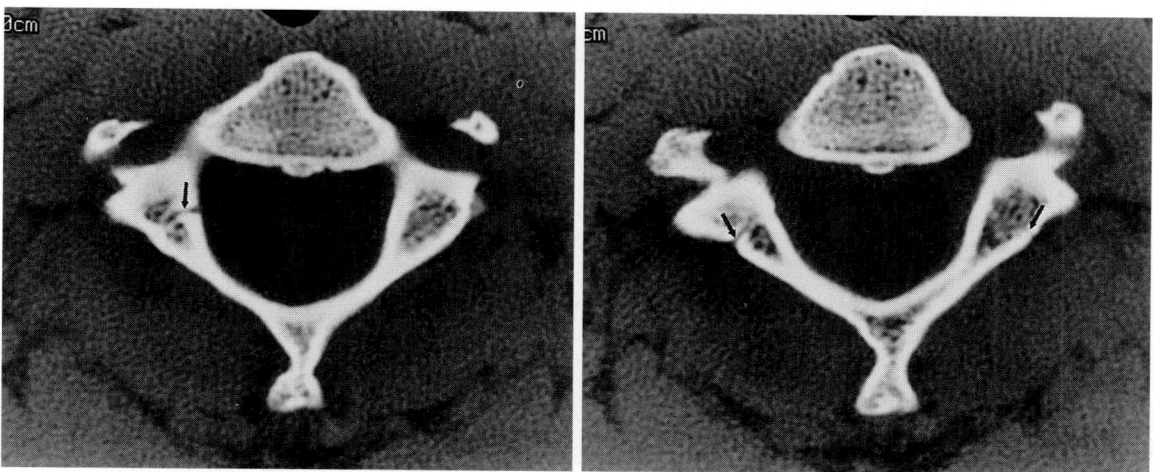

Figure 3–156. Clefts in the laminae of C2 can be confused with fractures on CT.

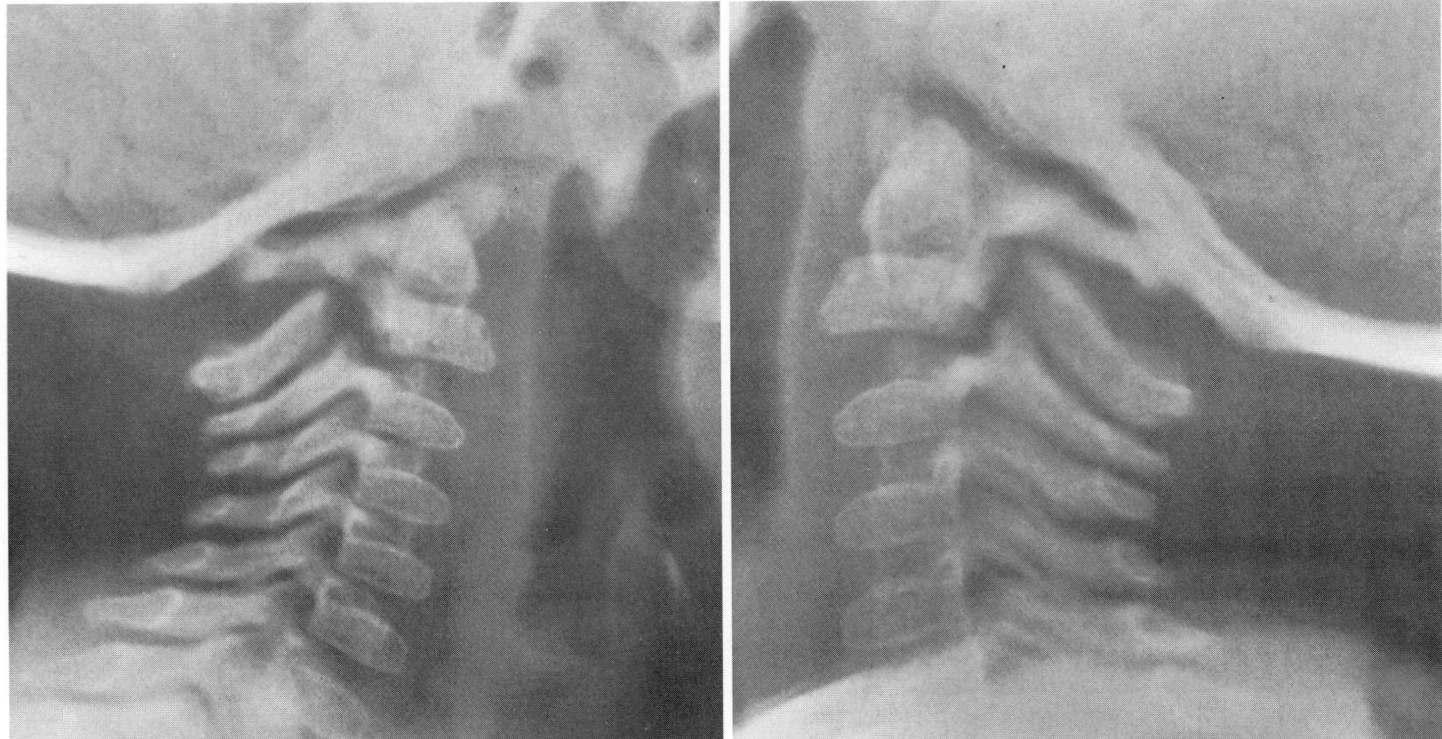

Figure 3–157. Two 1-year-old children with spondylolysis of C2 originally diagnosed as hangman's fractures. Hangman's fracture is very uncommon in children, but spondylolysis of C2 is not. CT confirmation should be obtained to make the differentiation in the emergency situation. (Refs: Parisi M et al: Hangman's fracture or primary spondylolysis: A patient and a brief review. *Pediatr Radiol* 21:367, 1991; Riebel G, Bayley JC: A congenital defect resembling the hangman's fracture. *Spine* 16:1240, 1991; Smith JT et al: Persistent synchondrosis of the second cervical vertebra simulating hangman's fracture in a child. *J Bone Joint Surg* 75A:228, 1993; Mondschein J, Karasick D: Spondylolysis of the axis vertebra. *Am J Roentgenol* 172:556, 1999.)

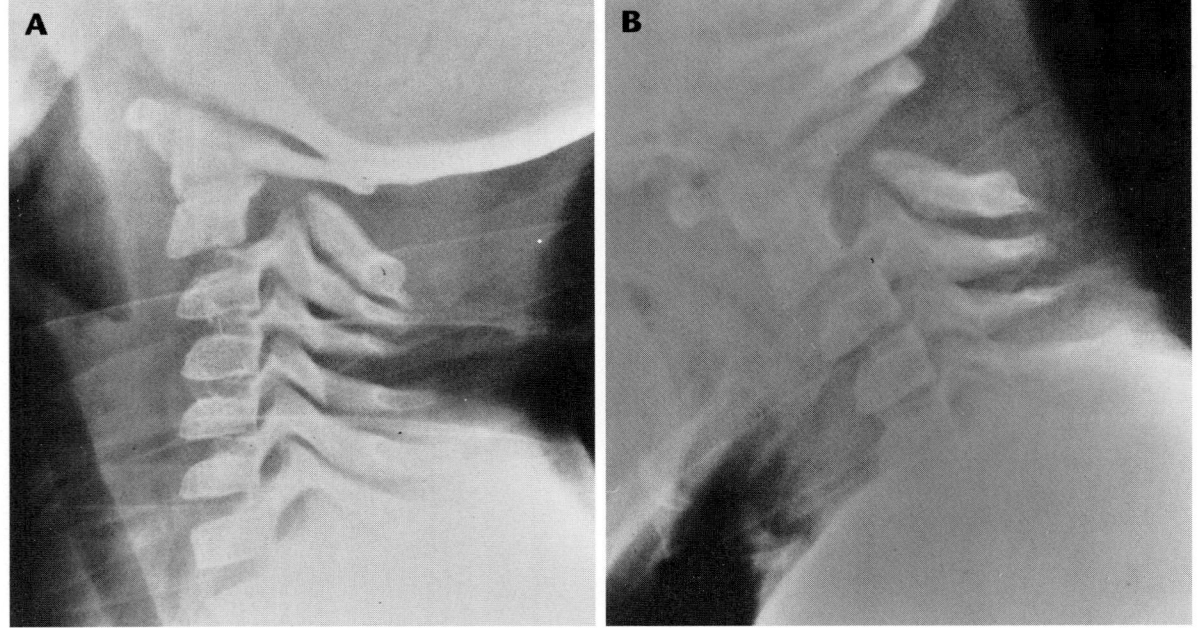

Figure 3–158. Spondylolysis of C2 in a Down syndrome 3-year-old showing spondylolisthesis on flexion. **A,** Neutral position. **B,** Flexion.

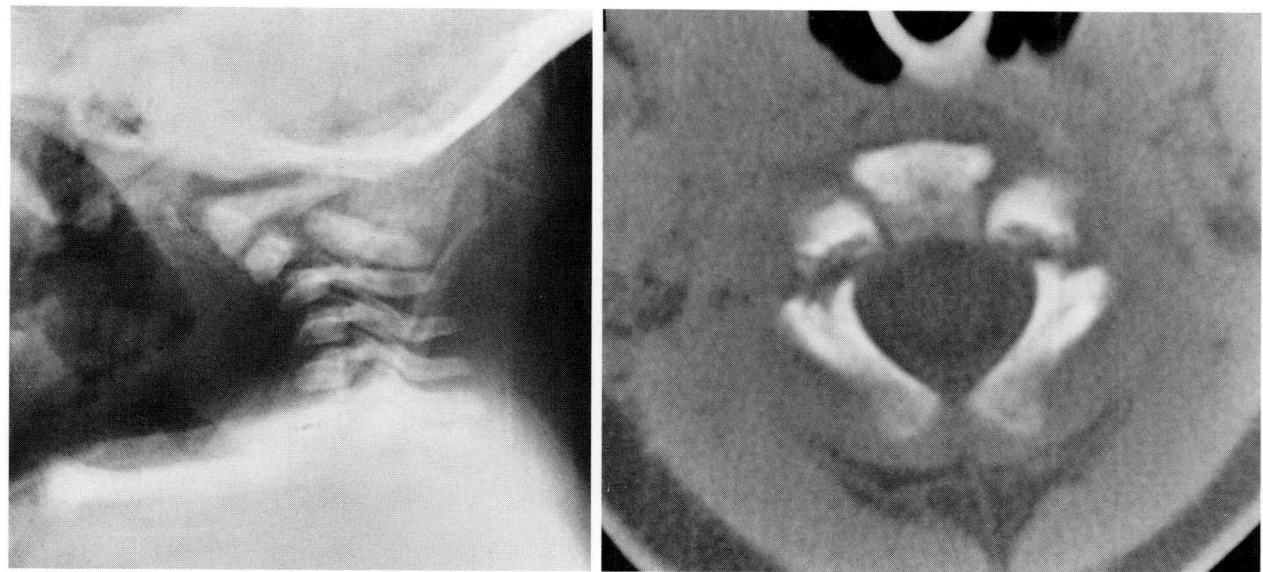

Figure 3–159. Spondylolysis of C2 in a 2-month-old child. Note that spondylolisthesis may occur with this entity and does not necessarily denote prior trauma.

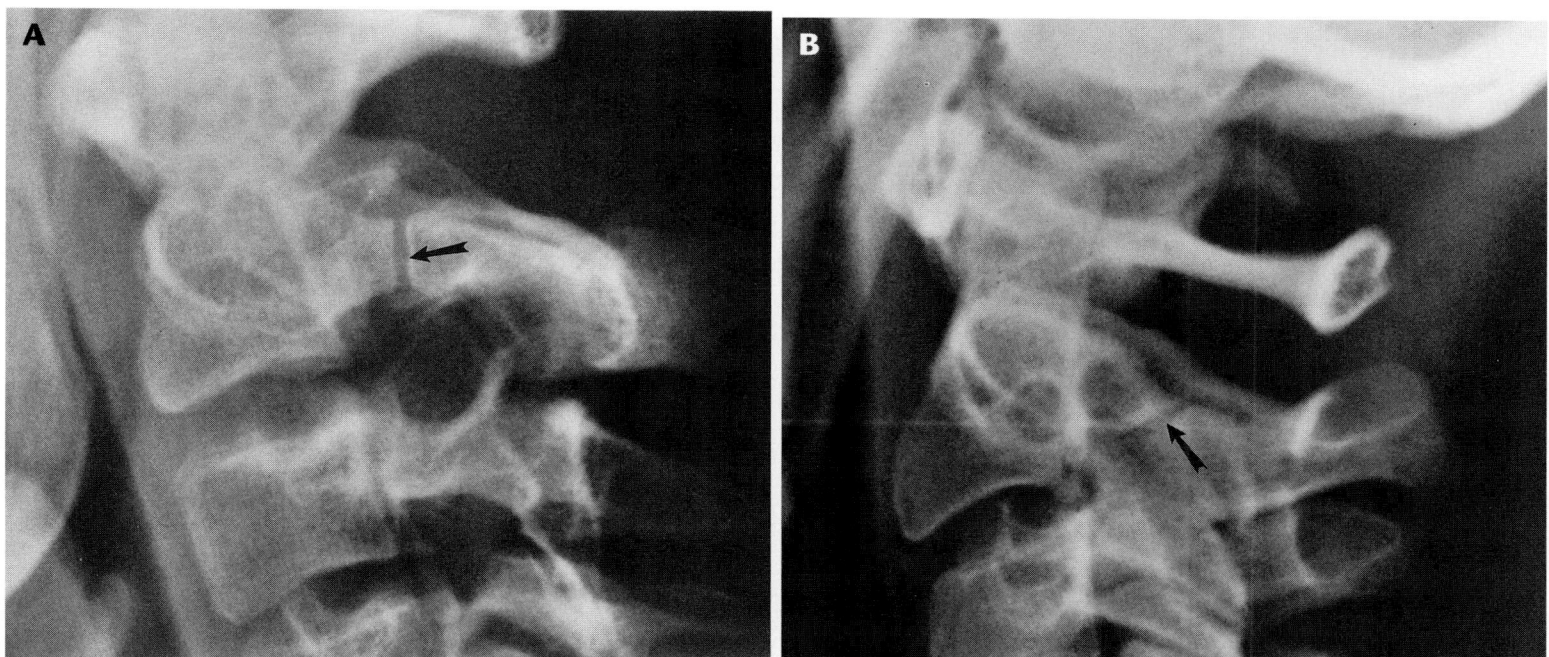

Figure 3–160. A, B, Two examples of spondylolysis of C2 in adults.

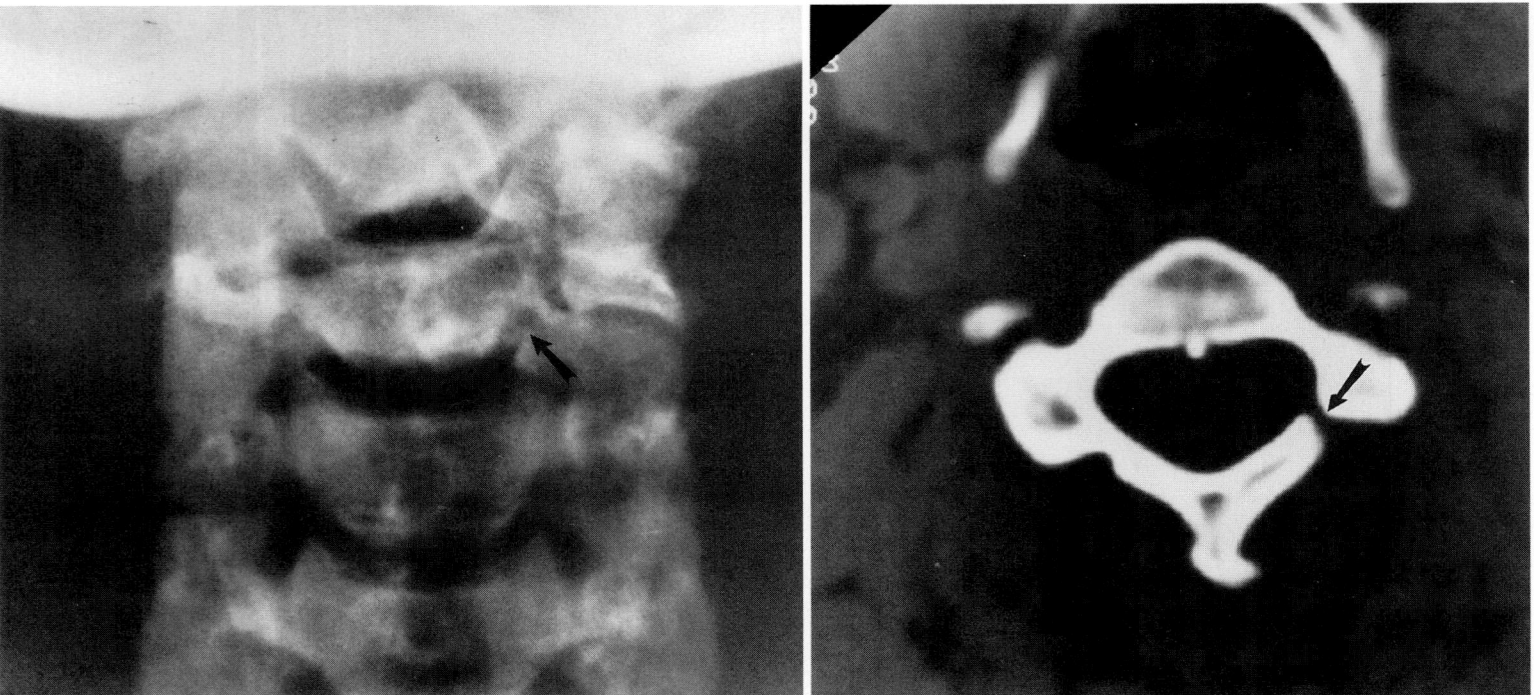

Figure 3–161. Spondylolysis of C3 with hypoplasia of the left lateral mass.

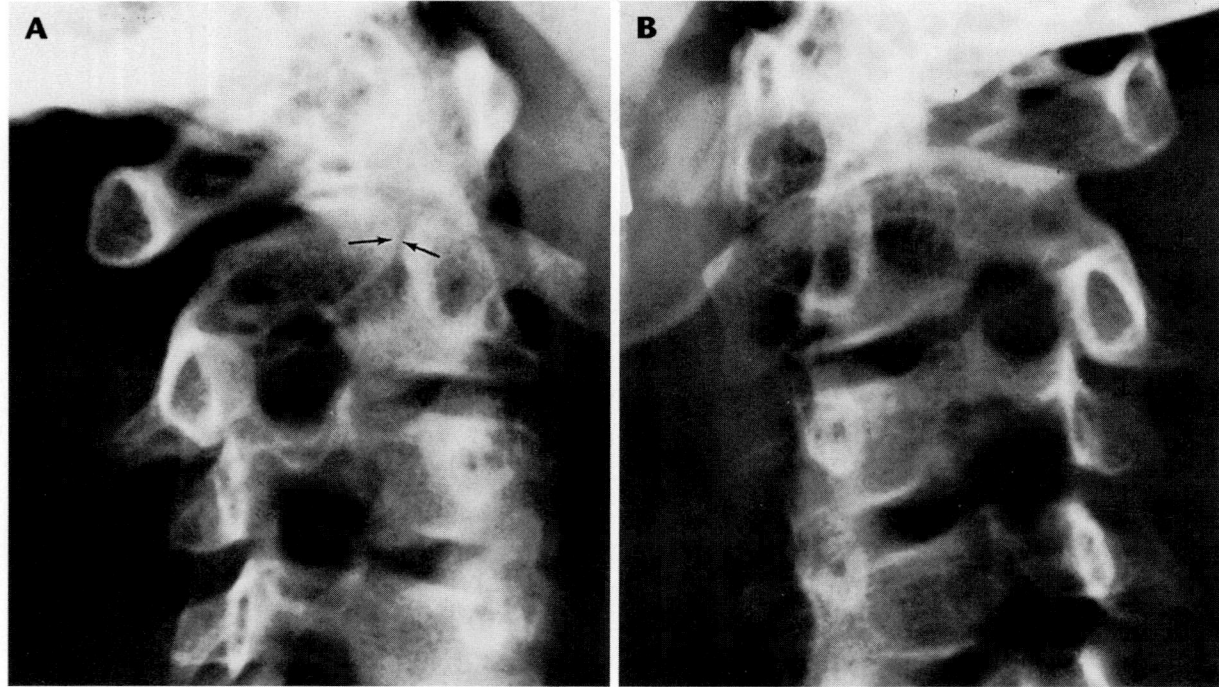

Figure 3–162. A, Unilateral closure defect in the lamina on the left side of C2.
B, Opposite side shown for comparison.

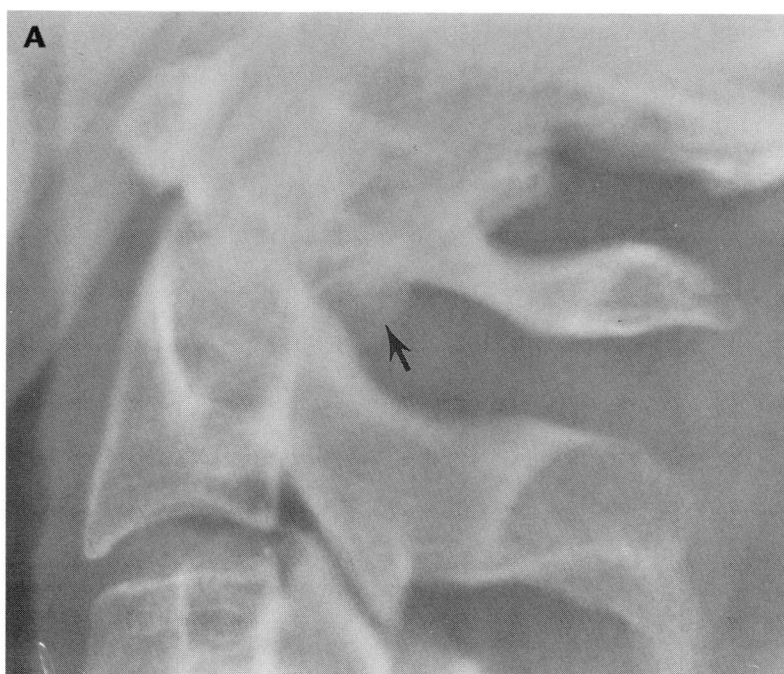

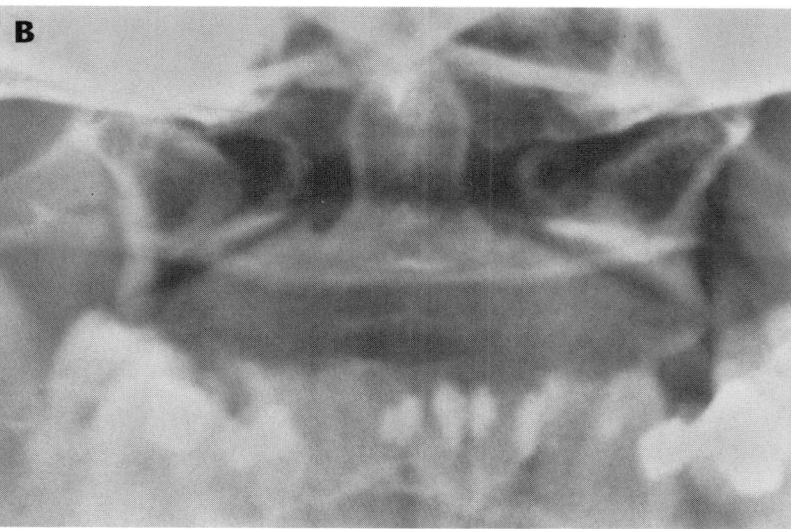

Figure 3–163. A, Facet between C1 and C2 seen as osseous mass as the result of rotation. **B,** Frontal view shows no abnormality.

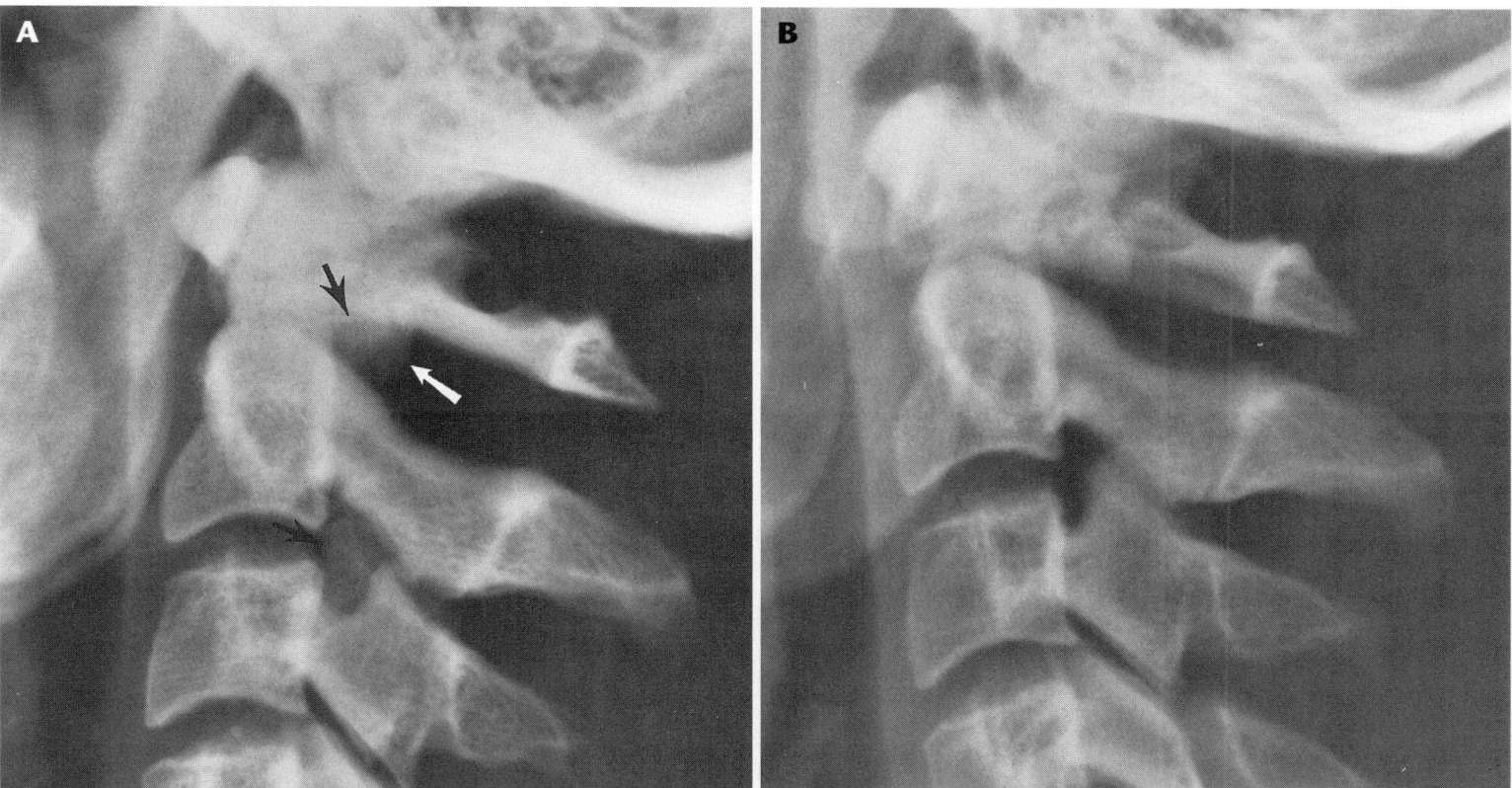

Figure 3–164. A, Simulated lesions between C1, C2, and C3, produced by rotation. **B,** Improved positioning eliminates the shadows.

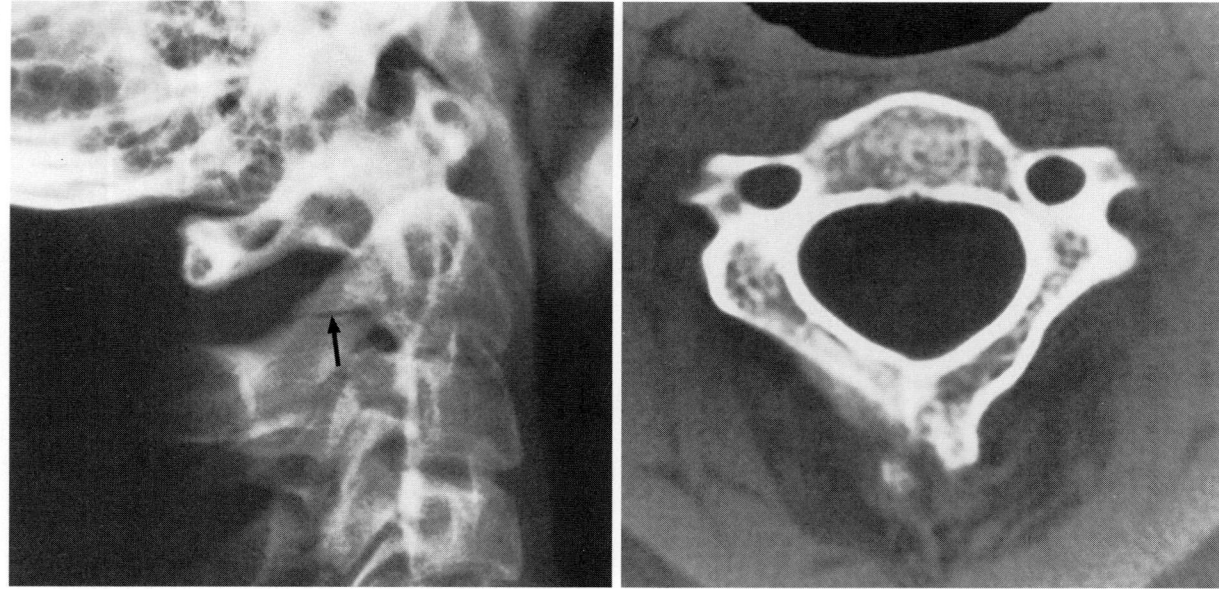

Figure 3–165. *Left,* Simulated fracture of the neural arch of C2, produced by rotation. *Right,* CT shows no fracture.

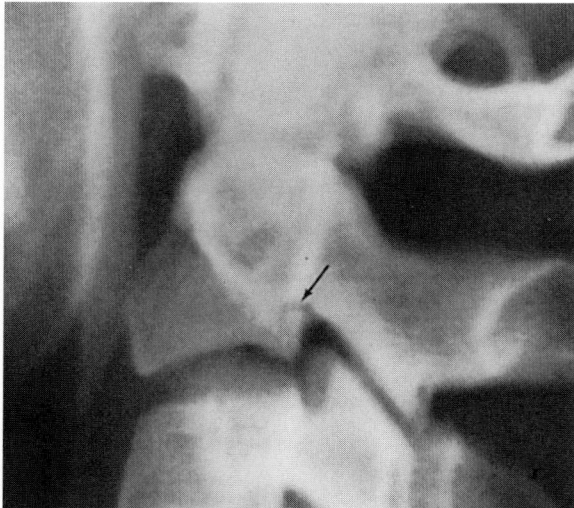

Figure 3–166. Simulated fracture of C2, produced by slight rotation with superimposition of the superior articular process on the vertebral body.

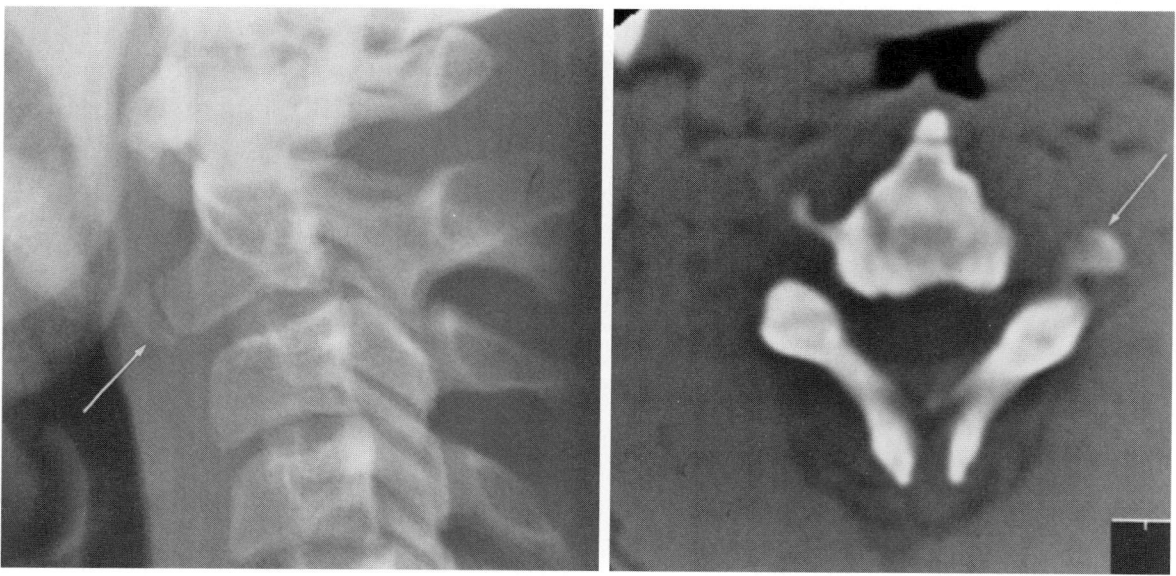

Figure 3–167. Unusual development of C2, with ossicle arising from anterior vertebral body.

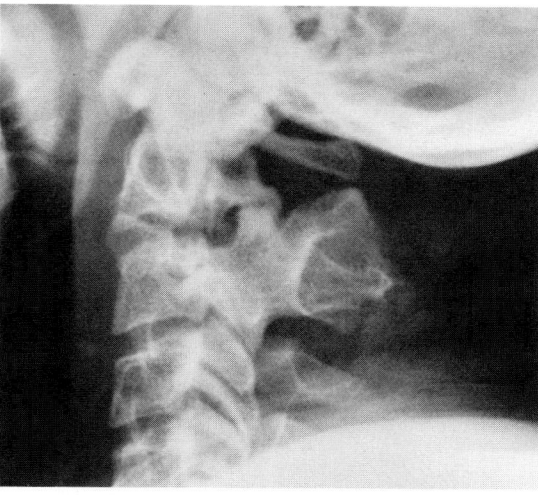

Figure 3–168. Hypoplasia of C2 with hypertrophy of the posterior elements of C3 and an anomalous articulation with the neural arch of C3.

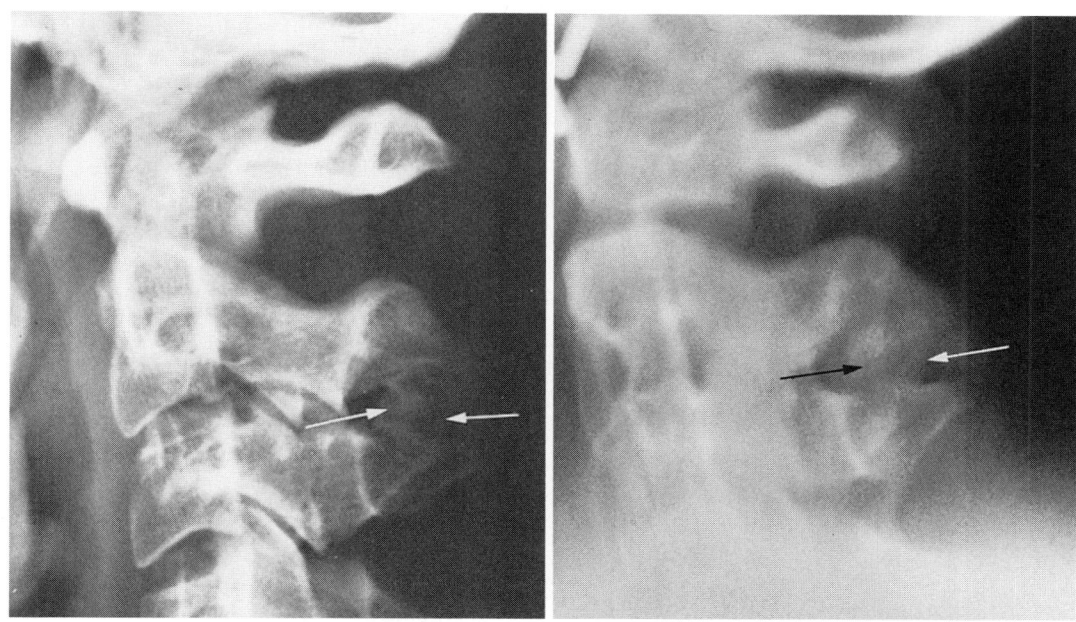

Figure 3–169. Anomalous ossicle between the spinous processes of C2 and C3. *Left,* Plain film. *Right,* Tomogram.

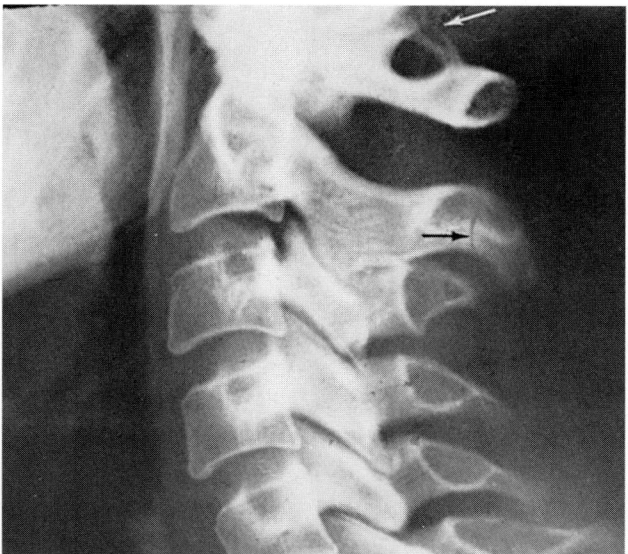

Figure 3–170. Fissure in the spinous process of C2, simulating a fracture. The *upper arrow* indicates the arcuate foramen.

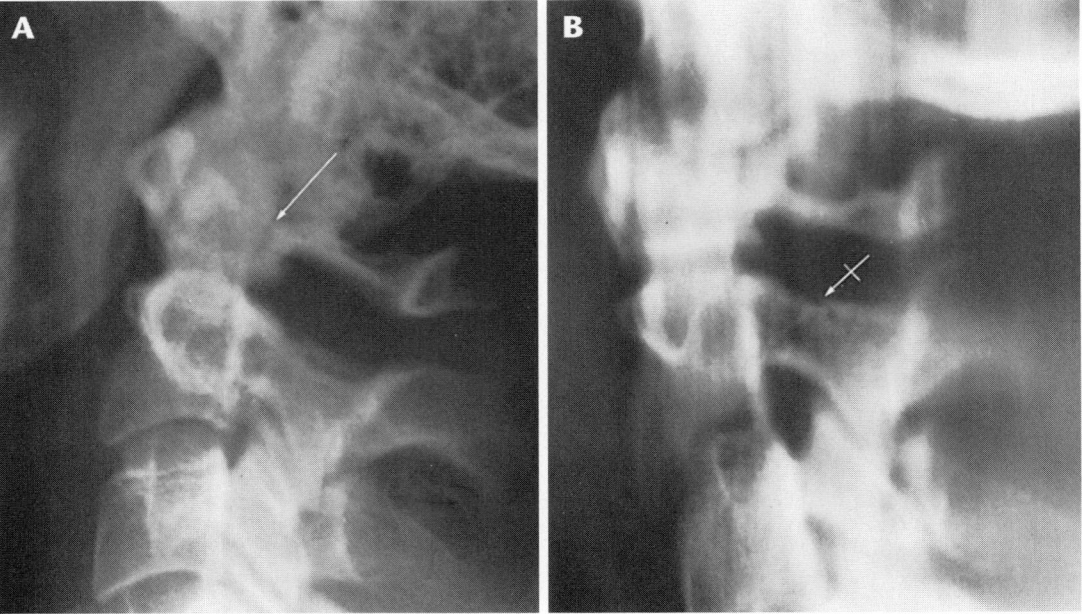

Figure 3–171. **A,** Simulated fracture produced by Mach effect of the odontoid process. **B,** Tomogram shows no fracture of C1. Note the pseudofracture of C2 (↔).

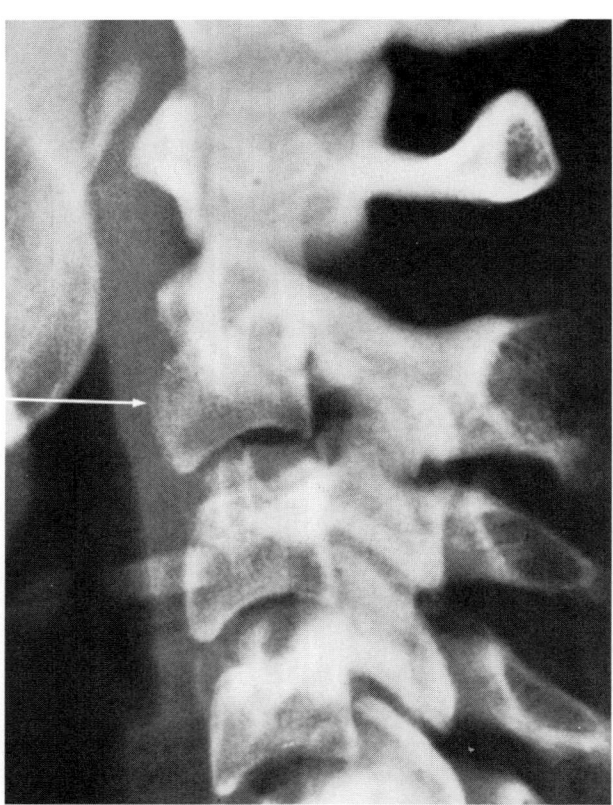

Figure 3–172. In some patients, the C2 vertebra is larger in its inferior portions than the adjacent C3 vertebra, giving a pseudo "fat C2 sign" that indicates a vertical C2 body fracture. (Refs: Bohrer SP: Pseudosigns in cervical spine trauma radiology. *Contemp Diagn Radiol* 12:13, 1989; Smoker WRK, Dolan KD: The "fat C2": A sign of fracture, *Am J Roentgenol* 148:609, 1989.)

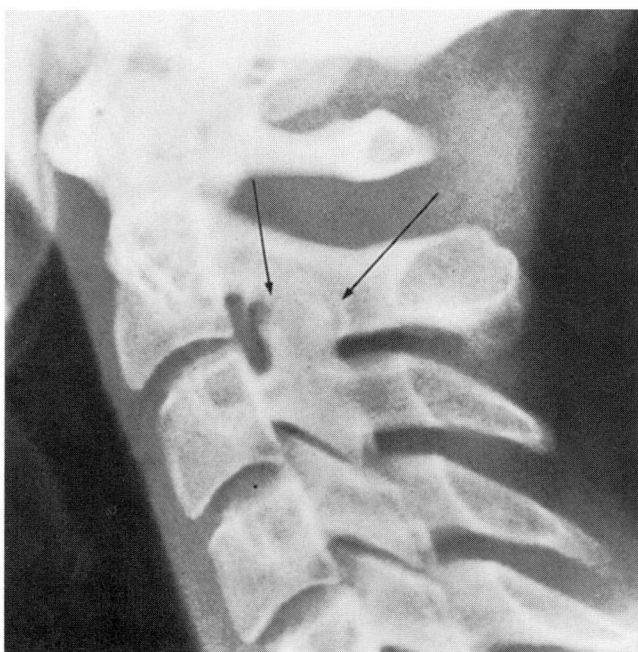

Figure 3–173. Anomalous articulation between C2 and C3.

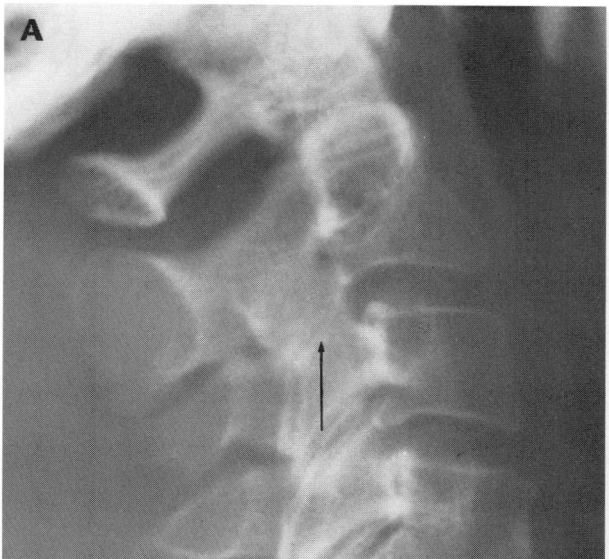

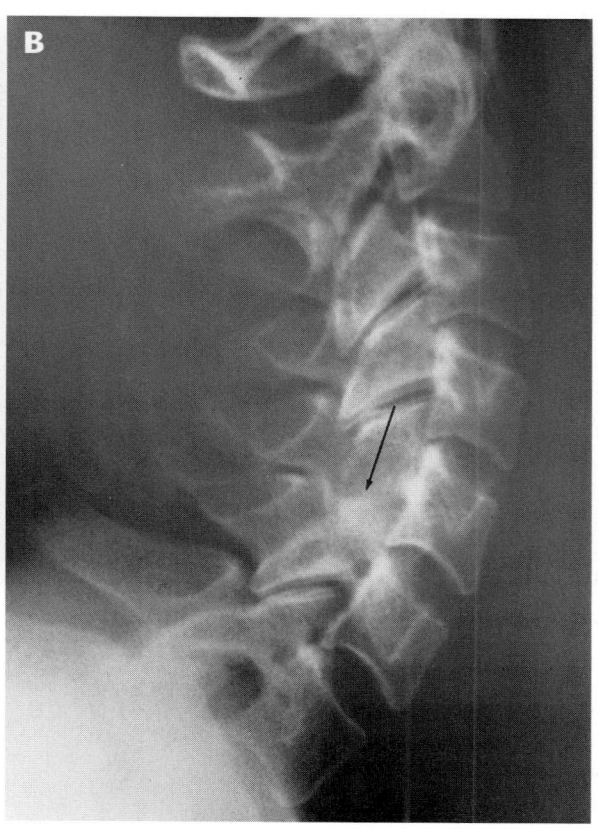

Figure 3–174. A, Simulated fusion of posterior elements of C2 and C3, produced by rotation. **B,** Repeat film shows no abnormality at C2–C3, but apparent fusion appears at C5 and C6. In some patients this pseudofusion is the result of oblique orientation of the facets with reference to the x-ray beam. (Ref: Massengill AD et al. C2–C3 facet joint "pseudofusion." *Skeletal Radiol* 26:27, 1997.)

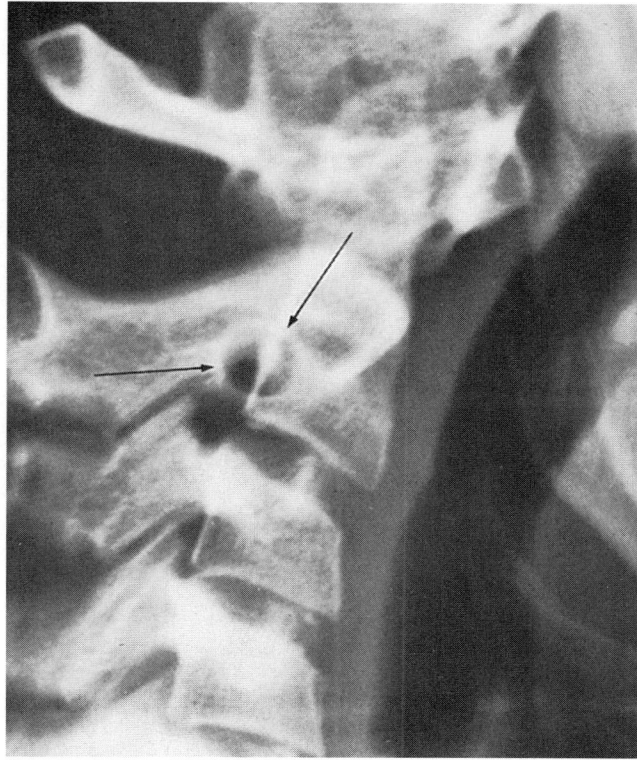

Figure 3–175. The foramen transversarium. The central density is a portion of the vertebra projected through the lucency of the foramen.

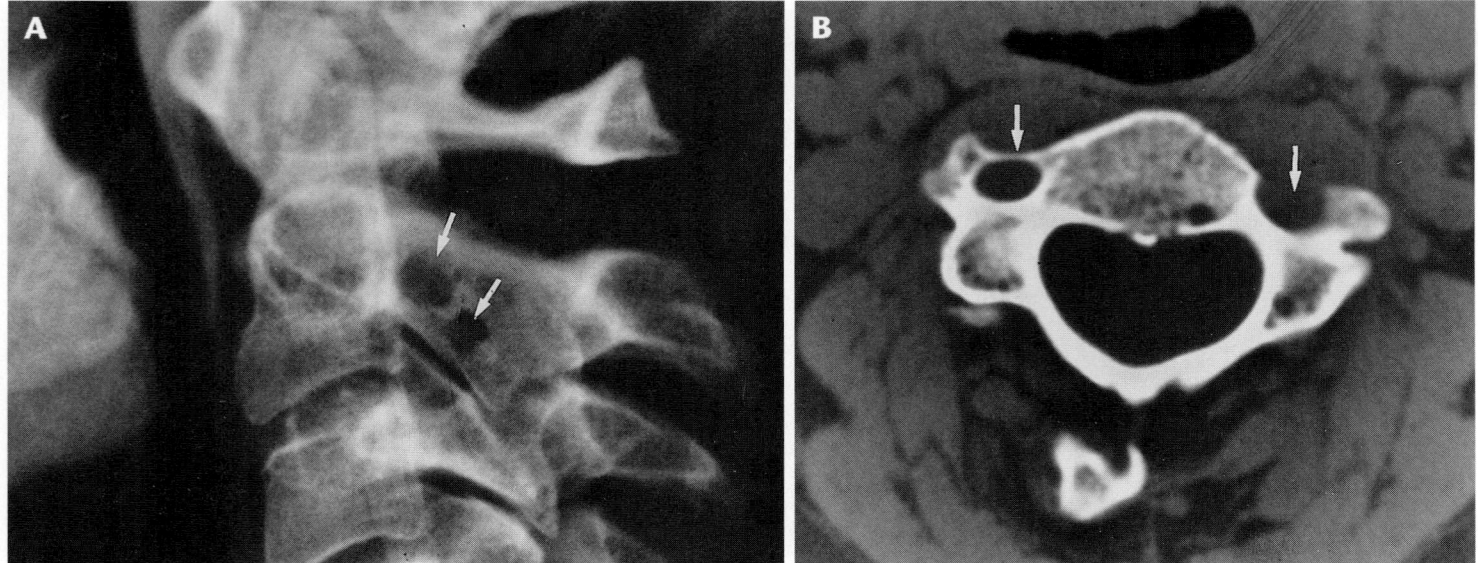

Figure 3–176. A, Asymmetric foramina transversarium producing unusual appearance of posterior elements *(arrows).* **B,** CT demonstrates incomplete foramen on left.

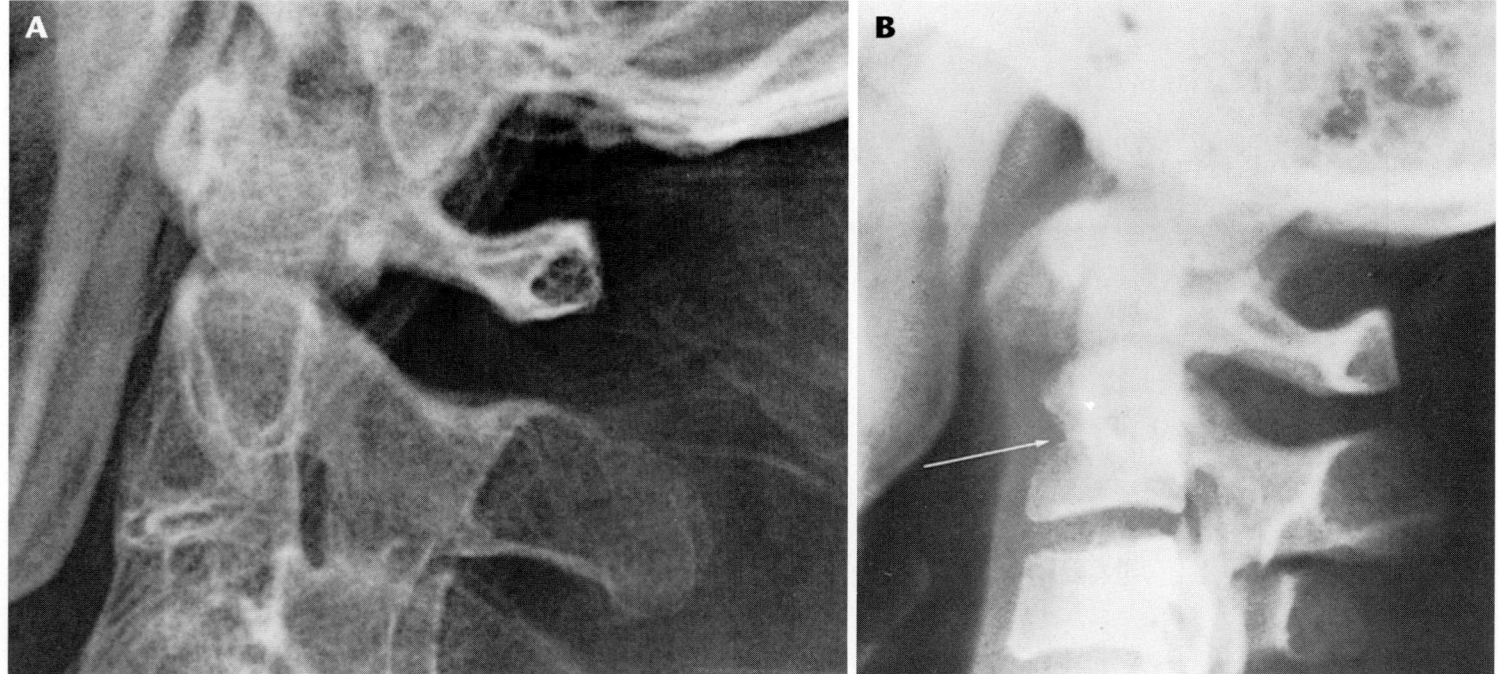

Figure 3–177. A, Nonsegmented C2–C3 with characteristic calcification in the rudimentary disk. **B,** Developmental cleft in the anterior aspect of C2.

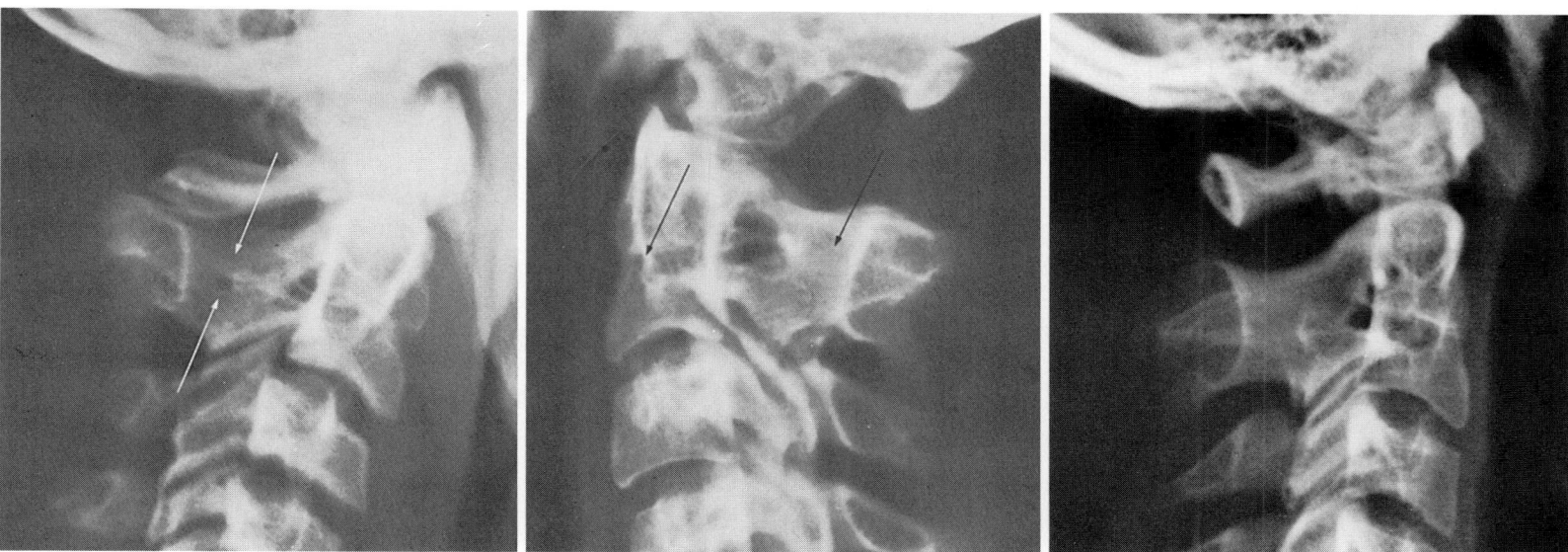

Figure 3–178. Three examples of incomplete segmentation of commonly called *congenital block vertebra*. Occasionally, this may predispose the patient to early degenerative spondylosis at the next lower intervertebral disc. (Ref: de Graaff R: Vertebrae C2–C3 in patients with cervical myelopathy. *Acta Neurochir* 61:111, 1982.)

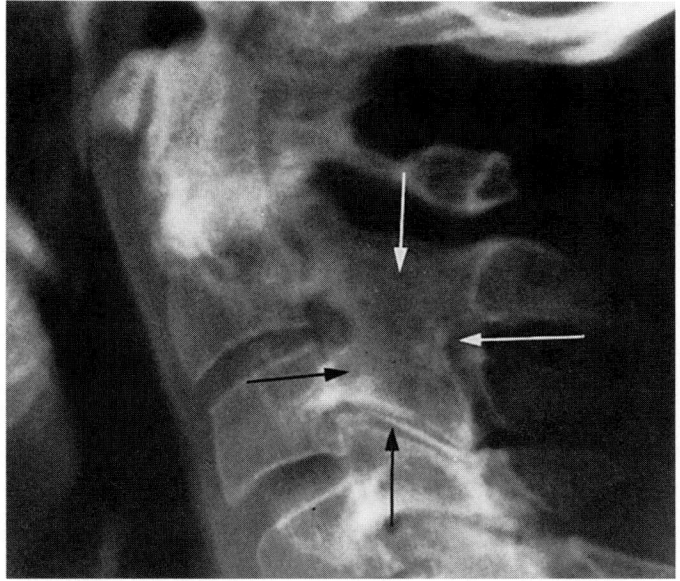

Figure 3–179. Failure of segmentation of the neural arches of C2 and C3.

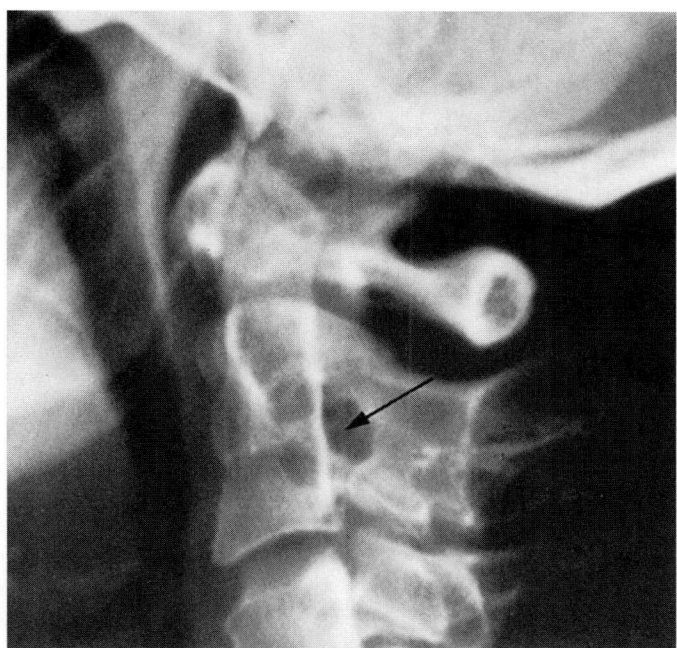

Figure 3–180. Incomplete segmentation of C2–C3 with a huge irregular foramen between the neural arches.

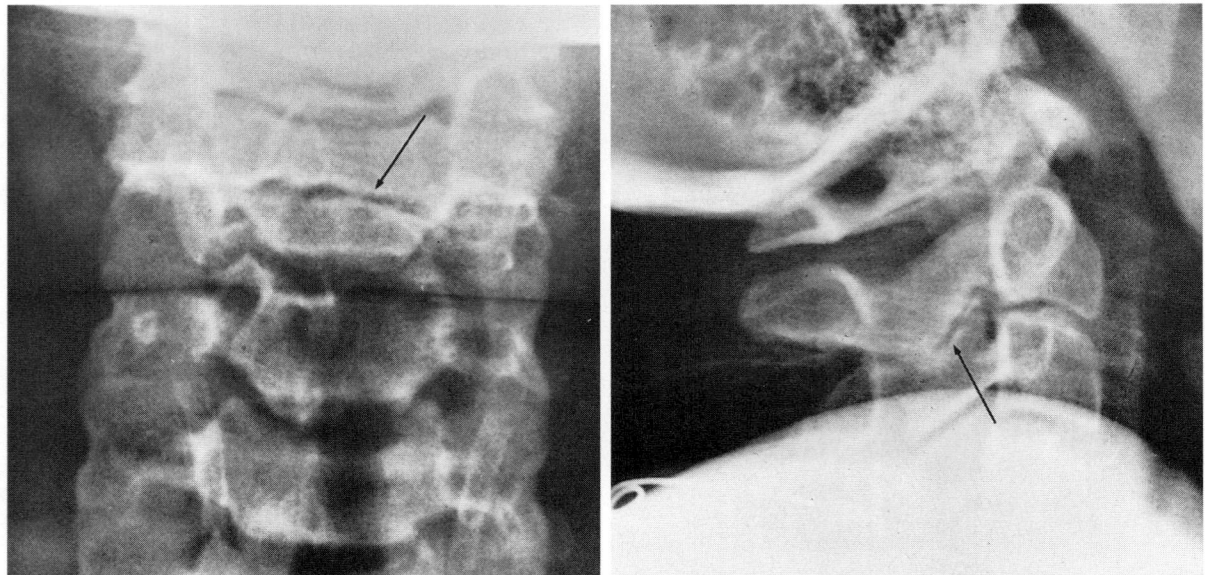

Figure 3–181. Partial segmentation of C2–C3, originally diagnosed as a fracture.

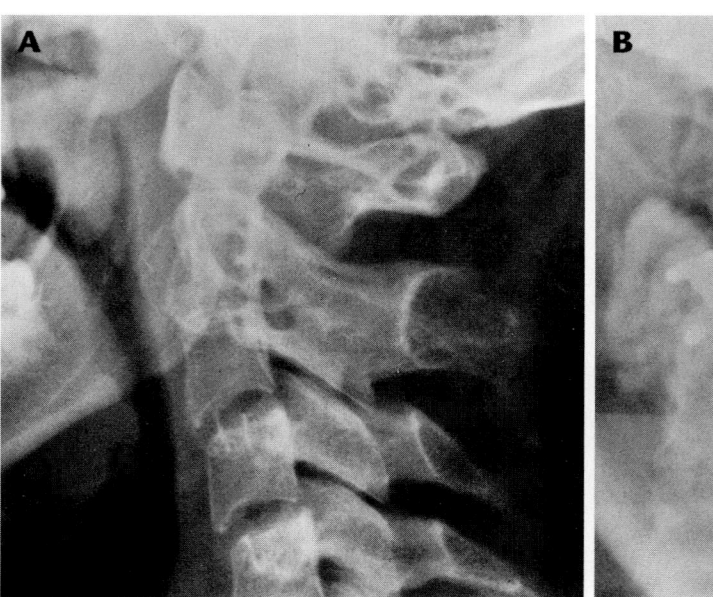

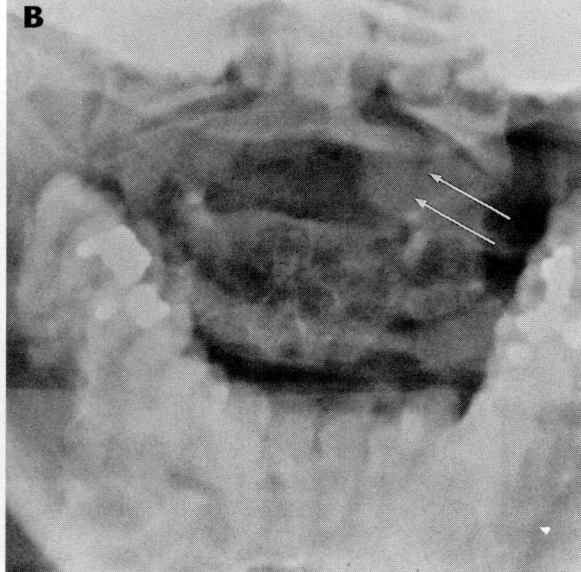

Figure 3–182. A, B, Block vertebrae are often associated with defects in architecture. Note the failure of fusion of the lateral mass of C2 in the AP film **(B)**. Rarely this anomaly may be associated with radiculopathy. (Ref: Okada K et al: Cervical radiculopathy associated with an anomaly of the cervical vertebrae. *J Bone Joint Surg* 70A:1399, 1988.)

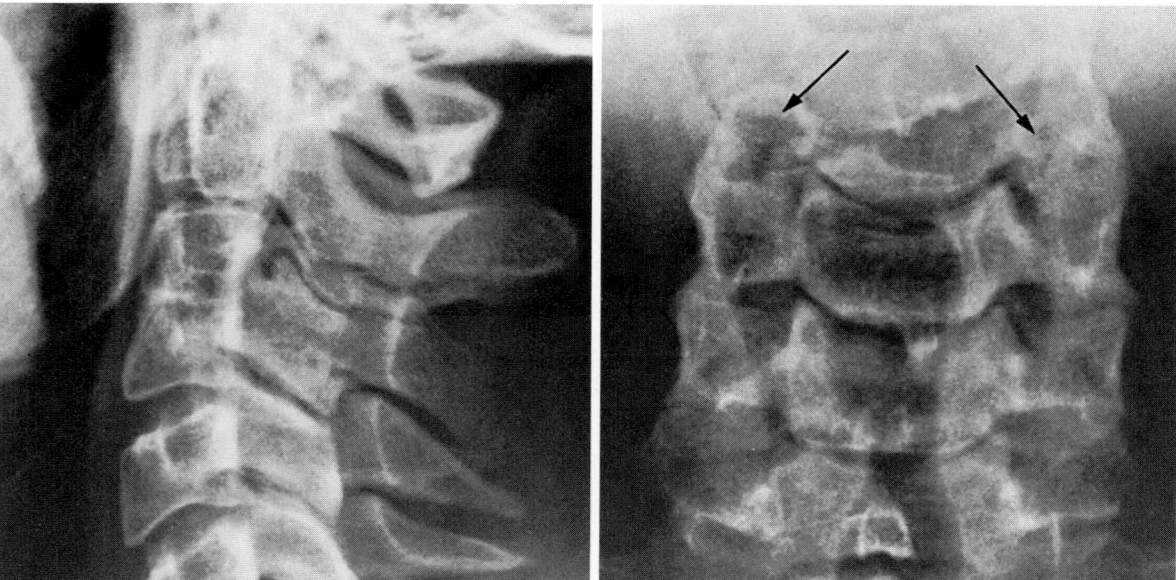

Figure 3–183. Nonsegmentation of C3 and C4 with asymmetric development of the pedicles.

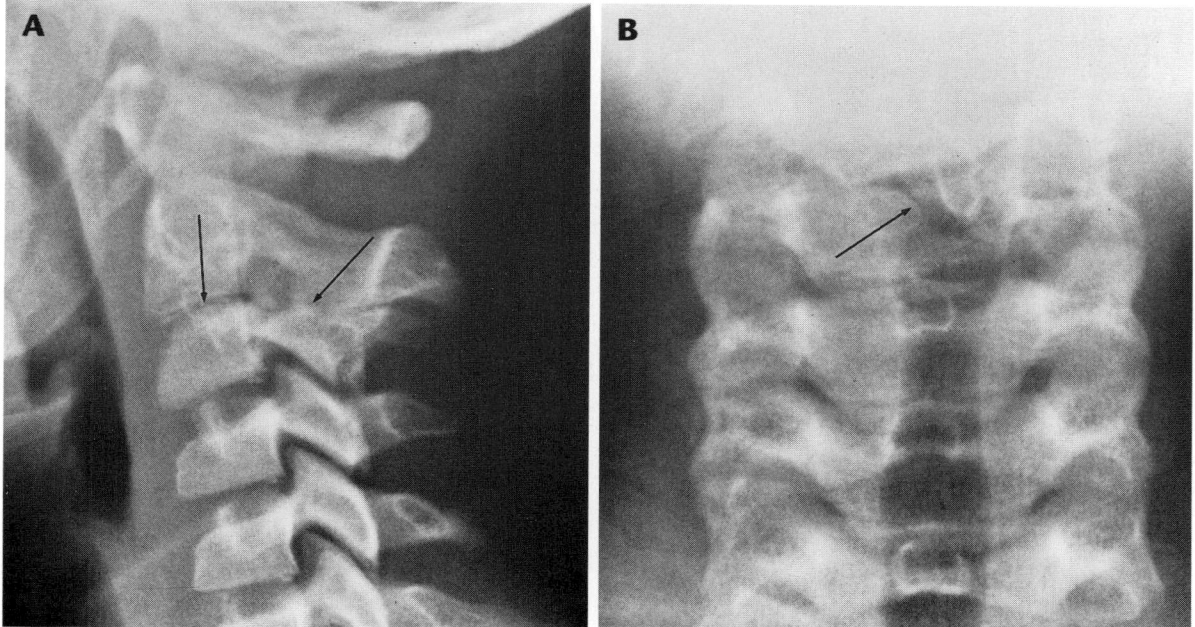

Figure 3–184. Partial segmentation of C2–C3 **(A)** with spina bifida **(B),** seen in a 9-year-old child.

Figure 3–185. Pseudosubluxation of C2 on C3 in a 6-year-old boy **(A)**. This is the normal area of maximum movement in the child; pseudosubluxation is regularly seen in flexion. A view with the head in neutral position **(B)** shows normal relationships. (Ref: Jacobson G, Beeckler HH: Pseudosubluxation of the axis in children. *Am J Roentgenol* 82:472, 1959.)

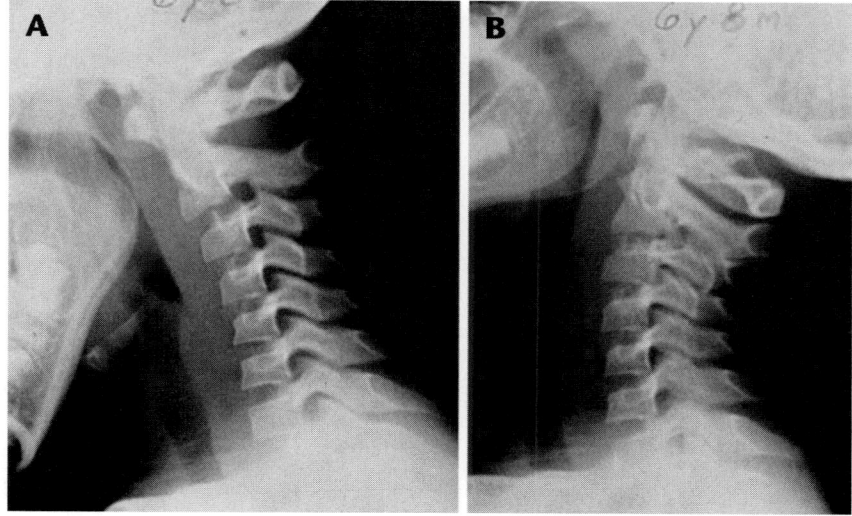

Figure 3–186. Another example of pseudosubluxation of C2 on C3 in a 4-year-old boy. Note the neck in flexion. The posterior cervical line is useful in differentiating true subluxation from pseudosubluxation of C2 on C3, see Figure 3–193. (Ref: Swischuk LE: Anterior displacement of C2 in children: Physiologic or pathologic. *Radiology* 122:759, 1977.)

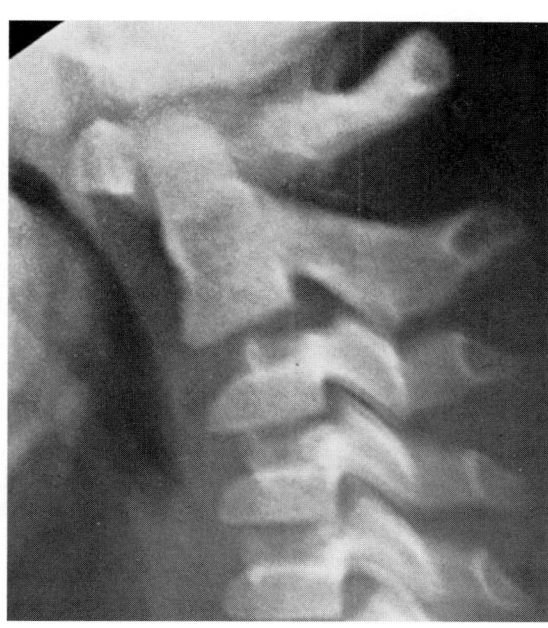

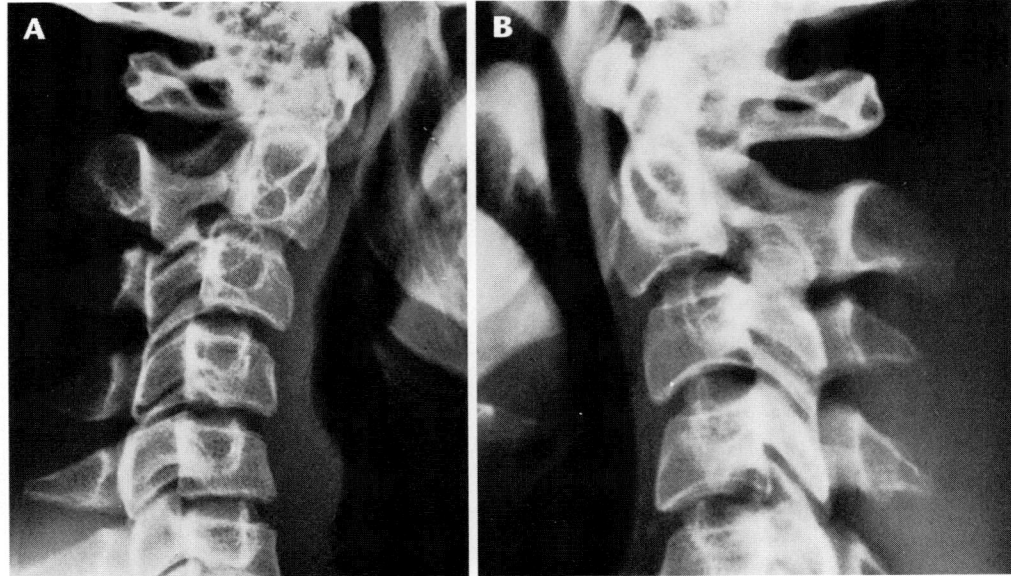

Figure 3–187. Physiologic subluxation of C2 on C3 may also occur in adults. **A,** 20-year-old man. **B,** 34-year-old woman. (Ref: Harrison RB et al: Pseudosubluxation of the axis in young adults. *J Can Assoc Radiol* 31:176, 1980.)

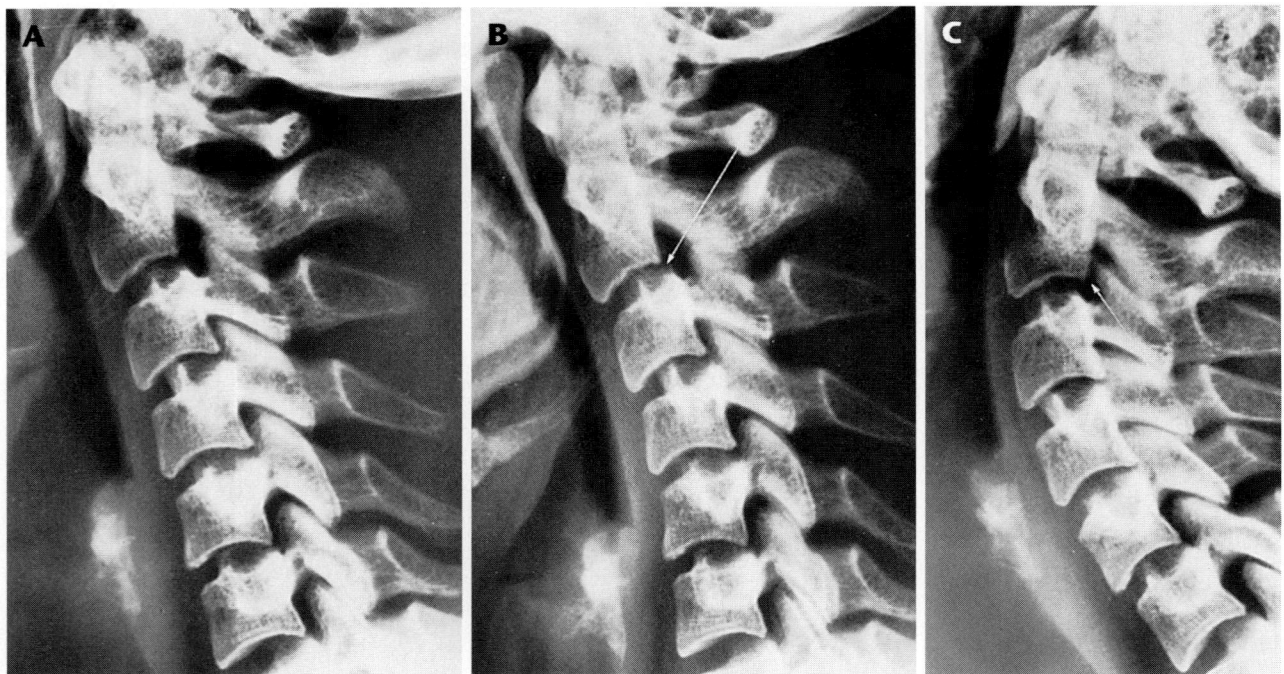

Figure 3–188. Physiologic subluxation may occasionally be seen in cervical extension as well as in flexion, as in this 20-year-old man. **A,** Neutral position. **B,** Flexion. **C,** Extension. (Ref: Harris JH: Radiographically subtle soft tissue injuries of the cervical spine. *Curr Probl Diagn Radiol* 18:166, 1989.)

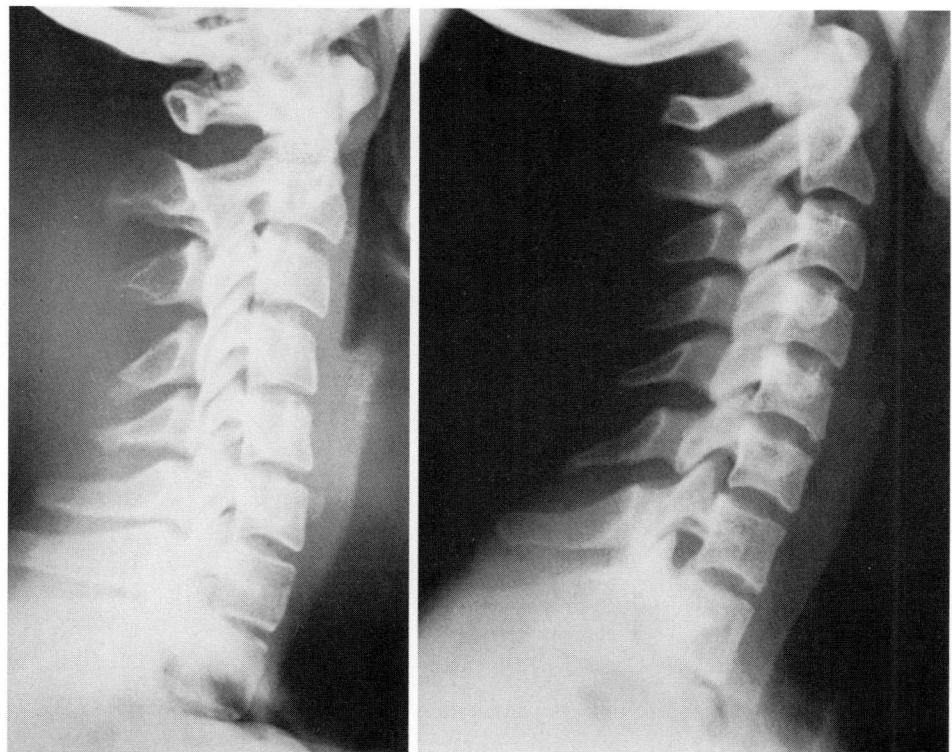

Figure 3–189. Normal variations in the curvature of the cervical spine, depending on head position in the same patient on the same day. Such variations should not necessarily be taken as evidence of posttraumatic muscle spasm.

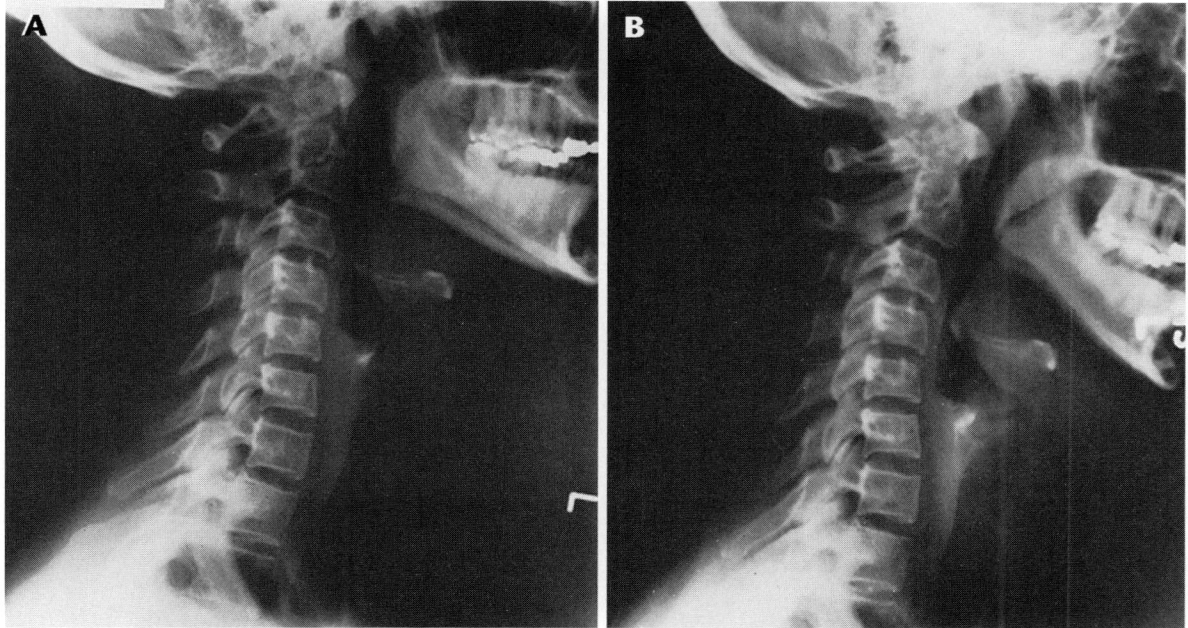

Figure 3–190. Normal cervical spine. **A,** Neutral position. **B,** Flexion. Note the striking, alteration in curvature that can be produced with only slight alteration in head position.

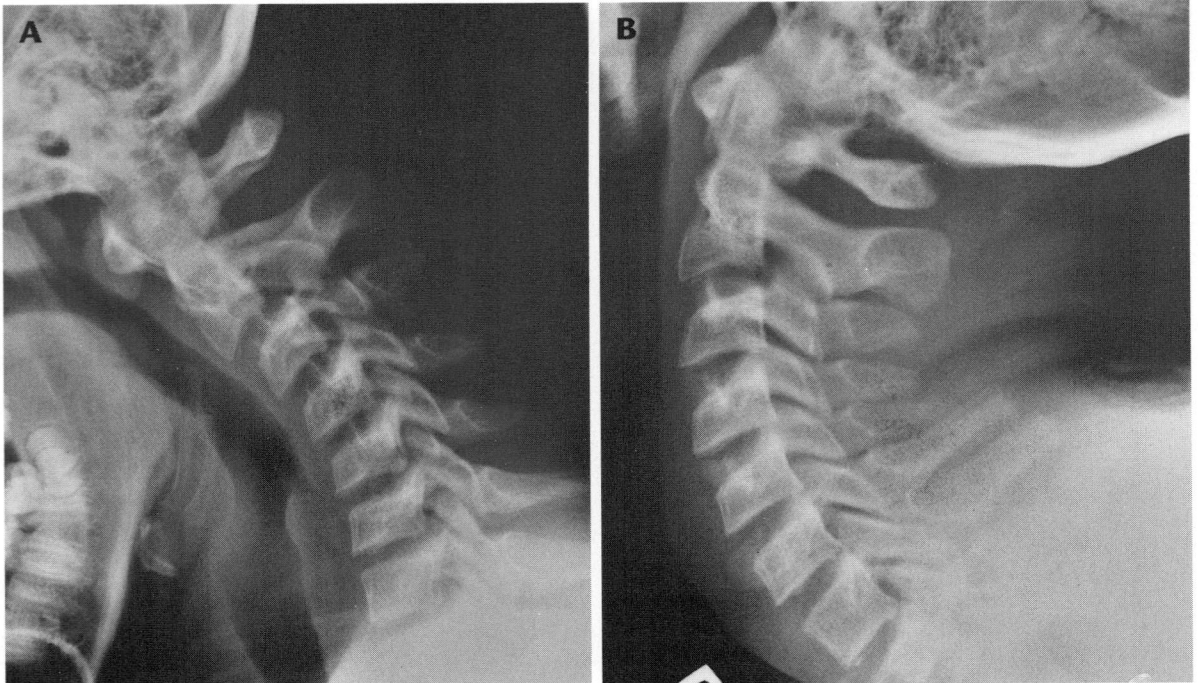

Figure 3–191. Marked physiologic subluxation of C2 on C3, C3 on C4, and C4 on C5 with flexion in a 13-year-old boy. Note that the spinolaminar line is intact. **A,** Flexion. **B,** Extension.

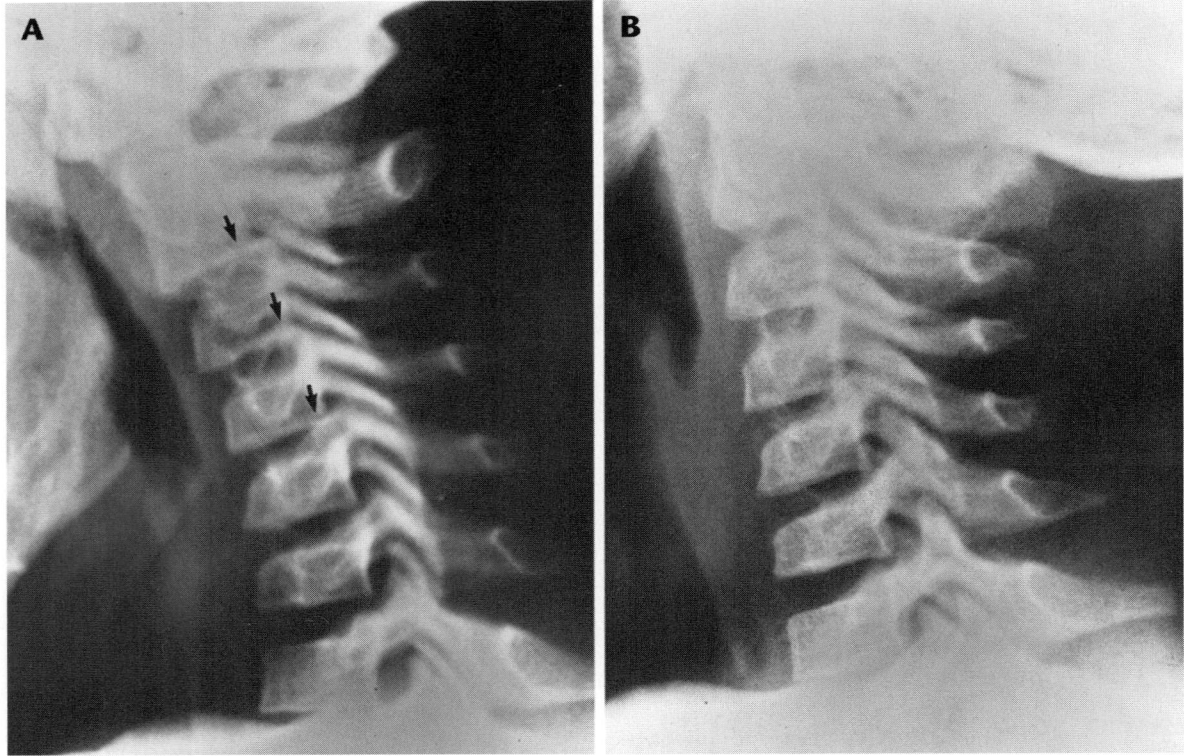

Figure 3–192. Physiologic subluxation may occur at multiple levels in flexion, particularly in children. **A,** Note the anterior subluxation of C2 on C3, C3 on C4, and C4 on C5 in a child. Posterior cervical line is intact. **B,** Normal alignment in neutral position. (Ref: Swischuk LE: The cervical spine in childhood. *Curr Probl Diagn Radiol* 13:10, 1984.

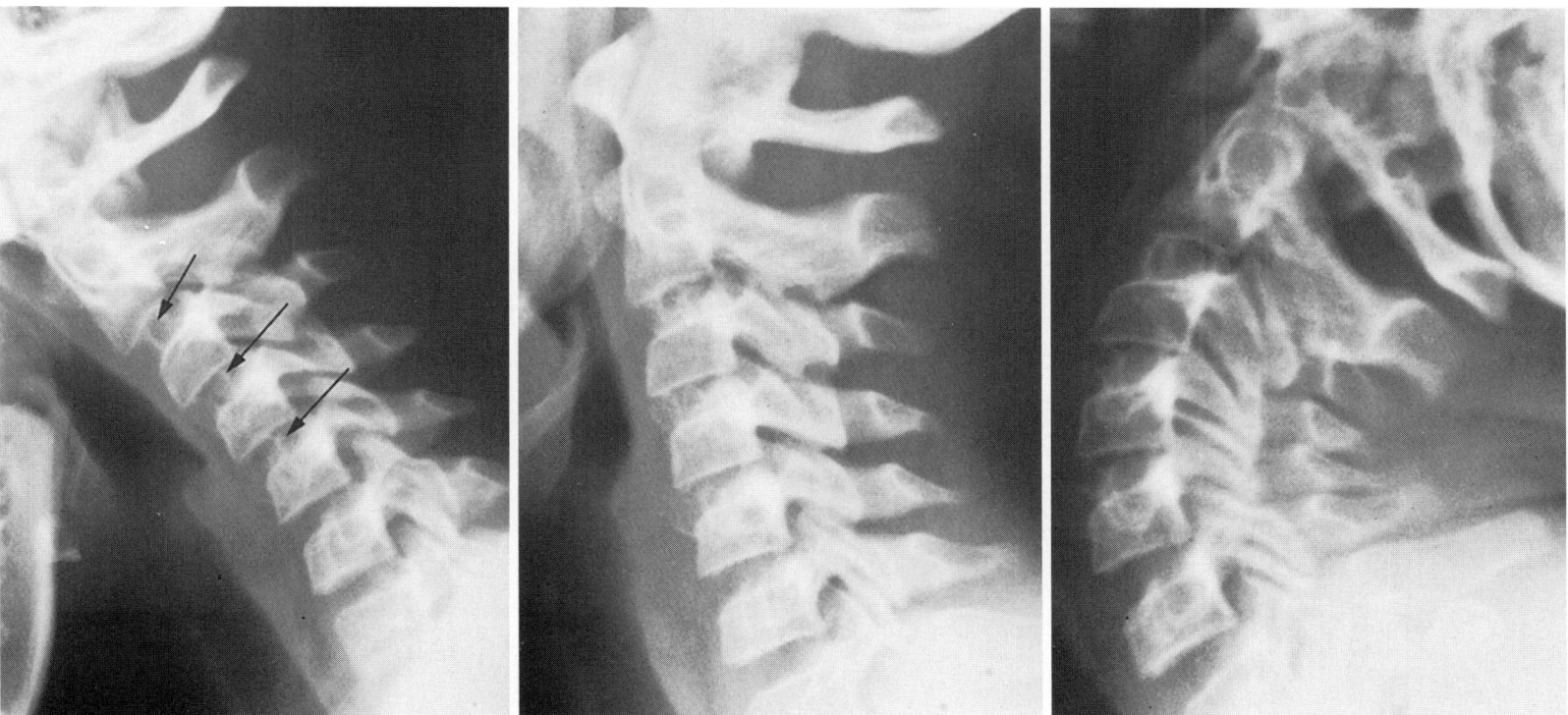

Figure 3–193. *Left,* Multiple physiologic subluxations on flexion in 9-year-old boy. *Center,* Neutral position. *Right,* Extension.

Figure 3–194. Physiologic subluxation of C2 on C3 and C3 on C4 in a 17-year-old boy on flexion.

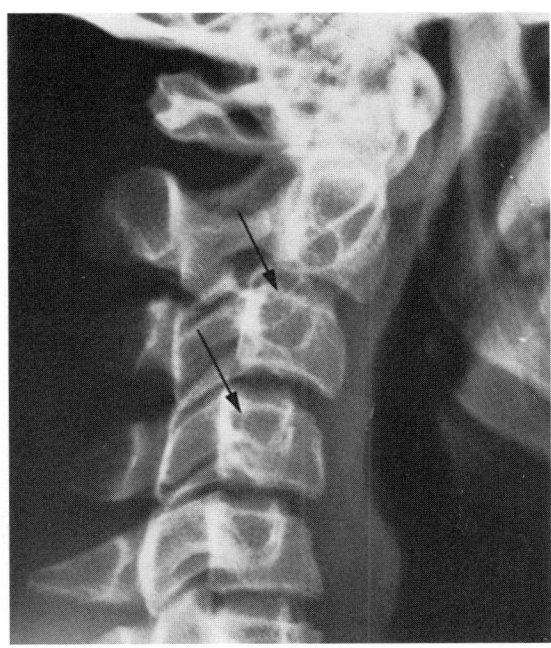

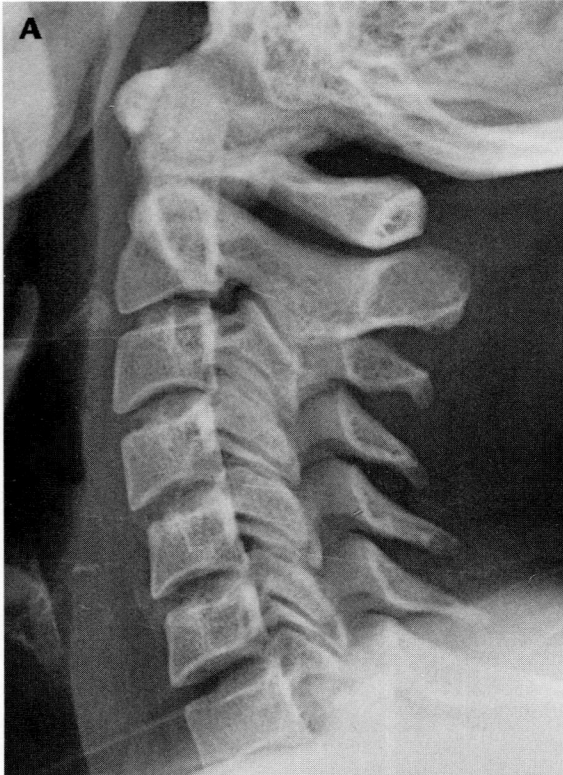

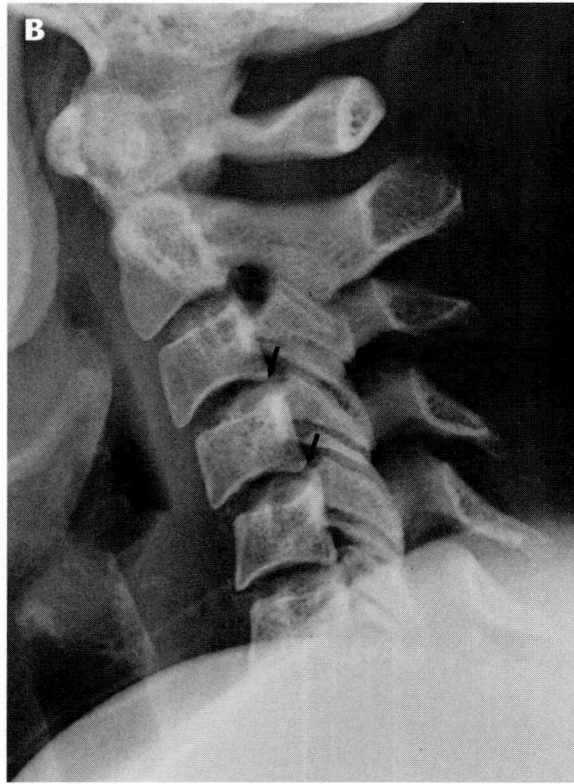

Figure 3–195. Physiologic subluxation of C2 on C3 and C3 on C4 in a 29-year-old pregnant woman, possibly related to relaxing hormone. **A,** Neutral position. **B,** Flexion.

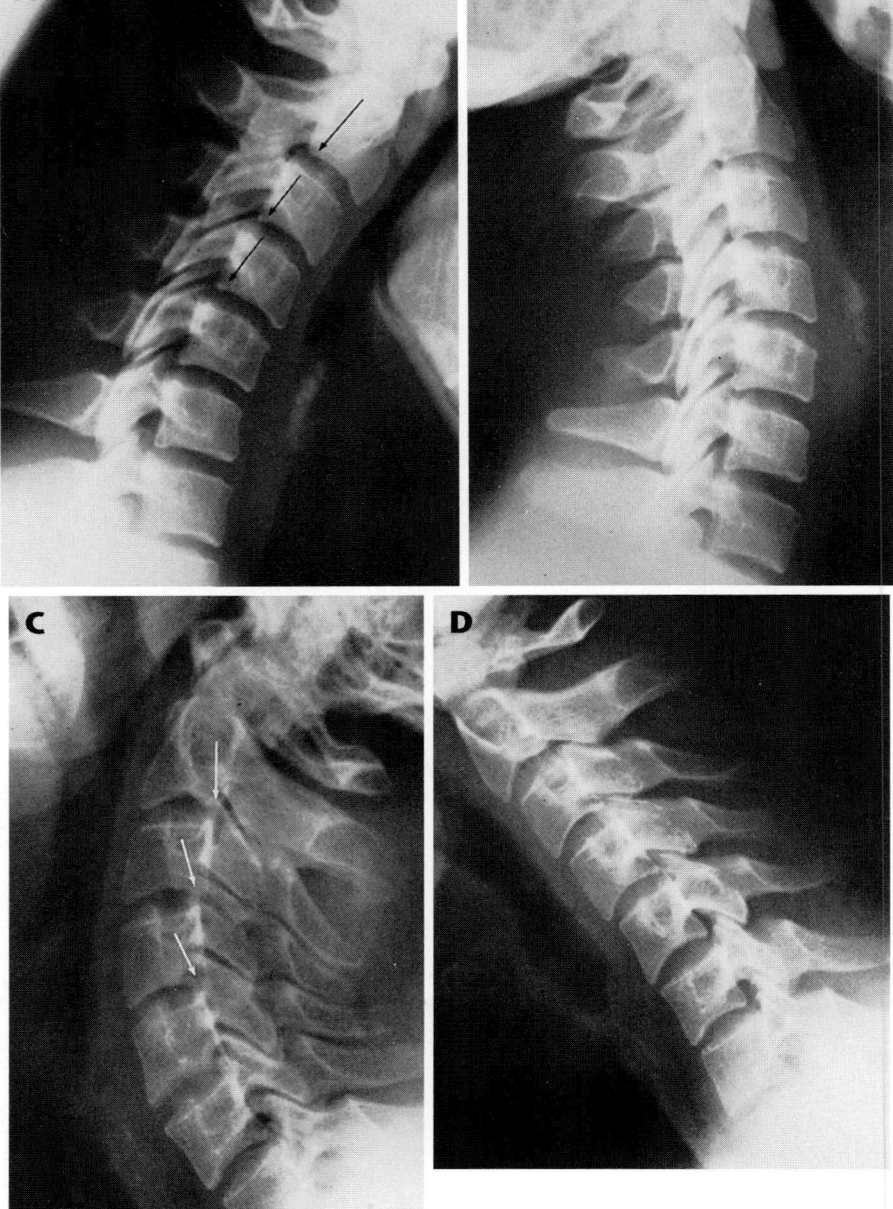

Figure 3–196. A and **B,** Physiologic anterior "slipping" of cervical vertebrae on flexion (**A**) and correction on extension (**B**). **C** and **D,** Physiologic posterior "slipping" of cervical vertebrae on extension (**C**) and correction on flexion (**D**). These minor degrees of "malalignment" with extremes of motion are not necessarily abnormal in themselves, particularly if the "slipping" occurs at multiple levels in continuity. (Ref: Scher AT: Anterior subluxation: An unstable position. *Am J Roentgenol* 133:275, 1979.)

Figure 3–197. A, An example of the simulated fracture of the posterior neural arch of C3, produced by rotation. **B,** Corrected position. No fracture is seen.

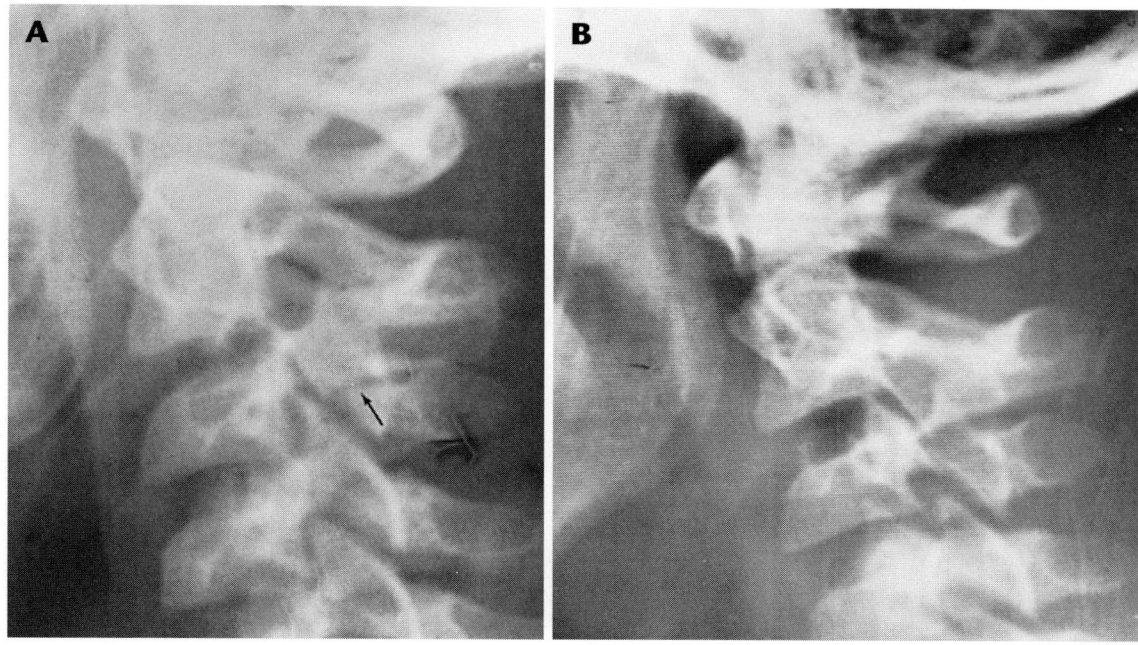

Figure 3–198. A, Simulated fracture of the posterior neural arch of C3, produced by rotation. **B,** Corrected position. No fracture is seen.

Figure 3–199. A, Simulated fracture of the neural arch of C3, produced by rotation. **B,** Repeat examination with correction of rotation shows restitution to normal appearance. Note also the absence of a lordotic curve in **A.** This is a common variation, especially between the ages of 8 and 16 years. (Ref: Cattell HS, Filtzer DL: Pseudosubluxation and other normal variations in the cervical spine in children. *J Bone Joint Surg* 47A:1295, 1965.)

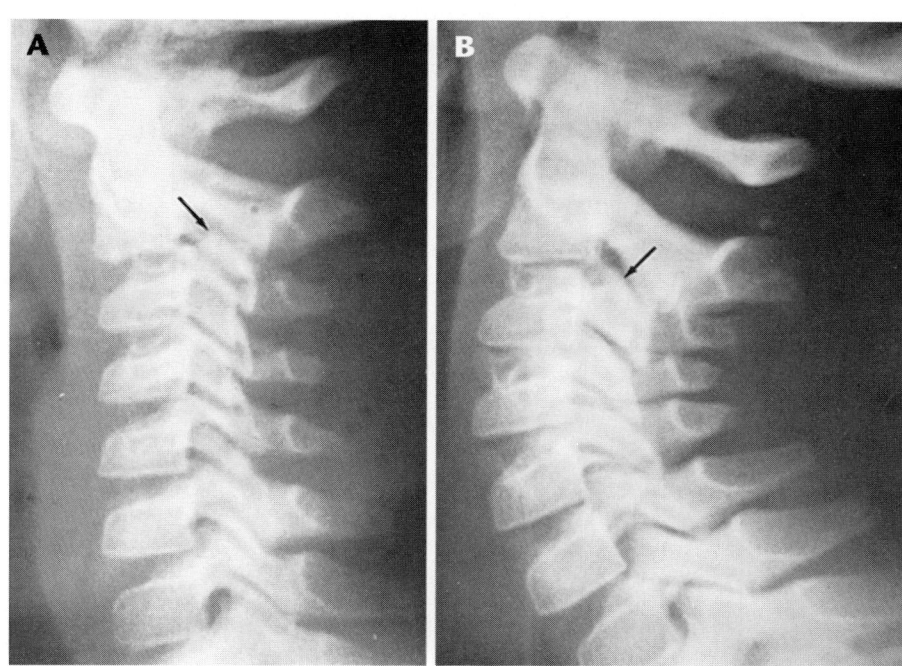

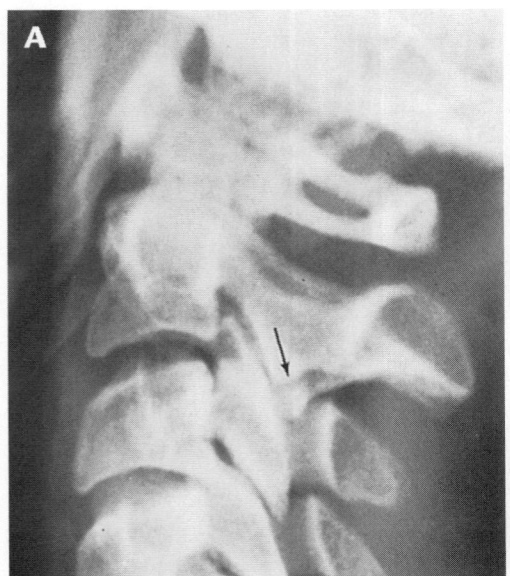 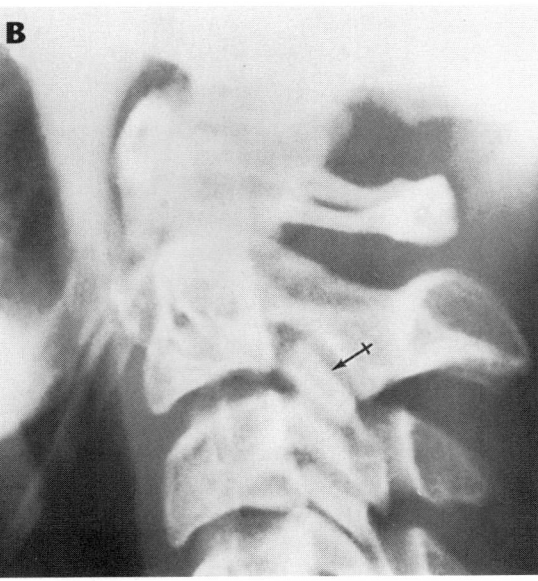

Figure 3–200. A, Pseudofracture of the neural arch of the type shown in Figure 3–198 (→). **B,** Repeat film shows disappearance of the pseudofracture shown in **A** and the appearance of the pseudofracture shown in the preceding figure (↦).

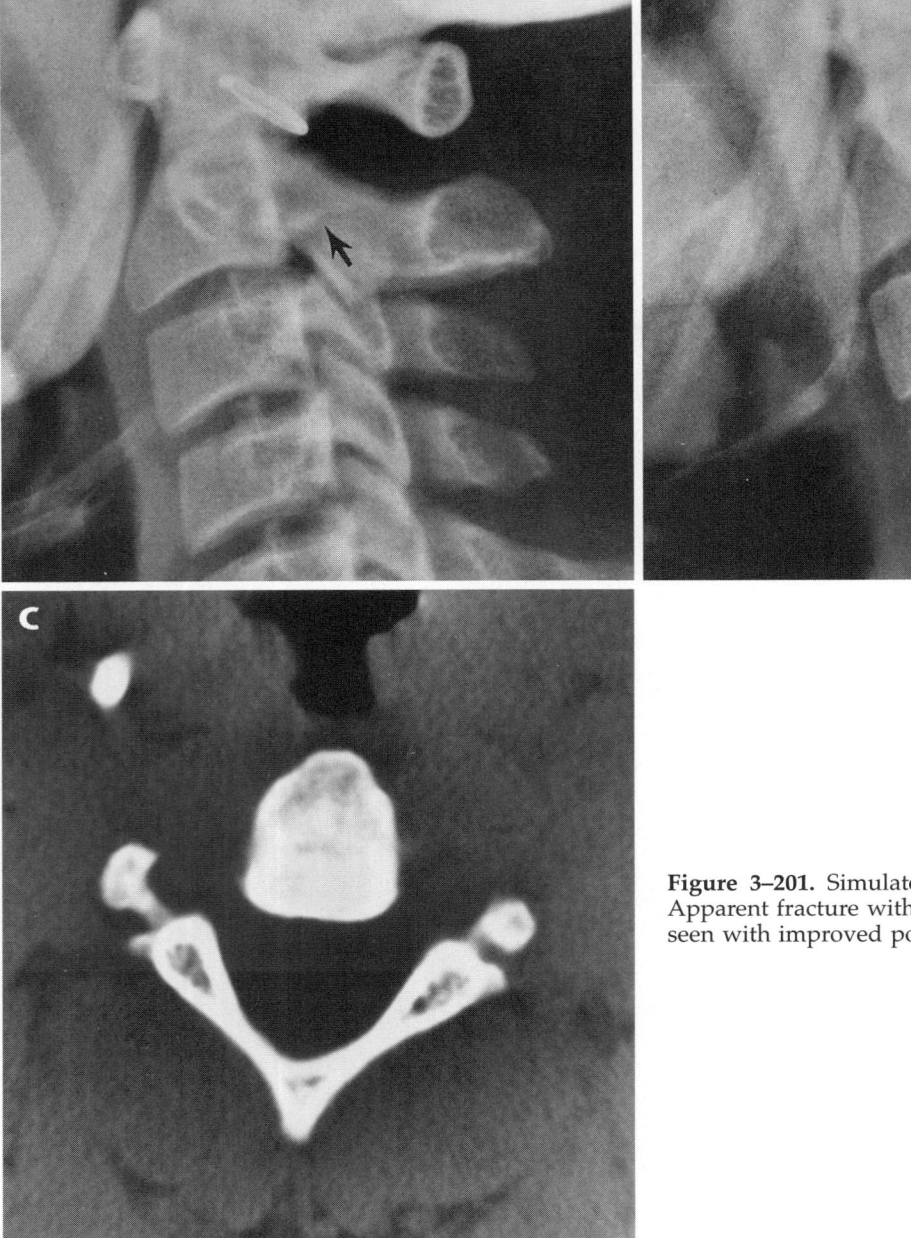

Figure 3–201. Simulated fracture of C2 produced by rotation. **A,** Apparent fracture with slight rotation. **B,** Suspected lesion not seen with improved positioning. **C,** CT shows no abnormality.

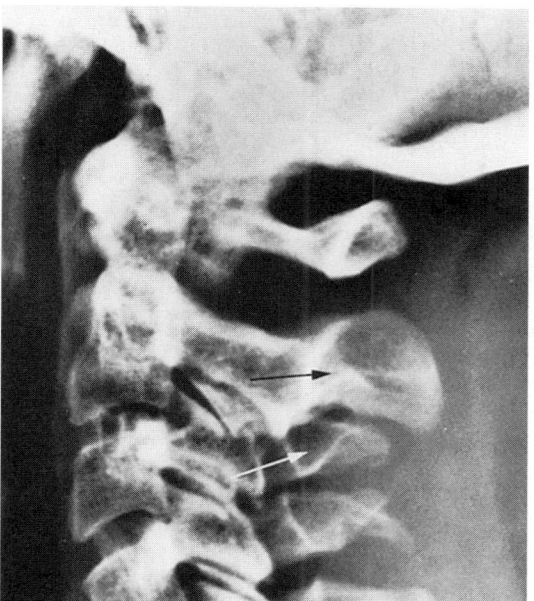

Figure 3–202. Backward "displacement" of the spinolaminal line at C2 is a normal variation in both children and adults and should not be mistaken for evidence of subluxation. (Ref: Kattan K: Backward "displacement" of the spinolaminal line at C2: A normal variation. *Am J Roentgenol* 129:289, 1977.)

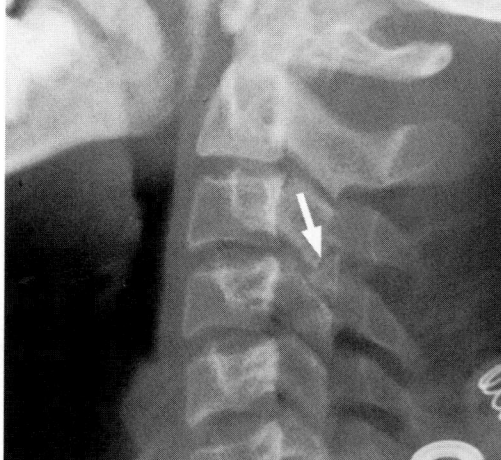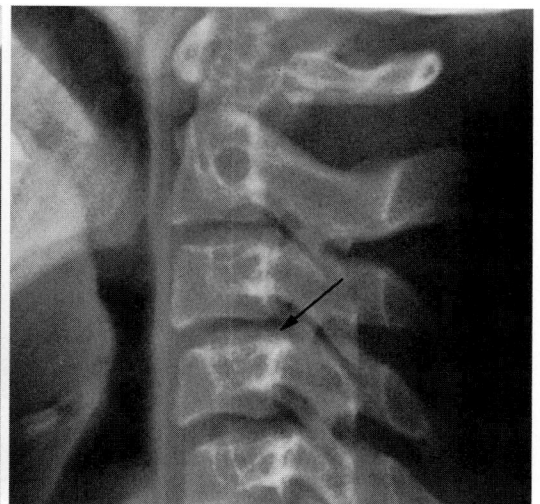

Figure 3–203. *Left,* pseudofracture of the inferior articulating process of C3. *Right,* true lateral shows that the pseudofracture is due to the overlapping shadows of the inferior articulating processes.

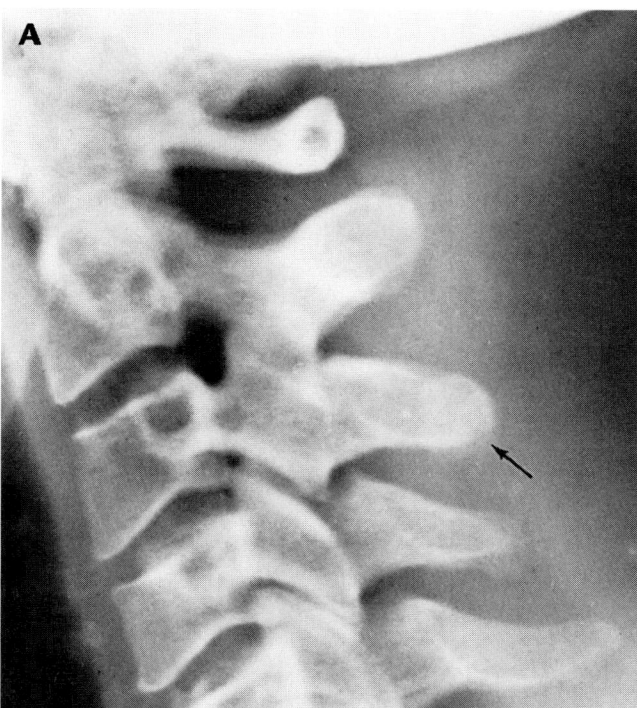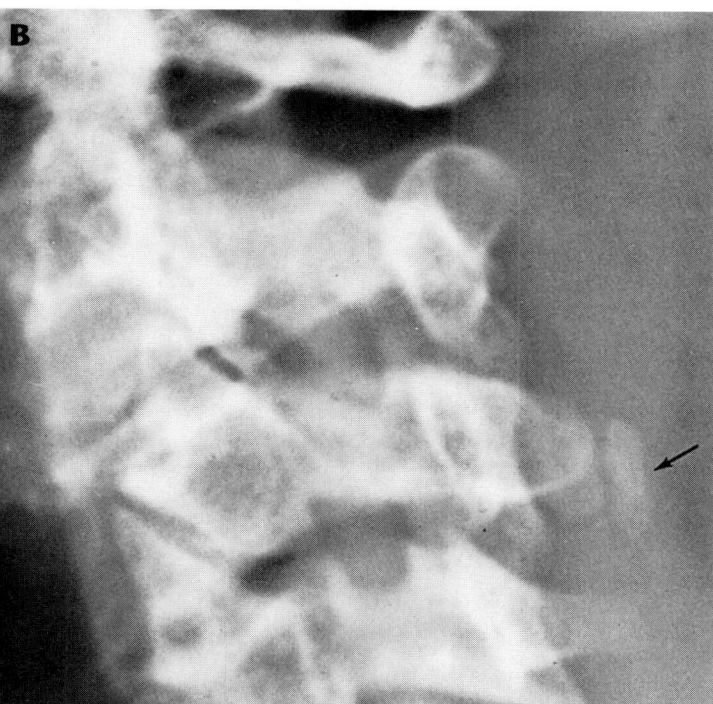

Figure 3–204. Accessory ossification centers at the tip of the spinous process of C3. **A,** Lateral projection. **B,** Oblique projection.

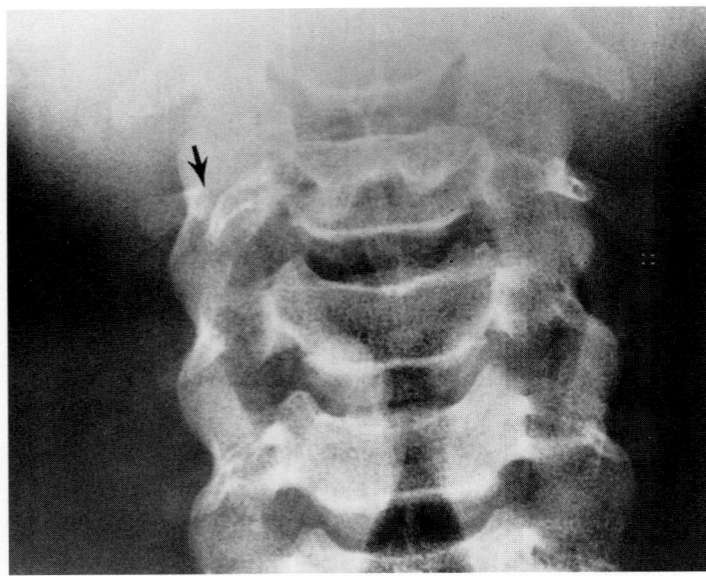

Figure 3–205. Ununited traverse process of C3.

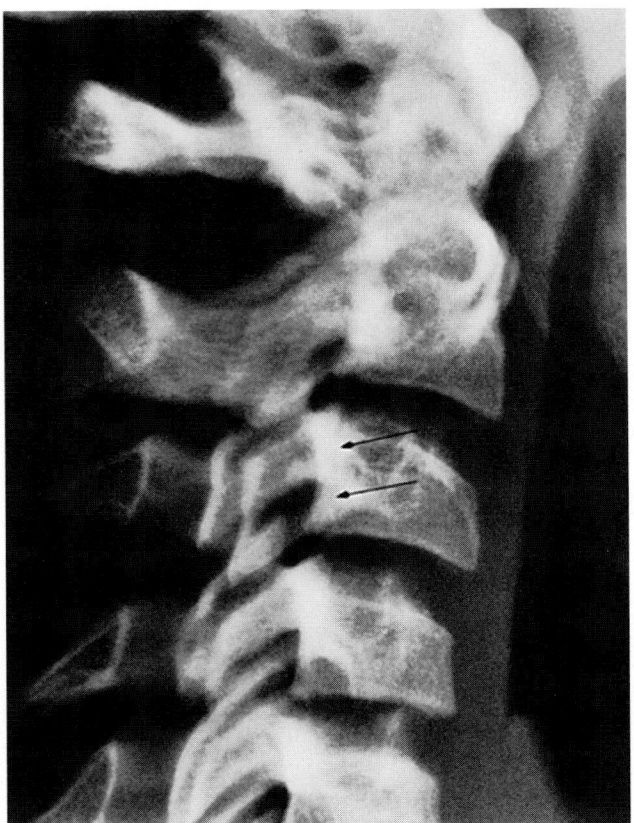

Figure 3–206. Simulated fracture of C3 caused by rotation.

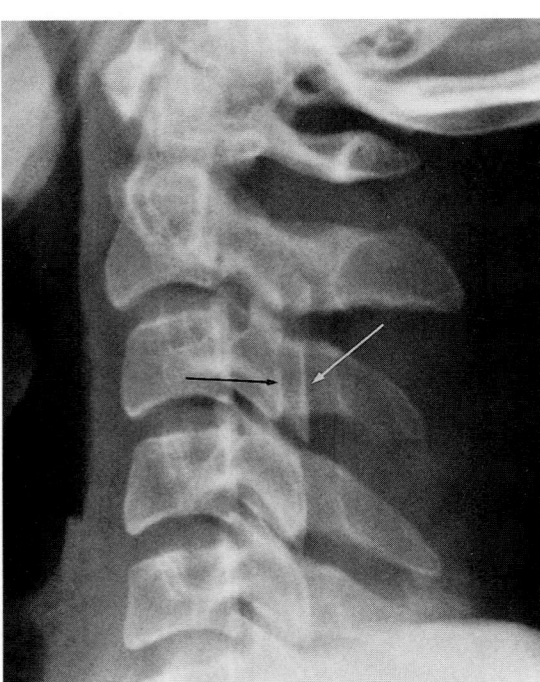

Figure 3–207. Simulated rotary dislocation of C3 resulting from positioning. Note that the facets are in proper relationship above and below.

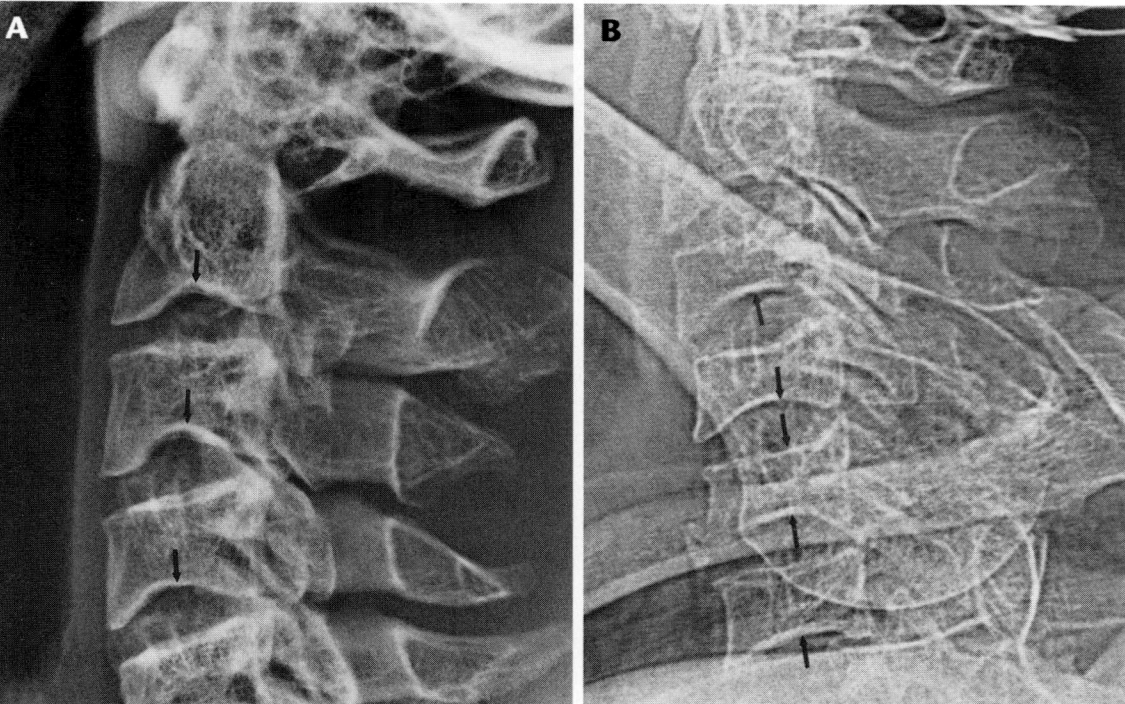

Figure 3–208. Two examples of notochordal remnants of the cervical spine. **A,** Notochordal remnants at C2–C4. **B,** Notochordal remnants at C2–C6.

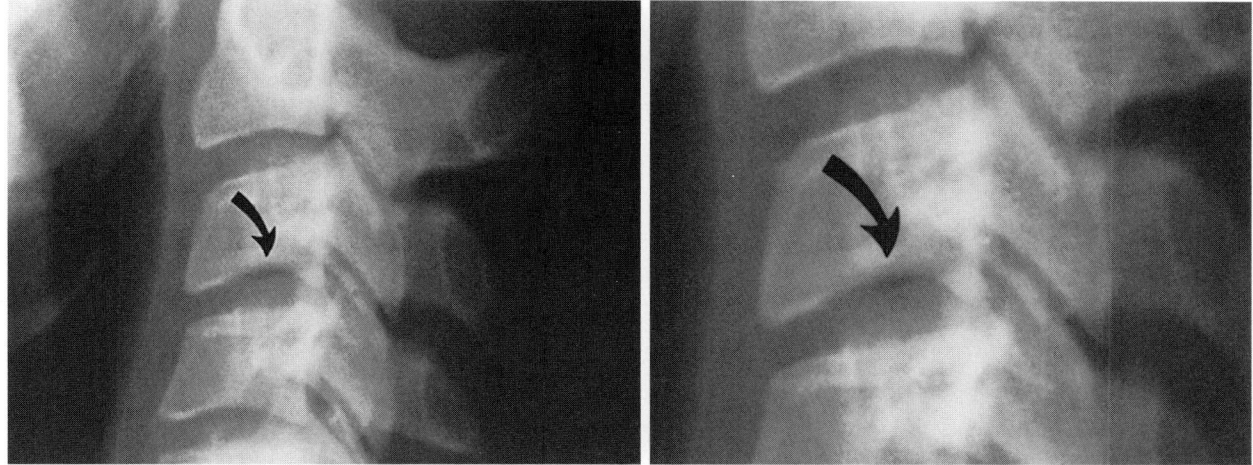

Figure 3–209. Two examples of the pseudovacuum of the cervical intervertebral disc related to the Mach band phenomenon. This should not be confused with a true vacuum sign of an intervertebral disc injury. (Ref: Daffner RH, Gehweiler JA: Pseudovacuum of the cervical intervertebral disc. *Am J Roentgenol* 137:737, 1981.)

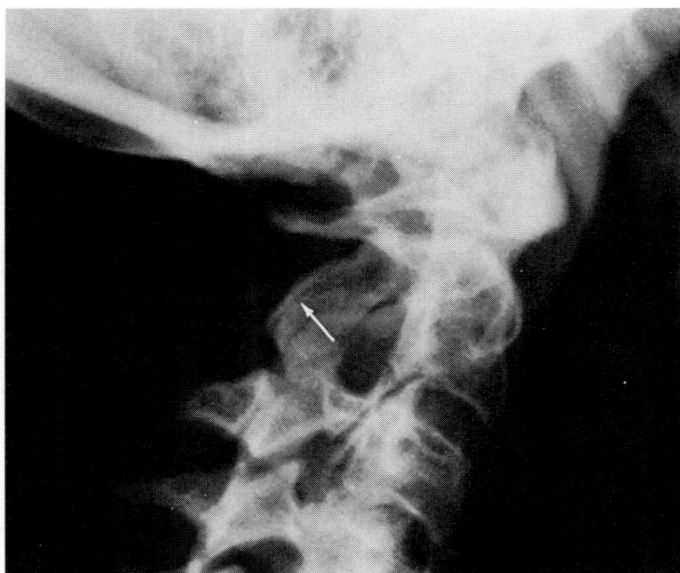

Figure 3–210. Absence of the posterior elements of C2.

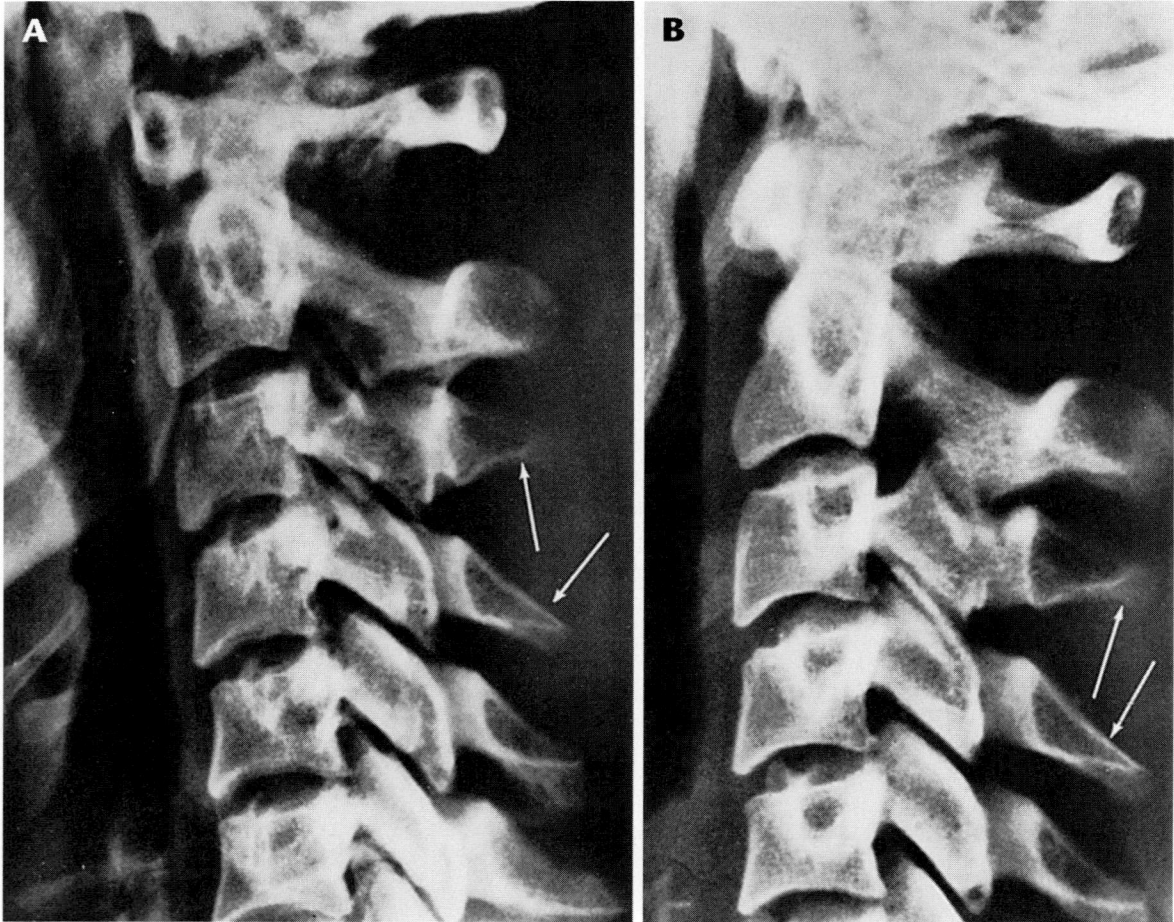

Figure 3–211. Wide spacing between spinous processes of C3 and C4, which might be misconstrued as evidence of flaring caused by soft tissue injury. Note the lack of change between flexion **(A)** and neutral position **(B)**. This pseudofanning occurs most commonly at C3–C4. (Ref: Bohrer SP: Pseudosigns in cervical spine trauma radiology. *Contemp Diagn Radiol* 12:13, 1989.

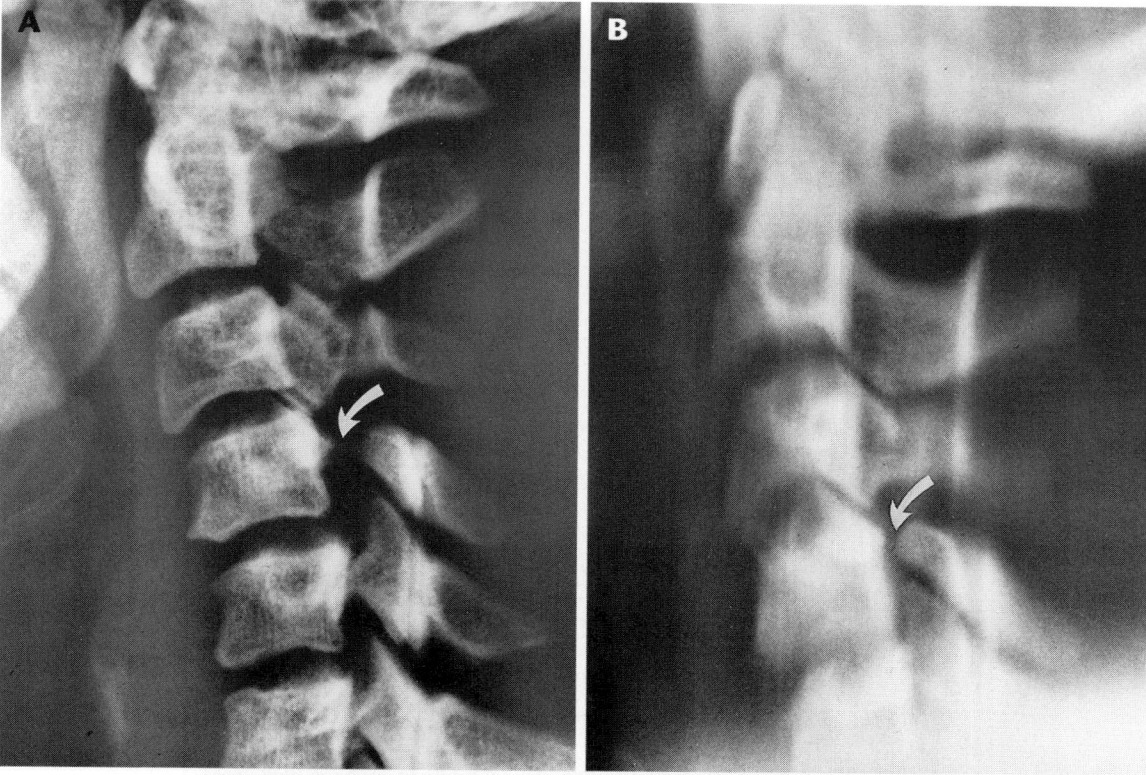

Figure 3–212. Spondylolysis of the neural arch of C4, simulating a fracture. **A,** Plain film, lateral. **B,** Tomogram. **C,** CT scan. (Ref: Forsberg DA: Cervical spondylolysis. *Am J Roentgenol* 154:751,1990.)

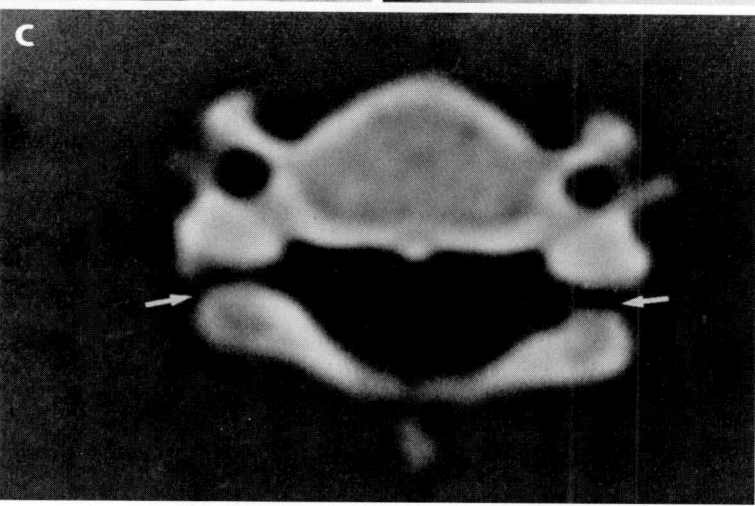

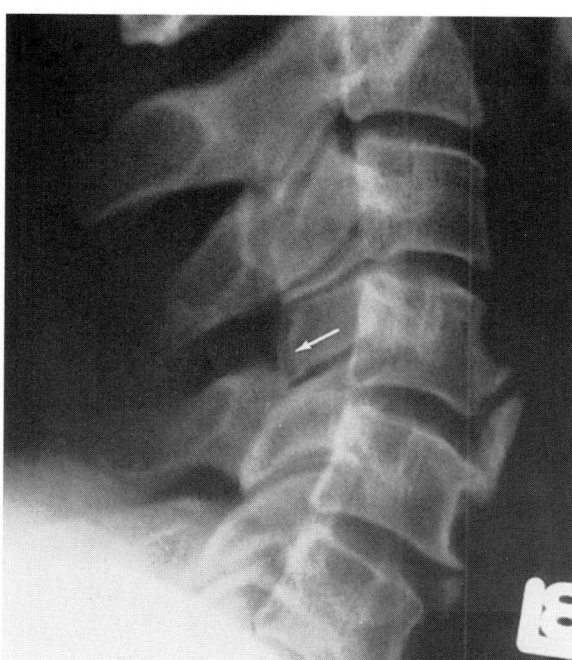

Figure 3–213. Absence of portions of the posterior arch of C4.

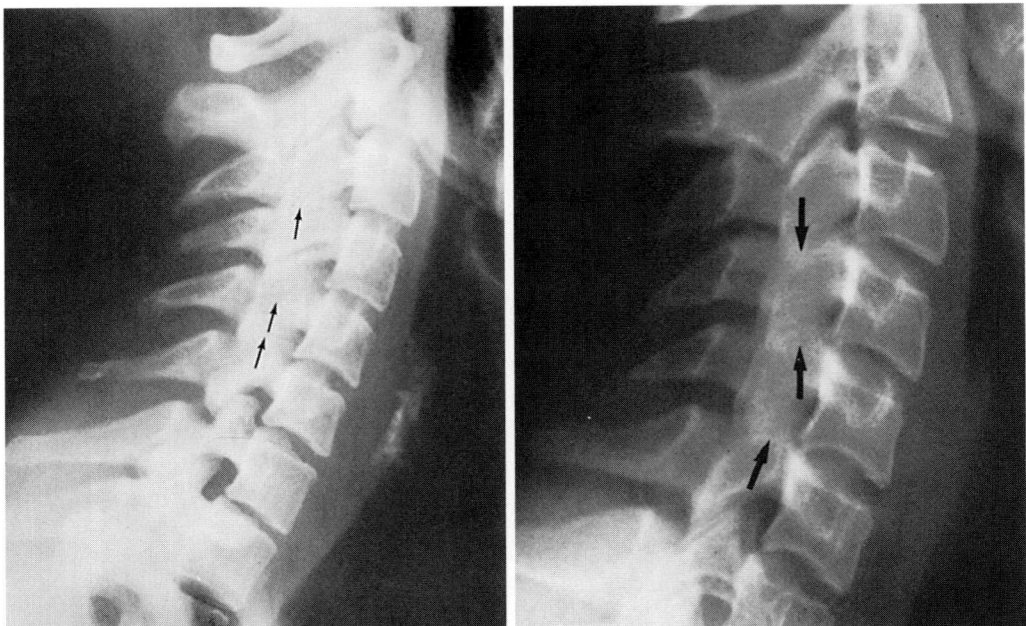

Figure 3–214. Two examples of simulated fusion of the apophyseal joints, produced by projection.

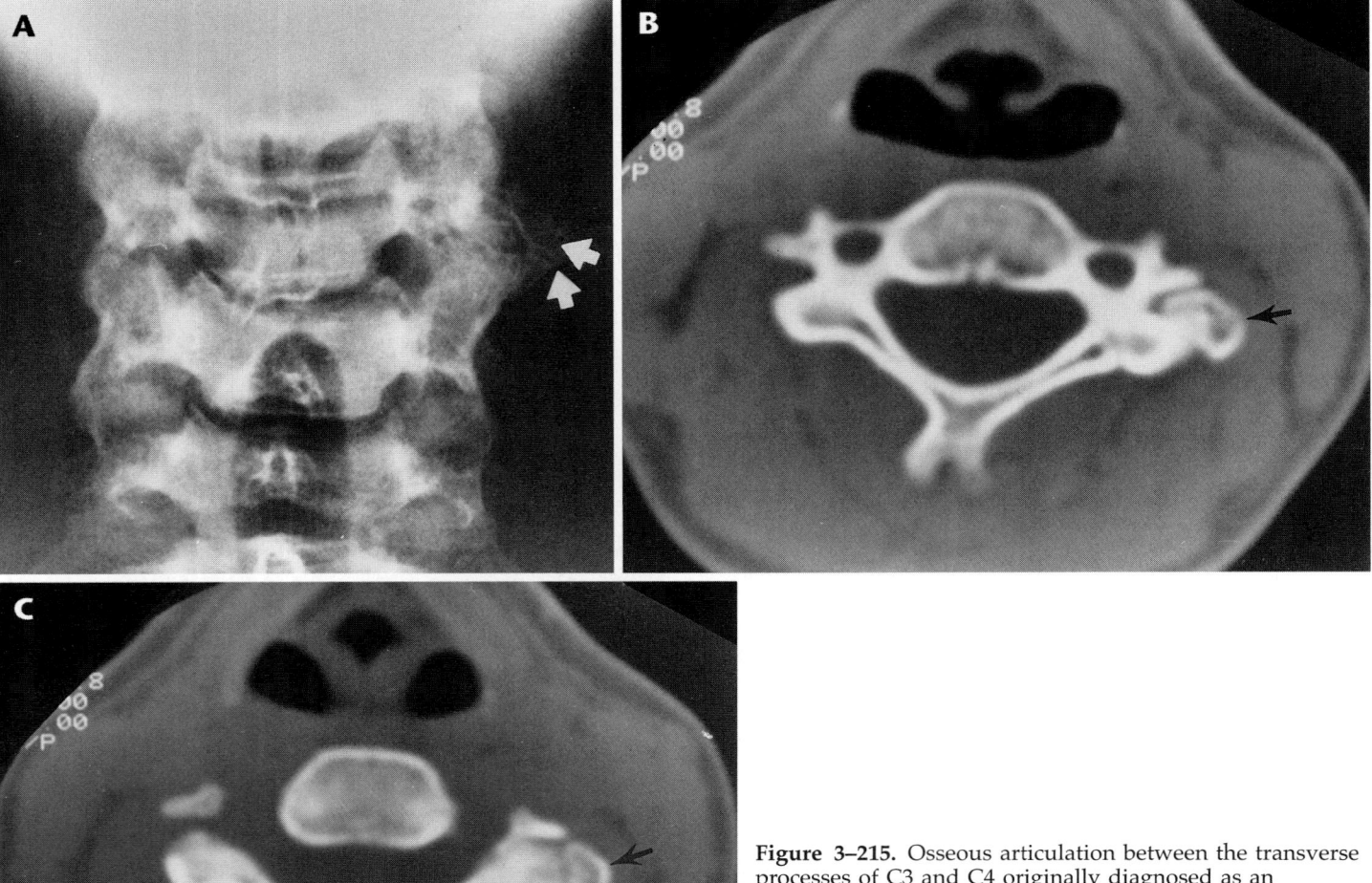

Figure 3–215. Osseous articulation between the transverse processes of C3 and C4 originally diagnosed as an osteochondroma. **A,** Anteroposterior view. **B,** CT of C3; **C,** CT of C4.

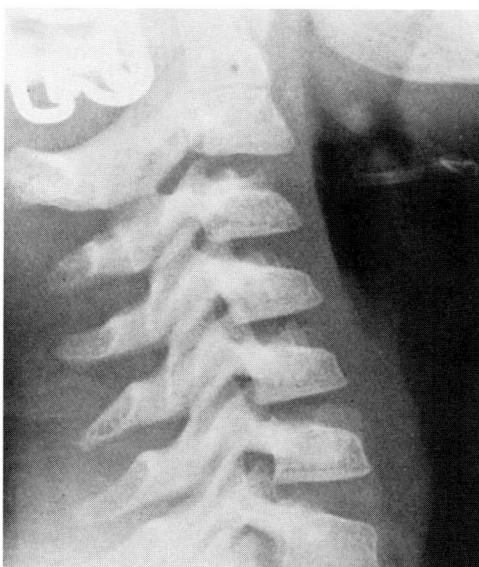

Figure 3–216. Normal wedge shape of juvenile cervical vertebral bodies, which should not be confused with compression fracture.

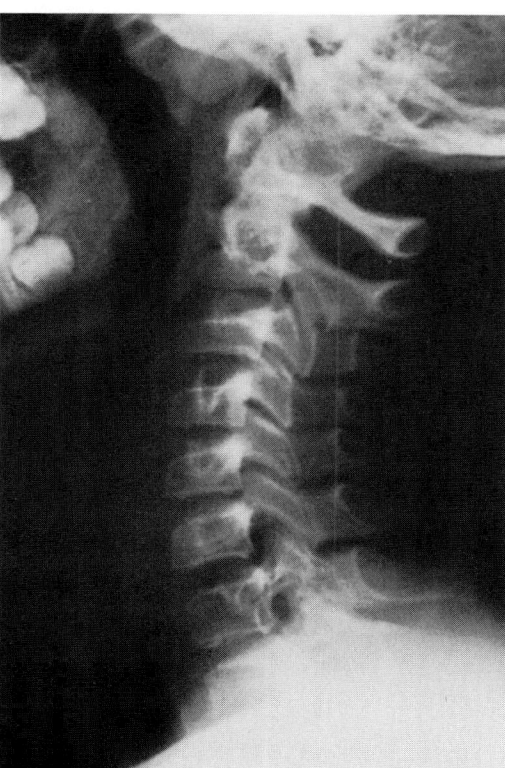

Figure 3–217. Wedge-shaped vertebral bodies in a 13-year-old boy. Note particularly the marked wedging of C3, mistaken for a compression fracture (Ref: Swischuk LE et al: Wedging of C3 in infants and children: Usually a normal finding and not a fracture. *Radiology* 188:523–526, 1993.)

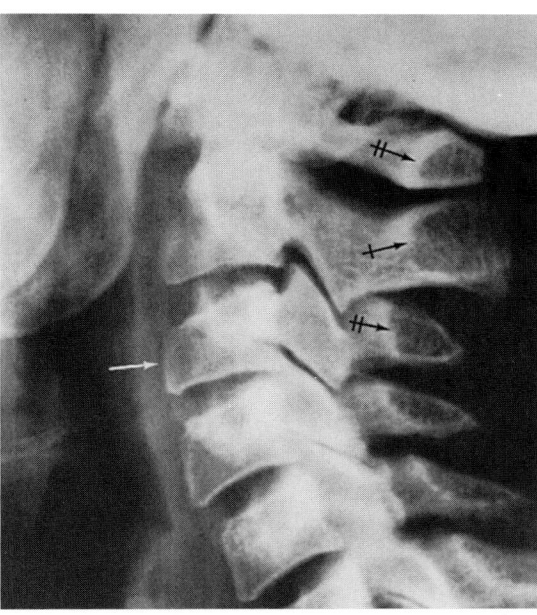

Figure 3–218. Normal retention of wedged configuration of C3 in a 54-year-old woman. Note also that the base of the spinous process of C2 (⟶) lies slightly posterior to that of C1 and C3 (⫽⟶). This is a normal variation that may be seen in children as well and should not be mistaken for evidence of subluxation. (Ref: Kattan KR: Backward "displacement" of the spinolaminal line at C2: A normal variation. *Am J Roentgenol* 129:289, 1977.)

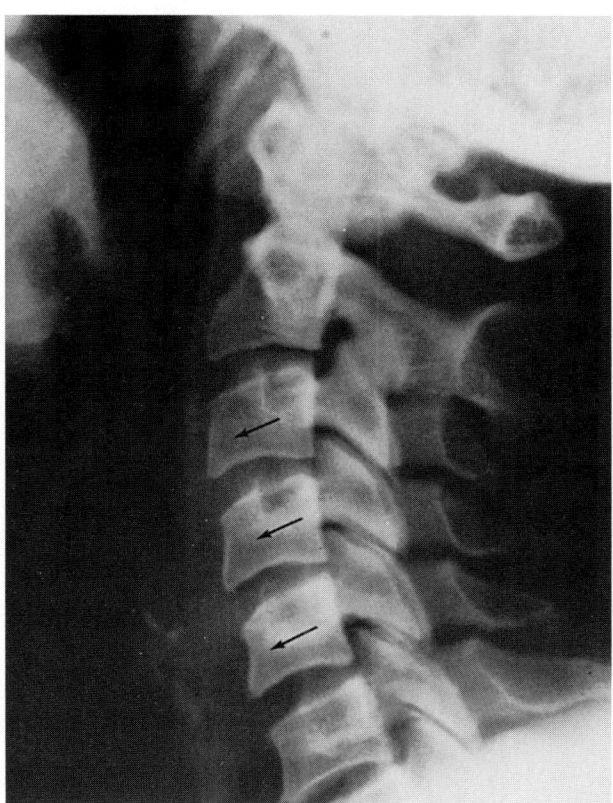

Figure 3–219. Normal retention of wedged configuration of C3, C4, and C5 in an adult.

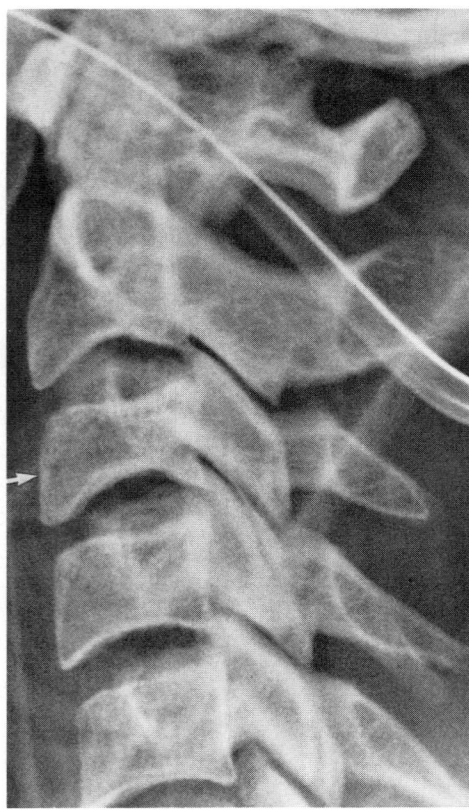

Figure 3–220. Unusual configuration of C3. Tomography showed no evidence of a fracture.

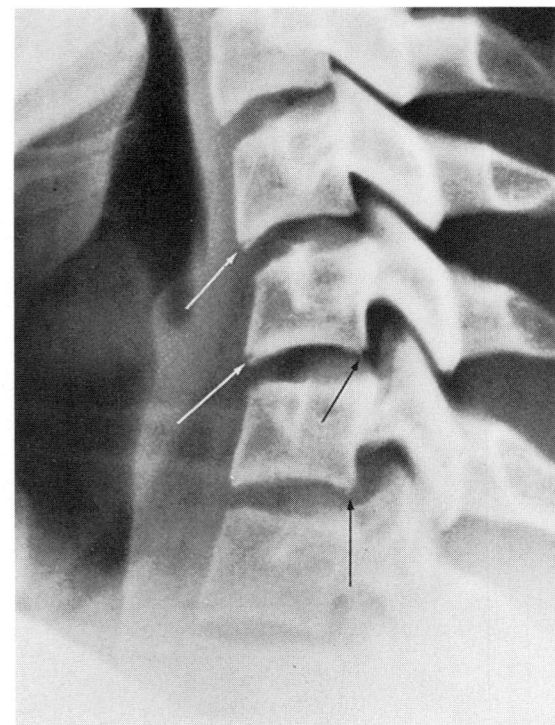

Figure 3–221. Anterior and posterior ring apophyses of the vertebrae. (Ref: Anni G, Hudson JM: Posterior ring apophyses of the cervical spine. *Am J Roentgenol* 139:383, 1982.)

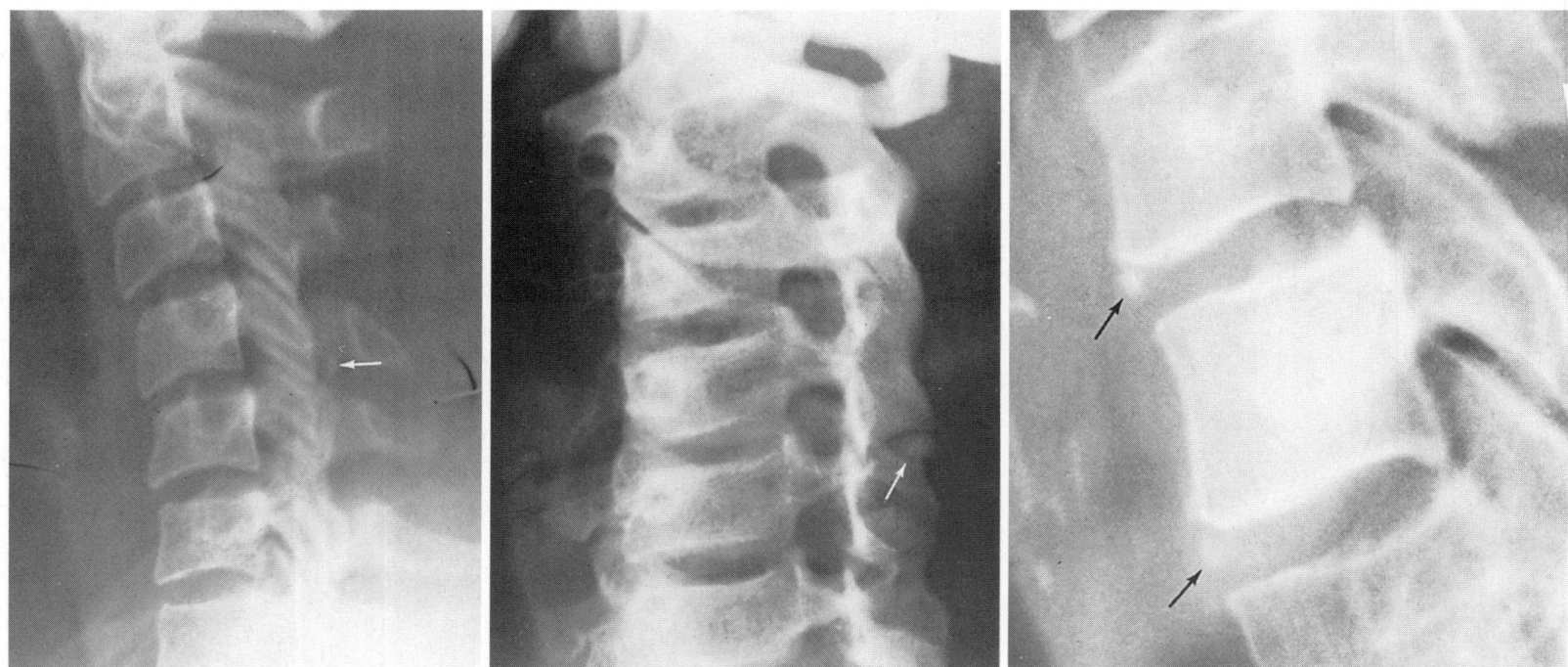

Figure 3–222. Ununited ossification centers at the inferior articular process of C4 (*left* and *center*). Ununited ossification centers of the fifth and sixth cervical vertebrae, which simulate fracture (limbus vertebrae) (*right*).

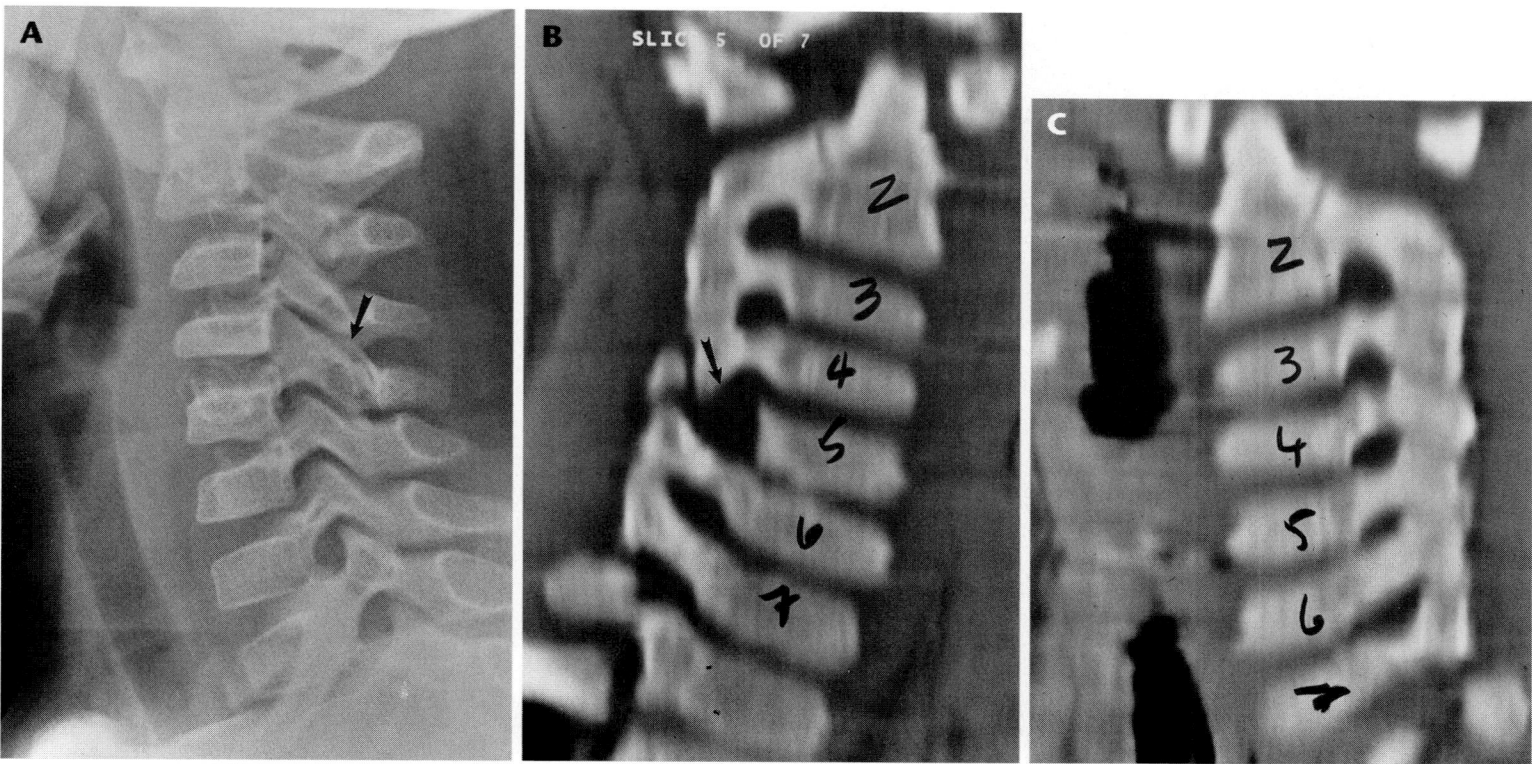

Figure 3–223. Simulated jumped facet at C4 produced by absent pedicle on the right. **A,** Lateral projection. **B,** Reformatted CT showing absent pedicle. **C,** Reformatted CT of opposite side.

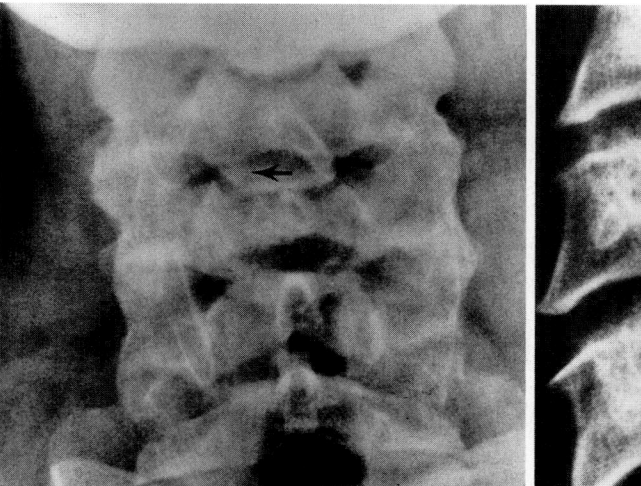
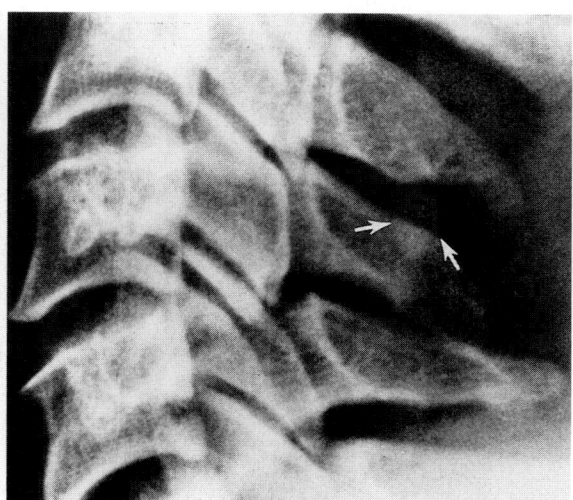

Figure 3–224. Bifid spinous process of C4 with failure of union of the right limb.

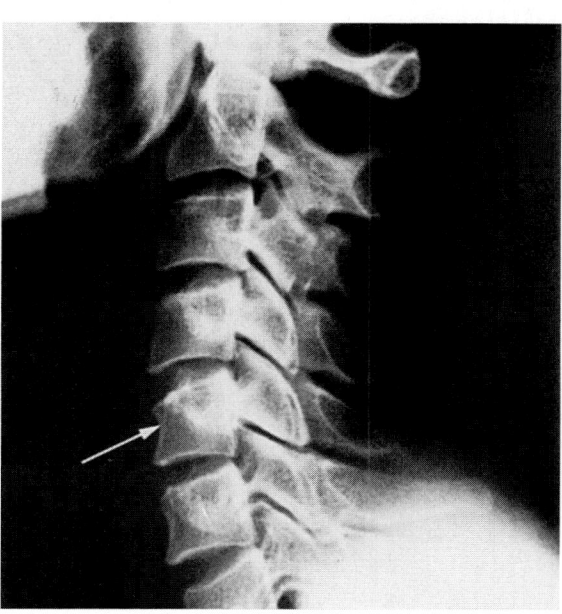

Figure 3–225. Normal wedged appearance of C5 in a 33-year-old man that should not be mistaken for a compression fracture. Note the absence of condensation of bone or buckling of the anterior cortex. (Refs: Kattan K, Pais MJ: Some borderlands of the cervical spine. *Skeletal Radiol* 8:1, 1982; Kim KS et al: Pitfalls in plain film diagnosis of cervical spine injuries: False positive interpretation. *Surg Neurol* 25:381, 1986.)

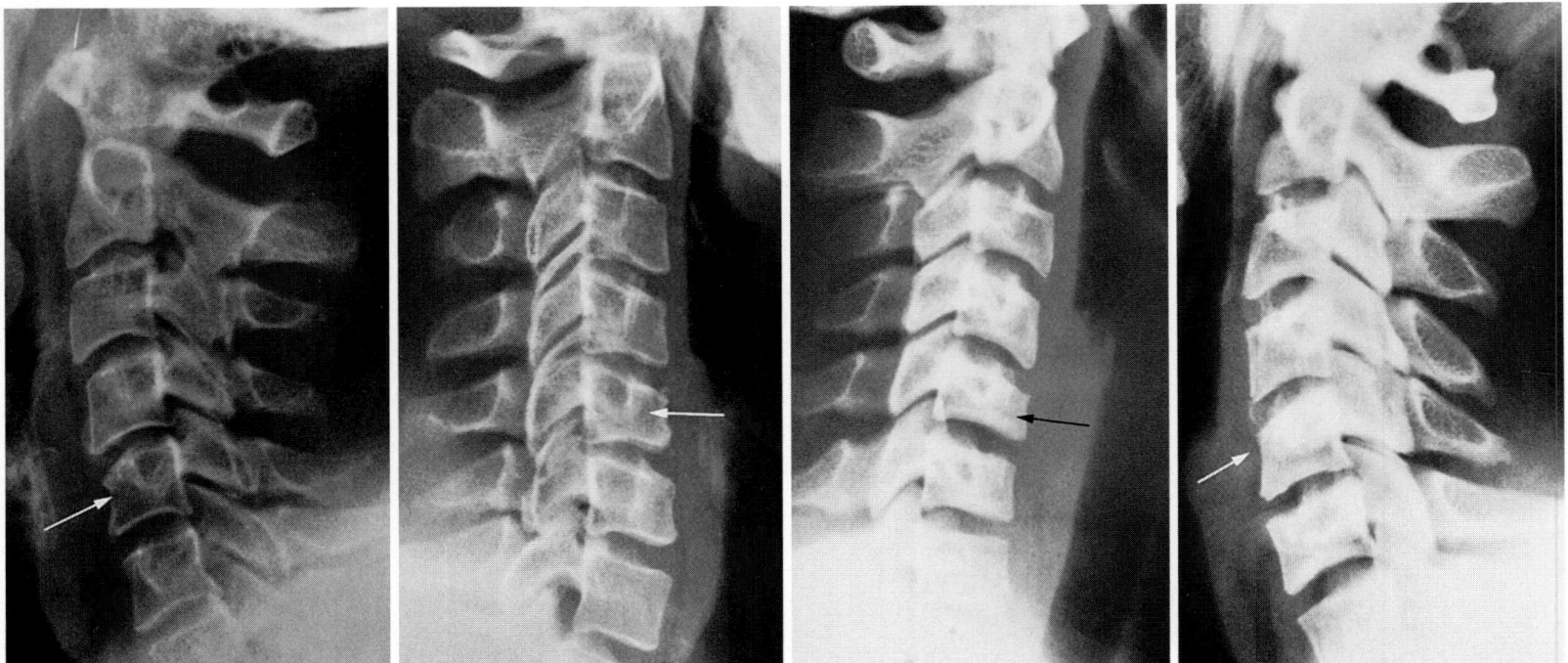

Figure 3–226. Four additional examples of unusual configurations of C5 that might be misconstrued as evidence of trauma.

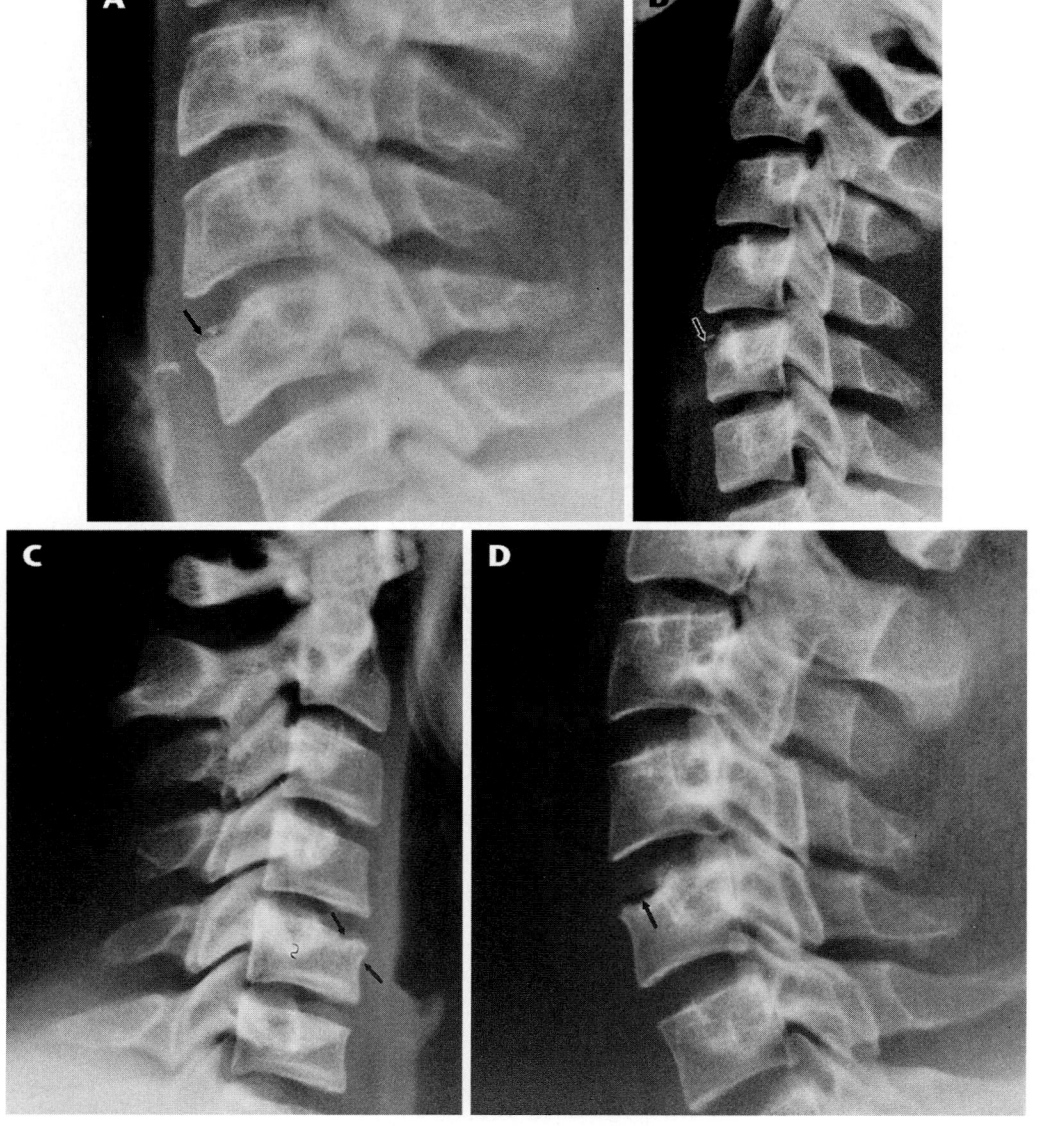

Figure 3–227. A–D, Four examples of simulated fractures of C5 in young patients without symptoms in this location, caused by Schmorl's nodes. Note the gas in the anterior aspect of the disc in **D**. It is possible that these anterior disc herniations may produce the wedged configuration of C5 in adults illustrated in the preceding two figures. (Ref: Paajanen H et al: Disc degeneration in disease. *Skeletal Radiol* 18:523, 1989.)

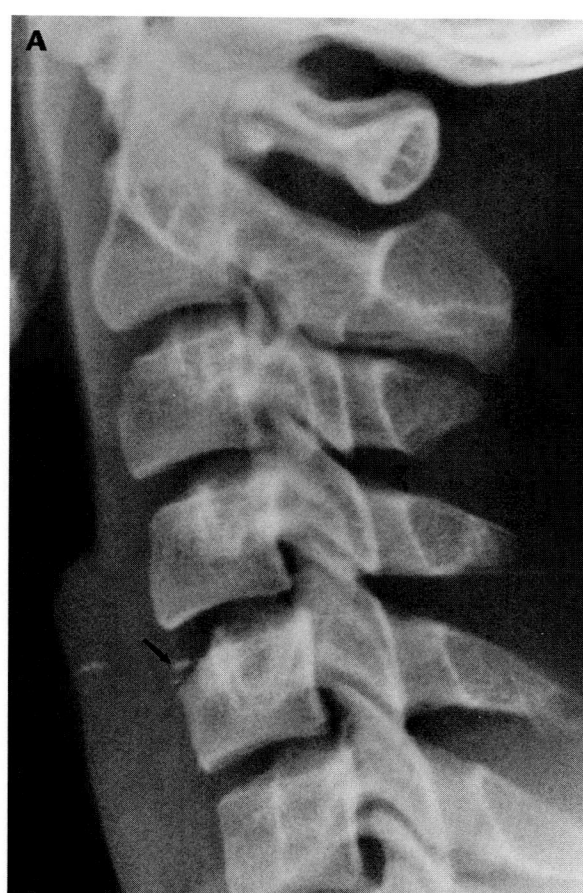

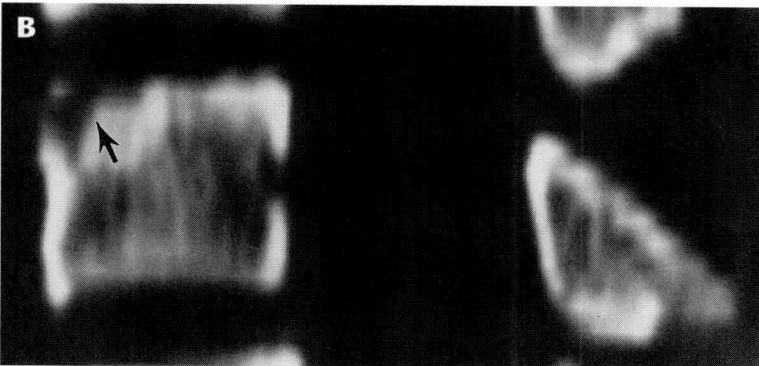

Figure 3–228. A, B, The same entity as in Figure 3–227 demonstrated by reformatted CT.

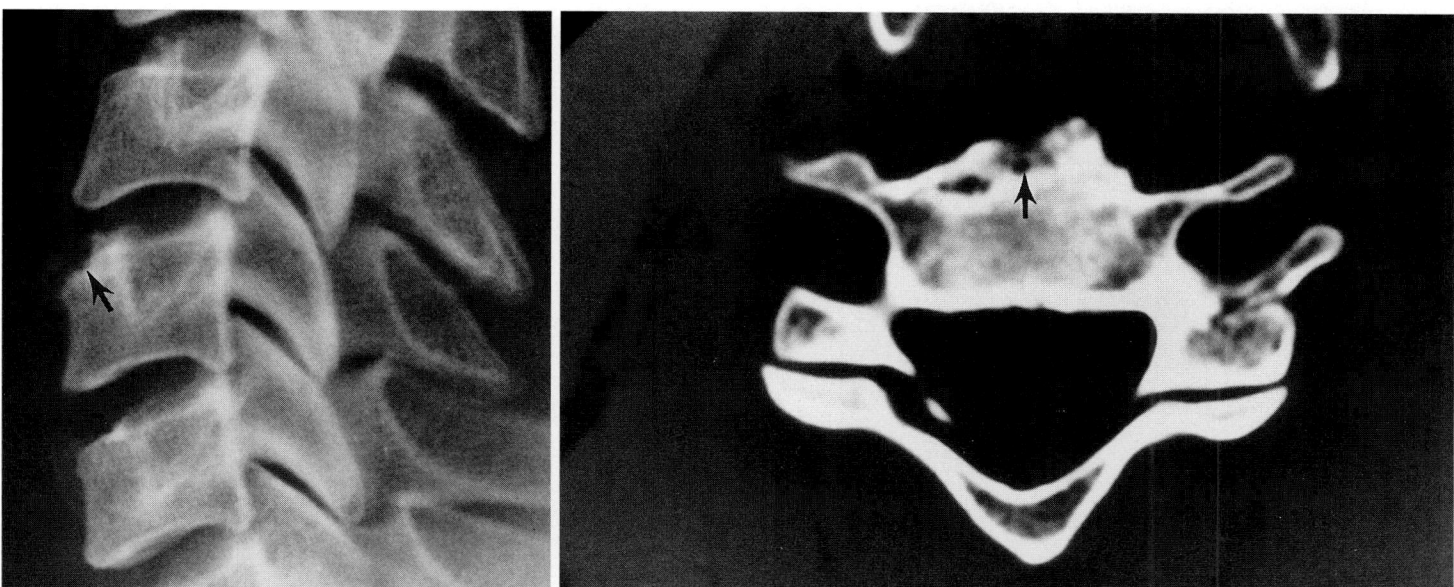

Figure 3–229. The same entity as the preceding figure with axial CT demonstration.

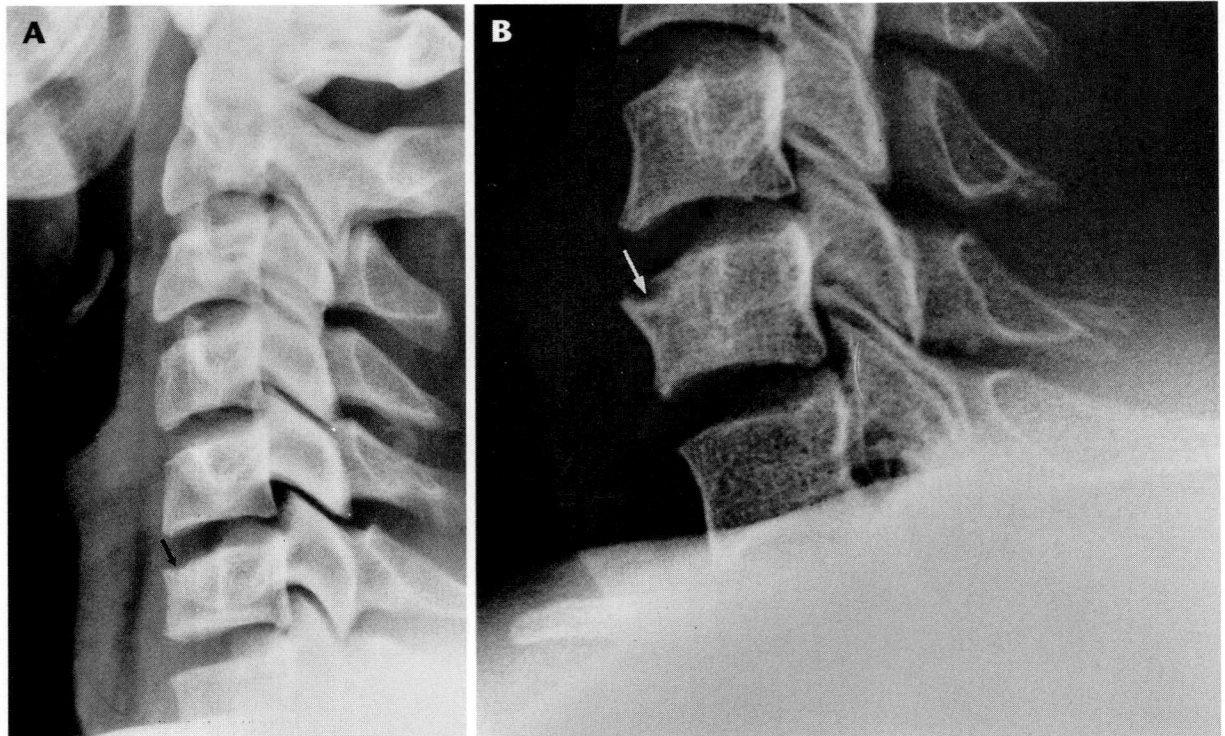

Figure 3–230. A, B, Contour defects at C6 similar to those of Figures 3–226 through 3–229.

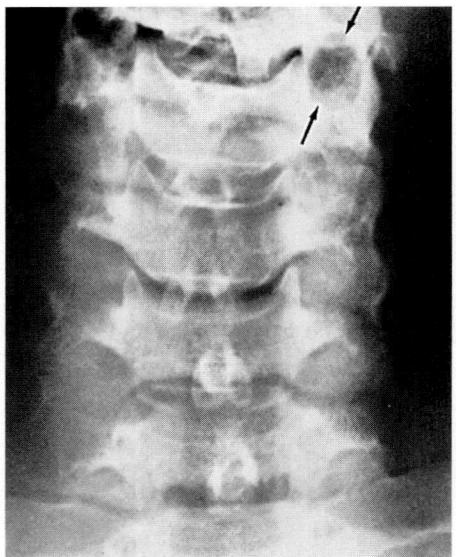

Figure 3–231. Simulated destructive lesion of the third and fourth cervical vertebrae, produced by slight rotation at the time of filming.

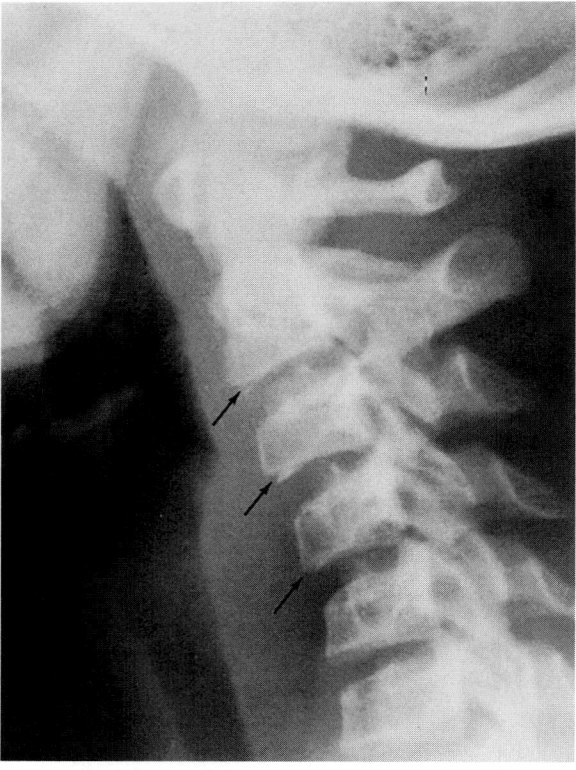

Figure 2–232. The normal secondary ossification centers of the vertebrae in a 14-year-old boy.

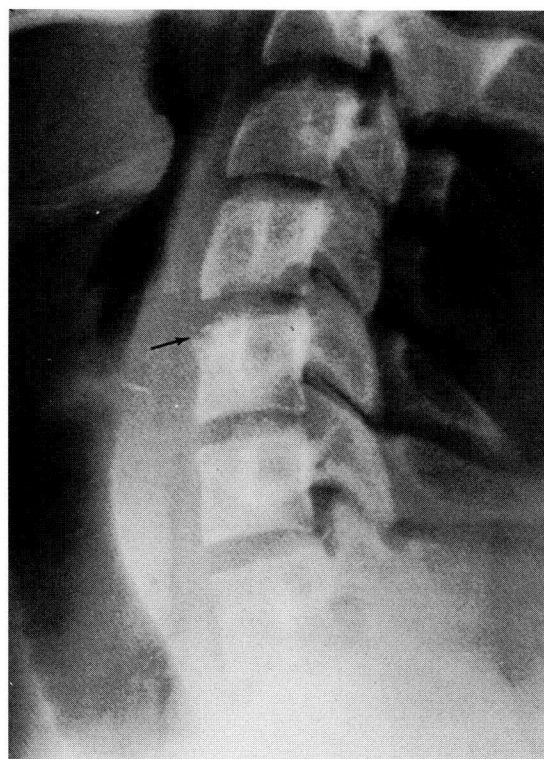

Figure 3–233. Closing secondary ossification centers in a 16-year-old boy.

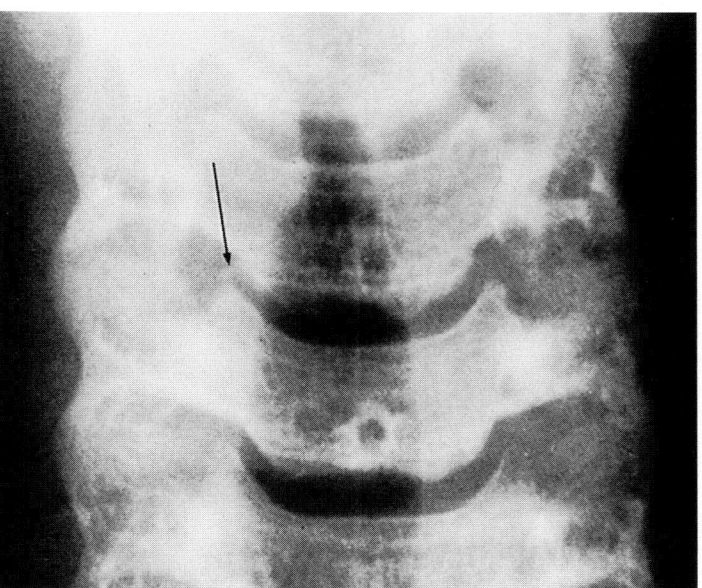

Figure 3–234. Unfused uncinate apophysis, which might be mistaken for a fracture. (Ref: Shaft RE et al: Lateral hyperflexion injuries of the cervical spine. *Skeletal Radiol* 3:73, 1978.)

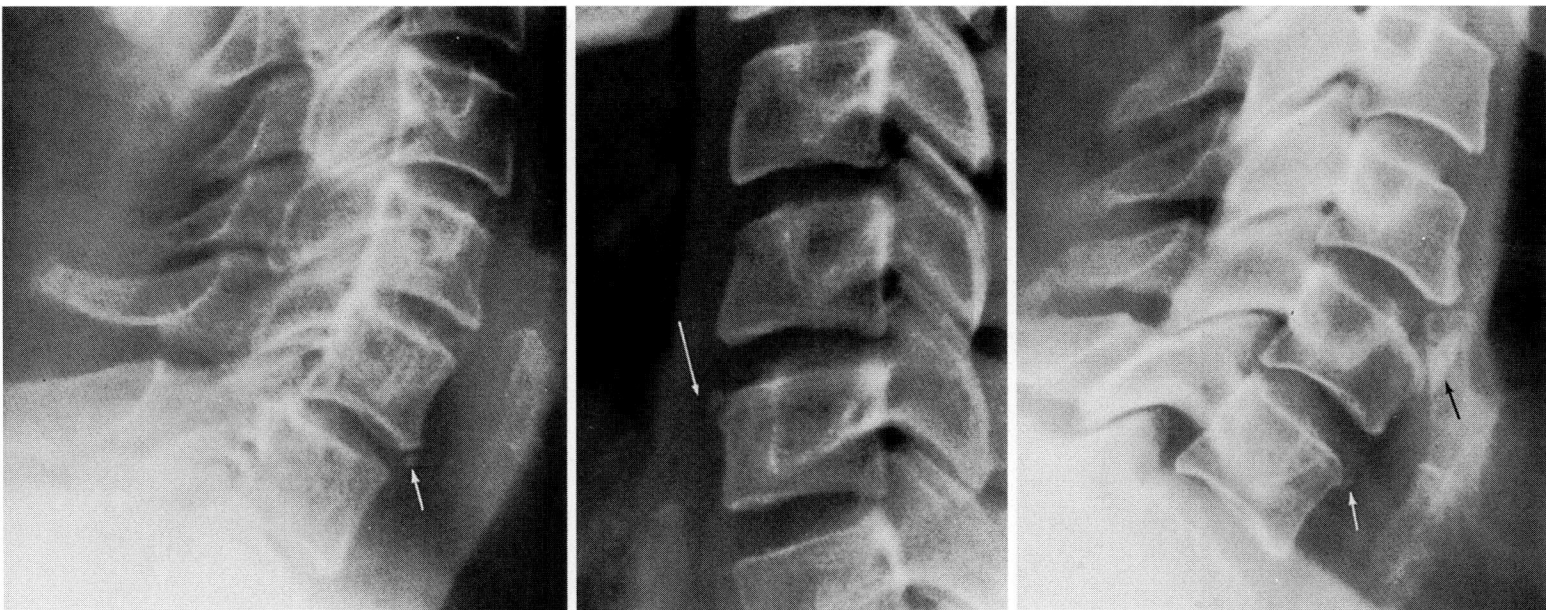

Figure 3–235. Three examples of cervical limbus vertebrae. When these elements appear in adult life they probably represent calcification in the annulus fibrosus secondary to stress. (Ref: Kerns S et al: Annulus fibrosus calcification in the cervical spine: Radiologic-pathologic correlation. *Skeletal Radiol* 15:605, 1978.)

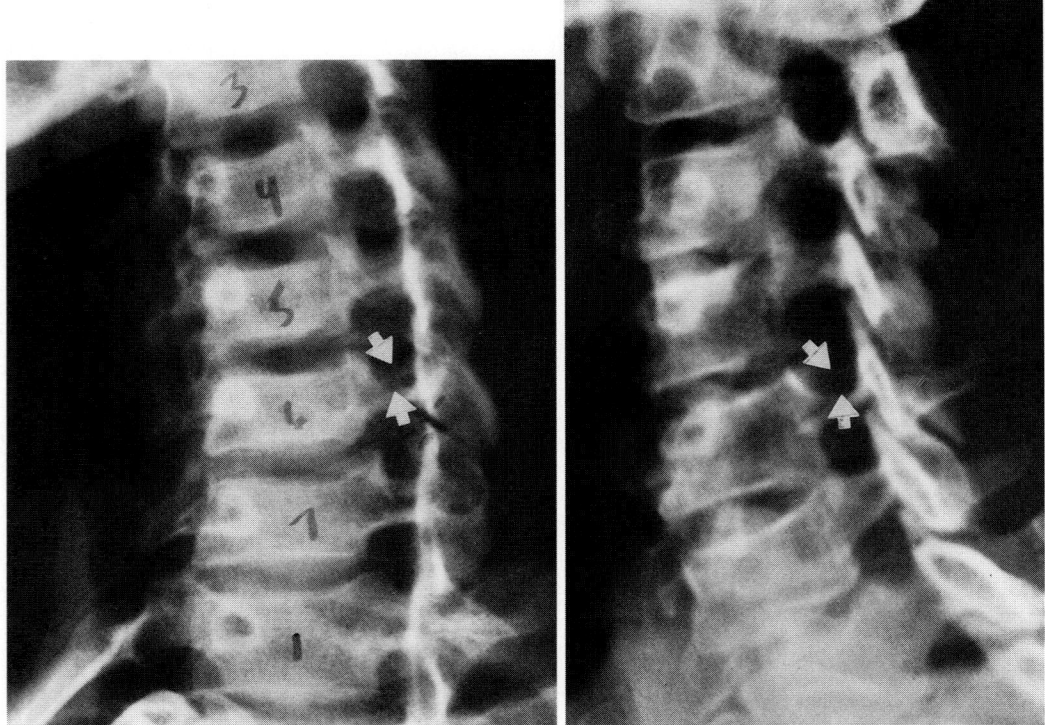

Figure 3–236. Two examples of pseudoenlargement of the neutral foramen as a result of superimposition of the foramina on both sides. Note the two margins of pedicle *(arrows)*.

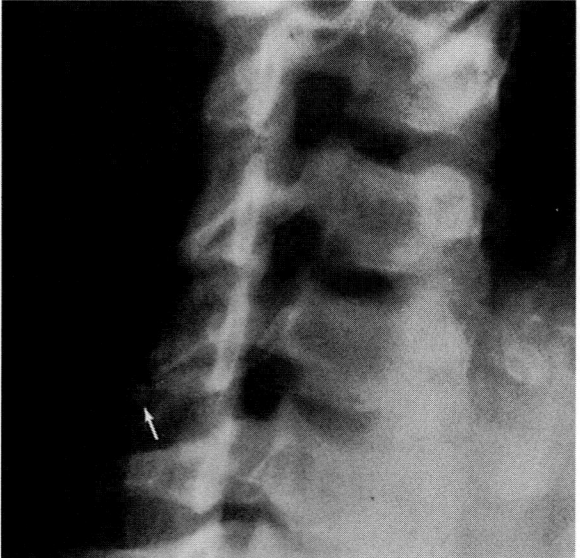

Figure 3–237. Ununited ossification center of the inferior articular process of C5.

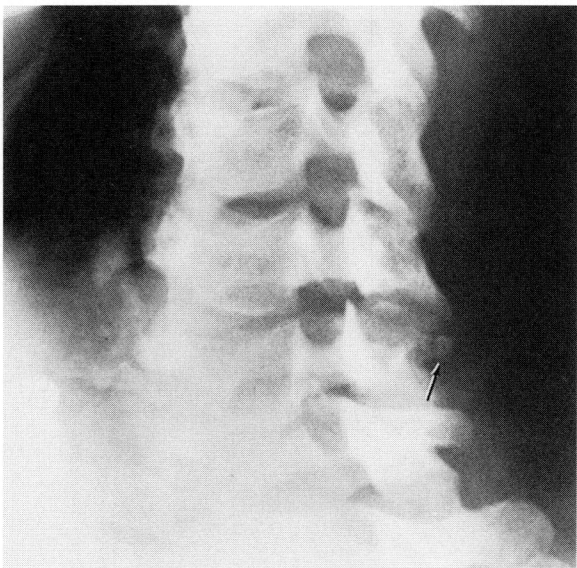

Figure 3–238. Ununited ossification center of the inferior articular process of C6.

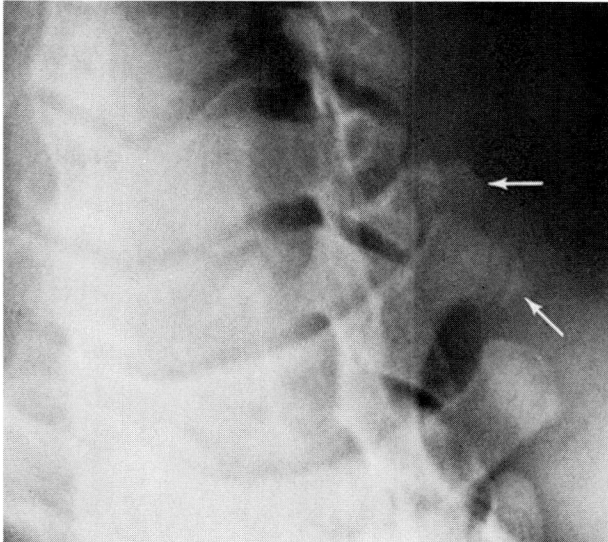

Figure 3–239. Ununited ossification centers of the transverse processes of the last two cervical vertebrae in a 38-year-old man.

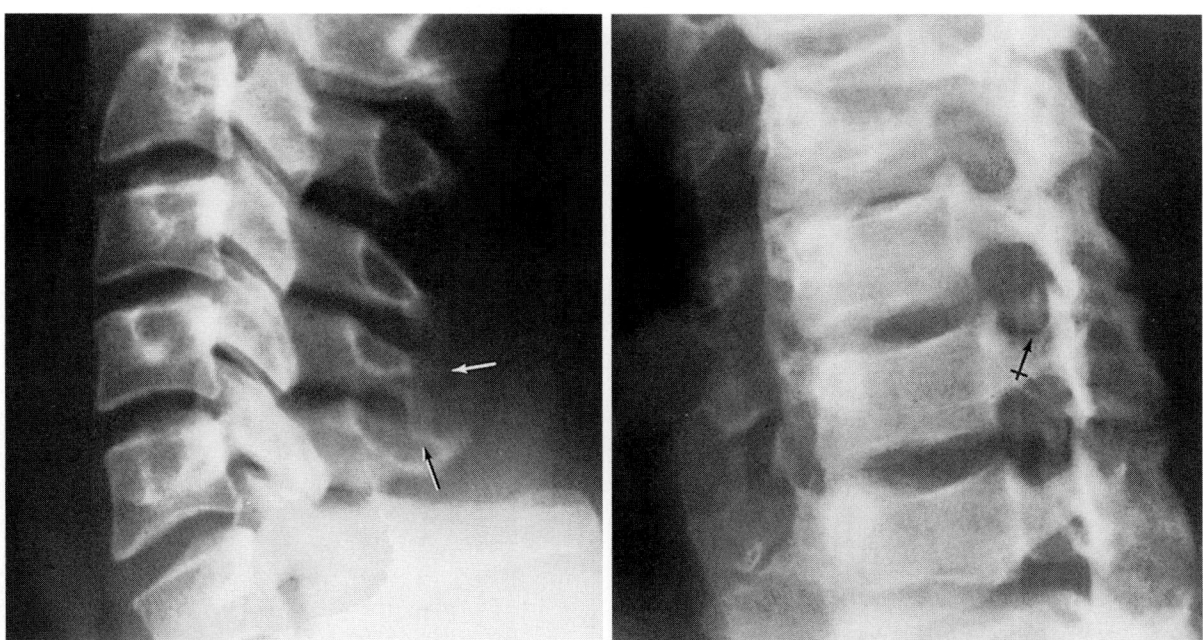

Figure 3–240. A bifid spinous process (→) can project into the neural foramen and simulate a fracture (↦).

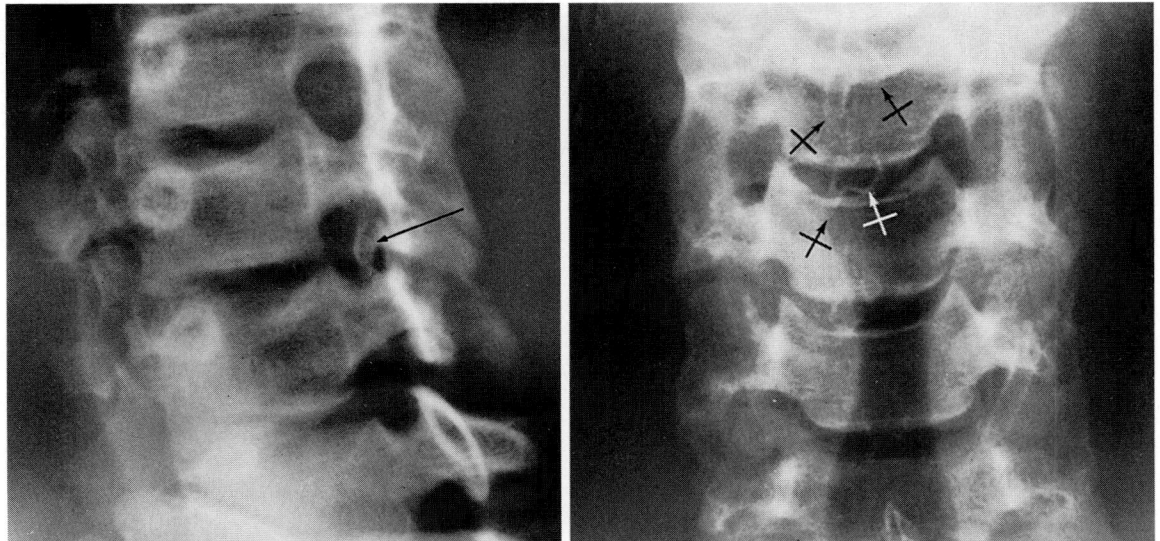

Figure 3–241. An example of the confusing appearance of the neural foramina (→), produced by bifid spinous processes (↦).

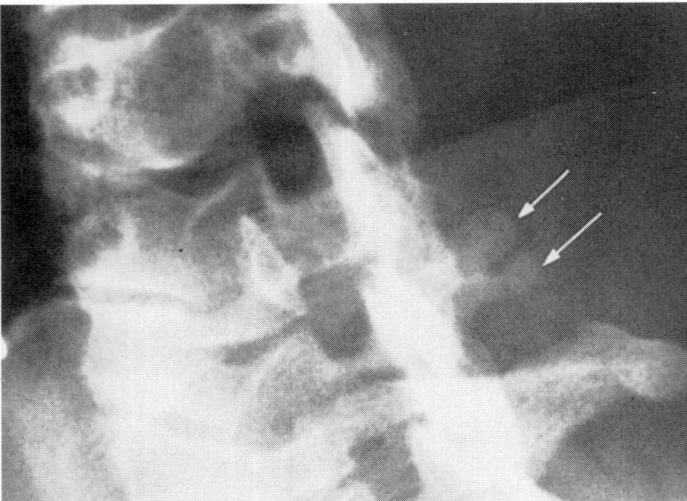

Figure 3–242. A bifid spinous process in the horizontal plane.

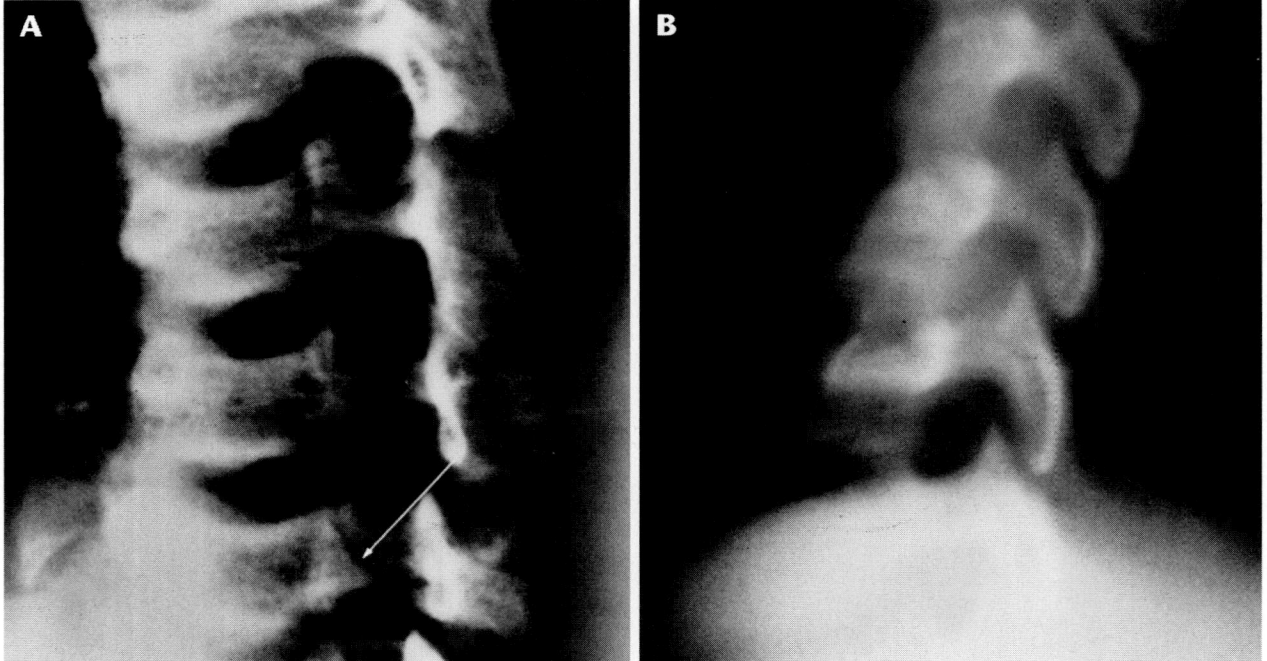

Figure 3–243. **A,** Facet seen in the oblique projection and mistaken for a fracture of the pedicle. **B,** Tomogram shows no fracture. (Ref: Zielinski CJ, Griffith JL: A joint shadow in the cervical spine presenting as a vertebral body fracture. *Spine* 12:595, 1987.)

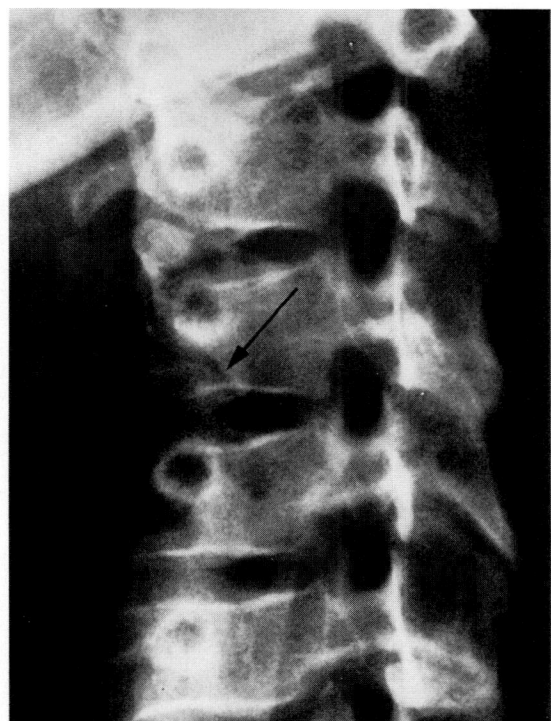

Figure 3–244. A facet resembling a fracture, seen in the oblique projection.

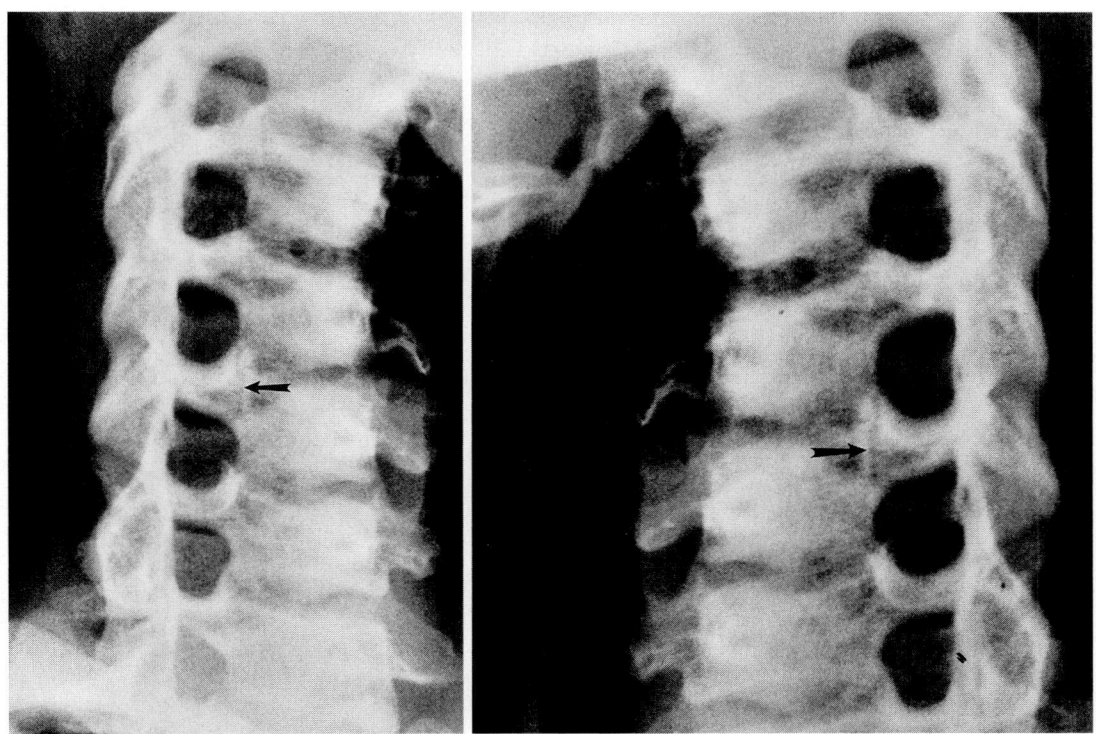

Figure 3–245. Abortive spondylolysis of C5.

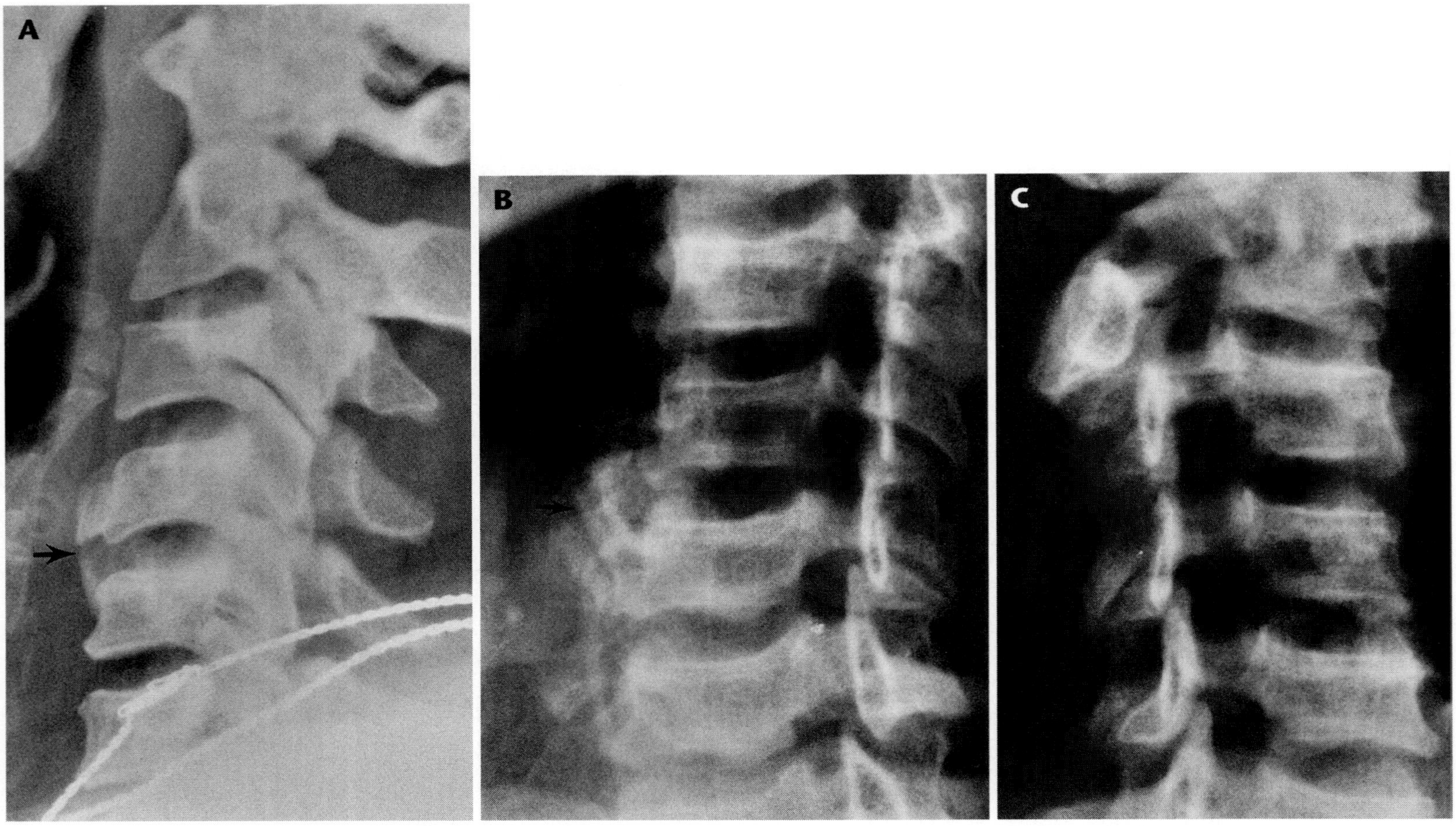

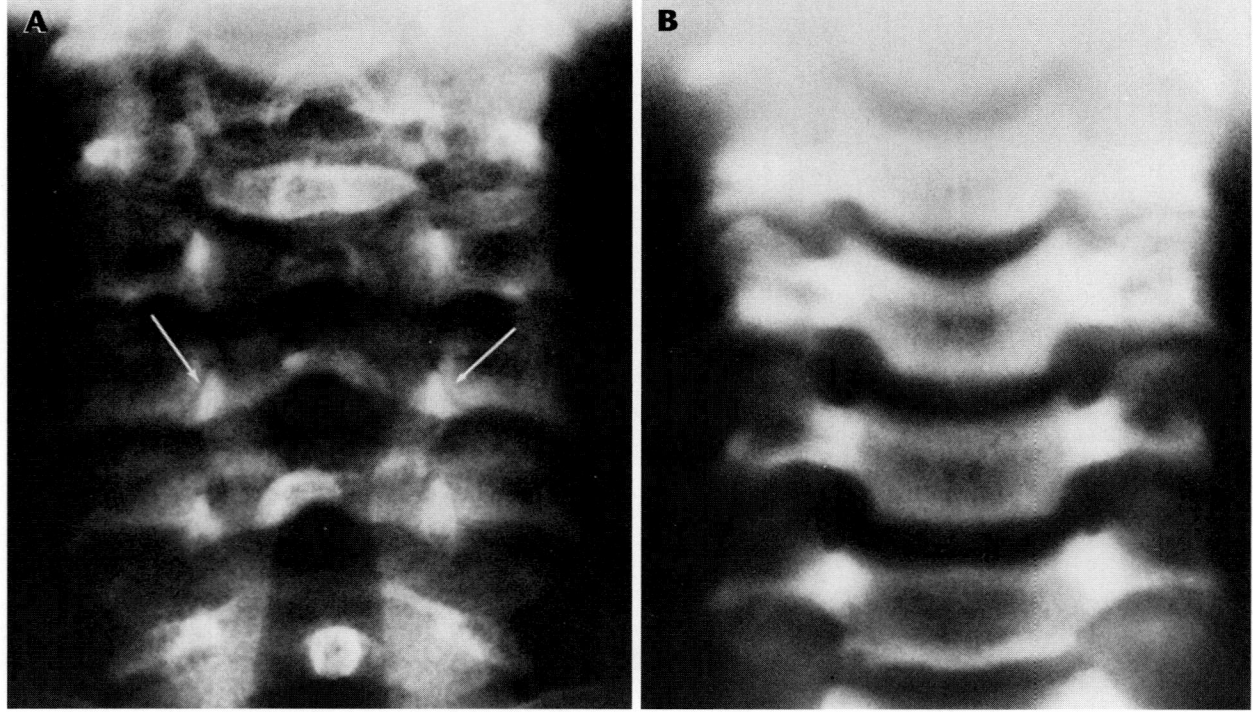

Figure 3–246. Anomalous articulation between the transverse processes of C4 and C5. **A,** Lateral projection. **B,** Right posterior oblique. **C,** Left posterior oblique for comparison with **B.**

Figure 3–247. A, Simulated fractures of the laminae of C5, produced by facets. **B,** Tomogram shows no fracture.

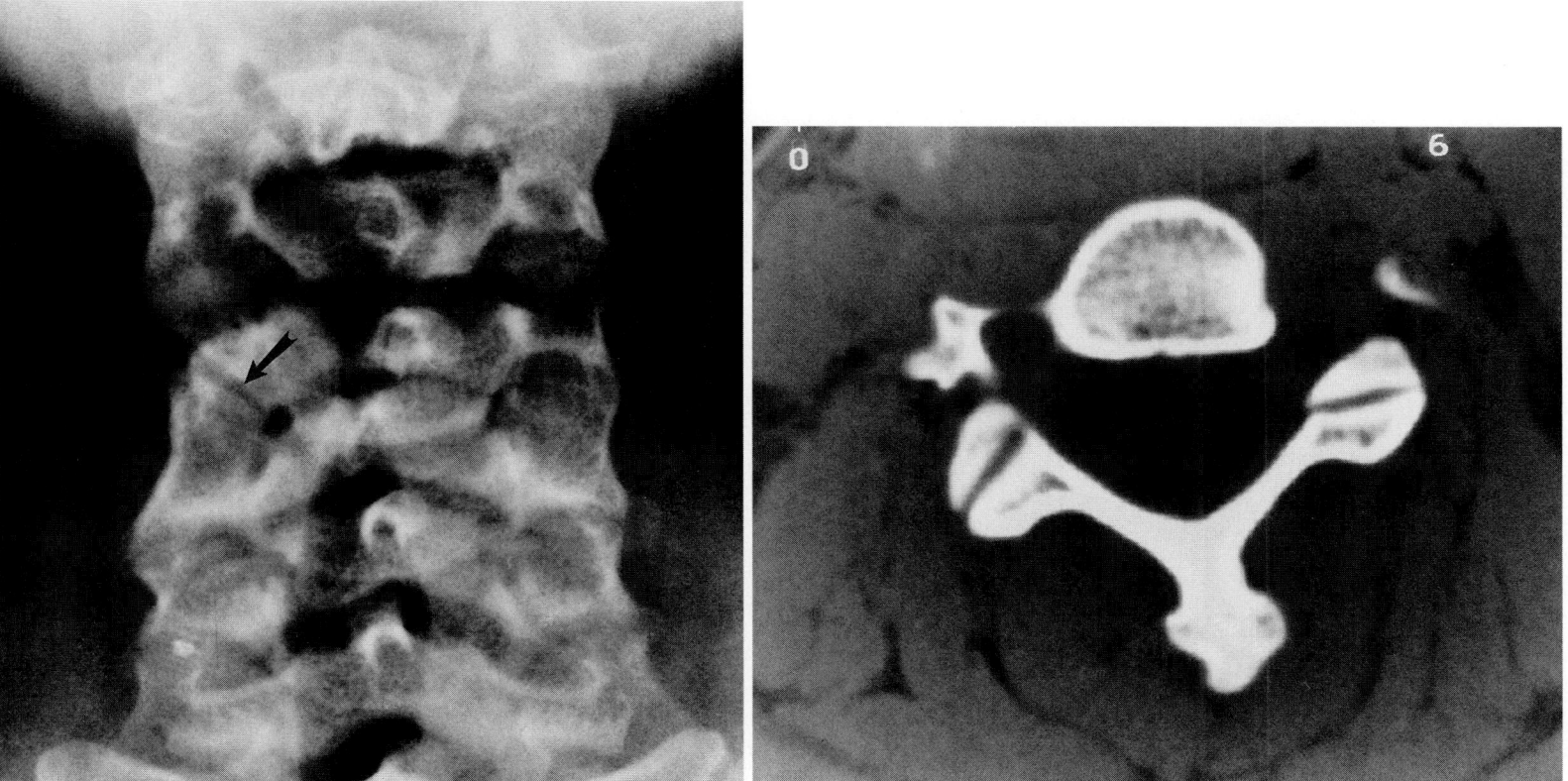

Figure 3–248. Simulated fracture of the right lateral mass of C5 resulting from a short lamina on that side. Note that the facets are not in the same plane and that the spinous process is not in the midline.

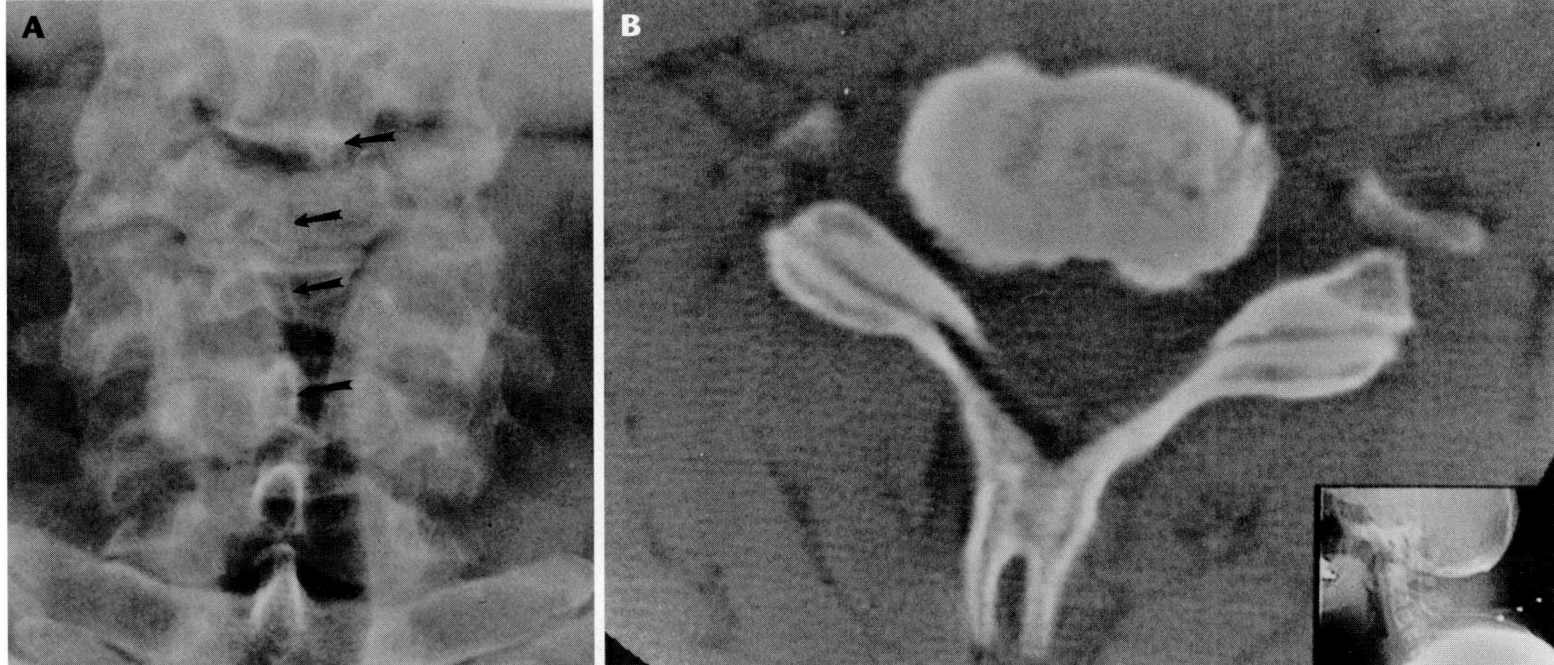

Figure 3–249. Developmental deviation of the spinous processes at C4 and C5. **A,** Anteroposterior projection. **B,** CT.

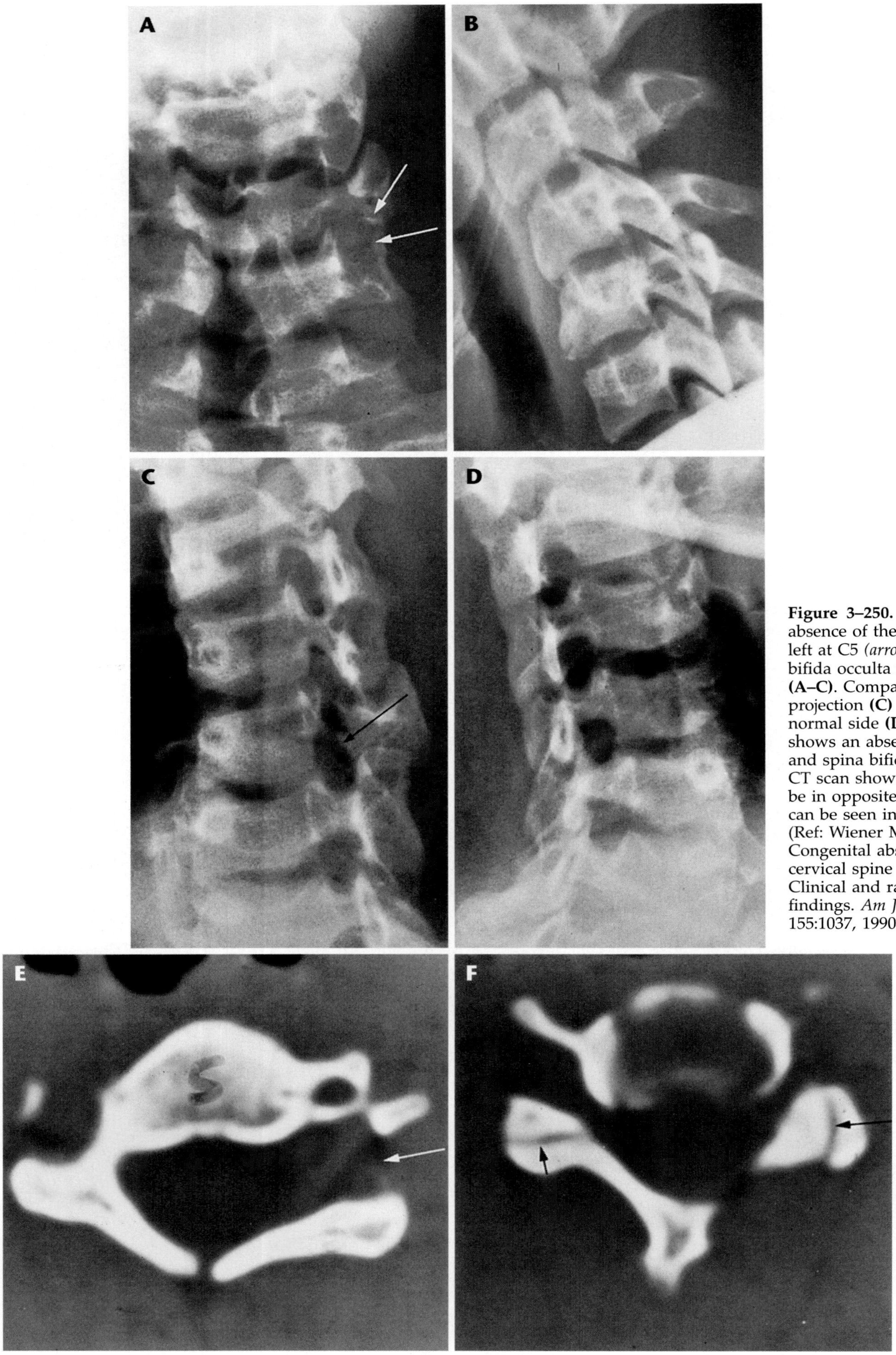

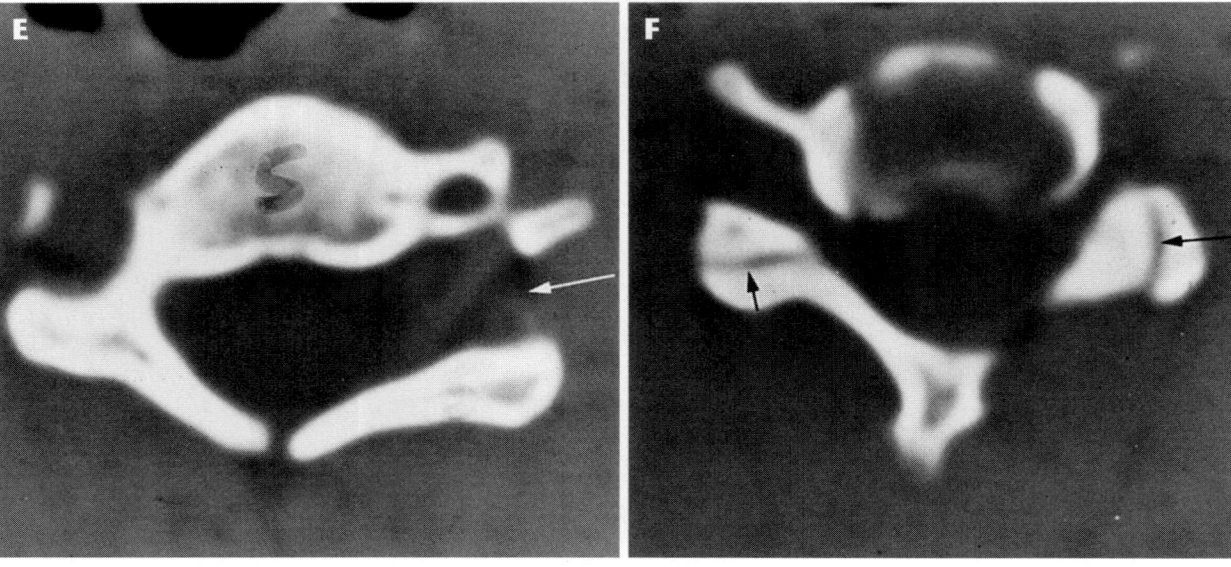

Figure 3–250. Congenital absence of the pedicle on the left at C5 *(arrows)*. A spina bifida occulta is also present **(A–C)**. Compare the oblique projection **(C)** with the normal side **(D)**. **E,** CT shows an absence of pedicle and spina bifida occulta. **F,** CT scan shows the facets to be in opposite planes. This can be seen in **A** as well. (Ref: Wiener MD et al: Congenital absence of a cervical spine pedicle: Clinical and radiologic findings. *Am J Roentgenol* 155:1037, 1990.)

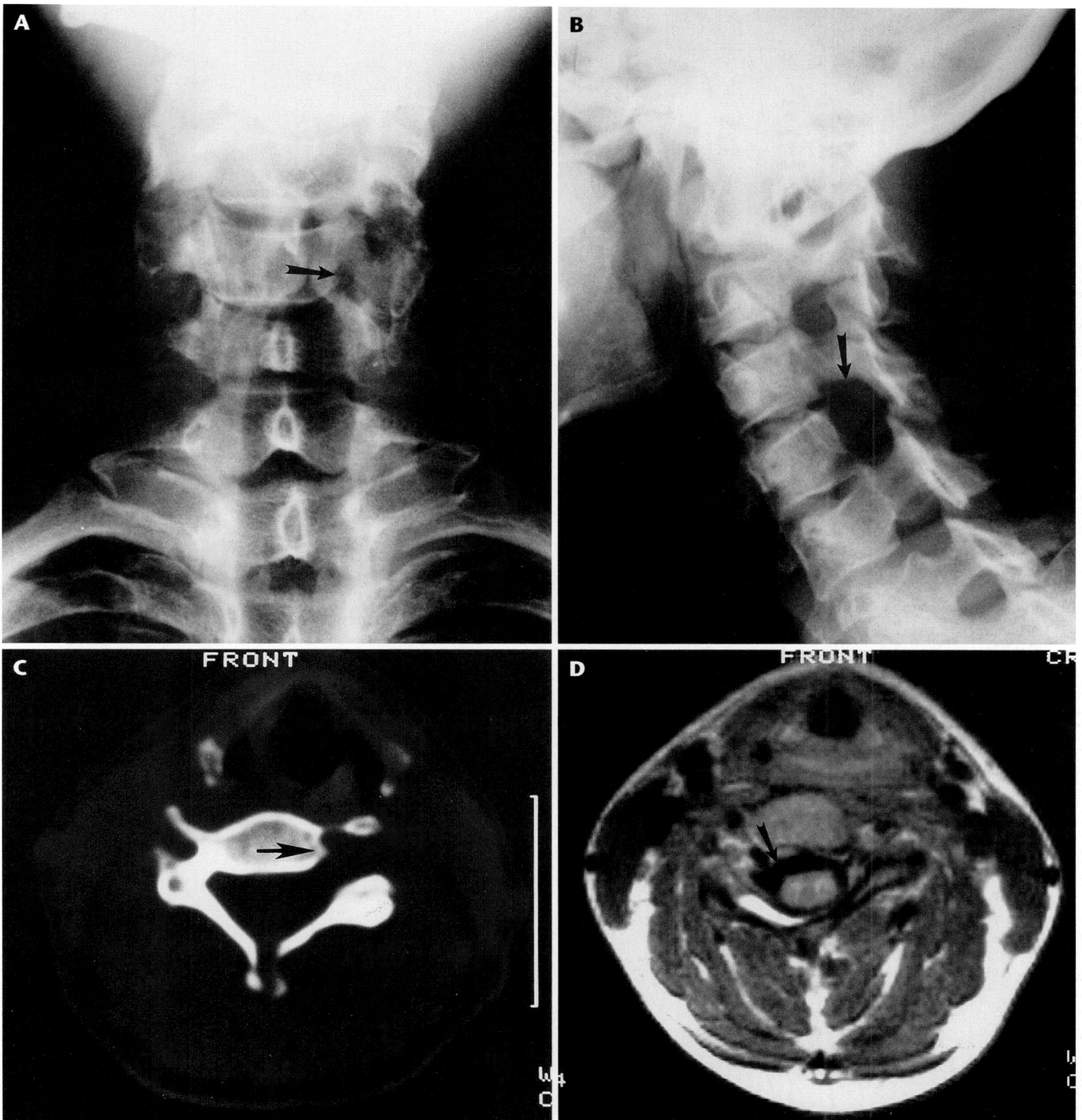

Figure 3–251. Absent pedicle at C5. **A** and **B,** AP and oblique views show a widened intervertebral foramen at C5 with absence of the pedicle on the left. **C,** CT shows an absence of the pedicle on the left as well as spina bifida of the spinous process. **D,** Axial T-1–weighted MRI scan of a similar case with an absence of the right pedicle shows widened cerebrospinal fluid space on the right. (Ref: Edwards MG: Imaging of the absent cervical pedicle syndrome. *Skeletal Radiol* 20:32, 1991.)

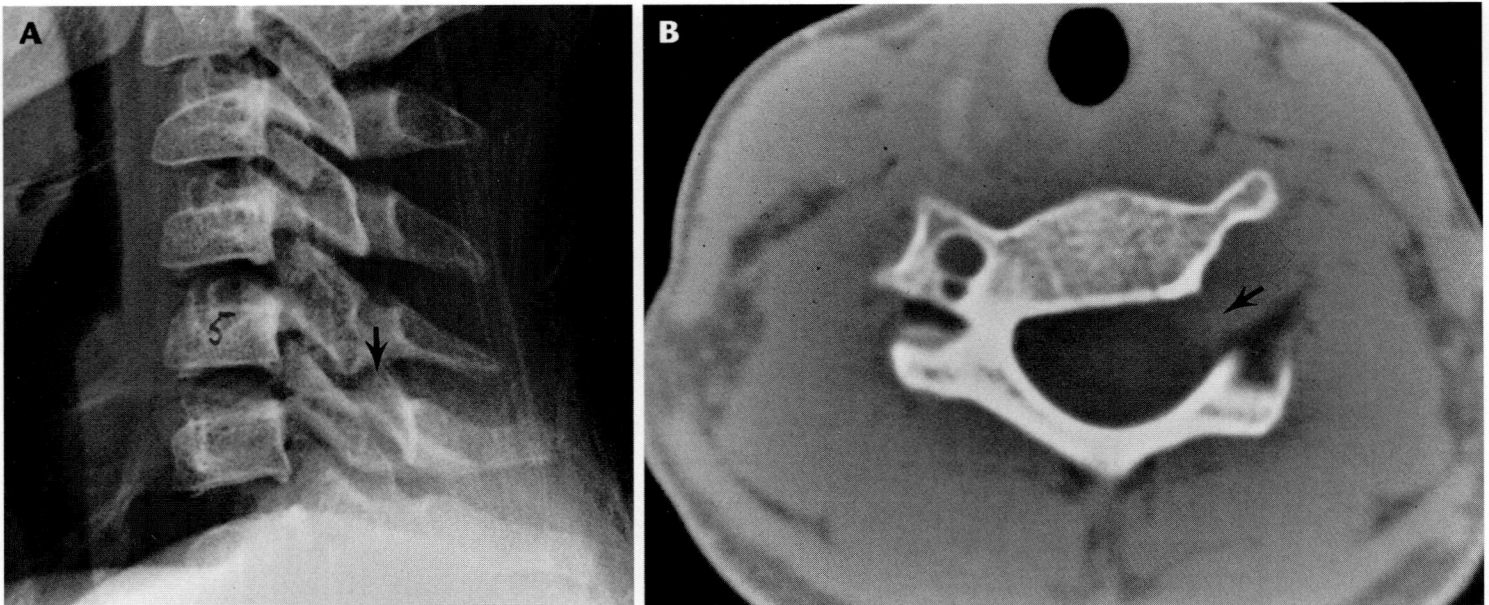

Figure 3–252. Simulated jumped facet at C6 produced by absent pedicle on the left side. **A,** Lateral projection. **B,** CT.

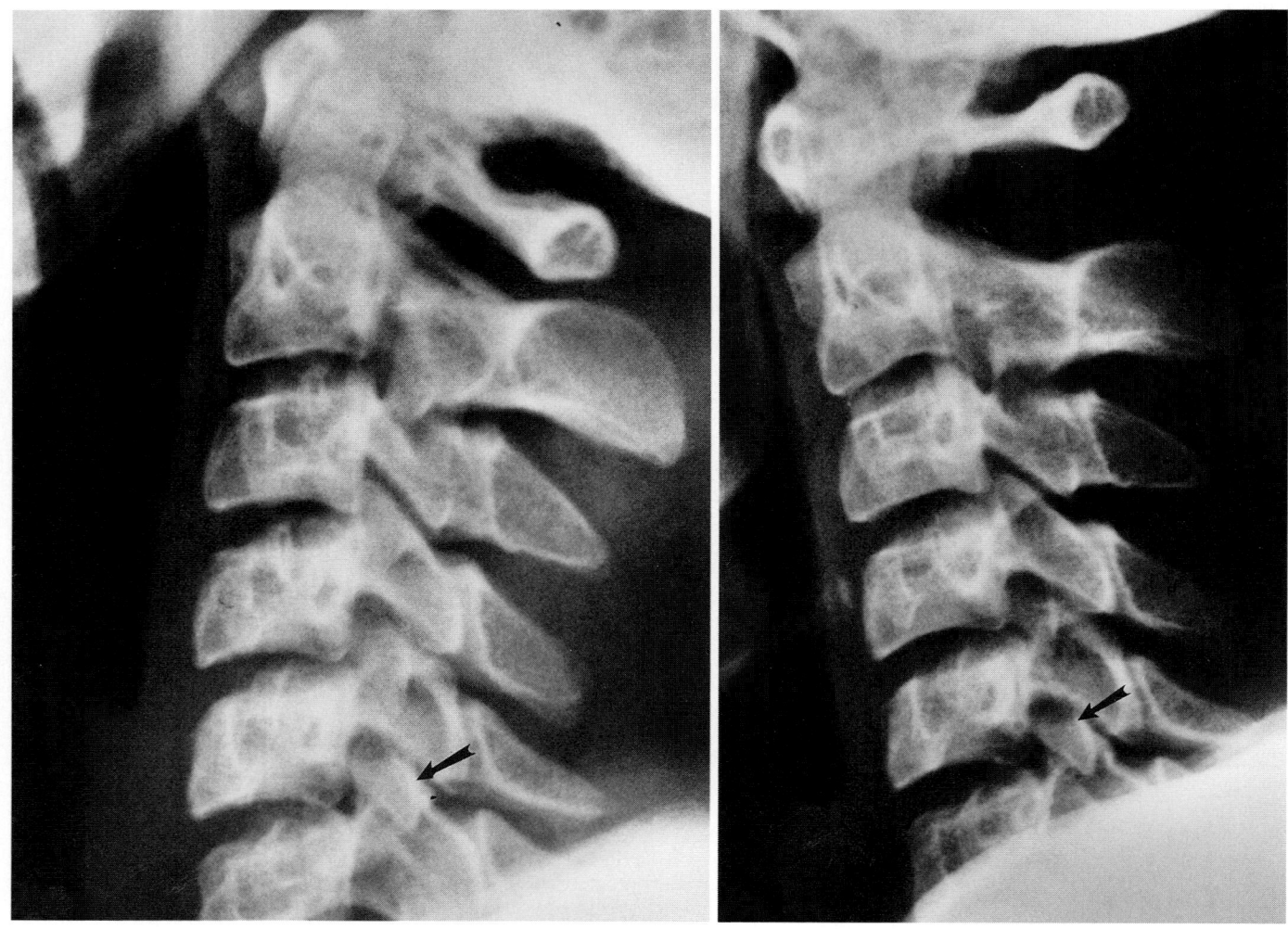

Figure 3–253. Two examples of a simulated facet fracture at C5, produced by rotation of the spine at the time of filming.

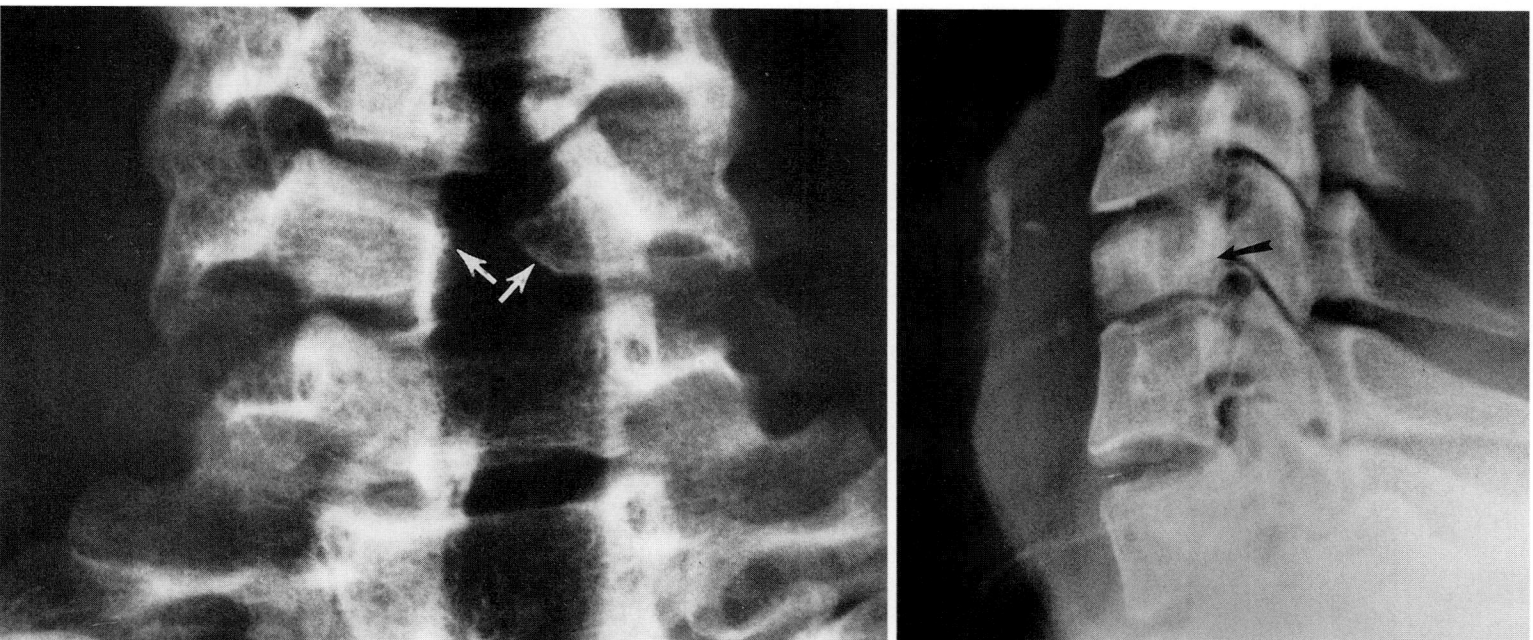

Figure 3–254. Hemivertebra (butterfly vertebra) at C6.

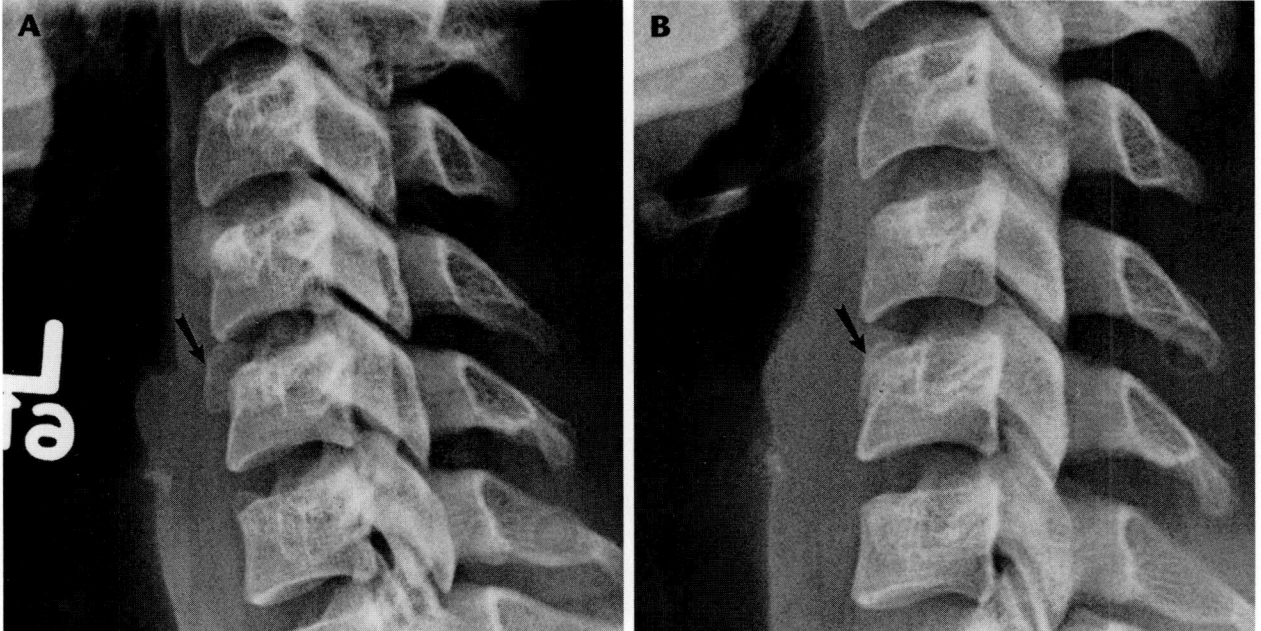

Figure 3–255. Simulated fracture of C5 due to elongated transverse process, more evident in **A** due to rotation and less evident in true lateral, **B**.

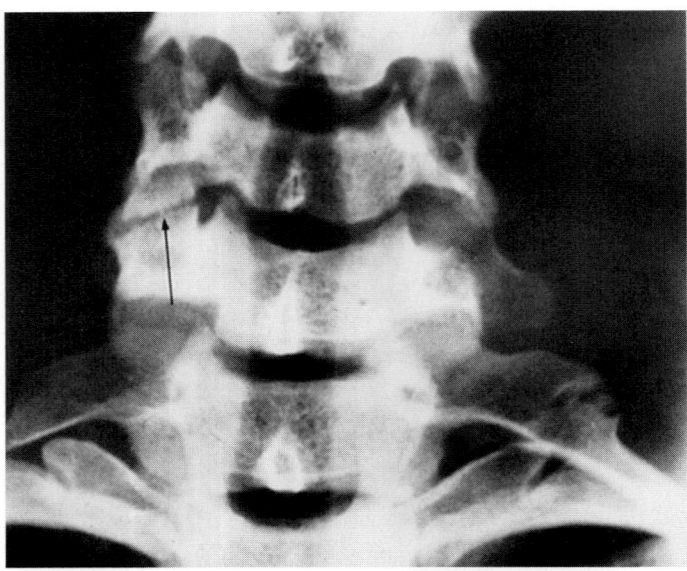
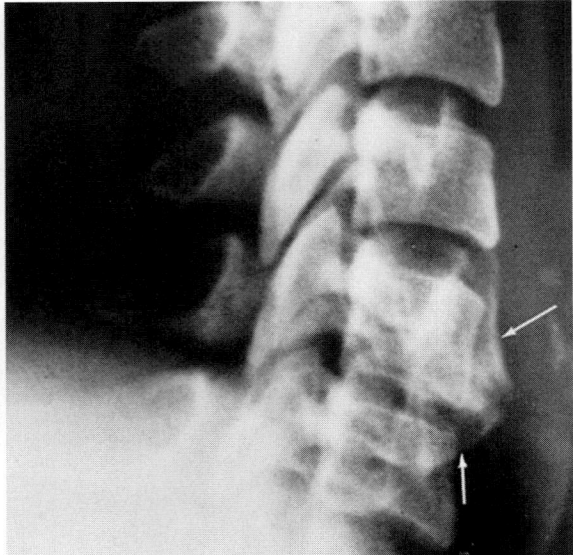
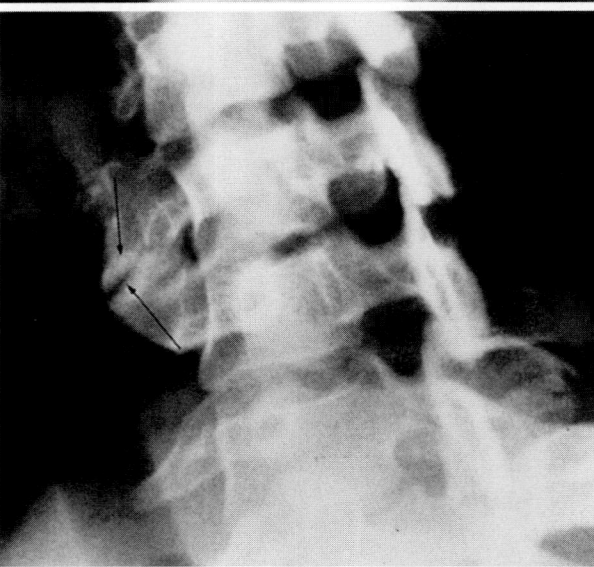

Figure 3–256. Anomalous articulation between transverse processes of C5 and C6 caused by elongation of the anterior tubercle. (Ref: Applebaum Y et al: Elongation of the anterior tubercle of a cervical vertebral transverse process: An unusual variant. *Skeletal Radiol* 10:265, 1983.)

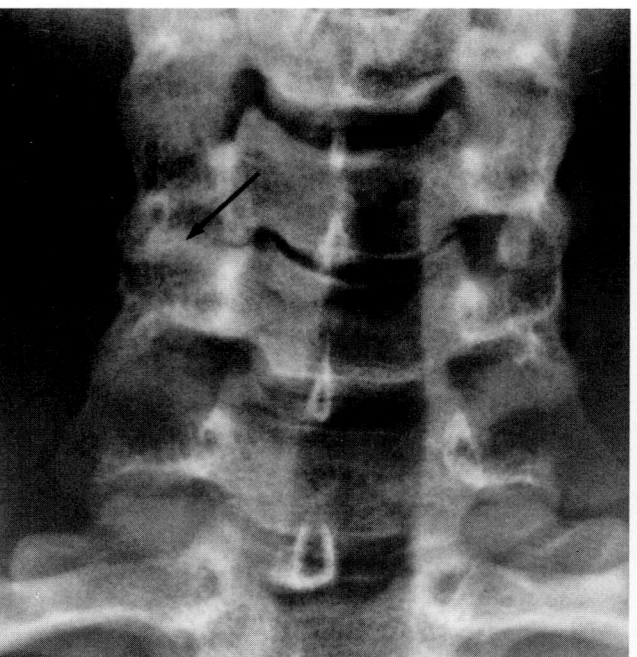
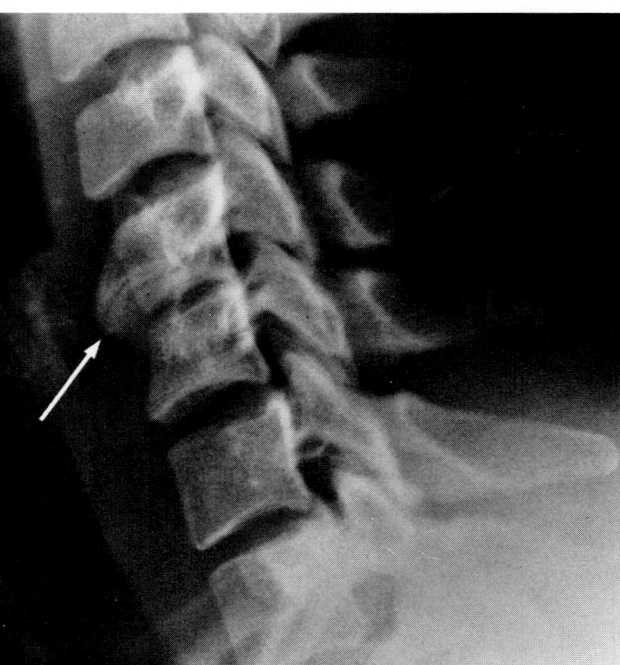

Figure 3–257. An anomalous articulation similar to that shown in Figure 3–256 between the transverse processes of C5 and C6 can be seen with incomplete segmentation of these two vertebral bodies.

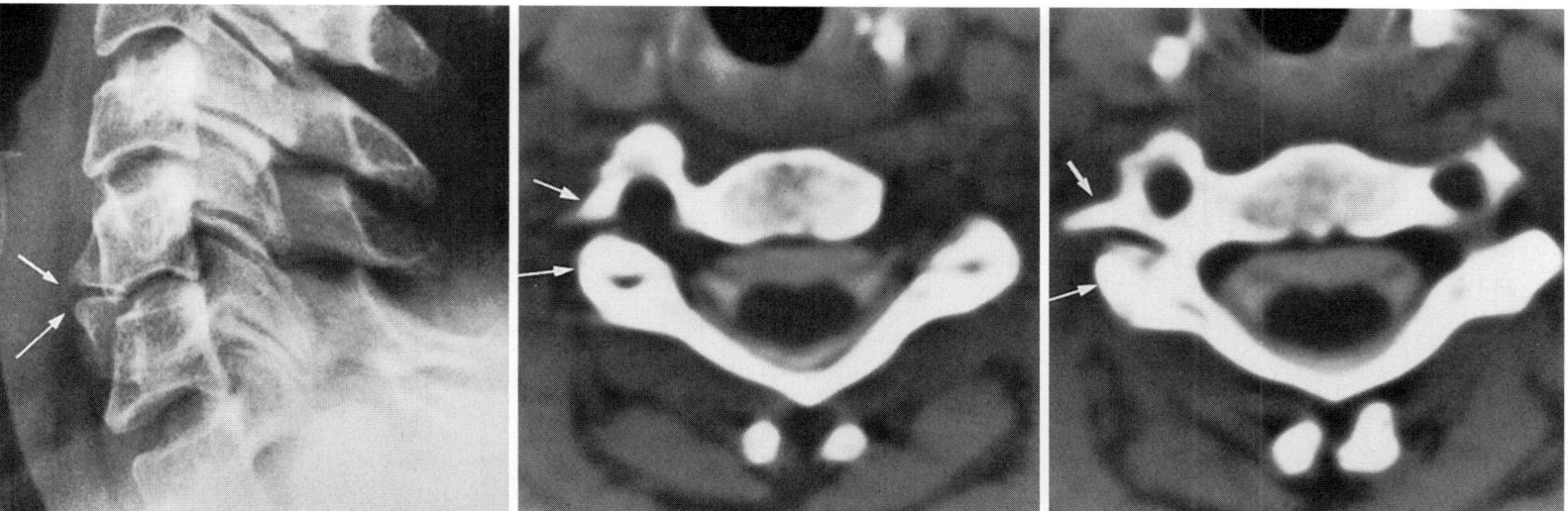

Figure 3–258. Anomalous articulation between the transverse processes of C5 and C6 similar to that of Figure 3–257 with CT myelogram confirmation *(arrows)*.

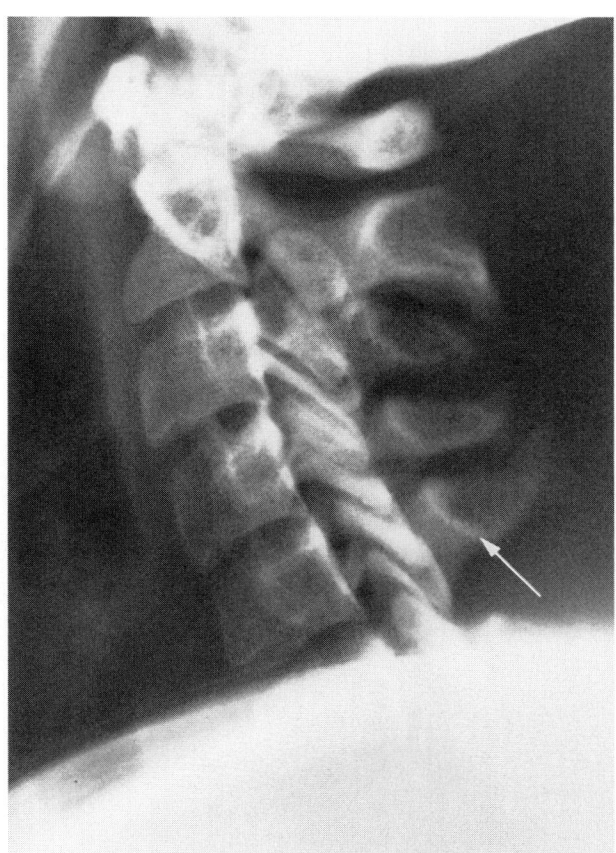

Figure 3–259. Uptilted spinous process of C5 might be misconstrued as evidence of soft tissue injury between C5 and C6.

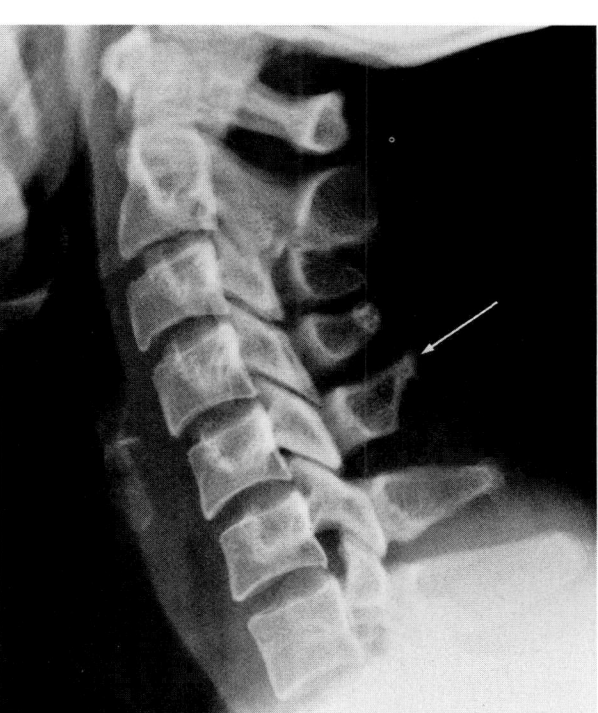

Figure 3–260. Upturned spinous process originally interpreted as evidence of ligamentous injury with flaring of the spinous processes.

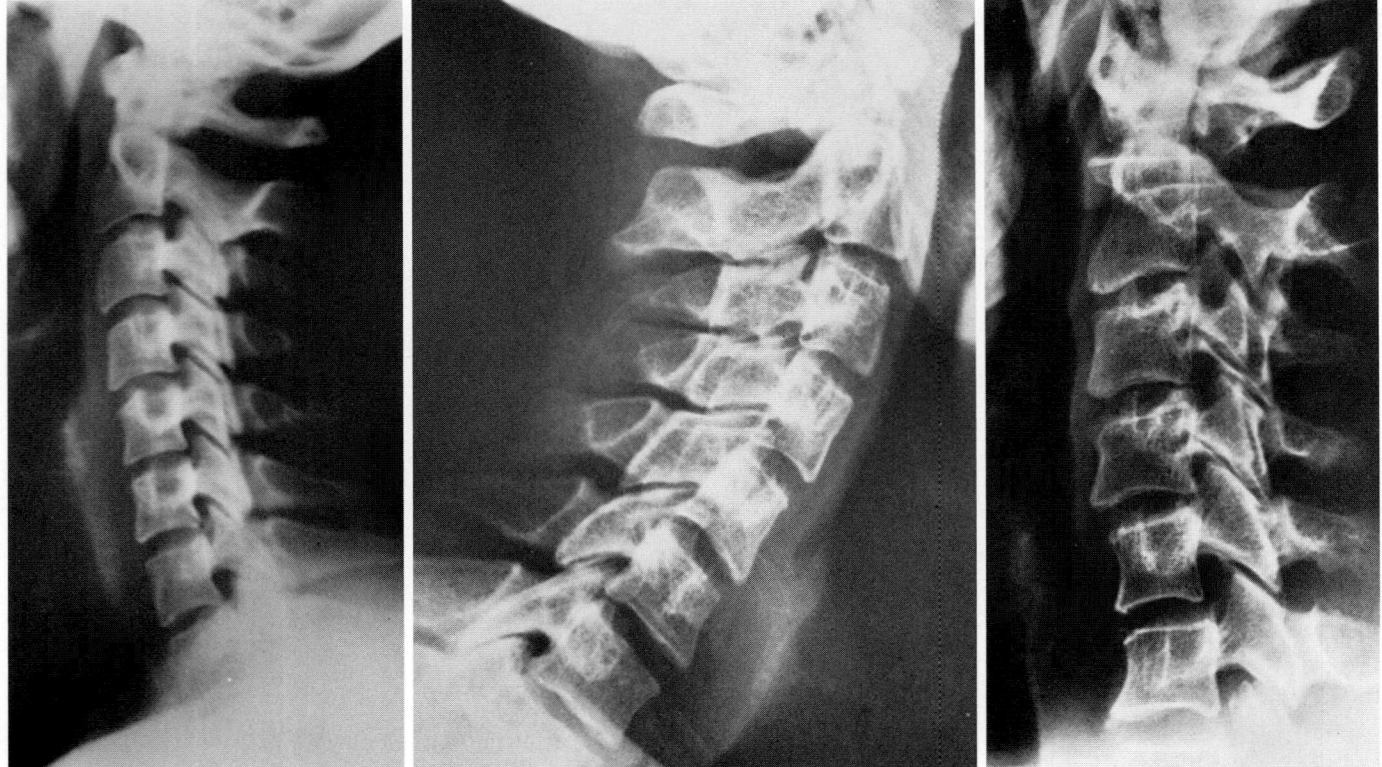

Figure 3–261. Three examples of the variability of vertebral body size in a given individual.

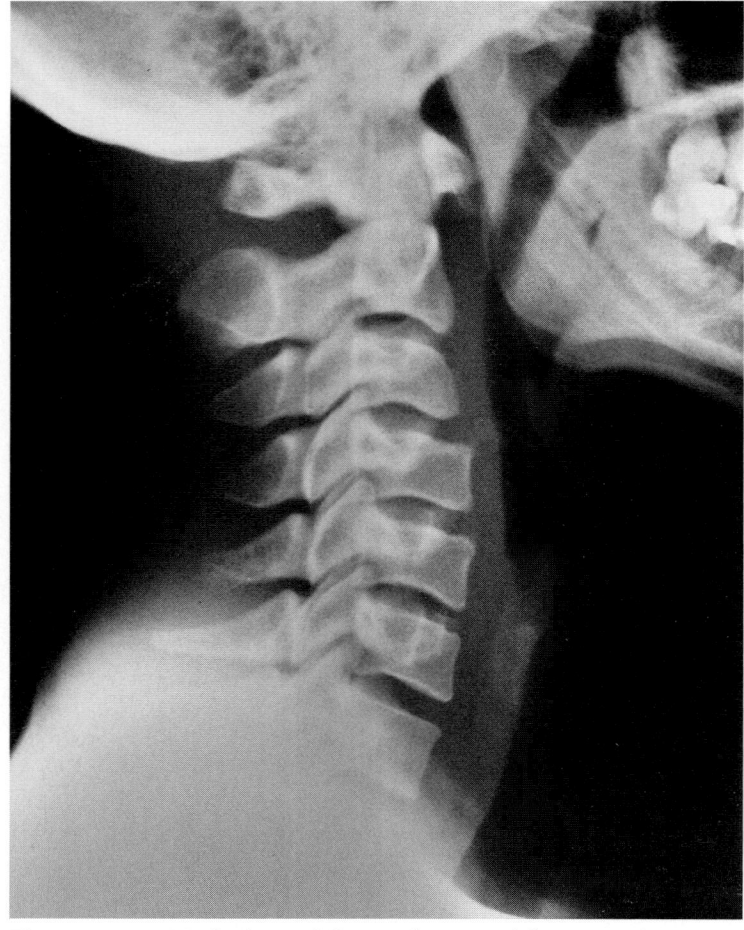

Figure 3–262. Marked variability in the size of the cervical vertebra.

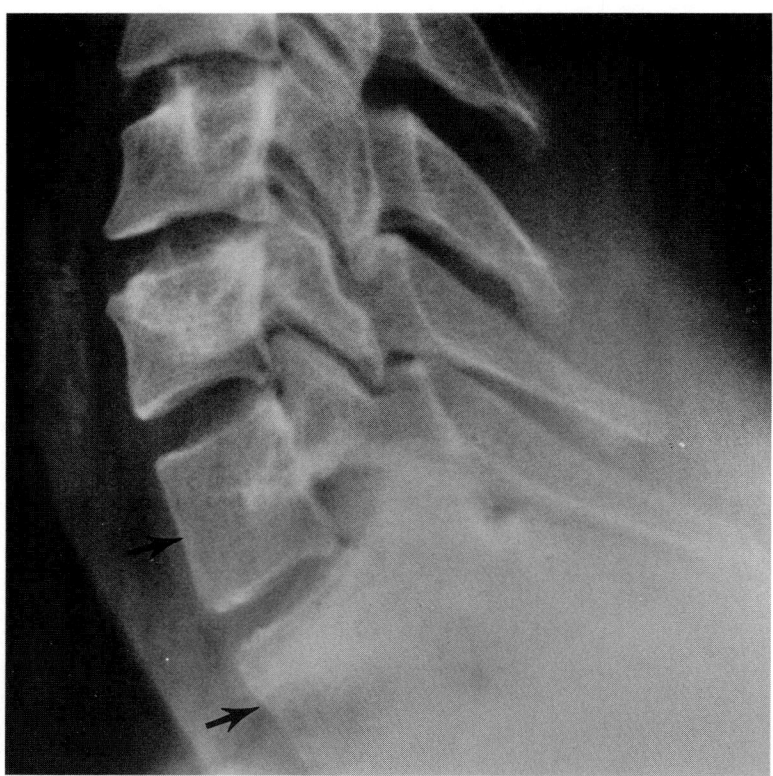

Figure 3–263. Unusually tall bodies of C6 and C7.

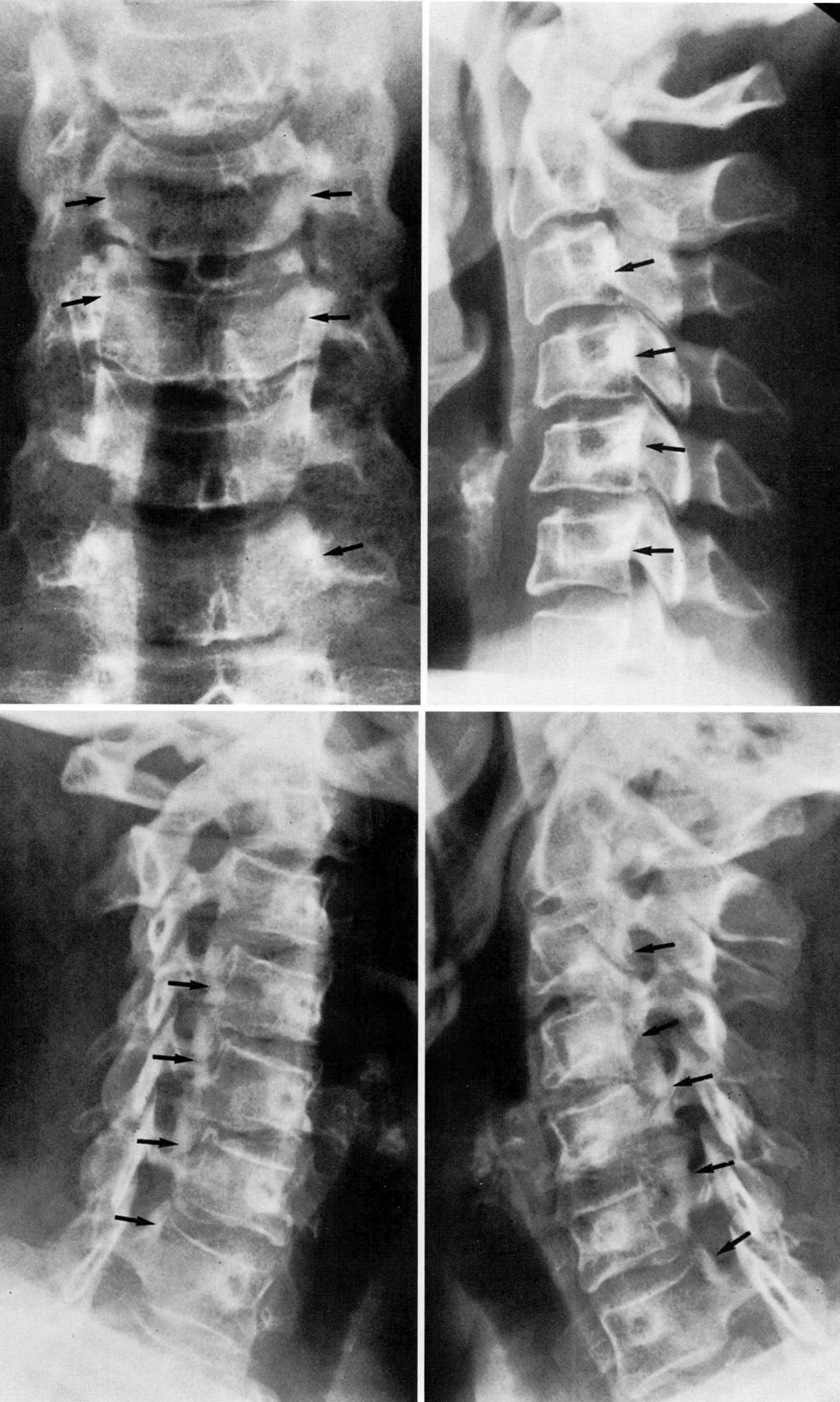

Figure 3–264. Sclerosis of the pedicles and posterolateral aspects of the vertebral bodies in a 36-year-old woman, best seen in the oblique projection. This is apparently not related to degenerative spondylosis.

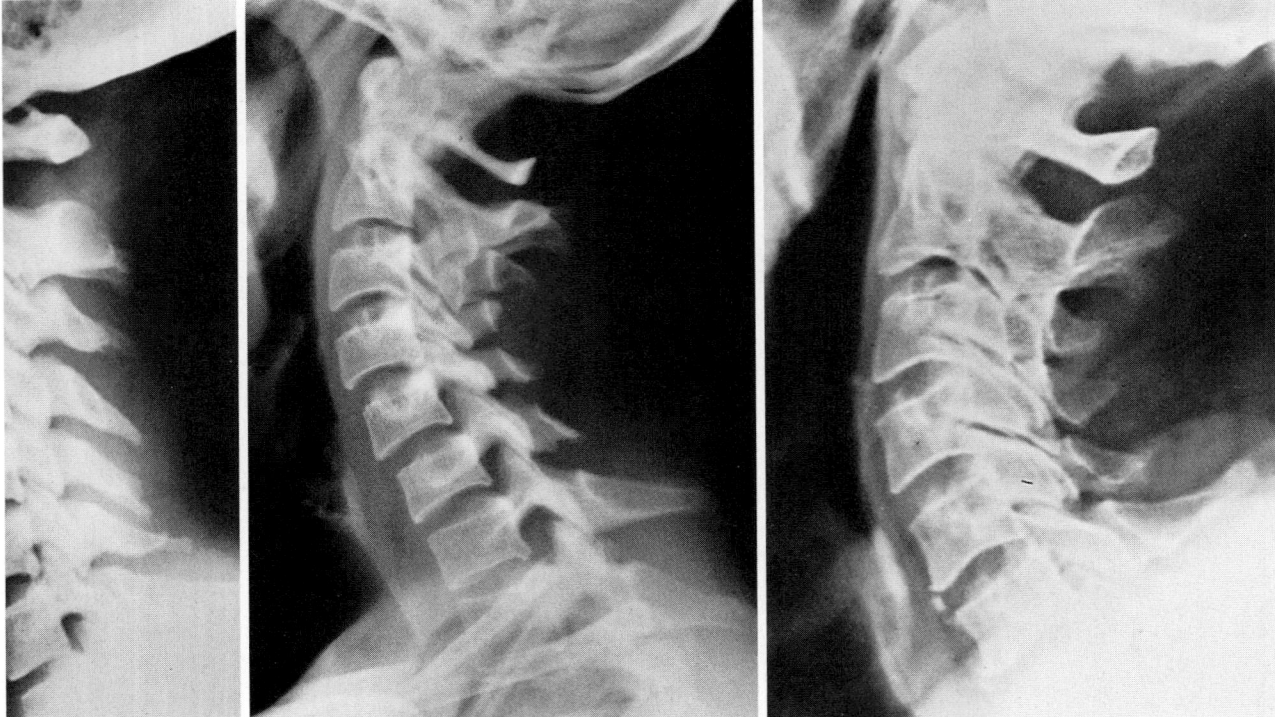

Figure 3–265. Three examples of the normal variability of size and configuration of spinous processes.

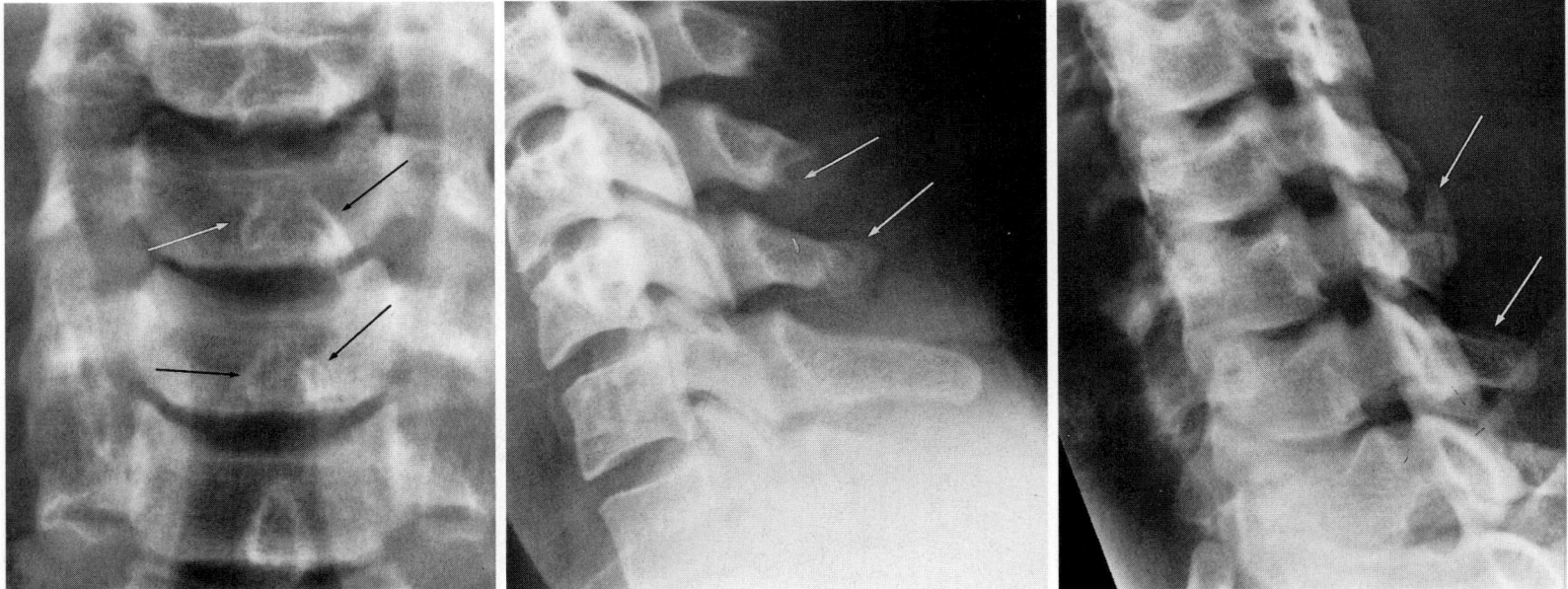

Figure 3–266. Bifid spinous processes of C5 and C6, which may be mistaken for fractures.

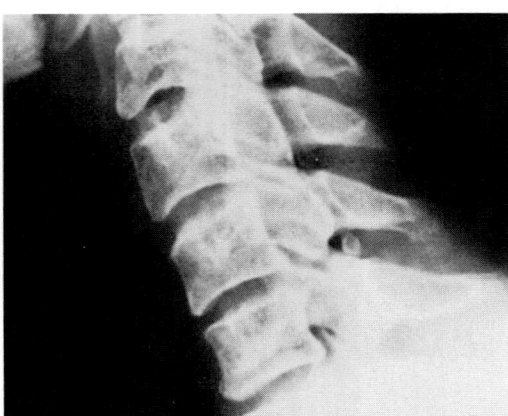

Figure 3–267. Ossicle between C5 and C6, probably ligamentous.

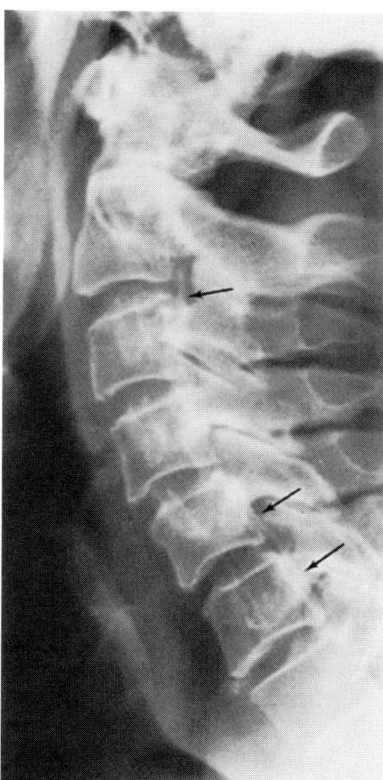

Figure 3–268. Calcification of the posterior longitudinal ligament. This may or may not be significant. (Ref: Minagi H, Gronner AT: Calcification of the posterior longitudinal ligament: A cause of cervical myelopathy. *Am J Roentgenol* 105:365, 1969.)

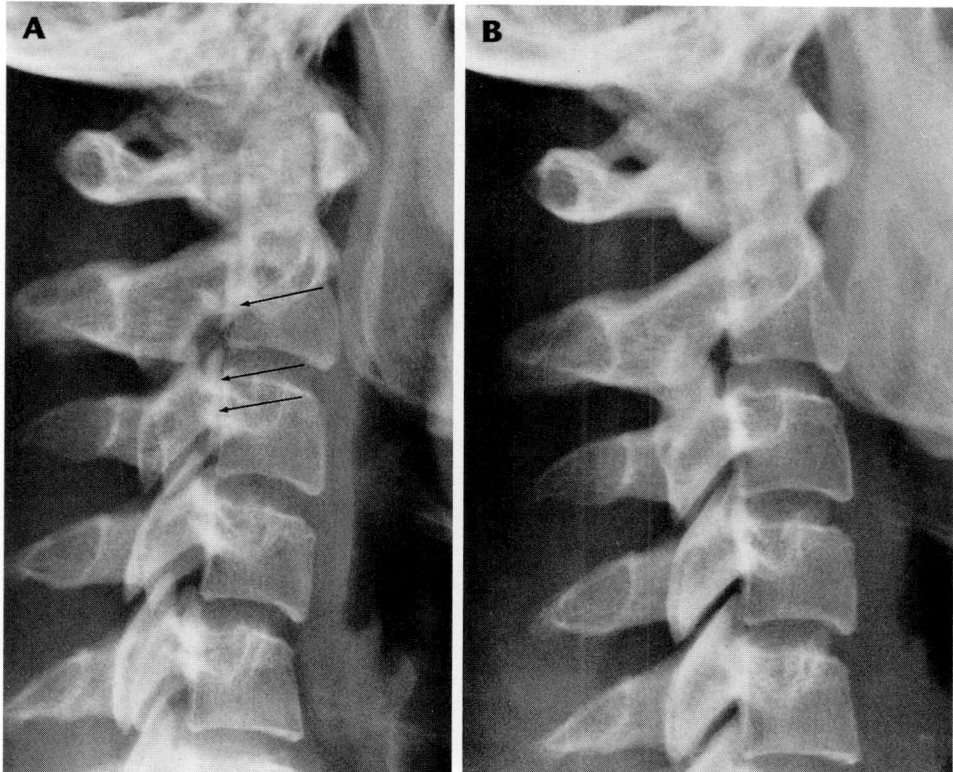

Figure 3–269. A, Simulated calcification of the posterior spinal ligament, produced by rotation. **B,** Not seen with correct positioning.

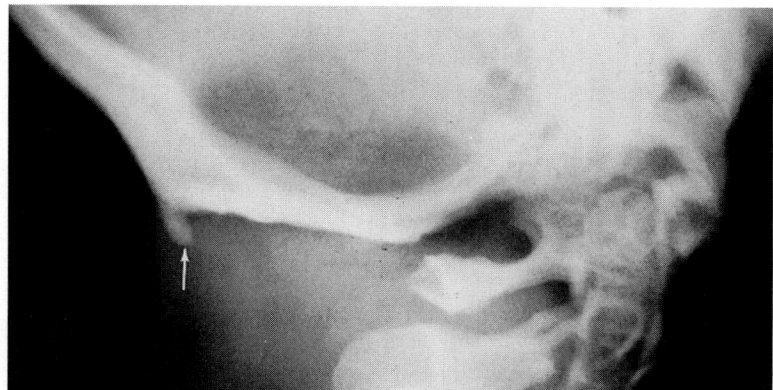

Figure 3–270. Calcification of the ligamentum nuchae at the base of the skull.

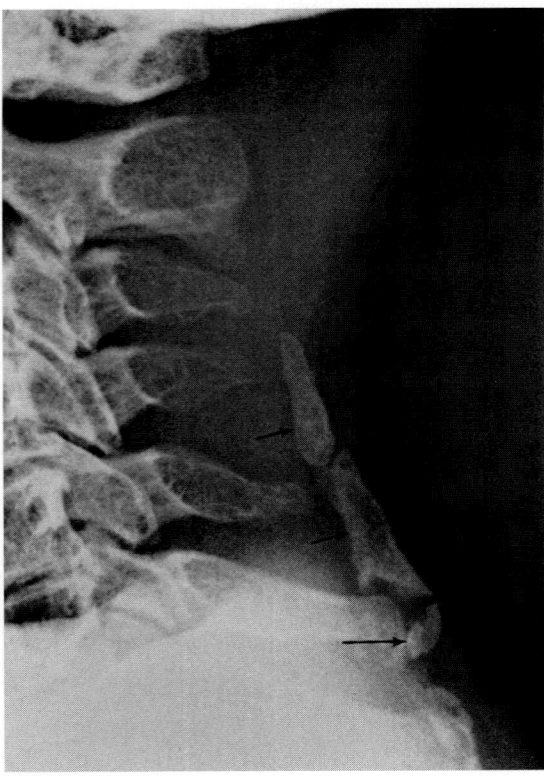

Figure 3–271. Huge ossified ligamentum nuchae.

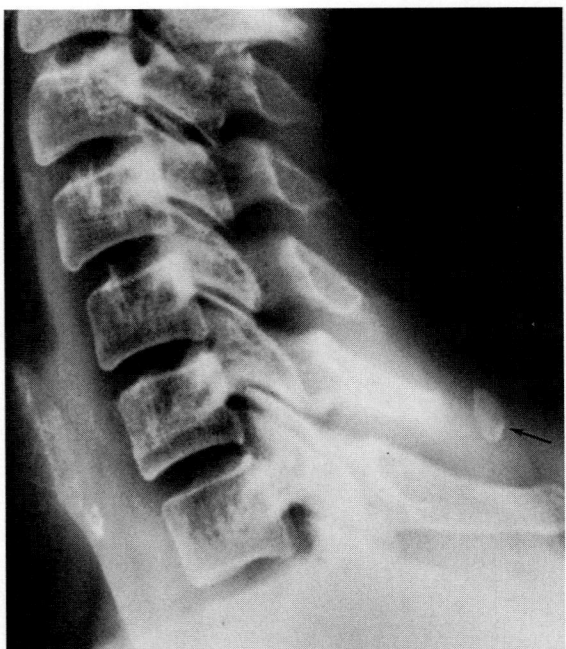

Figure 3–272. Calcification of the ligamentum nuchae.

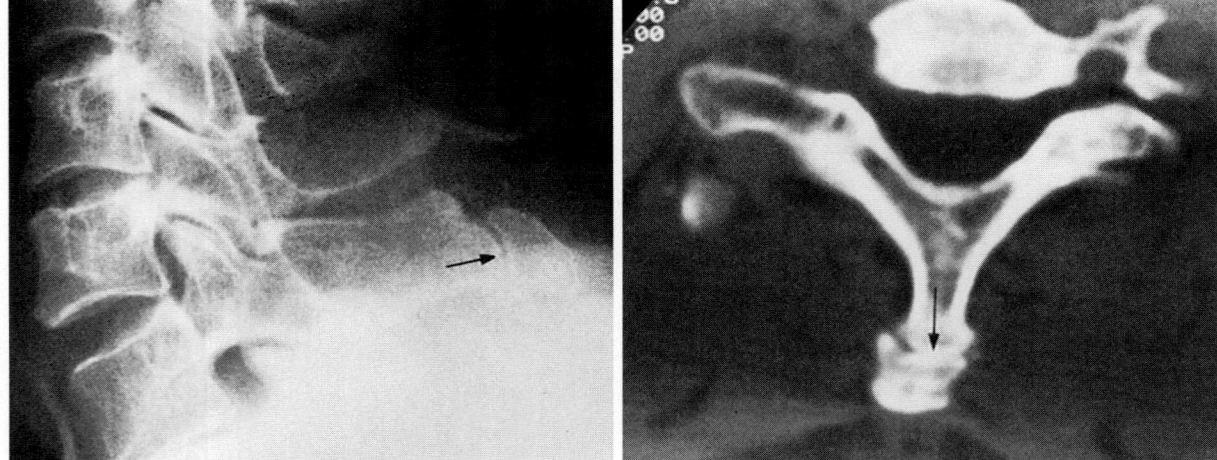

Figure 3–273. Ununited apophysis of the spinous process of C6 with an anomalous articulation.

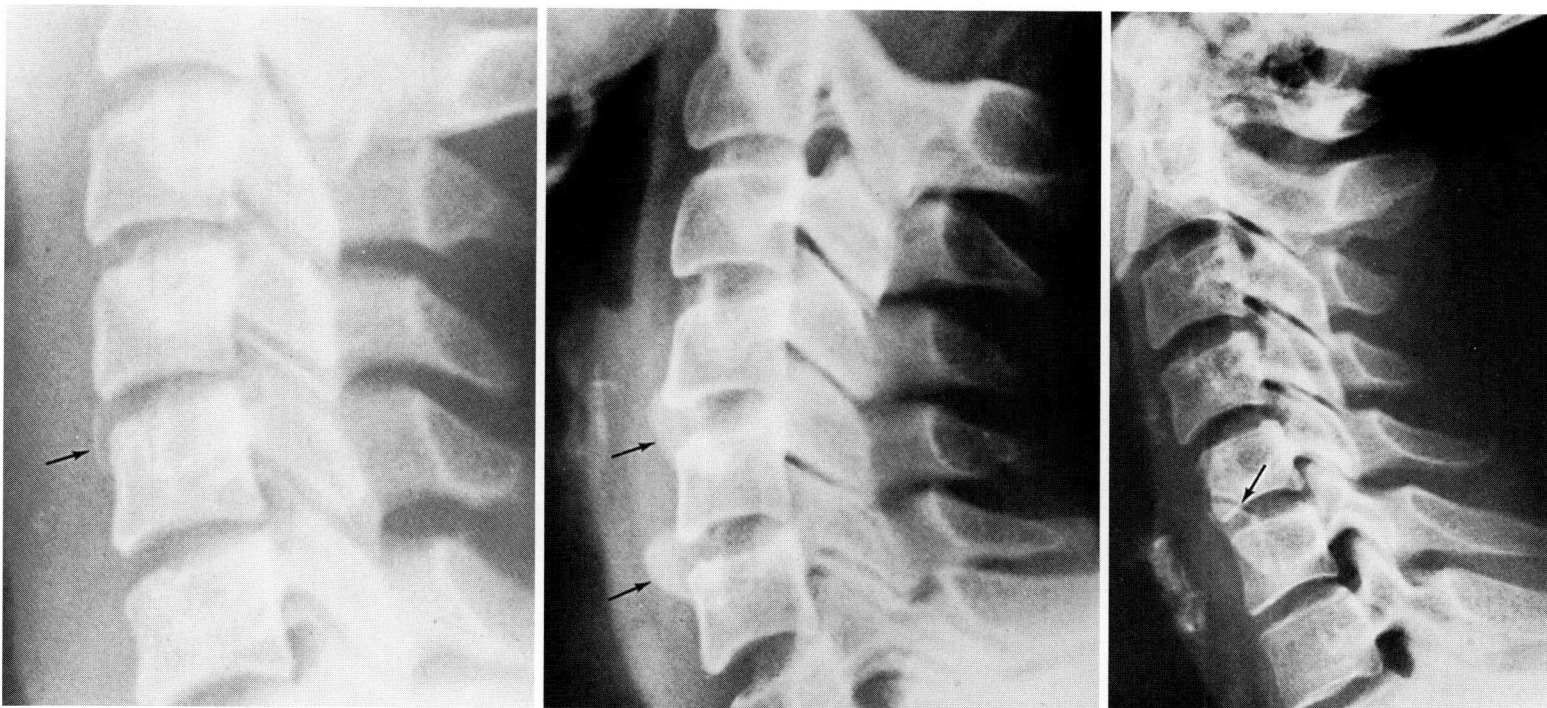

Figure 3–274. Three examples of normal elongation of the transverse process of C5 and C6, producing an unusual appearance anterior to the vertebral bodies (see Fig. 3–256). (Ref: Laypayowker MS: An unusual variant of the cervical spine. *Am J Roentgenol* 83:656, 1960.)

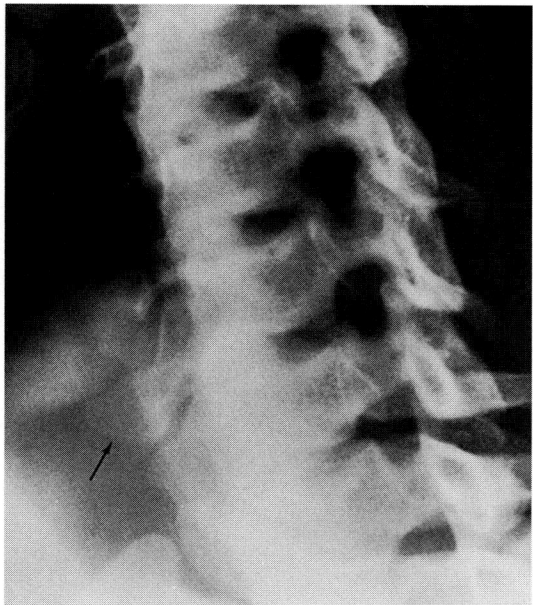

Figure 3–275. Oblique projection of the cervical spine showing the anterior tubercle of the transverse process, the structure responsible for the shadows in the preceding figure.

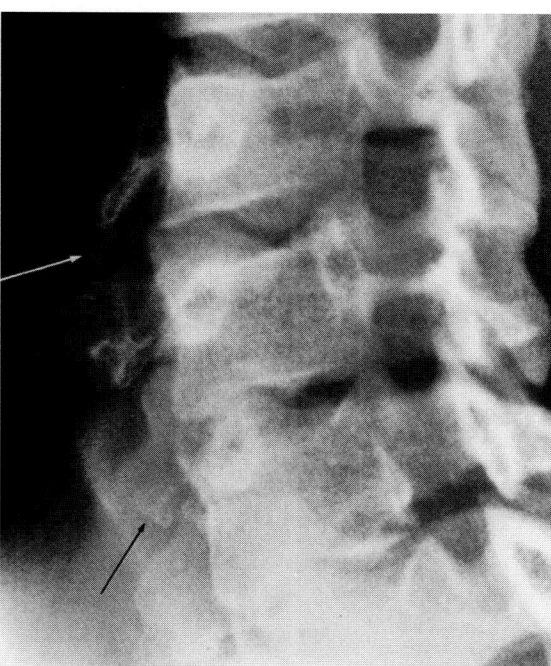

Figure 3–276. Large transverse processes with attempts to form ribs at C5 and C7.

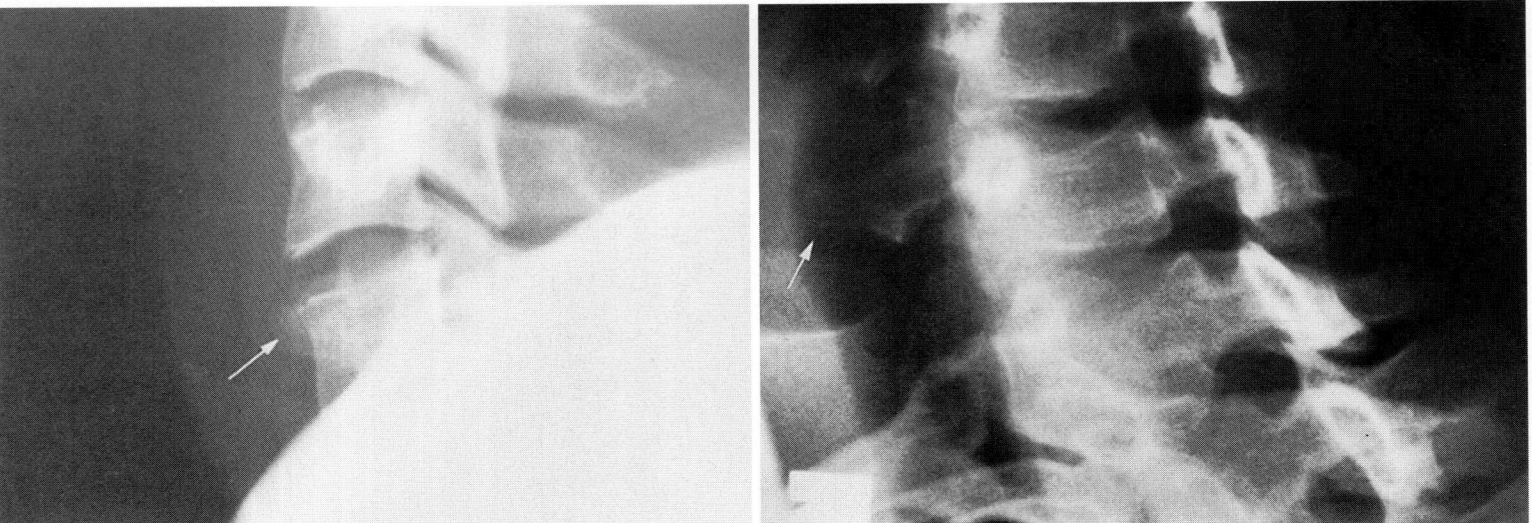

Figure 3–277. *Left*, Long transverse process of C6, simulating a fracture *(arrow)*. *Right*, Oblique projection shows the elongated transverse process *(arrow)*.

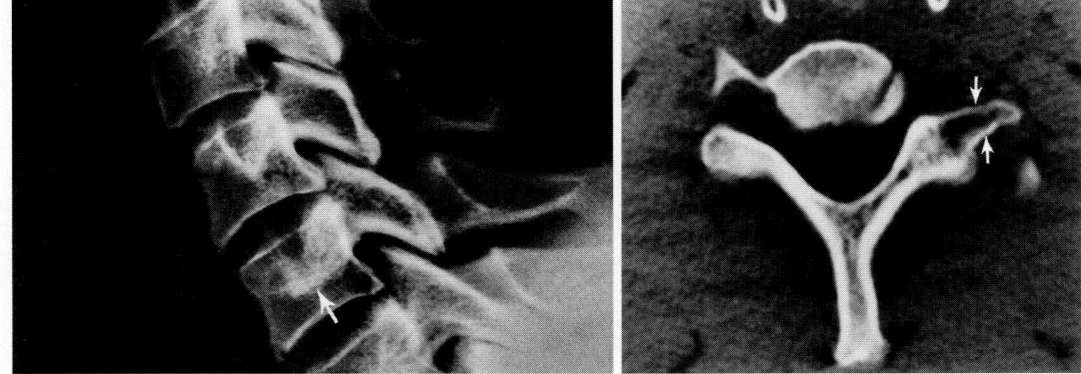

Figure 3–278. Increased density of the body of C6 produced by an enlarged and elongated transverse process on the left.

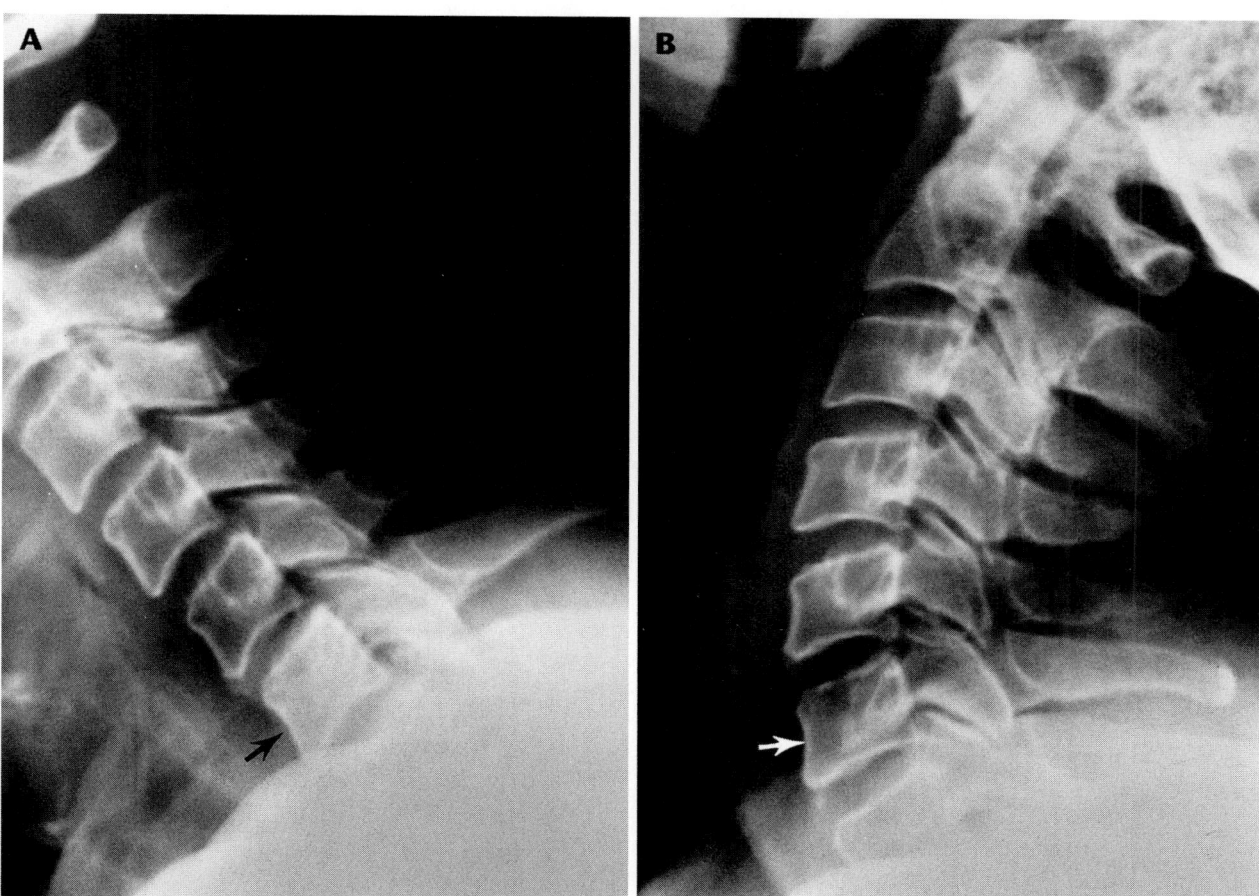

Figure 3–279. A, Increased density of C6 produced by overlying soft tissues. **B,** Density disappears when the cervical spine is extended and reduces the soft tissue overlying the vertebra.

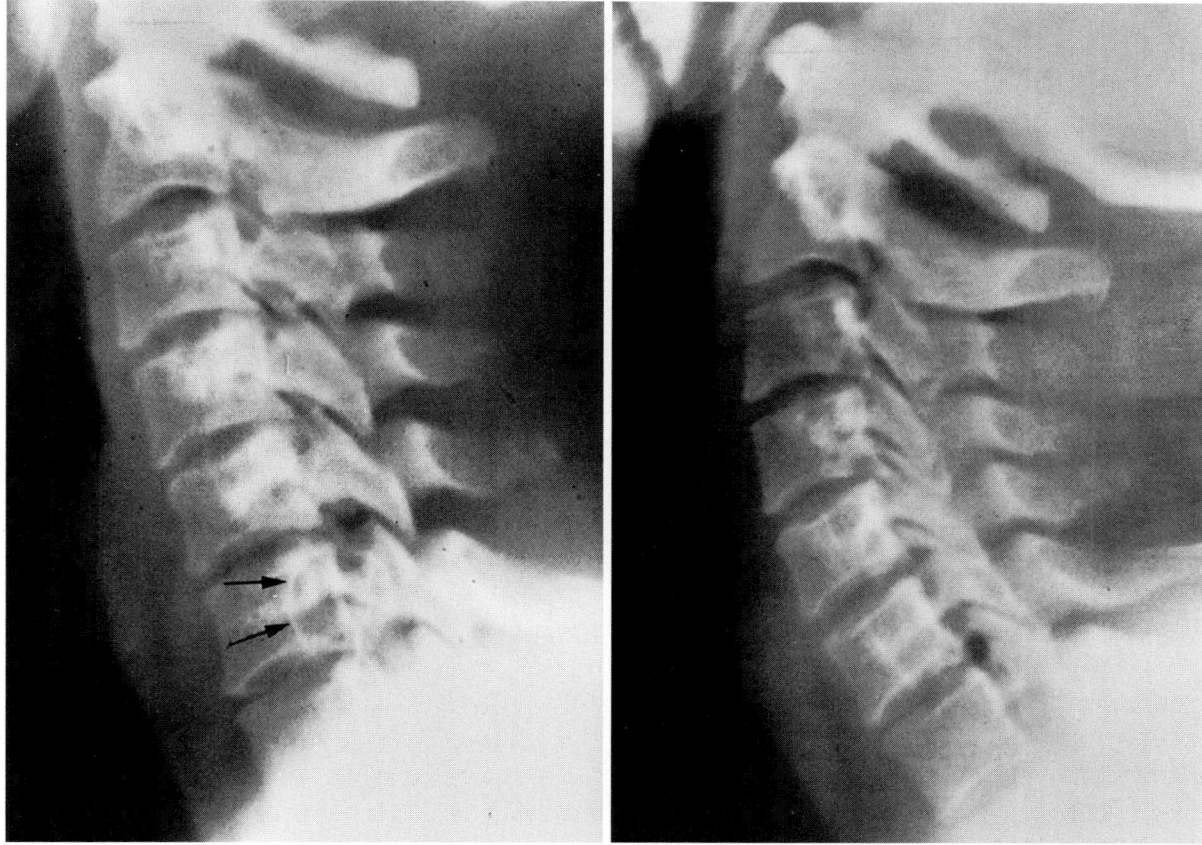

Figure 3–280. *Left,* Ringlike shadow produced by lateral elements of the vertebra with slight rotation at the time of filming. *Right,* True lateral projection does not show the ring shadow.

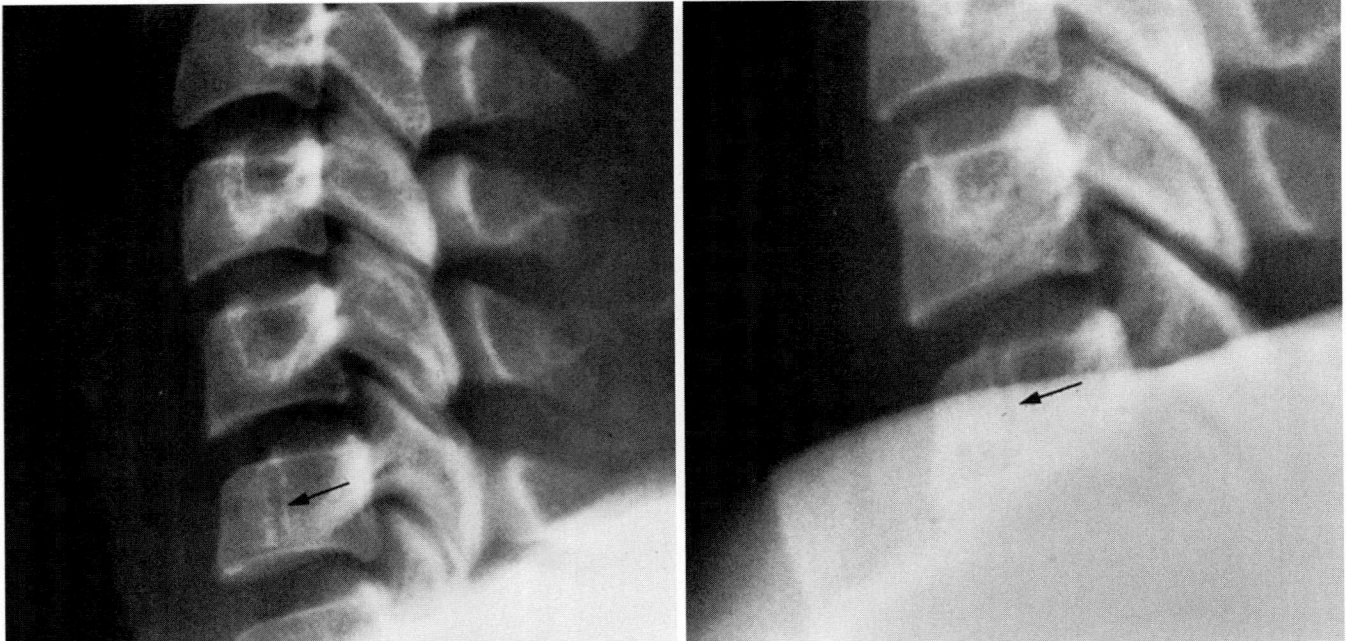

Figure 3–281. Simulated fractures of vertebral bodies produced by the shadows of the transverse processes.

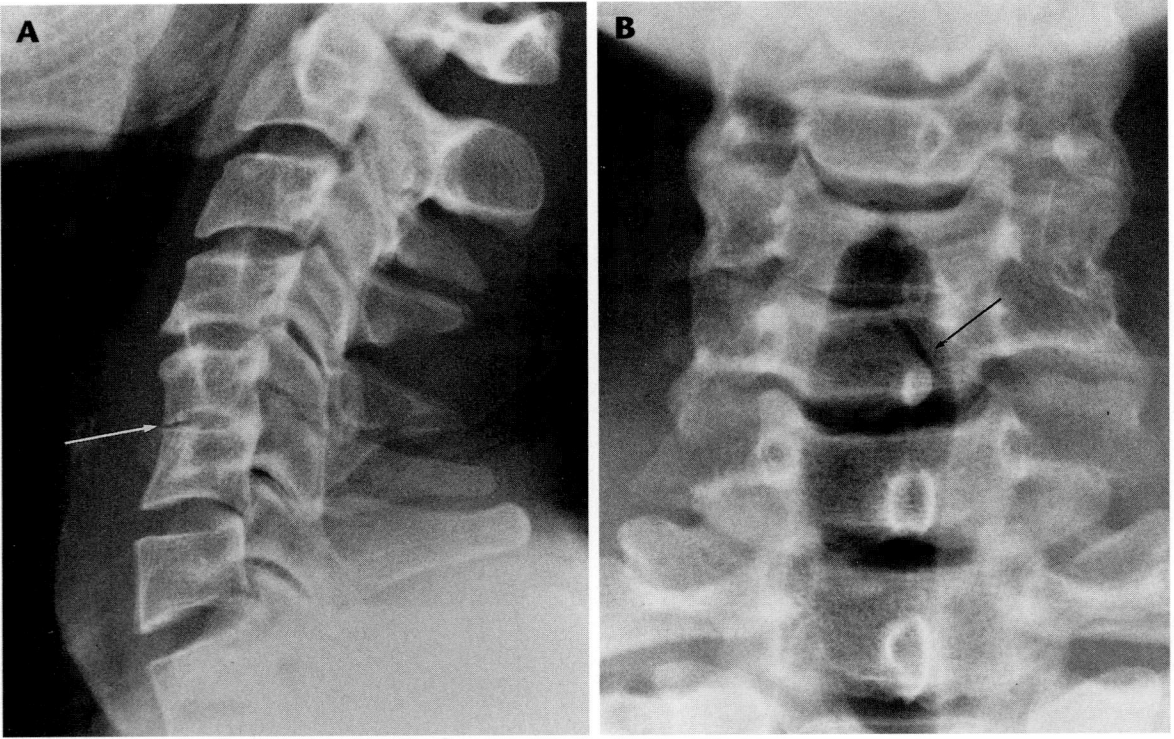

Figure 3–282. Block vertebrae at C5–C6 with spina bifida.

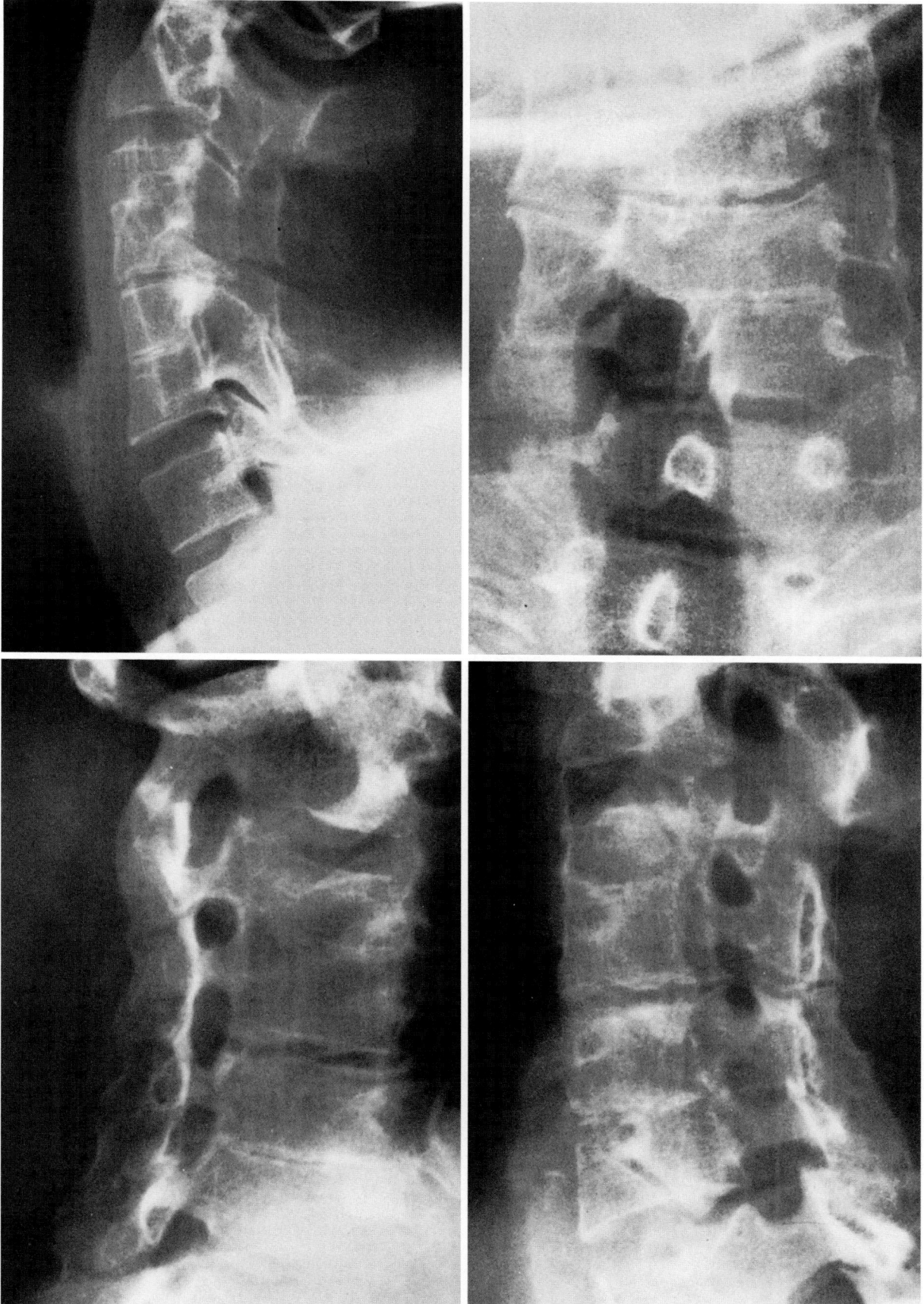

Figure 3–283. Nonsegmented vertebrae at C3–C4 and C5–C6. Oblique projection shows resulting deformity of intervertebral foramina.

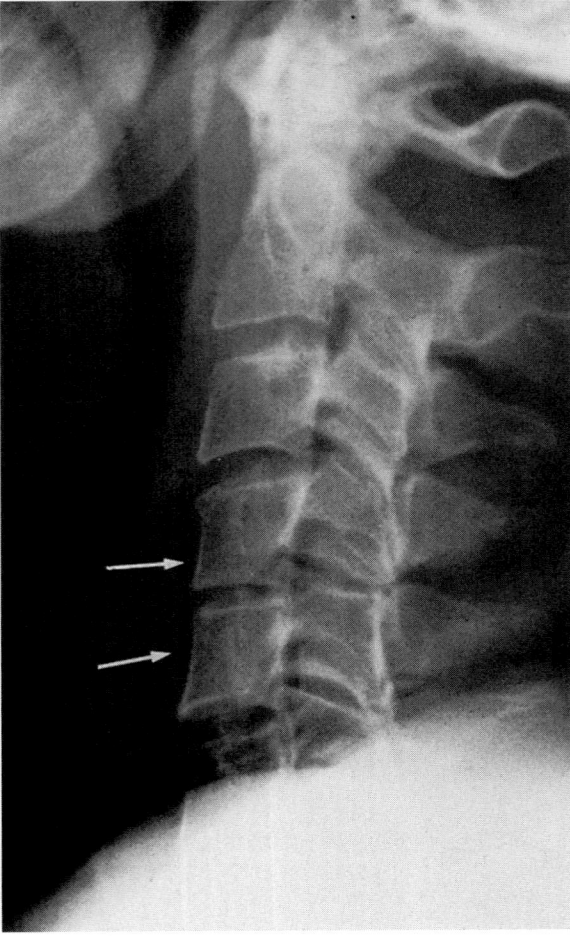

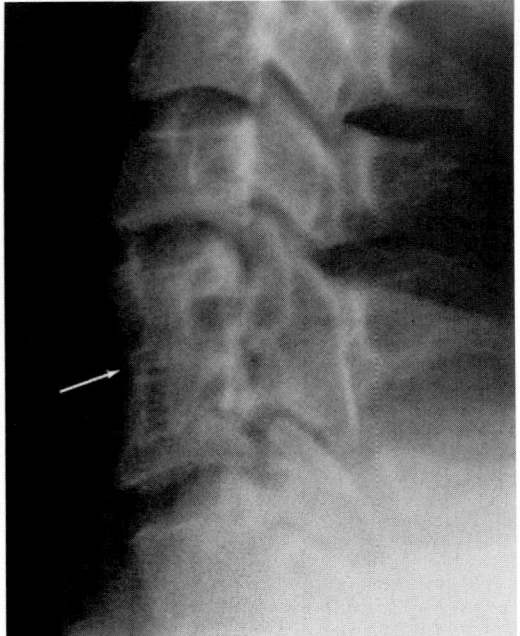

Figure 3–285. Failure of segmentation of C5–C6.

Figure 3–284. Partial segmentation error at C4–C5. Note the underdevelopment of the vertebral bodies.

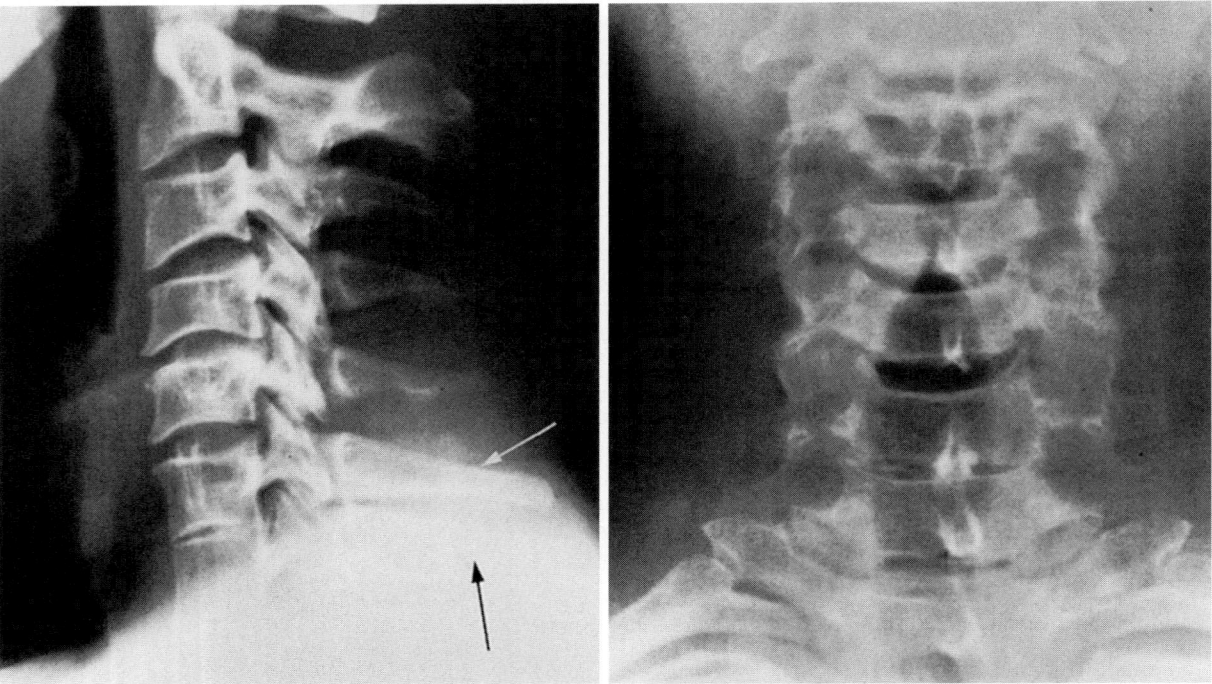

Figure 3–286. Block vertebrae of C6–C7 with marked elongation of the spinous processes.

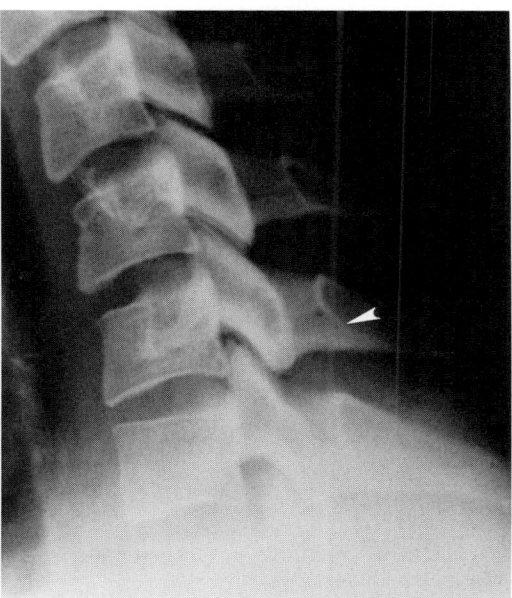

Figure 3–287. Posterior tilt of the spinolaminal line of C6, which should not be confused with the effect of an intraspinal lesion.

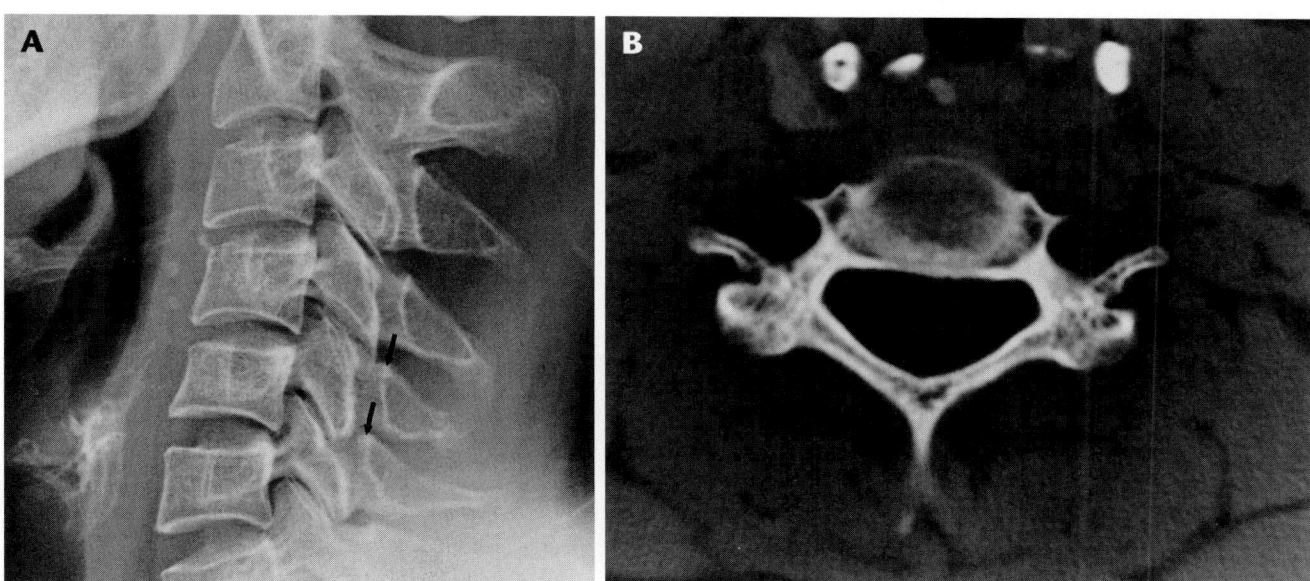

Figure 3–288. Failure of the spinolaminar line at C6 in the absence of fracture, a variation of normal. **A,** Lateral projection. **B,** CT.

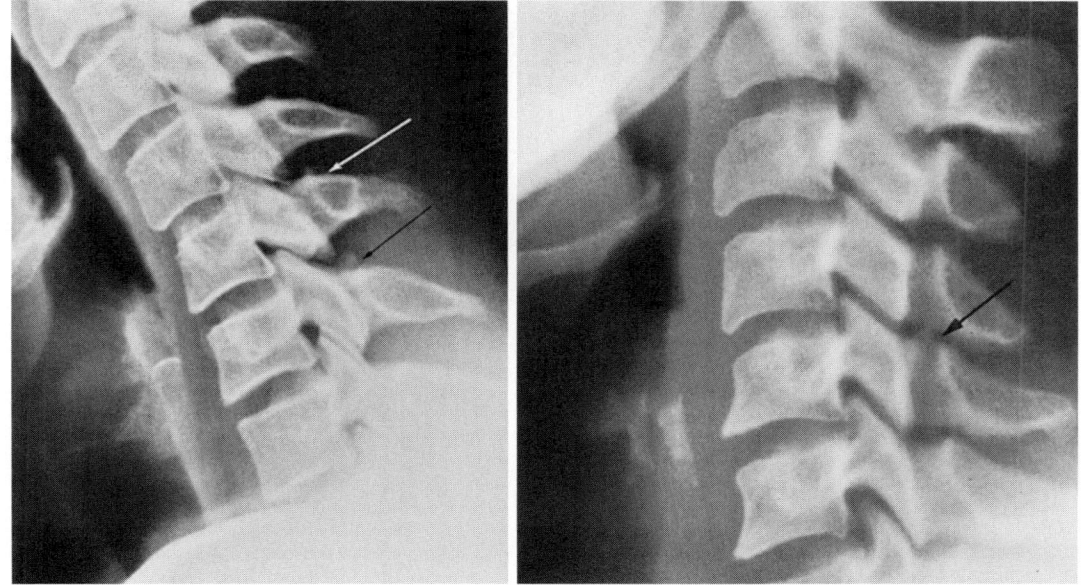

Figure 3–289. Two examples of developmental spurlike processes arising from the posterior portion of the neural arches of C5 and C6.

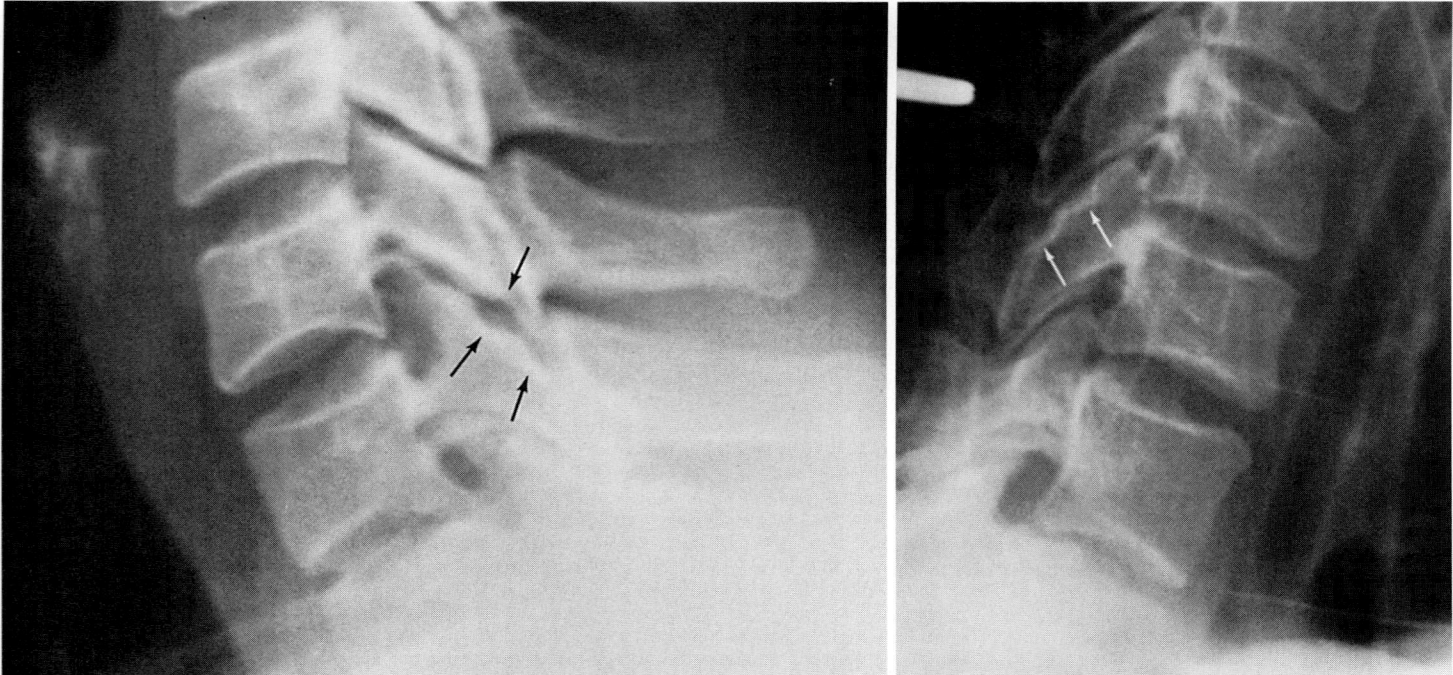

Figure 3–290. Two examples of normal notching of the apophyseal joint surfaces of the lower cervical spine, not to be mistaken for erosion or fracture. (Ref: Keats TE, Johnstone WH: Notching of the lamina of C-7: A proposed mechanism. *Skeletal Radiol* 7:273, 1982.)

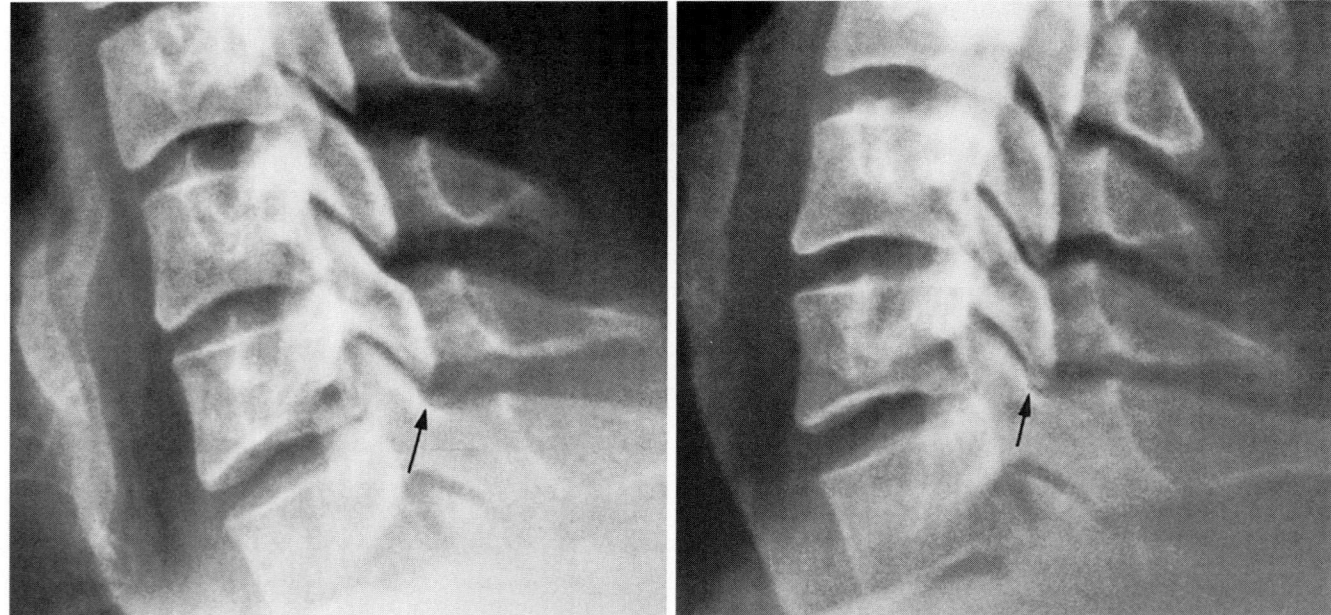

Figure 3–291. *Left,* The laminar notch at C7. *Right,* In extension, note how the inferior articular process fits into the notch.

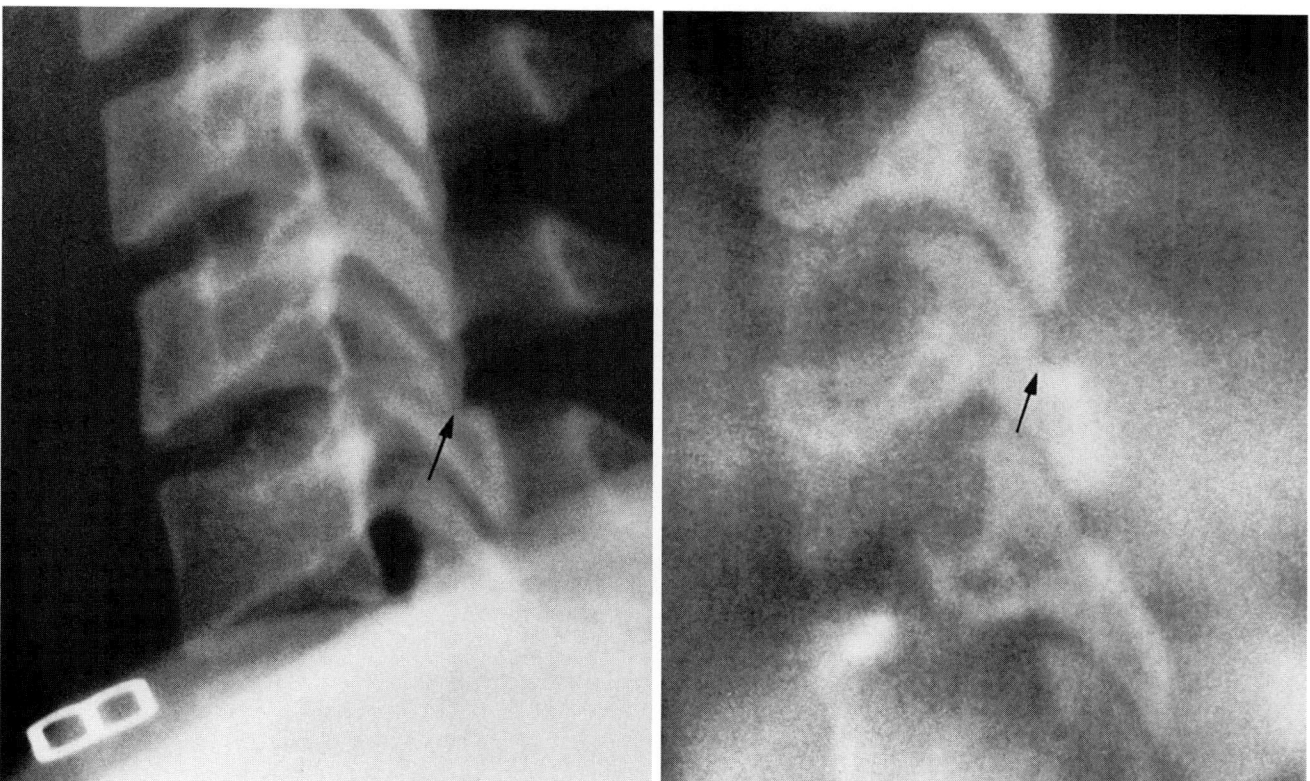

Figure 3–292. *Left,* The laminar notch at C7, which was mistaken for a fracture. *Right,* Tomogram shows no fracture.

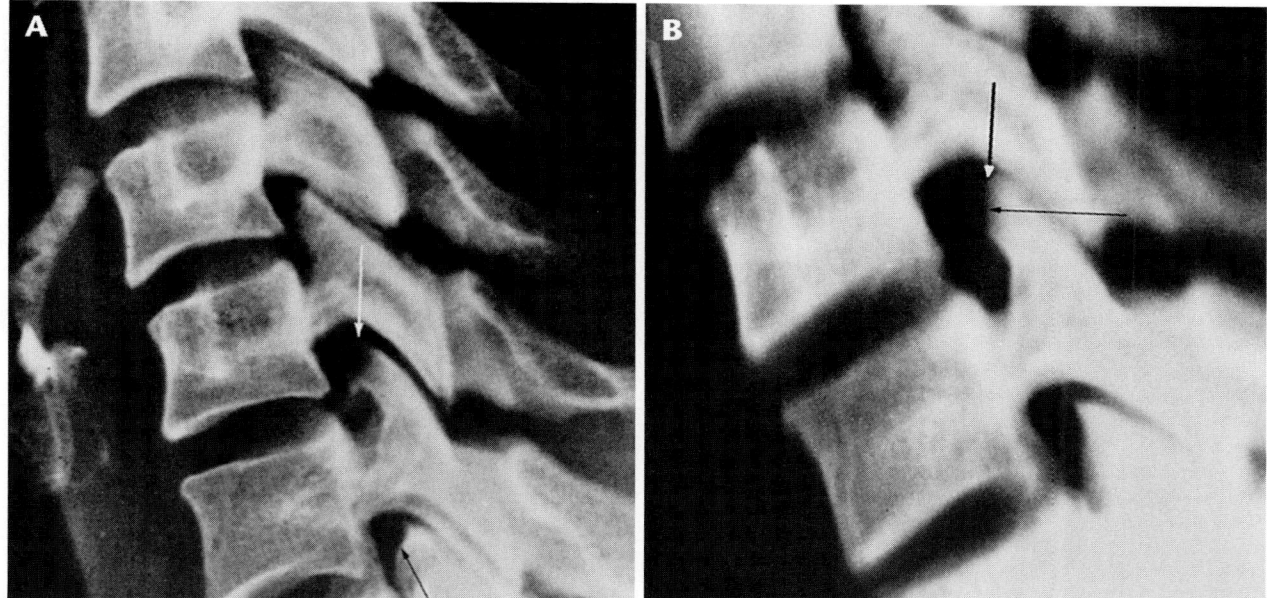

Figure 3–293. Notches in the superior extremity of the superior articulating processes of C6 and C7, presumably developmental, detected as an incidental finding. **A,** Plain film. **B,** Tomogram.

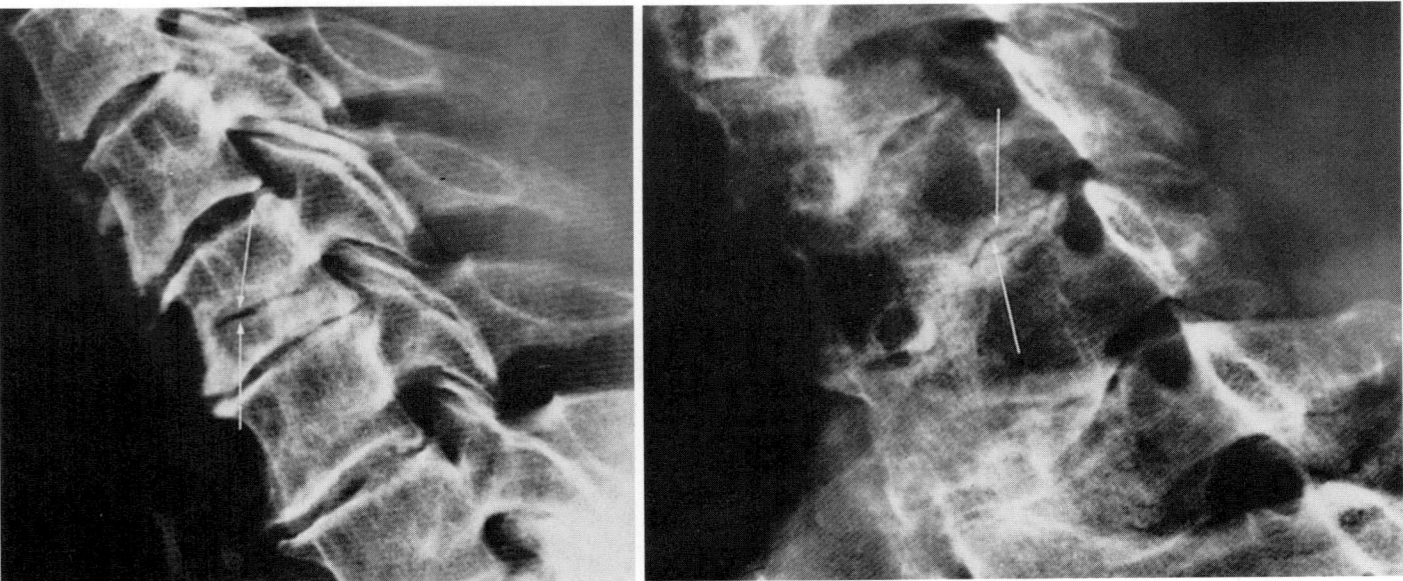

Figure 3–294. Simulated fracture of C5 produced by uncovertebral joint degeneration. (Ref: Goldberg RP et al: The cervical split: A pseudofracture. *Skeletal Radiol* 7:267, 1982.)

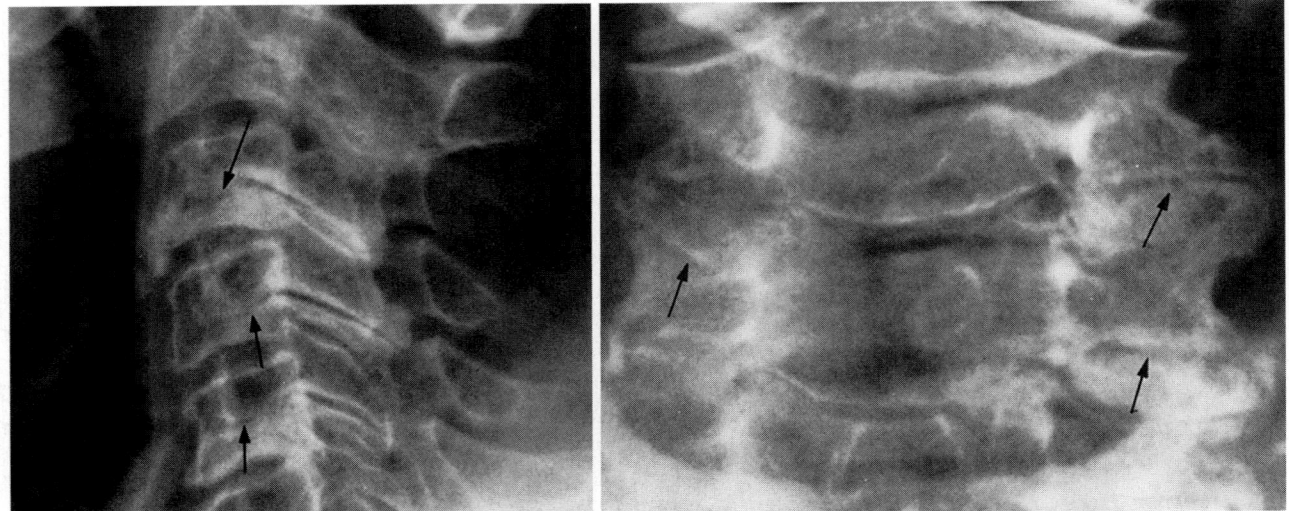

Figure 3–295. Multiple pseudofractures produced by degeneration of the facet and uncovertebral joints, and by rotation in the lateral projection.

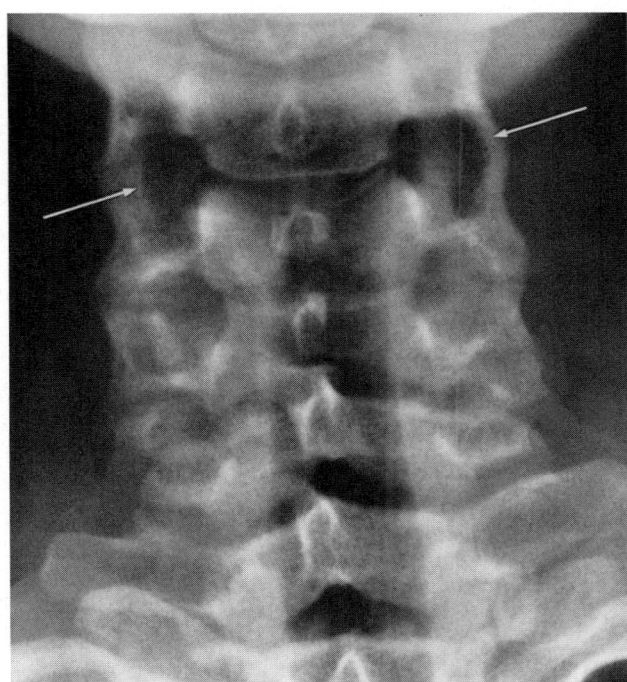

Figure 3–296. Air in the pyriform sinuses simulating destructive lesions of the cervical spine.

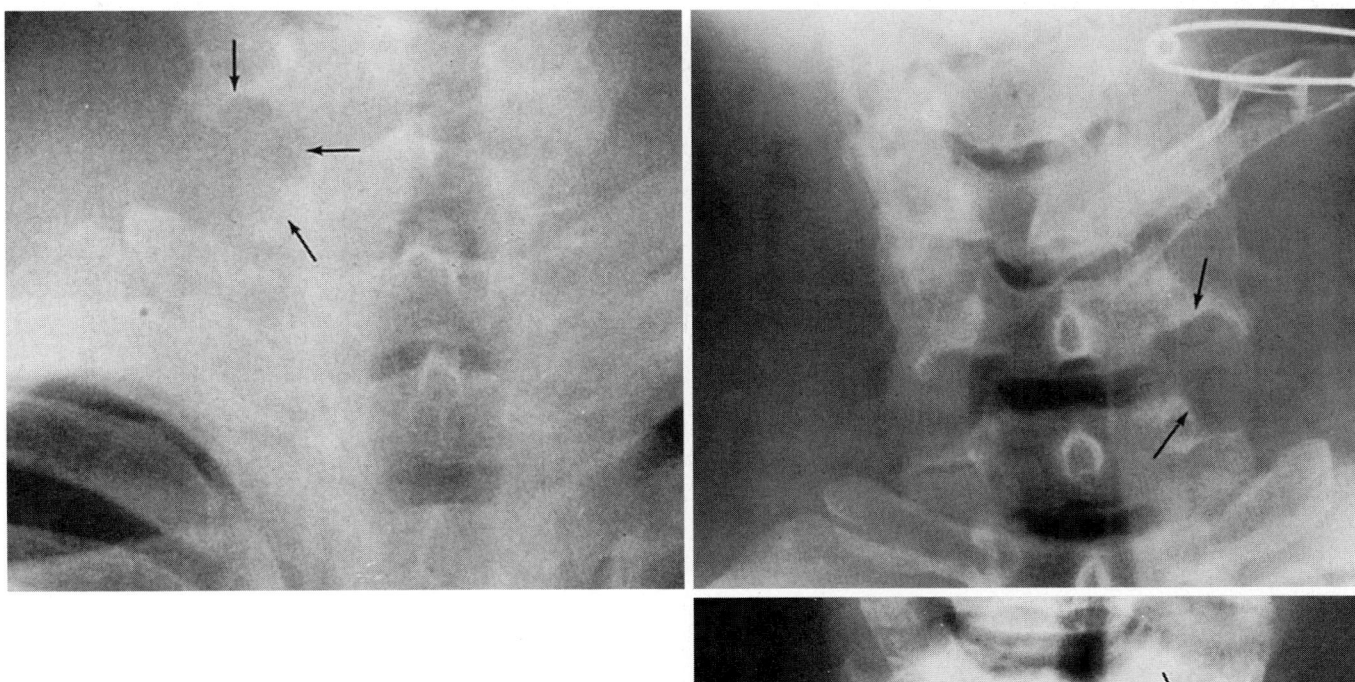

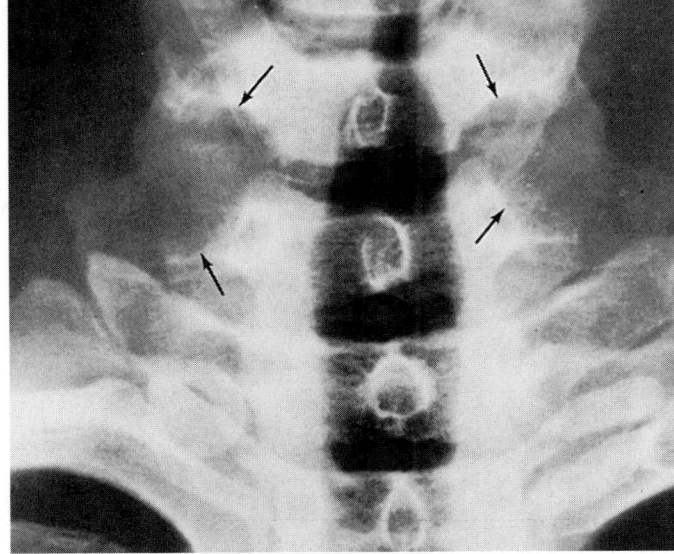

Figure 3–297. Three examples of simulated destructive lesions of the lower cervical spine, produced by projection.

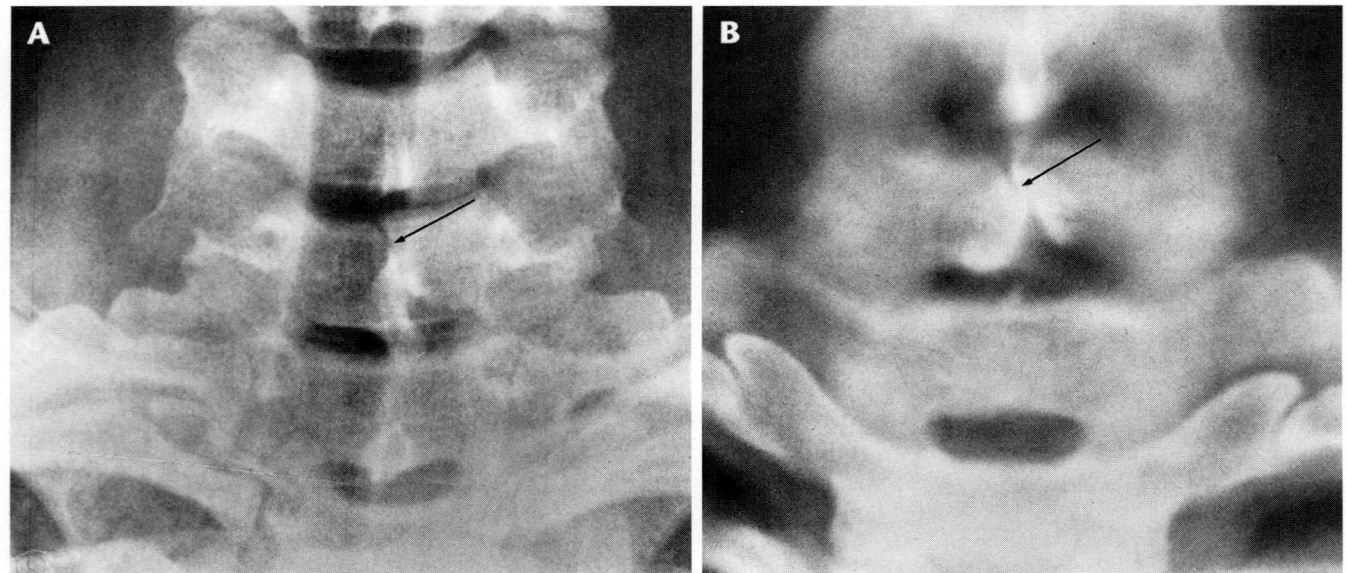

Figure 3–298. Spina bifida of C7 simulating a fracture. **A,** Plain film.
B, Tomogram.

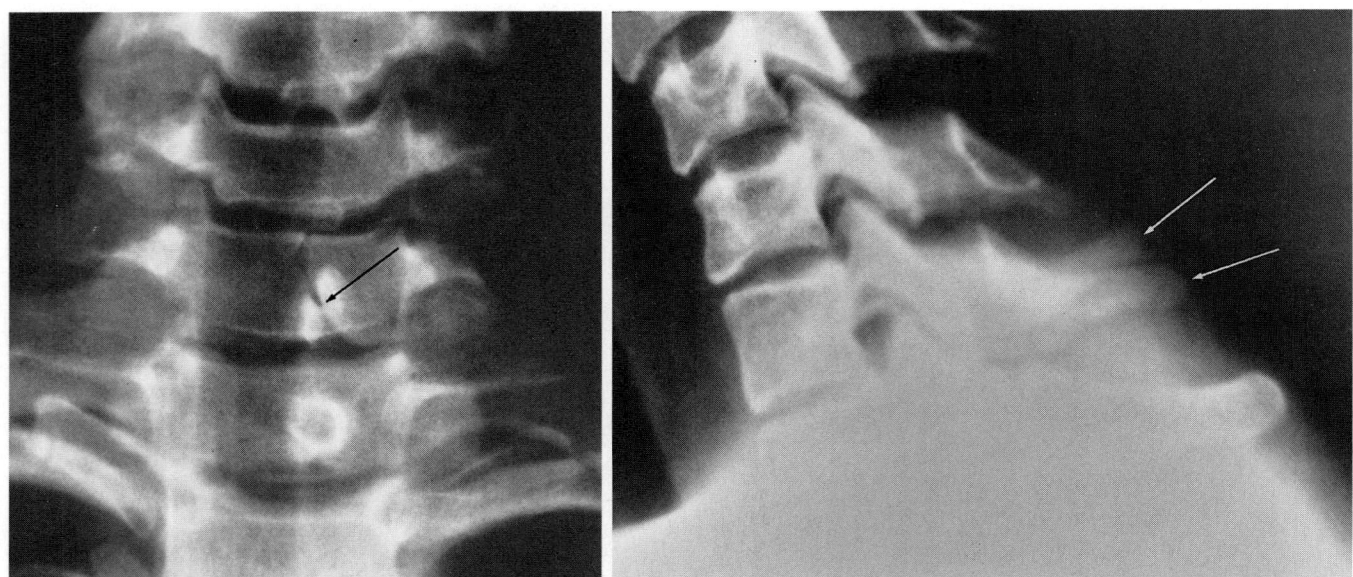

Figure 3–299. Spina bifida of C7 with double spinous processes.

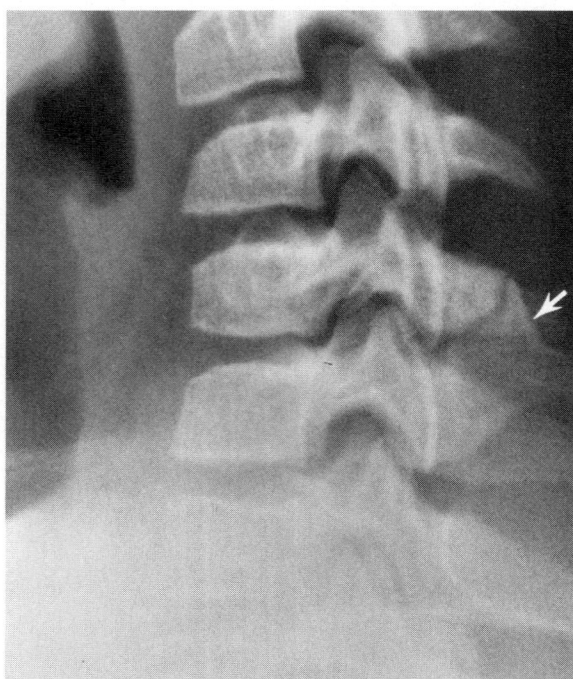

Figure 3–300. Anomalous bridge between the spinous processes of C6 and C7.

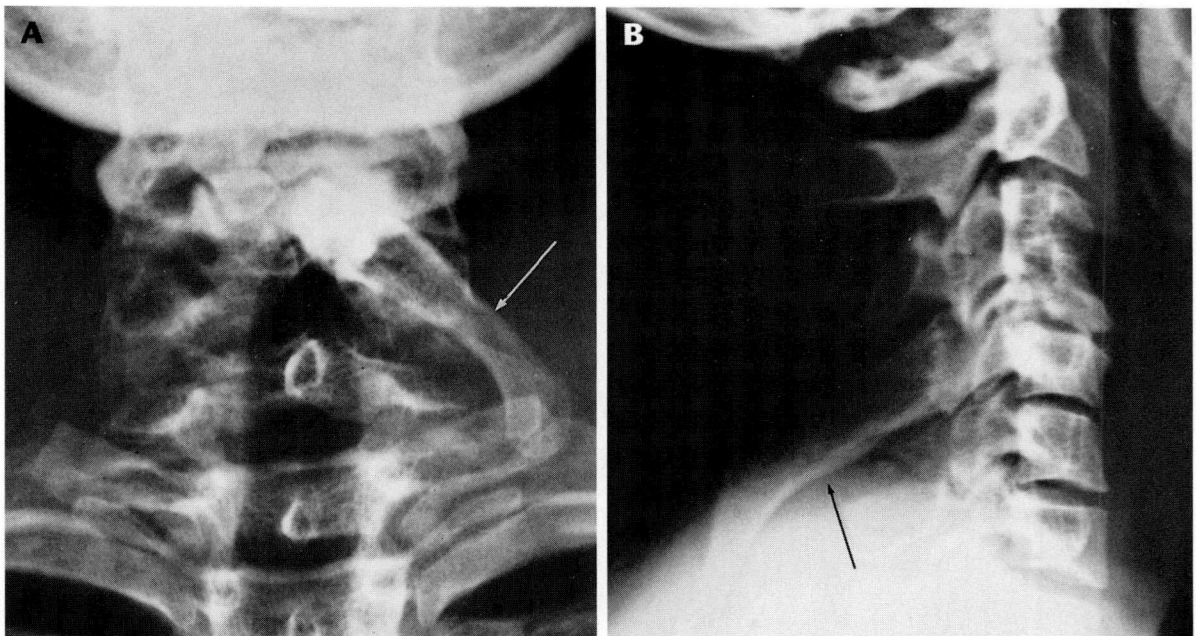

Figure 3–301. The omovertebral bone between C5 and T1, unassociated with Sprengel's deformity.

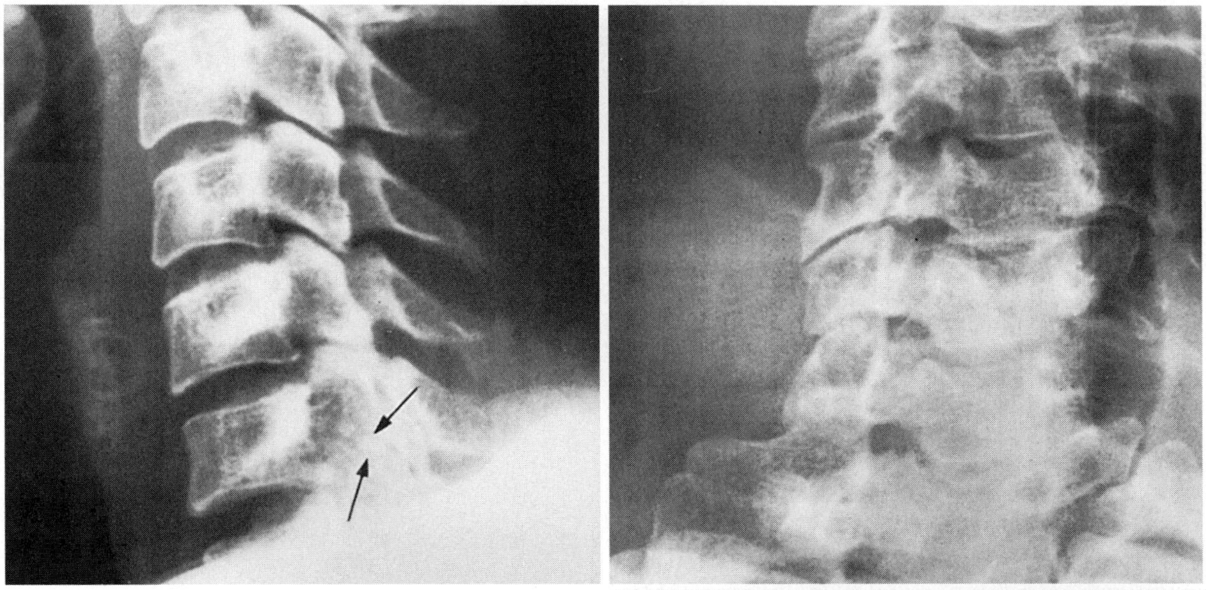

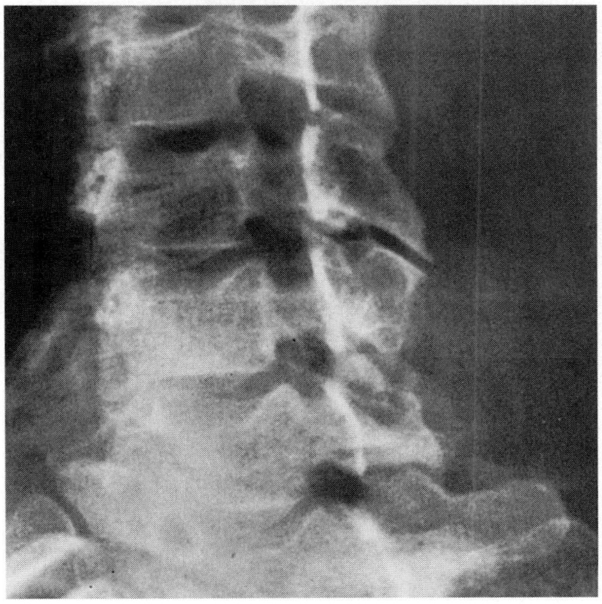

Figure 3–302. *Top left,* The lateral elements of C6 projected slightly caudad show two apophyseal joints that were misinterpreted as fractures. *Top right and bottom,* Oblique projections show no abnormality.

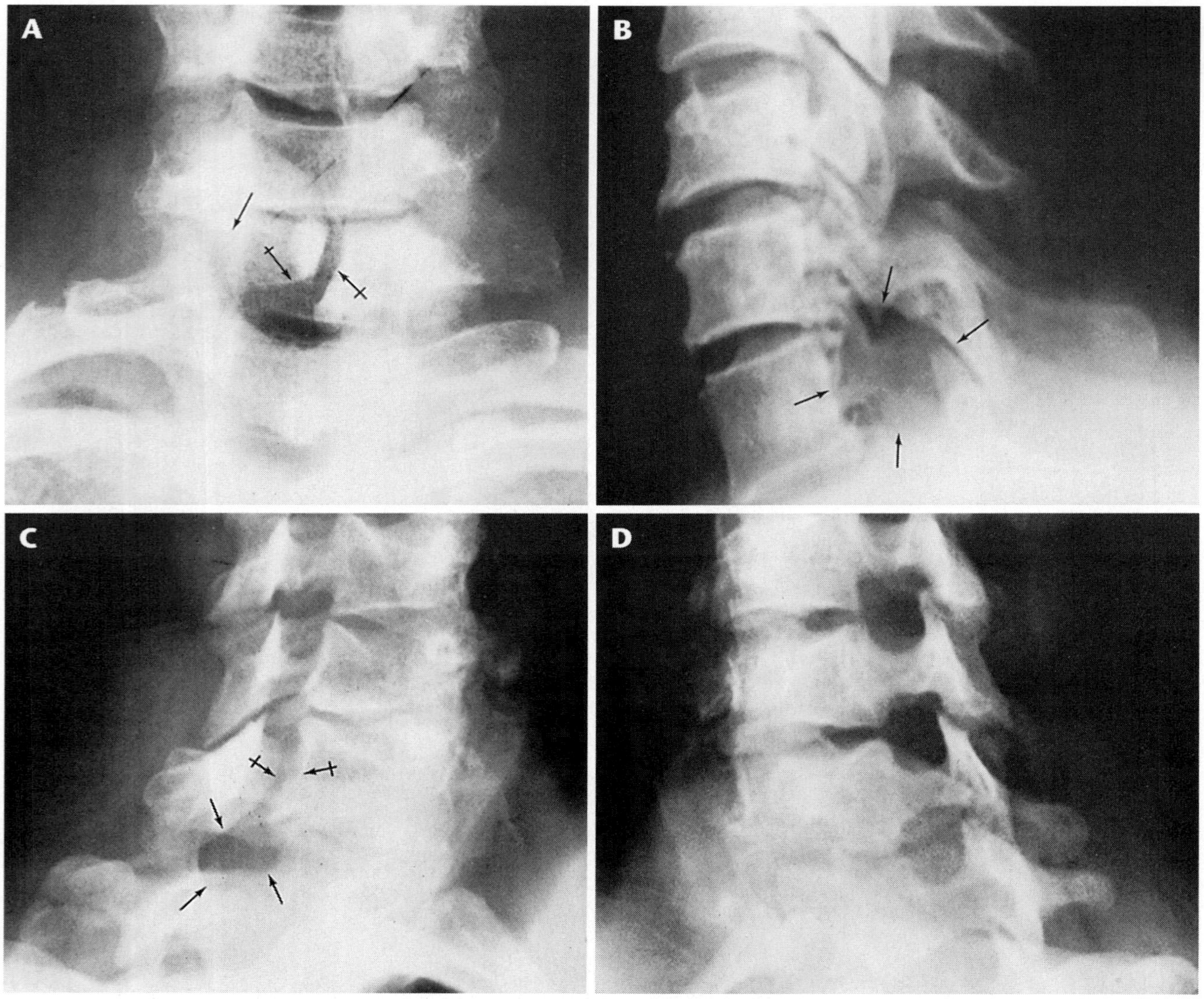

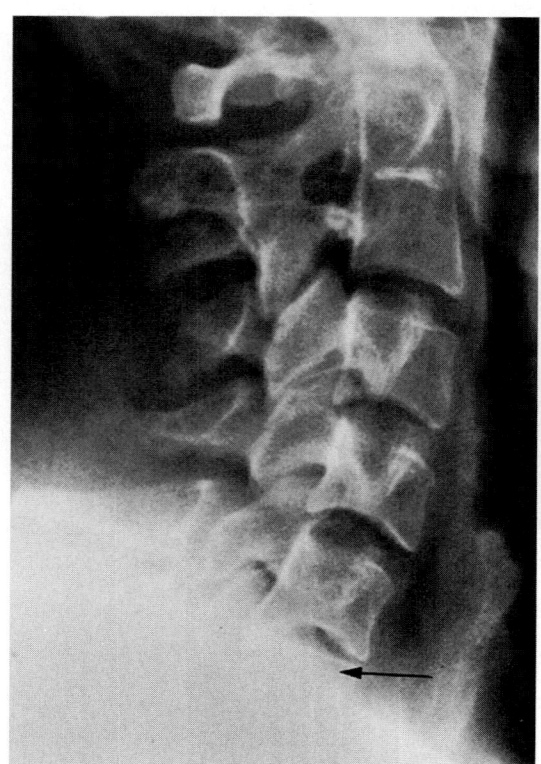

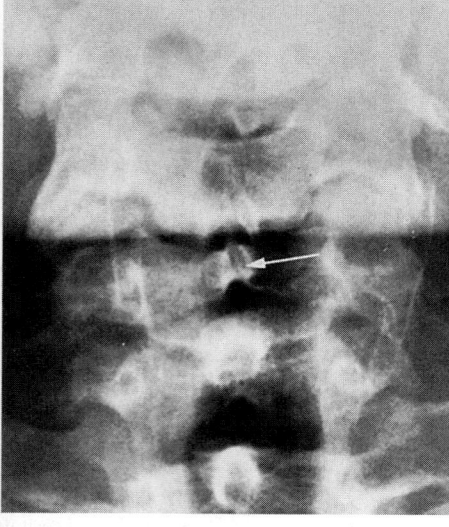

Figure 3–303. Congenital absence of the C7 pedicle on the right (←). A spina bifida occulta is also present (↔) **(A–C)**. Compare oblique projection **(C)** with normal side **(D)**. This congenital lesion may be mistaken for an acquired one (see Fig. 3–251). (Refs: Chapman M: Congenital absence of cervical pedicle. *Skeletal Radiol* 1:65, 1976; and Van Dijk Azn R et al: The absent cervical pedicle syndrome. *Neuroradiology* 29:69, 1987.)

Figure 3–304. *Left,* Partial nonsegmentation of C6 and C7, which was mistaken for acquired narrowing of the intervertebral disc in a 35-year-old man. C2 and C3 are also nonsegmented. *Right,* The spina bifida occulta at C6 indicates the developmental nature of the finding at C6 and C7 *(arrow).*

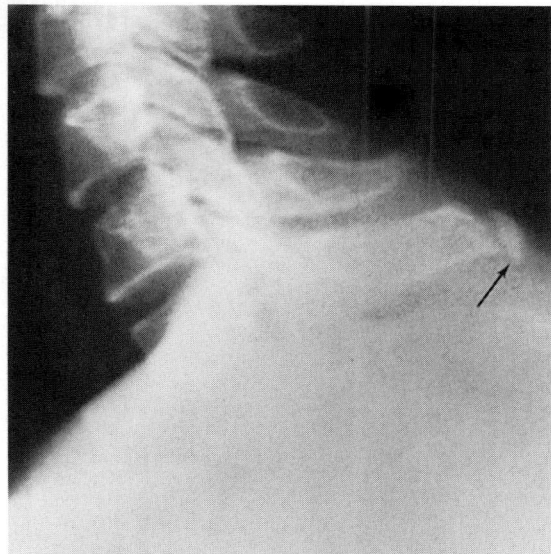

Figure 3–305. Failure of union of the apophysis of the tip of the spinous process of C7 simulating a fracture.

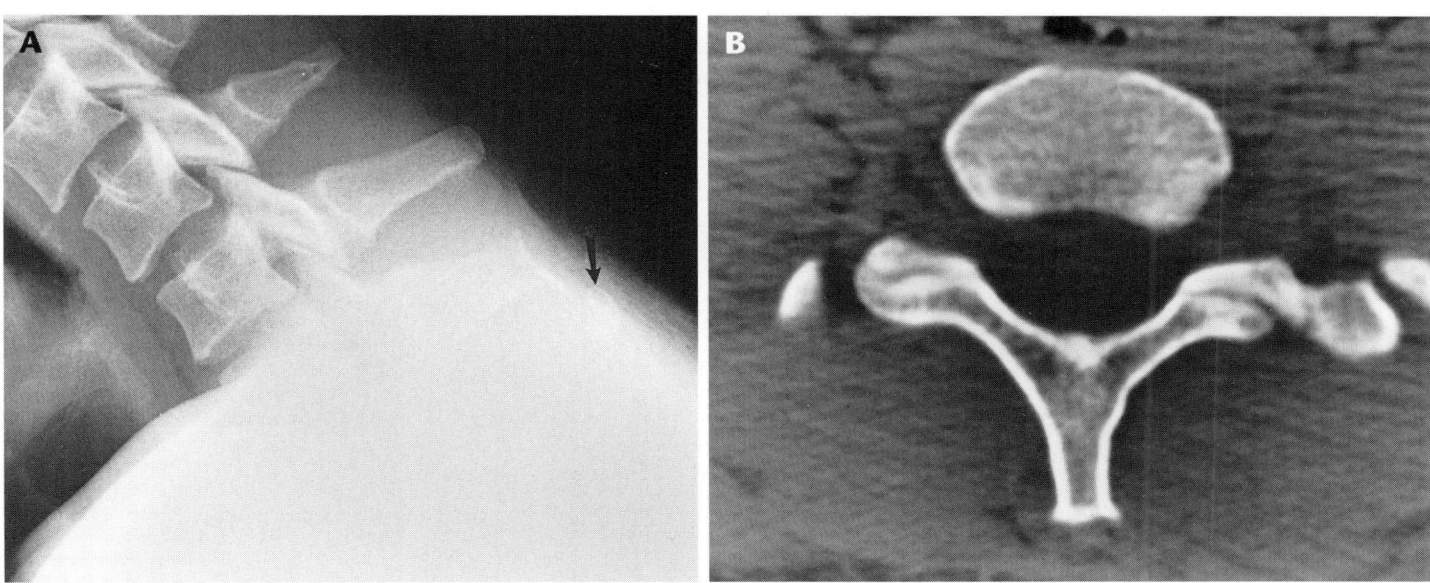

Figure 3–306. Failure of union of the apophysis of the tip of the spinous process of C7 with inferior displacement of the apophysis. **A,** Lateral projection. **B,** CT shows truncation of the spinous process.

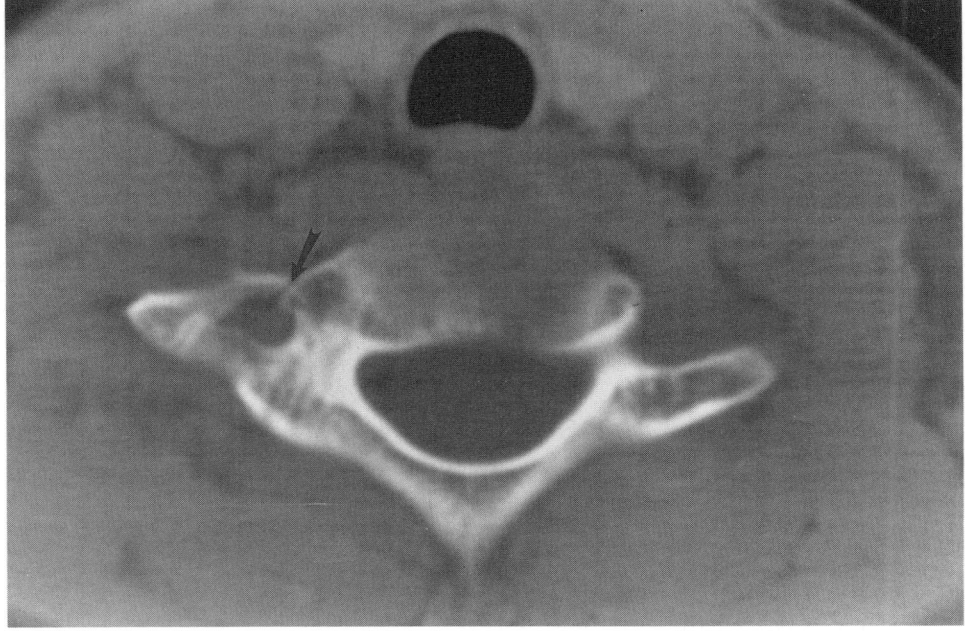

Figure 3–307. Closure defect in the foramen transversarium at C7.

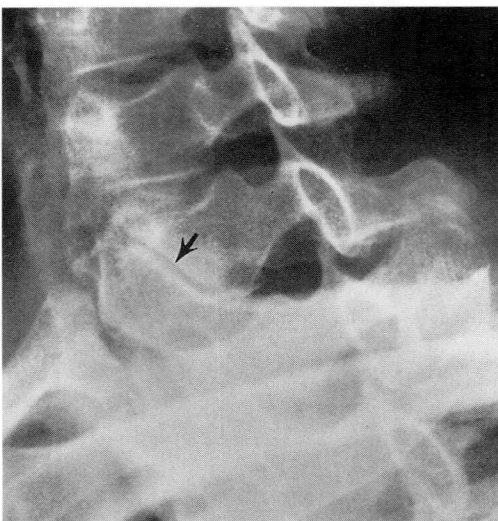

Figure 3–308. The facet between C7 and T1.

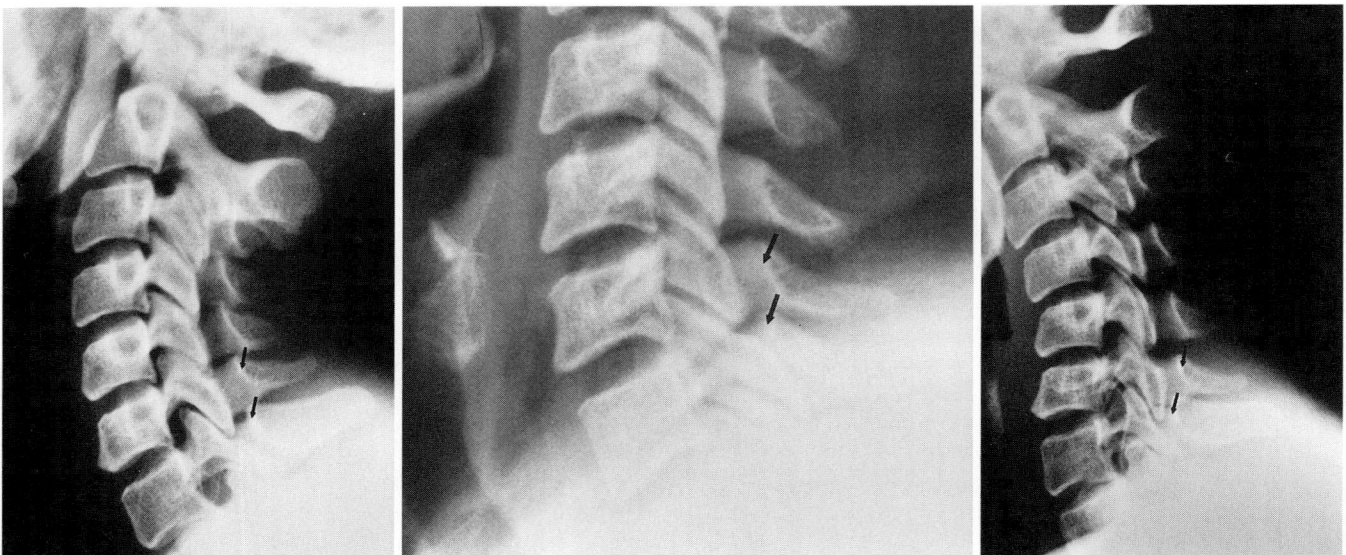

Figure 3–309. Three examples of failure of the posterior laminar line at C7 in the absence of fracture, a variation of normal. This variant may be associated with incomplete segmentation of the cervical vertebrae. (Ref: Ehara S: Relationship of elongated anterior tubercle to incomplete segmentation in the cervical spine. *Skeletal Radiol* 25:243, 1996.)

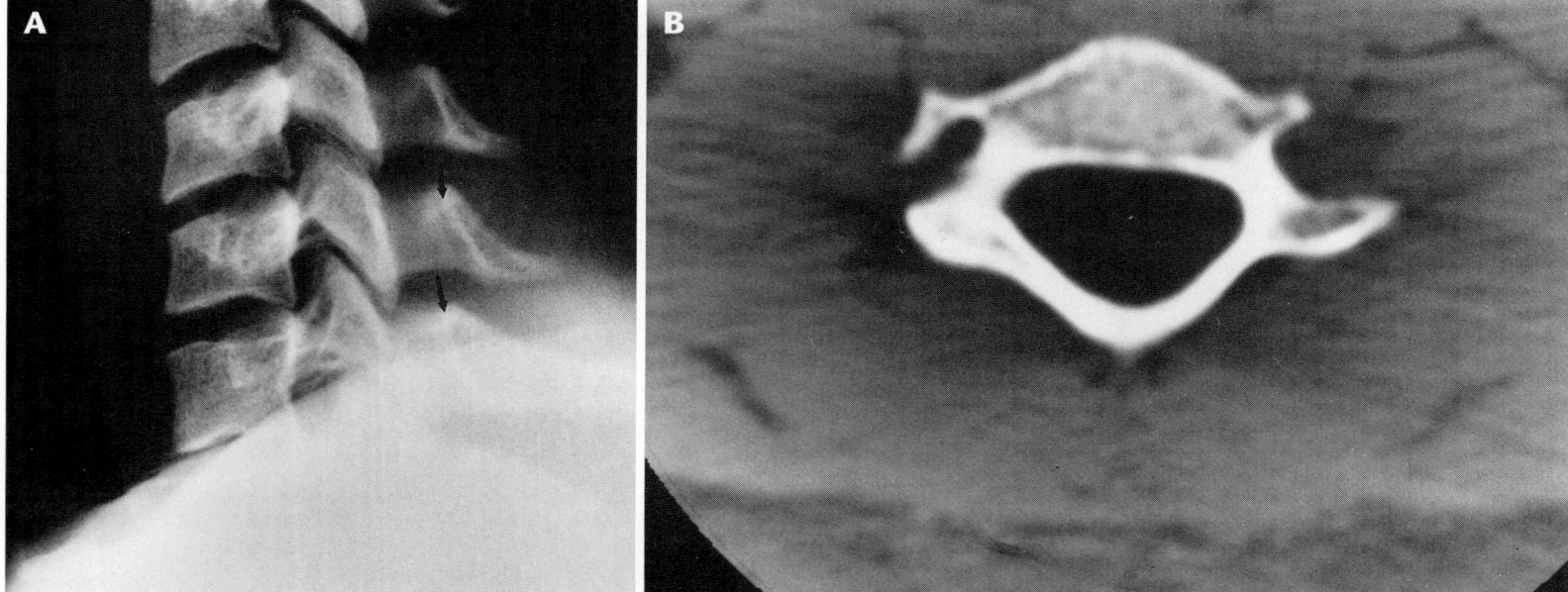

Figure 3–310. A, Marked failure of the posterior laminar line at C7. **B,** CT shows no fracture.

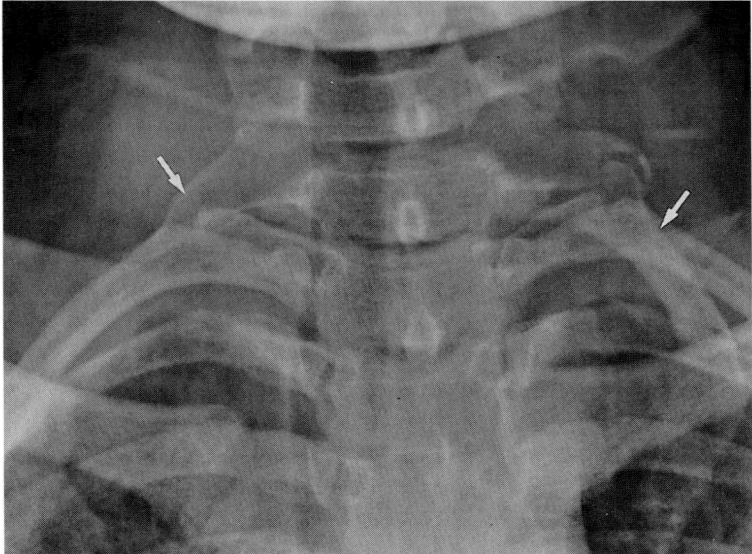

Figure 3–311. Cervical rib on the left and elongated transverse process on the right at C7.

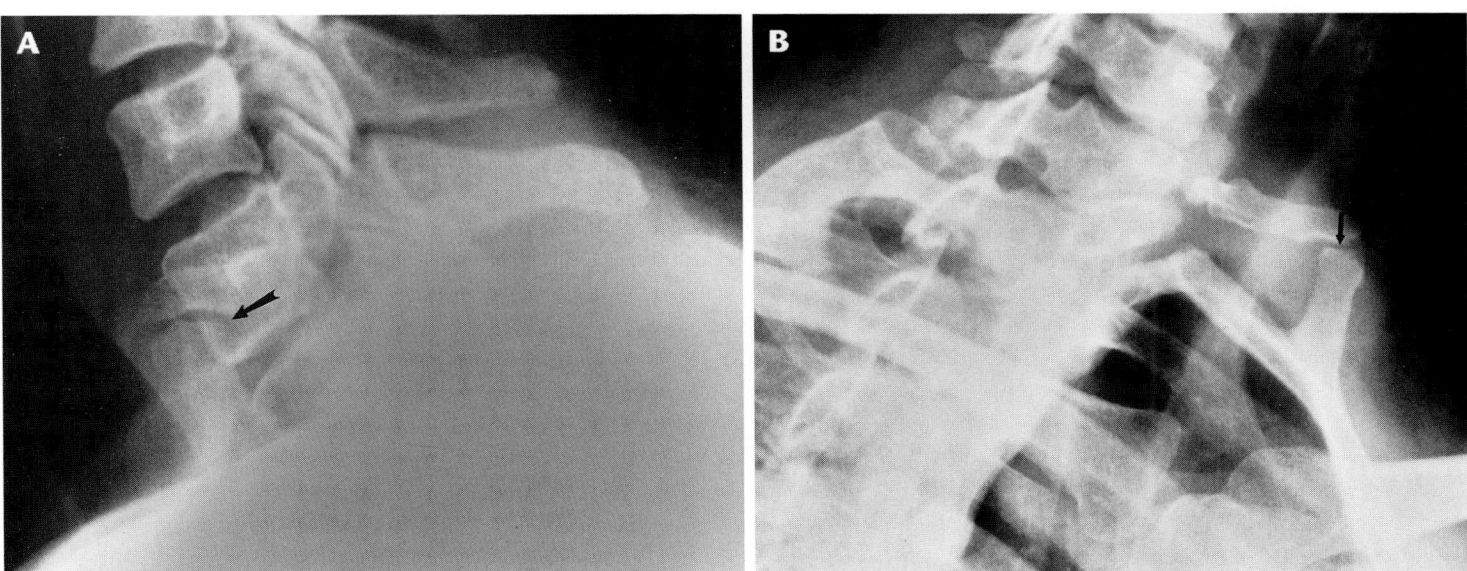

Figure 3–312. Cervical rib on the left articulating with the first rib. **A,** Lateral projection. **B,** Oblique projection.

The Thoracic Spine

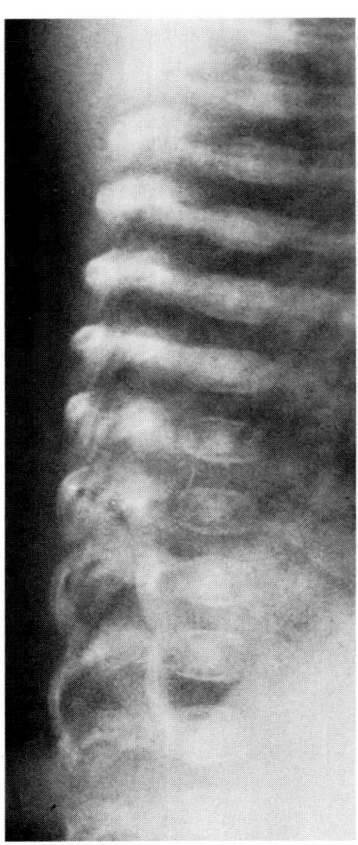

Figure 3–313. The normal "bone in bone" appearance of the thoracic vertebrae in a neonate.

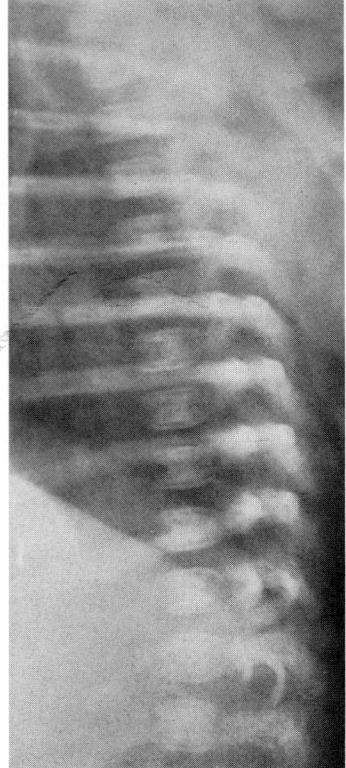

Figure 3–314. Normal thoracic spine of a 1-month-old baby. The "bone in bone" appearance is present, and the large central notches on the anterior surface of the vertebrae are normal at this age.

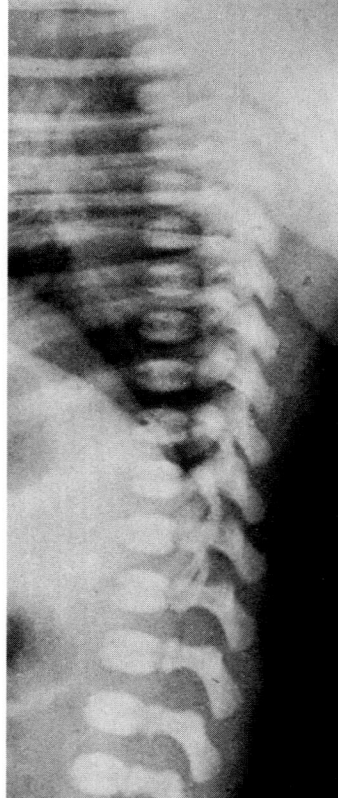

Figure 3–315. Normal neonatal thoracic spine, showing "sandwich" appearance as a result of large venous sinuses.

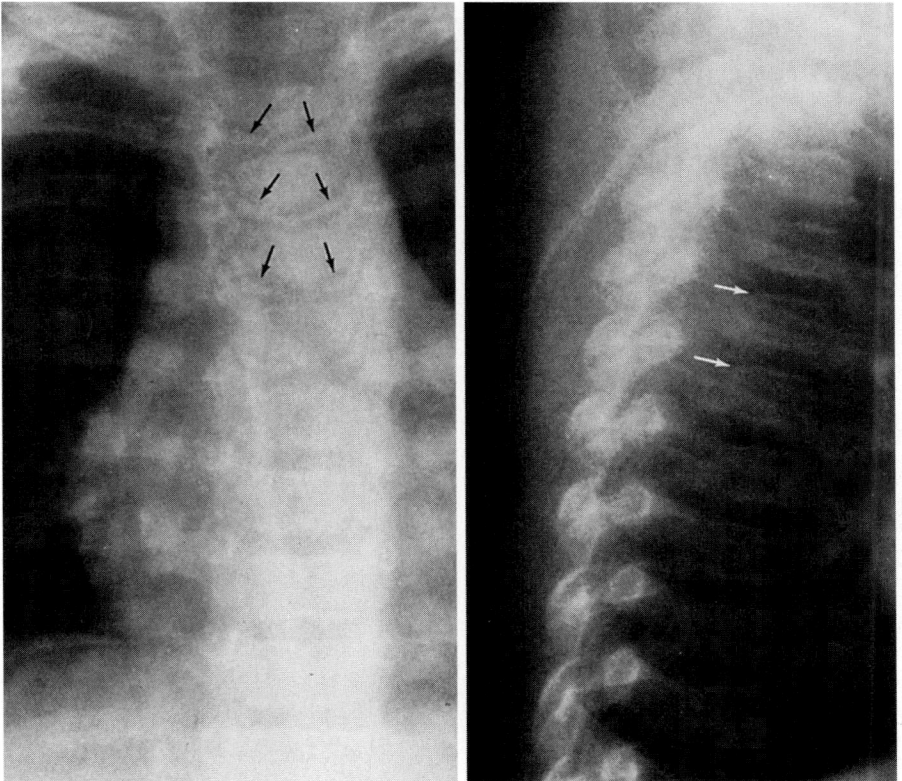

Figure 3–316. The dense end plates of the vertebral bodies produce an unusual appearance in the frontal film of a 4-month-old child.

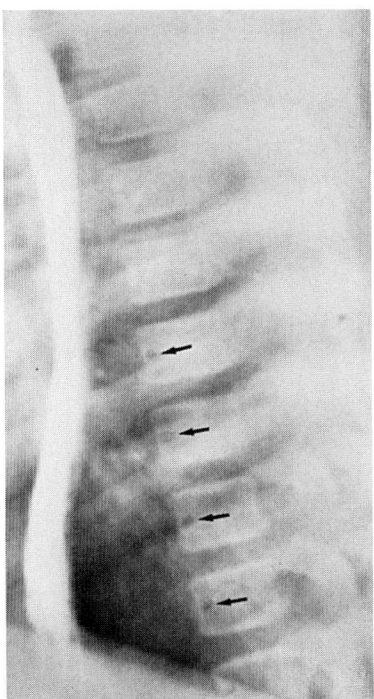

Figure 3–317. Prominent residual venous sinus "holes" in older child's thoracic spine.

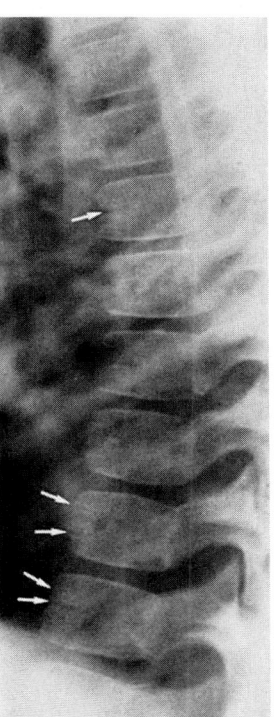

Figure 3–318. Normal thoracic spine of a 5-year-old child. The vascular stripes in the center of the anterior portion of the vertebral body and the notches in the anterior corners of the vertebrae are normal at this age.

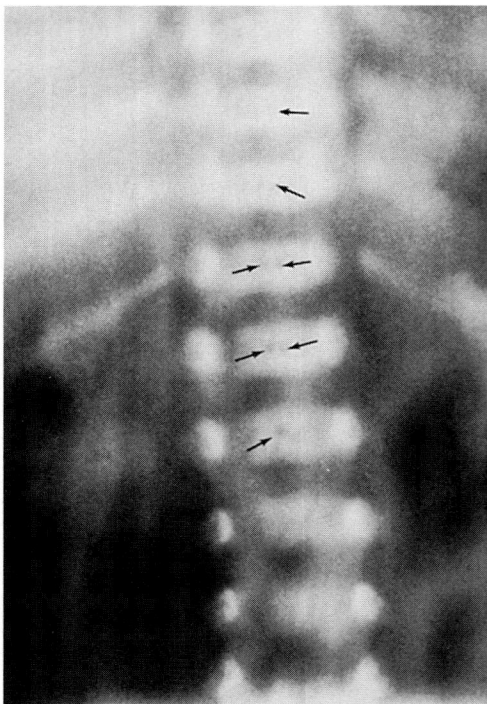

Figure 3–319. The appearance of the venous grooves in the frontal projection of a newborn.

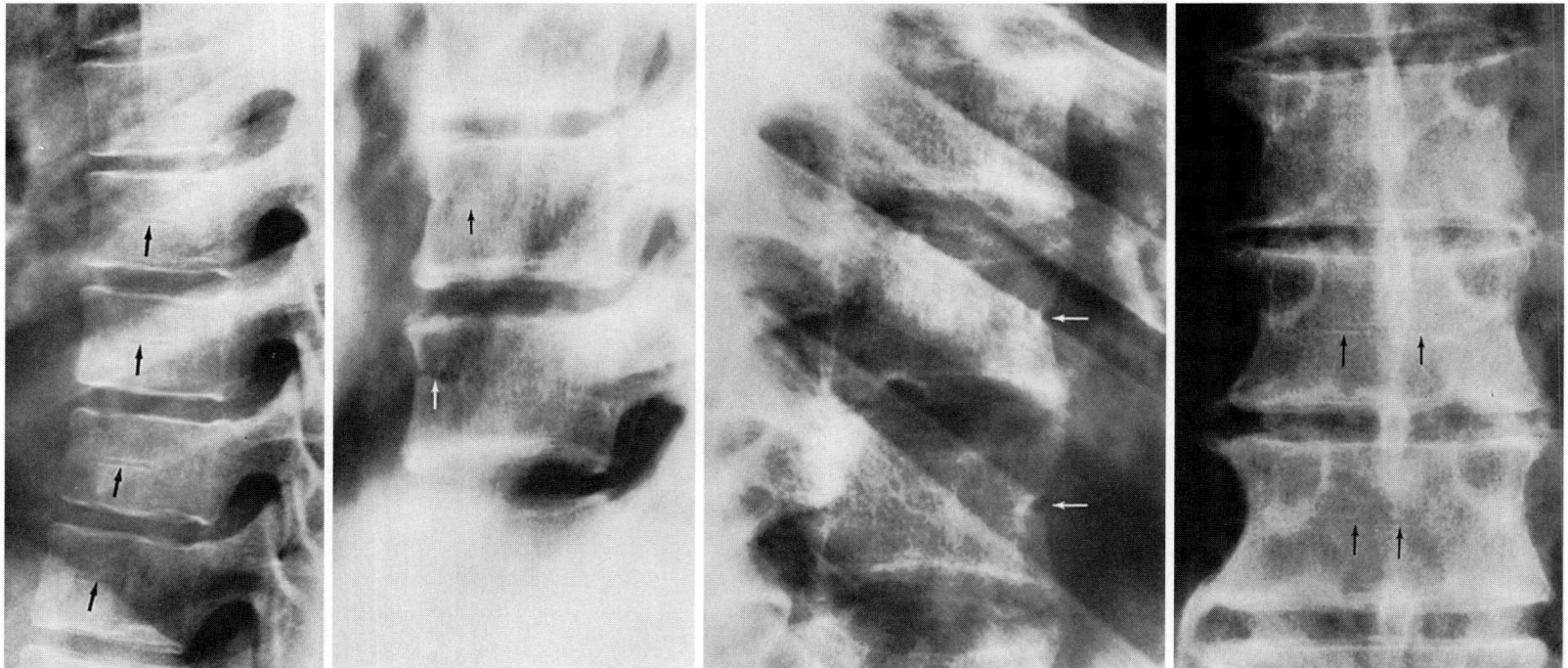

Figure 3–320. Four examples of residual venous sinus grooves in adults.

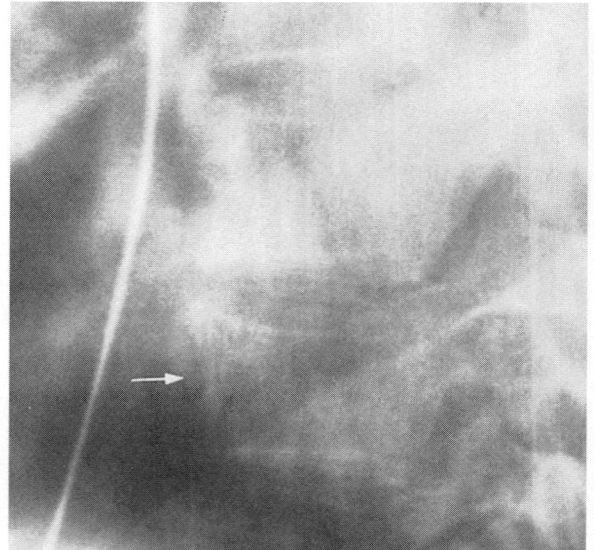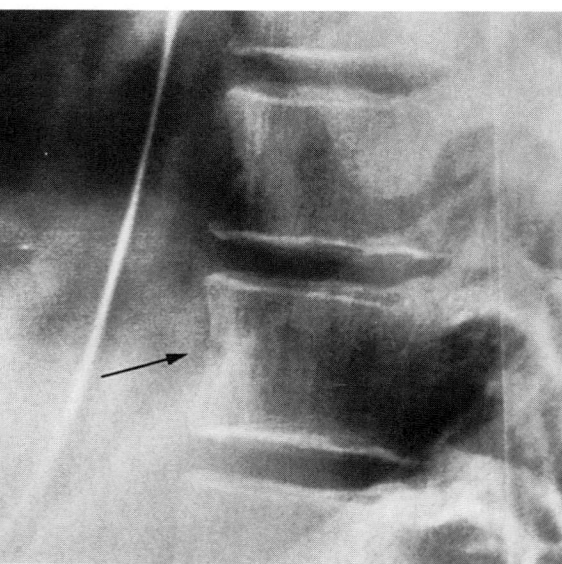

Figure 3–321. *Left,* Residual venous sinus grooves may add to the impression of a compression fracture in a poorly positioned lateral projection. Better lateral projection (*right*) shows no fracture.

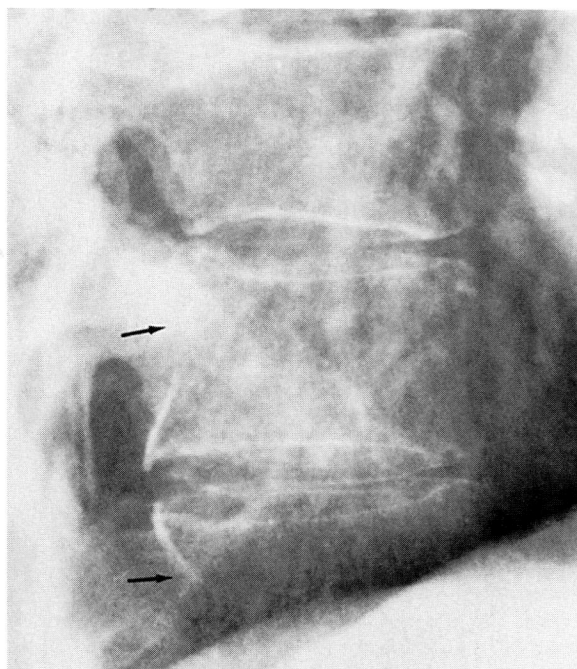

Figure 3–322. Persistence of the posterior vascular notch in a 33-year-old man.

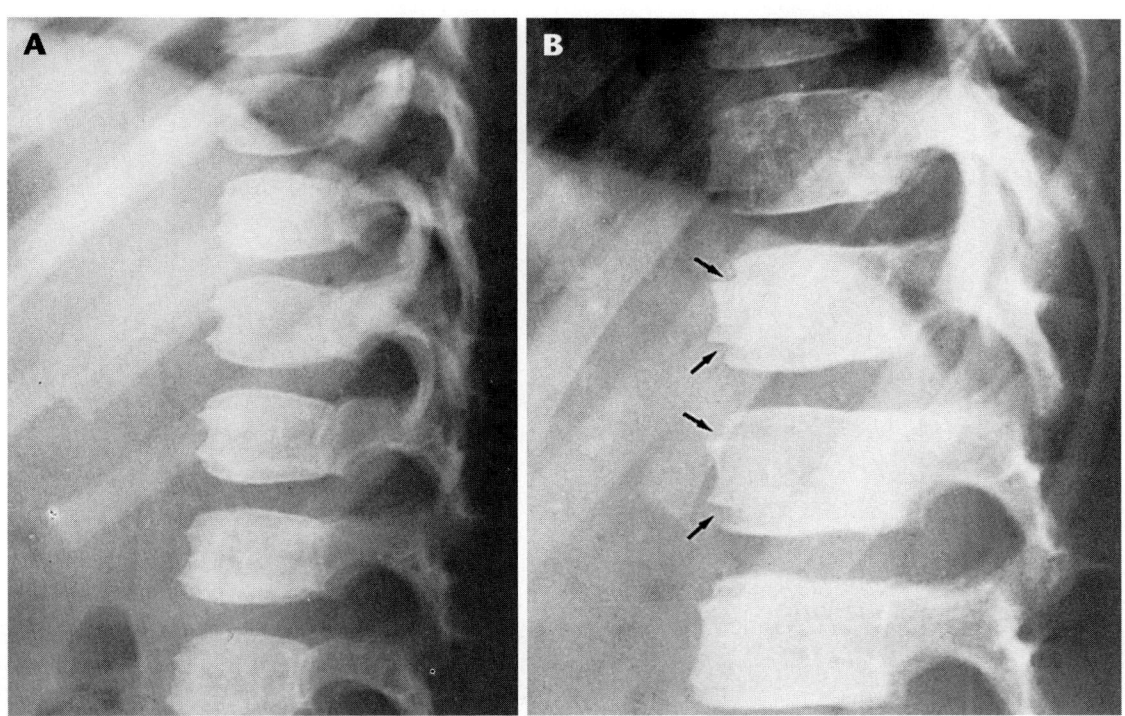

Figure 3–323. Normal "step" defects on the anterior surfaces of juvenile vertebrae. **A,** A 4-year-old child. **B,** A 7-year-old child.

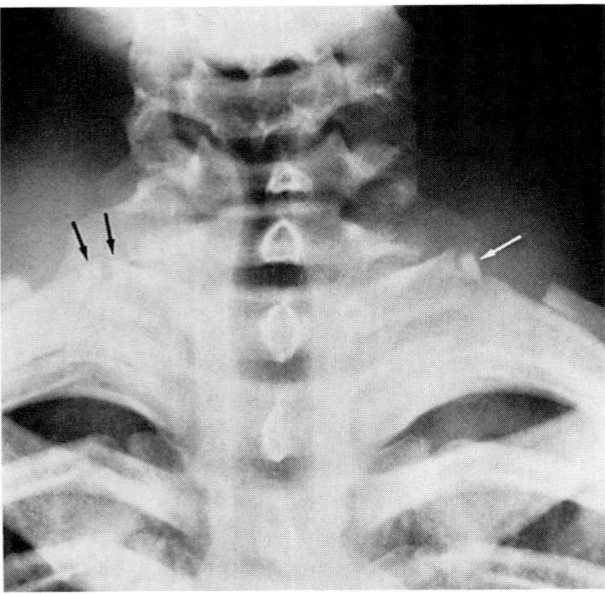

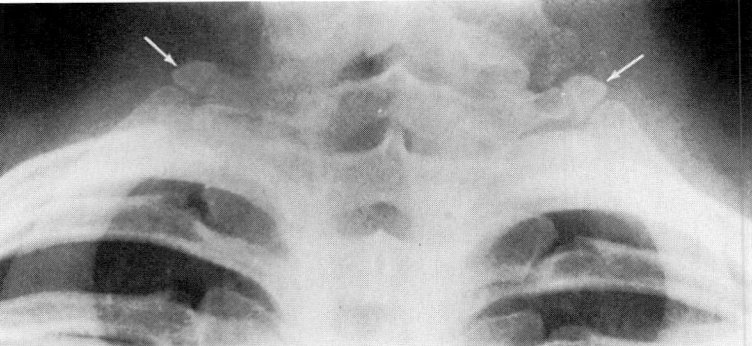

Figure 3–325. Nonunited ossification centers at the distal ends of the transverse processes of T1 in an adult.

Figure 3–324. Ossification centers at the distal ends of the transverse processes of T1 in an adolescent.

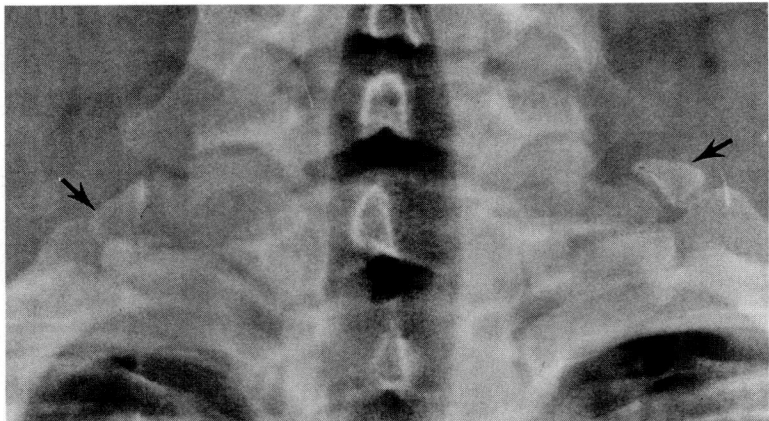

Figure 3–326. Unfused ossification centers of the transverse processes of T1.

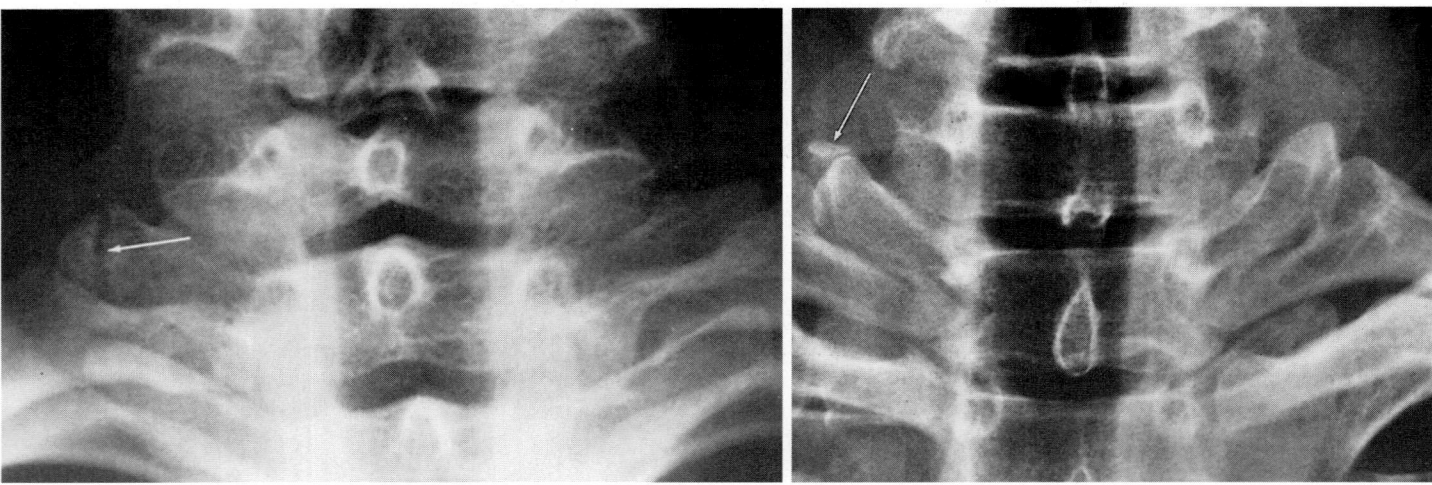

Figure 3–327. Two examples of unilateral persistence of the ossification centers of the transverse processes in young adults.

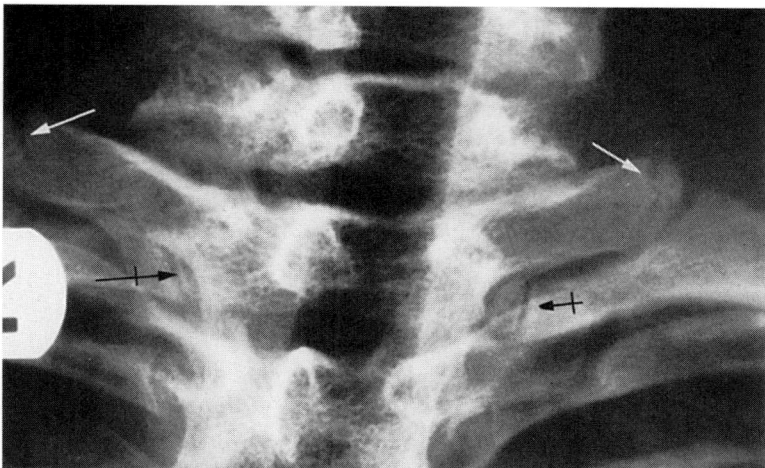

Figure 3–328. Unfused apophysis of the transverse processes of T1 (←) and at the medial ends of the first ribs (↔) in a 14-year-old boy.

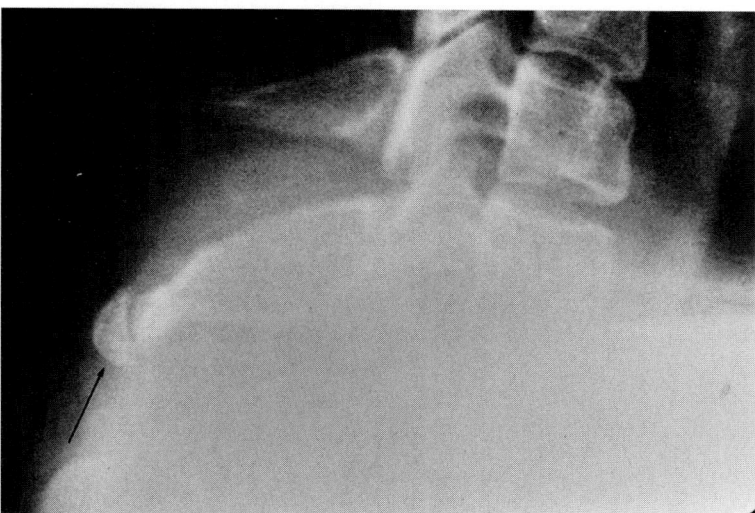

Figure 3–329. Failure of union of the apophysis for the tip of the spinous process of T1.

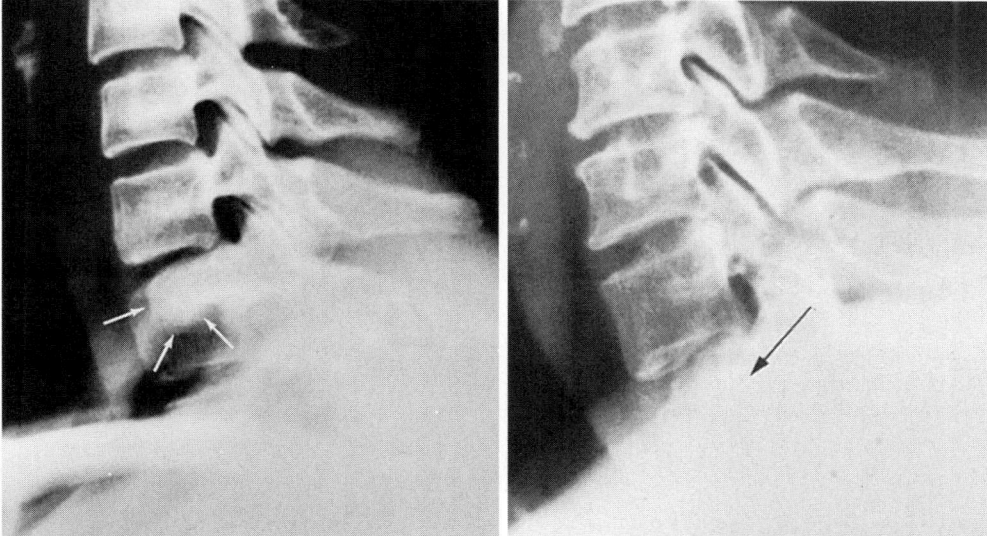

Figure 3–330. Two examples of how the lateral elements of T1 produce apparent sclerosis of a portion of the vertebral body and may simulate a metastatic deposit.

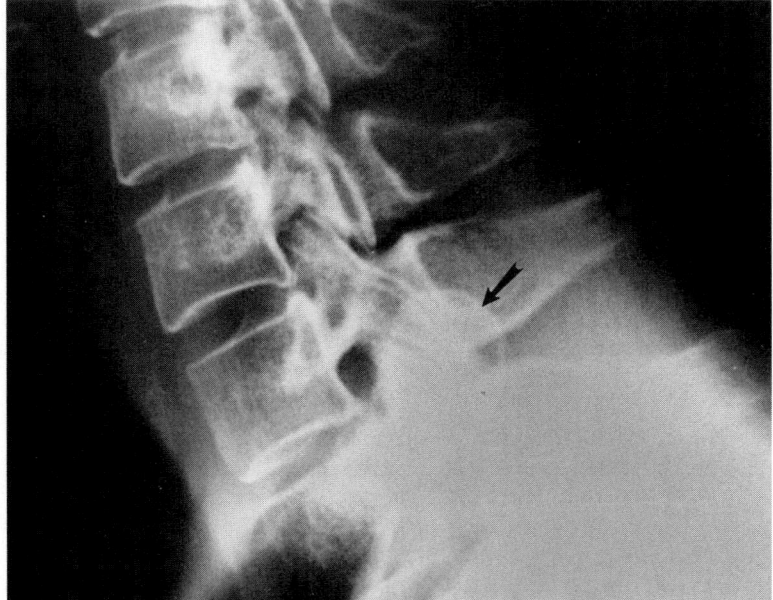

Figure 3–331. Ringlike shadow produced by the lateral elements of the vertebra with slight rotation.

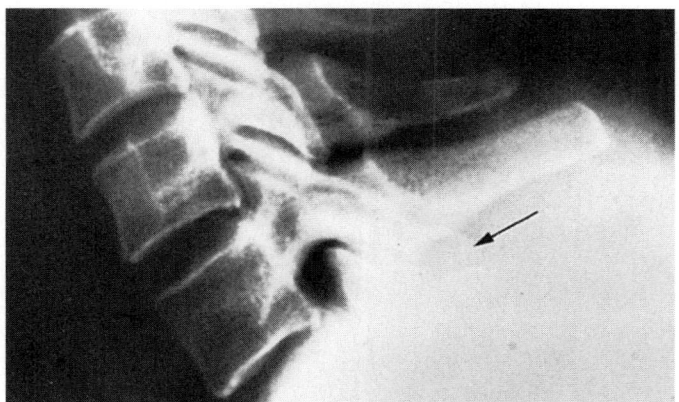

Figure 3–332. Shadow produced by the normal posterior angulation of the transverse process of T1.

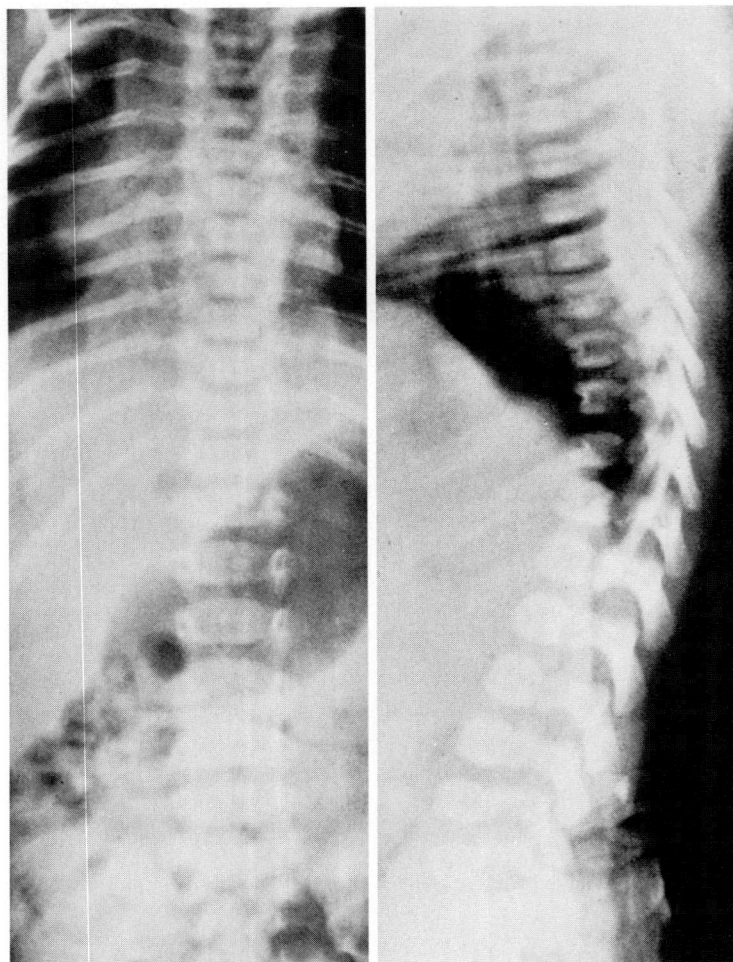

Figure 3–333. Apparent narrowing of interpedicular distance at the thoracolumbar junction in a 2-week-old infant produced by the normal thoracolumbar kyphosis and resultant magnification effect.

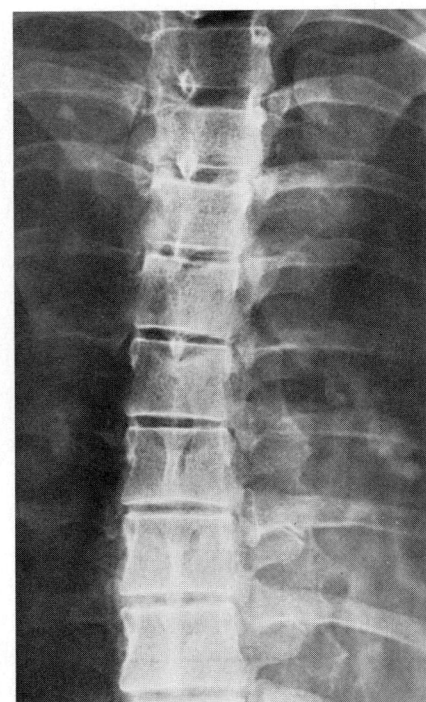

Figure 3–334. Narrow pedicles in a young woman on a developmental basis.

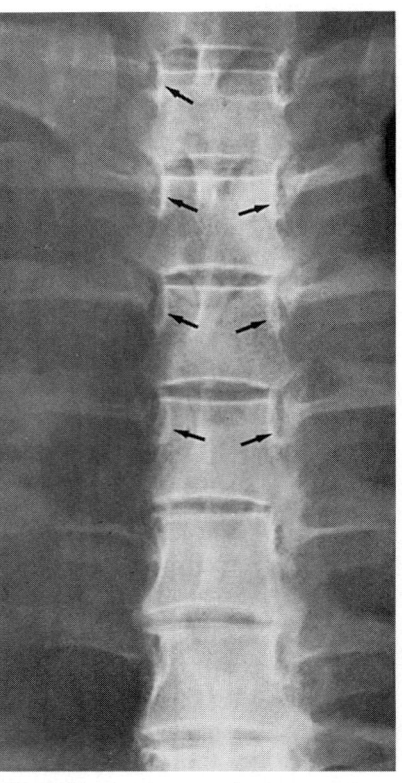

Figure 3–335. Delicate bone structure in a young woman with thin pedicles, simulating pedicular erosion.

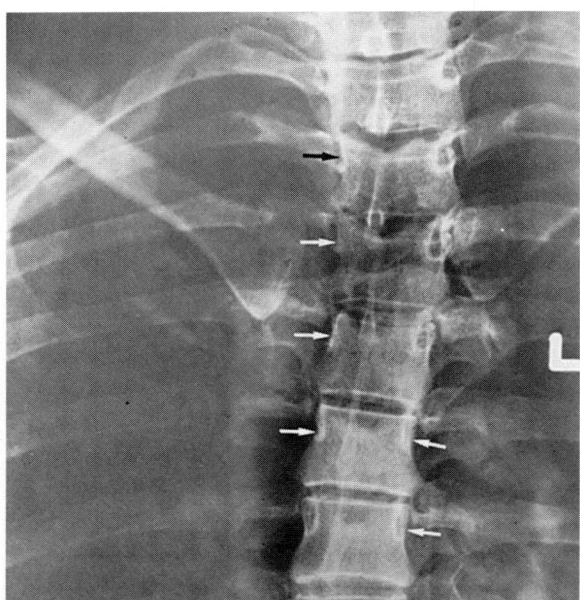

Figure 3–336. Minor scoliosis, producing simulated pedicle erosion.

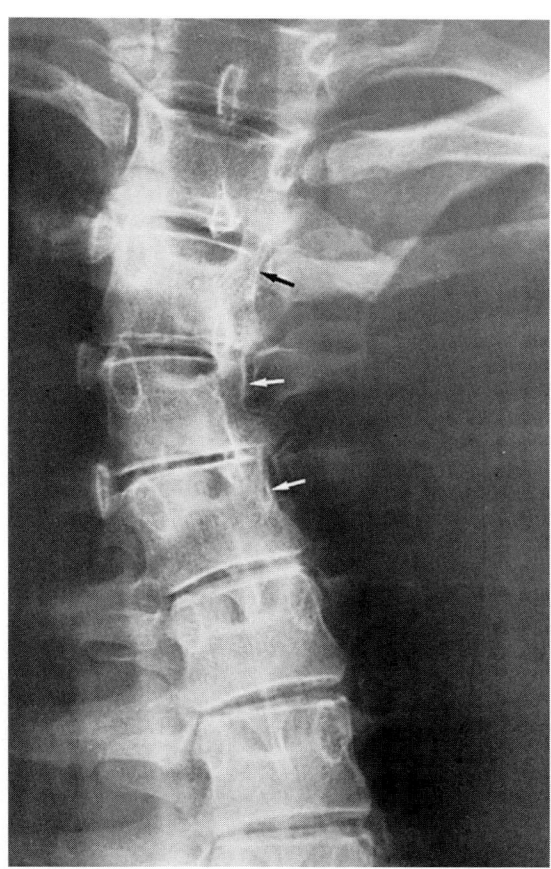

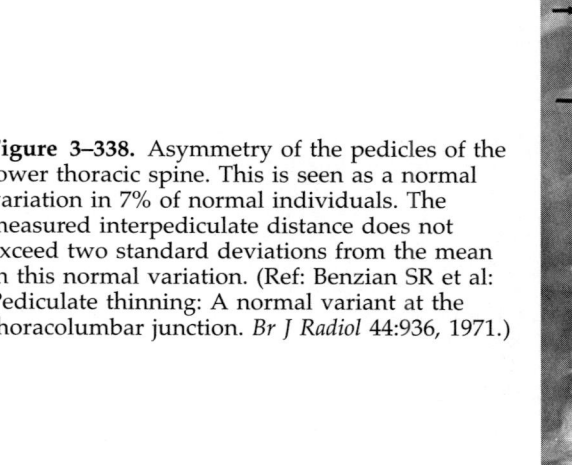

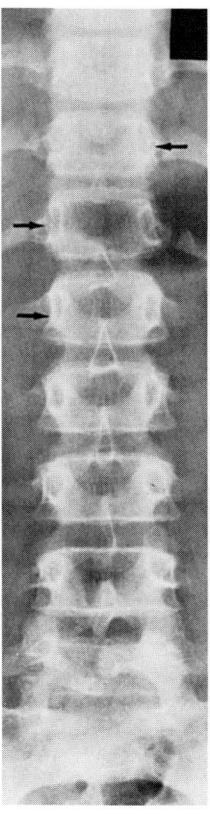

Figure 3–338. Asymmetry of the pedicles of the lower thoracic spine. This is seen as a normal variation in 7% of normal individuals. The measured interpediculate distance does not exceed two standard deviations from the mean in this normal variation. (Ref: Benzian SR et al: Pediculate thinning: A normal variant at the thoracolumbar junction. *Br J Radiol* 44:936, 1971.)

Figure 3–337. Localized scoliosis simulating pedicle erosion.

Figure 3–339. Pedicle thinning at the thoracolumbar junction may be extreme and may even be associated with concave medial borders. The absence of pertinent clinical findings should suggest this recognized normal variation. (Ref: Charlton OP et al: Pedicle thinning at the thoracolumbar junction: A normal variant, *Am J Roentgenol* 134:825, 1980.)

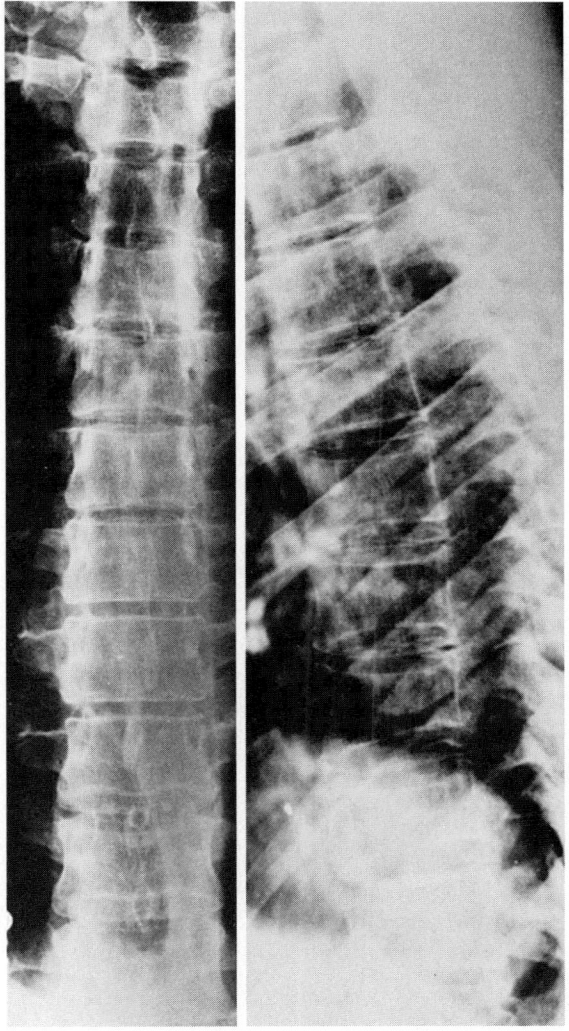

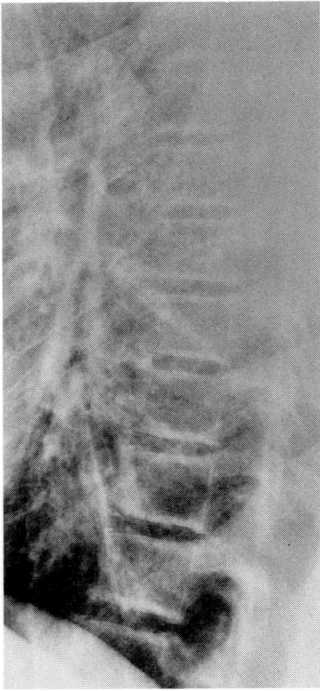

Figure 3–340. Sclerotic vertebral end plates in a healthy 14-year-old boy.

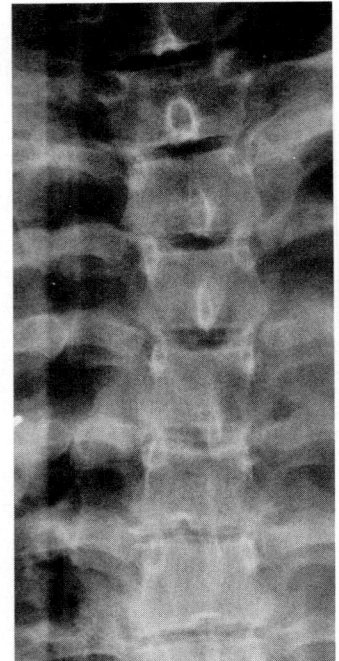

Figure 3–341. Magnification of the upper thoracic vertebra caused by kyphosis.

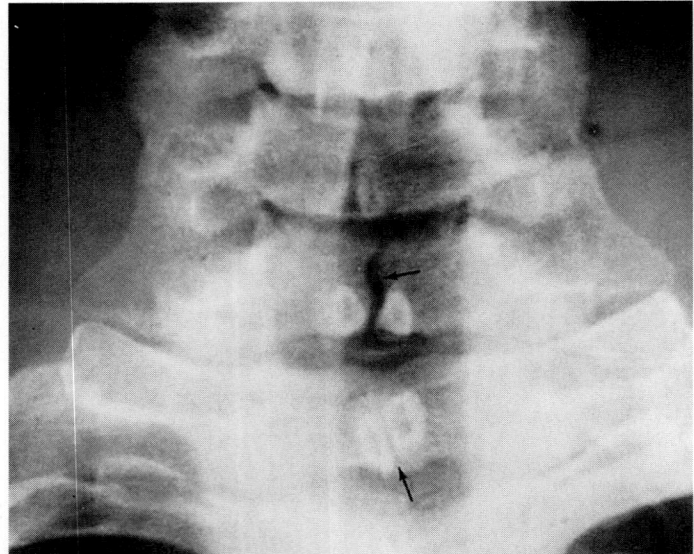

Figure 3–342. Spina bifida occulta of C7 and T1 with double spinous processes.

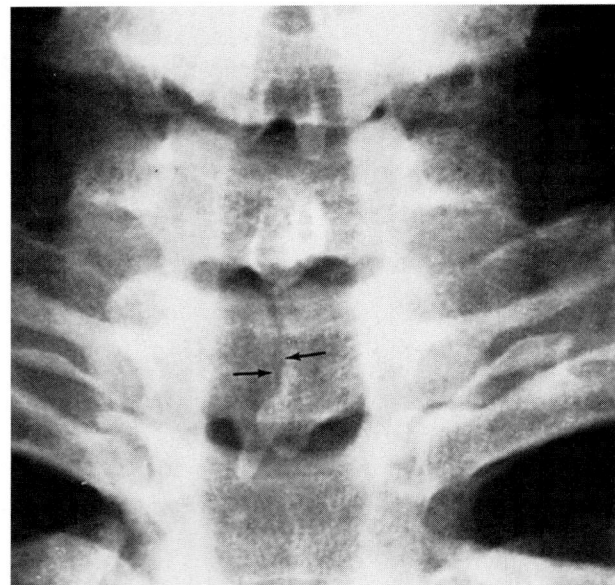

Figure 3–343. Spina bifida of T1 simulating a fracture.

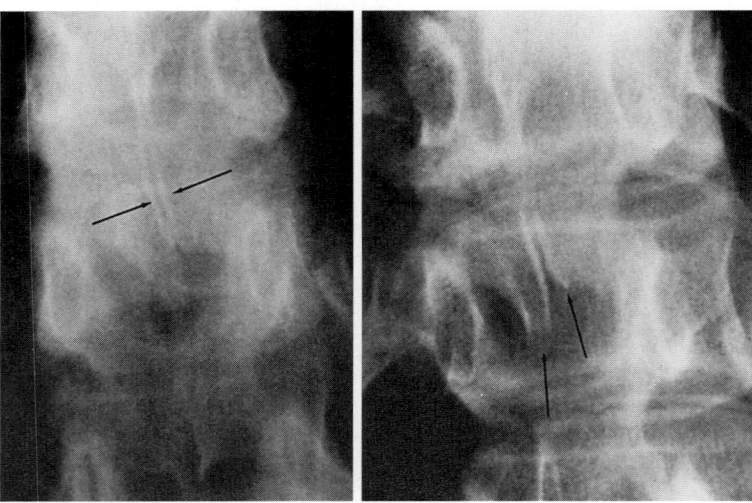

Figure 3–344. Spina bifida of the spinous process of T12.

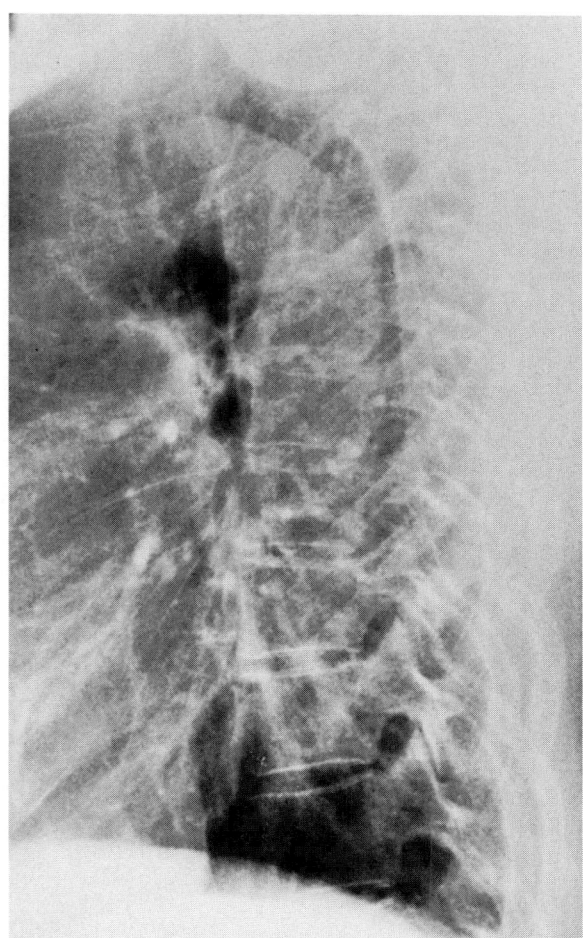

Figure 3–345. Thoracic lordosis, a normal variation, in a 54-year-old man.

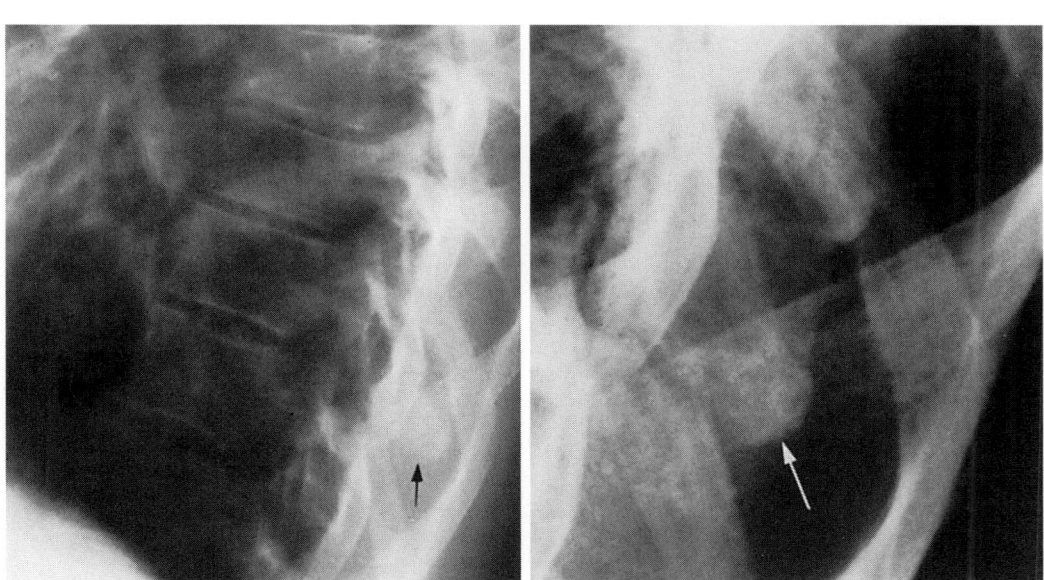

Figure 3–346. *Left,* Bulbous spinous process of T11 simulating a mass. *Right,* Detailed view shows identity of the shadow.

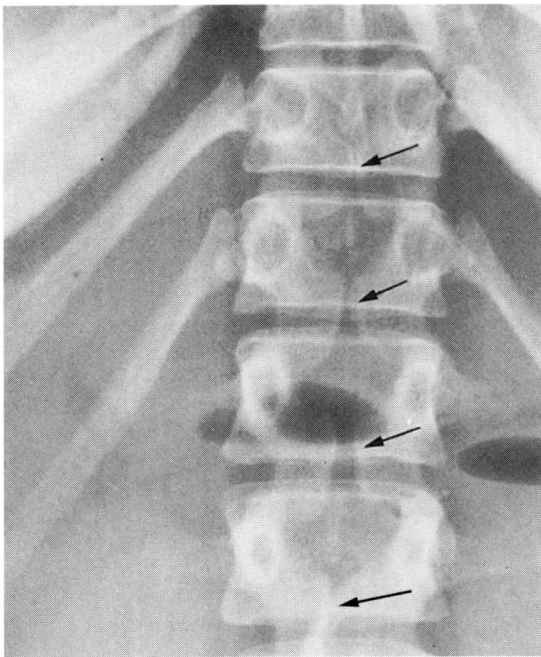

Figure 3–347. Spina bifida occulta of T11 and T12, and L1 and L2.

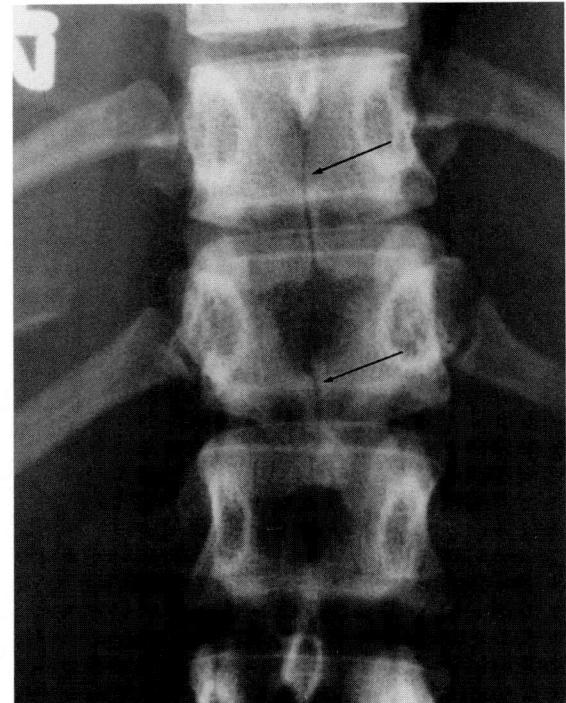

Figure 3–348. Spina bifida of T11 and T12.

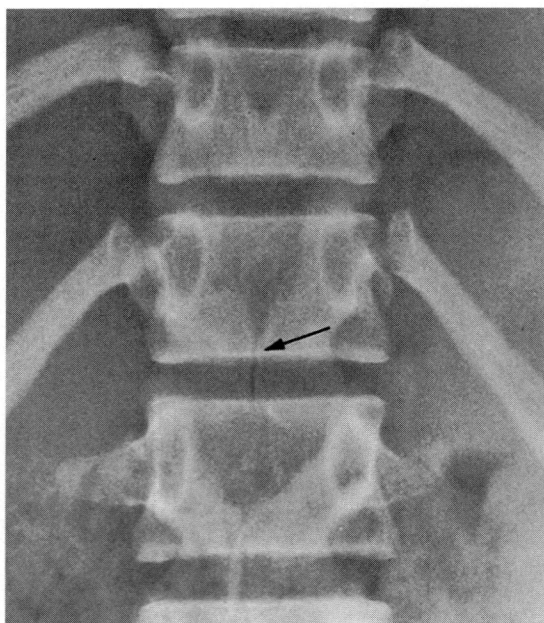

Figure 3–349. Spina bifida occulta of T12.

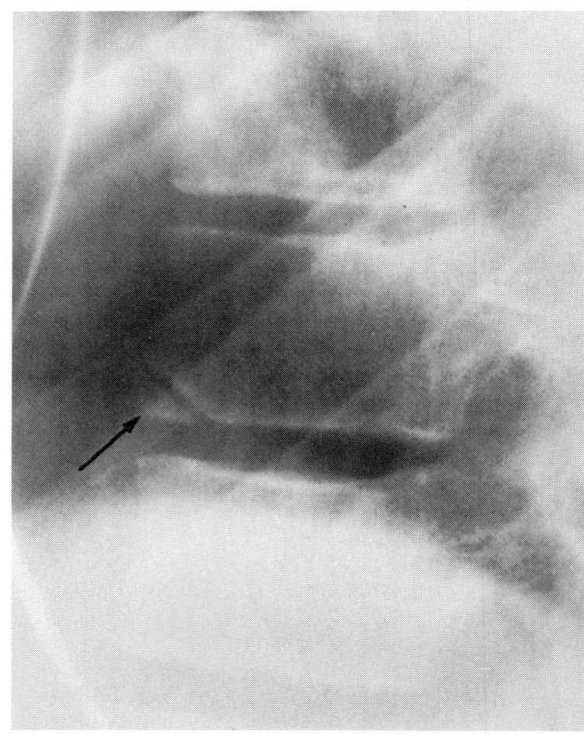

Figure 3–350. Limbus vertebra at T10 in a 24-year-old man.

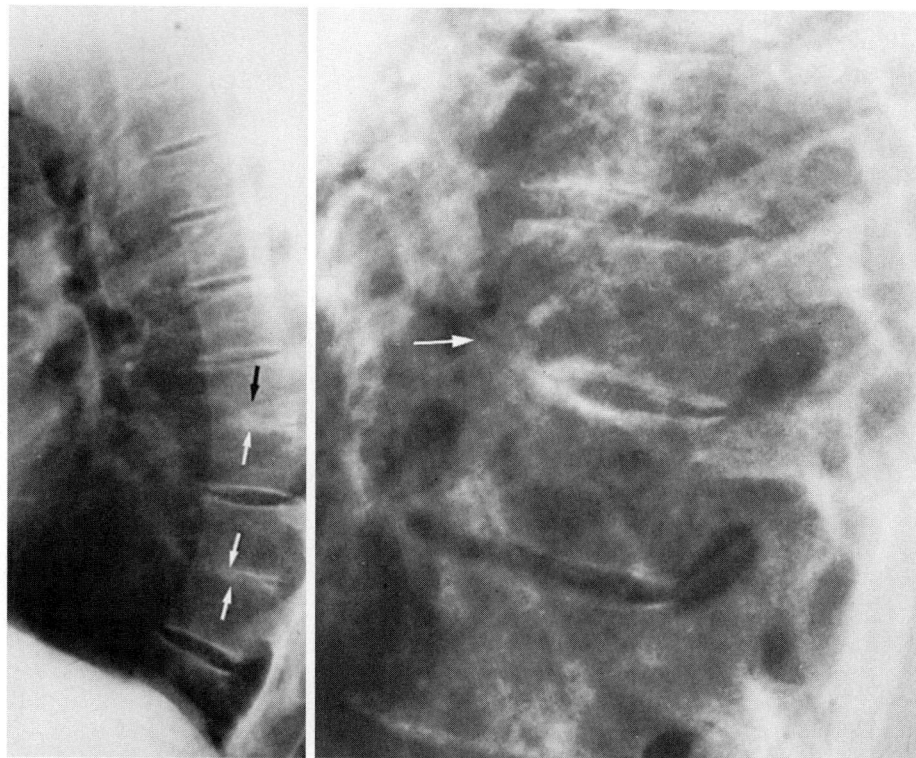

Figure 3–351. Two examples of failure of segmentation of the thoracic vertebrae. Partial development of the intervertebral discs is seen. This should not be confused with the effects of inflammatory spondylitis.

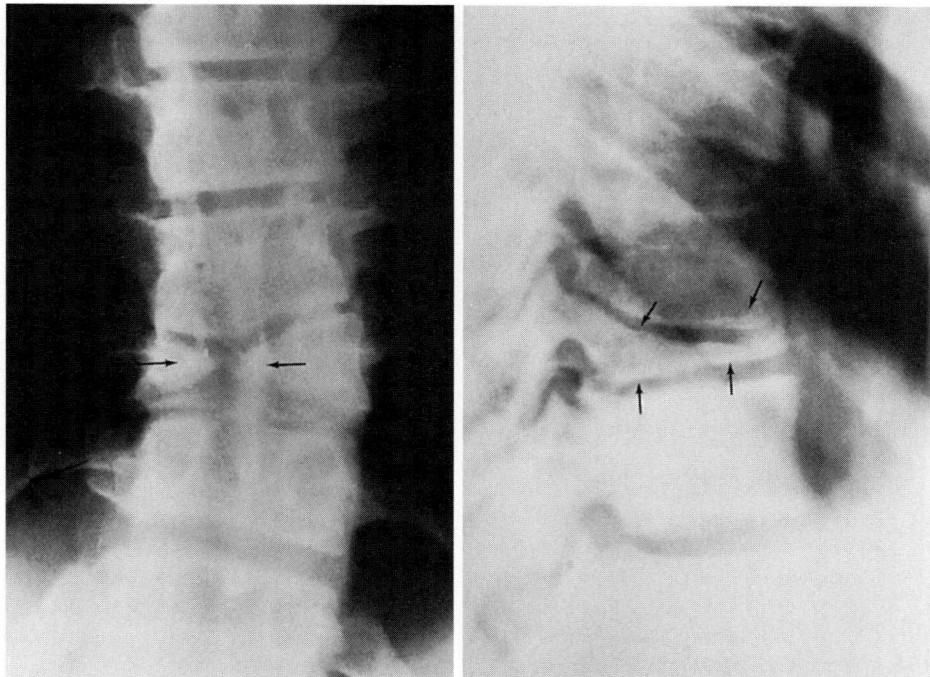

Figure 3–352. Congenital butterfly vertebra. Note overgrowth of the adjacent vertebra.

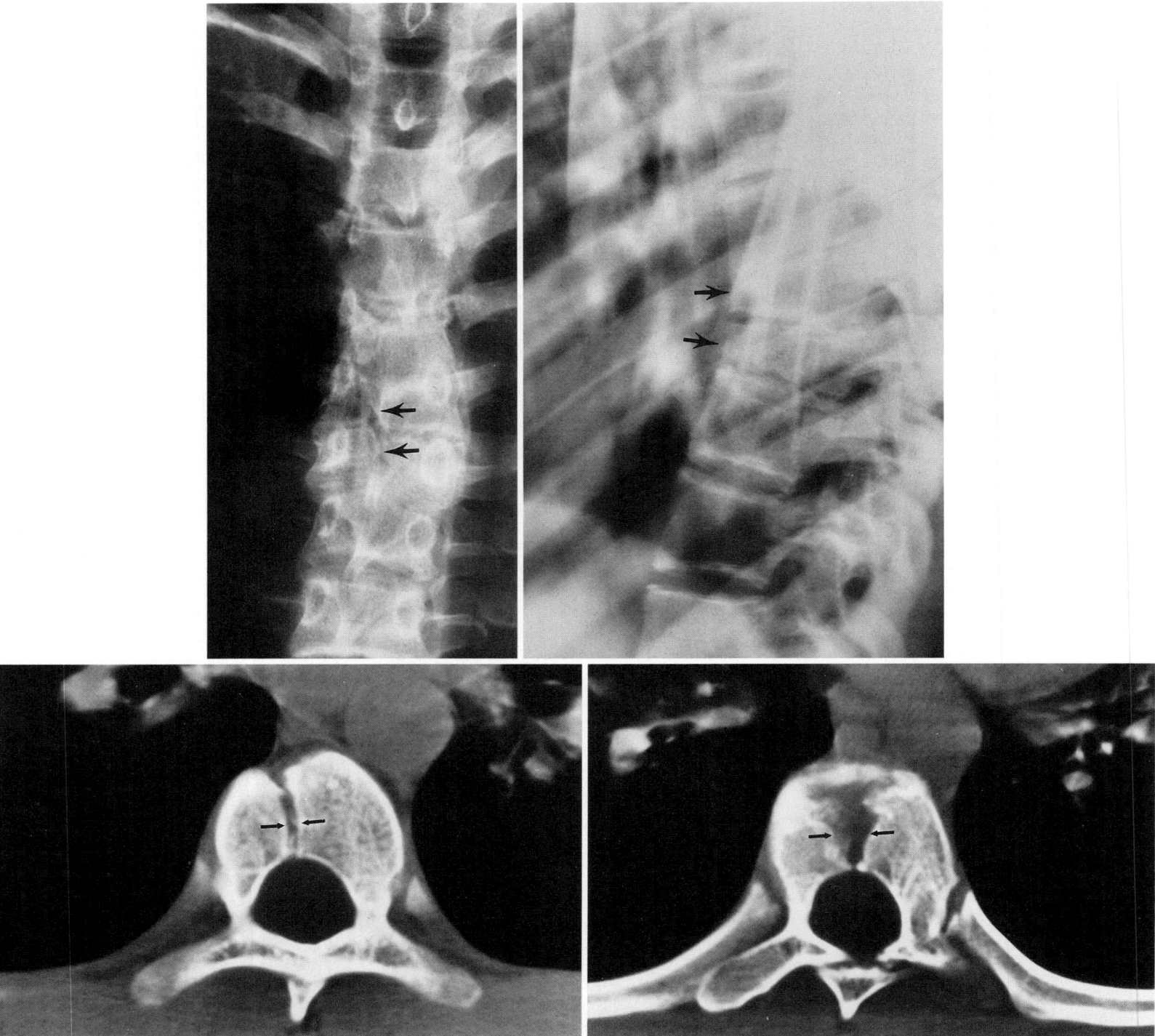

Figure 3–353. Butterfly vertebrae at T6 and T7.

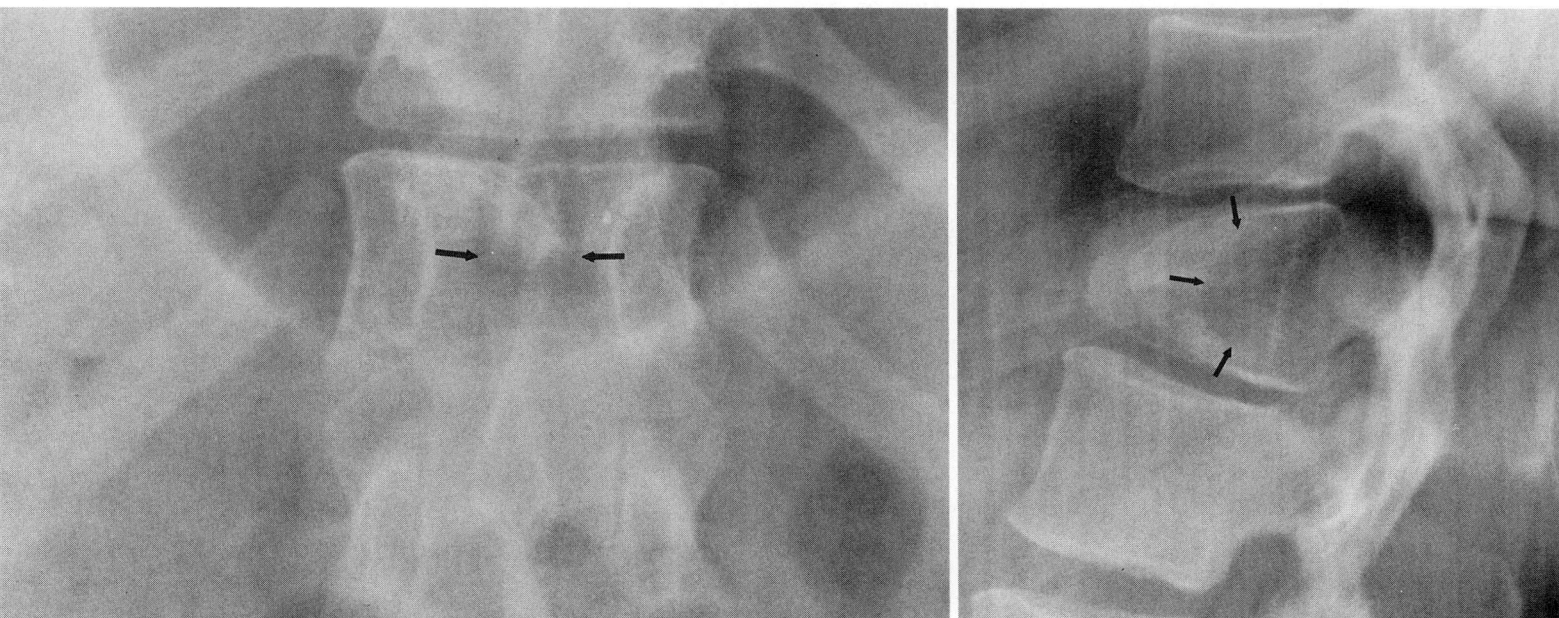

Figure 3–354. Butterfly vertebra at T12 simulating a lucent lesion in the lateral projection.

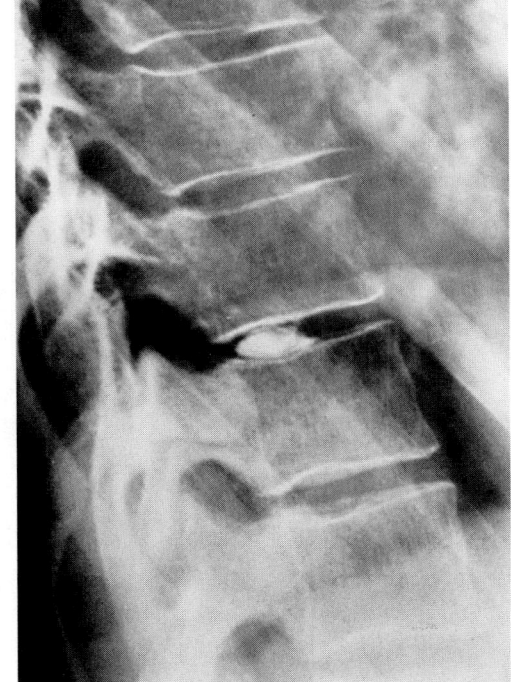

Figure 3–355. Asymptomatic calcification of the nucleus pulposus in a young adult. This is generally asymptomatic. When it occurs in the cervical region in children, it may be associated with signs and symptoms but is self-limited. (Ref: Melnick JC, Silverman FN: Intervertebral disk calcification in childhood. *Radiology* 80:399, 1963.)

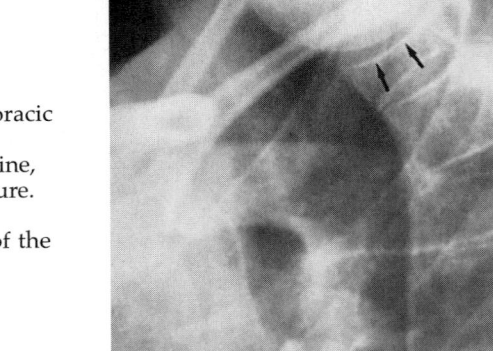
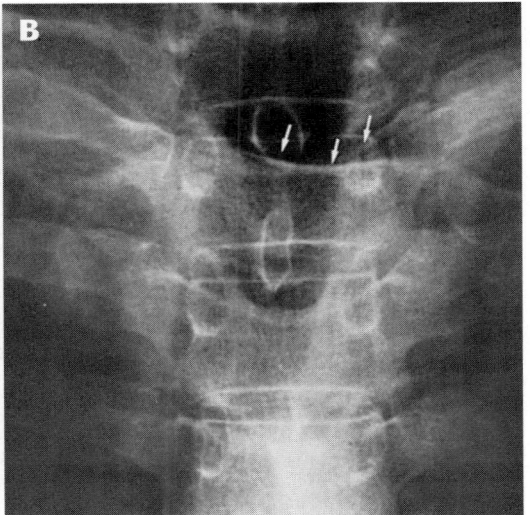

Figure 3–356. Pseudofractures of the thoracic spine. **A,** Superimposition of the glenoid process of the scapula on the thoracic spine, simulating a vertebral compression fracture. **B,** Pseudofracture of the second thoracic vertebra, produced by superimposition of the superior margin of the manubrium.

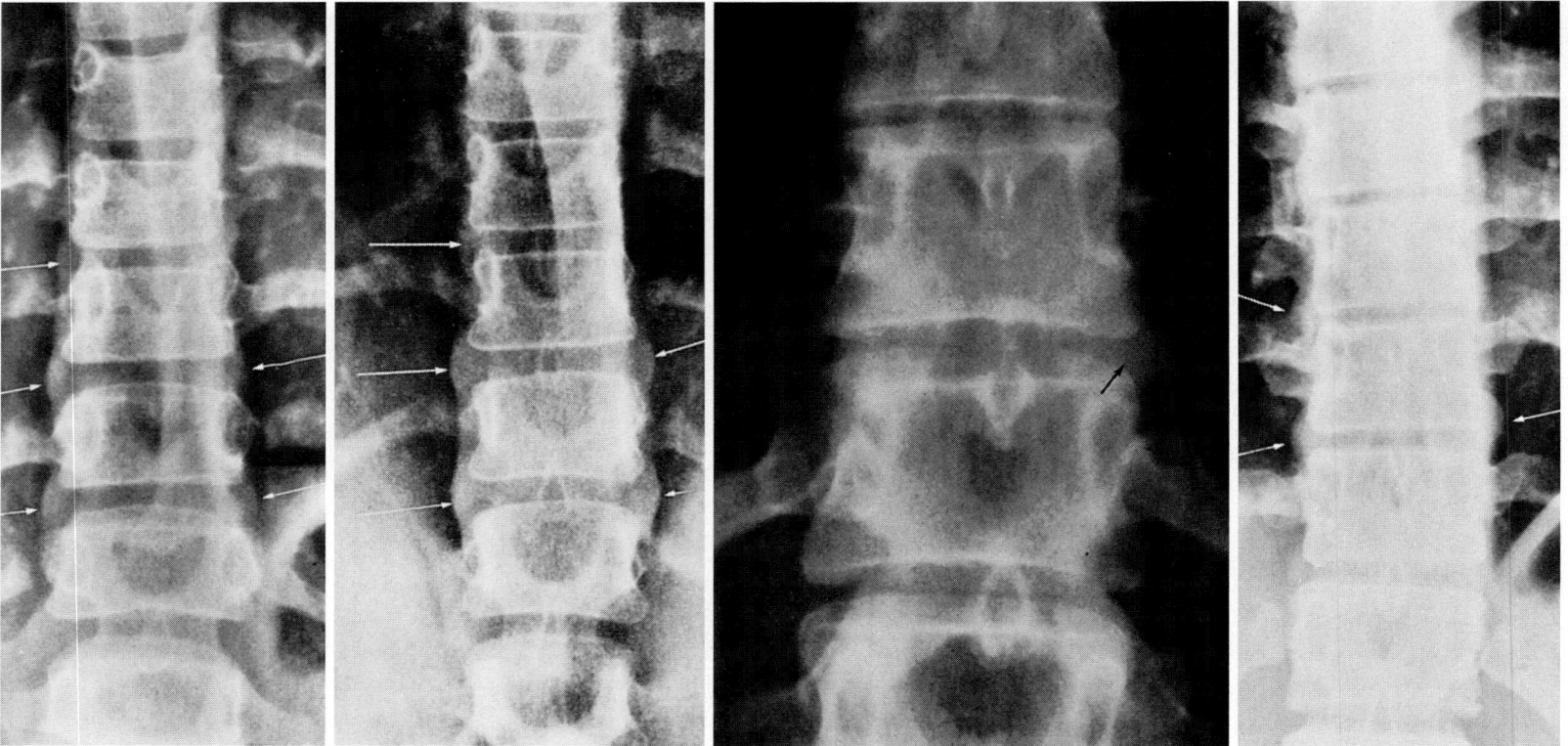

Figure 3–357. Four examples of how the facet joints of the spine may simulate bulging annuli or paraspinous masses.

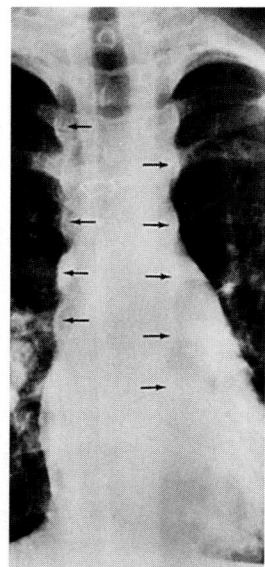

Figure 3–358. "Bumpy spine" produced by hypertrophy of the costovertebral articulations.

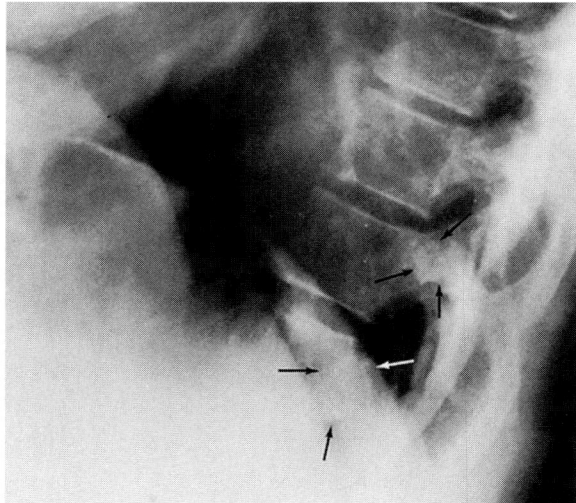

Figure 3–359. Simulated nodule produced by slight thickening of the bone at the superior aspect of the area where the two laminae join to form the spinous process. (Ref: Shortsleeve MJ, Foster SC: Pulmonary nodule. *Radiology* 131:311, 1979.)

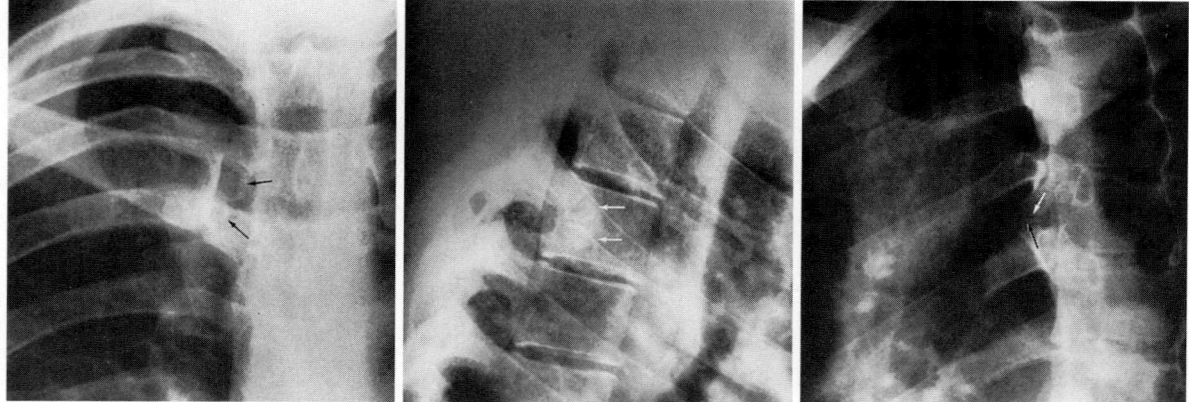

Figure 3–360. Atypical jointlike union of the transverse processes at the level of T4 and T5.

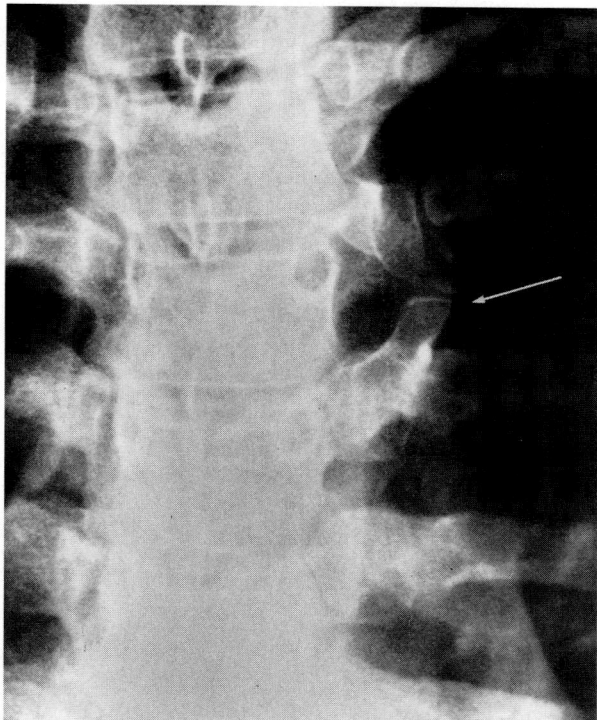

Figure 3–361. Anomalous articulation between the transverse processes of T3 and T4.

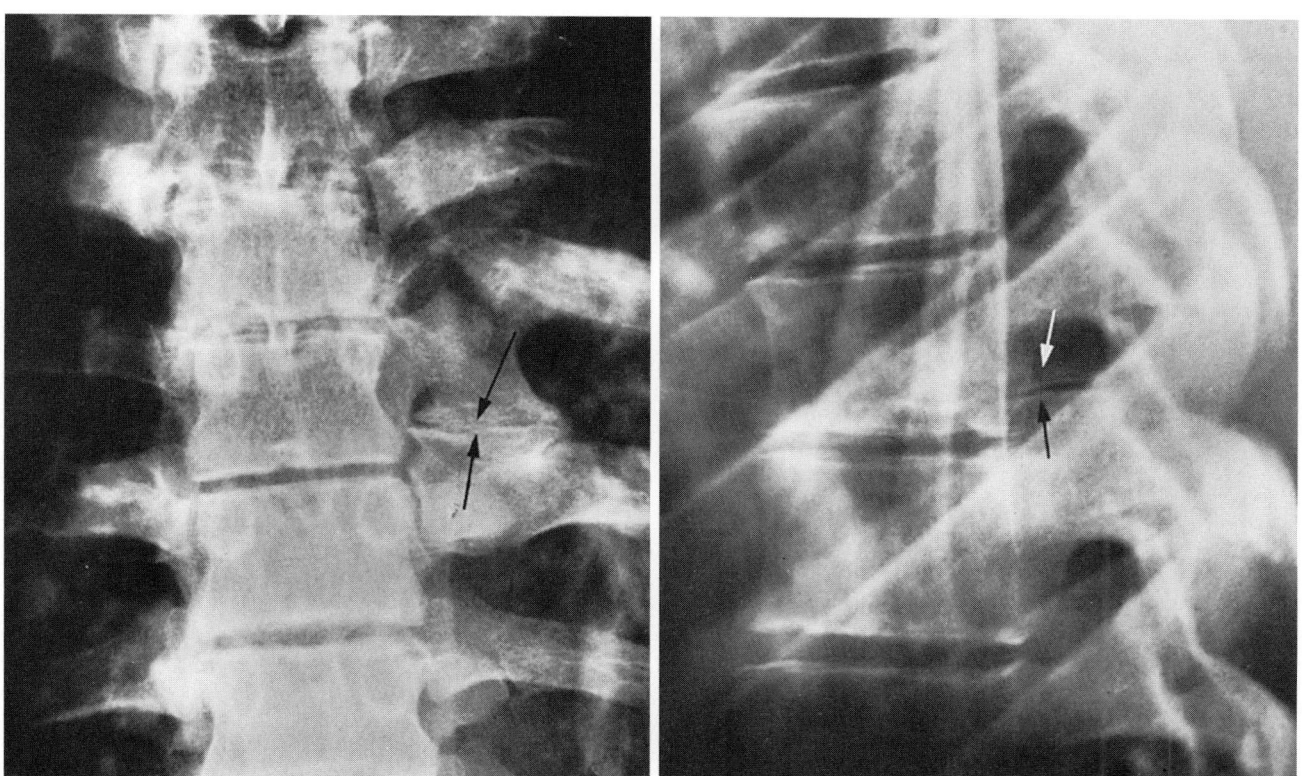

Figure 3–362. Anomalous articulation between T5 and T6 that can be seen in the lateral projection as well.

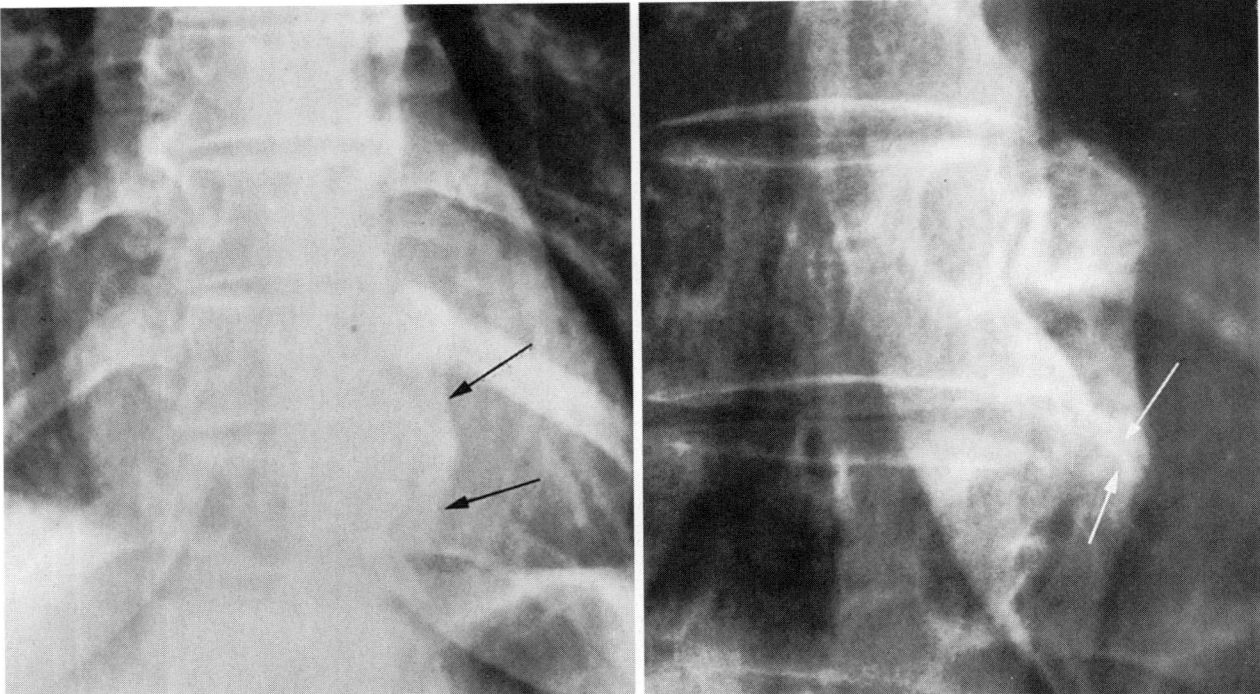

Figure 3–363. *Left,* Anomalous articulation between the transverse processes of T11 and T12, which was mistaken for a mediastinal mass. *Right,* Spot film shows the anomalous articulation.

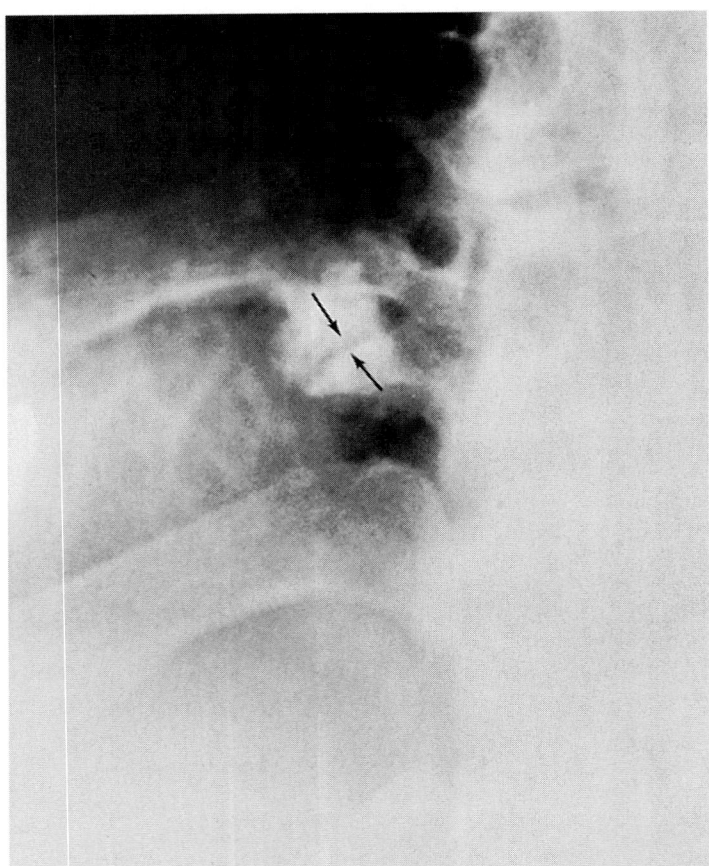

Figure 3–364. Anomalous articulation between the rib and the adjacent transverse process.

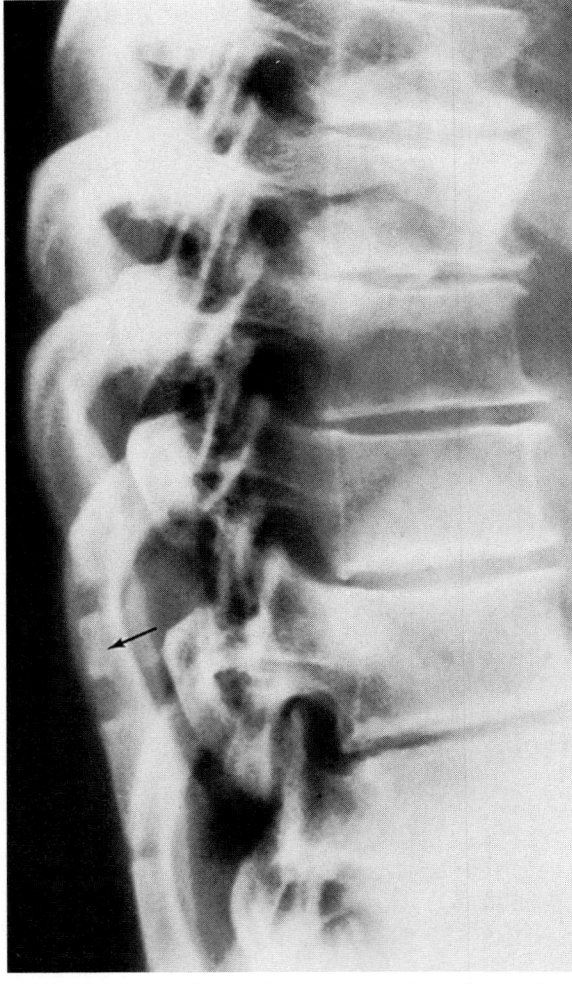

Figure 3–365. Apparent destructive lesion of the rib, produced by superimposition of the spinous process *(arrow).*

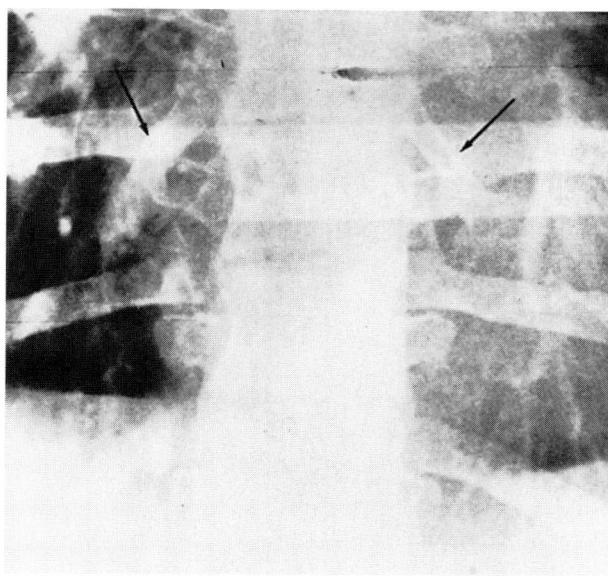

Figure 3–366. Bilateral styloid processes of T9.

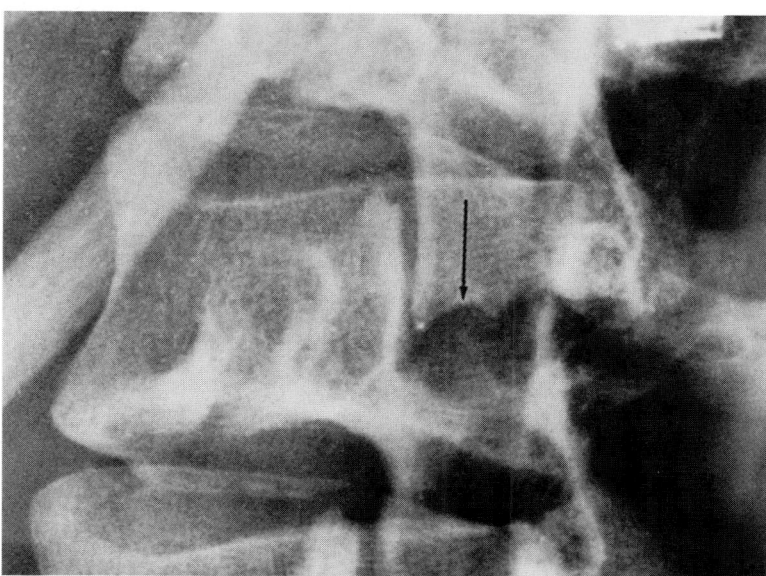

Figure 3–367. Developmental notch in the inferior articulating process of T12 is a common anatomic variant at this level.

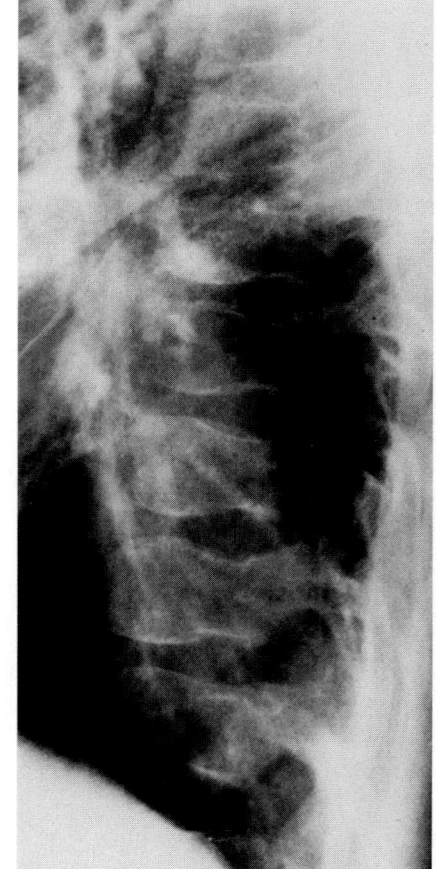

Figure 3–368. Thoracic notochordal remnants in a 15-year-old boy.

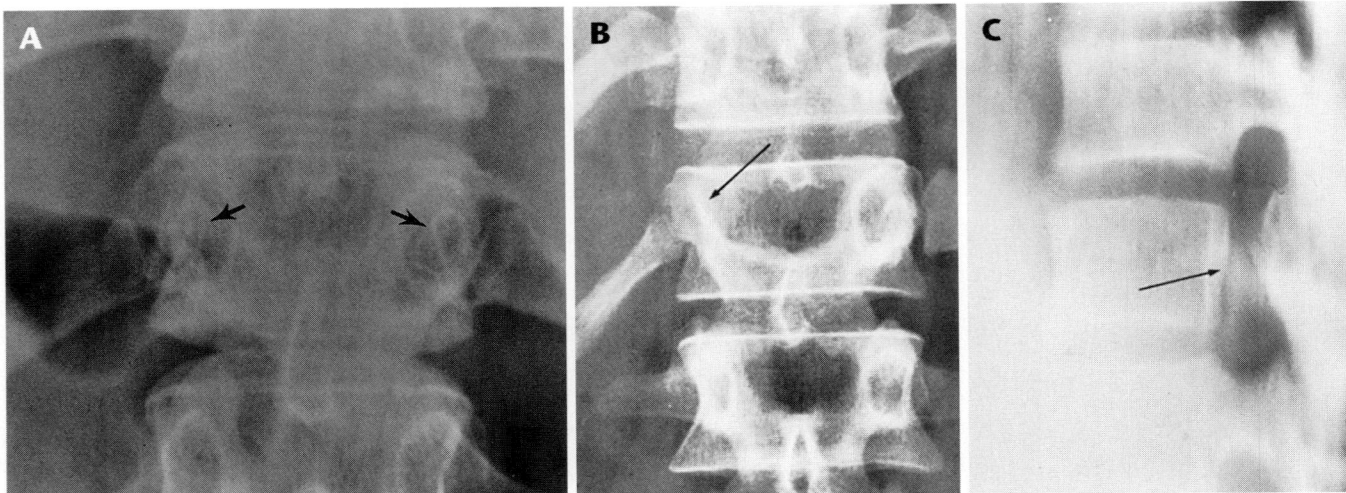

Figure 3–369. A, Target pedicle of T12. This appearance is produced by superimposition of the shadows of the inferior and lateral tubercules on the shadow of the pedicle. **B,** Absent pedicle at T12. Frontal film shows absence of the pedicular ring shadow. **C,** Absent pedicle at T12. Tomogram shows incomplete shadows of the pedicles as seen above and below. (Refs: Ehara S et al: Target pedicle of T-12: Radiologic-anatomic correlation. *Radiology* 174:871, 1990; Manaster BJ, Norman A: CT diagnosis of thoracic pedicle aplasia. *J Comput Assist Tomogr* 7:1090, 1983; Lederman RA, Kaufman RA: Complete absence and hypoplasia of pedicles of the thoracic spine. *Skeletal Radiol* 15:219, 1986.)

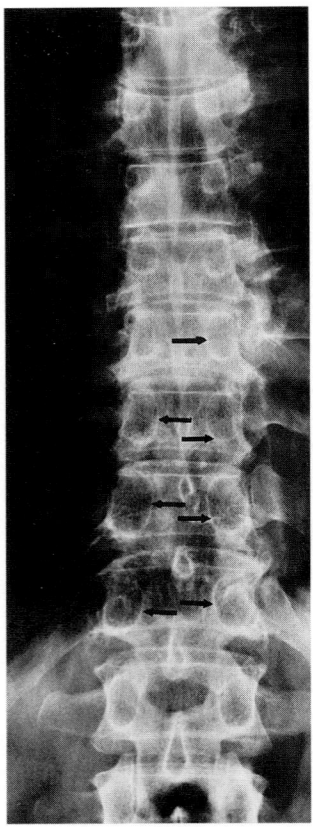

Figure 3–370. Huge thoracic pedicles.

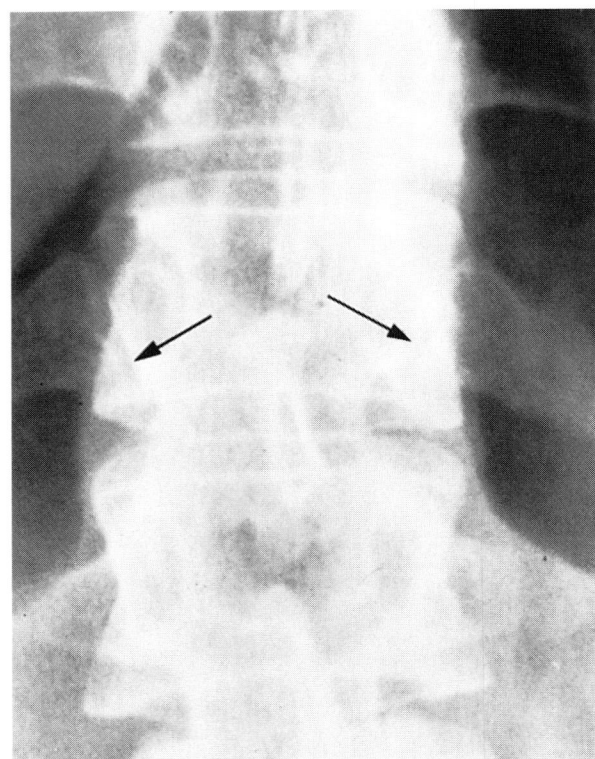

Figure 3–371. The costovertebral articulation superimposed on the body of T12.

The Lumbar Spine

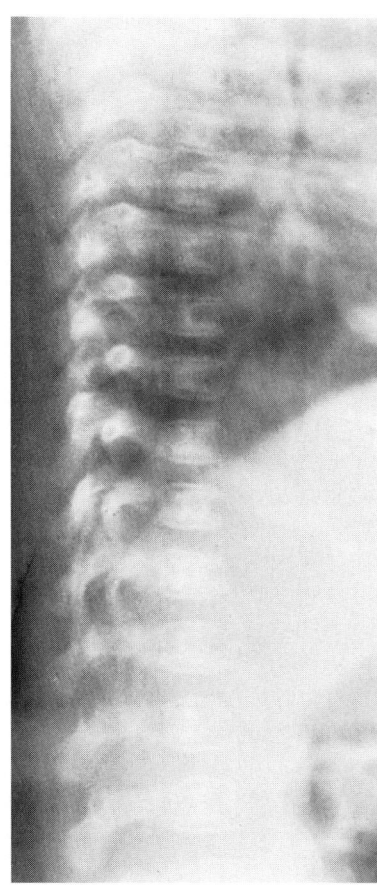

Figure 3–372. The normal "bone in bone" appearance of the neonate.

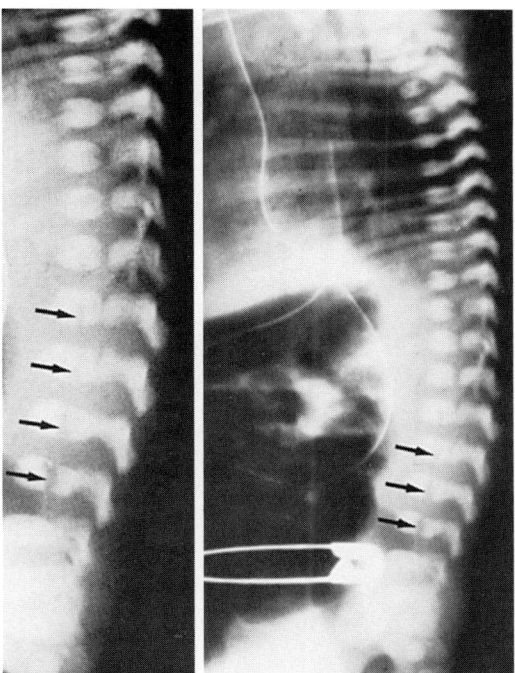

Figure 3–373. Two examples of coronal cleft vertebrae in neonates. These occur more commonly in males and most often in the lumbar region.

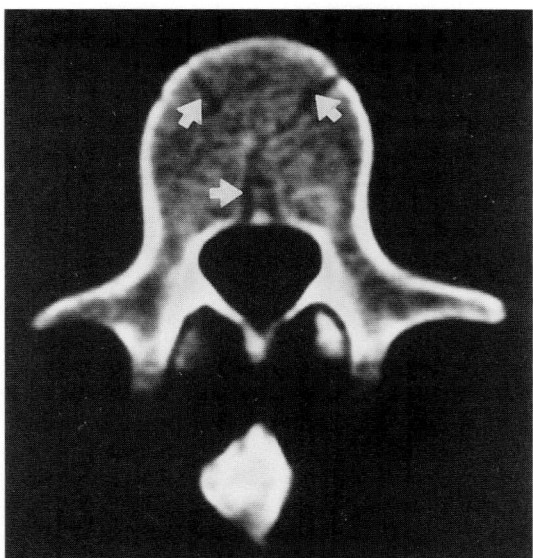

Figure 3–374. Normal vascular channels of the lumbar vertebral body by CT.

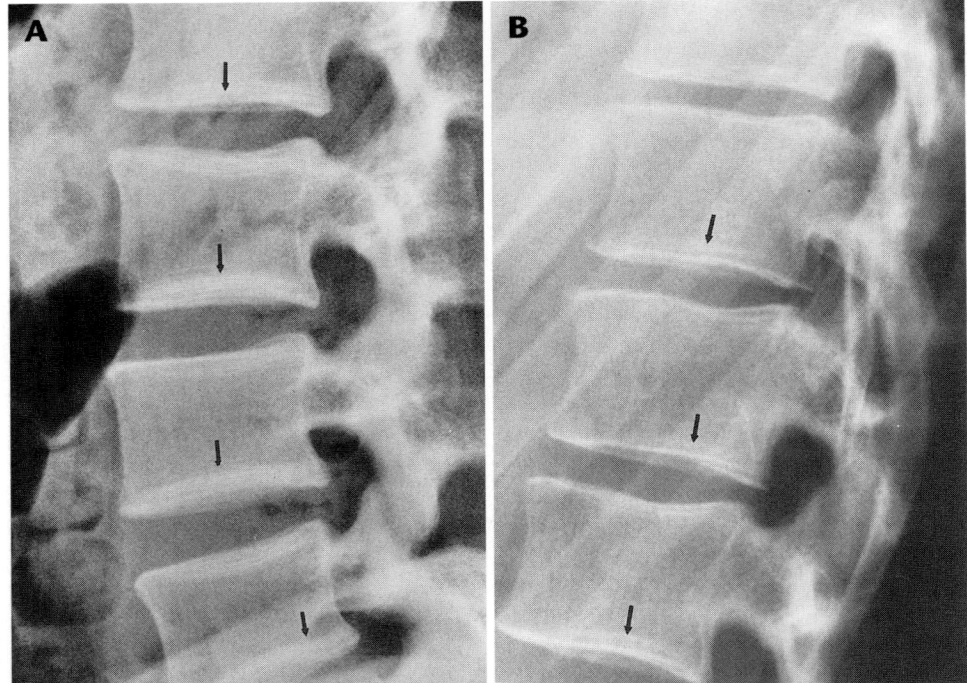

Figure 3–375. Two examples of "growth lines" in the lumbar vertebra. **A,** 19-year-old man. **B,** 38-year-old-man.

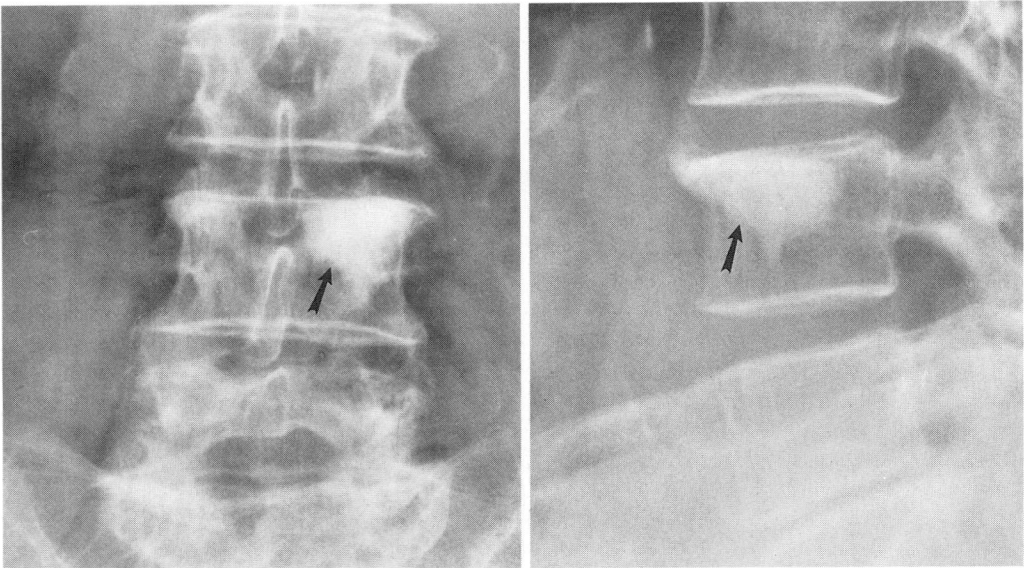

Figure 3–376. Lumbar bone island. (Ref: Resnik D et al: Spinal enostosis [bone islands]. *Radiology* 147:373, 1983.)

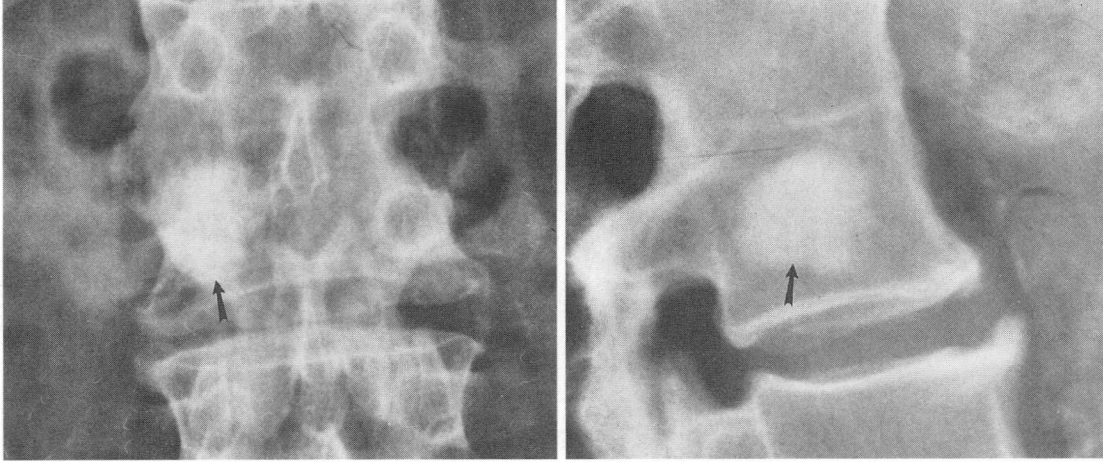

Figure 3–377. Lumbar bone island.

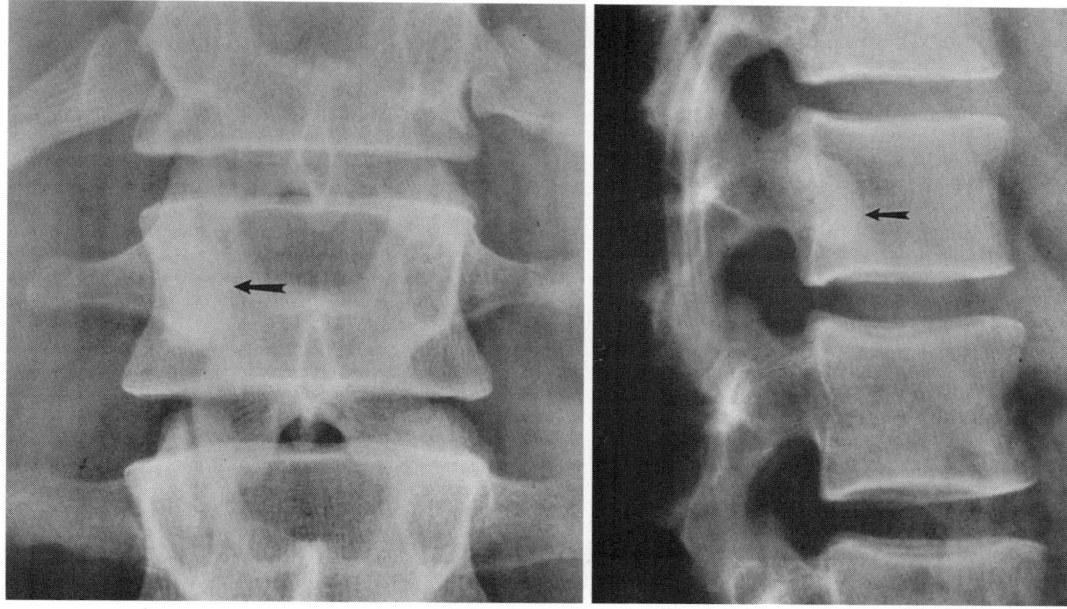

Figure 3–378. Lumbar bone island.

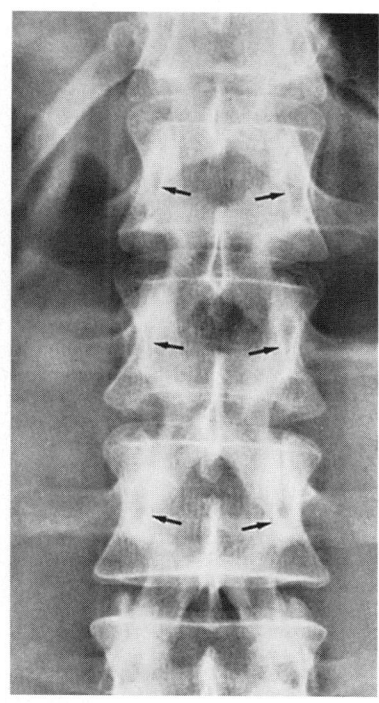

Figure 3–379. Normal variation in pedicle size. The interpediculate distance in this variation does not exceed two standard deviations from the mean (see Figs. 3–380 and 3–381). (Ref: Benzian SR et al: Pediculate thinning: A normal variant of the thoracolumbar junction. *Br J Radiol* 44:936, 1971.)

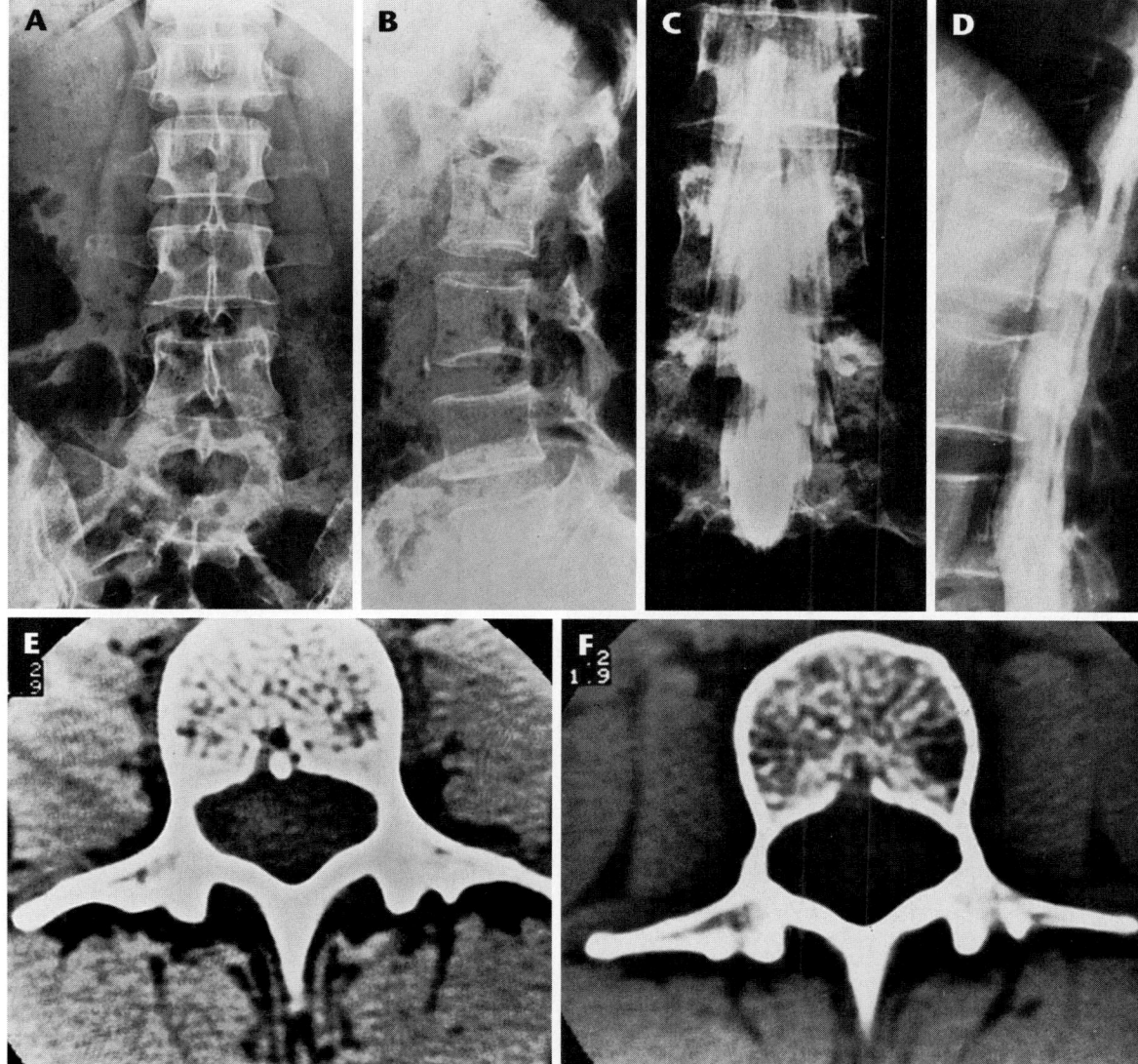

Figure 3–380. Congenitally wide thoracolumbar spinal canal unassociated with neurologic signs or symptoms. **A** and **B,** Plain film—large canal with thin pedicles. **C** and **D,** Myelogram large dural sac. **E** and **F,** CT scans—large spinal canal (see Fig. 3–3). (Ref: Patel NP et al: Radiology of lumbar vertebral pedicles: Variants, anomalies and pathologic conditions. *Radiographics* 7:101, 1987.)

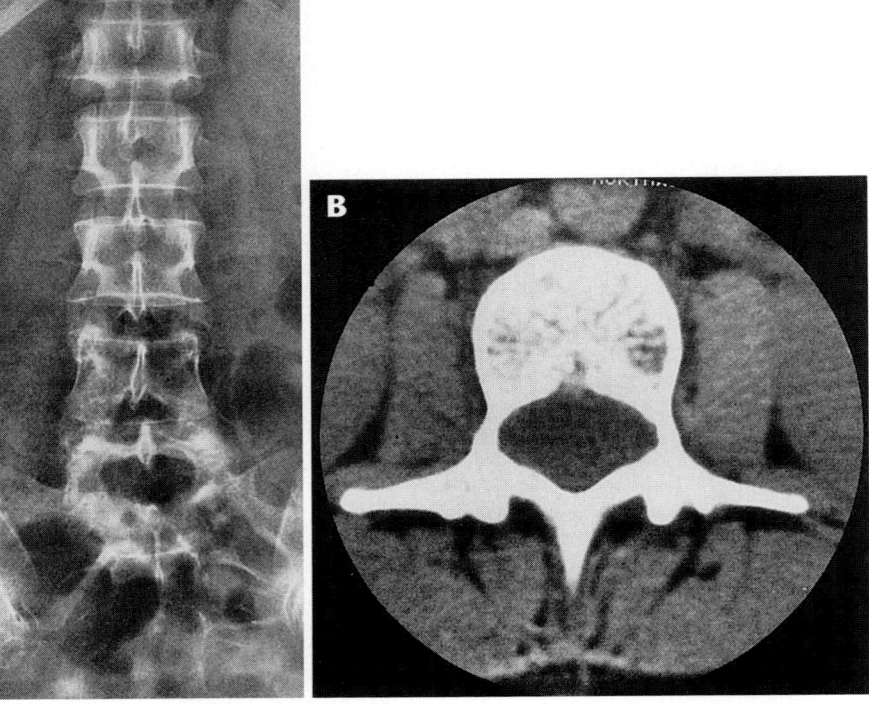

Figure 3–381. Another example of thin lumbar pedicles as a normal variant. **A,** Anteroposterior view shows flat pedicles with medial concavity and wide interpediculate distance throughout the lumbar spine. **B,** CT scan at L2 shows the thin pedicles. There is no intraspinal mass. Myelogram showed a large dural sac. (Ref: Atlas S et al: Roentgenographic evaluation of thinning of the lumbar pedicles. *Spine* 18:1190, 1993.)

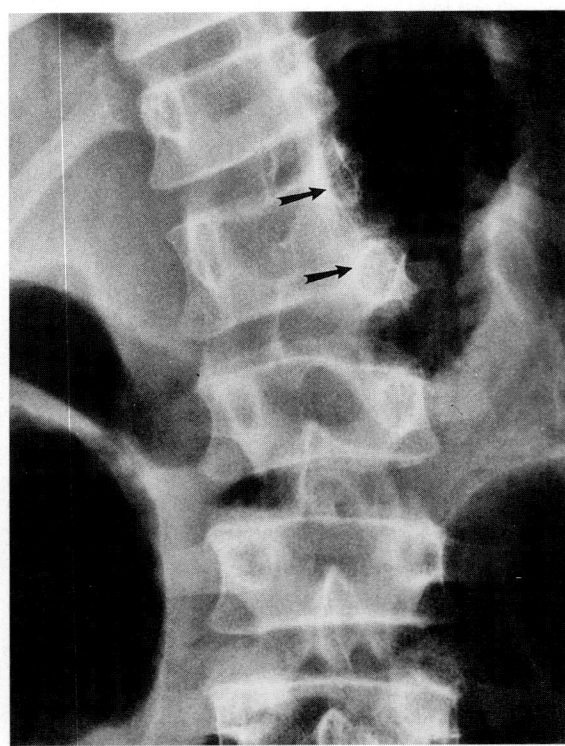

Figure 3–382. Duplication of the pedicles of L1.

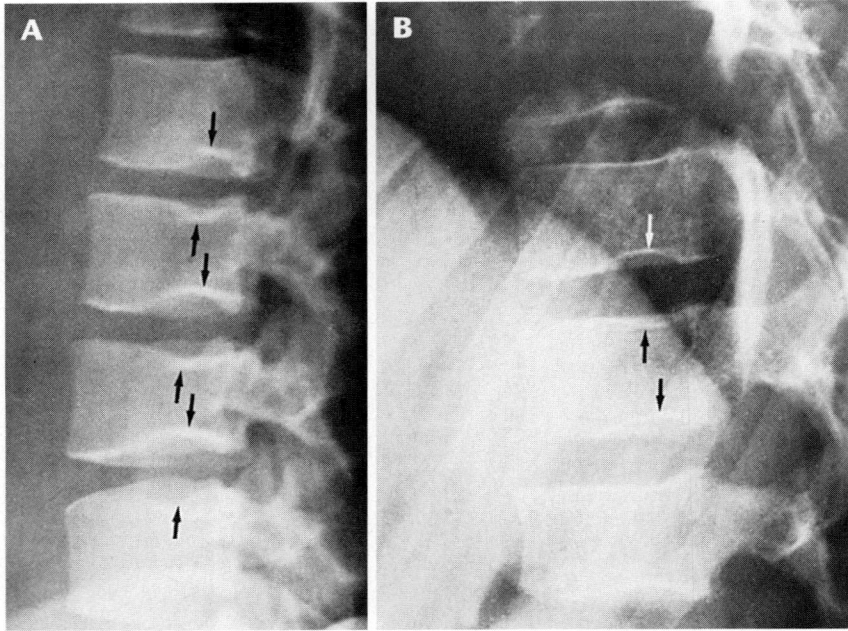

Figure 3–383. Two examples of end plate depressions secondary to notochordal remnants. Indentations of this type in the end plates of normal vertebrae of young people indicate the site of the notochordal recession into the intervertebral disc. They should be differentiated from Schmorl's nodes. **A,** A 27-year-old man. **B,** A 12-year-old girl. (Ref: Dietz GW, Christensen EE: Normal "Cupid's bow" contour of the lower lumbar vertebrae. *Radiology* 121:577, 1976.)

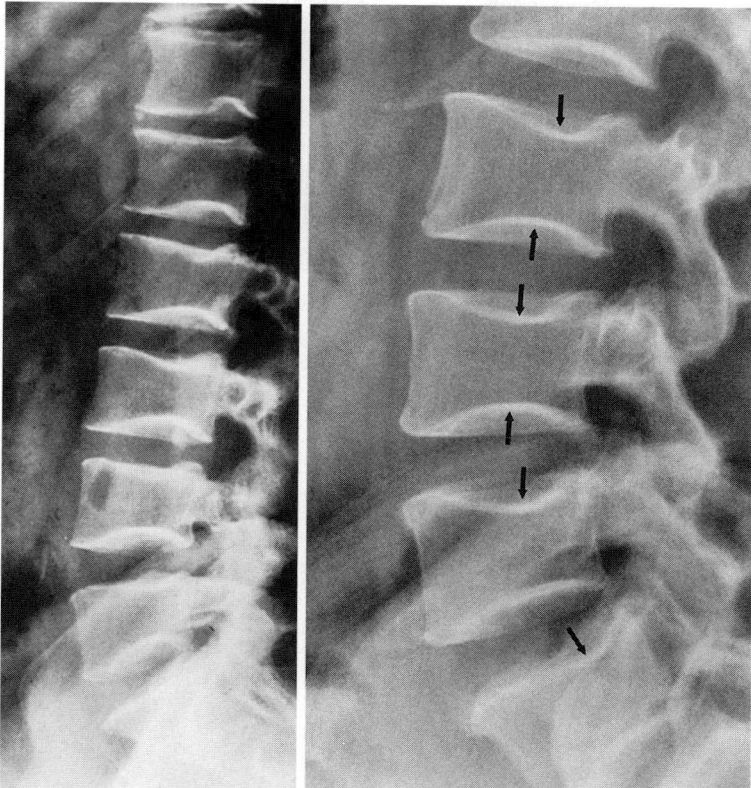

Figure 3–384. Two examples of notochordal remnants producing balloon discs. (Ref: Tsuji H et al: Developmental balloon discs of the lumbar spine in healthy subjects. *Spine* 10:907, 1985.)

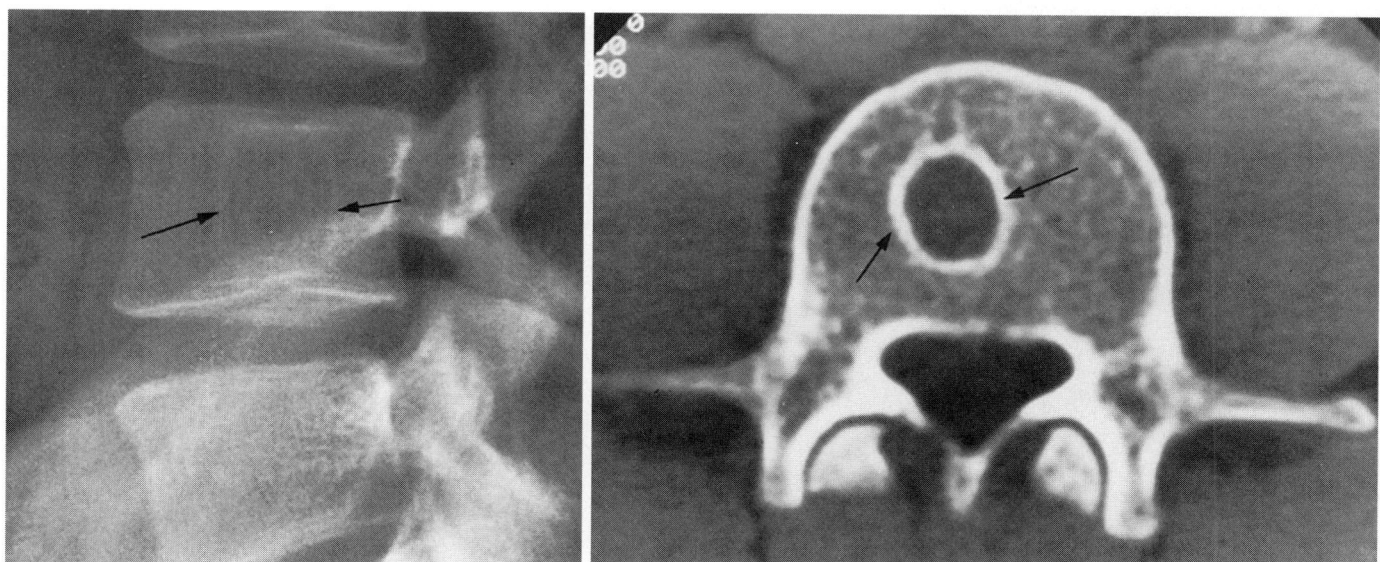

Figure 3–385. Central radiolucency within the body of L4, an incidental finding probably representing a notochordal remnant.

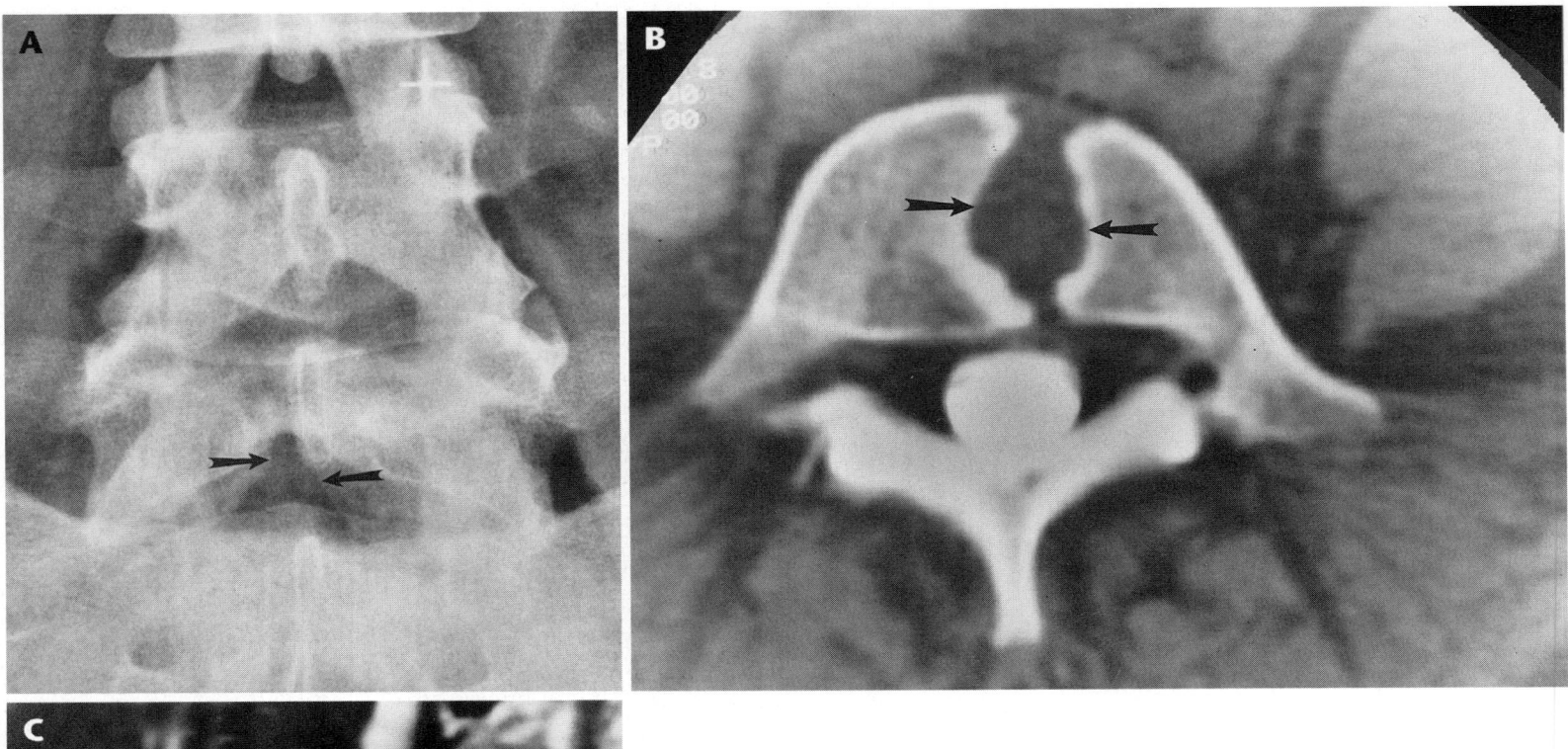

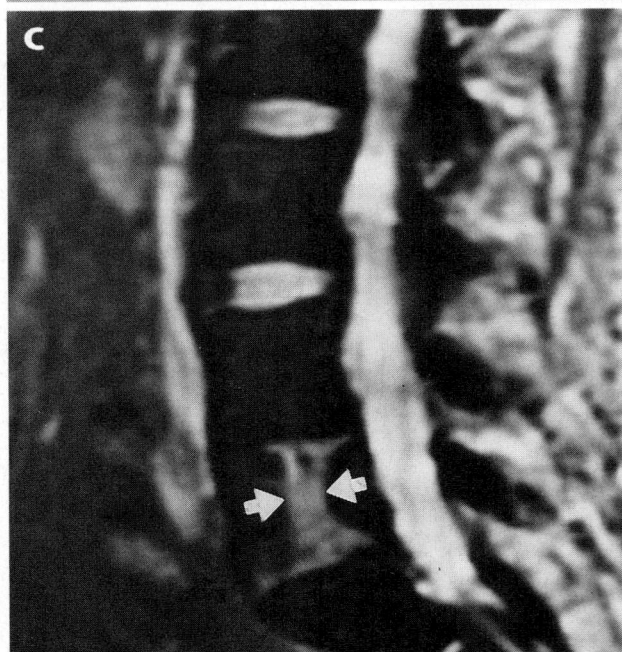

Figure 3–386. Notochordal remnant at L5. **A,** Anteroposterior film shows a defect in the vertebral body. **B,** CT scan shows a central defect. **C,** T2–weighted MR image shows a high signal in the area of defect similar to that of the intervertebral discs.

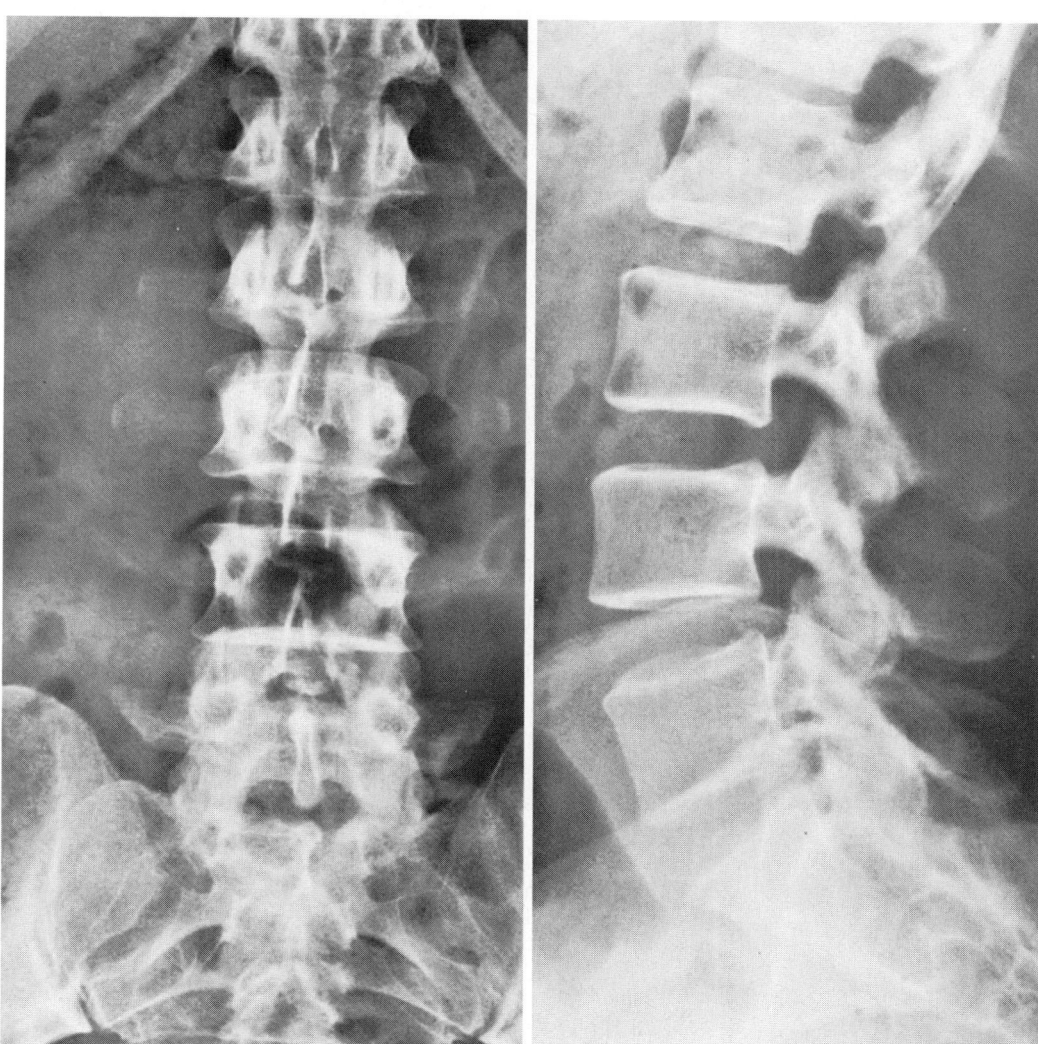

Figure 3–387. Unusually tall intervertebral discs in a 31-year-old woman.

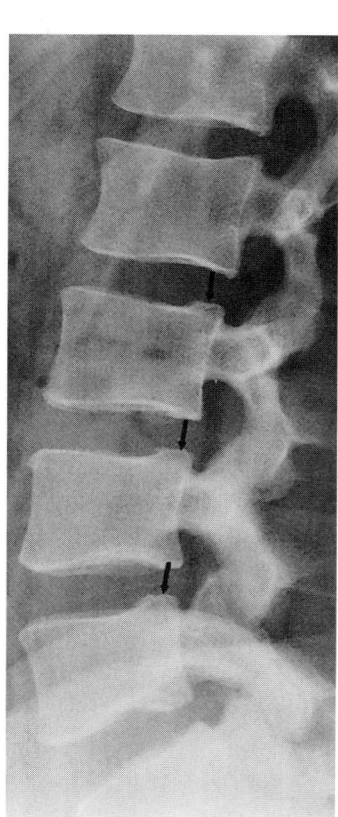

Figure 3–388. Unusual contour of the posterior aspect of the superior end plates of the lumbar vertebra.

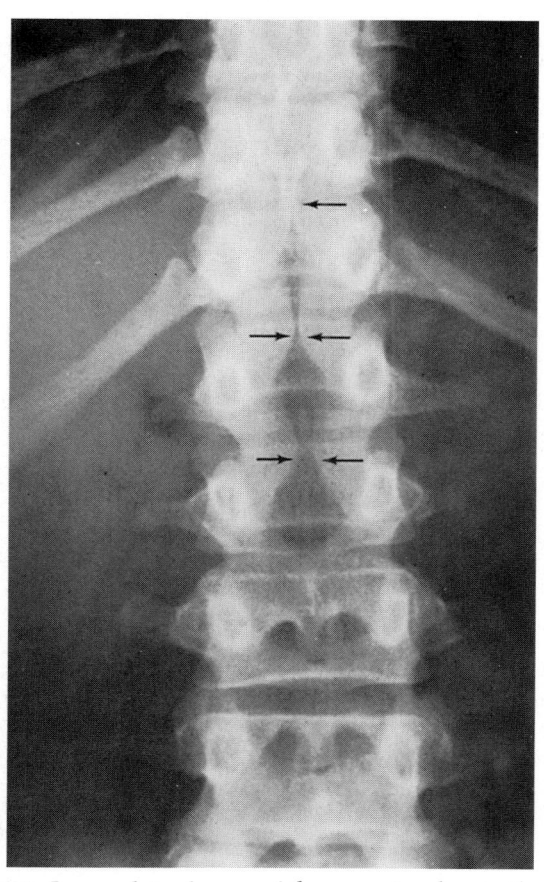

Figure 3–389. Incomplete closure of the neural arches in the lower dorsal and upper lumbar spine.

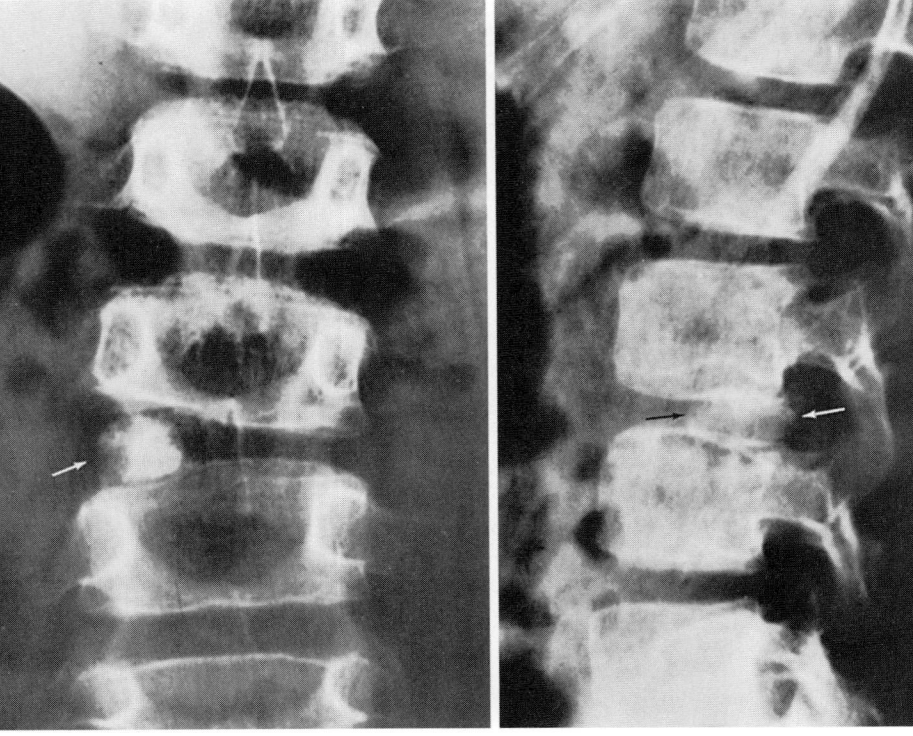

Figure 3–390. Partial hemivertebra that was mistaken for a calcified intervertebral disc. Note the deformities of adjacent vertebral bodies.

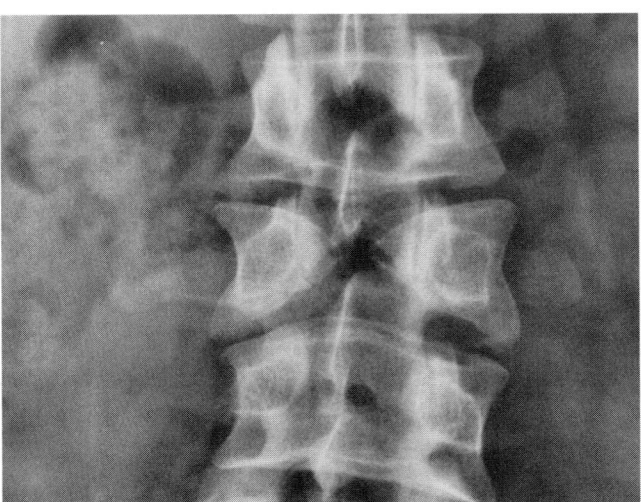

Figure 3–391. "Butterfly" lumbar vertebra.

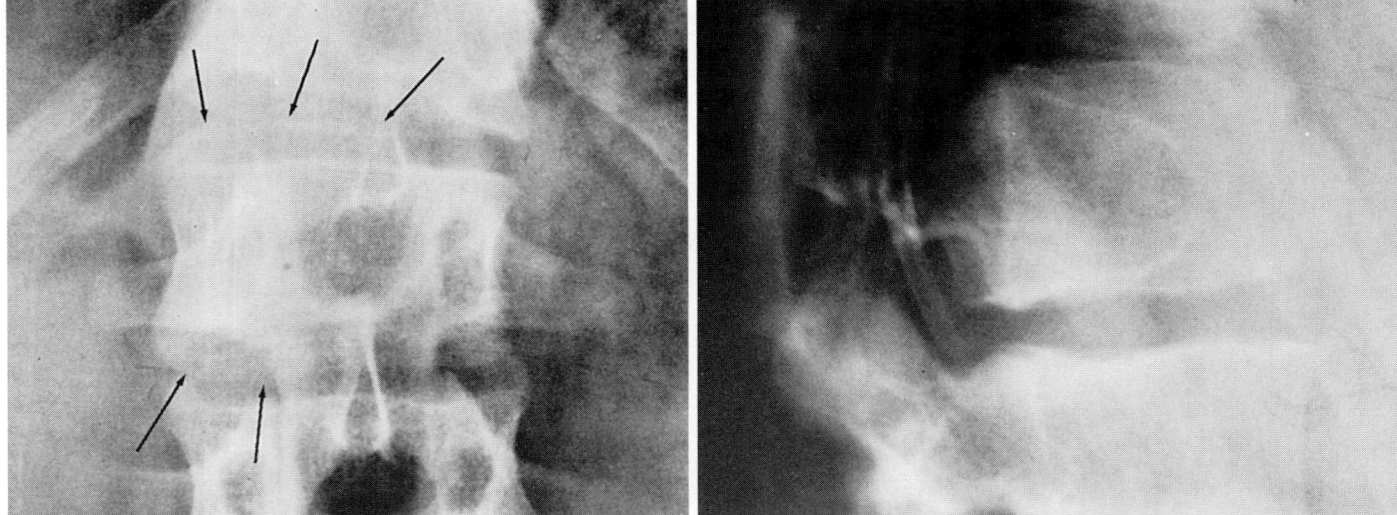

Figure 3–392. Hypoplastic vertebra on the left, originally misinterpreted as a lytic lesion of the vertebra. Note that in the frontal plane, vertebral end plates are seen only on the patient's right side (*arrows*).

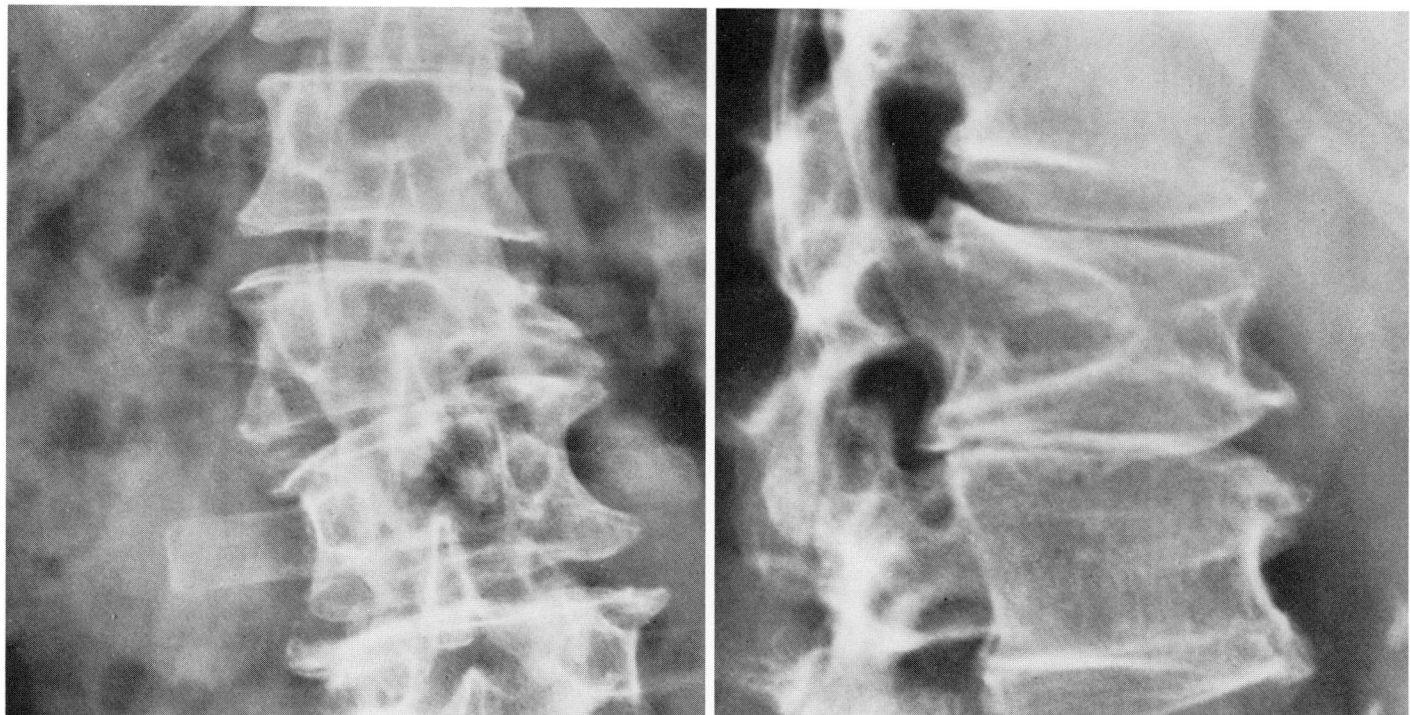

Figure 3–393. Another case of hypoplastic vertebra on the left, with more obvious changes than in Figure 3–392. Note the hypoplastic pedicle on the patient's left side. (Ref: McMaster MJ, David CV: Hemivertebra as a cause of scoliosis. *J Bone Joint Surg* 68B:588, 1986.)

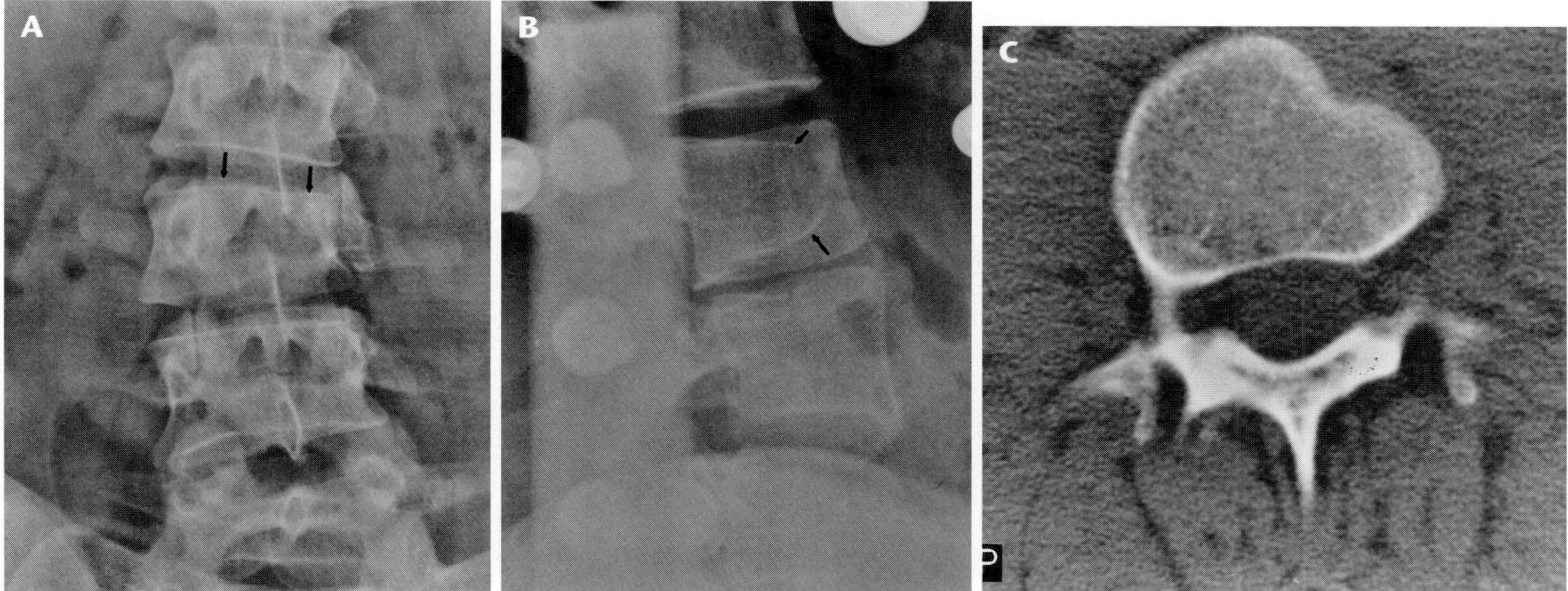

Figure 3–394. Hypoplastic vertebra producing the characteristic appearance in the lateral projection. **A,** Anteroposterior projection. **B,** Lateral projection. **C,** CT.

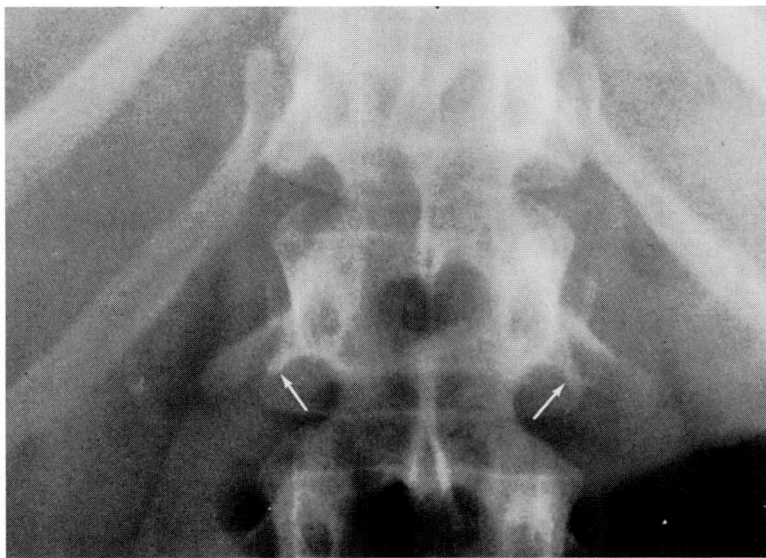

Figure 3–395. Bilateral styloid processes of L1.

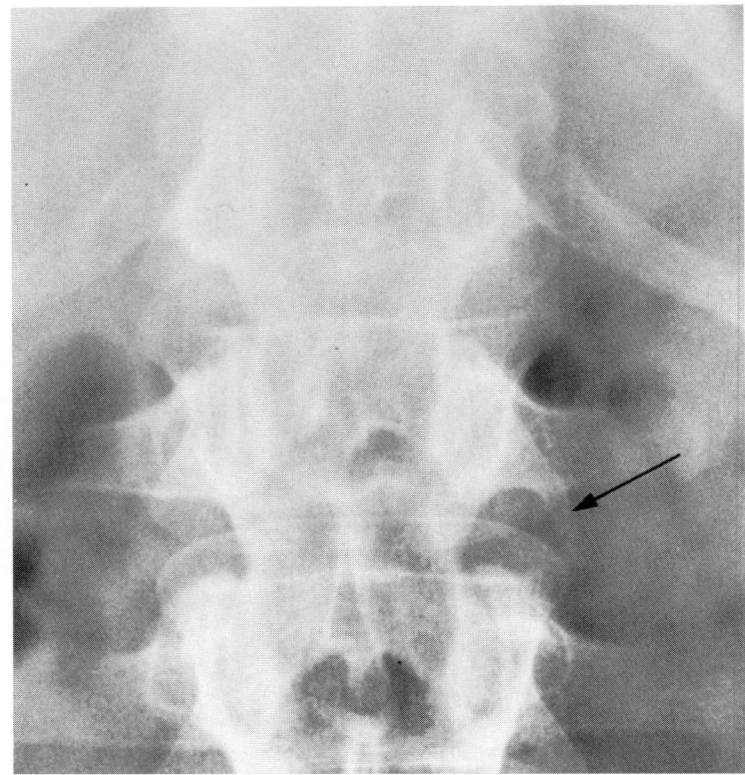

Figure 3–396. Unilateral styloid process of L1.

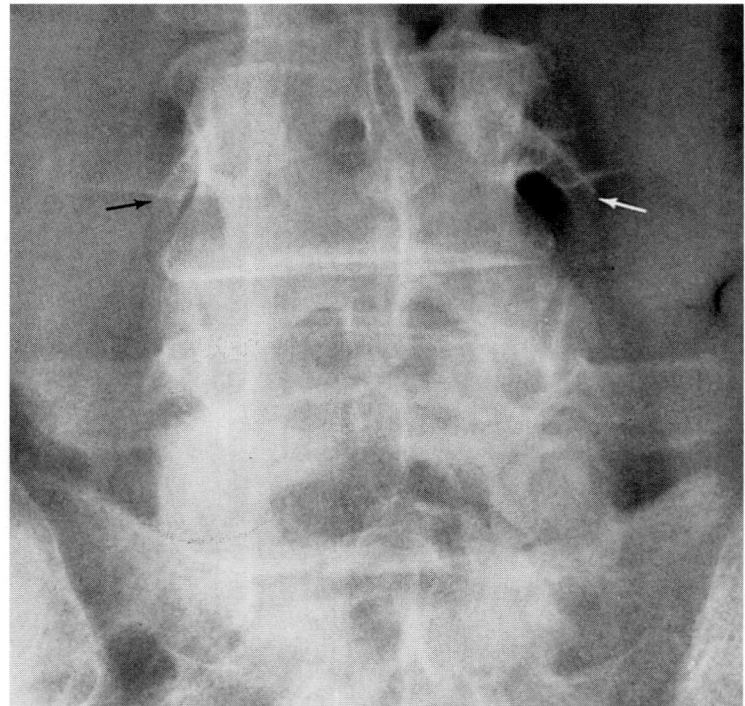

Figure 3–397. Bilateral styloid process of L4. These accessory processes arise posterior to the base of the superior articular facet.

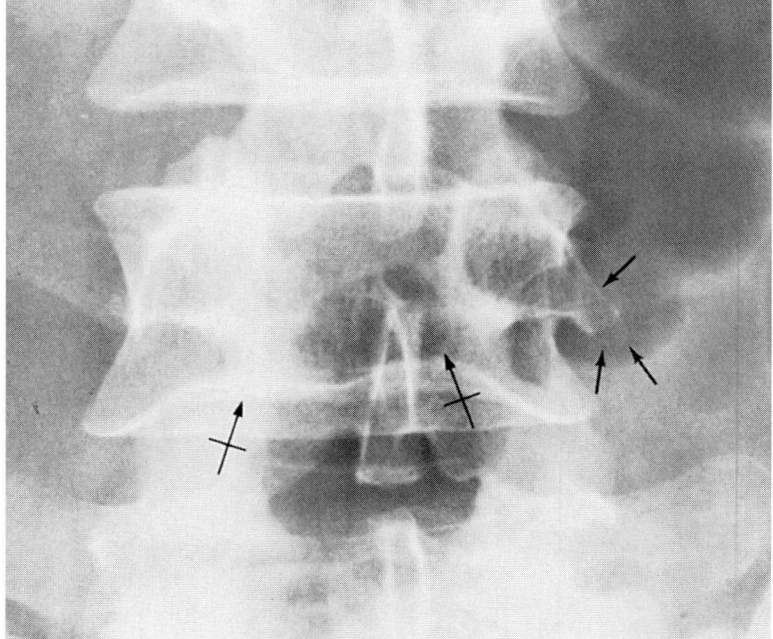

Figure 3–398. Unilateral styloid process of L4 (←). Note normal "Cupid's bow" configuration of inferior plate of L4 (↦), a normal variation. (Ref: Dietz GW, Christensen EE: Normal "Cupid's bow" contour of the lower lumbar vertebrae. *Radiology* 121:577, 1976.)

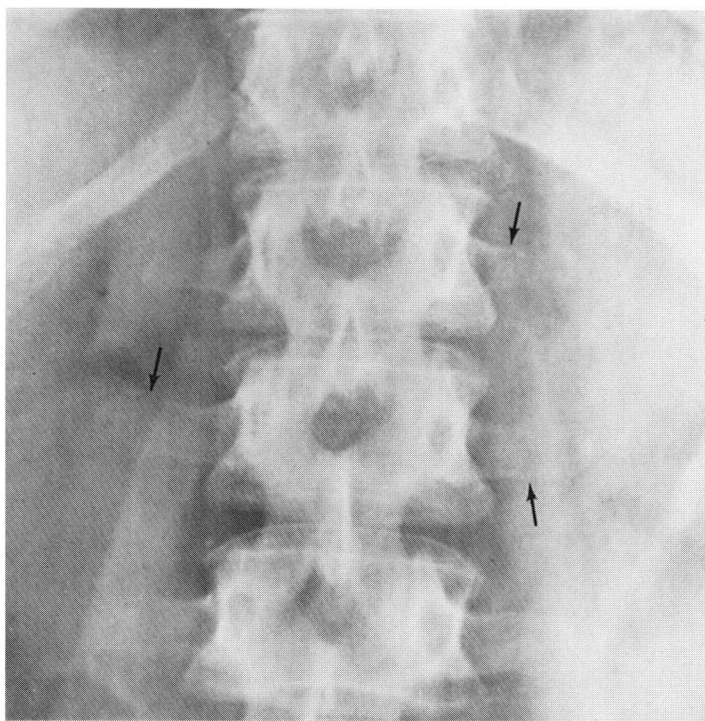

Figure 3–399. Simulated fractures of the transverse processes, produced by the crossing shadow of the psoas muscle.

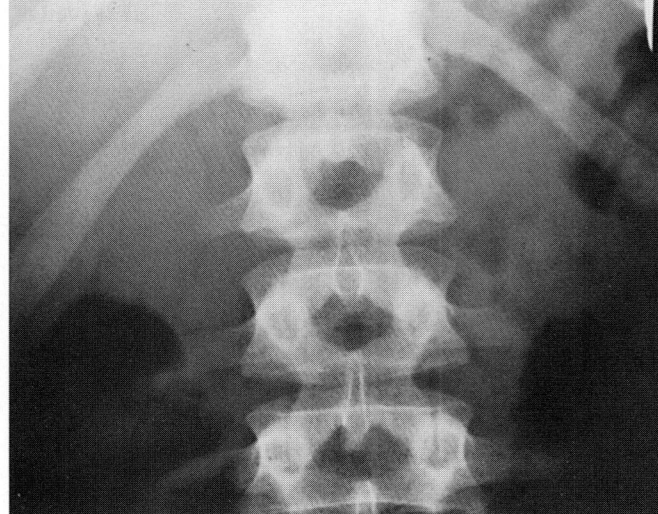

Figure 3–400. Absence of the transverse process of the left side of L1.

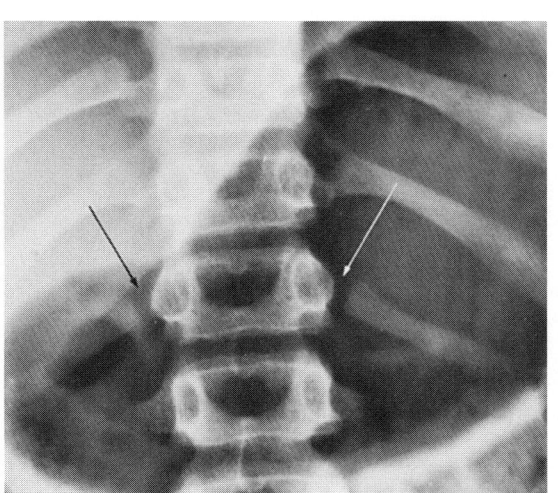

Figure 3–401. Unconnected ribs at L1 bilaterally.

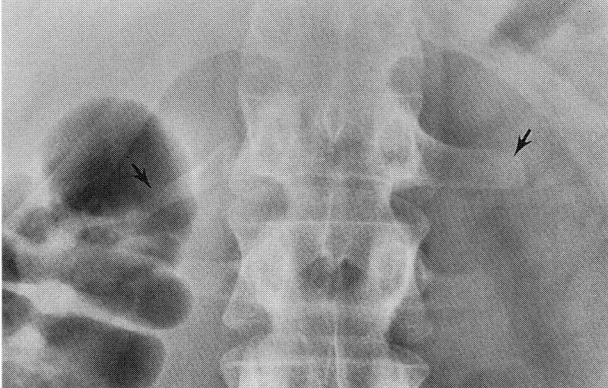

Figure 3–402. Asymmetric development of L1 with a rib on the right and a transverse process on the left.

Figure 3–403. Failure of union of the L1 transverse process with the vertebral body.

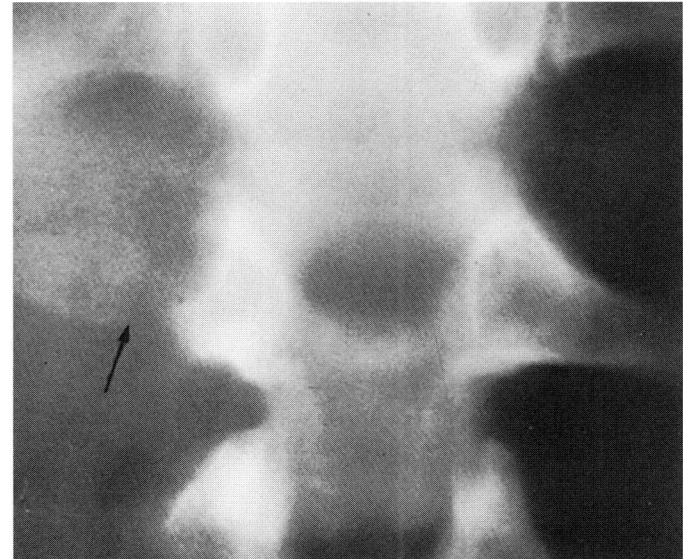

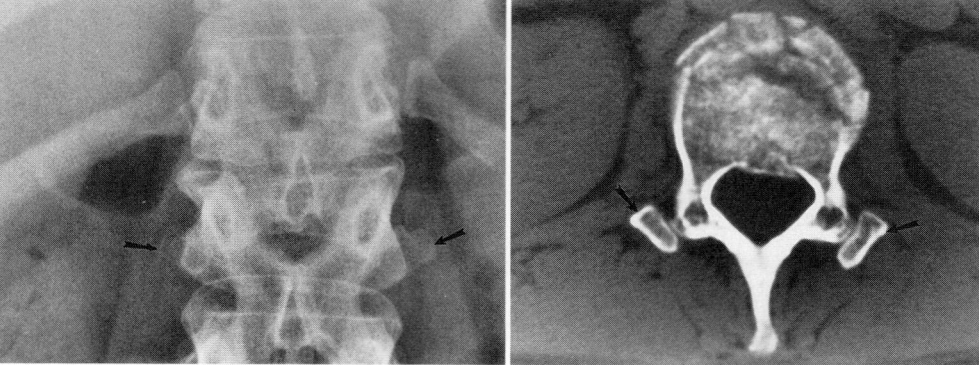

Figure 3–404. Ununited transverse process of L1. Note attenuated sites of origin from the neural arch. The patient has an acute fracture of the vertebral body.

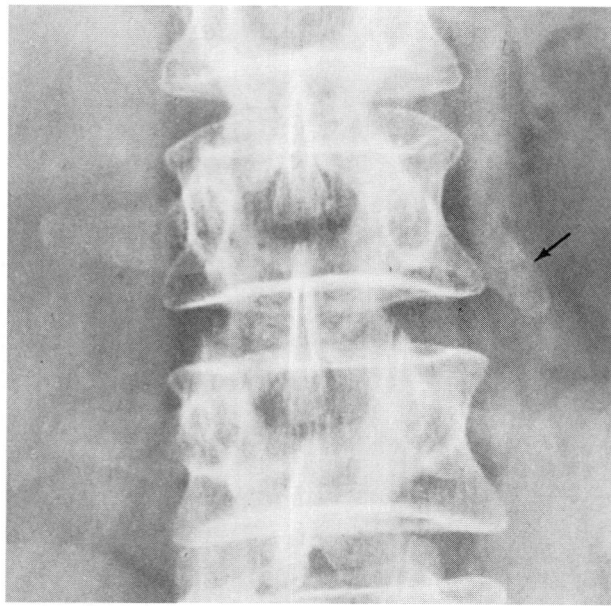

Figure 3–405. Ptotic transverse process of L3. This variant may easily be mistaken for a fracture.

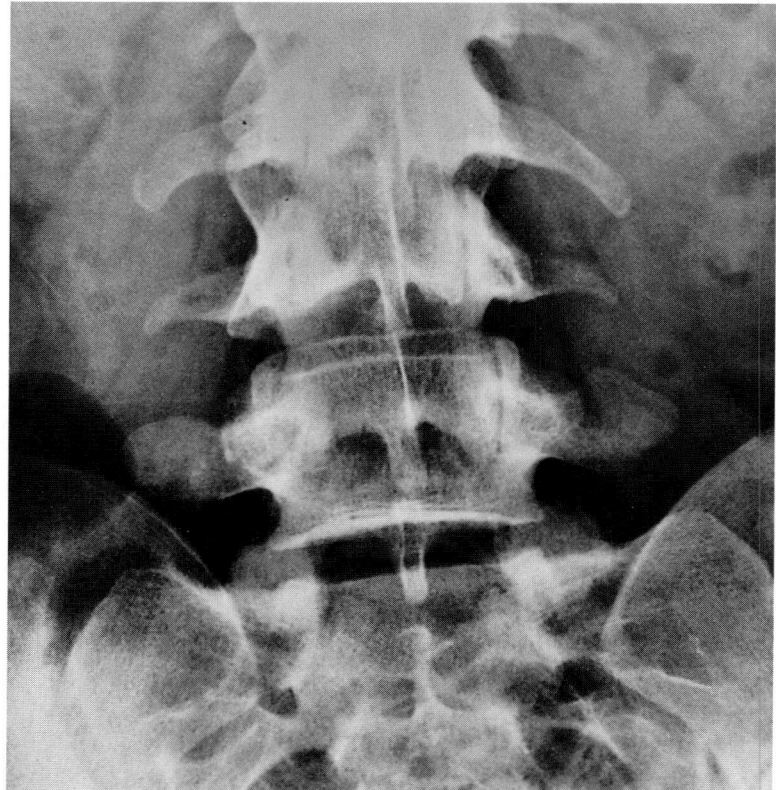

Figure 3–406. Ptotic transverse processes.

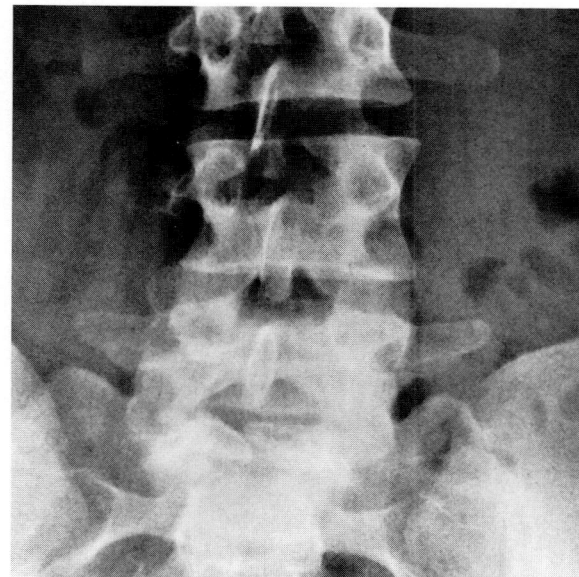

Figure 3–407. Congenital absence of the transverse process on the left side of L4.

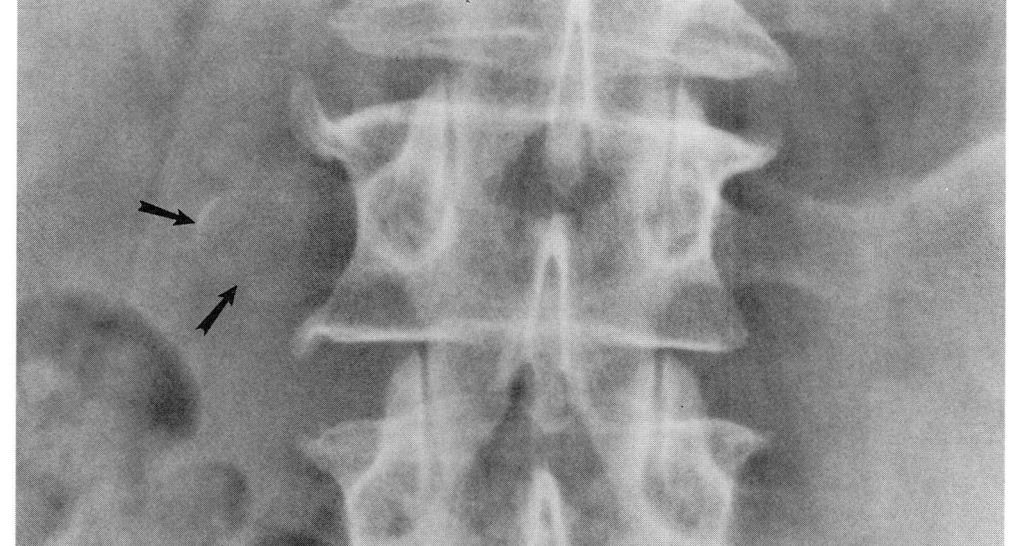

Figure 3–408. Asymmetric transverse processes with an enlarged process on the right that was mistaken for a biliary calculus.

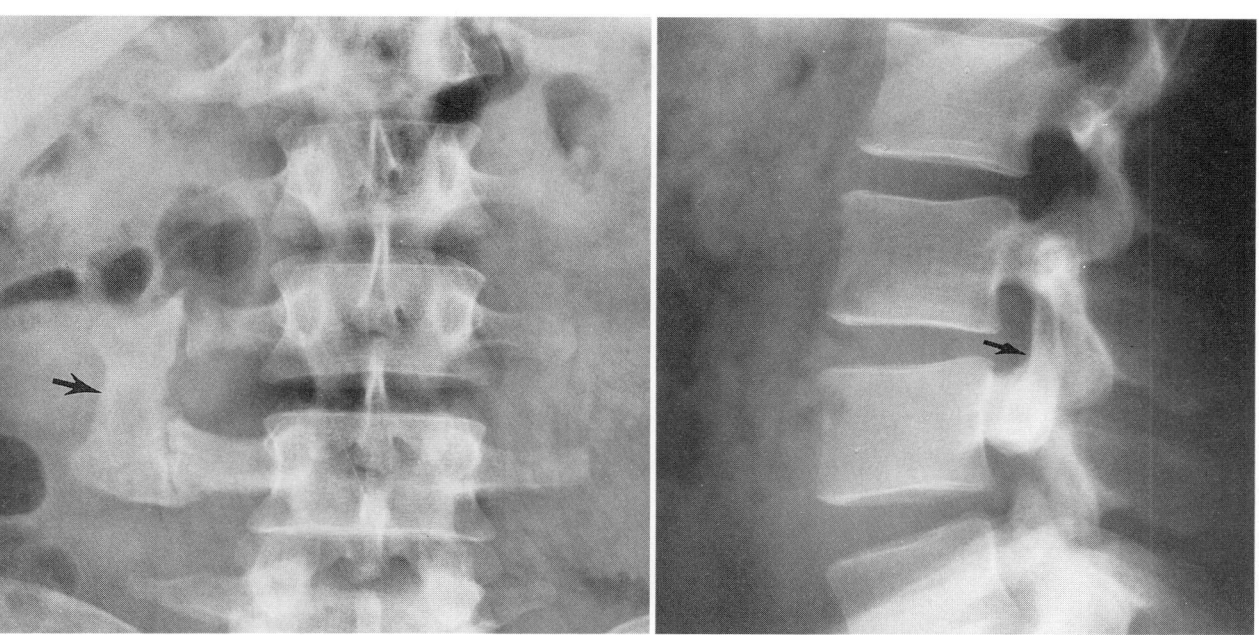

Figure 3–409. Developmental bridge between the transverse processes of L3 and L4.

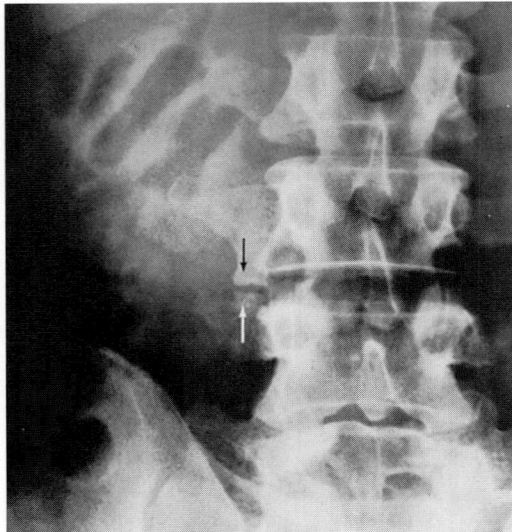

Figure 3–410. Anomalous articulation between the transverse processes of L3 and L4.

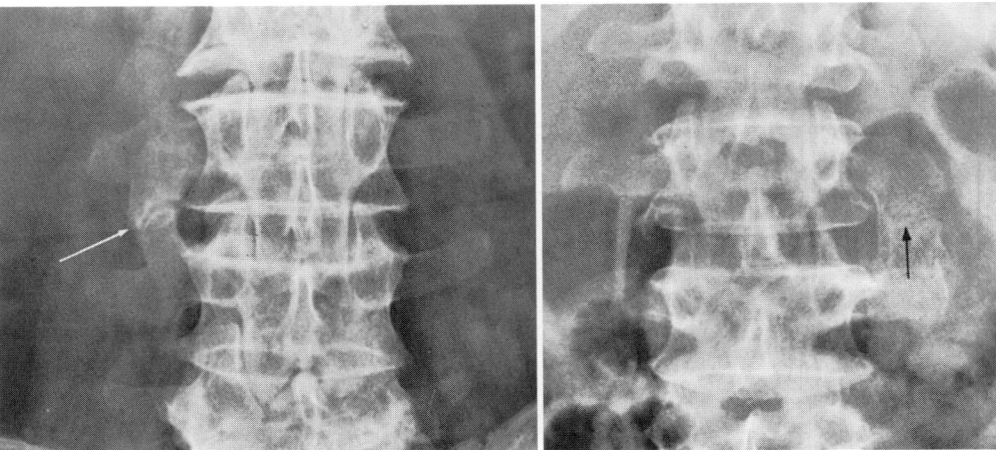

Figure 3–411. Two examples of pseudarthrosis between the transverse processes of L3 and L4. (Ref: Yoslow W, Becker MH: Osseous bridges between the transverse processes of the lumbar spine: Report of three cases and review of the literature. *J Bone Joint Surg* 50A:513, 1968.)

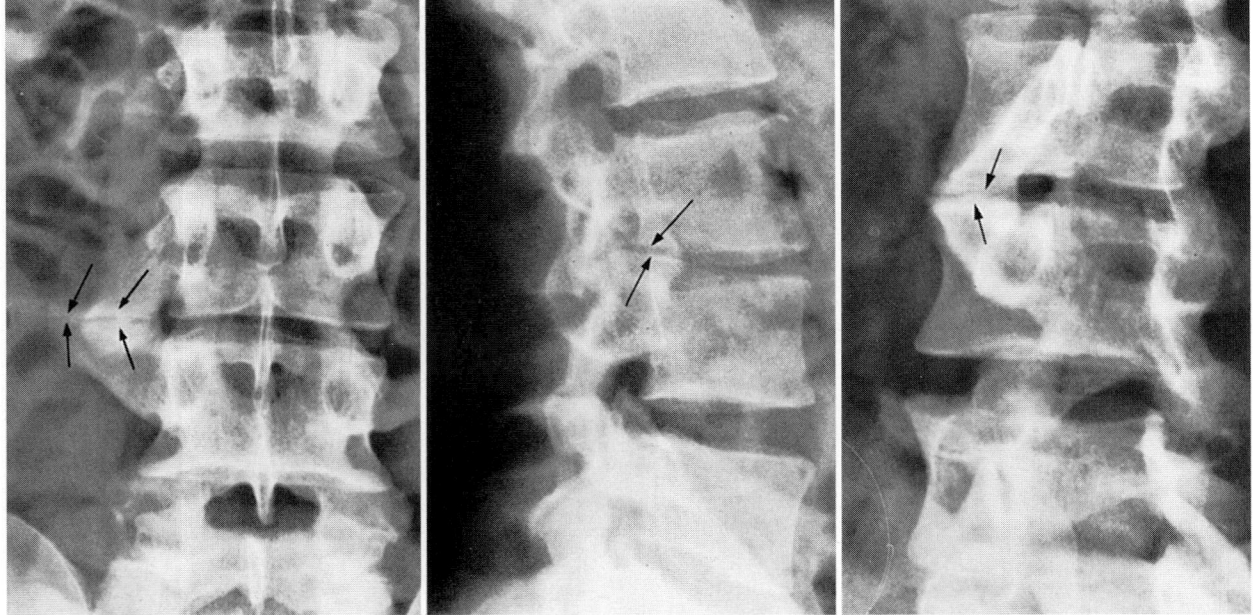

Figure 3–412. Very large anomalous articulation between the transverse processes of L3 and L4. *Left,* AP projection. *Center,* Lateral projection. *Right,* Oblique projection.

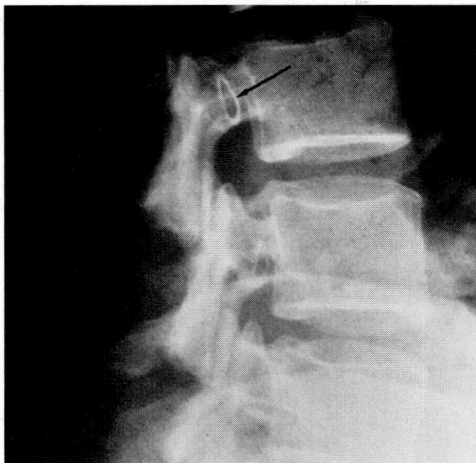

Figure 3–413. Transverse process of L3 seen in cross-section.

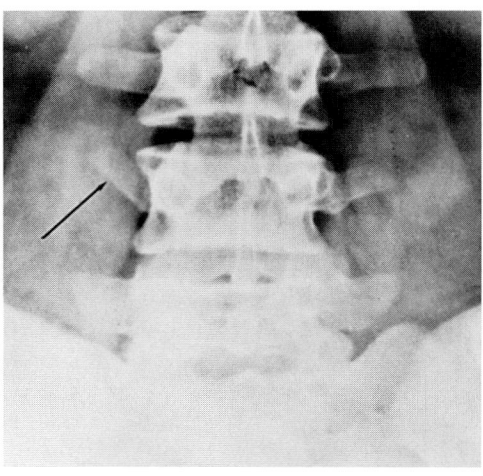

Figure 3–414. Cephalad-directed transverse process of L4.

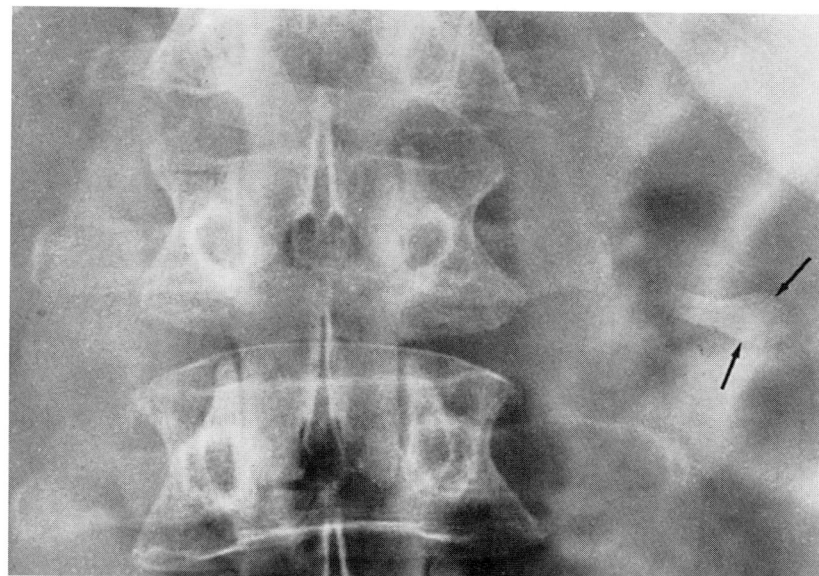

Figure 3–415. Abortive rib formation at L2.

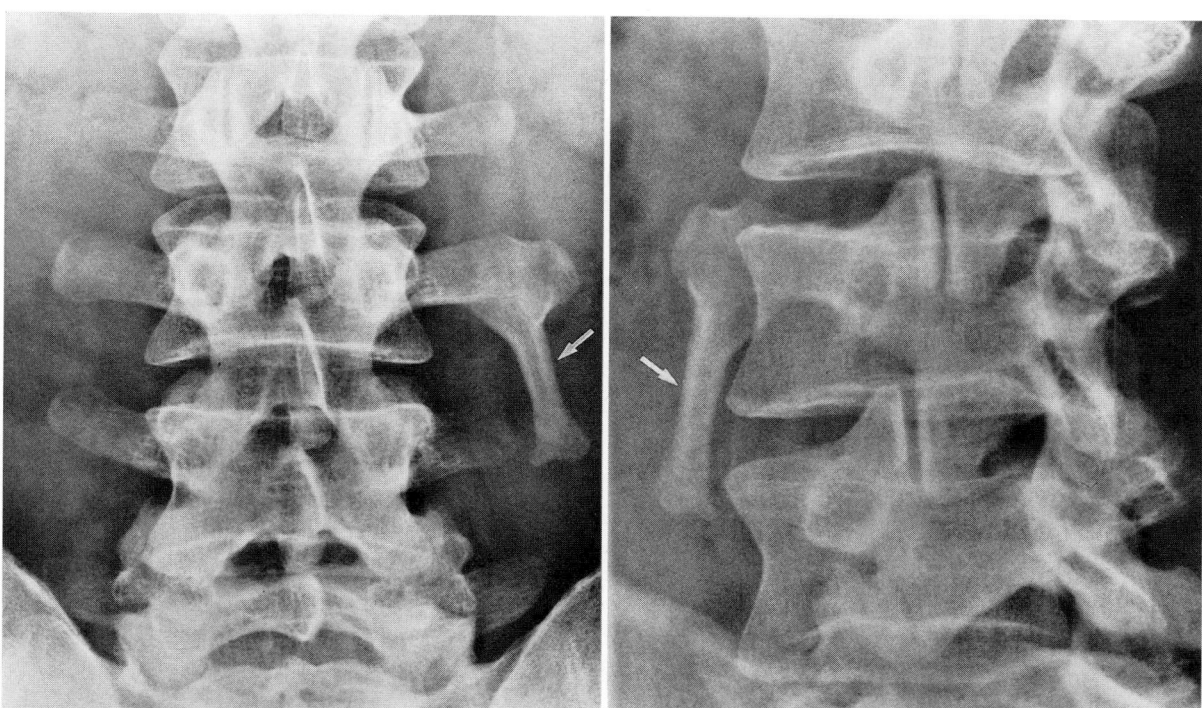

Figure 3–416. Lumbar rib. (Courtesy of Dr. Gary M. Guebert.)

Figure 3–417. Large osseous bridge between L1, L2, and L3 in a patient with no history of trauma, simulating a lumbar rib.

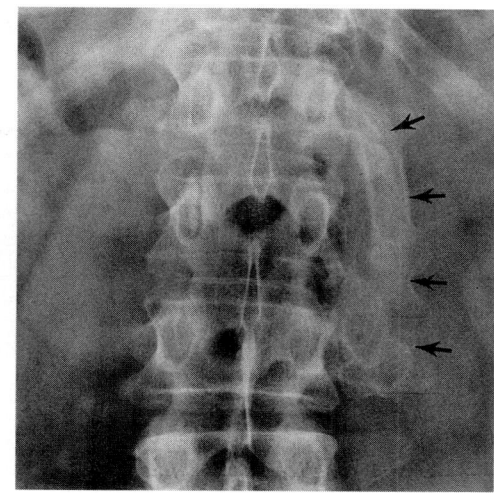

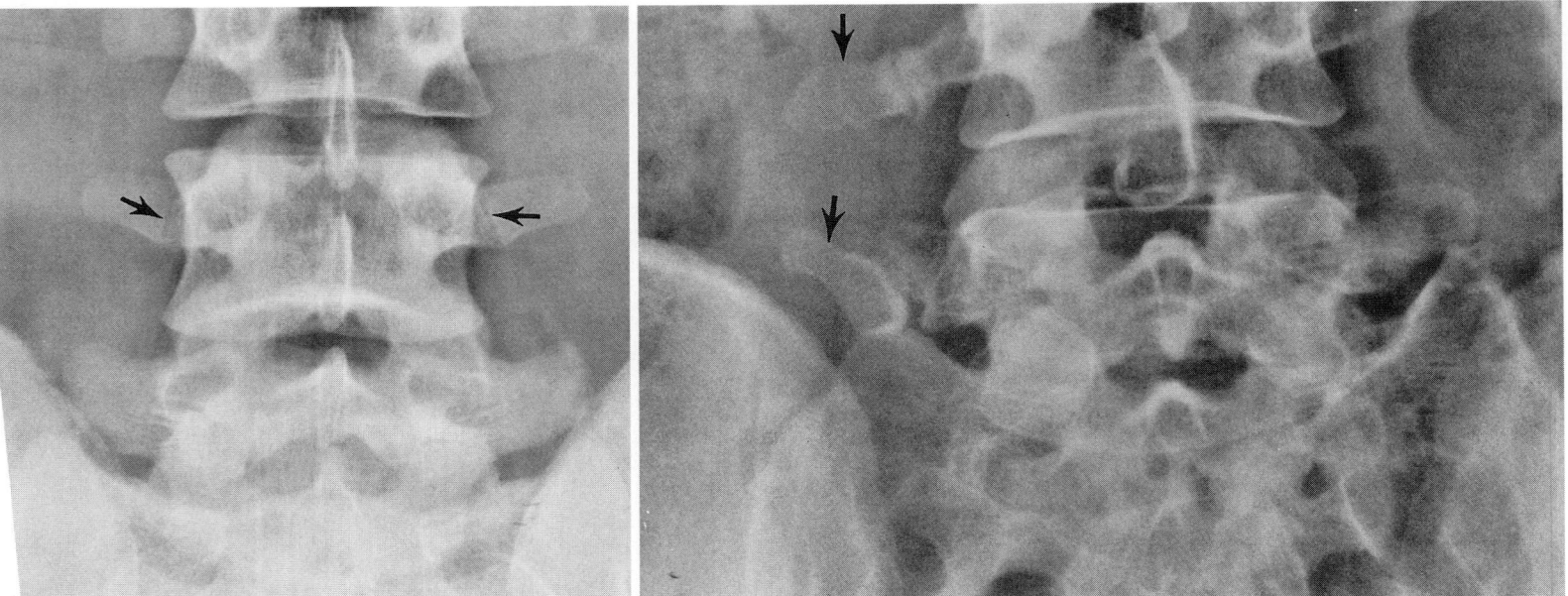

Figure 3–418. Two examples of lumbar ribs.

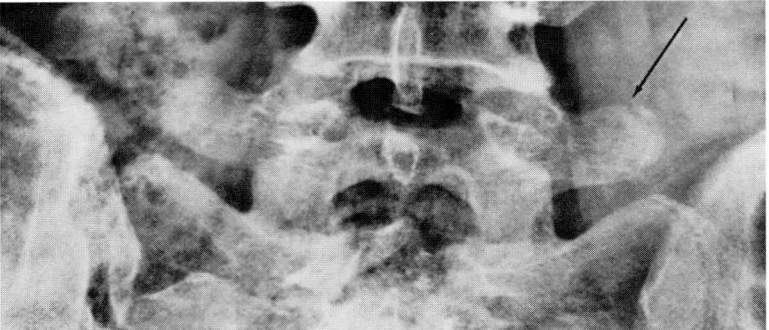

Figure 3–419. Persistence of the apophysis of the transverse process of L5.

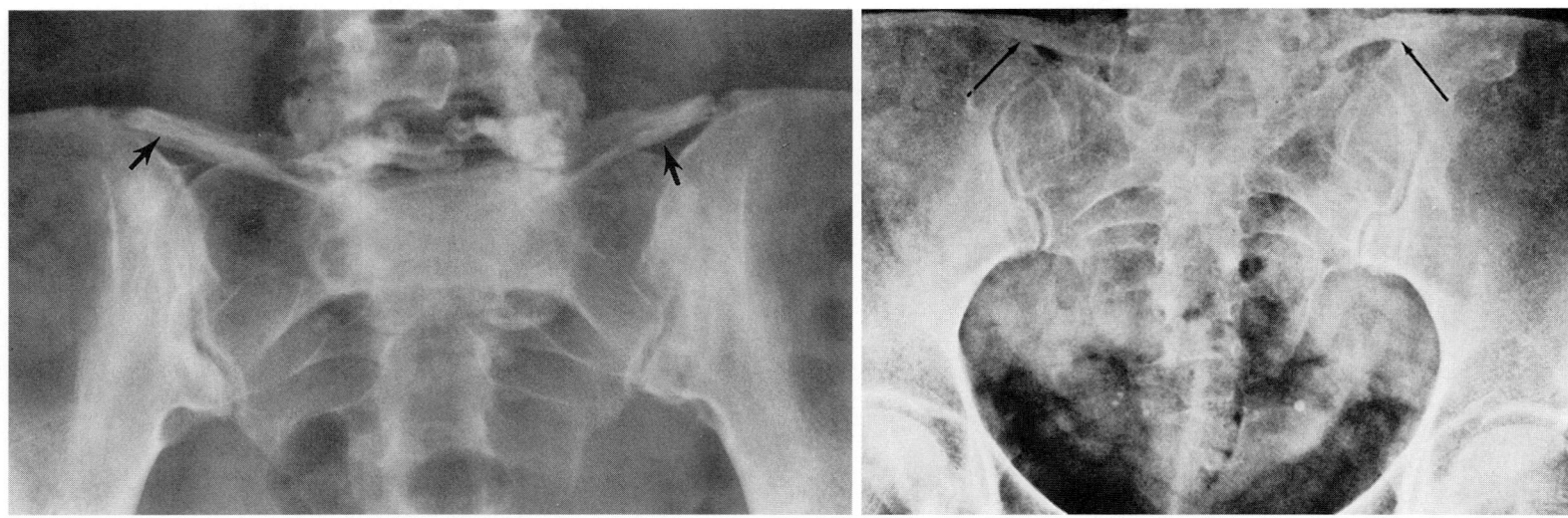

Figure 3–420. Two examples of heavy calcification of the iliolumbar ligaments.

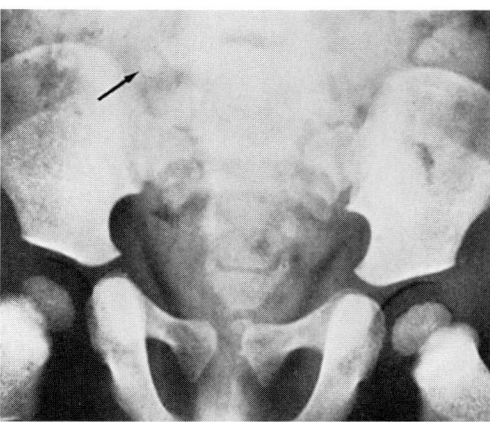

Figure 3–421. Separate ossification center for transverse process of L5.

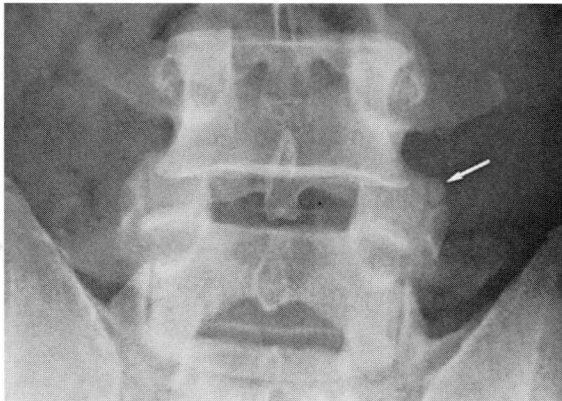

Figure 3–422. Ununited secondary ossification center of the end of the superior articulating process of L5.

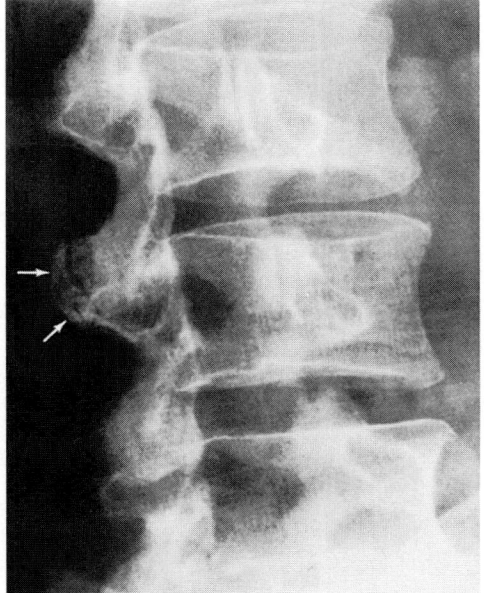

Figure 3–423. Persistent apophysis of the mamillary process of L4.

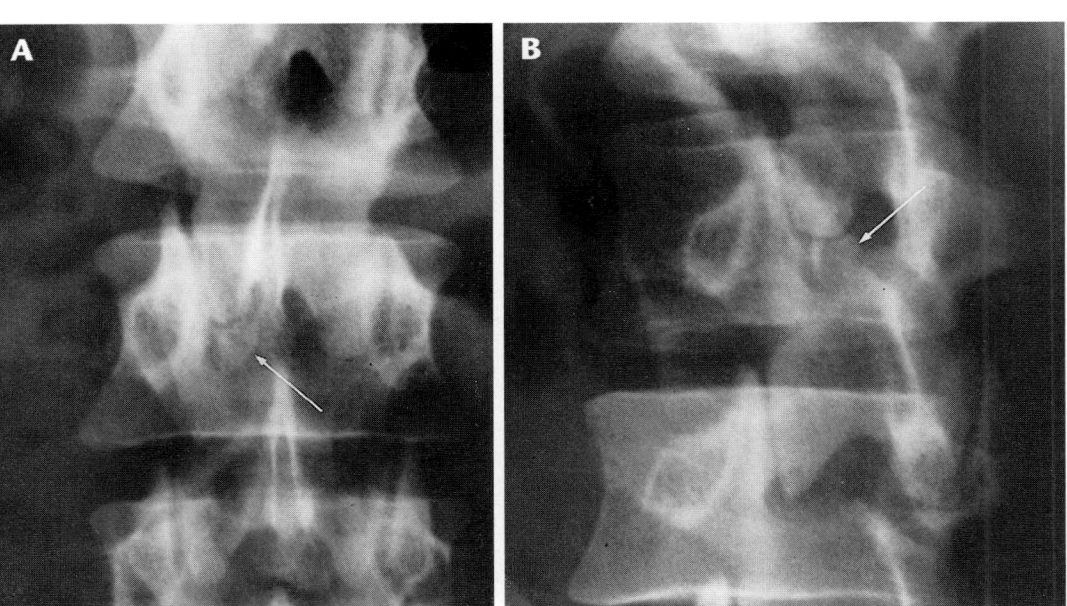

Figure 3–424. Ununited ossification center of the end of the inferior articulating process of L3, which may be mistaken for a fracture. **A,** Frontal projection. **B,** Oblique projection.

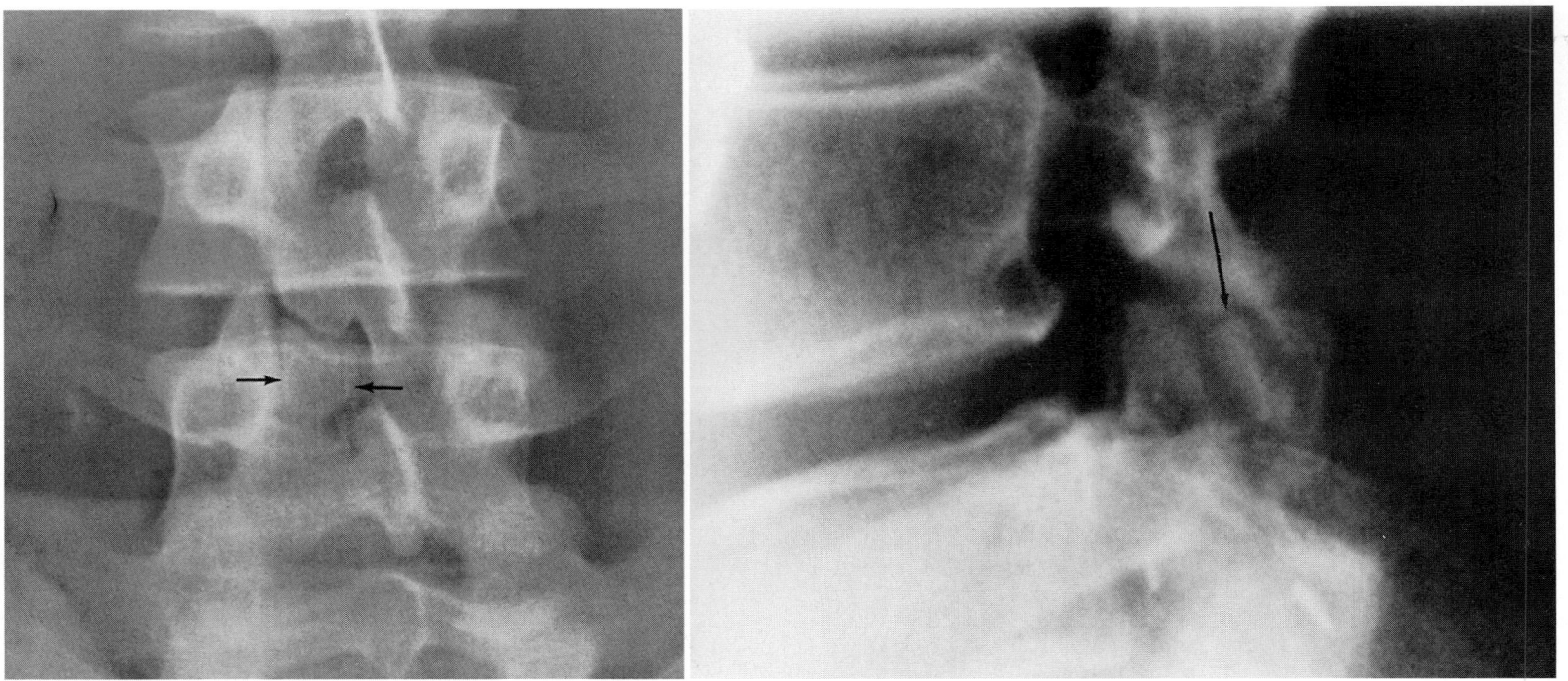

Figure 3–425. Ununited ossification center of the inferior articulating process of L3.

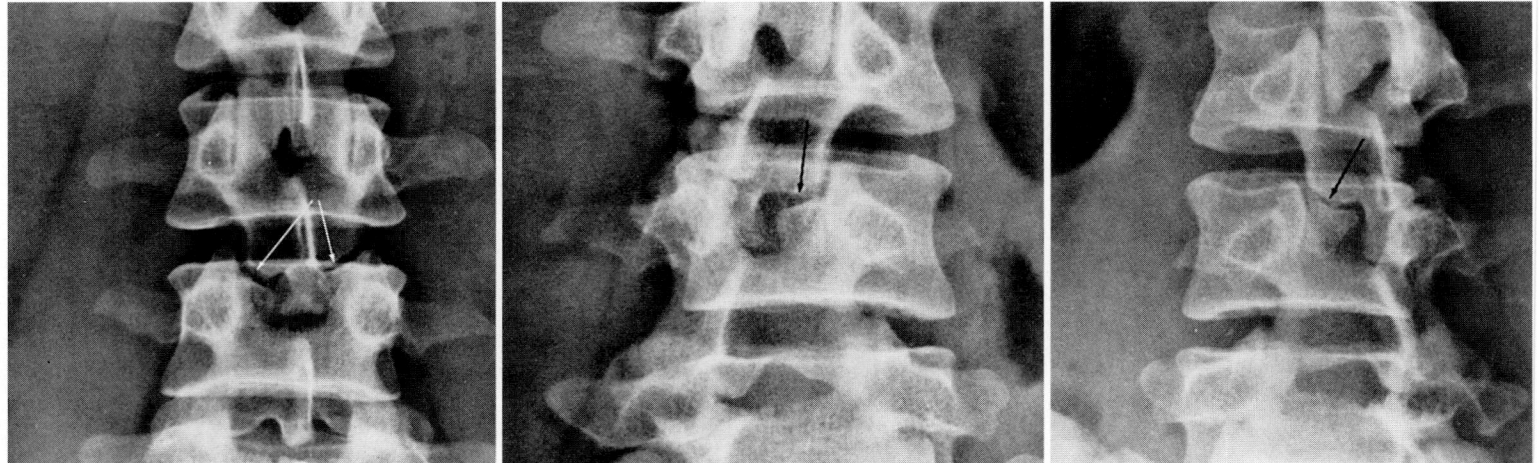

Figure 3–426. Bilateral failure of union of the ossification centers of the inferior articulating process of L3.

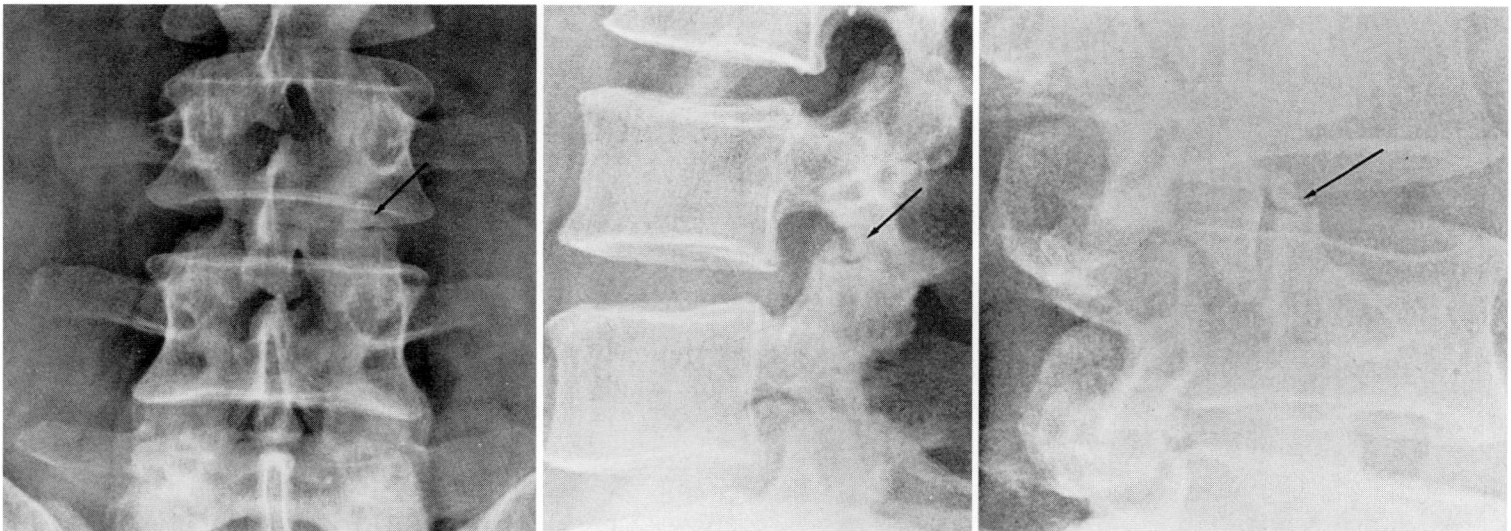

Figure 3–427. Failure of fusion of the ossification center of the superior articulating process of L4.

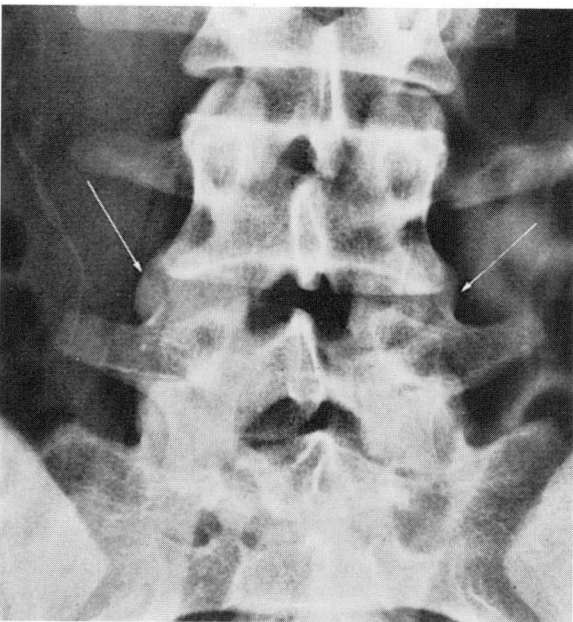

Figure 3–428. The facets between L4 and L5, simulating an osseous or soft tissue mass.

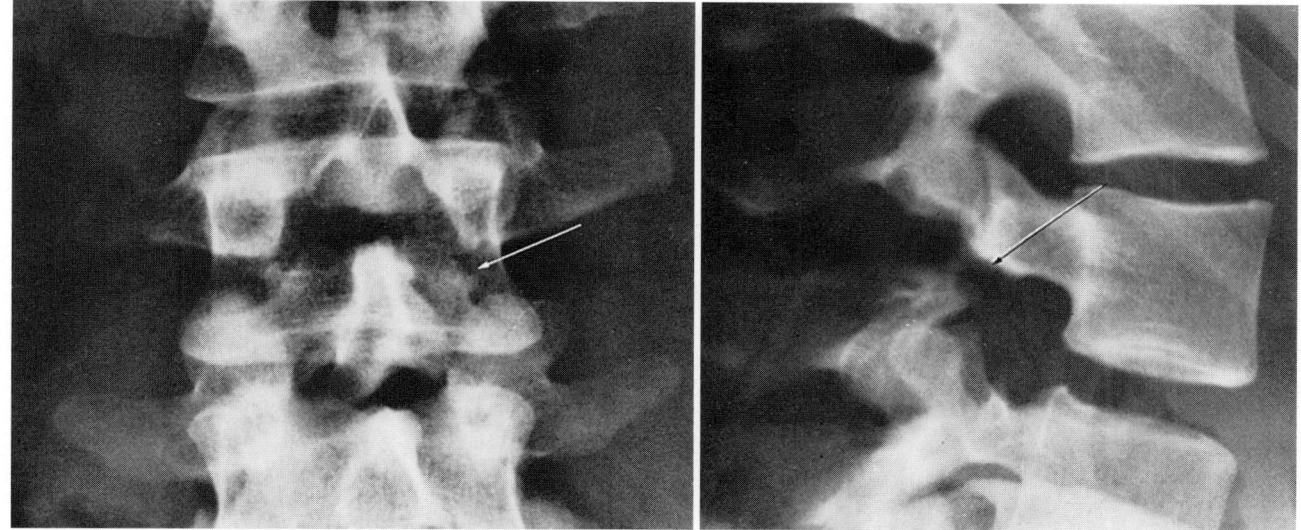

Figure 3–429. Absence of the inferior articulating process of L3. (Refs: Arcomano JP, Karas S: Congenital absence of the lumbosacral articular processes. *Skeletal Radiol* 8:133, 1982; Phillips MR, Keagy RD: Congenital absence of lumbar articular facets with computerized axial tomography documentation. *Spine* 13:676, 1988.)

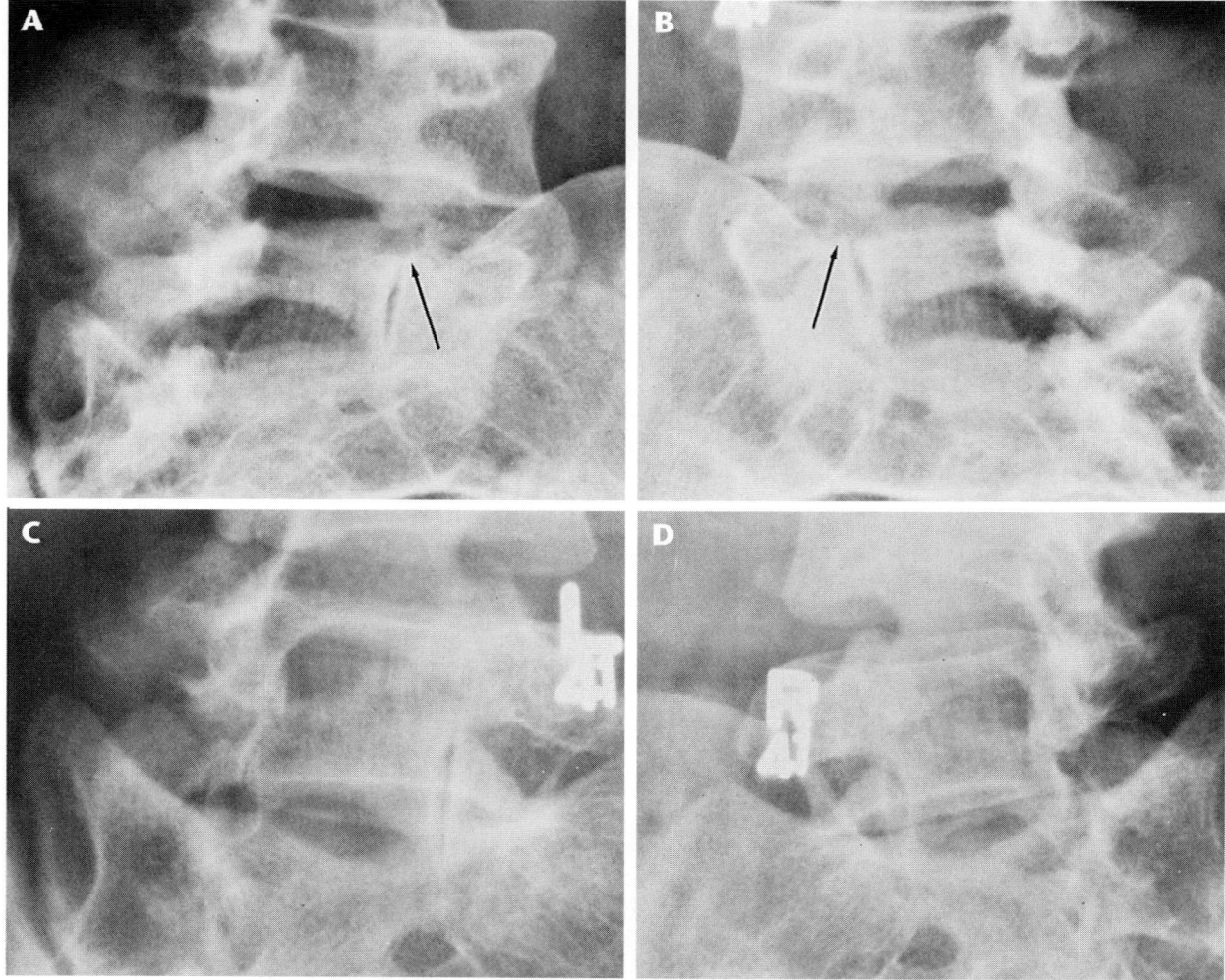

Figure 3–430. A and **B,** Apparent bilateral spondylolysis of L5 caused by projection. **C** and **D,** Films made with 15-degree cephalad angulation show no spondylolysis.

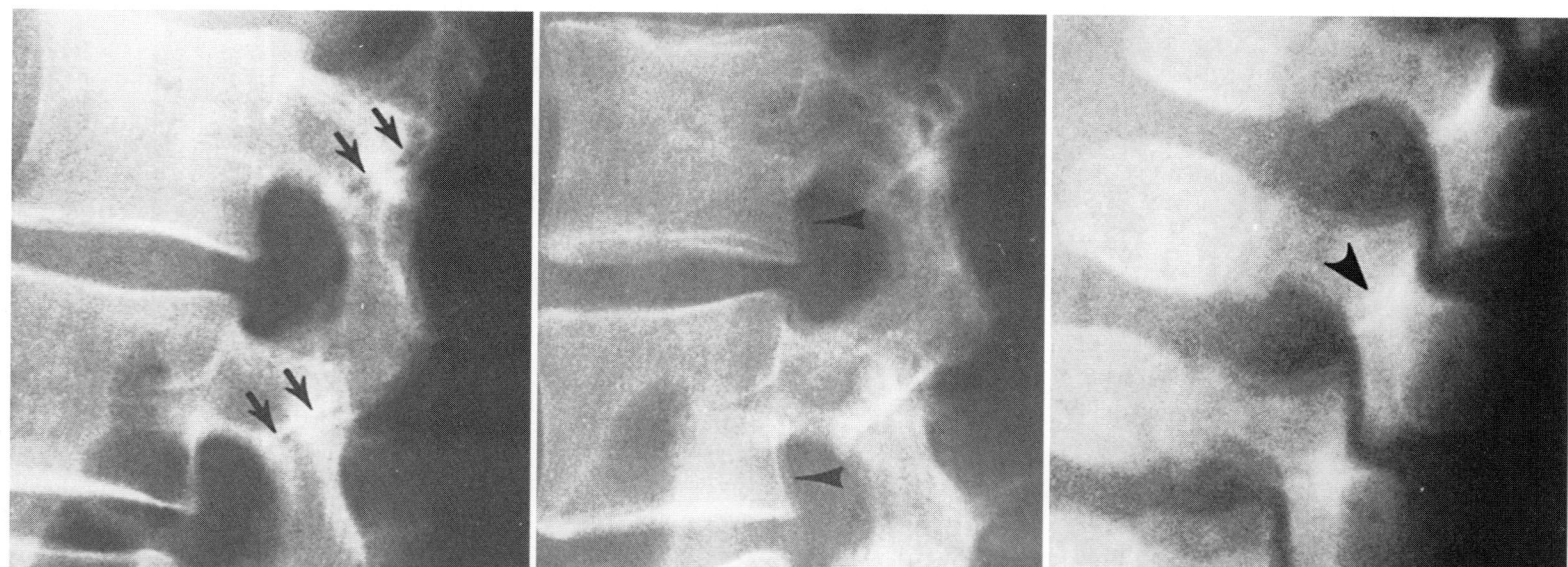

Figure 3–431. Pseudospondylolysis is seen at L2 and L3 in perfectly positioned lateral projections and results from superimposition of the transverse processes. *Left,* Pseudospondylolysis at L2 and L3 in a true lateral projection. *Center,* The defects disappear when a minor degree of obliquity is present. *Right,* Pseudospondylolysis in an infant. (From El-Khoury GY et al: Pseudospondylolysis. *Radiology* 139:72, 1981.)

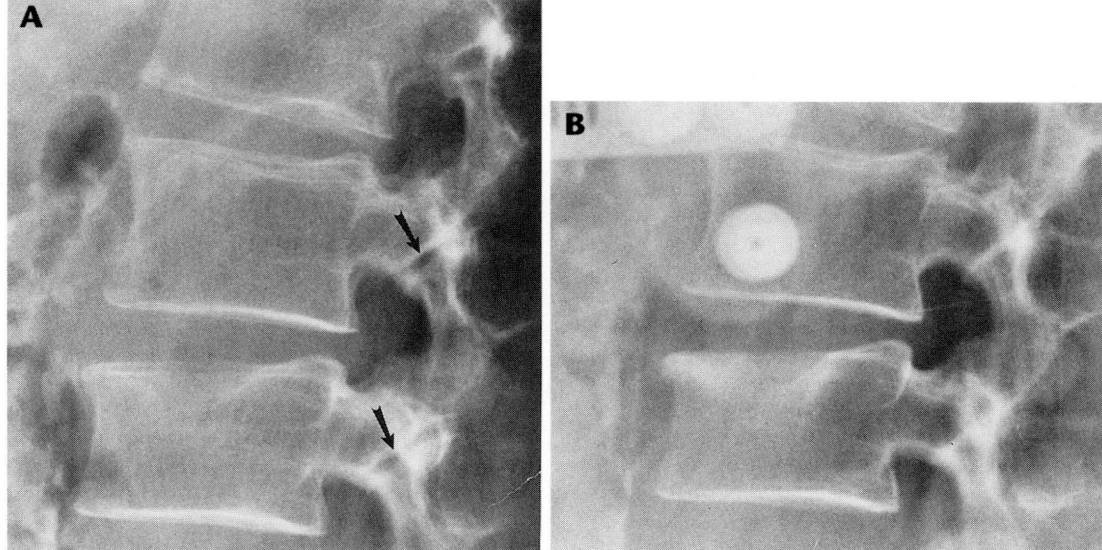

Figure 3–432. A, B, Pseudospondylolysis at L2 and L3 in a 54-year-old man with slight rotation at a time of filming, corrected by better positioning **(B).**

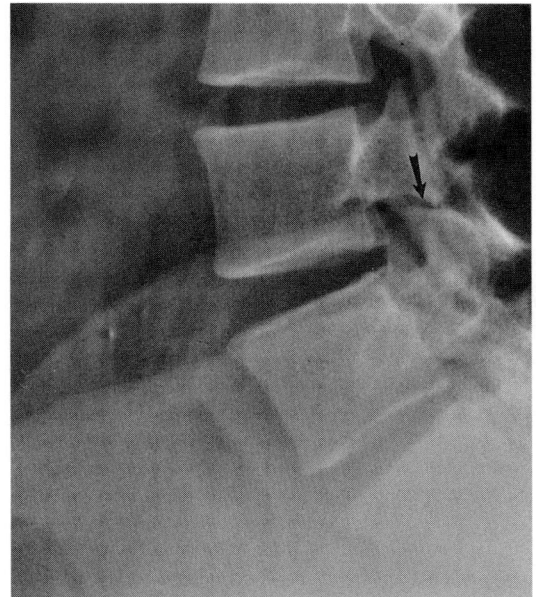

Figure 3–433. Simulated spondylolysis of L4 caused by superimposition of the shadow of the crest of the ilium.

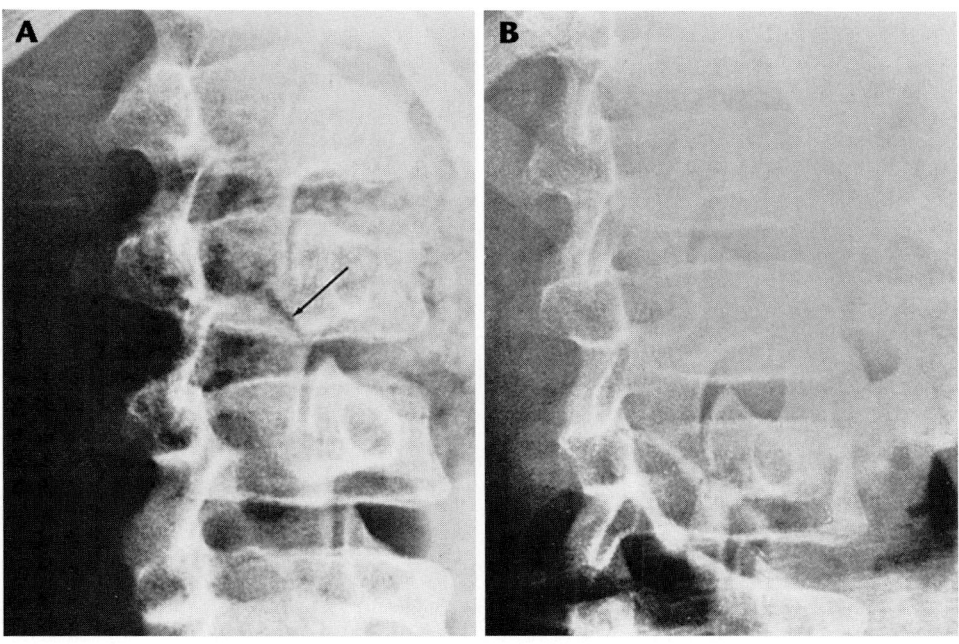

Figure 3–434. A, Bowel gas simulating spondylolysis of L2. **B,** Repeated examination clarifies the issue.

Figure 3–435. "Pig snout" pedicle results from superimposition of the shadows of the pedicle and an unusual downward projection of the distal end of the transverse process. (Courtesy of Dr. WE Litterer.) (Ref: Patel NP et al: Radiology of lumbar vertebral pedicles: variants, anomalies and pathologic conditions. *Radiographics* 7:101, 1981.)

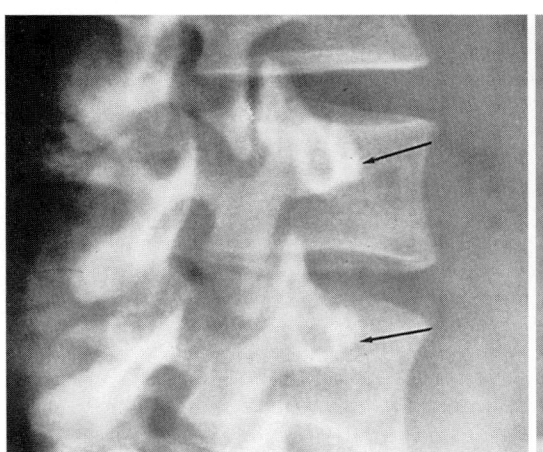
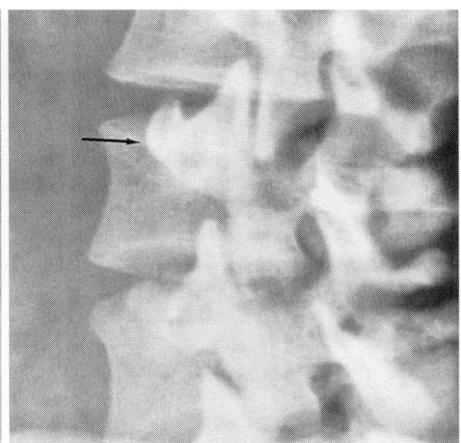

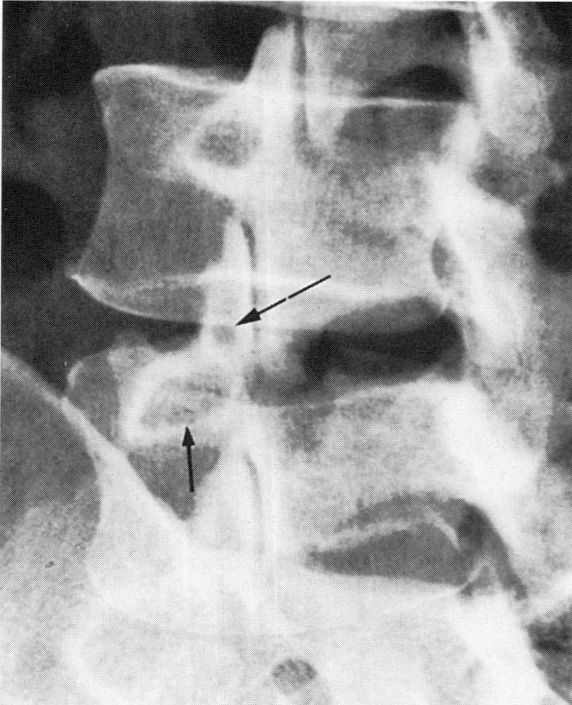

Figure 3–436. The two-eyed Scotty dog. The second "eye" is created by a prominent mamillary process. (Ref: Resnik CS et al: The two-eyed Scotty dog: a normal anatomic variant. *Radiology* 149:680, 1983.)

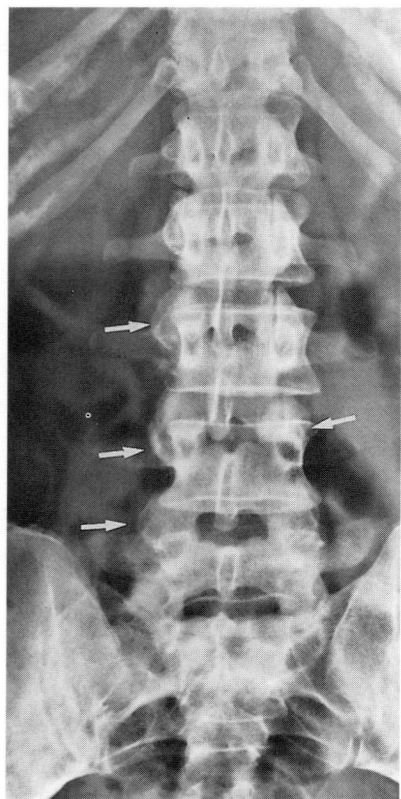

Figure 3–437. Asymmetry of the facets of the lumbar spine simulating masses.

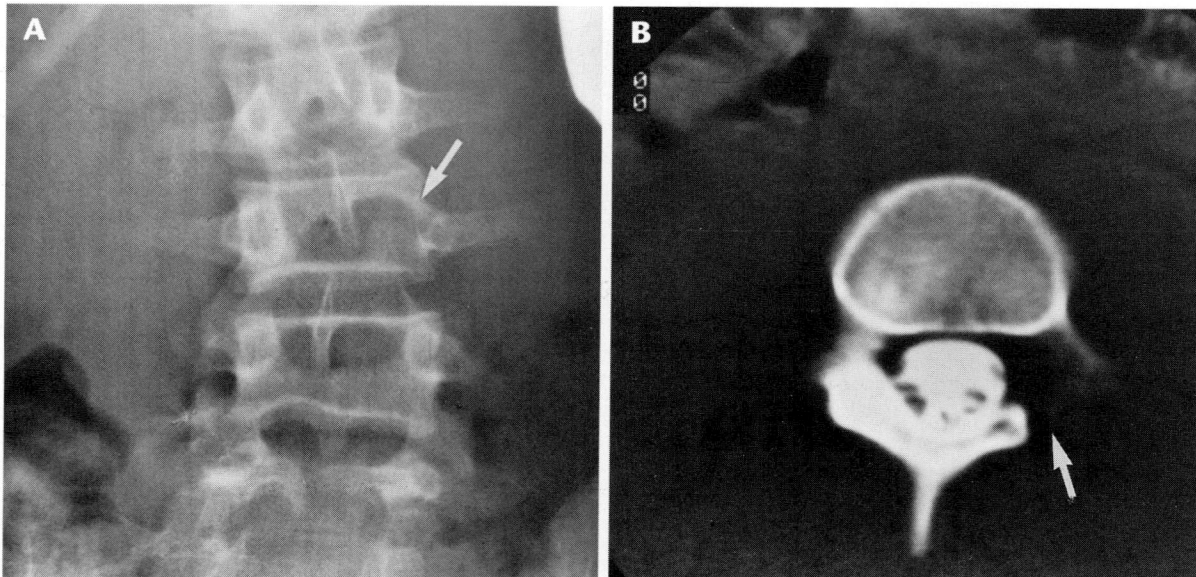

Figure 3–438. Congenital absence of the left pedicle of L3. **A,** Plain film. **B,** CT scan. (Ref: Wortzman G, Steinhardt MI: Congenitally absent lumbar pedicle: a reappraisal. *Radiology* 152:713, 1984.)

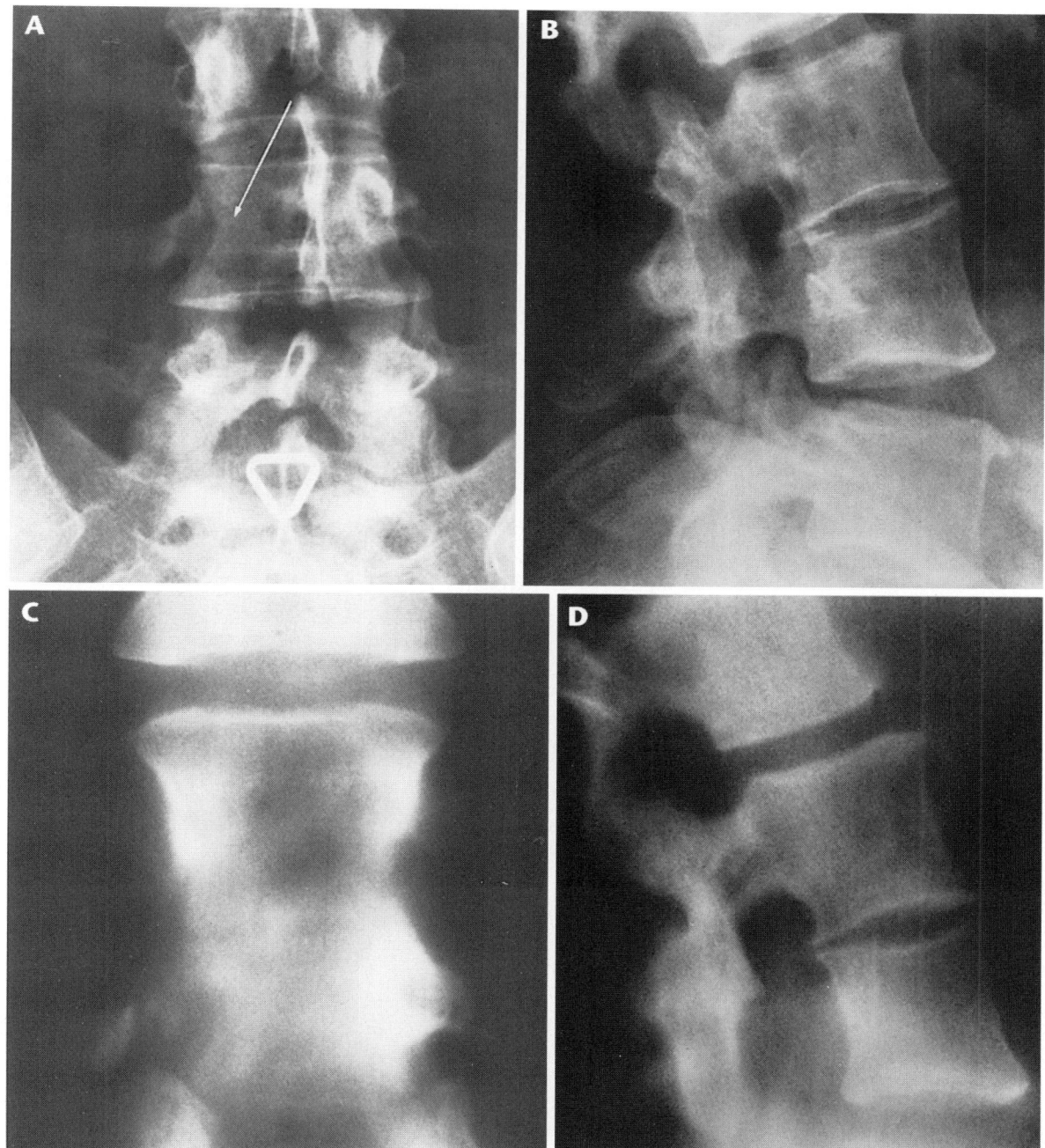

Figure 3–439. Congenital absence of the pedicle on the right side of L4 with incomplete segmentation of L3 and L4. **A** and **B,** Plain films. **C** and **D,** Tomograms. Note the huge intervertebral foramen in **D.** (Ref: MacLeod S, Hendry GMA: Congenital absence of a lumbar pedicle. *Pediatr Radiol* 12:207, 1982.)

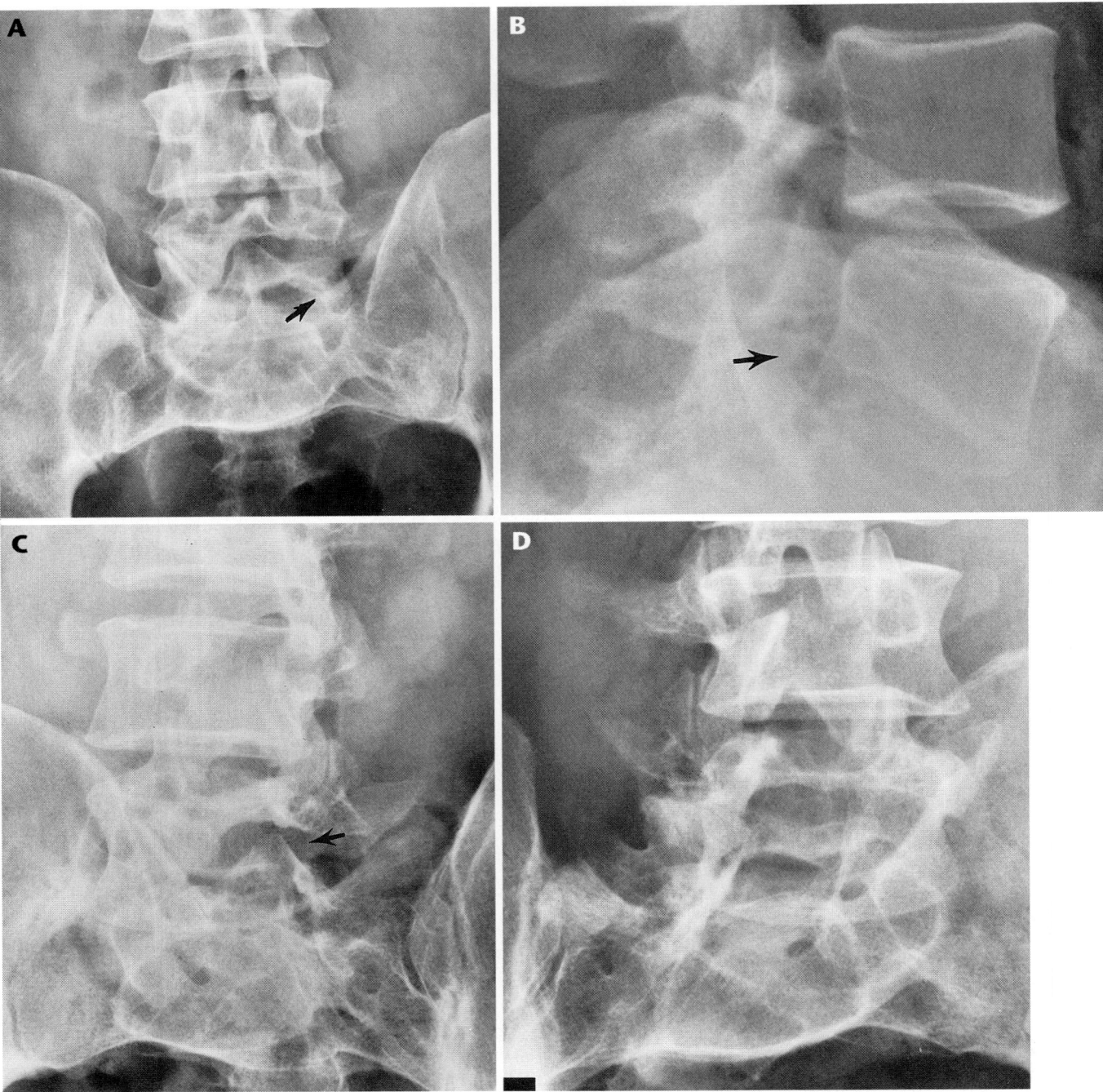

Figure 3–440. Absence of the lamina of L5 on the left. **A,** Anteroposterior. **B,** Lateral. **C,** Right posterior oblique. **D,** Left posterior oblique.

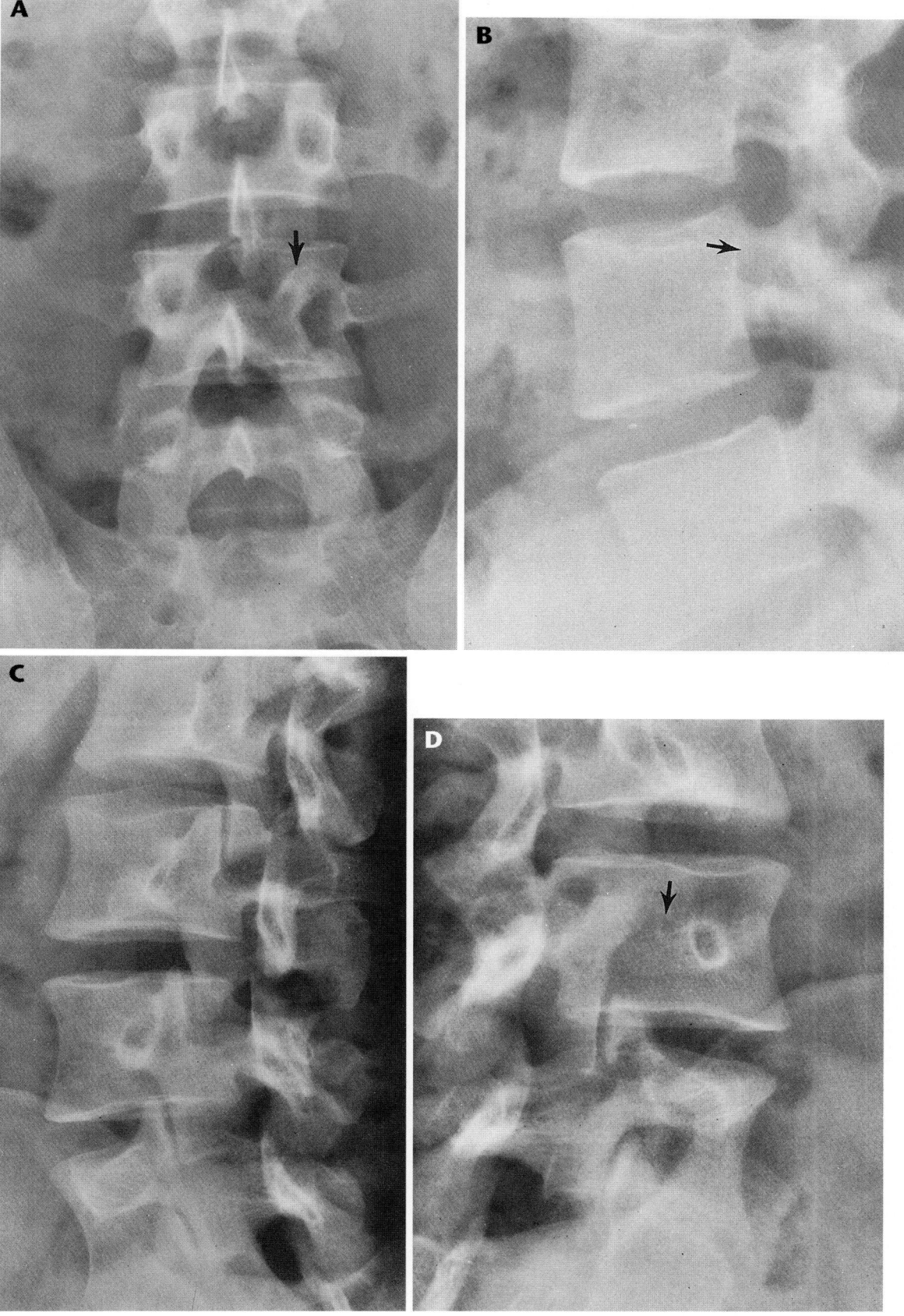

Figure 3–441. Absence of the lamina on the left of L4. Note that the pedicle on the right is enlarged. **A,** Anteroposterior. **B,** Lateral. **C,** Right posterior oblique. **D,** Left posterior oblique.

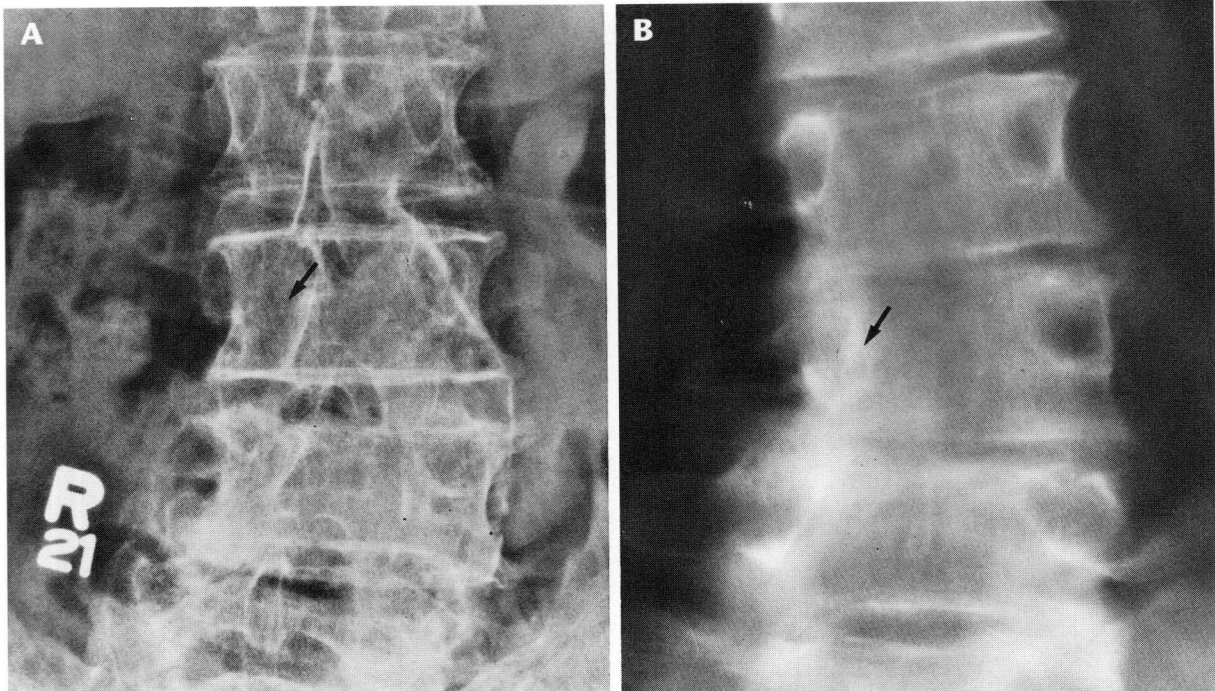

Figure 3–442. A, Simulated destruction of the pedicle on the right side of L4, produced by scoliosis. **B,** Tomogram shows pedicle to be intact.

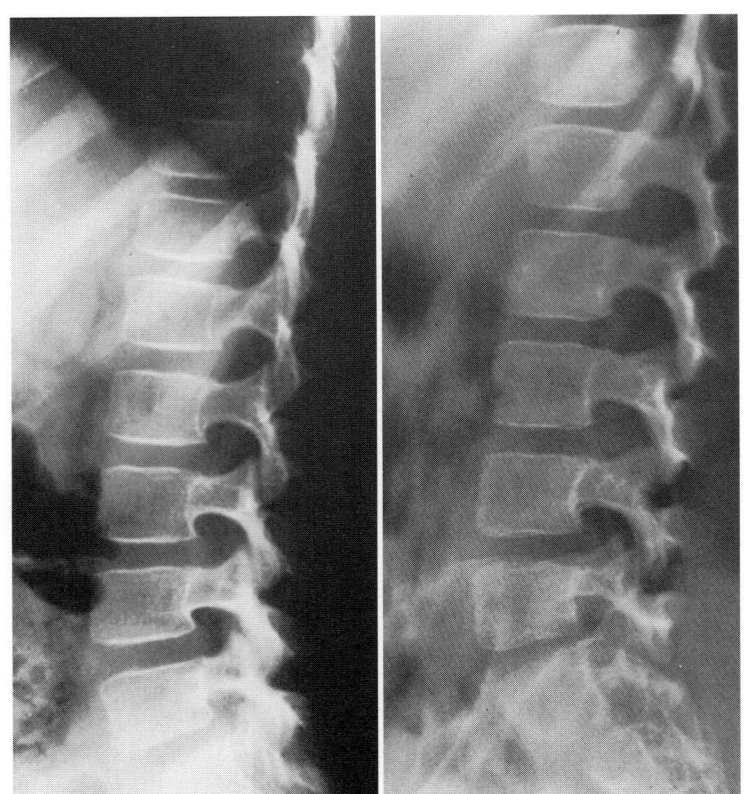

Figure 3–443. Scalloping of the posterior aspects of the vertebral bodies may be seen as a normal variant, particularly in childhood. *Left,* 6-year-old. *Right,* 10-year-old.

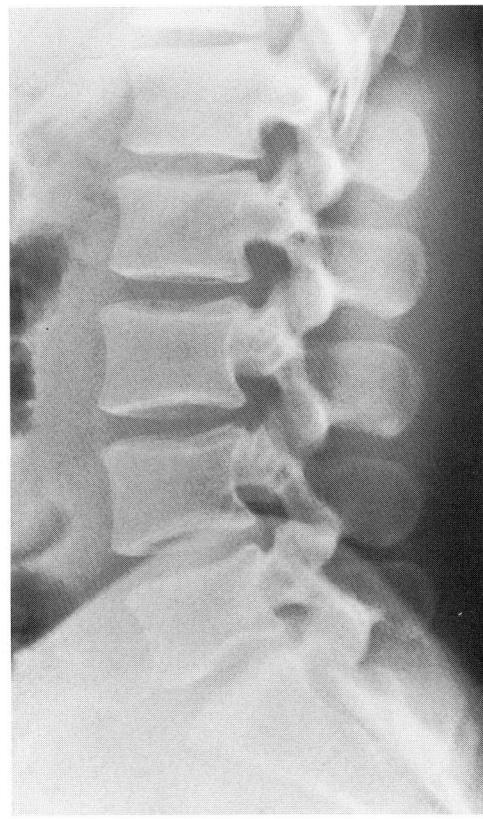

Figure 3–444. Scalloping of the posterior aspects of the vertebral bodies in an asymptomatic 21-year-old man. This variation may also be seen in patients with spinal stenosis.

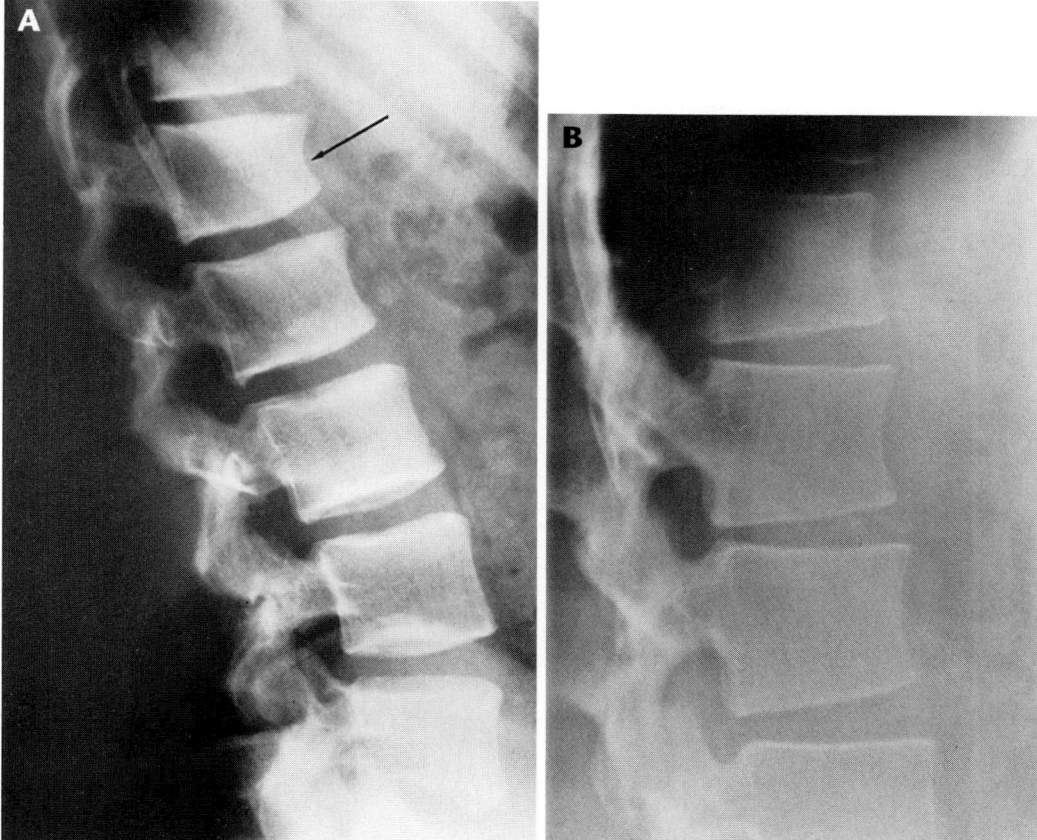

Figure 3–445. A, The bodies of T12 and L1 are often slightly wedge-shaped.
B, Another example of normal wedging of the bodies of T12, L1, and L2.

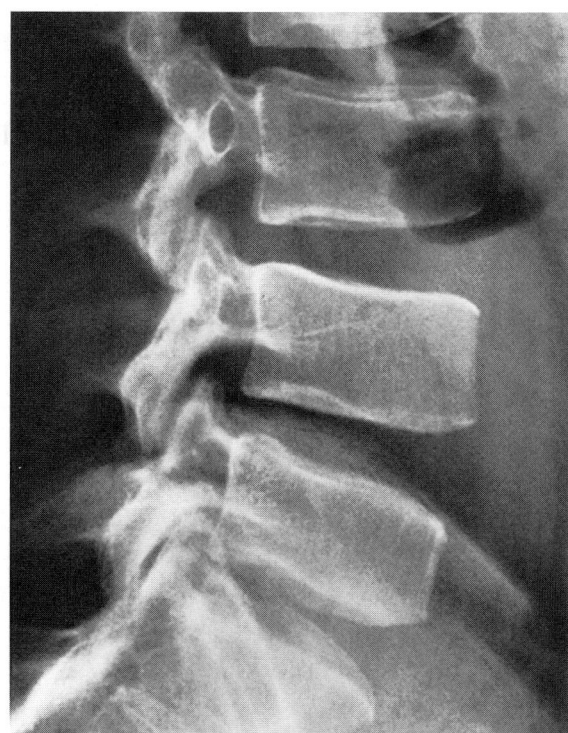

Figure 3–446. Long lumbar vertebrae.

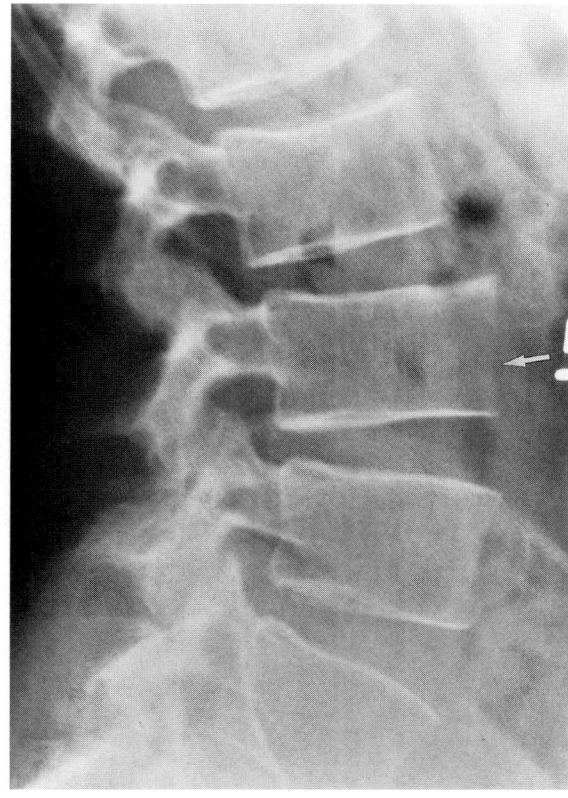

Figure 3–447. Oversized lumbar vertebra.

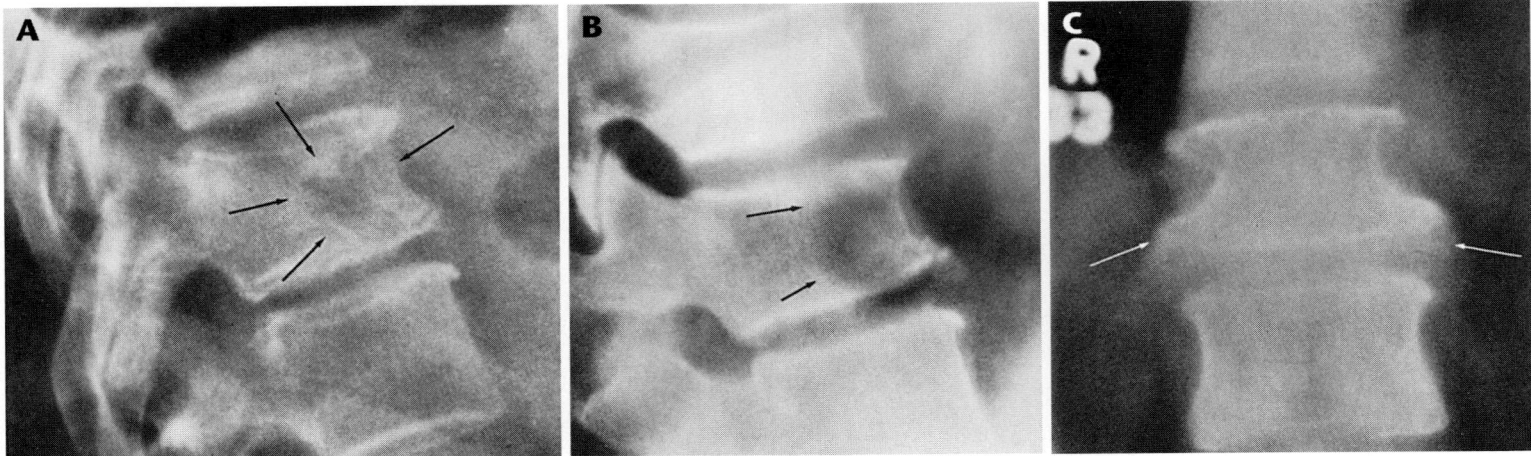

Figure 3–448. Spurred osteoporotic vertebra may produce an appearance suggesting pathologic destruction. **A,** Plain film. **B** and **C,** Tomograms. (Ref: Wagner A: "Spurious" defect of the lumbar vertebral body. *Am J Roentgenol* 135:1095, 1980.)

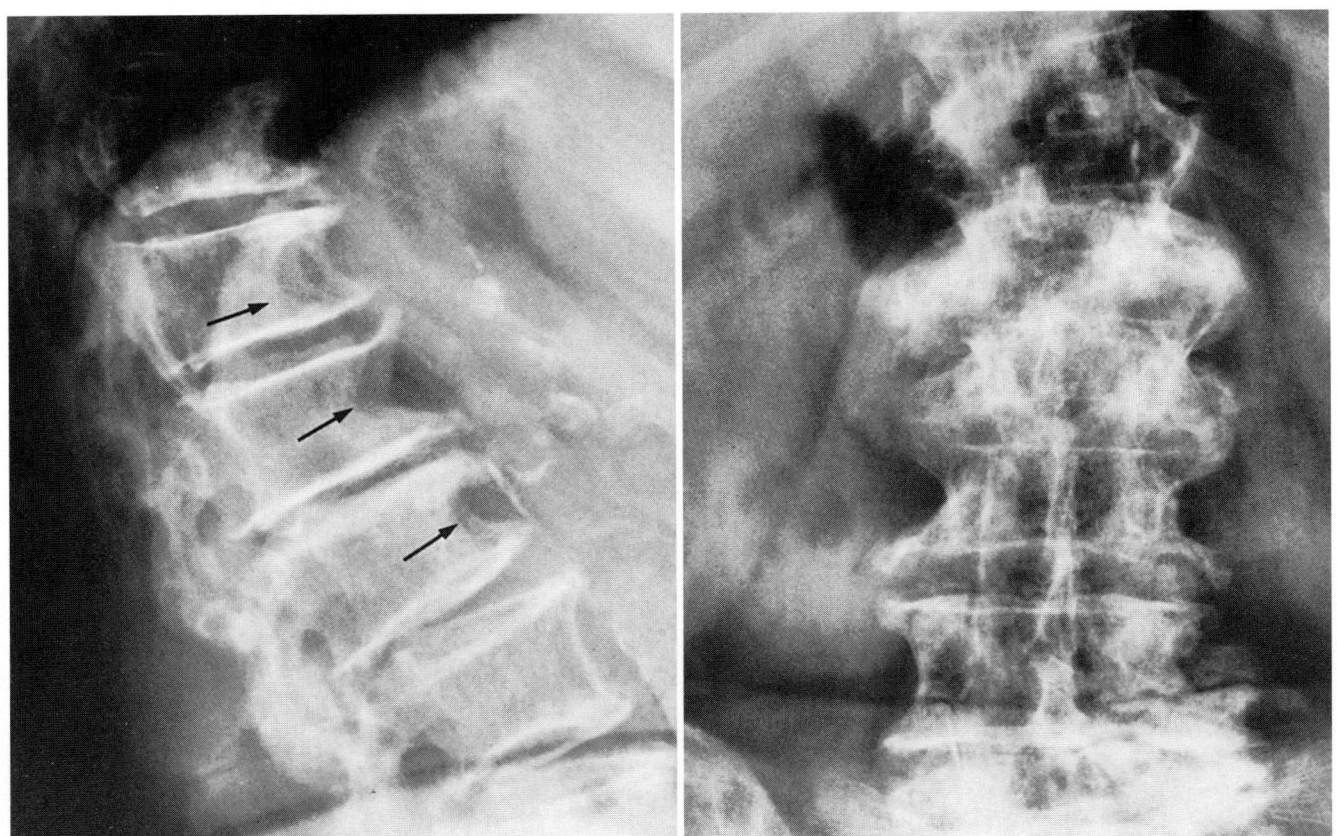

Figure 3–449. Multiple spurious defects of the lumbar spine in an 83-year-old woman.

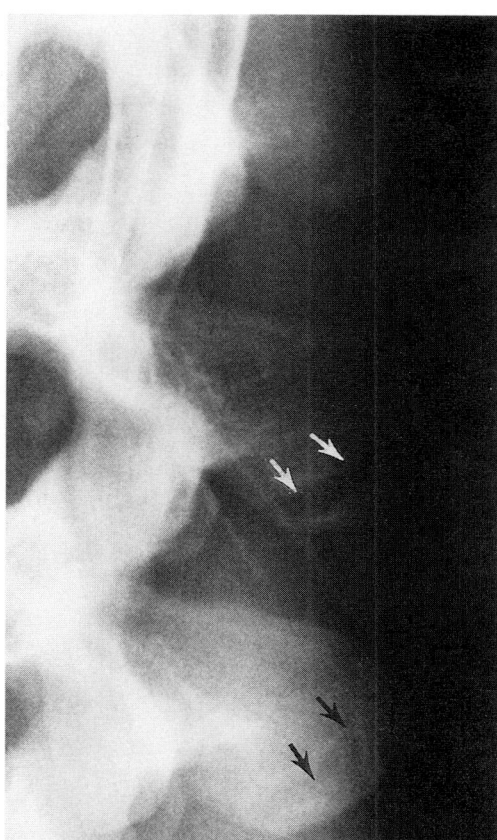

Figure 3–450. The closing apophyses of the spinous processes of the lumbar spine in a 22-year-old man.

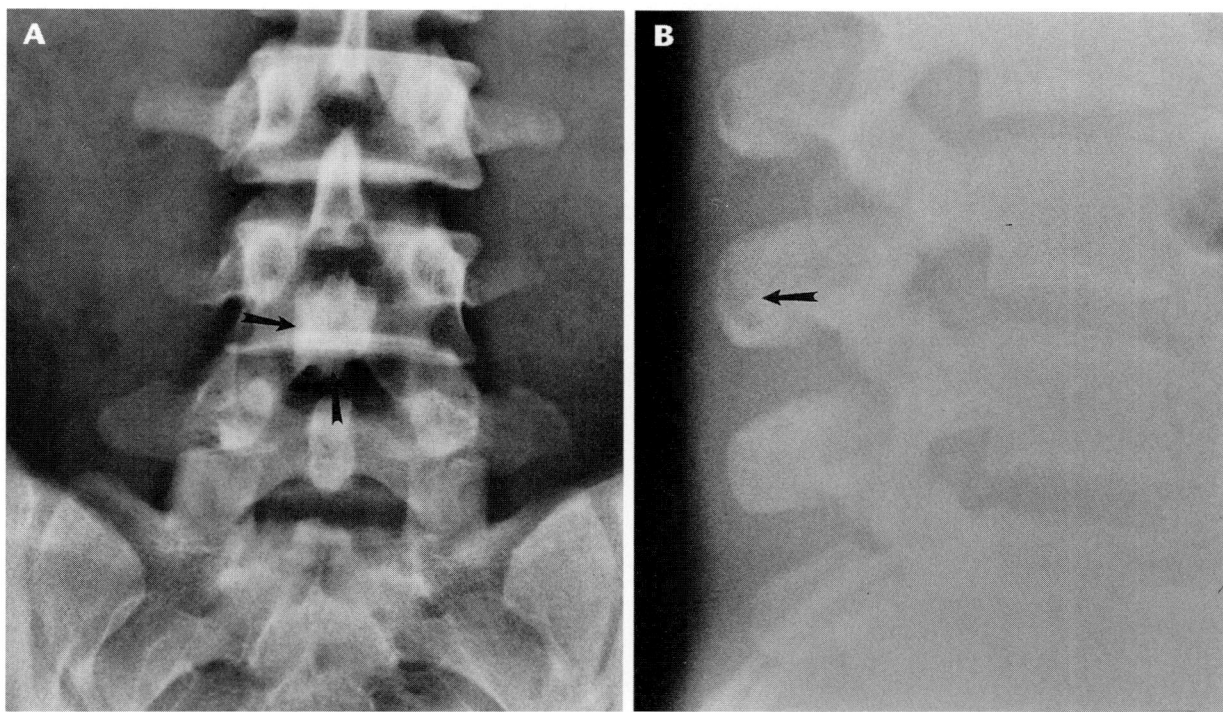

Figure 3–451. Sclerosis of the spinous process of L4, as an incidental finding. **A,** Anteroposterior projection. **B,** Lateral projection.

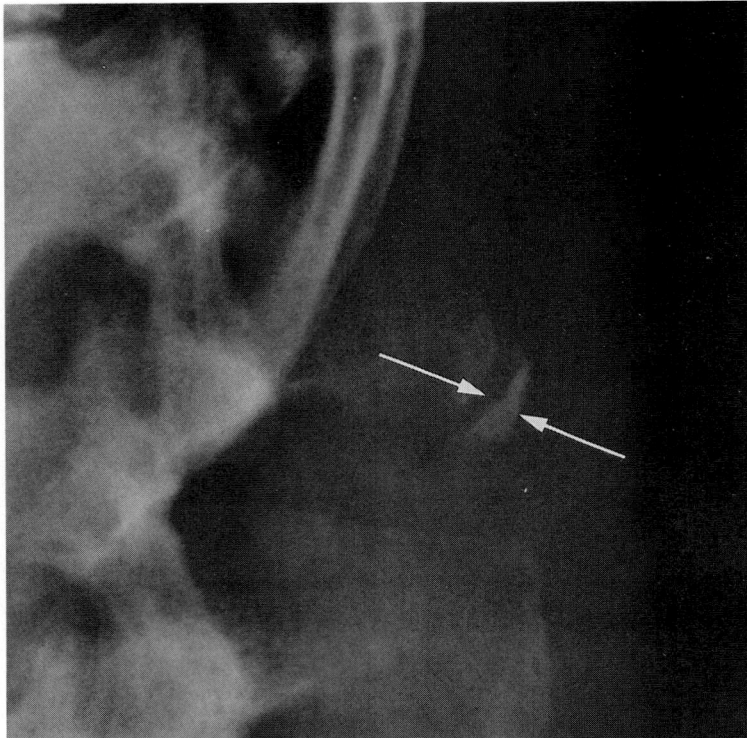

Figure 3–452. Ununited apophysis of the spinous process of L1.

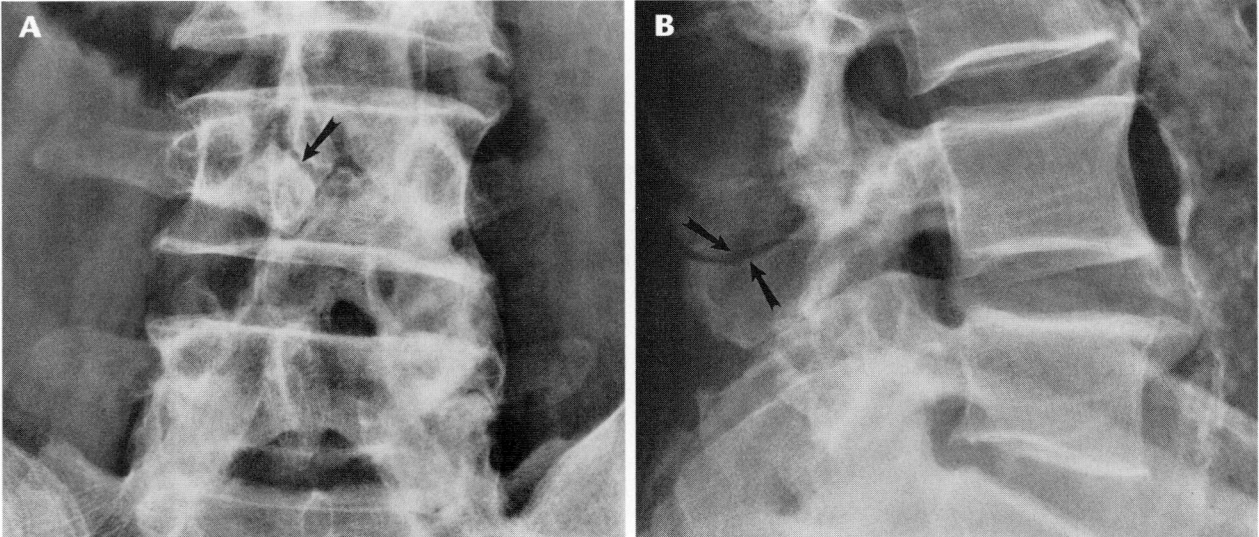

Figure 3–453. A, B, Bifid spinous process of L4.

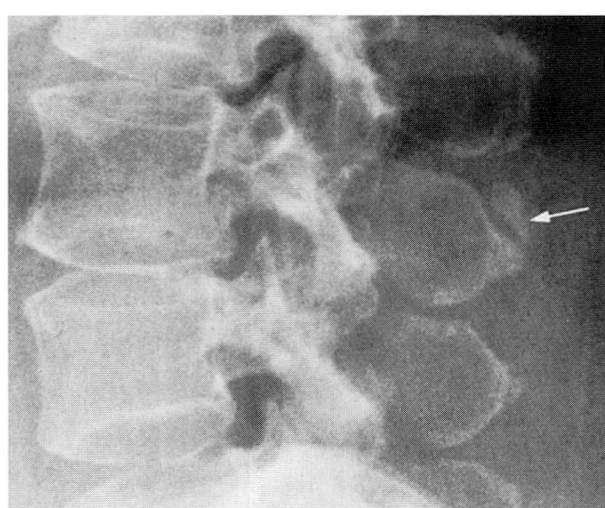

Figure 3–454. Calcification of the interspinous ligament in an 81-year-old man. These calcifications are an aging phenomenon and should not be mistaken for an avulsion fracture. (Ref: Scapinelli R: Localized ossifications in the supraspinous and interspinous ligaments in adult man. *Rays (Rome)* 13:29, 1988.)

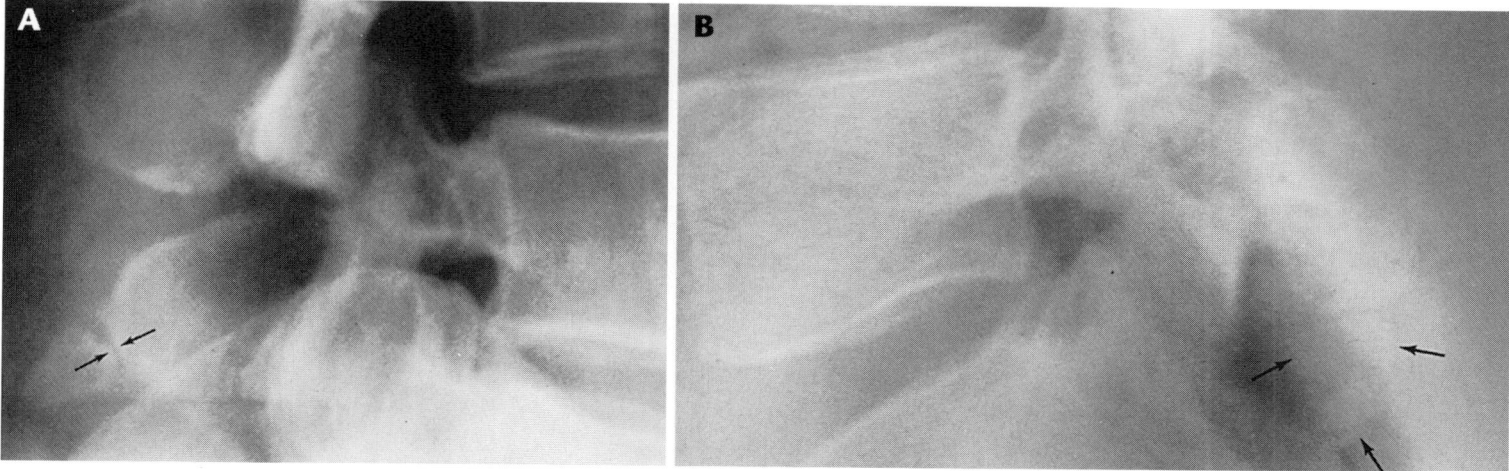

Figure 3–455. A, B, Two examples of failure of union of the ossification centers of the tip of the L5 spinous process.

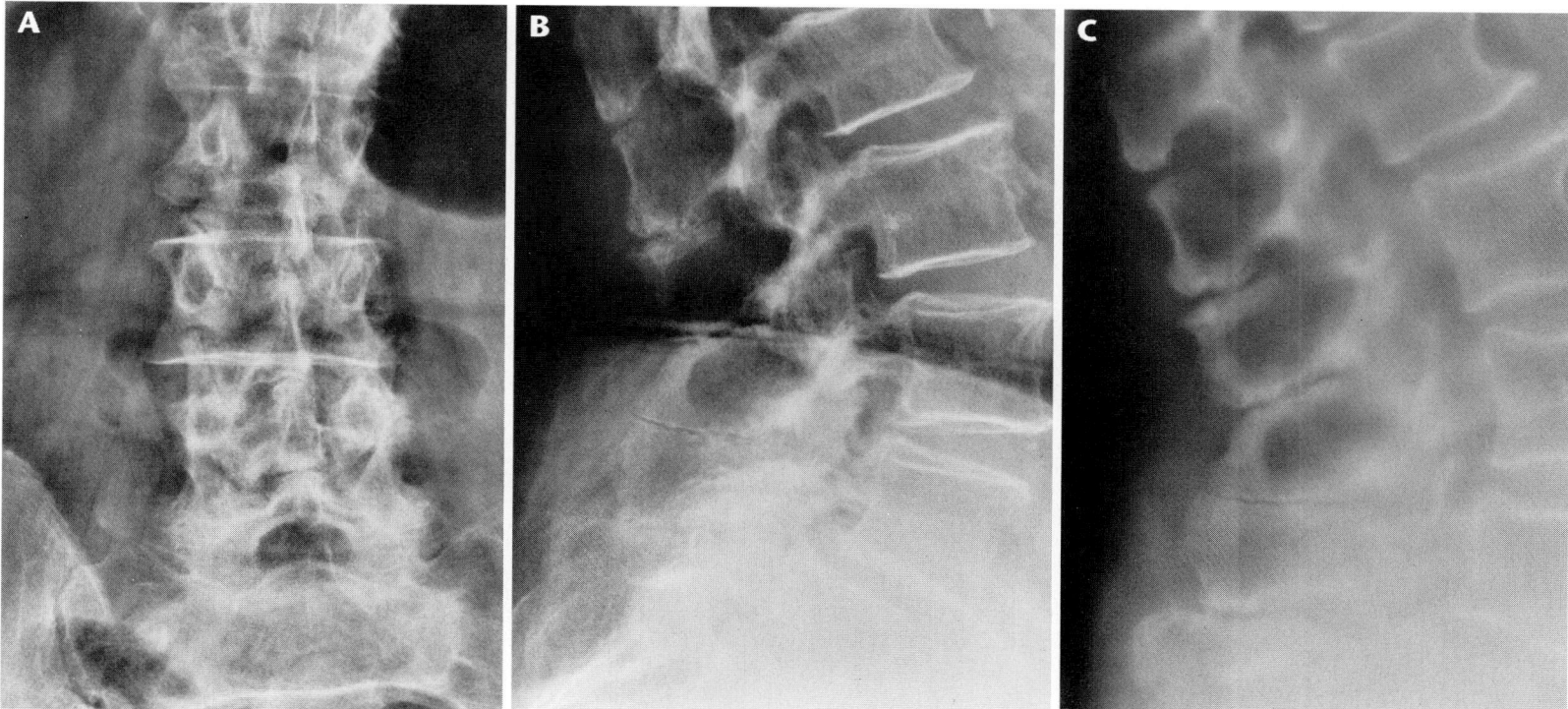

Figure 3–456. Degenerative changes in the lumbar spinous processes with aging. With marked lordosis and loss of height of the intervertebral discs, the spinous processes come into articulation and eventually develop hypertrophic degenerative changes in these pseudarthroses. This has been termed *kissing spinous processes* or Baastrup's disease and may be symptomatic. **A,** Anteroposterior view shows enlargement of the spinous processes, particularly at L4. **B,** The posterior articulation and the enlarged spinous processes produce an unusual appearance that might be mistaken for bone destruction. **C,** Tomogram shows the sclerosis of the margins of the spinous processes and the relative radiolucency of the nonarticulating portions. (Ref: Jacobson HG et al: The "swayback" syndrome. *Am J Roentgenol* 79:672, 1958.)

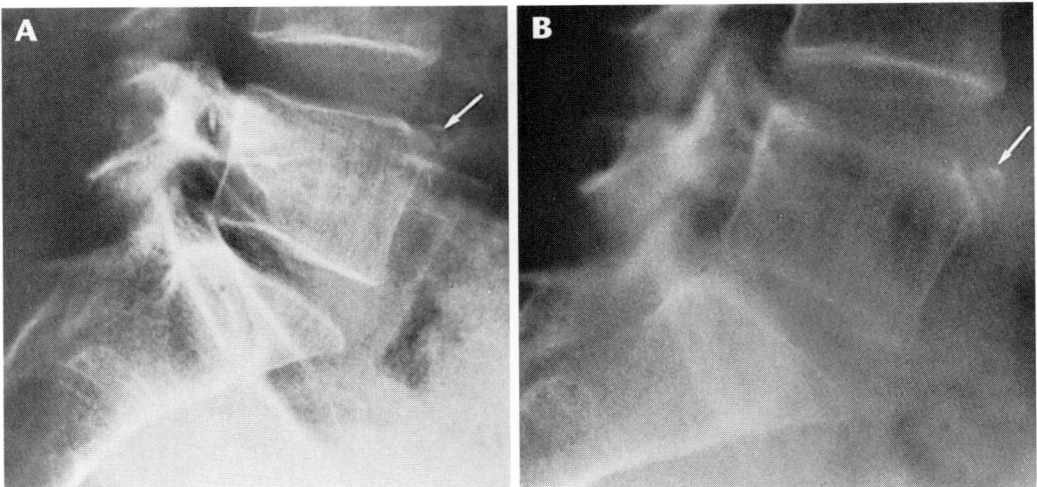

Figure 3–457. Ununited secondary ossification center (limbus vertebra), simulating a fracture of L5. **A,** Plain film. **B,** Laminagram. There is evidence to suggest that limbus vertebrae are the result of intravertebral disc herniation. (Refs: Kozlowski K: Anterior intravertebral disc herniations in children: Unrecognized chronic trauma to the spine. *Australas Radiol* 23:67, 1979; Henales V et al: Intervertebral disc herniations [limbus vertebrae] in pediatric patients: Report of 15 cases. *Pediatr Radiol* 23:608, 1993.)

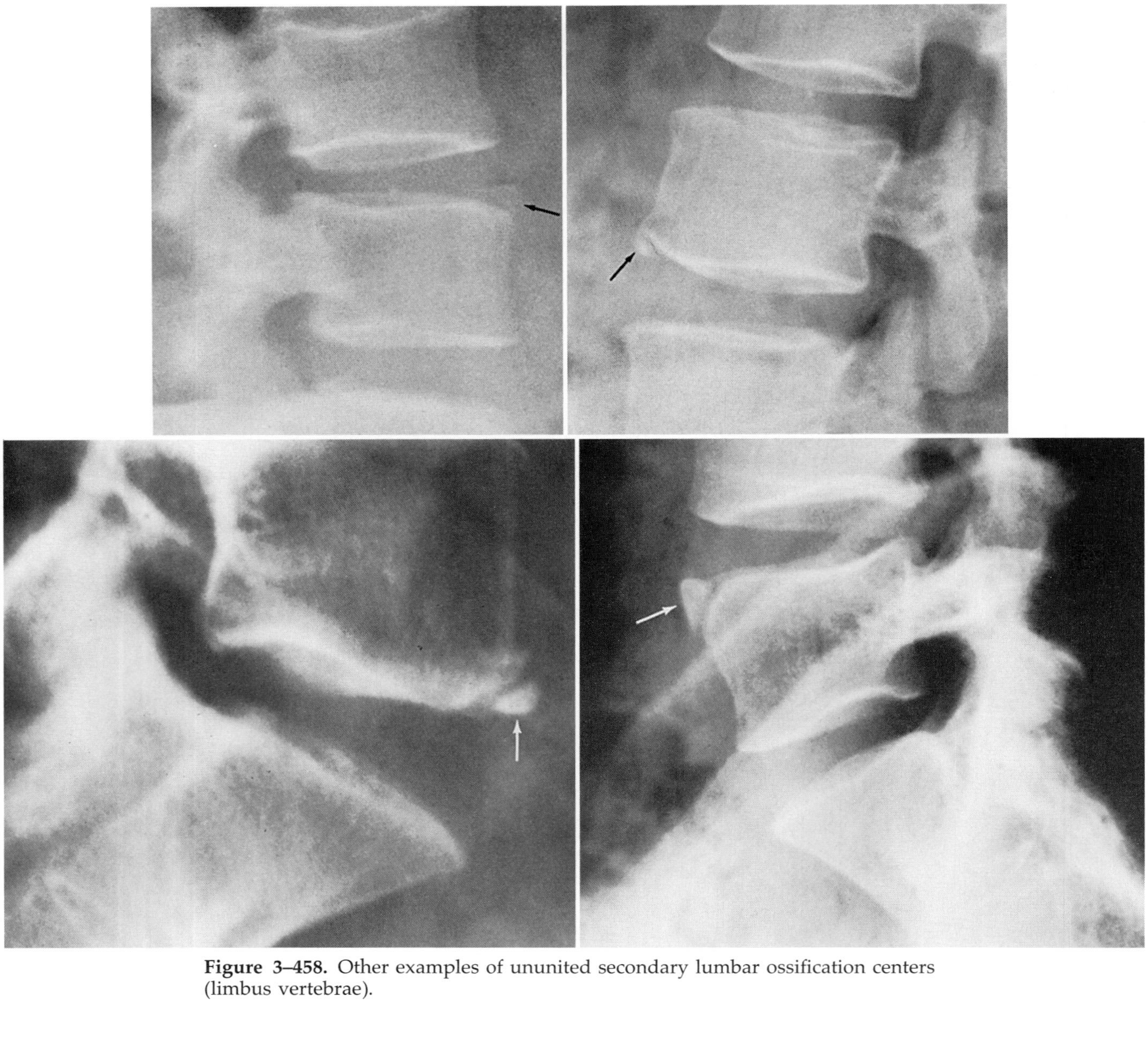

Figure 3–458. Other examples of ununited secondary lumbar ossification centers (limbus vertebrae).

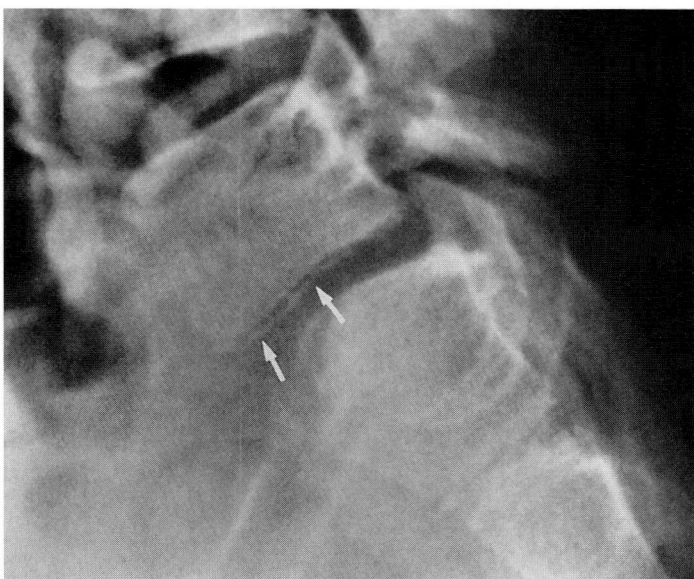

Figure 3–459. The ring apophysis of L5 seen in its entirety in an 8-year-old girl.

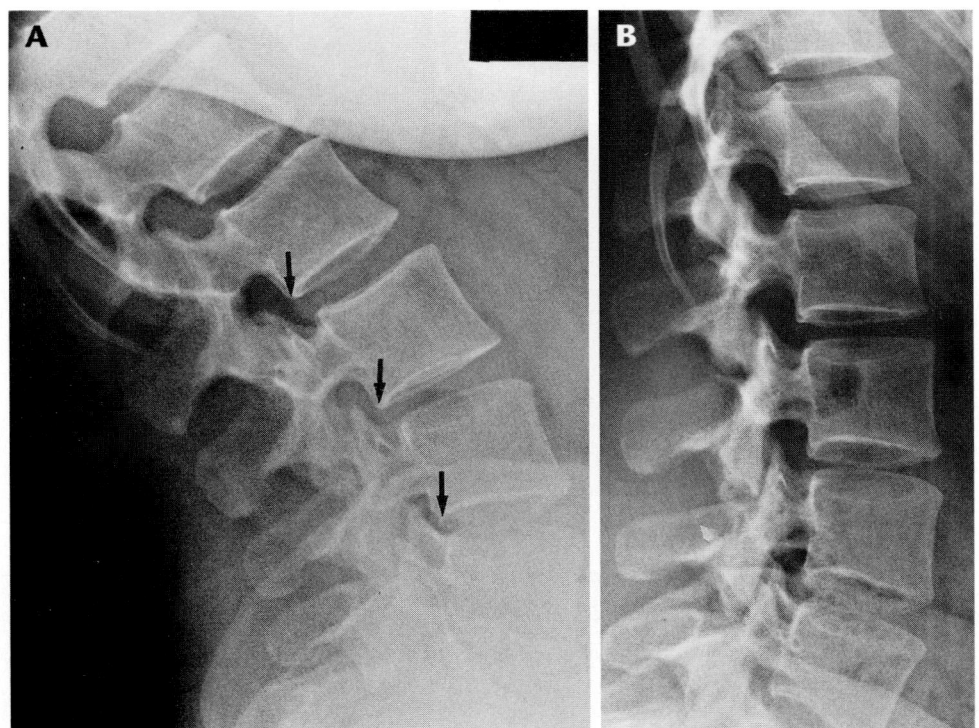

Figure 3–460. A, Normal posterior "stepping" of lumbar vertebrae on extension. **B,** Normal alignment in neutral position.

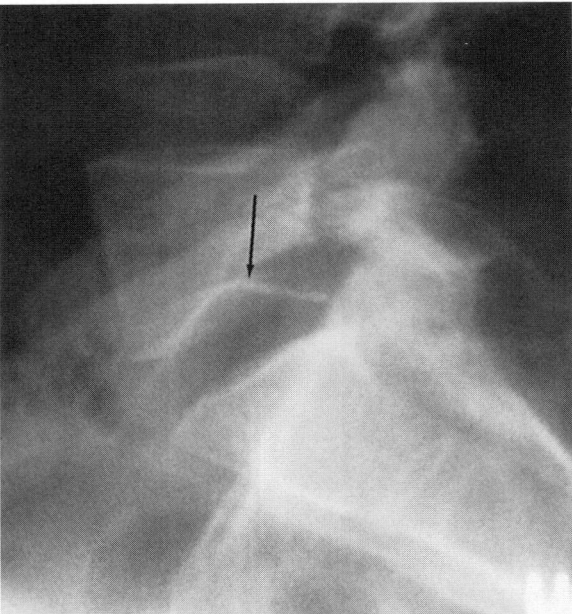

Figure 3–461. Wedge shape of L5 and bowing of the inferior end plates are normal variations and not reflections of pathology. (Ref: Dietz GW, Christensen EE: Normal "cupid's bow" contour of the lower lumbar vertebrae. *Radiology* 121:577, 1976.)

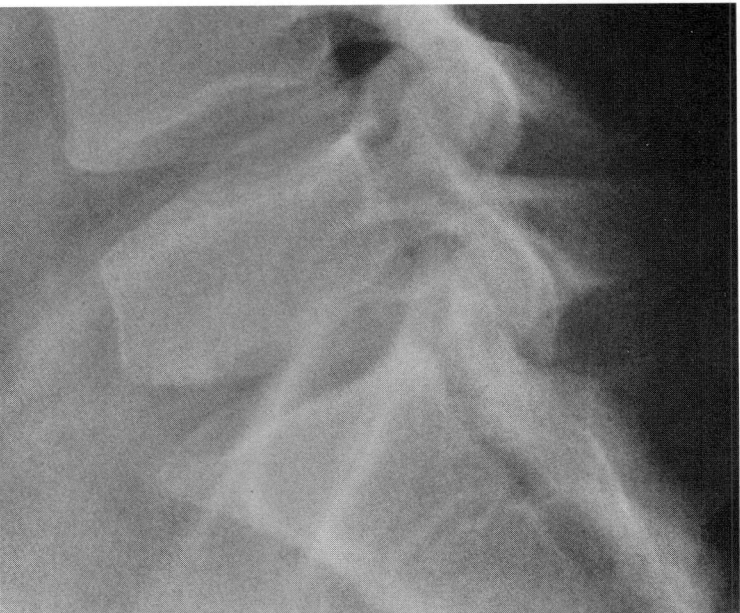

Figure 3–462. Wedged configuration of L5 with no history of prior trauma and no evidence of fracture.

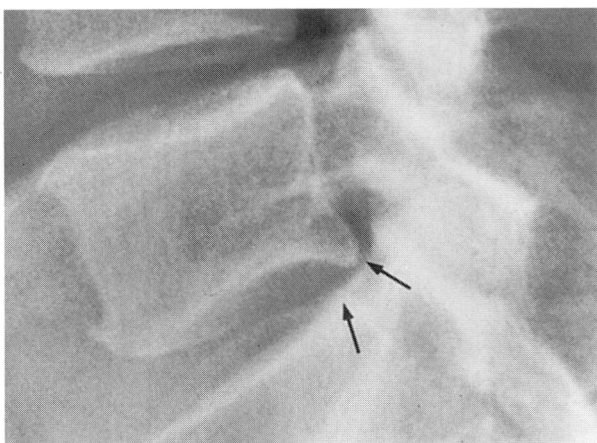

Figure 3–463. Apparent reverse spondylolisthesis of L5 on S1. The apparent displacement is usually due to errors in positioning. In some individuals, it results from the fact that the anteroposterior diameter of the superior surface of the sacrum is smaller than the inferior surface of the fifth lumbar vertebra. The anterior relationships are more reliable. (Ref: Melamed A, Ansfield DJ: Posterior displacement of lumbar vertebrae. *Am J Roentgenol* 58:307, 1947.)

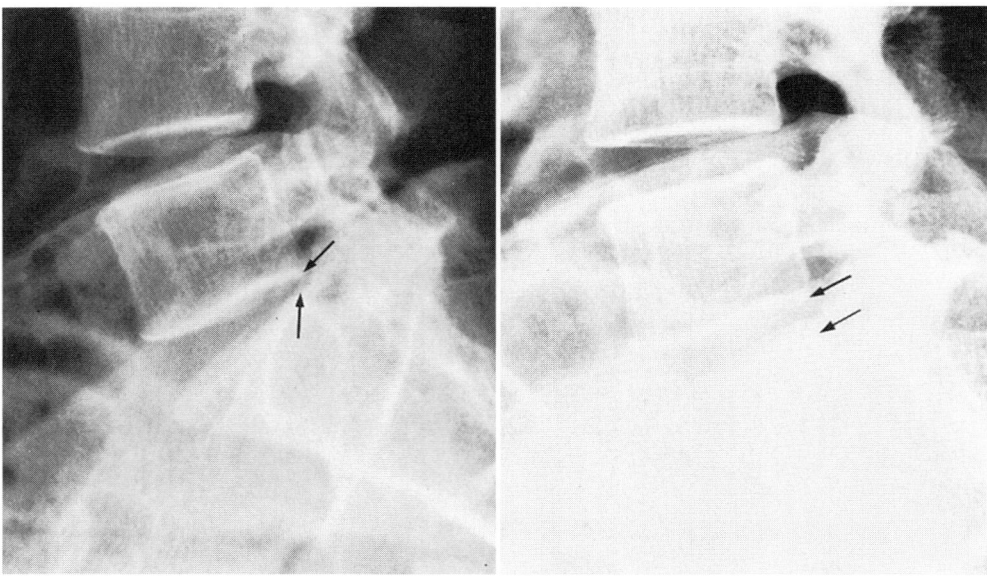

Figure 3–464. *Left,* Apparent retrospondylolisthesis of L5 on S1 as a result of rotation. *Right,* True lateral projection shows normal relationships.

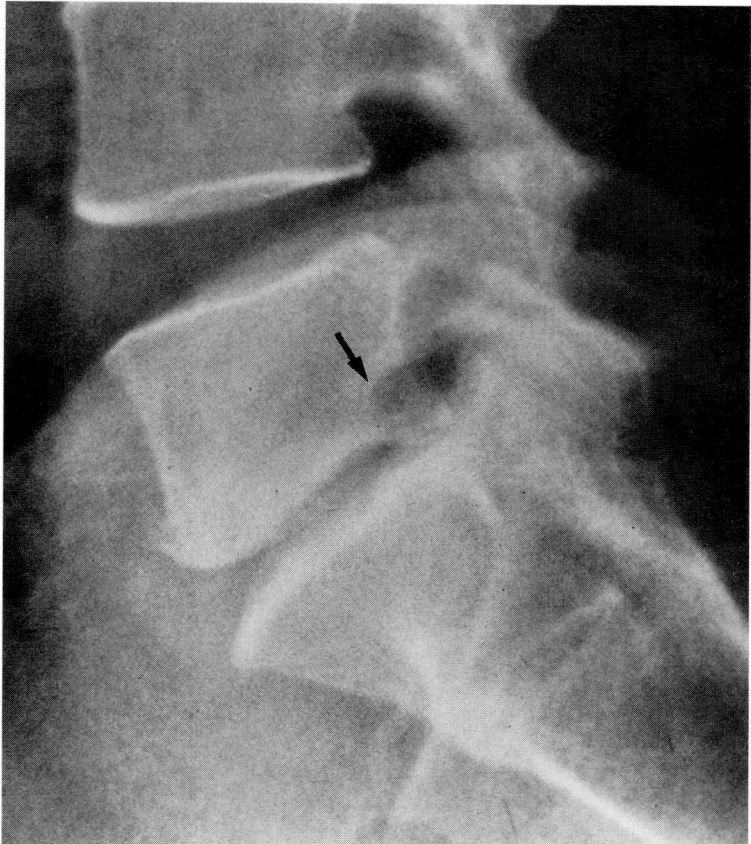

Figure 3–465. Simulated defect produced by the neural arch of L5. A CT scan showed a herniated nucleus but no defect in the vertebral body.

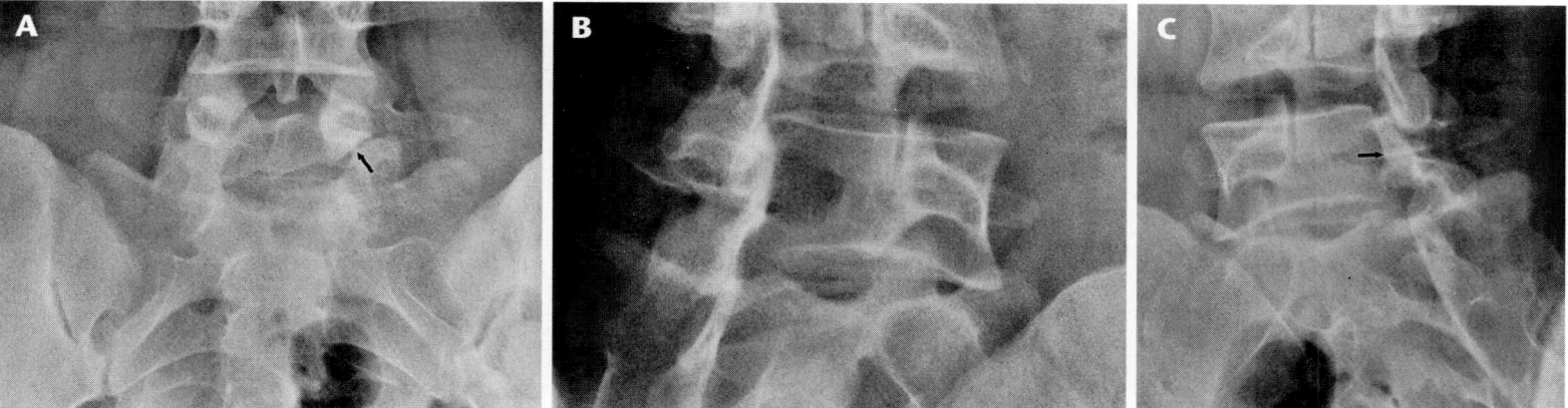

Figure 3–466. Simulated spondylolysis of L5 on the left by short inferior articulating process seen in **C**. **A,** Anteroposterior projection. **B,** Left oblique. **C,** Right oblique.

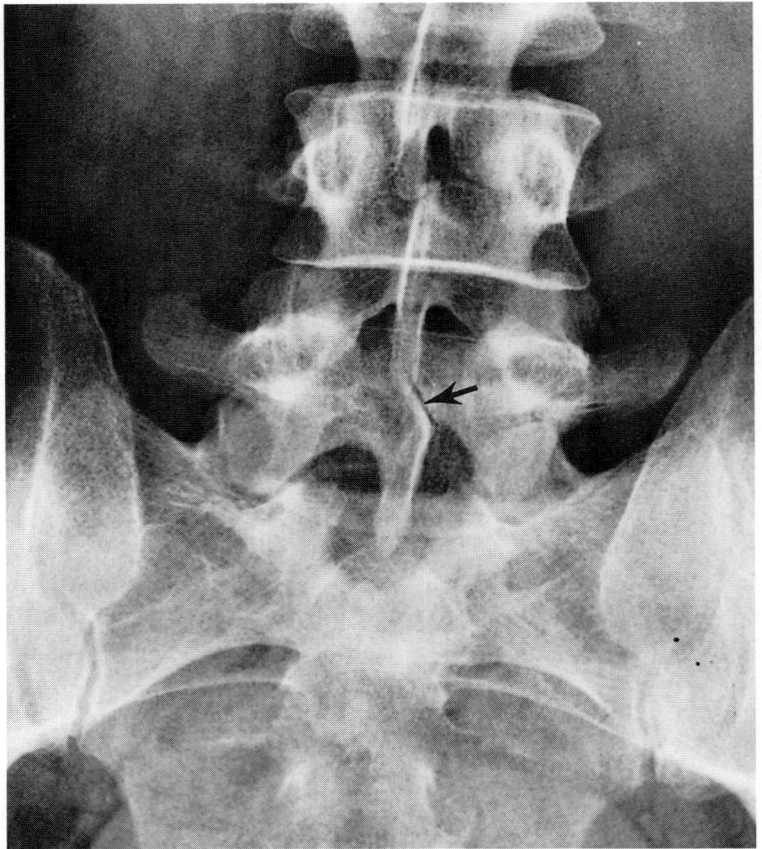

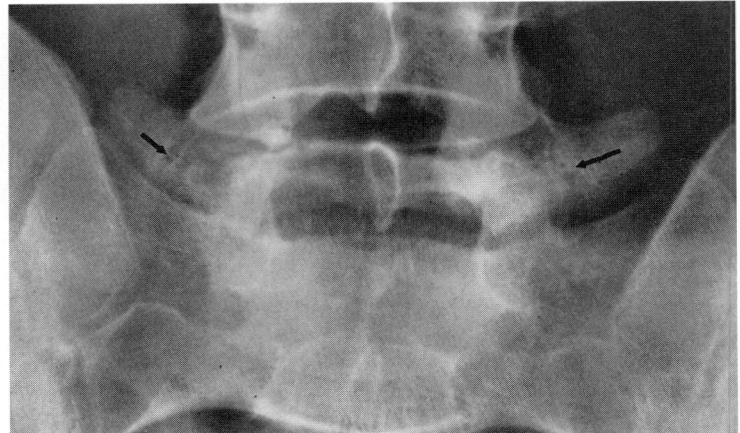

Figure 3–468. Anomalous ribs at L5.

Figure 3–467. Spina bifida occulta of L5, off center, which might be confused with a fracture.

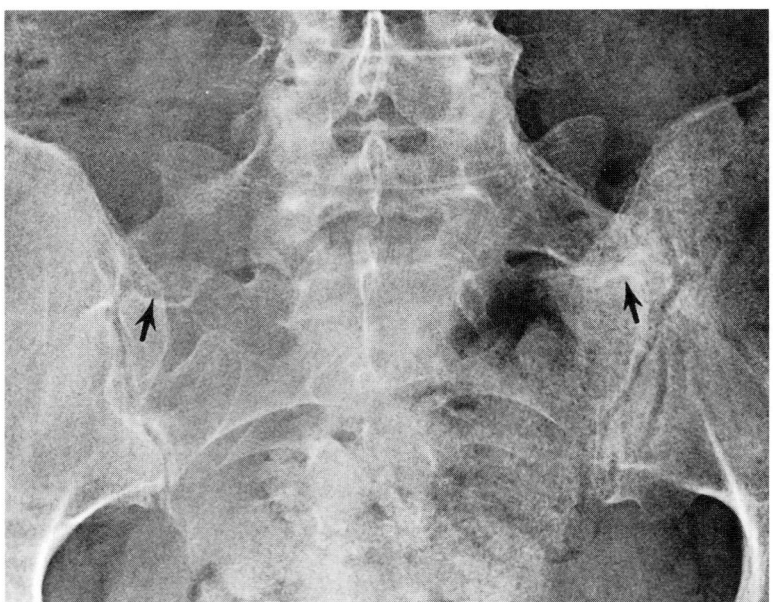

Figure 4–469. Bilateral sacralization of L5 with anomalous articulations with the sacrum.

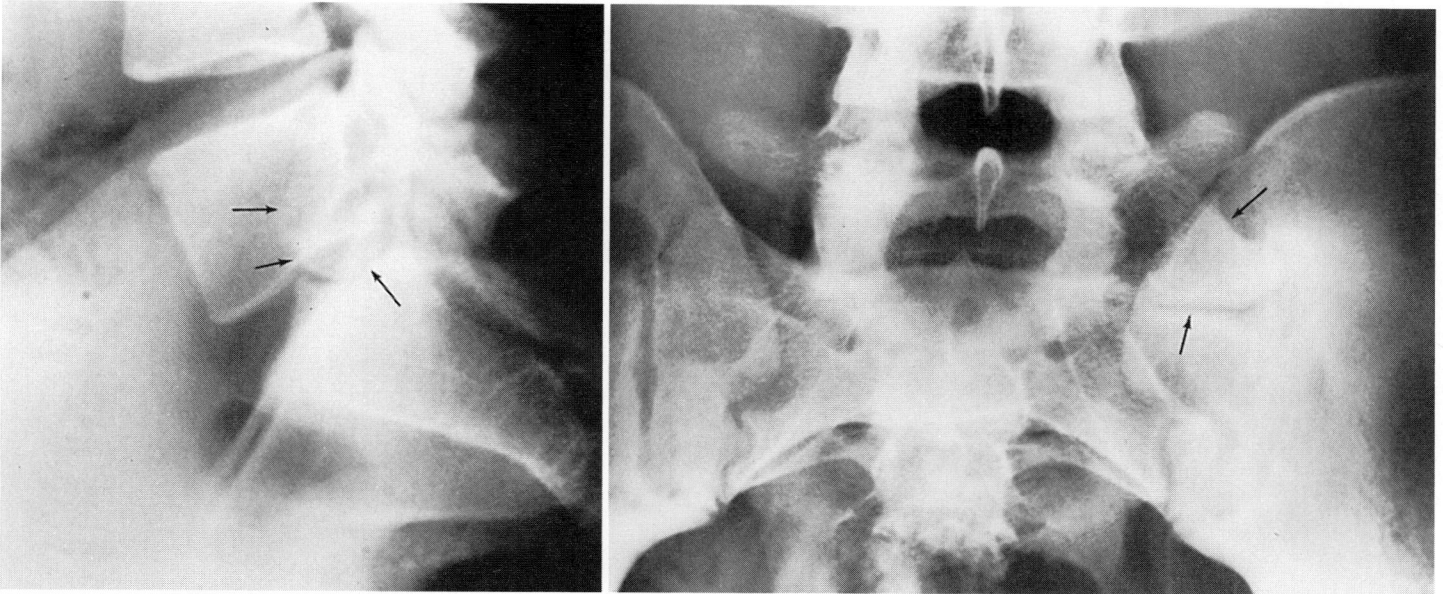

Figure 3–470. Unilateral sacralization of L5 on left side. Note the additional density created in the lateral projection. The anomalous articulation should not be mistaken for a fracture.

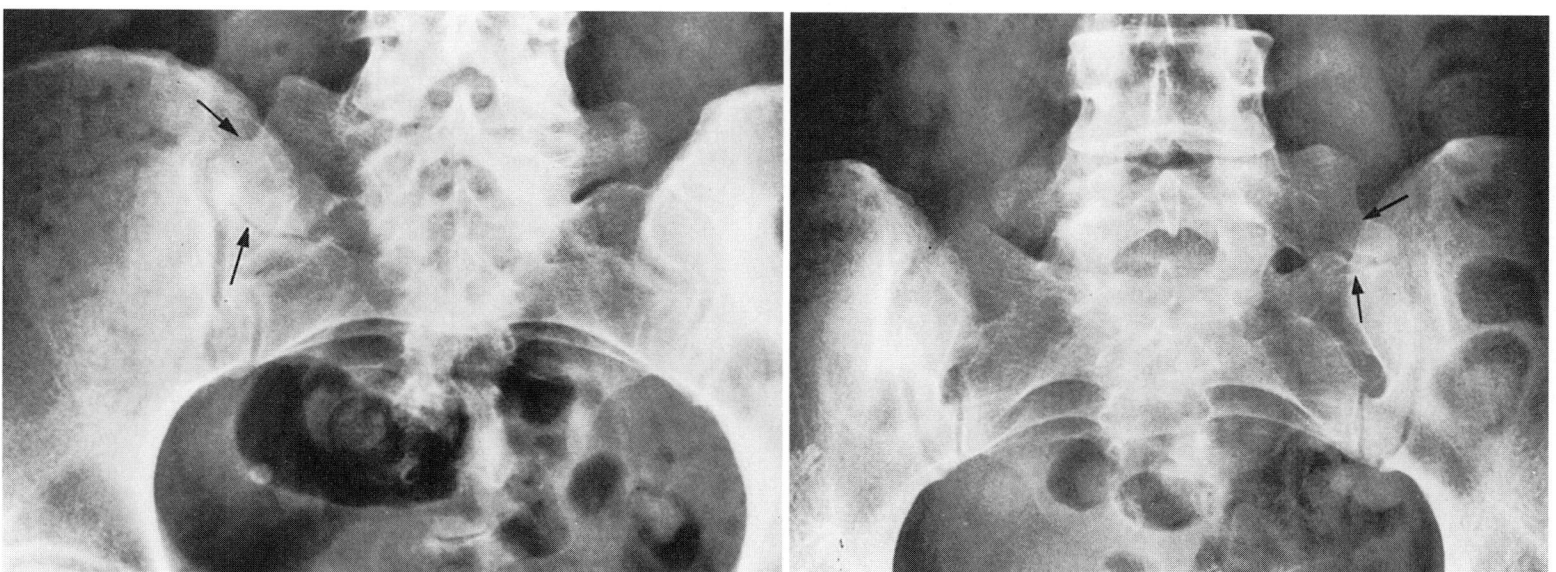

Figure 3–471. Two other examples of anomalous articulations between L5 and the sacrum. This anatomic arrangement is essentially unstable and may become symptomatic. (Ref: Jonsson B et al: Anomalous lumbosacral articulations and low-back pain, *Spine* 14:831, 1989.)

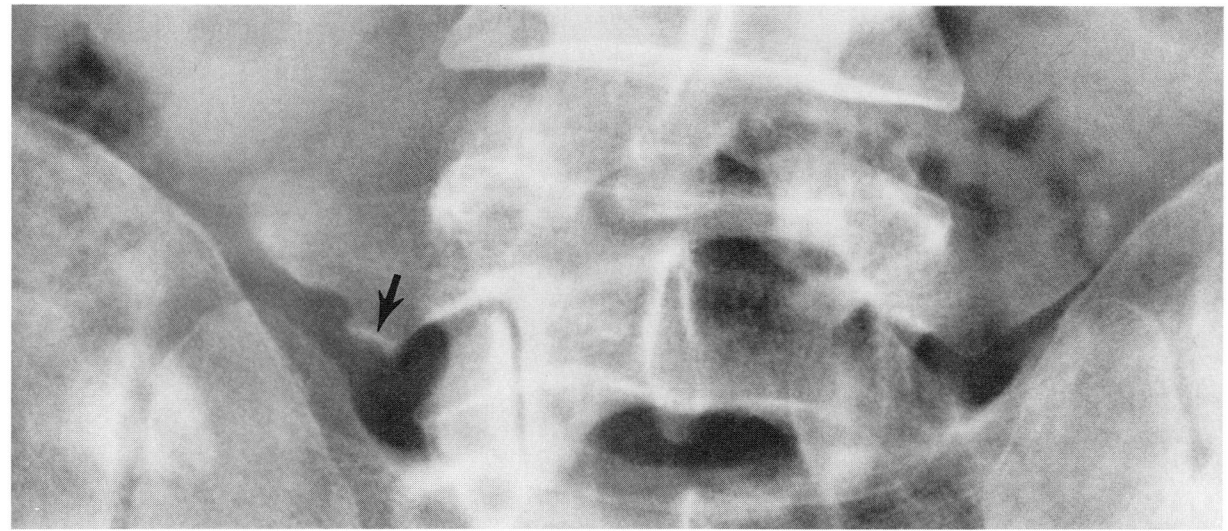

Figure 3–472. Partial formation of an anomalous articulation of L5 with the sacrum.

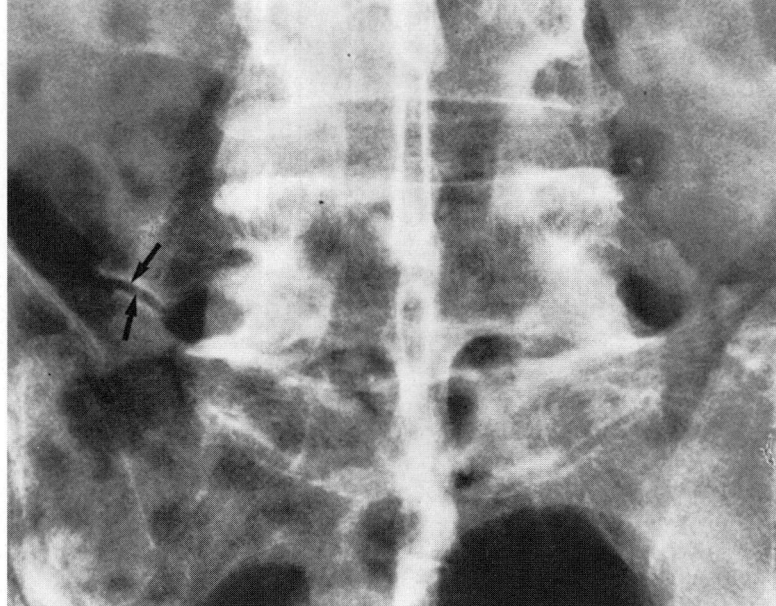

Figure 3–473. Anomalous articulation between the transverse process of L5 and the adjacent sacrum.

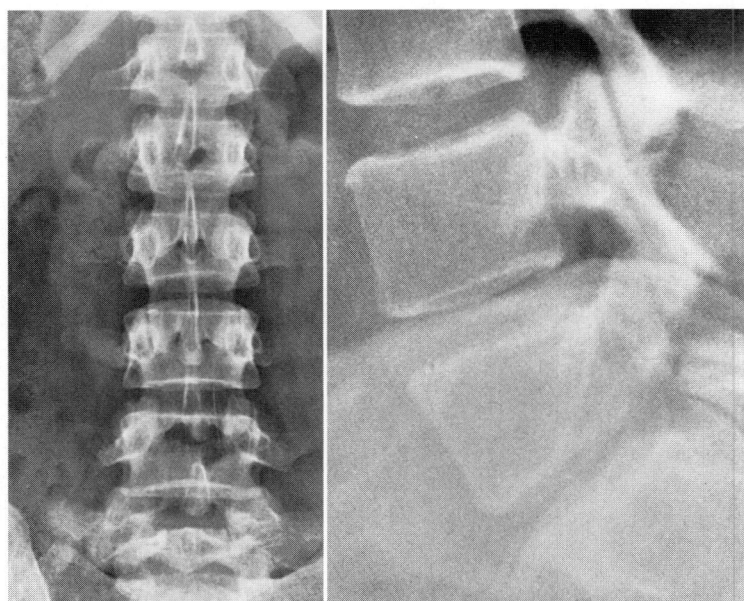

Figure 3–474. Patients with transitional vertebrae often have a significantly narrower lumbosacral disc than those with no transitional features. This narrowing does not imply disc degeneration. This finding is illustrated in this patient with six lumbar vertebrae. (Ref: Nicholson AA et al: The measured height of the lumbosacral disc in patients with and without transitional vertebrae. *Br J Radiol* 61:454, 1988.)

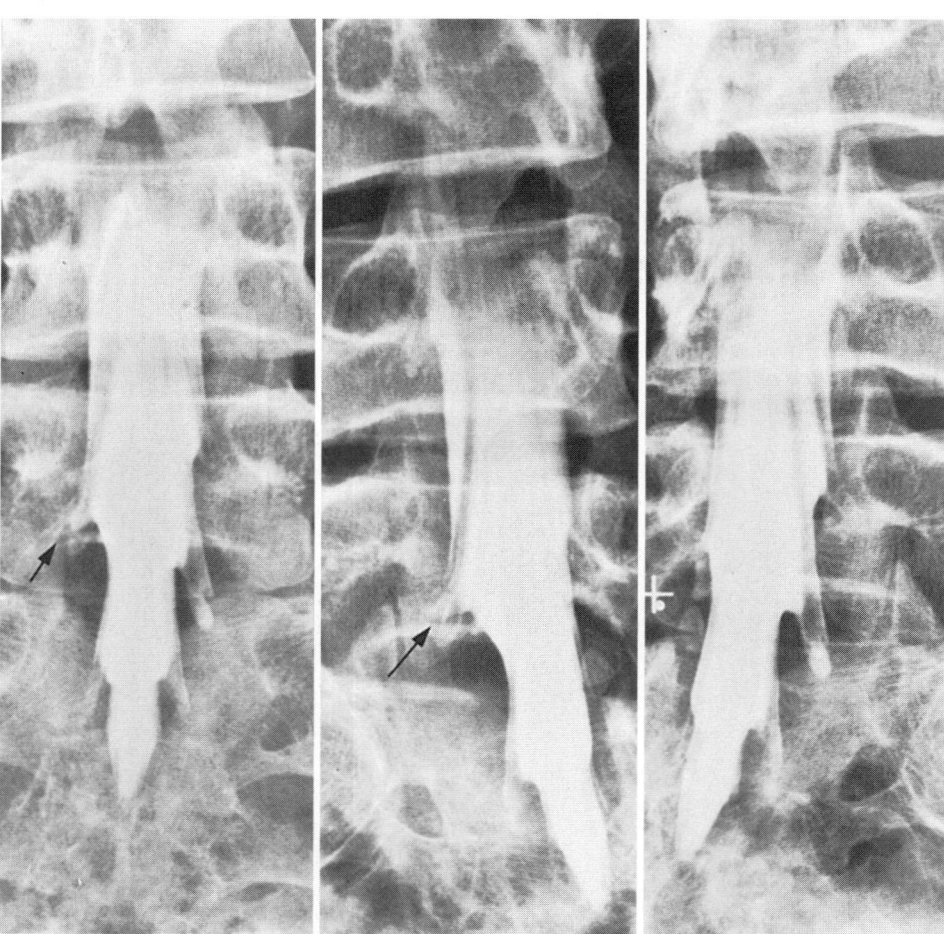

Figure 3–475. Conjoined lumbosacral nerve roots may be mistaken for the impressions of a disc herniation. Two root sleeves are demonstrated by metrizamide myelography. (Ref: Cail WS, Butler AB: Conjoined lumbosacral root sleeves. *Surg Neurol* 20:113, 1983.)

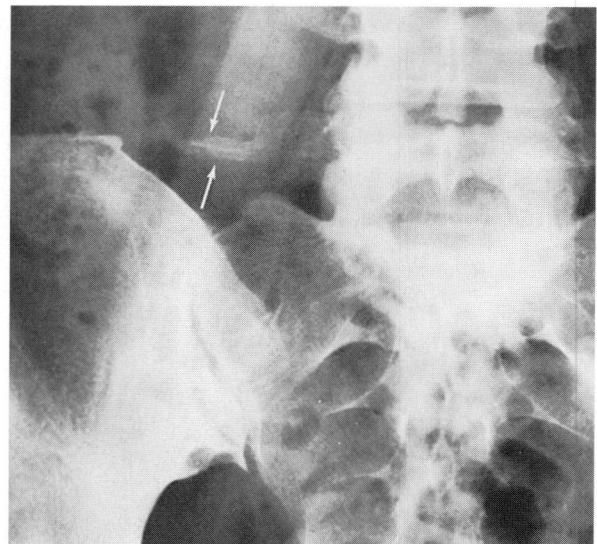

Figure 3–476. Calcification of the iliolumbar ligament.

The Sacrum

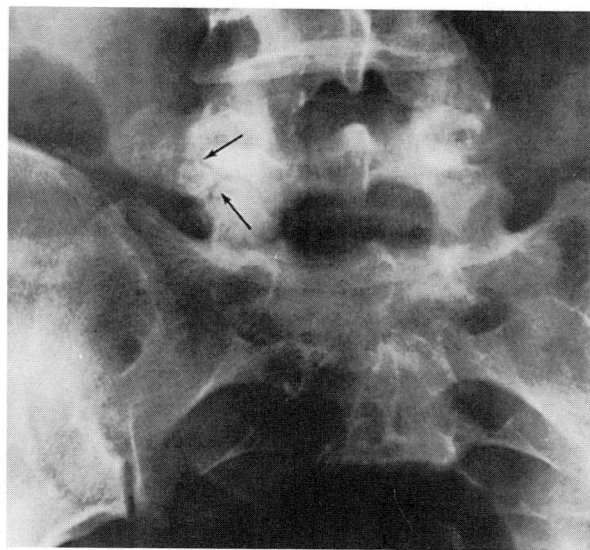

Figure 3–477. An ununited ossification center for the superior articulating facet of S1.

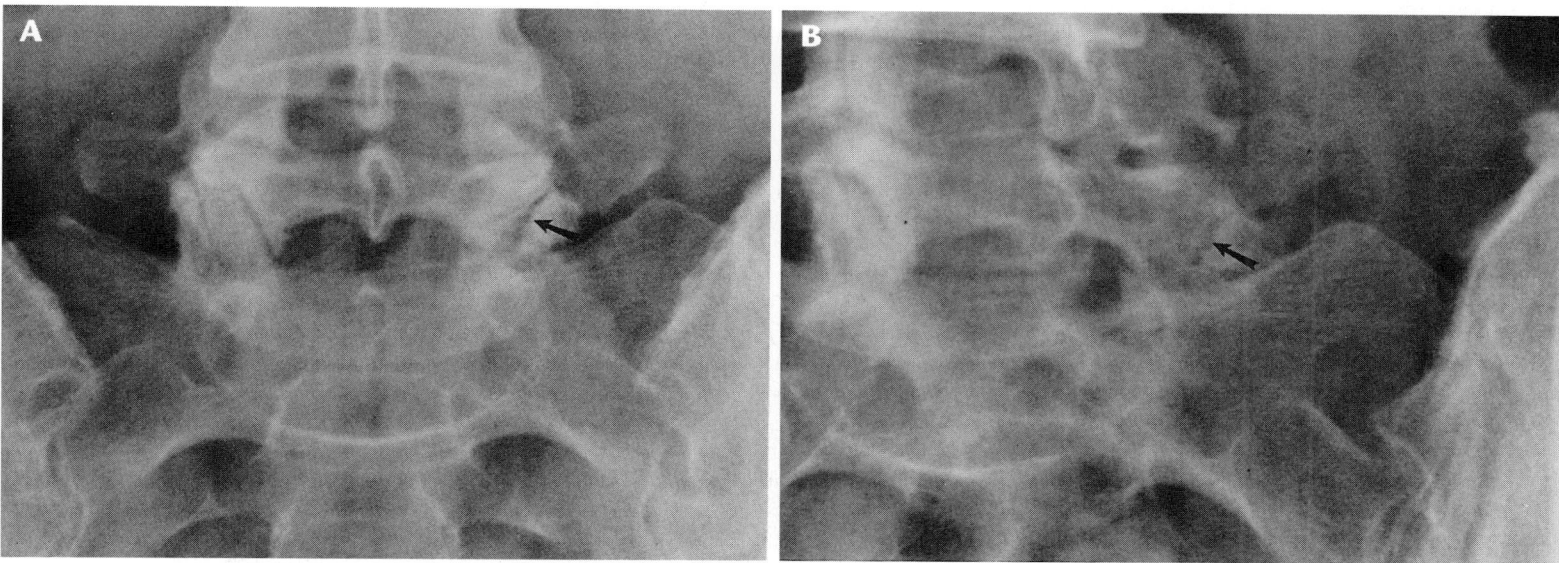

Figure 3–478. Another example of an unfused ossification center for the superior facet of S1, not to be mistaken for a fracture. **A,** Anteroposterior projection. **B,** Right oblique.

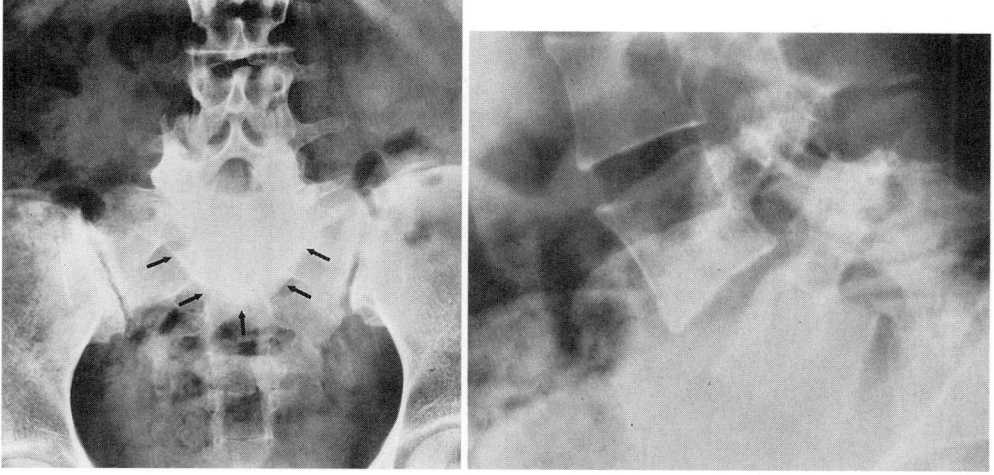

Figure 3–479. Marked lumbar lordosis may simulate the "Napoleon's hat sign" of spondylolisthesis of L5 in the frontal projection.

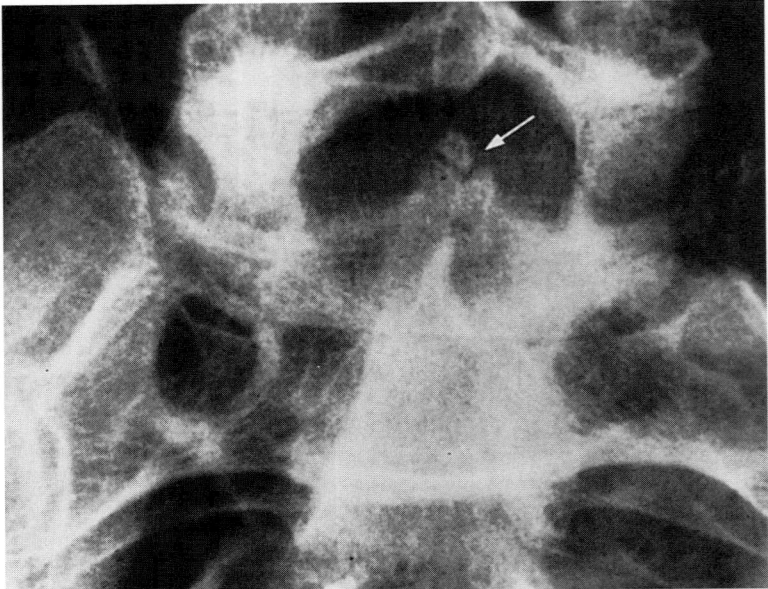

Figure 3–480. Ununited ossification center for the spinous process of S1.

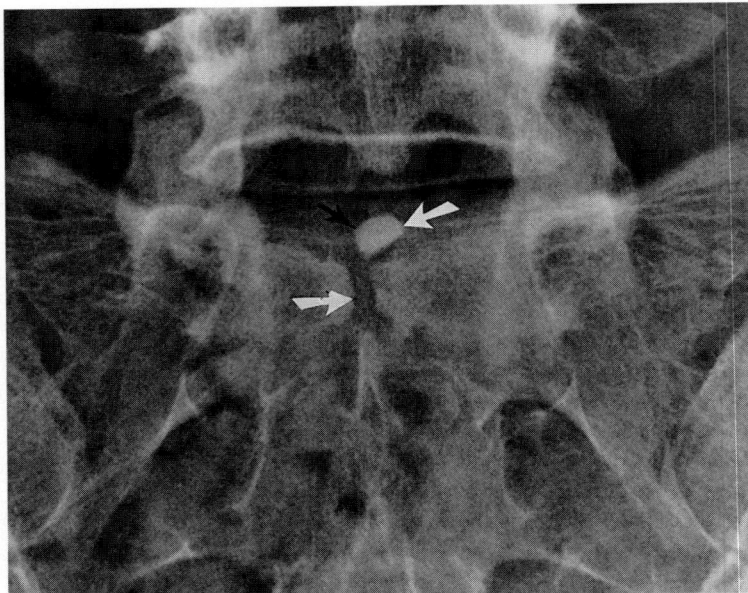

Figure 3–481. Ununited ossification center for the spinous process of S1 associated with spina bifida occulta.

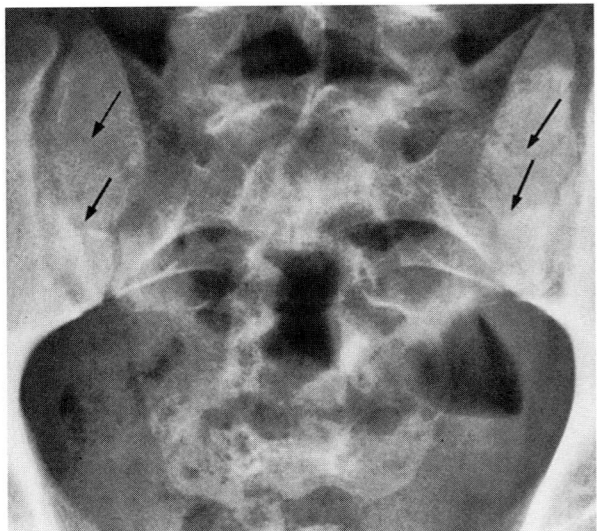

Figure 3–482. The alae of the sacral vertebrae in a 15-year-old boy.

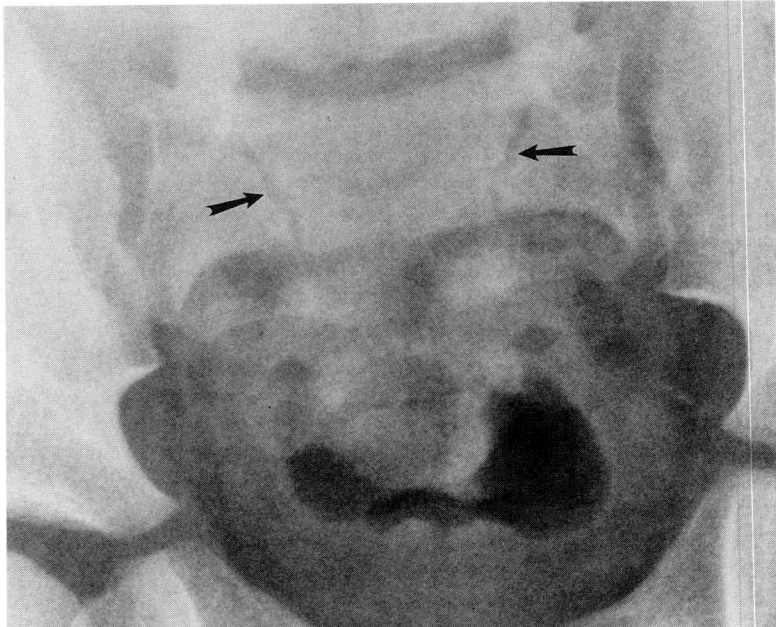

Figure 3–483. The synchondrosis between the body and alae of the sacrum in a 3-year-old child. These usually close between ages 1 and 7.

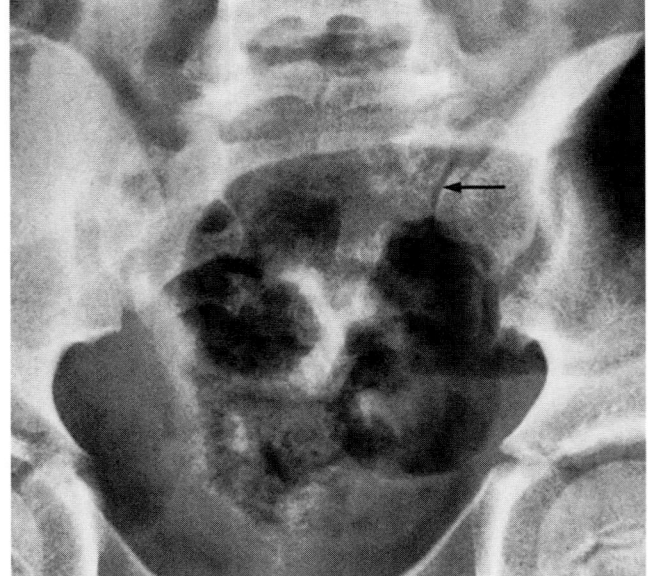

Figure 3–484. The same phenomenon seen in Figure 3–483 persisting in a 9-year-old boy.

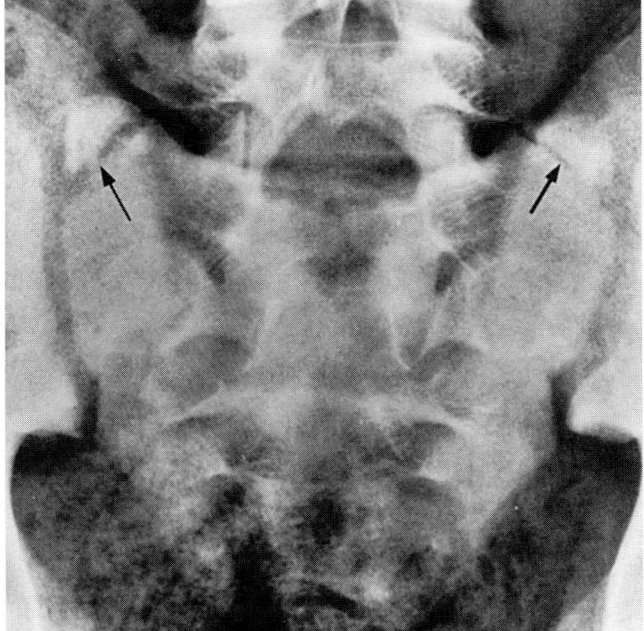

Figure 3–485. Accessory ossification centers for the sacral alae in a 15-year-old boy.

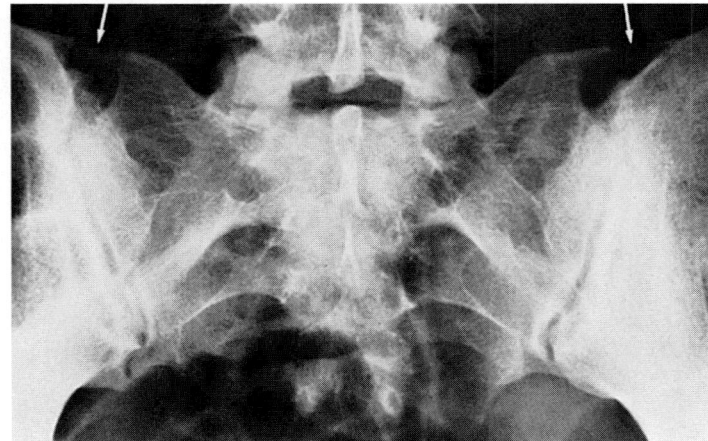

Figure 3–486. "Angel-wing" sacrum, produced by calcification in the iliosacral ligaments.

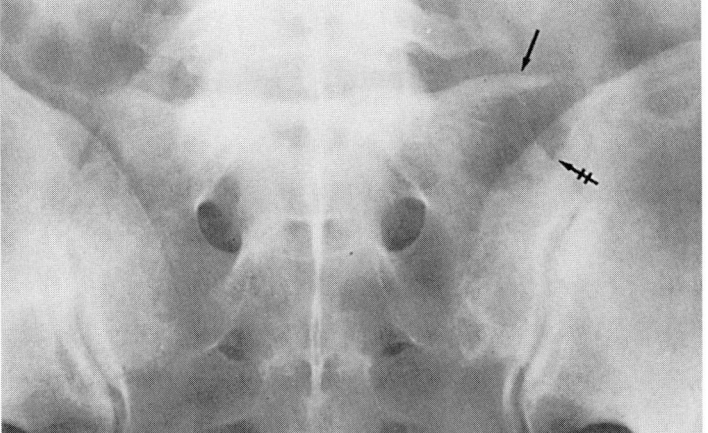

Figure 3–487. Calcification of the iliosacral ligament. Note simulation of a destructive lesion in the sacrum immediately below, produced by overlying colonic gas (⊬).

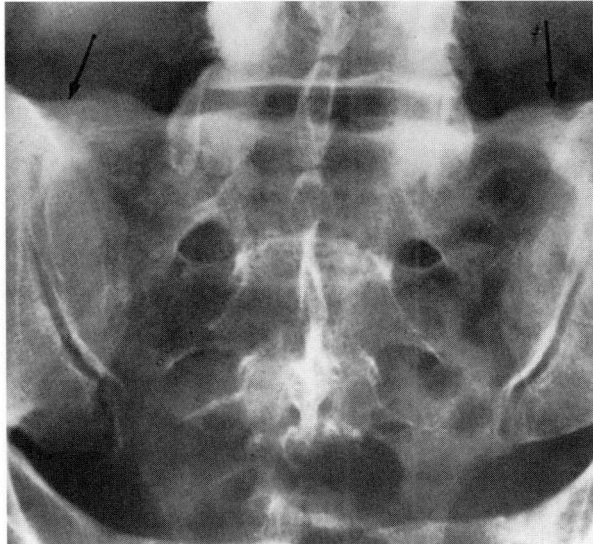

Figure 3–488. Calcification of the iliosacral ligaments.

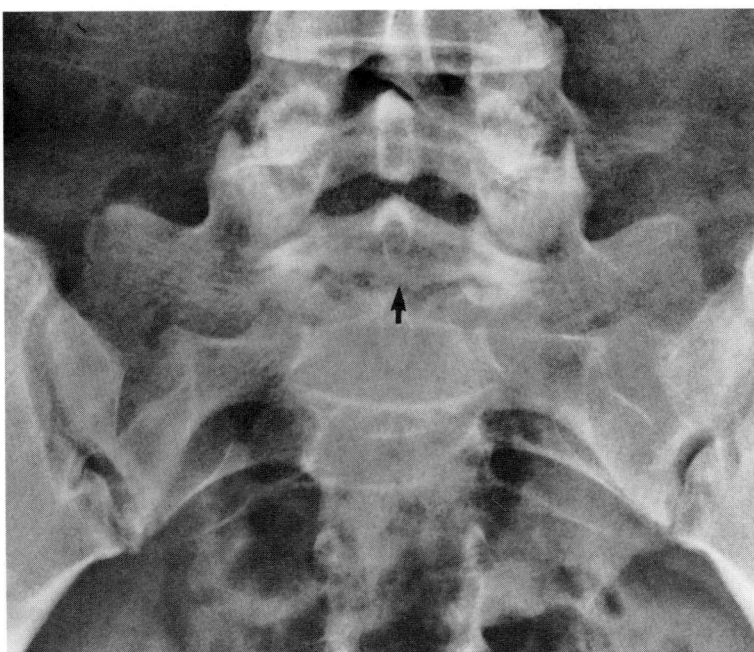

Figure 3–489. Lumbarized S1 with residual disc *(arrow)*.

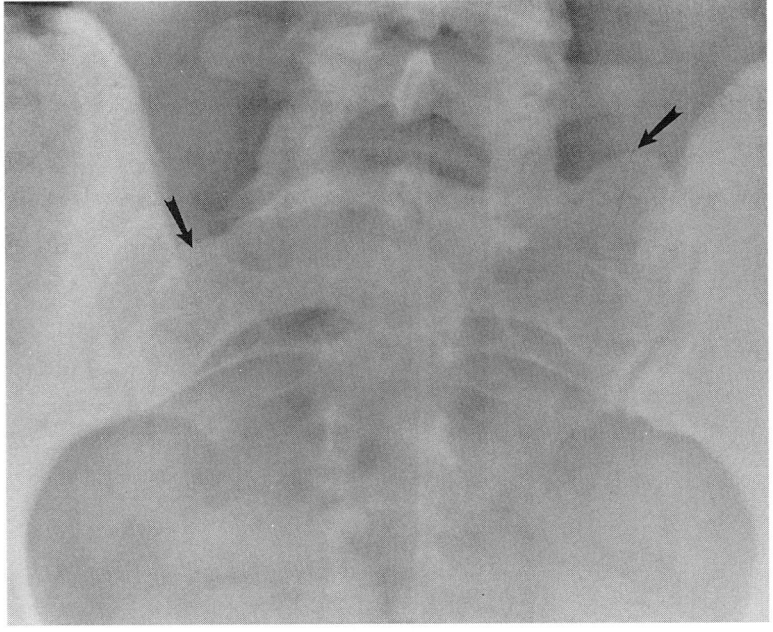

Figure 3–490. Developmental absence of the right ala of S1.

335

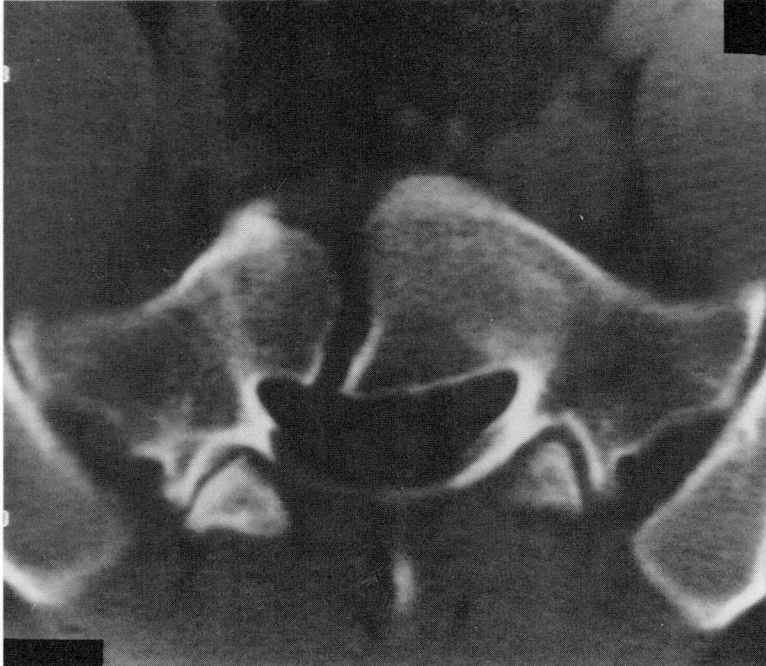

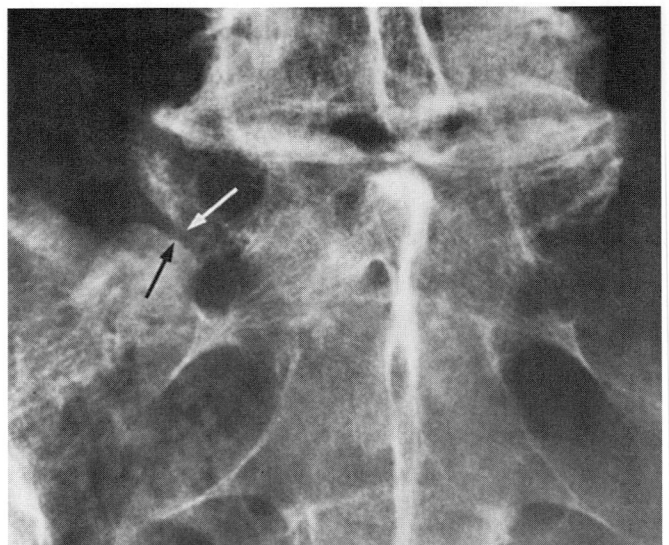

Figure 3–492. Unilateral anomalous articulation between S1 and S2.

Figure 3–491. Midline cleft of S1, probably related to persistence of the notochord.

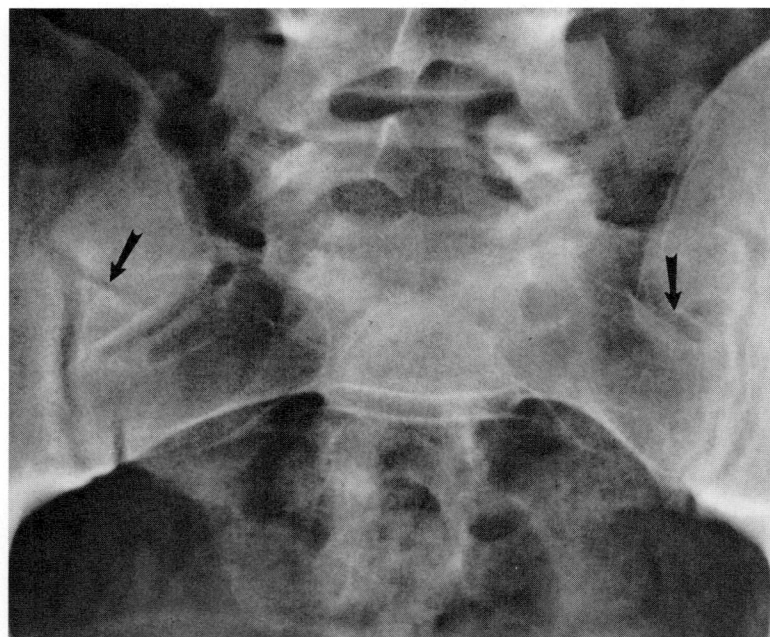

Figure 3–493. Failure of fusion of the lateral elements of the sacrum producing "accessory sacroiliac joints."

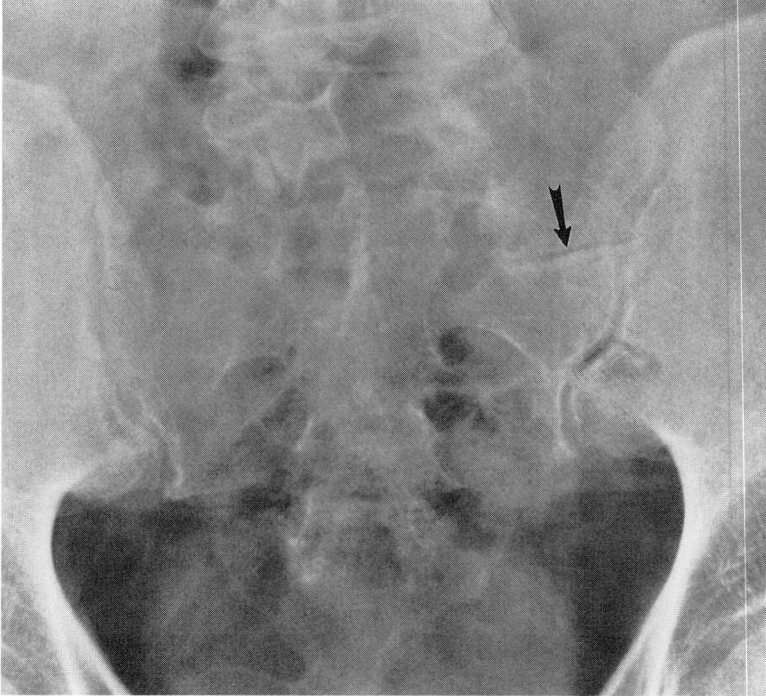

Figure 3–494. The same entity as in preceding figure seen unilaterally.

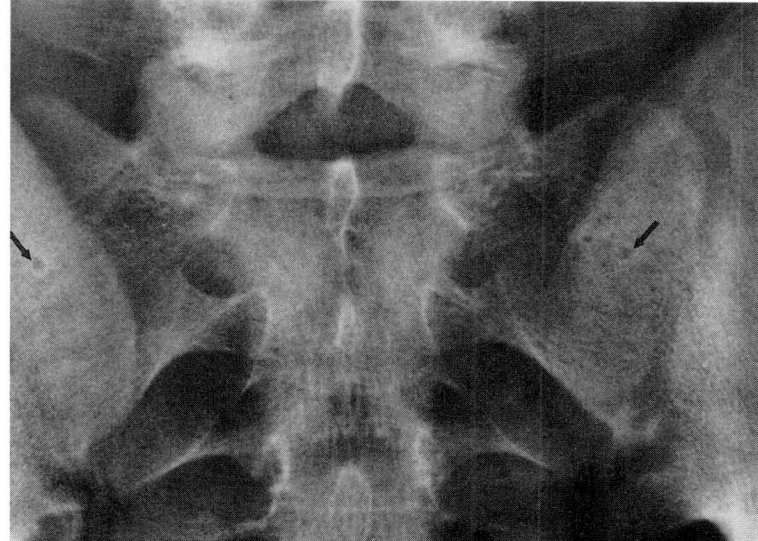

Figure 3–495. Nutrient foramina of the sacral alae in an 8-year-old boy.

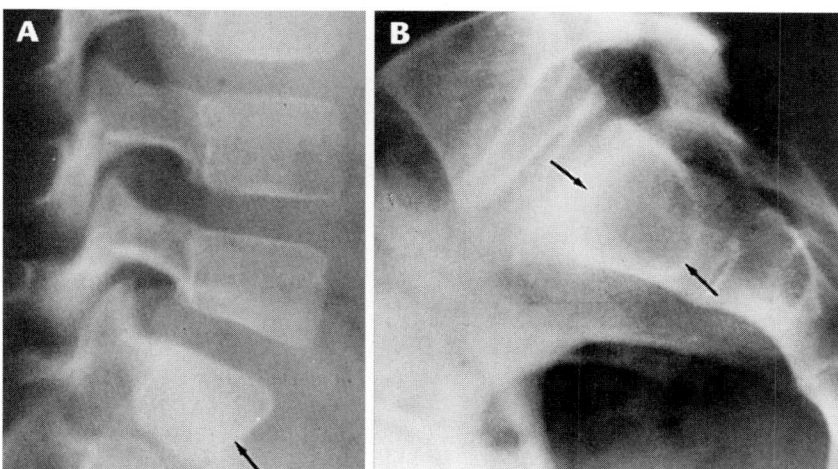

Figure 3–496. Normal variations in the appearance of the first sacral segment. **A,** Normal relative increase in density in a 2-year-old boy. This is at times mistaken for osteosclerosis. **B,** Pseudocyst of the sacrum *(arrow)* in a young adult as a result of the large amount of cancellous bone, with the suggestion of a similar appearance in the second sacral segment.

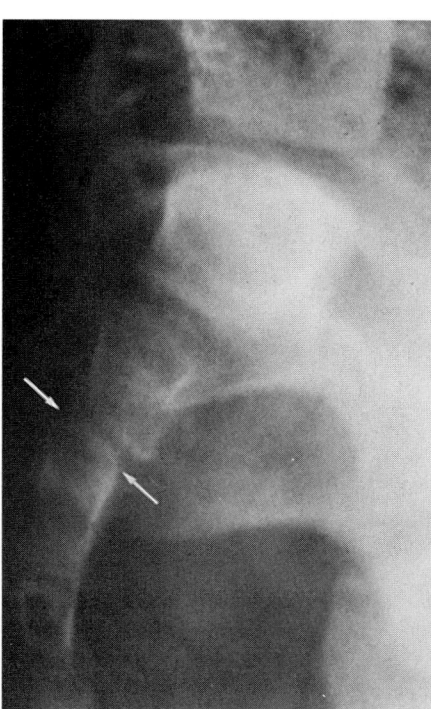

Figure 3–497. Simulated fracture of the sacrum in a young child. This appearance of the second and third sacral segments is not unusual in children.

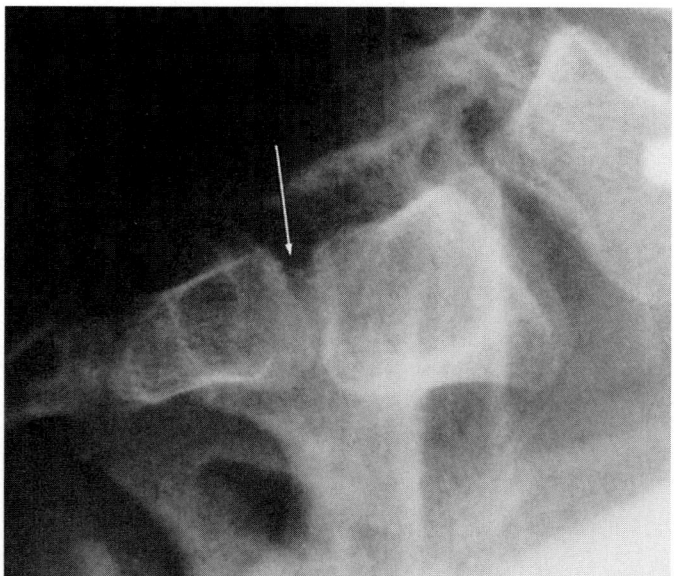

Figure 3–498. Widening of the posterior aspect of the S1–S2 interspace, a variation in development in youth that may be mistaken for a destructive lesion. (Ref: Cacciarelli AA: Posterior widening of the S1-2 interspace in children: A normal variant of sacral development. *Am J Roentgenol* 129:305, 1977.)

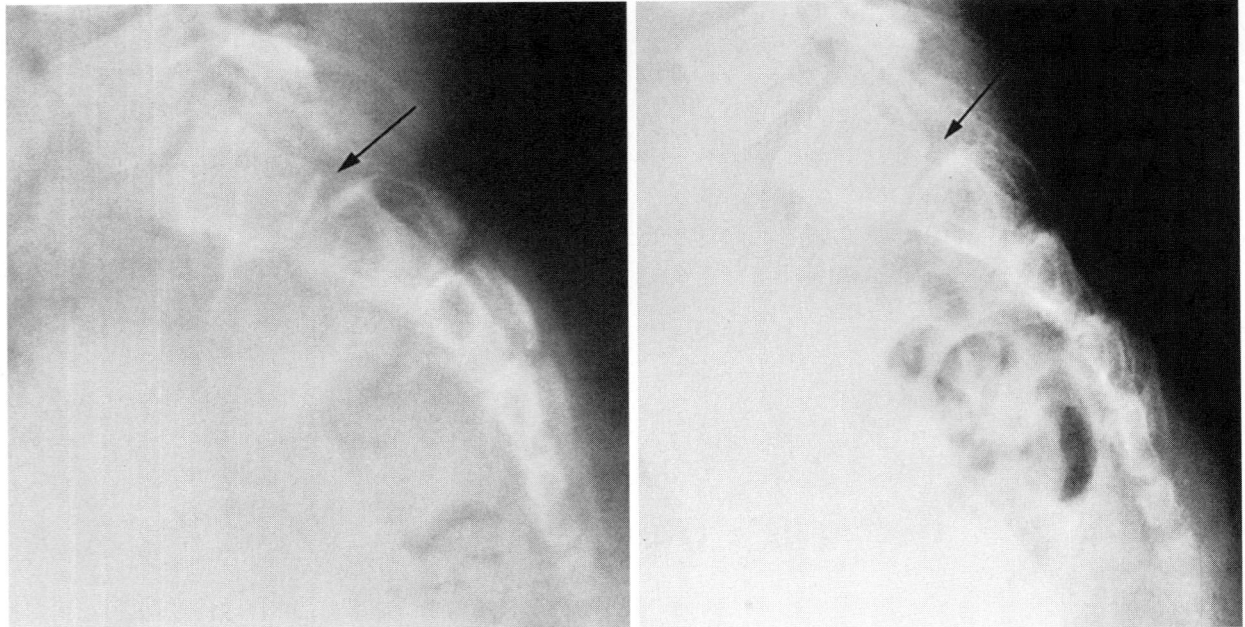

Figure 3–499. *Left,* The wide posterior aspect of the S1–S2 interspace misdiagnosed as a fracture in a 13-year-old boy following paddling with a board. *Right,* Follow-up film made 3 months later shows no change.

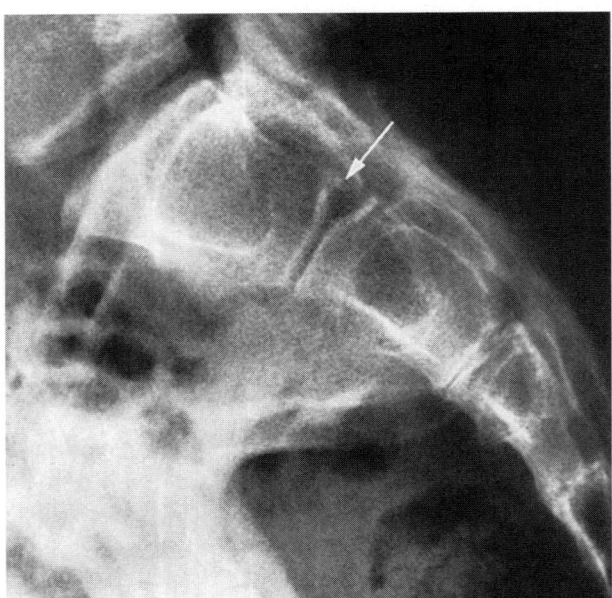

Figure 3–500. The S1–S2 posterior widening in a 15-year-old boy. At this age the end plates are better defined.

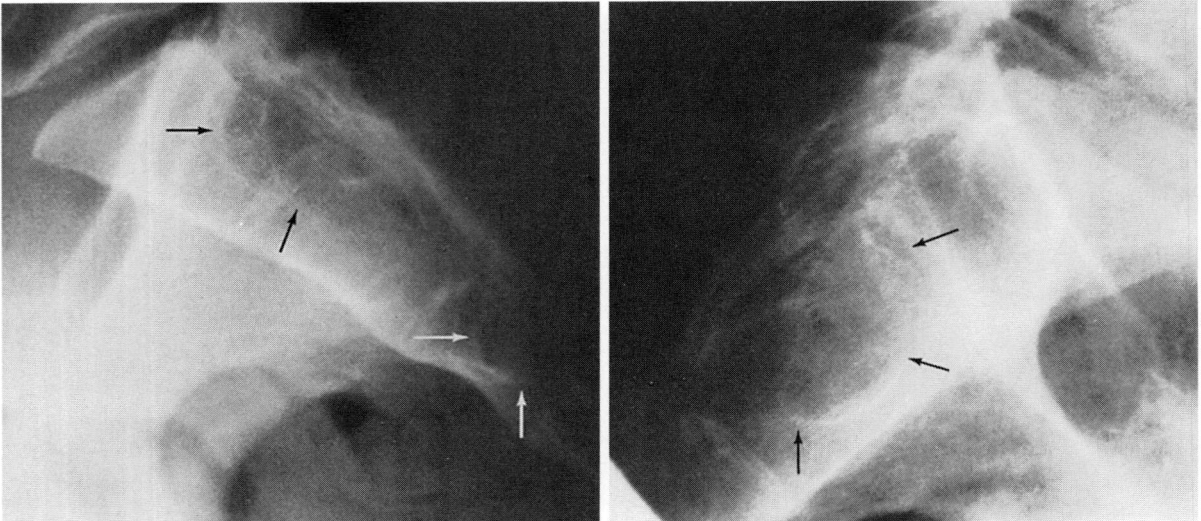

Figure 3–501. Apparent cystic lesions of the sacrum, produced by the shadows of the fossae cribrosa of the sacrum. (Ref: Kreyenbühl W, Hessler C: A variation of the sacrum on the lateral view. *Radiology* 109:49, 1973.)

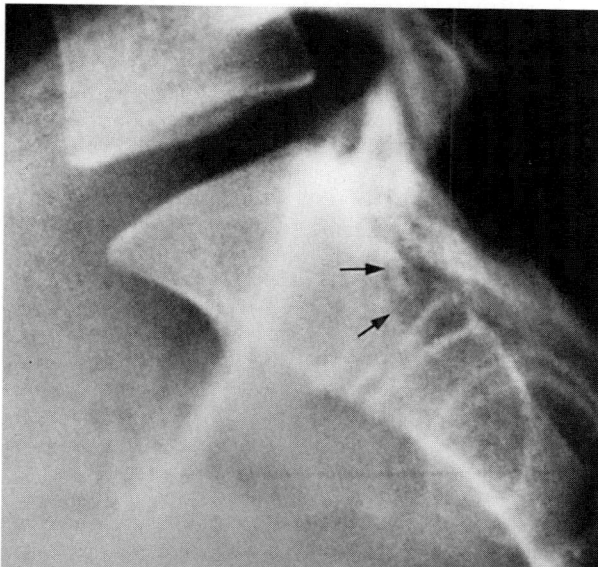

Figure 3–502. Lucency in posterior aspect of S1 in a 16-year-old boy simulating a destructive lesion, similar to Figure 3–501.

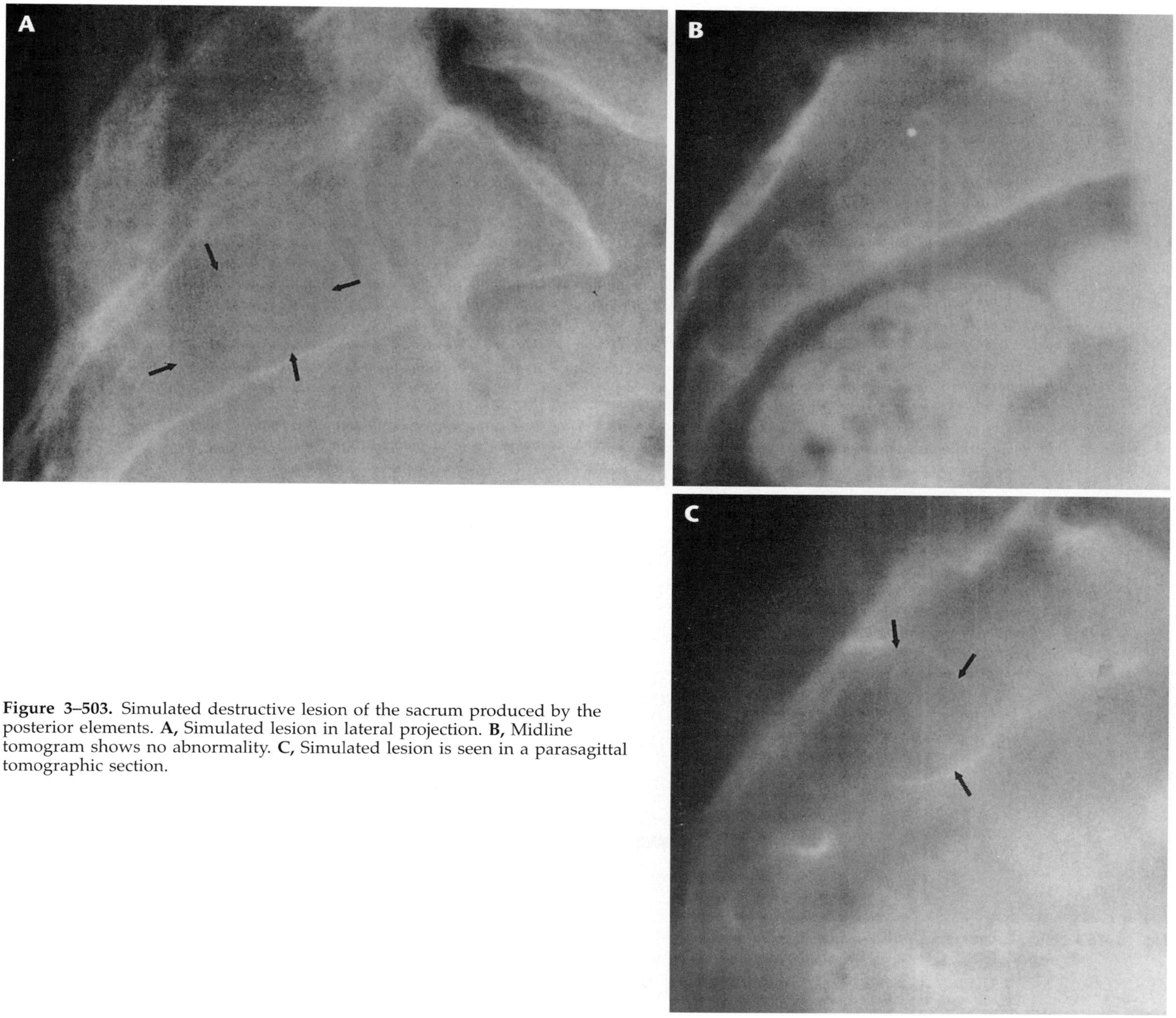

Figure 3–503. Simulated destructive lesion of the sacrum produced by the posterior elements. **A,** Simulated lesion in lateral projection. **B,** Midline tomogram shows no abnormality. **C,** Simulated lesion is seen in a parasagittal tomographic section.

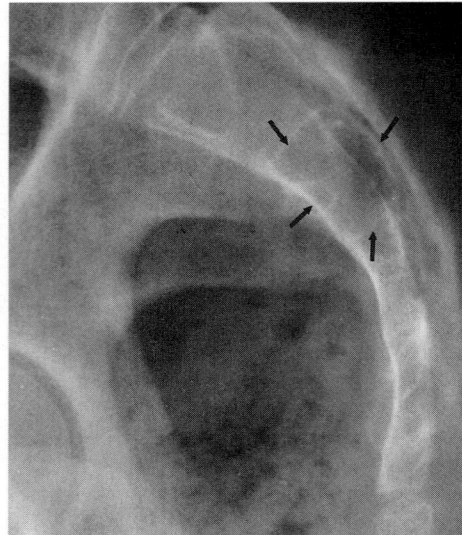

Figure 3–504. An additional example of simulated sacral lesions, as in Figure 3–503.

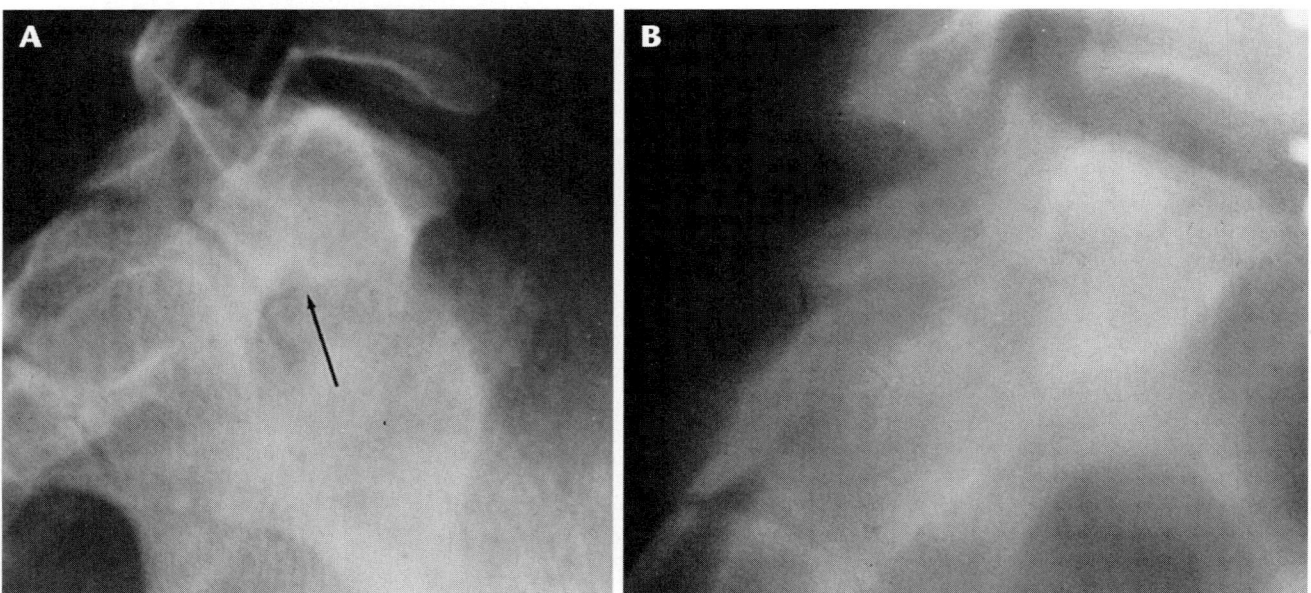

Figure 3–505. A, Simulated destructive lesion of S1 caused by rotation at time of filming. B, Tomogram shows no abnormality.

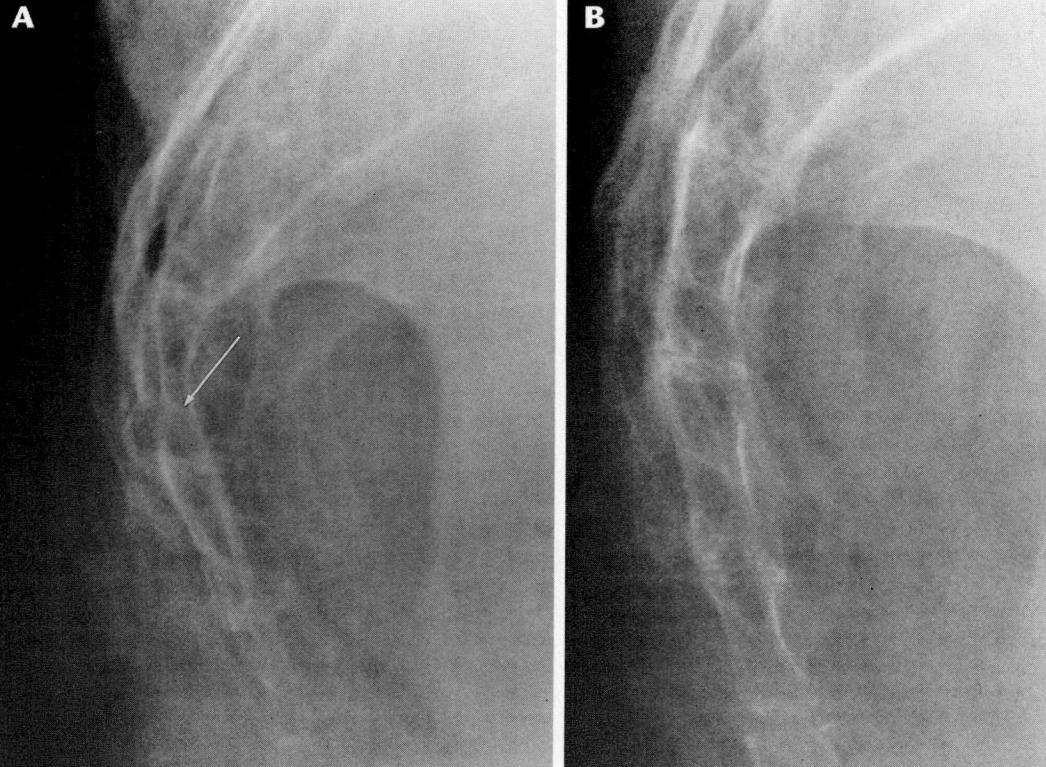

Figure 3–506. A, Simulated destructive lesion of the sacrum produced by the fossae cribrosa and rotation. B, True lateral projection shows no abnormality.

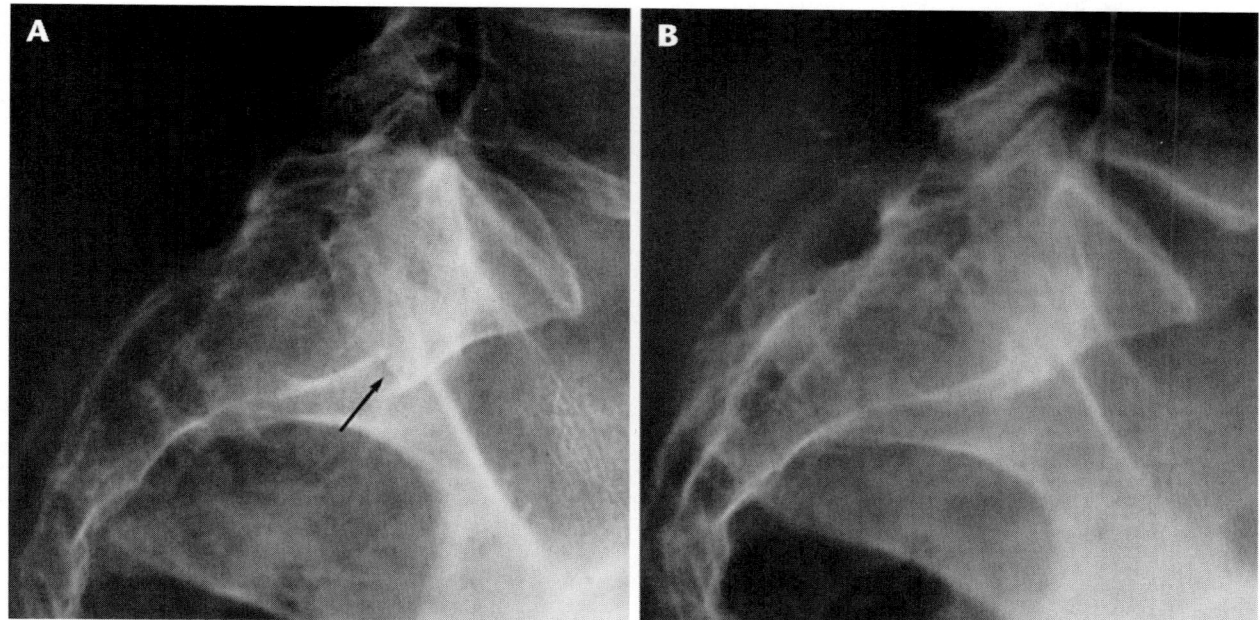

Figure 3–507. A, Apparent fracture of the sacrum caused by rotation at the time of filming. **B,** Repeat film shows no abnormality.

Figure 3–508. Large posterior elements of the fourth and fifth sacral segments.

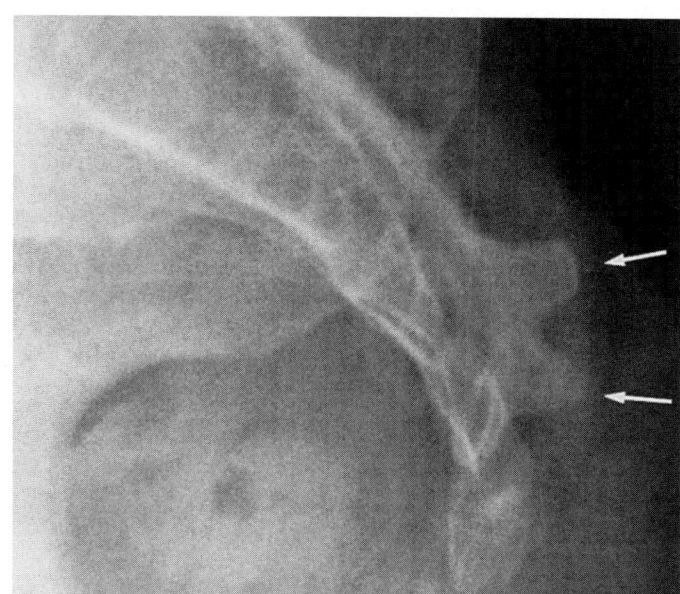

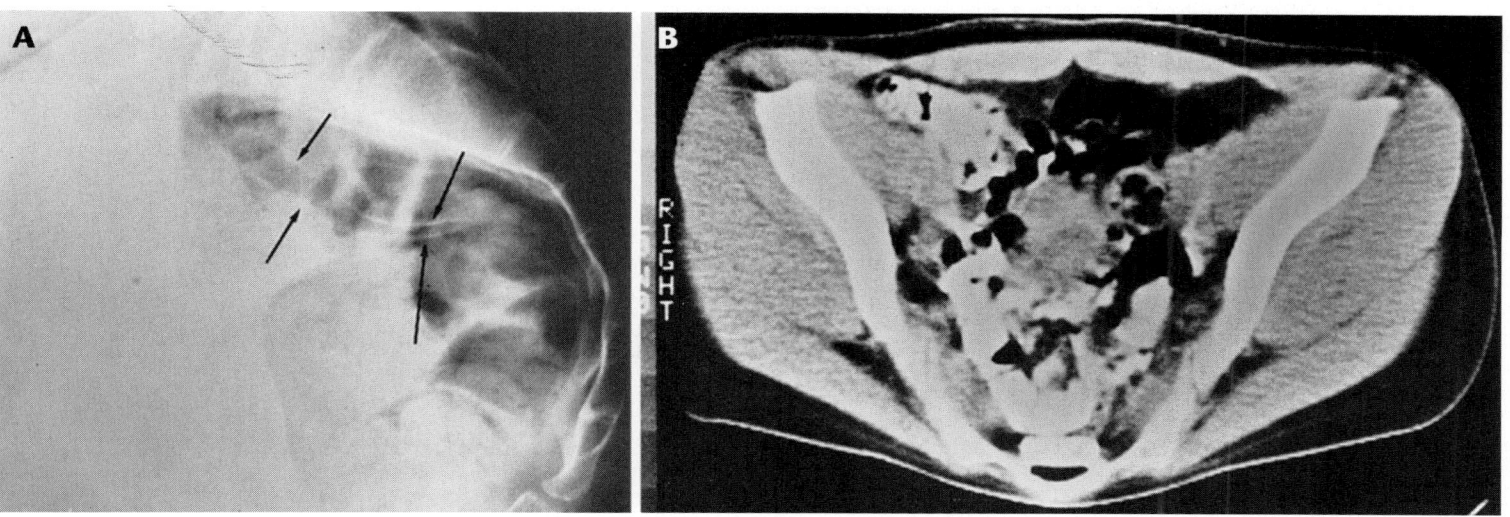

Figure 3–509. A, Unusually deep sacral curve, which results in apparent expansile lesions with shell-like margins. **B,** CT shows no intrinsic lesion of the sacrum.

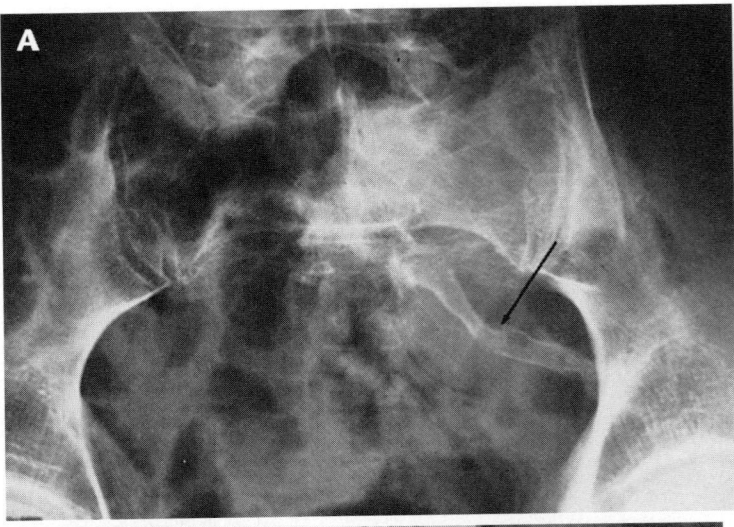

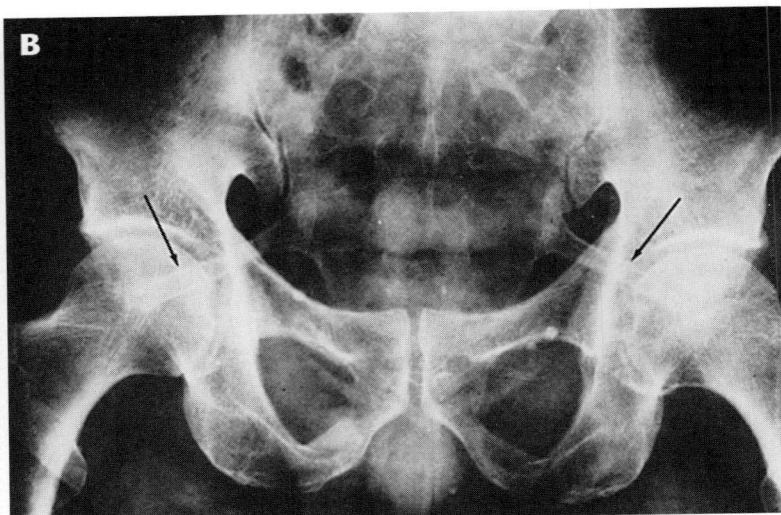

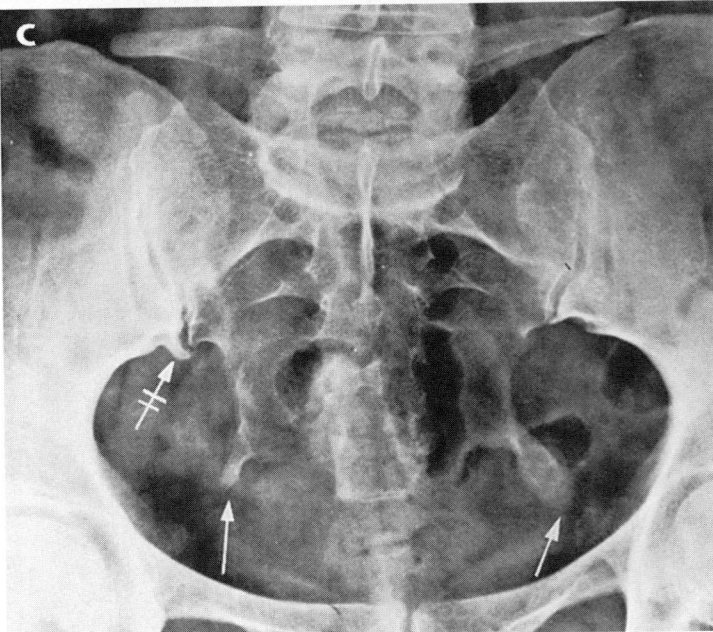

Figure 3–510. Sacral ribs. **A,** Unilateral. **B,** Bilateral. **C,** Bilateral and asymmetric sacral ribs. Note also calcification in the iliolumbar ligaments and ilial spur at the right sacroiliac joint (⫣). (Ref: Halloran W: Sacral ribs. *Q Bull Northwestern Univ Med School* 34:304, 1960.)

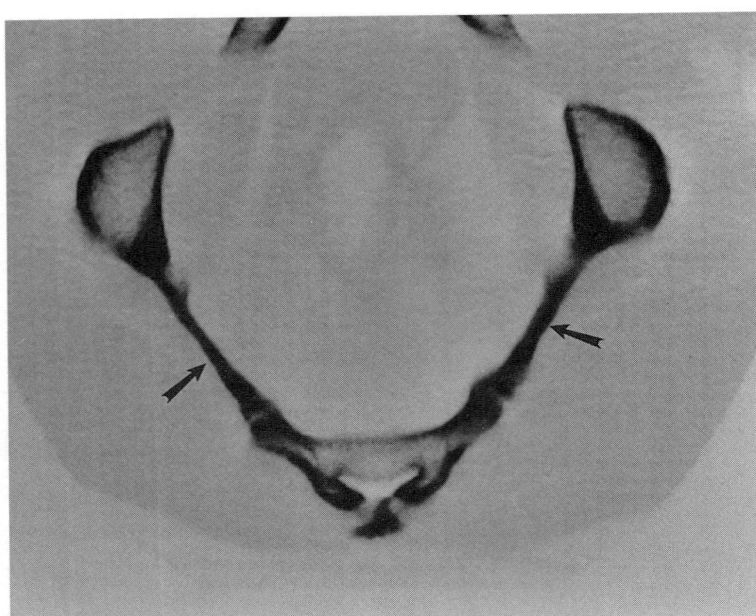

Figure 3–511. Sacral ribs by CT.

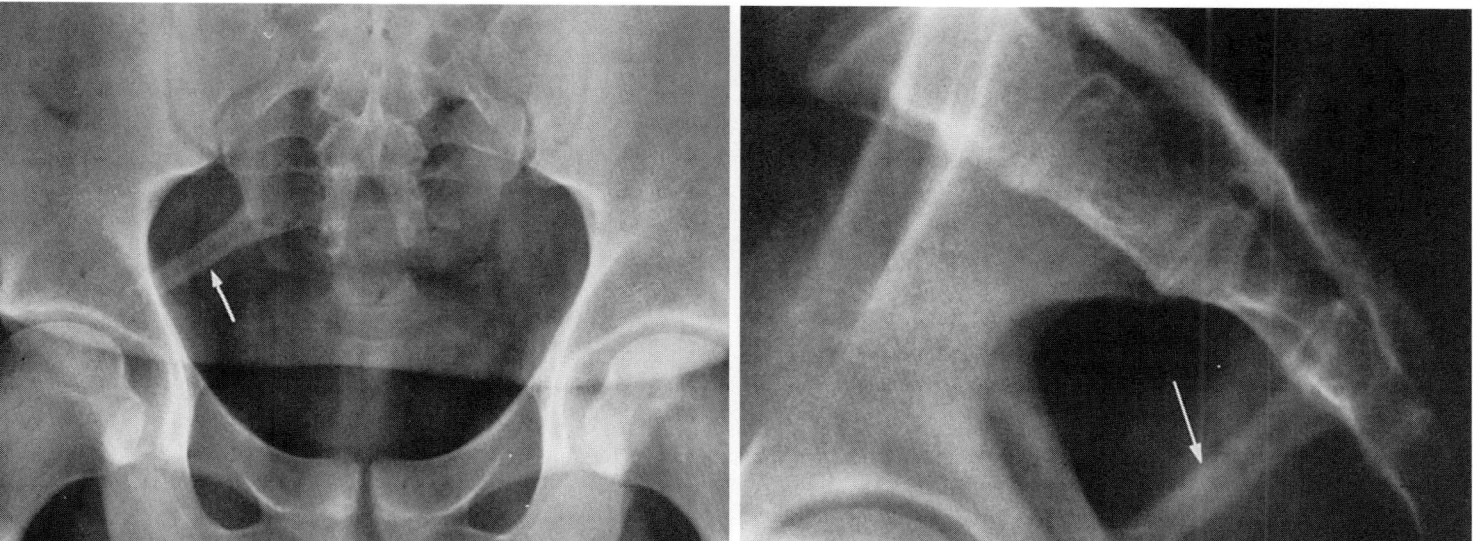

Figure 3–512. Unilateral sacral rib also seen in lateral projection.

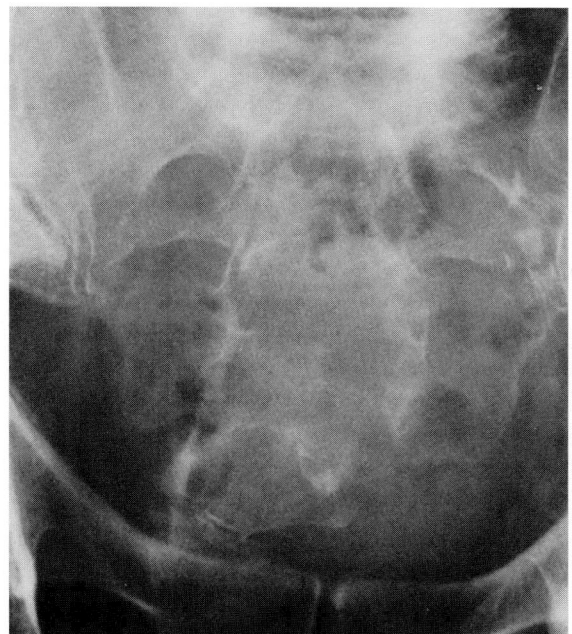

Figure 3–513. Scoliosis of the sacrum and coccyx.

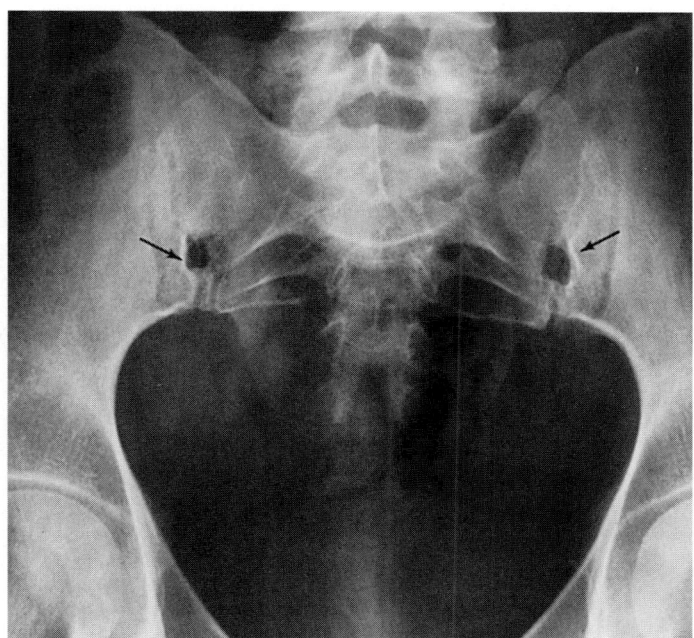

Figure 3–514. Normal foraminal shadows in the sacrum.

Figure 3–515. Developmental defects in the ala of the sacrum.

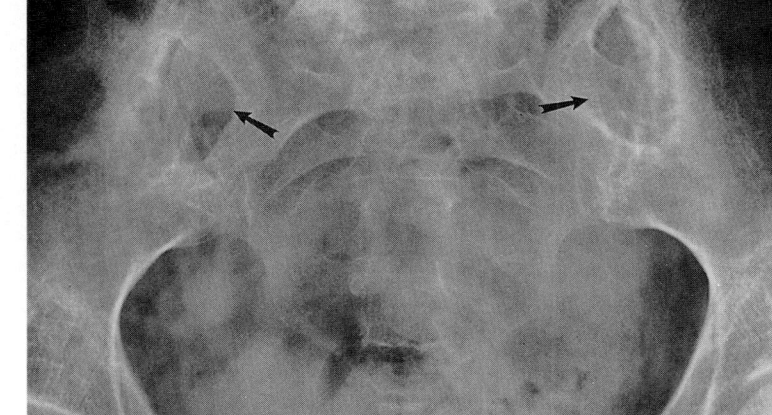

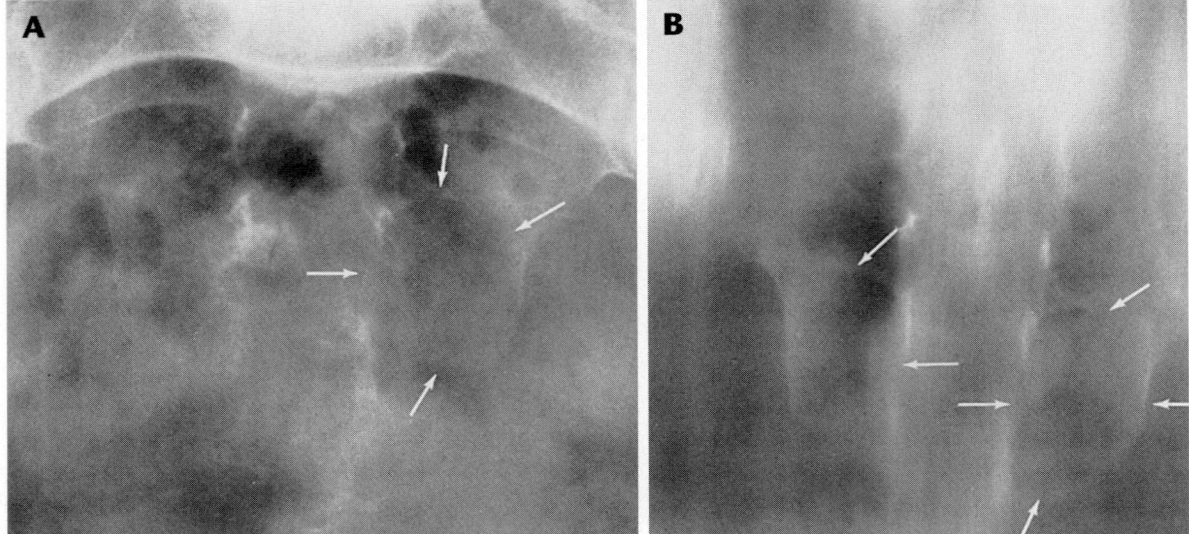

Figure 3–516. Simulated destructive lesions of the wings of the sacrum produced by the foramina of the sacrum. Bowel gas may accentuate this appearance as well. **A,** Plain film. **B,** Tomogram.

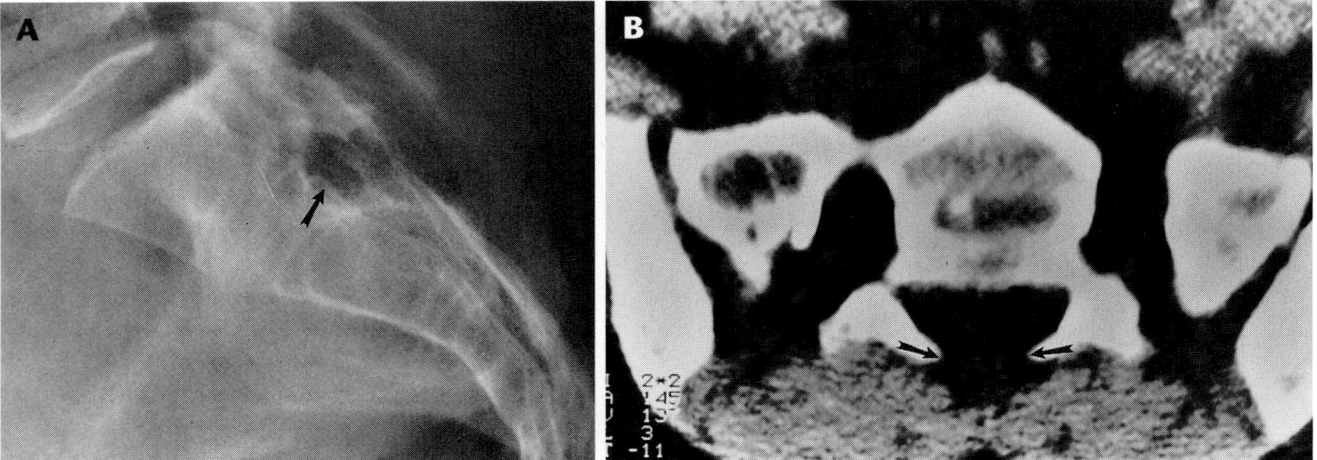

Figure 3–517. Simulated destructive lesion of the sacrum resulting from spina bifida occulta of S1. **A,** Lateral projection. **B,** CT.

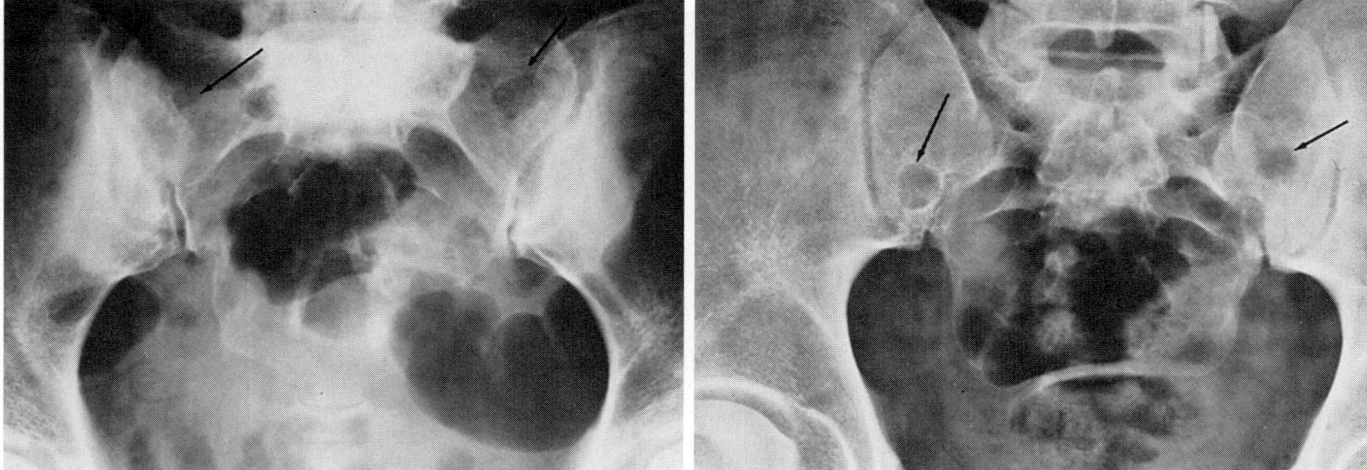

Figure 3–518. Two examples of fossae in the sacral wings simulating destructive lesions.

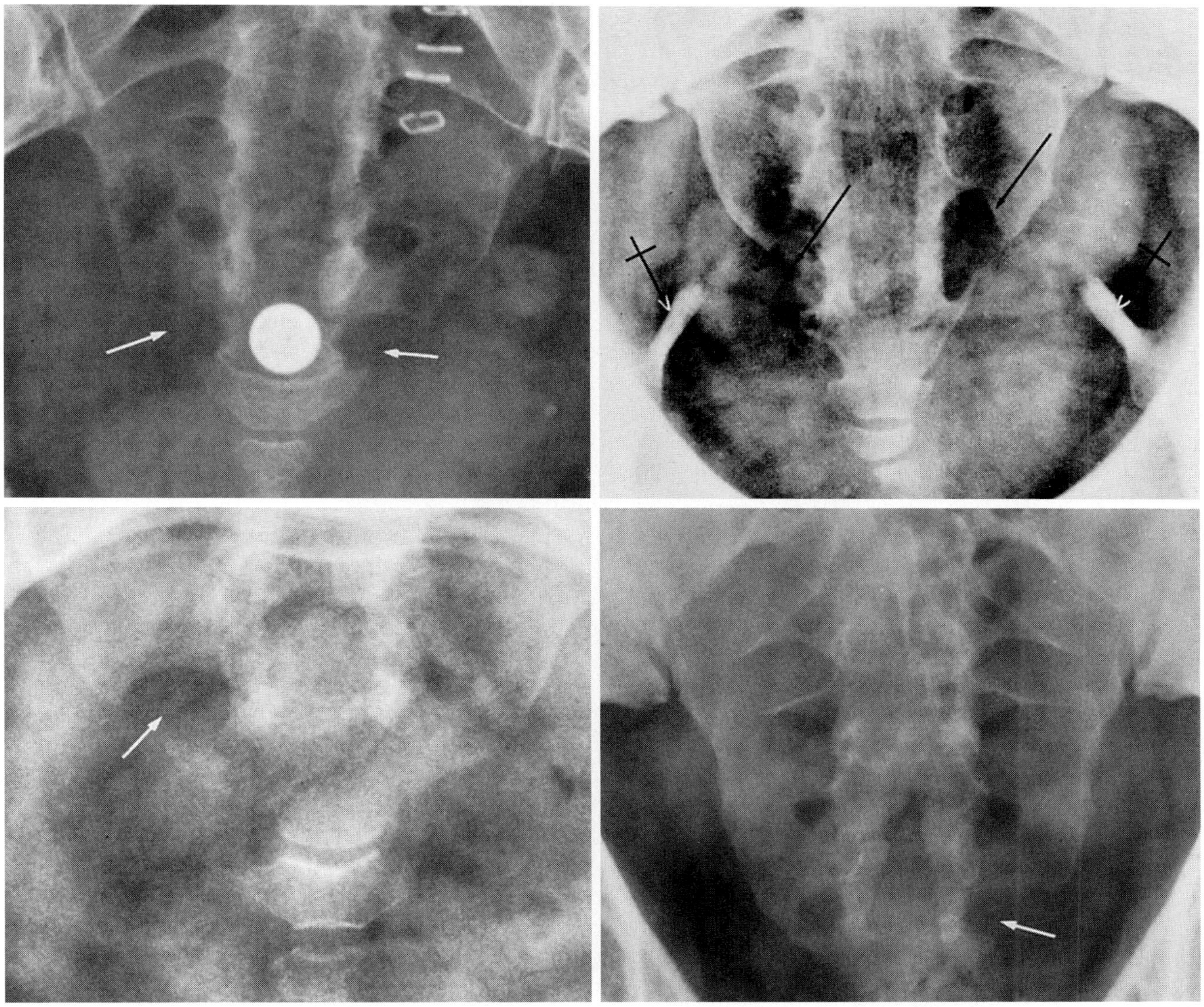

Figure 3–519. Developmental variations in the sacrum. *Top left,* Symmetric defects
(→). *Top right,* Asymmetric defects (→). Calcification is present in the sacrospinal
ligaments (↔). *Bottom,* Other asymmetric defects.

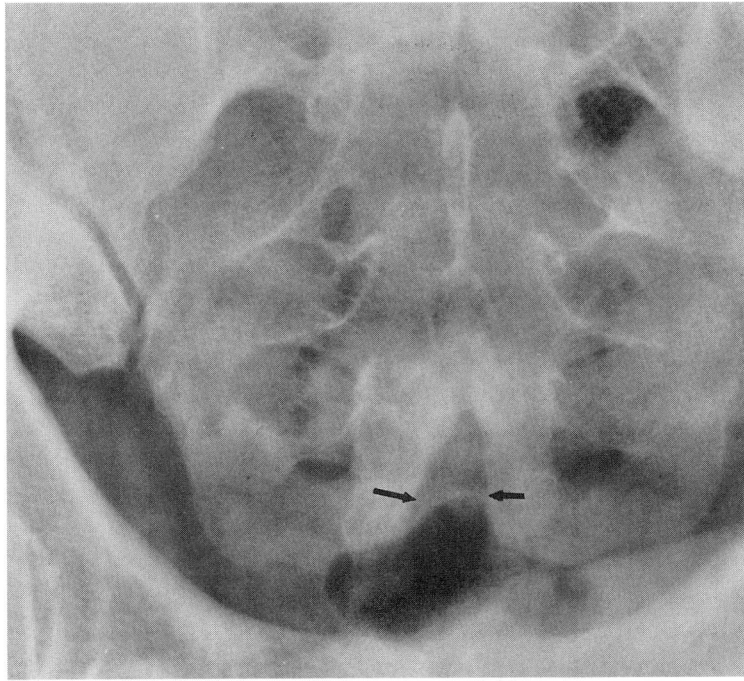

Figure 3–520. Open sacral canal.

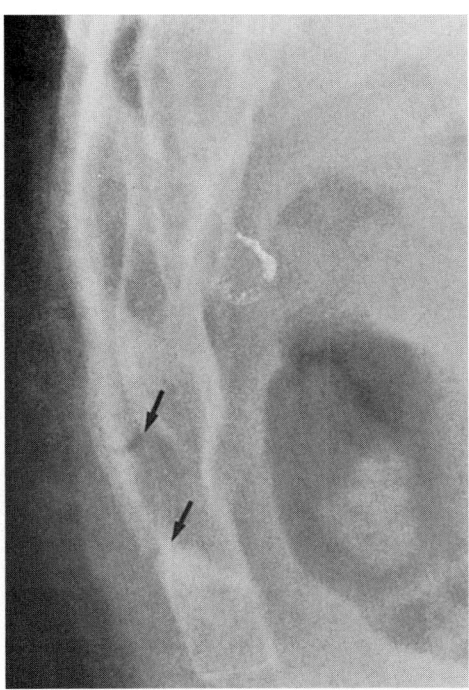

Figure 3–521. Fusion lines of the sacral segments simulating fractures.

The Coccyx

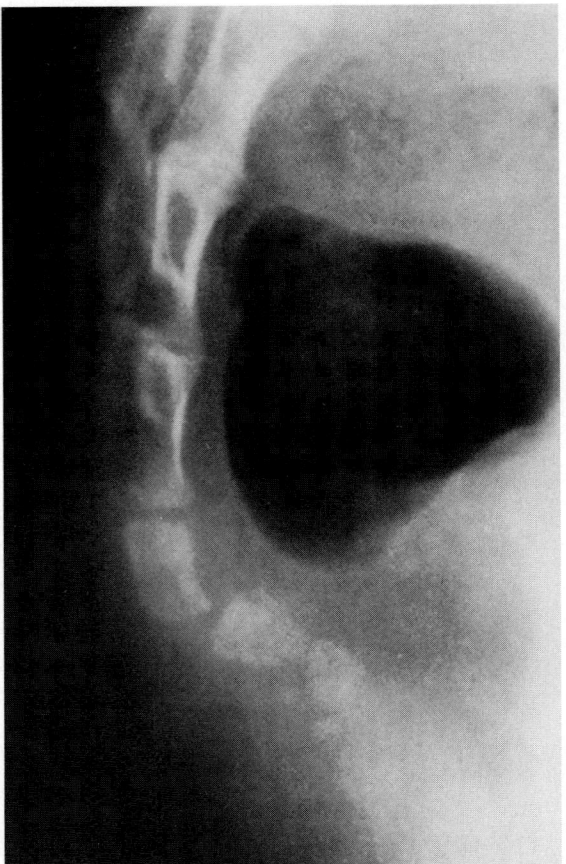

Figure 3–522. Normal anterior angulation of the coccyx. The position of the coccyx is not useful, in itself, in the identification of trauma. (Ref: Postaccini F, Massolrio M: Idiopathic coccygodynia: Analysis of 51 operative cases and a radiographic study of the normal coccyx. *J Bone Joint Surg* 65A:1116, 1983.)

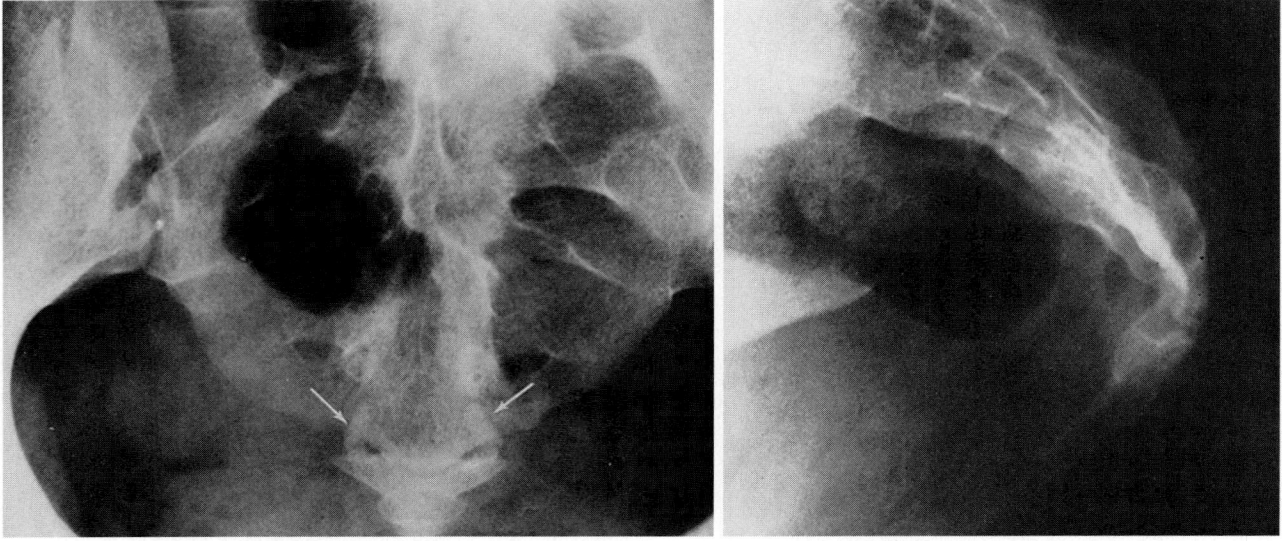

Figure 3–523. Anterior angulation of the coccyx. Note portions of the posterior arch of the distal portion of the sacrum, which might be mistaken for a fracture (*arrows*).

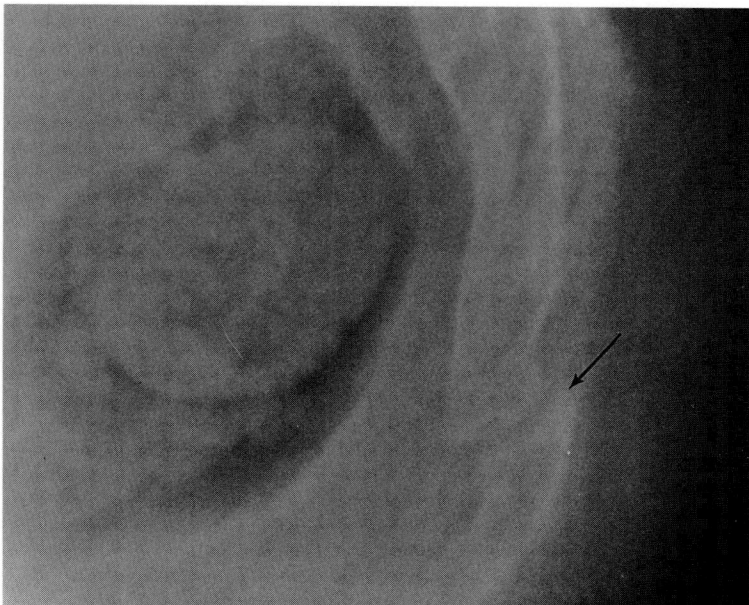

Figure 3–524. Posterior position of the coccyx with reference to the distal end of the sacrum is a normal variation and not indicative of dislocation.

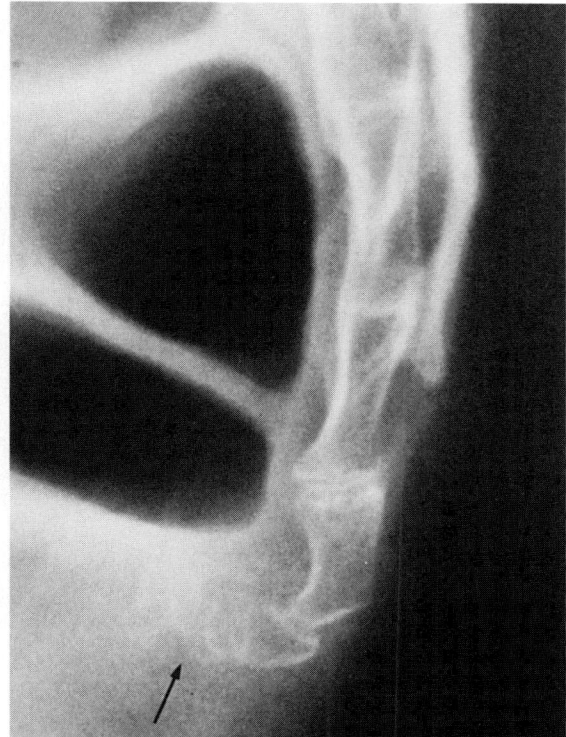

Figure 3–525. Marked anteflexion of the coccyx.

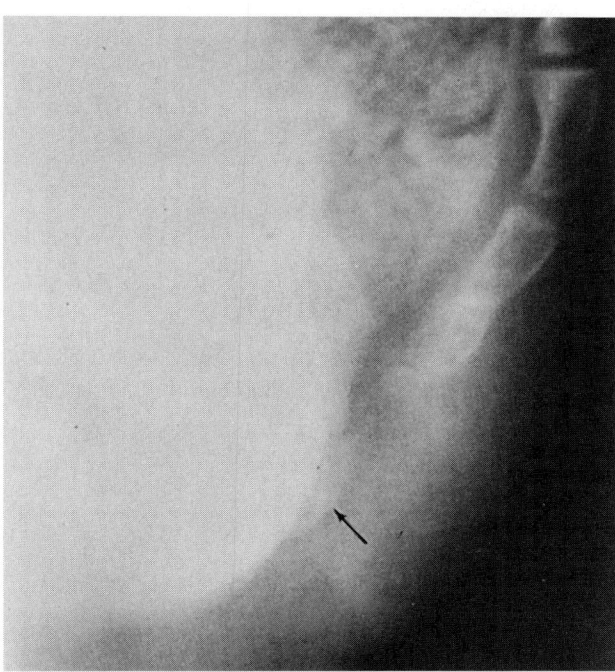

Figure 3–526. The ischial apophysis in a 15-year-old boy, not to be confused with a fracture of the tip of the coccyx.

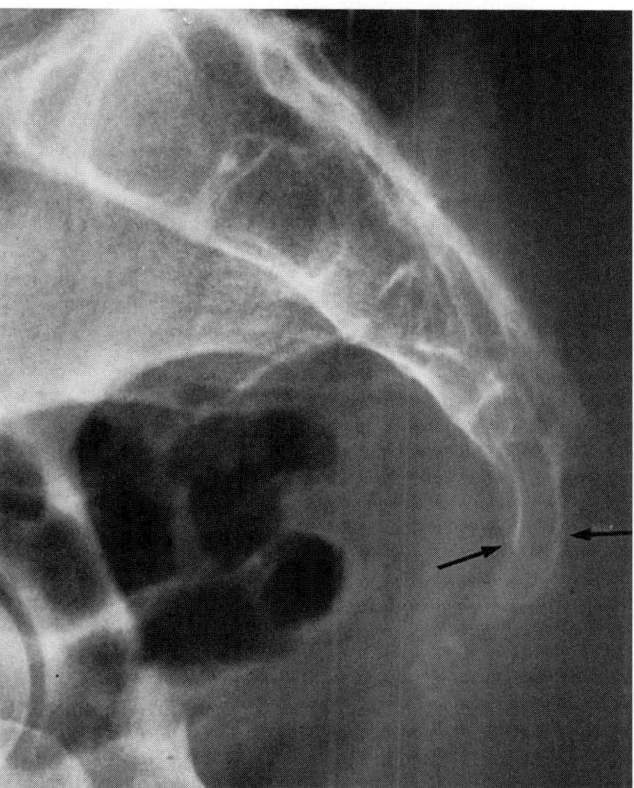

Figure 3–527. The junction of the coccyx and the last sacral segmen mistaken for a fracture.

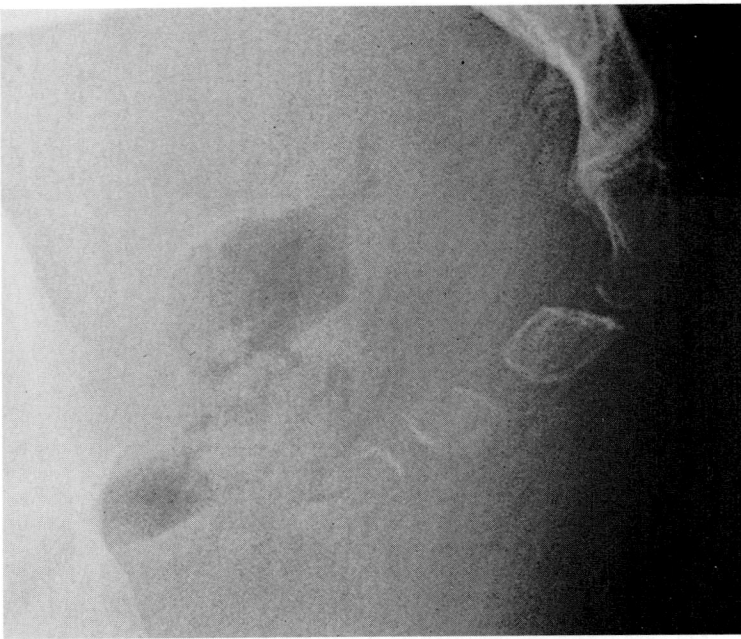

Figure 3–528. "Floating coccyx."

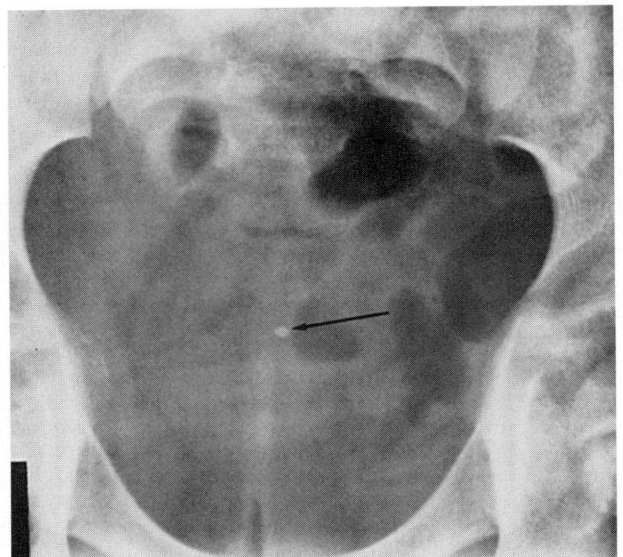

Figure 3–529. The ossification center for the first coccygeal segment in a 10-year-old child, which should not be confused with a calculus or enterolith.

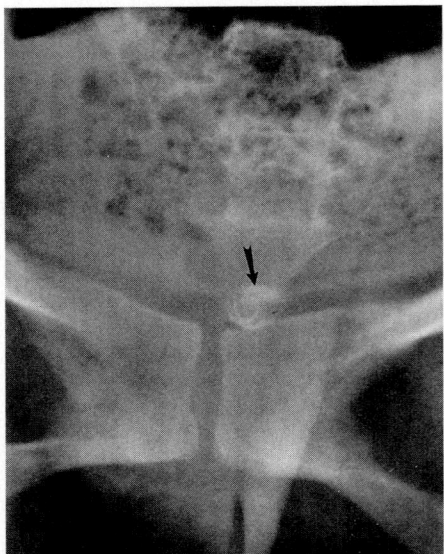

Figure 3–530. Axial view of the coccyx, which may simulate a calculus.

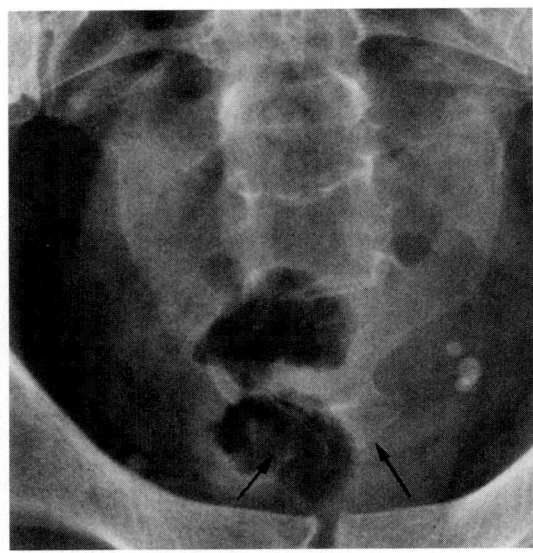

Figure 3–531. Congenital bifid coccyx.

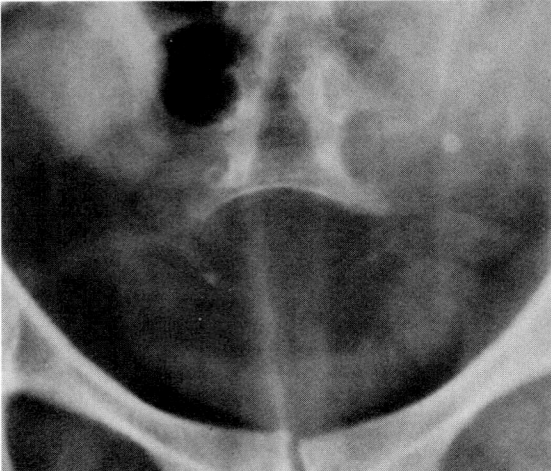

Figure 3–532. Congenital absence of the coccyx and anomalous development of the distal end of the sacrum.

The Sacroiliac Joints

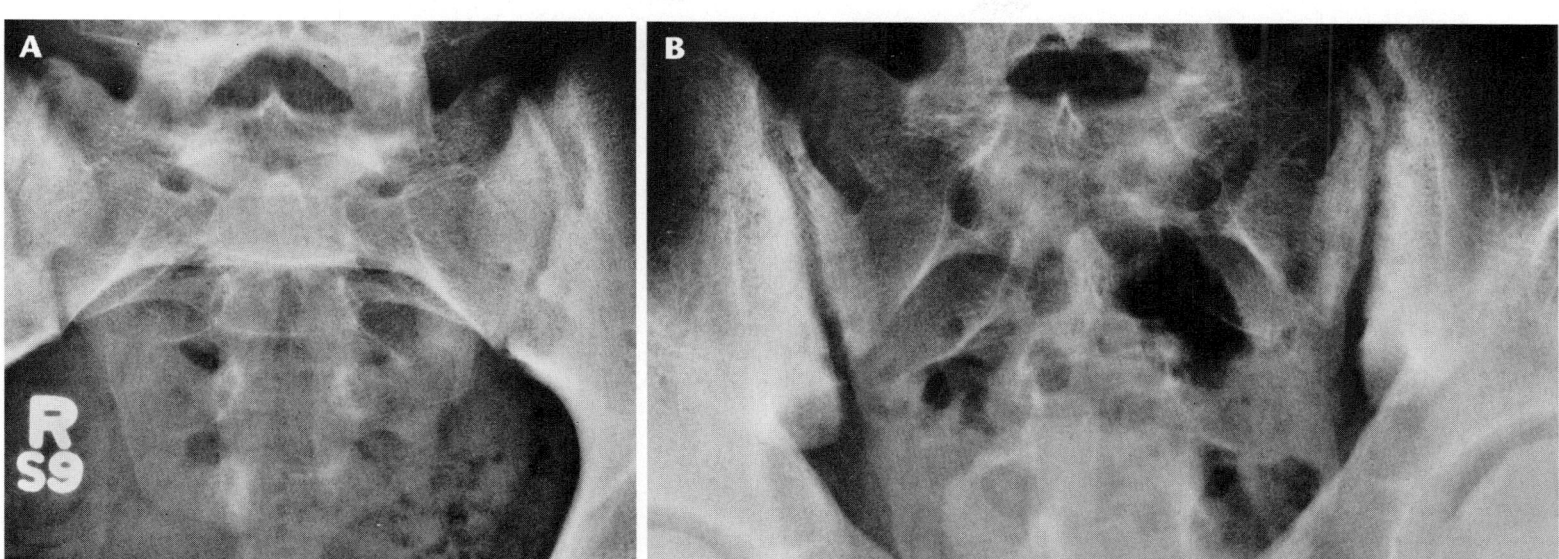

Figure 3–533. The sacroiliac joints in the adolescent are normally wide and irregular. These normal alterations should not be confused with the findings of ankylosing spondylitis. **A,** Standard anteroposterior view of pelvis. **B,** Sacroiliac projection with 30-degree cephalad angulation of the tube (Ferguson's projection).

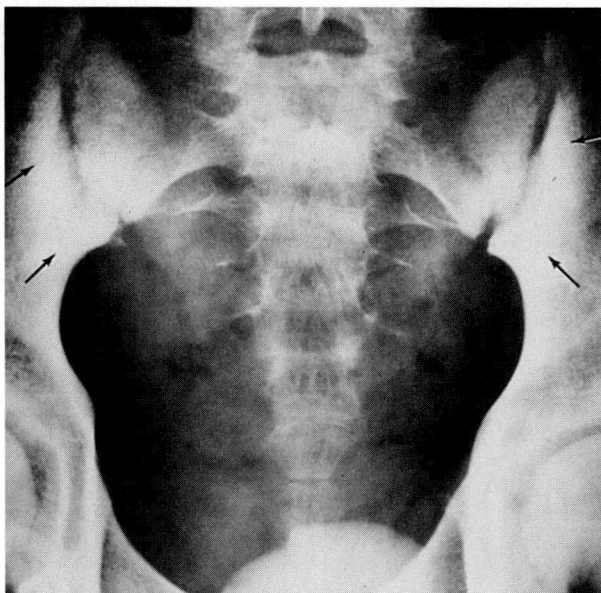

Figure 3–534. Normal sclerosis and irregularity of the sacroiliac joints in a 14-year-old boy, resembling the changes of ankylosing spondylitis.

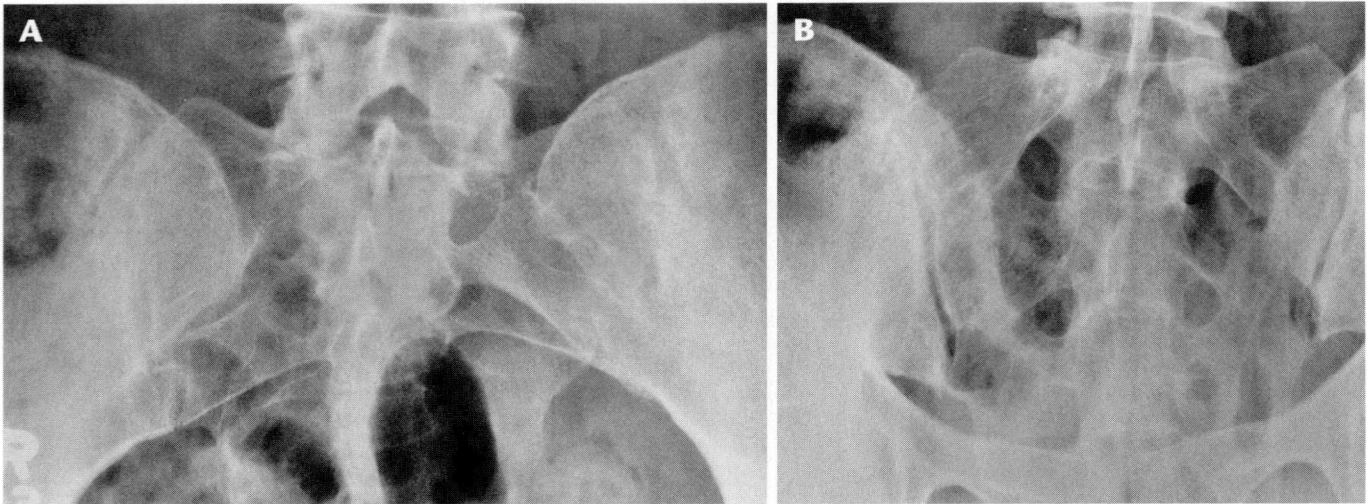

Figure 3–535. A, Simulated obliteration of the sacroiliac joints suggesting ankylosing spondylitis. **B,** Normal appearance of sacroiliac joints on Ferguson's view. The frontal view of the pelvis cannot always be relied upon to depict the true state of the sacroiliac joints.

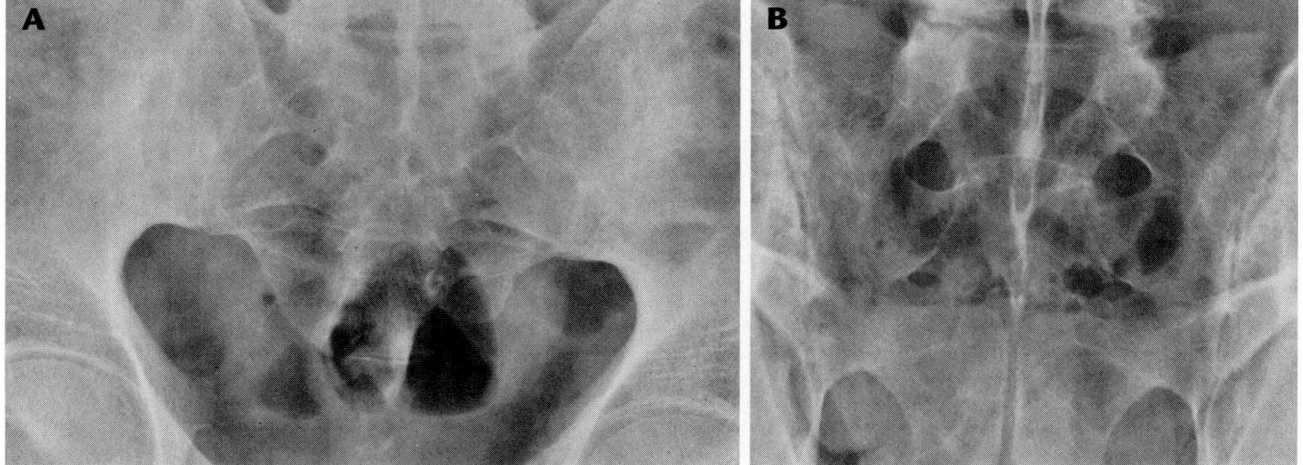

Figure 3–536. A, Erroneous diagnosis of ankylosing spondylitis based on appearance of the sacroiliac joints. **B,** Ferguson's view shows no abnormality.

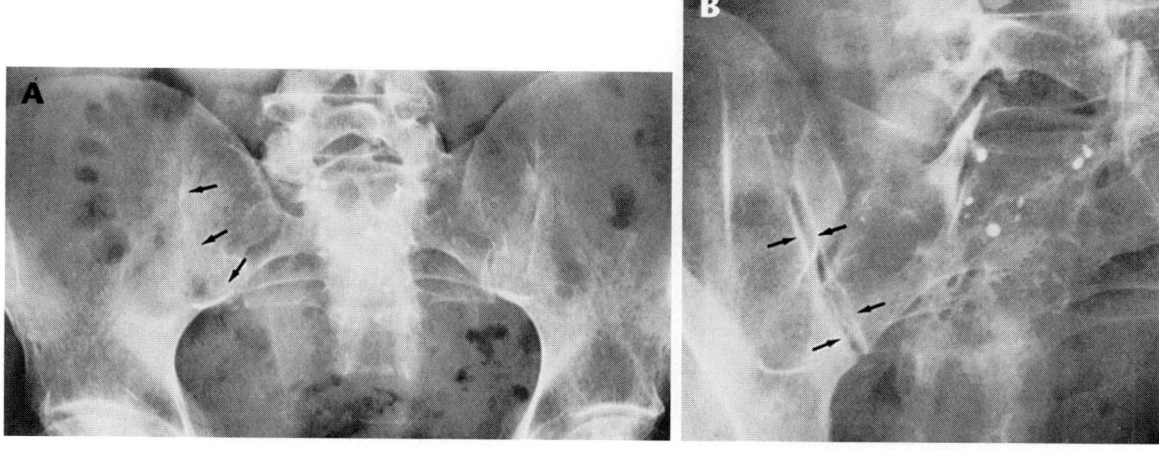

Figure 3–537. **A,** Simulated obliteration of the sacroiliac joint caused by slight rotation. This can be clarified by oblique projection of the sacroiliac joint **(B).**

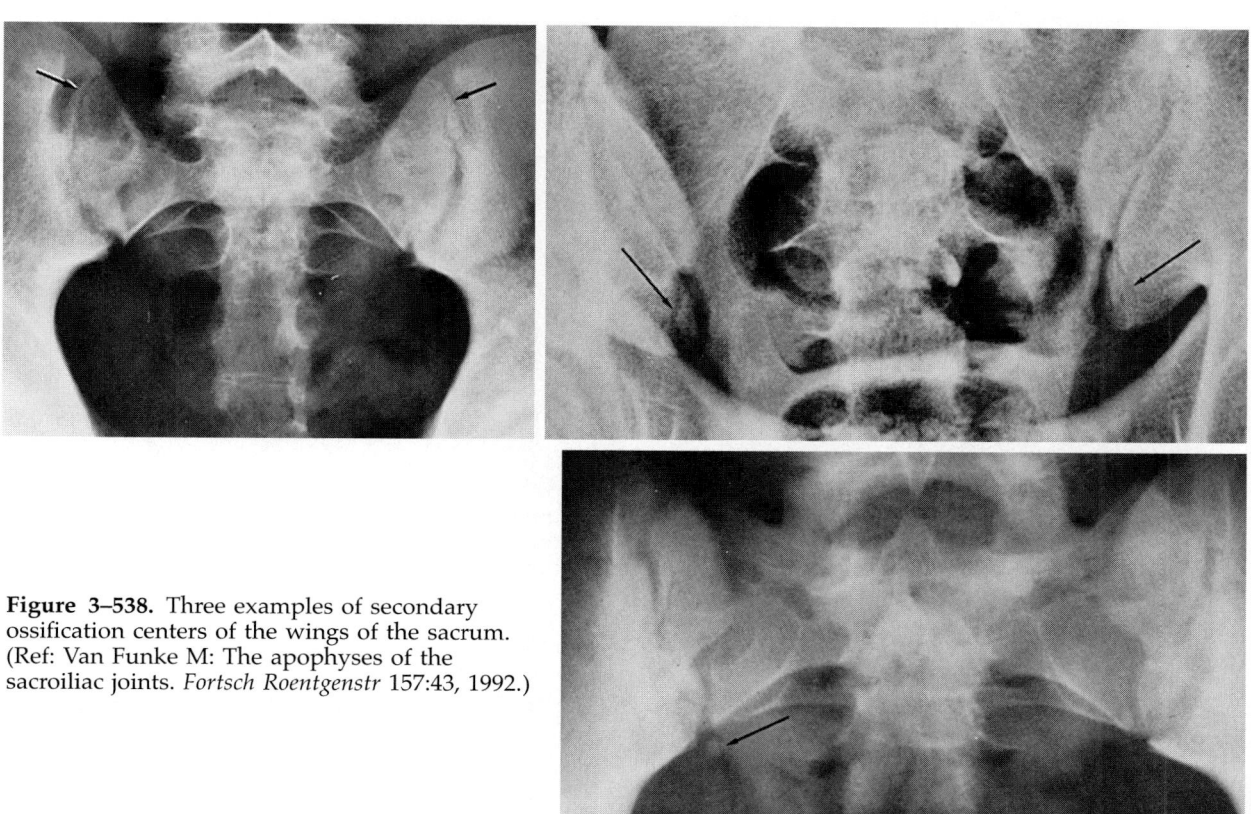

Figure 3–538. Three examples of secondary ossification centers of the wings of the sacrum. (Ref: Van Funke M: The apophyses of the sacroiliac joints. *Fortsch Roentgenstr* 157:43, 1992.)

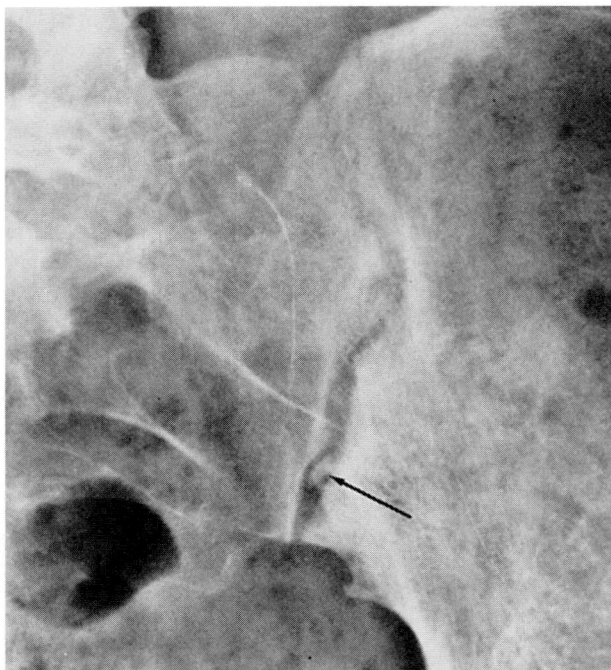

Figure 3–539. Persistence of a secondary center of ossification of the sacrum in a 25-year-old woman.

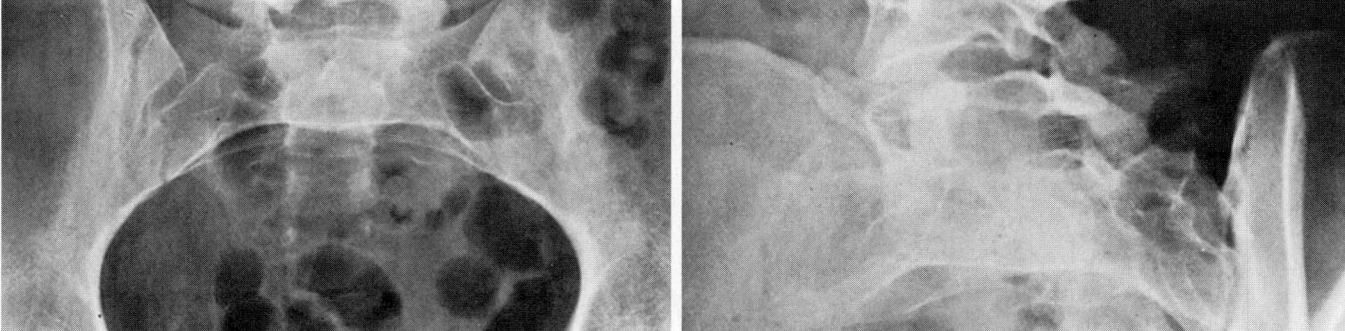

Figure 3–540. *Left,* Apparent absence of the left sacroiliac joint caused by different plane of orientation of the joint compared with the patient's right side. *Right,* Oblique projection shows an intact left sacroiliac joint.

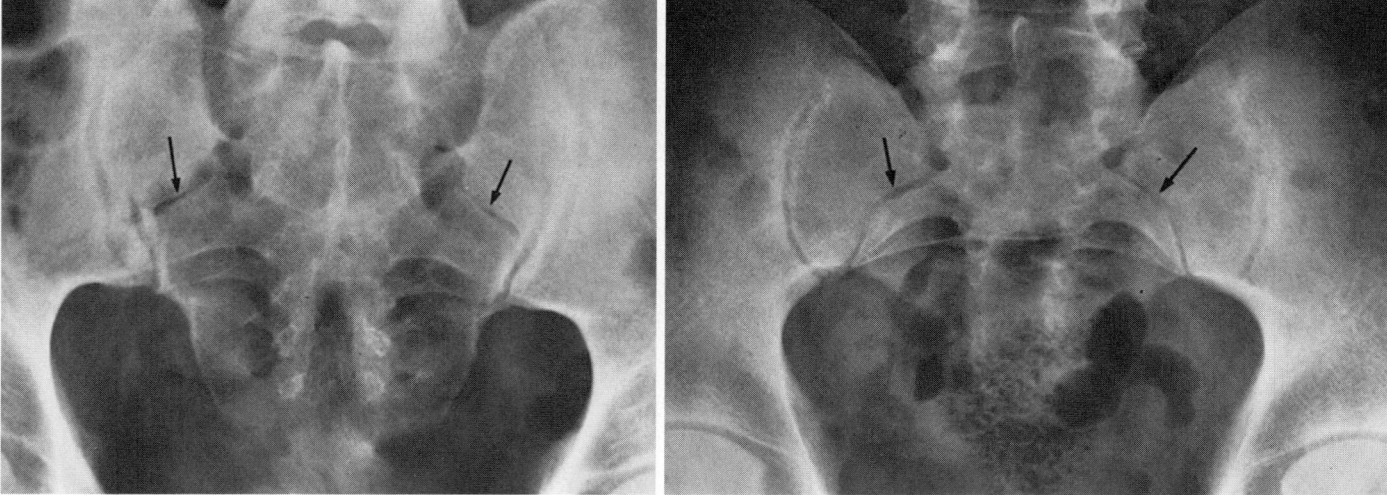

Figure 3–541. Two examples of bilateral accessory sacroiliac joints. (Ref: Ehara S et al: The accessory sacroiliac joint: A common anatomic variant. *Am J Roentgenol* 150:857, 1988.)

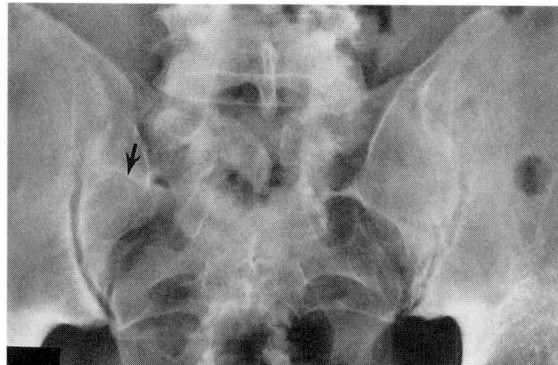

Figure 3–542. Secondary sacroiliac joint on the right. Note the unusual clarity of the right sacroiliac joint compared with the left.

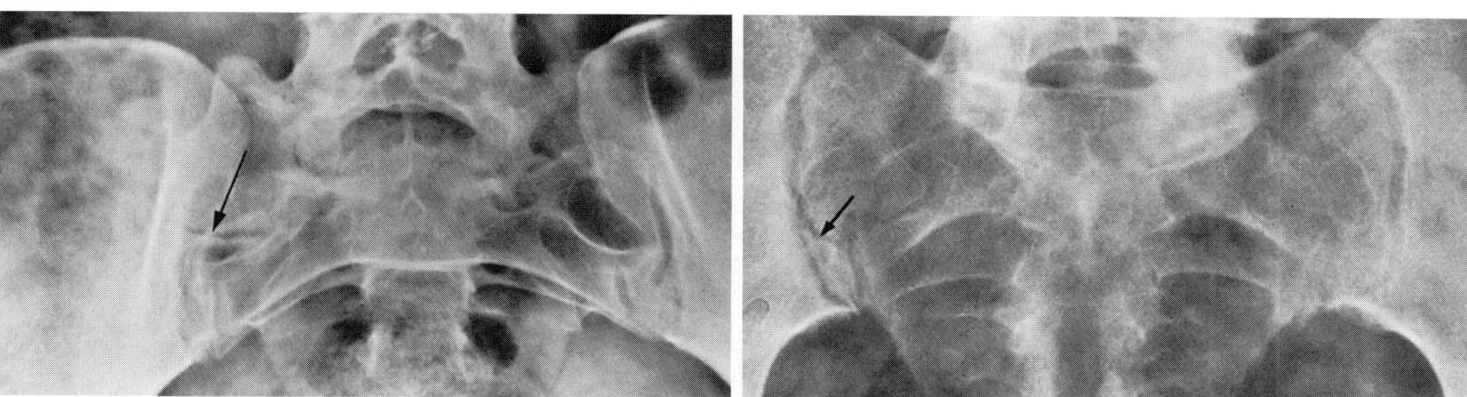

Figure 3–543. Unilateral accessory sacroiliac joints that might be mistaken for fractures.

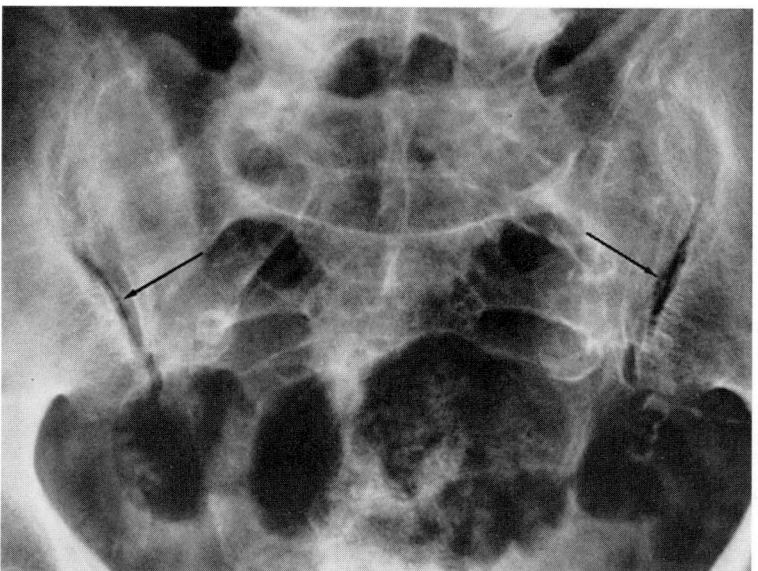

Figure 3–544. Vacuum phenomena in the sacroiliac joints.

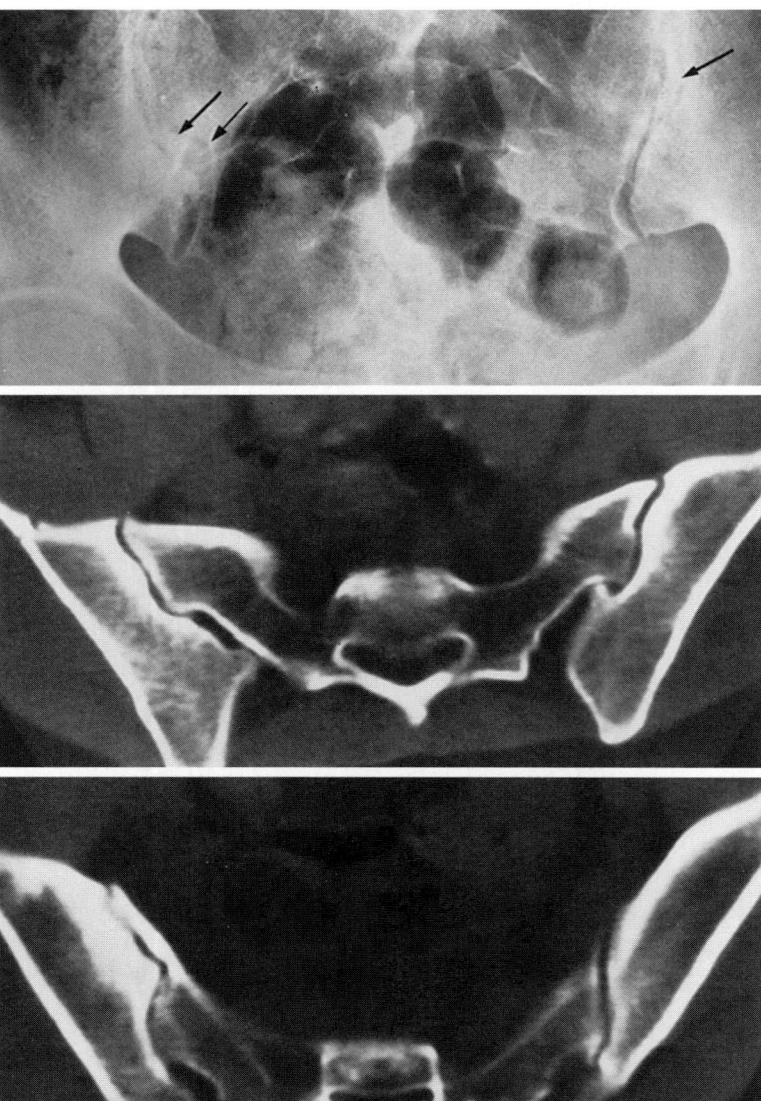

Figure 3–545. Variations in development of the sacroiliac joints *(top).* CT scans illustrate the normal asymmetries to better advantage *(center* and *bottom).*

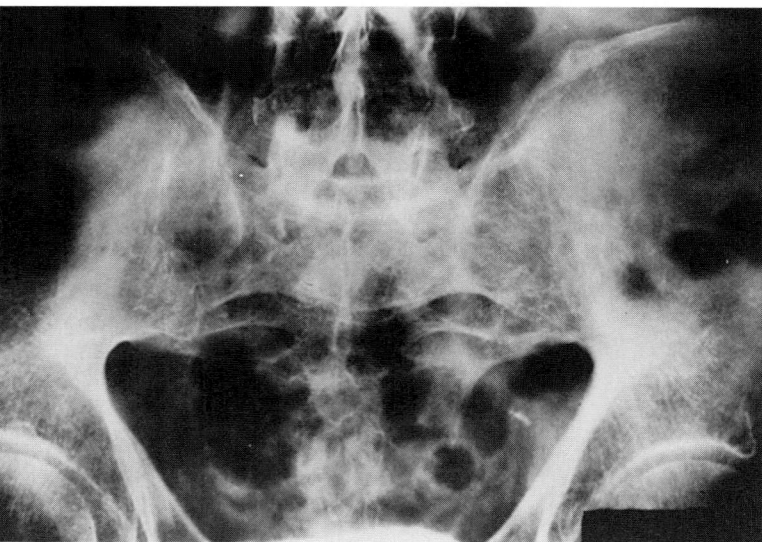

Figure 3–546. Obliteration of the sacroiliac joints in a 73-year-old man. This phenomenon apparently may occur in the absence of inflammatory spondylitis. (Ref: Resnick D et al: Clinical and radiographic abnormalities in ankylosing spondylitis: A comparison of men and women. *Radiology* 119:293, 1976.)

CHAPTER

4

The Pelvic Girdle

The Ilium

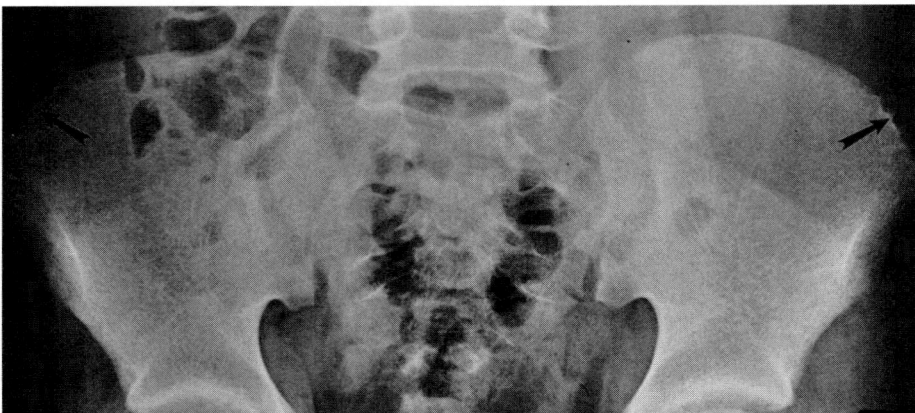

Figure 4–1. Normal irregularity of the iliac crest in a 9-year-old boy. This appearance is typical before the development of the secondary ossification center for the crest of the ilium.

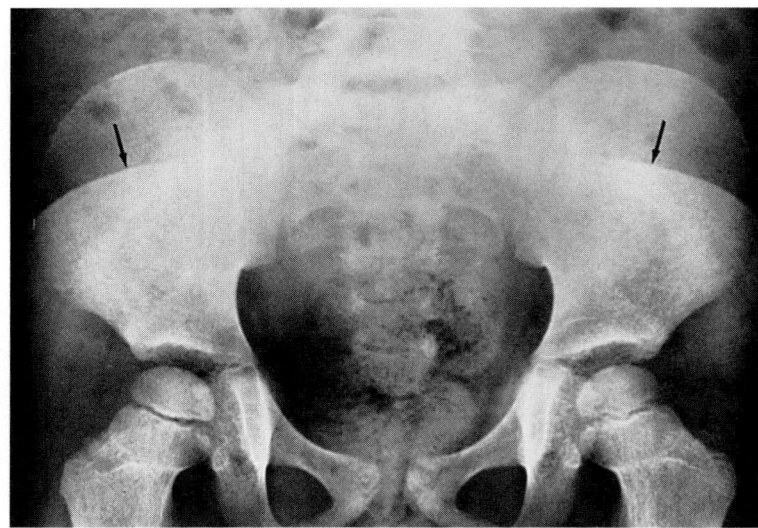

Figure 4–2. "Double" iliac wings produced by the shadow of the buttocks.

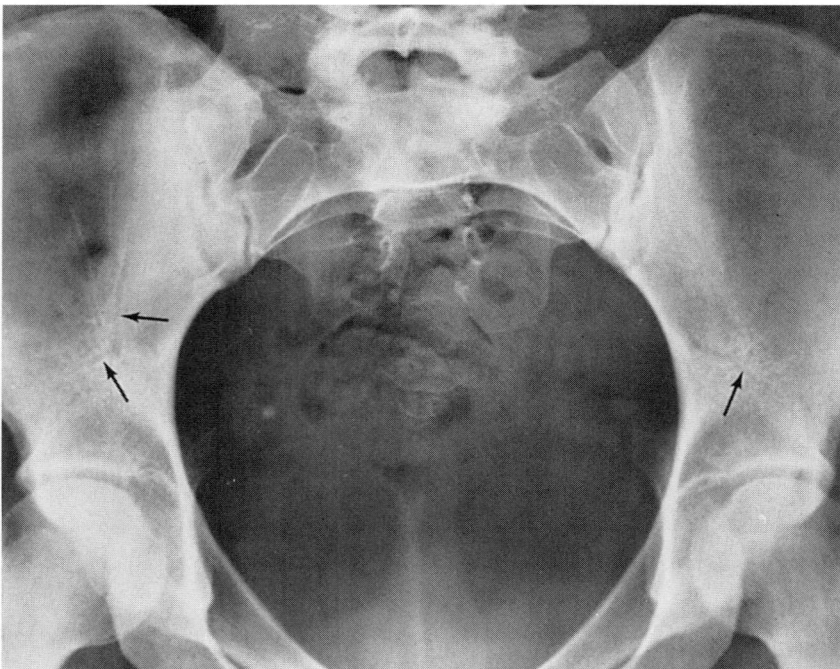

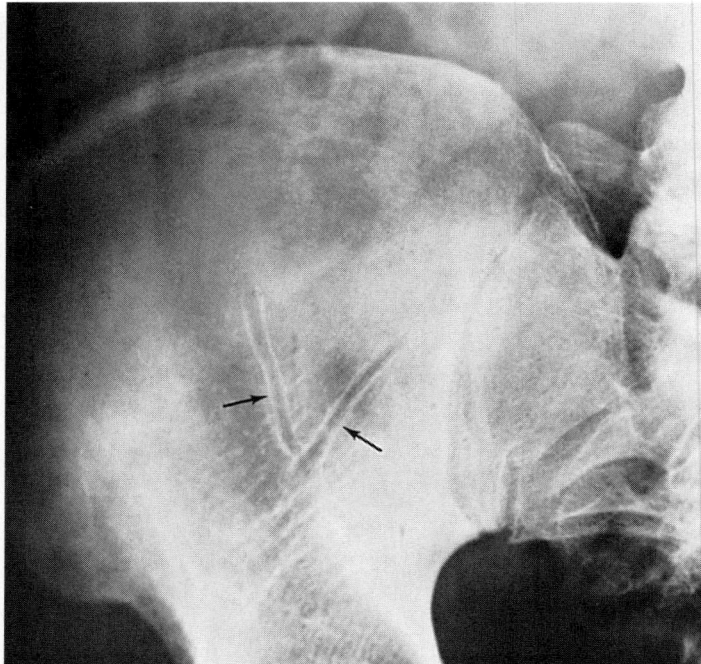

Figure 4–3. Examples of the grooves for the nutrient arteries of the ilium.

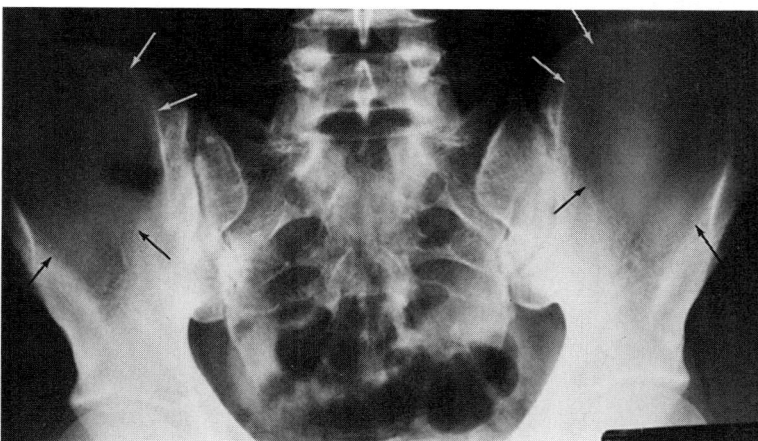

Figure 4–4. Normal lucency of the iliac fossae, which may resemble a cystic lesion in bone.

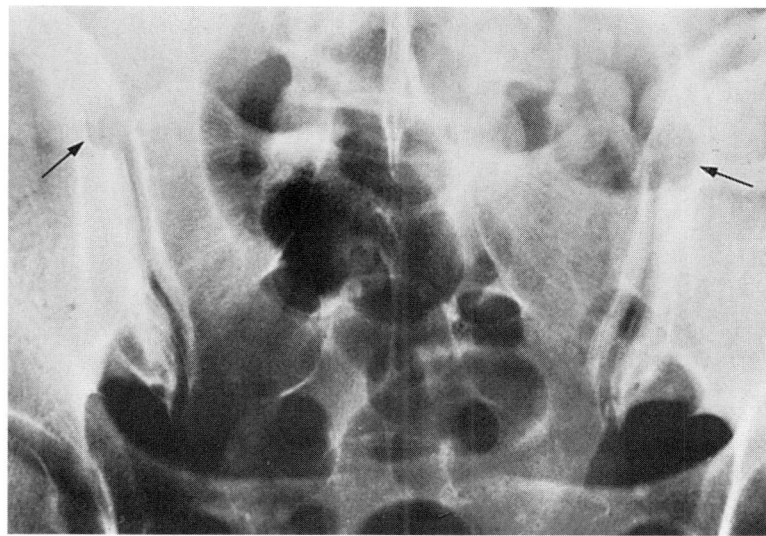

Figure 4–5. Unusual fossae in the ilia in a 37-year-old man.

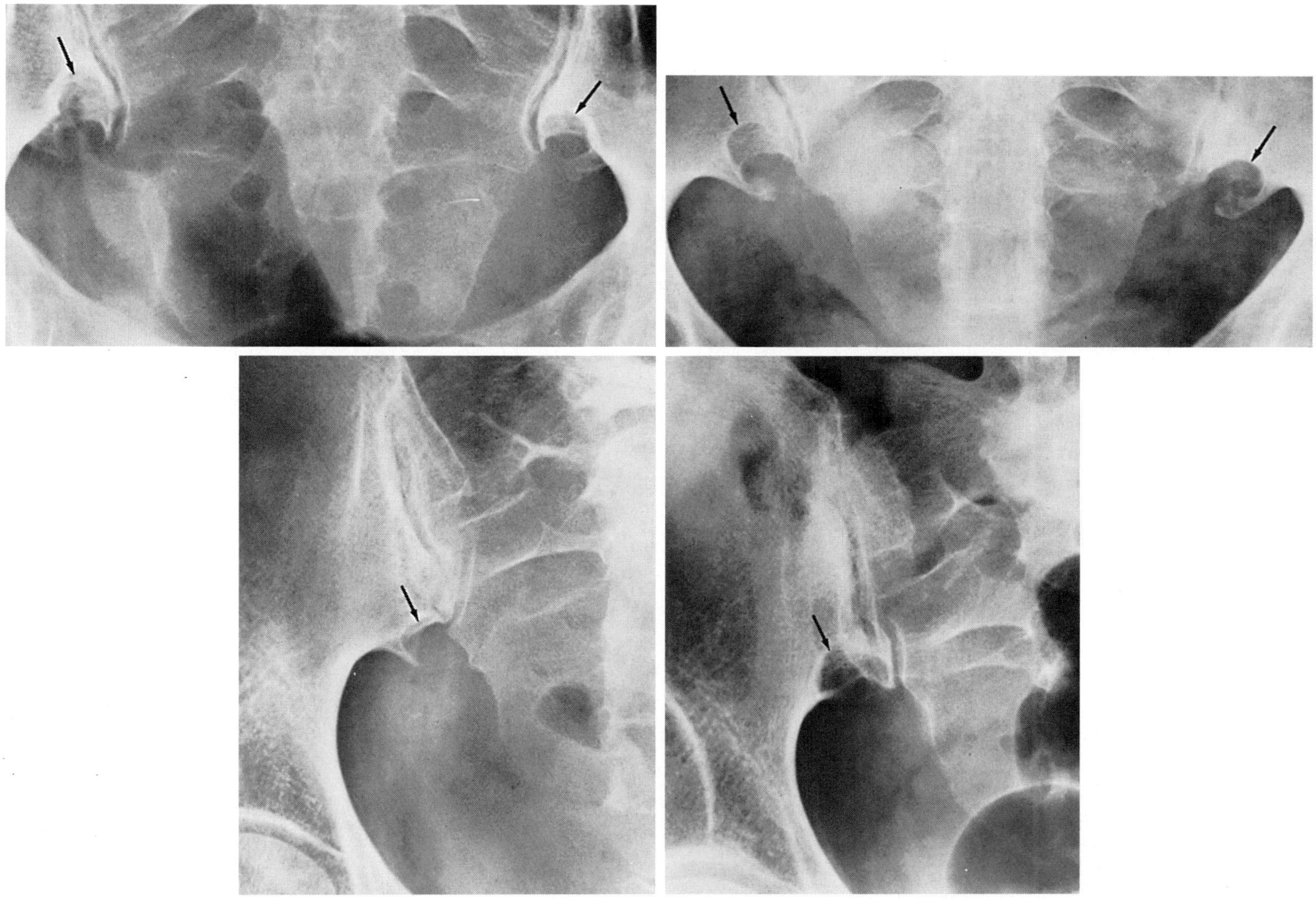

Figure 4–6. Examples of the preauricular sulcus (paraglenoid). This groove is due to resorption of bone at the insertion of the anterior sacroiliac ligament in response to stress. It is characteristic of the female pelvis and is not necessarily symptomatic. Very deep sulci are found only in parous women. (Refs: Dee PM: The preauricular sulcus. *Radiology* 140:354, 1981; Schemmer D et al: Radiology of the paraglenoid sulcus. *Skeletal Radiol* 24:205, 1994.)

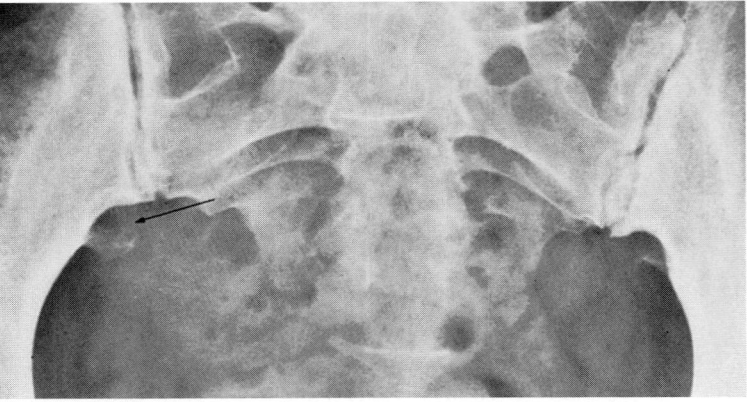

Figure 4–7. Unusual preauricular sulcus with asymmetry with opposite side.

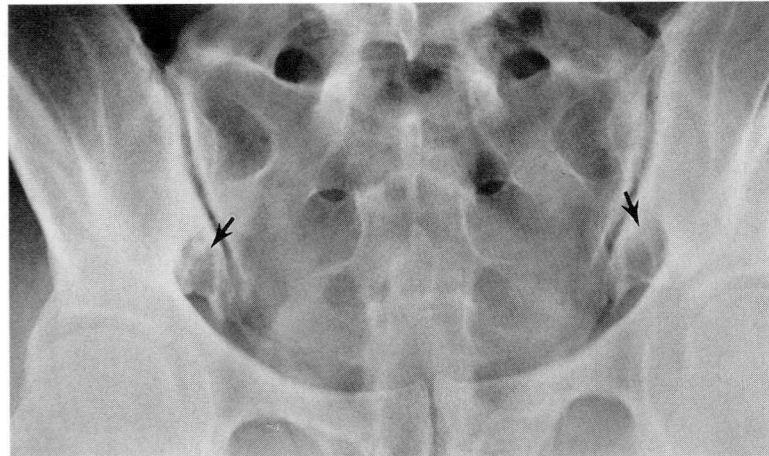

Figure 4–8. Paraglenoidal sulci simulating destructive lesions on the Ferguson view.

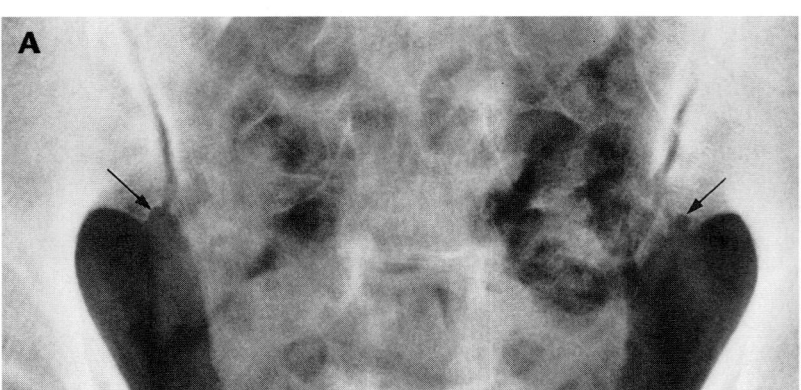

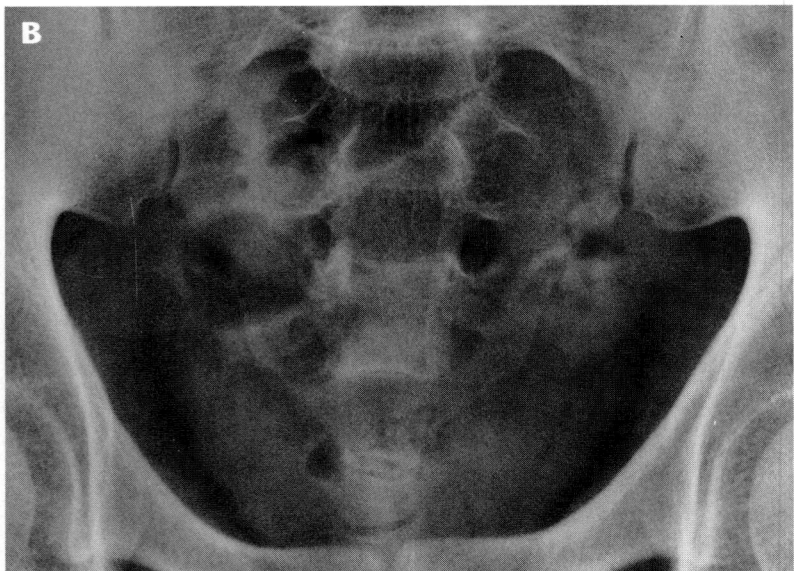

Figure 4–9. Small notches in the ilia in males, similar to the paraglenoidal sulci. **A,** 17-year-old boy. **B,** 50-year-old man.

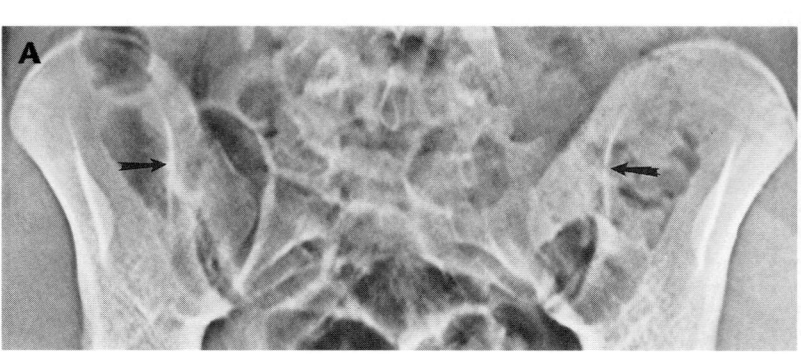

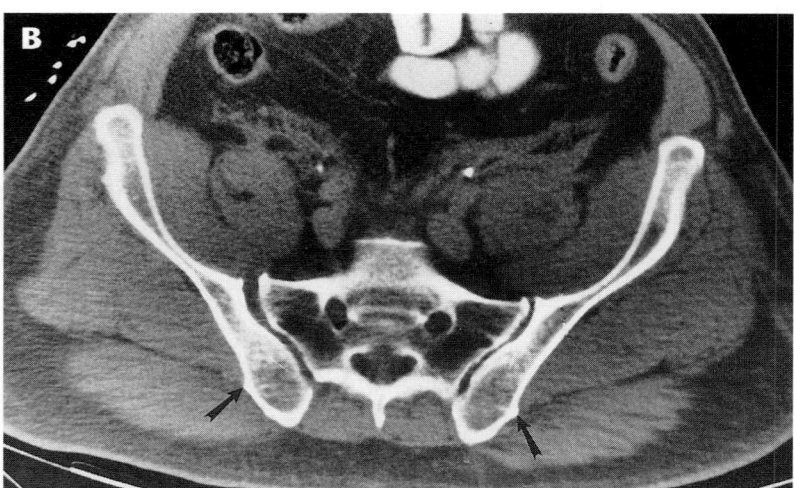

Figure 4–10. A, Crest between the insertions of the gluteus maximus and erector spinae muscles. **B,** CT showing the location of the crest.

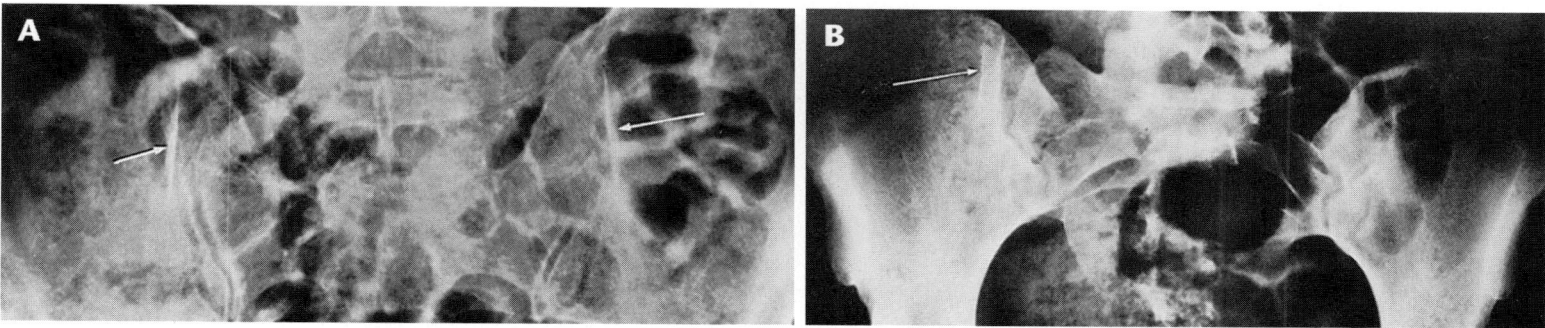

Figure 4–11. The crest illustrated in the preceding figure seen bilaterally in **A** and unilaterally in **B**, the latter originally misinterpreted as a fracture.

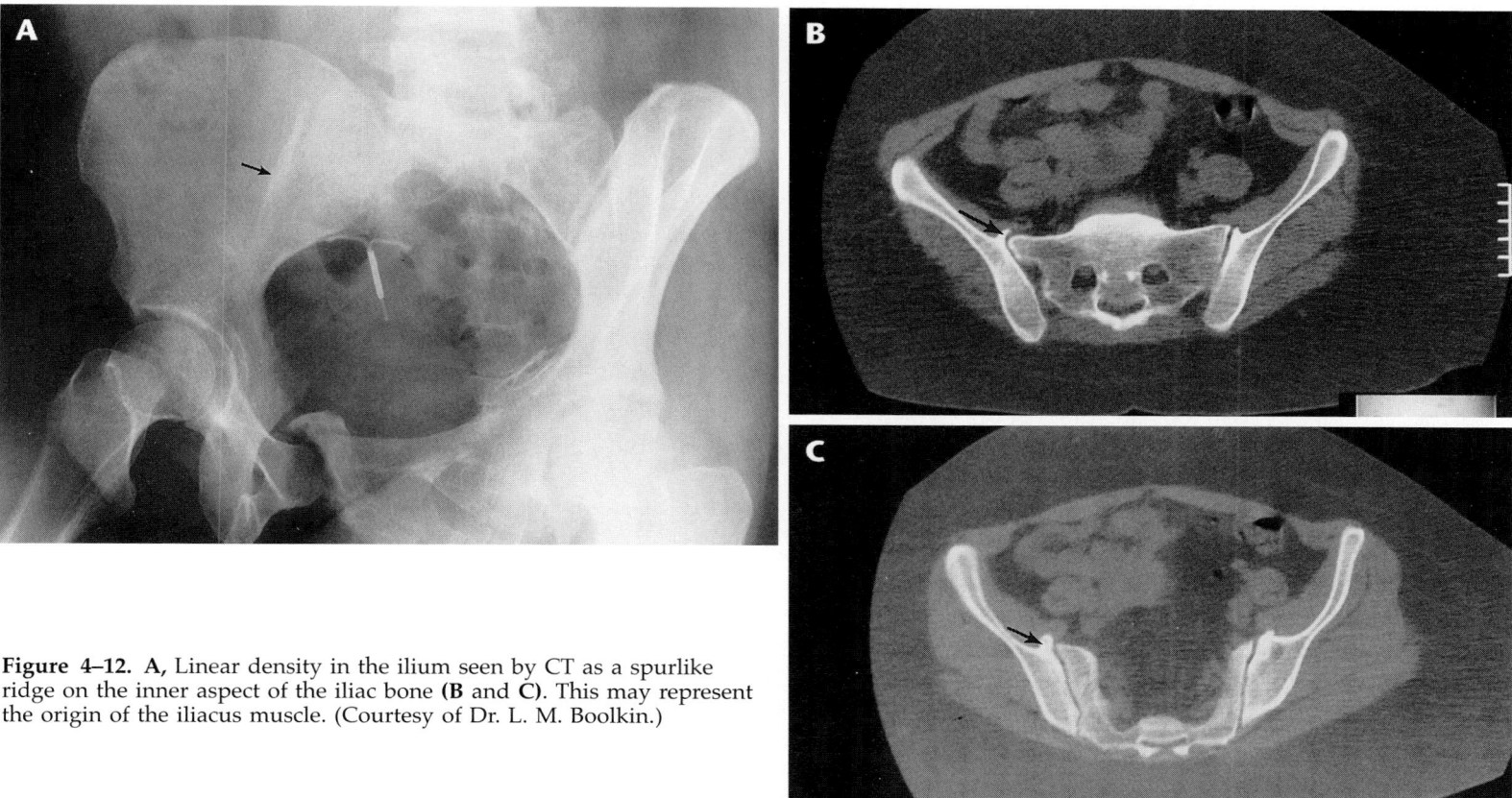

Figure 4–12. A, Linear density in the ilium seen by CT as a spurlike ridge on the inner aspect of the iliac bone **(B** and **C)**. This may represent the origin of the iliacus muscle. (Courtesy of Dr. L. M. Boolkin.)

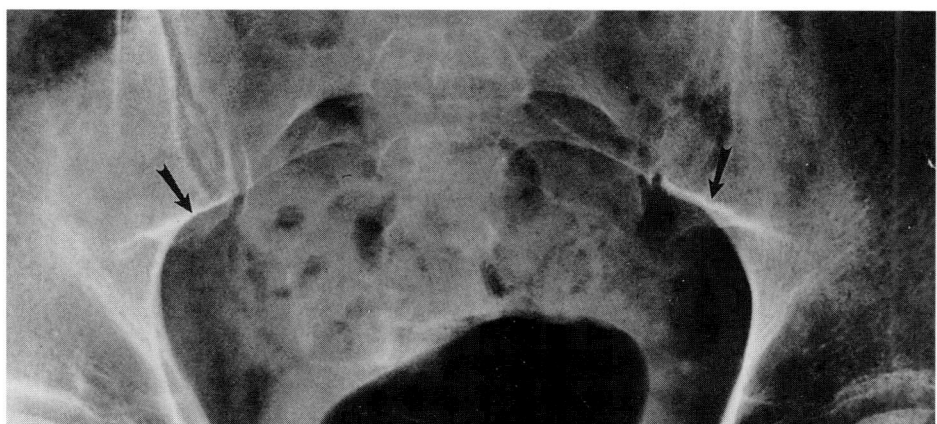

Figure 4–13. Dense white lines probably representing the roofs of the sciatic foramina.

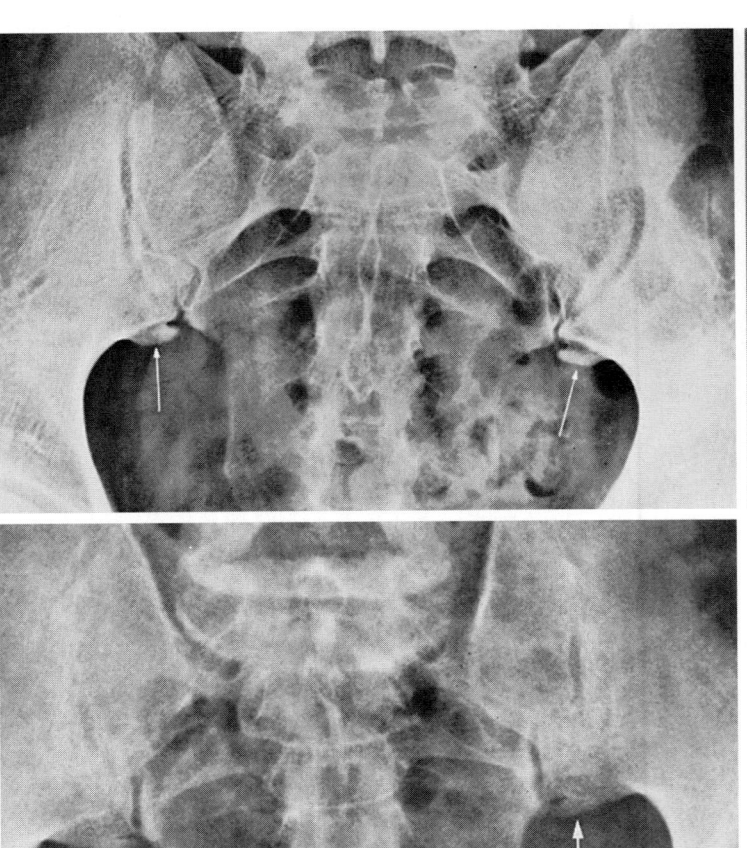
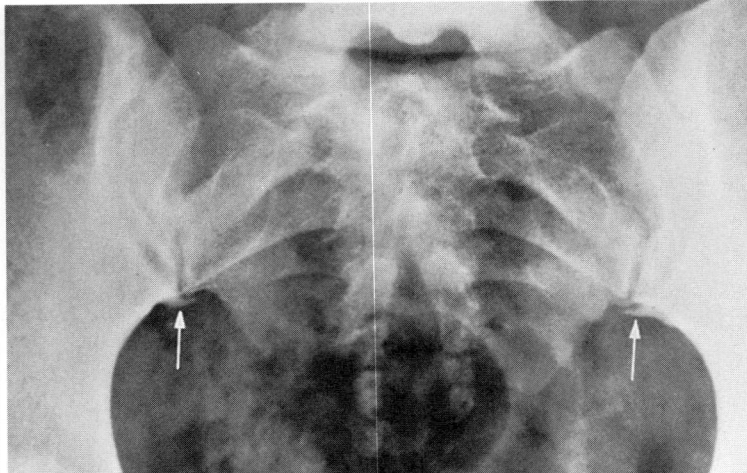

Figure 4–14. Developmental spurs at the inferior aspect of the sacroiliac joints. *Top left*, 30-year-old man. *Top right*, 30-year-old woman. *Bottom*, 55-year-old man.

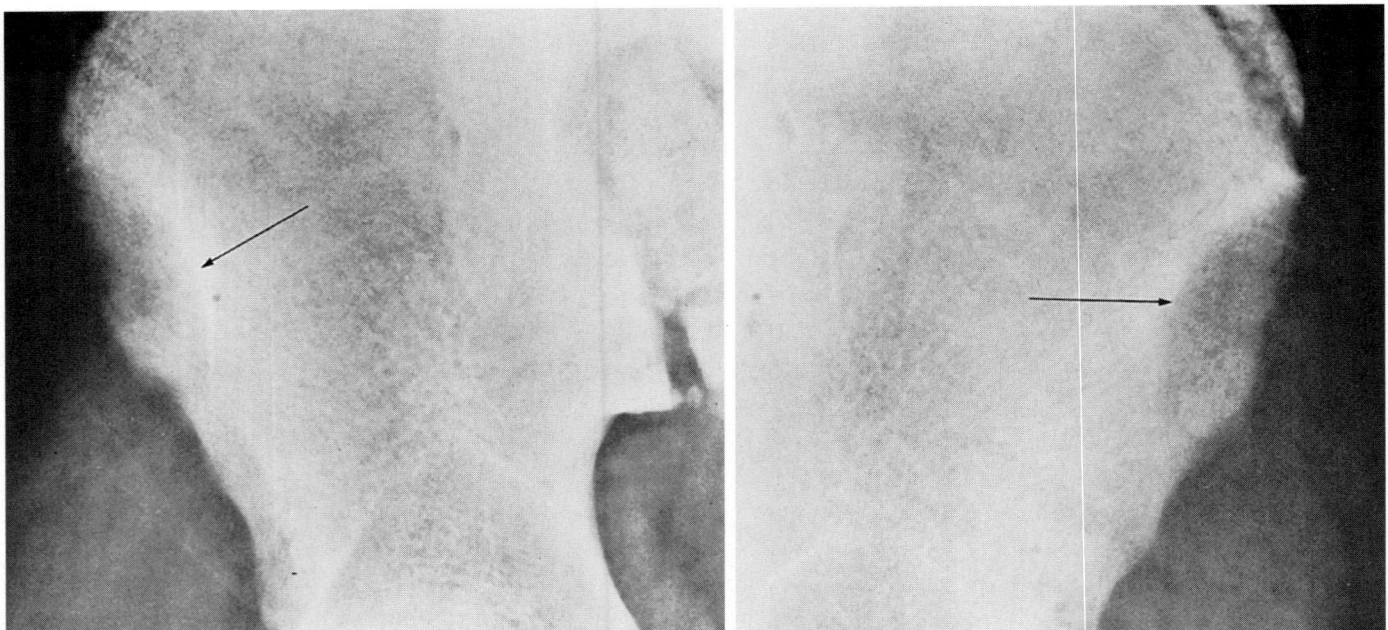

Figure 4–15. Irregular ossification of the ilium seen in adolescents, representing the origins of the sartorius muscle. These areas may mimic destructive lesions.

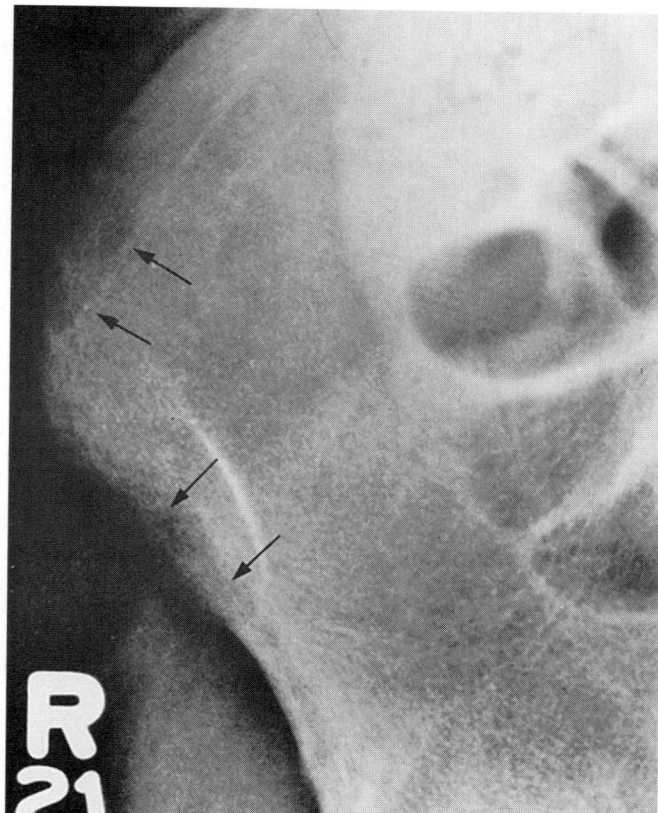

Figure 4–16. The same entity seen in the preceding figure, with more localized radiolucencies.

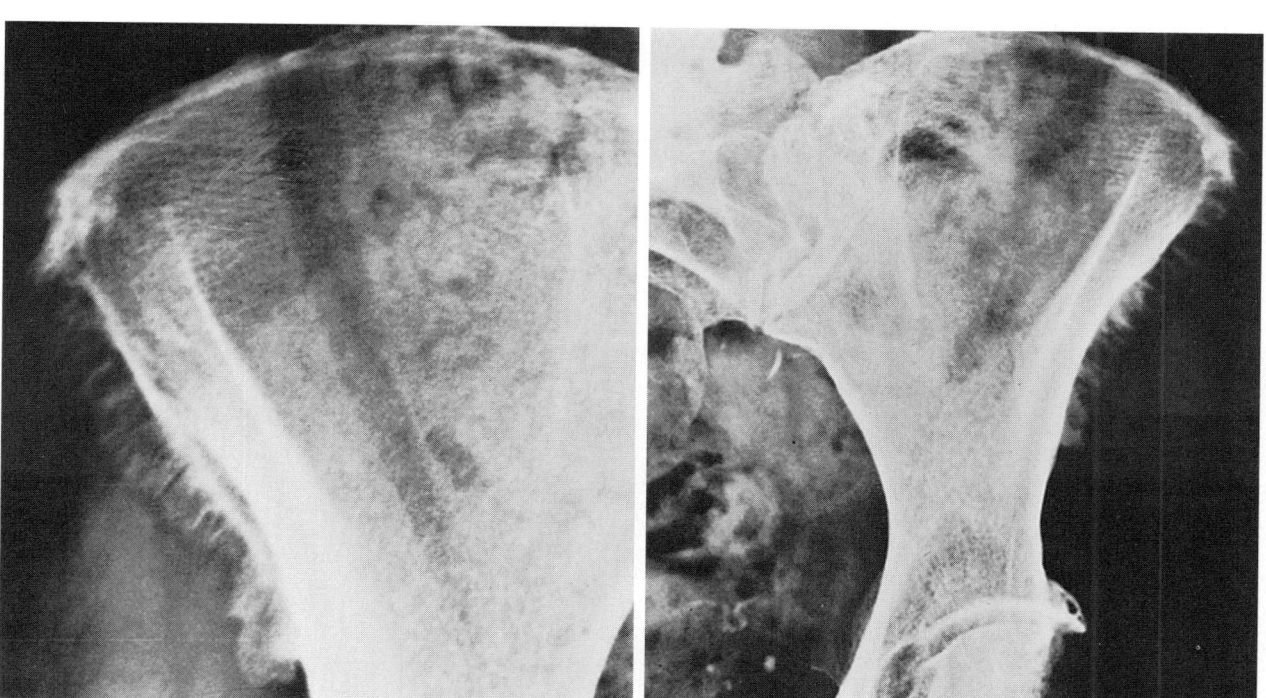

Figure 4–17. Spurring of muscle attachments at the ilium, seen in aged individuals.

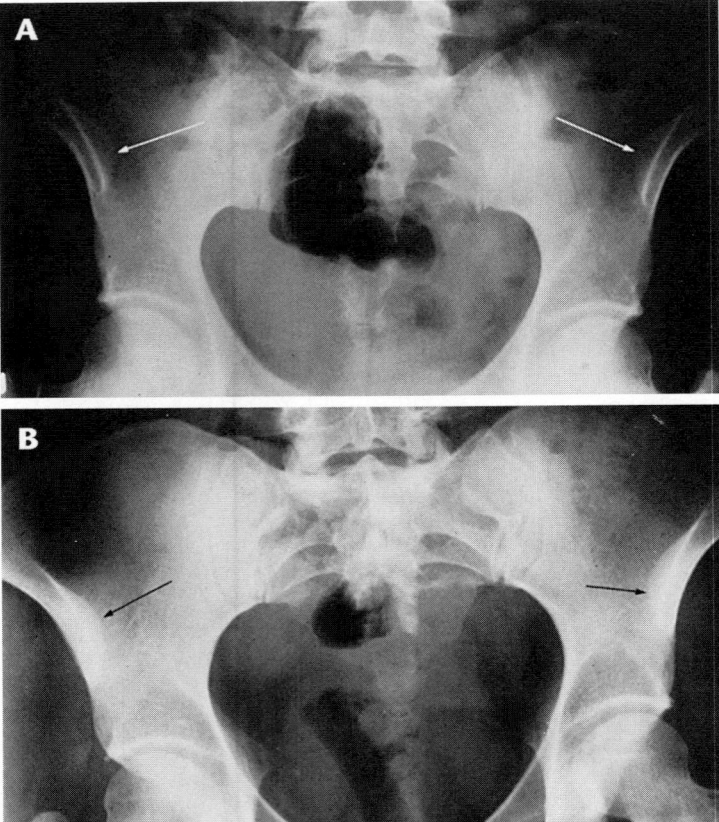

Figure 4–18. A, Flanges on the edge of the ilium, which may simulate sclerotic lesions **(B).**

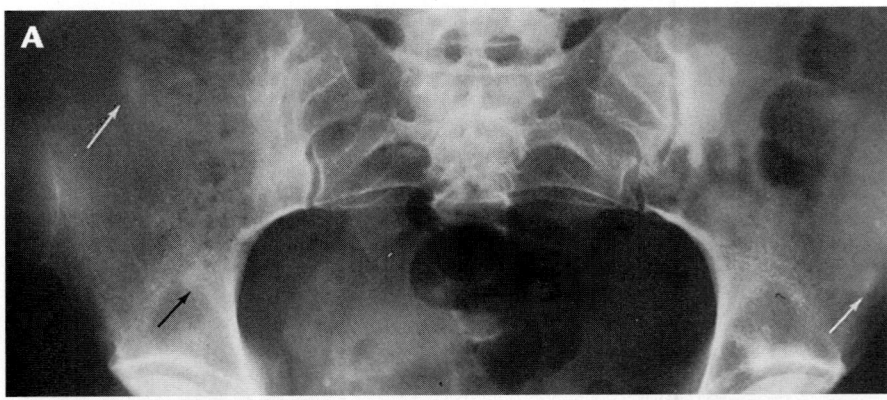

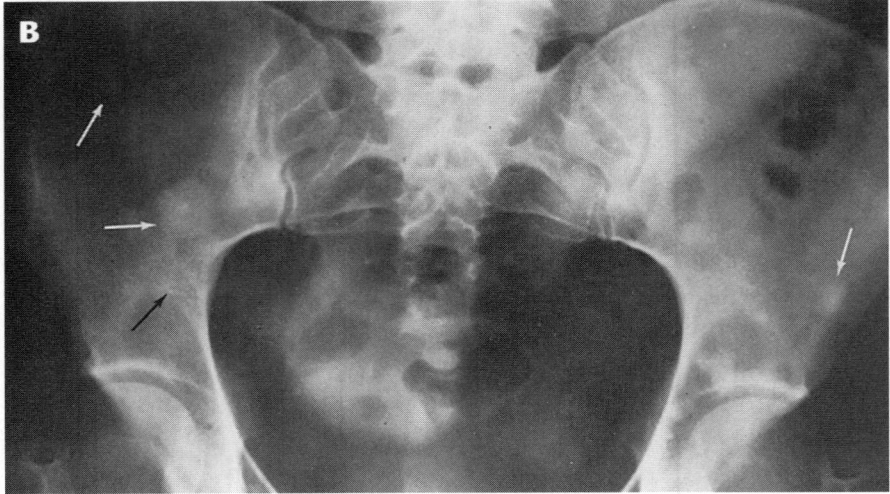

Figure 4–19. Growing bone islands in a normal male. There is a 4-year interval between **A** and **B**. (Ref: Blank N, Lieber A: The significance of growing bone islands. *Radiology* 85:508, 1965.)

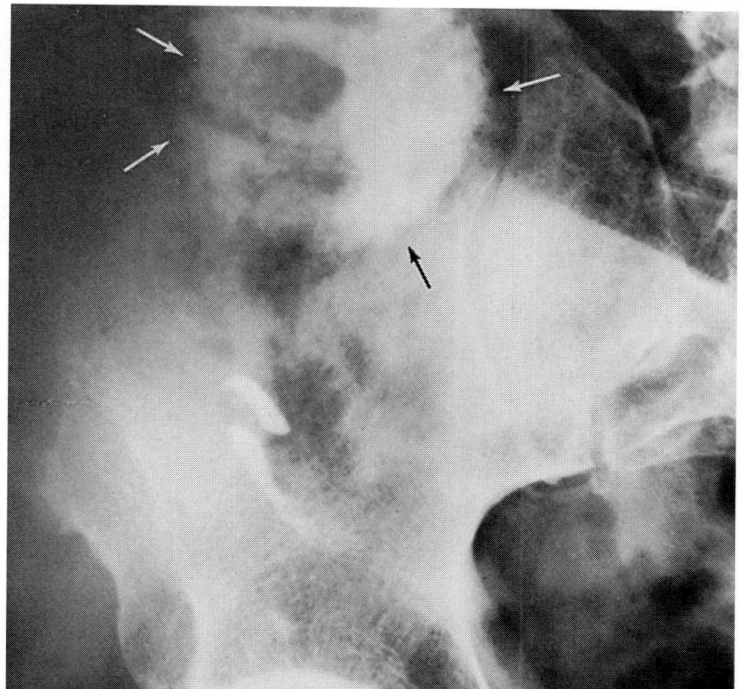

Figure 4–20. Giant bone island in a 60-year-old man. (Refs: Smith J: Giant bone islands. *Radiology* 107:35, 1973; Ehara S et al: Giant bone island: Computed tomography findings. *Clin Imag* 13:231, 1989.)

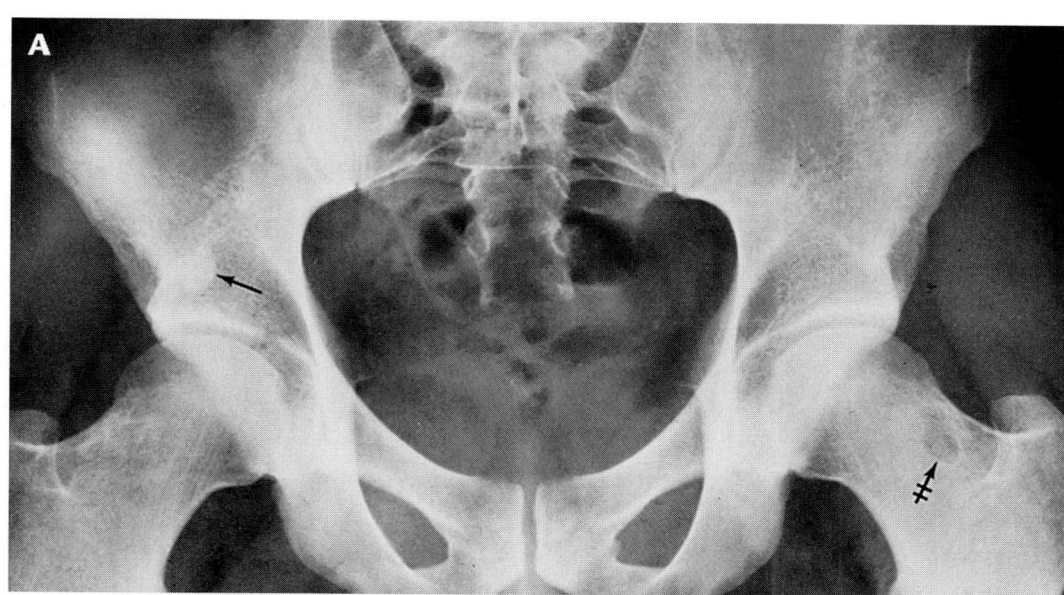

Figure 4–21. Iliac bone islands. **A,** Bone island in a 27-year-old man (←). These are common in the ilium, may grow, and occasionally disappear. They are of no clinical significance. A ring lesion (herniation pit) is present in the left femoral neck (⇇). **B,** Growing bone island in a young woman. **C,** Nine years later, the bone island has increased in size. (Ref: Kim SK, Barry WF Jr: Bone islands. *Radiology* 90:77, 1968.)

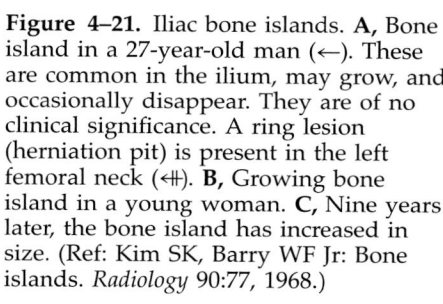

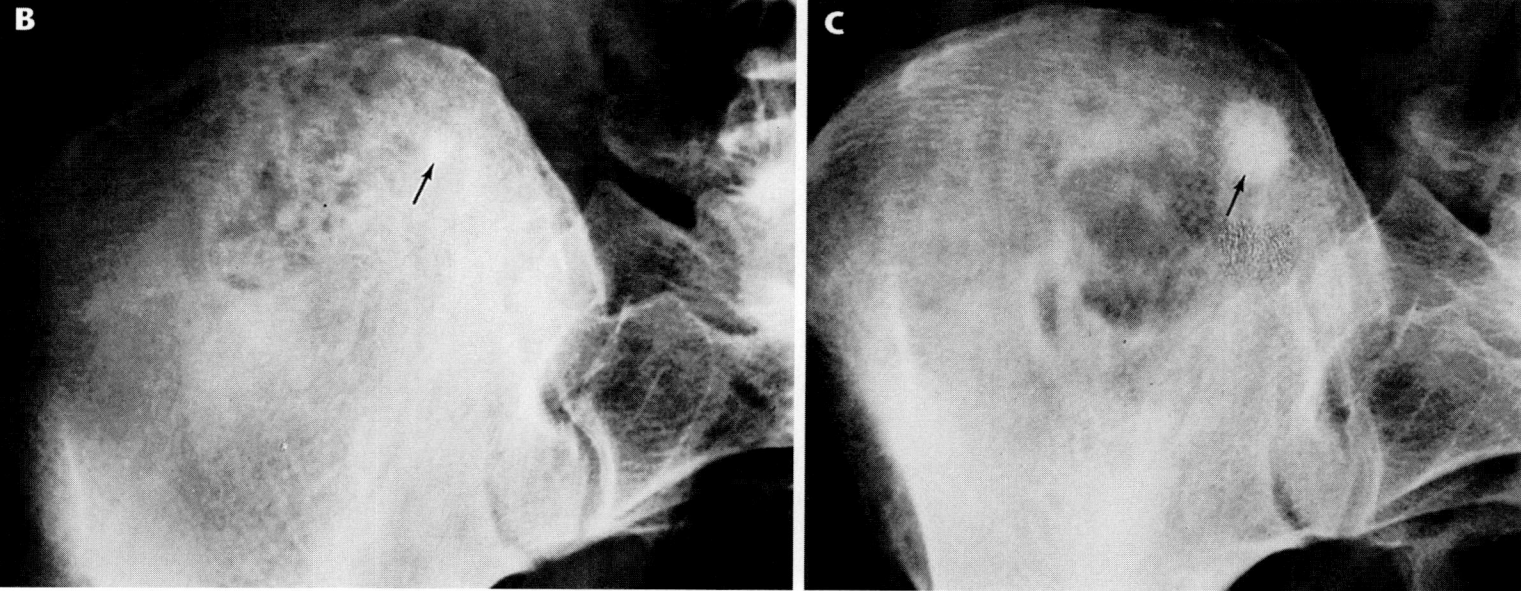

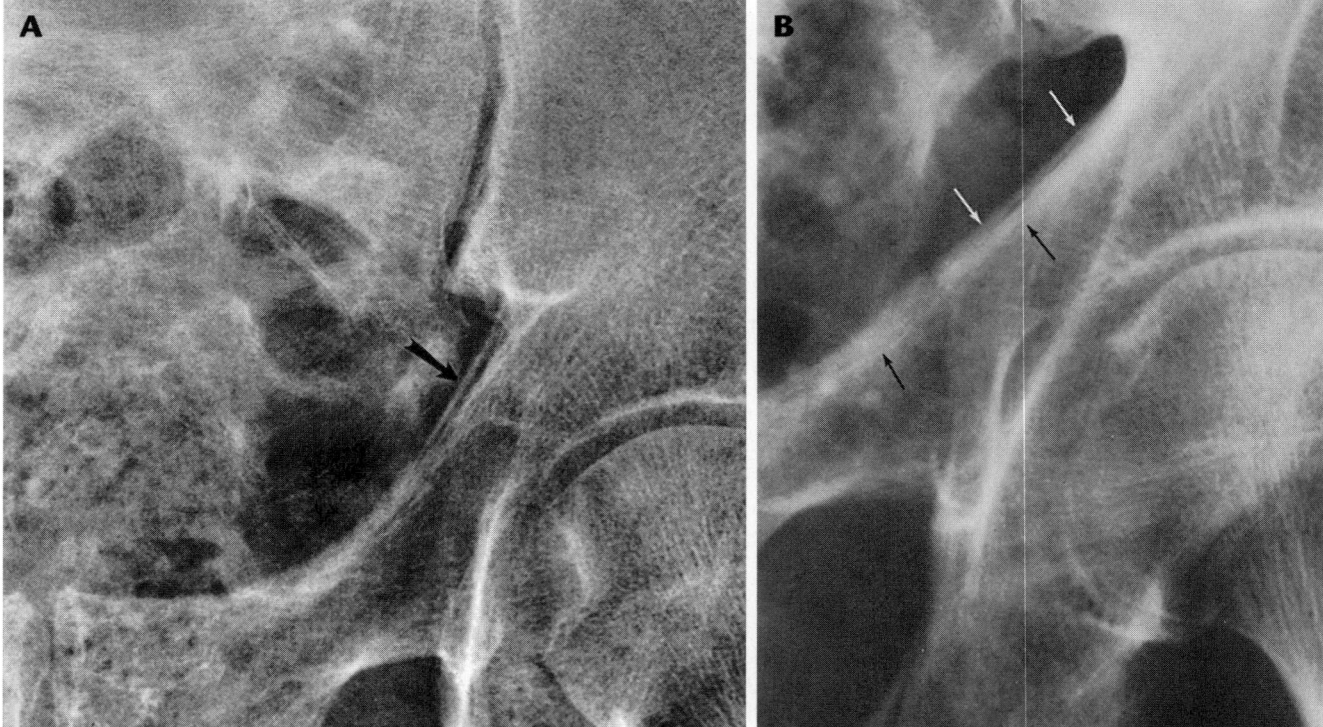

Figure 4–22. A, B, Two examples of normal aging changes in the pelvic brim. This alteration in elderly patients may be mistaken for periostitis or Paget's disease (→).

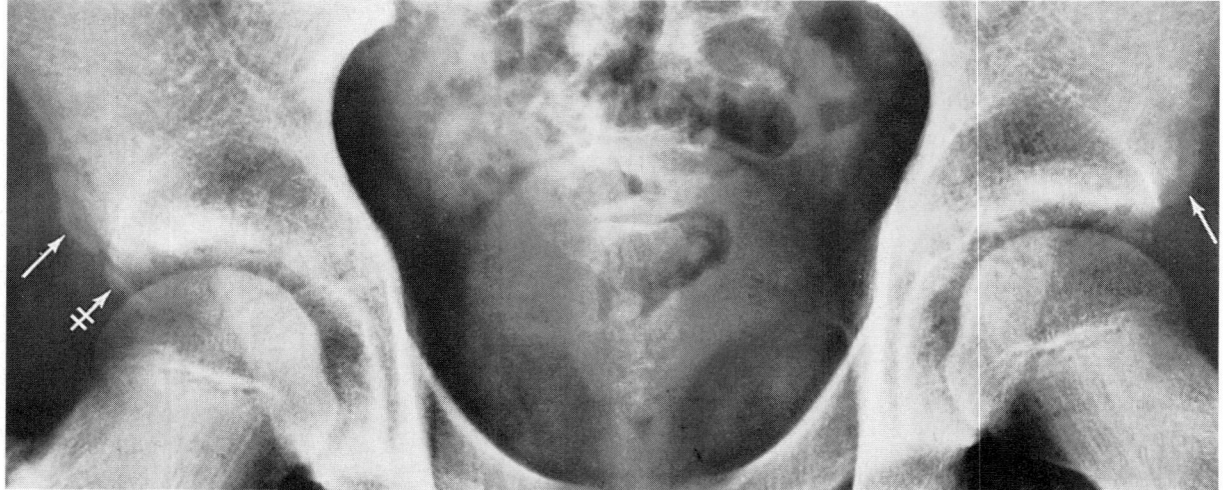

Figure 4–23. Ossification center for the anterior inferior iliac spine (←) and acetabular rim (⊀) in a 13-year-old boy.

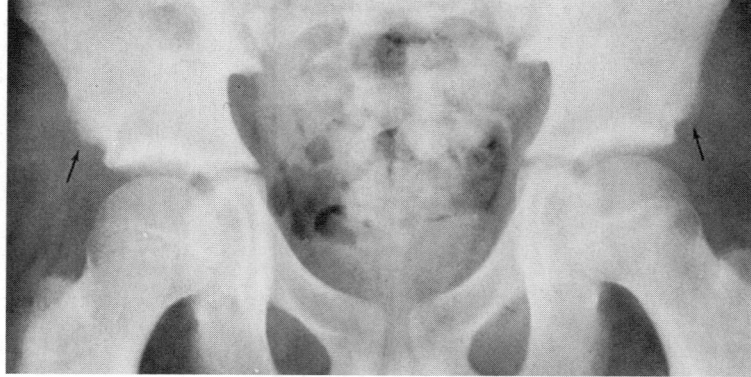

Figure 4–24. Prominent anterior inferior iliac spines in a 12-year-old boy.

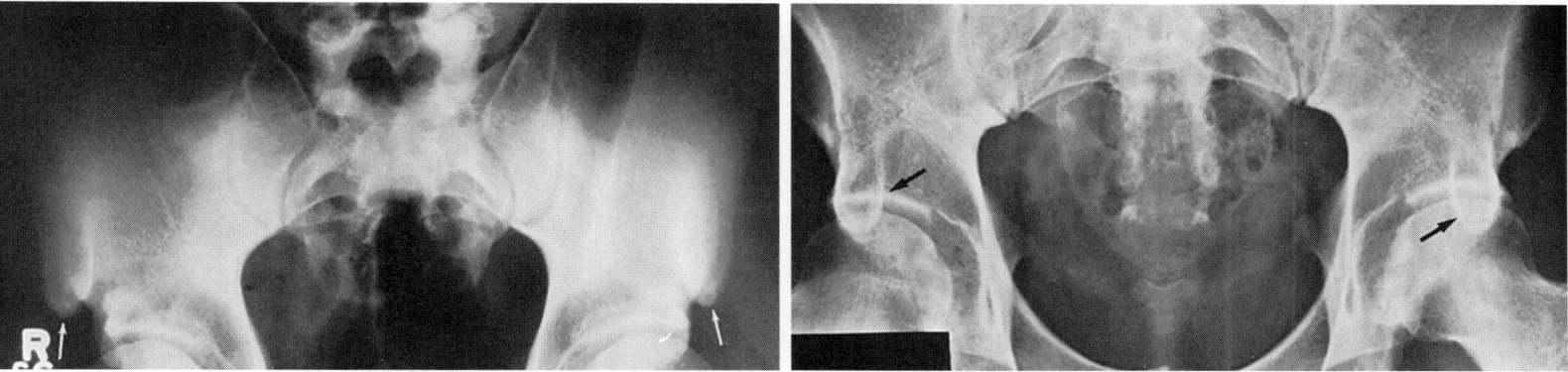

Figure 4–25. Two examples of pelvic "ears," a normal variant of development.

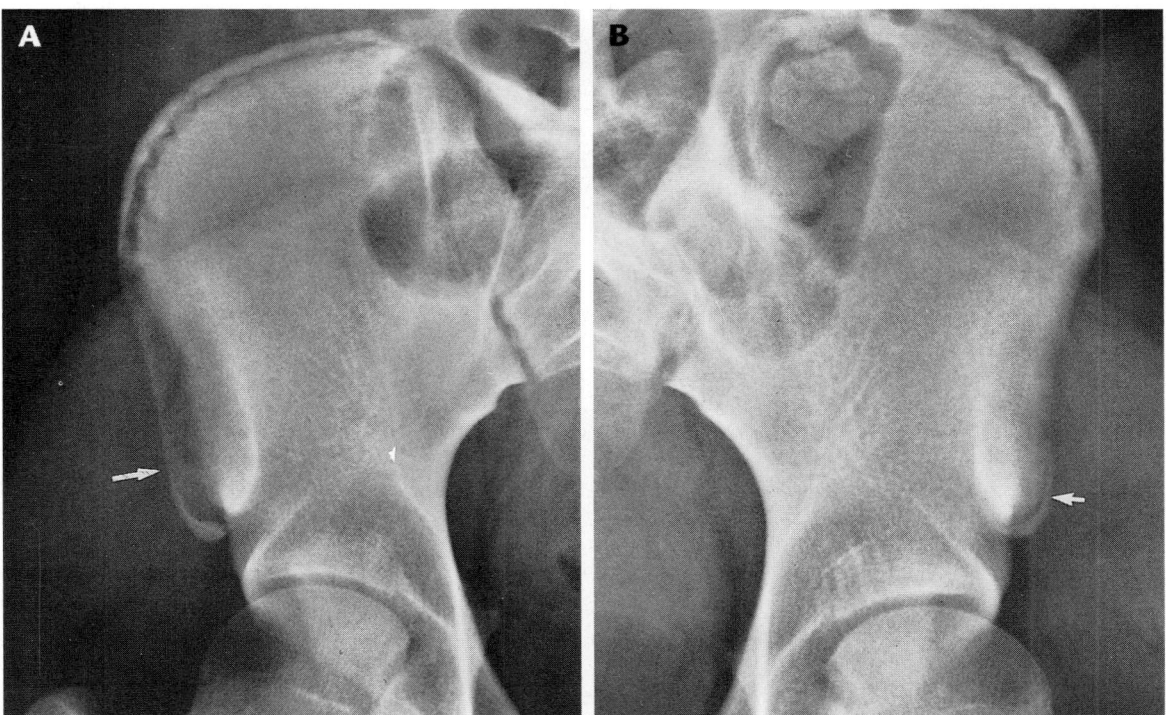

Figure 4–26. A, B, The development of pelvic "ears" is secondary to these long caudad extensions of the iliac apophyses seen in a 15-year-old boy.

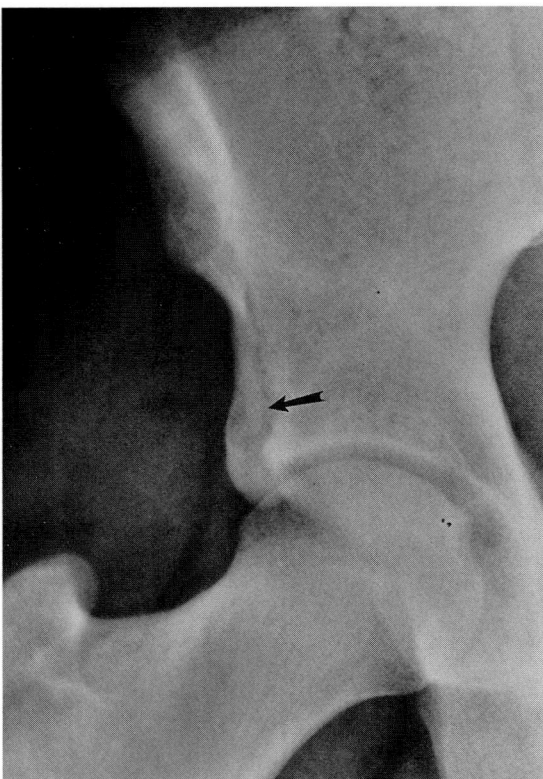

Figure 4–27. Partial closure of the apophyses illustrated in the preceding figure should not be mistaken for evidence of trauma.

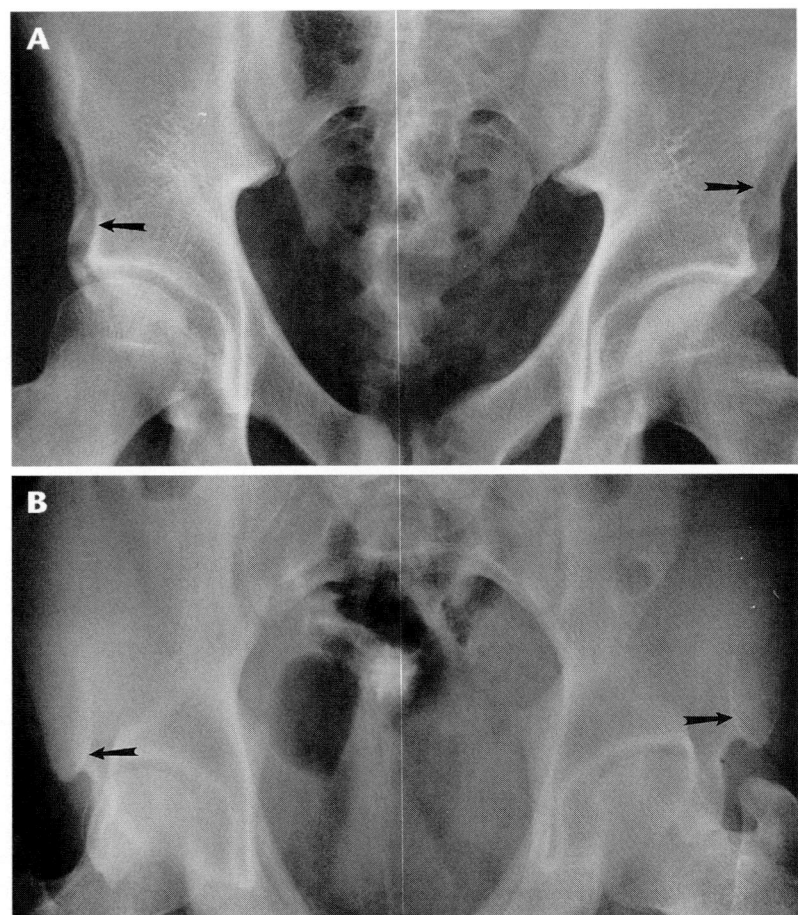

Figure 4–28. A, Large pelvic "ears" may be mistaken for a fracture in the anteroposterior view of the pelvis. **B,** Pelvic "ears" demonstrated in pelvic inlet view.

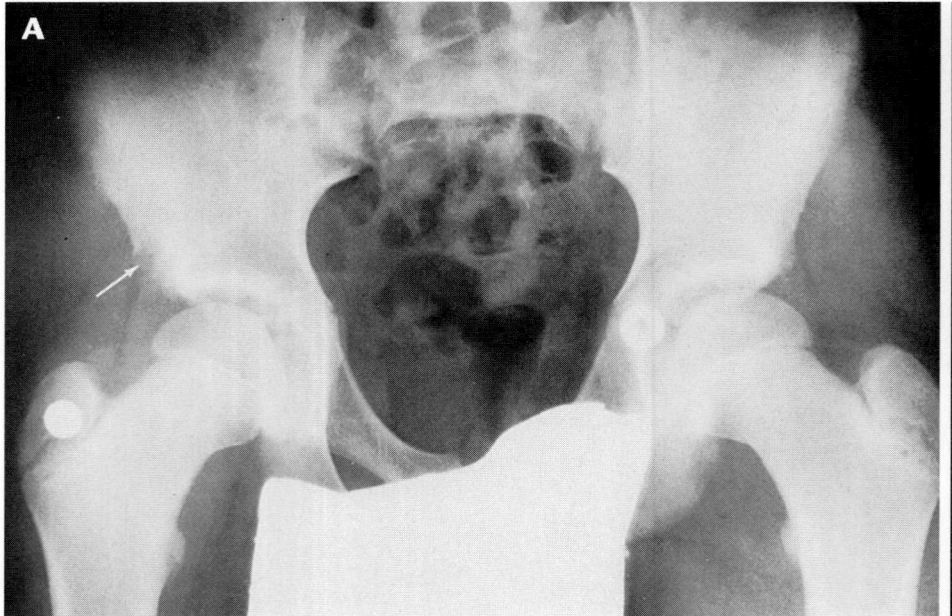

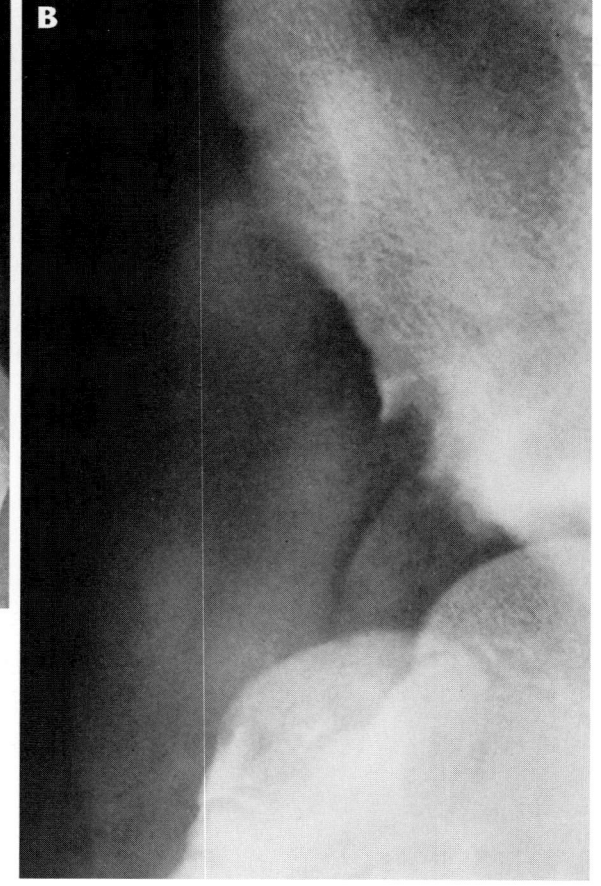

Figure 4–29. A, Irregularity of the anterior inferior iliac spine in an adolescent boy. This represents a "tug" lesion at the insertion of the rectus femoris muscle and should not be mistaken for the changes of neoplasm. **B,** Enlargement of area of interest. Note that the muscle planes are not disturbed. (Ref: Murray RO, Jacobson HG: *The radiology of skeletal disorders,* 2nd ed. New York, Churchill Livingstone, 1977, p. 274.)

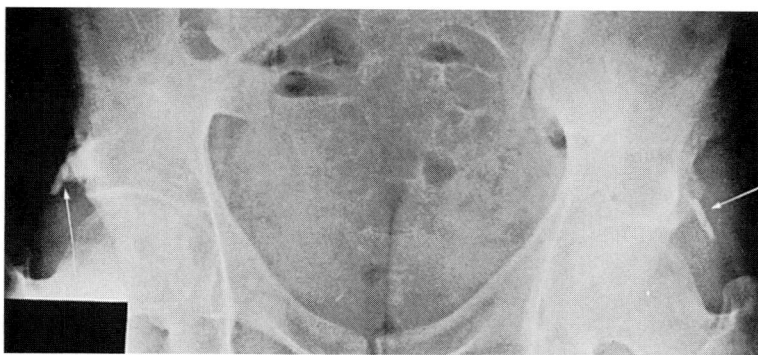

Figure 4–30. Old healed avulsive lesions of the anterior inferior iliac spines.

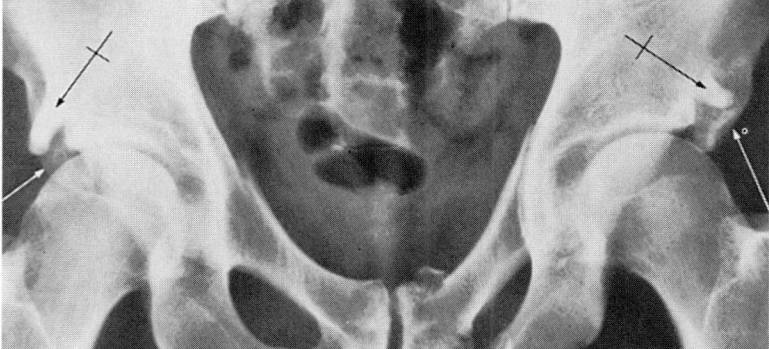

Figure 4–31. Combined pelvic "ears" (→) and healed "avulsive" lesions (↦) of the anterior inferior iliac spine in a 24-year-old man with pelvic fractures.

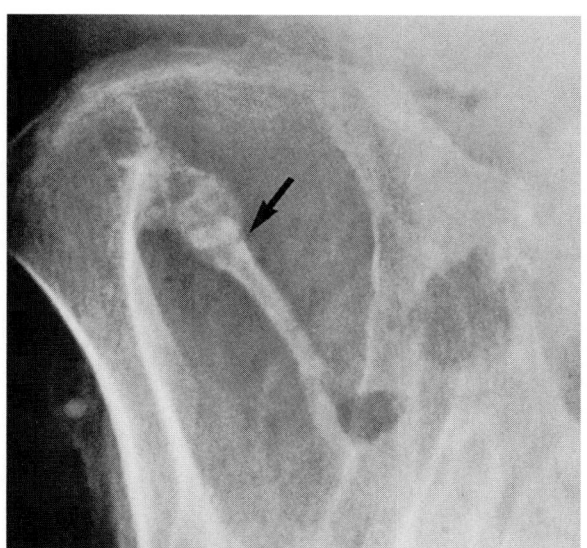

Figure 4–32. An iliac rib (pelvic digit), a developmental anomaly. Note pseudoarticulation (←). (Ref: Greenspan A, Norman A: The "pelvic digit"—An unusual developmental anomaly. *Skeletal Radiol* 9:118, 1982.)

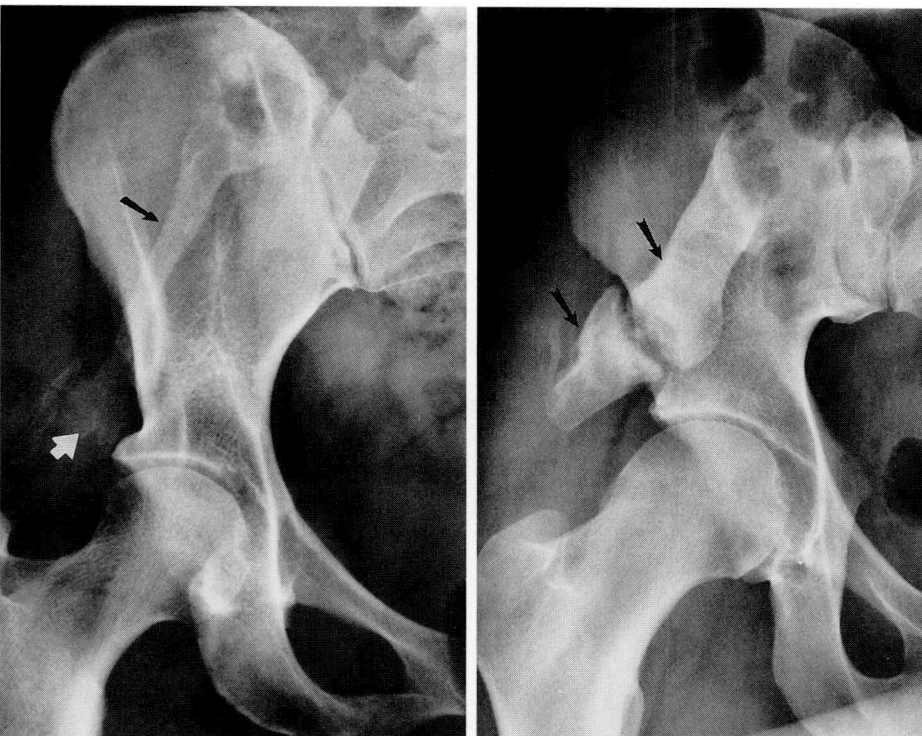

Figure 4–33. Two additional examples of pelvic digits. (Ref: Granieri GF, Bacarini L. The pelvic digit. *Skeletal Radiol* 25:723, 1996.)

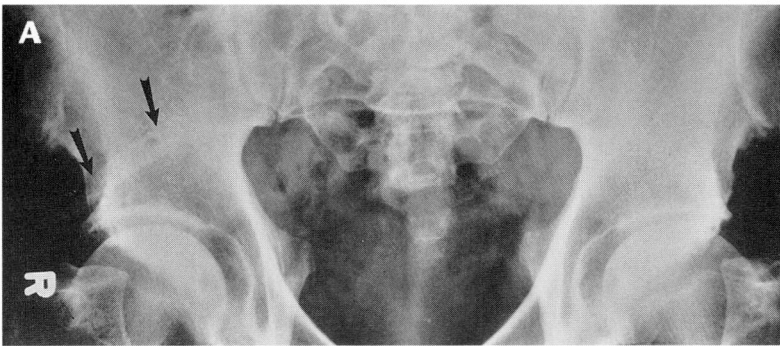

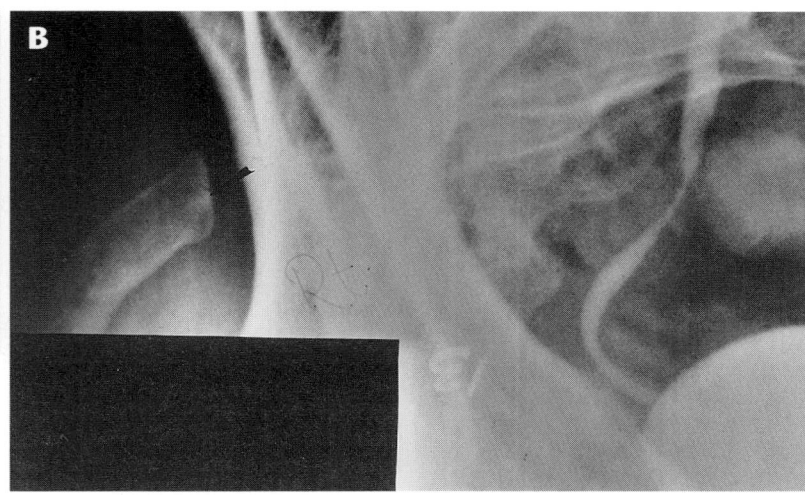

Figure 4–34. Pelvic digit with large extrailiac component. **A,** Frontal projection. **B,** Left posterior oblique projection.

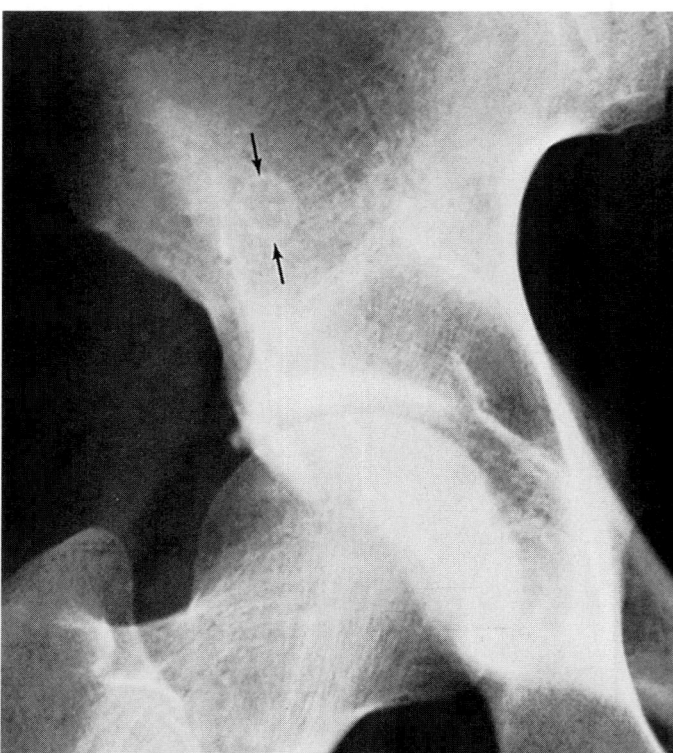

Figure 4–35. Ring-like lesion of the ilium in a 31-year-old man. This is probably a developmental defect in the bone and is of no clinical significance.

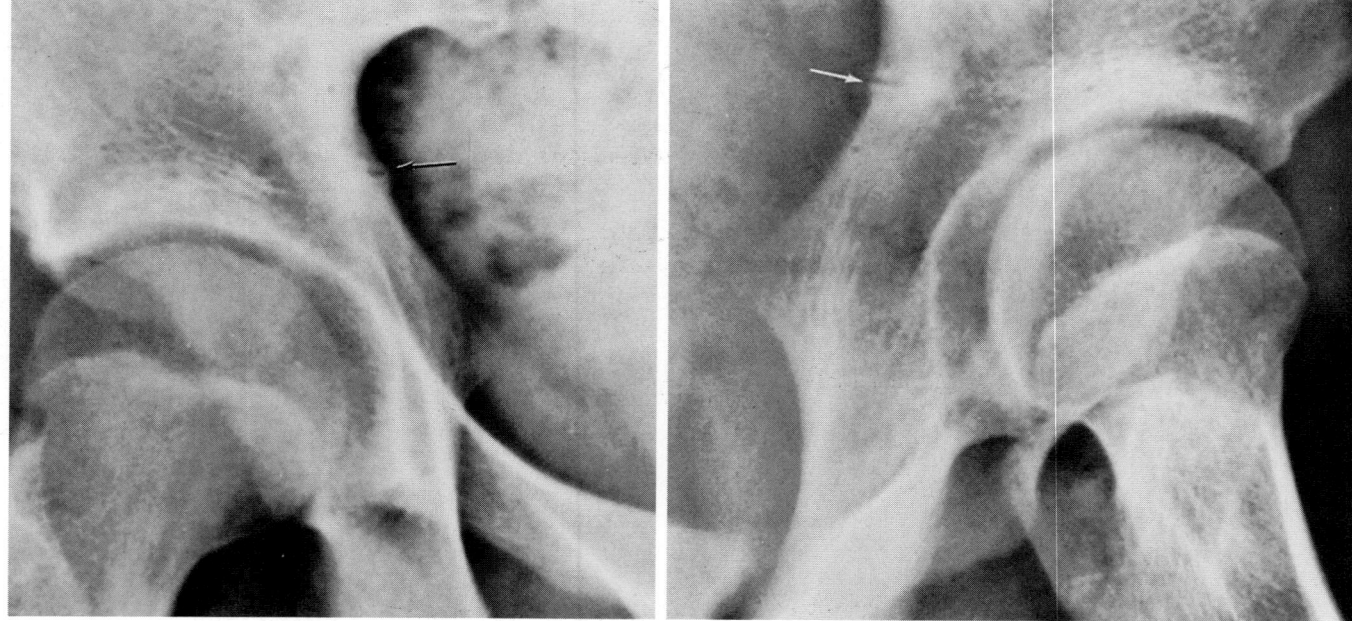

Figure 4–36. Remnants of the synchondrosis between the ilium and ischium in a 12-year-old girl.

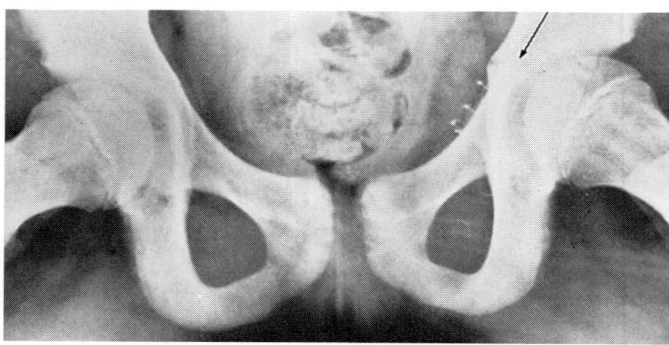

Figure 4–37. Asymmetric closure of the synchondrosis between the ilium and ischium in an 8-year-old girl, misinterpreted as a fracture.

The Pubis and Ischium

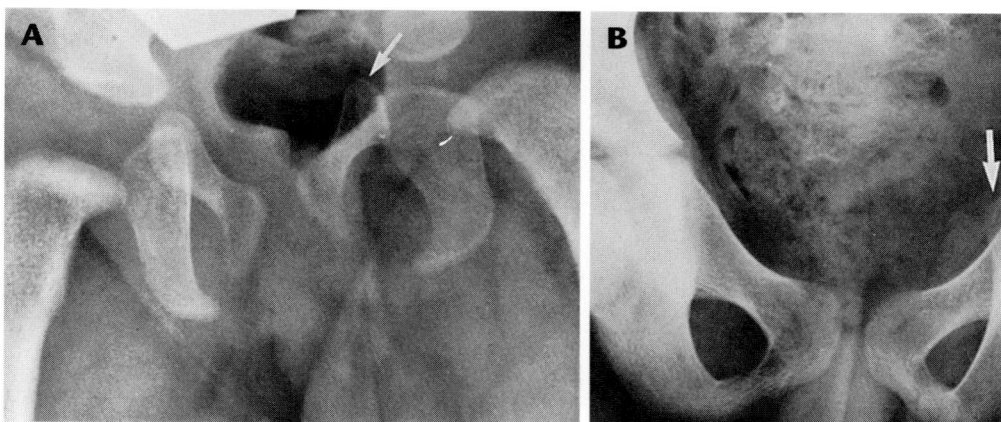

Figure 4–38. Faulty positioning with rotation may simulate medial protrusion of the ischium and a fracture through the triradiate cartilage in a normal immature pelvis. **A,** Infant. **B,** Older child. (Ref: Shipley RT et al: Artifact of projection simulating a pelvic fracture. *Am J Roentgenol* 141:479, 1983.)

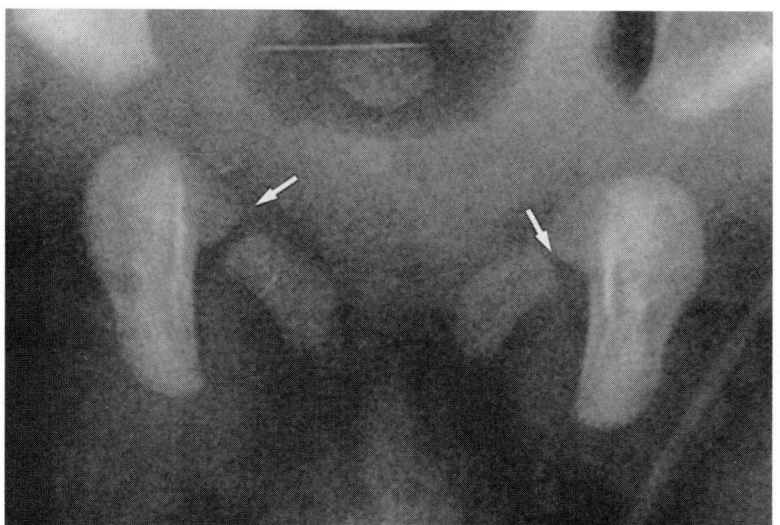

Figure 4–39. Duplicate ossification centers of the pubis in a 3-day-old child. See following figure.

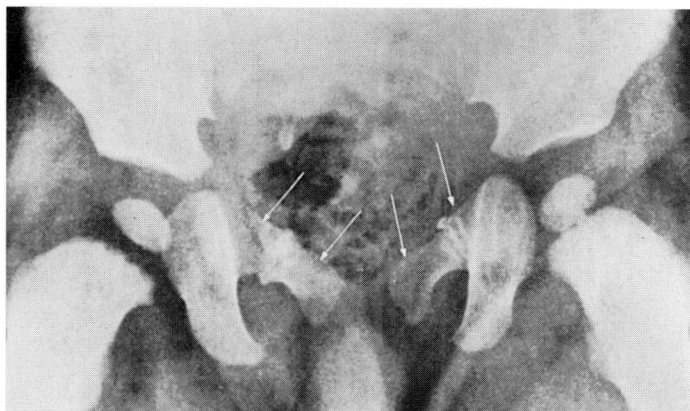

Figure 4–40. Double ossification centers of the pubis in a 3-month-old child. This appearance should not be mistaken for evidence of child abuse. (Ref: Caffey J, Madell SH: Ossification of the pubic bones at birth. *Radiology* 67:346, 1956.)

Figure 4–41. Duplicate ossification center seen unilaterally.

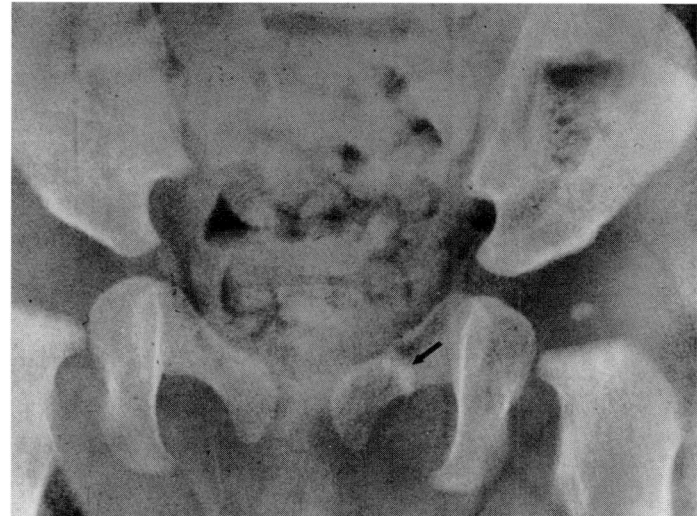

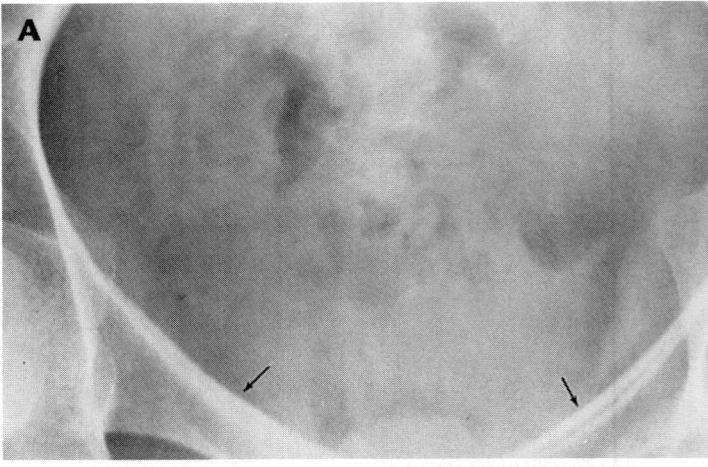

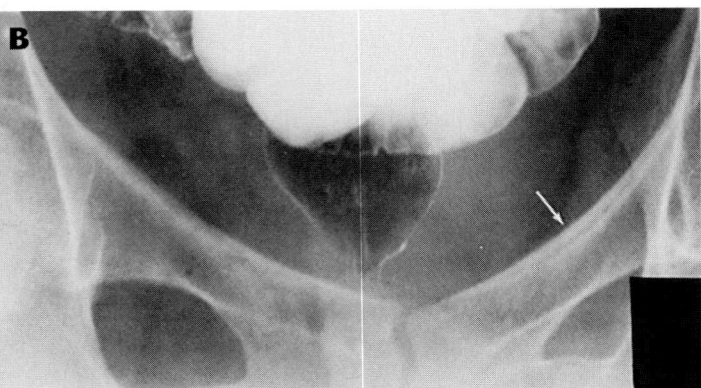

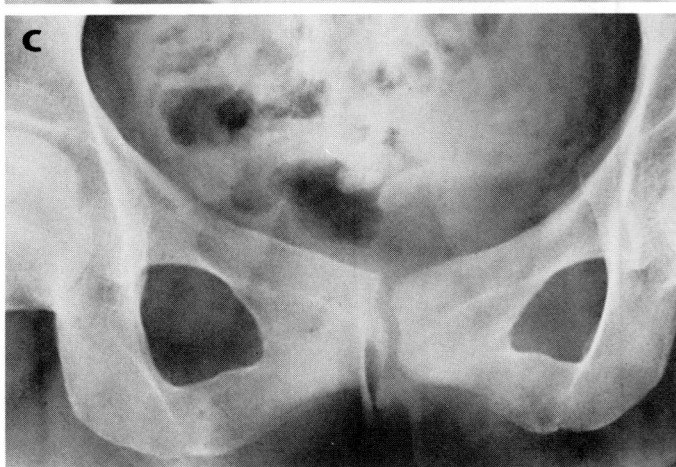

Figure 4–42. Cephalad angulation of the beam may produce a double contour of the upper aspects of the superior pubic rami, which may be mistaken for periosteal proliferation. **A,** Marked cephalad angulation. **B,** Less cephalad angulation. **C,** Perpendicular projection shows only a single contour of the bone.

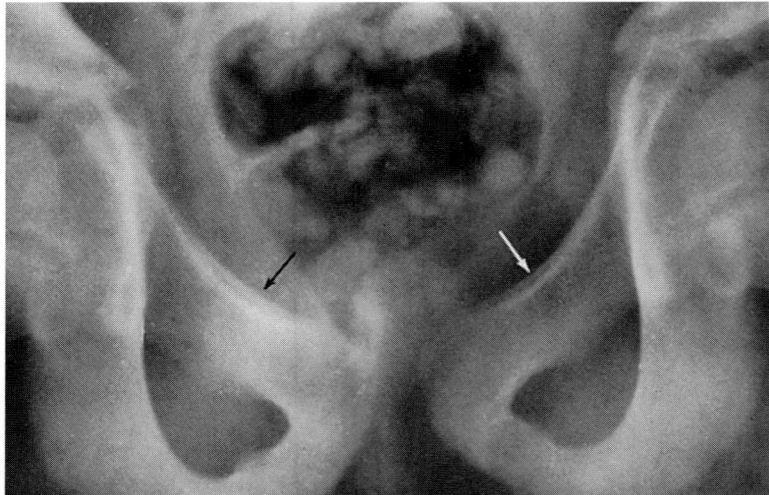

Figure 4–43. Simulated periosteal proliferation of the superior rami of the pubis in an 8-year-old as a result of cephalad angulation of the beam.

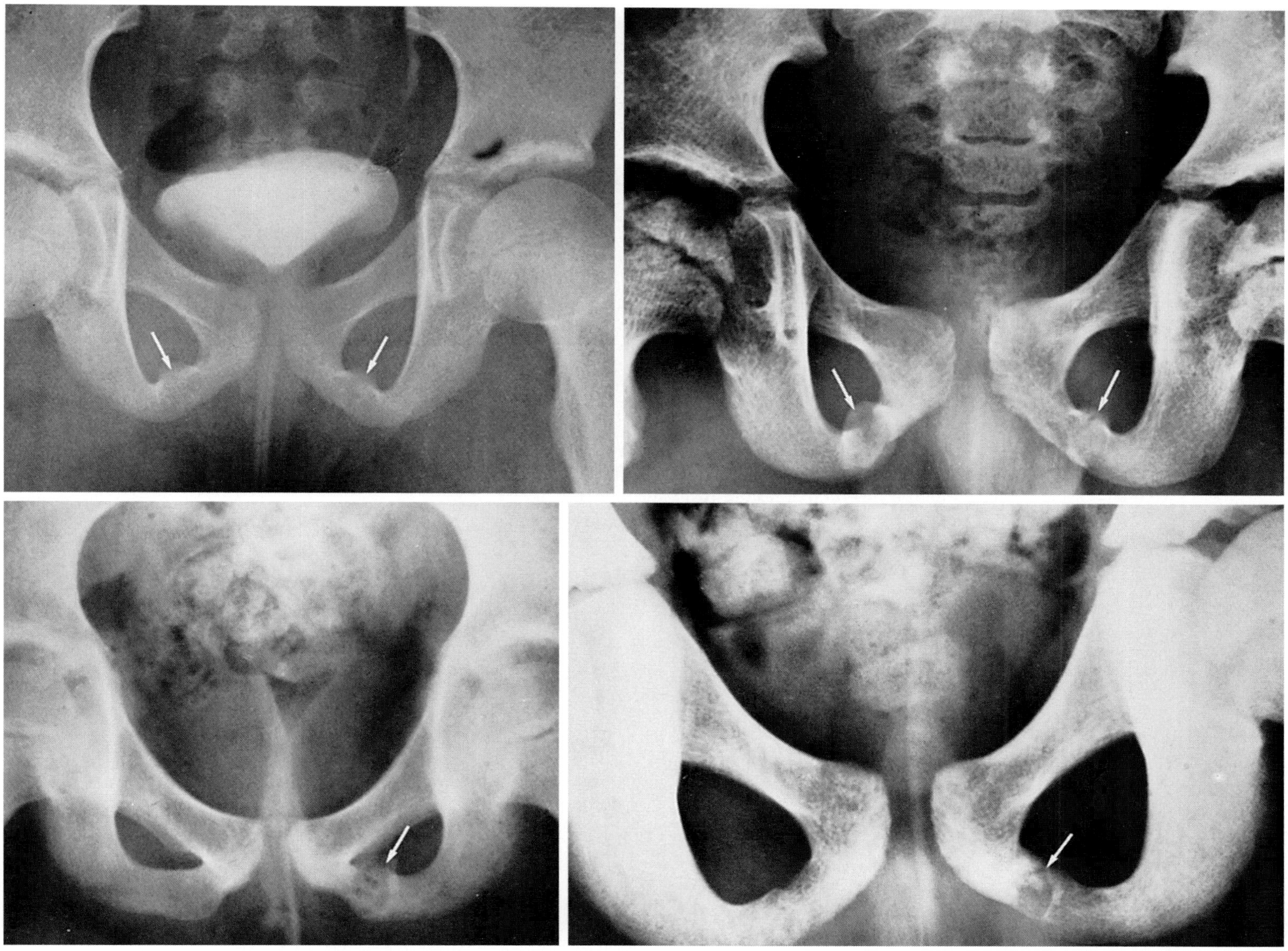

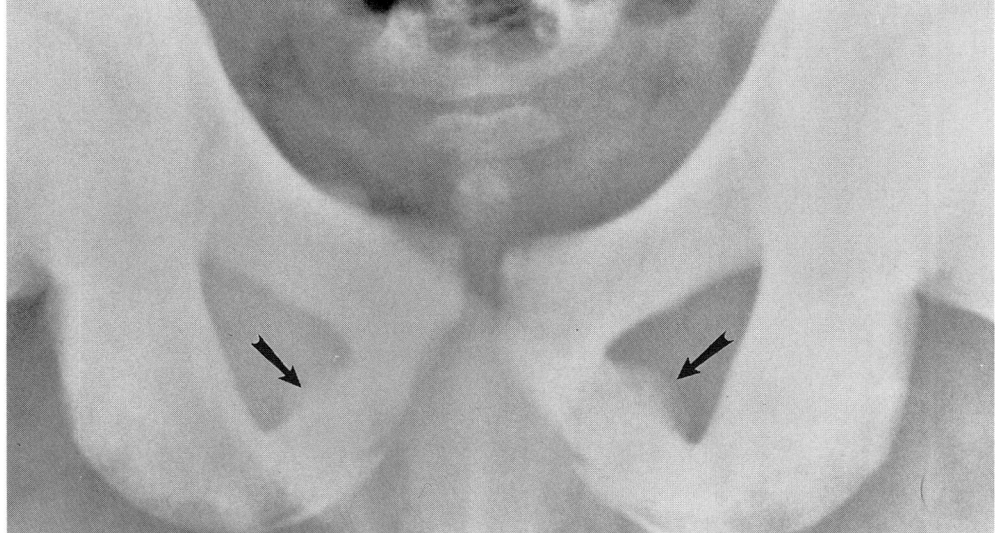

Figure 4–44. Normal variations and asymmetry in closure of the ischiopubic synchondrosis. These are normal phenomena and should not be mistaken for evidence of osteochondrosis.

Figure 4–45. Delayed closure of the ischiopubic synchondroses in a healthy 15-year-old boy. This usually closes between 4 and 8 years of age.

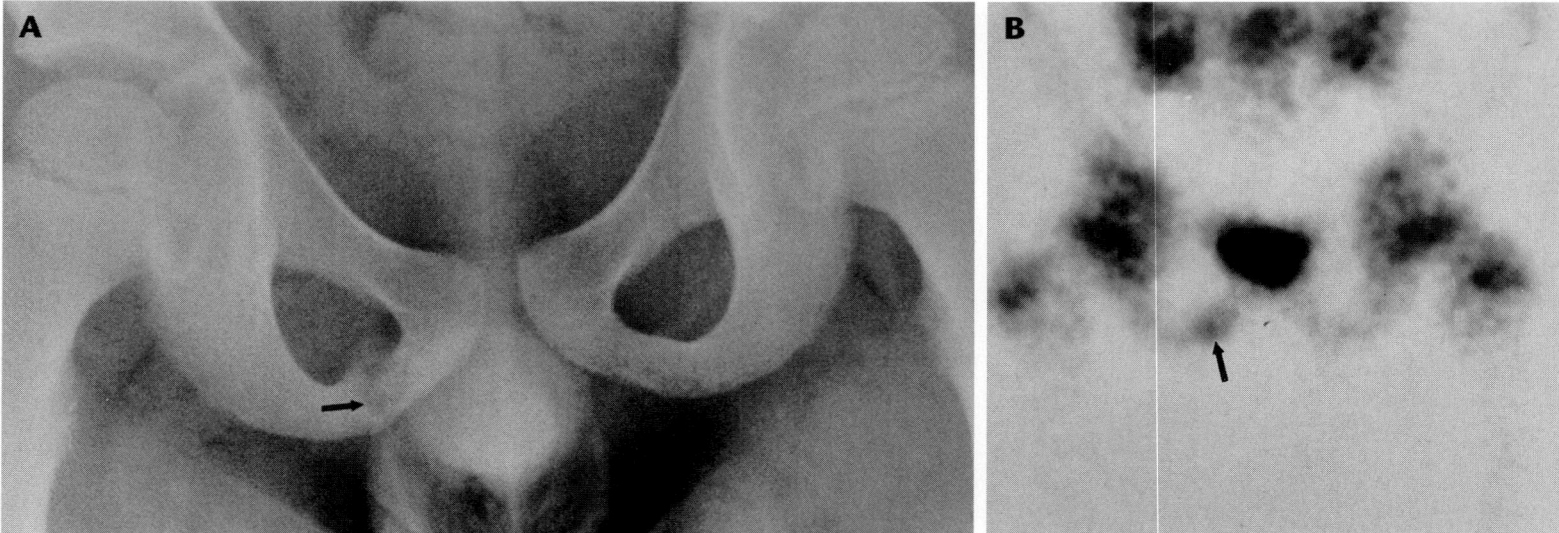

Figure 4–46. Normal open ischiopubic synchondrosis in a 6-year-old boy thought to represent a destructive lesion. **A,** Plain film. **B,** Nuclear scan.

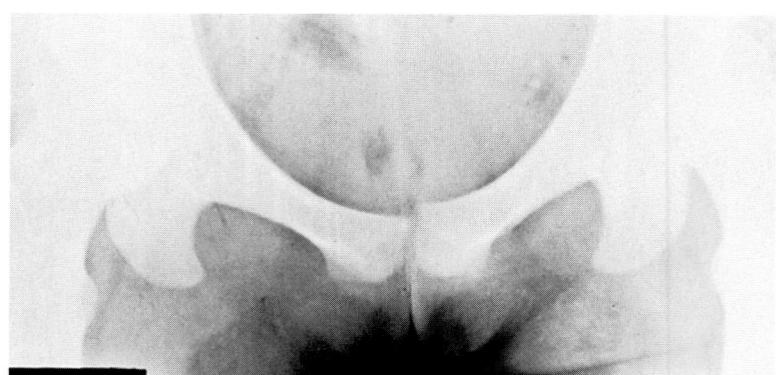

Figure 4–47. Incomplete development of the obturator rings in an otherwise healthy woman.

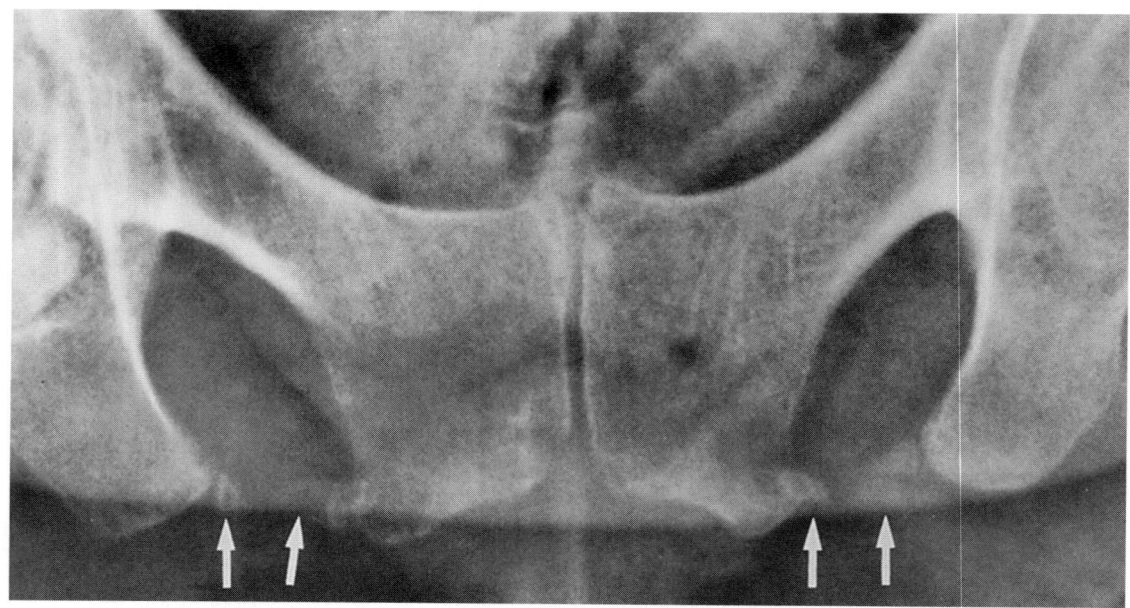

Figure 4–48. Incomplete closure of the ischiopubic synchondroses in a 72-year-old woman. Note accessory ossification centers in gaps *(arrows)*. (Ref: Sandomenico C, Tamburrini O: Bilateral accessory ossification center of the ischiopubic synchondroses in a female infant. *Pediatr Radiol* 10:253, 1981.)

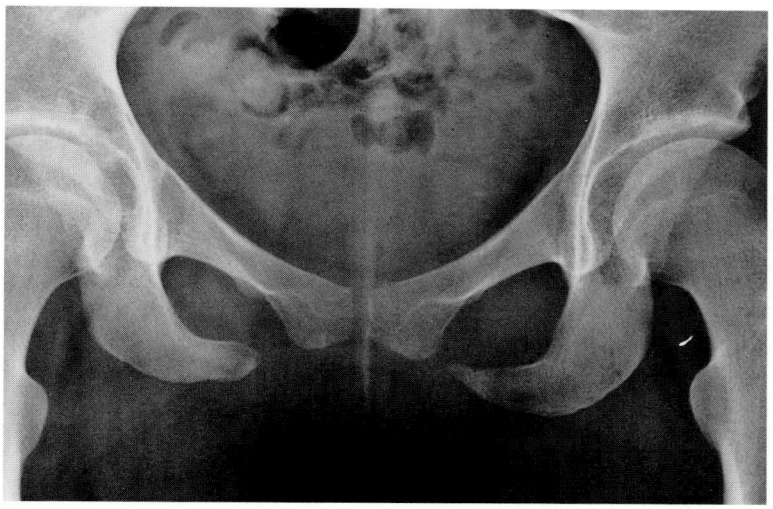

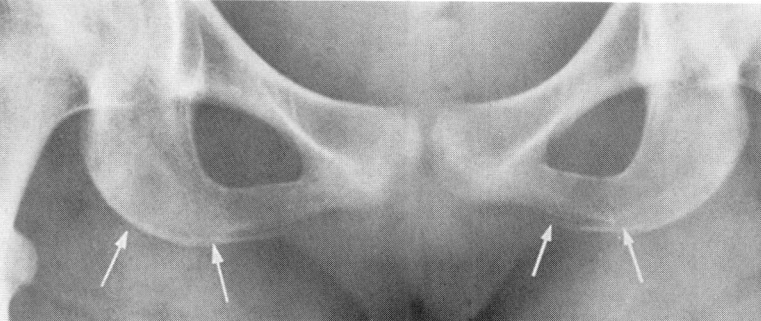

Figure 4–50. The normal ischial apophyses in a 20-year-old woman.

Figure 4–49. Failure of closure of the ischiopubic synchondroses in a healthy 21-year-old woman.

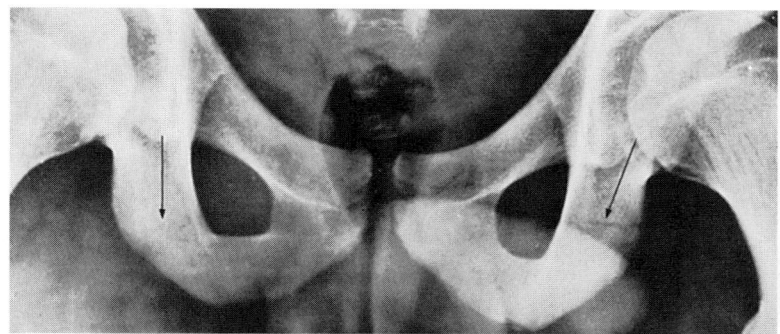

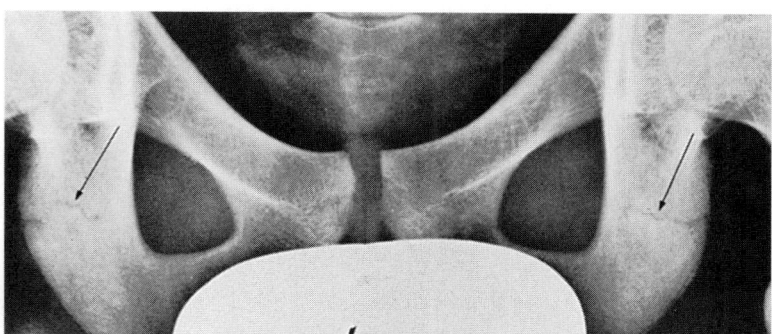

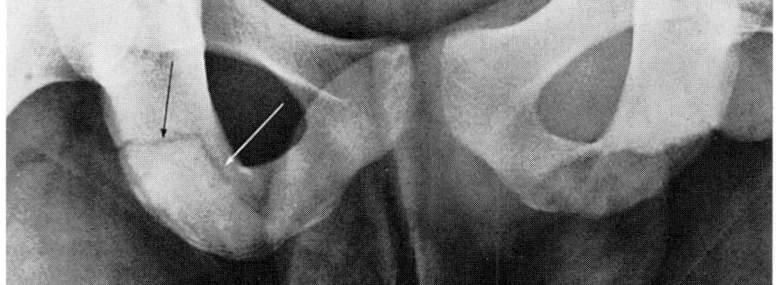

Figure 4–51. The ischial apophysis seen en face may simulate a fracture in adolescence.

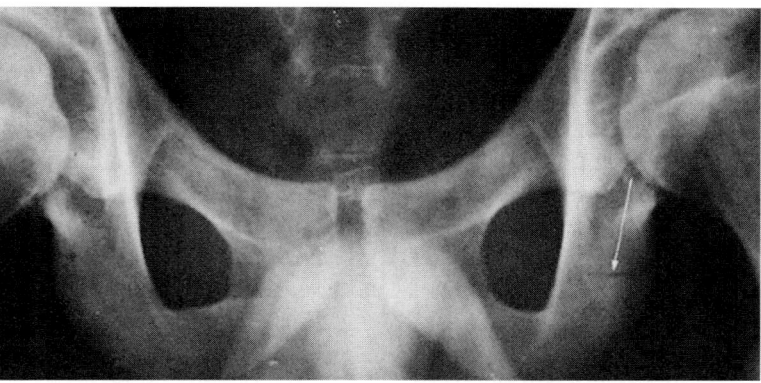

Figure 4–52. The ischial apophysis seen en face unilaterally.

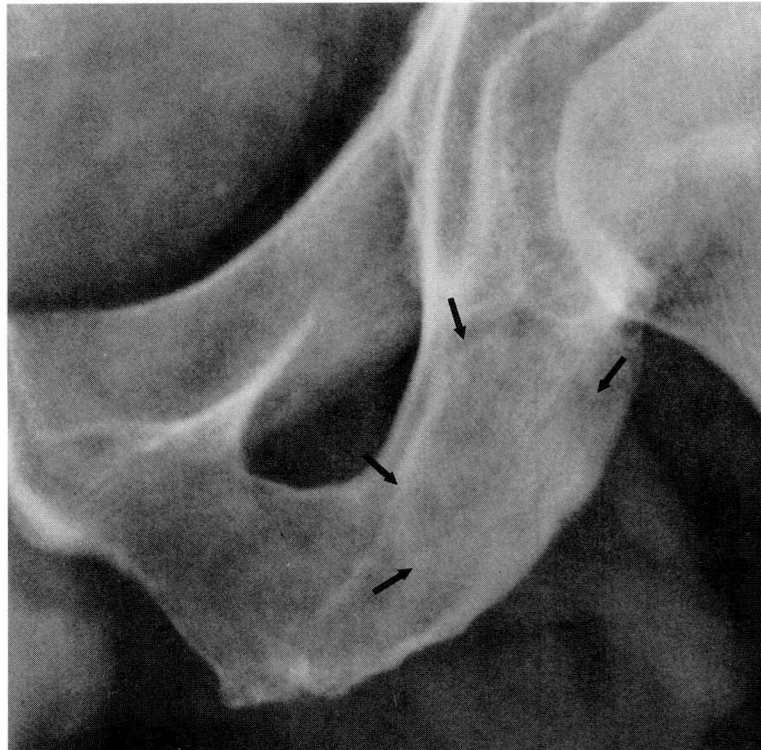

Figure 4–53. The closed ischial apophysis.

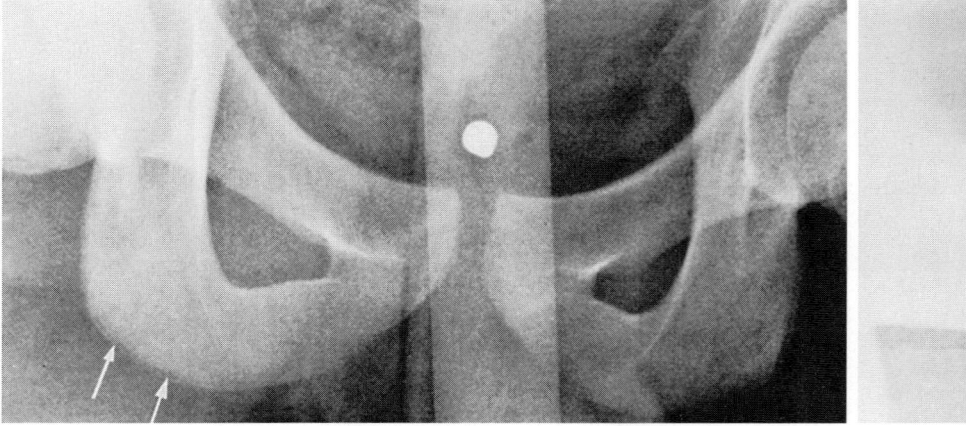
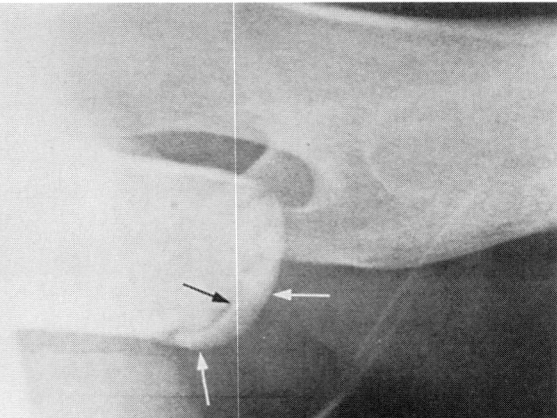

Figure 4–54. An unusual presentation of the ischial apophysis in the lateral projection of the hip in a 13-year-old boy. *Left,* AP view shows only the margin of the apophysis. *Right,* Apophysis seen in lateral projection of the hip.

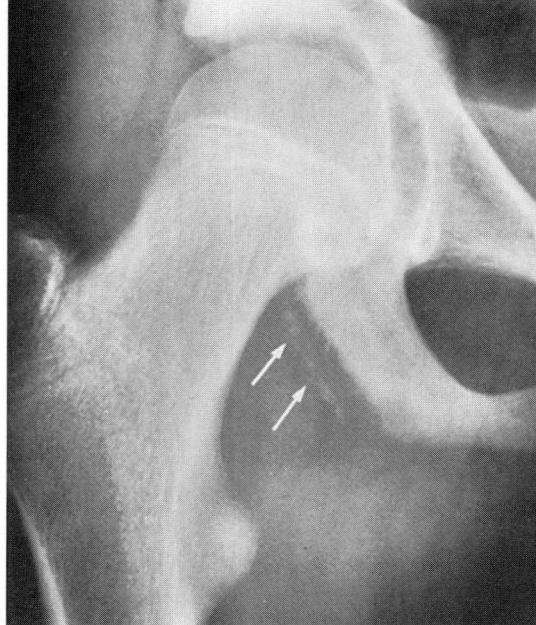

Figure 4–55. Prominent ischial apophysis in an asymptomatic 12-year-old boy.

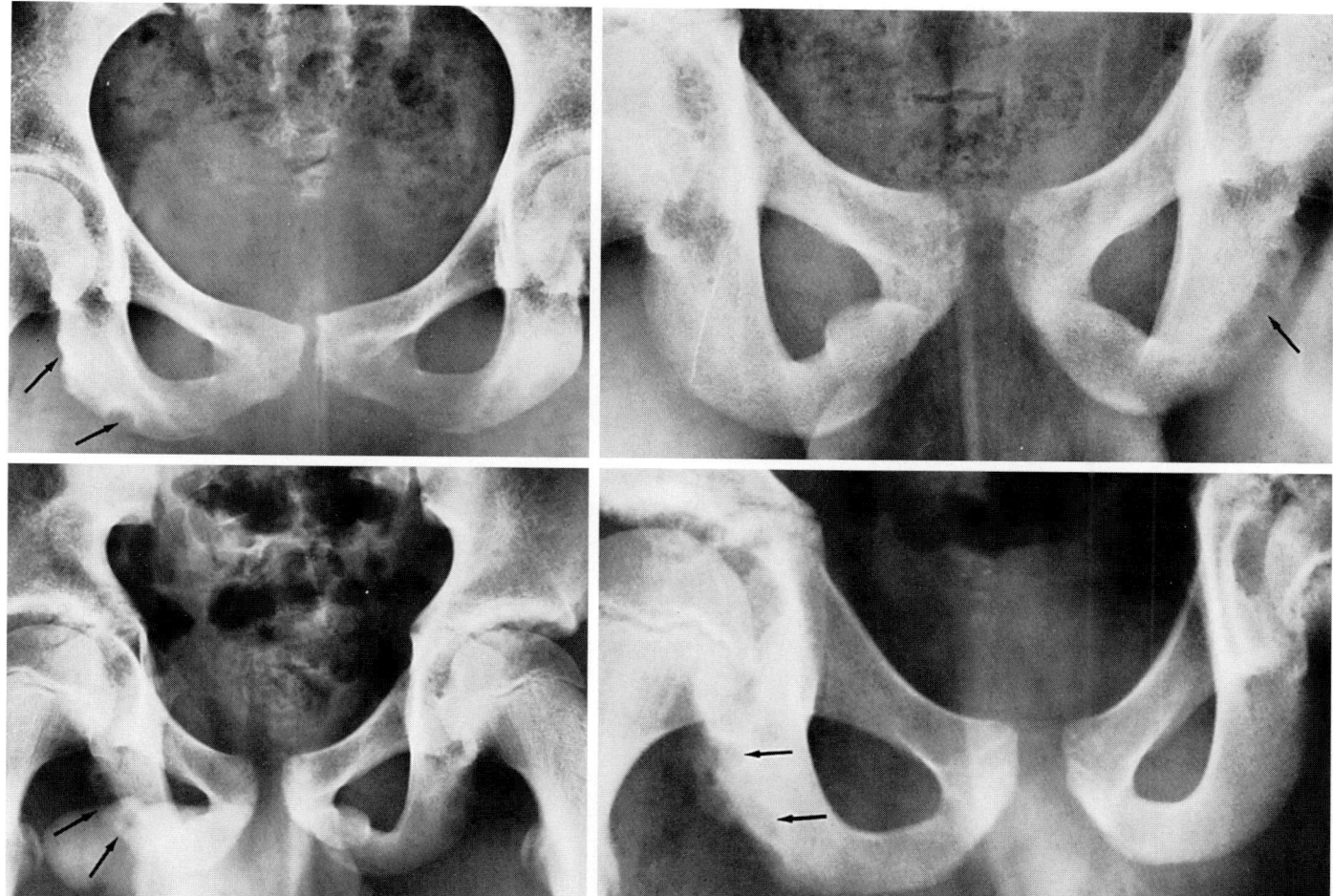

Figure 4–56. Normal irregularities of ossification of the ischia in adolescent children. These changes are usually asymmetric and disappear with increasing age. These alterations represent "tug" lesions caused by the pull of the hamstring muscles on the apophyses.

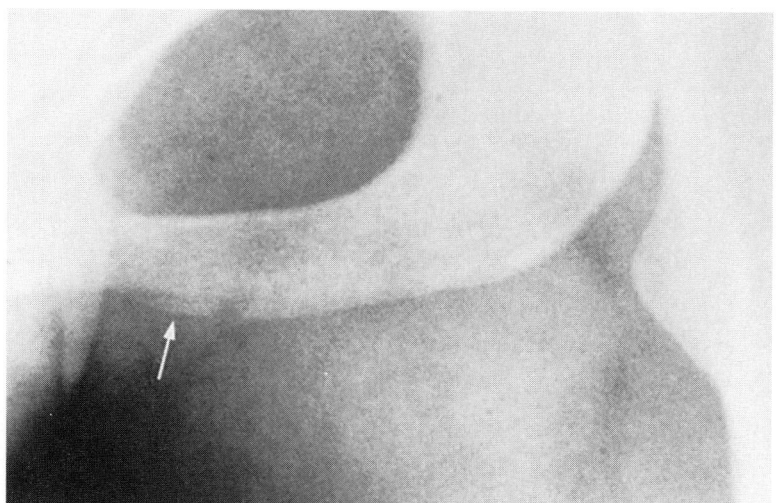

Figure 4–57. Remnant of the ischial apophysis in a 22-year-old woman.

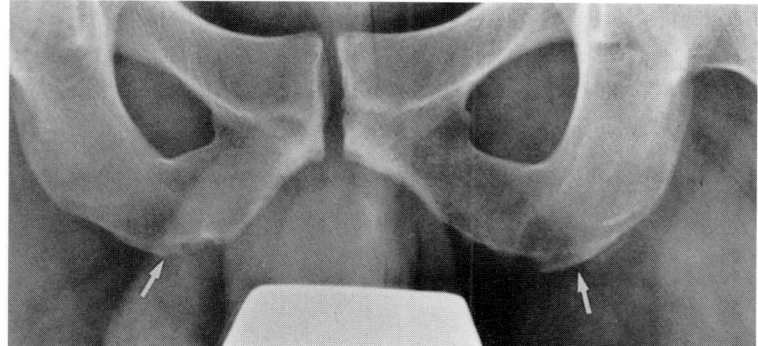

Figure 4–58. Fused ischial apophyses in a 26-year-old man.

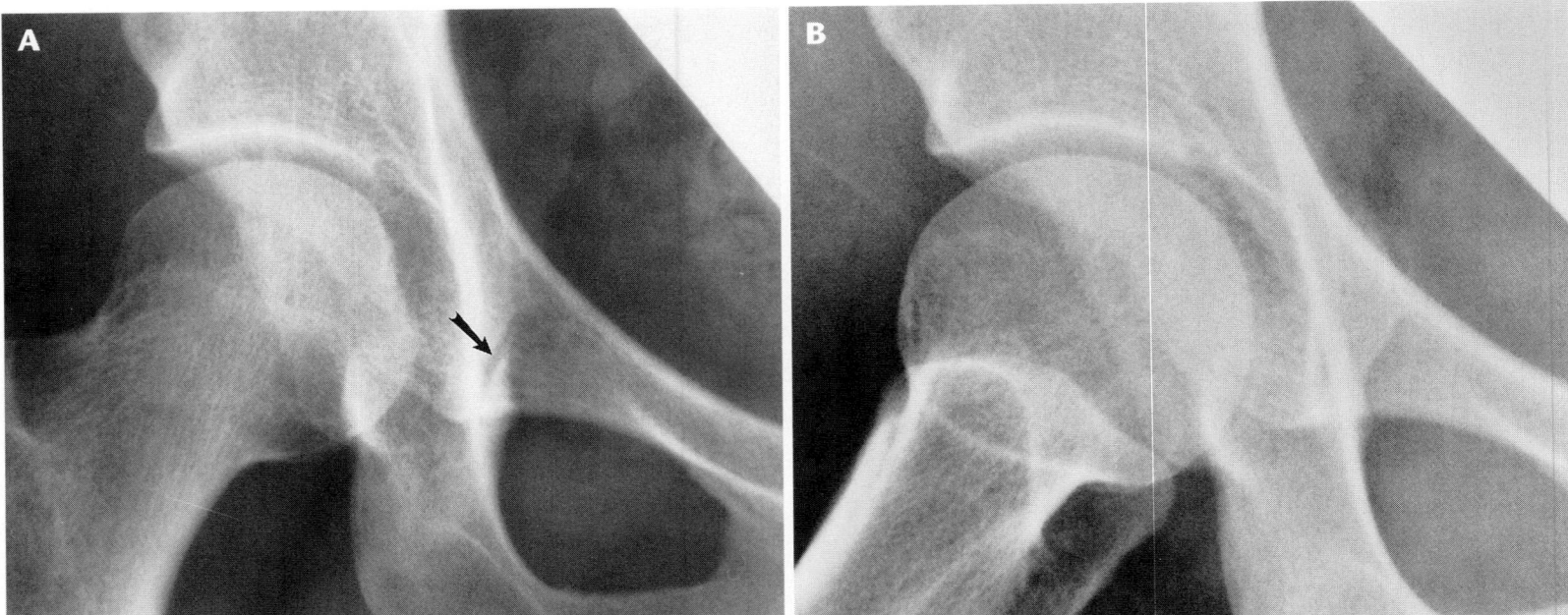

Figure 4–59. A, Simulated fracture of the ischium produced by superimposition of the ischial spine with hip in internal rotation. **B,** Not seen with hip in external rotation.

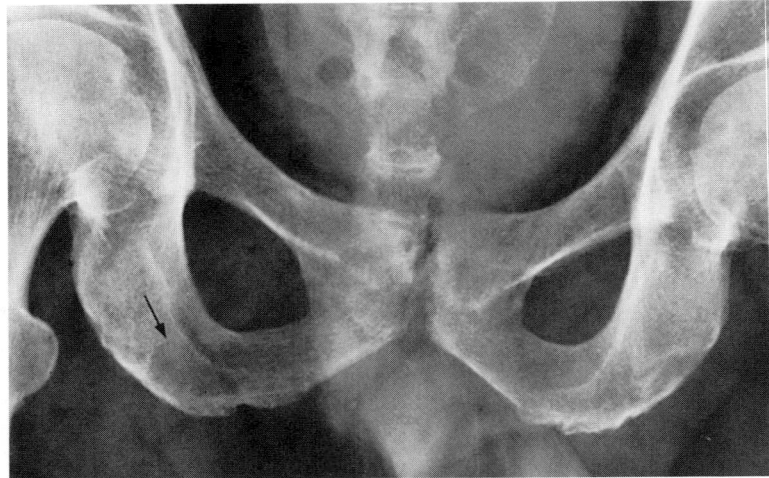

Figure 4–60. Simulated destructive lesion in the ischium produced by edge of the ischial tuberosity. The same phenomenon is present to a lesser degree on the opposite side.

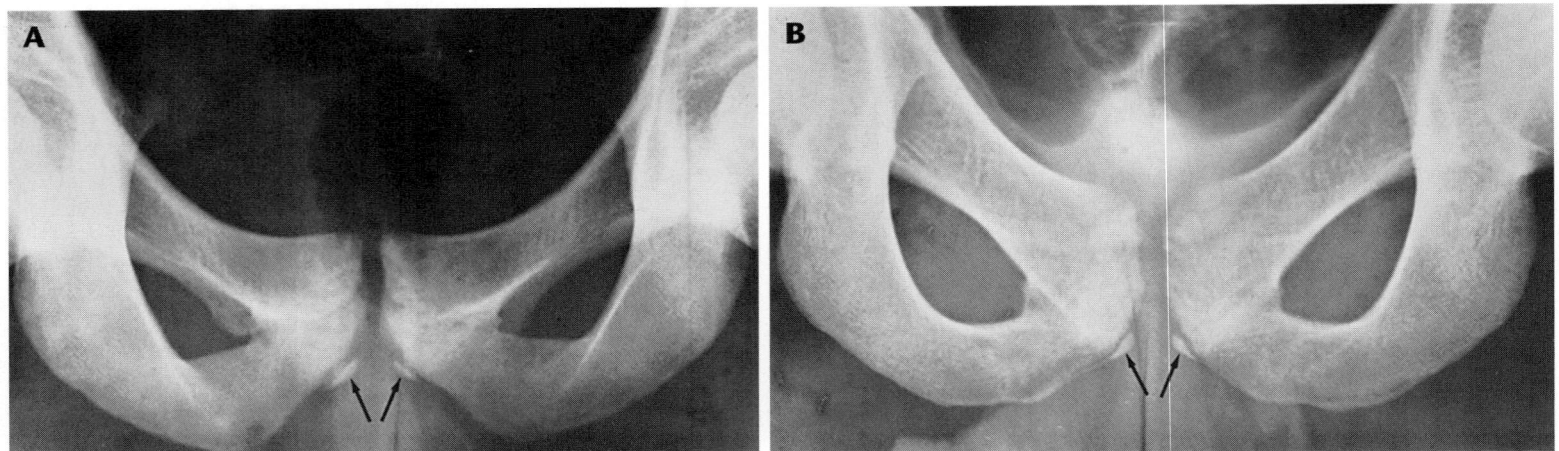

Figure 4–61. Accessory ossification centers at the symphysis pubis. **A,** 19-year-old man. **B,** 20-year-old man.

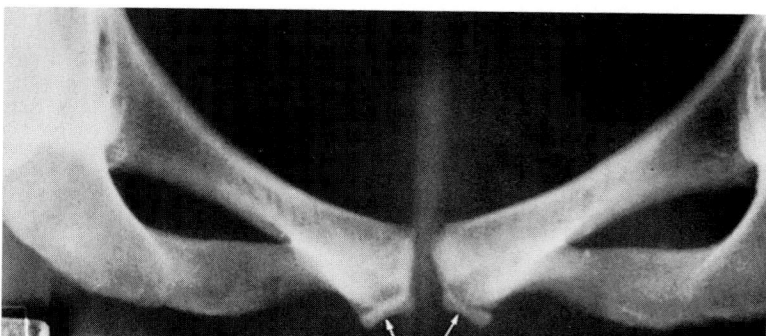

Figure 4–62. Ununited inferior pubic ossification centers in a 25-year-old woman.

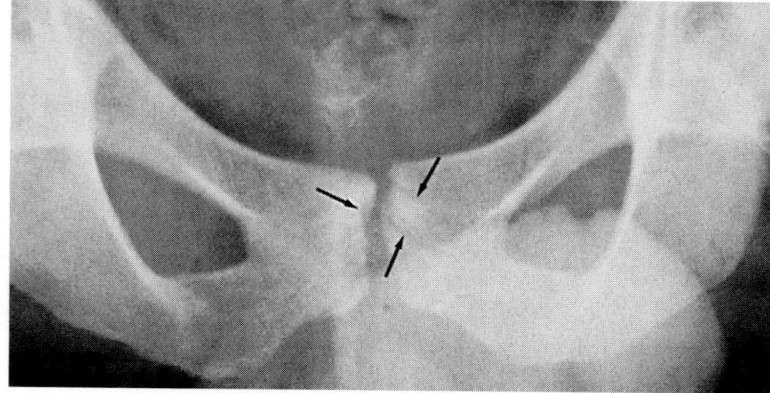

Figure 4–63. Normal irregular ridges on the medial aspects of the pubic bones in a 22-year-old man.

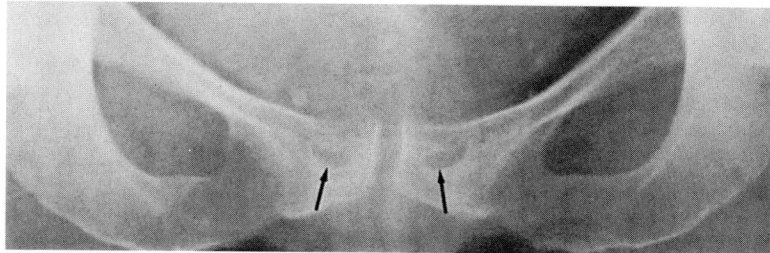

Figure 4–64. Simulated cysts of the symphysis pubis produced by areas of thin bone below the superior ramus of the pubis.

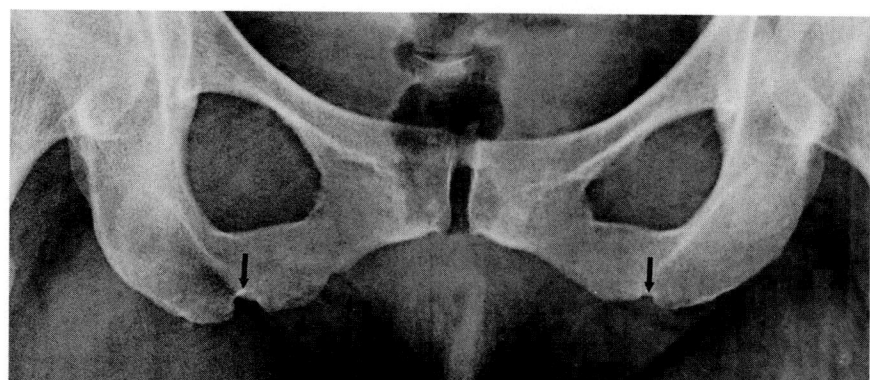

Figure 4–65. Developmental notches at the closed ischiopubic junctions.

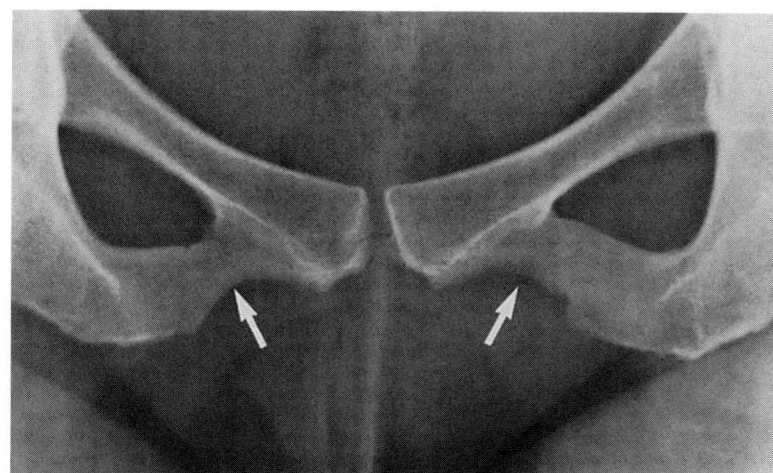

Figure 4–66. Fossae in the inferior rami of the pubis.

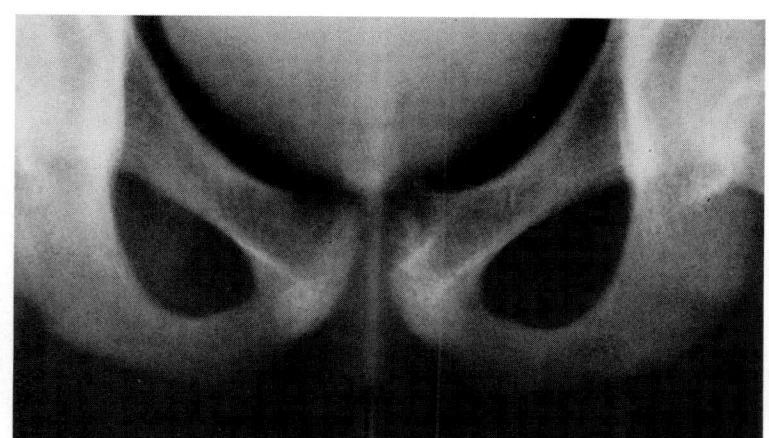

Figure 4–67. Normal irregularities of the margins of the symphysis pubis in a 12-year-old girl.

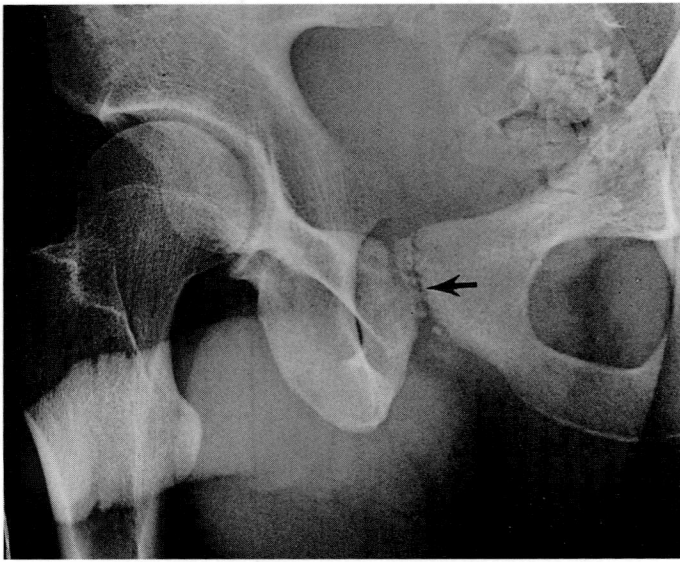

Figure 4–68. Normal developmental irregularities of the symphysis pubis in an 18-year-old man.

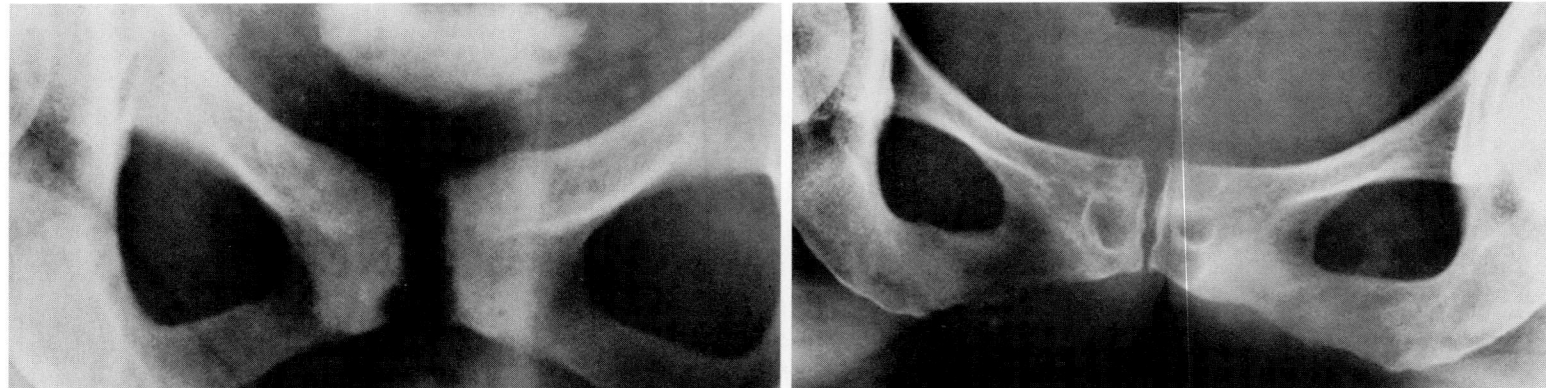

Figure 4–69. Postpartum changes in the symphysis pubis.

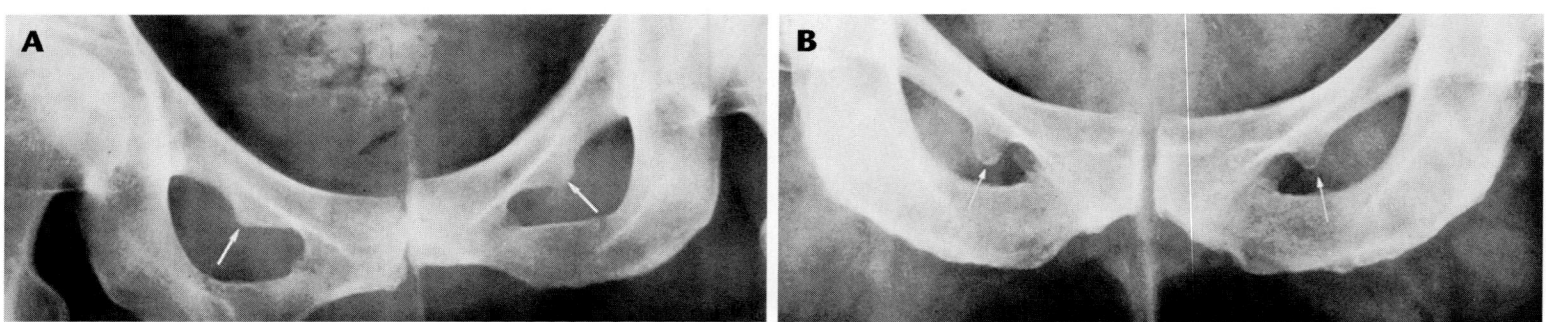

Figure 4–70. A, B, Pubic spurs are a common normal variation in development. The malalignment of the symphysis in **A** is a postpartum alteration.

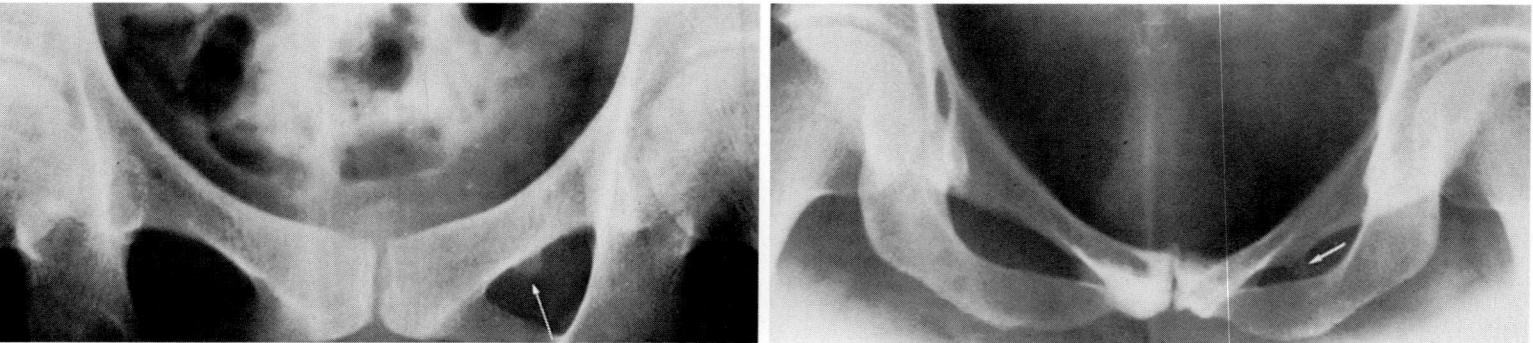

Figure 4–71. Unilateral pubic spurs. The condensing changes around the symphysis and the irregularity of the symphyseal margins are postpartum changes.

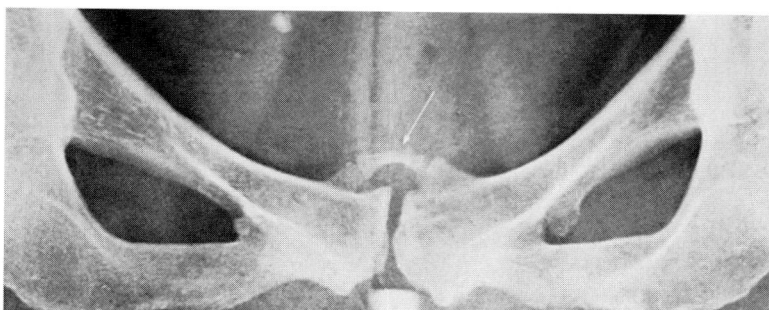

Figure 4–72. Ossification of the suprapubic ligament in a 42-year-old woman.

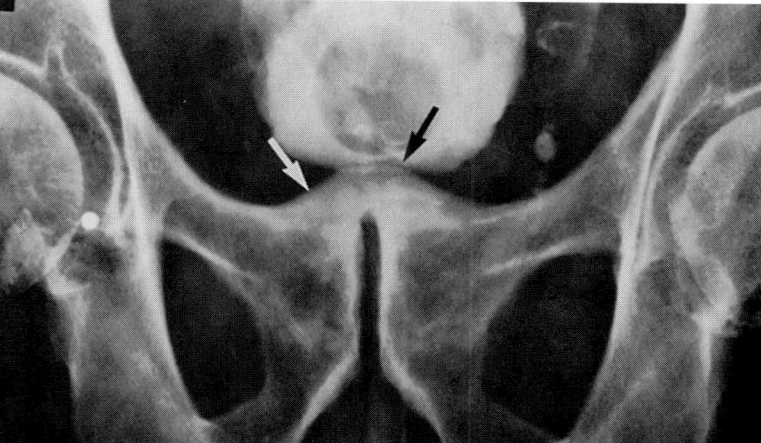

Figure 4–73. Ossification of the suprapubic ligament in a 74-year-old man.

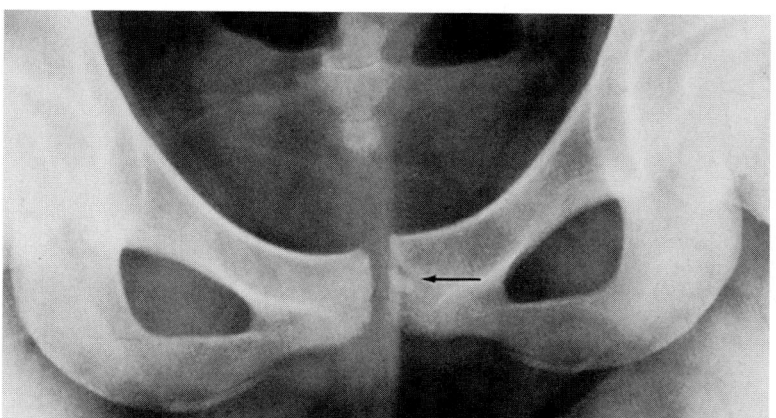

Figure 4–74. Normal malalignment of the symphysis pubis in a 14-year-old girl. The lower margin of the symphysis is a more reliable indicator of the level than the upper margin. (Ref: Vix VA, Ryu CY: The adult symphysis pubis: normal and abnormal. *Am J Roentgenol* 112:517, 1971.) Note also the accessory ossification center in the margin of the left side of the symphysis. Such accessory centers are common in the juvenile symphysis *(arrow)*.

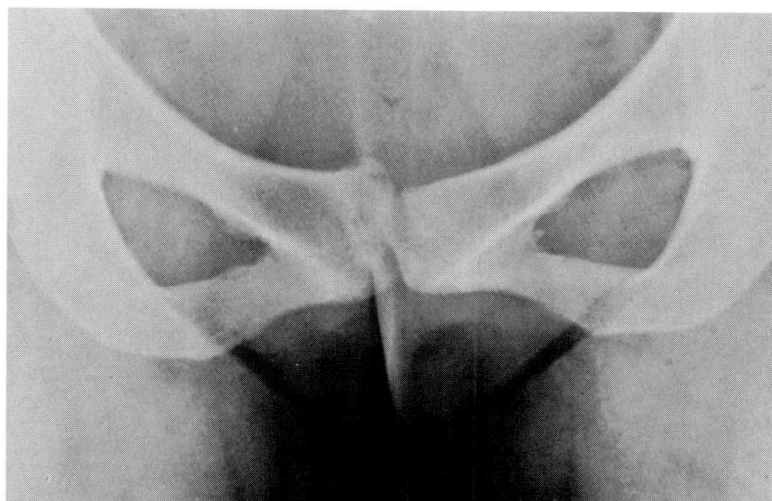

Figure 4–75. Normal malalignment and irregularities of the symphysis pubis in a 21-year-old woman.

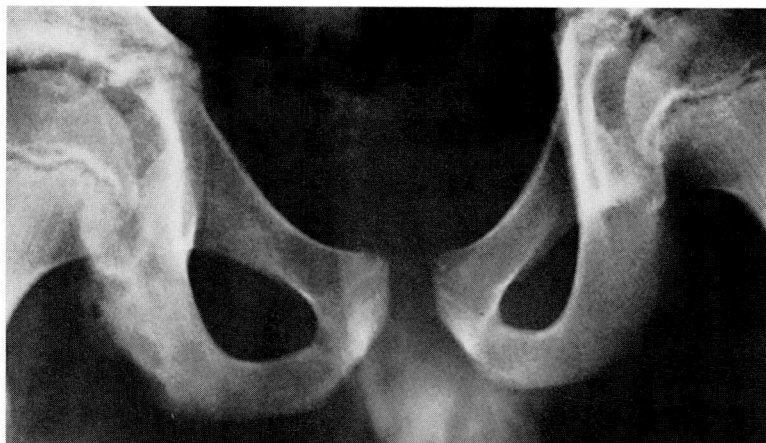

Figure 4–76. Developmentally wide symphysis pubis in a 12-year-old boy.

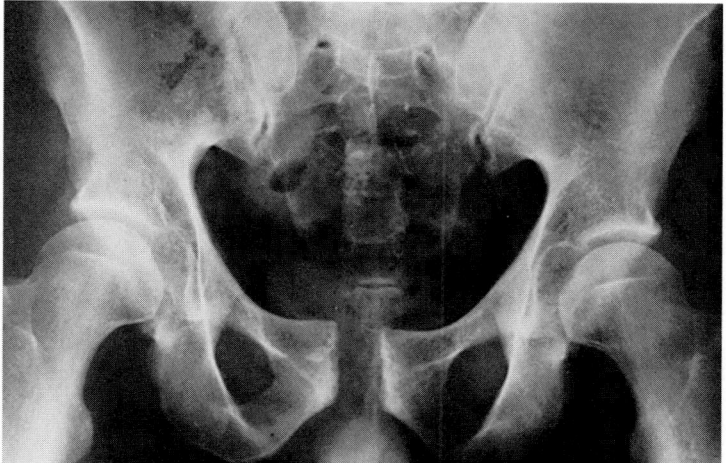

Figure 4–77. Congenitally wide symphysis pubis in a young man with no history of trauma or developmental defect. This is a rare isolated variant. (Ref: Muecke EC, Currarino G: Congenital widening of the pubic symphysis: Associated clinical disorders and roentgen anatomy of affected bony pelvis. *Am J Roentgenol* 103:179, 1968.)

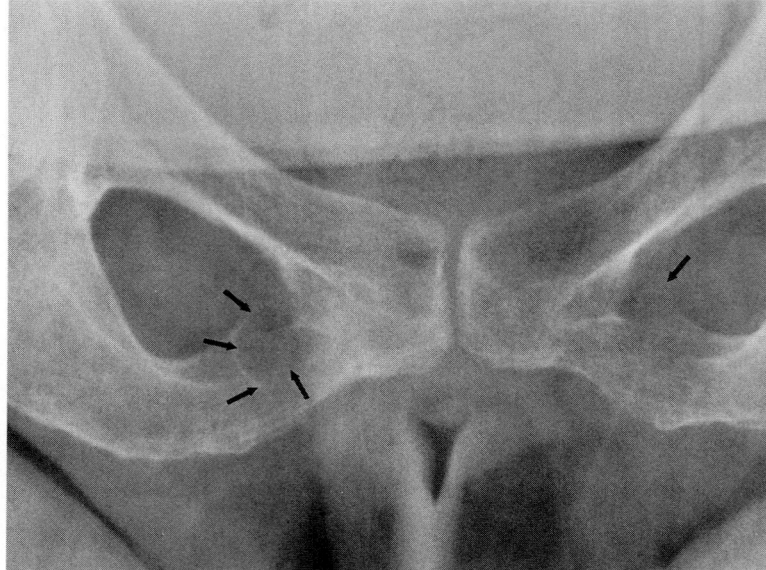

Figure 4–78. Simulated cyst of the pubis resulting from spurs in the obturator foramen. Note spur on opposite side as well.

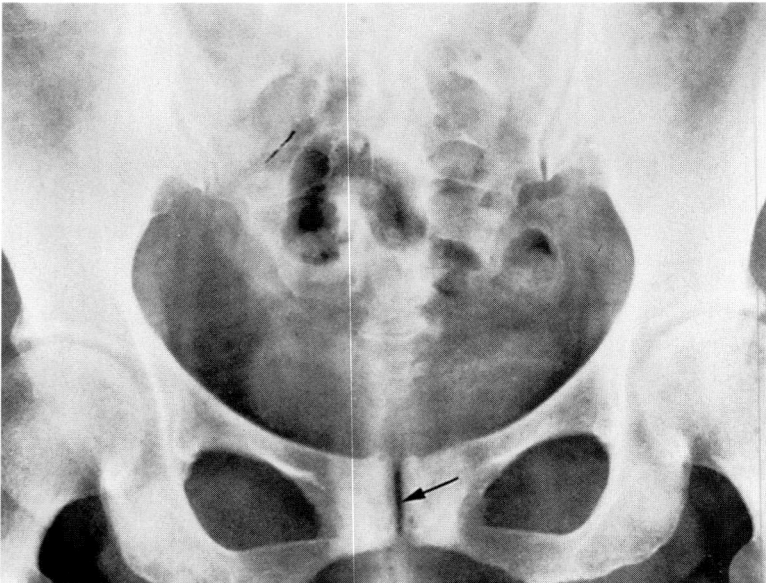

Figure 4–79. Postpartum symphyseal changes in the symphysis pubis with vacuum phenomenon.

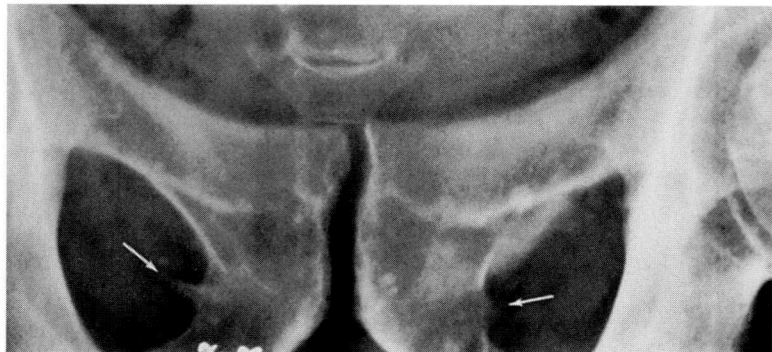

Figure 4–80. Spurs in the obturator foramen arising from the pubis, a finding usually seen in the elderly.

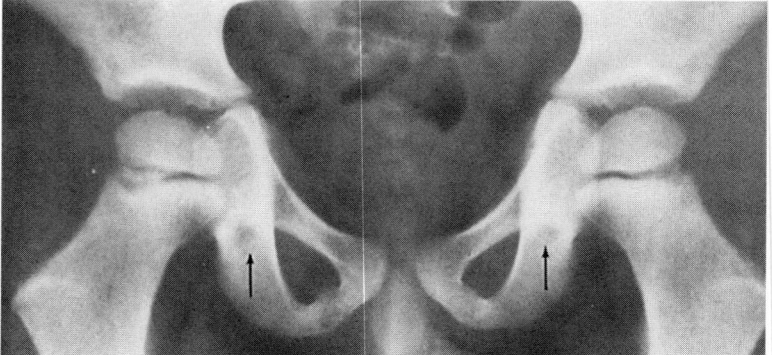

Figure 4–81. Discrete radiolucencies in the ischia produced in part by the crossing shadow of the pubis. These are seen in children and adults.

The Acetabulum

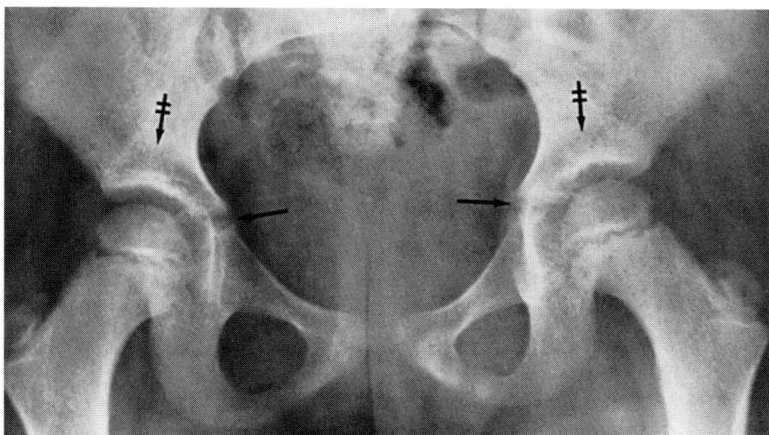

Figure 4–82. Normal protrusio acetabuli (←) in a 7-year-old girl. This is a normal phenomenon seen in children from about 4 to 12 years of age. Note also the normal radiolucent patches above the acetabula (←╫). (Ref: Alexander C: The aetiology of primary protrusio acetabuli. *Br J Radiol* 38:567, 1965.)

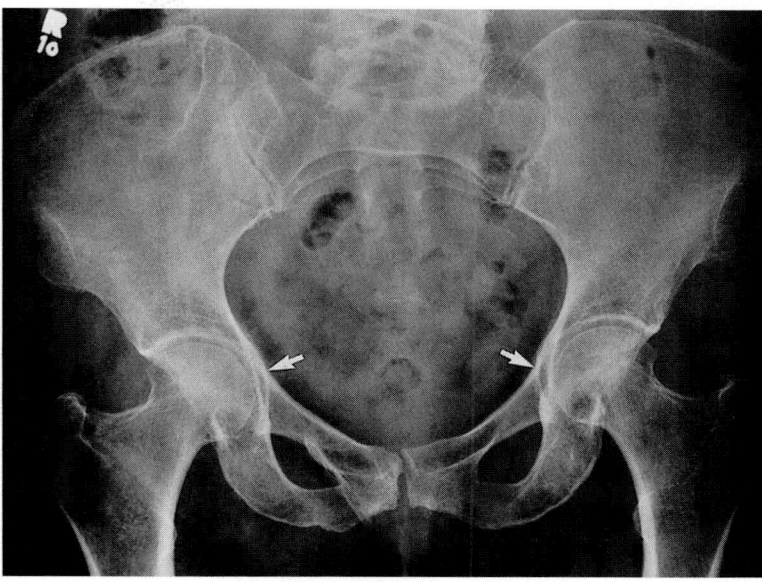

Figure 4–83. Mild protrusio acetabuli may be seen as a normal variation. The distance between the medially located acetabular line and the laterally located ilioischial line may be up to 6 mm in women and 3 mm or more in men. (Ref: Resnick D: *Diagnosis of bone and joint disorders*, 3rd ed., Philadelphia, WB Saunders, 1995, p. 4310.)

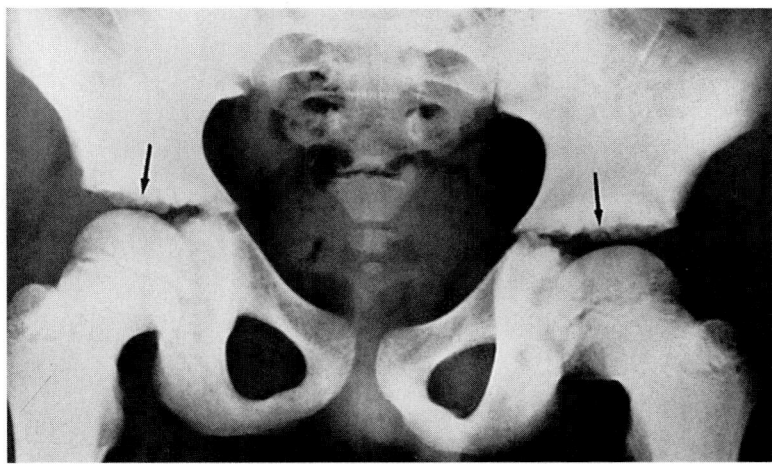

Figure 4–84. Normal irregularity of the acetabular roofs in a young child. This appearance is normal between the ages of 7 and 12 years.

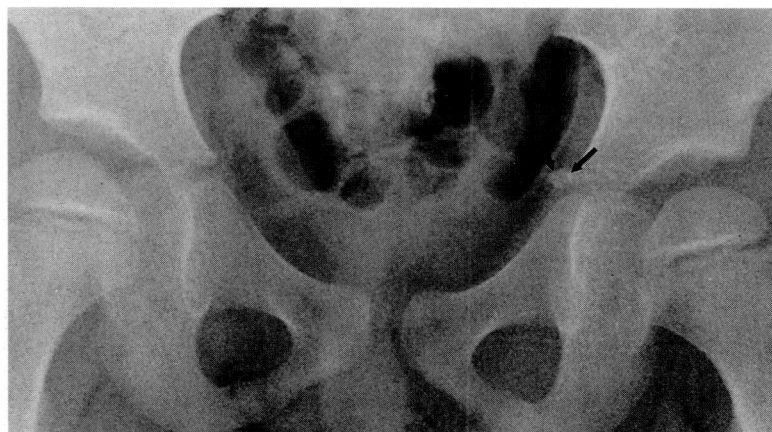

Figure 4–85. Ossicle at the triradiate cartilage in a 5-year-old boy.

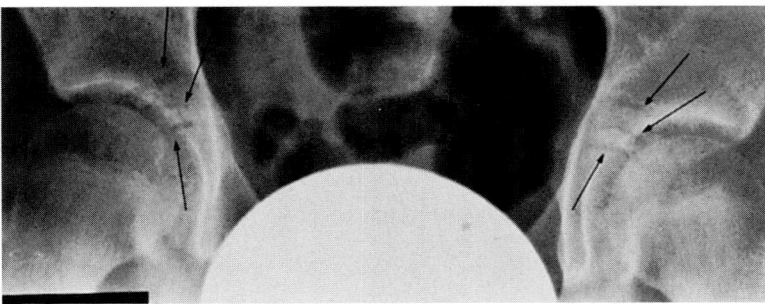

Figure 4–86. Chondroid stripes in the acetabula in a 12-year-old girl. This is a common finding in adolescents.

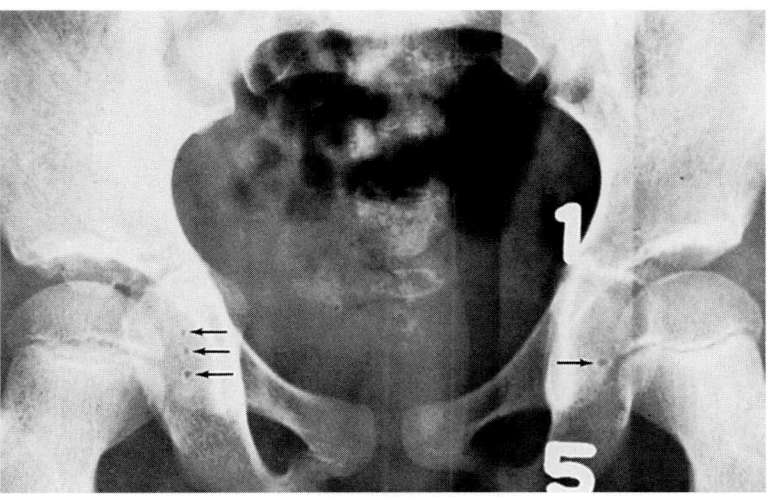

Figure 4–87. Normal nutrient foramina, multiple on the patient's right side and single on his left side.

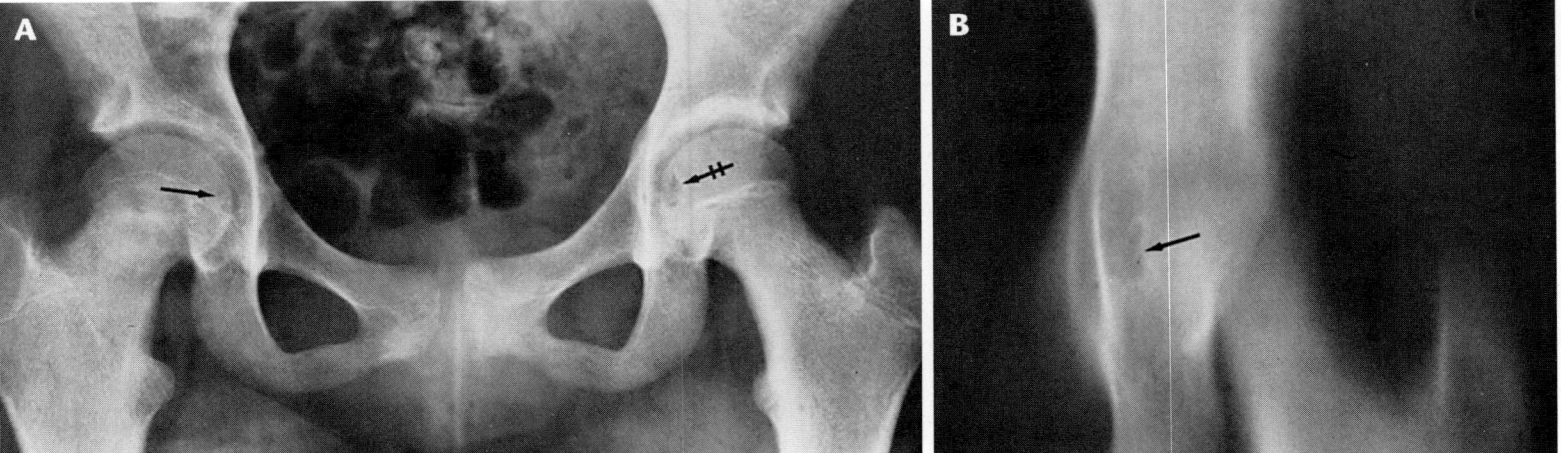

Figure 4–88. Pit for nutrient vessels in acetabulum (←). If completely superimposed on the femoral head, this shadow may simulate a destructive lesion (⇇). **A,** Plain film. **B,** Tomogram.

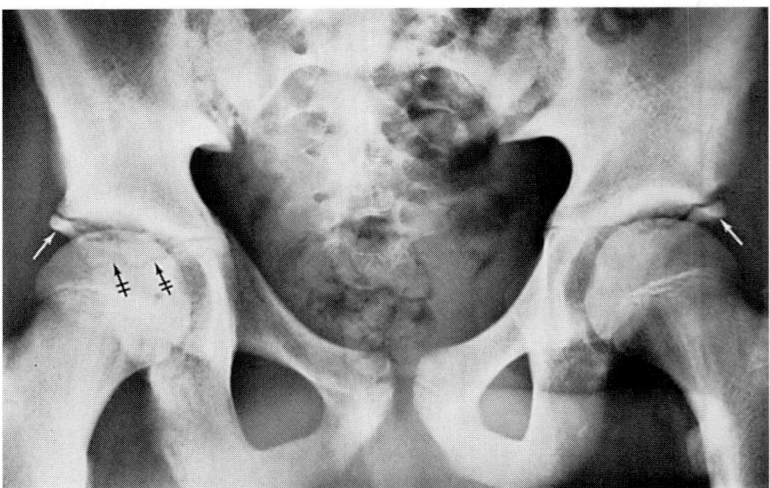

Figure 4–89. Accessory ossification centers in the superior portions of the acetabula (os acetabuli marginalis superior) in a 14-year-old boy (←). Note also additional ossification centers in the acetabula at lower level (⇇). These centers usually fuse solidly with the contiguous portions of the ilium. (Ref: Caffey J: *Pediatric x-ray diagnosis,* 9th ed. Chicago, Mosby, 1993, p. 178.)

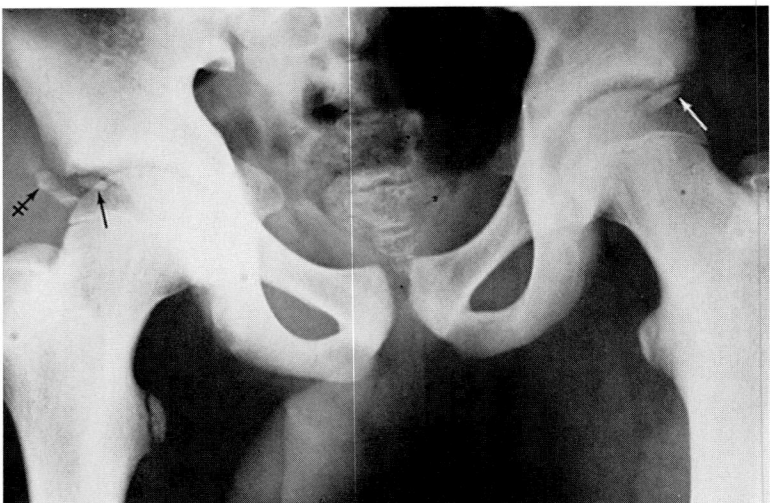

Figure 4–90. Accessory ossification centers (←) in a 14-year-old boy, with additional centers laterally (⇇).

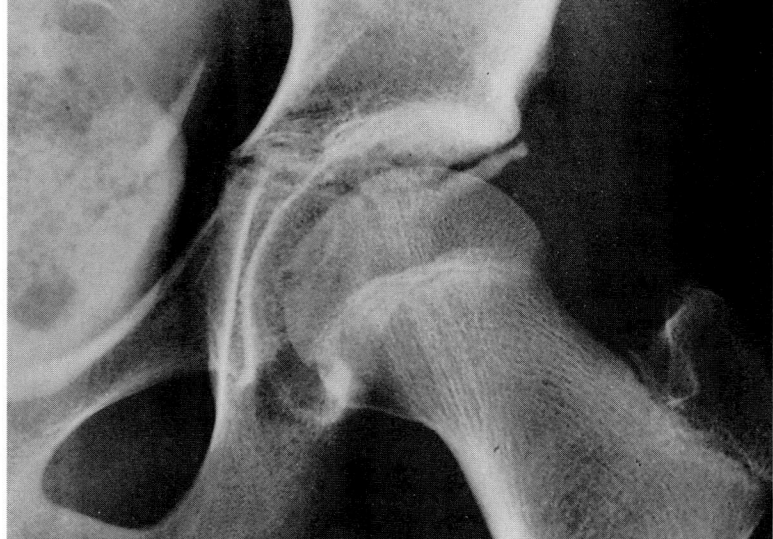

Figure 4–91. A nice demonstration of the secondary ossification centers of the acetabulum.

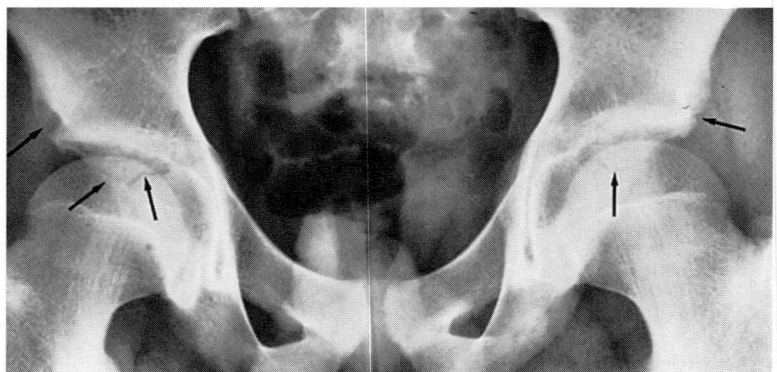

Figure 4–92. Partial union of secondary ossification centers of the acetabula in the adolescent (←).

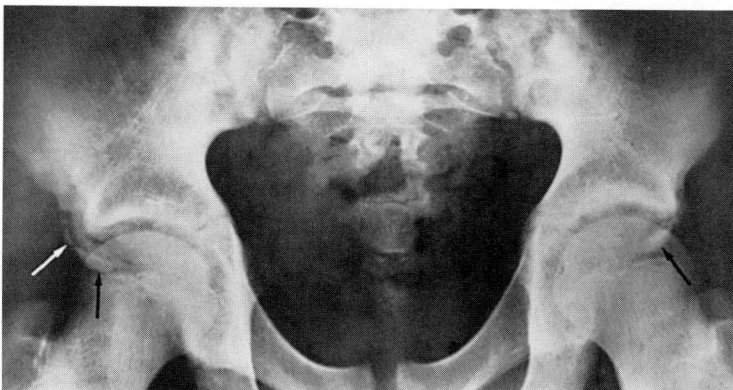

Figure 4–93. Additional example of multiple accessory ossification centers of the acetabula in a 14-year-old girl.

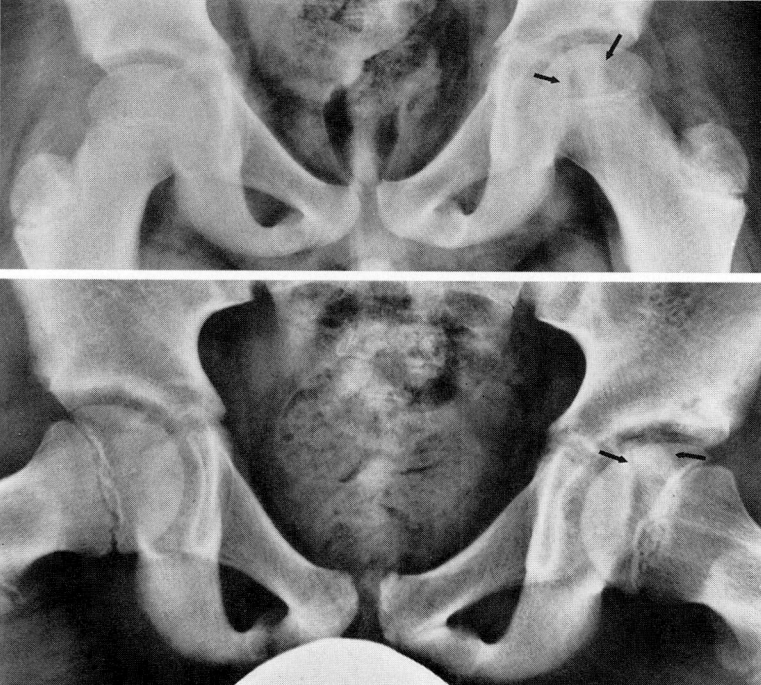

Figure 4–94. Unusual appearance of the left femoral head in a 6-year-old girl as a result of irregular closure of secondary ossification centers of the acetabulum.

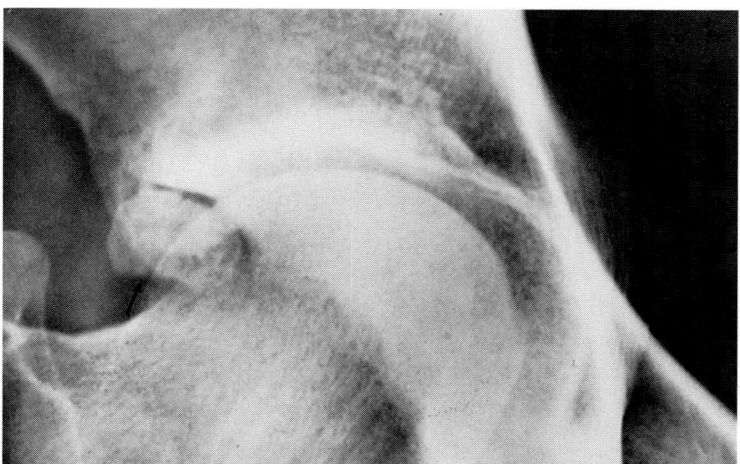

Figure 4–95. An os acetabuli marginalis superior, persisting as a separate ossicle into adult life. These persistent ossification centers are commonly called os acetabuli.

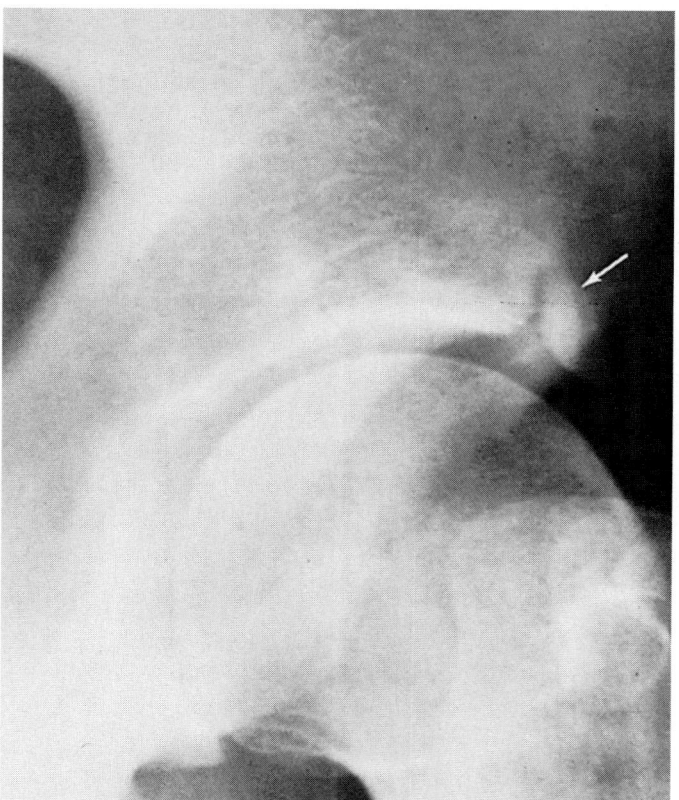

Figure 4–96. An os acetabuli marginalis superior, persisting into adult life in a 22-year-old man.

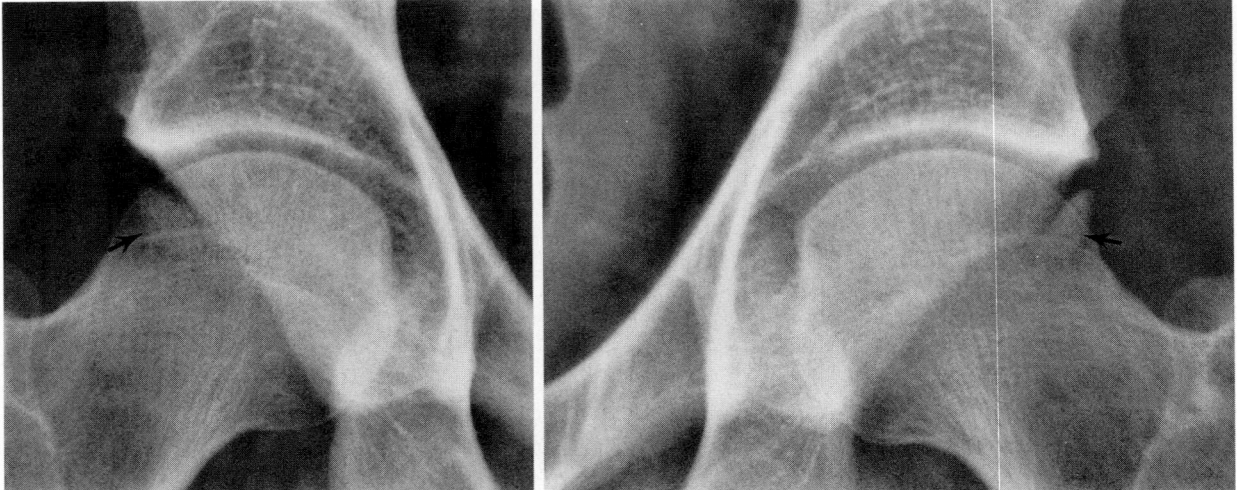

Figure 4–97. Bilateral os acetabuli marginalis superior in a 25-year-old man.

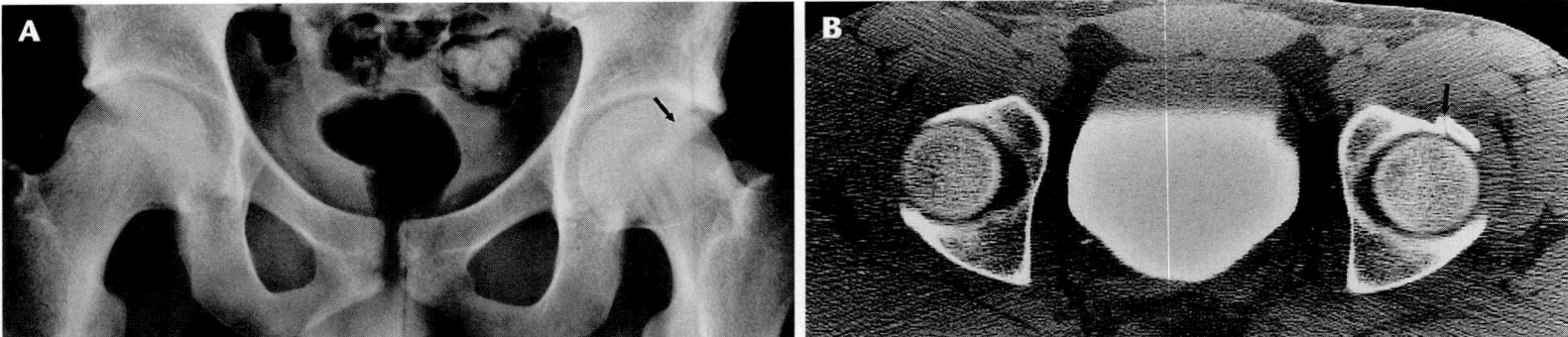

Figure 4–98. A, Persistent os acetabuli marginalis superior misdiagnosed as a fracture. **B,** CT shows the ossicle of the anterior lip of the acetabulum.

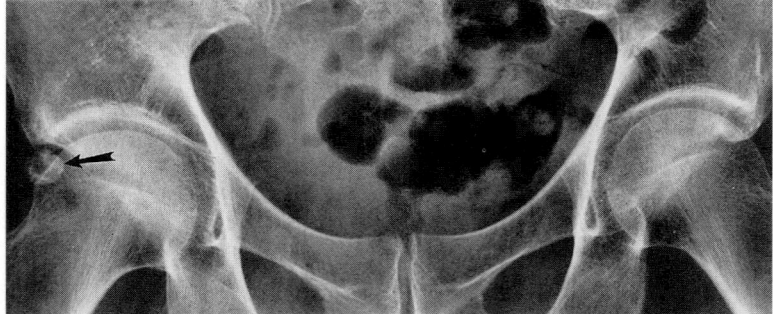

Figure 4–99. The os acetabuli on the right. Note the corresponding appearance on the left.

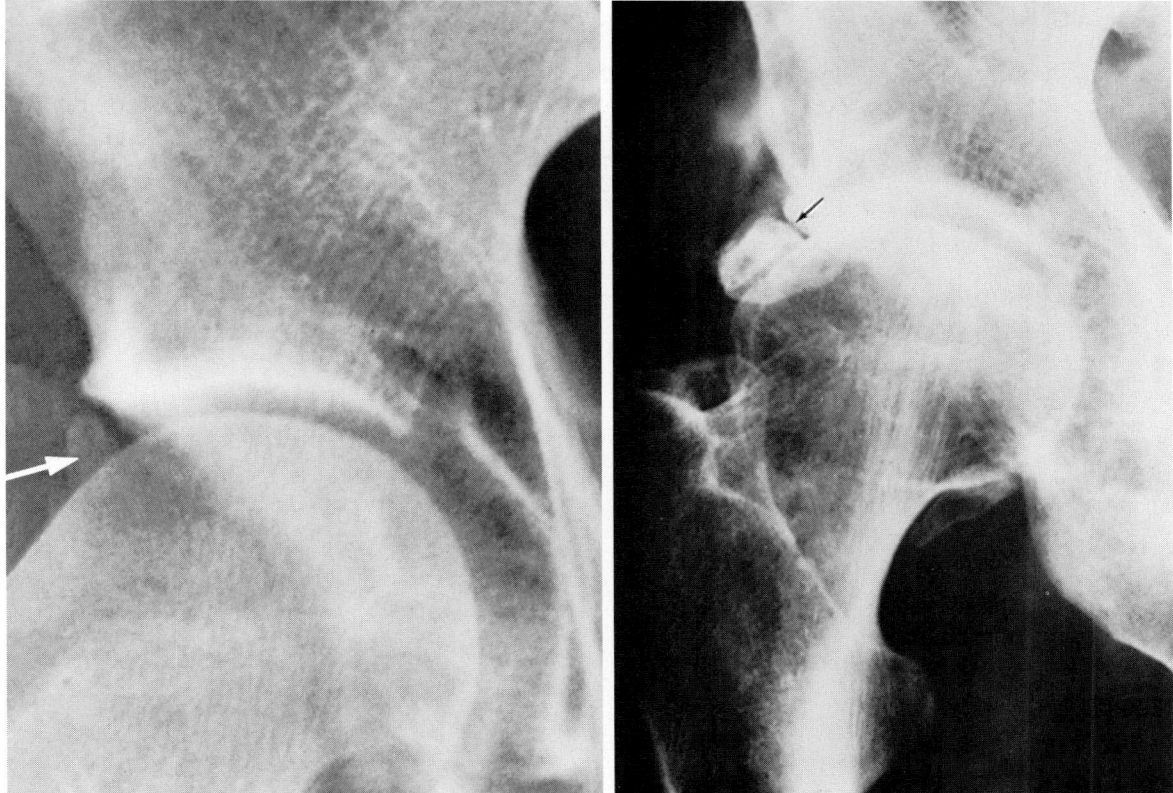

Figure 4–100. Two examples of the os acetabuli. This ossicle should be distinguished from calcification in the rectus femoris tendon insertion. (Ref: Kawashima A et al: Paraacetabular periarthritis calcarea: Its radiographic manifestations. *Skeletal Radiol* 17:476, 1988.)

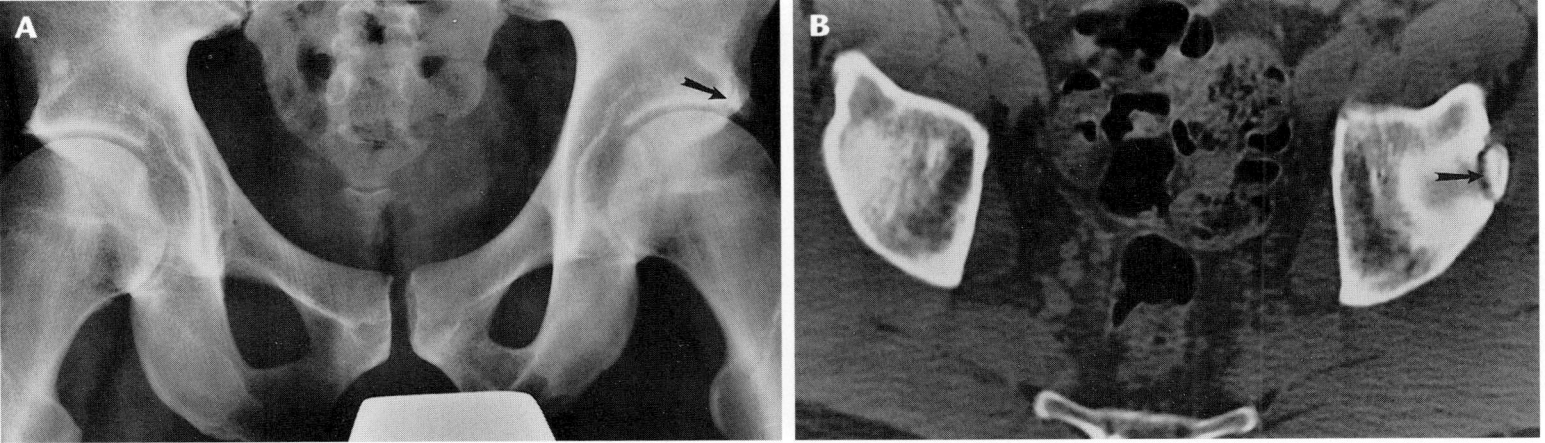

Figure 4–101. The os acetabulum by CT. **A,** Plain film. **B,** CT.

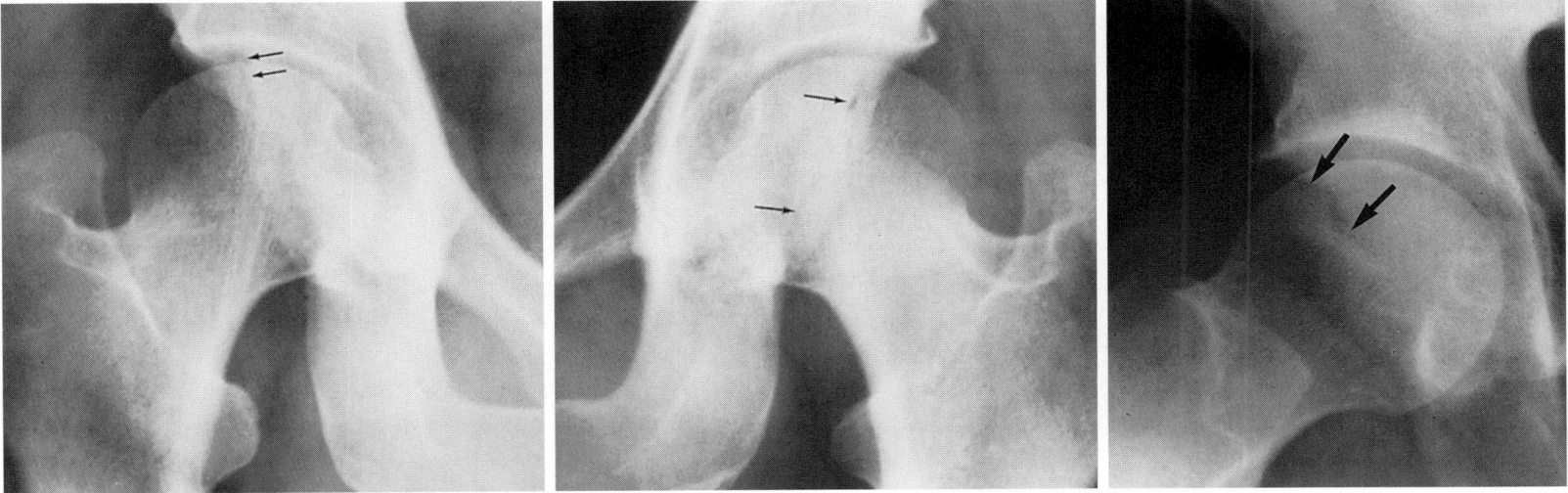

Figure 4–102. Three examples of persistence of all or portions of secondary ossification centers of the acetabulum in adults. These may be mistaken for fractures.

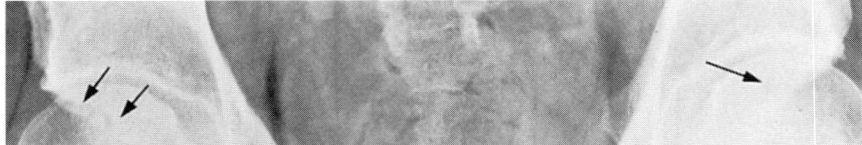

Figure 4–103. Incomplete closure of the os acetabuli marginalis superior, producing apparent radiolucencies in the heads of the femurs in a 32-year-old man.

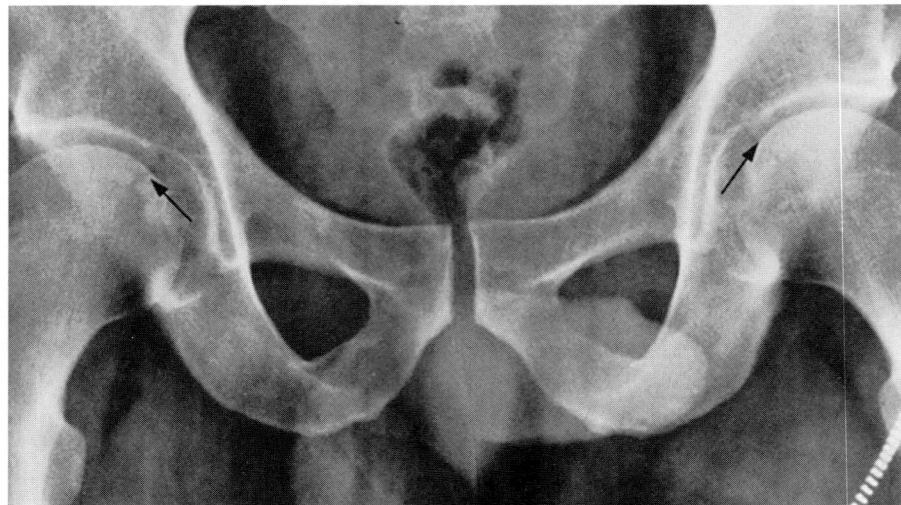

Figure 4–104. Incomplete closure of the ossification centers of the acetabulum simulating fractures in a 40-year-old man.

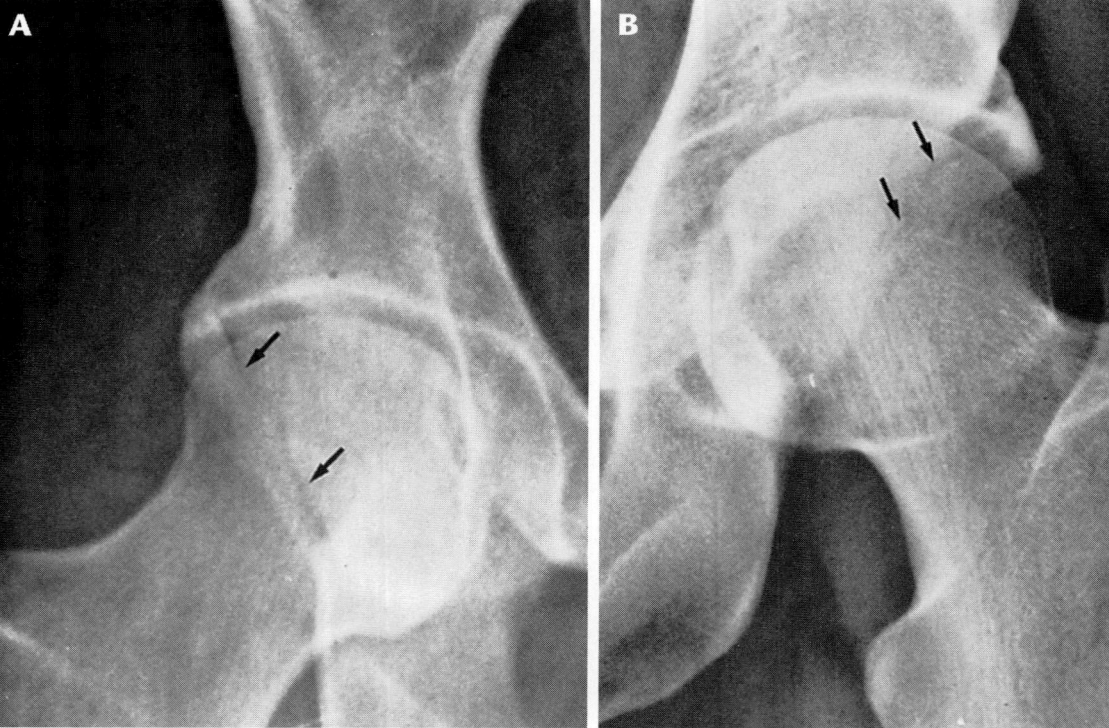

Figure 4–105. A, Another example of the accessory center of ossification of the posterior lip of the acetabulum simulating a fracture in a 32-year-old woman. **B,** A similar but less marked appearance is present in opposite hip.

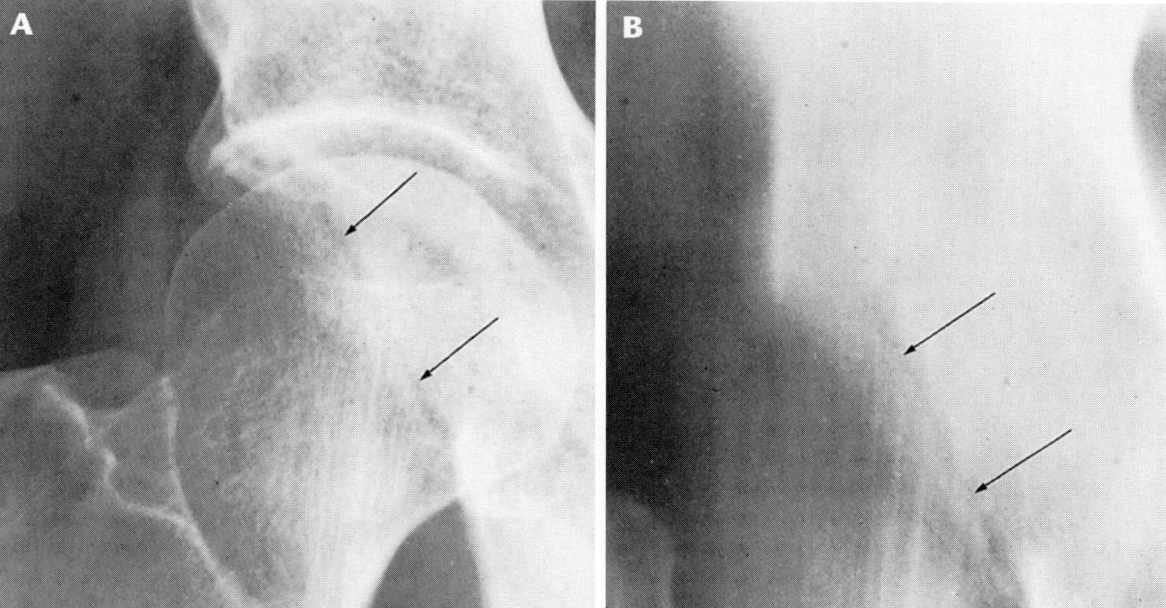

Figure 4–106. Persistence of a secondary center of ossification of the posterior lip of the acetabulum, which was mistaken for a fracture. **A,** Conventional film. **B,** Tomogram.

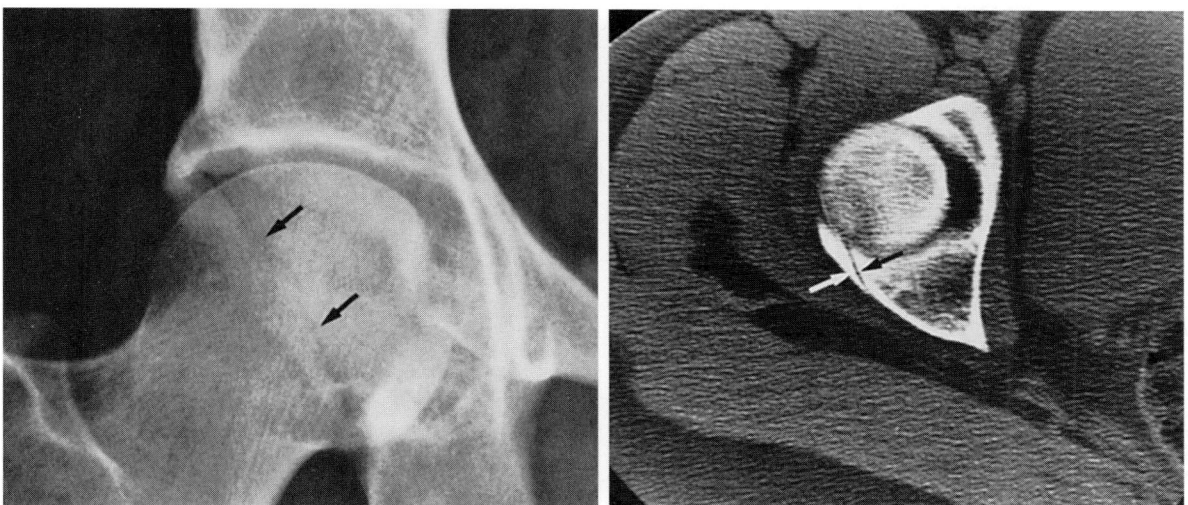

Figure 4–107. The same entity as in the preceding two figures with CT confirmation.

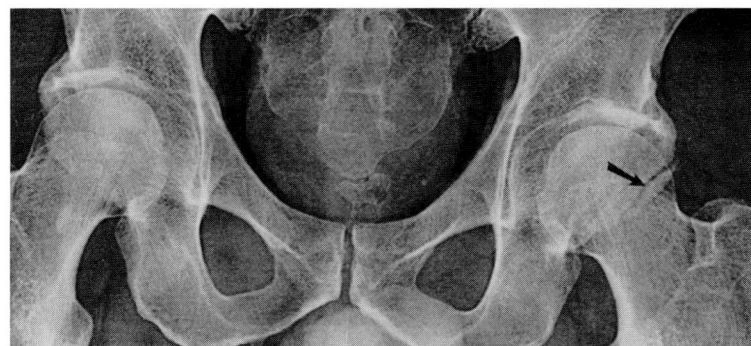

Figure 4–108. Unilateral ununited apophysis on the left.

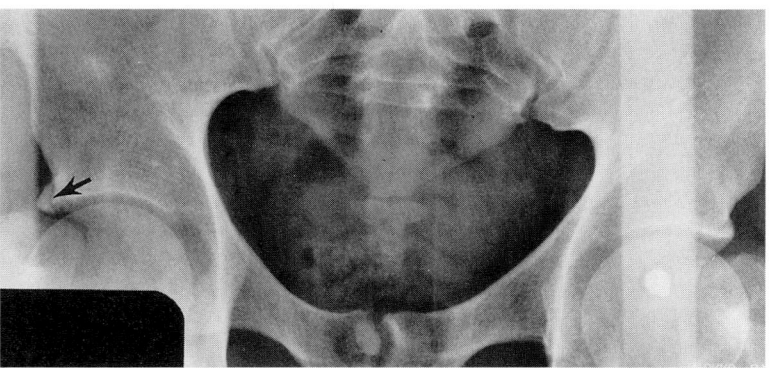

Figure 4–109. Ununited apophysis on the right in a 20-year-old man.

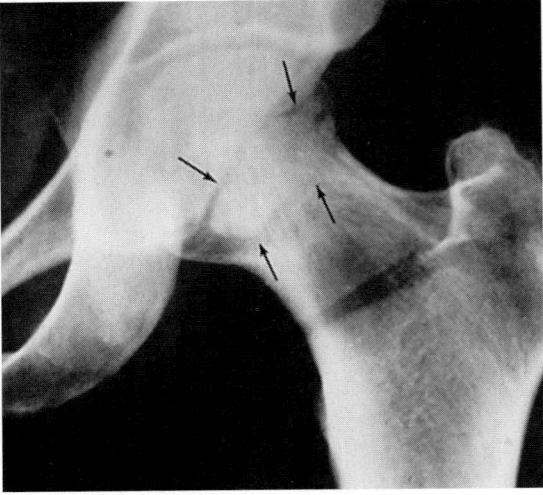

Figure 4–110. A large accessory bone at the posterior margin of the acetabulum.

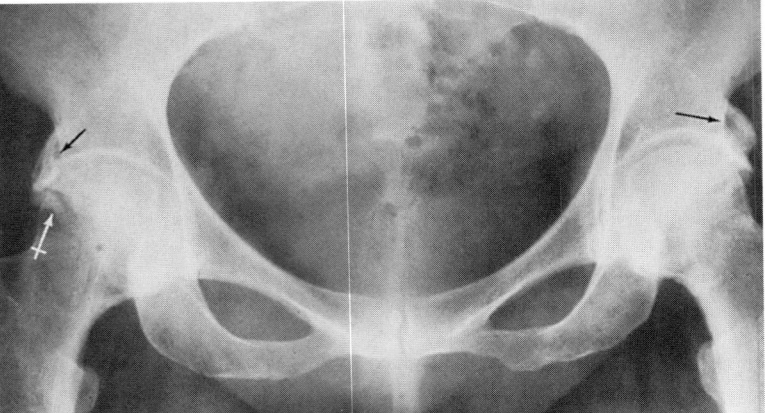

Figure 4–111. Spurlike margins of the acetabulum (→). Note the ununited ossification center (↦).

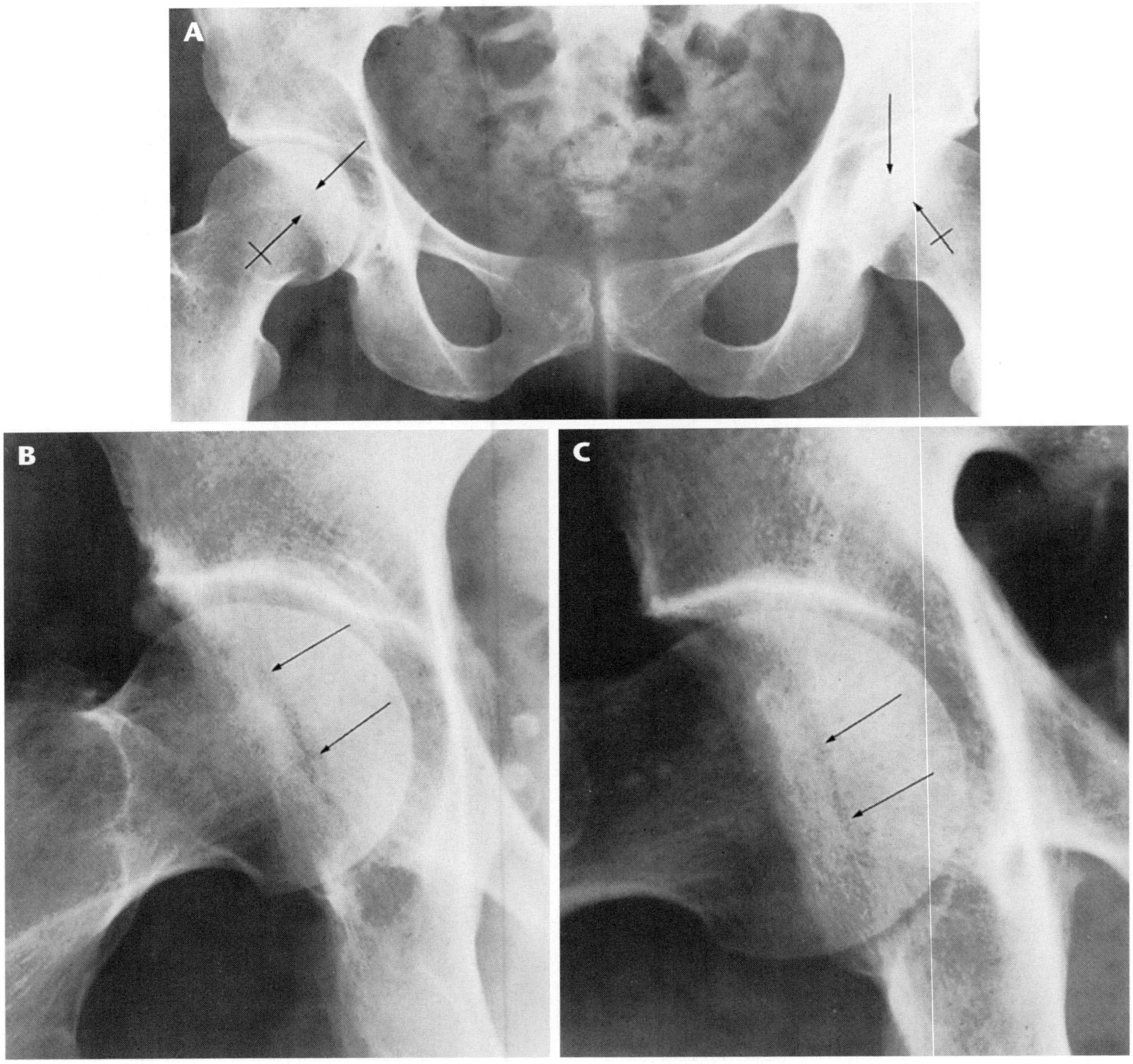

Figure 4–112. A, The anterior lip of the acetabulum (→) and the posterior lip (↦) may be identified in most individuals. Between them, there is a relative radiolucency, best seen on the patient's right side. **B** and **C,** The lucent interval in these two patients produces an appearance simulating a fracture of the posterior wall of the acetabulum (See Figs. 4–105 through 4–107.)

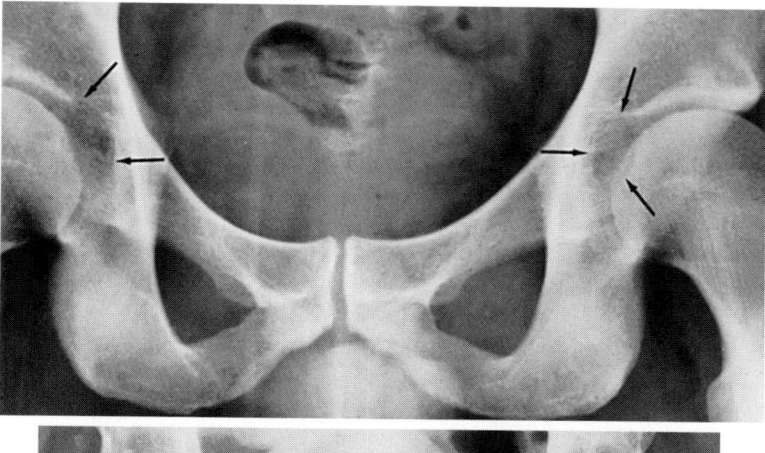

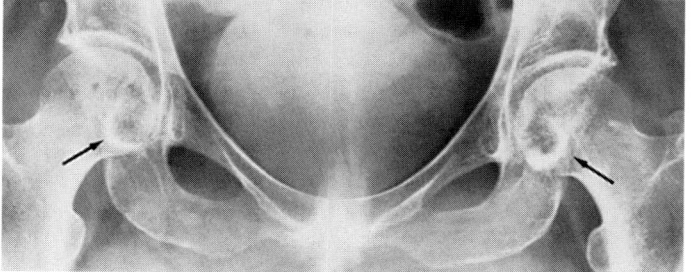

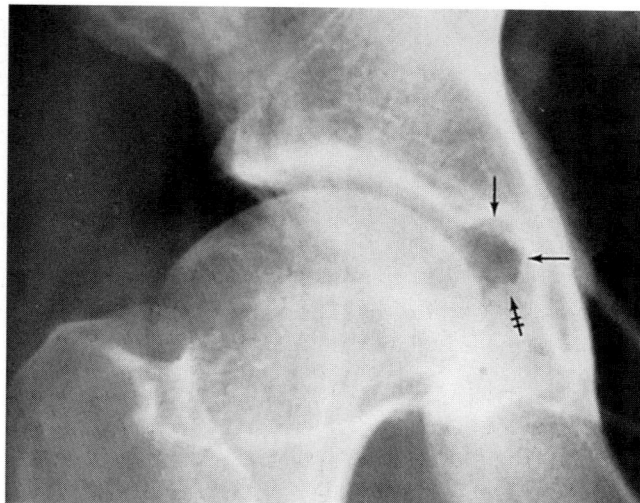

Figure 4–114. Simulated destructive lesion of the acetabulum (←) caused by an undulation in the anterior margin of the acetabulum coupled with superimposition of the shadow of the ischium (⇇). This might be mistaken for a lesion on the apex of the acetabulum.

Figure 4–113. Apparent defects in the acetabulum as a result of projection and not anatomic alteration.

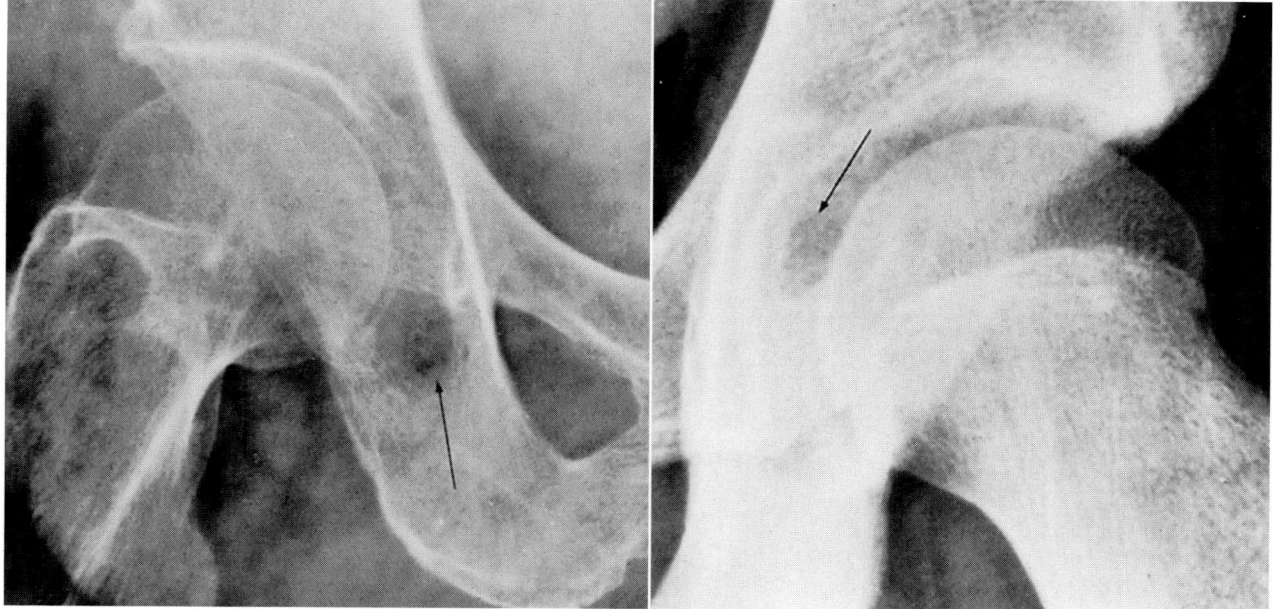

Figure 4–115. Two other examples of fossae (different patients), which should not be mistaken for pathologic processes. Bilateral symmetry is helpful.

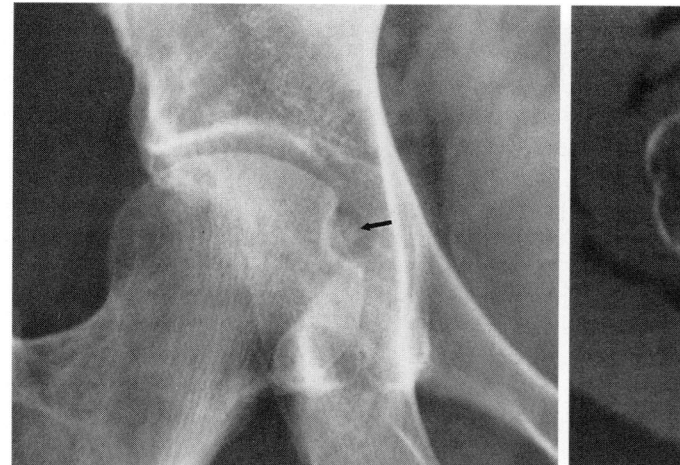

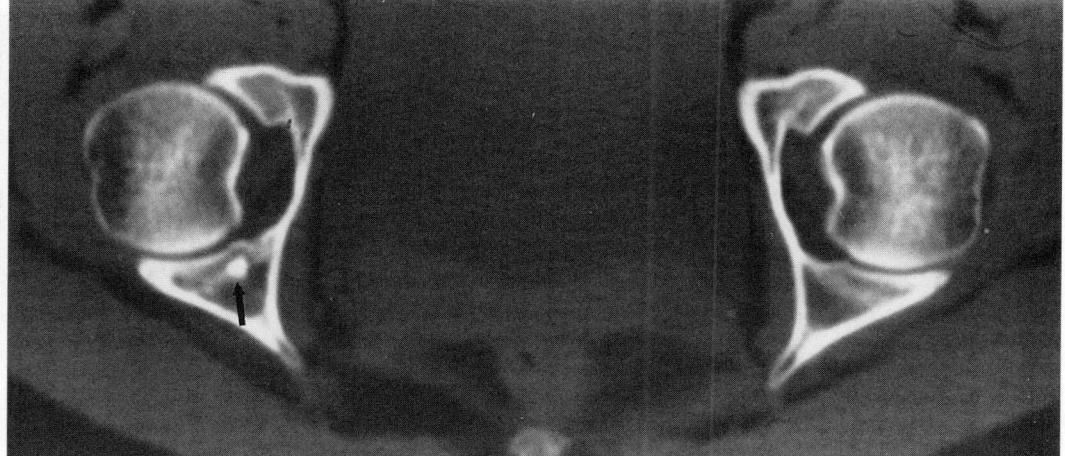

Figure 4–116. Bone island in the ischium simulating a foveal lesion.

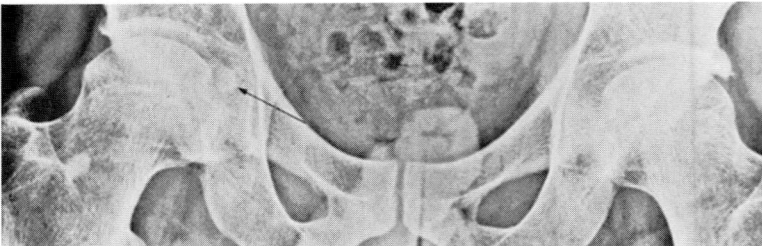

Figure 4–117. A bone island in the acetabulum.

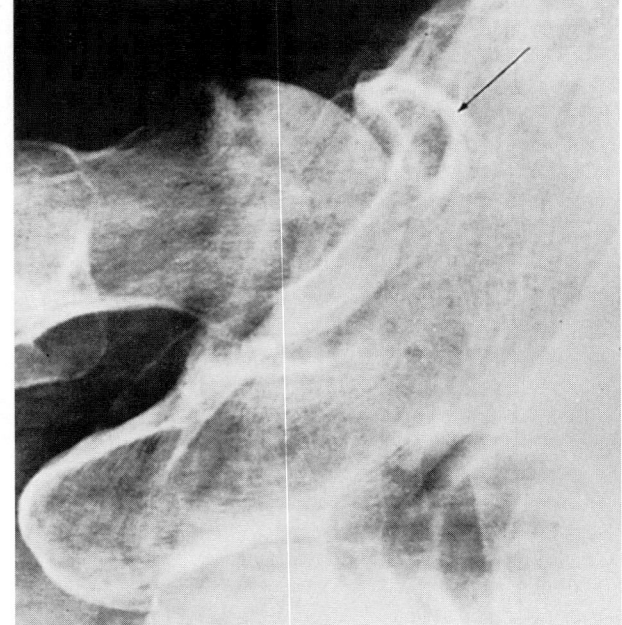

Figure 4–118. In the lateral projection of the hip, the superior margin of the acetabulum may simulate a cyst.

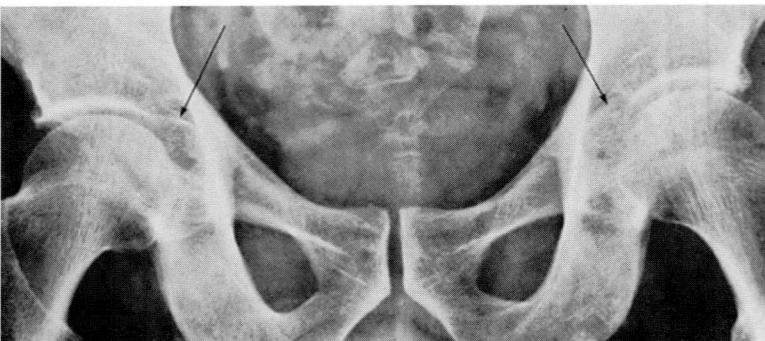

Figure 4–119. The roofs of the acetabula may project asymmetrically in normal individuals.

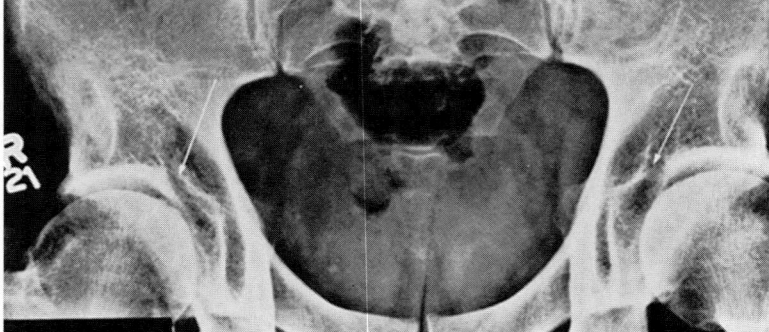

Figure 4–120. The superior acetabular notch is the result of an accessory fossa in the apex of the acetabulum and is of no significance. (Ref: Johnstone WH et al: The anatomic basis for the superior acetabular roof notch: "Superior acetabular notch." *Skeletal Radiol* 8:25, 1982.)

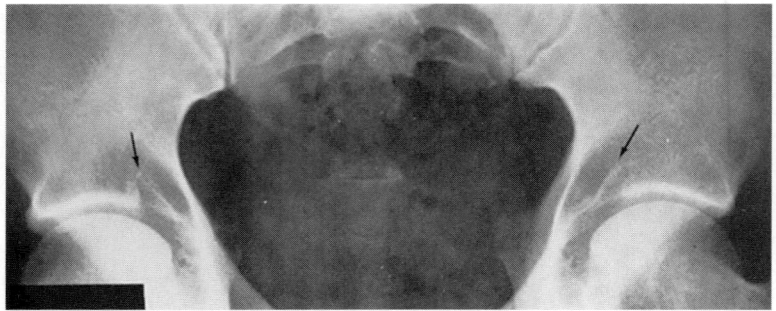

Figure 4–121. Marked notching of the roof of the acetabulum.

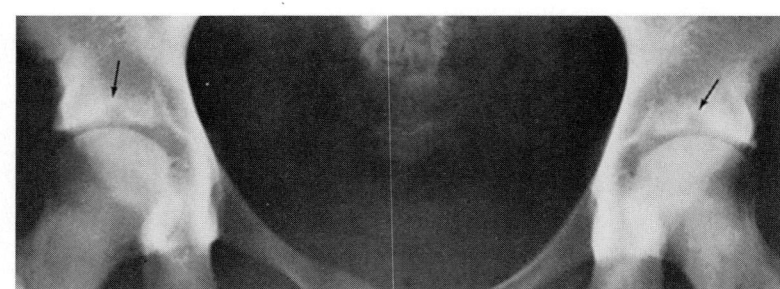

Figure 4–122. Unusual second lateral notch in the roof of the acetabulum in a young woman. (Courtesy of Dr. W. B. Guilford.)

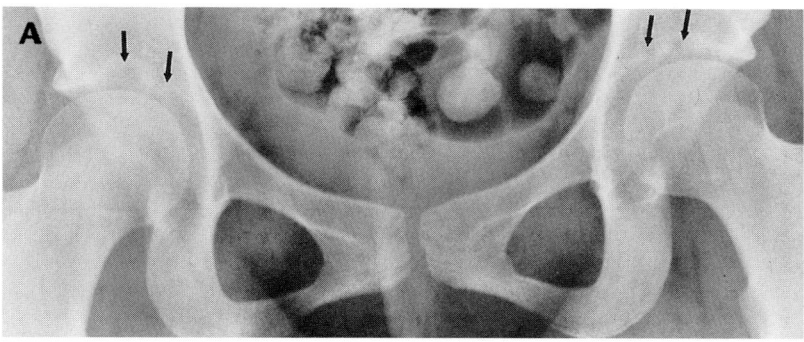
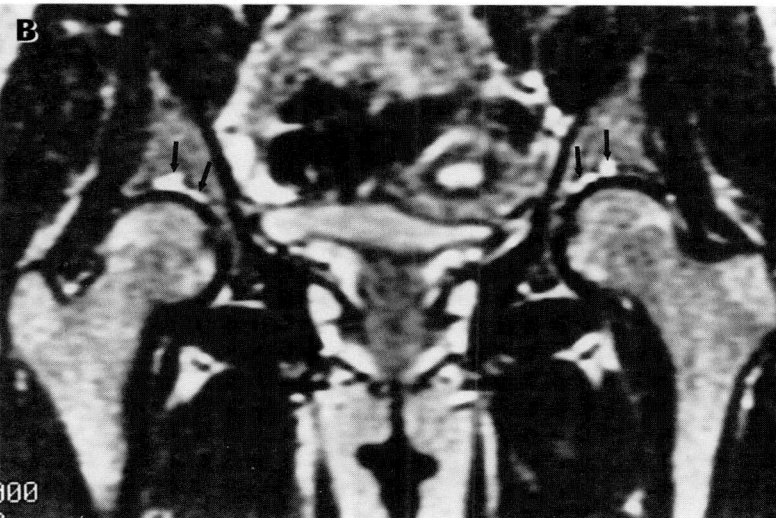

Figure 4–123. The acetabular notches demonstrated by MRI. **A,** Plain film. **B,** T-2–weighted image shows fluid signal in the notches as anticipated.

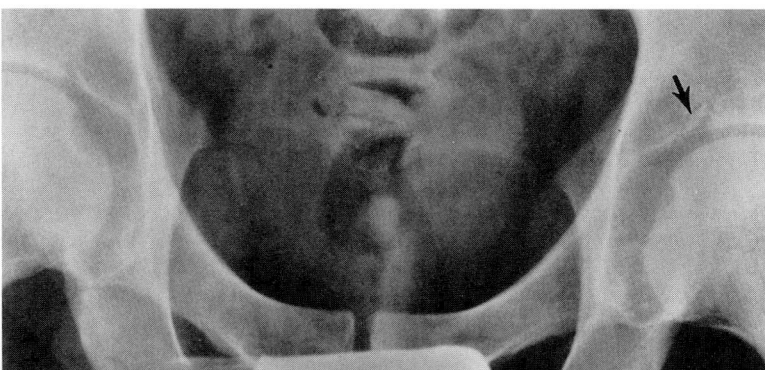

Figure 4–124. Variation in appearance of the acetabular notch on the left.

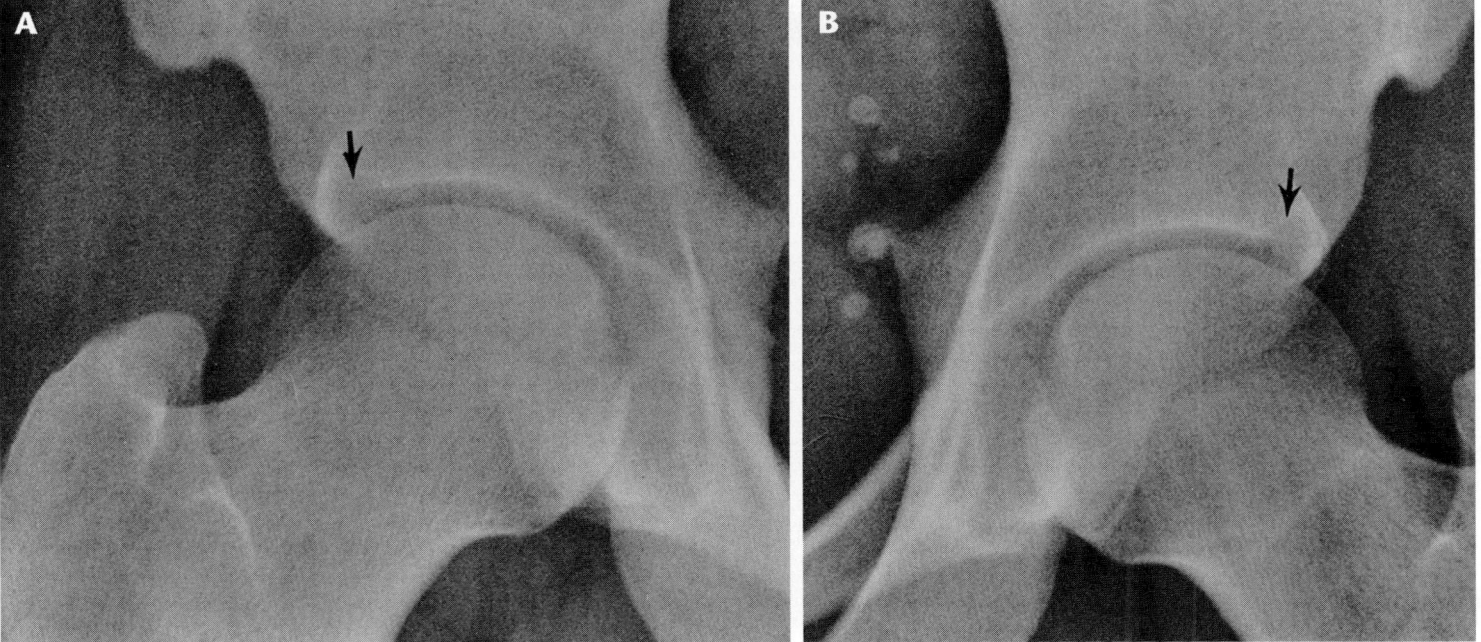

Figure 4–125. A, B, Bilateral laterally placed acetabular notches.

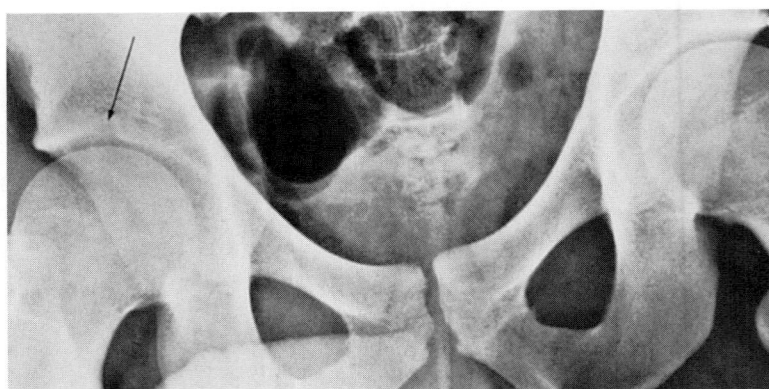
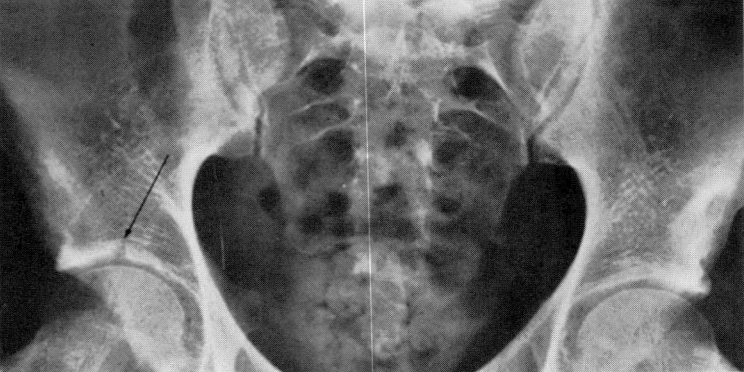

Figure 4–126. Two examples of asymmetric lateral acetabular notches, which are also probably due to fossae in the acetabulum.

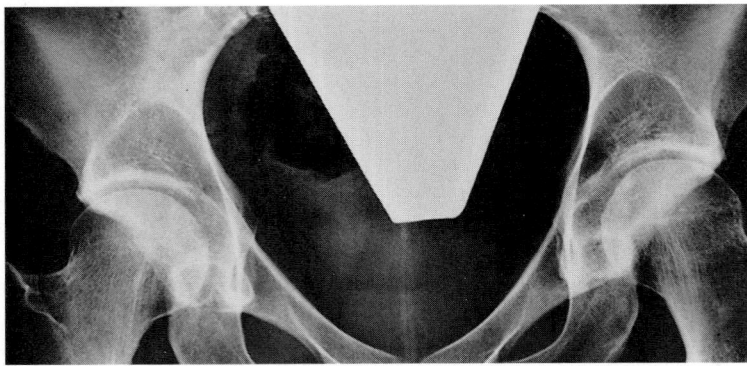

Figure 4–127. Exaggeration of the normal triangle of radiolucency above the acetabula. The slight difference in density is due to rotation as evidenced by the asymmetry of the obturator foramina.

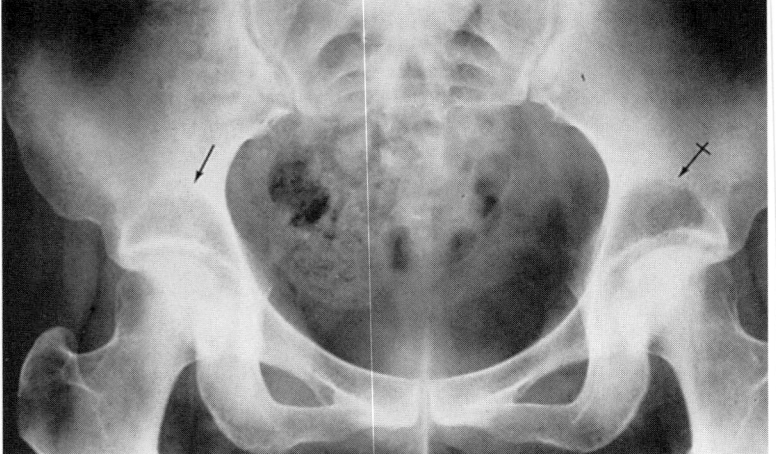

Figure 4–128. Normal triangular area of lucency above the acetabulum (→). This is normally bilaterally symmetric. The greater radiolucency is due to metastatic neoplasm (↦). Note lack of rotation at time of filming.

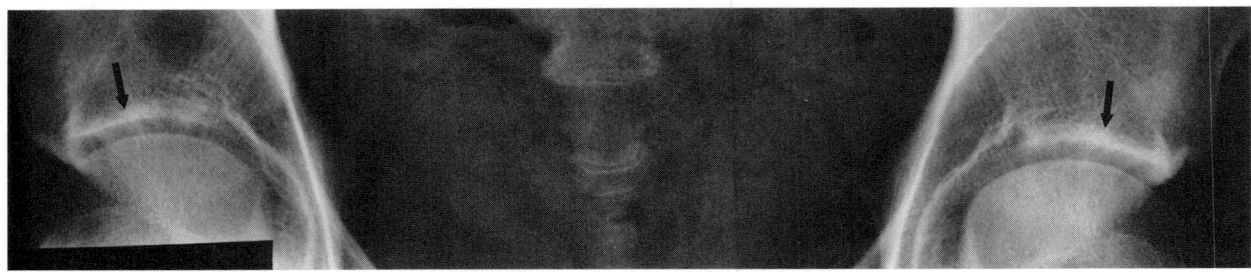

Figure 4–129. Normal asymmetry in the density of the roofs of the acetabula in a 30-year-old man, not to be confused with the changes of degenerative arthritis. Note symmetry of the joint width.

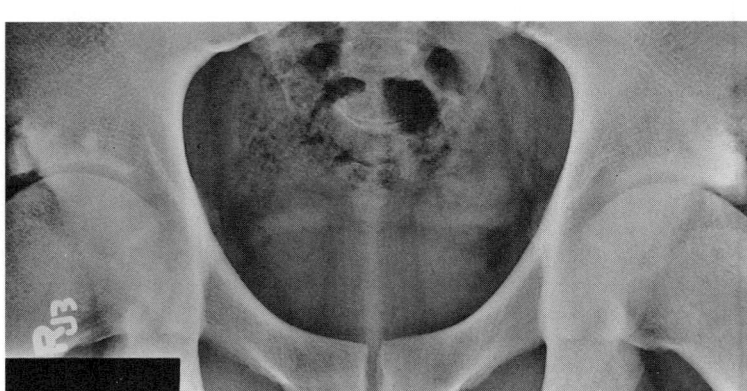

Figure 4–130. Exaggeration of the normal acetabular roof sclerosis without joint disease. Note the os acetabulum on the patient's right side.

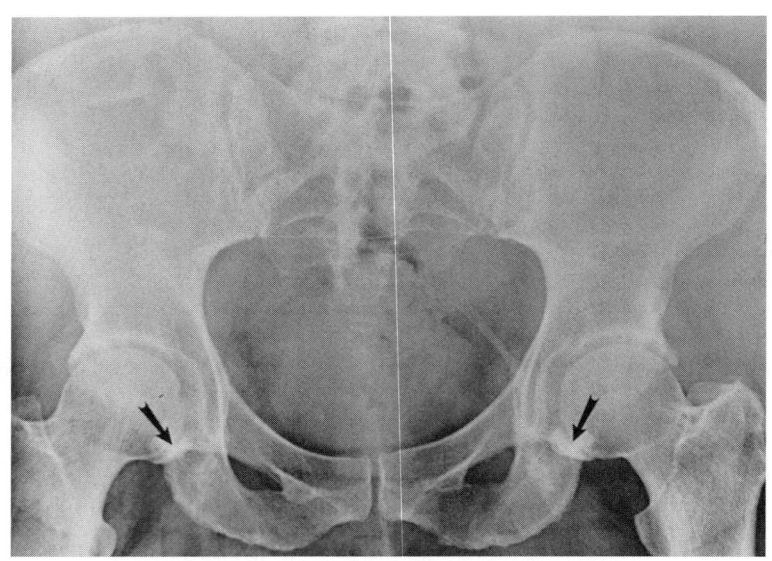

Figure 4–131. Sclerosis of the inferior lips of the acetabula without degenerative joint disease. Note enthesopathy at upper lips of the acetabula and at the iliac crests.

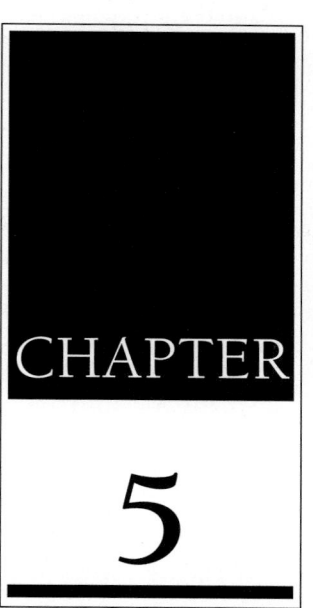

CHAPTER 5

The Shoulder Girdle and Thoracic Cage

The Scapula

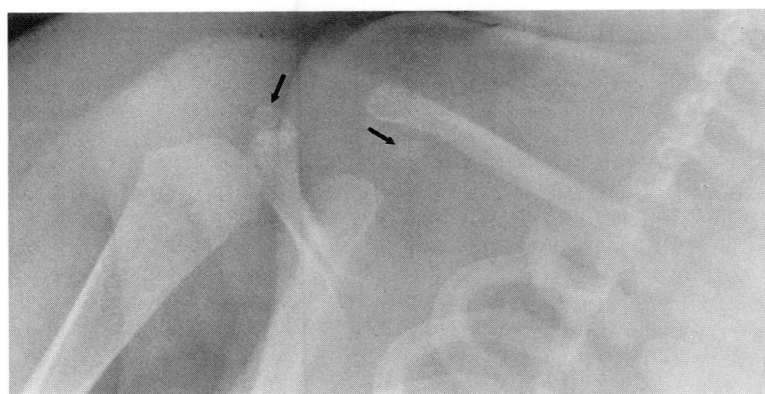

Figure 5–1. Premature appearance of the ossification centers of the acromion and coracoid in a 1-month-old child. The coracoid process is not usually seen until the third month or later, and the secondary center for the acromion is not usually seen until 10 to 12 years of age.

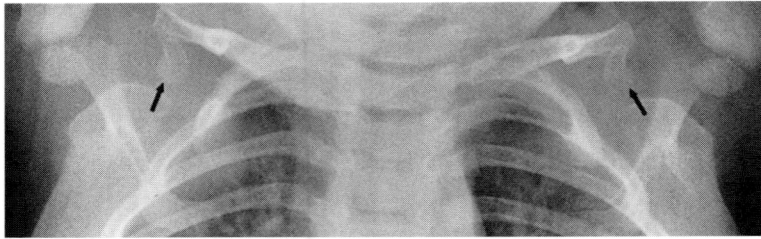

Figure 5–2. The coracoid processes seen as separate bones in a 2-year-old child.

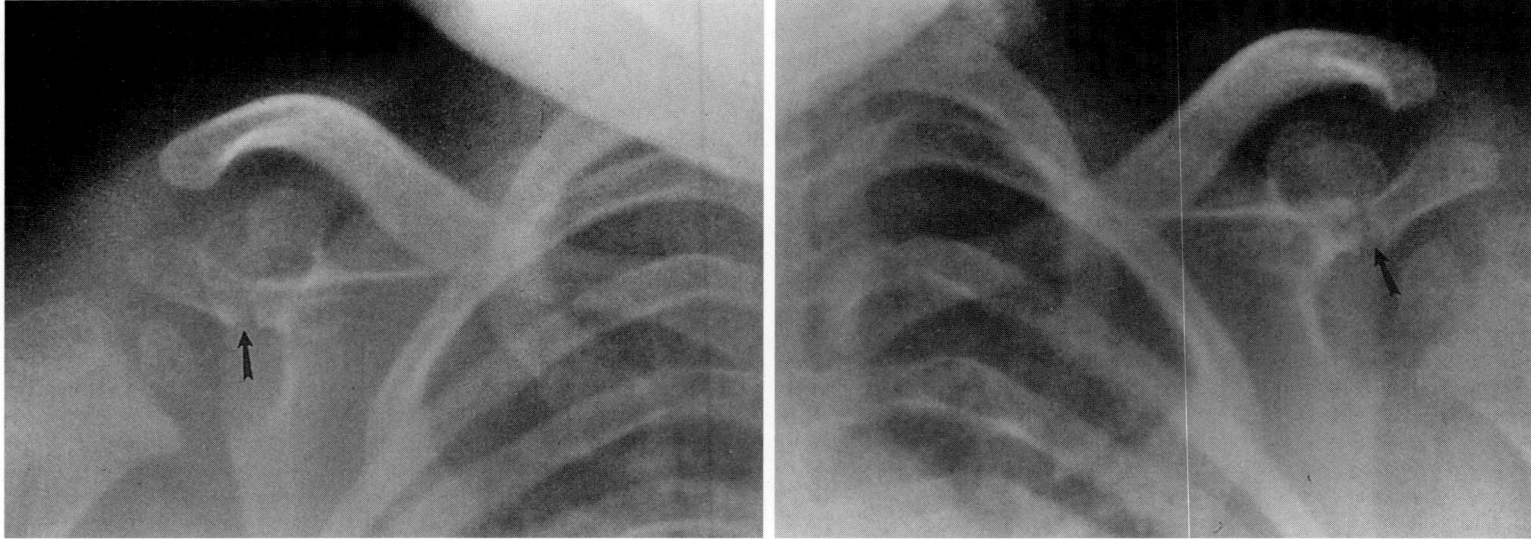

Figure 5–3. Development of the acromion processes as separate centers in a 1-year-old girl. Not to be mistaken for the acromial fracture associated with child abuse. (Ref: Currarino G, Prescott P: Fractures of the acromion in young children and a description of a variant in acromial ossification which may mimic a fracture. *Pediatr Radiol* 24:251, 1994.)

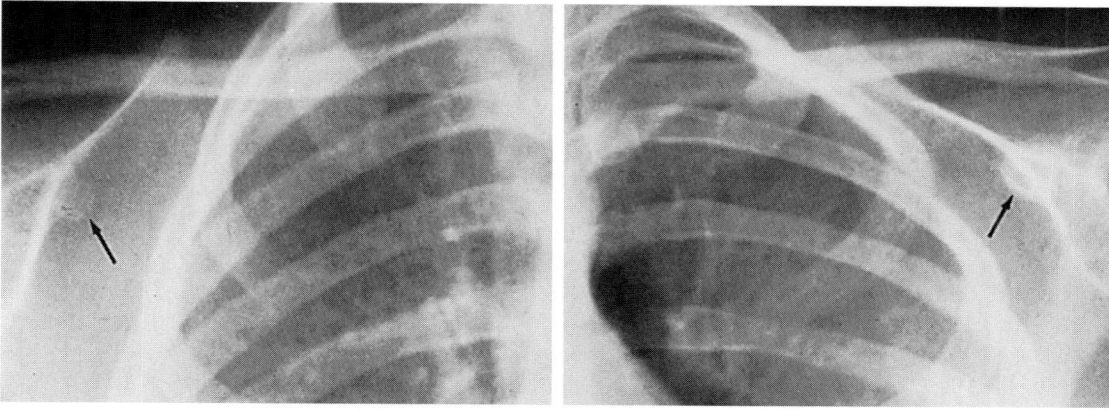

Figure 5–4. Normal appearance of the ossification centers of the coracoid processes in a 5-year-old boy.

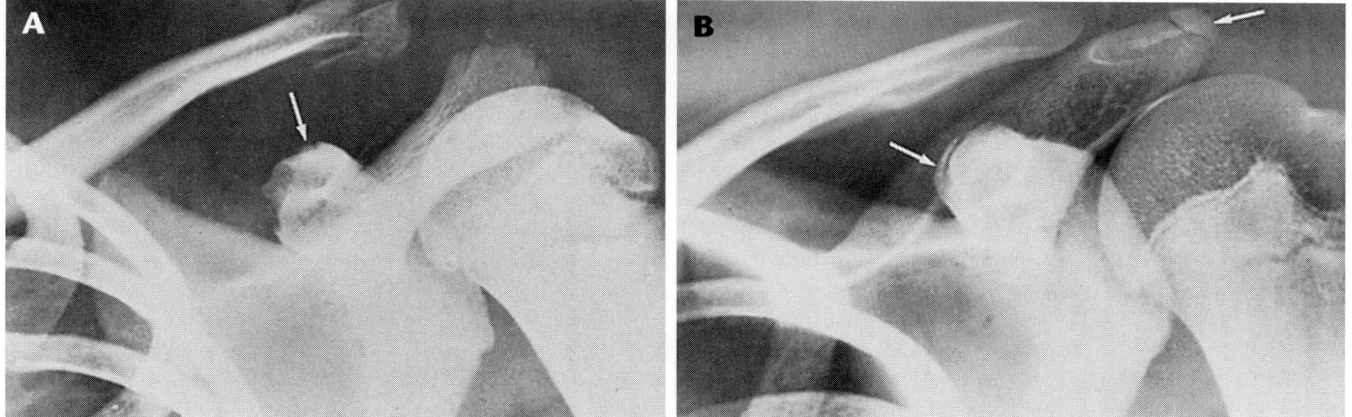

Figure 5–5. Normal appearance of the coracoid processes during growth. **A,** 13-year-old boy before appearance of the secondary ossification center. **B,** 15-year-old boy. Note secondary ossification centers for coracoid and acromion processes.

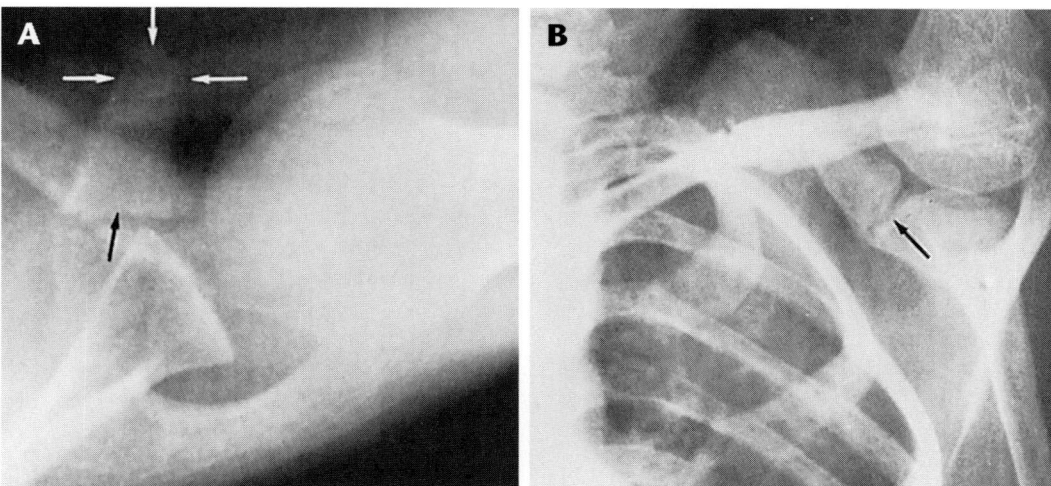

Figure 5–6. Appearance of the ossification center of the coracoid process in adolescence before fusion occurs. It may be mistaken for a fracture. **A,** Axillary projection. **B,** Arm elevated.

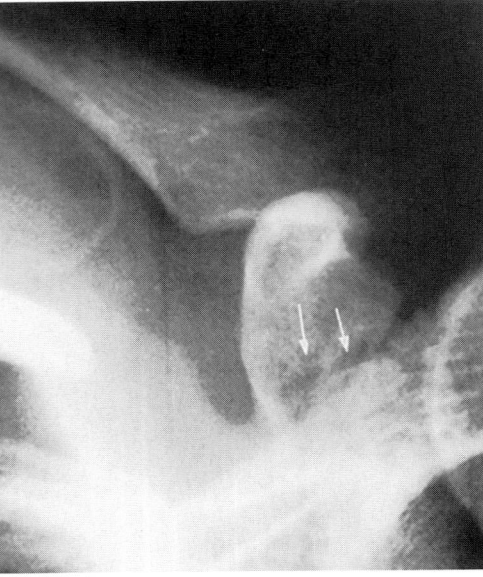

Figure 5–7. The apophysis of the coracoid process mistaken for a fracture in a 14-year-old boy.

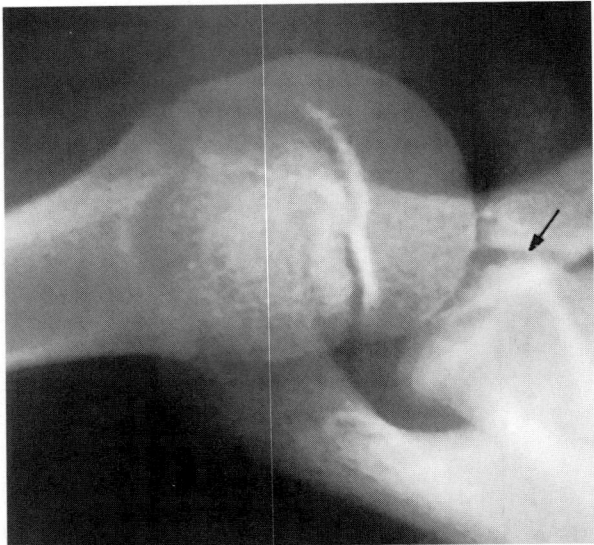

Figure 5–8. The synchondrosis of the base of the coracoid in a 15-year-old boy that simulates a cleft in the glenoid, as seen in axillary projection.

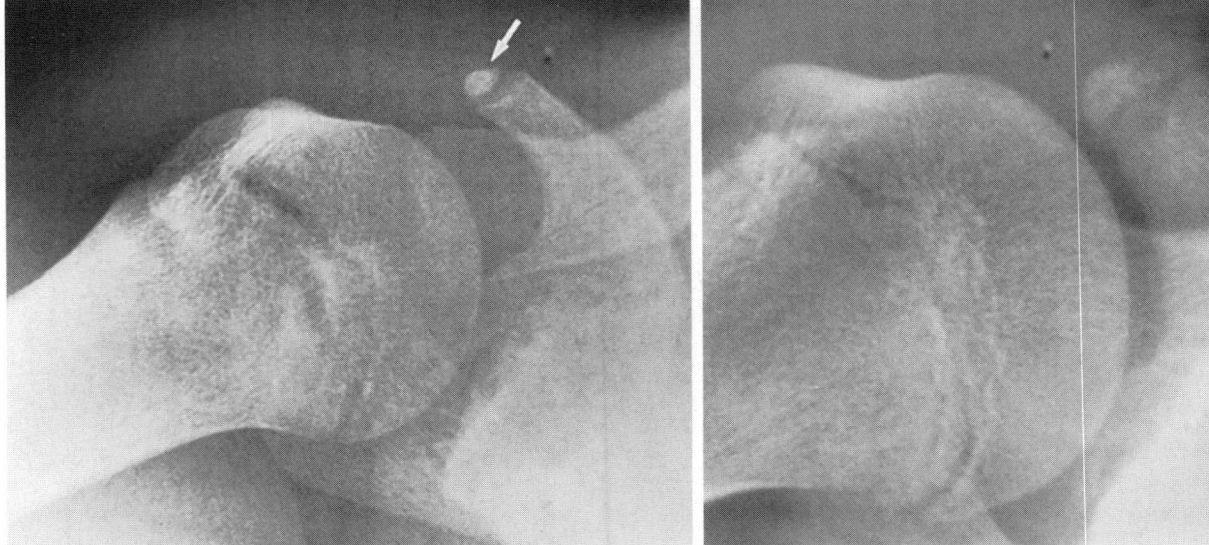

Figure 5–9. Two examples of the secondary apophysis of the tip of the coracoid process.

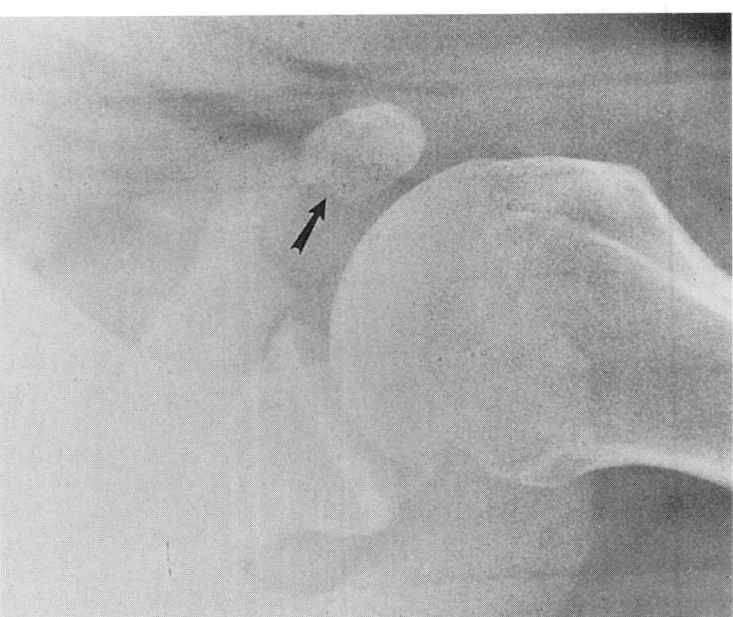

Figure 5–10. Failure of union of the secondary apophysis of the coracoid persisting as a separate bone, the coracoid bone.

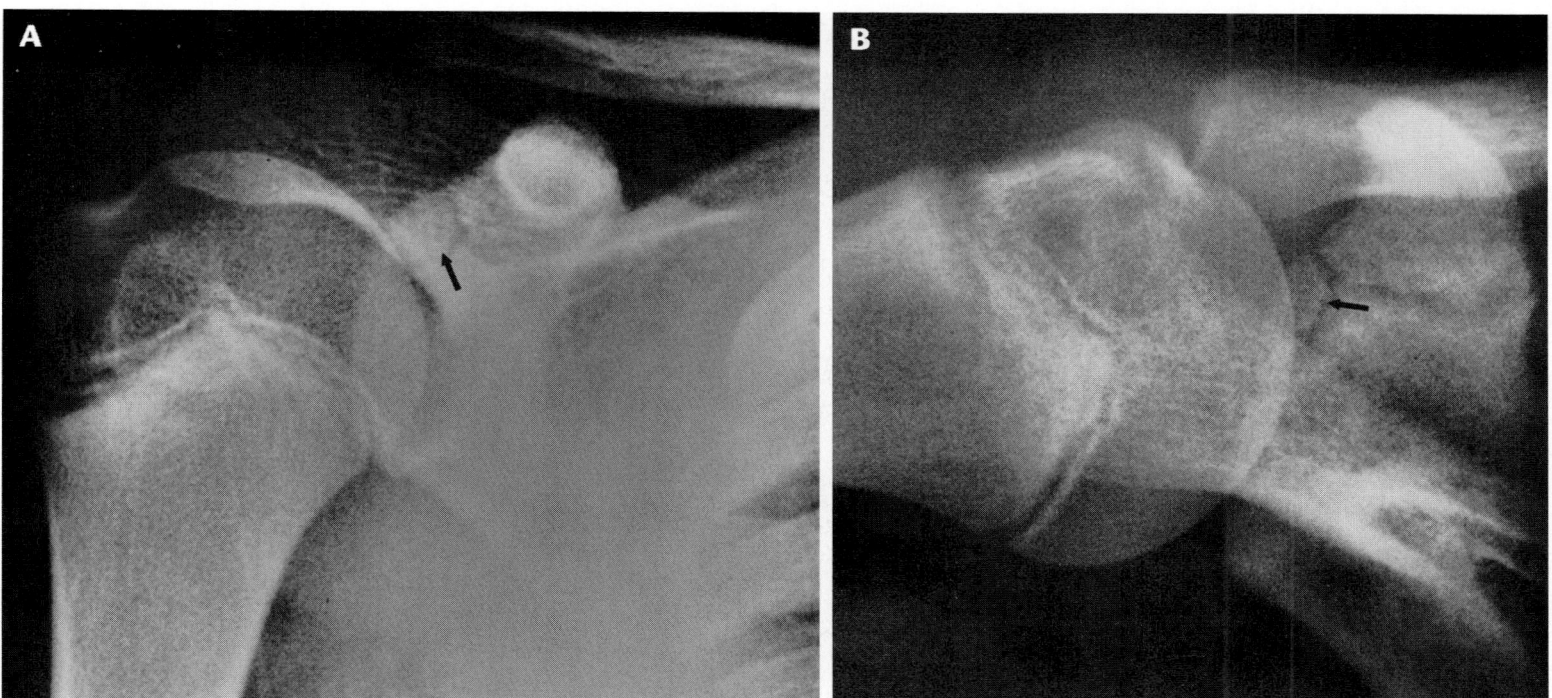

Figure 5–11. Accessory ossification center at the synchondrosis at the base of the coracoid in a 14-year-old boy. **A,** Anteroposterior projection. **B,** Abduction film.

Figure 5–12. The same entity described in the preceding figure.

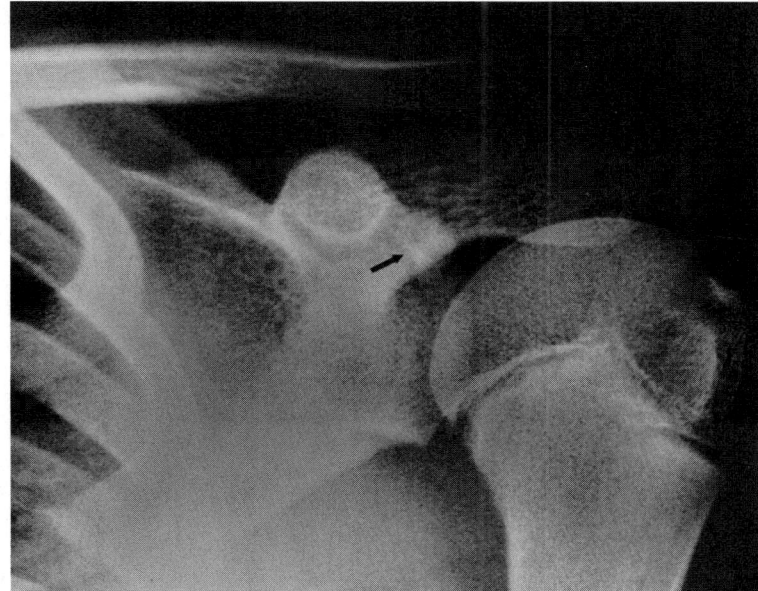

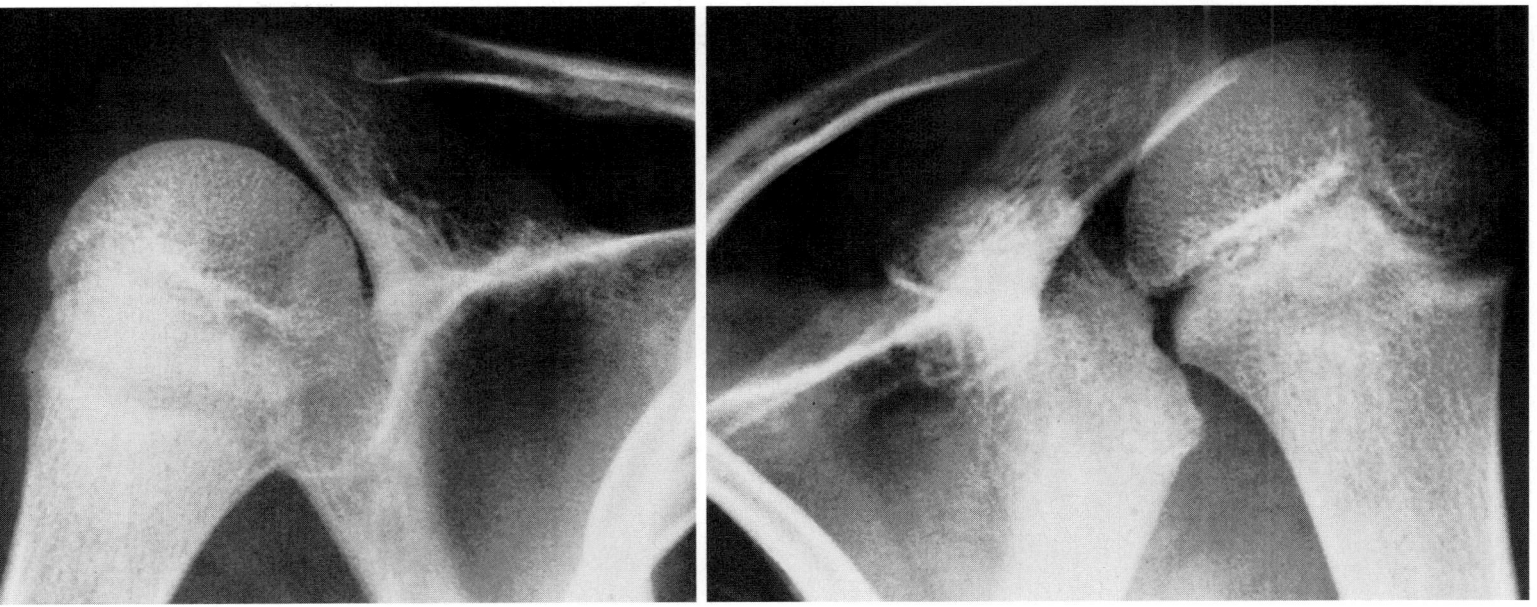

Figure 5–13. Unusually long and stout acromion processes in a 6-year-old boy.

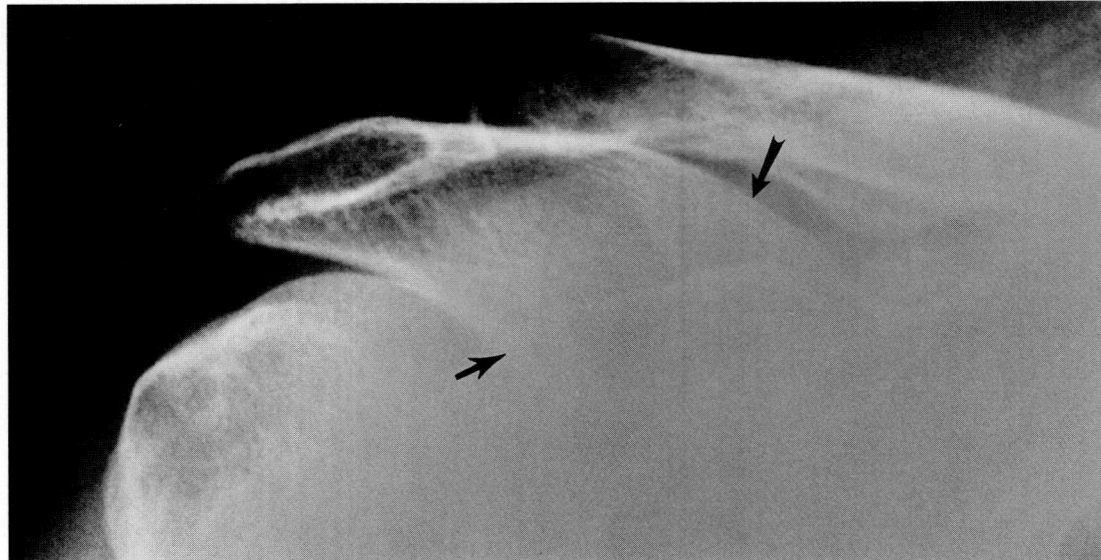

Figure 5–14. Unusually stout acromion in an adult.

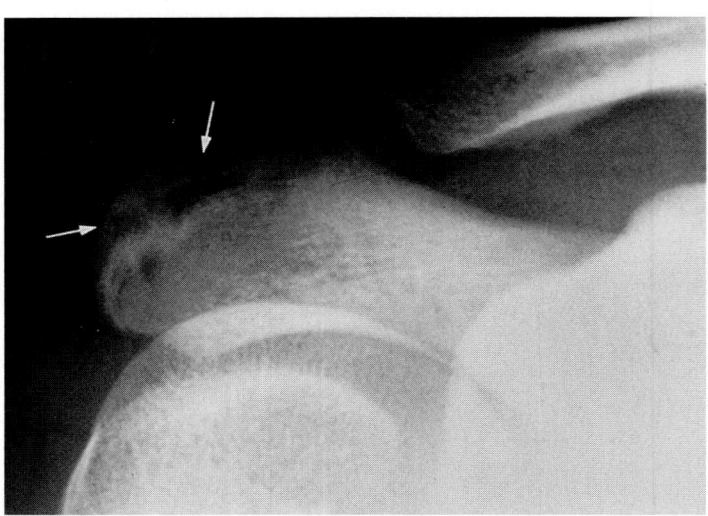

Figure 5–15. The normal closing acromial apophysis in a 13-year-old boy. The irregularity of the apophyseal line is normal. The distal end of the acromion ossifies irregularly in infants and may be misinterpreted as evidence of child abuse. (Ref: Kleinman PK, Spevak MR: Variations in acromial ossification simulating infant abuse in victims of sudden infant death syndrome. *Radiology* 180:185, 1991.)

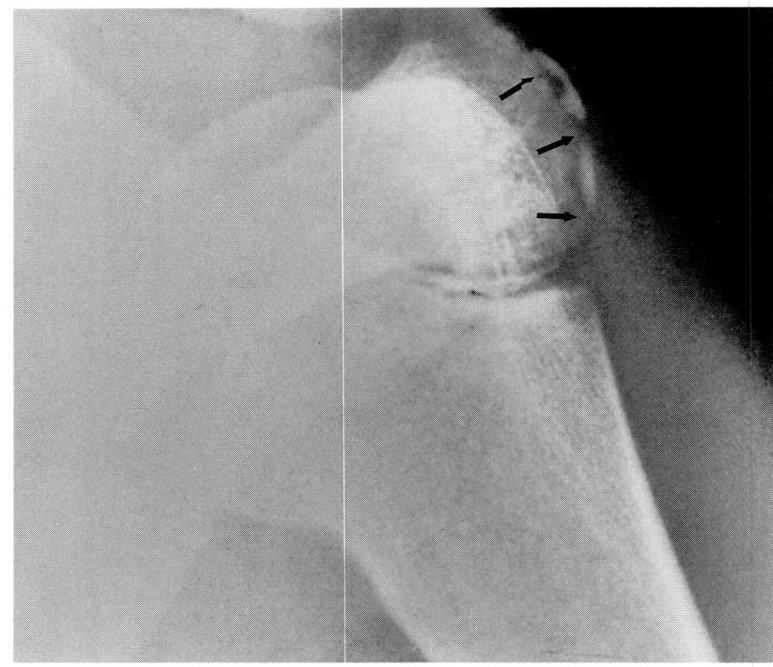

Figure 5–16. Normal irregularity of the acromion in a 12-year-old boy, which was mistaken for a pathologic process.

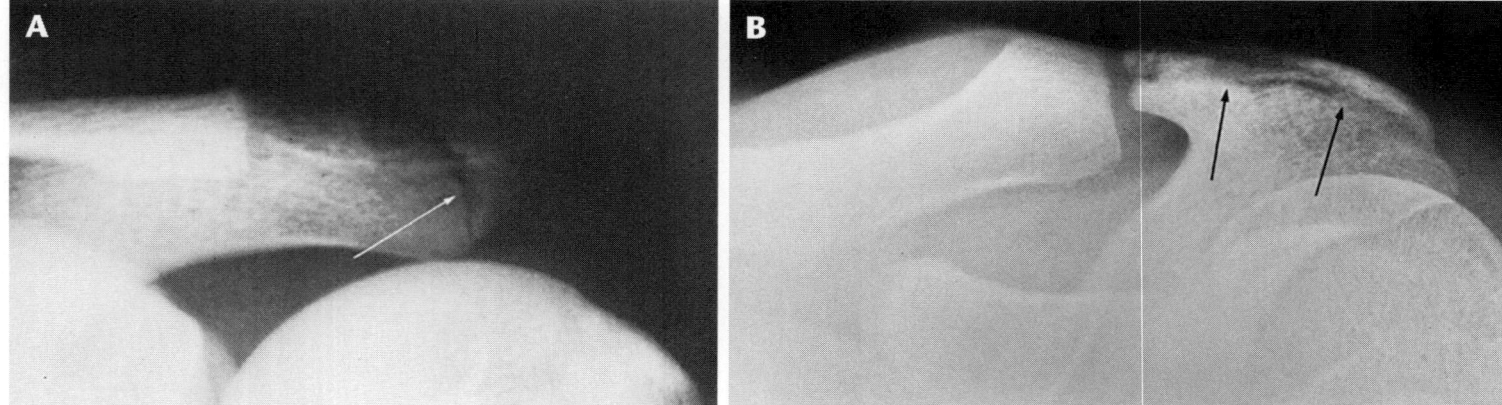

Figure 5–17. A, B, Normal closing acromial apophyses. Note the irregular mineralization and density of the center in **B.**

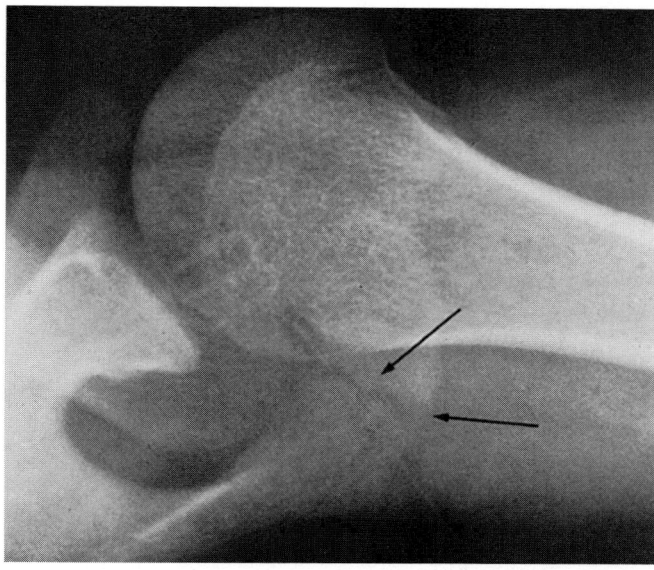

Figure 5–18. The apophysis of the acromion in a 14-year-old boy, shown in axillary projection. This closes at 18 to 20 years of age.

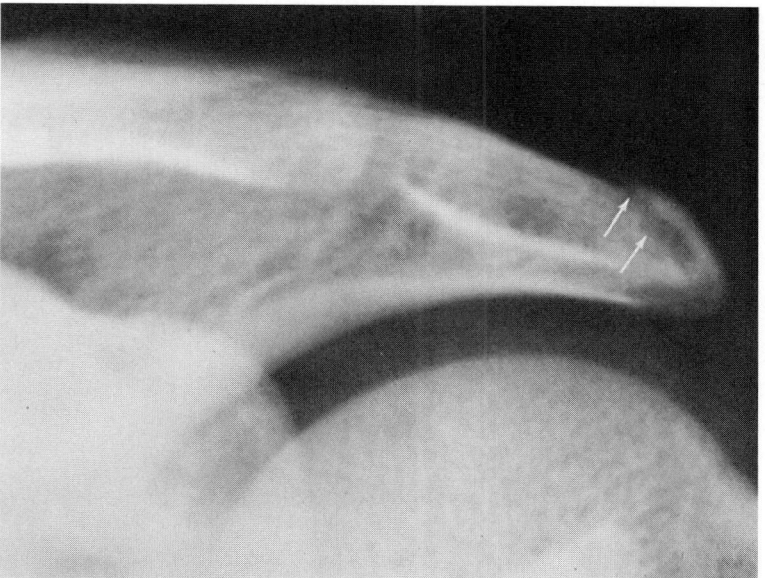

Figure 5–19. Remnant of the line of closure of secondary ossification center for the acromion in an 18-year-old man.

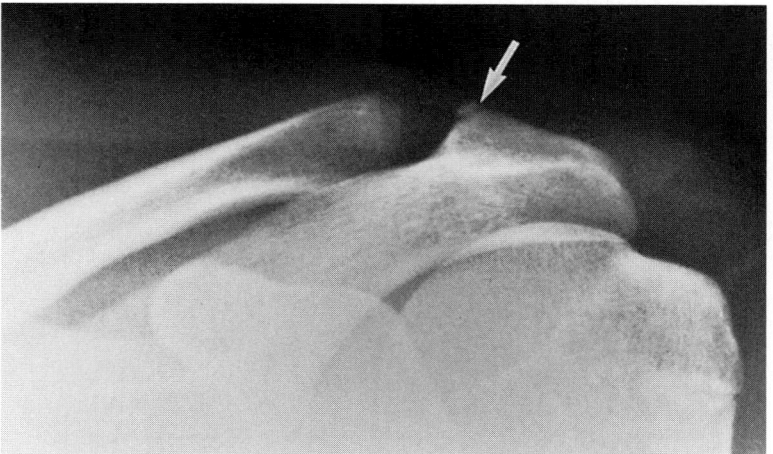

Figure 5–20. Persistent apophysis of the acromion in a 17-year-old boy. The opposite side was closed.

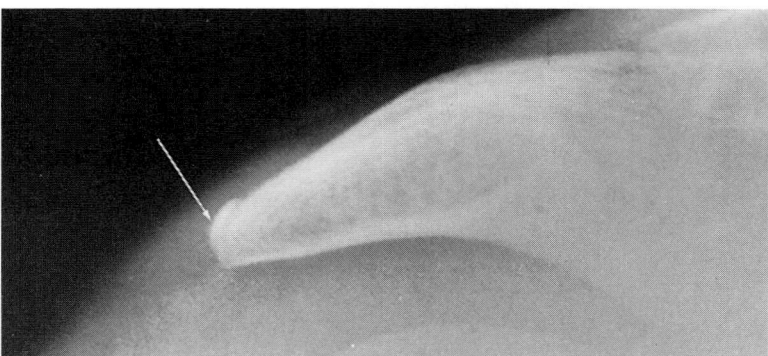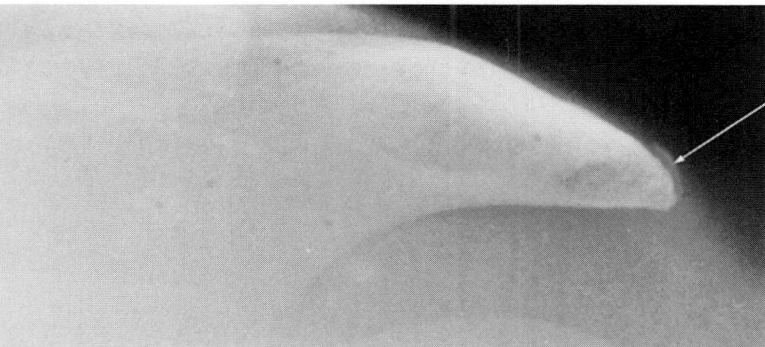

Figure 5–21. The apophysis of the end of the acromion in a 16-year-old boy should not be mistaken for a fracture.

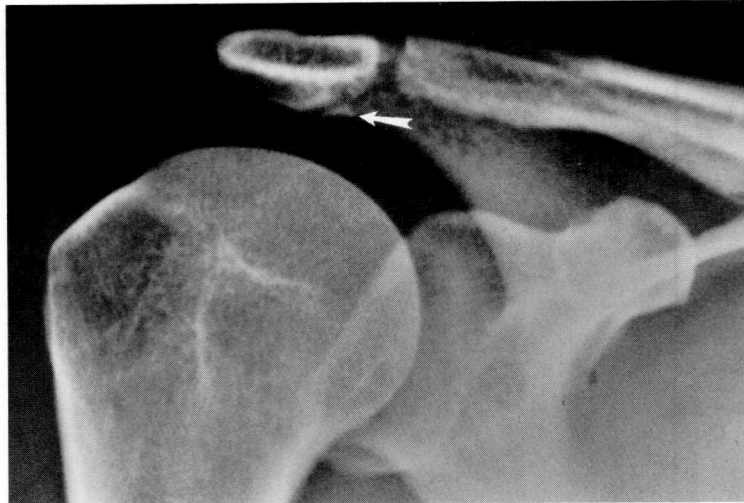

Figure 5–22. Ununited accessory ossification center for the acromion in a 38-year-old man.

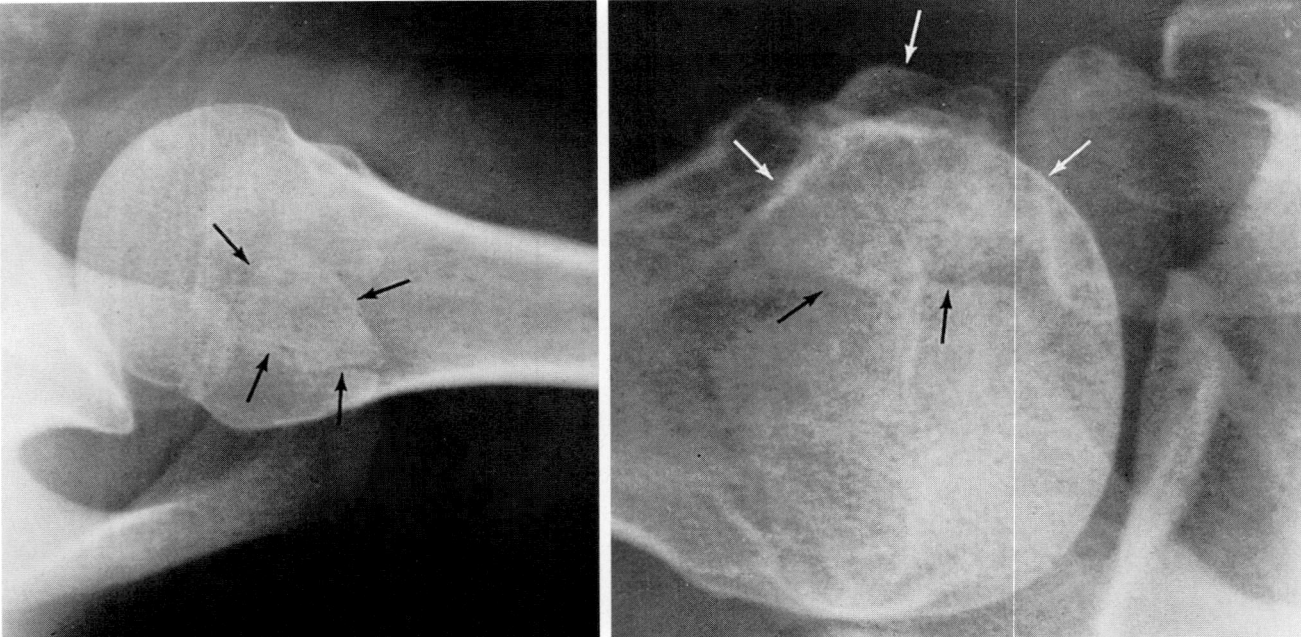

Figure 5–23. Two examples of the os acromiale. This secondary ossification center persists into adult life as a separate bone and is often mistaken for a fracture of the acromion process when seen in the axillary projection. It is usually, but not invariably, bilateral. (Refs: Park JG et al: Os acromiale associated with rotator cuff impingement: MR imaging of the shoulder. *Radiology* 193:255, 1994; Edelson JG et al: Os acromiale. *J Bone Joint Surg* 75B:551, 1993.)

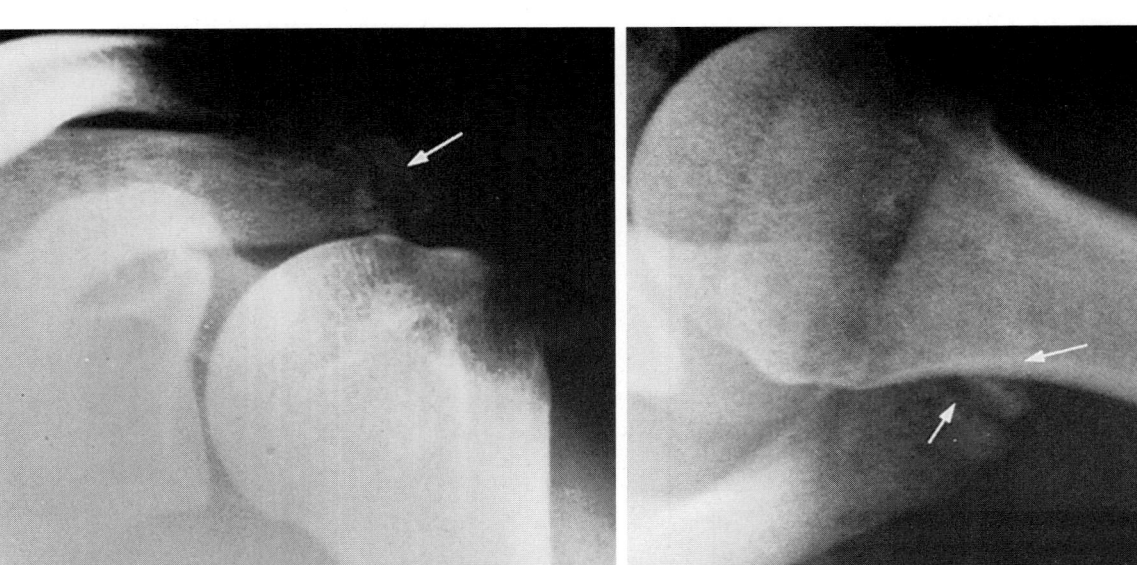

Figure 5–24. The os acromiale may occasionally be seen in the frontal projection *(left)* as well as in the axillary projection *(right)*.

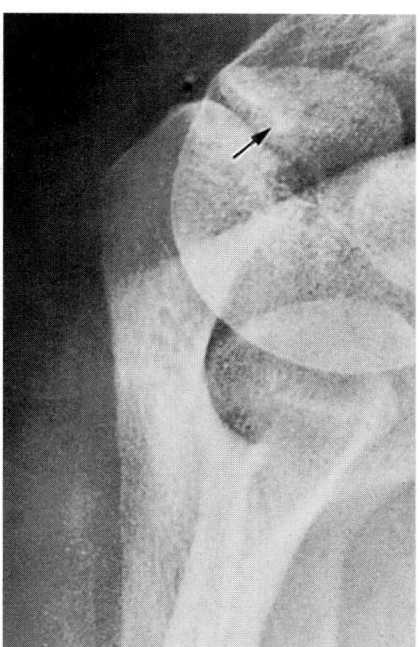

Figure 5–25. The os acromiale seen in the tangential view of the scapula.

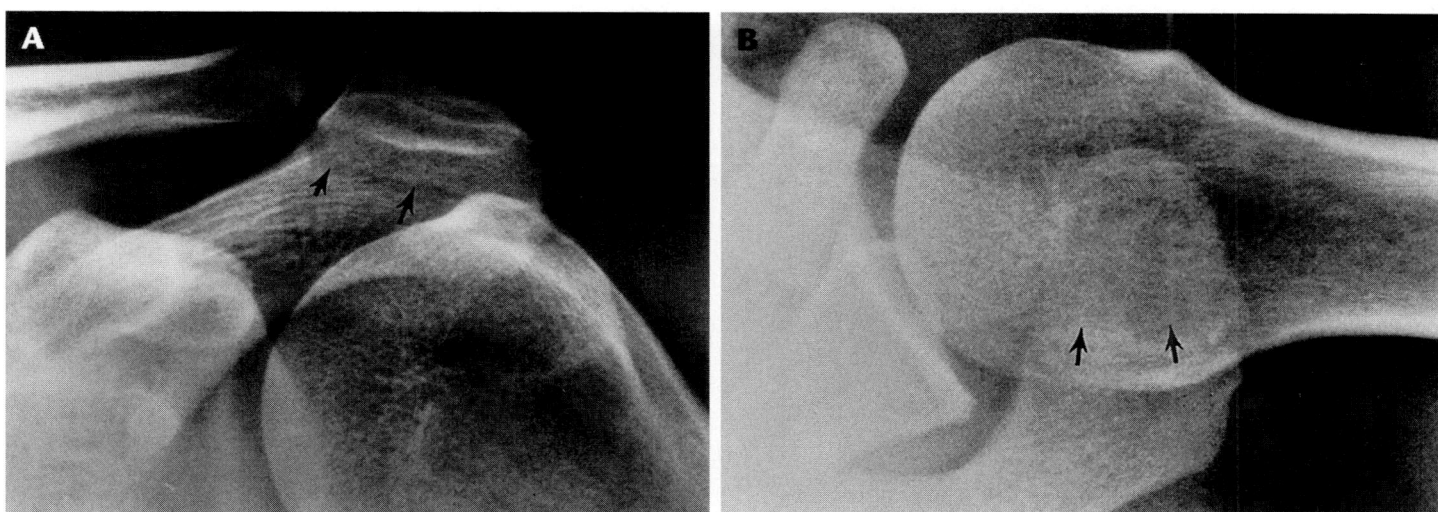

Figure 5–26. A, Os acromiale visible on frontal film simulating a fracture. **B,** Axillary projection demonstrates the os acromiale.

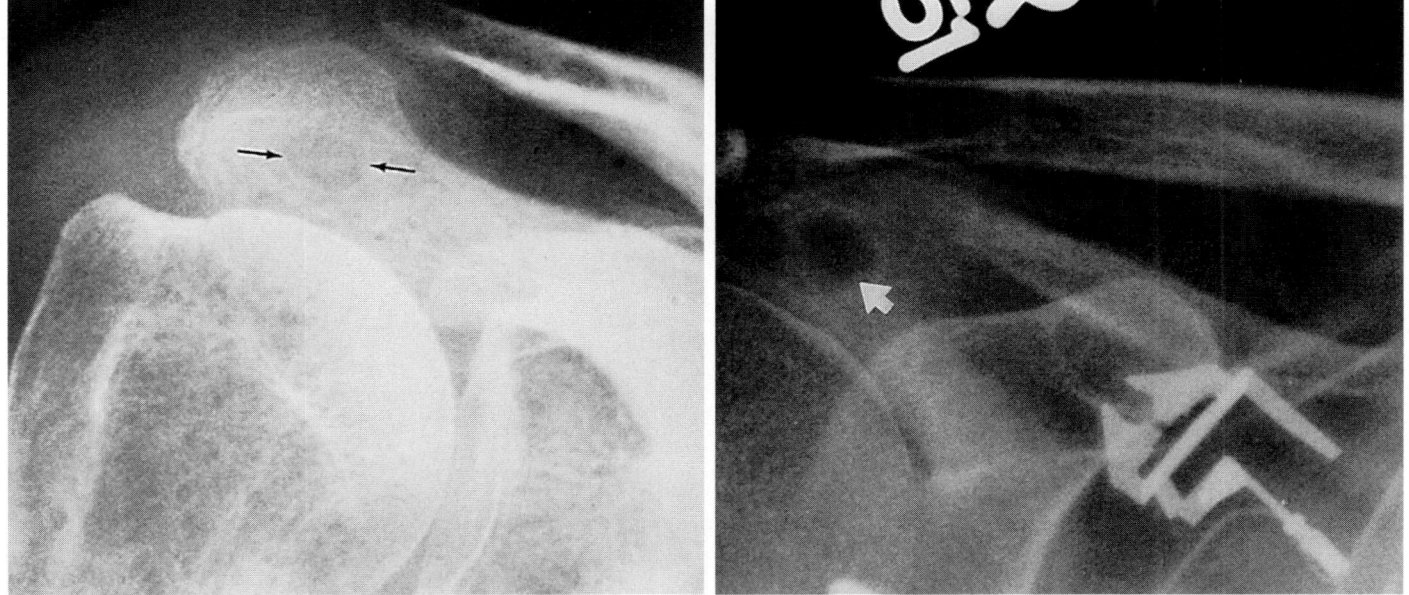

Figure 5–27. Normal fossae in the acromion process, simulating a destructive lesion.

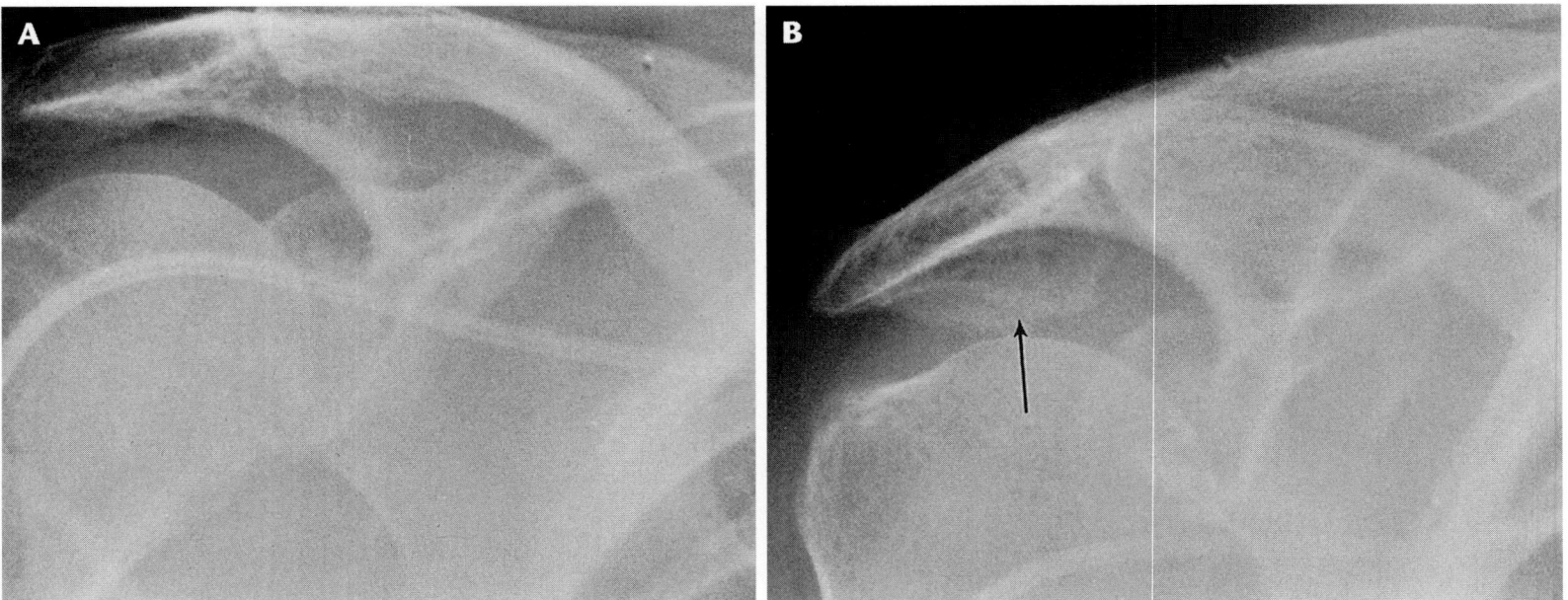

Figure 5–28. Acromial pseudospur produced by positioning. **A,** Anteroposterior projection. **B,** Patient has assumed a kyphotic position. (Refs: Cone RO et al: Shoulder impingement syndrome: Radiographic evaluation. *Radiology* 1150:29, 1984; Jim YF et al: Shoulder impingement syndrome. *Skeletal Radiol* 21:449, 1992.)

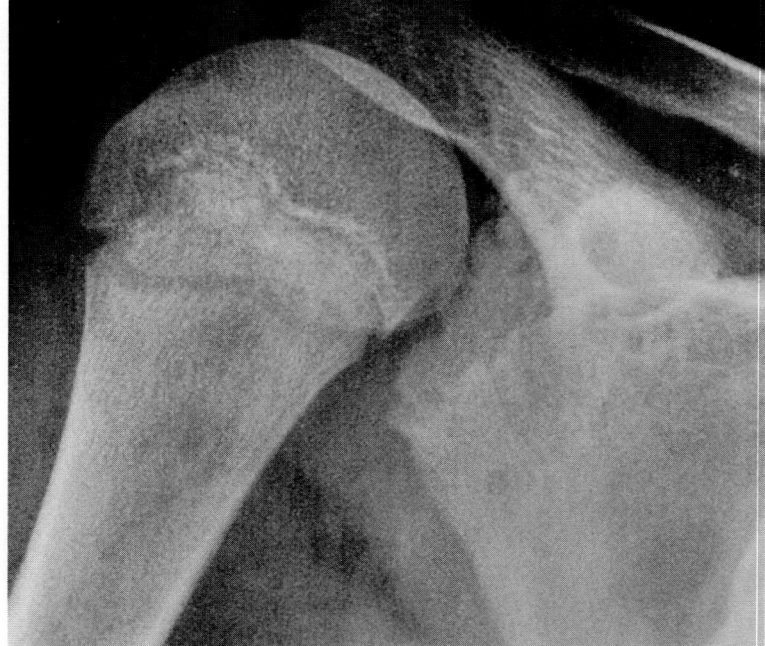

Figure 5–29. 13-year-old boy showing the normal irregularity of the glenoid seen before the secondary centers develop.

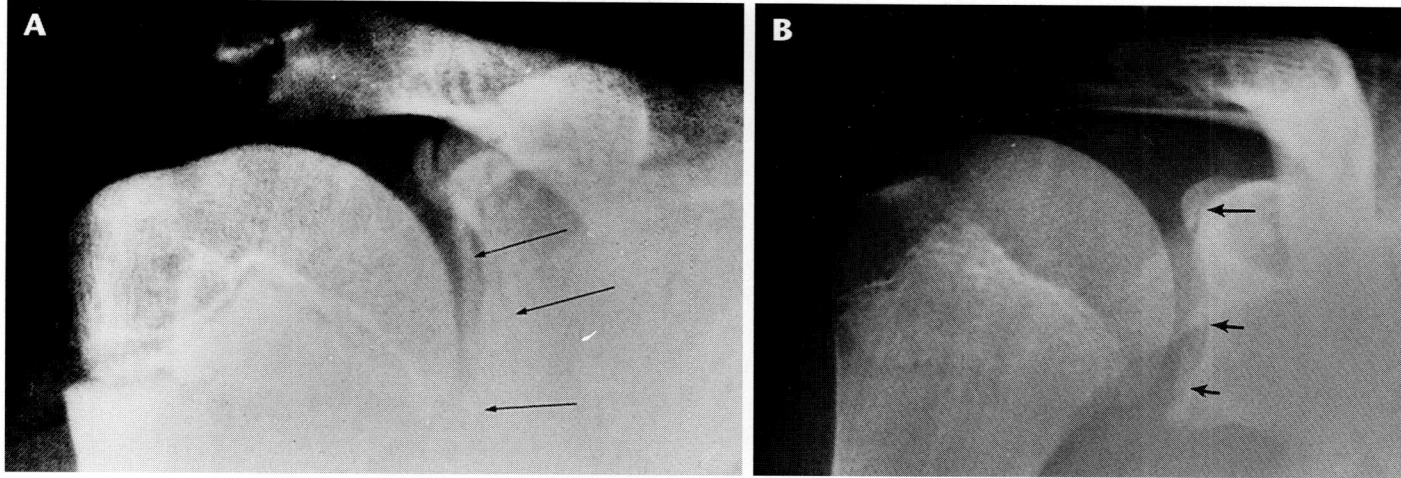

Figure 5–30. The ring apophysis of the glenoid fossa in children. **A,** 8-year-old boy. **B,** 13-year-old boy.

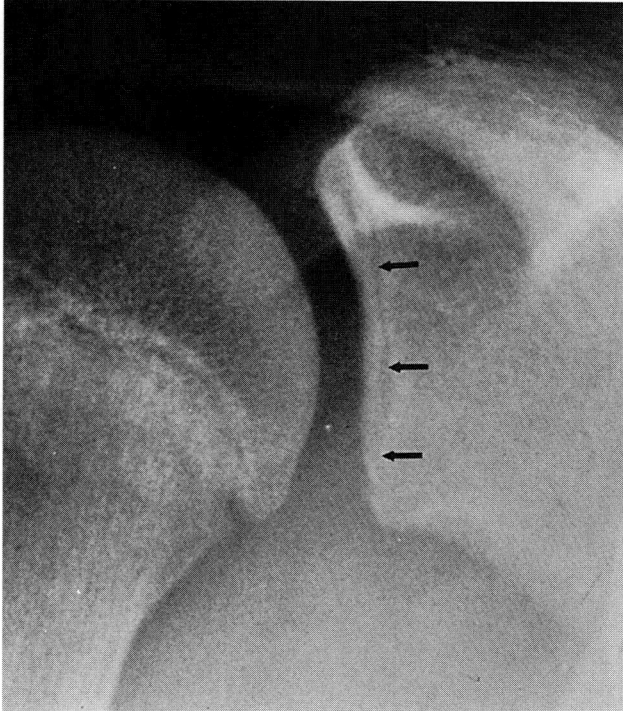

Figure 5–31. The ring apophysis of the glenoid in a 10-year-old boy.

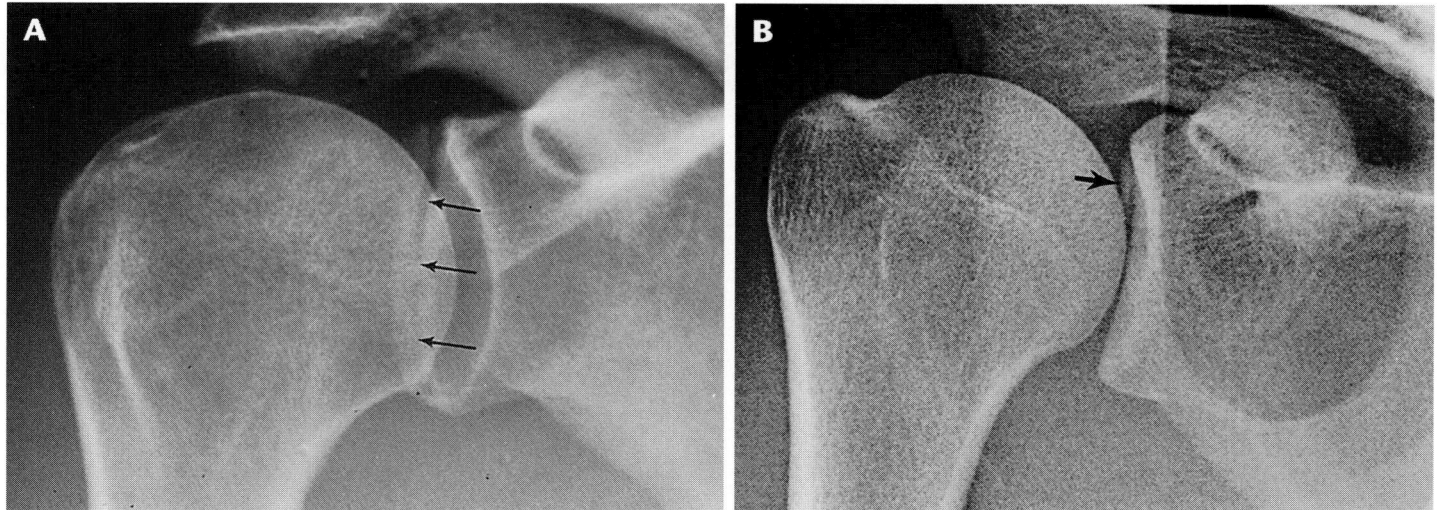

Figure 5–32. Two examples of remnants of the ring apophysis in adults.

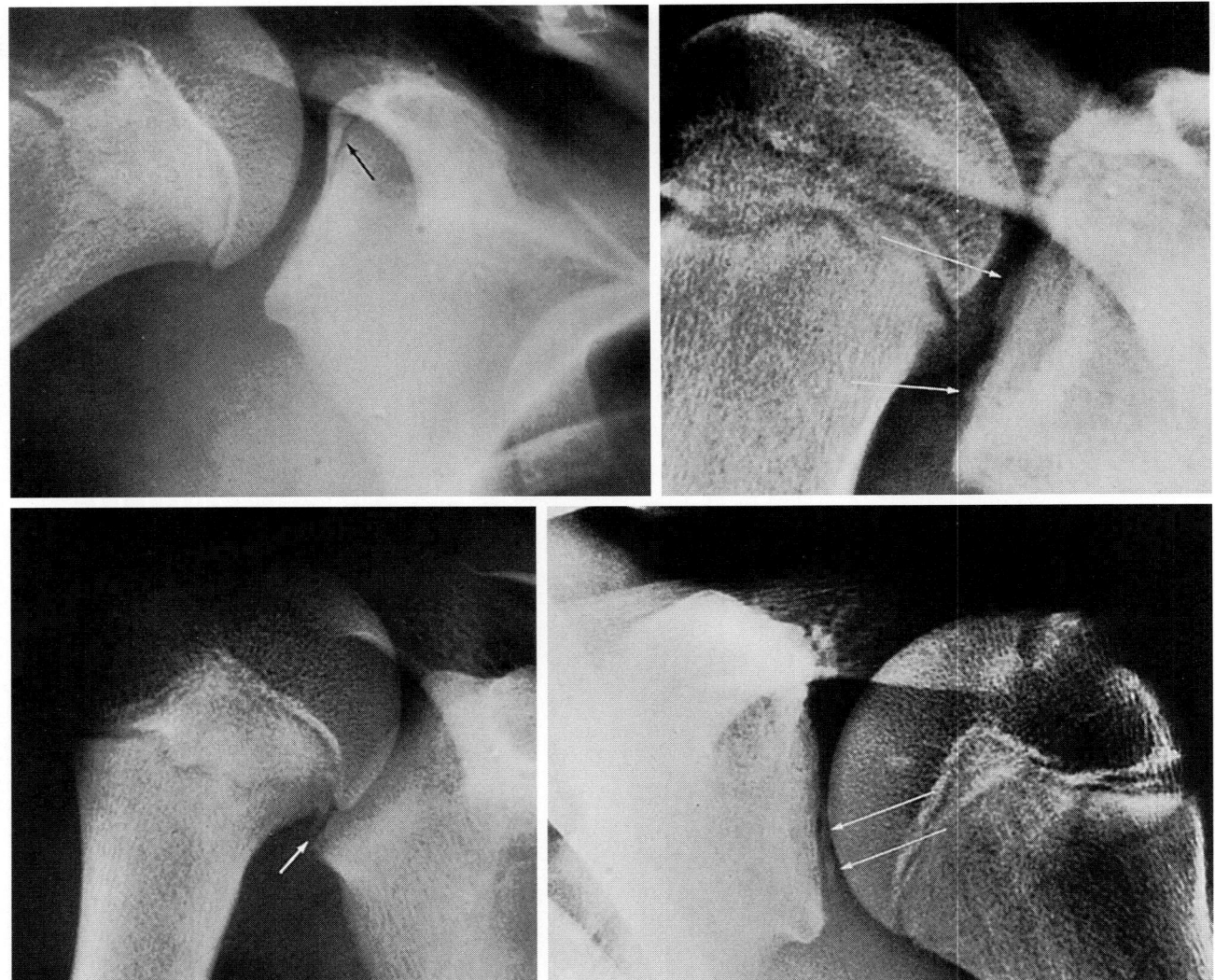

Figure 5–33. Secondary ossification centers for the glenoid, which should not be mistaken for fractures. (Ref: Ogden JA, Phillips SB: Radiology of postnatal skeletal development. VII. The scapula. *Skeletal Radiol* 9:157, 1983.)

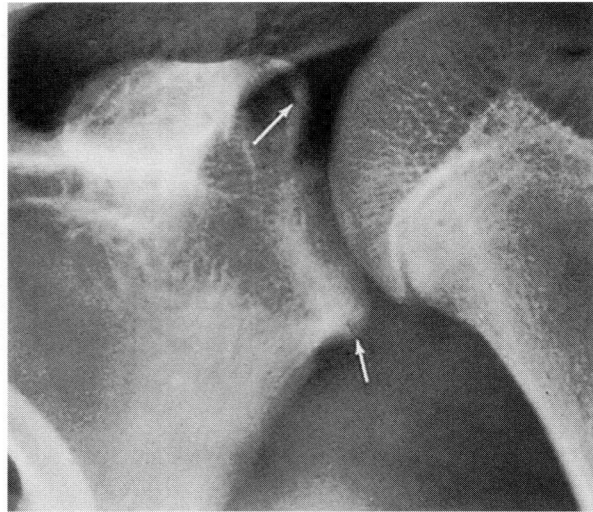

Figure 5–34. Secondary centers of ossification of the glenoid. Note the large apophysis at the superior margin.

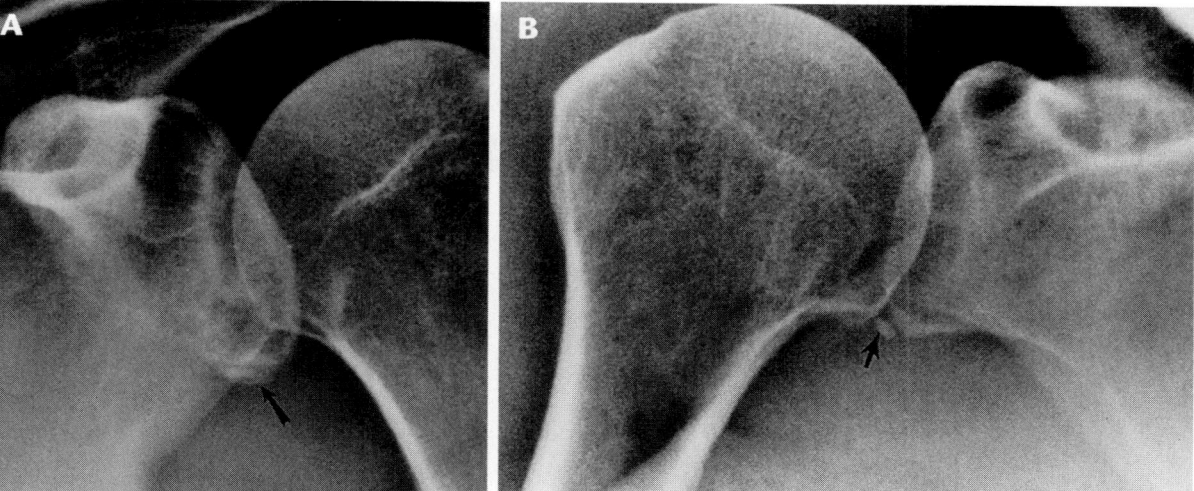

Figure 5–35. Ossicle at inferior aspect of the glenoid fossa as a remnant of the ring apophysis. **A,** 32-year-old man. **B,** 57-year-old man.

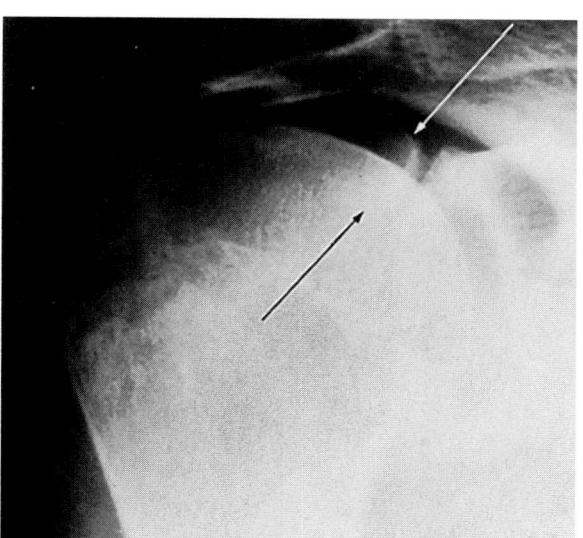

Figure 5–36. Failure of fusion of the apophysis at the superior margin of the glenoid in an adult.

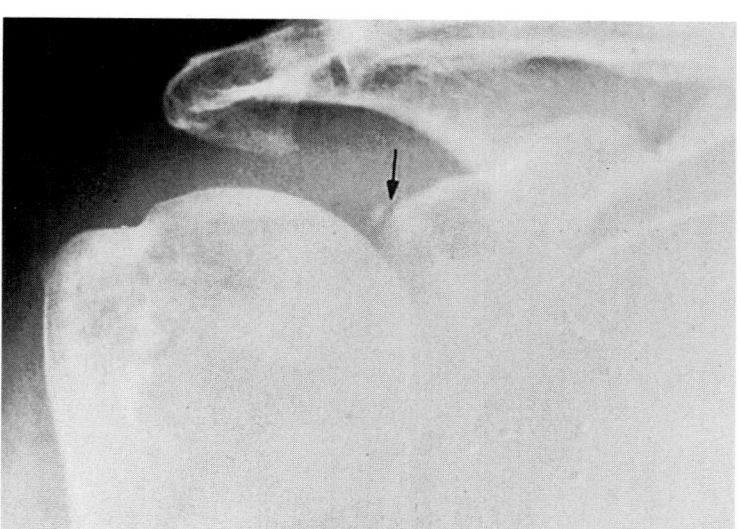

Figure 5–37. Small ossicle at the superior margin of the glenoid in an adult, similar to that in Figure 5–36. This may be mistaken for calcific tendonitis of the long head of the biceps tendon. (Ref: Goldman AB: Calcific tendinitis of the long head of the biceps brachii distal to the glenohumeral joint. *Am J Roentgenol* 153:1011, 1989.)

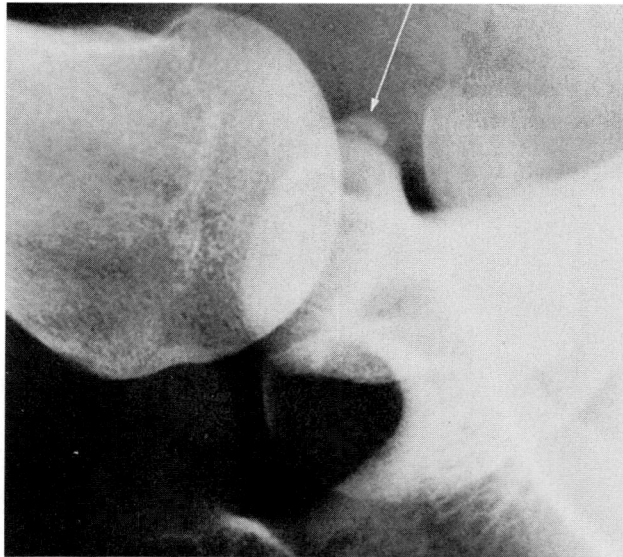

Figure 5–38. Ununited portion of the glenoid apophysis seen in the axial projections may be mistaken for a fracture fragment.

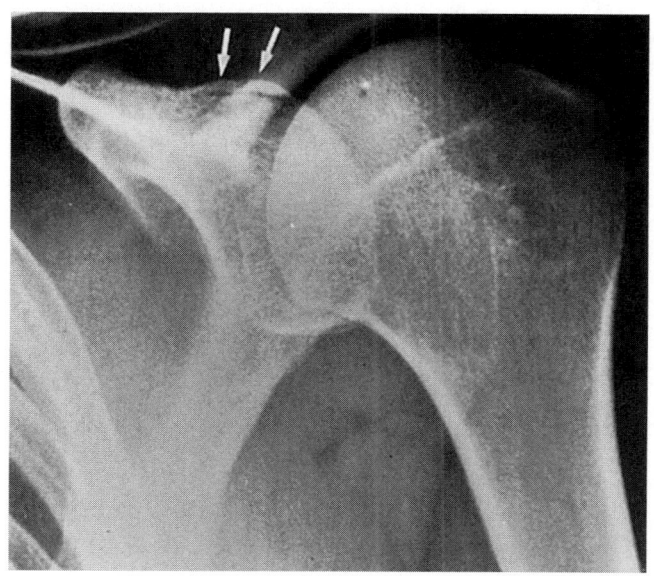

Figure 5–39. Persistence of the glenoid apophysis in an adult.

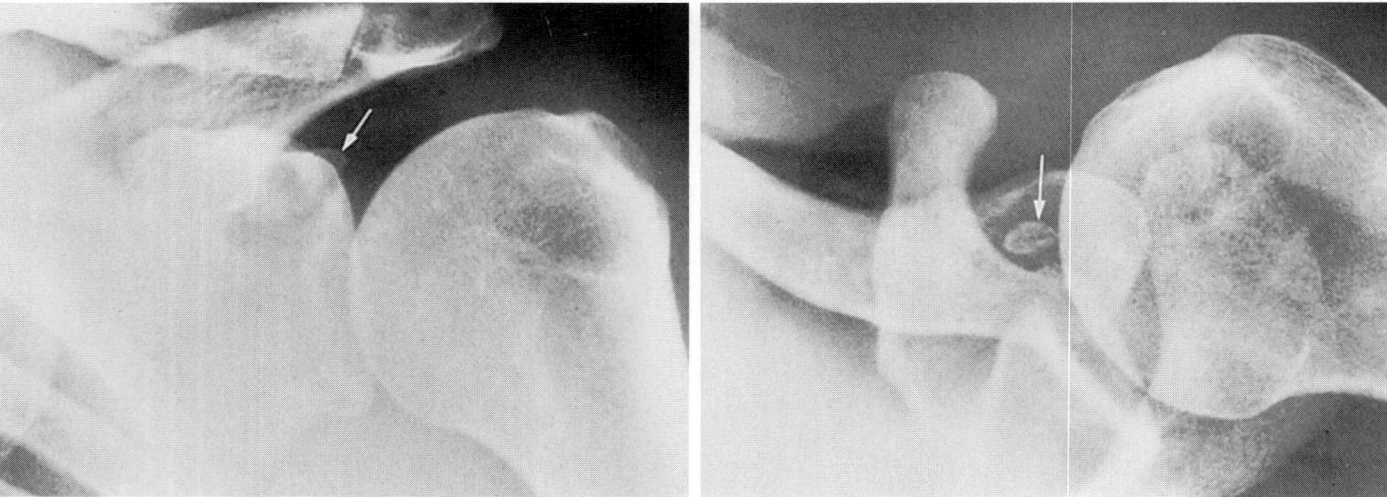

Figure 5–40. Small ossicle at the margin of the glenoid fossa that may represent a remnant of the apophysis. *Left,* Frontal projection. *Right,* Axillary projection.

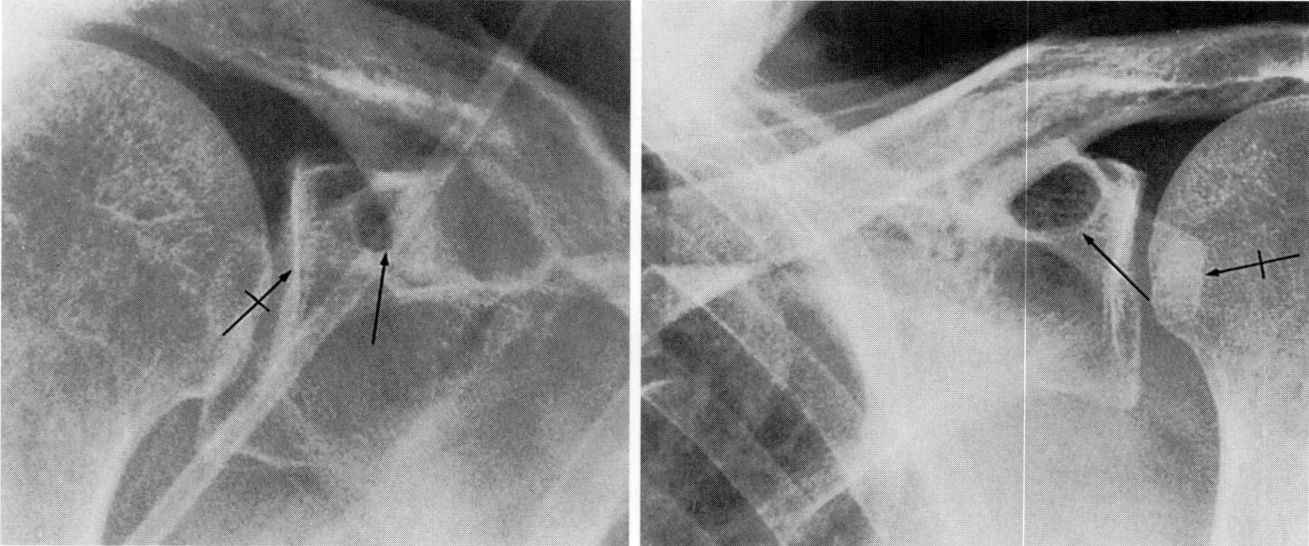

Figure 5–41. Apparent lucencies in the neck of the scapula caused by end-on projection of the coracoid (←). Note the position of coracoid tip (↔).

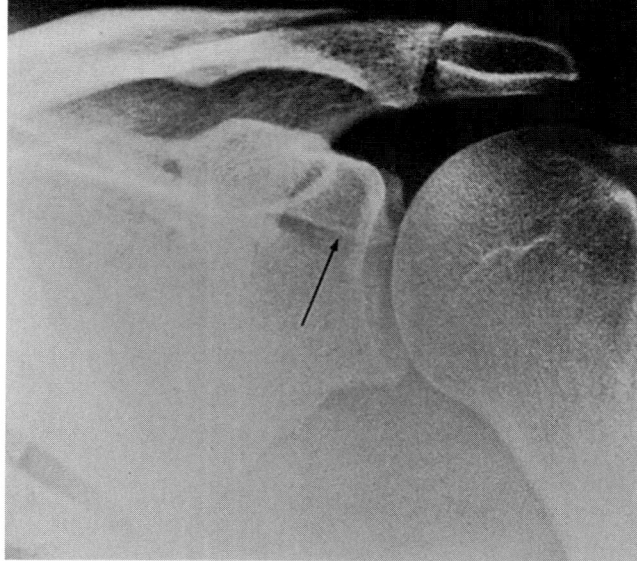

Figure 5–42. The coracoid process seen in the oblique projection of the shoulder.

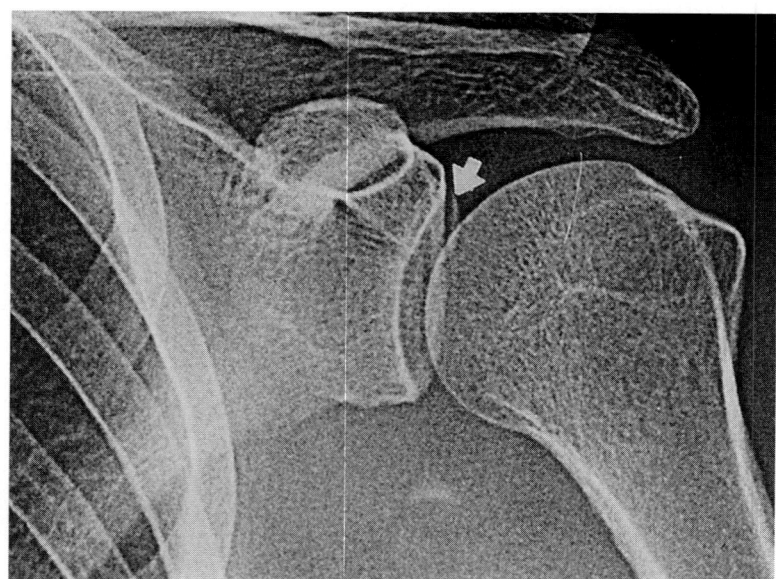

Figure 5–43. The coracoid process projected over the glenoid, simulating a fracture.

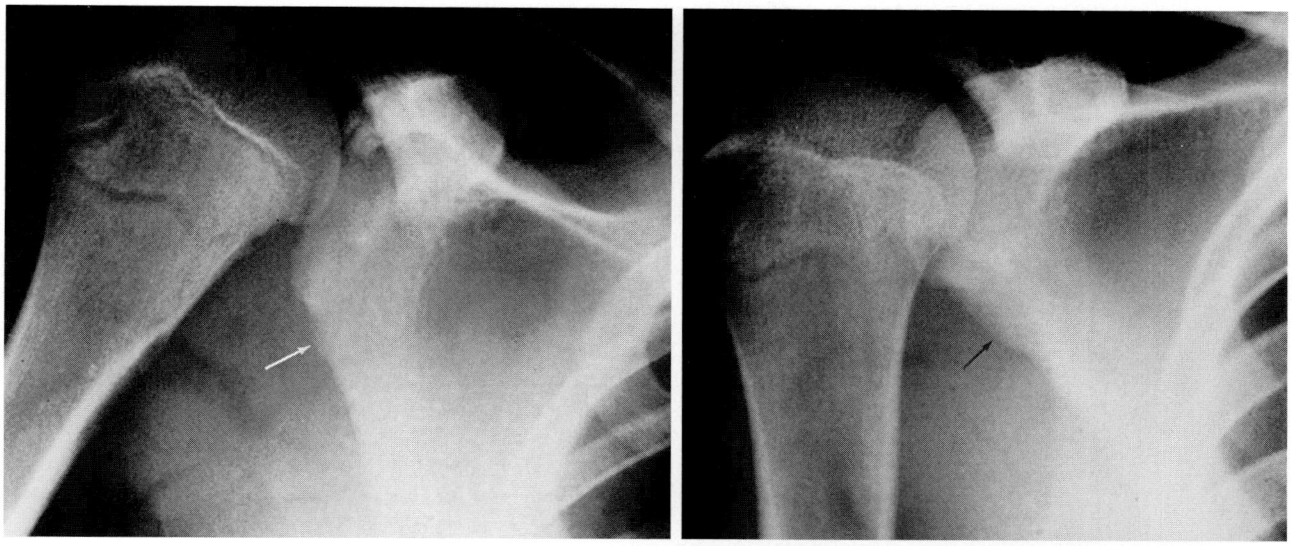

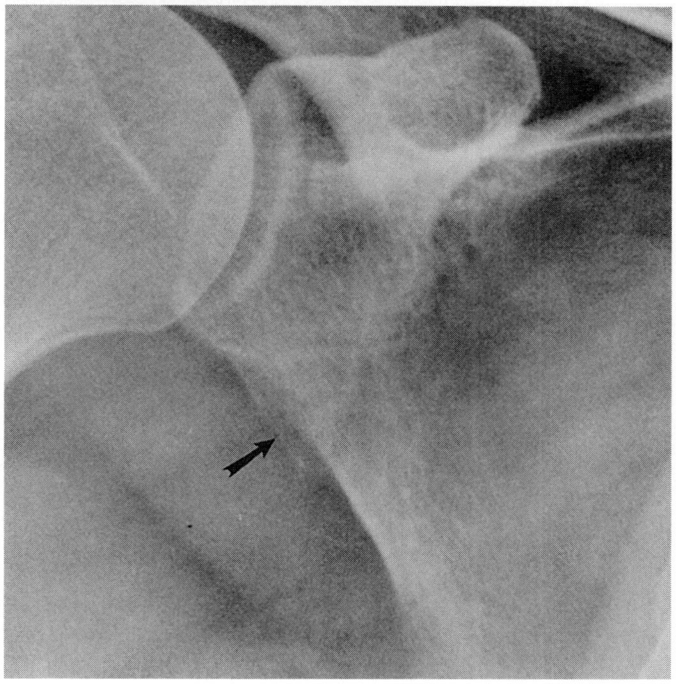

Figure 5–44. Normal excrescences of the lower margin of the neck of the scapula, which may be mistaken for periostitis.

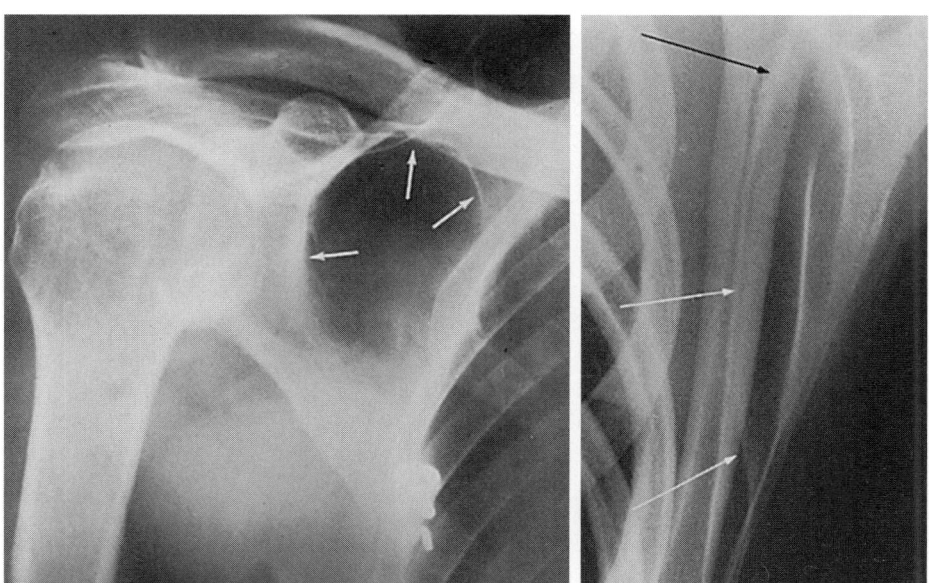

Figure 5–45. Normal radiolucency of the wing of the scapula, which may resemble a cystic lesion.

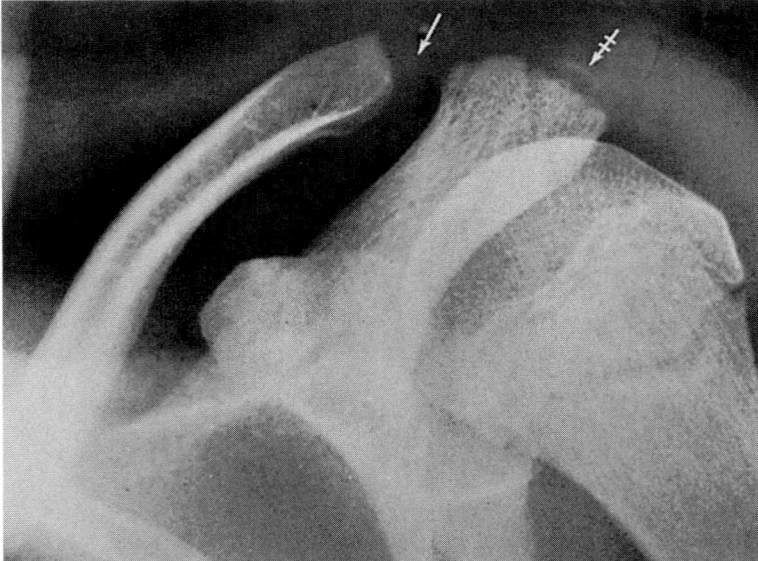

Figure 5–46. Normally wide acromioclavicular joint and apparent malalignment in a 14-year-old girl (←). This appearance, if not compared with the opposite side, may be mistaken for an acromioclavicular separation. Note also the secondary ossification center for the tip of the acromion process (↤⊞).

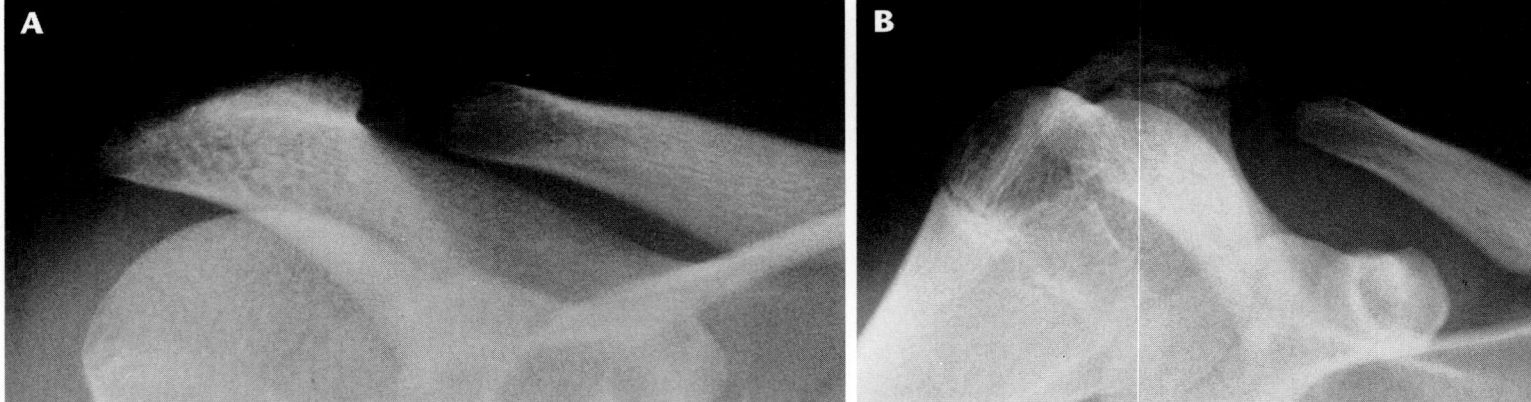

Figure 5–47. Apparent widening of the acromioclavicular joint by positioning. **A,** Anteroposterior projection with internal rotation. **B,** 30-degree right posterior oblique projection with external rotation.

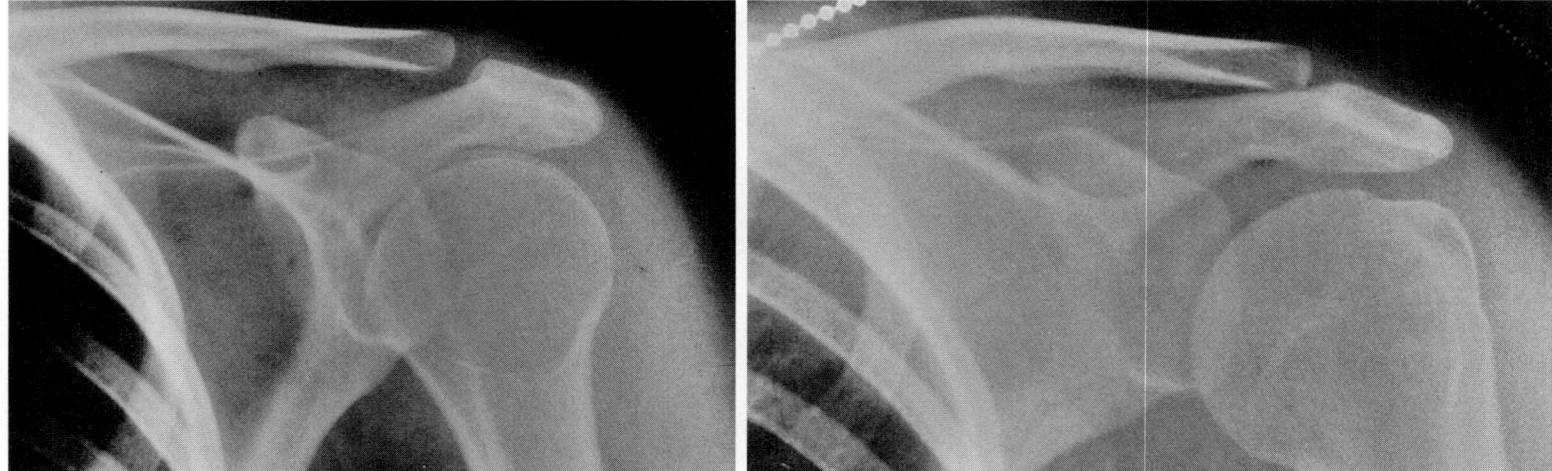

Figure 5–48. Same phenomenon as the preceding illustration. Note also apparent malalignment of the clavicle and acromion, *right*.

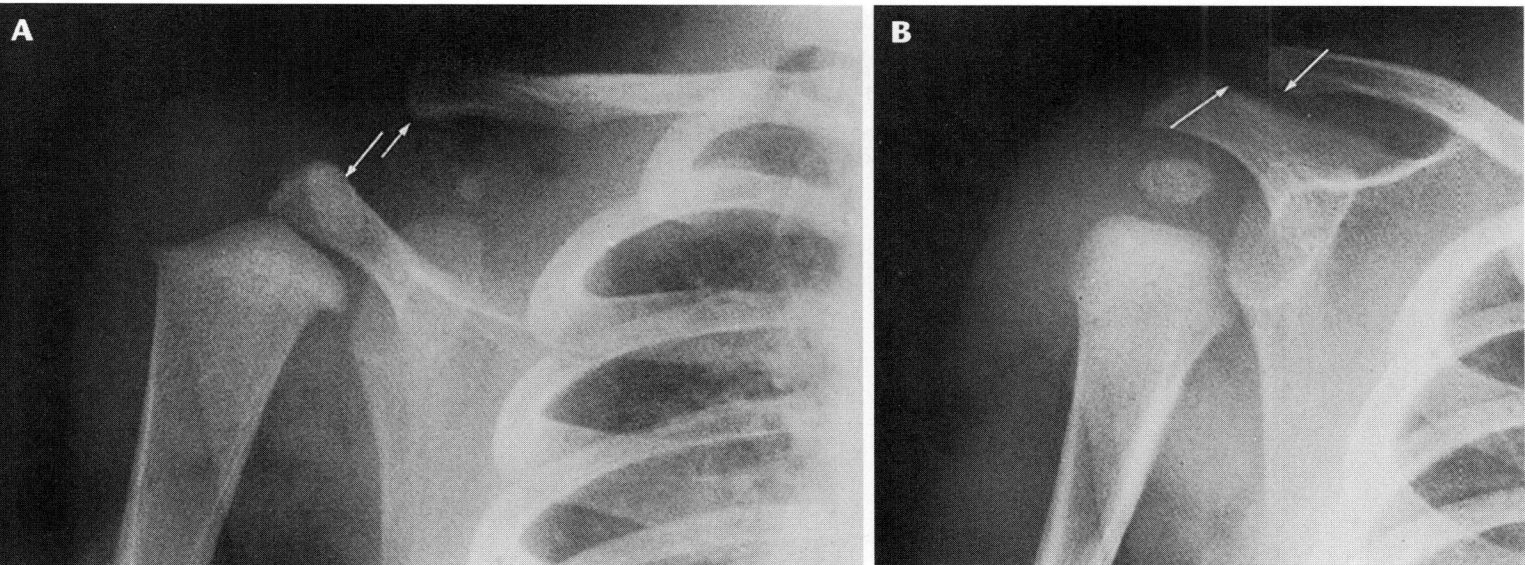

Figure 5–49. Positioning of the arms in children may produce an appearance simulating acromioclavicular separation. **A,** External rotation. **B,** Internal rotation.

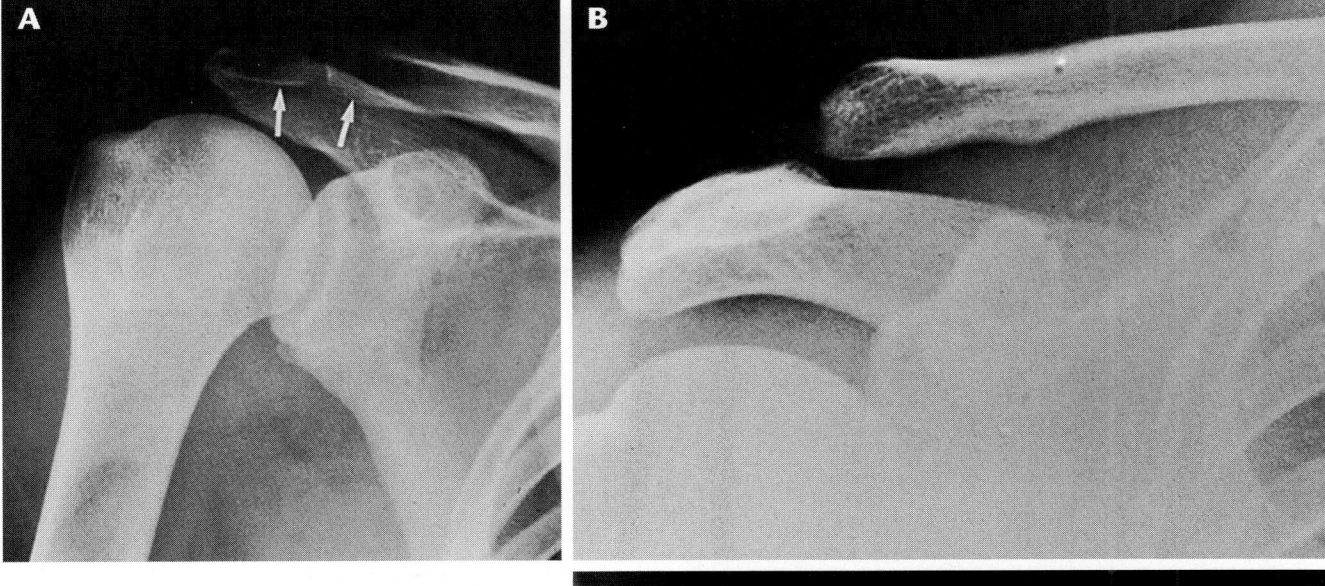

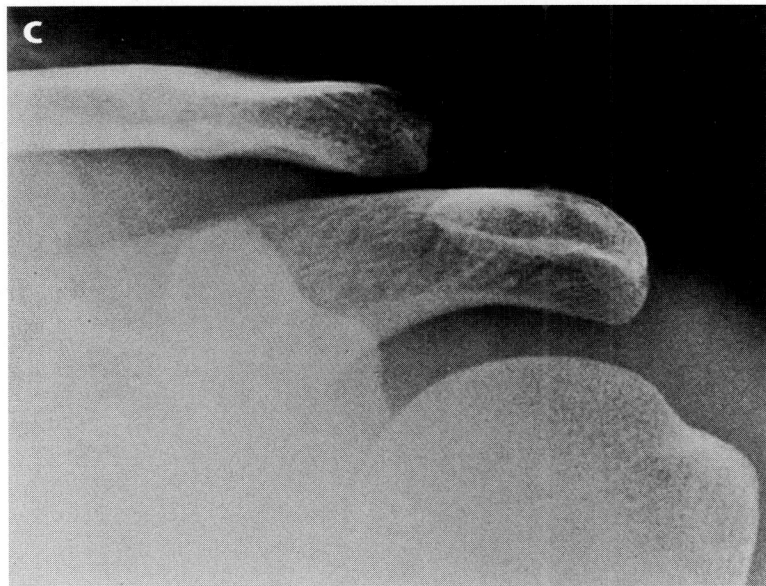

Figure 5–50. Variations in configuration of the acromioclavicular joint. **A,** In most normal individuals the inferior aspect of the clavicle is at the same level as the inferior aspect of the acromion. **B** and **C,** In a small percentage of normal individuals the distal end of the clavicle lies above or below the acromion (in this case above) and might be interpreted as an acromioclavicular separation. This variation emphasizes the value of examining both sides. (Refs: Urist MR: Complete dislocations of the acromioclavicular joint. *J Bone Joint Surg* 28:813, 1946; Pettrone FA, Nirschl RP: Acromioclavicular dislocation. *Am J Sports Med* 6:160, 1978.)

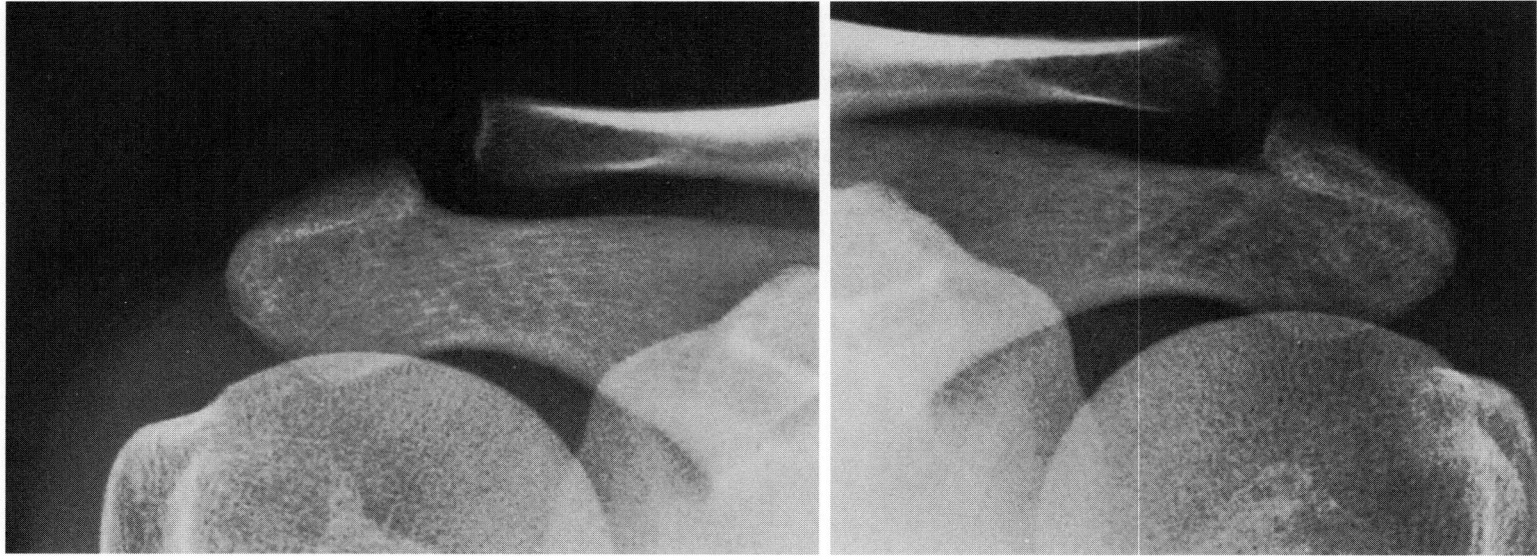

Figure 5–51. Another example of normal but apparently dislocated acromioclavicular joints. Note also the unusual width of the joint.

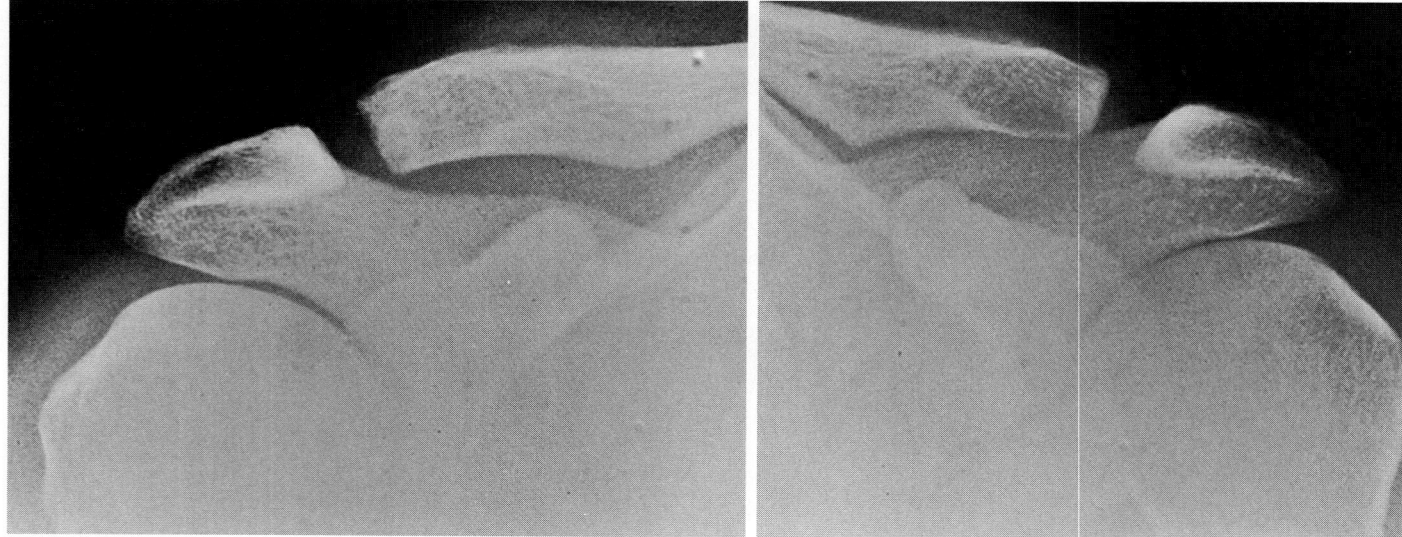

Figure 5–52. Unusually wide acromioclavicular joints in a normal individual. These measurements exceed the quoted normal range. Examination of both shoulders will resolve this problem. (Refs: Petersson CJ, Redlund-Johnell I: Radiographic joint space in normal acromioclavicular joint. *Acta Orthop Scand* 54:431, 1983; Kern JW, Harris JH: Case 752, normal variant of the acromion simulating grade I acromioclavicular separation. *Skeletal Radiol* 21:419, 1992.)

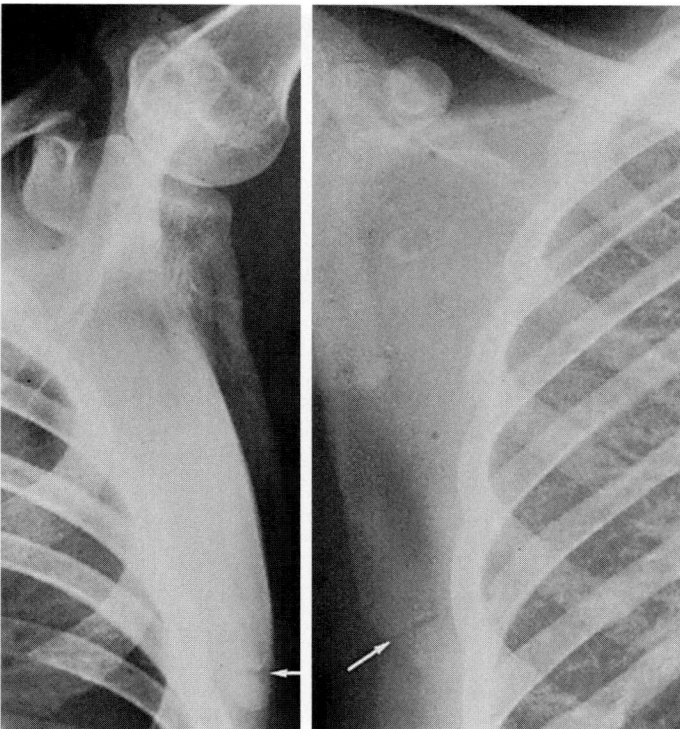

Figure 5–53. Two examples of secondary ossification centers (infrascapular bone) of the inferior angle of the scapula in 16-year-old boys. These usually fuse by 20 years of age.

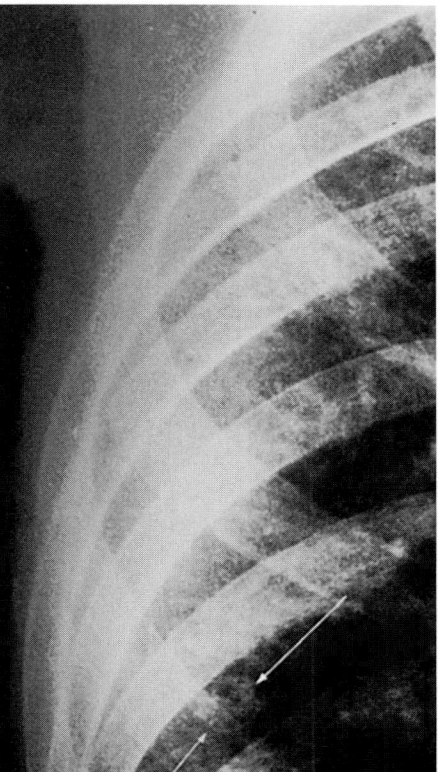

Figure 5–54. An infrascapular bone that was mistaken for a lung lesion.

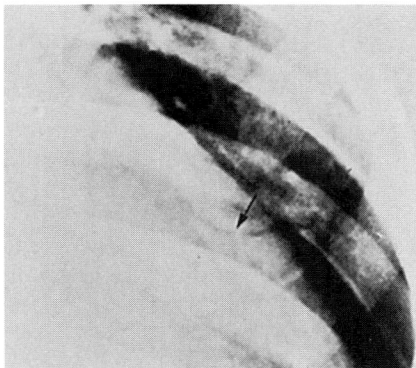

Figure 5–55. An infrascapular bone simulating a rib fracture.

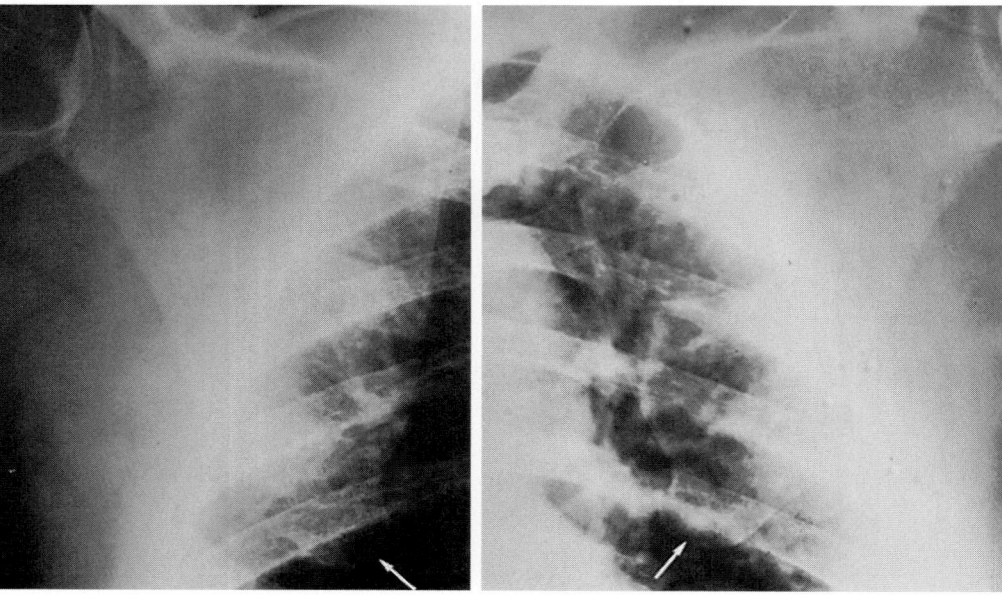

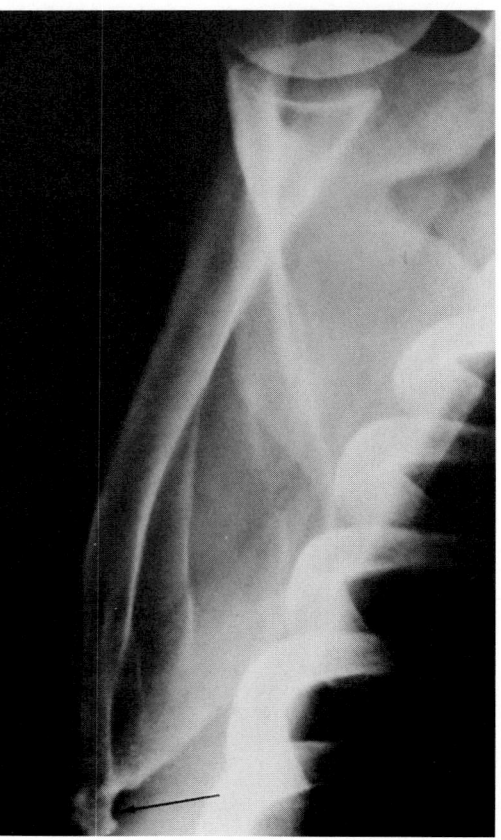

Figure 5–56. Hooklike configuration of the distal angles of the scapula.

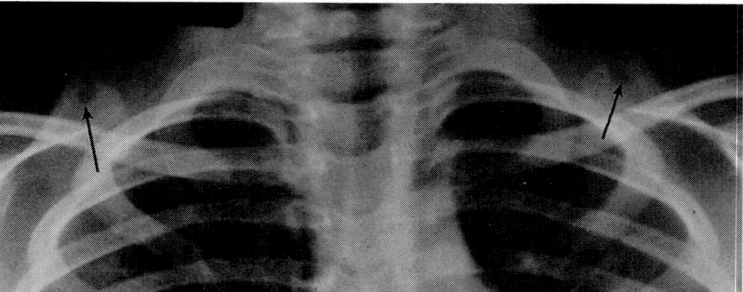

Figure 5–57. Developmental notchlike defects on the superior margin of the scapulae.

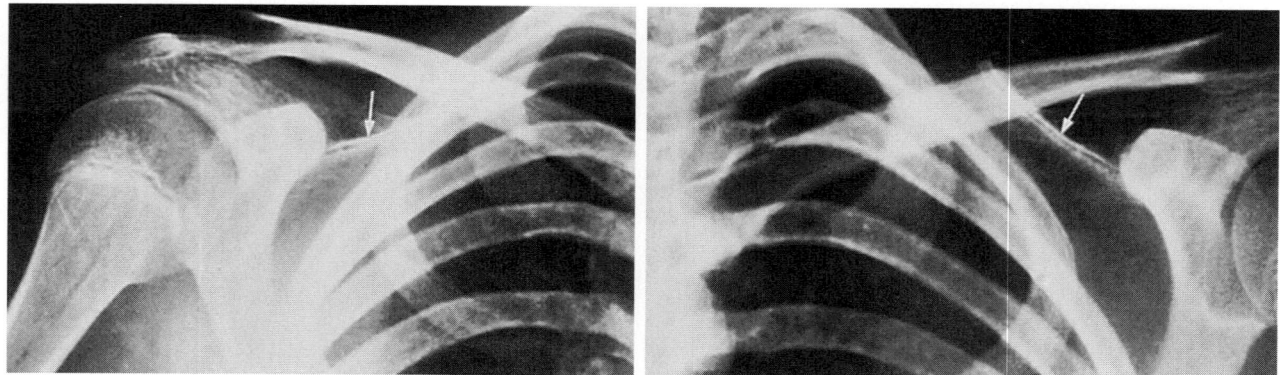

Figure 5–58. Double cortical lines of the scapular spine in a 3-year-old child.

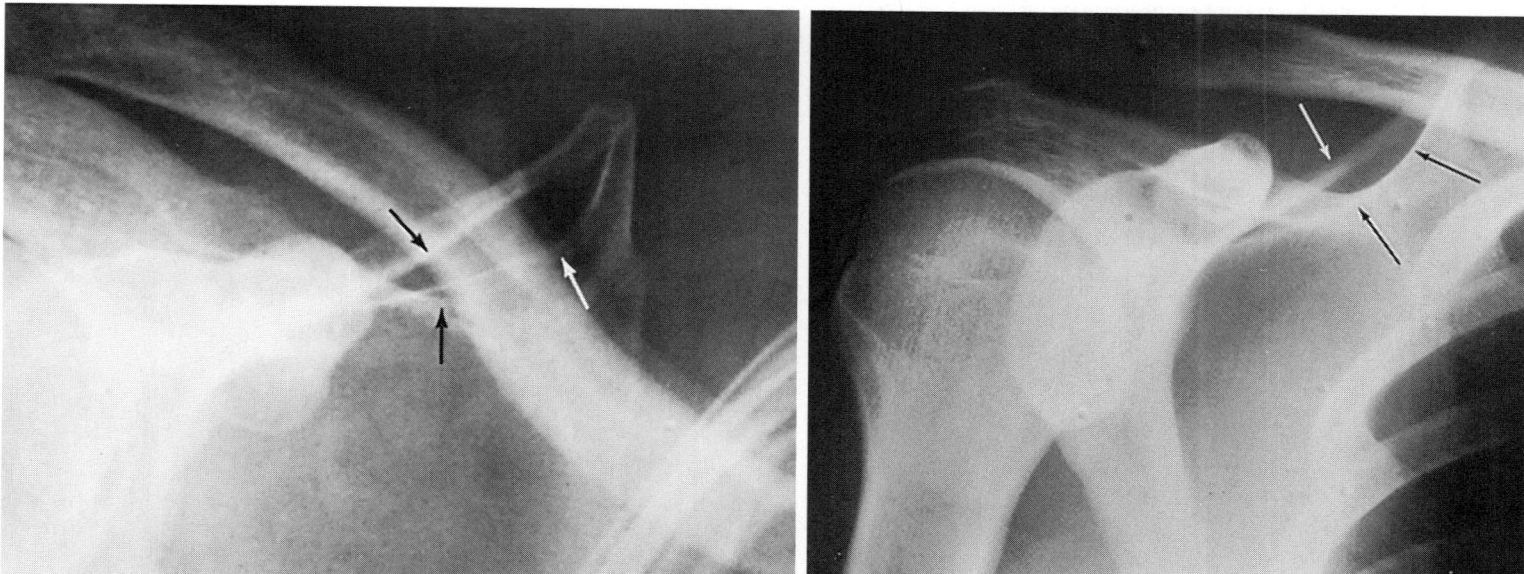

Figure 5–59. Clasplike cranial margin of the scapula, which produces a pseudoforamen. The thin sheet of bone that forms the fossa supraspinatus appears to be absent. (Ref: Goldenberg DB, Brogdon BG: Congenital anomalies of the pectoral girdle demonstrated by chest radiography. *J Can Assoc Radiol* 18:472, 1967.)

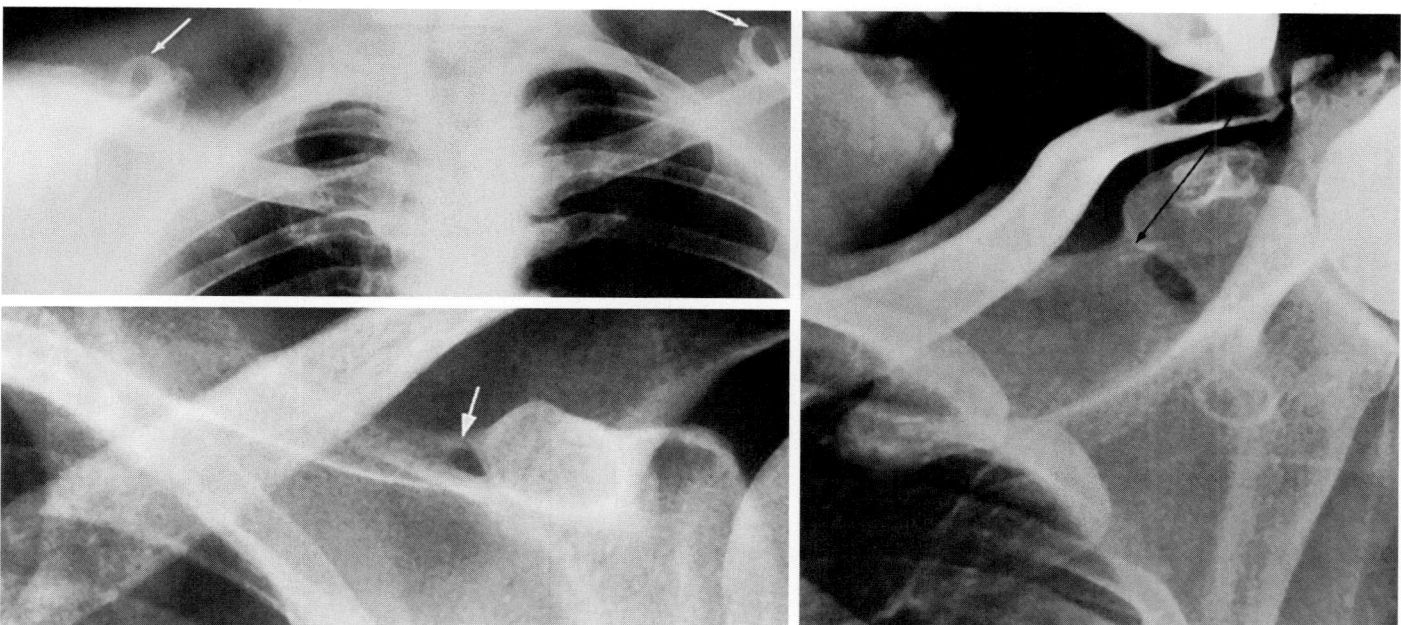

Figure 5–60. Examples of calcification of the transverse superior ligament of the scapula. (Ref: Kohler A, Zimmer EA: *Borderlands of normal and early pathologic findings in skeletal radiography*, 4th ed. New York, Thieme Medical, 1993, p. 216.)

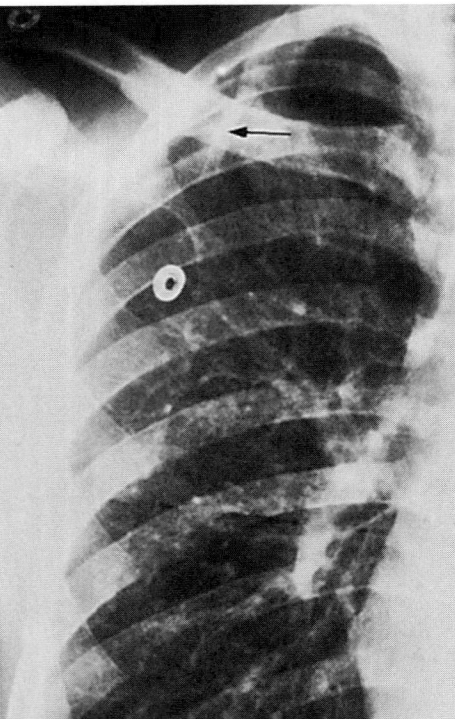

Figure 5–61. The superior end of the body of the scapula simulating a fracture fragment.

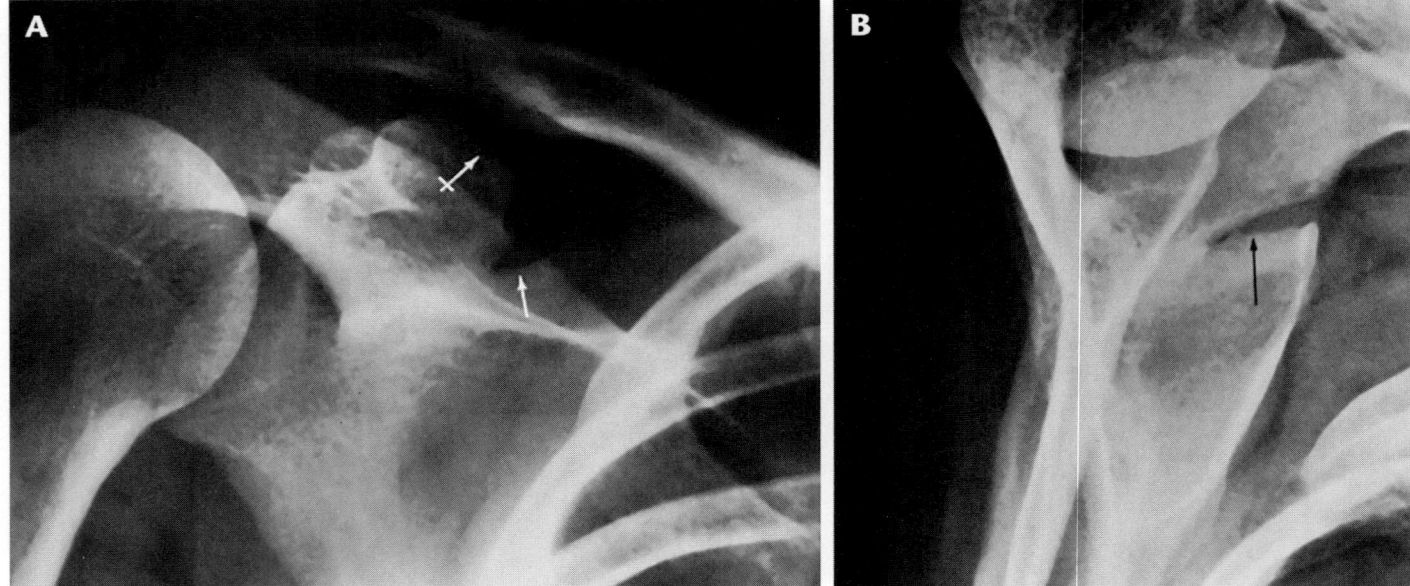

Figure 5–62. A, B, Deep notch on the superior margin of the scapula (→). Note also partial formation of a coracoclavicular articulation (↔) in **A.**

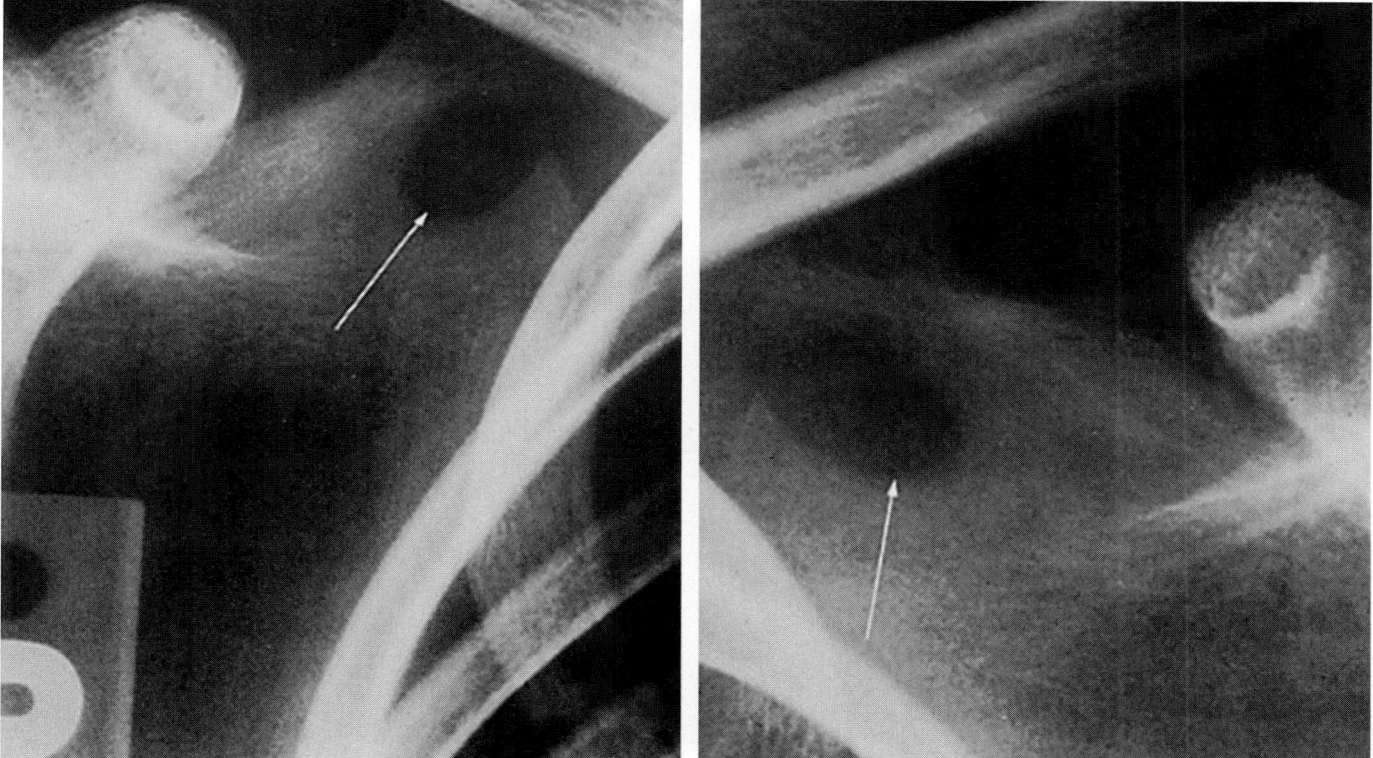

Figure 5–63. Foramina-like defects in the superior border of the scapula.

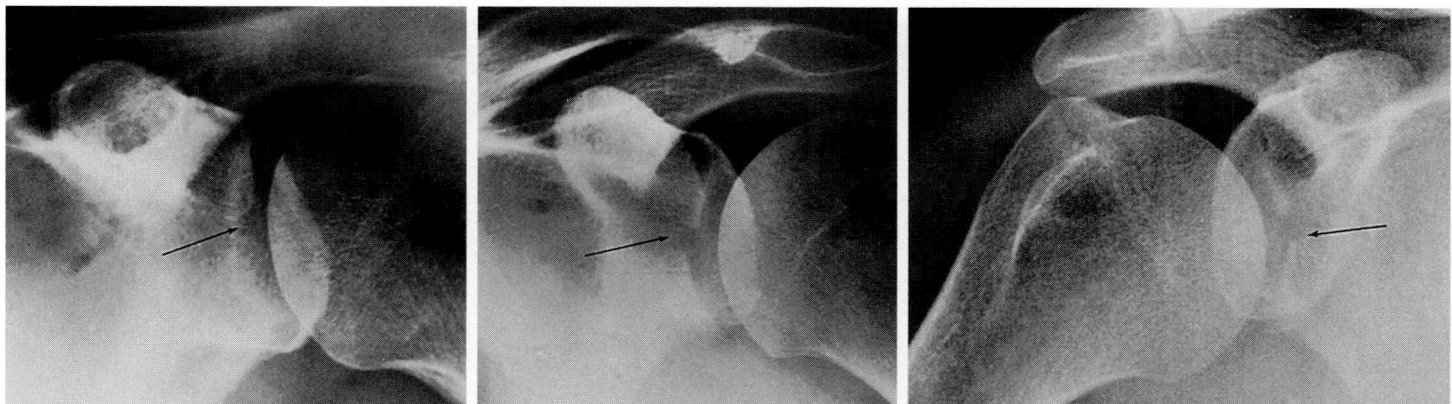

Figure 5–64. Three examples of developmental defects in the glenoid. These may be similar in origin to the acetabular notch.

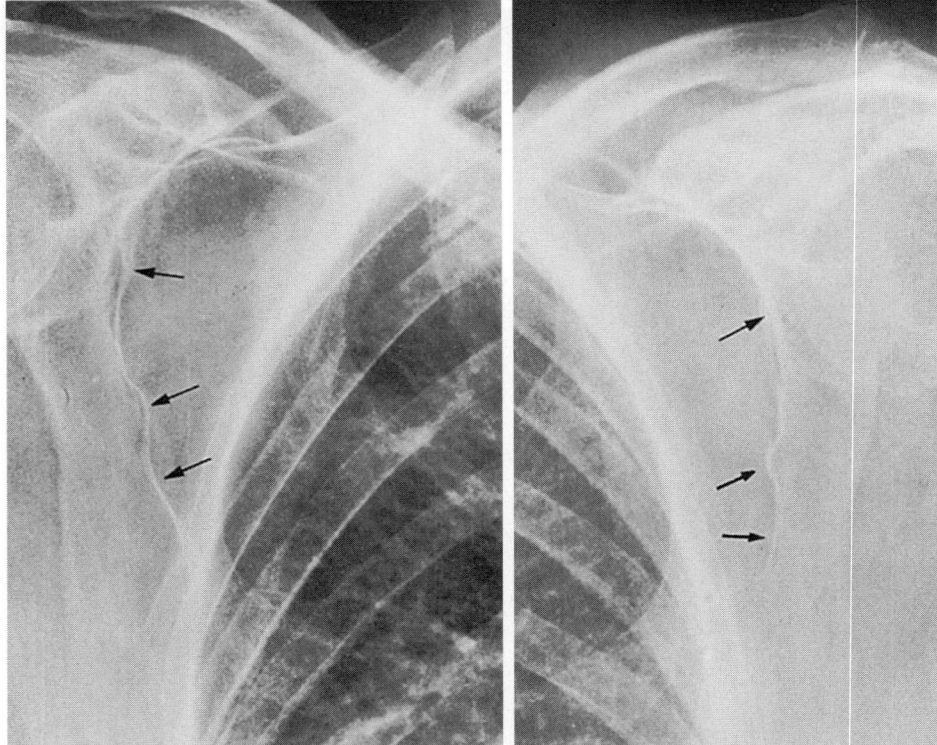

Figure 5–65. Sclerotic margins of the scapular fossae.

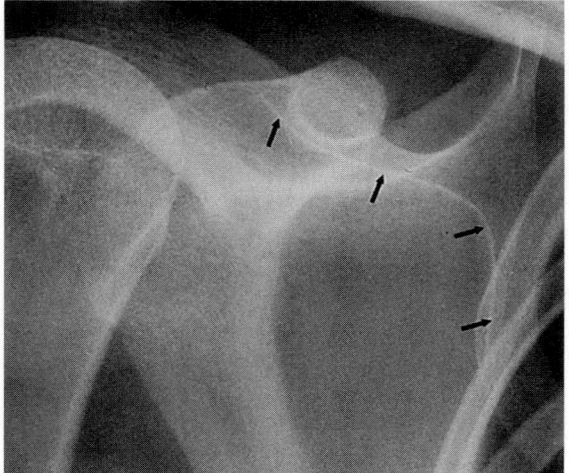

Figure 5–66. The margin of the scapular fossa simulating a wire or catheter.

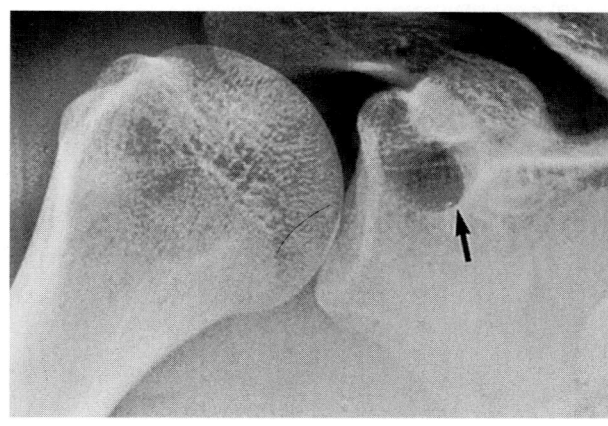

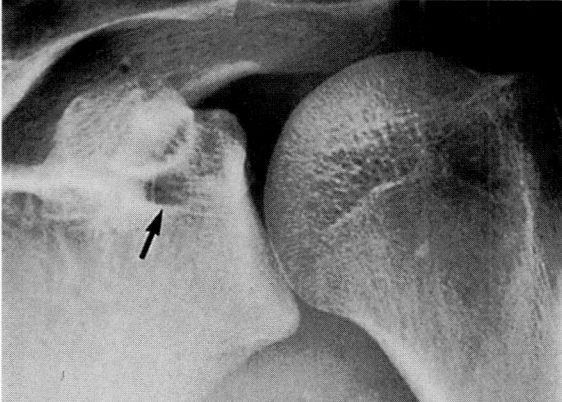

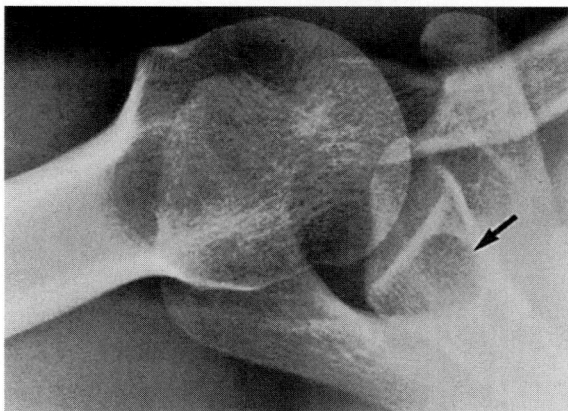

Figure 5–67. Normal lucencies in the neck of the scapula that may be mistaken for destructive lesions. They probably represent the lucency of the cancellous bone of the glenoid marginated by the coracoid process.

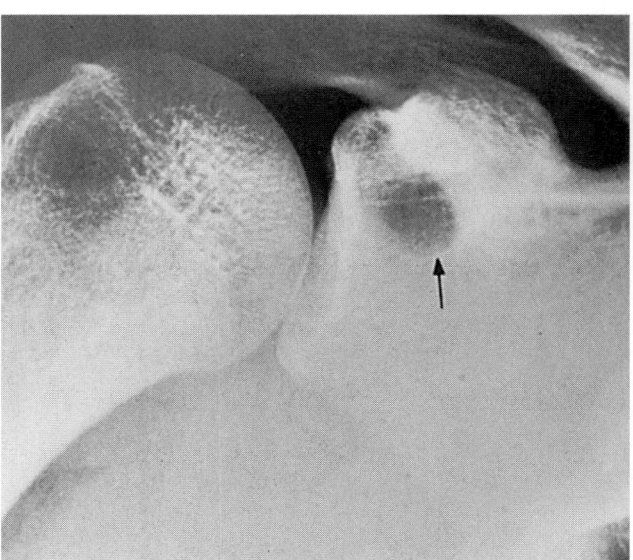

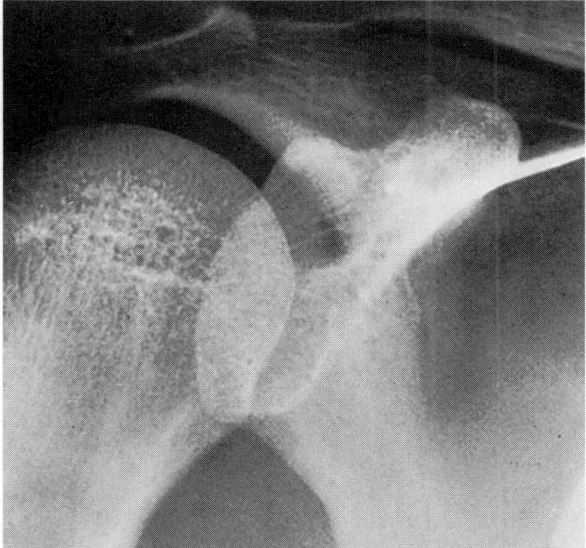

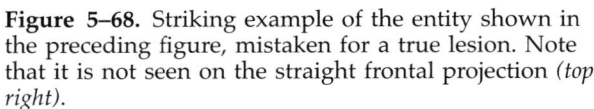

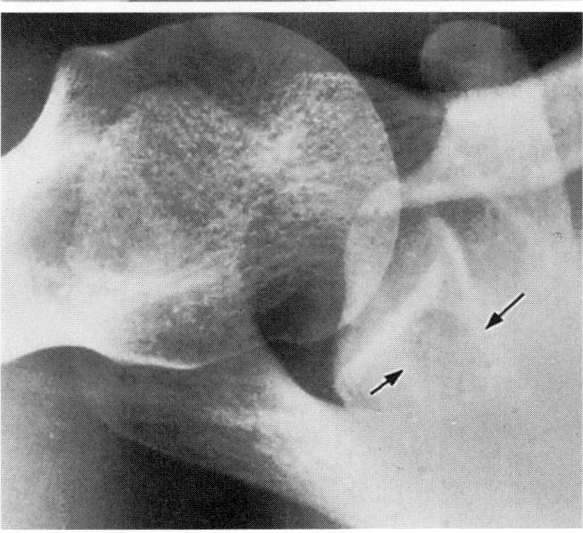

Figure 5–68. Striking example of the entity shown in the preceding figure, mistaken for a true lesion. Note that it is not seen on the straight frontal projection *(top right)*.

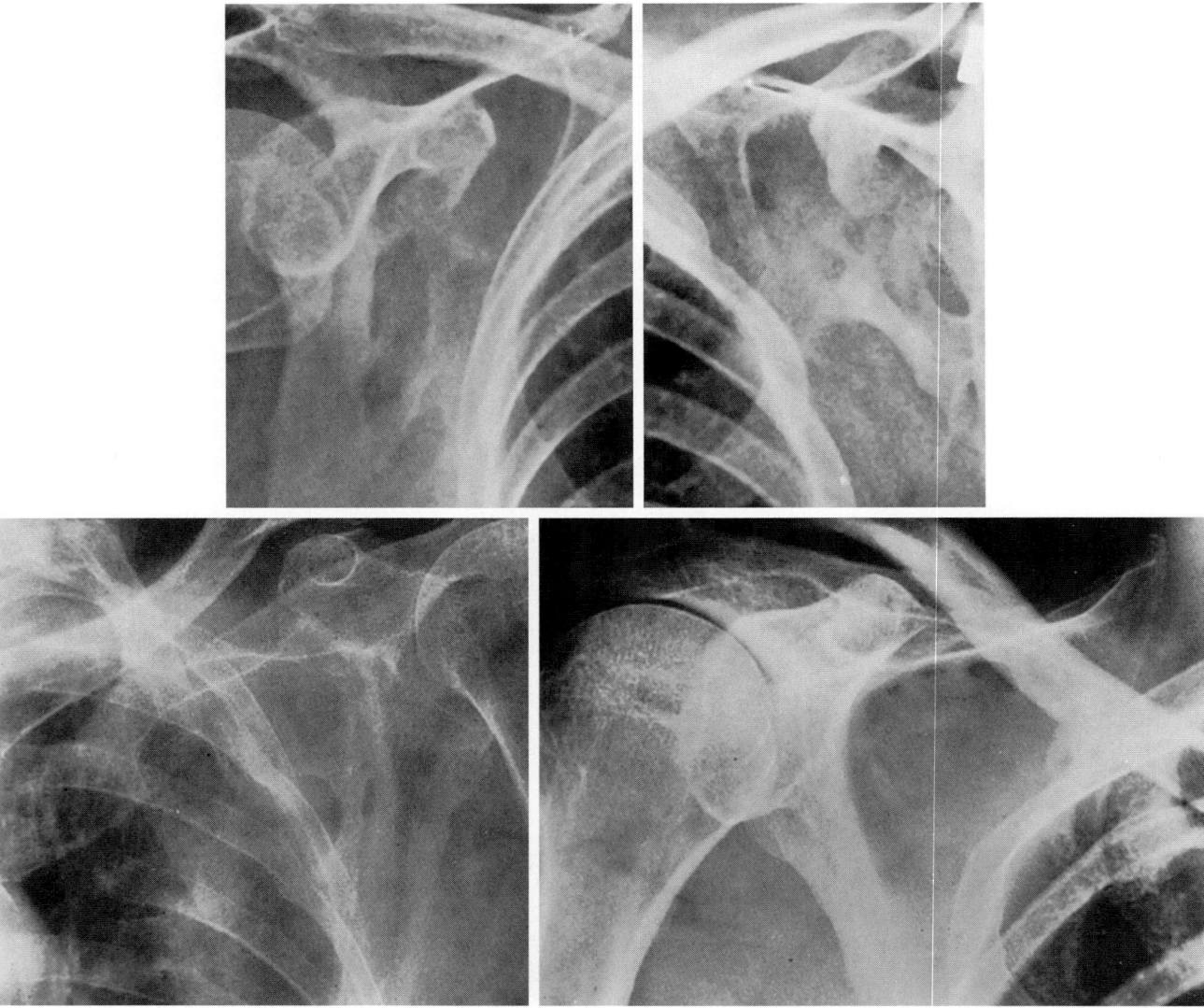

Figure 5–69. Developmental defects of the scapula that may be mistaken for a pathologic process. (Refs: Cigtay OS, Mascatello VJ: Scapular defects: A normal variation. *Am J Roentgenol* 132:239, 1979; Pate D et al: Scapular foramina. *Skeletal Radiol* 14:270, 1985.)

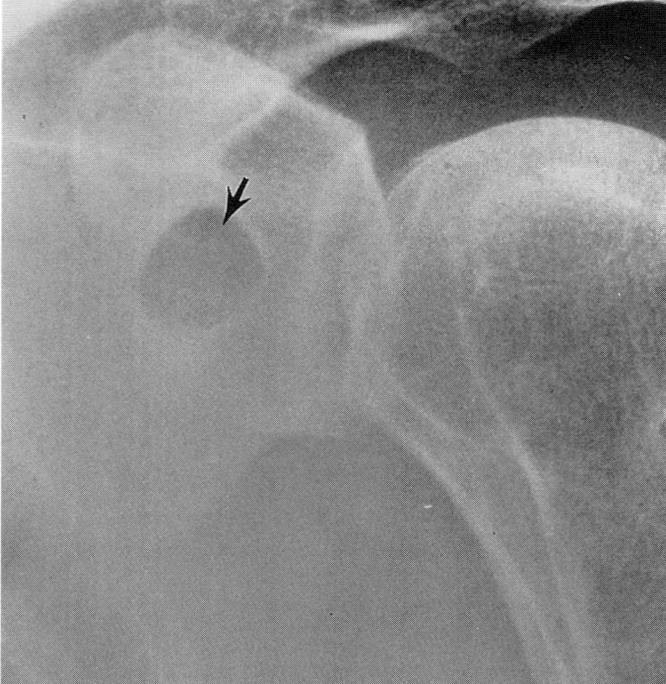

Figure 5–70. Fossa in the neck of the scapula.

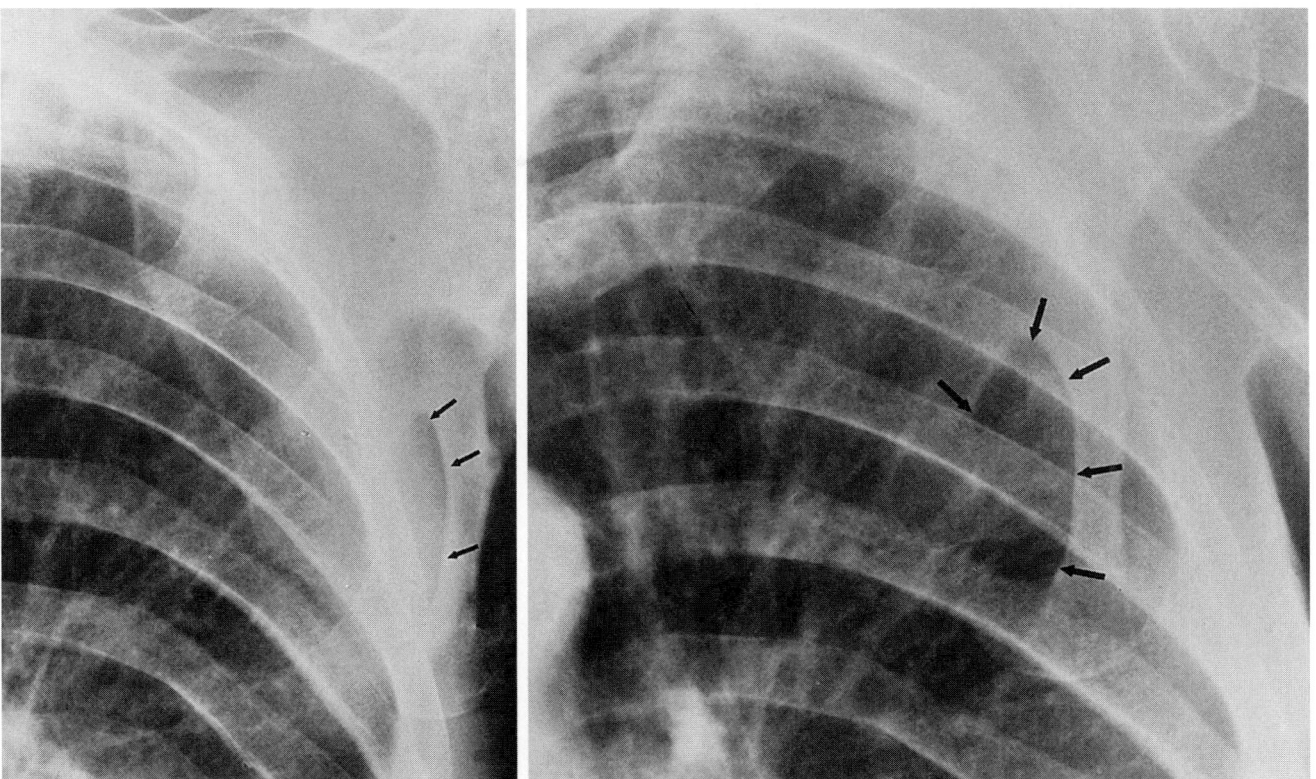

Figure 5–71. Foramen in the wing of the scapula.

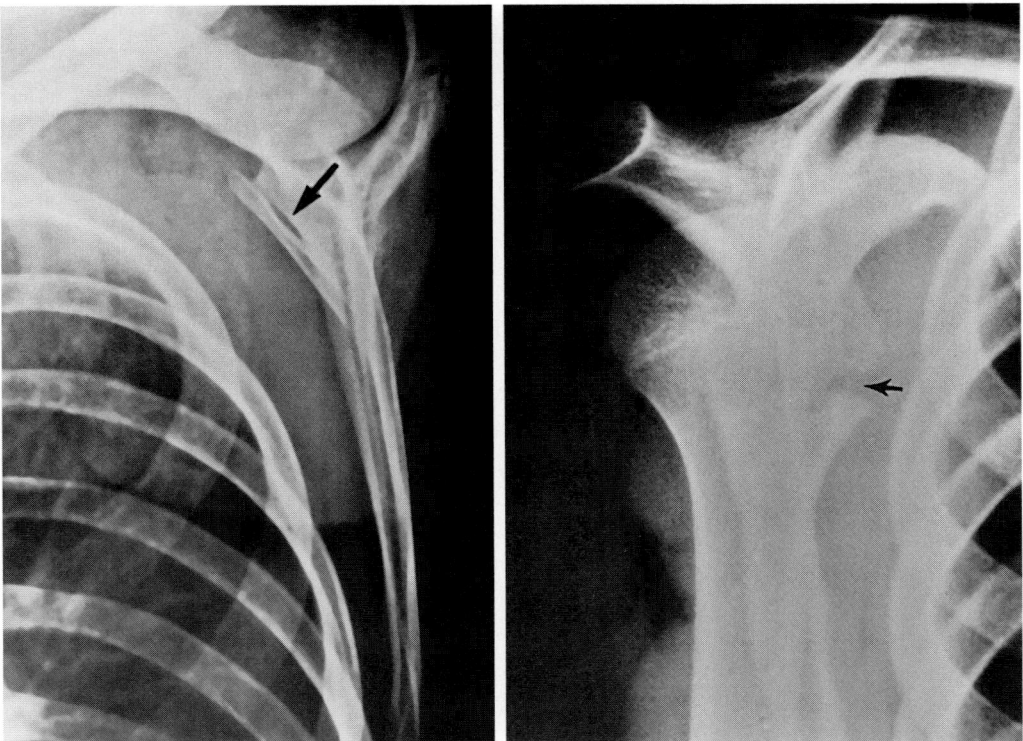

Figure 5–72. Simulated fractures of the scapula by a superimposition of the free margin of the scapula.

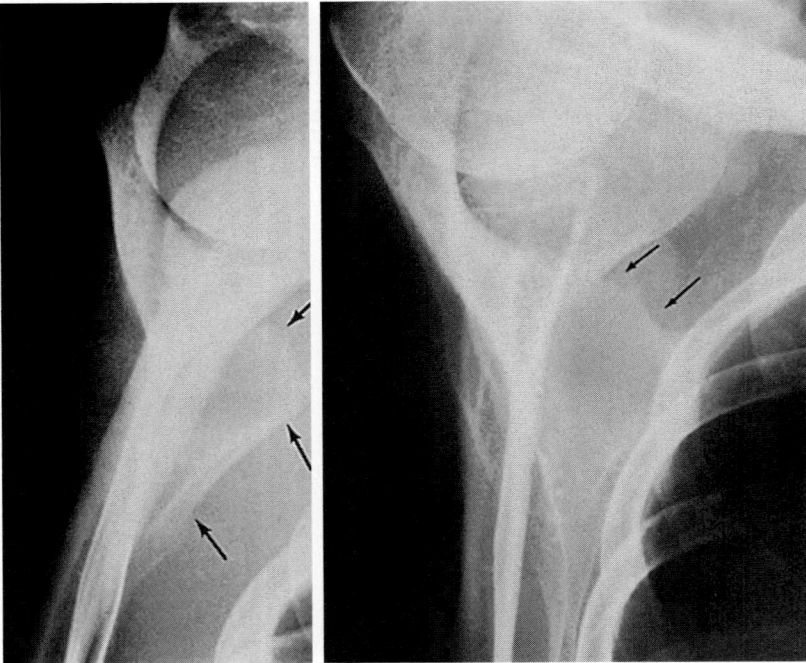

Figure 5–73. Tangential views of the scapula with simulated fractures produced by the overlapping shadow of the free border on the body of the scapula.

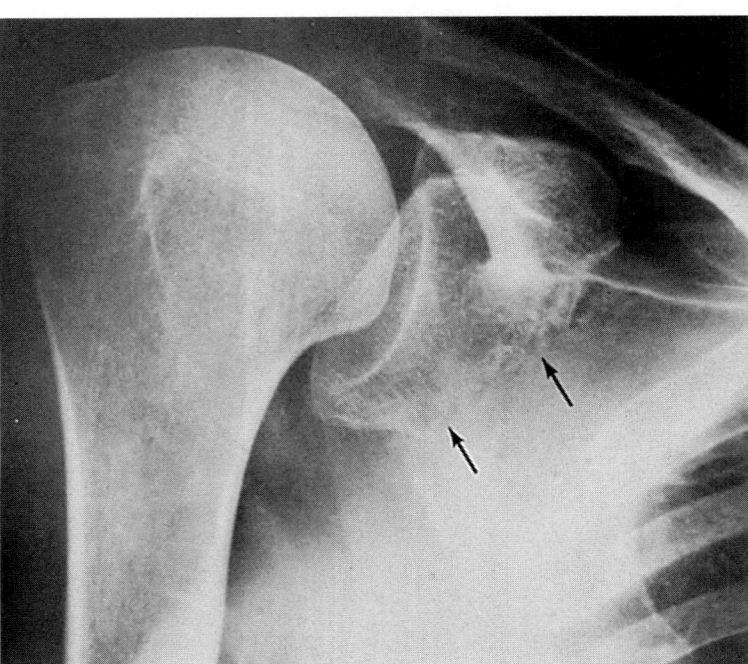

Figure 5–74. Simulated fracture of the neck of the scapula, produced by trabecular pattern.

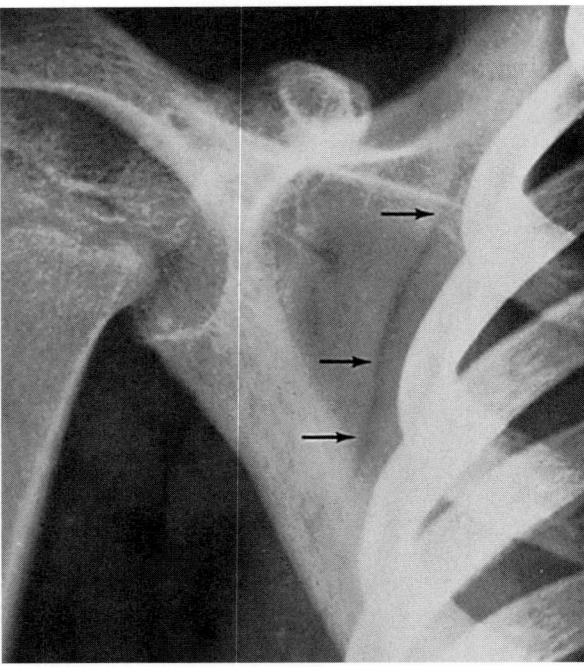

Figure 5–75. Fat stripe of chest wall simulating a fracture of the scapula.

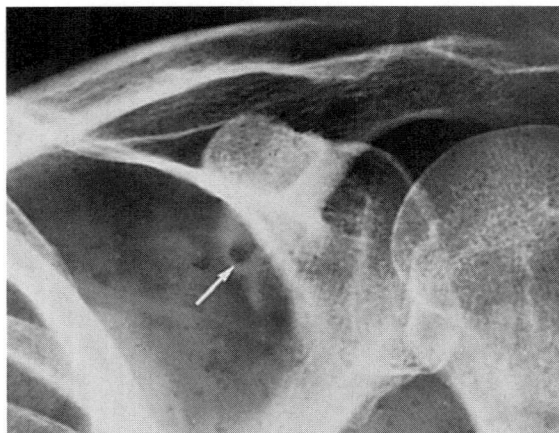

Figure 5–76. Large nutrient foramen of the scapula.

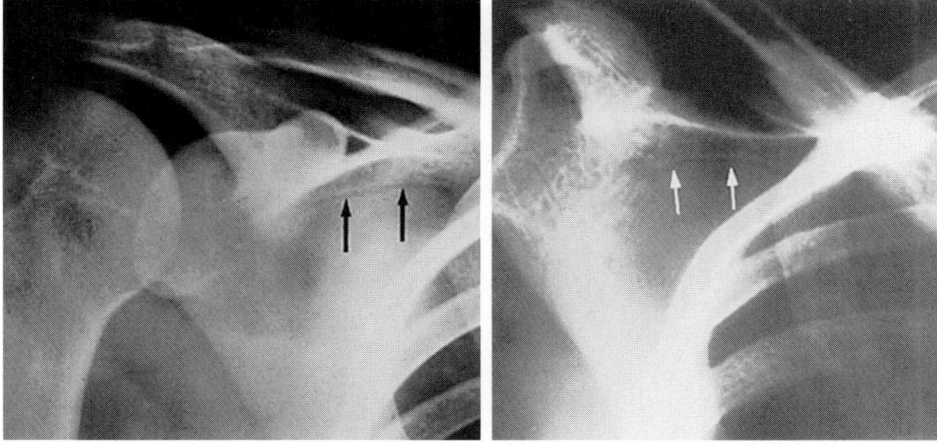

Figure 5–77. Two examples of vascular channels that might be mistaken for fracture.

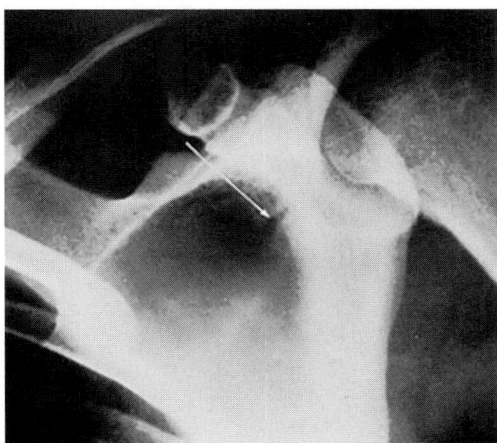

Figure 5–78. Vascular groove in the neck of the scapula.

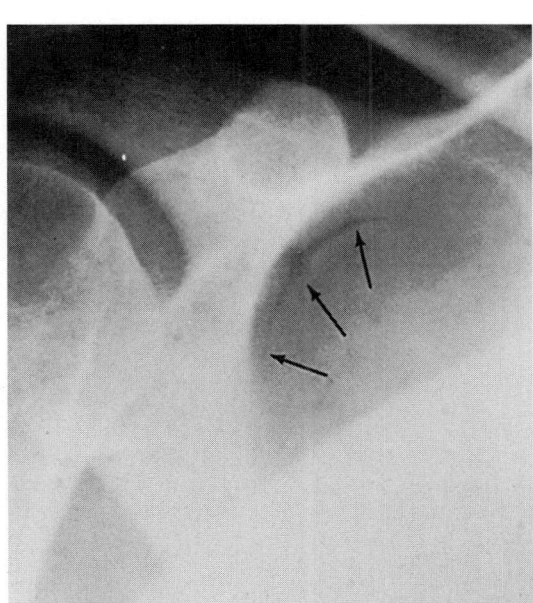

Figure 5–79. Prominent vascular channel in the wing of the scapula.

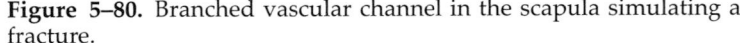

Figure 5–80. Branched vascular channel in the scapula simulating a fracture.

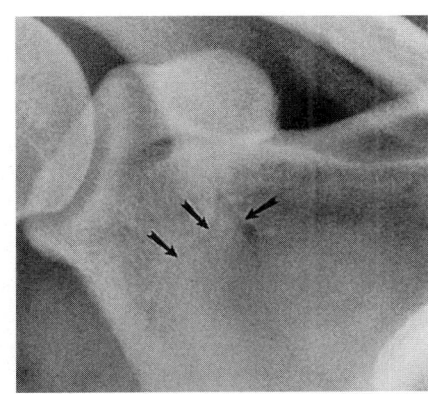

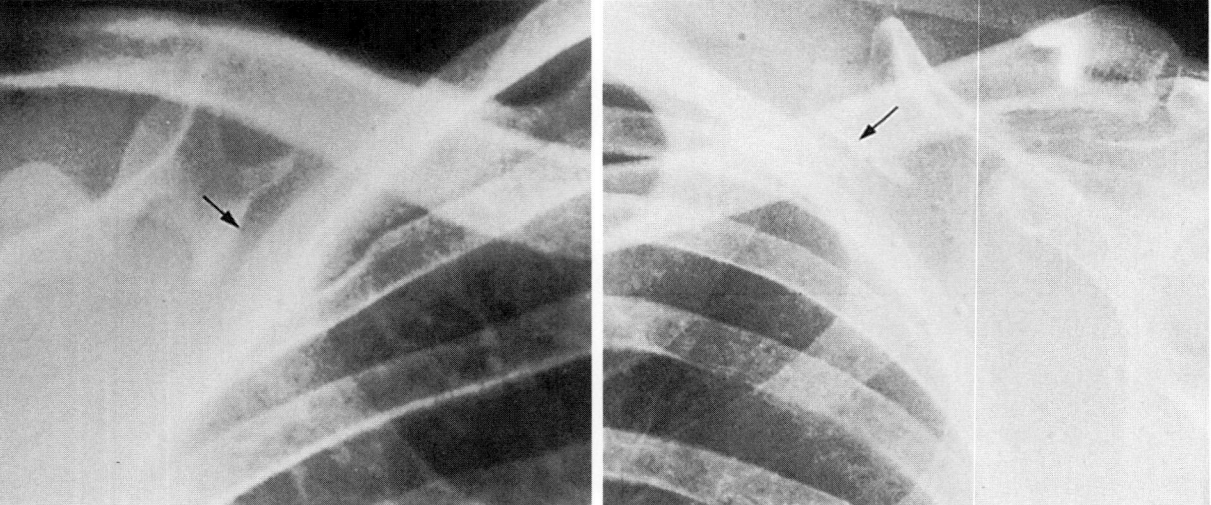

Figure 5–81. Two examples of articulations between the scapula and adjacent ribs.

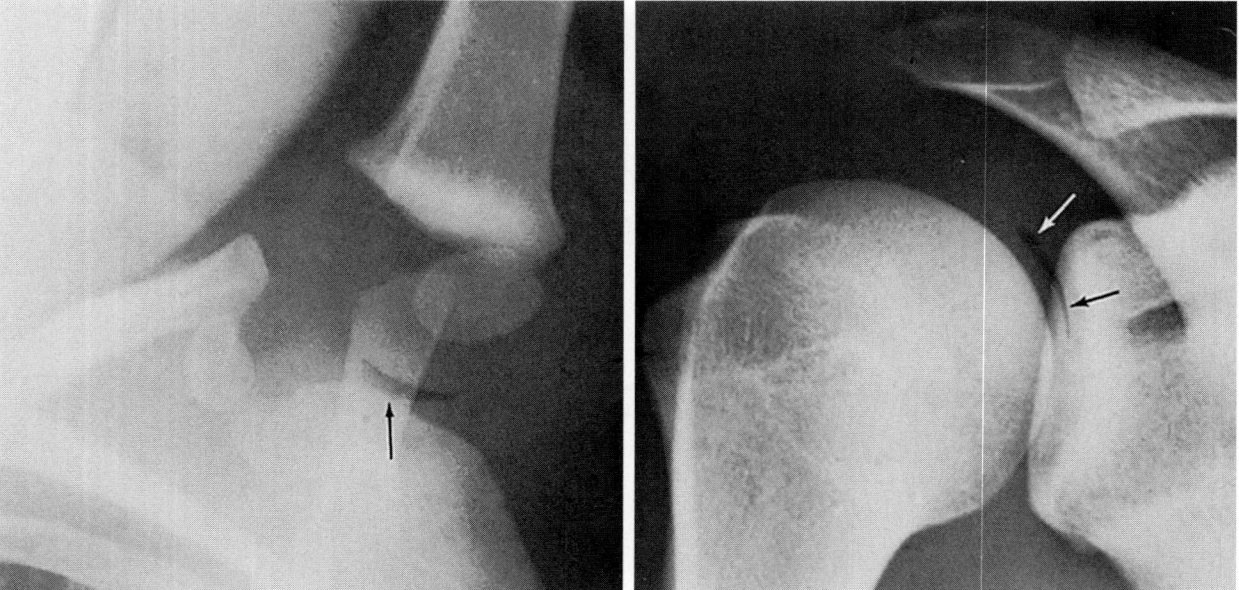

Figure 5–82. Examples of the normal "vacuum" phenomenon in the shoulder joint.

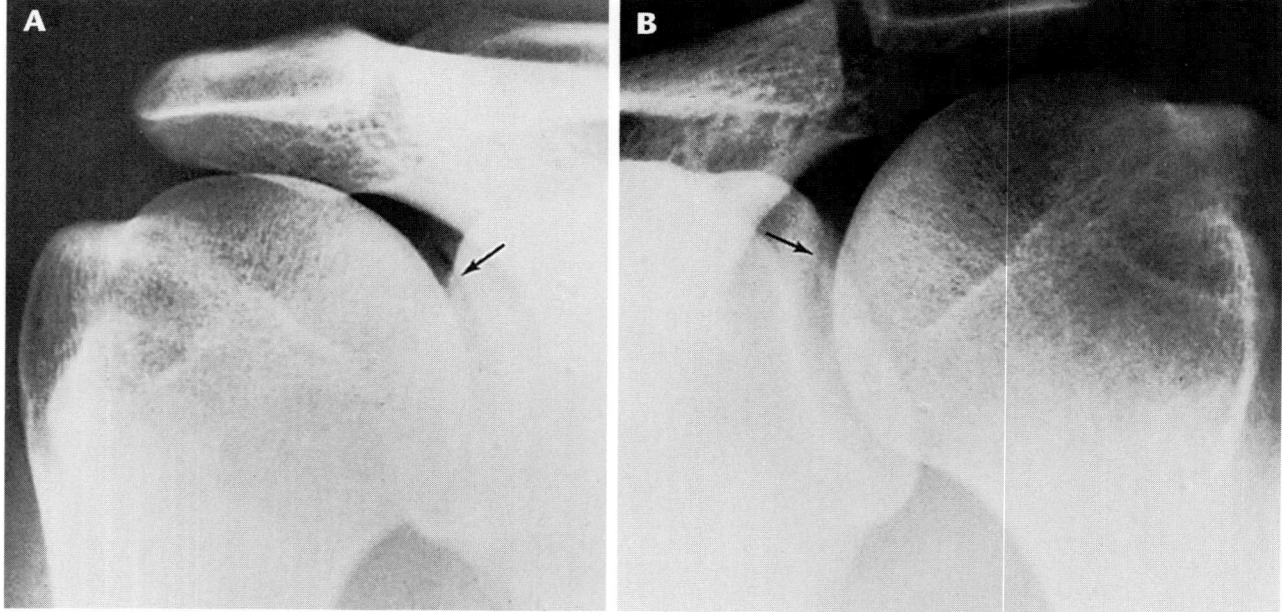

Figure 5–83. A, B, "Vacuum" phenomenon in both shoulder joints. When the lucency is seen overlying only bone, as in **B,** it may be mistaken for fracture.

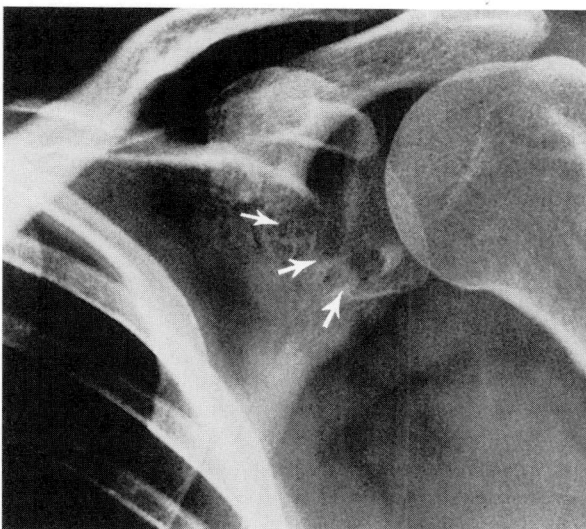

Figure 5–84. Marked accentuation of the trabecular pattern of the scapula in a 49-year-old woman. CT and MRI showed no abnormality.

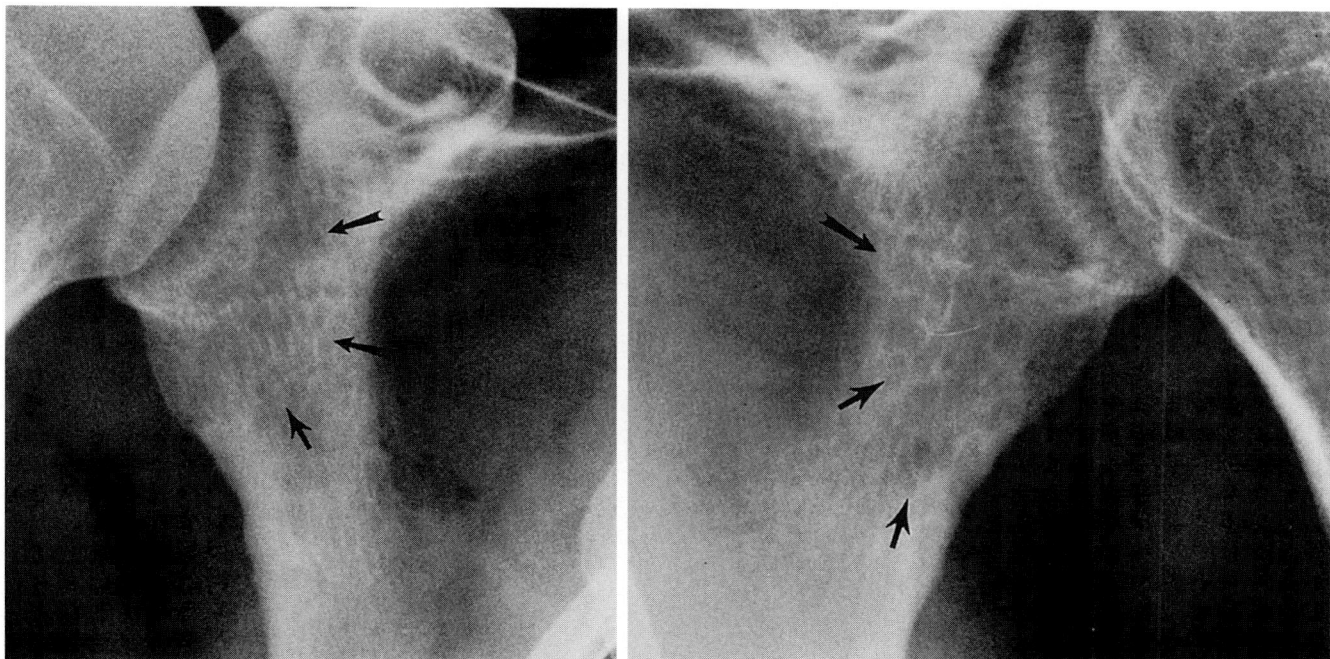

Figure 5–85. Similar but less marked example of the entity illustrated in the preceding figure, seen here in a 32-year-old man.

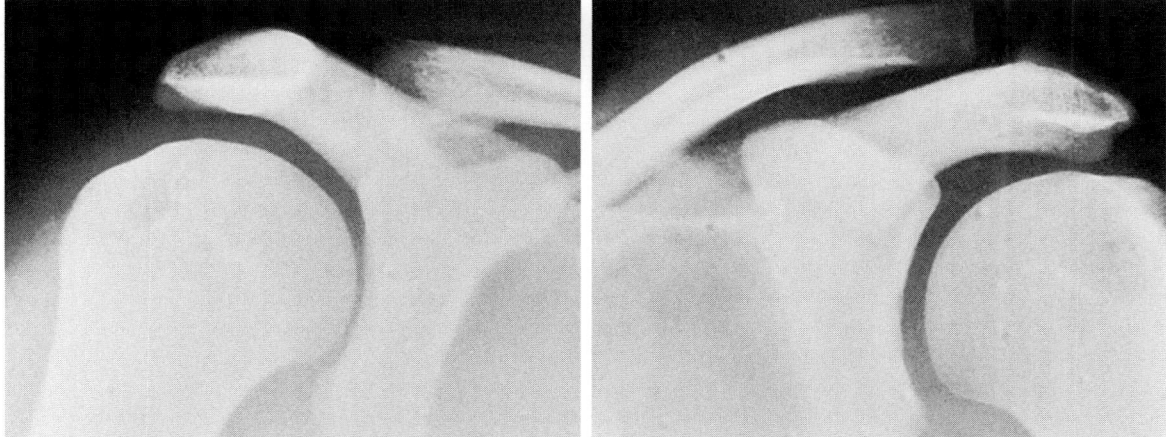

Figure 5–86. Dysplastic scapulae with wide acromioclavicular joints and large, shallow glenoid fossae. (Refs: Resnick D et al: Bilateral dysplasia of the scapular neck. *Am J Roentgenol* 139:387, 1982; Trout TE, Resnick D: Glenoid hypoplasia and its relationship to instability. *Skeletal Radiol* 25:37, 1996.)

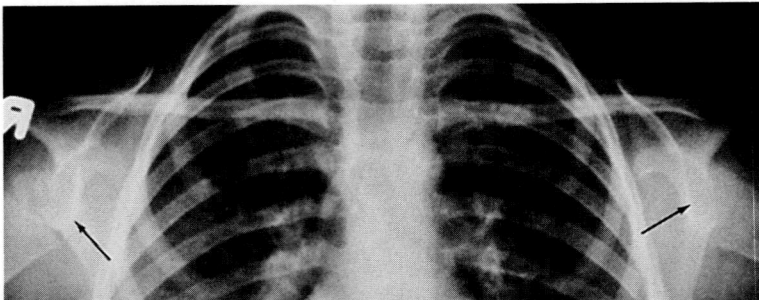

Figure 5–87. Conventional positioning of the arms for chest radiography may produce an appearance simulating dislocations of the shoulders in children.

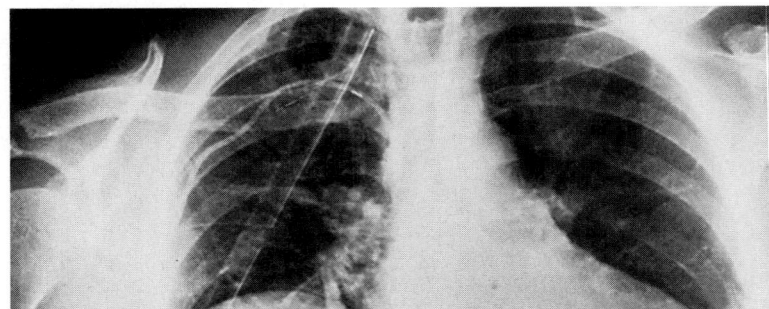

Figure 5–88. *Left,* Simulated dislocation of the right shoulder secondary to positioning in an elderly individual.

The Clavicle

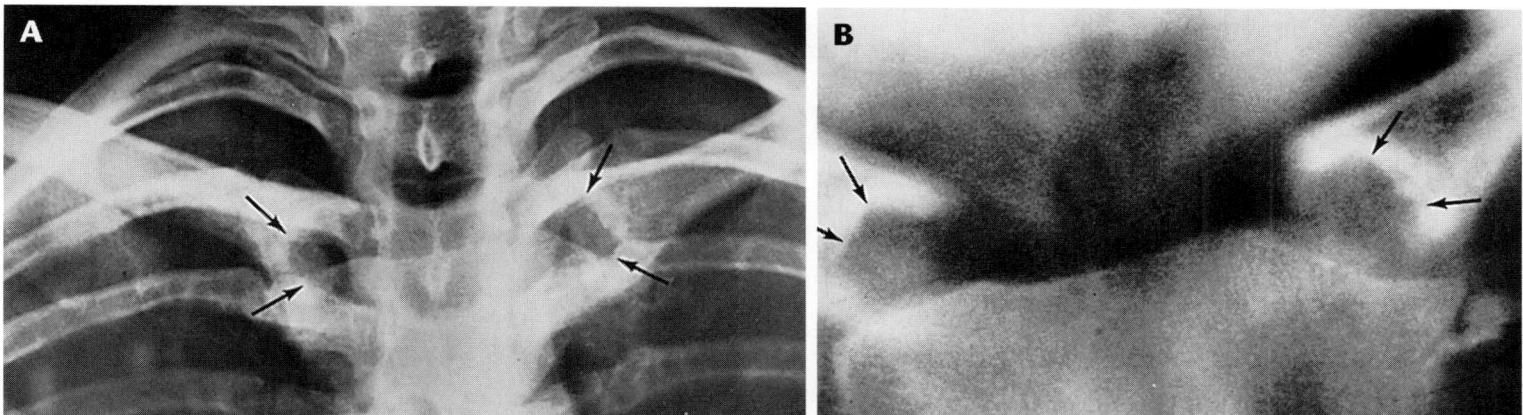

Figure 5–89. Normal irregular appearance of the medial ends of the clavicles in an 18-year-old man. This appearance, before completion of development, may be misinterpreted as evidence of disease. **A,** Plain film. **B,** Tomogram.

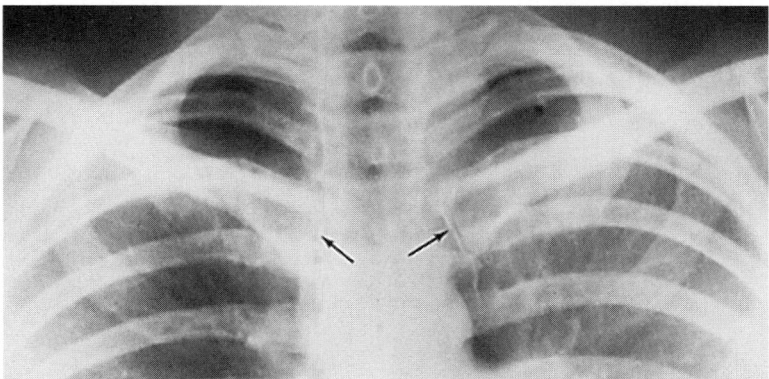

Figure 5–90. Secondary ossification centers of the medial ends of the clavicles in a 20-year-old man.

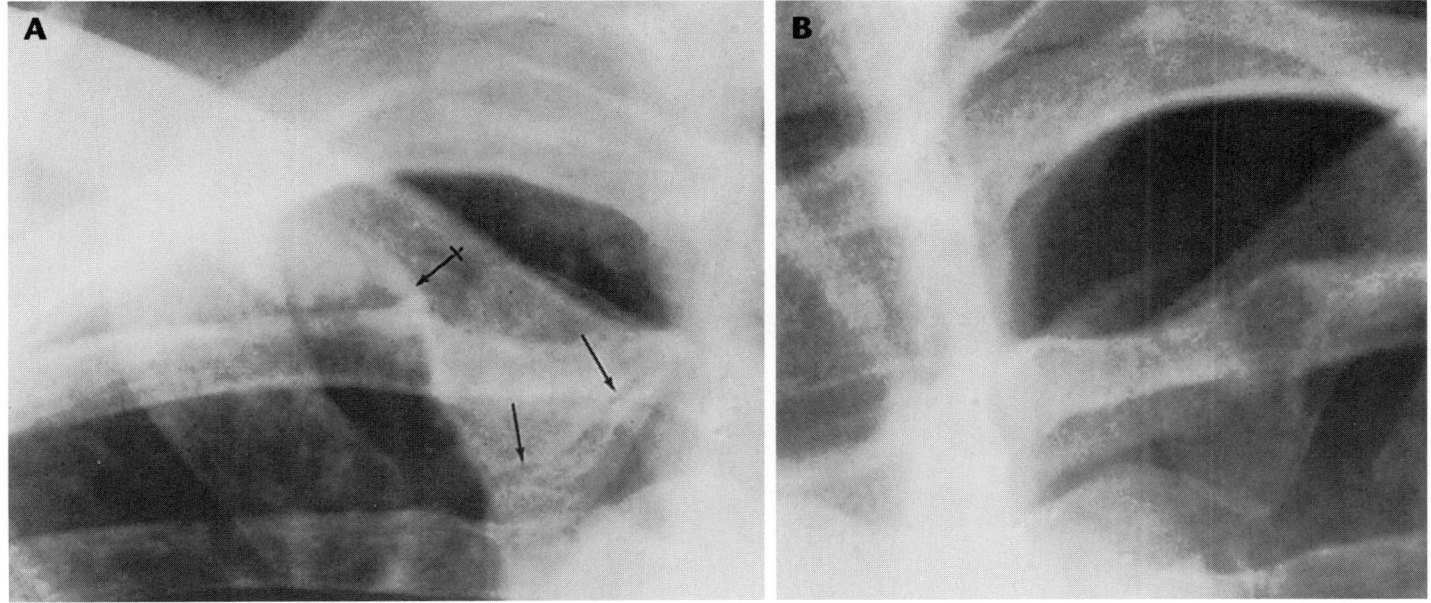

Figure 5–91. Asymmetric closure of secondary ossification centers of medial ends of clavicles in a 21-year-old man. **A,** Open apophysis (→). **B,** Closed apophysis. Note also deep rhomboid fossa in **A** (↦).

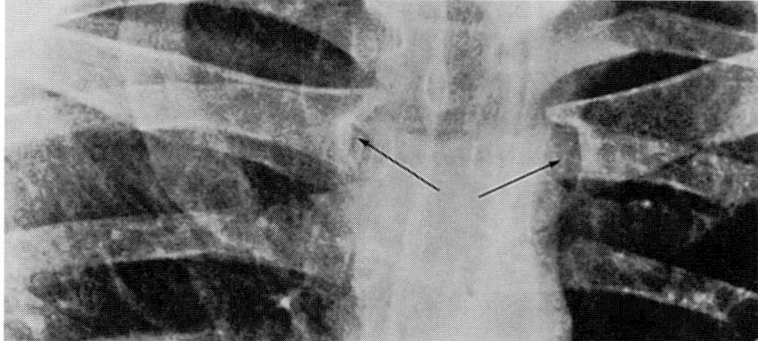

Figure 5–92. Failure of the medial ends of the clavicles to develop completely in an otherwise normal adult.

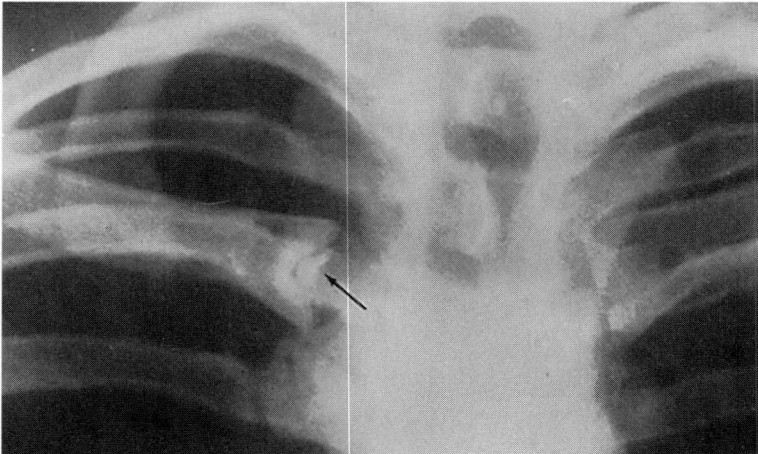

Figure 5–93. An ununited ossification center for the medial end of the clavicle, which has persisted as a separate ossicle. Note cupped juvenile configuration of the adjacent end of the clavicle in contrast to the opposite side.

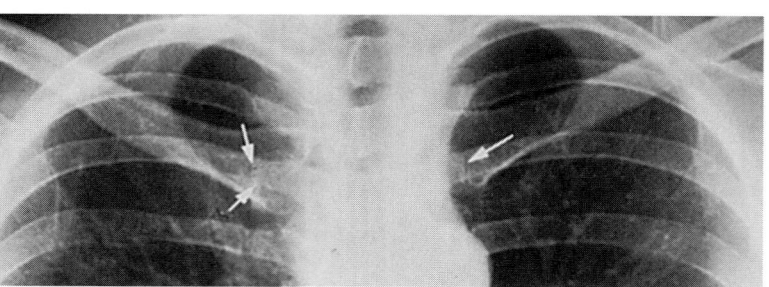

Figure 5–94. Normal asymmetry of the medial ends of the clavicles.

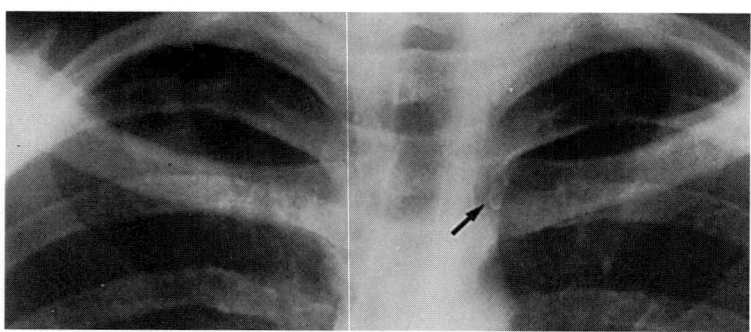

Figure 5–95. An accessory ossicle at the medial end of the clavicle.

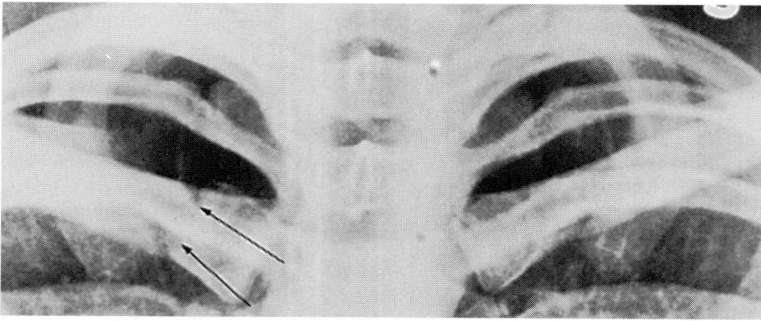

Figure 5–96. Simulated fracture of the medial end of the clavicle produced by overlapping shadows of the transverse processes, rhomboid fossa, and ribs.

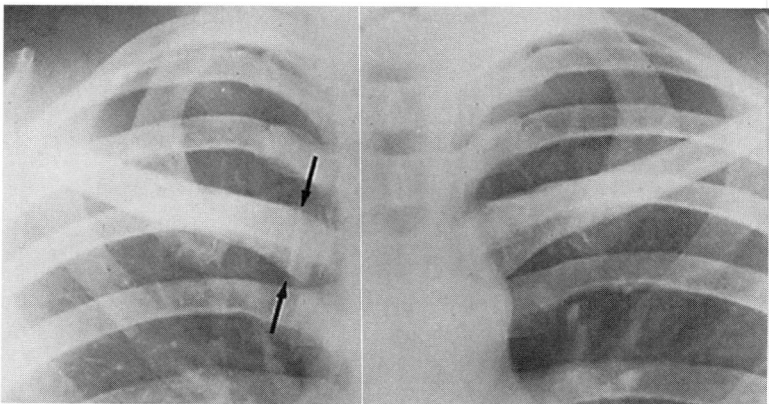

Figure 5–97. A dense closed epiphyseal line in an adult, simulating a fracture with overriding.

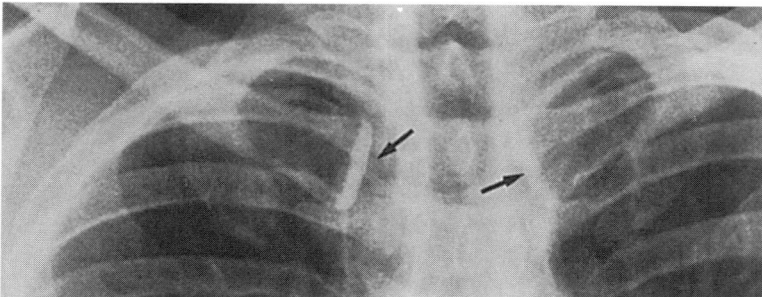

Figure 5–98. Sclerosis of the medial ends of the clavicle in a healthy 41-year-old man.

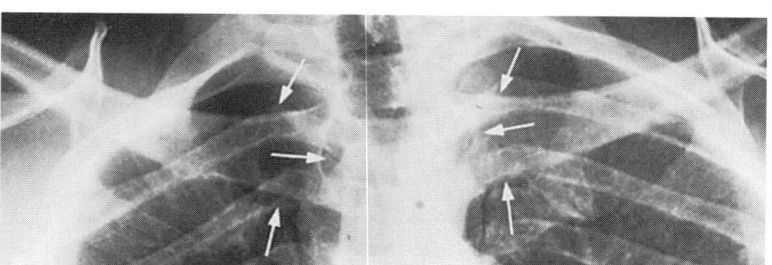

Figure 5–99. Unusually stout medial ends of the clavicles with cupping of the articular surfaces.

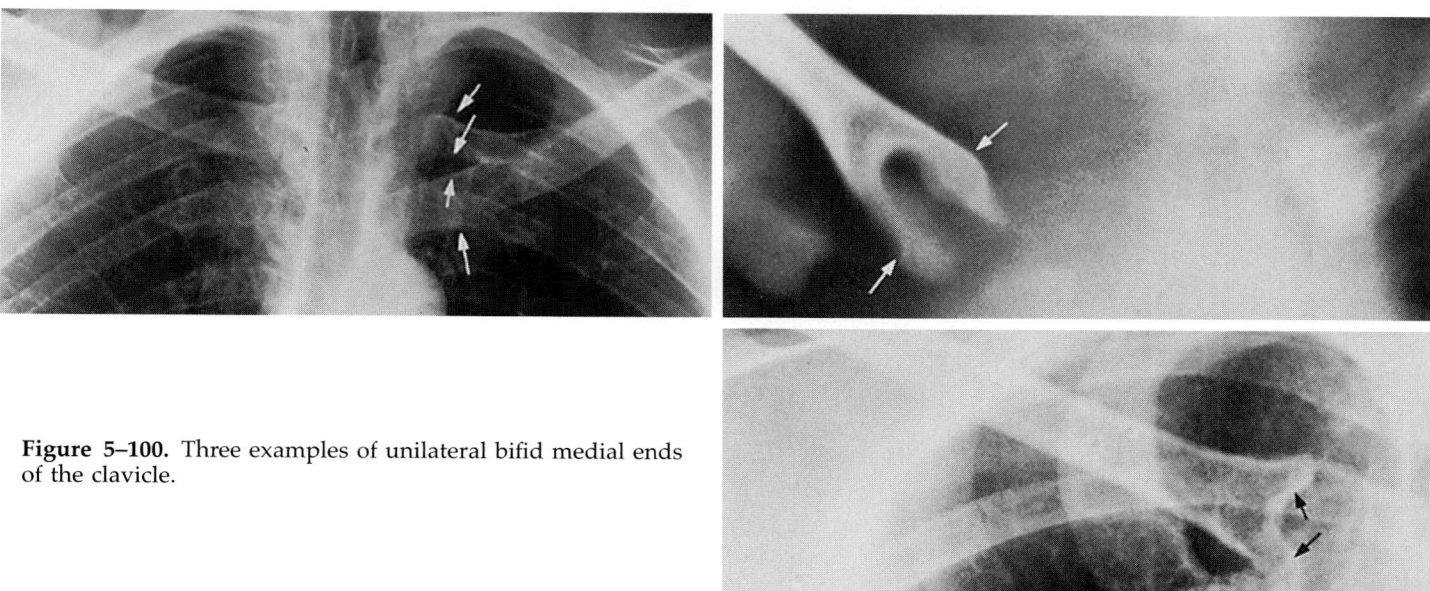

Figure 5–100. Three examples of unilateral bifid medial ends of the clavicle.

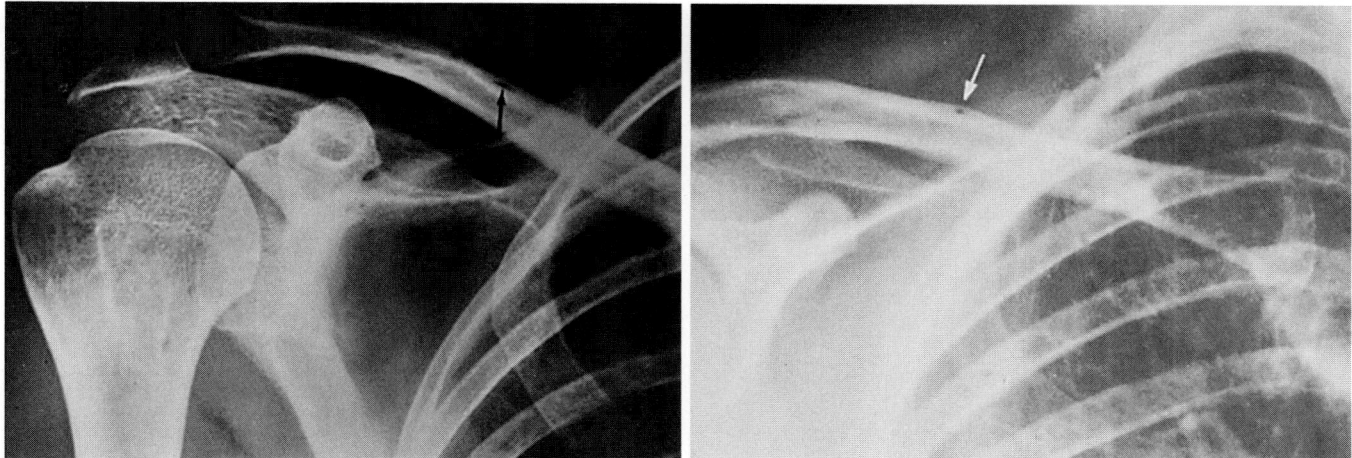

Figure 5–101. Two examples of the canal for the middle supraclavicular nerve.

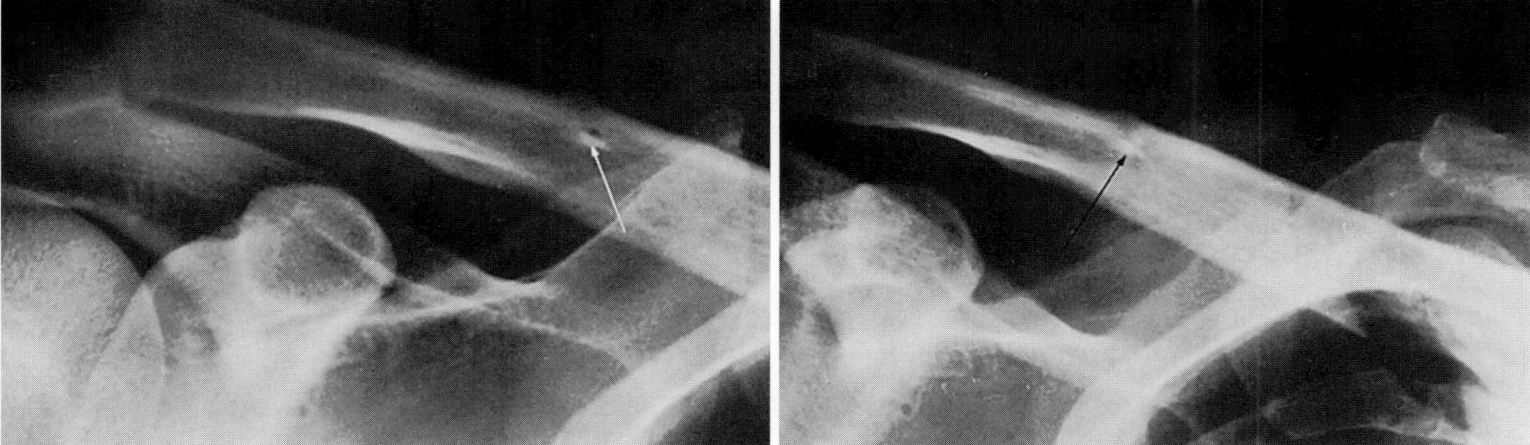

Figure 5–102. The canal for the supraclavicular nerve mistaken for a fracture in a 43-year-old man.

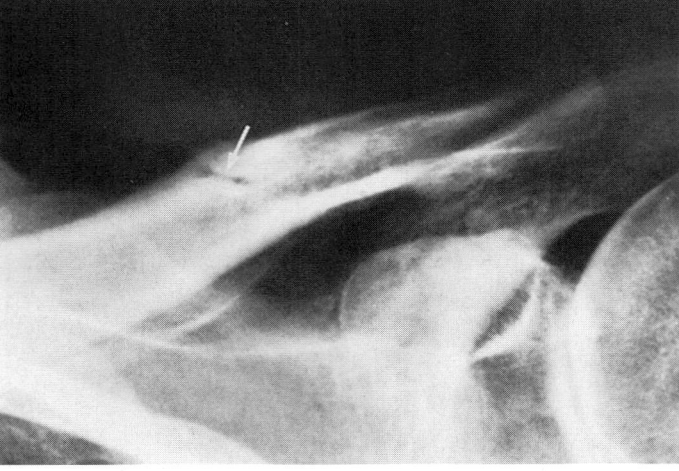

Figure 5–103. The canal for the middle supraclavicular nerve mistaken for fracture in a 70-year-old man.

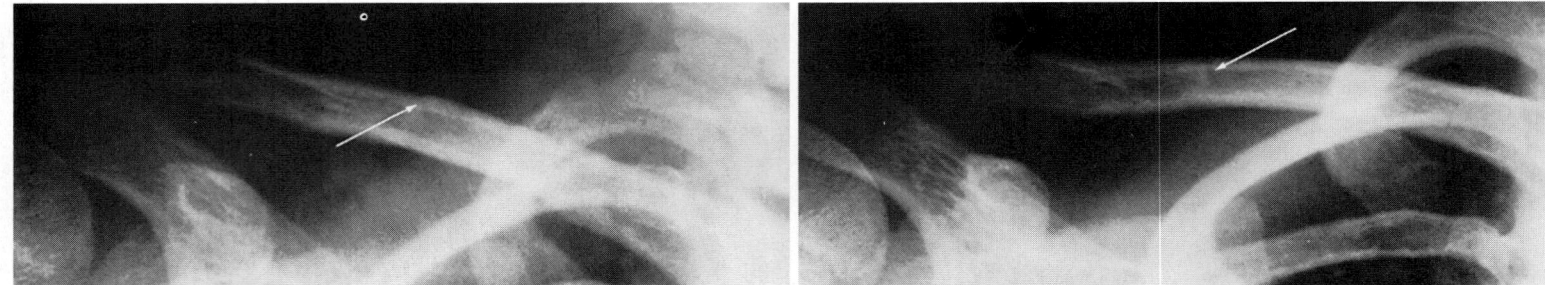

Figure 5–104. The canal for the supraclavicular nerve mistaken for a fracture in a 5-year-old boy.

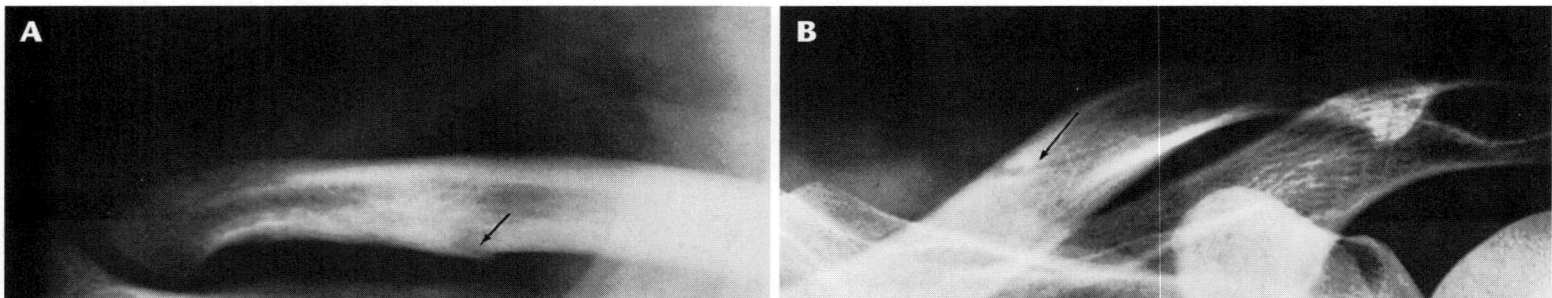

Figure 5–105. The nutrient canal of the clavicle is usually located posteriorly and not seen but may appear on the inferior border. (Ref: Ogdon TA et al: Radiology of postnatal skeletal development. III. The clavicle. *Skeletal Radiol* 4:196, 1979.)

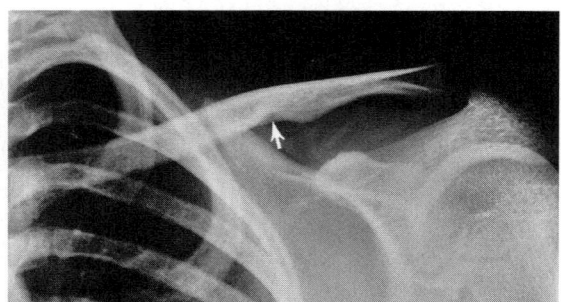

Figure 5–106. The fossa at the entry point of the nutrient vessel and the canal of the nutrient vessel is nicely demonstrated in this patient.

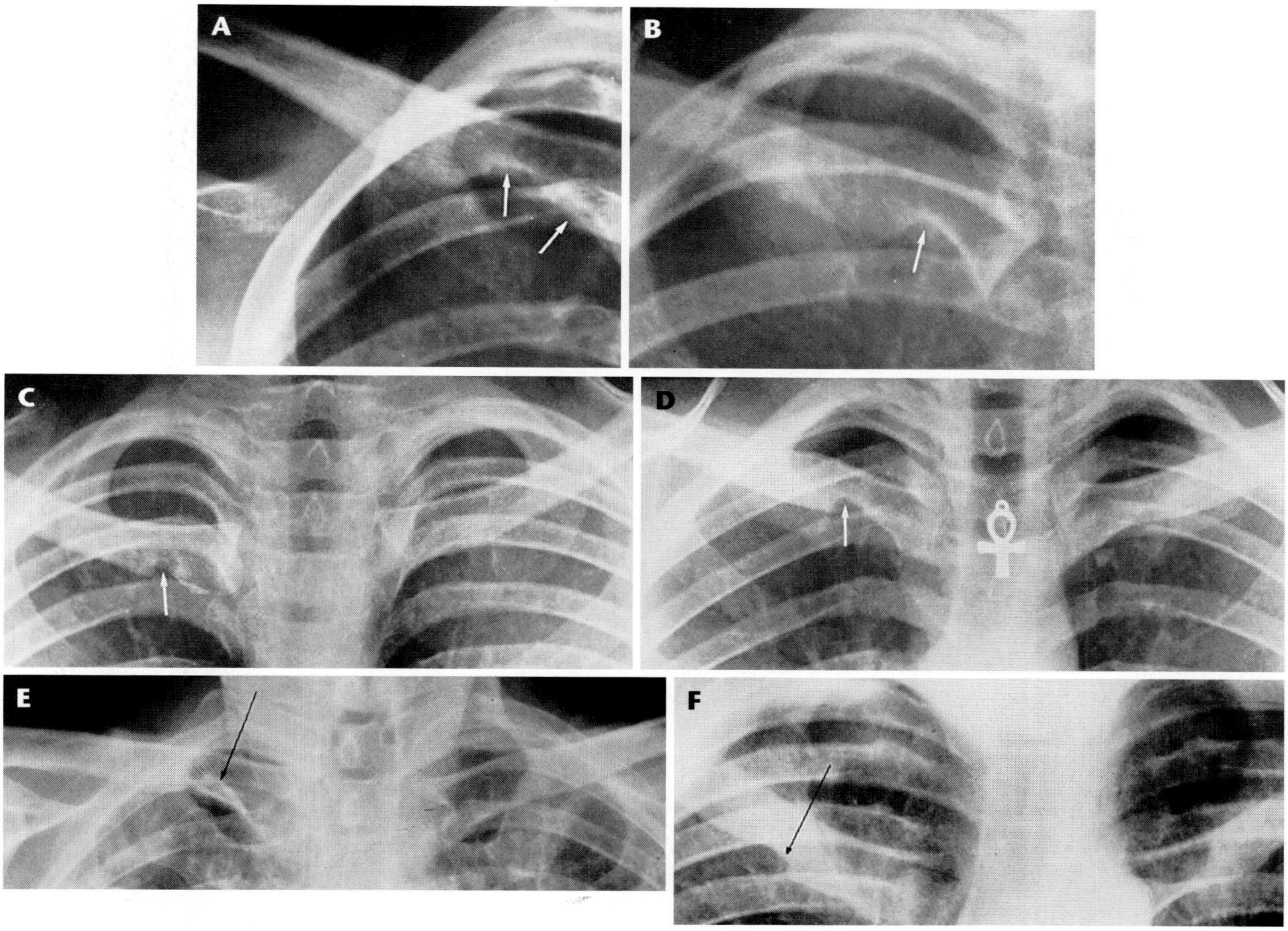

Figure 5–107. Examples of rhomboid fossa, the site of attachment of the rhomboid ligament between the first rib and the clavicle. Note how it may simulate bone destruction and the fact that it is not necessarily bilaterally symmetric.

Figure 5–108. An exostosis-like extension of the clavicle at the usual site of the rhomboid fossa.

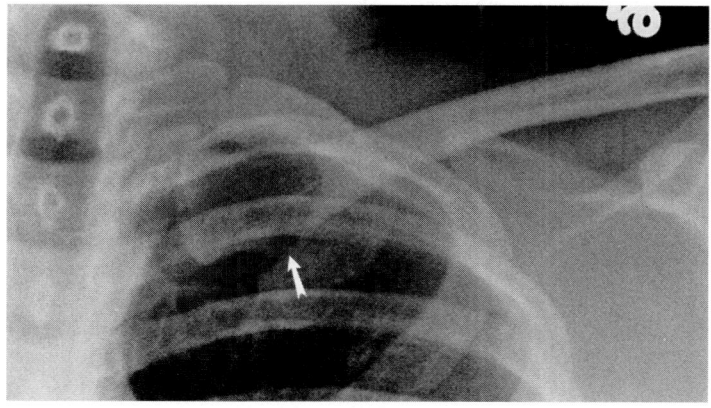

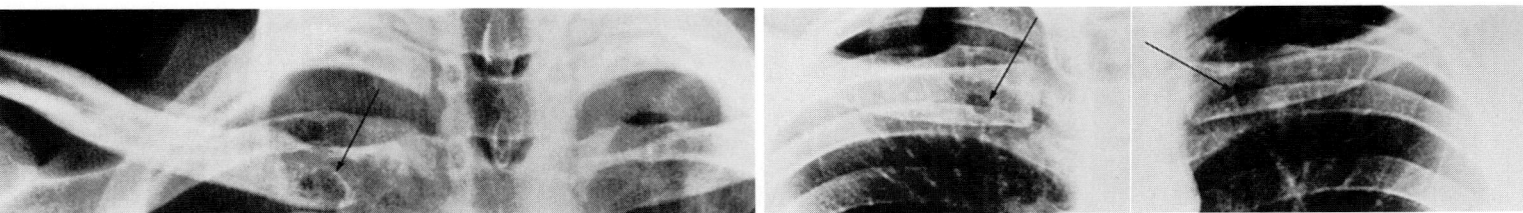

Figure 5–109. Rhomboid fossae, which could be mistaken for cavitary lesions in lung.

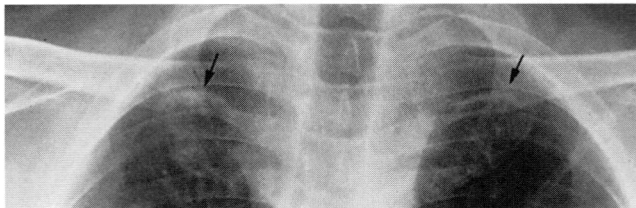

Figure 5–110. Bilateral rhomboid fossae simulating apical pneumothoraces.

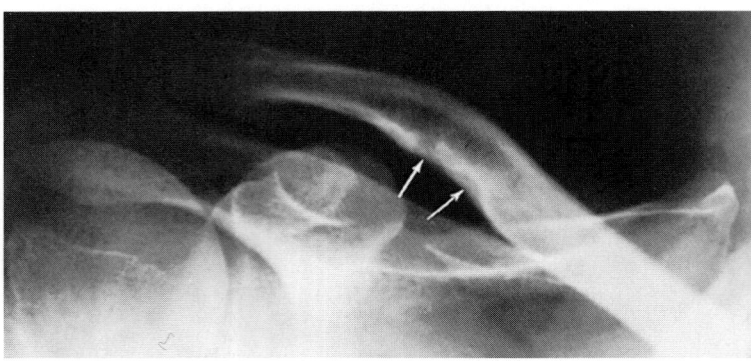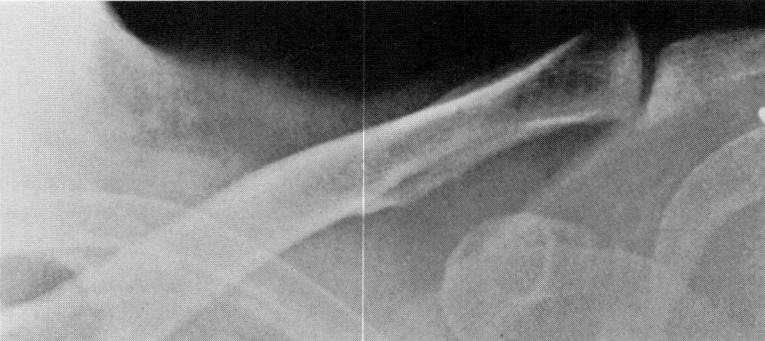

Figure 5–111. Grooves for the insertion of the coracoclavicular ligament.

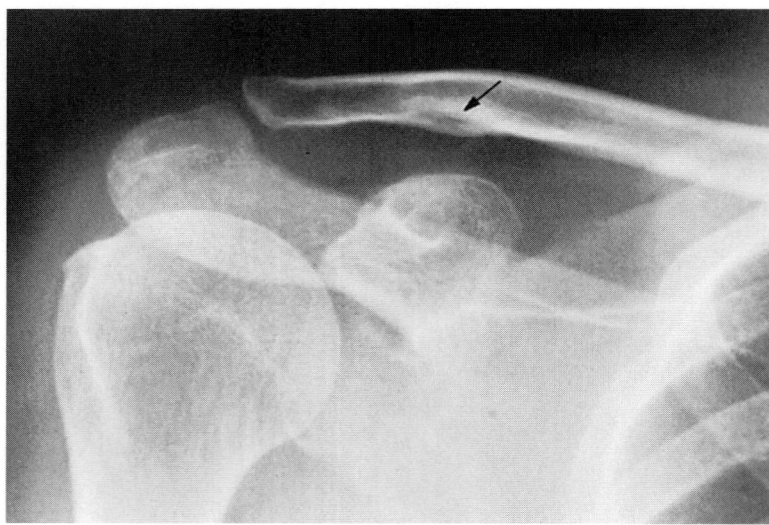

Figure 5–112. Groove for the coracoclavicular ligament simulating an erosion.

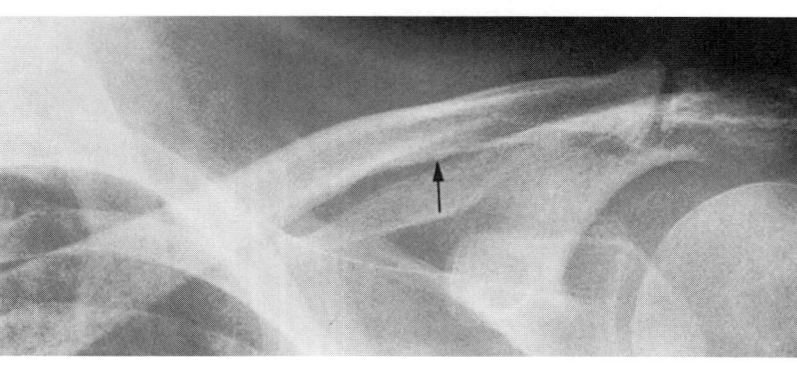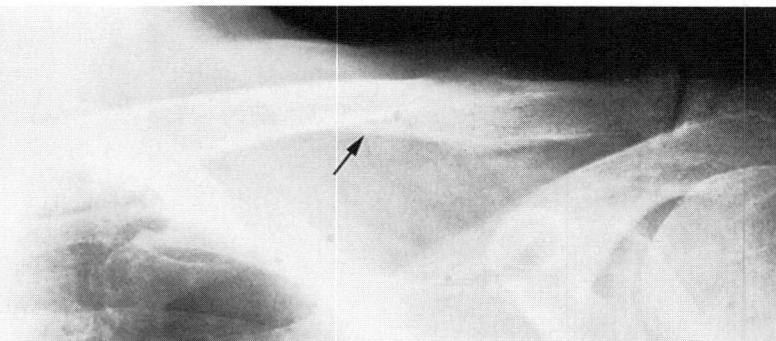

Figure 5–113. Groove for the insertion of the coracoclavicular ligament mistaken for a fracture. *Left,* External rotation. *Right,* Internal rotation.

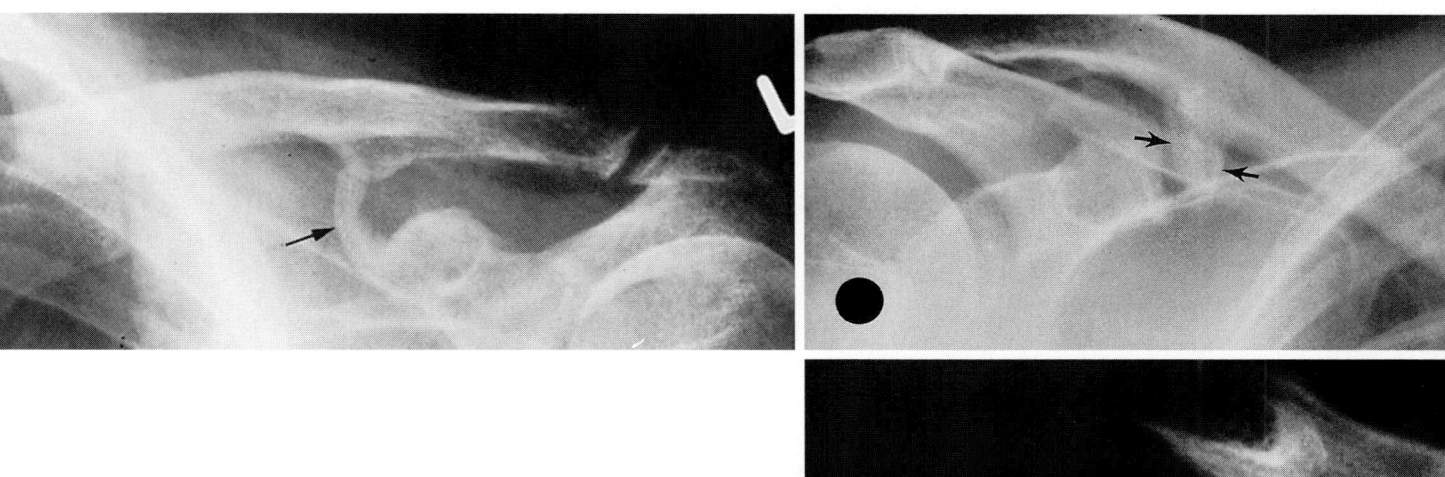

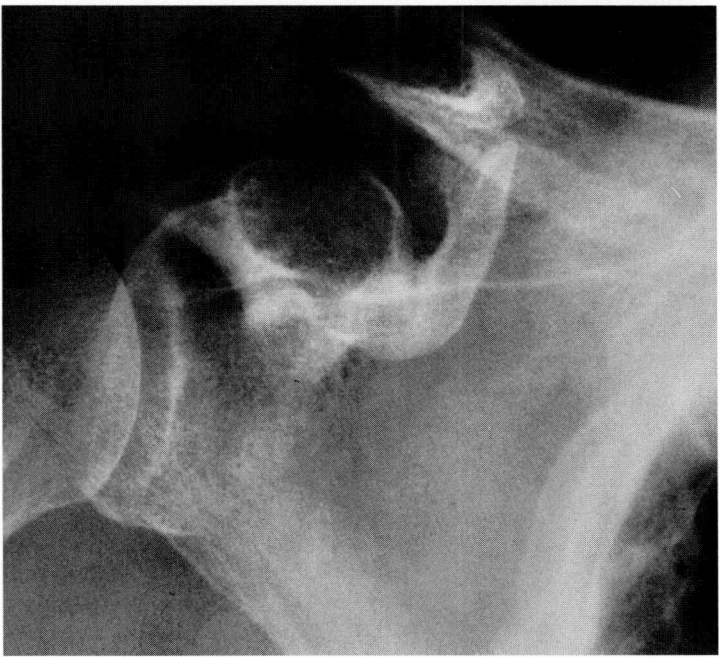

Figure 5–114. Three examples of ossification of the coracoclavicular ligament.

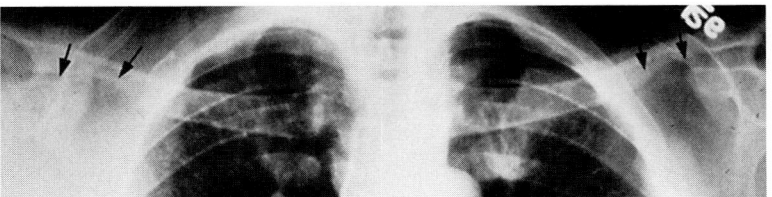

Figure 5–115. Examples of deep fossae in the distal portions of the clavicle probably representing the origin of the deltoid muscle.

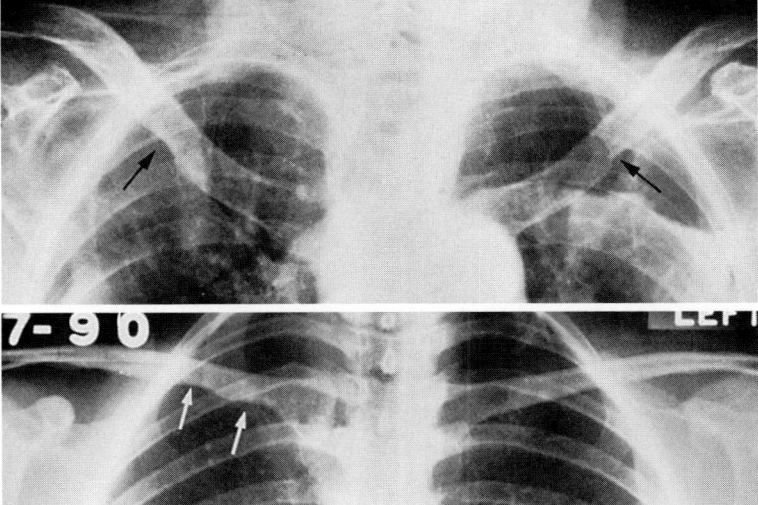

Figure 5–116. Examples of wavy inferior margins of the clavicles thought to be related to the subclavian arteries. *Top,* Bilateral. *Bottom,* Unilateral on the right. It has also been suggested that this configuration may be the product of rotation of the clavicle with aging. (Refs: Levin B: The unilateral wavy clavicle. *Skeletal Radiol* 19:519, 1990; Freiberger RH: Letter to the editor. *Skeletal Radiol* 20:192, 1990.)

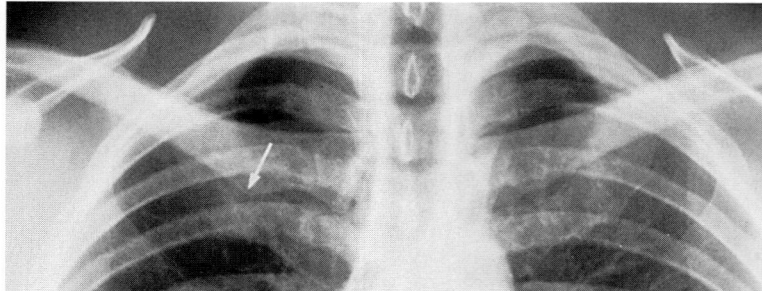

Figure 5–117. Abortive articulation between the clavicle and the first rib.

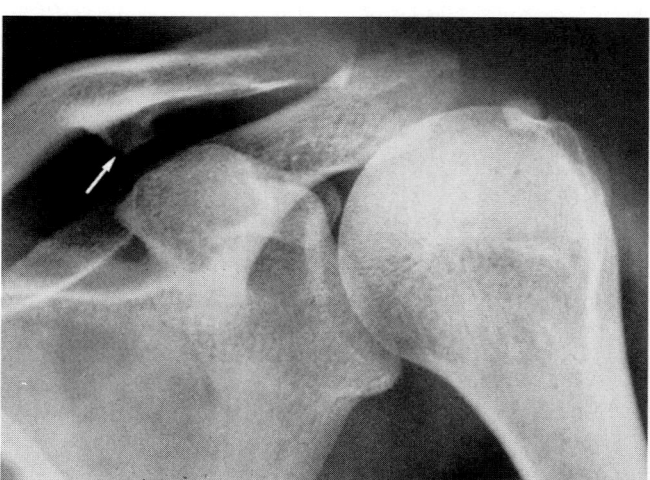

Figure 5–118. Three examples of the coracoclavicular joint, an anomalous articulation that develops in the coracoclavicular ligament and is usually of no clinical significance. (Ref: Haramati N et al: Coracoclavicular joint: Normal variant in humans. *Skeletal Radiol* 23:117, 1994.)

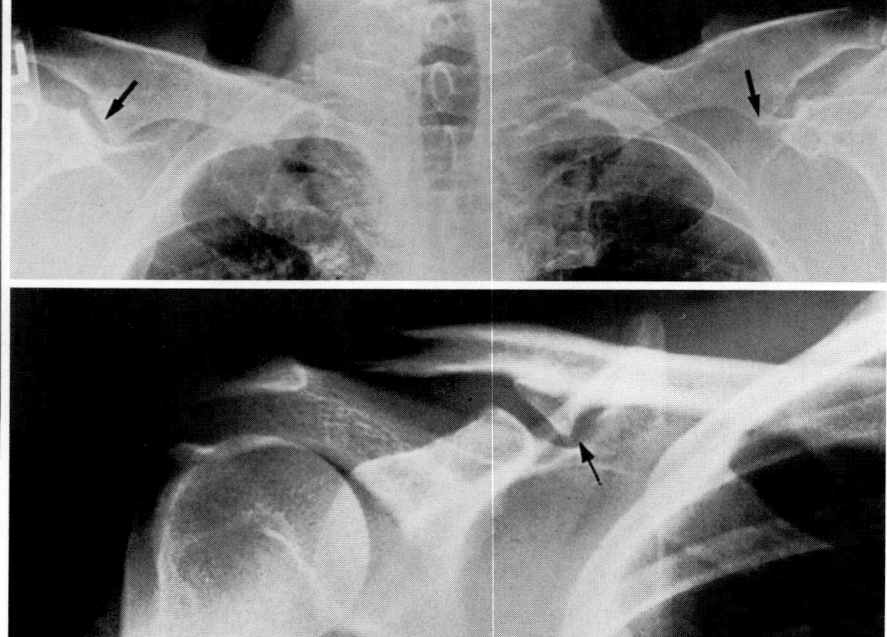

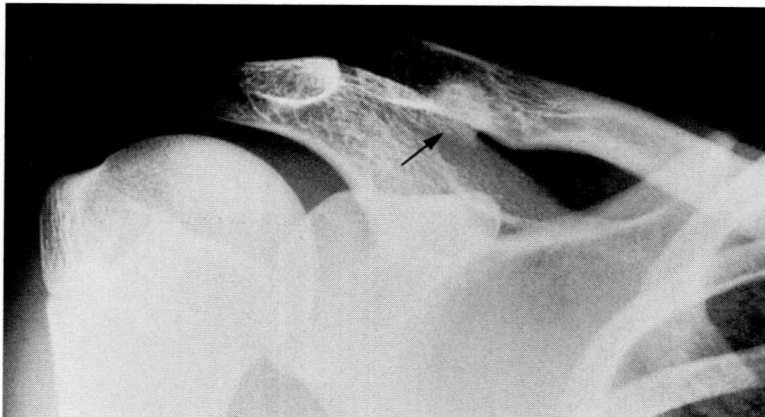

Figure 5–119. Developing coracoclavicular articulation in a 9-year-old child.

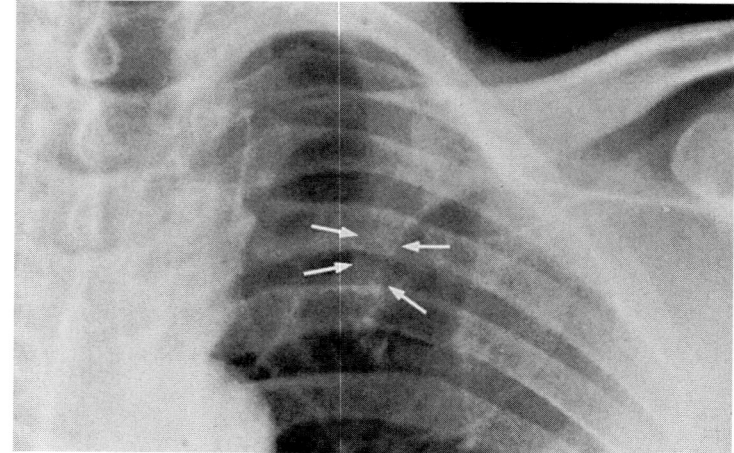

Figure 5–120. The costoclavicular joint, an anomalous articulation between the clavicle and the anterior aspect of the first rib. (Ref: Redlund-Johnell I: The costoclavicular joint. *Skeletal Radiol* 15:25, 1986.)

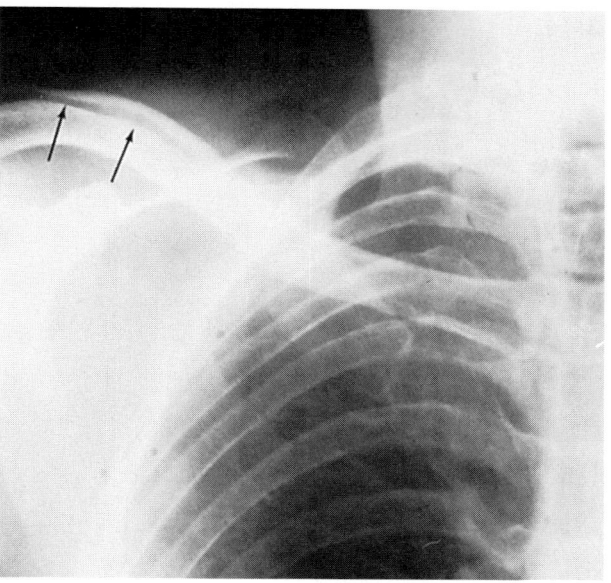

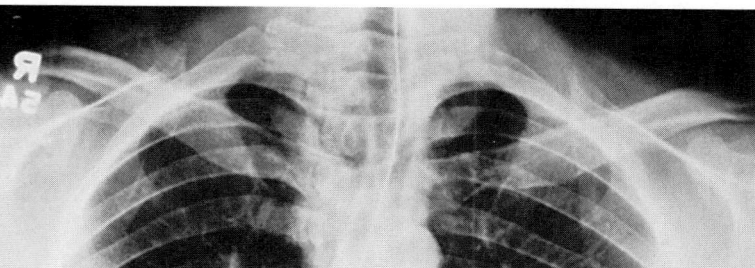

Figure 5–122. Unusually stout clavicular shafts in contrast to the medial and distal portions.

Figure 5–121. Unusual appearance of the clavicle, produced by overlapping shadow of the scapula.

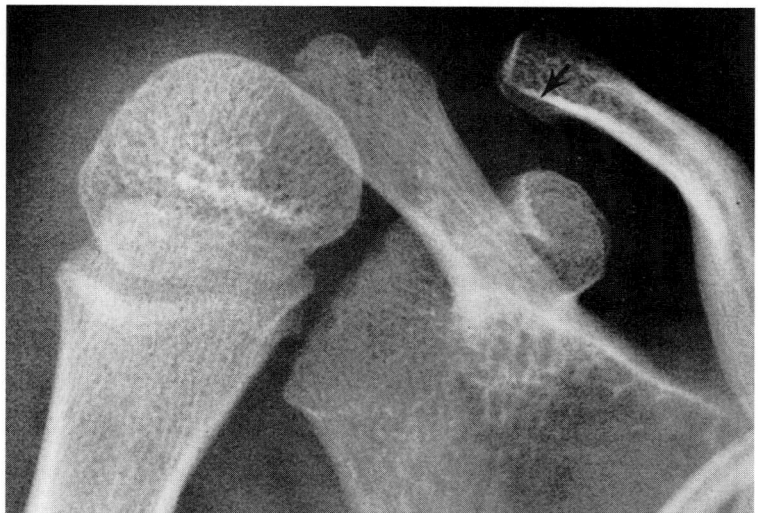

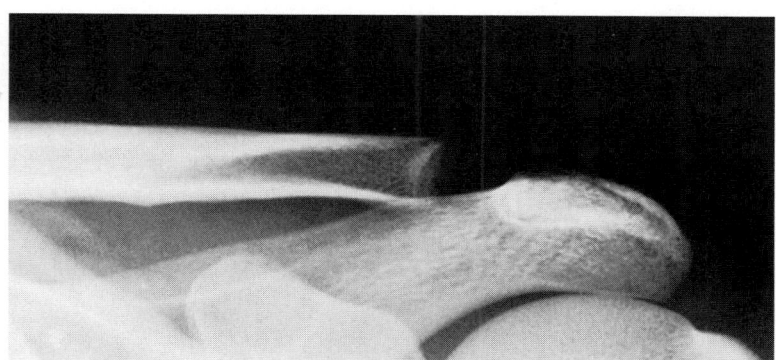

Figure 5–124. Irregular appearance of the distal end of the clavicle before growth is completed in a 16-year-old.

Figure 5–123. Normal flange on the distal end of the clavicle in a 4-year-old boy.

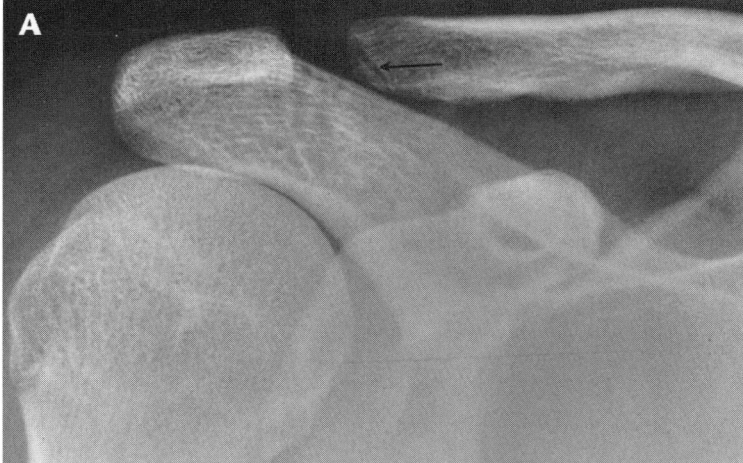

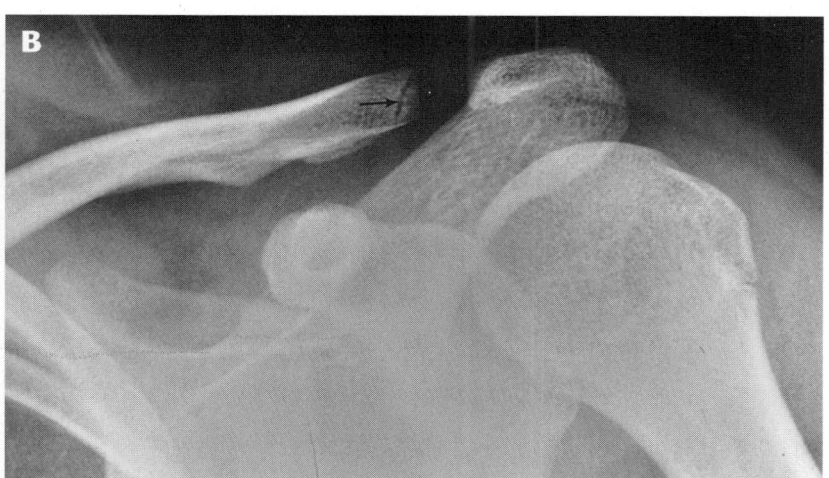

Figure 5–125. A, B, Bilateral simulated fractures of the distal ends of the clavicles in a 16-year-old boy.

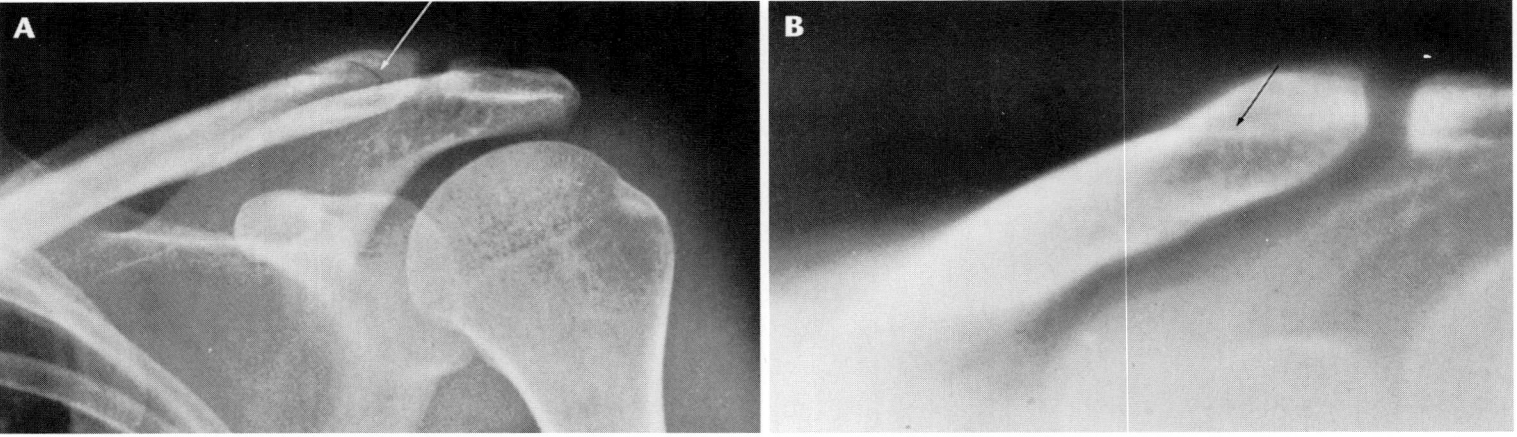

Figure 5–126. Simulated fracture of the distal end of the clavicle produced by a bony flange. **A,** Plain film. **B,** Tomogram.

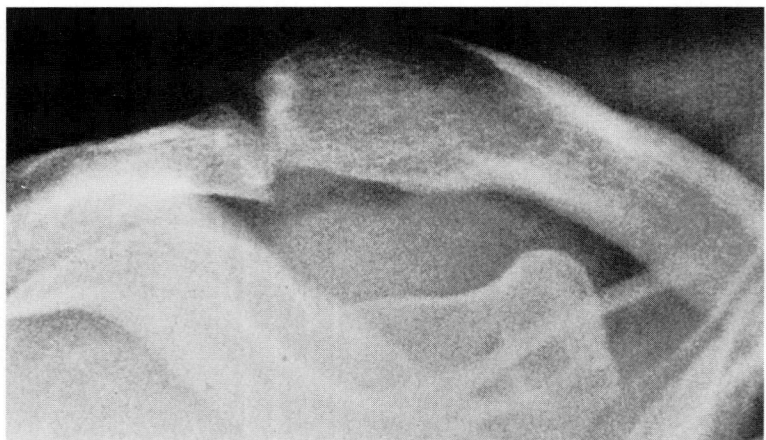

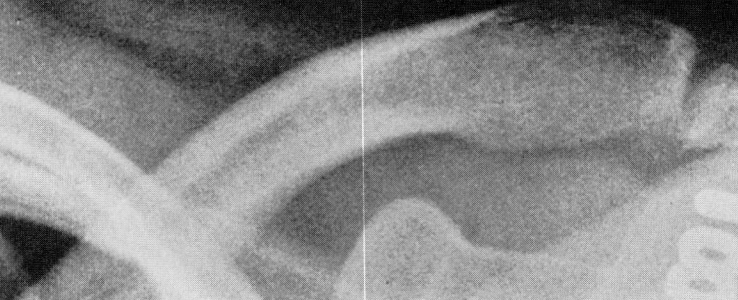

Figure 5–127. Large distal ends of the clavicles may have a cyst-like appearance because of the large amount of cancellous bone.

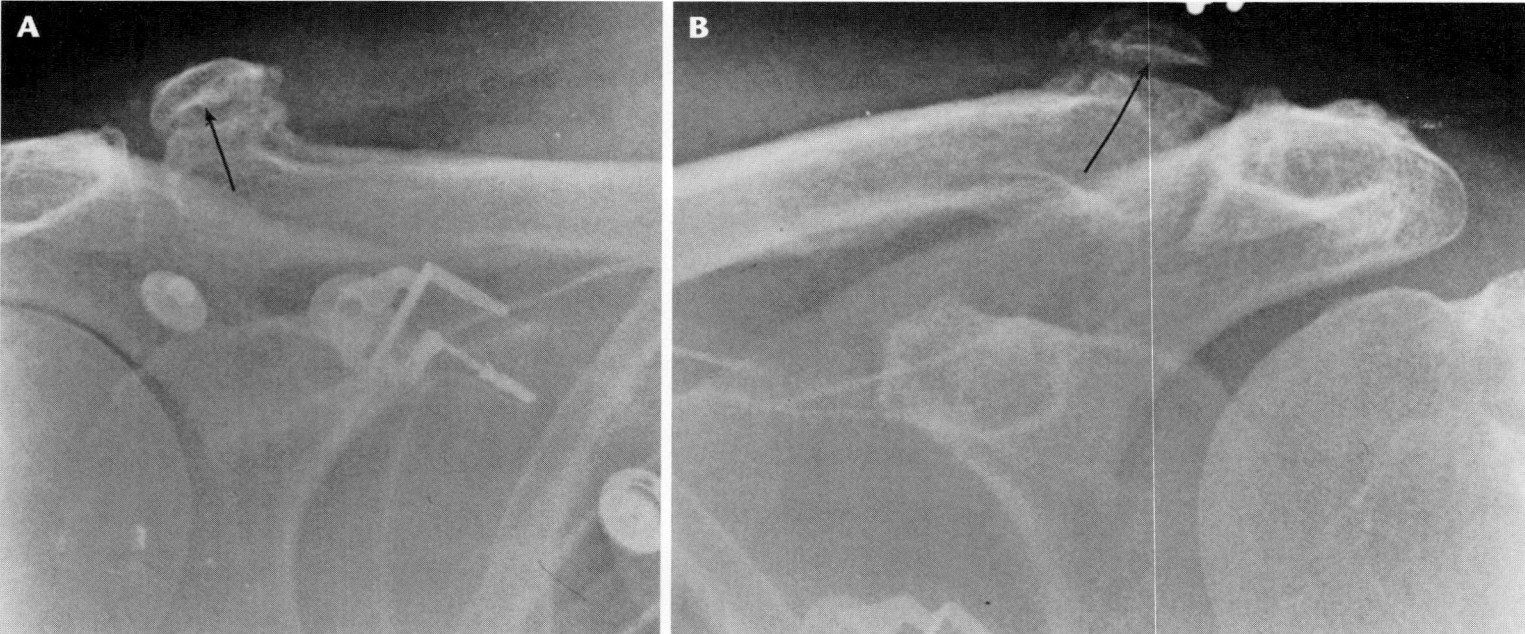

Figure 5–128. A, B, Unusual ossicles on the superior aspects of both clavicles in a 60-year-old man.

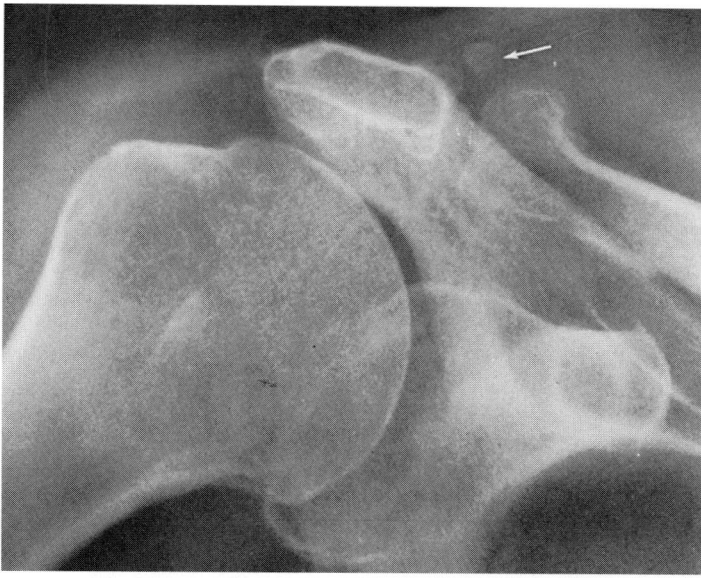

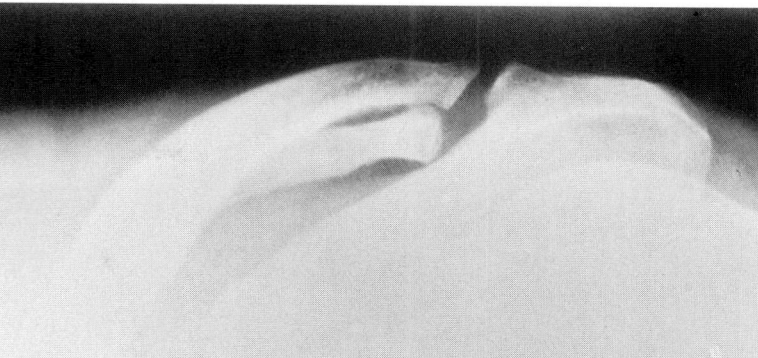

Figure 5–130. Duplication of the distal end of the clavicle. (Ref: Twig HL, Rosenbaum RC: Duplication of the clavicle. *Skeletal Radiol* 6:281, 1981.)

Figure 5–129. An accessory ossicle in the acromioclavicular joint.

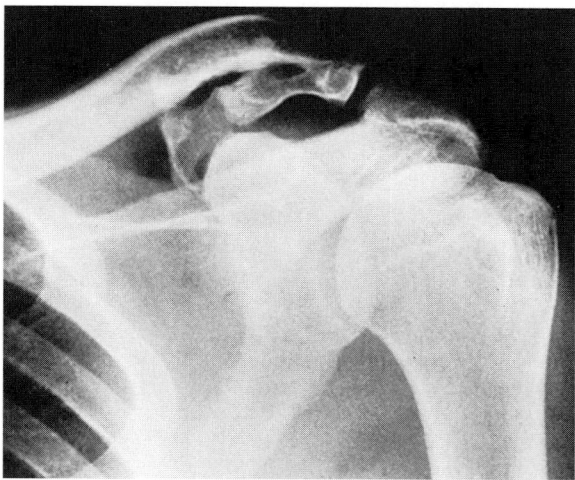

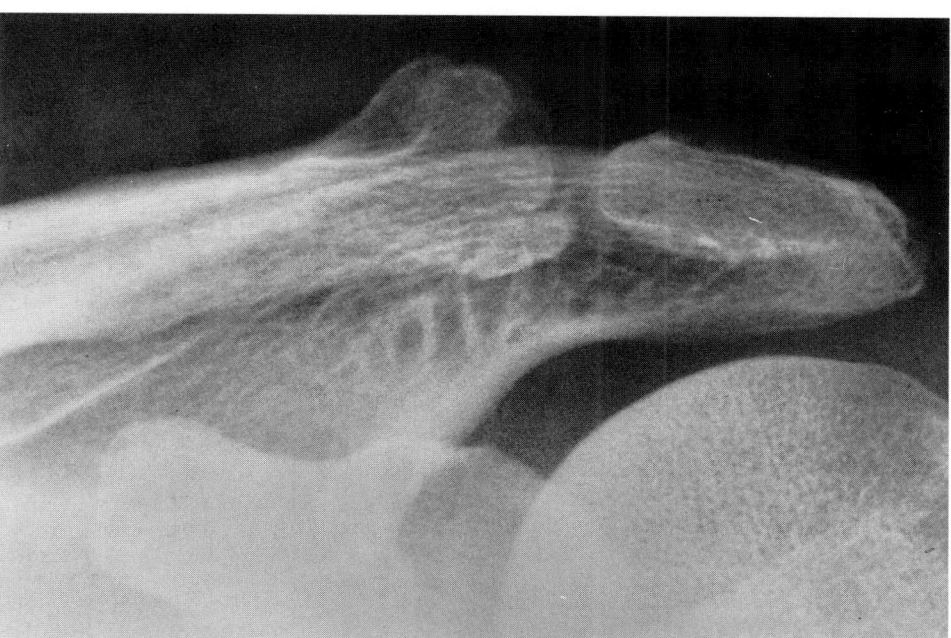

Figure 5–131. Unusual duplication anomaly of the distal end of the clavicle. This appearance may also be simulated by ossification in the coracoclavicular ligament. (Ref: Schubert F: Duplication of the clavicle or ossification in the coracoclavicular ligament. Australas Radiol 41:70, 1997.)

Figure 5–132. Unusual configuration of the distal end of the clavicle.

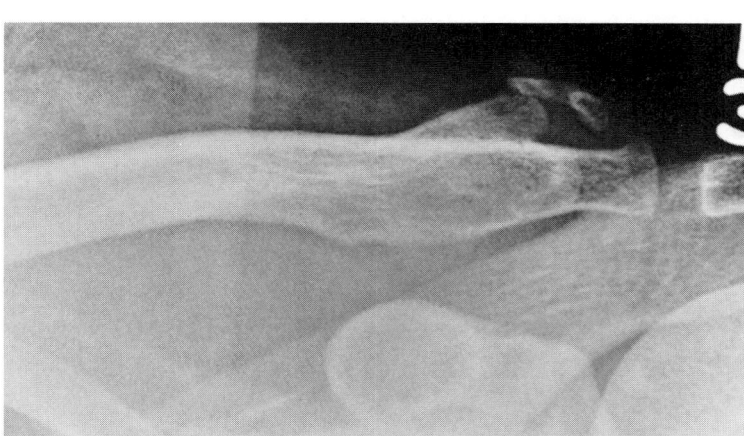

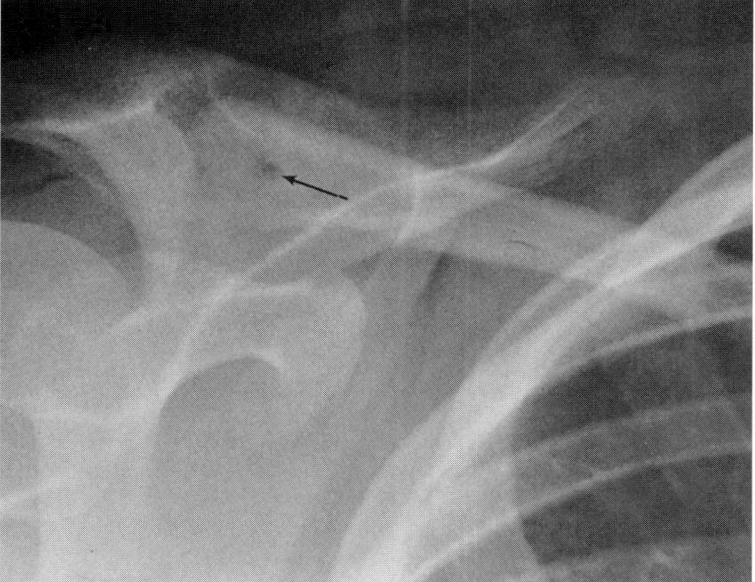

Figure 5–133. Partial duplication of the distal end of the clavicle.

Figure 5–134. Fish-mouth configuration of the distal end of the clavicle. This was present bilaterally.

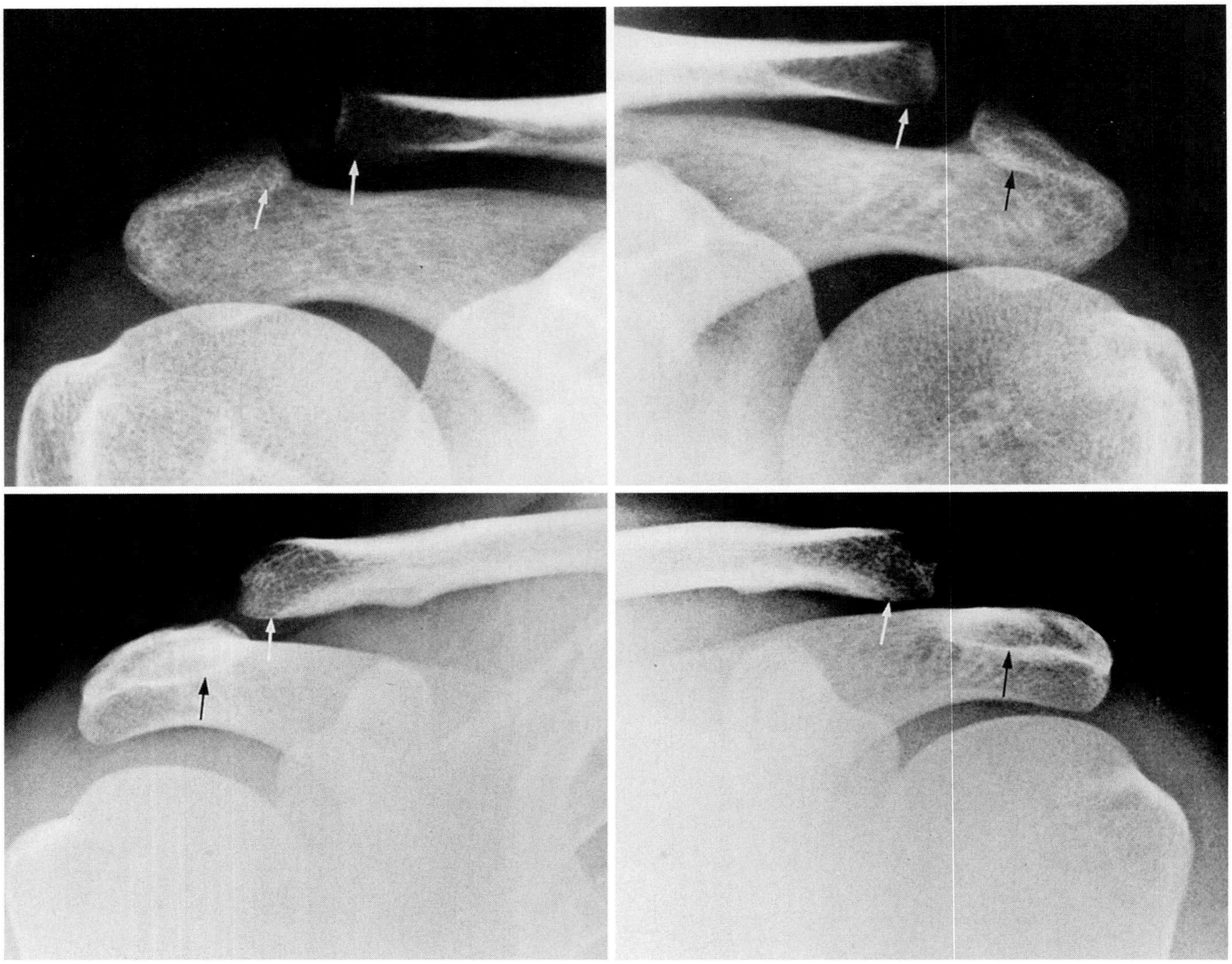

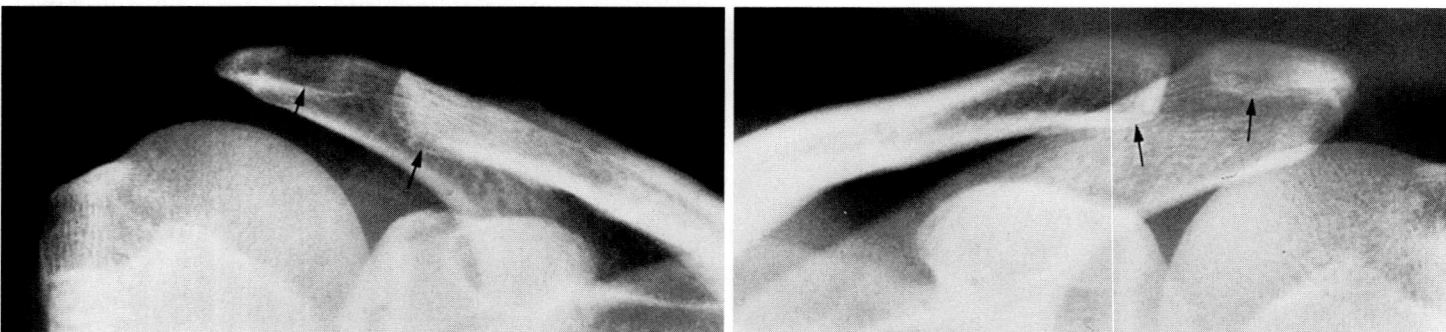

Figure 5–135. There is wide normal variation in the alignment of the acromion and the clavicle. The inferior margin of the clavicle aligns with the lower margin of the acromion in 81% of patients. The clavicle projects above the acromion in 7%, below the acromion in 7%, and overrides the acromion in 5%. Both sides should be examined routinely to detect these variations. *Top,* Bilateral cephalad position of distal ends of the clavicles in relationship to the acromion. *Bottom,* Very marked example of the same entity. (Ref: Keats TE, Pope TL: The acromioclavicular joint: Normal variation and diagnosis of dislocation. *Skeletal Radiol* 17:159, 1988.)

Figure 5–136. Bilateral caudad position of the distal ends of the clavicles in relationship to the acromion.

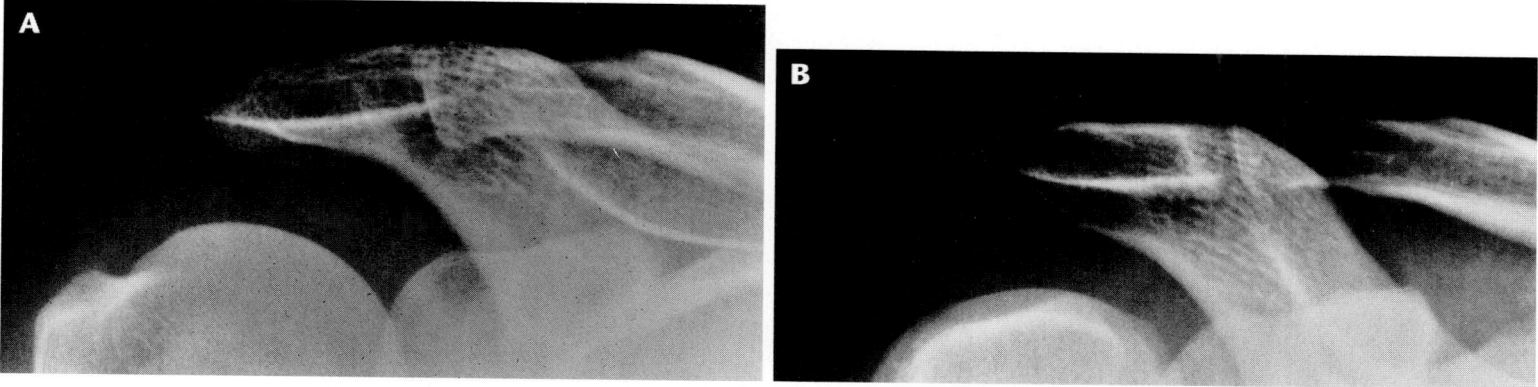

Figure 5–137. Apparent inferior displacement of the distal end of the clavicle in external rotation in right posterior oblique position **(A)** and normal relationship of the clavicle to the acromion in the internal rotation view made in anteroposterior projection **(B)**. This phenomenon is the result of foreshortening of the clavicle and its superimposition on the acromion.

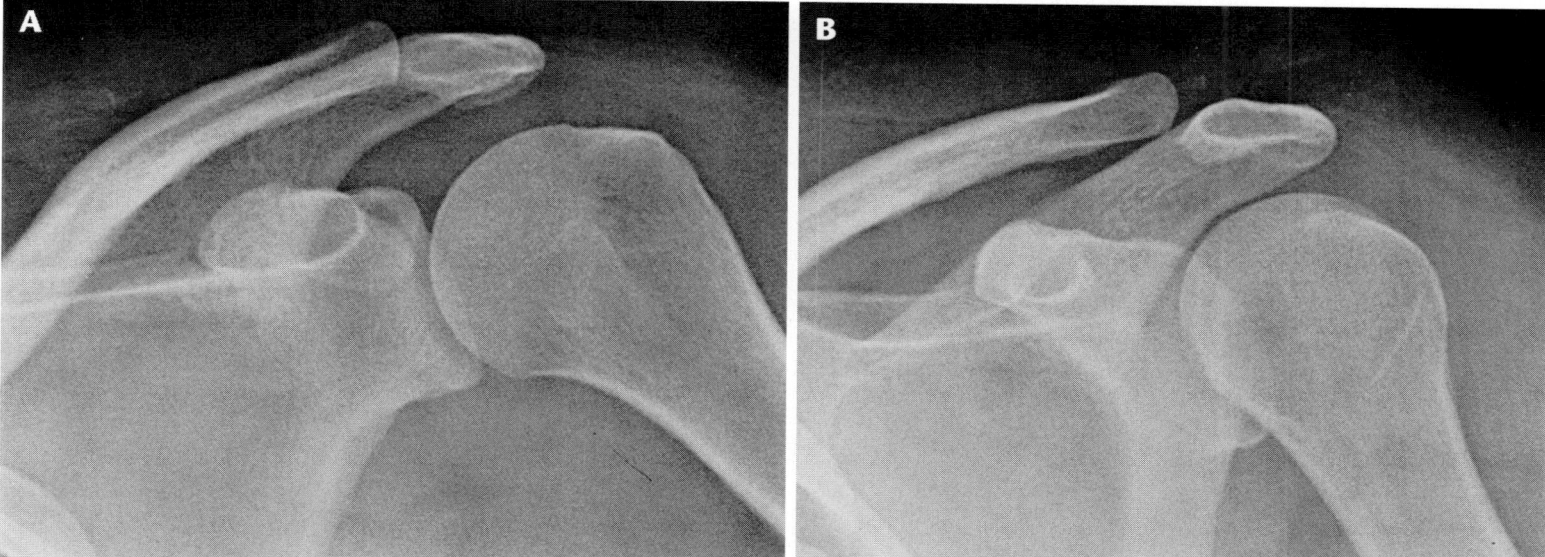

Figure 5–138. Apparent change in orientation of the clavicle at the acromioclavicular joint with rotation of the shoulder. **A,** External rotation. **B,** Internal rotation.

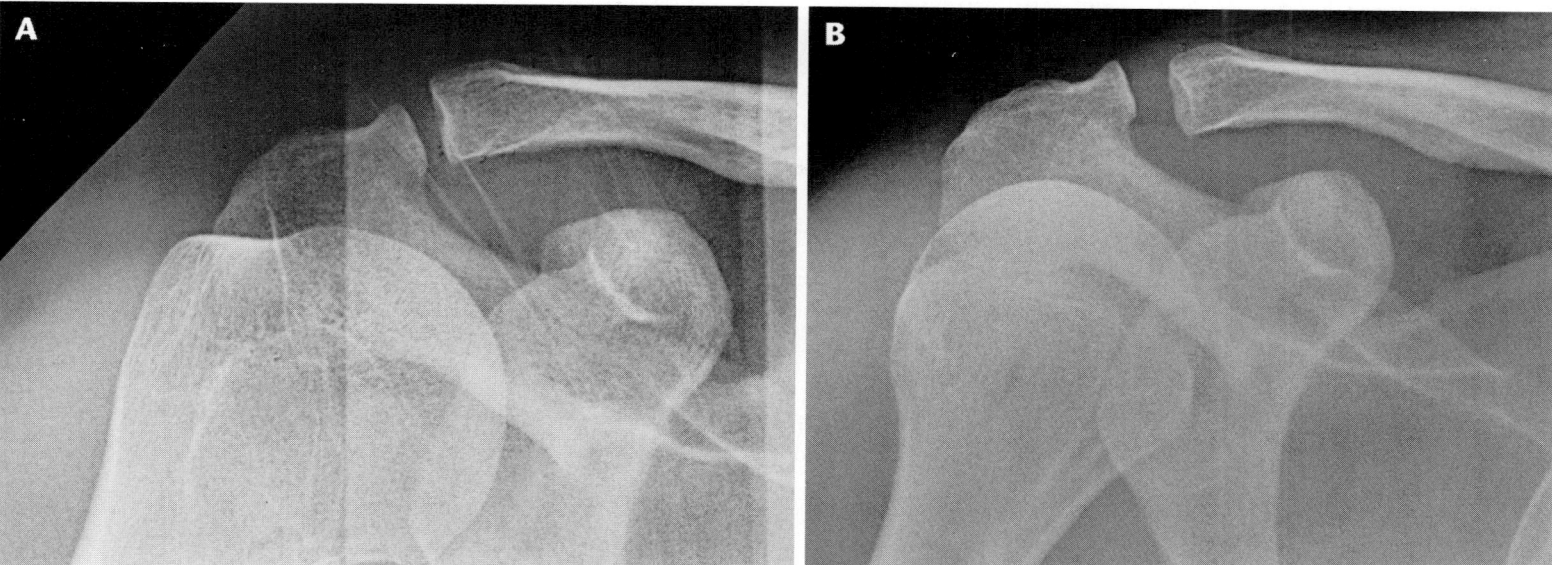

Figure 5–139. Apparent changes in the width of the acromioclavicular joint with rotation of the shoulder. **A,** External rotation. **B,** Internal rotation.

The Sternum

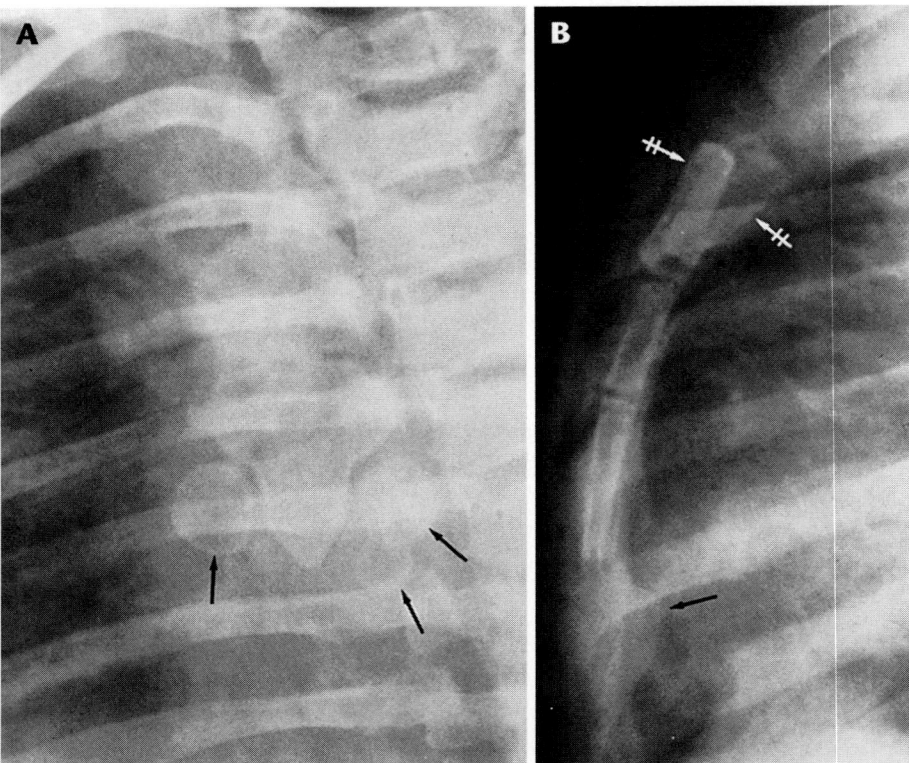

Figure 5–140. Variations in development of the sternum. **A** and **B,** Accessory ossification centers for the body of the sternum in a 5-month-old girl. (→) These, as well as duplication of the manubrial centers, may be seen in the lateral projection (⧺). (Ref: Ogden JA et al: Radiology of postnatal skeletal development. II. The manubrium and sternum. *Skeletal Radiol* 4:189, 1979.)

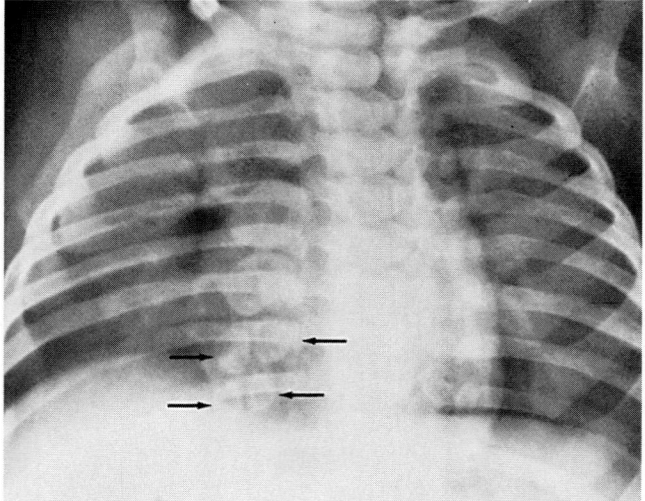

Figure 5–141. Duplication of the ossification centers of the lower portion of the body of the sternum in an 11-month-old child.

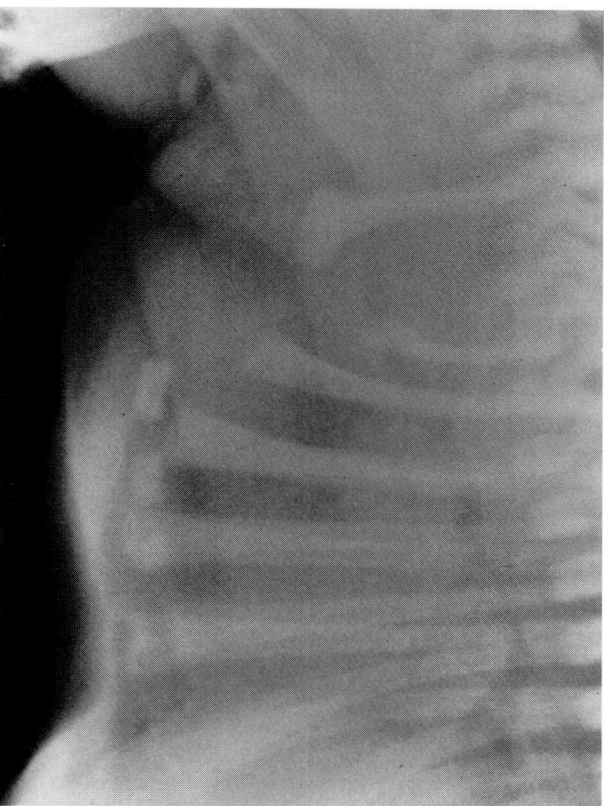

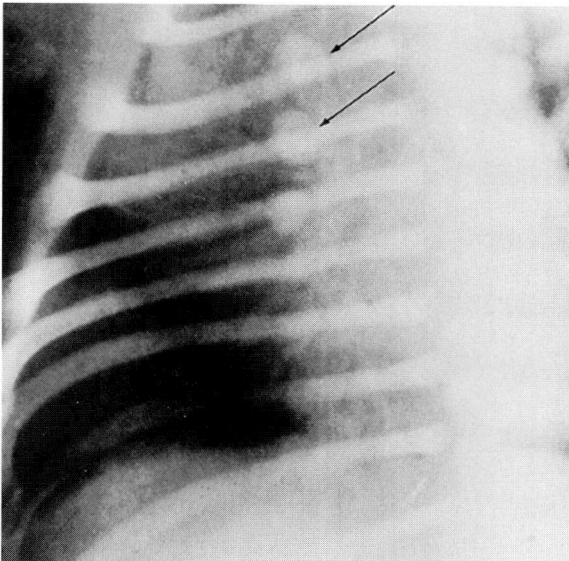

Figure 5–143. The sternal ossification centers superimposed on the ribs in a badly positioned chest film, simulating healing rib fractures.

Figure 5–142. Delayed appearance of the ossification center of the manubrium in a neonate.

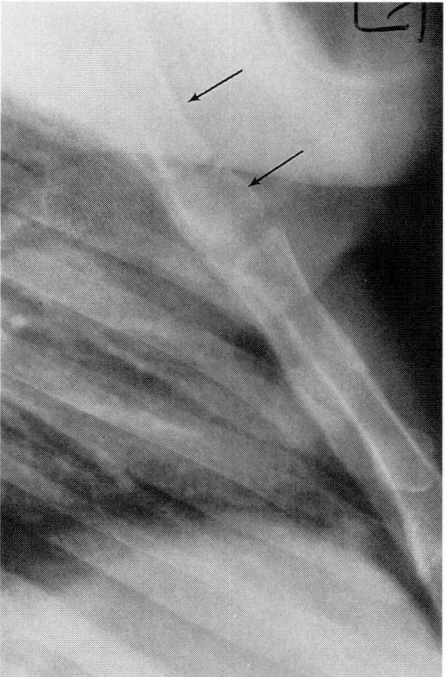

Figure 5–144. Double ossification centers of the manubrium in a normal 5-month-old boy. This is frequently seen in Down syndrome but also occurs as a normal variant.

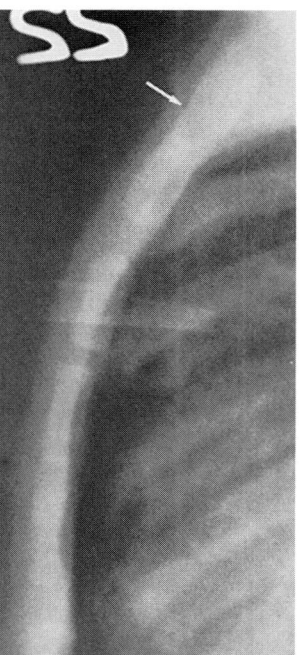

Figure 5–145. Double ossification centers of the manubrium in an adult.

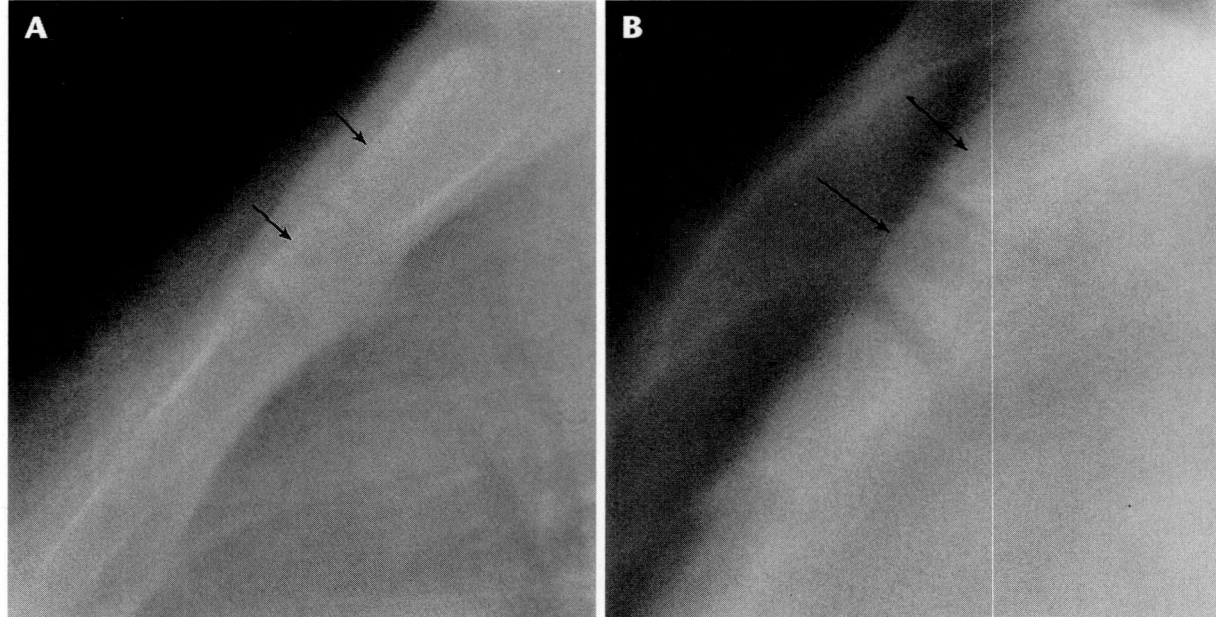

Figure 5–146. Double ossification centers of the manubrium in a 13-year-old boy mistaken as a fracture. **A,** Plain film. **B,** Tomogram.

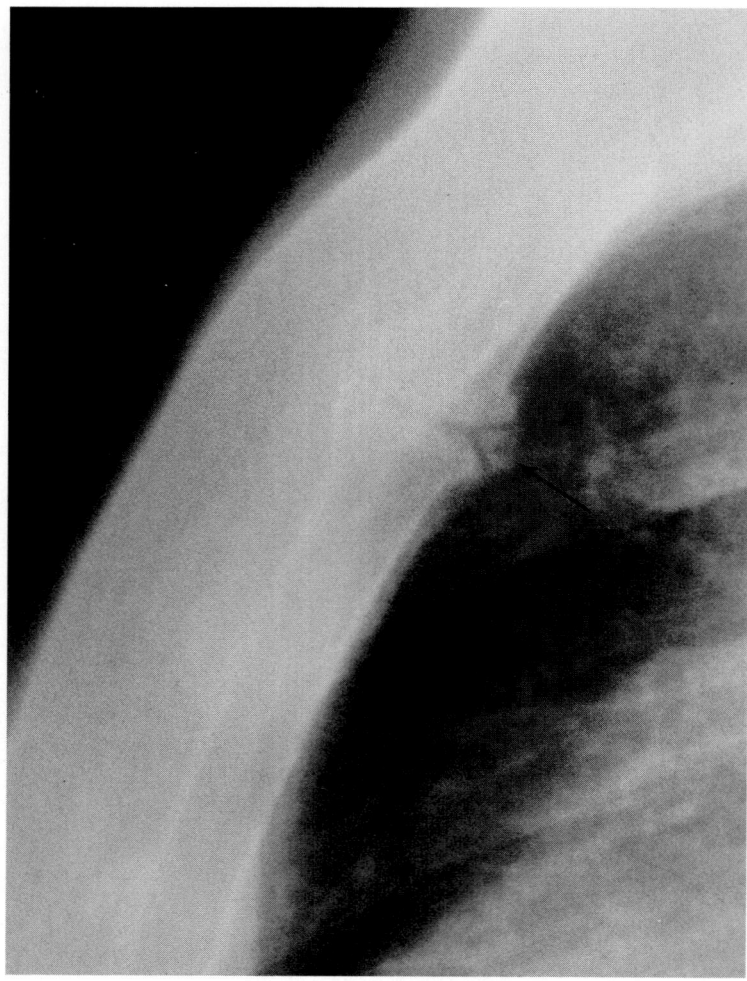

Figure 5–147. Ossicle at the sternomanubrial joint, probably degenerative in origin.

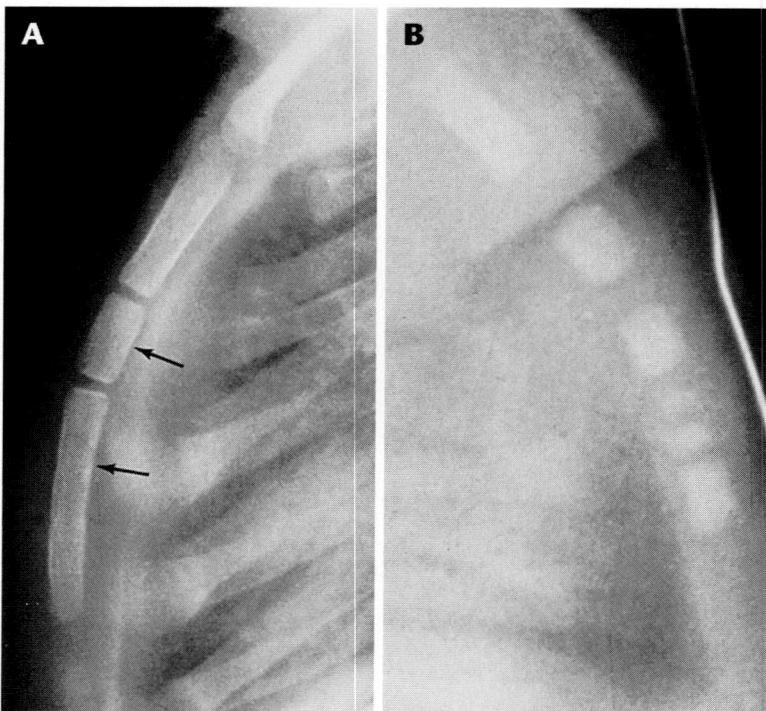

Figure 5–148. Variations in development of the sternum. **A,** Development of the body of the sternum from only two centers. **B,** Marked variability in size of the centers of ossification of the body of the sternum.

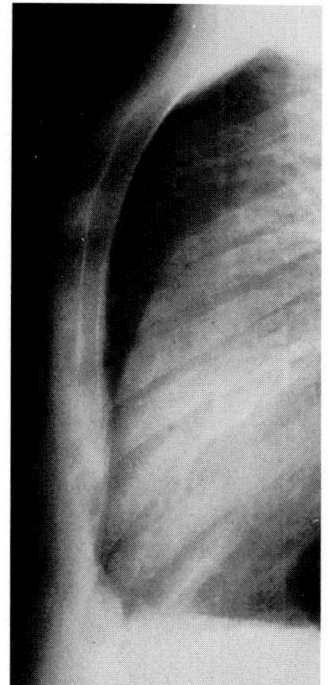

Figure 5–149. Nonsegmentation of the sternum in a 30-year-old man, probably secondary to premature fusion of centers.

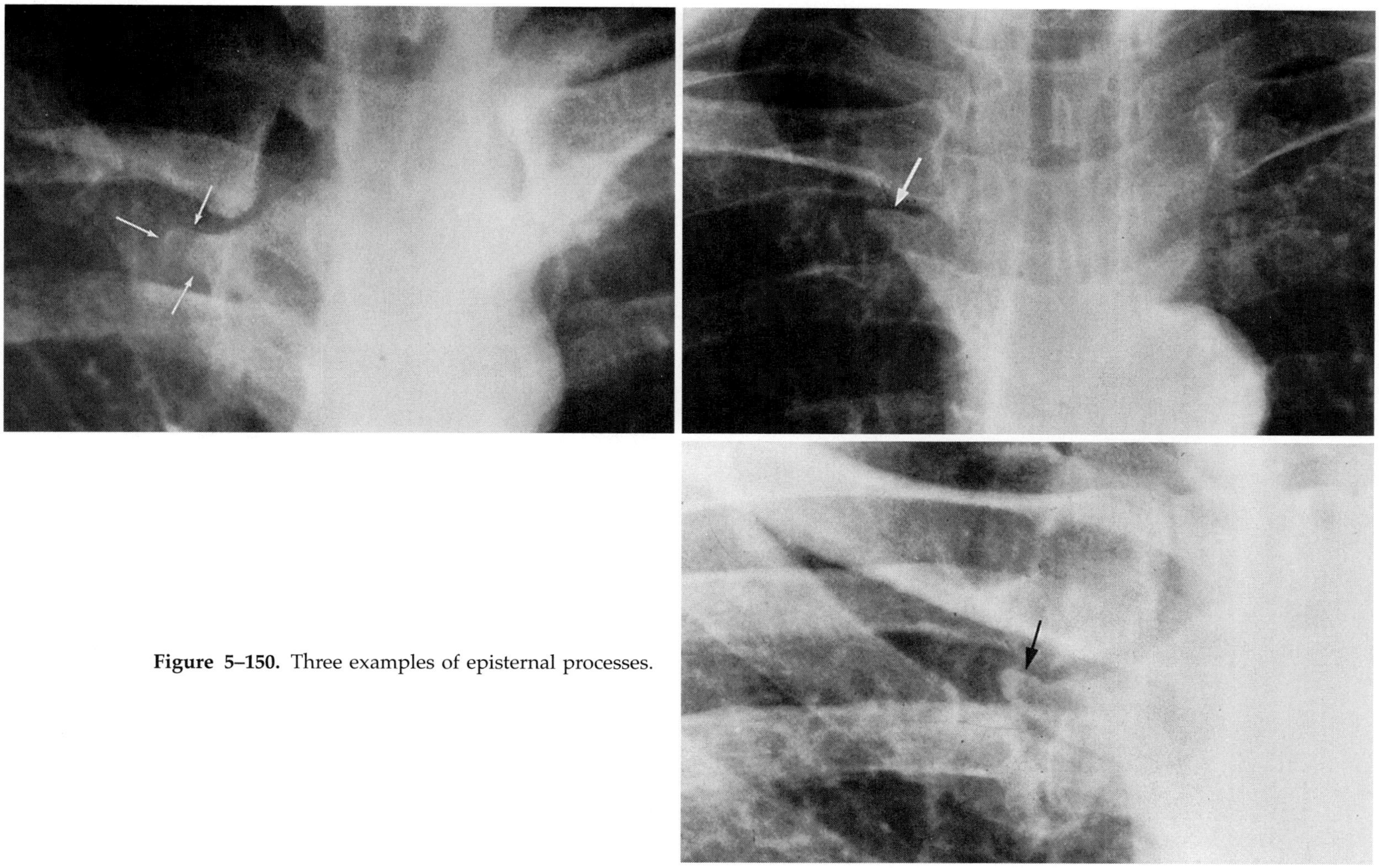

Figure 5–150. Three examples of episternal processes.

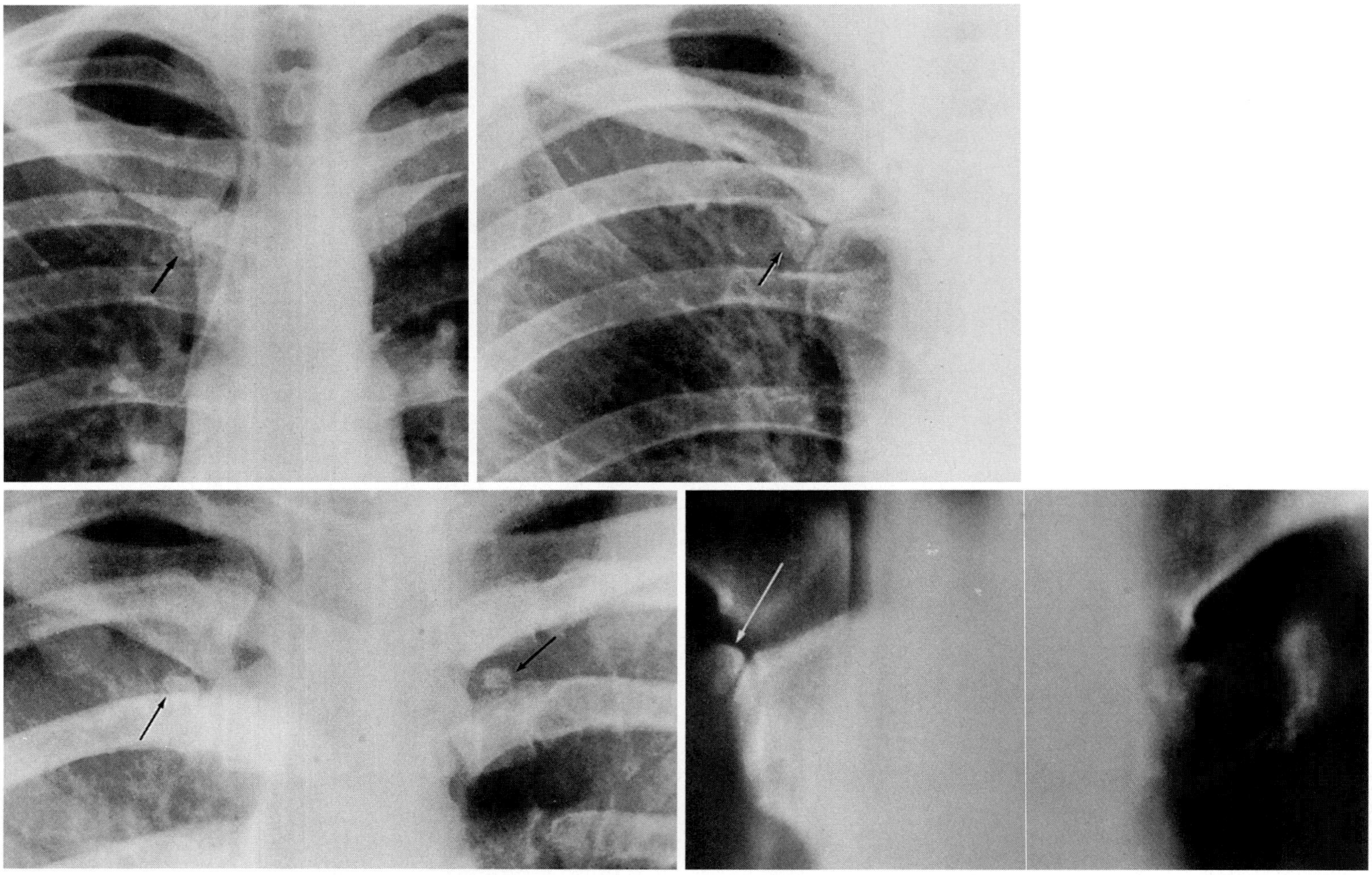

Figure 5–151. Examples of episternal bones in adults. (Refs: Brown WH: Episternal bones. *Radiology* 75:116, 1960; Stark P et al: Episternal ossicles. *Radiology* 165:143, 1987.)

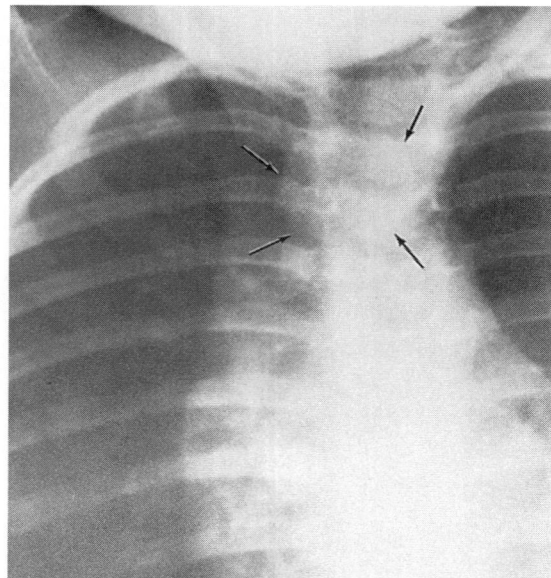

Figure 5–152. The manubrium in an 11-month-old child, mistaken for a mediastinal mass.

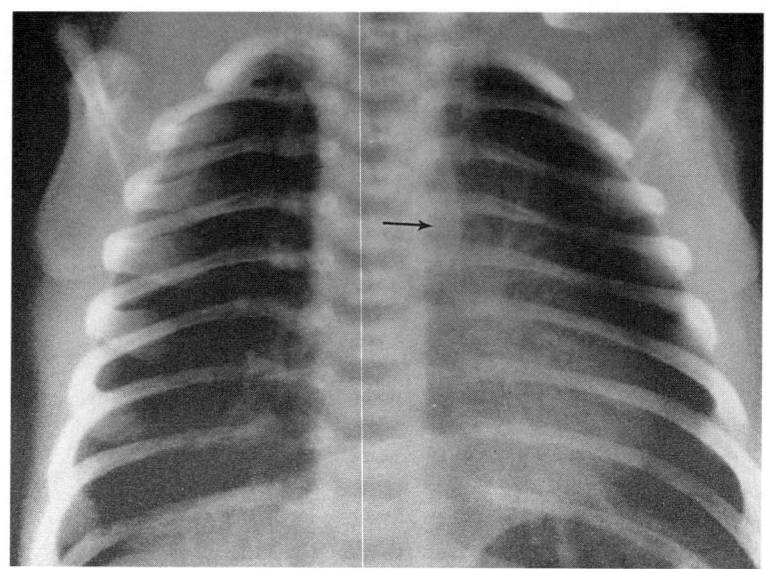

Figure 5–153. The manubrium may simulate a mass, produced by slight rotation of the patient.

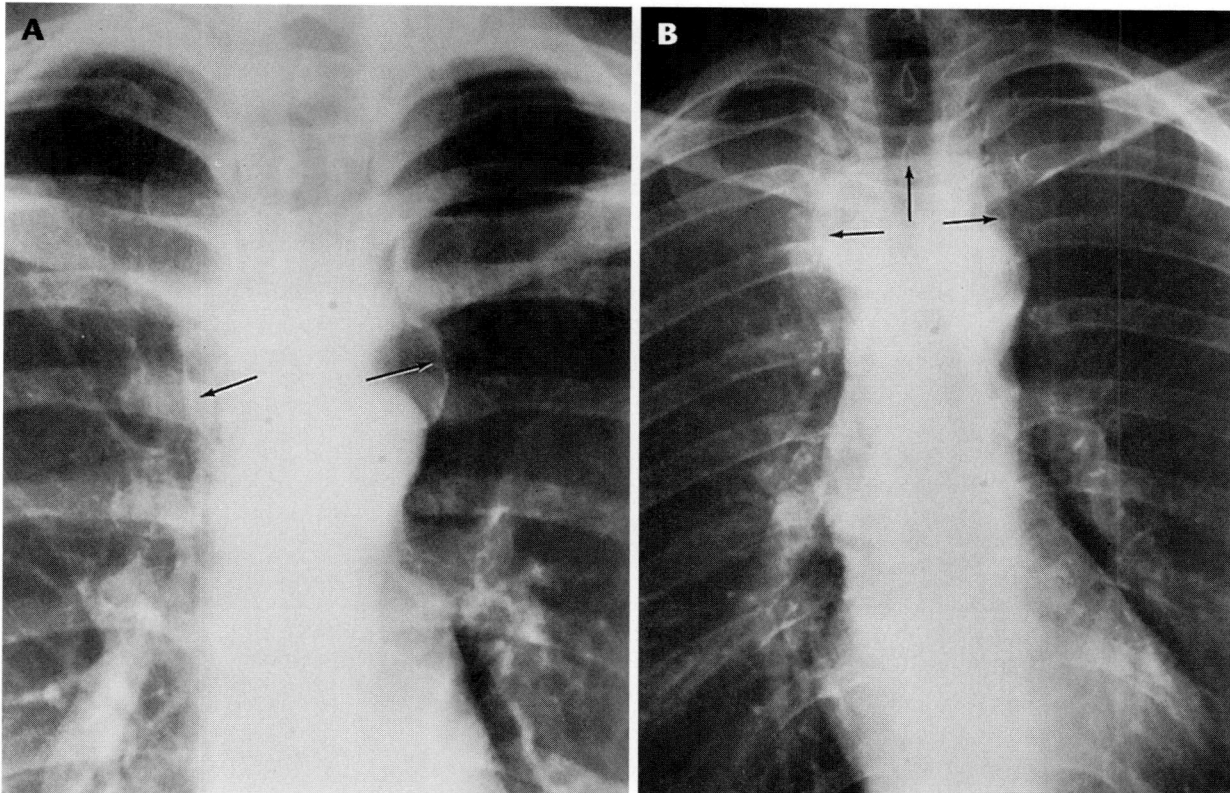

Figure 5–154. A, B, The manubrium in adults resembling mediastinal masses. Note in **A** the sclerosis of the borders of the manubrium, which may suggest a mass lesion with a calcified border.

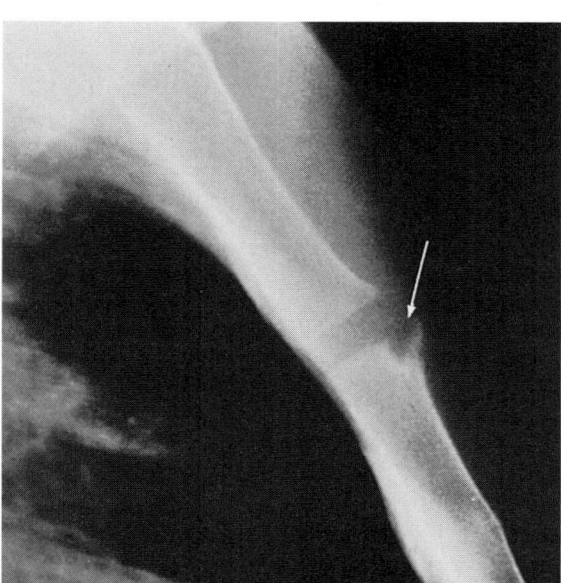

Figure 5–155. Developmental irregularity of the superior margin of the sternum at the sternomanubrial joint in an adolescent boy. Defects of this type have been likened to Schmorl's nodes of the spine. (Ref: Kohler A, Zimmer EA: Borderlands of normal and early pathologic findings. *Skeletal radiography,* 4th ed. New York, Thieme Medical, 1993, p. 236.)

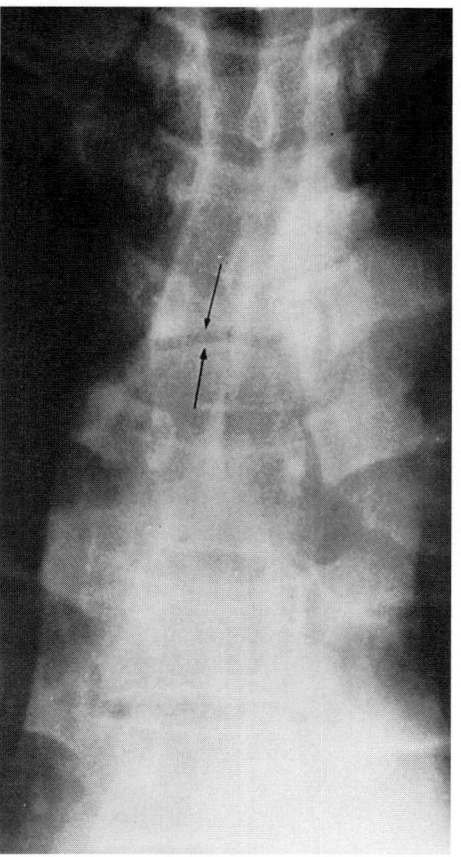

Figure 5–156. The sternomanubrial joint may simulate a fracture of the dorsal spine in the frontal plane.

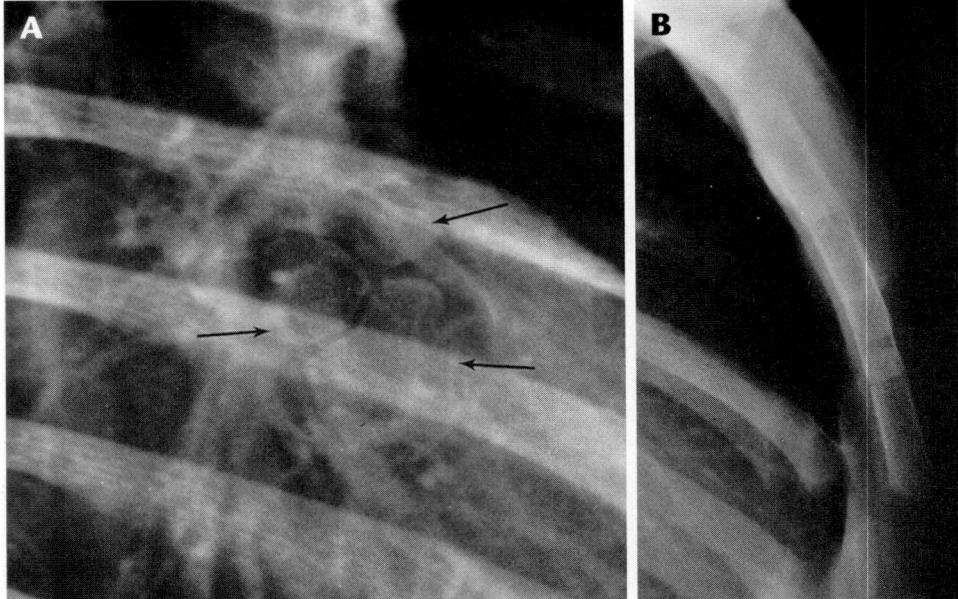

Figure 5–157. Anomalous development of the sternal segments in haphazard alignment in an 11-year-old boy. **A,** Oblique projection. **B,** Lateral projection.

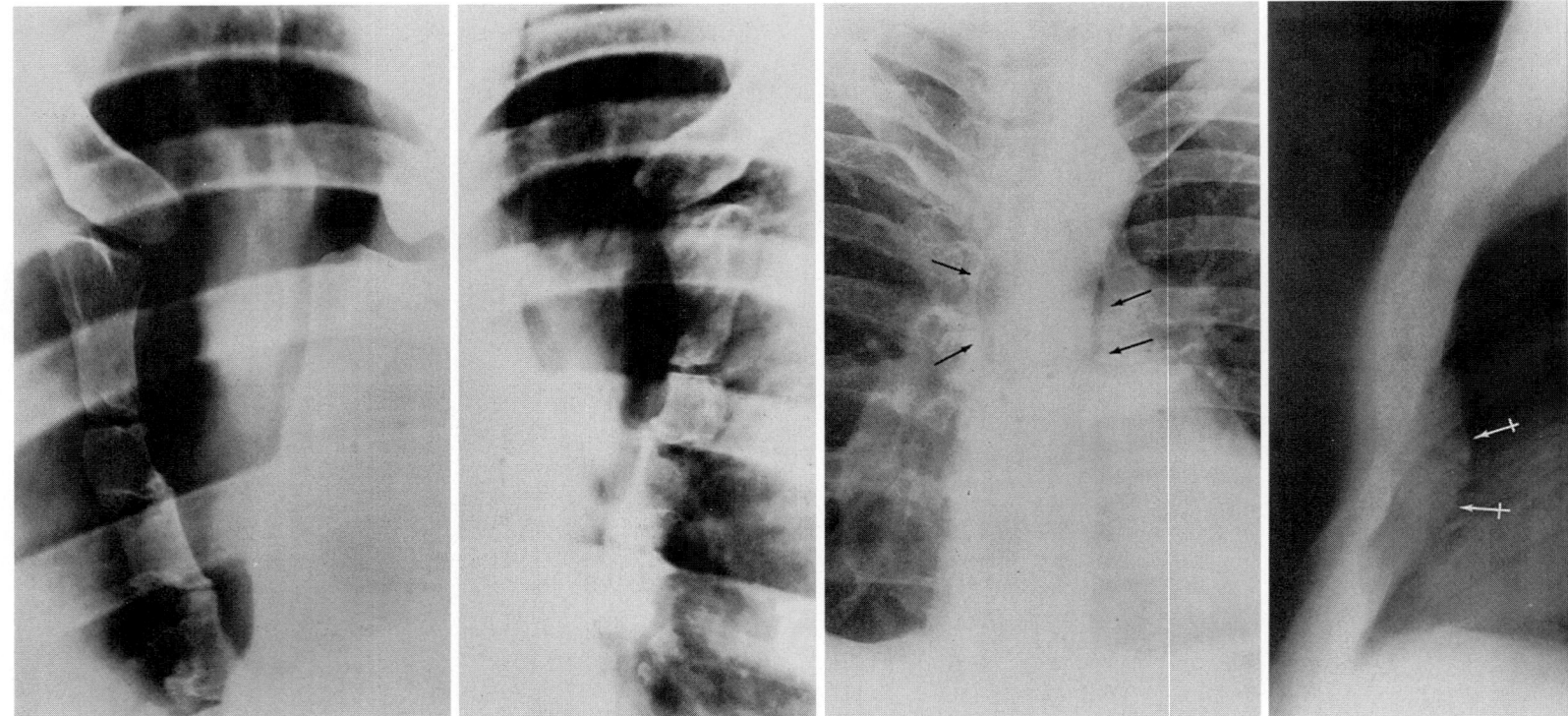

Figure 5–158. Congenital bifid sternum, an unusual variant. Note the radiolucency in the midline in the frontal chest film (→) and the mass effect in the lateral film (↔). (Courtesy of Dr. W. P. Brown.) (Ref: Larsen LL, Ibach HF: Complete congenital fissure of the sternum. *Am J Roentgenol* 87:1062, 1962.)

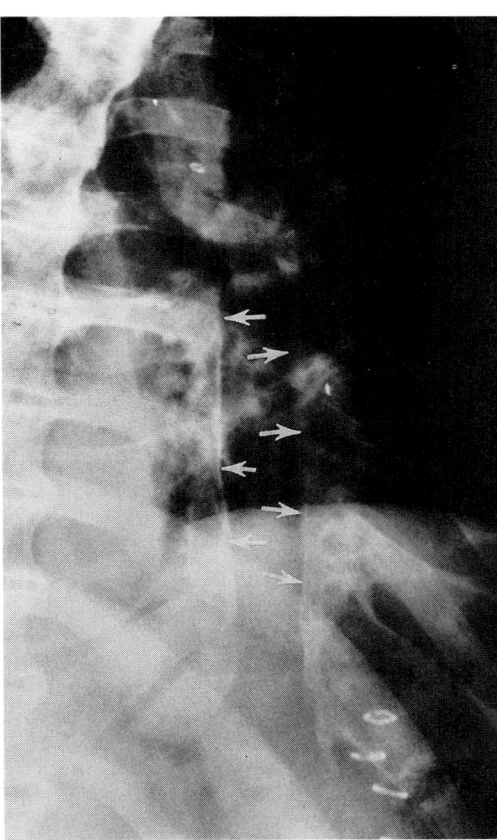

Figure 5–159. Bifid sternum.

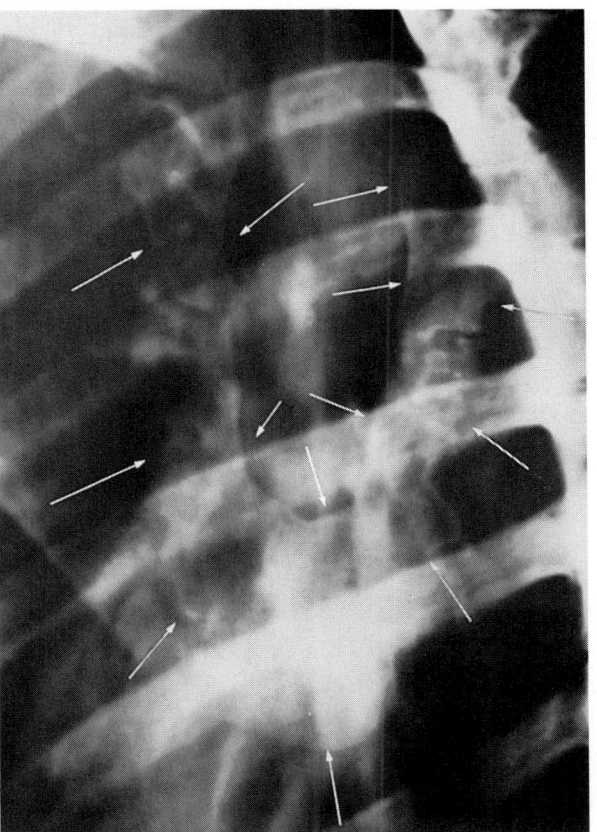

Figure 5–160. Partial bifid sternum with union at distal end. (Courtesy of Dr. W. E. Litterer.)

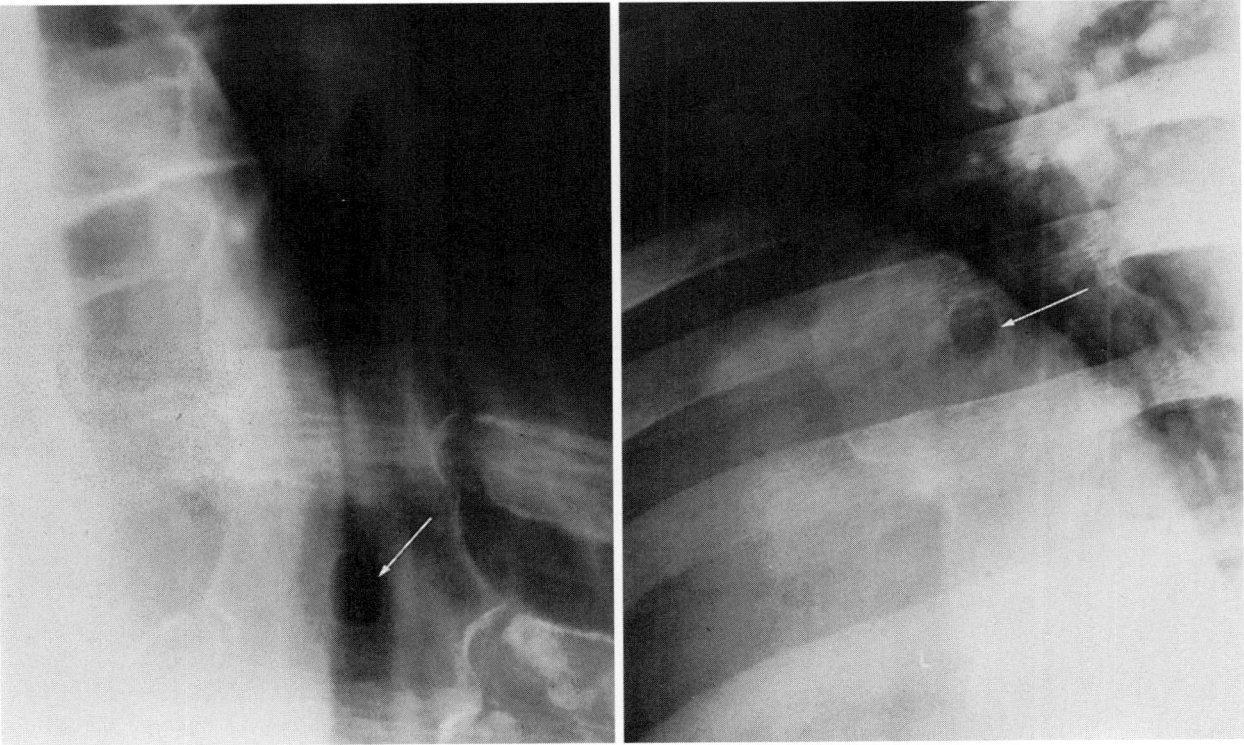

Figure 5–161. Two examples of sternal foramina, a finding of no significance. (Ref: Resnik CS, Brower AC: Midline circular defect of the sternum. *Radiology* 130:657, 1979.)

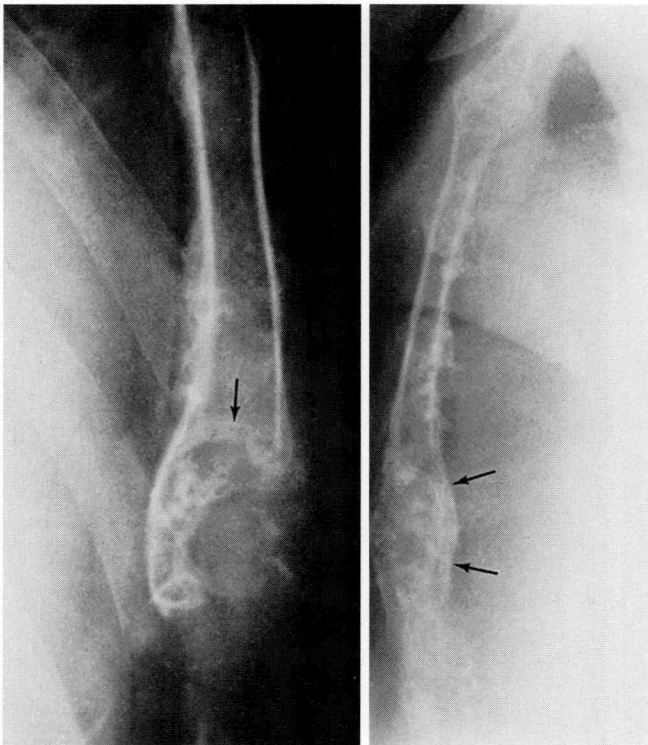

Figure 5–162. Variations in configuration of the xiphoid process and calcified costal cartilage, simulating destructive or neoplastic lesions of the sternum, particularly if there are symptoms referable to this area. (From Keats TE: Four normal anatomic variations of importance to radiologists. *Am J Roentgenol* 78:89, 1957.)

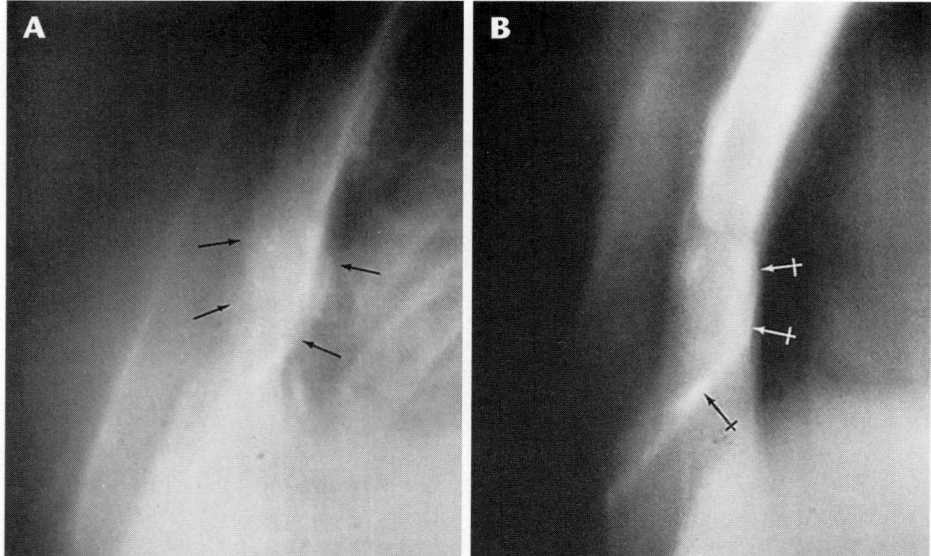

Figure 5–163. A, Plain film. Simulated mass lesion of the sternum produced by the xiphoid process and calcified costal cartilage (→). **B,** Tomogram. Note posterior curvature of the xiphoid process, which contributes to this misleading appearance (↦).

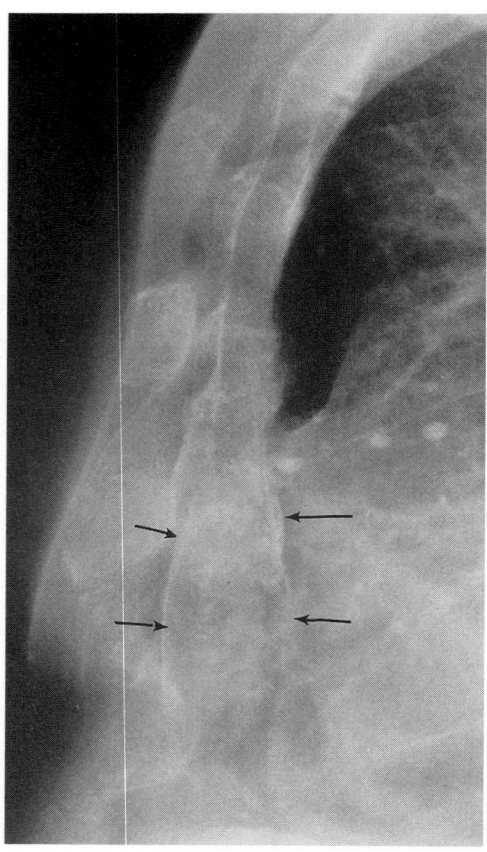

Figure 5–164. Costal cartilage simulating a mass at the xiphoid.

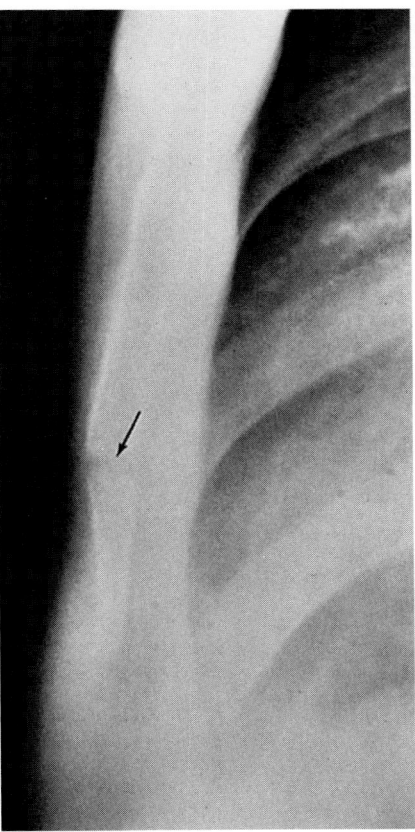

Figure 5–165. The normal junction of the xiphoid process and body of the sternum, not to be mistaken for a fracture.

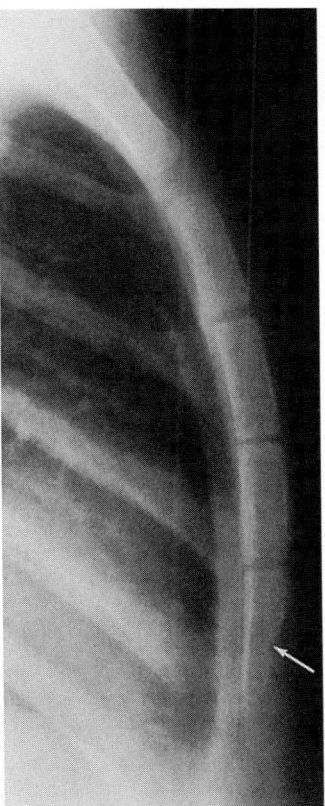

Figure 5–166. Indentation on anterior surface of the last sternal segment.

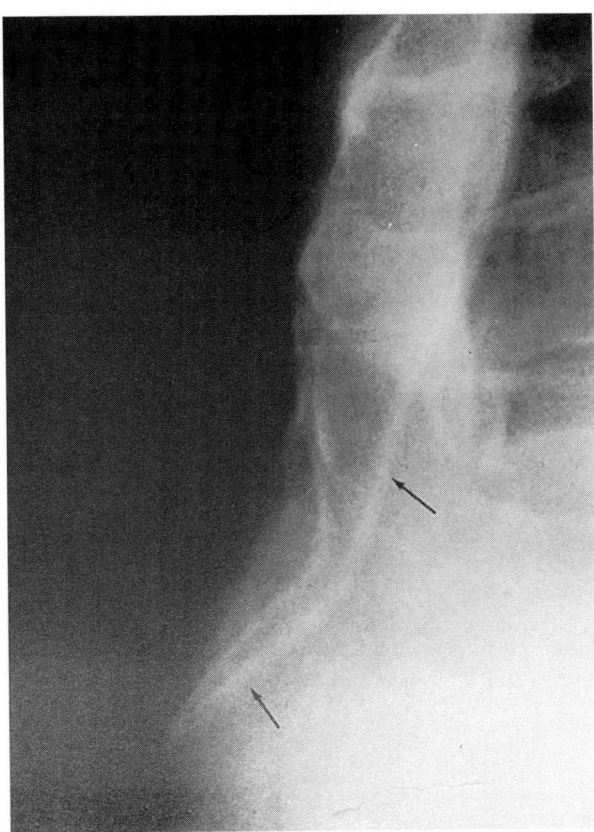

Figure 5–167. Marked anterior flexion of the xiphoid process.

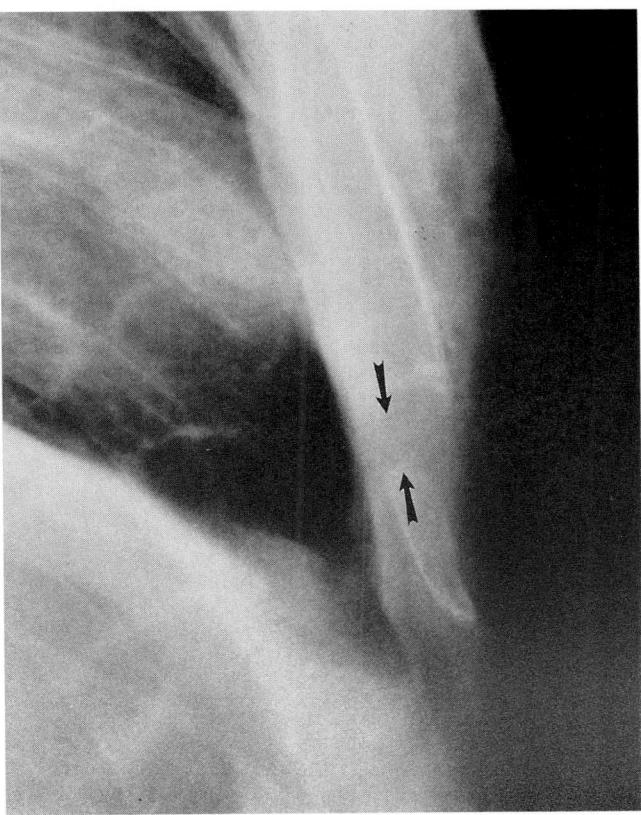

Figure 5–168. Gap between the sternum and xiphoid simulating a fracture dislocation.

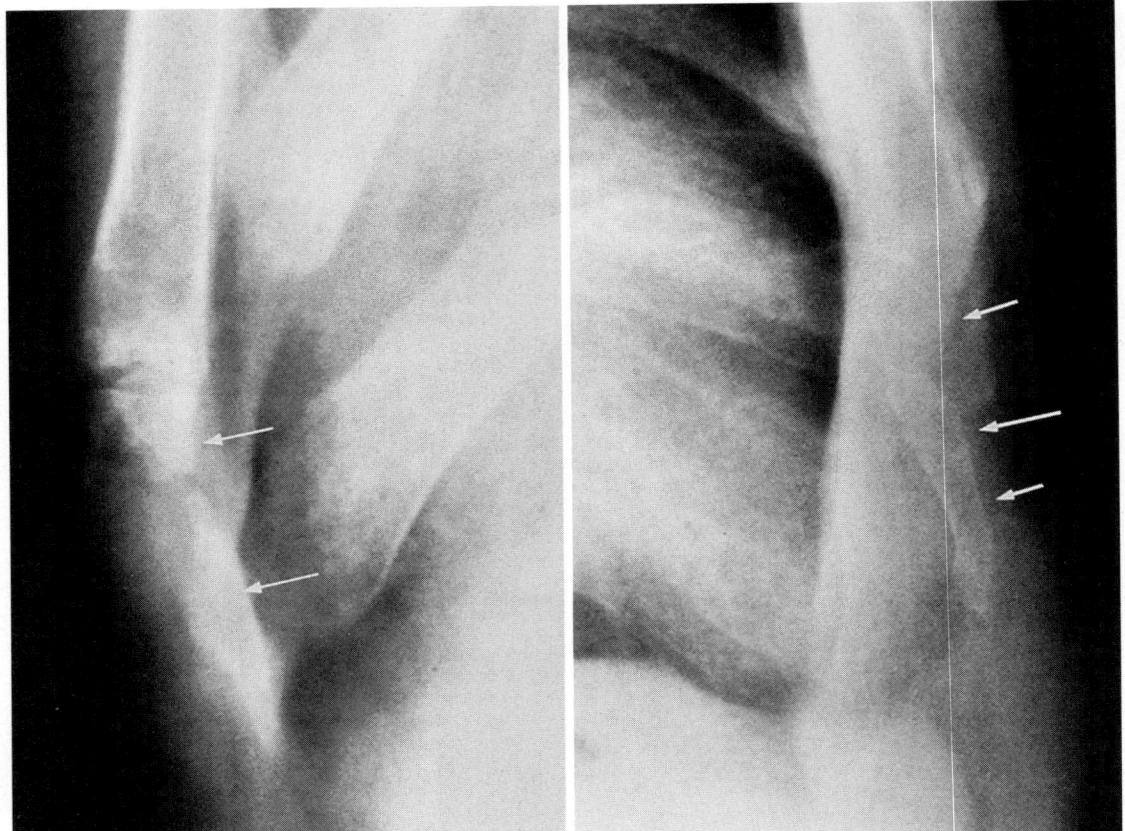

Figure 5–169. Unusual partitioned xiphoid processes.

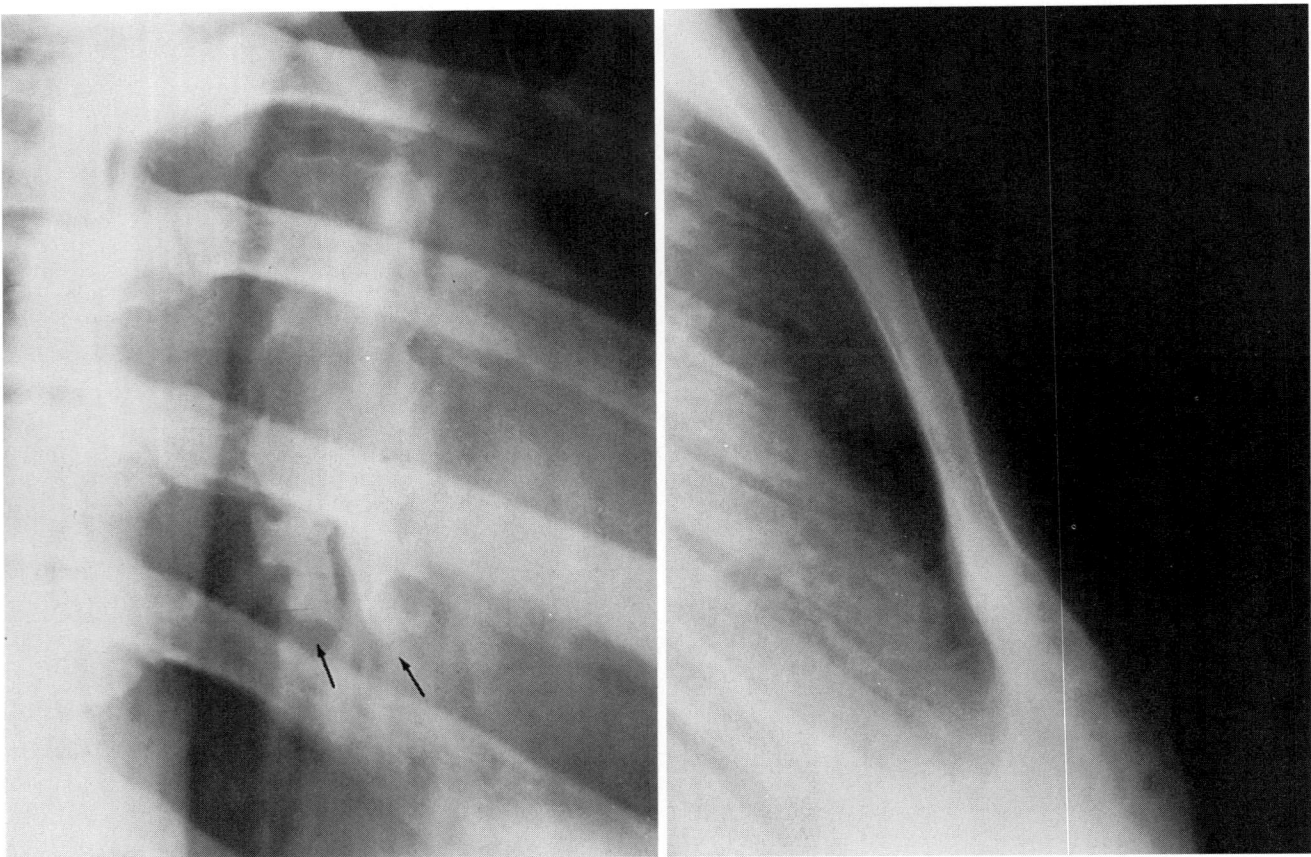

Figure 5–170. Bifid xiphoid process.

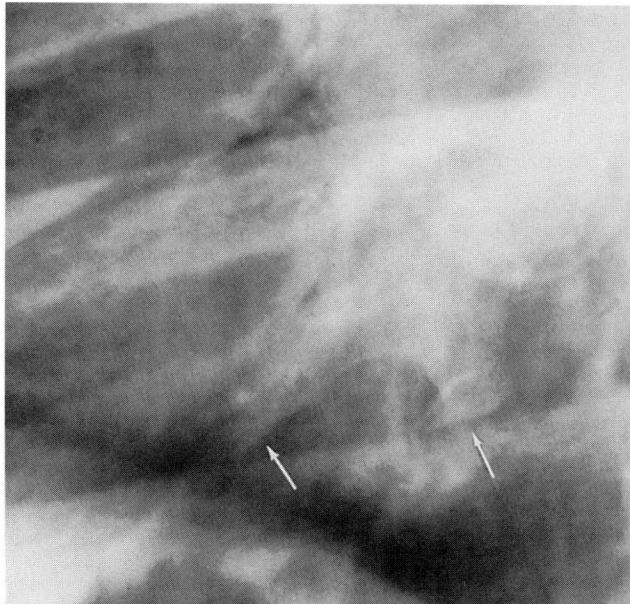

Figure 5–171. Bifid xiphoid process with one limb directed anteriorly.

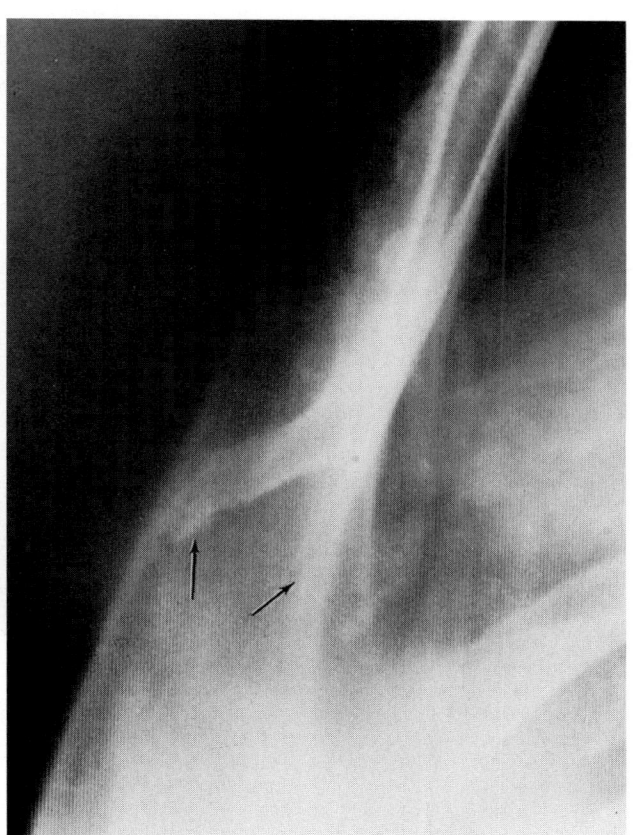

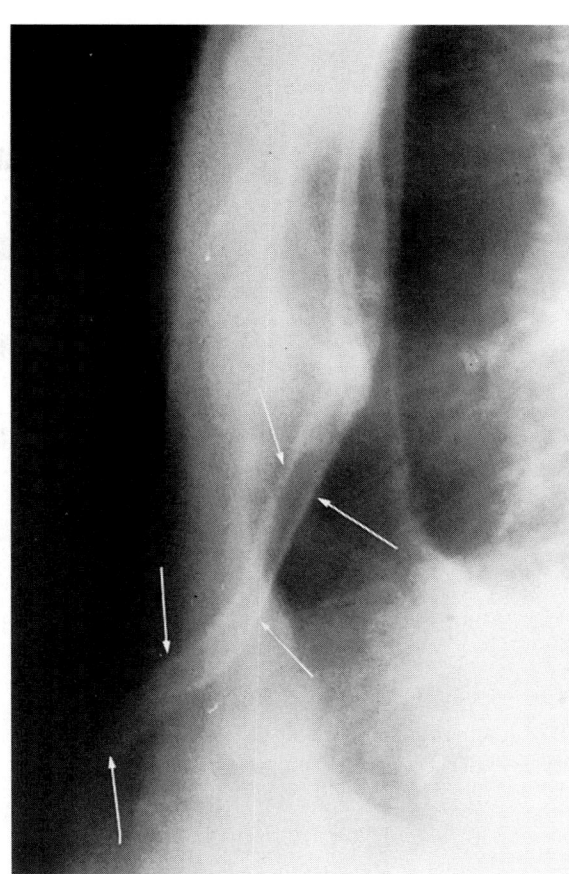

Figure 5–172. Elongated xiphoid process directed anteriorly. This type of xiphoid may be jointed as well. The anterior direction may produce an apparent epigastric mass on clinical examination. (Ref: Sanders PC, Knight RW: Radiologic appearance of the xiphoid process presenting as an upper abdominal mass. *Radiology* 141:489, 1981.)

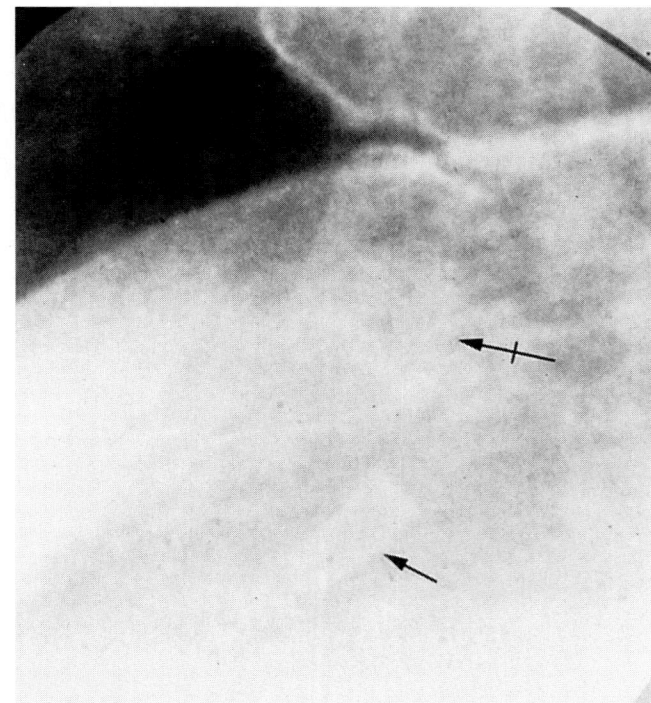

Figure 5–173. Accessory center (←) for the xiphoid process (⟵⟶).

The Ribs

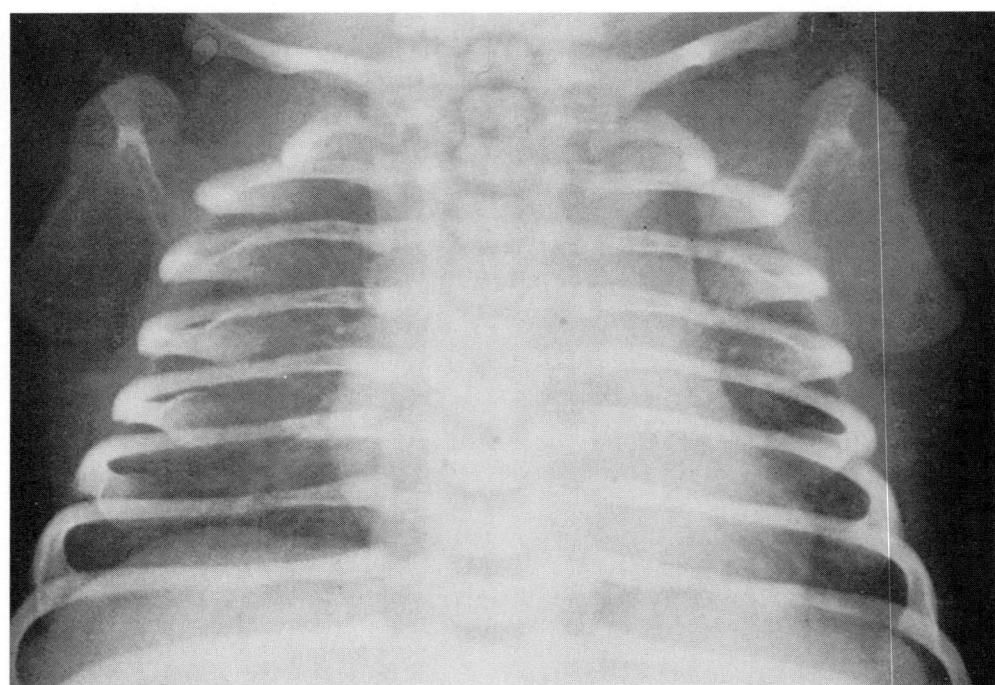

Figure 5–174. Simulated cupping of the anterior ends of the ribs produced by lordotic projection.

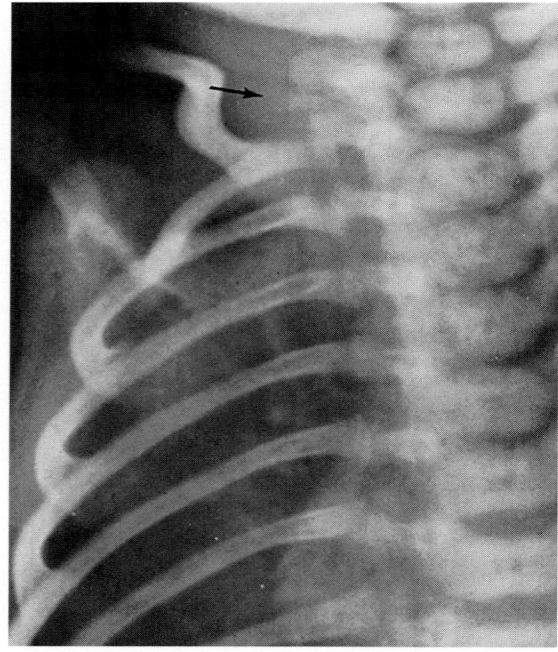

Figure 5–175. Cervical rib in a 2-week-old infant.

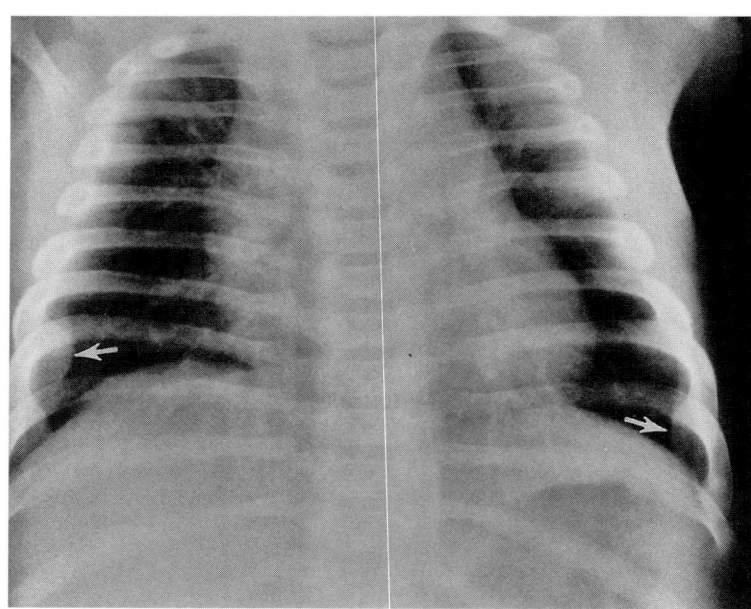

Figure 5–176. Large anterior ends of the ribs simulating extrapleural masses in an 8-month-old infant.

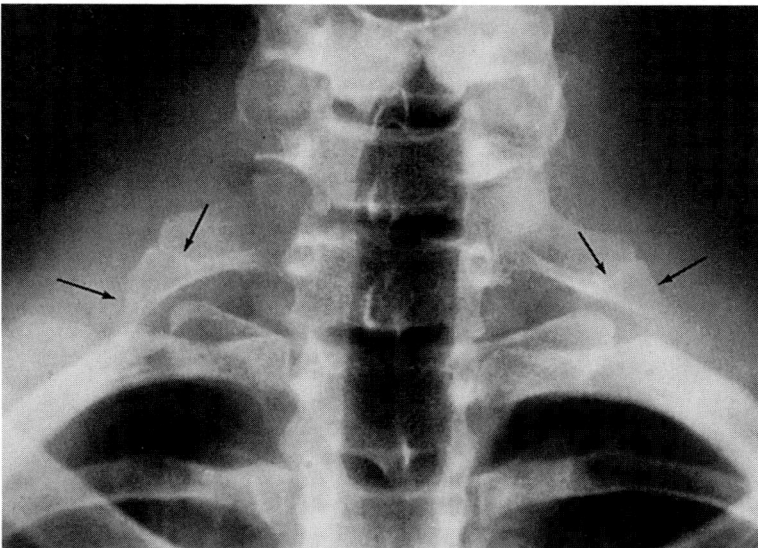

Figure 5–177. Well-developed cervical ribs in an adult.

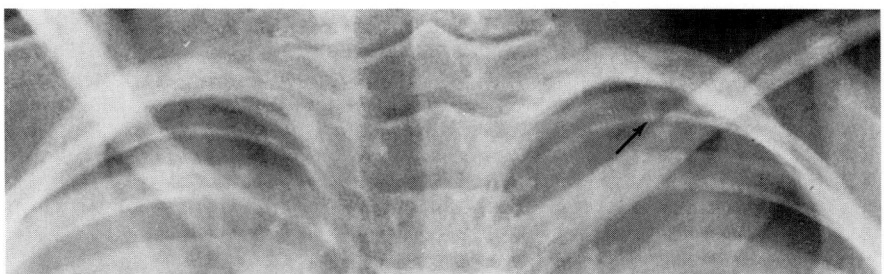

Figure 5–178. The anterior end of a cervical rib simulates a parenchymal lesion.

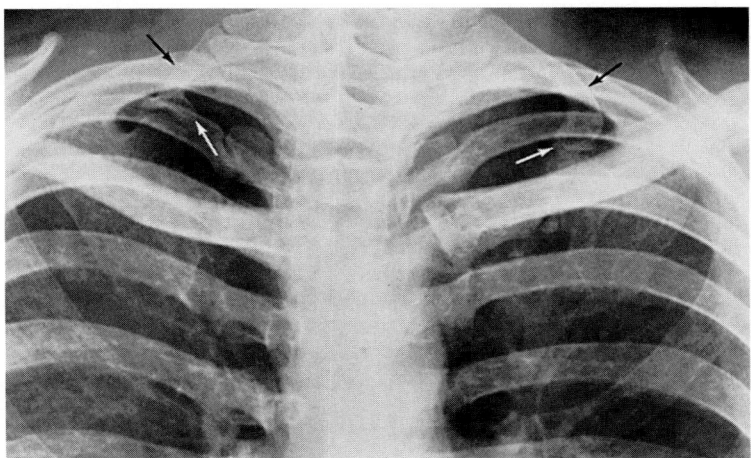

Figure 5–179. Large bilateral cervical ribs, which articulate with the first ribs.

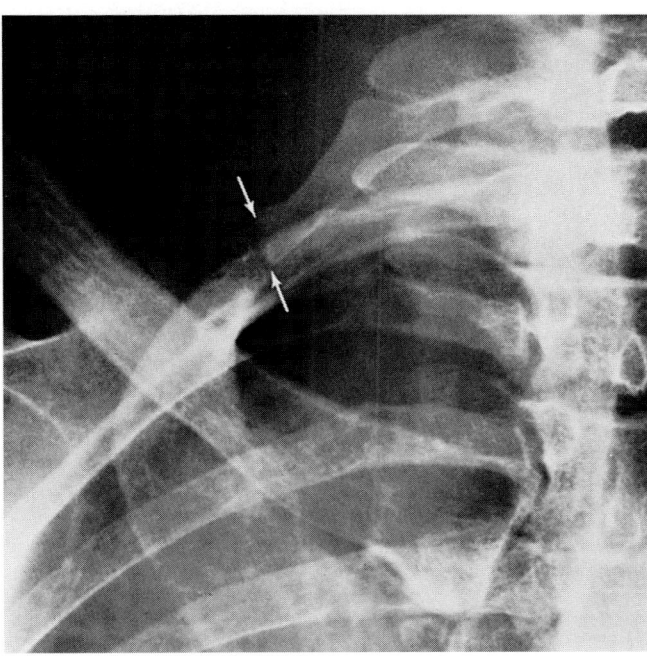

Figure 5–180. Cervical rib articulating at its distal end with an additional bony element.

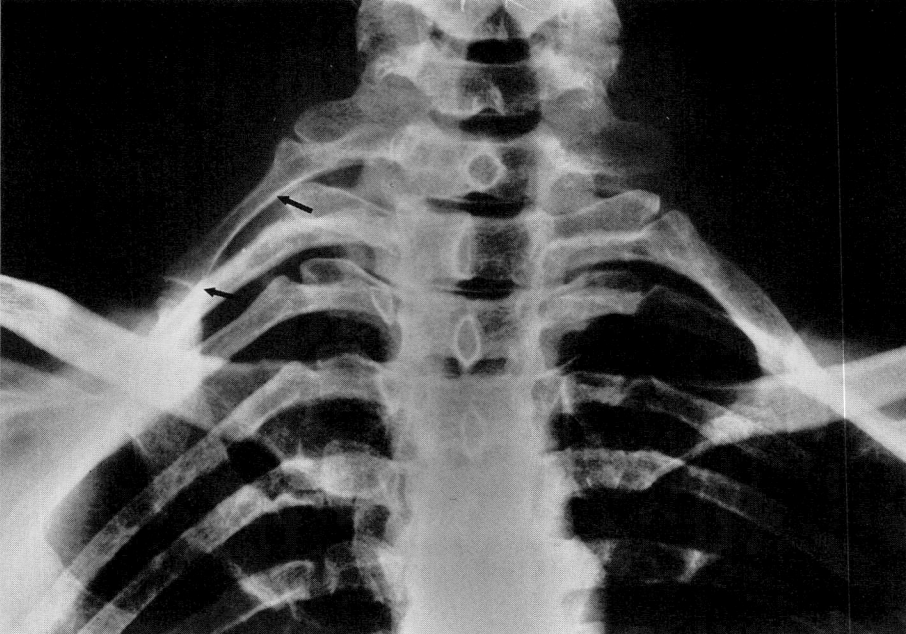

Figure 5–181. Right cervical rib with articulation with the first rib.

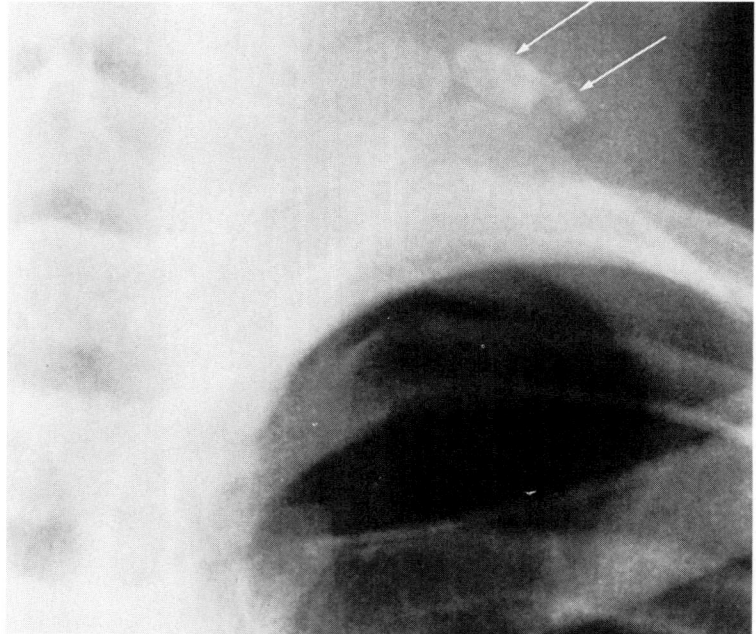

Figure 5–182. Accessory rib elements at transverse process of T1.

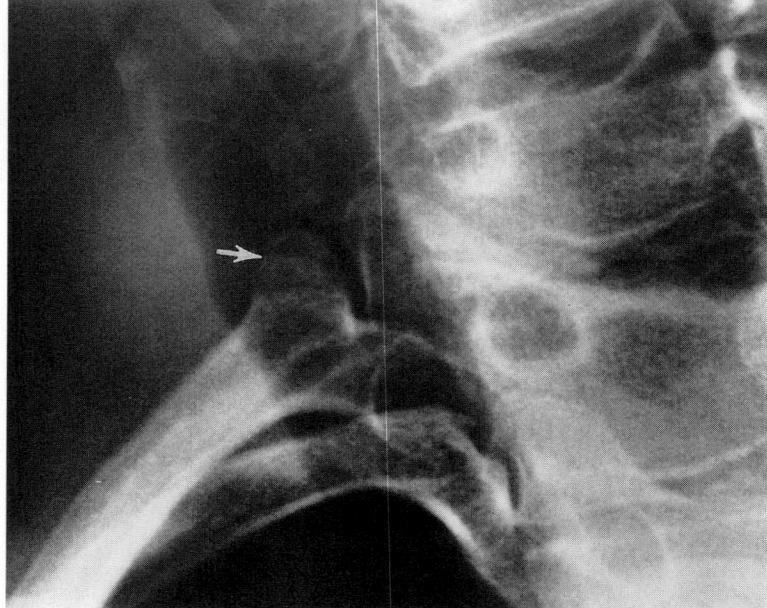

Figure 5–183. Ununited apophysis of the first rib in a 28-year-old man.

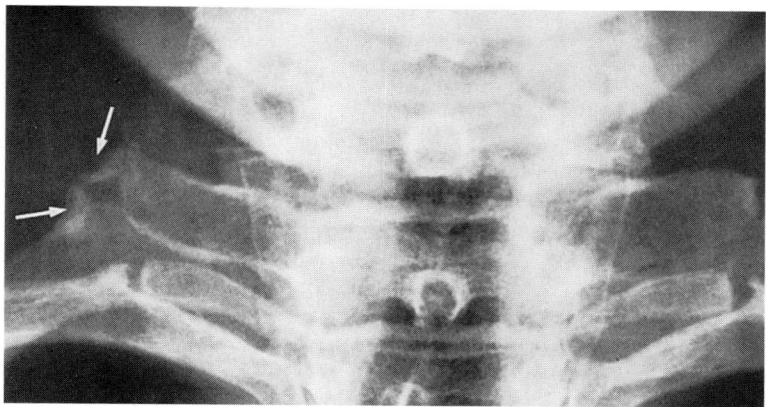

Figure 5–184. Jointed ligamentous calcifications between the transverse process of T1 and the first rib.

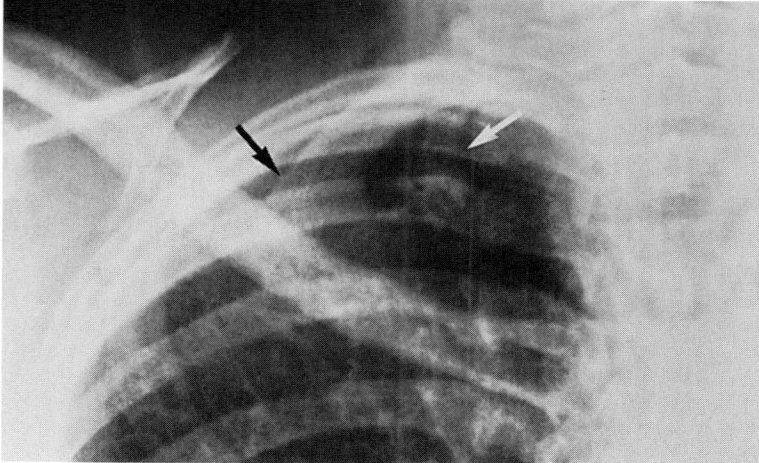

Figure 5–185. This patient presented with a hard right supraclavicular mass, which is explained by the anomalous arrangement of the first and second ribs. Such variants may efface the supraclavicular fossa and simulate a mass. (Ref: Fakhry SM, Thomas CG Jr: Pseudotumor of the supraclavicular fossa. *South Med J* 79:822, 1986.)

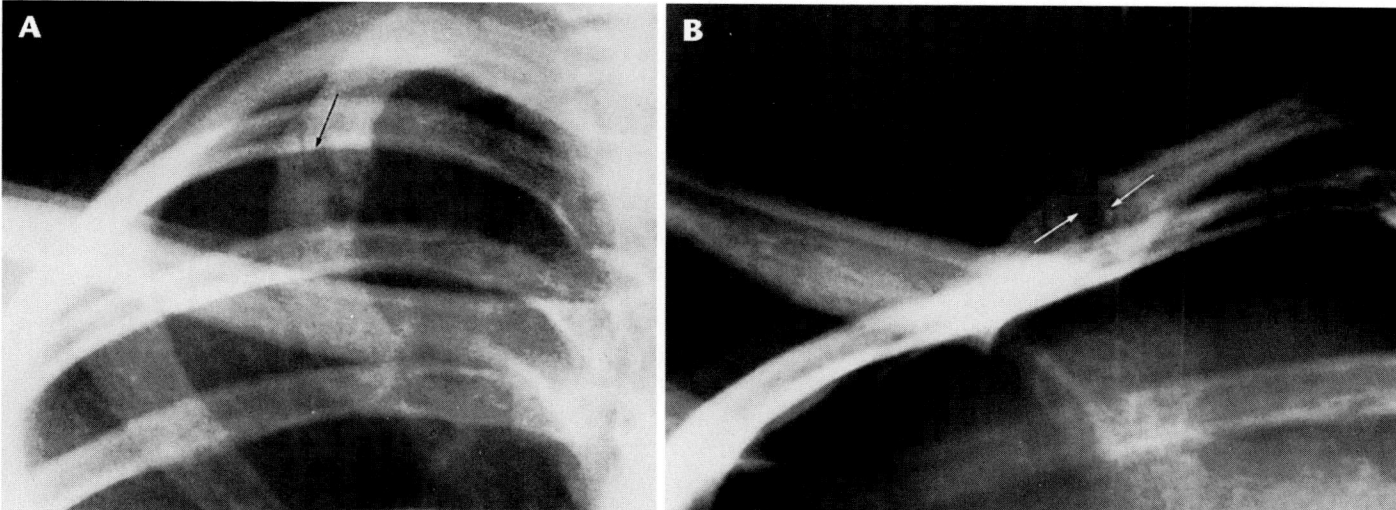

Figure 5–186. Anomalous articulation in the first ribs, simulating a fracture in **A** and a mass lesion in **B**.

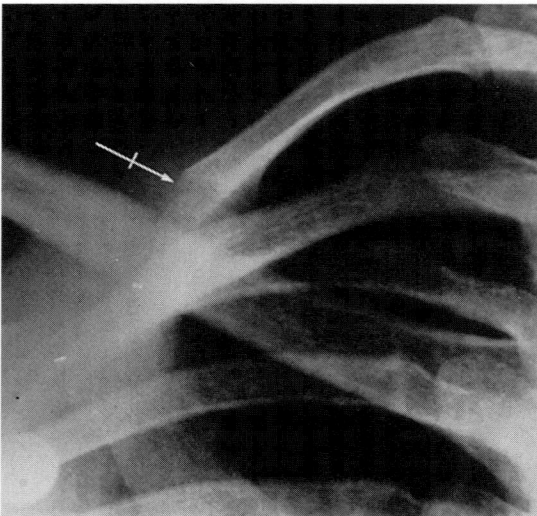

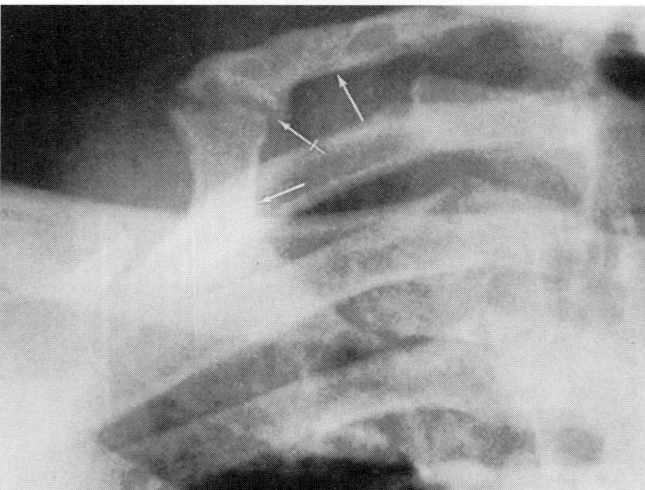

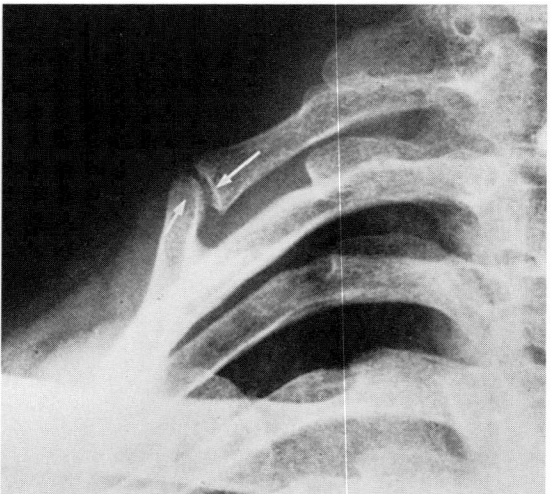

Figure 5–187. Three examples of anomalous articulations in the midportion of the first ribs, simulating a fracture (↔).

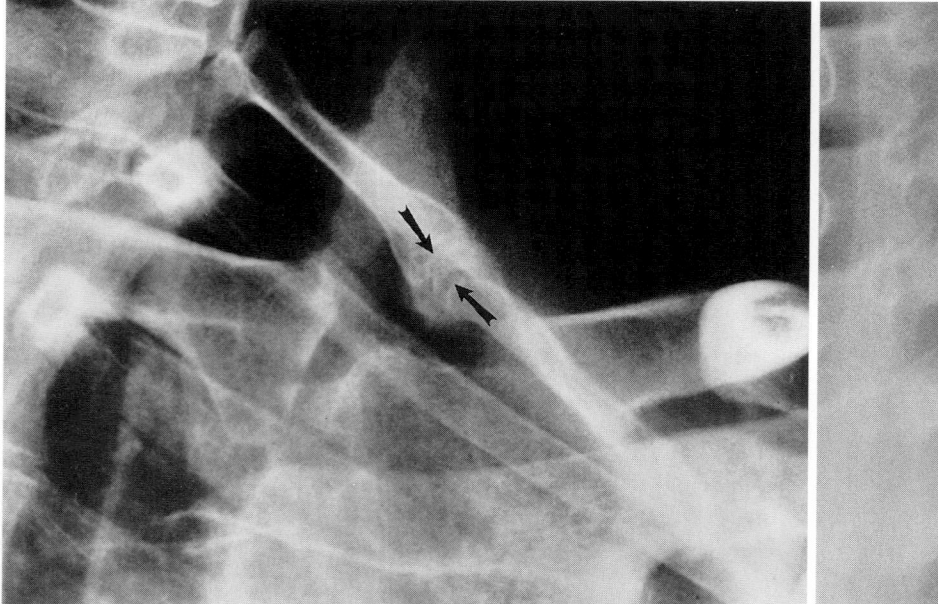

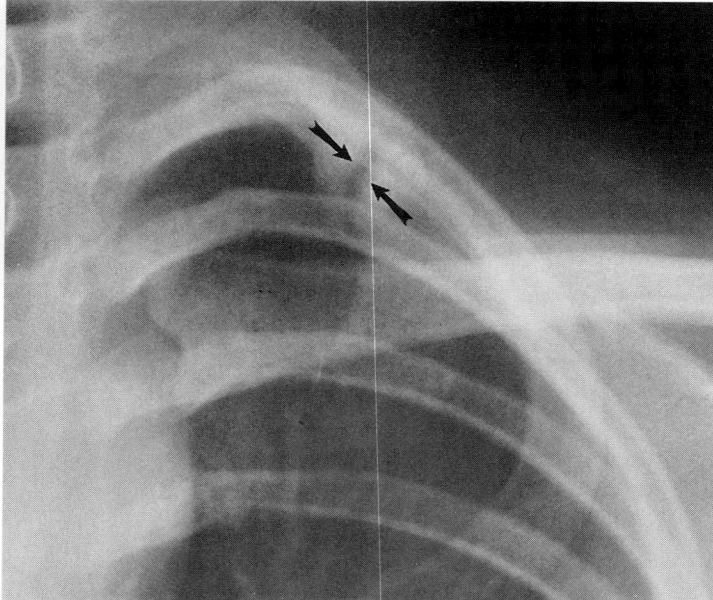

Figure 5–188. Two examples of anomalous articulations in the first rib on the left.

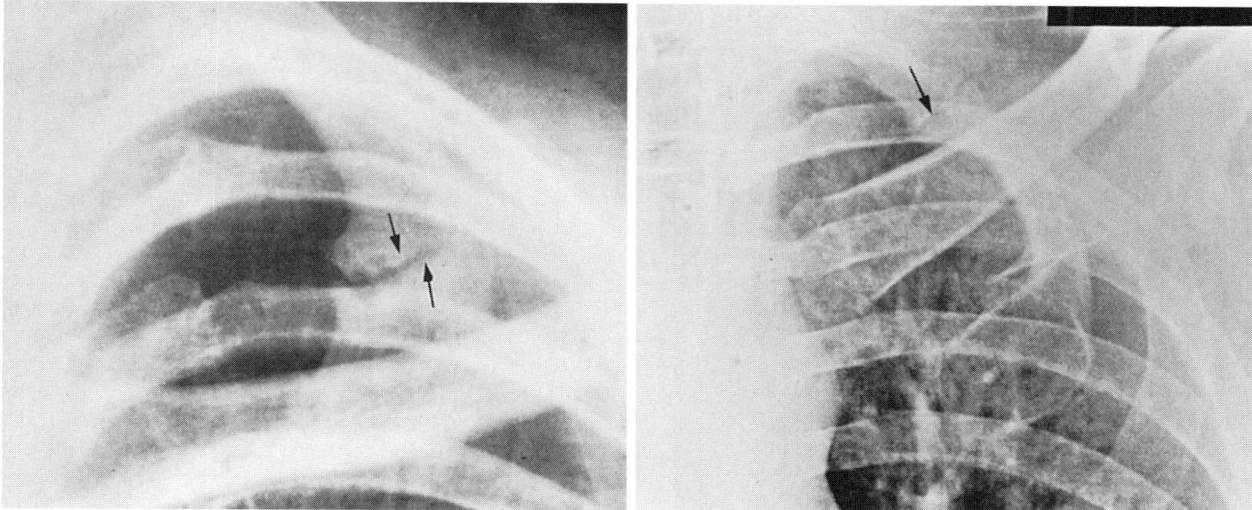

Figure 5–189. Anomalous articulations in the left first rib.

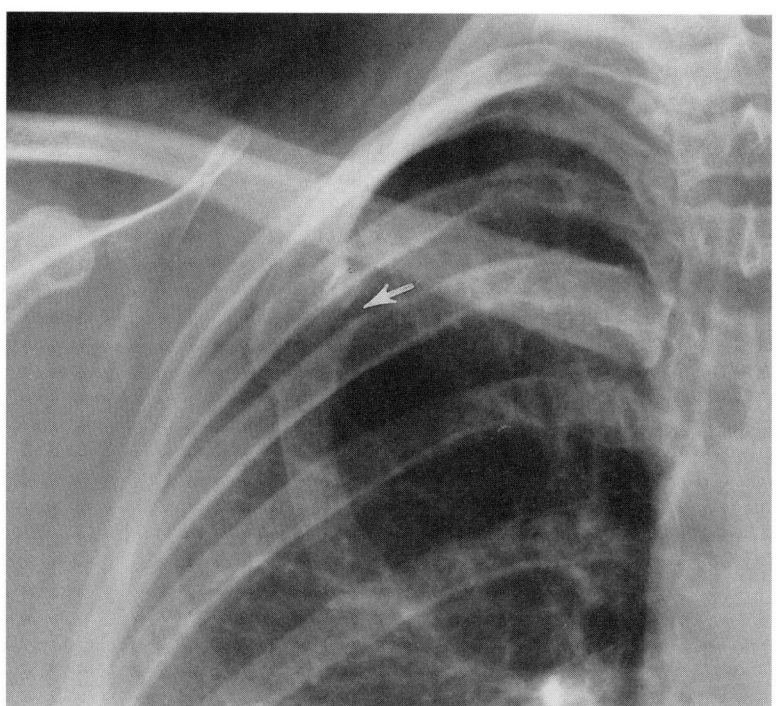

Figure 5–190. Jointed second rib.

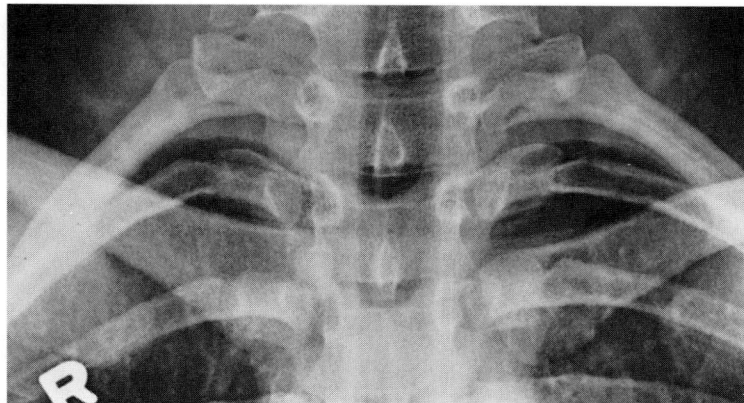

Figure 5–191. Striking increase in density of the first ribs in a normal 29-year-old man.

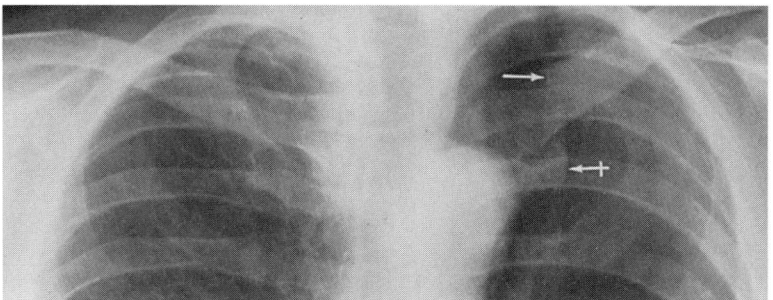

Figure 5–192. Anomalous development of the first rib (→) with the costal cartilage ununited to the rib (↦).

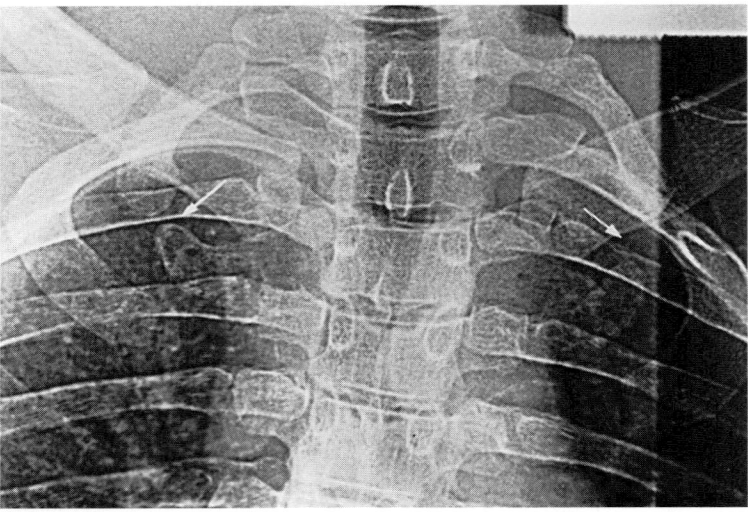

Figure 5–193. Bilateral failure of the first costal cartilages to unite with the first rib.

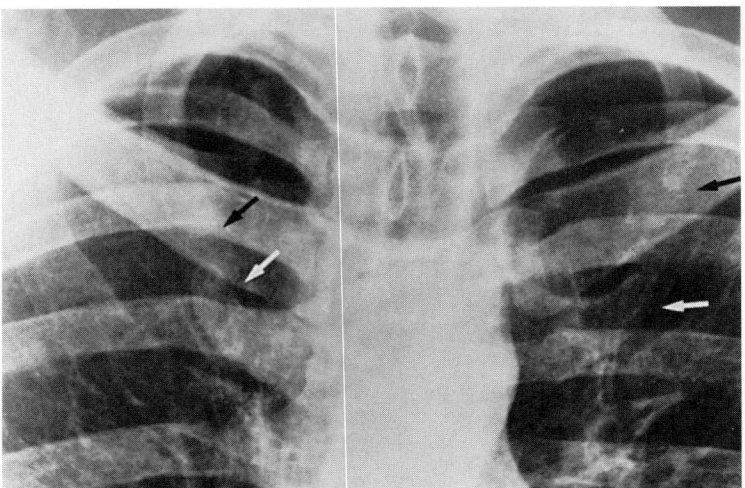

Figure 5–194. Failure of first ribs to join costal cartilages.

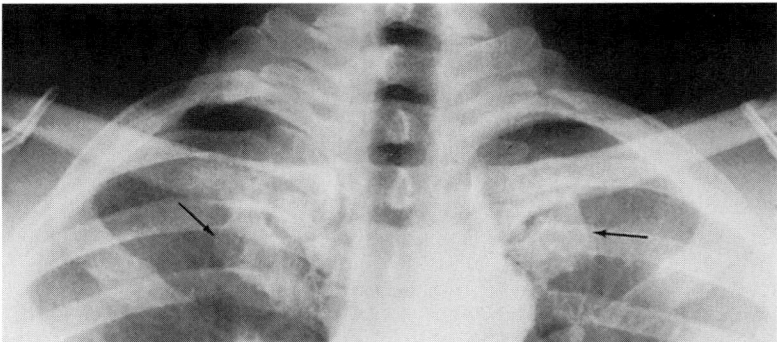

Figure 5–195. Developmental absence of the first ribs. Note that the costal cartilages have formed even in the absence of the ribs *(arrows)*.

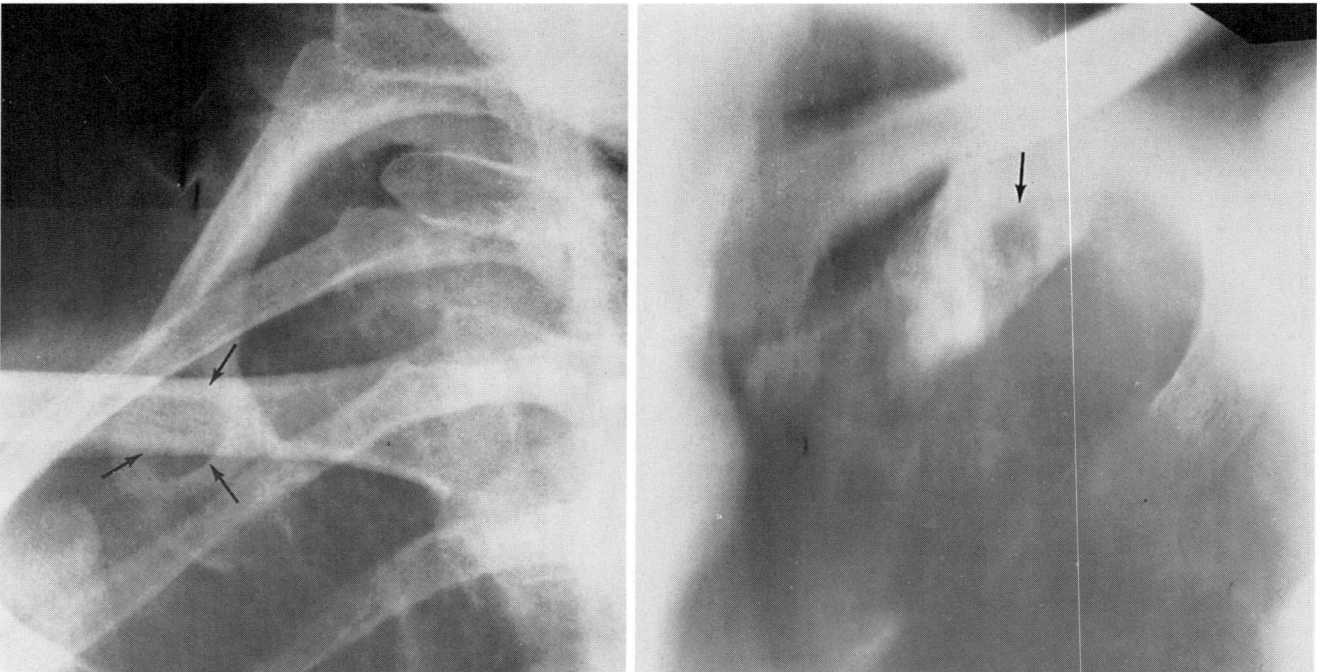

Figure 5–196. Two examples of normal areas of lucency in the anterior ends of the first ribs. These may be unilateral or bilateral, are fairly constant in their location, and should not be confused with areas of bone destruction.

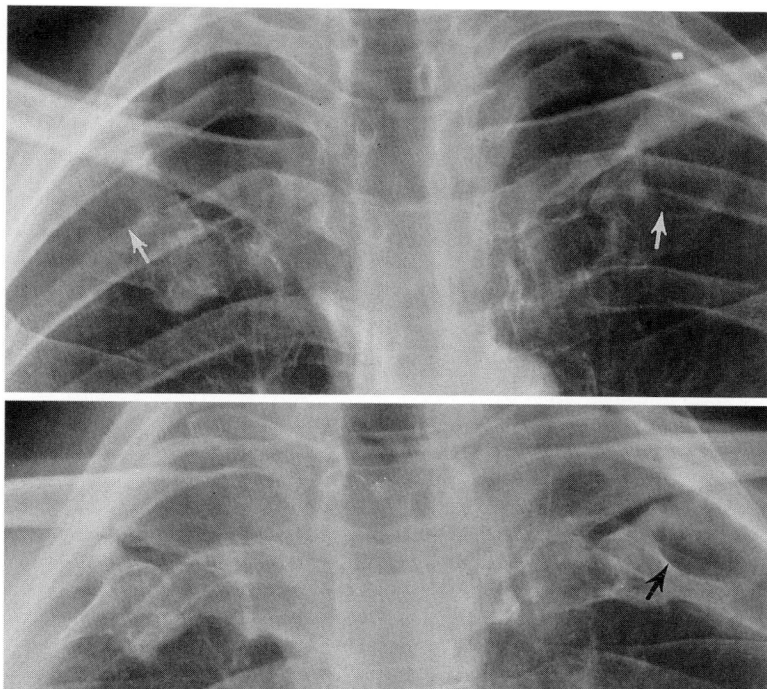

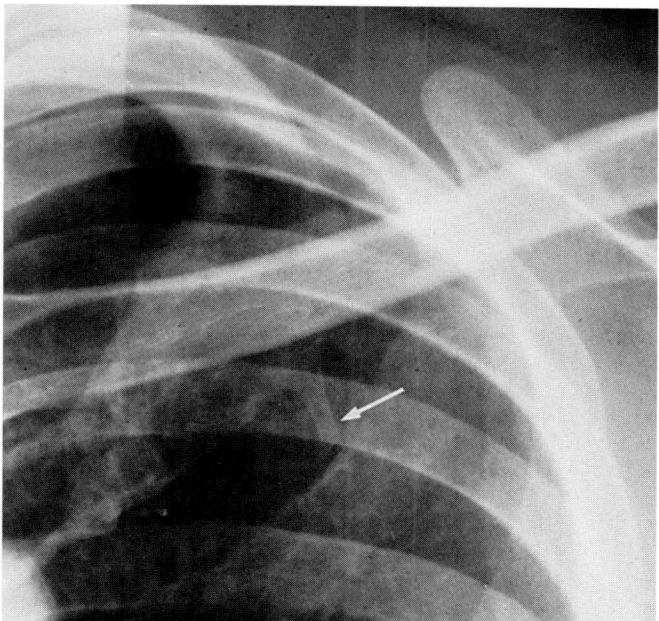

Figure 5–198. Spurlike process arising from the anterior portion of the first rib.

Figure 5–197. Huge fossae in the anterior ends of the first ribs, as in preceding illustration.

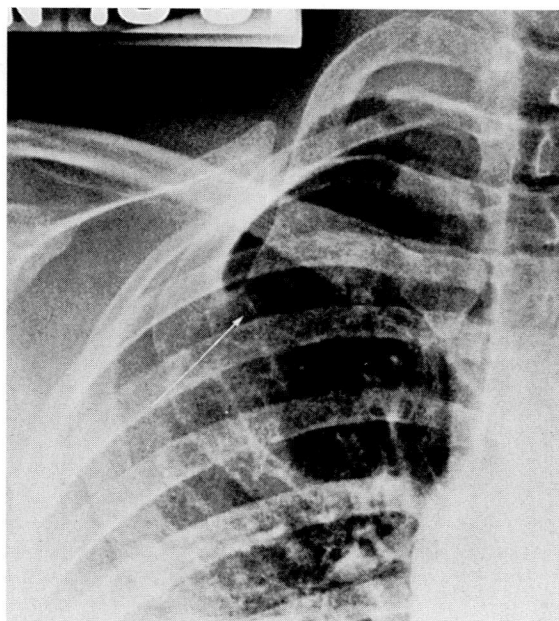

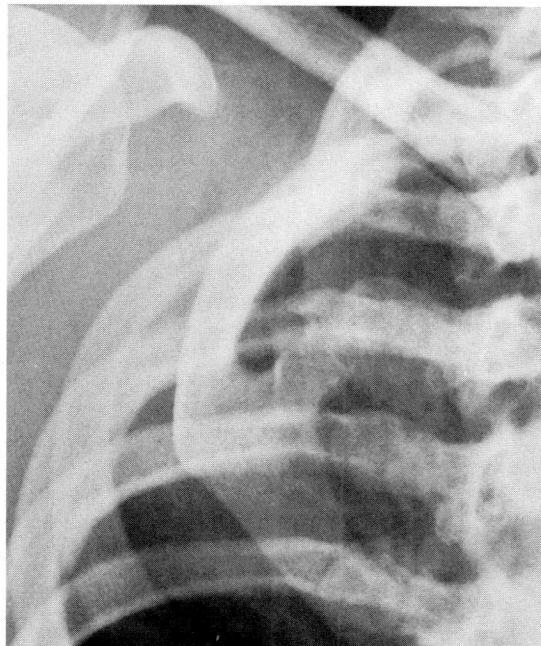

Figure 5–199. Fusion of the anterior portions of the first and second ribs.

Figure 5–200. Developmental fusion between the anterior ends of the first and second ribs.

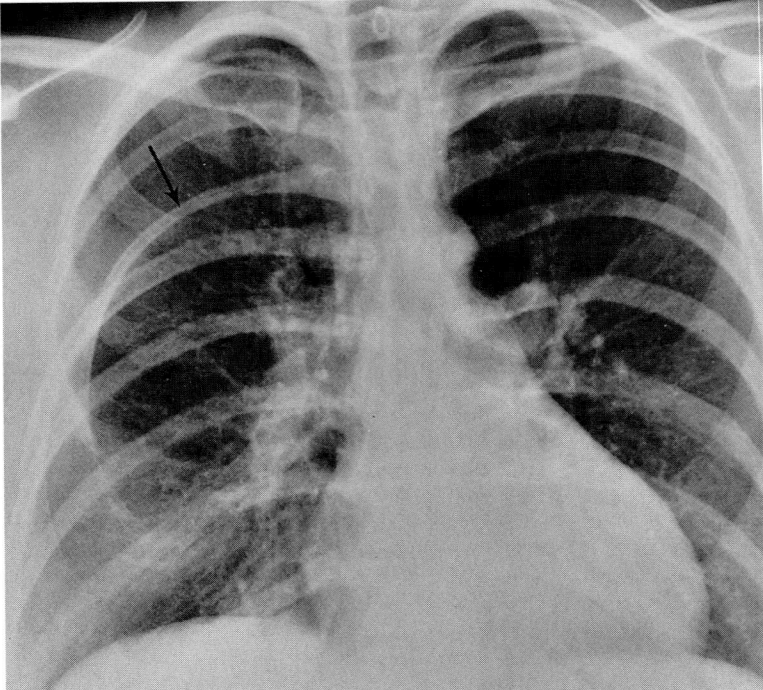

Figure 5–201. Anomalous development of the right fifth rib that might simulate a pneumothorax.

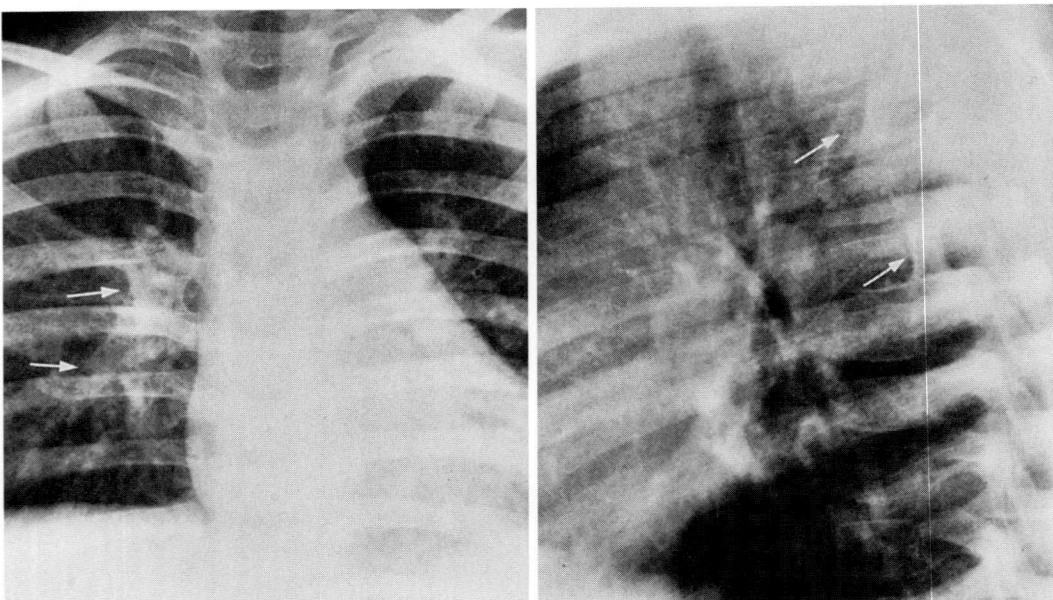

Figure 5–202. Fusions of the posterior portions of the right fifth, sixth, and seventh ribs, which can be seen in the lateral projection as well.

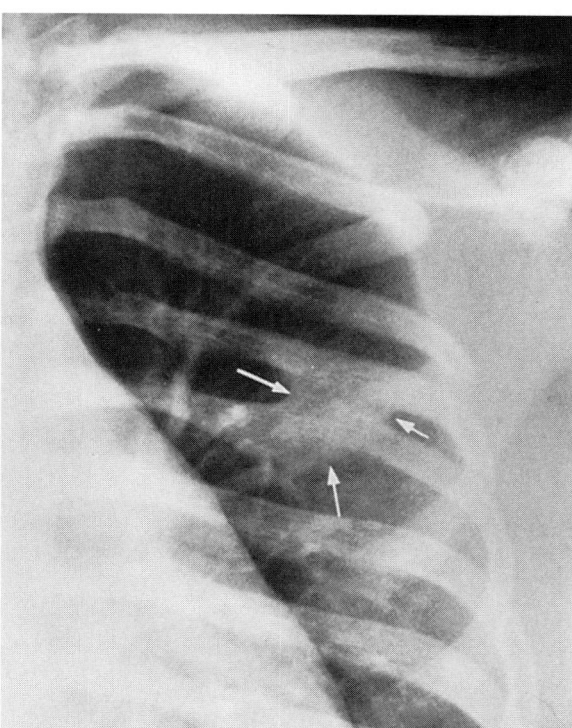

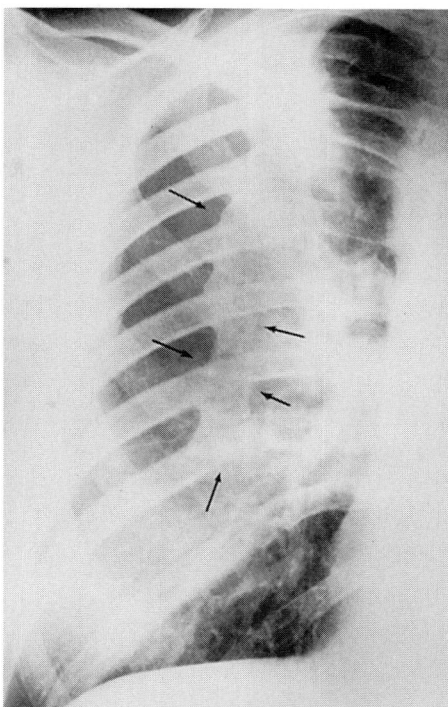

Figure 5–203. Fusion of the posterior portion of the fourth and fifth ribs in a 12-year-old boy.

Figure 5–204. Extensive developmental fusions of the posterior ribs.

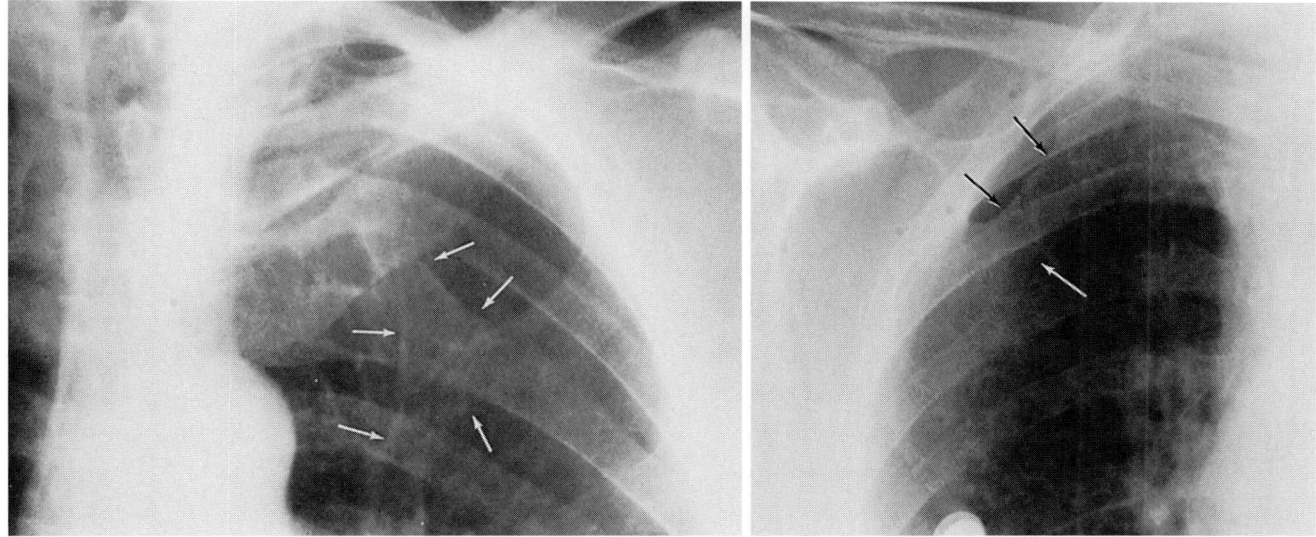

Figure 5–205. Localized developmental fusions of portions of the posterior ribs may simulate parenchymal lesions or pneumothorax.

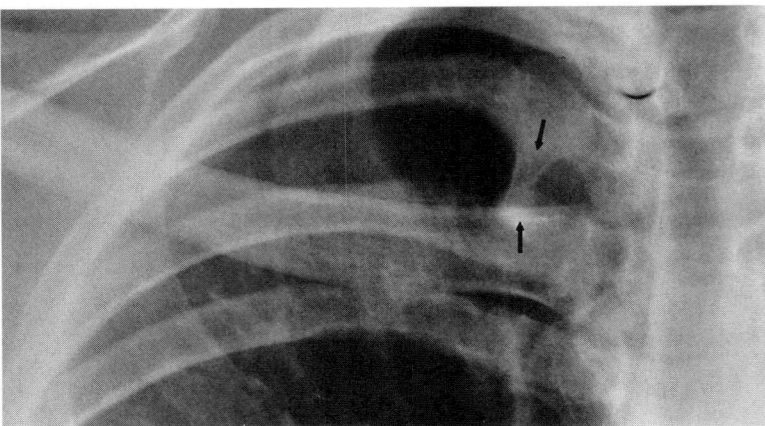

Figure 5–206. An osseous bridge between the posterior portions of the third and fourth ribs.

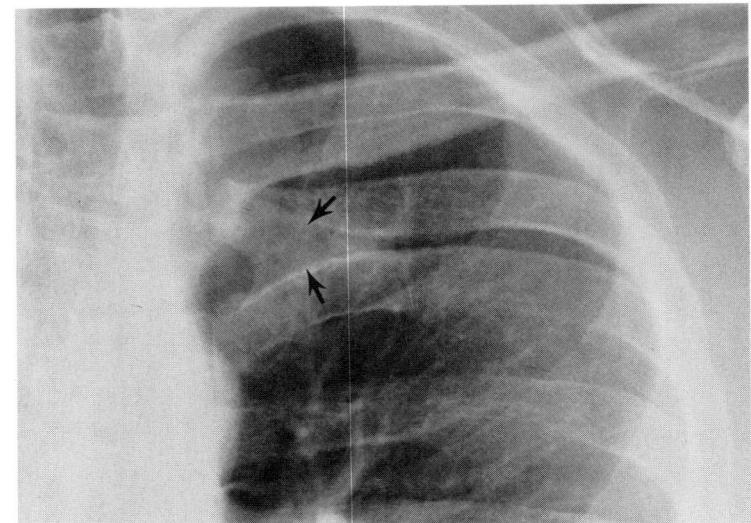

Figure 5–207. Fusion between posterior portions of the fourth and fifth ribs.

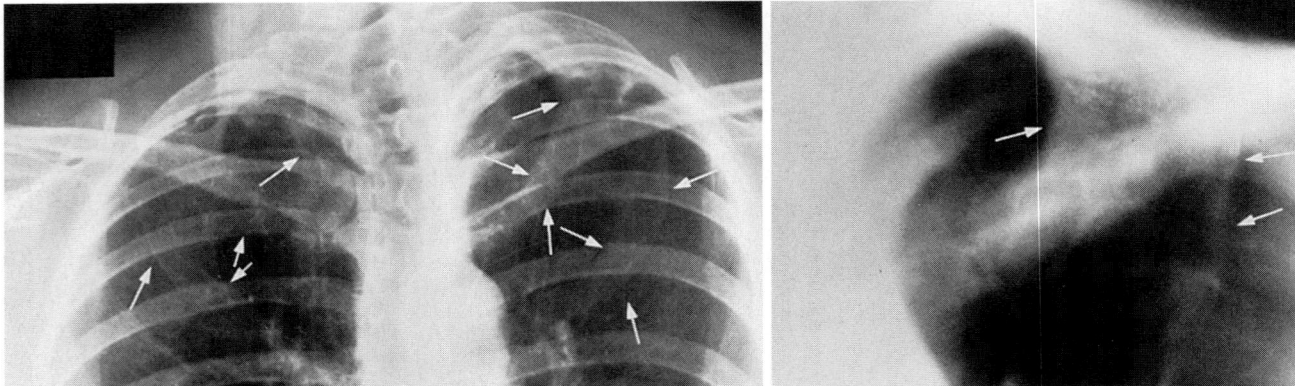

Figure 5–208. Large first rib with bifurcated anterior end mistaken for a mass lesion. *Left,* Plain film. *Right,* Tomogram.

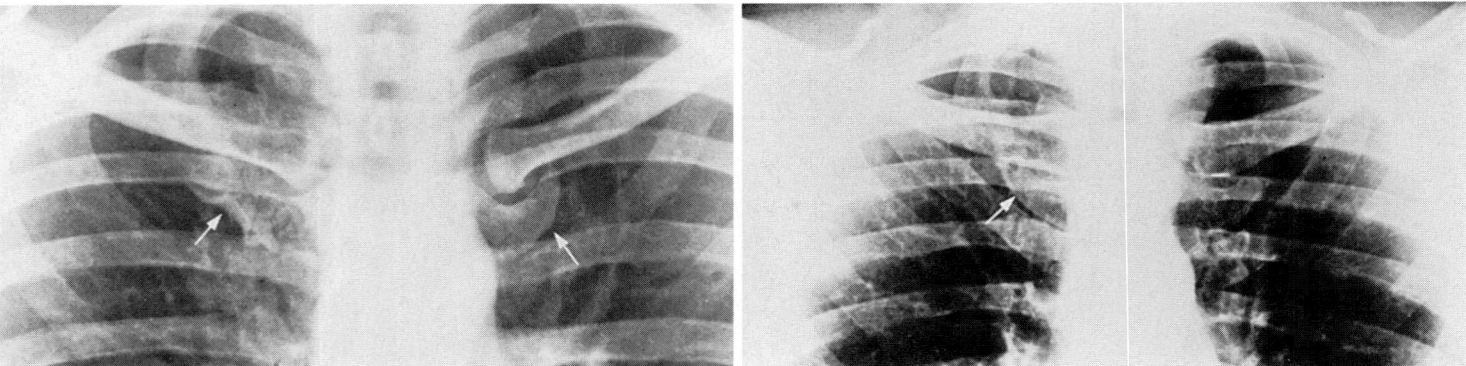

Figure 5–209. Variations in development of the costal cartilages of the first ribs.

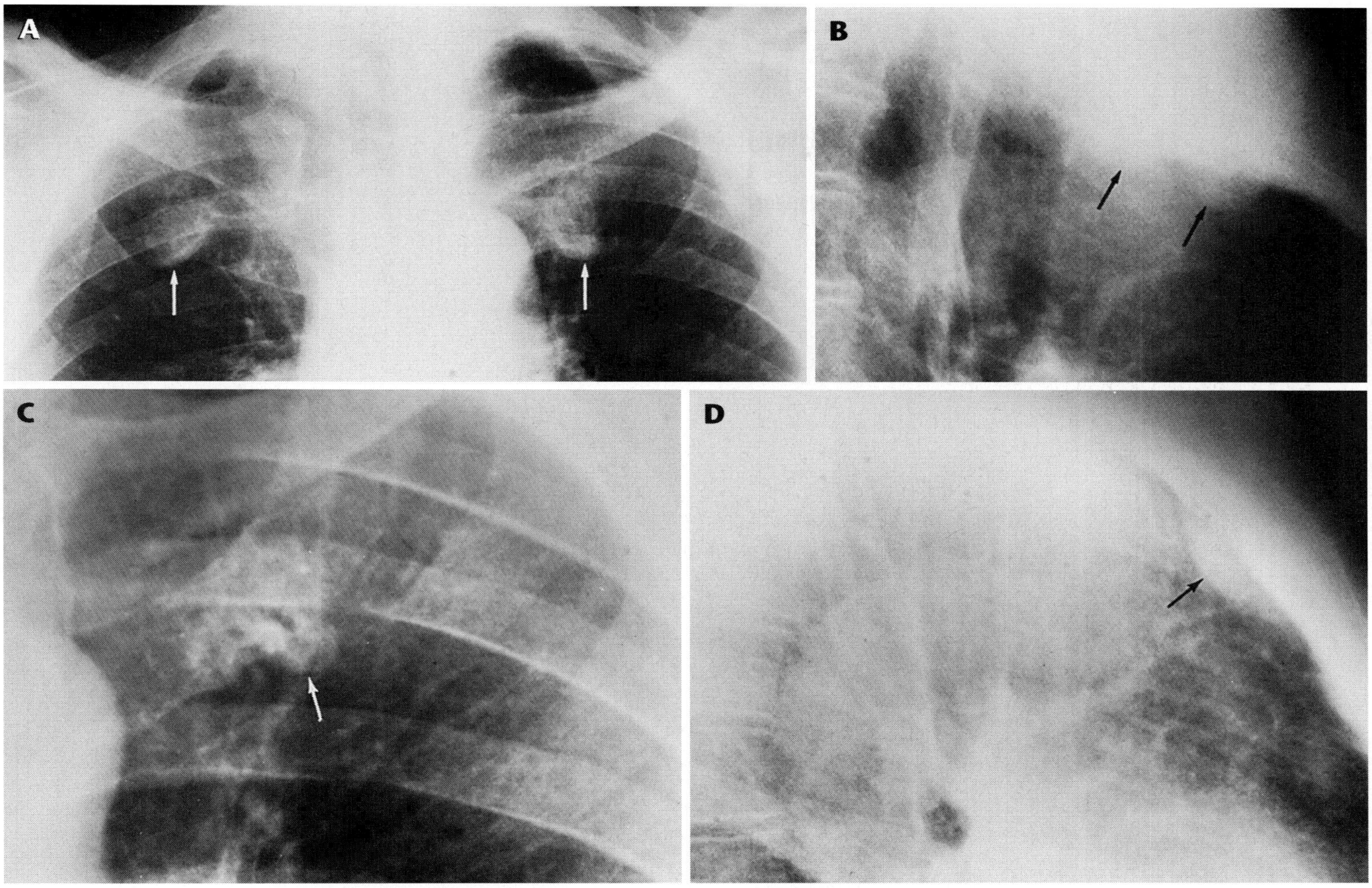

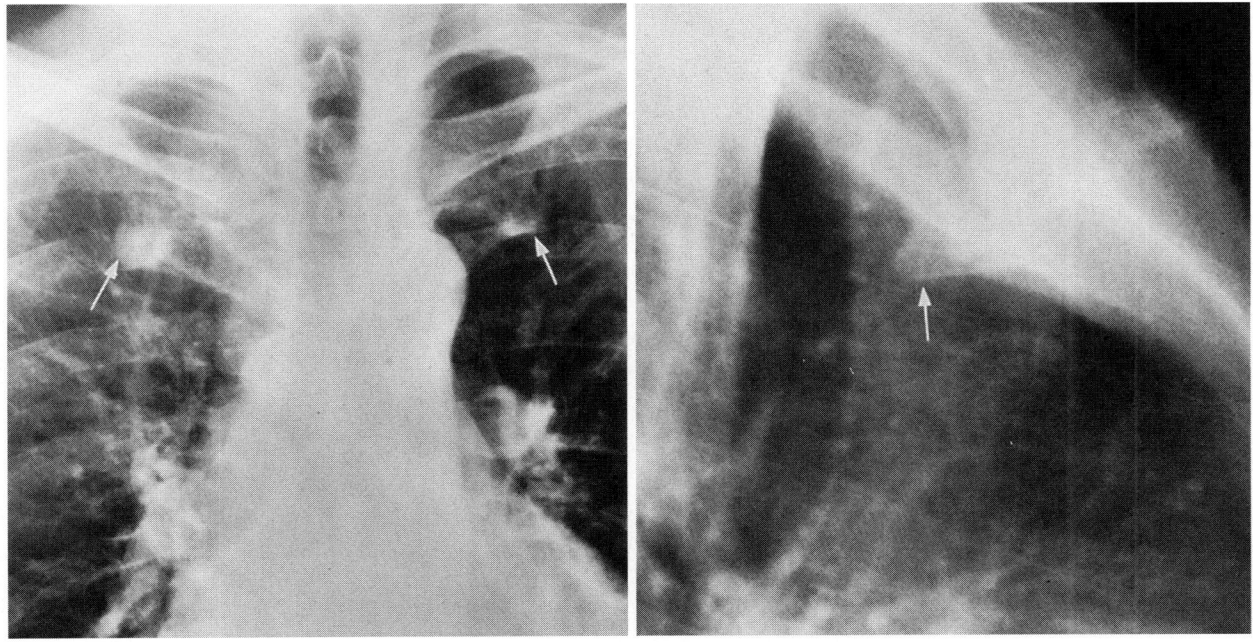

Figure 5–210. Very large calcified costal cartilages simulate an intrathoracic lesion in both projections. **A** and **B,** 74-year-old man. **C** and **D,** 58-year-old man. The first sternocostal joint may be classified as either a synchondrosis or a synostosis, but a joint cavity lateral to the first sternocostal joint may be present. (Ref: Schils JP et al: Sternocostal joints: Anatomic, radiographic and pathologic features in adult cadavers. *Invest Radiol* 24:596, 1989.)

Figure 5–211. Very large hypertrophied costal cartilage of the first ribs with marked intrathoracic extension seen in lateral projection.

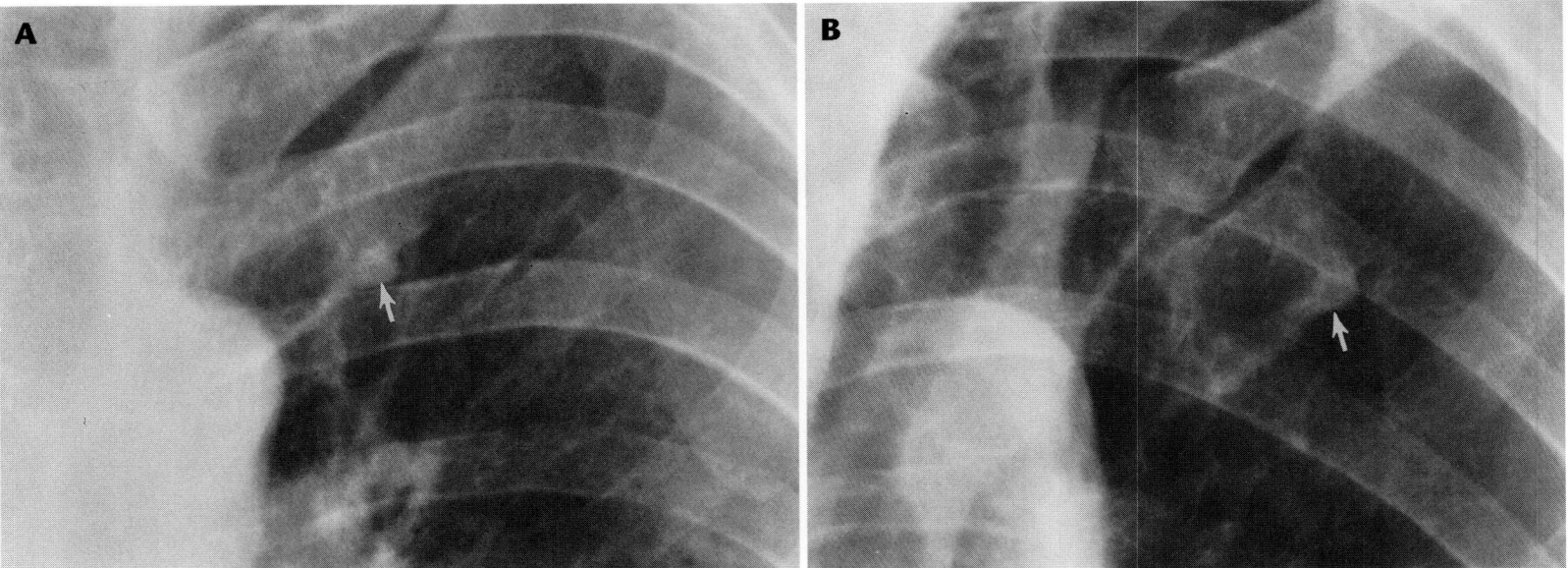

Figure 5–212. Nodular calcification of the costal cartilage of the first rib simulating a lesion in lung.

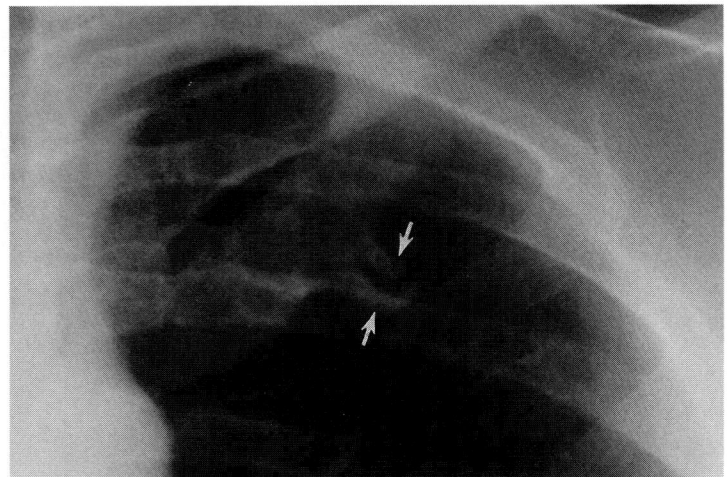

Figure 5–213. Spurs at the first costochondral junction.

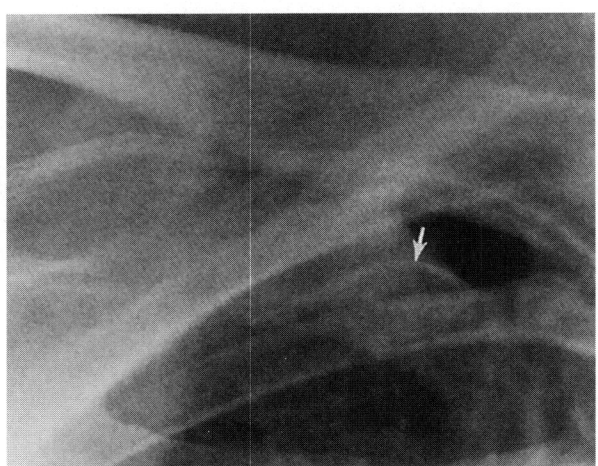

Figure 5–214. The costochondral junction simulating a pneumothorax.

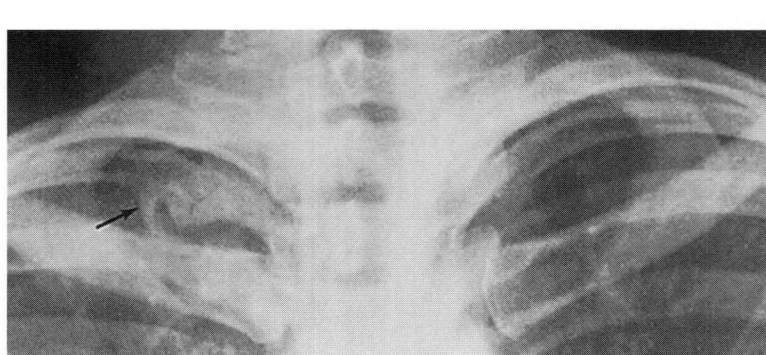

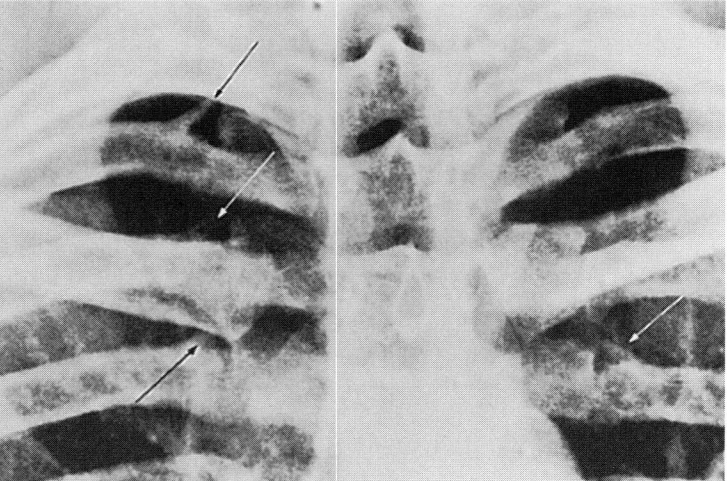

Figure 5–215. Developmental spurs at the costovertebral junctions.

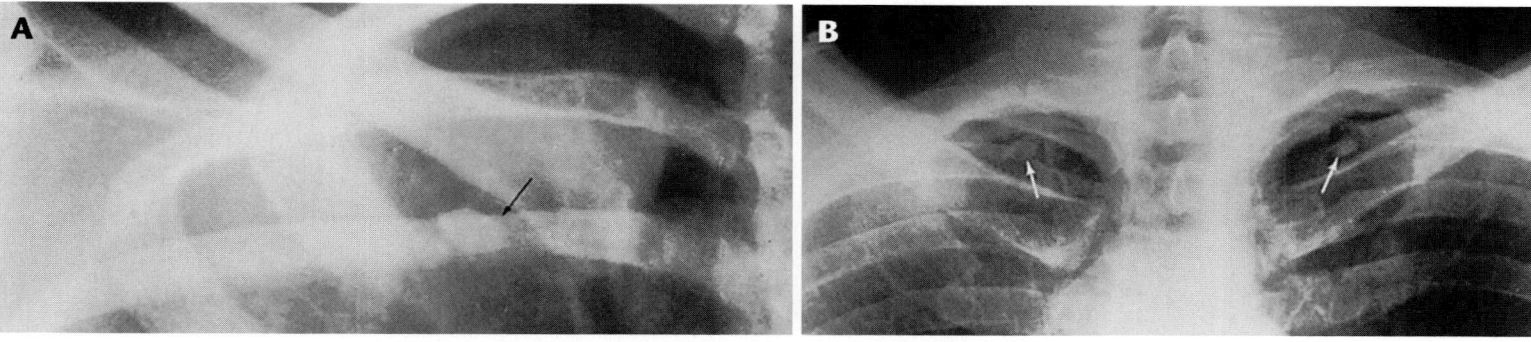

Figure 5–216. Ossicles related to rib ends. **A,** Anterior rib end. **B,** Posterior rib end.

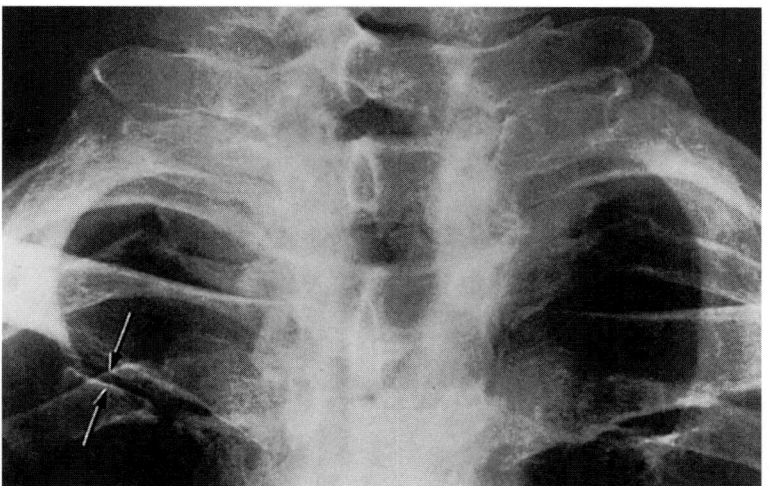

Figure 5–217. The costoclavicular joint. This joint is a variant of the ligamentous connection between the medial end of the clavicle and the first rib. (From Redlund-Johnell I: The costoclavicular joint. *Skeletal Radiol* 15:25, 1986.)

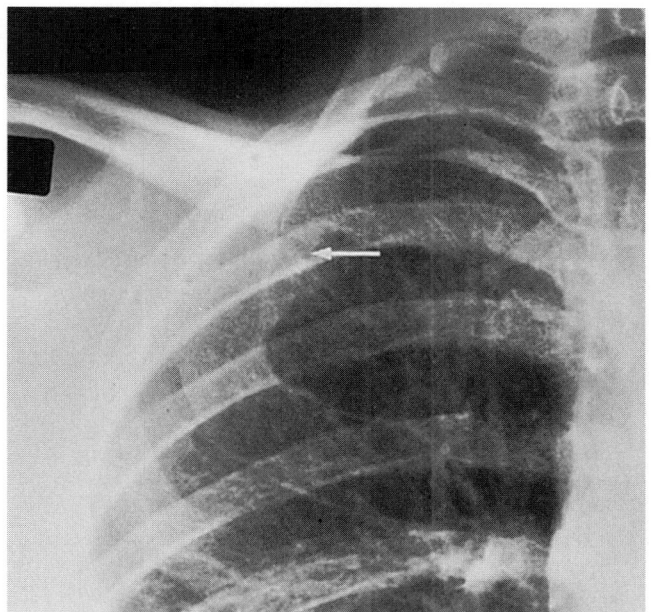

Figure 5–218. Articulation between the first and second ribs.

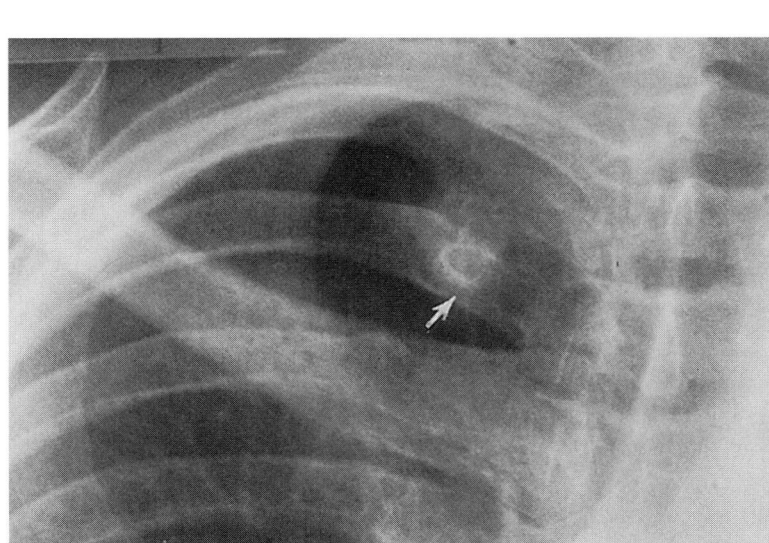

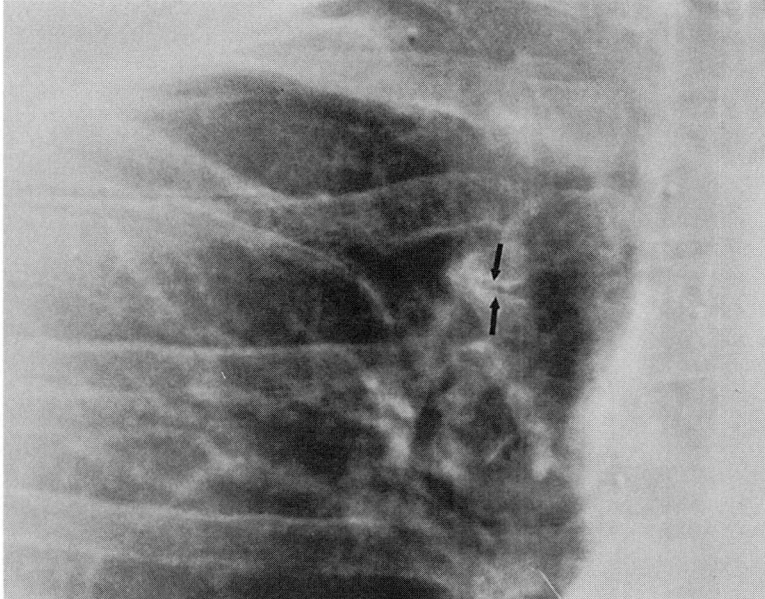

Figure 5–219. Articulation between the posterior aspects of the third and fourth ribs mistaken for a parenchymal lesion. **A,** Posteroanterior projection. **B,** Right posterior oblique projection.

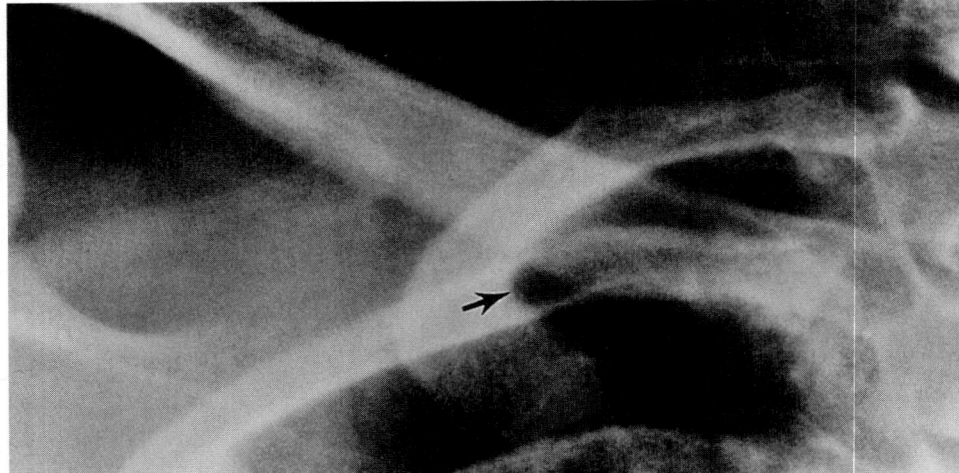

Figure 5–220. Superimposition of the clavicle and first rib simulating a destructive lesion in the second rib.

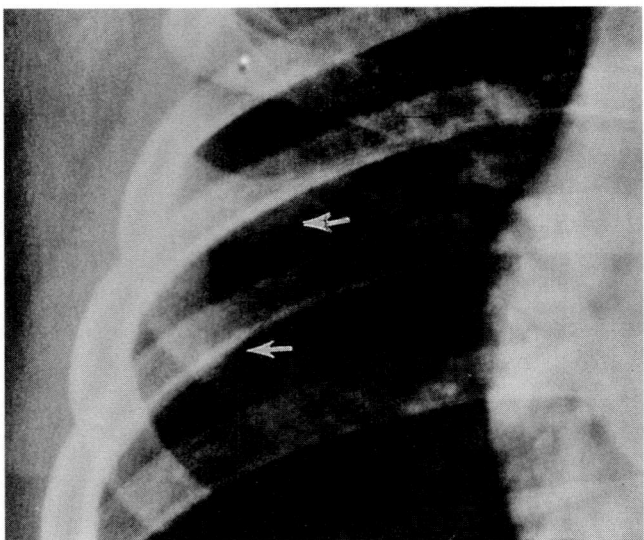

Figure 5–221. Bifid anterior end of the fourth rib.

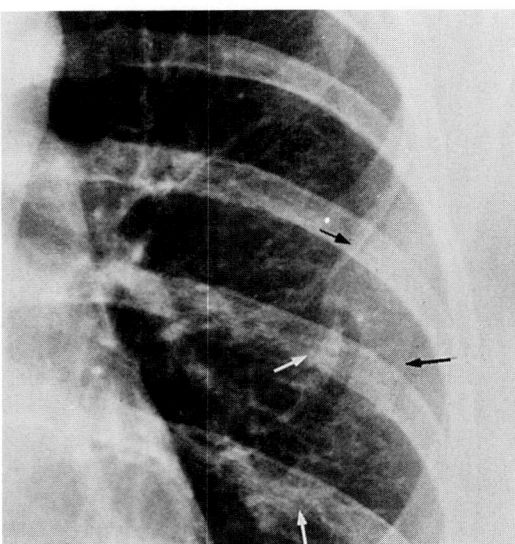

Figure 5–222. Anomalous development of the anterior end of the fourth rib.

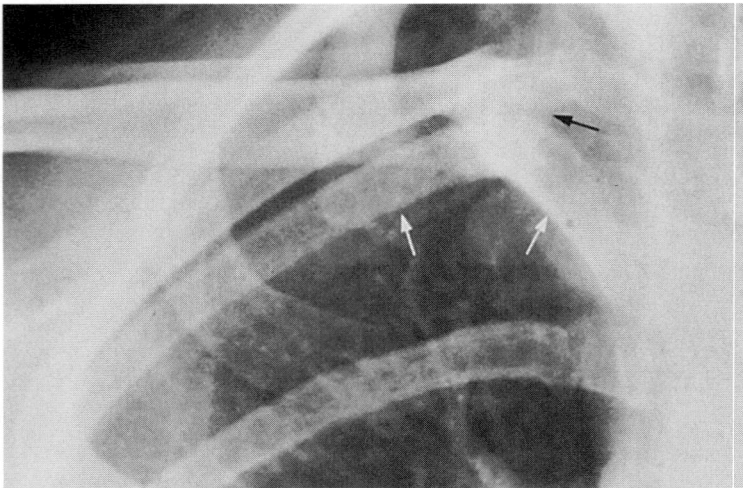

Figure 5–223. Marked cephalad angulation of the fourth rib *(white arrows)* with fusion to the adjacent third rib *(black arrow)*.

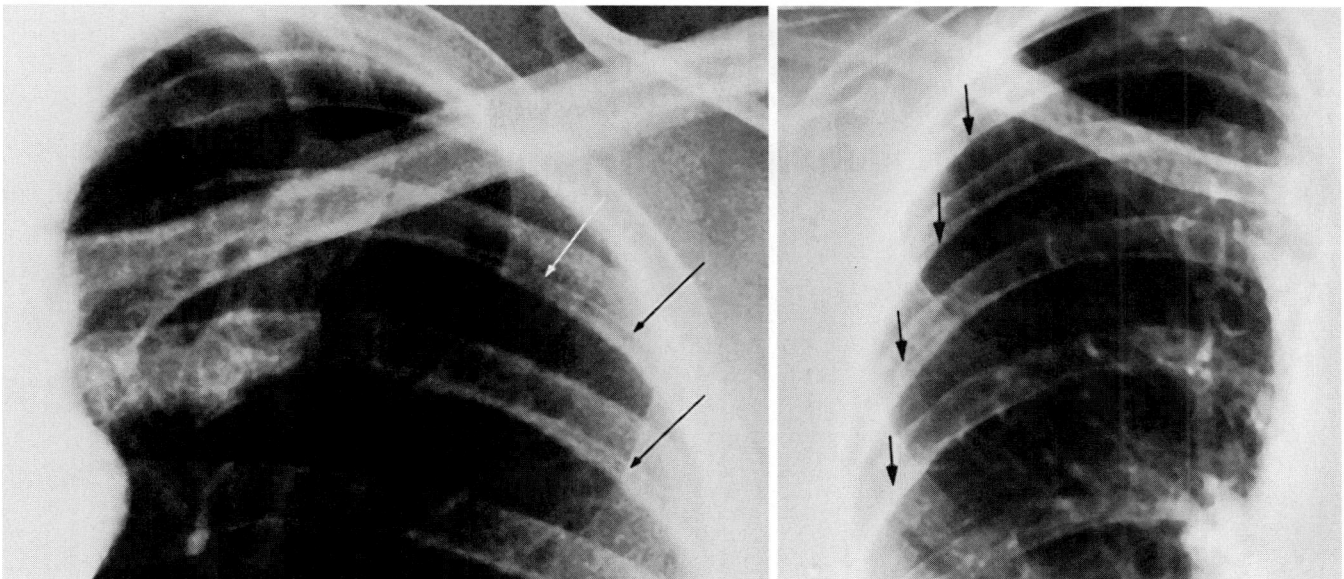

Figure 5–224. Grooves in the lower margins of the ribs, which might be mistaken for the lung edge of a pneumothorax.

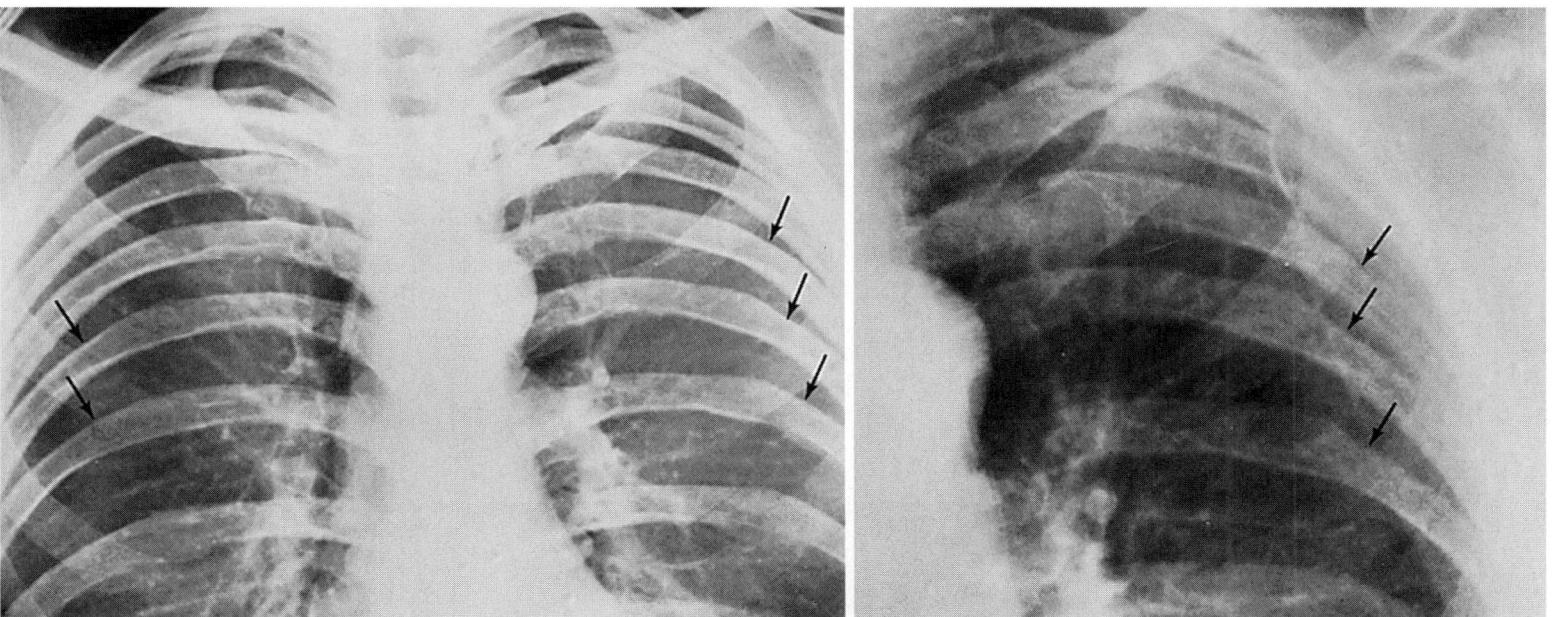

Figure 5–225. Two examples of pseudoerosion of the ribs. Loss of bone from the superior aspects of the ribs may be seen in a variety of pathologic processes, particularly in connective tissue diseases, but may also be seen in normal individuals with increasing age. (Ref: Keats TE: Superior marginal rib defects in restrictive lung disease. *Am J Roentgenol* 124:449, 1975.)

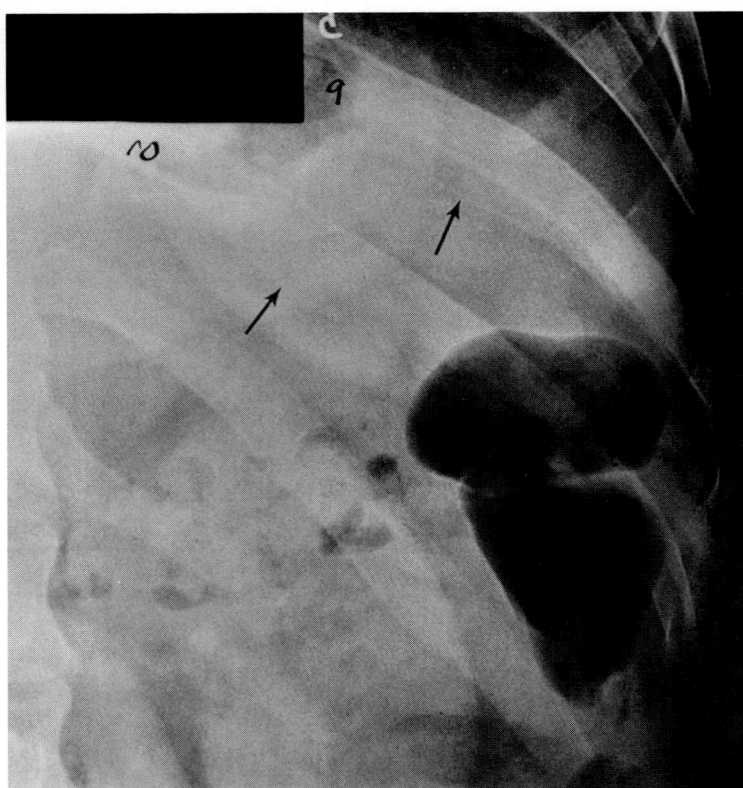

Figure 5–226. This thin flange of bone will also result in an apparent fusiform appearance of the rib, which should not be misinterpreted as a pathologic process.

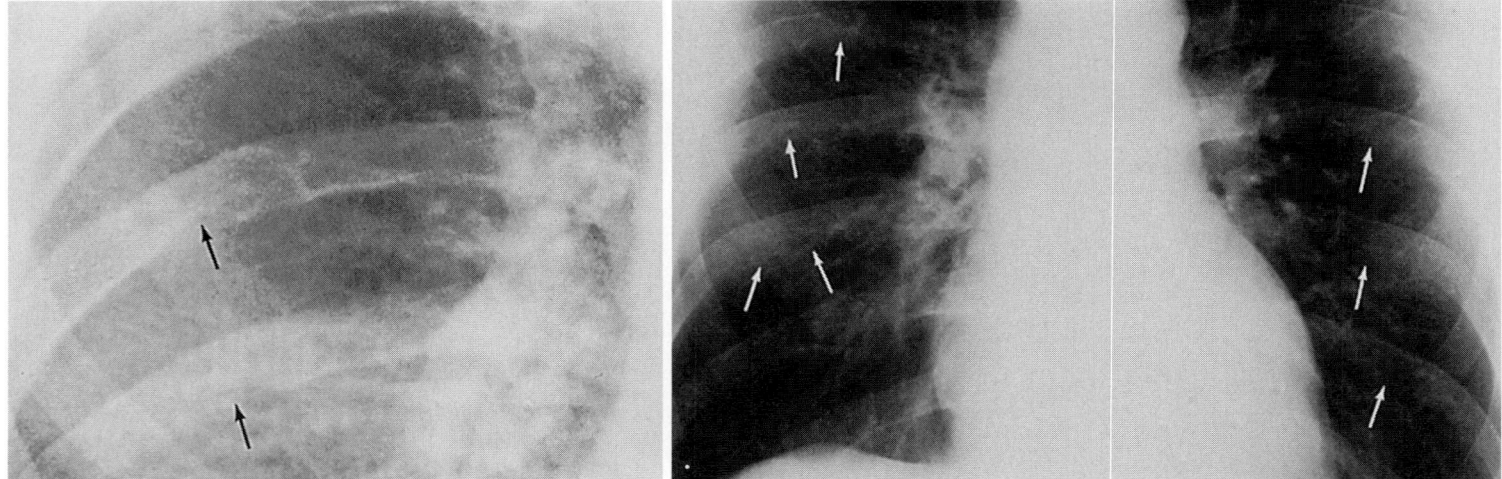

Figure 5–227. Two examples of simulated destruction of the inferior aspects of the posterior portions of the middle ribs. This variation is commonly seen and is due to the thin flange of bone at the lower portions of these ribs.

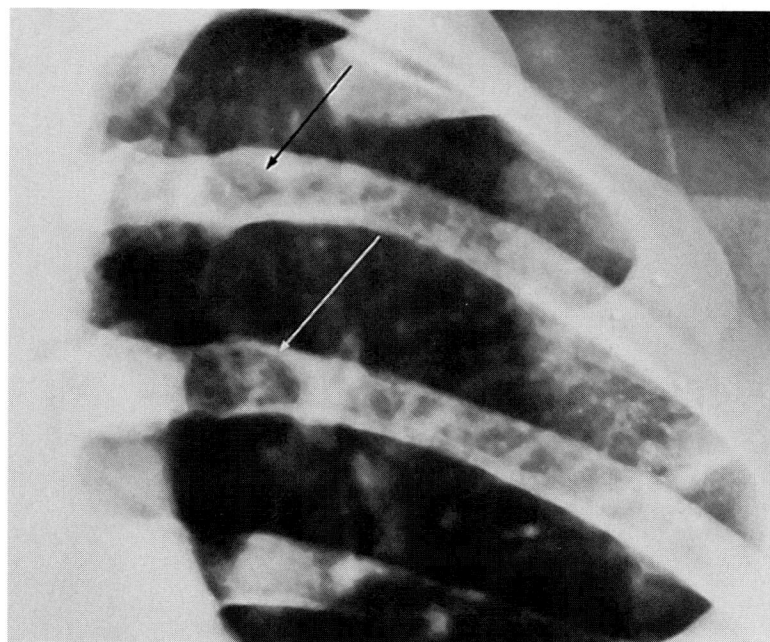

Figure 5–228. Simulated "cysts" of proximal rib ends produced by cancellous bone.

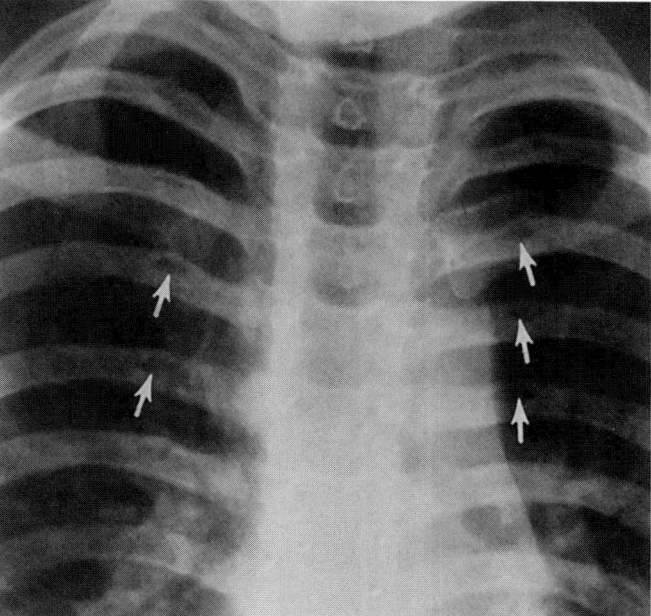

Figure 5–229. Lucencies in the tubercles of the proximal ends of the ribs.

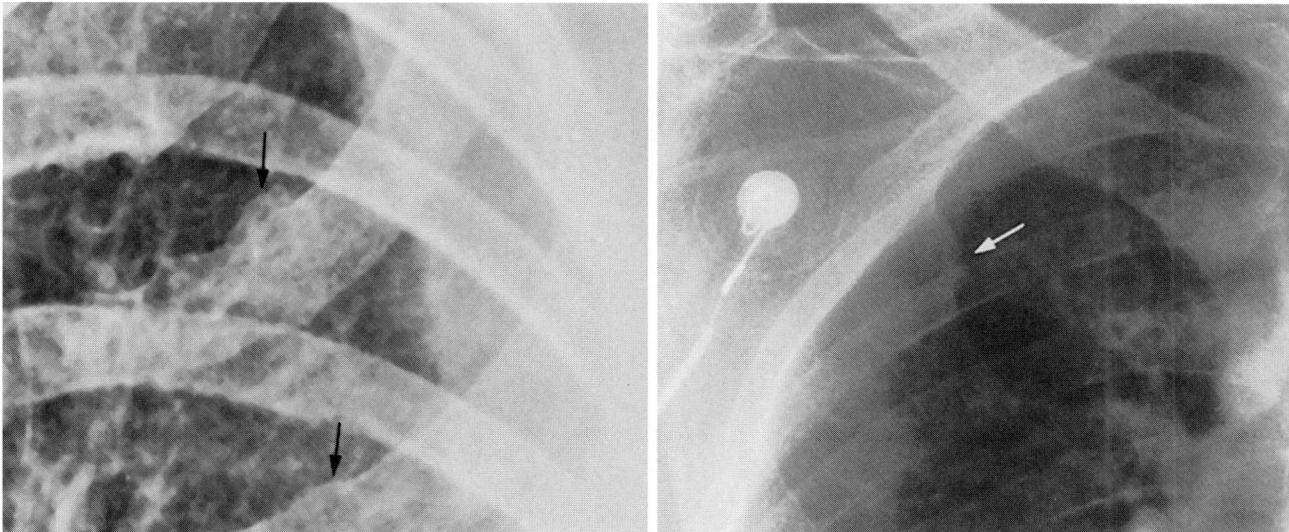

Figure 5–230. Localized protuberances on the anterior aspects of the second and third ribs.

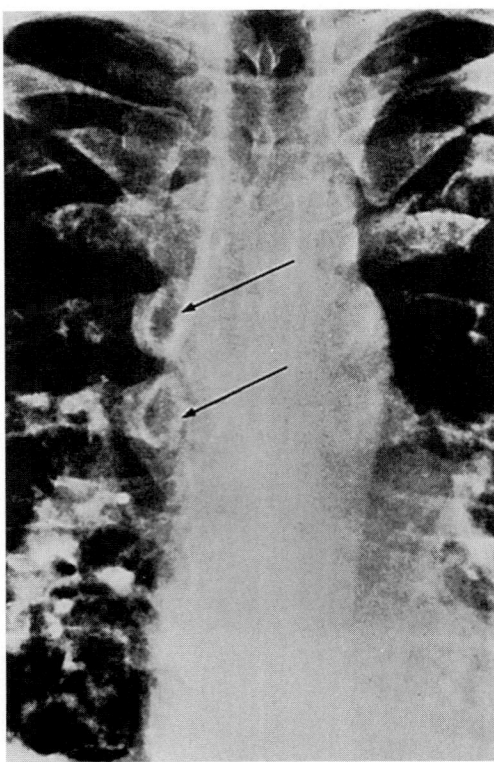

Figure 5–231. Enlarged costovertebral articulations produced by hypertrophic changes.

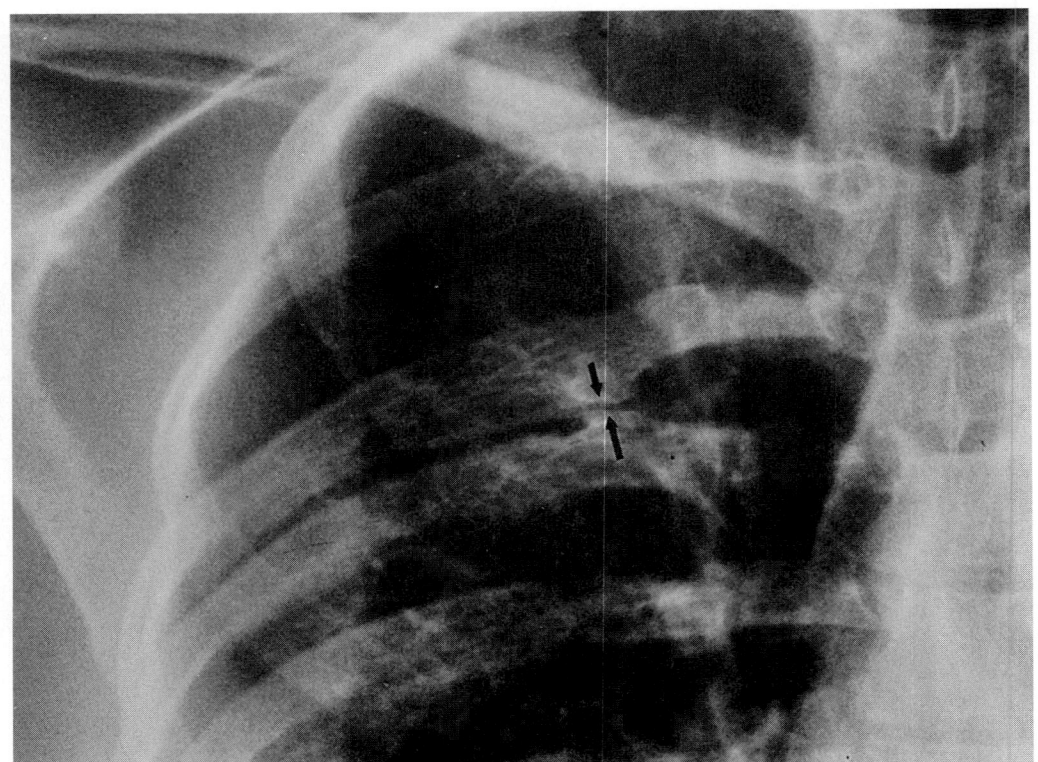

Figure 5–232. Articulation between two ribs.

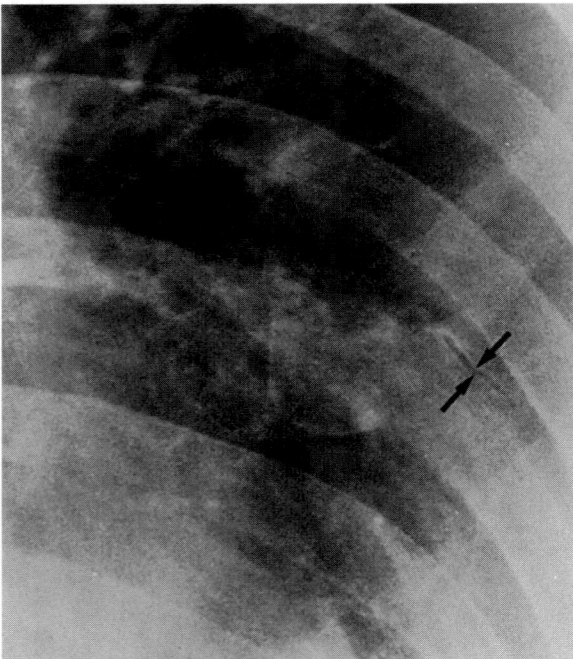

Figure 5–233. Articulation between two ribs.

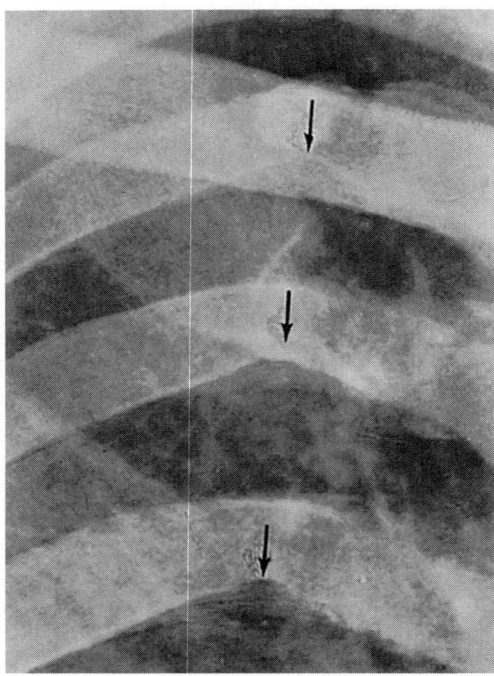

Figure 5–234. Normal exaggeration of the curve of the necks of the ribs, simulating rib notching.

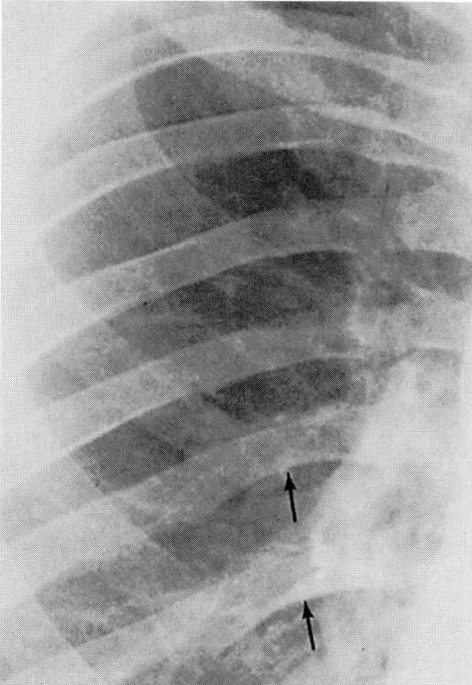

Figure 5–235. Normal exaggeration of curvature of the necks of the lower ribs.

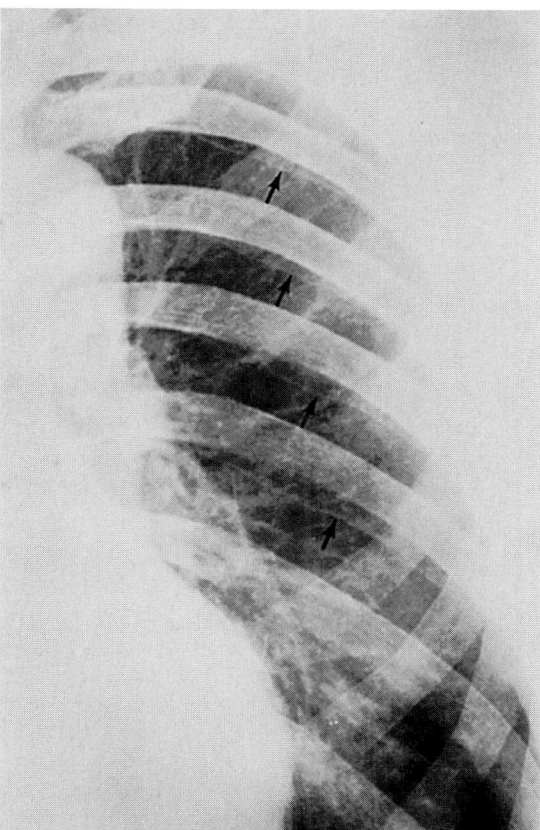

Figure 5–236. Companion shadows along lower rib margins produced by thin bony flanges.

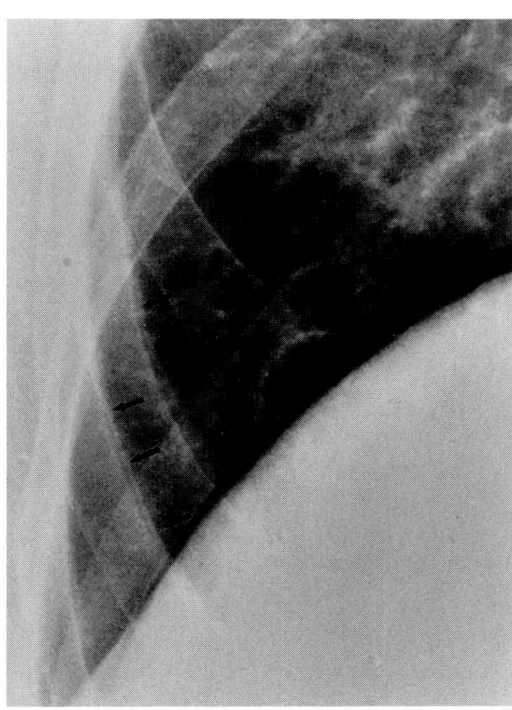

Figure 5–237. Soft tissue companion shadows of the upper margins of the lower anterior ribs.

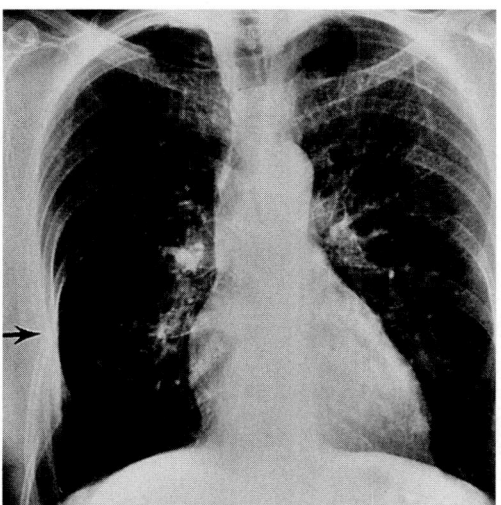

Figure 5–238. Developmental variation in contour of midchest with a tucklike configuration of the ribs. This variant is probably due to the presence of developmentally short ribs, which are often seen in the sixth, seventh, and eighth ribs. (Ref: Sheflin JF: Short ribs. *Am J Roentgenol* 165:1548, 1995.)

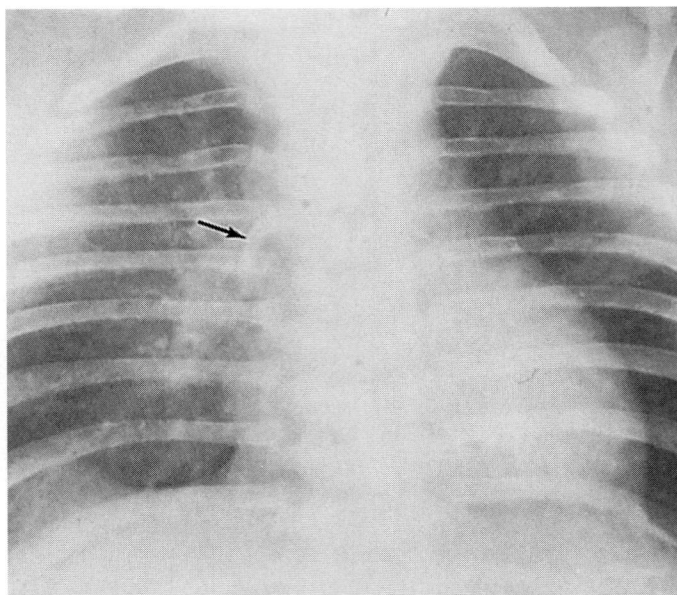

Figure 5–239. Intrathoracic rib. A rare anomaly of no clinical significance. (Ref: Weinstein AS, Mueller CF: Intrathoracic rib. *Am J Roentgenol* 94:587, 1965.)

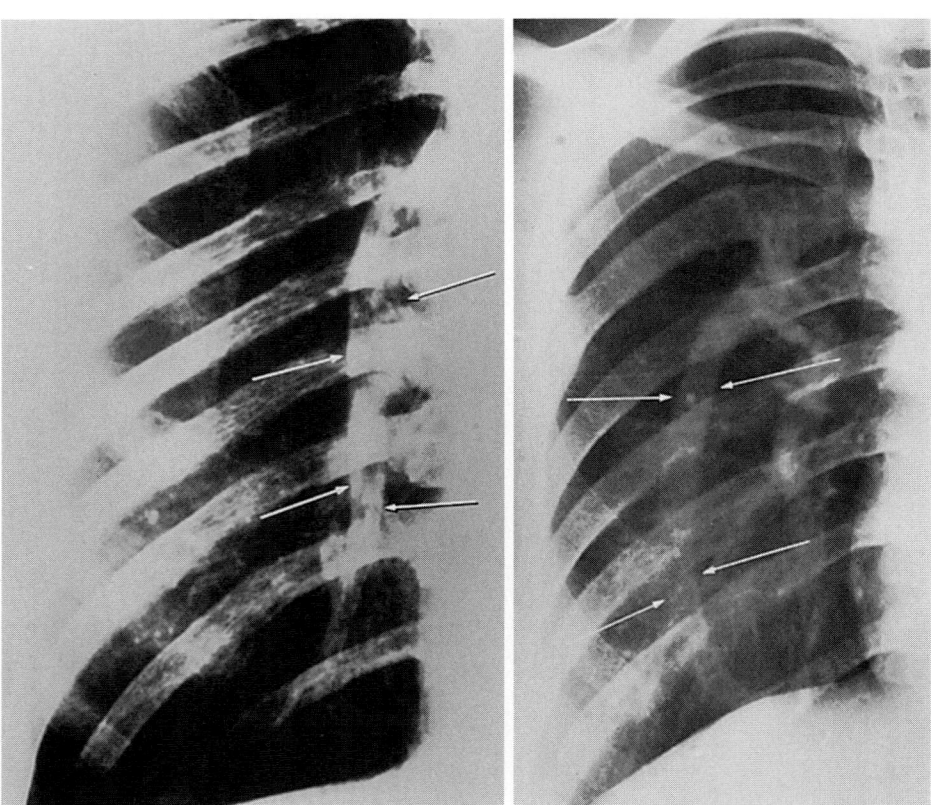

Figure 5–240. Two additional examples of intrathoracic ribs.

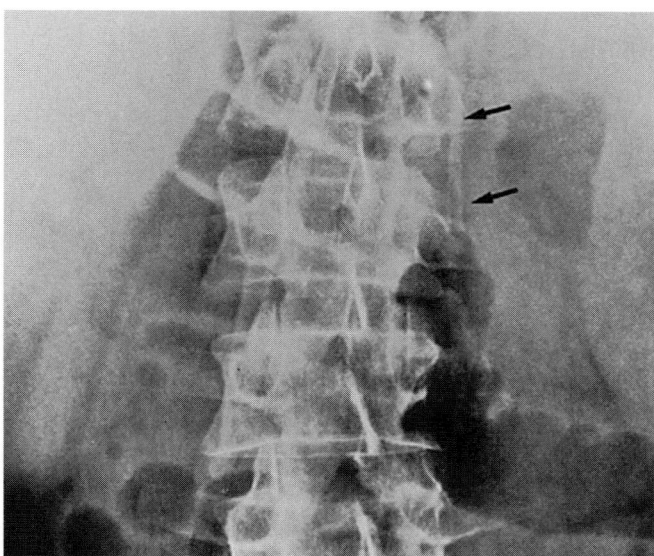

Figure 5–241. Intra-abdominal rib.

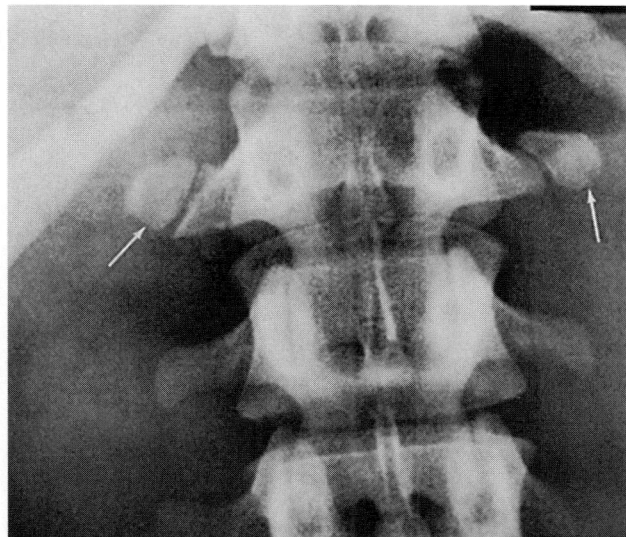

Figure 5–242. Anomalous development of the twelfth ribs.

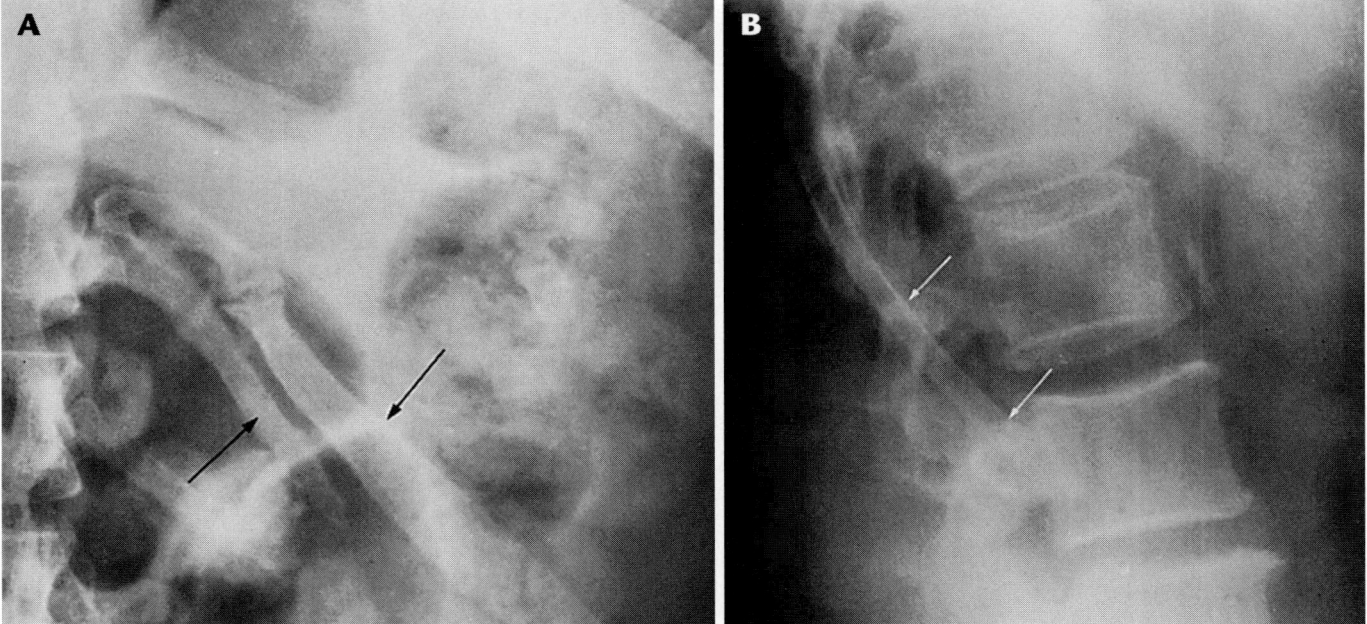

Figure 5–243. A, Duplication of the left eleventh rib. **B,** These ribs take a marked intra-abdominal course.

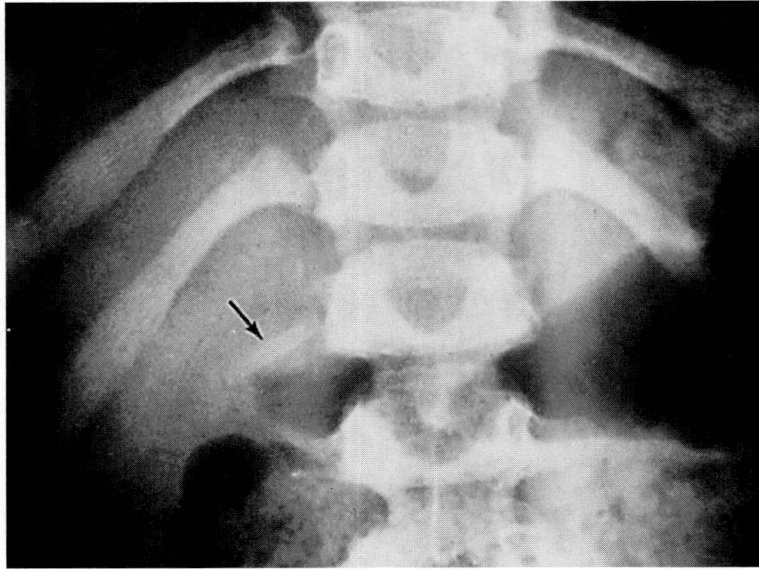

Figure 5–244. Unilateral development of the twelfth rib.

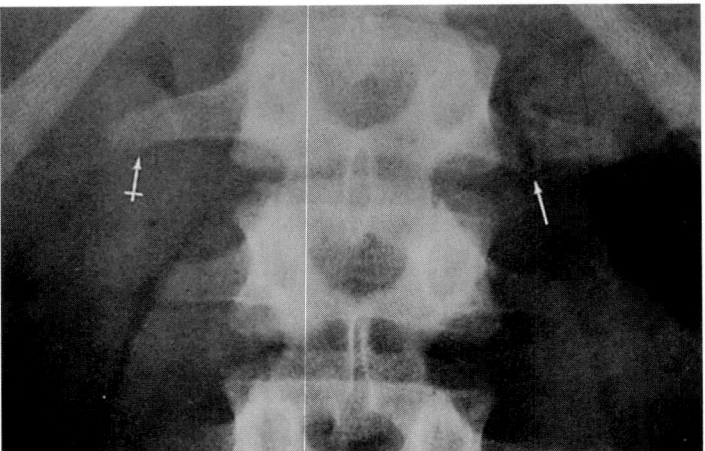

Figure 5–245. Unilateral development of the twelfth rib, simulating a fracture (→). Note the elongated transverse process on the opposite side (↦).

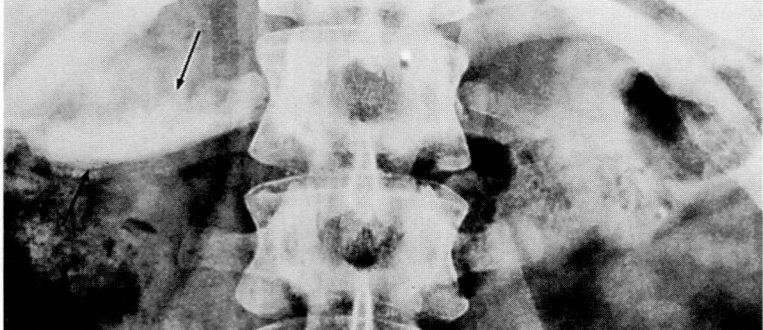

Figure 5–246. Gastric contents simulating sclerotic lesion of the rib.

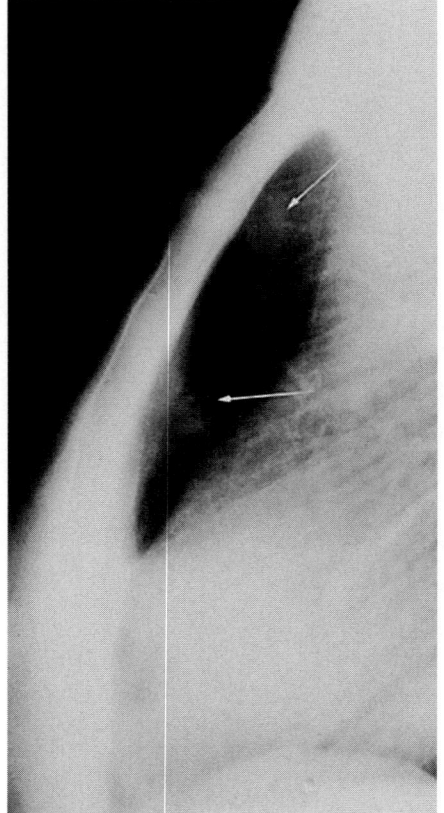

Figure 5–247. Anterior rib ends simulating nodular lesions in lung.

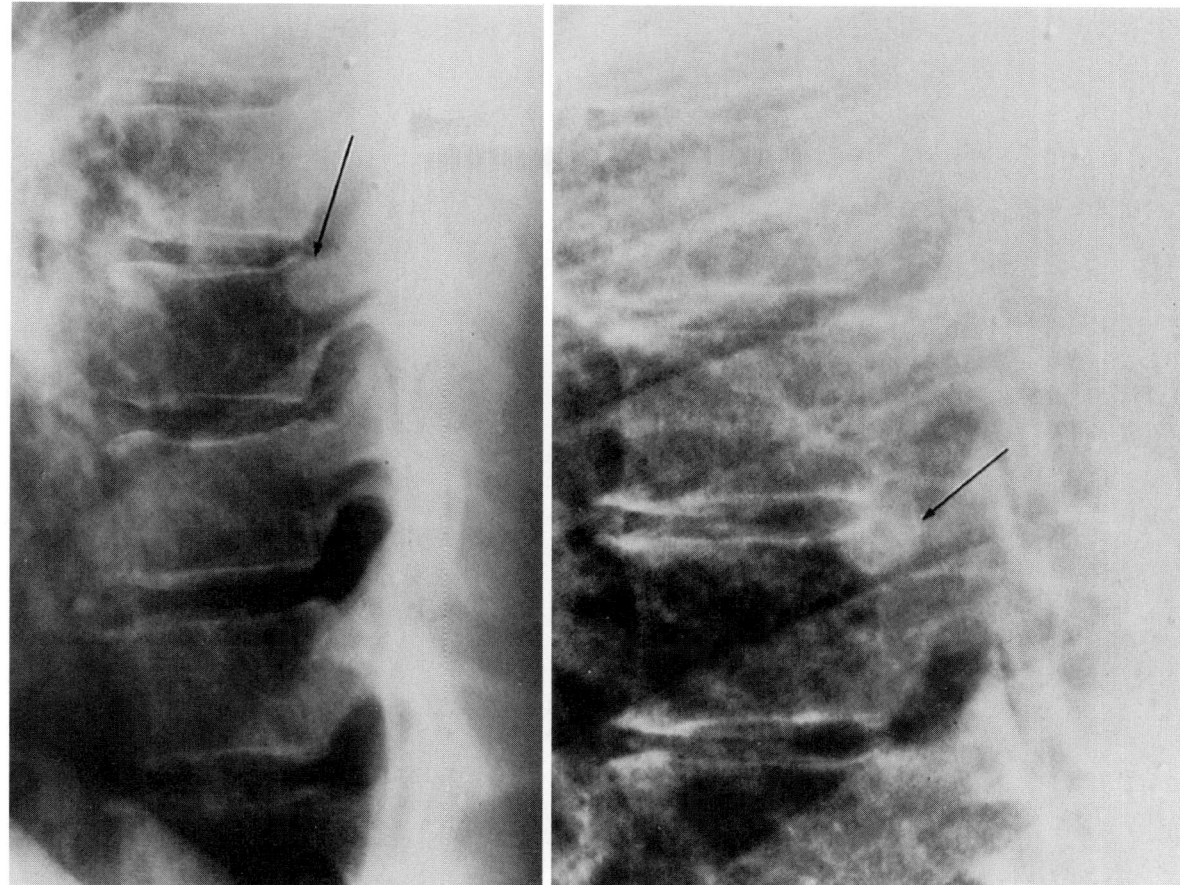

Figure 5–248. Two examples of the spinal transverse process simulating a pulmonary nodule. (Ref: Shortsleeve MJ, Foster SC: Pulmonary pseudonodule. *Radiology* 131:311, 1979.)

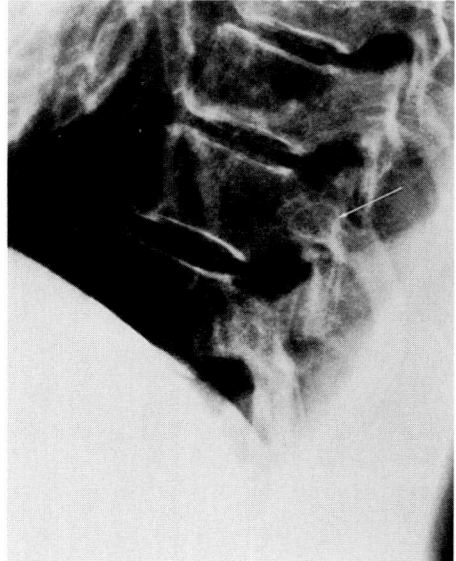

Figure 5–249. Transverse process in cross-section, simulating cavitary lung lesion.

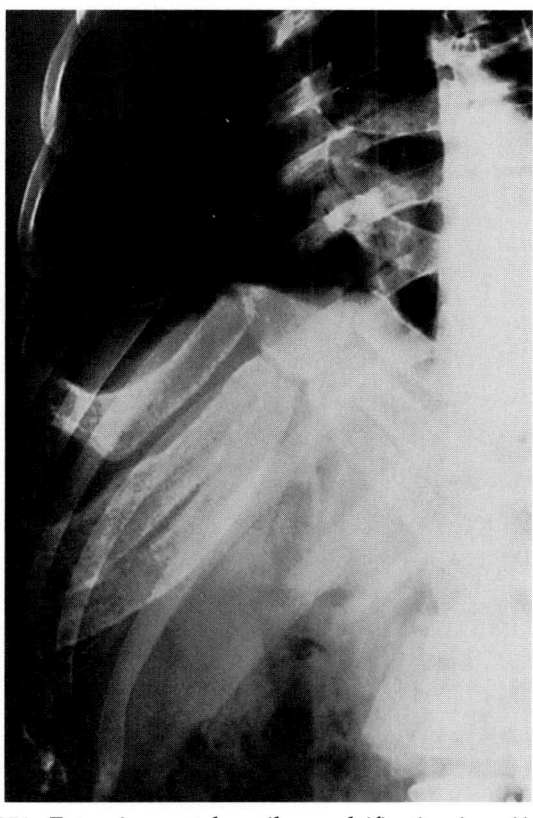

Figure 5–250. Extensive costal cartilage calcification in a 41-year-old man.

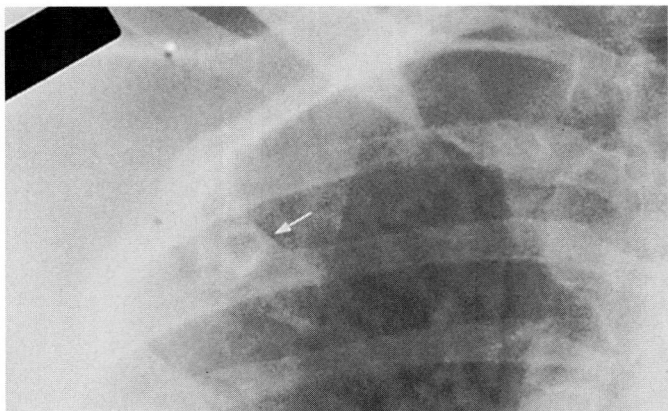

Figure 5–251. Ring-shaped costal cartilage calcification simulating cavitary lesion in lung.

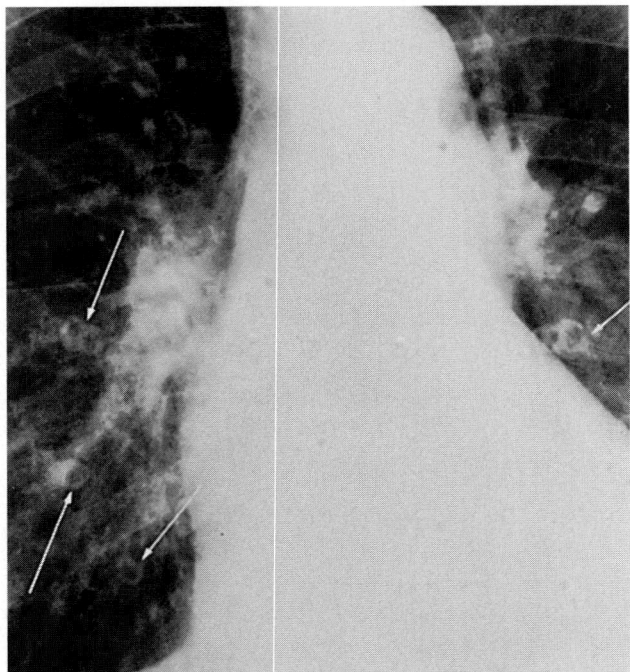

Figure 5–252. Circular costal cartilage calcification, suggesting cavitary lesions in lung.

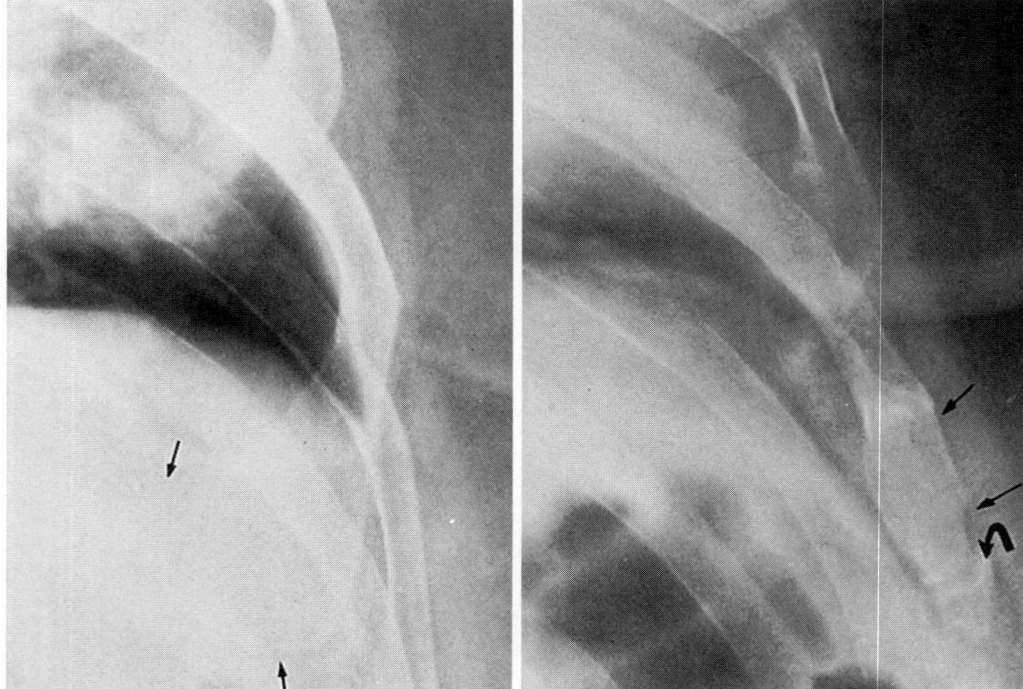

Figure 5–253. Calcified costal cartilage misinterpreted as a metastatic deposit. The cartilage is jointed (←). *Left,* Frontal projection. *Right,* Oblique projection.

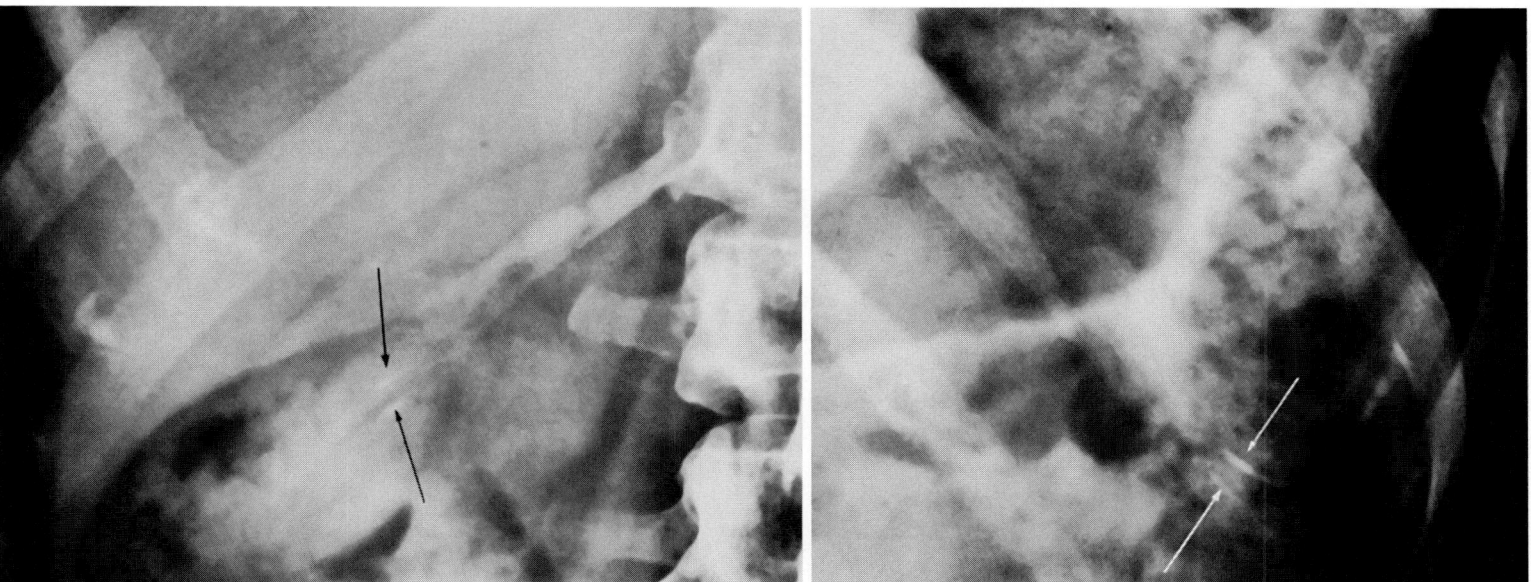

Figure 5–254. Costal cartilage calcification, simulating vascular calcification.

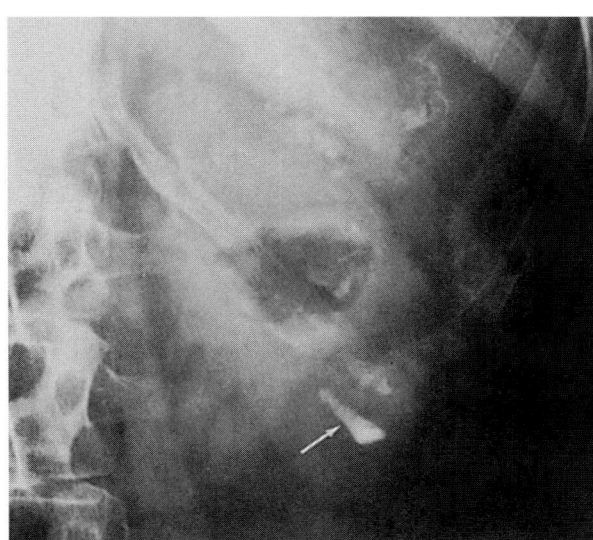

Figure 5–255. Linear costal cartilage calcification overlying the left kidney may be mistaken for a renal calculus.

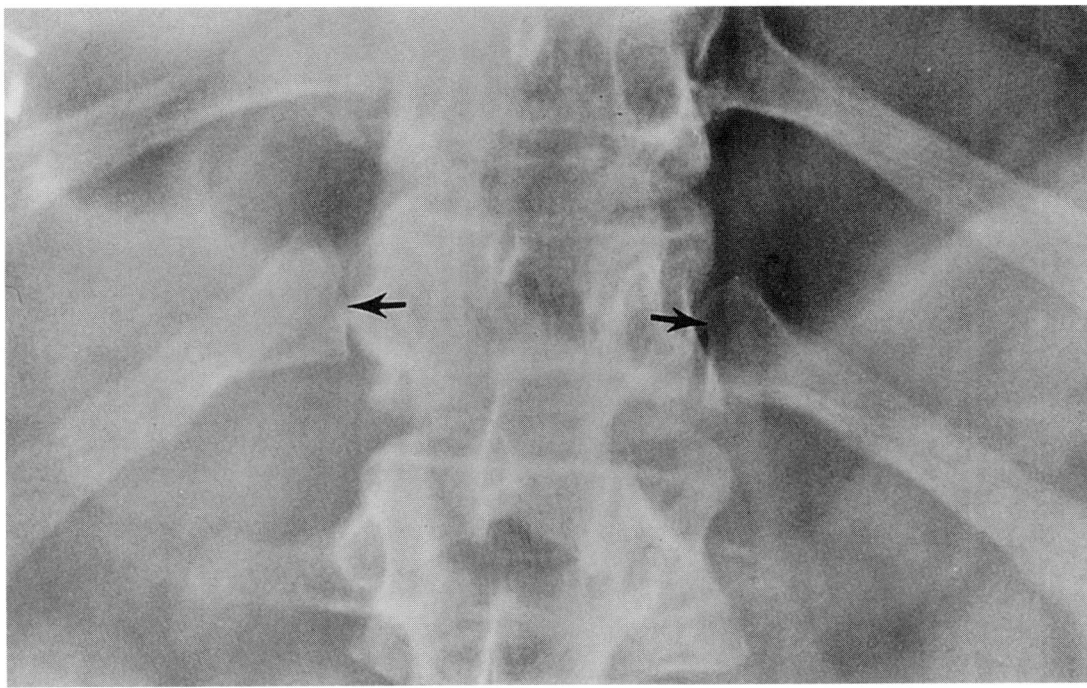

Figure 5–256. Simulated dislocations of the twelfth ribs by inability to visualize the transverse processes.

CHAPTER

6

The Upper Extremity

The Humerus

The Proximal Portion of the Humerus

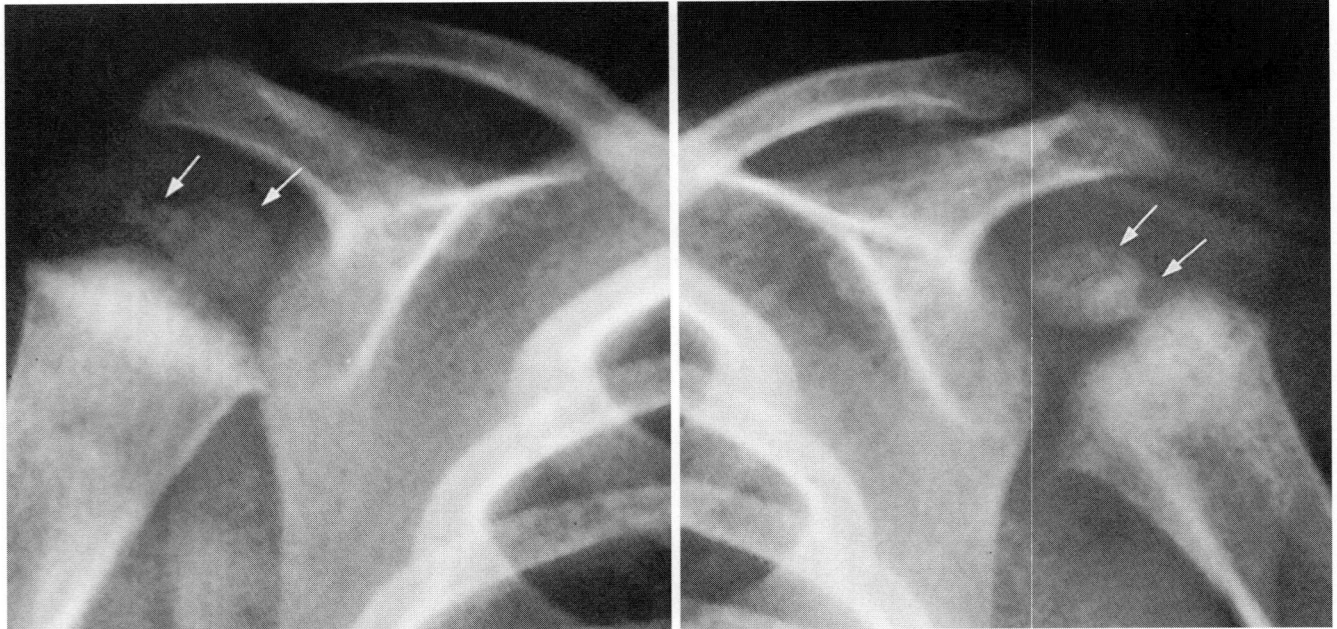

Figure 6–1. Bilateral duplicated capital humeral epiphyses in a 13-month-old child.

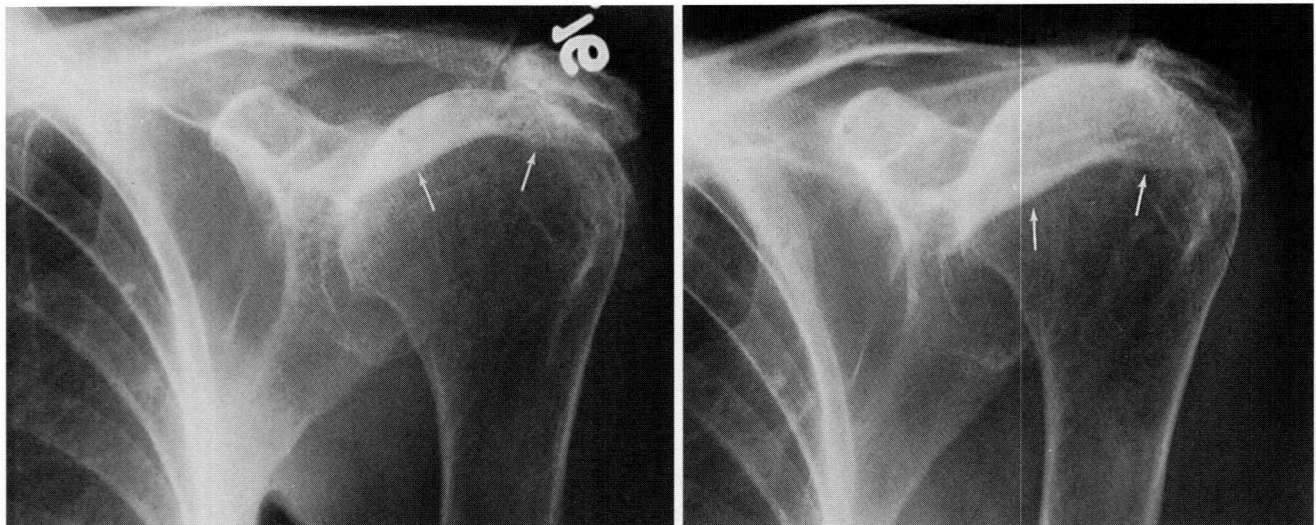

Figure 6–2. Simulated aseptic necrosis of the humeral head in an elderly patient, produced by overlapping of the shadows of the humeral head and scapula. Note variation in width of dense area with changes in position of the shoulder. This appearance is accentuated by rotator cuff tear.

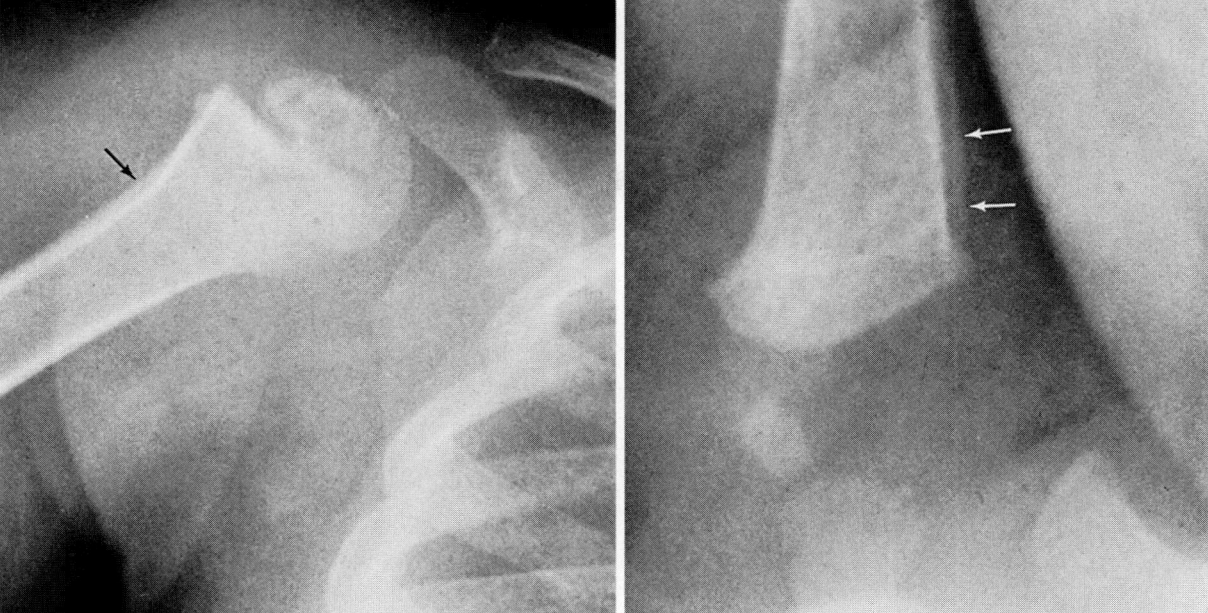

Figure 6–3. Two examples of simulated periostitis produced by the shadow of the bicipital groove in neonates, seen with the arm externally rotated or elevated.

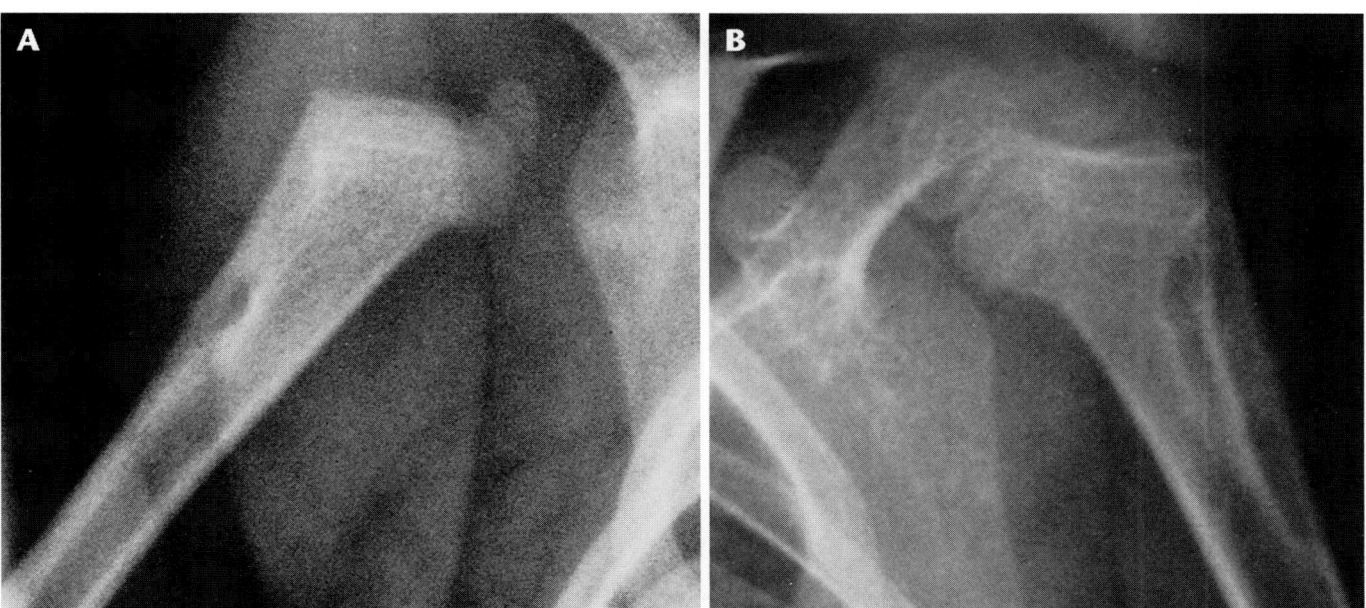

Figure 6–4. Deep bicipital grooves that may be mistaken for an abnormality. **A,** 7-month-old. **B,** 2-year-old.

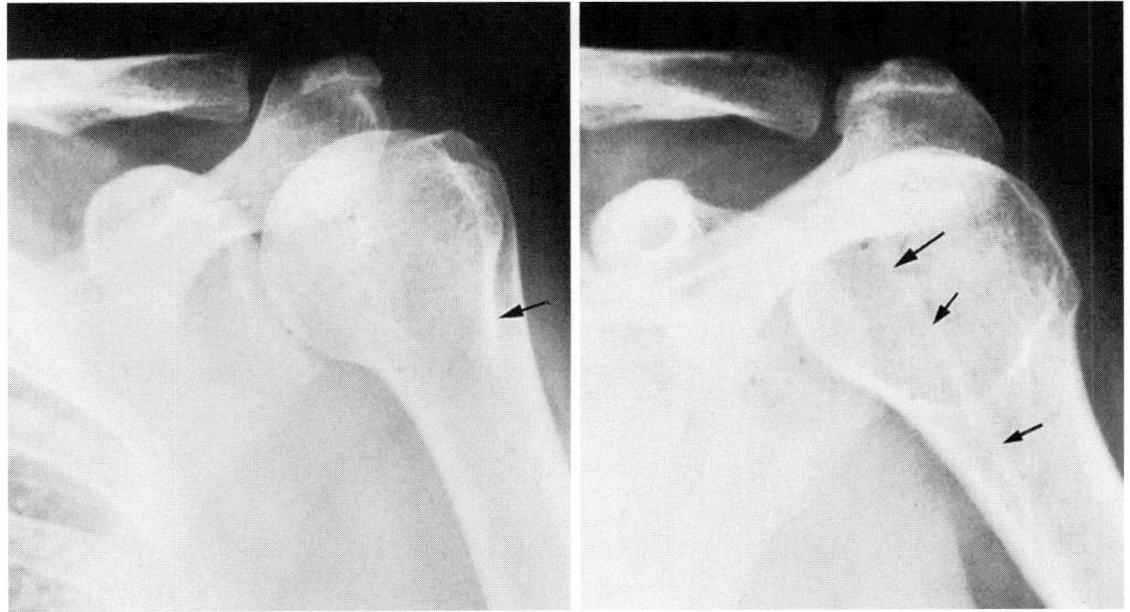

Figure 6–5. The shadows of the bicipital groove in an adult. *Left,* External rotation. *Right,* Internal rotation.

479

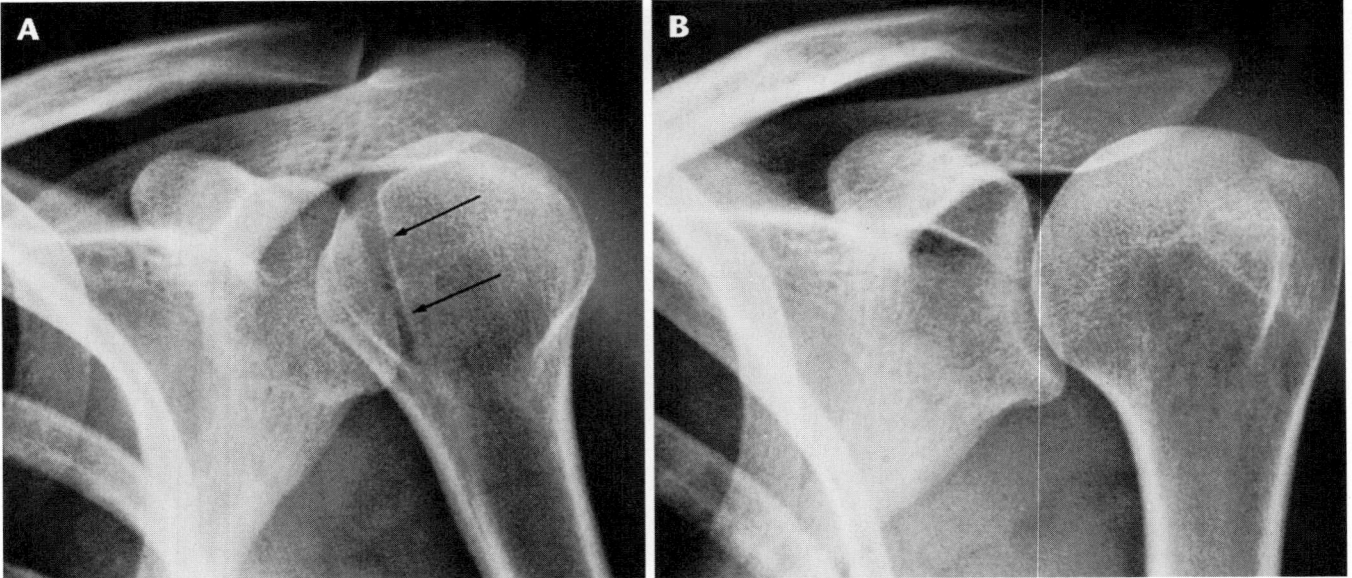

Figure 6–6. A, The bicipital groove in internal rotation should not be mistaken for an impaction fracture (trough sign). **B,** External rotation shows no abnormality.

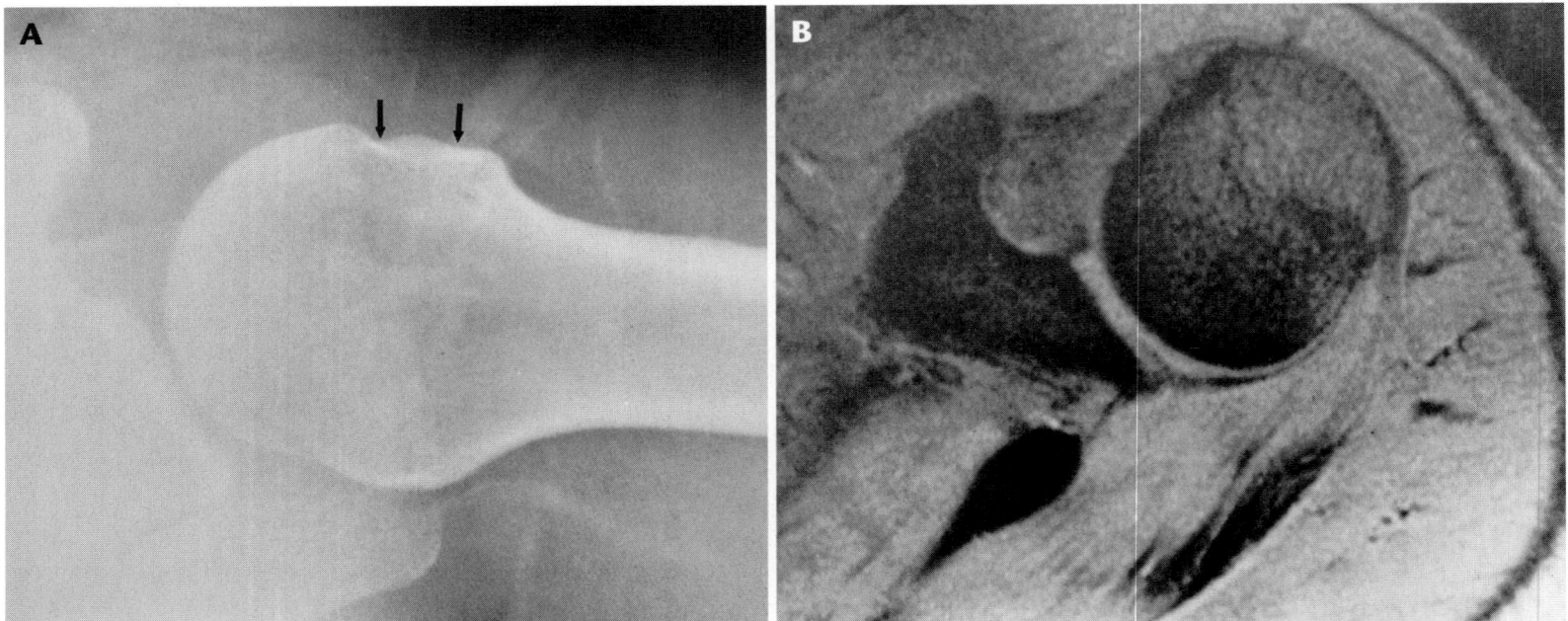

Figure 6–7. A, In the axillary projection, the anterior aspect of the humeral head may simulate a reverse Hill-Sach's impaction fracture. **B,** T-2–weighted MRI image shows no abnormality.

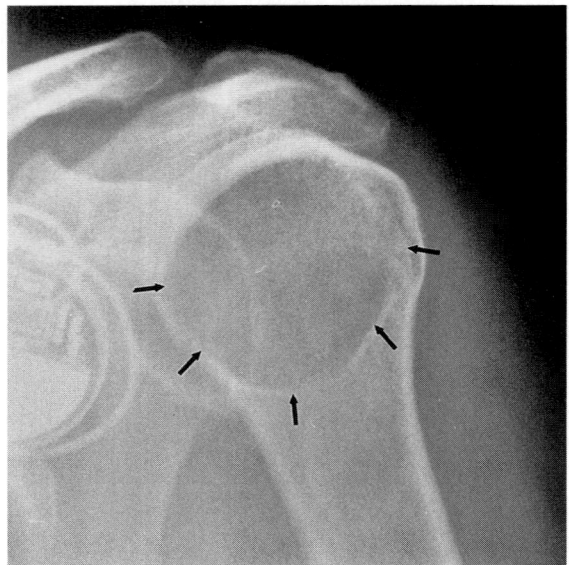

Figure 6–8. On internal rotation the humeral head may simulate a cystlike appearance.

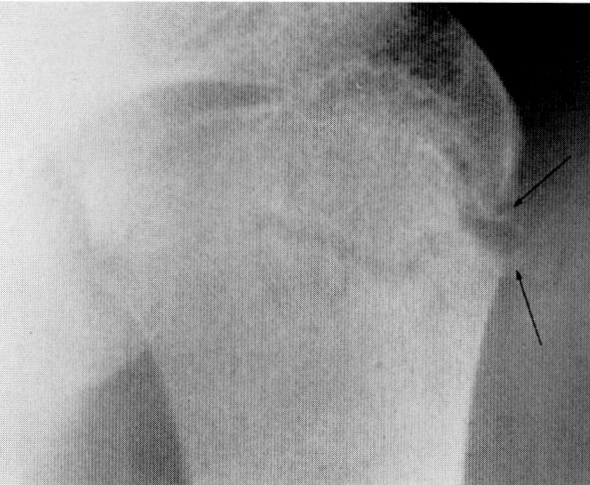

Figure 6–9. Beaking of the epiphyseal line in a 16-year-old boy. This beaking, particularly of the epiphysis, is seen elsewhere and should not be mistaken for an avulsion injury. (From Keats TE, Harrison RB: The epiphyseal spur. *Skeletal Radiol* 5:175, 1980.)

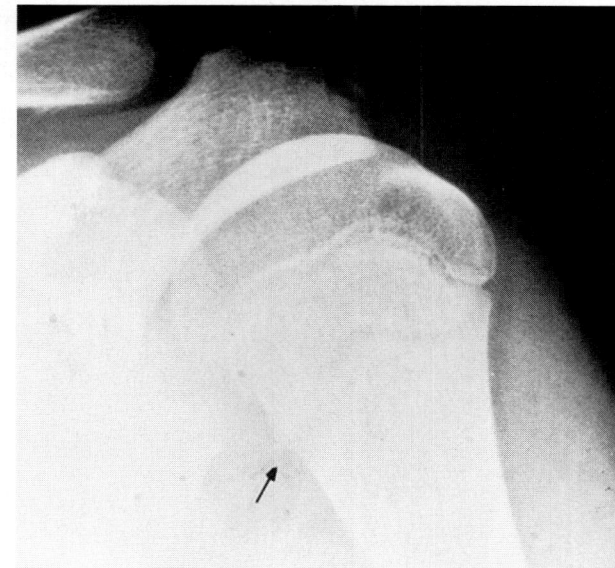

Figure 6–10. The lesser tuberosity in a 13-year-old boy seen in internal rotation.

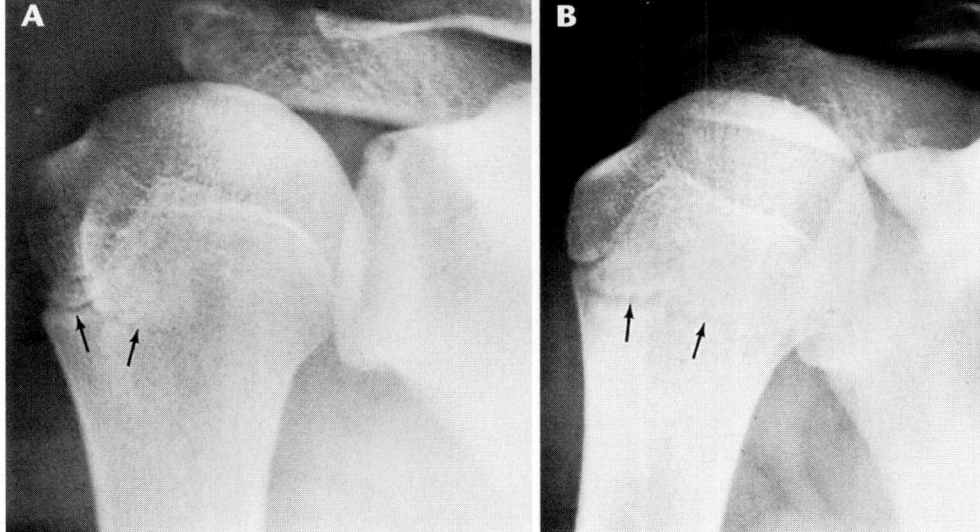

Figure 6–11. The normal epiphyseal lines of the proximal humerus in a 17-year-old boy. **A,** External rotation. **B,** Internal rotation. The epiphyseal line in **B** at times is mistaken for a fracture.

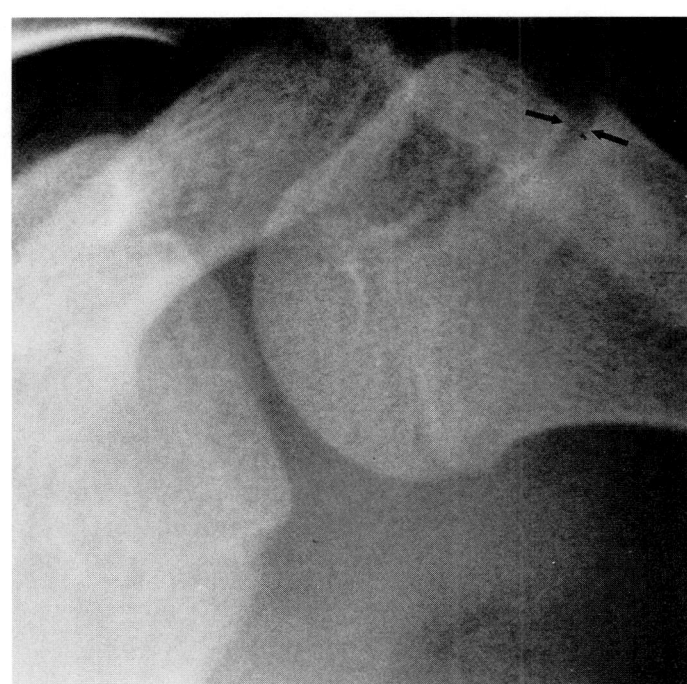

Figure 6–12. The lateral aspect of the epiphyseal line is normally quite wide and should not be mistaken for evidence of a fracture.

481

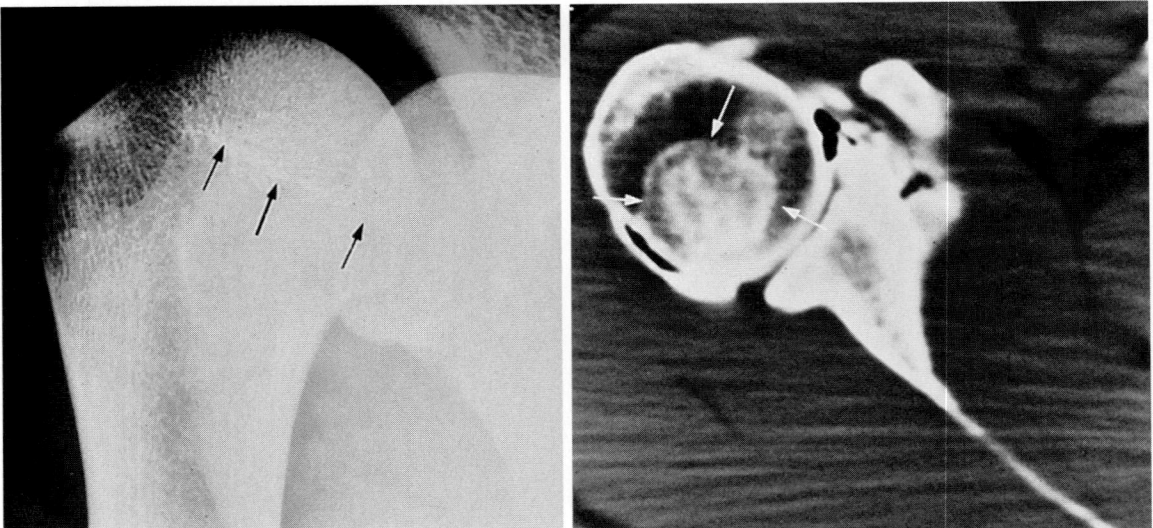

Figure 6–13. The closed epiphyseal line in an 18-year-old man simulates a lesion on CT.

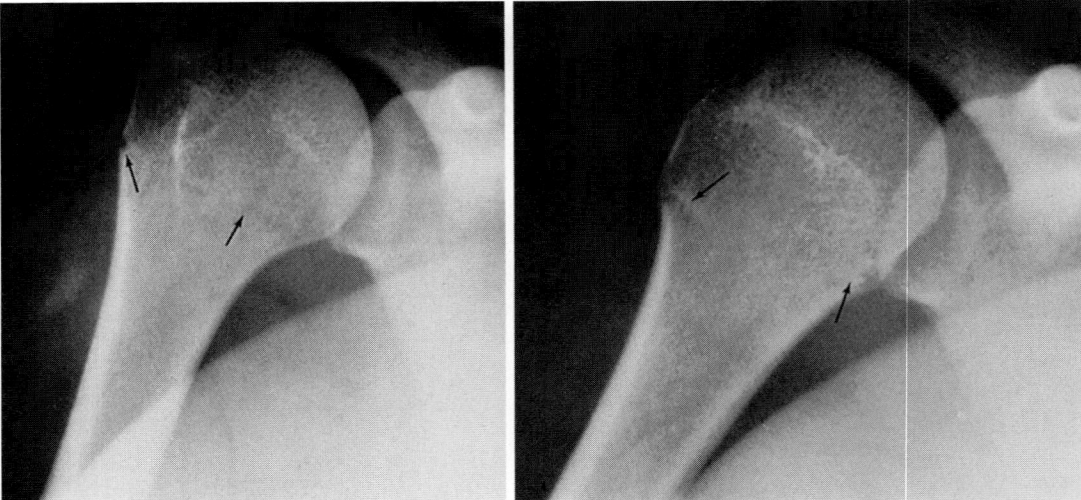

Figure 6–14. Residuals of the closing epiphyseal line in a 16-year-old boy.

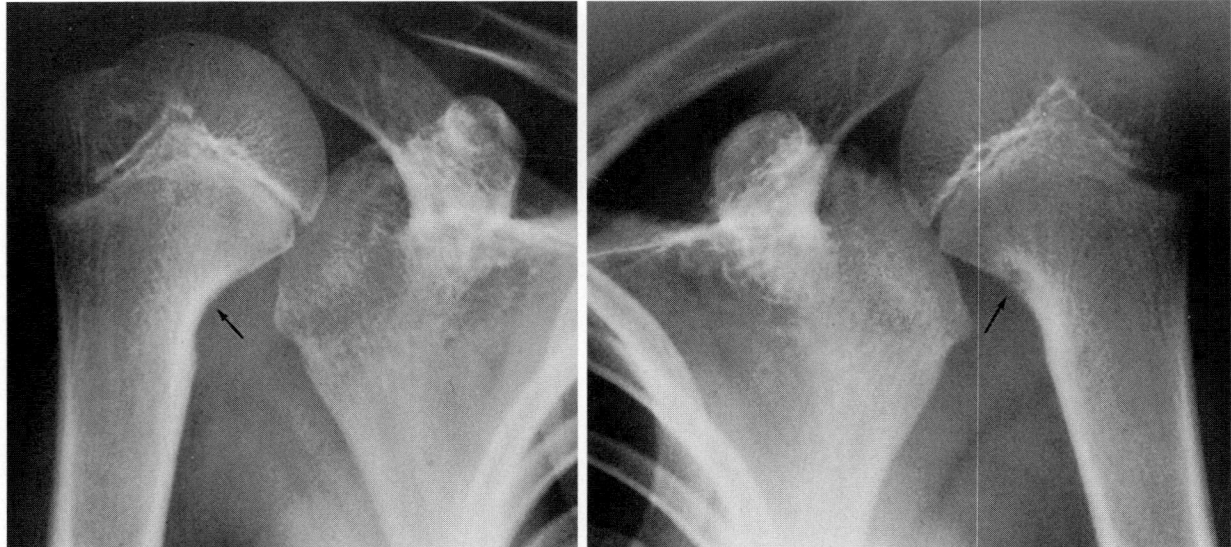

Figure 6–15. Bilateral upper humeral notches in an 11-year-old boy. These are seen in children between the ages of 10 and 16 years and represent a phase of growth. They are probably similar to the cortical lesions seen in the distal humerus, the distal end of the radius, the distal end of the femur, and the proximal end of the tibia. (Ref: Ozonoff MB, Zeiter FM Jr: The upper humeral notch: A normal variant in children. *Radiology* 113:669, 1974.)

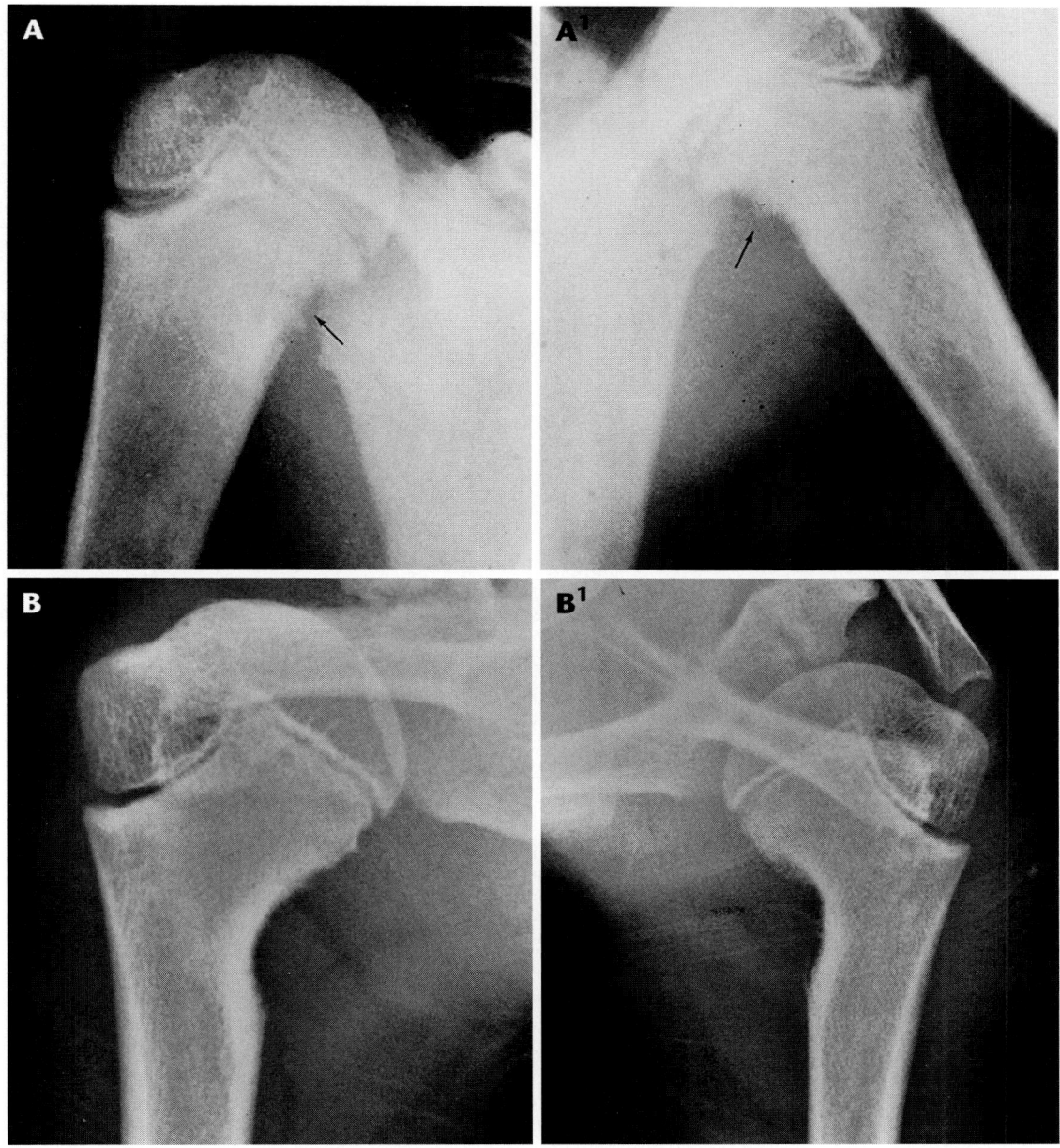

Figure 6–16. Other examples of upper humeral notches. **A** and **A¹**, 12-year-old boy. **B** and **B¹**, 12-year-old girl. Note how these variants may resemble the changes of malignancy.

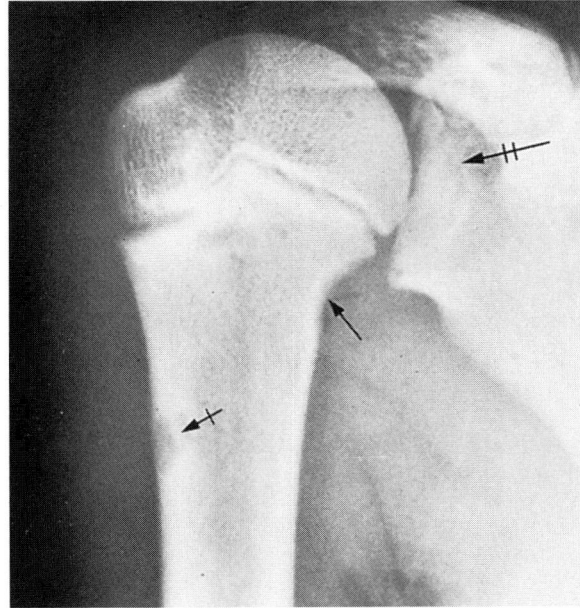

Figure 6–17. Upper humeral notch in a 13-year-old boy (←). Note also benign cortical defect (↔) and normal glenoid irregularities (↮).

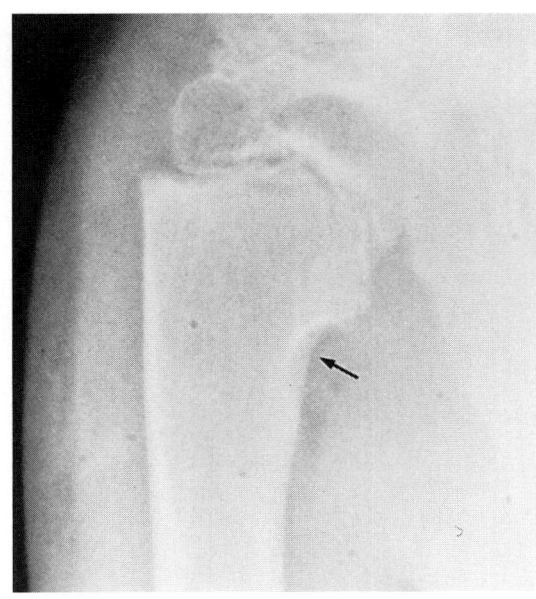

Figure 6–18. Very deep upper humeral notch in a 7-year-old boy.

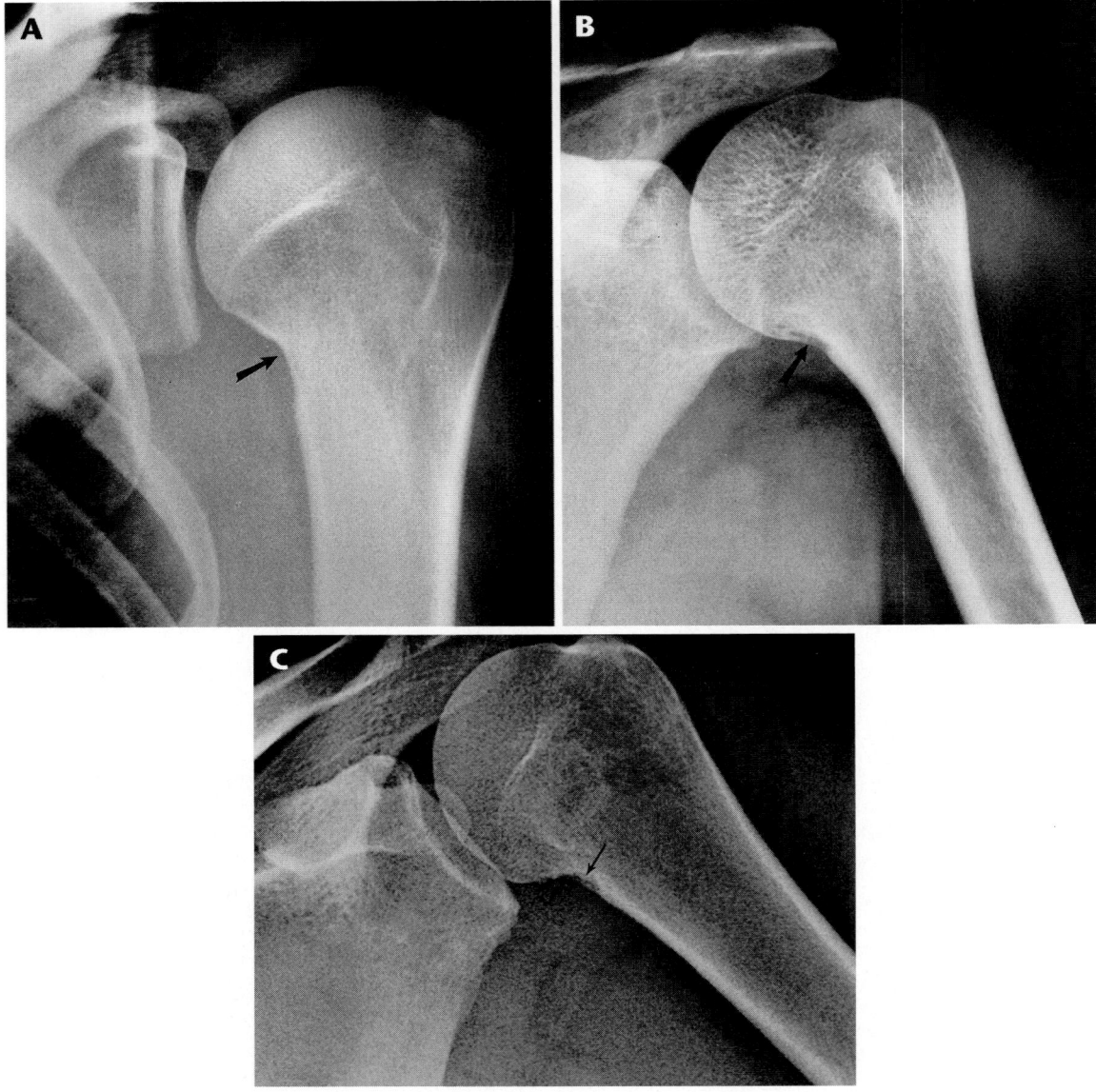

Figure 6–19. Residual upper humeral notches in adults. **A,** 28-year-old woman. **B,** 29-year-old woman. **C,** 35-year-old woman.

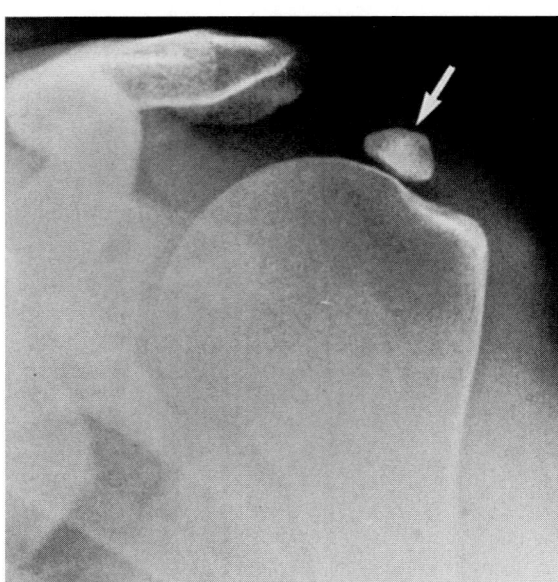

Figure 6–20. Unusual ossicle at the upper end of the humerus.

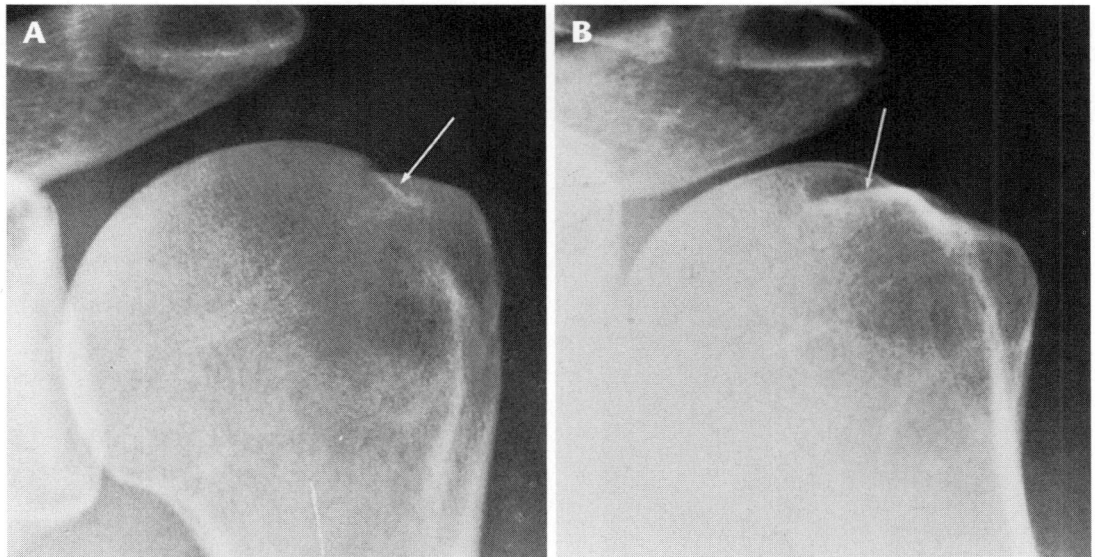

Figure 6–21. A, Simulated fracture of the greater tuberosity produced by positioning in external rotation. **B,** No fracture seen with internal rotation.

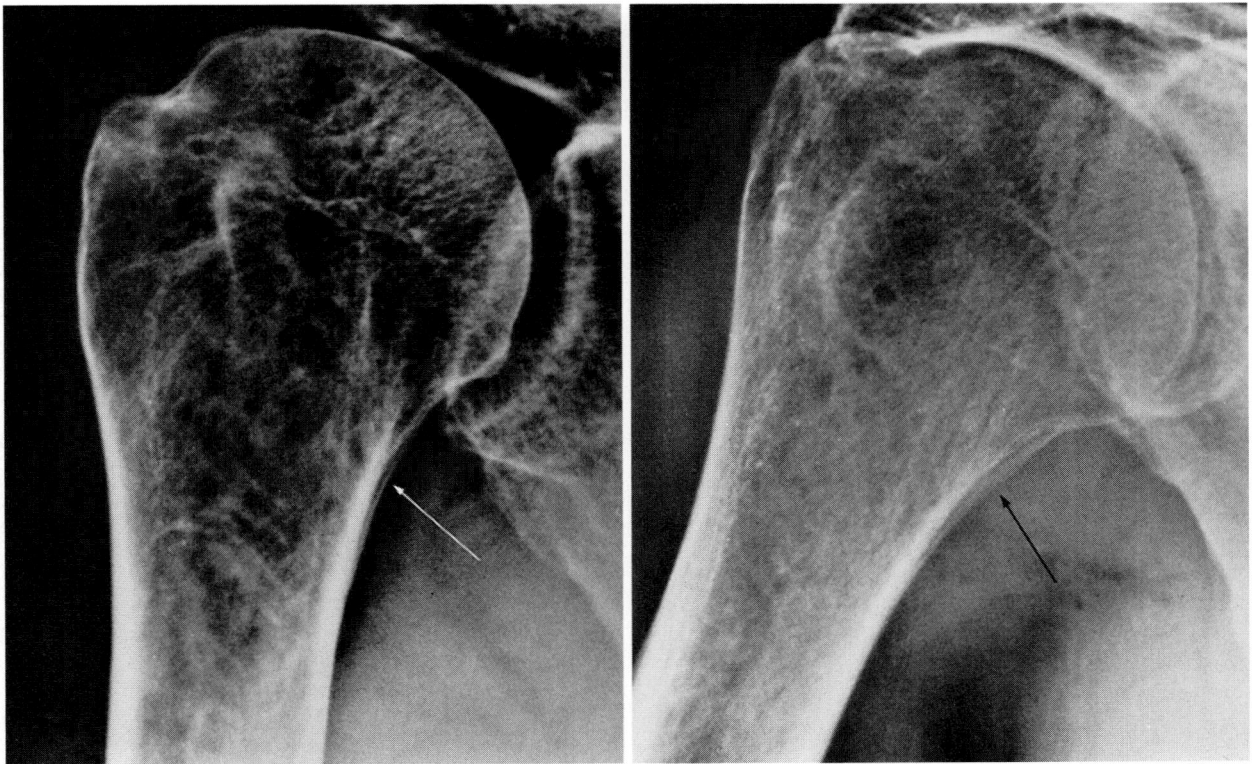

Figure 6–22. Two examples of how projection of the cortex of the humeral neck can simulate periostitis.

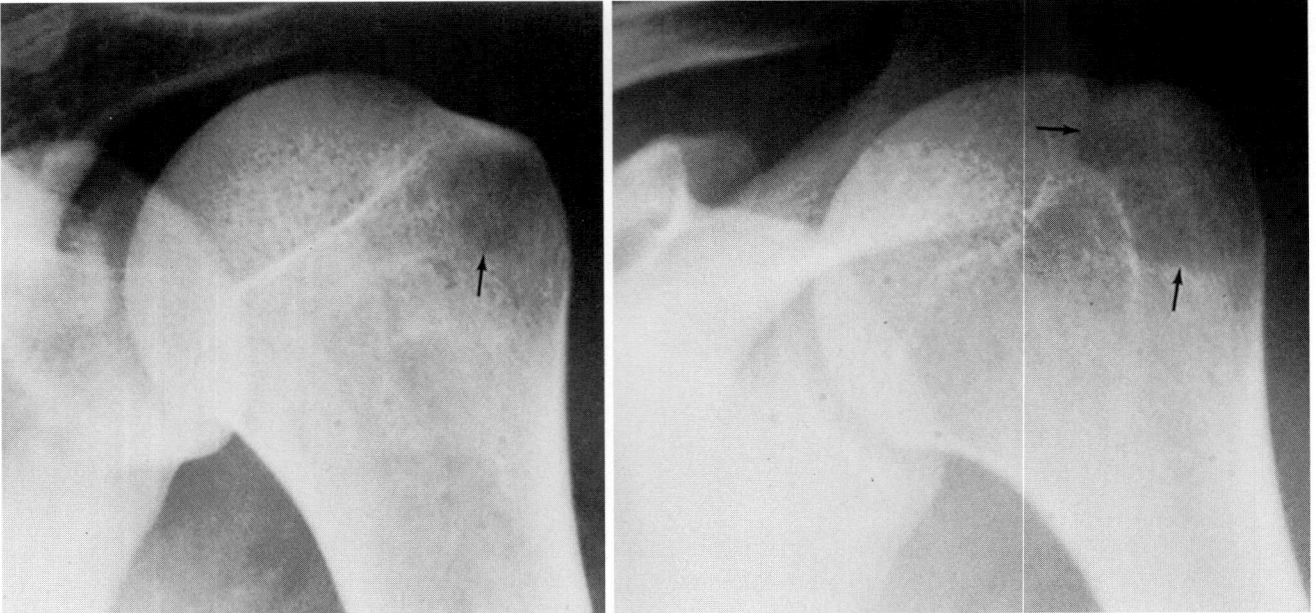

Figure 6–23. Examples of simulated destruction of the greater tuberosity. This appearance is the product of the lesser amount of cancellous bone present in this location. This is nicely demonstrated by MRI in the next figure. (Ref: Resnick D, Core RO: The nature of humeral pseudocysts. *Radiology* 150:27, 1984.)

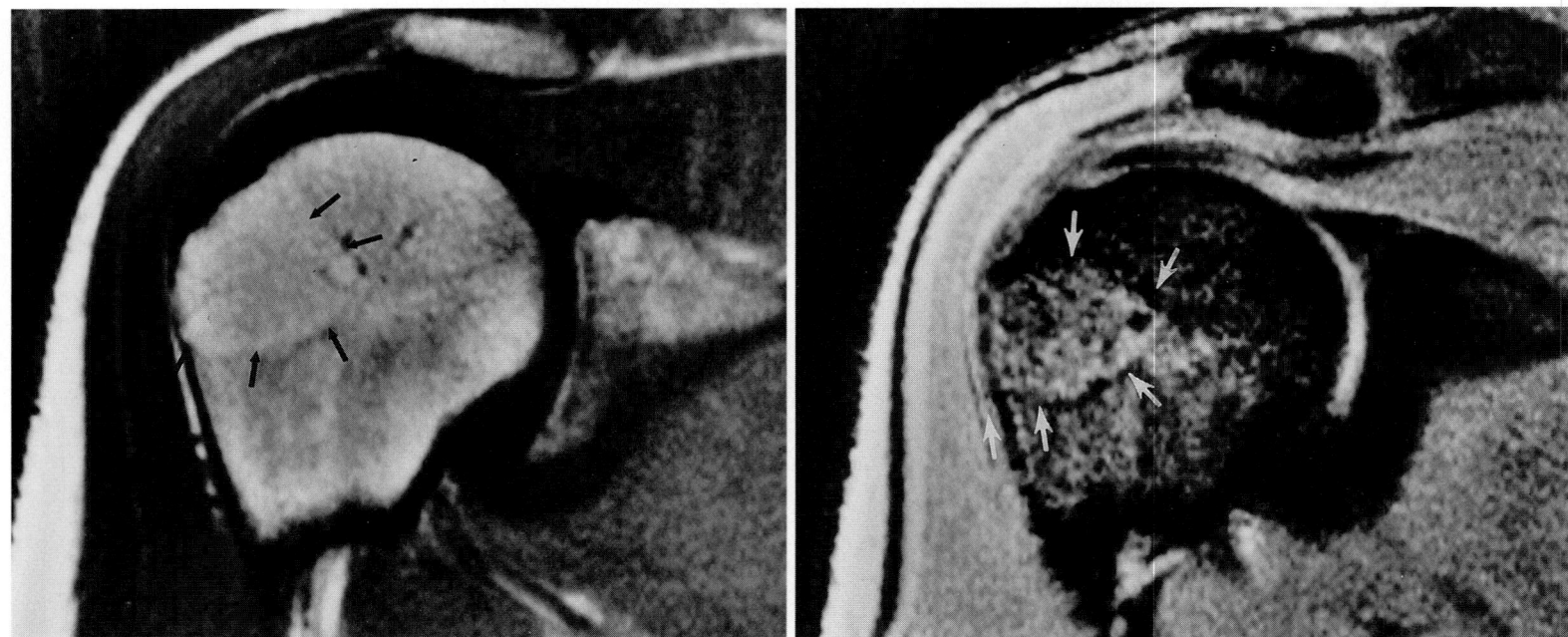

Figure 6–24. T-1– and gradient echo T-2–weighted images of the shoulder show the areas of cancellous bone in the greater tuberosity that result in the appearance shown in the preceding figure.

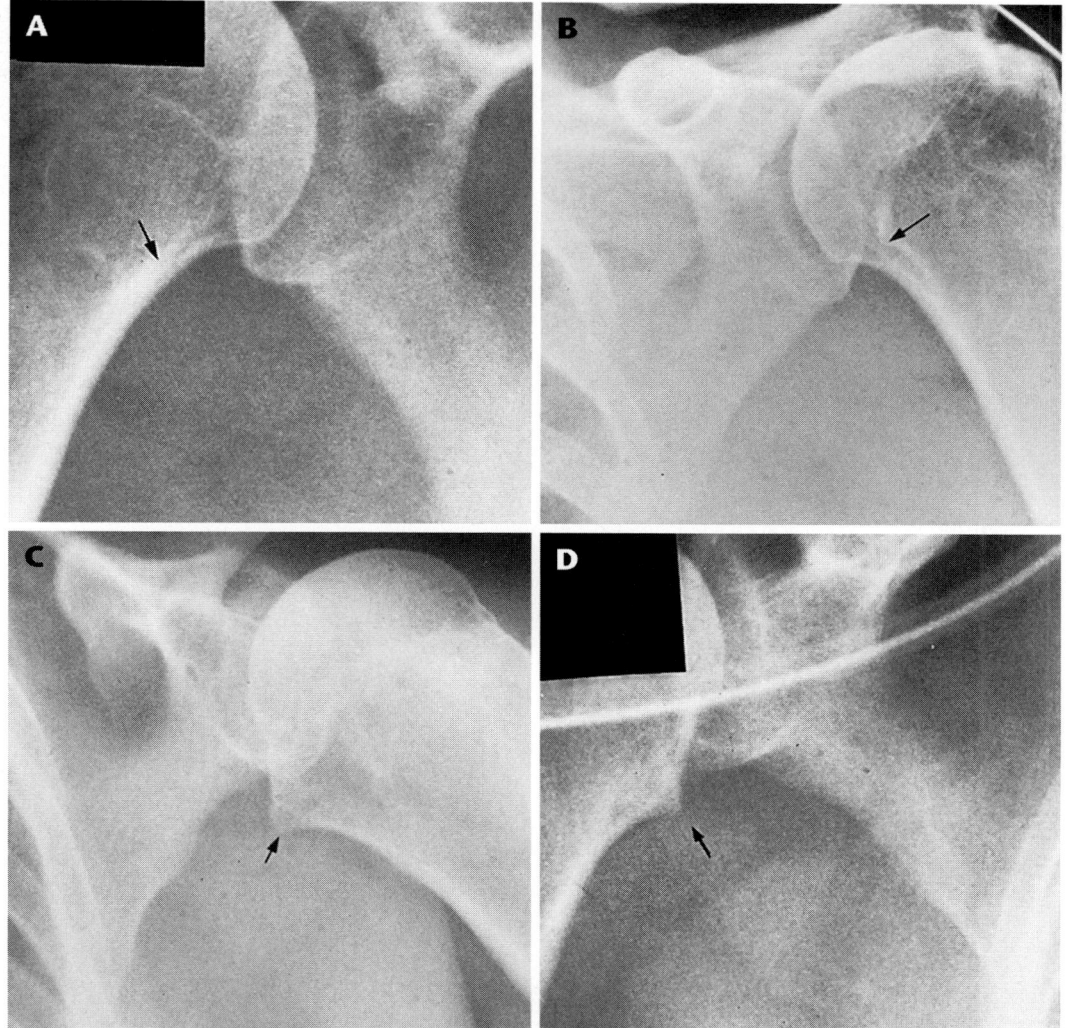

Figure 6–25. The lesser tuberosity seen in external rotation (**A** and **B**) and in internal rotation (**C** and **D**).

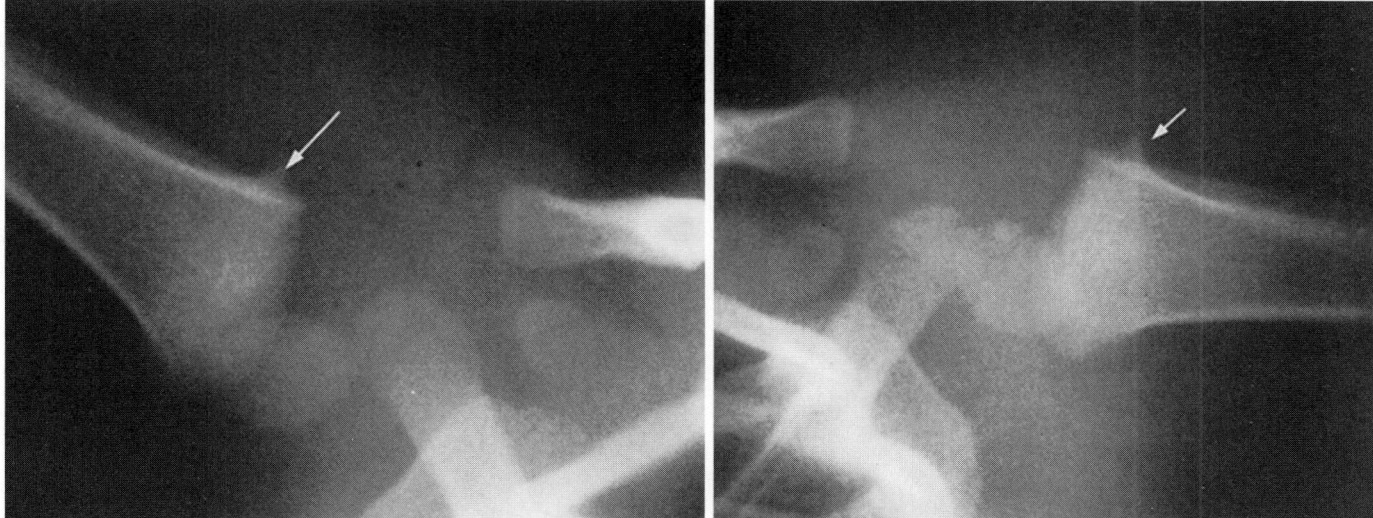

Figure 6–26. Metaphyseal spurs in a 19-month-old child. These are normal variants of growth.

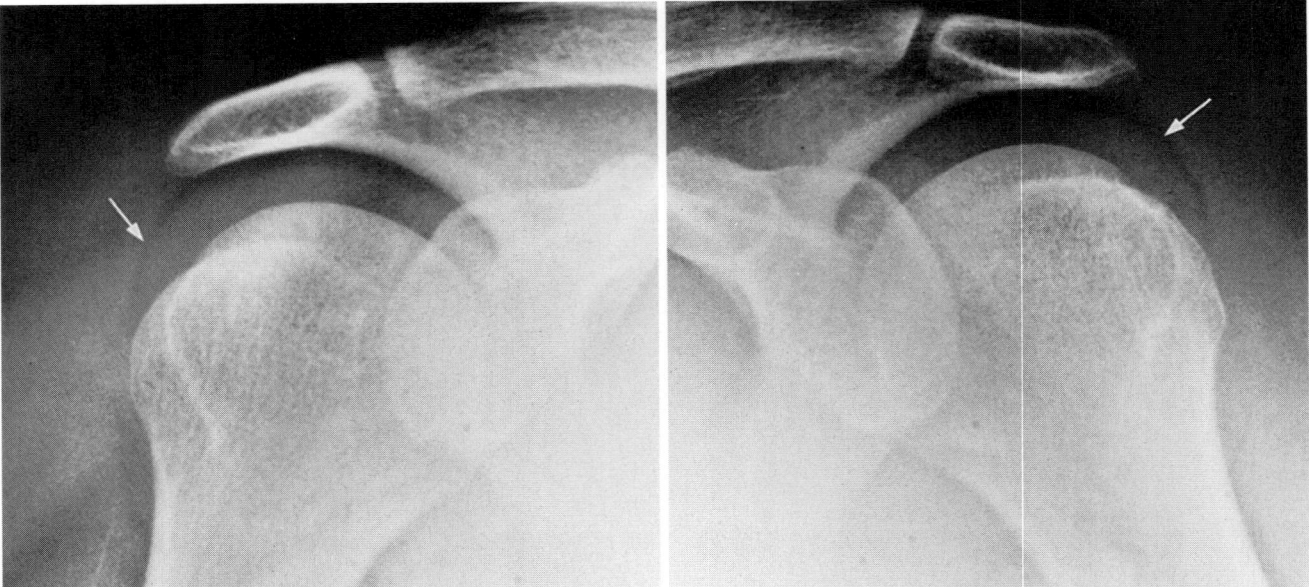

Figure 6–27. Bilateral visualization of the rotator cuff by surrounding fat in a 29-year-old man.

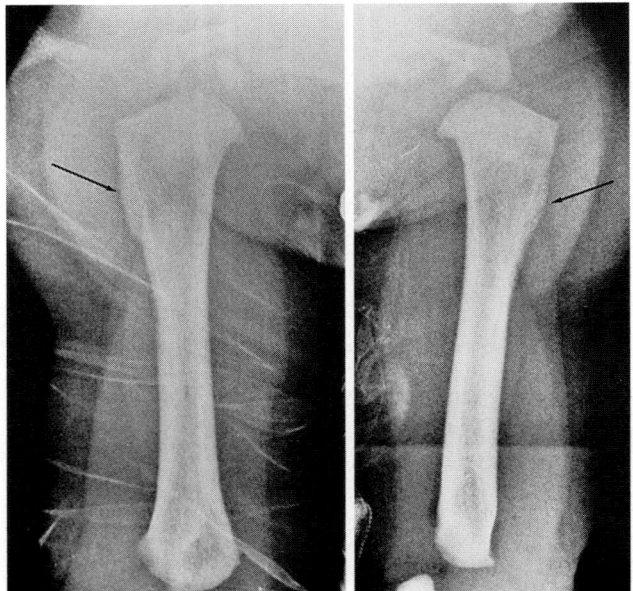

Figure 6–28. Cortical thickening underlying the deltoid muscle insertions in a 2-month-old child.

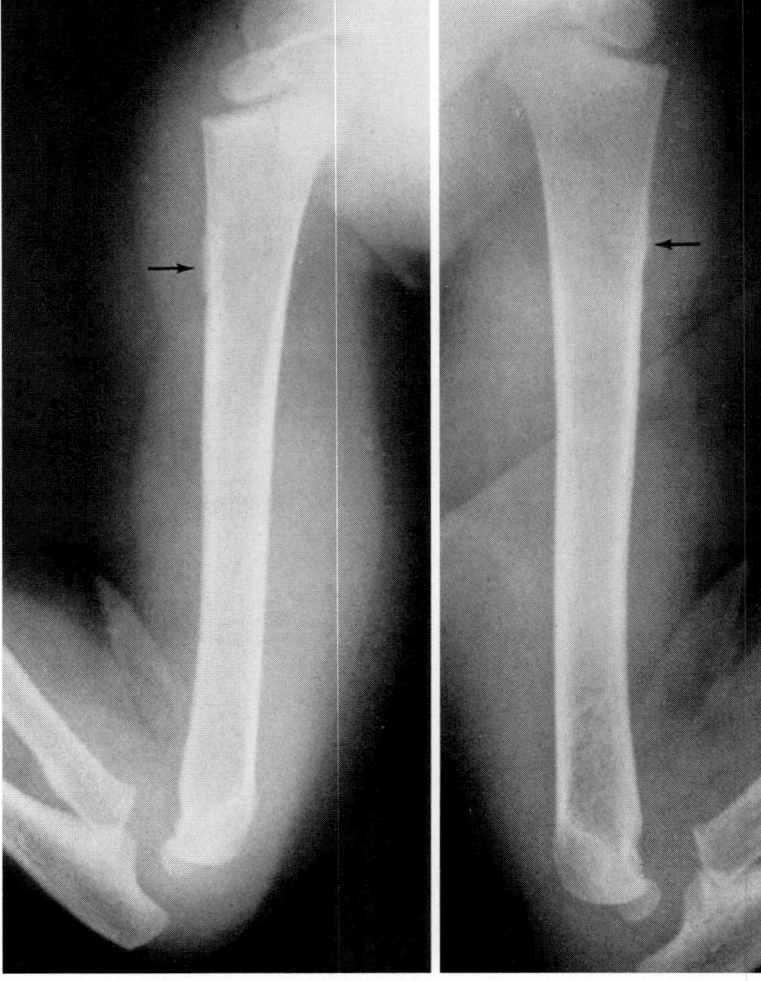

Figure 6–29. The insertion of the deltoid muscle in a 20-month-old child, which may simulate periostitis.

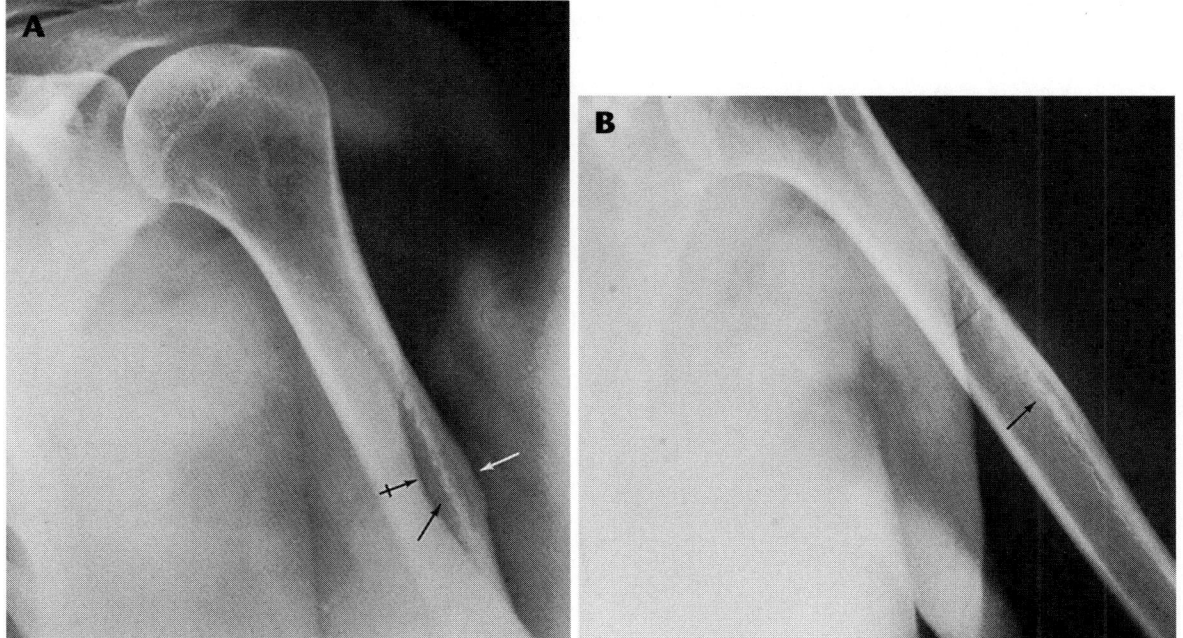

Figure 6–30. A, B, Prominent deltoid muscle insertion in two projections in a 50-year-old man (→). The medial shadow in **A** is a soft tissue fold (↦).

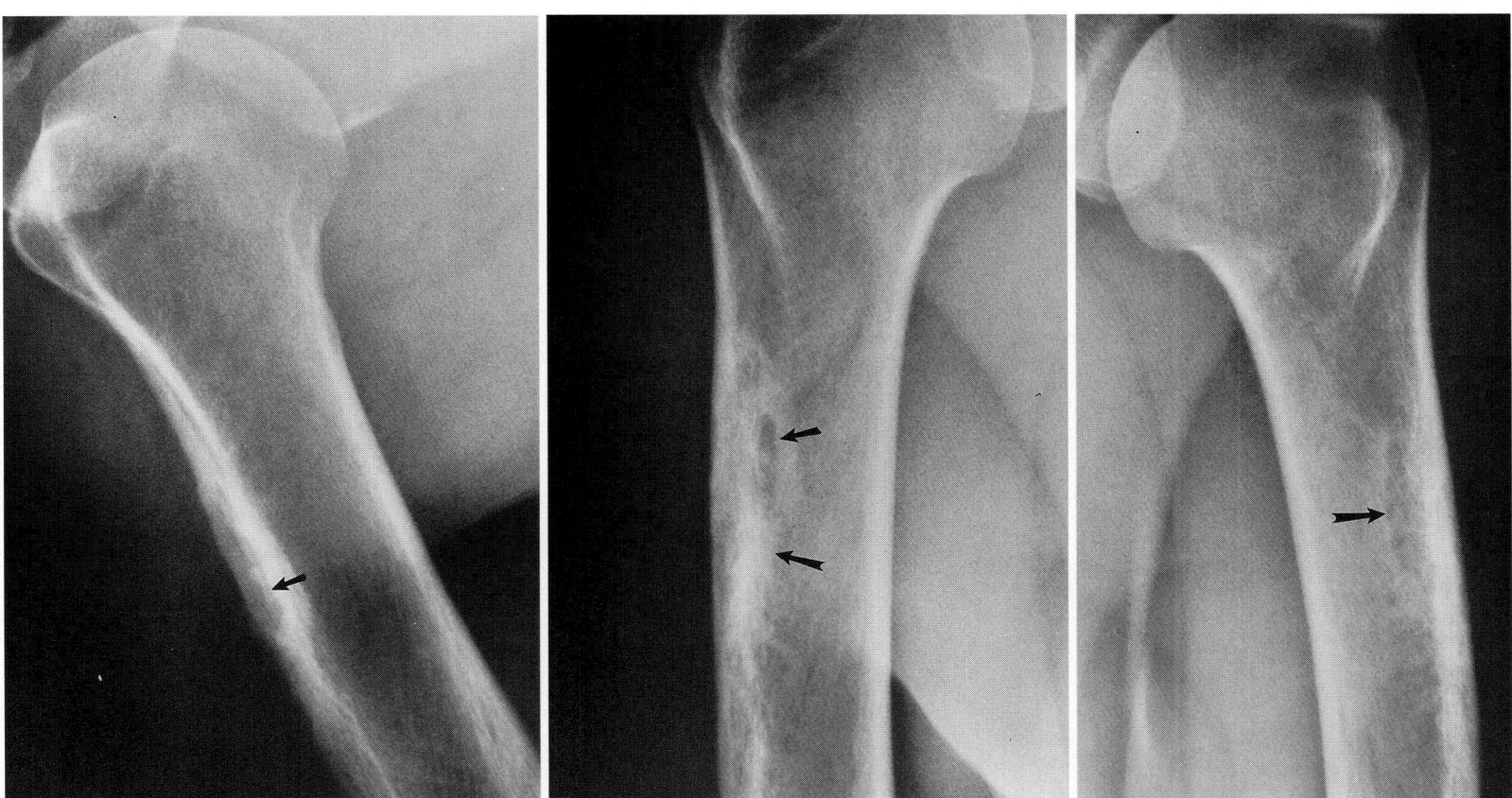

Figure 6–31. Unusually prominent deltoid muscle insertions seen bilaterally.

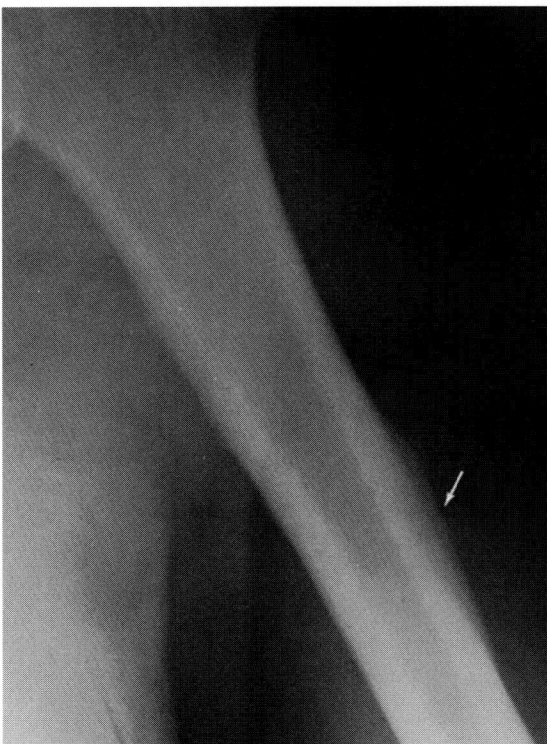

Figure 6–32. Deltoid muscle insertion that resembles periostitis.

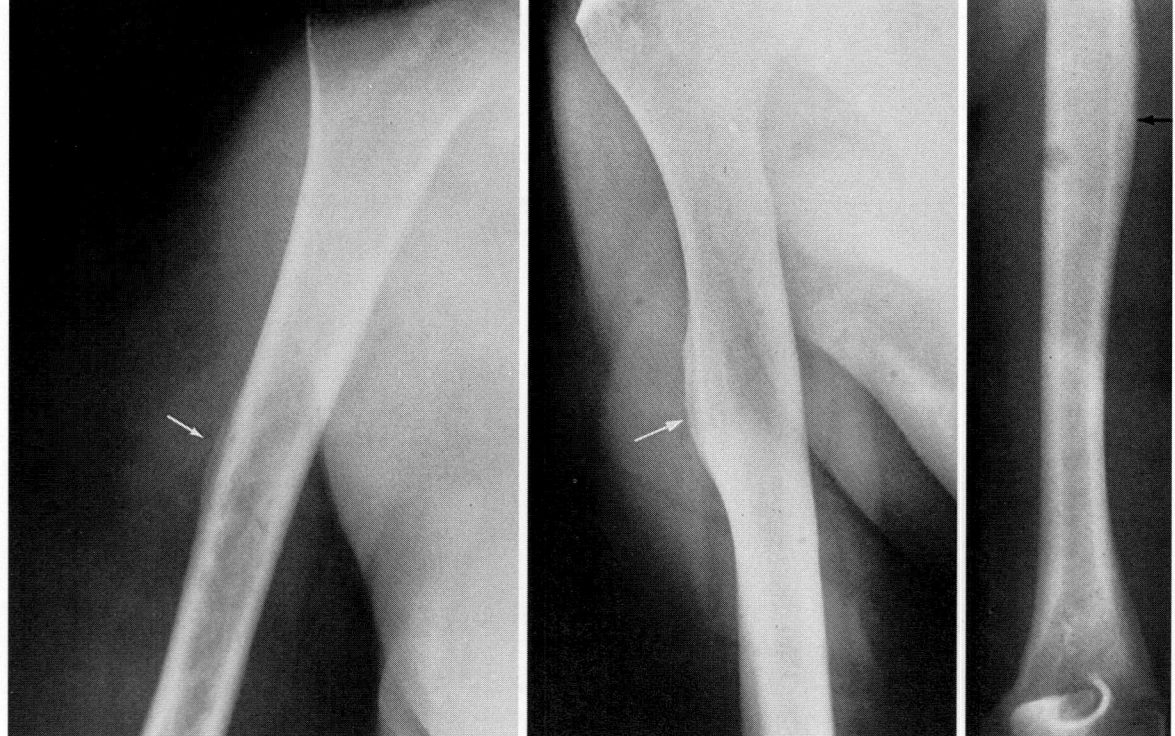

Figure 6–33. Localized cortical thickenings caused by a prominent deltoid muscle insertion.

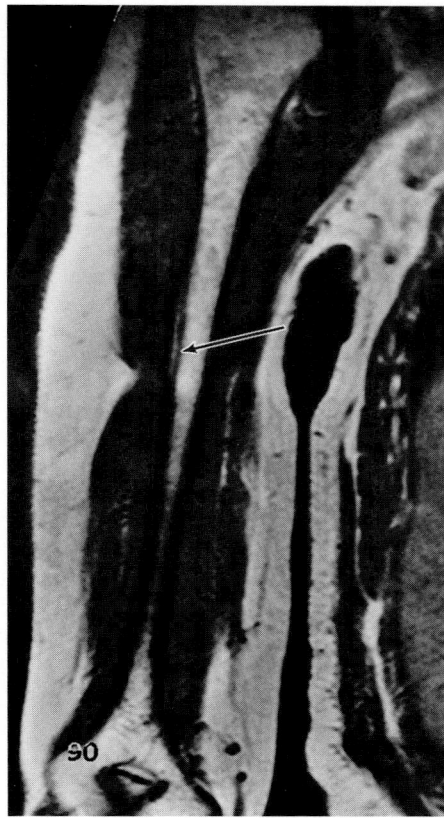

Figure 6–34. The deltoid insertion by T-1–weighted MRI.

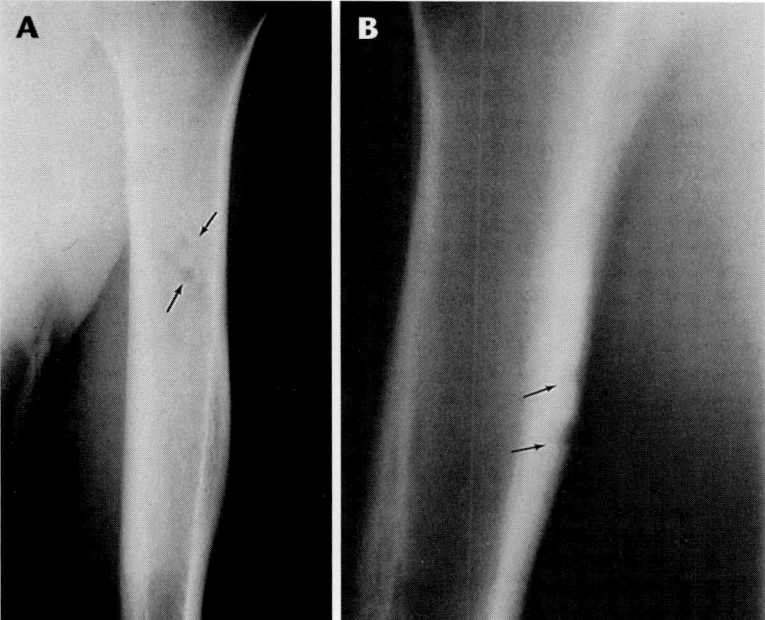

Figure 6–35. Radiolucencies produced by the insertion of the pectoralis major muscle. **A,** Plain film. **B,** Tomogram. (From Brower AC: Cortical defect of the humerus at the insertion of the pectoralis major. *Am J Roentgenol* 128:677, 1977.)

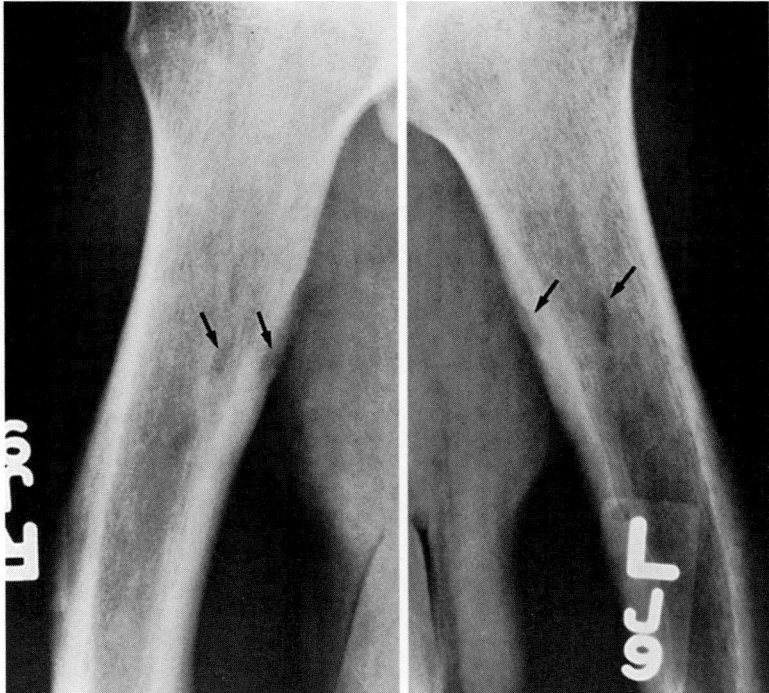

Figure 6–36. The same entity as in Figure 6–35 seen bilaterally in a heavily muscled 19-year-old man.

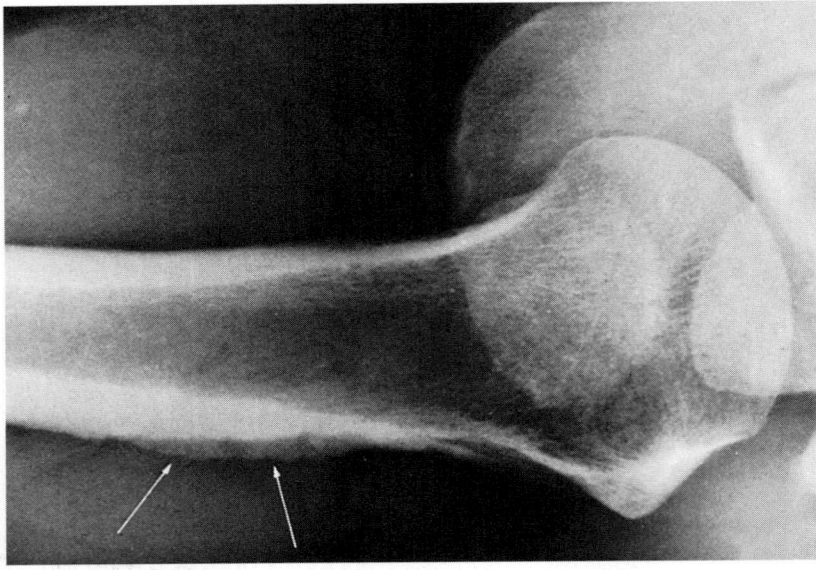

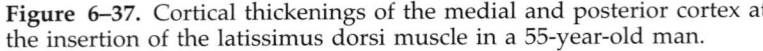

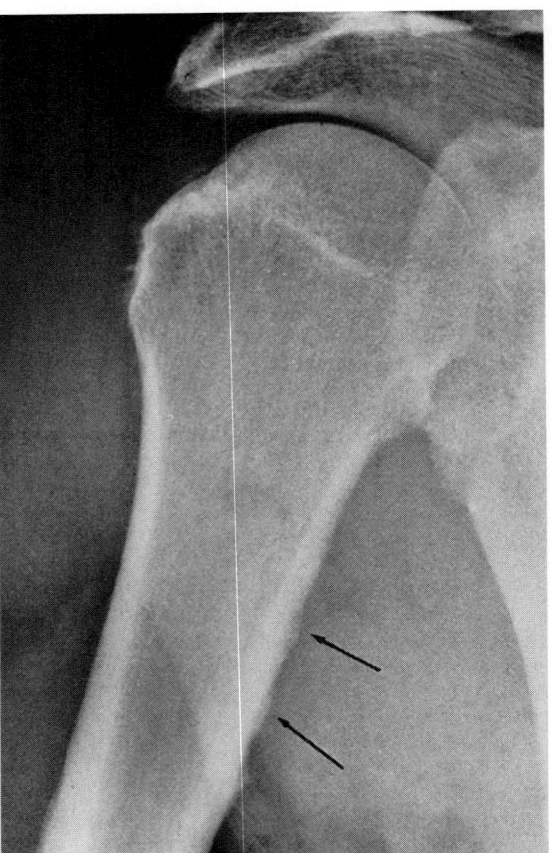

Figure 6–37. Cortical thickenings of the medial and posterior cortex at the insertion of the latissimus dorsi muscle in a 55-year-old man.

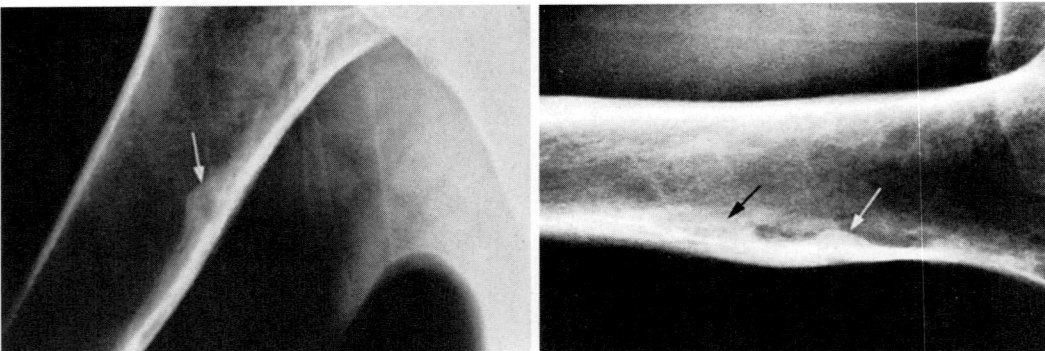

Figure 6–38. Latissimus dorsi muscle insertions in a 68-year-old man with endocortical thickenings.

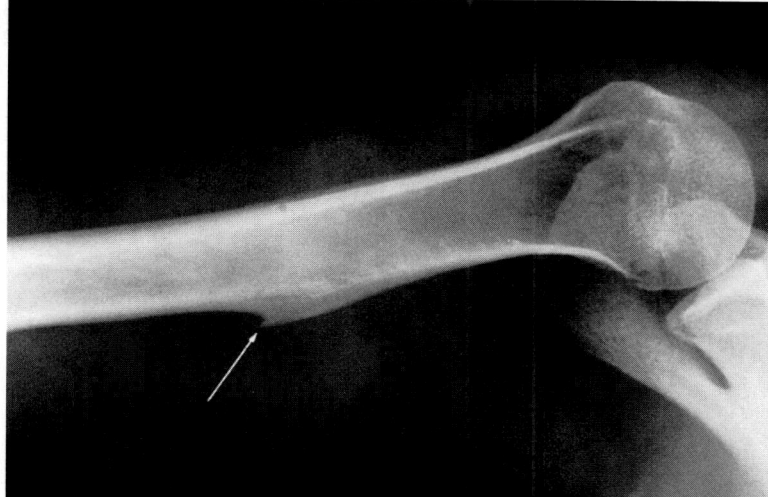

Figure 6–39. Spurlike insertion of the latissimus dorsi muscle.

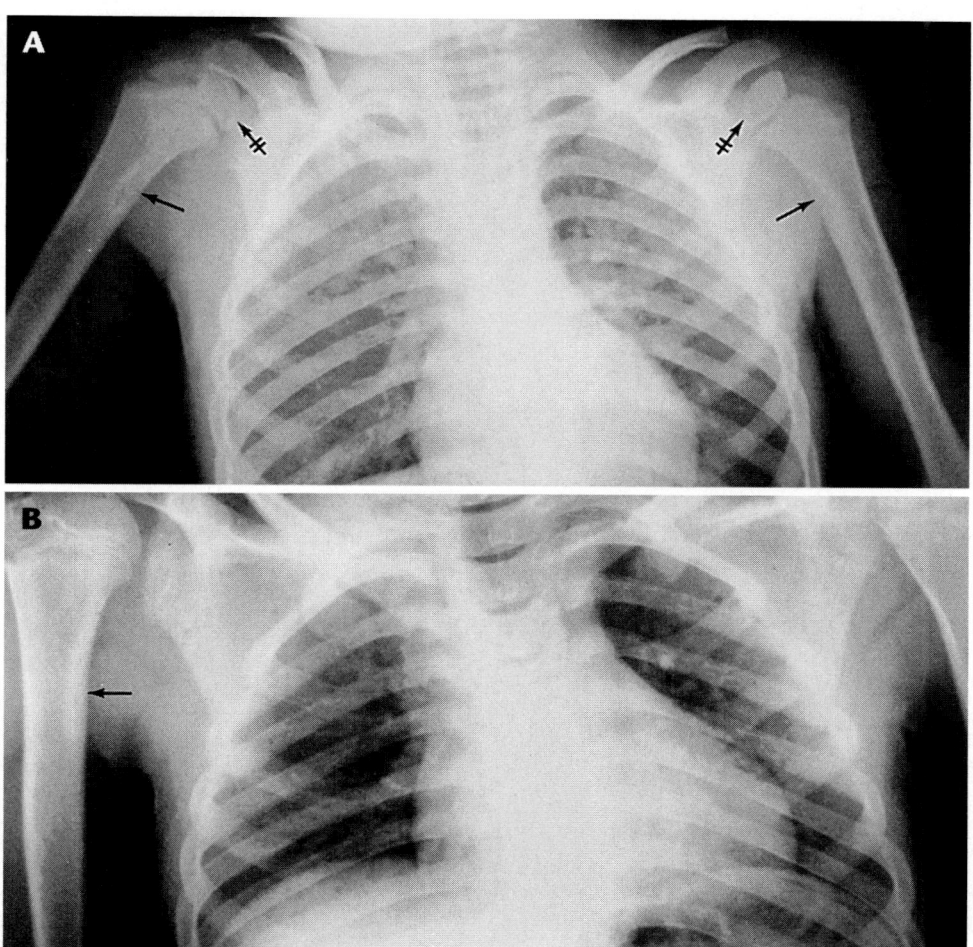

Figure 6–40. A, Benign cortical defects of the humerus in a 4-year-old child (←). Note also the location and appearance of the ossification centers for the greater tuberosity and head of the humerus at this age (⊣). **B,** 5 years later the cortical defect in the left humerus has disappeared; that on the right has left a sclerotic scar.

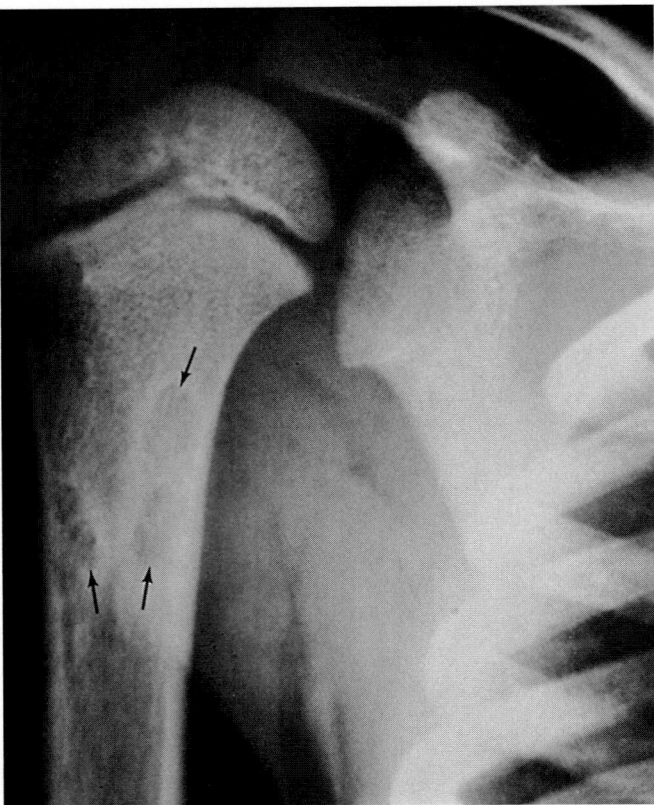

Figure 6–41. Multiple benign cortical defects of the proximal humerus. These fibrous lesions may be single or multiple and are of no clinical significance. (Ref: Caffey J: *Pediatric x-ray diagnosis*, 8th ed., Chicago, Mosby, 1985, p. 446.)

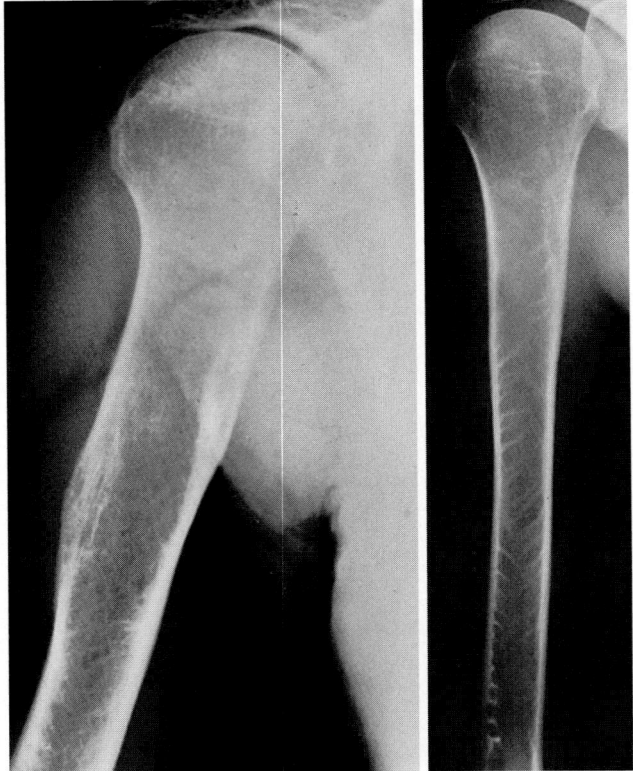

Figure 6–42. Two examples of "herringbone" trabecular pattern of the medullary cavity of the humerus.

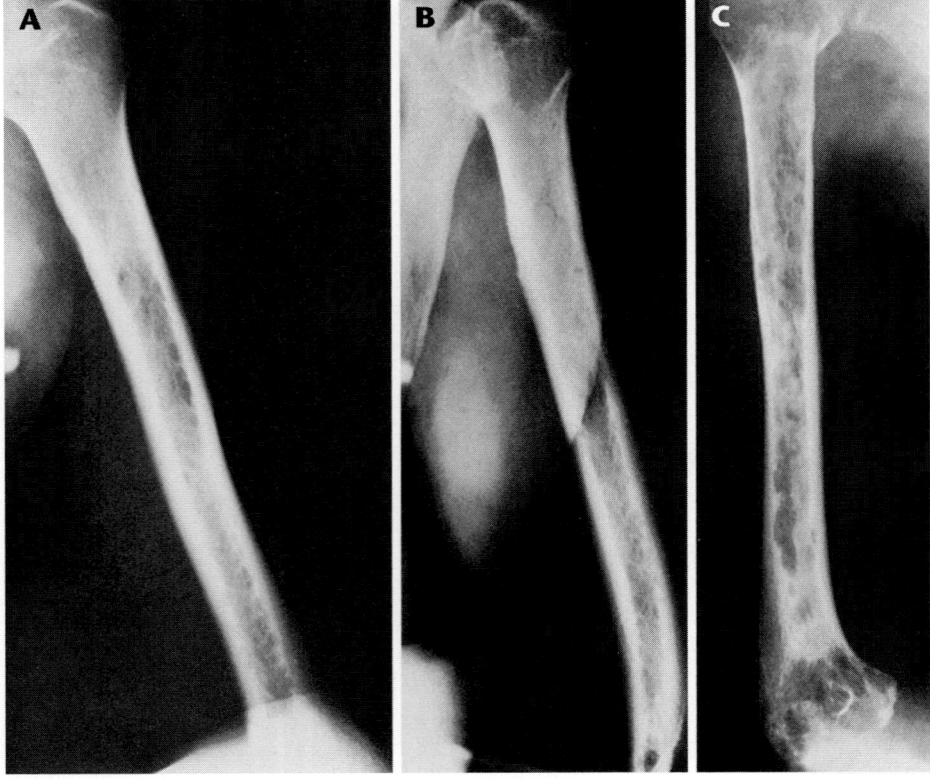

Figure 6–43. A and **B**, 26-year-old woman with "herringbone" medullary pattern of her left humerus. **C,** Her right humerus 2 weeks after casting for a fracture of the surgical neck. Note the peculiar type of deossification, which occurs in patients with this type of medullary trabecular pattern and resembles metastatic neoplasm or multiple myeloma. (Ref: Keats TE, Harrison RB: A pattern of posttraumatic demineralization of bone simulating permeative neoplastic replacement. *Skeletal Radiol* 3:113, 1978.) On close inspection this type of aggressive osteoporosis will show small cortical lucencies that will help differentiate it from malignant neoplastic permeation. (Ref: Helms CA, Munk PL: Pseudopermeative skeletal lesions. *Br J Radiol* 63:461, 1990.)

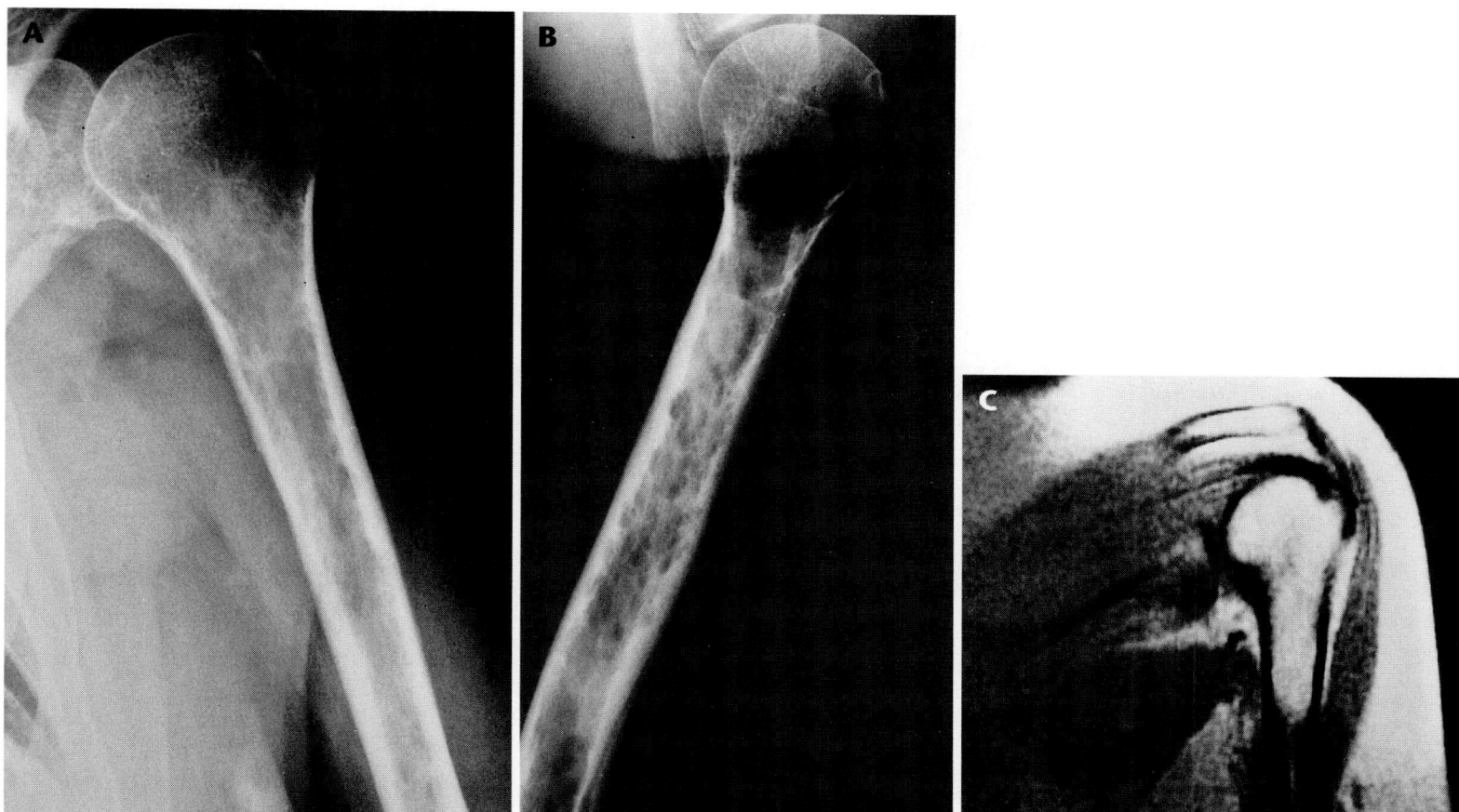

Figure 6–44. A and **B,** Another example of "aggressive" osteoporosis in a 50-year-old woman recently immobilized secondary to brain tumor. **C,** T-1–weighted MRI image shows normal fatty bone marrow.

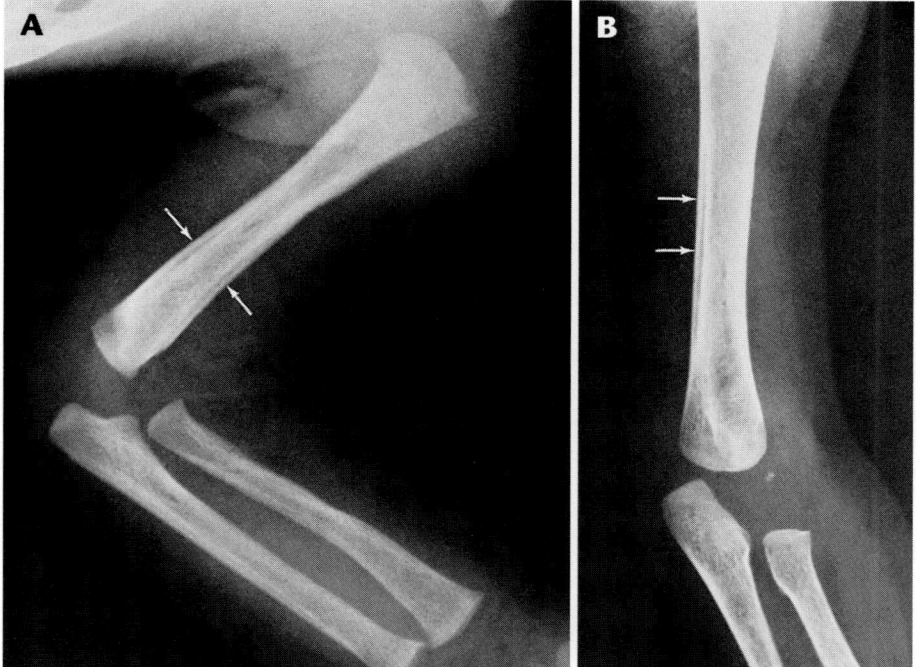

Figure 6–45. Two examples of physiologic "periostitis" of the newborn. **A,** 3-month-old infant. **B,** 8-month-old infant. This is not seen before 1 month of age and is usually symmetric in distribution, although not necessarily concentric, and may be seen in only one view. (Ref: Shopfner CE: Periosteal bone growth in normal infants: A preliminary report. *Am J Roentgenol* 97:154, 1966.)

The Distal Portion of the Humerus

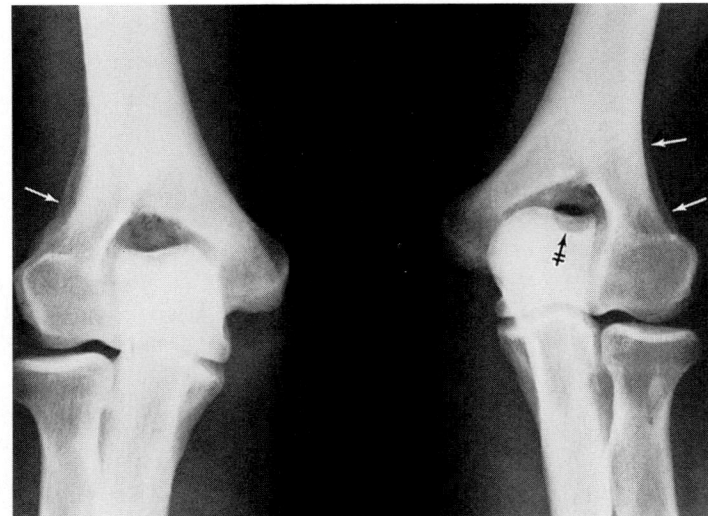

Figure 6–46. Normal thin flange of bone above the lateral epicondyle, which simulates periostitis (←). Note also the perforated olecranon fossa (⇇).

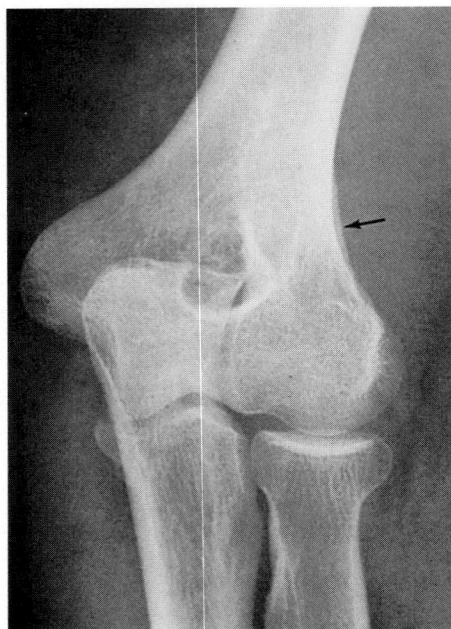

Figure 6–47. Simulated periostitis produced by the lateral epicondylar flange in another individual.

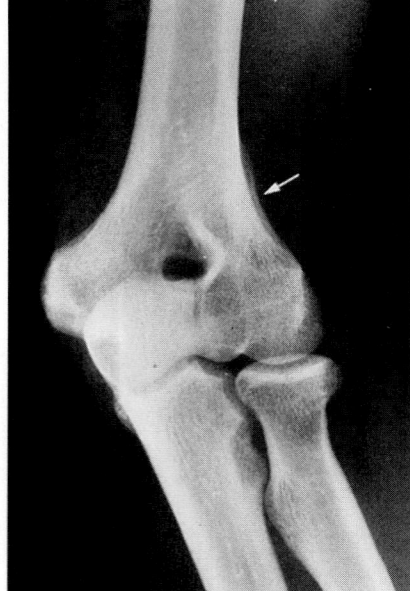

Figure 6–48. The epicondylar flange simulating a cortical fracture.

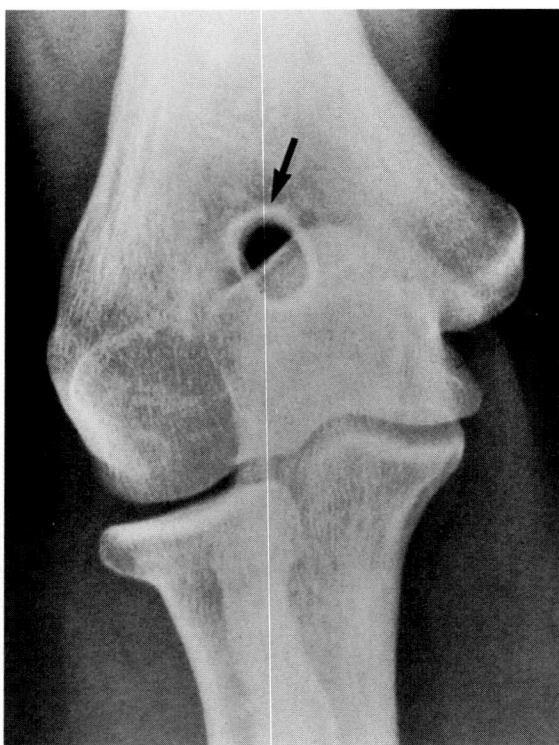

Figure 6–49. Olecranon foramen with marked sclerosis of its margins.

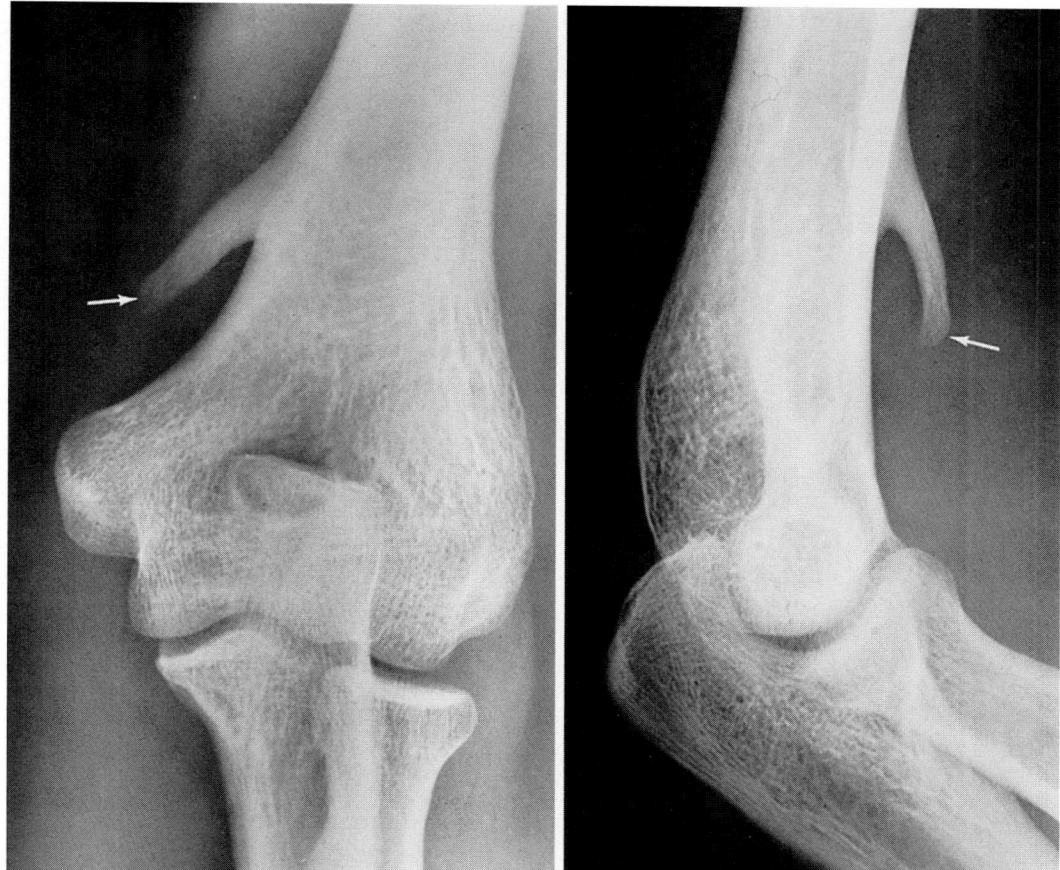

Figure 6–50. The supracondylar process. This vestigial structure is rarely associated with symptoms and occurs in about 1% of persons of European origin. Its axis is typically directed distally. (Ref: Barnard LB, McCoy SM: The supracondyloid process of humerus. *J Bone Joint Surg* 28:845, 1946.)

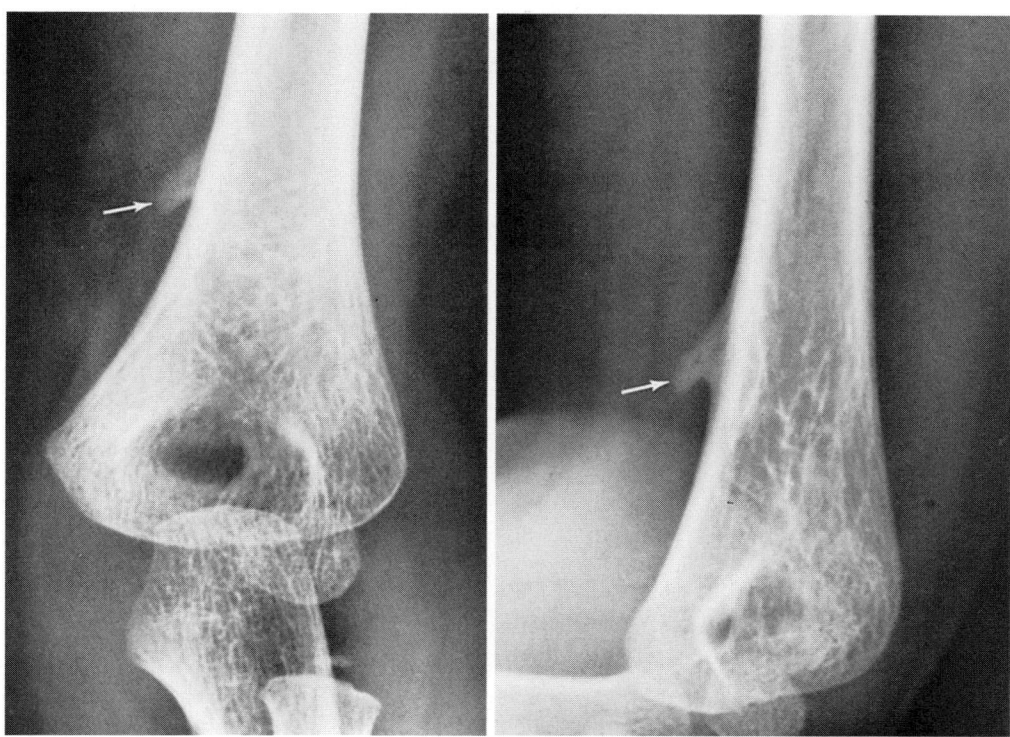

Figure 6–51. The supracondylar process in a 4-year-old boy.

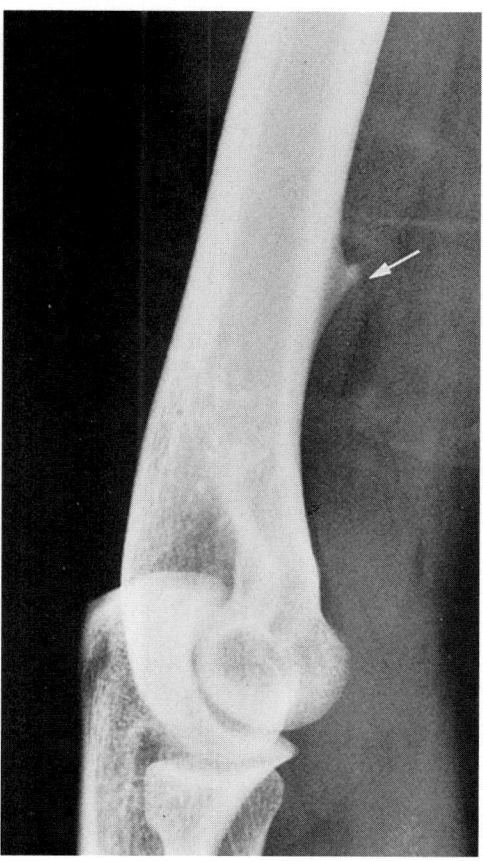

Figure 6–52. A supracondylar process directed cephalad rather than in the usual caudad direction.

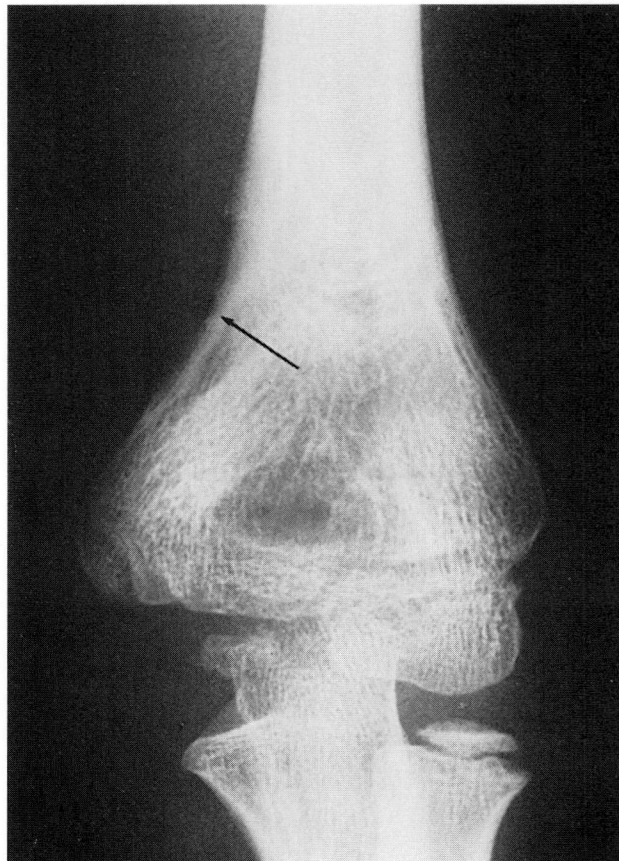

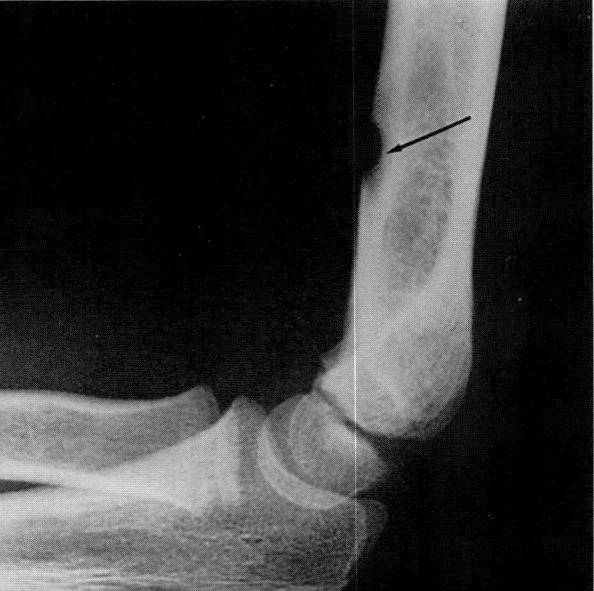

Figure 6–53. Developmental cortical notch on the medial cortex is of no significance. Its anatomic origin is uncertain.

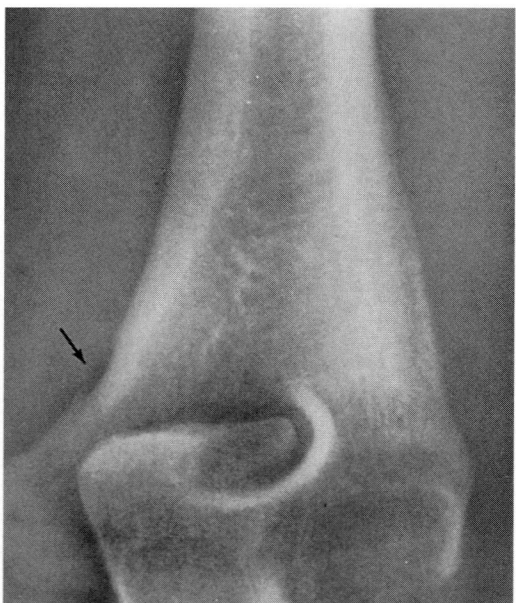

Figure 6–54. Another example of the humeral cortical notch.

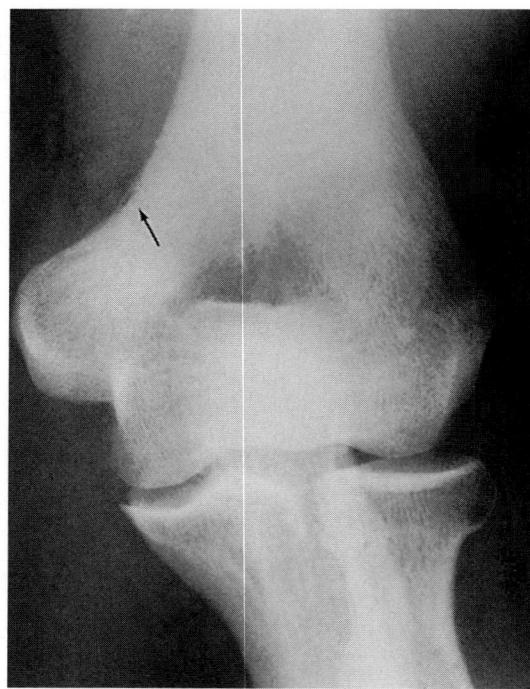

Figure 6–55. Developmental foramen above the medial epicondyle. Note its similarity to the notch in the preceding figure.

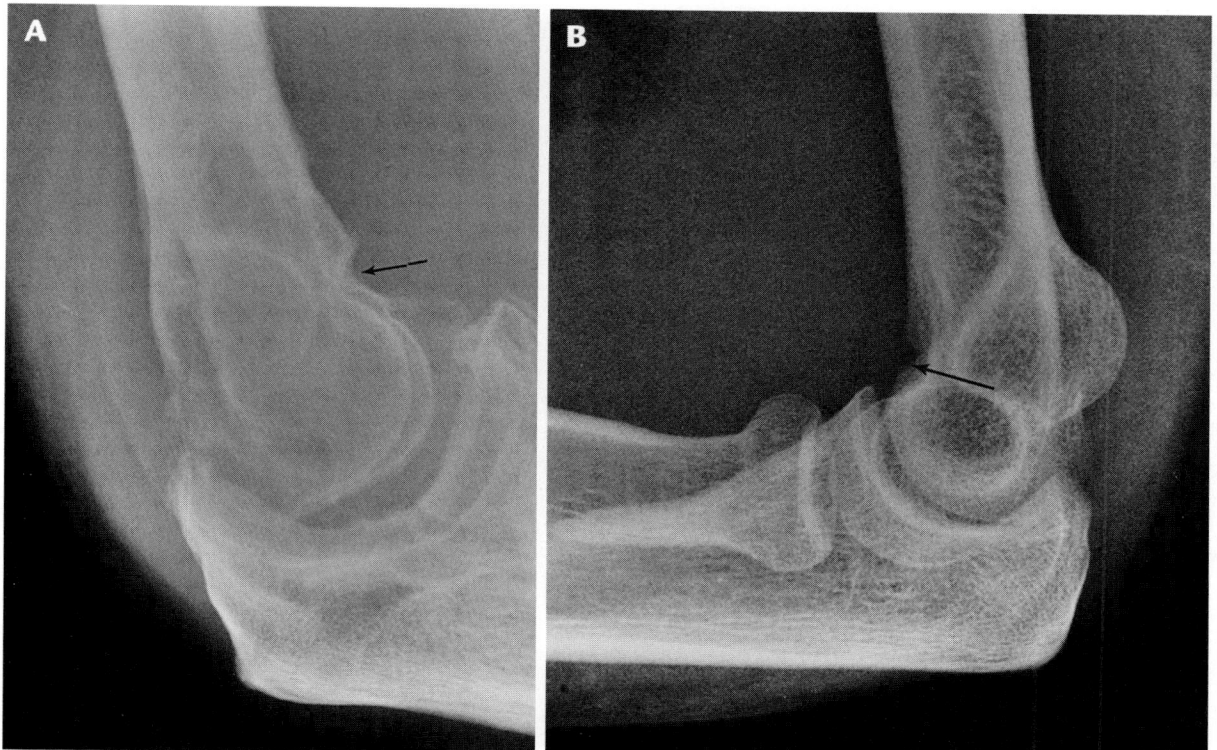

Figure 6–56. A, B, Two examples of small fossae on the anterior cortex of the distal humerus, probably developmental.

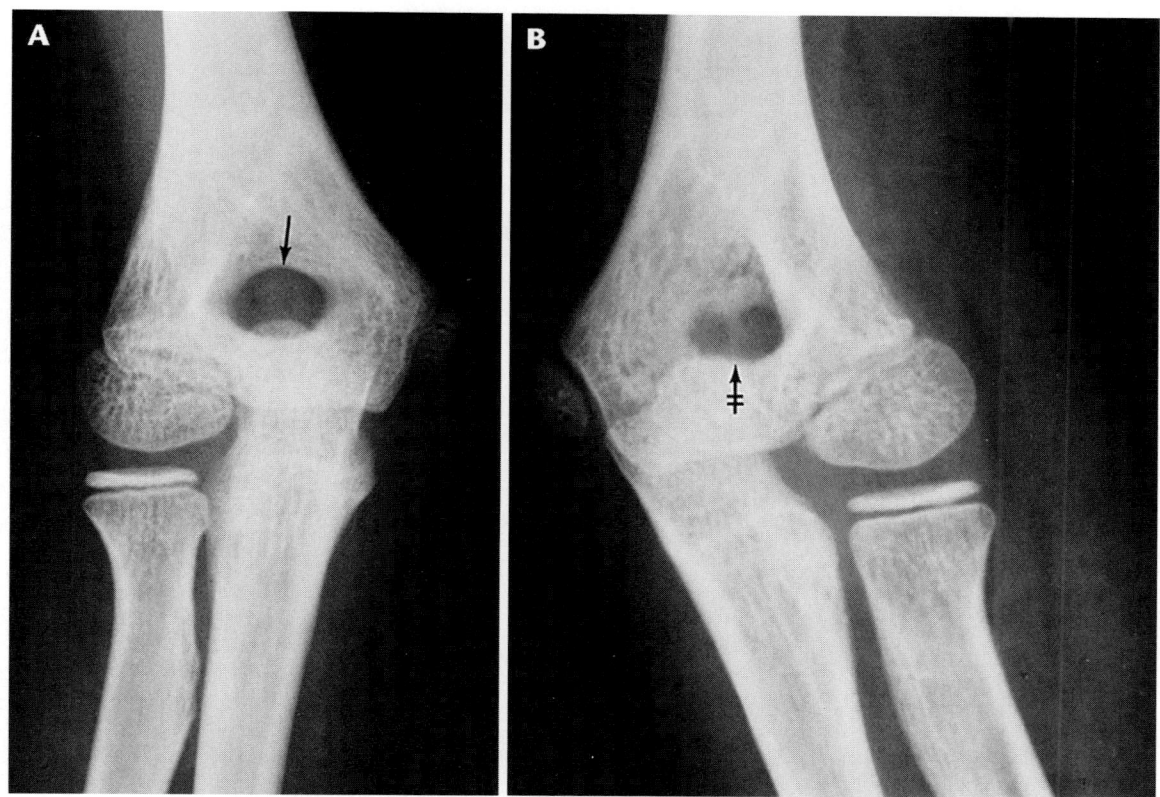

Figure 6–57. Variations in appearance of the olecranon fossa. **A,** Fossa is replaced by a complete foramen (←). **B,** Foramen is traversed by a bridge of bone (⊬).

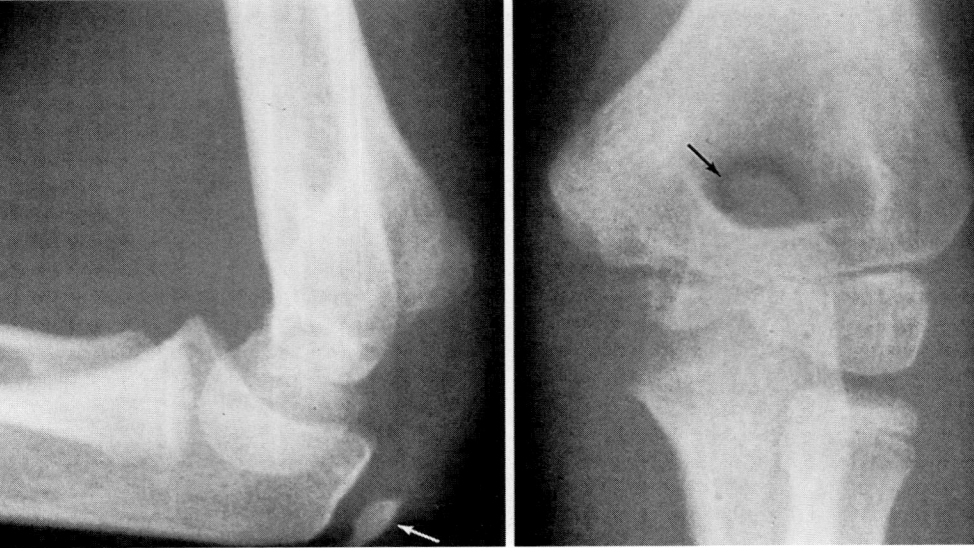

Figure 6–58. Simulated supratrochlear foraminal bone or fracture produced by the ossification center for the olecranon process in a 7-year-old girl.

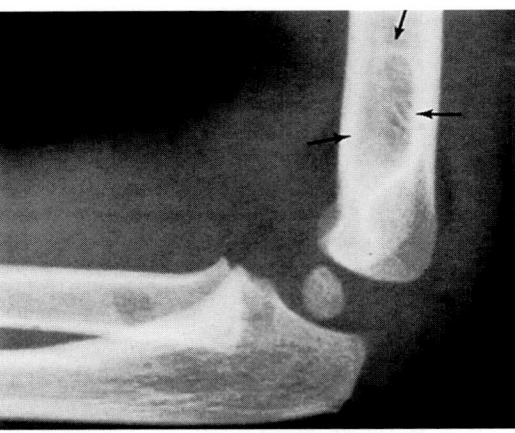

Figure 6–59. The normal rarefaction of bone of the distal humerus may simulate a cystic lesion in the lateral projection.

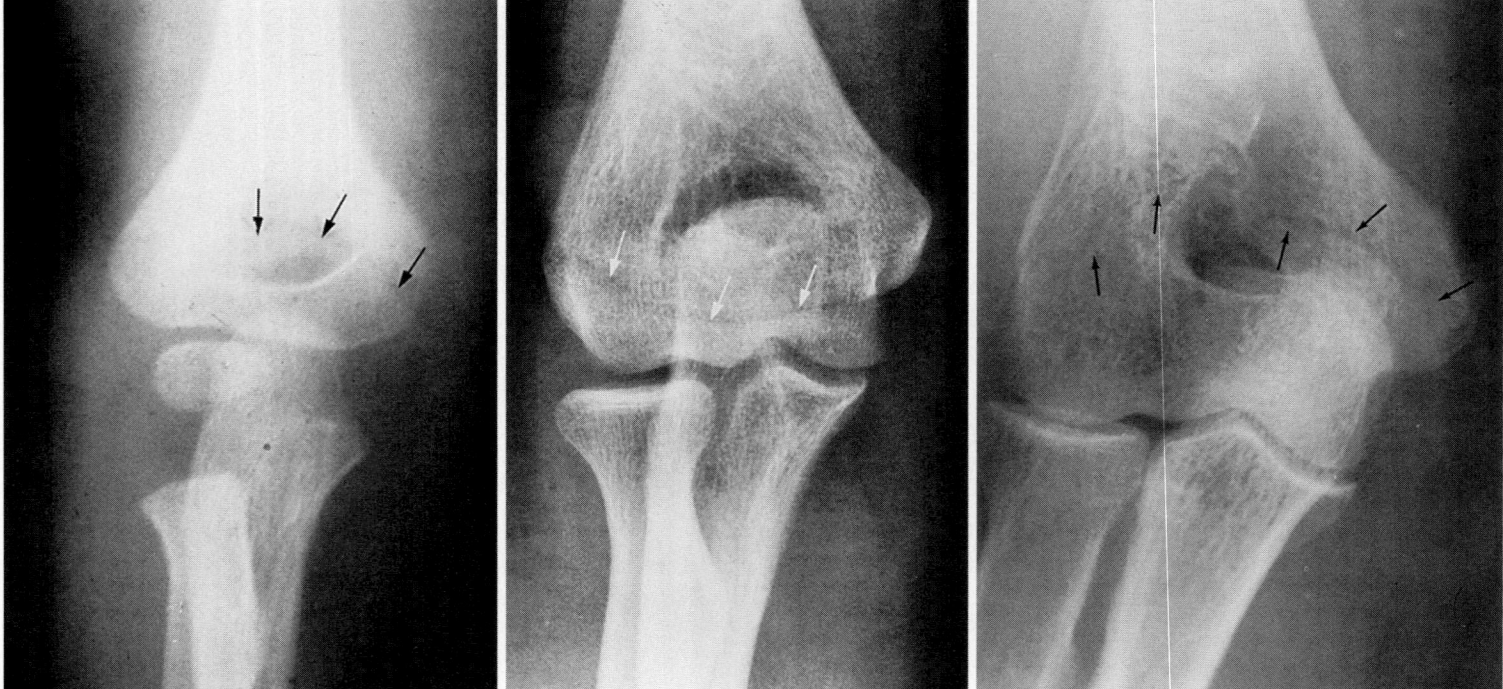

Figure 6–60. Simulated fractures produced by soft tissue folds.

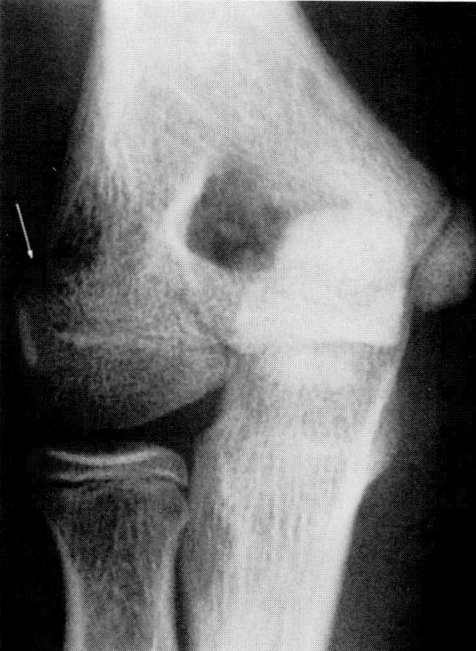

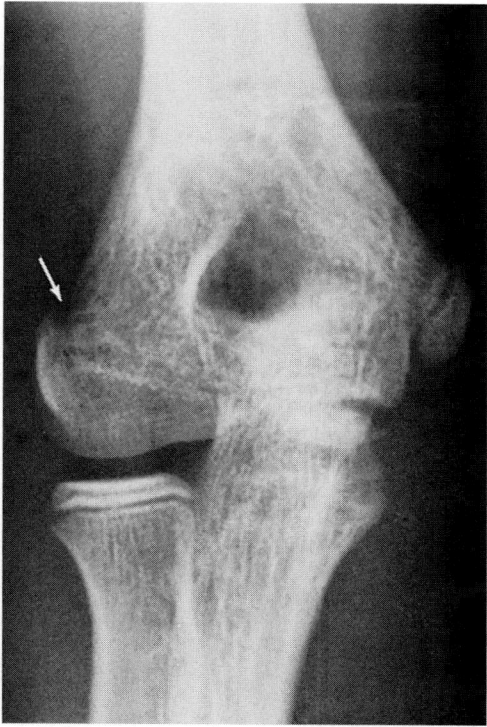

Figure 6–61. Apparent discontinuity of bone immediately above the epiphyseal line in a 12-year-old boy. This represents a variation in development of the metaphysis of a long bone in adolescence similar to the cortical lesions seen in the proximal end of the humerus, the distal radius, the distal end of the femur, and the proximal end of the tibia. This appearance may be misconstrued as evidence of dislocation of the epiphysis or a destructive lesion of the humerus. (Ref: Silberstein MJ et al: Some vagaries of the capitellum. *J Bone Joint Surg* 61A:244, 1979.)

Figure 6–62. The discontinuity seen in the preceding figure is now only minimally present in this 16-year-old boy, indicating the transient nature of this finding.

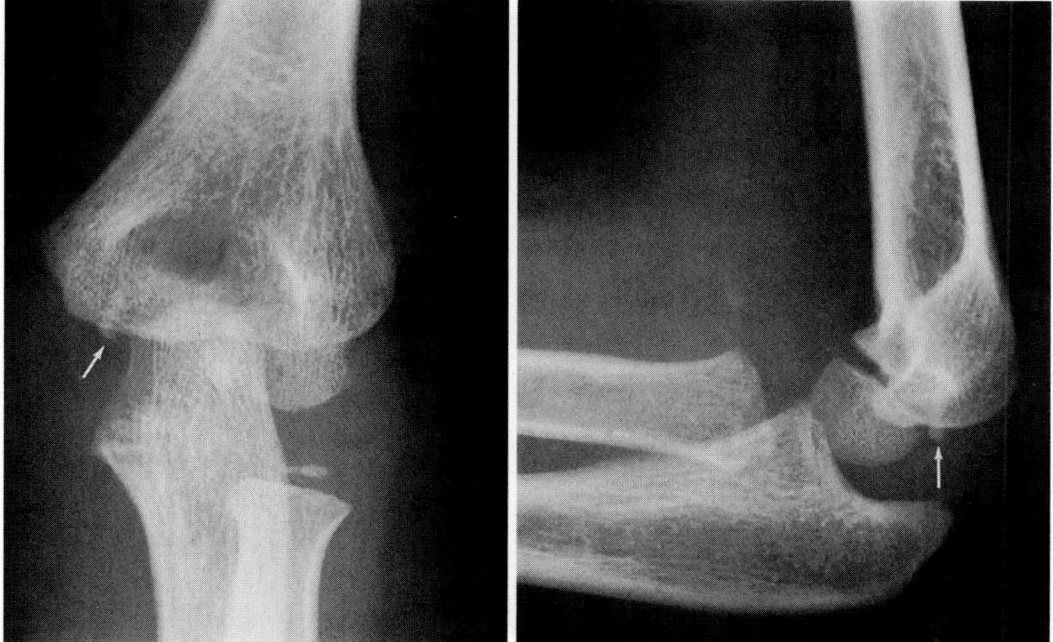

Figure 6–63. Early appearance of the ossification center for the trochlea in a 6-year-old girl. Rarely the trochlear ossification center may appear without evidence of a medial epicondylar center, as in this case. (Ref: Resnik CS, Hartenberg MA: Ossification centers of the pediatric elbow: A rare normal variant. *Pediatr Radiol* 16:254, 1986.)

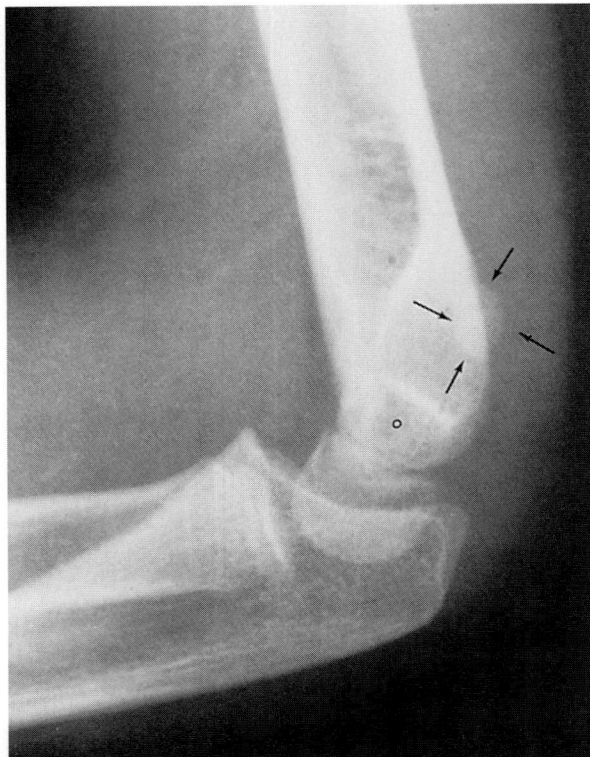

Figure 6–64. Normal appearance and position of the ossification center for the medial epicondyle in a 7-year-old boy.

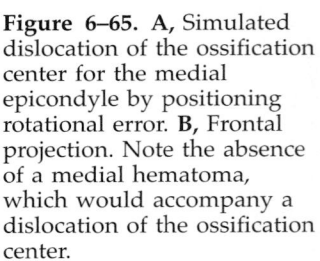

Figure 6–65. A, Simulated dislocation of the ossification center for the medial epicondyle by positioning rotational error. **B,** Frontal projection. Note the absence of a medial hematoma, which would accompany a dislocation of the ossification center.

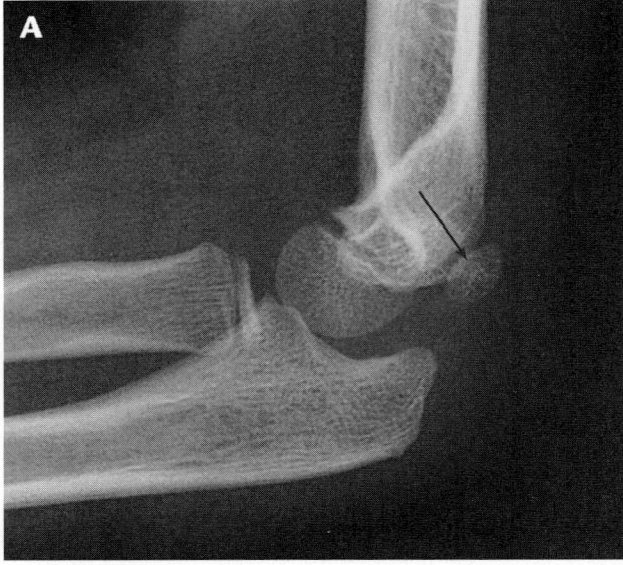

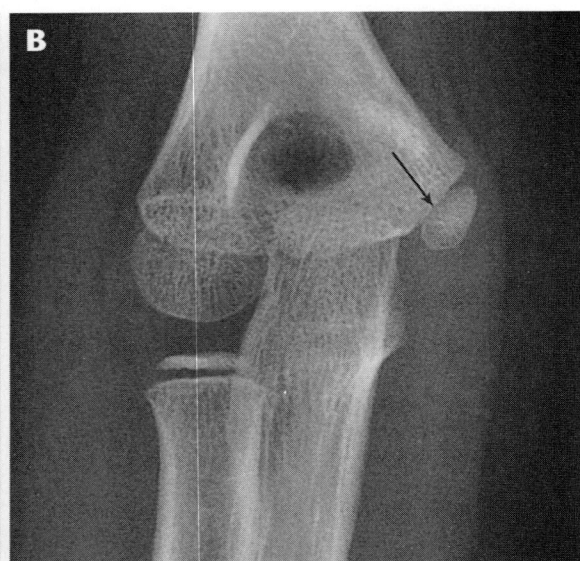

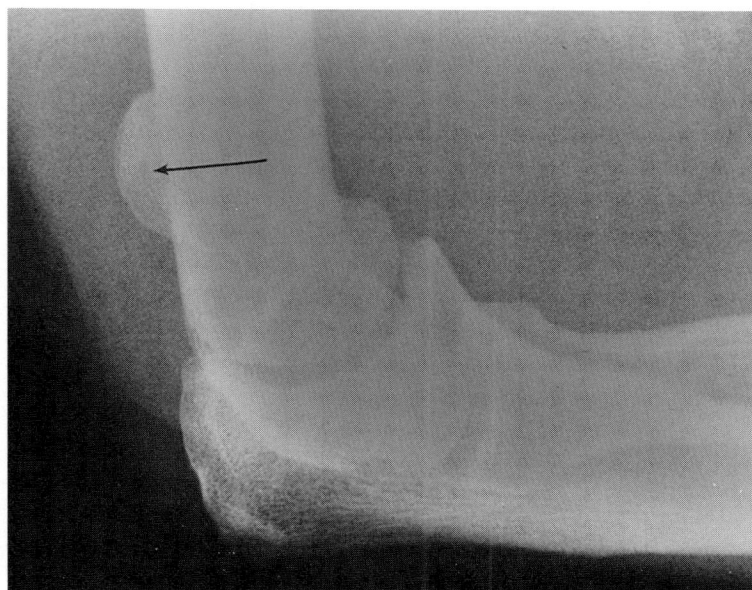

Figure 6–66. The medial epicondyle in the adult seen in off lateral projection.

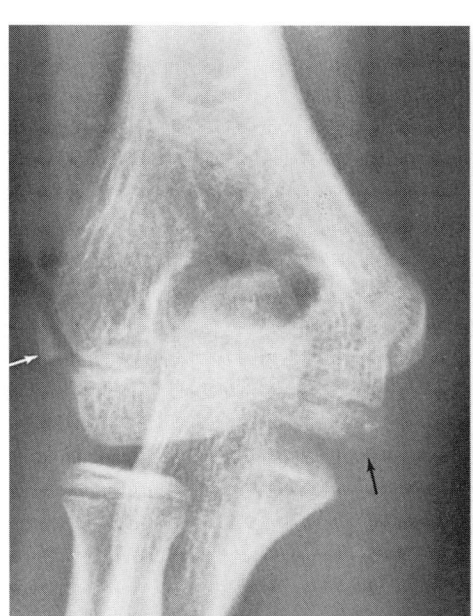
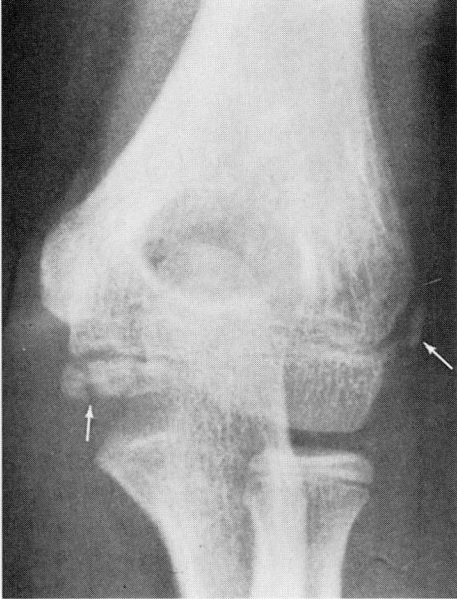

Figure 6–67. Normal irregularities and pseudofractures of the ossification centers of the distal humerus in a 10-year-old girl. Note the lack of bilateral symmetry of some of these defects.

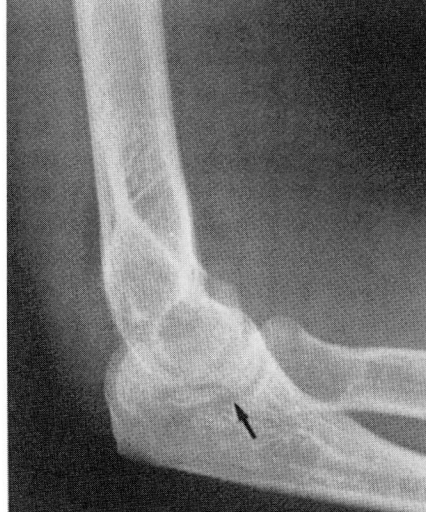
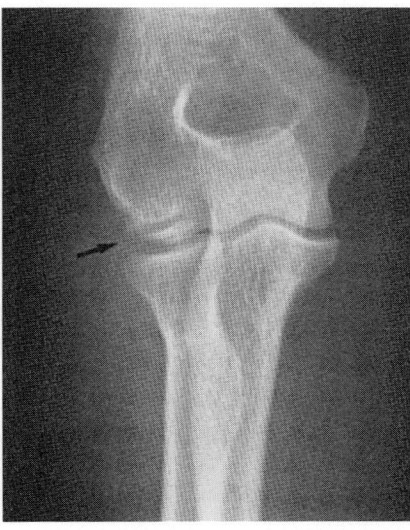
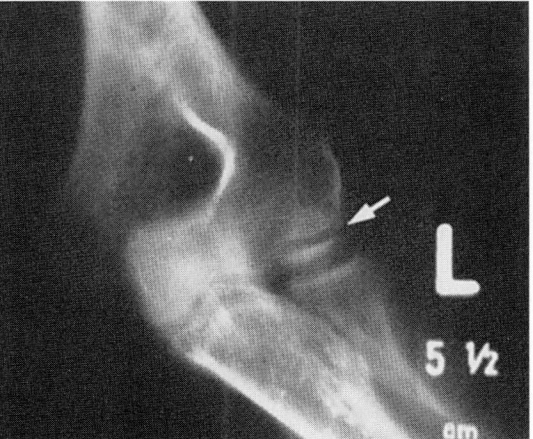

Figure 6–68. A persistent epiphysis of the capitellum in an adult. *Left* and *center*, Plain film. *Right*, Tomogram. (From Nuvemann M: Einseitig ausgebliebene Verschmelzung des capitulum humeri: Eine seltene manifestation der sogenannten persistierenden apophyse. *Fortschr Röntgenstr* 137:340, 1982.)

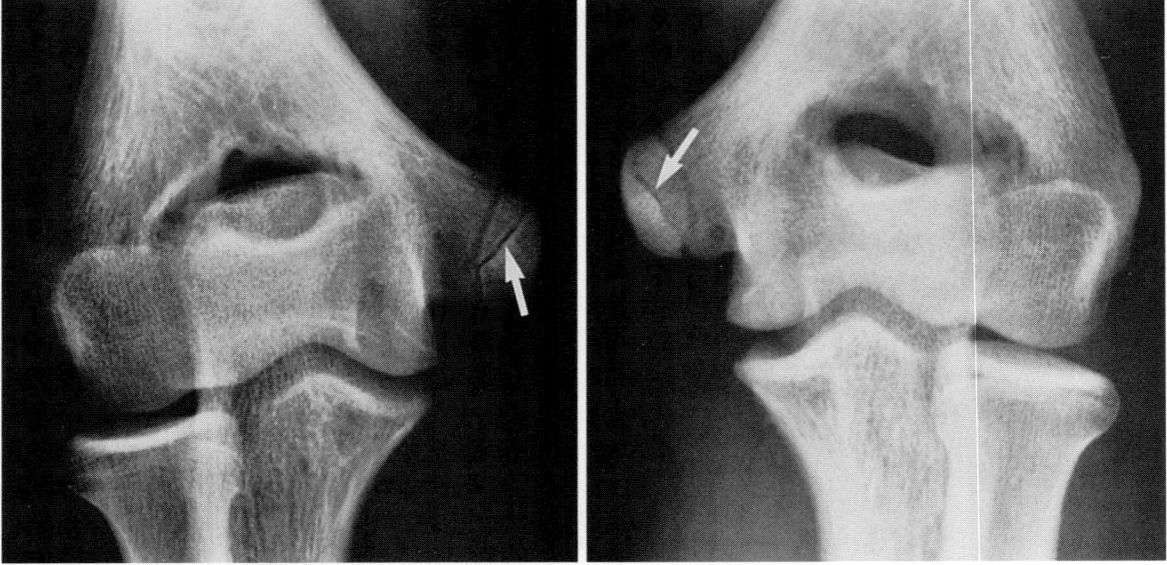

Figure 6–69. Bilateral cleft epiphyses for the medial epicondyle in a 15-year-old boy. The left elbow was immobilized for 2 weeks on the assumption that the cleft represented a fracture. (Ref: Harrison RB, Keats TE: Epiphyseal clefts. *Skeletal Radiol* 5:23, 1980.)

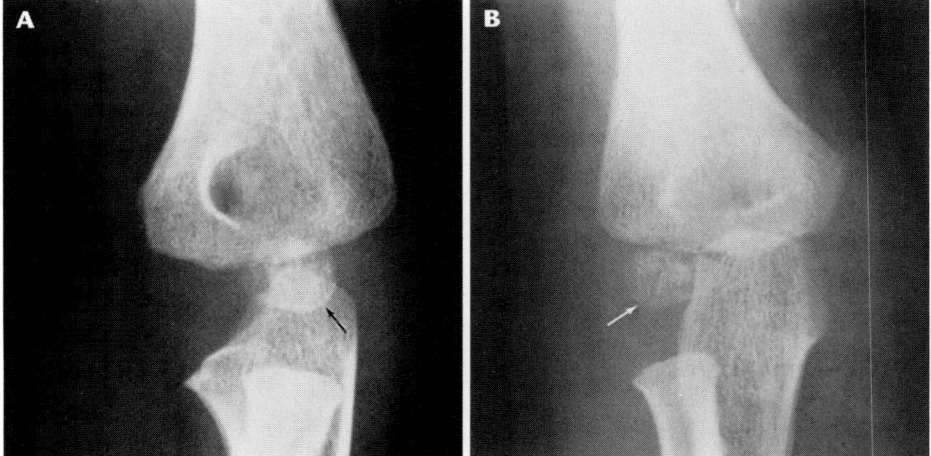

Figure 6–70. A, Apparent displacement of the ossification center for the capitellum as a result of poor positioning of the forearm. **B,** Proper position shows normal relationships.

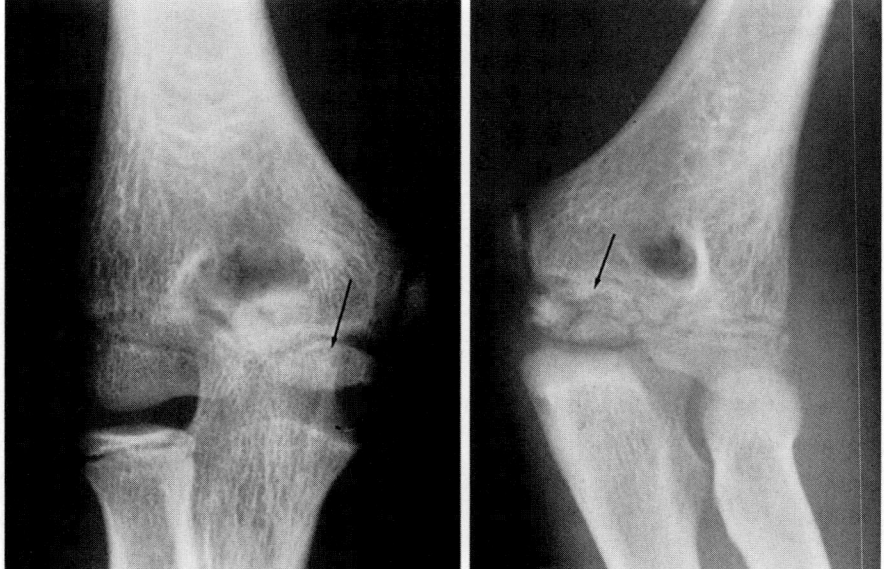

Figure 6–71. Marked asymmetry of ossification of the centers for the trochlea in an adolescent girl.

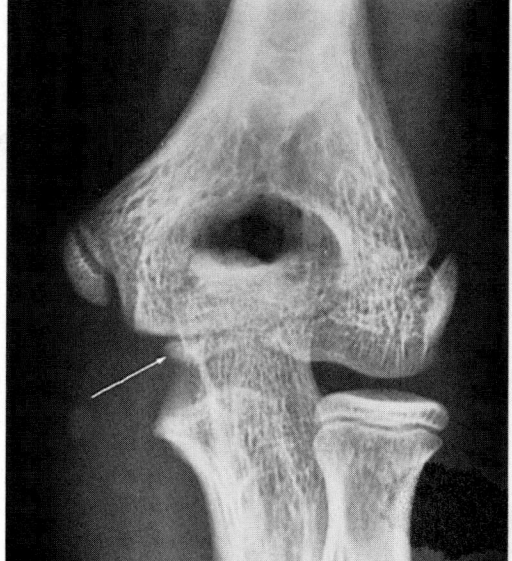
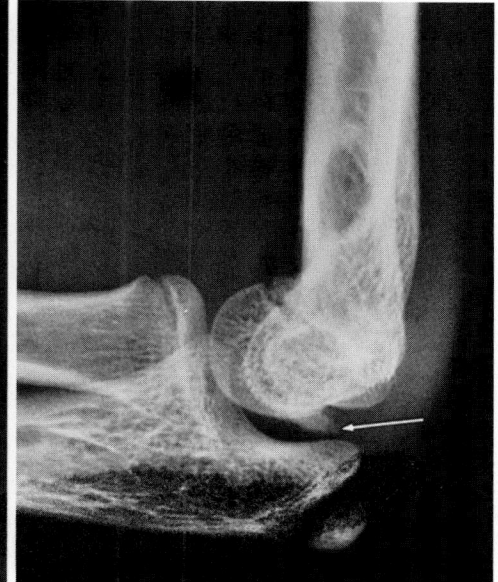

Figure 6–72. An example of how the epiphysis of the trochlea may be mistaken for a fracture in the lateral projection.

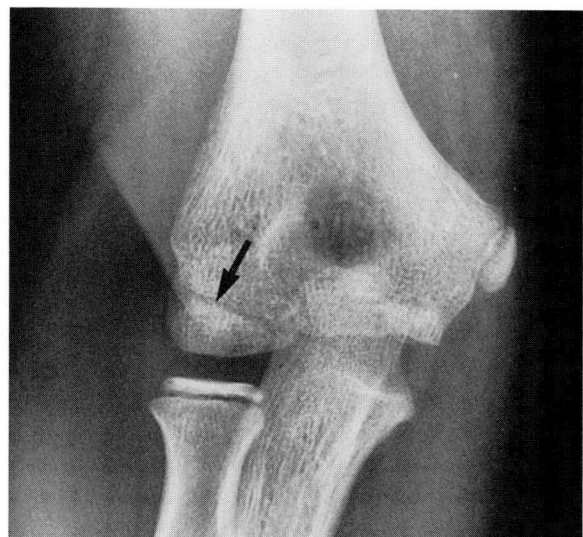
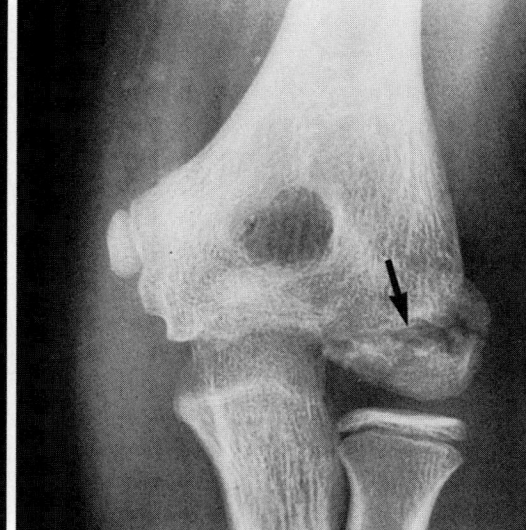

Figure 6–73. Asymmetric development of the epiphyses for the capitellum in a 12-year-old boy. Such normal asymmetries in architecture and rate of growth are particularly common in the elbow and should not be misconstrued as evidence of trauma.

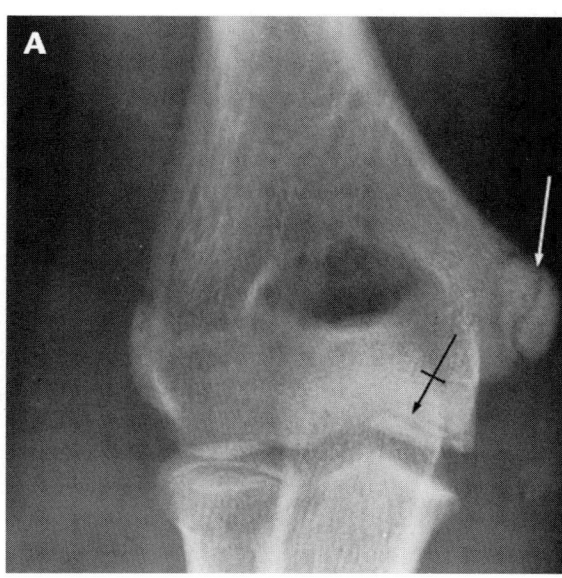
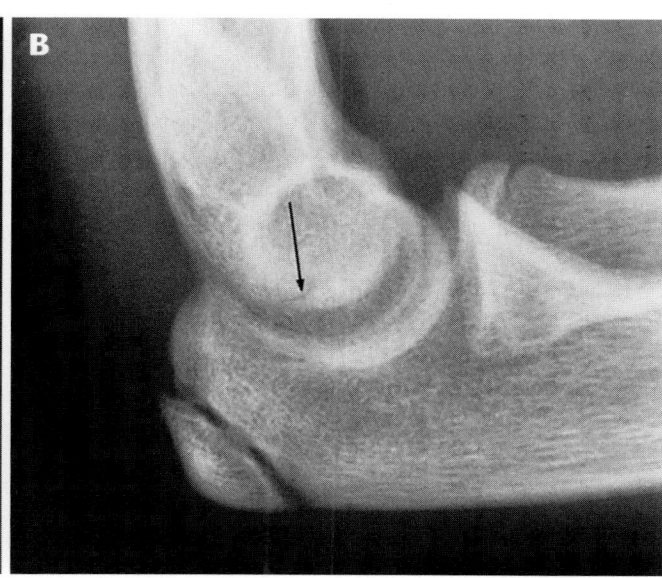

Figure 6–74. A, Simulated fracture of the ossification center of the medial epicondyle in a 14-year-old boy, produced by the superimposed radiolucent shadow of the growth plate between the ossification center and the bony side wall of the humerus (←). Note also the unusual appearance of the trochlea resulting from filming in a slight degree of flexion (↔). **B,** Note the radiolucency of the growth plate of the trochlea in lateral projection.

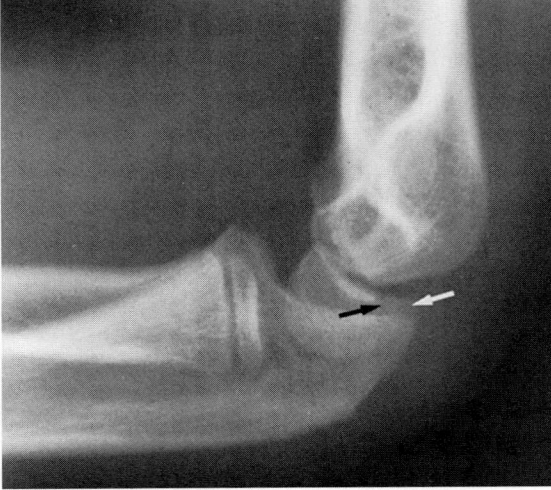

Figure 6–75. Normal irregularities in ossification of the capitellum, which should not be mistaken for a fracture.

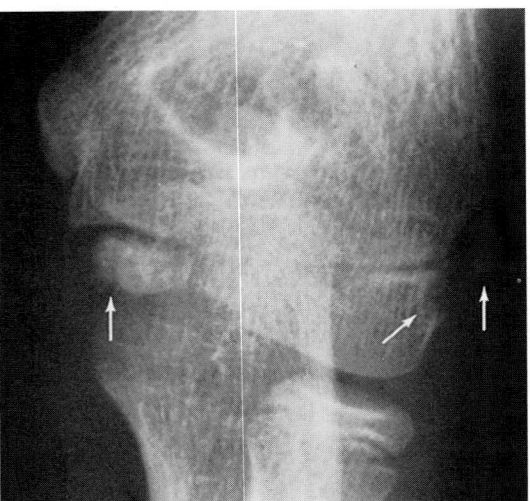

Figure 6–76. Several simulated fractures of the ossification centers of the distal humerus in an 11-year-old boy. Such irregularities of ossification are common.

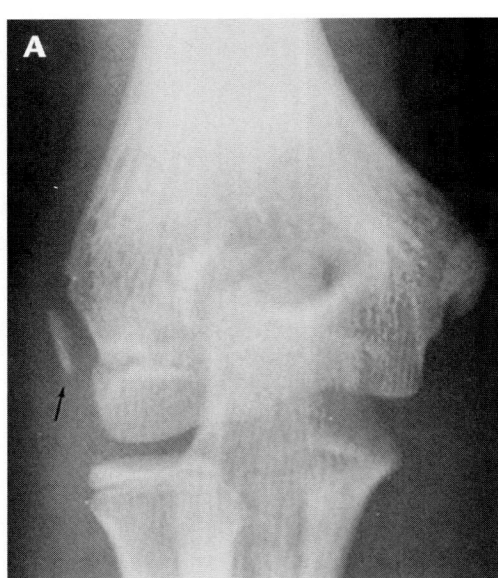

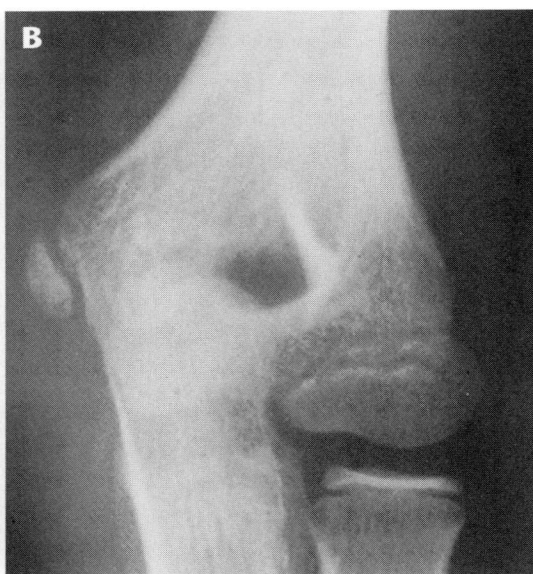

Figure 6–77. A, B, Normal asymmetry in development of ossification centers. Note absence of the ossification center for the lateral epicondyle in **B** in an 11-year-old girl. (Ref: Silberstein MJ et al: Some vagaries of the lateral epicondyle. *J Bone Joint Surg* 64A:444, 1982.)

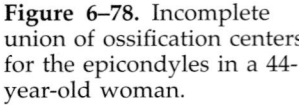

Figure 6–78. Incomplete union of ossification centers for the epicondyles in a 44-year-old woman.

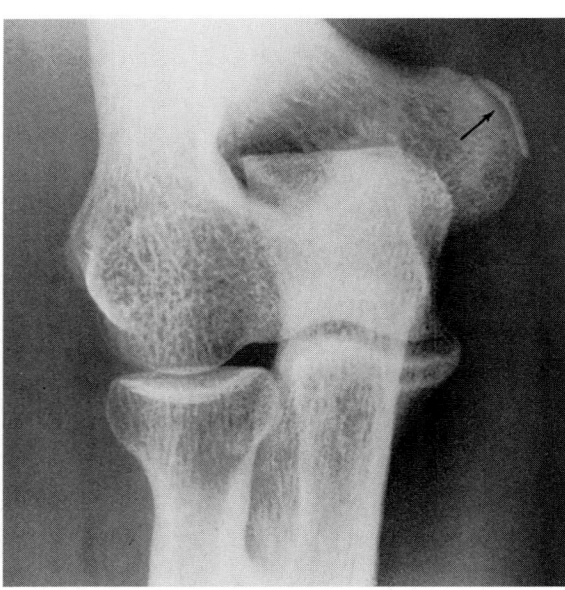

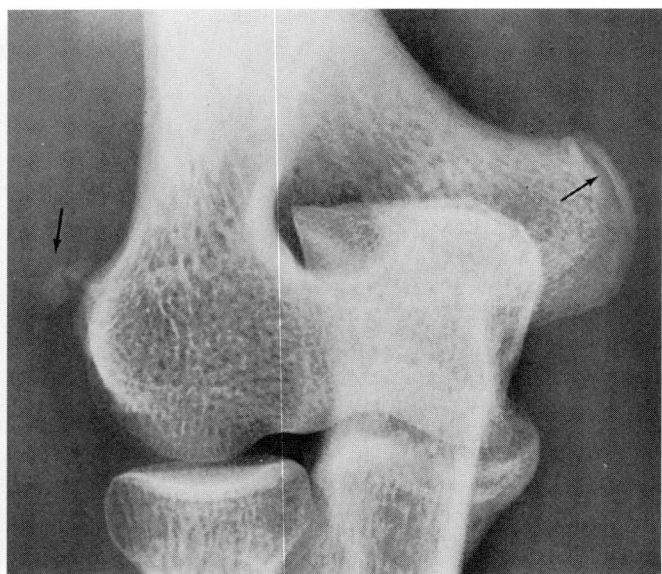

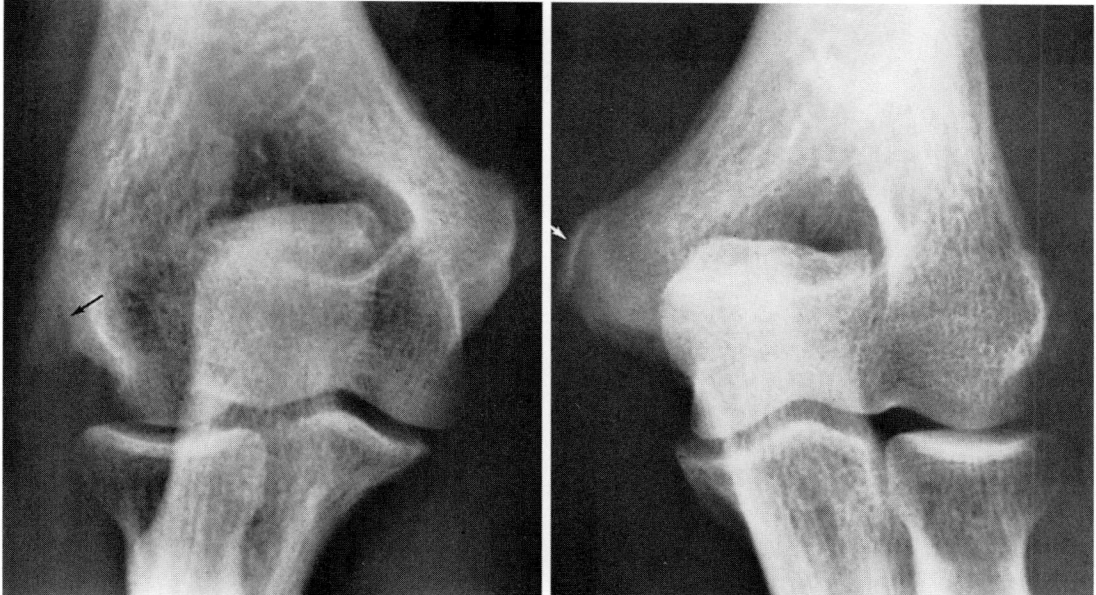

Figure 6–79. Incomplete union of the ossification centers of the epicondyles in a 54-year-old woman.

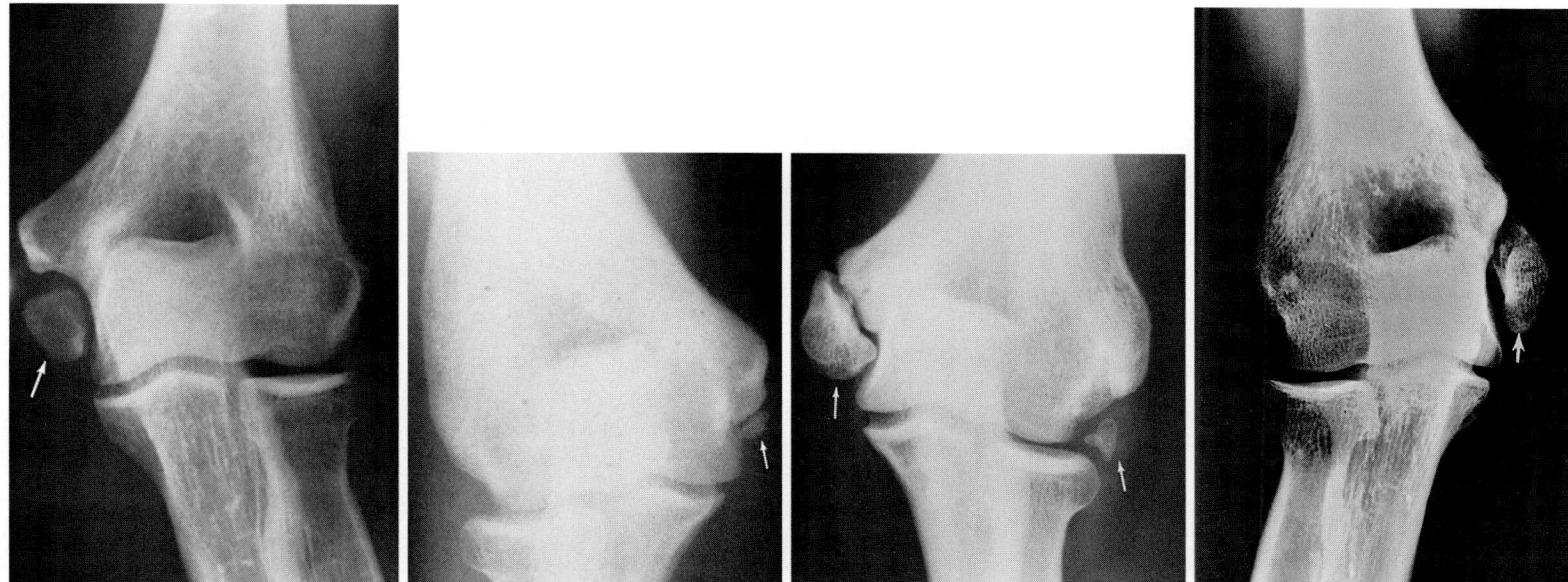

Figure 6–80. Examples of failure of union of ossification centers in adults.

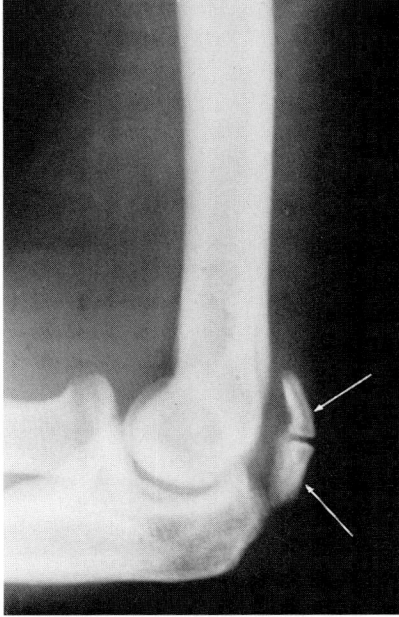

Figure 6–81. Patella cubiti, a sesamoid bone in the triceps tendon. (Ref: Kattan KR, Babcock DS: Bilateral patella cubiti. *Skeletal Radiol* 4:249, 1979.)

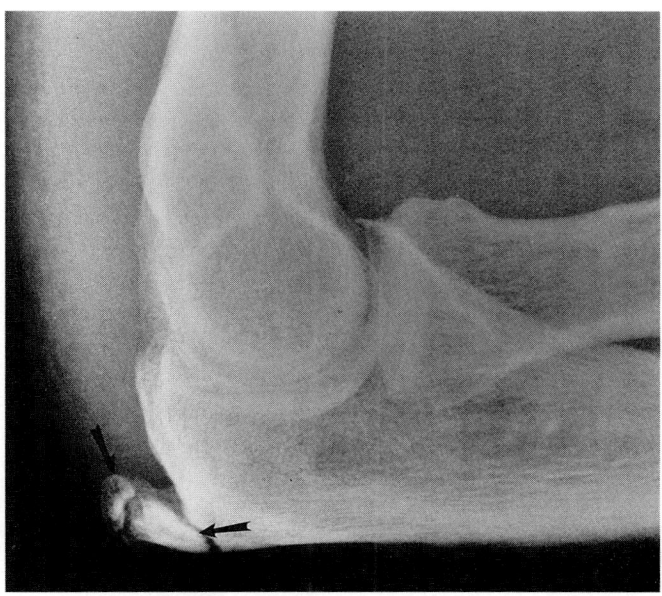

Figure 6–82. Patella cubiti in the inferior position.

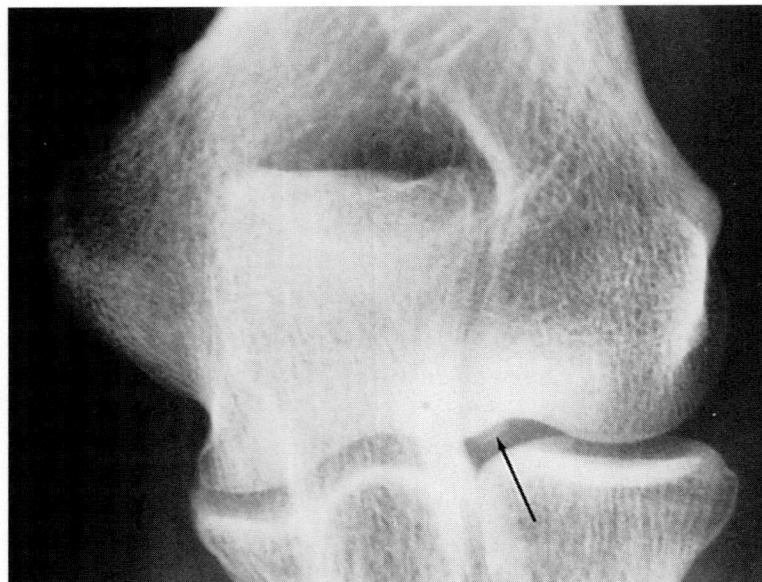

Figure 6–83. Projection of the middle eminence of the lower articular surface of the humerus.

Figure 6–84. Small bilateral ossicles related to the articular surface of the humerus. These may represent separate ossification centers for the middle eminence. Arthrograms indicate that they are enclosed in a lucent cartilage envelope.

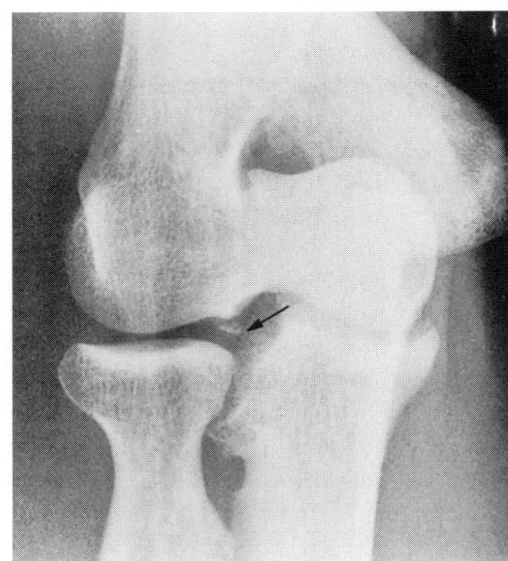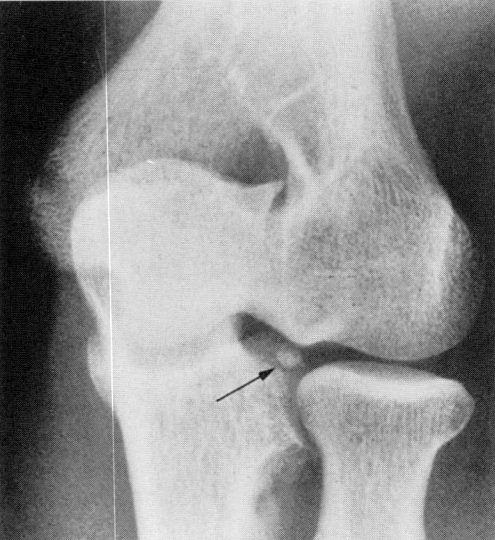

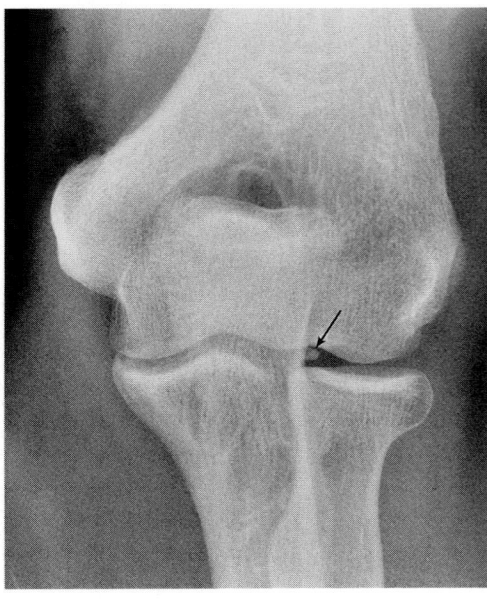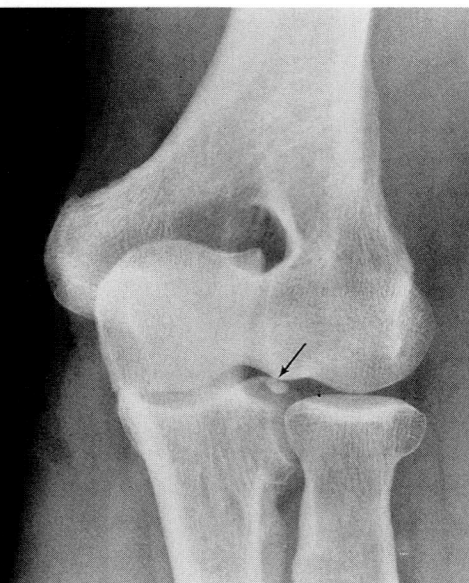

Figure 6–85. An additional example of the entity shown in the preceding figure.

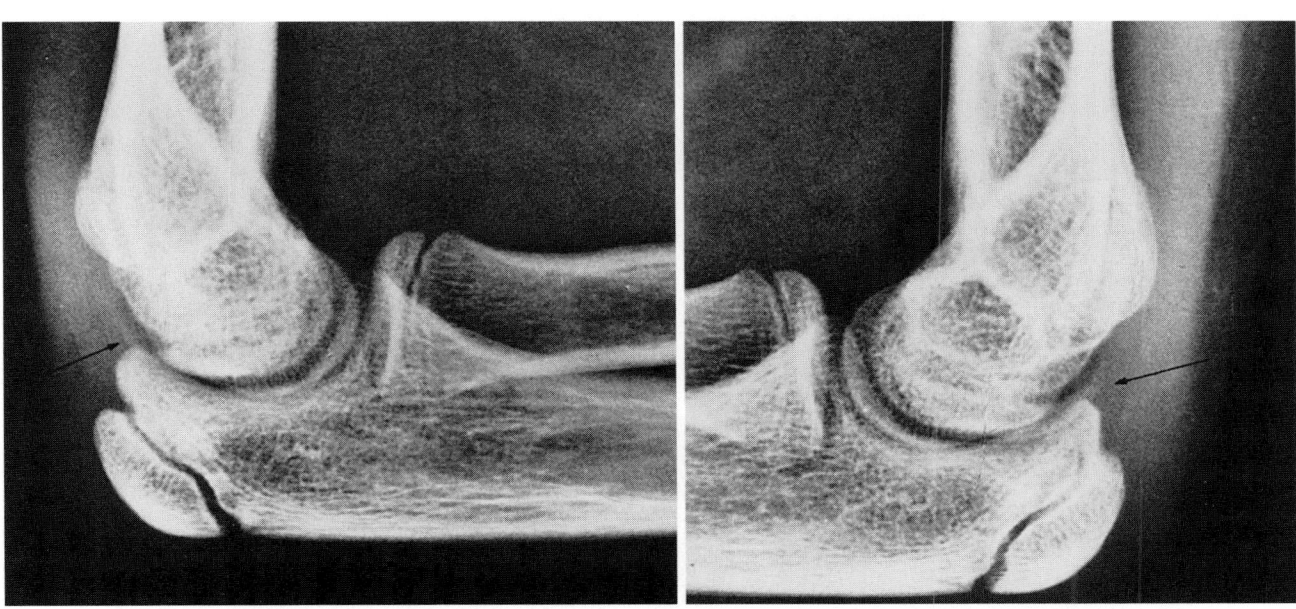

Figure 6–86. A, B, Two examples of paratrochlear bones at the lateral humeral condyle. (Ref: Schwartz GS: Bilateral antecubital ossicles (fabella cubiti) and other accessory bones of the elbow. *Radiology* 69:730, 1957.)

Figure 6–87. Spurlike shadows probably representing the edge of the capitellum in an 11-year-old boy.

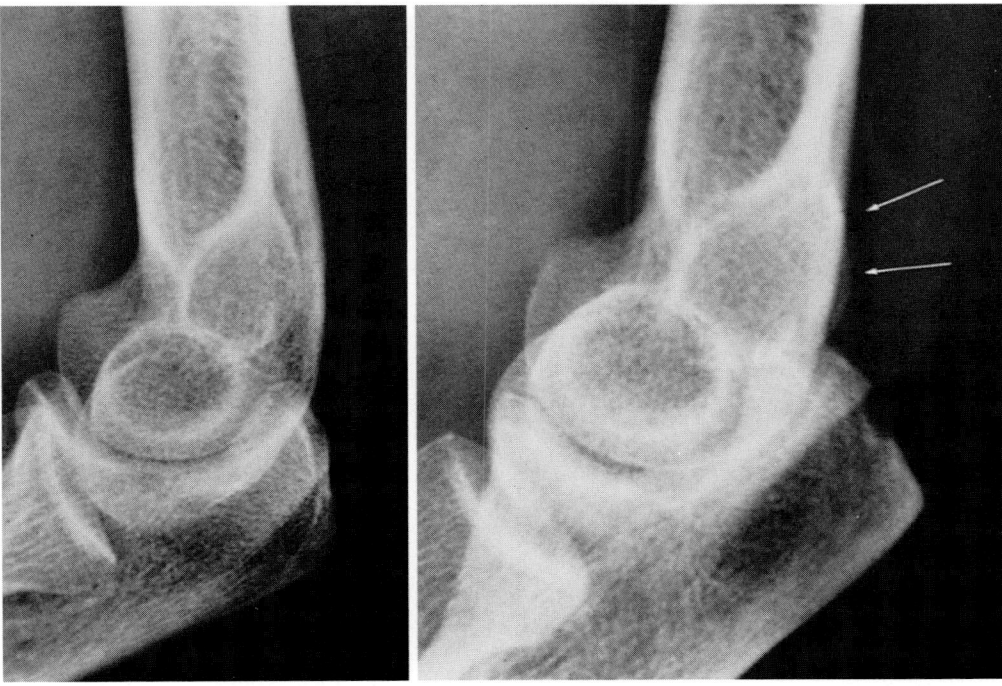

Figure 6–88. The posterior fat pad may be seen in some normal individuals with the elbow in extension. *Left*, Partial flexion. *Right*, Extension.

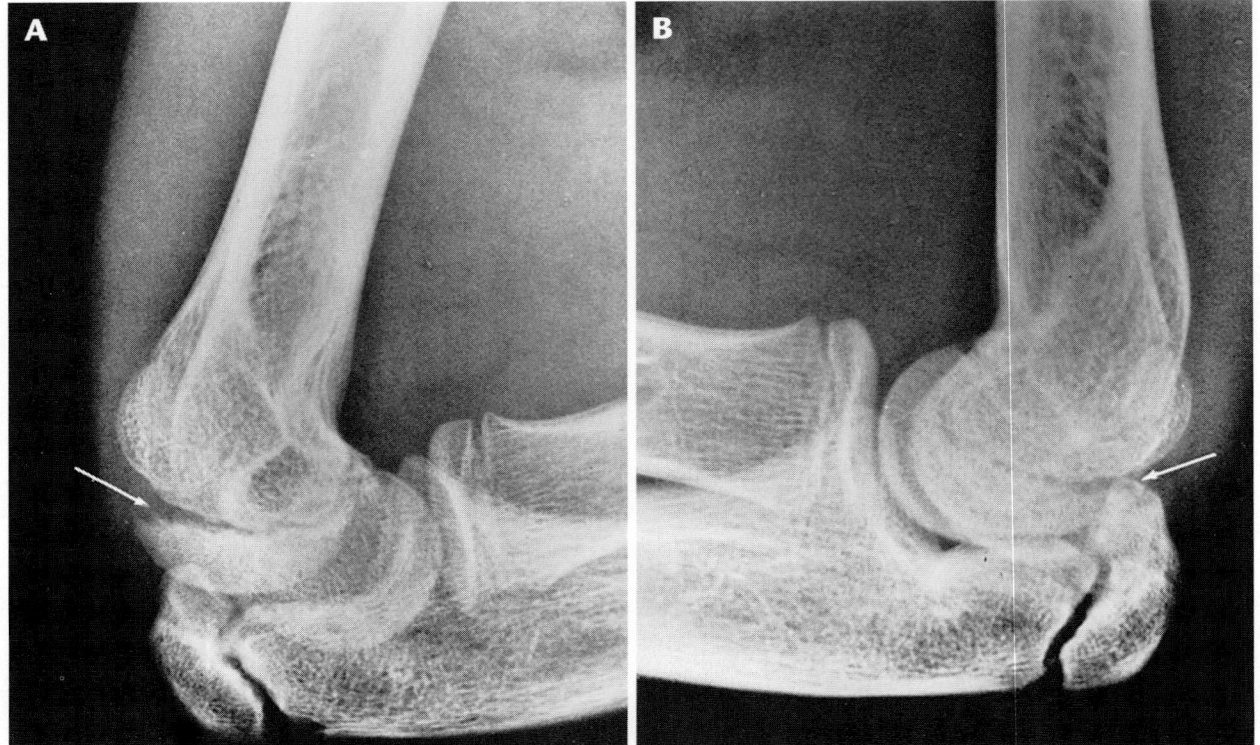

Figure 6–89. **A,** Simulated fracture through the epiphysis of the trochlea, produced by angulation of the beam. **B,** Comparison view of the opposite elbow in true lateral projection shows similar lucency without the simulated fracture.

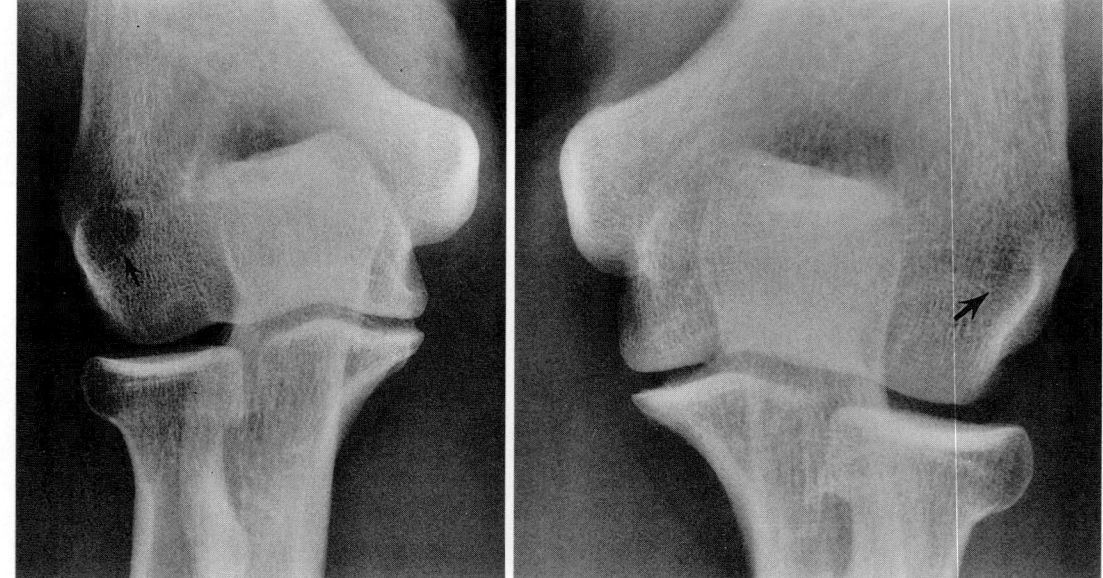

Figure 6–90. Circumscribed radiolucencies in metaphyses caused by fossae above the capitellum.

The Forearm

The Proximal Portion of the Forearm

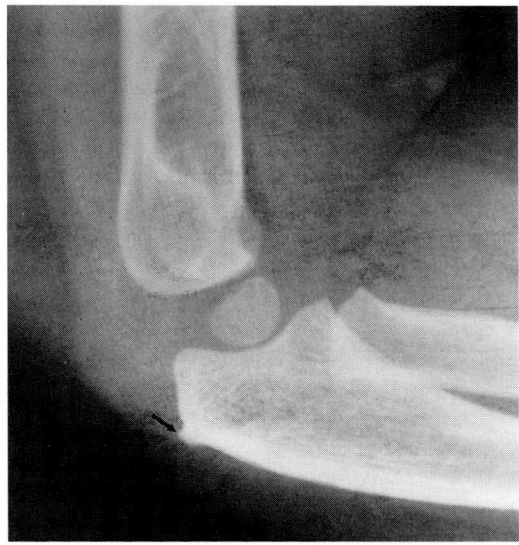

Figure 6–91. Spur at the olecranon in a 5-year-old child, probably representing modeling to receive the apophysis, which is not yet ossified.

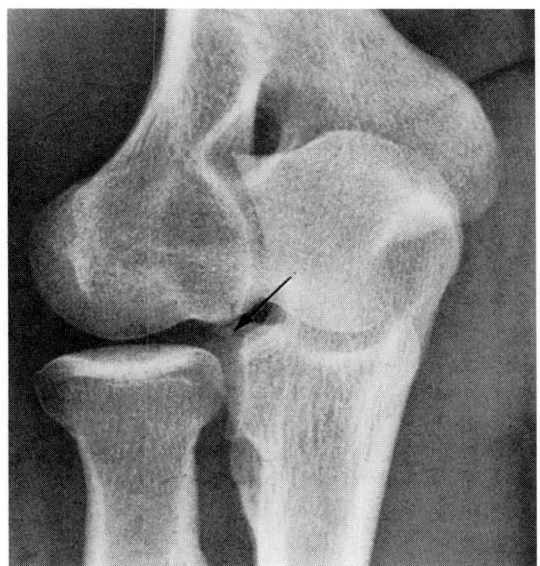

Figure 6–92. Probable bone island in the proximal portion of the ulna.

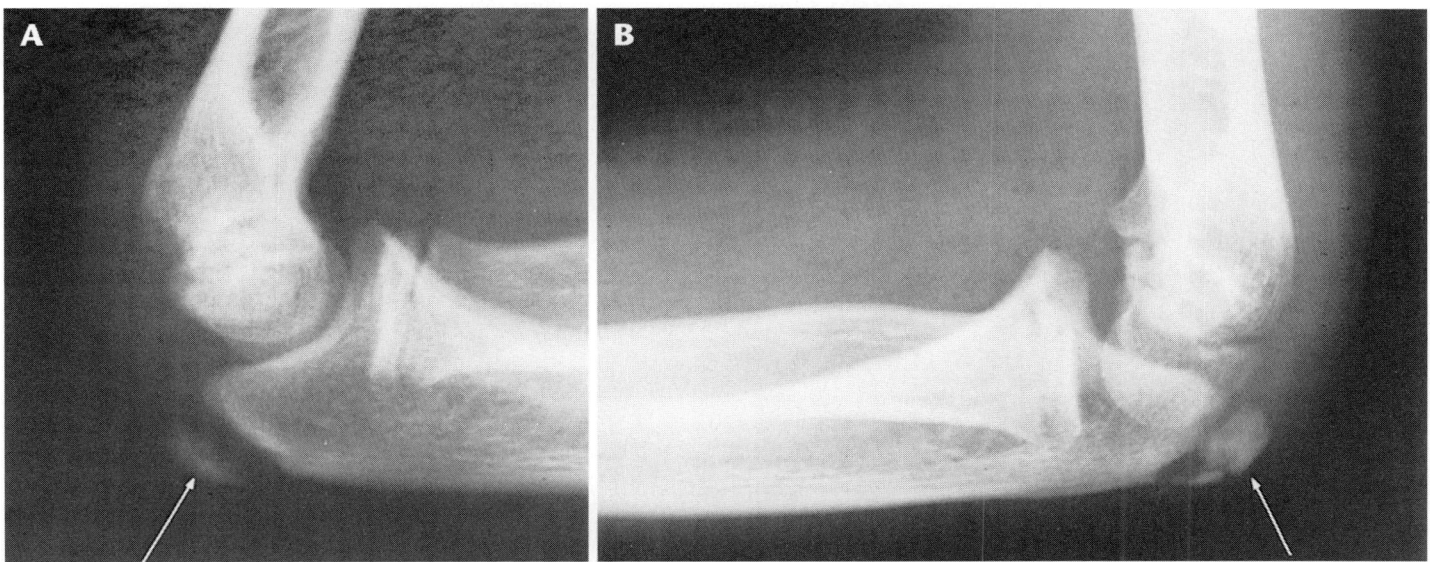

Figure 6–93. A, B, Normal asymmetry of development of the olecranon apophyses. Note irregular ossification in **B**.

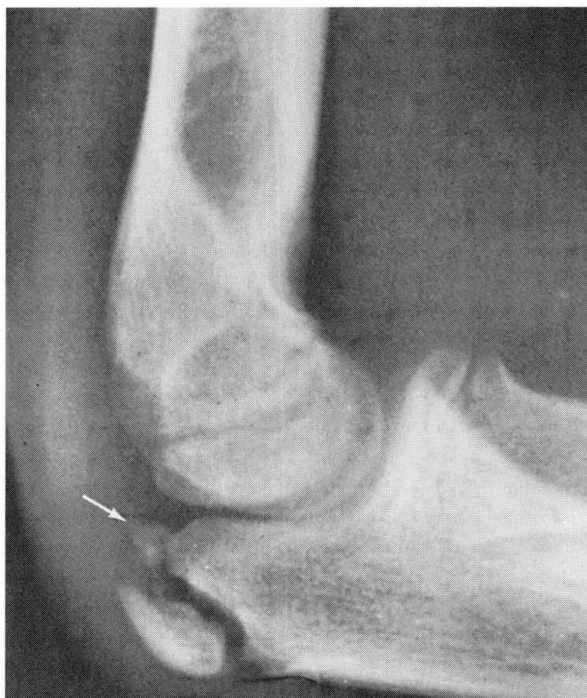

Figure 6–94. A separate nucleus of ossification for the olecranon process, not a fracture. (Ref: Silberstein MJ: Some vagaries of the olecranon. *J Bone Joint Surg* 63A:722, 1981.)

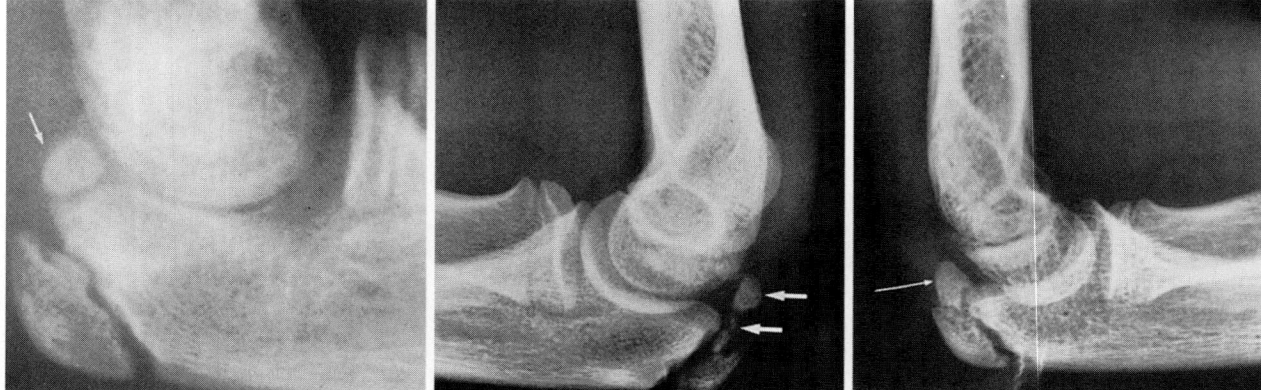

Figure 6–95. Other examples of separate apical nuclei of ossification for the olecranon process.

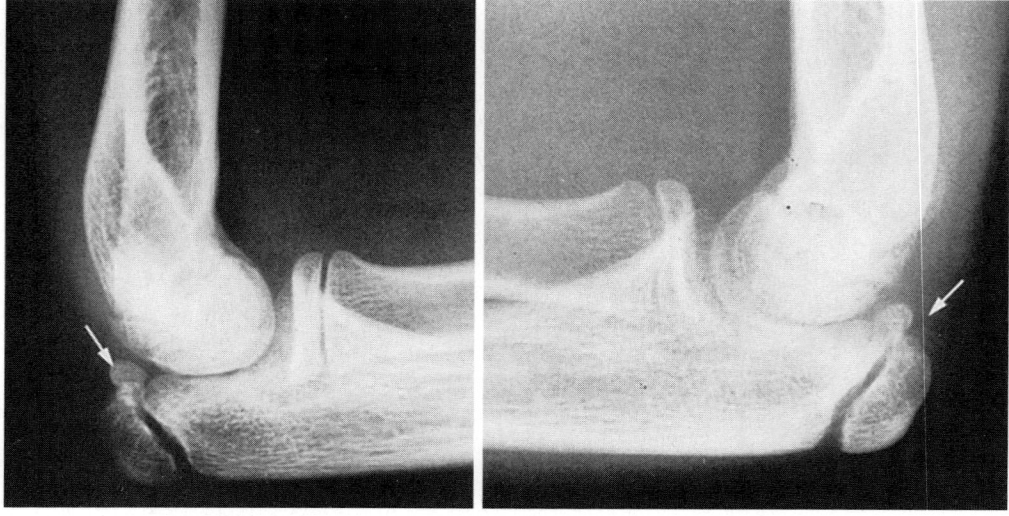

Figure 6–96. Bilaterally symmetric separate nuclei of ossification for the olecranon process in a 13-year-old boy.

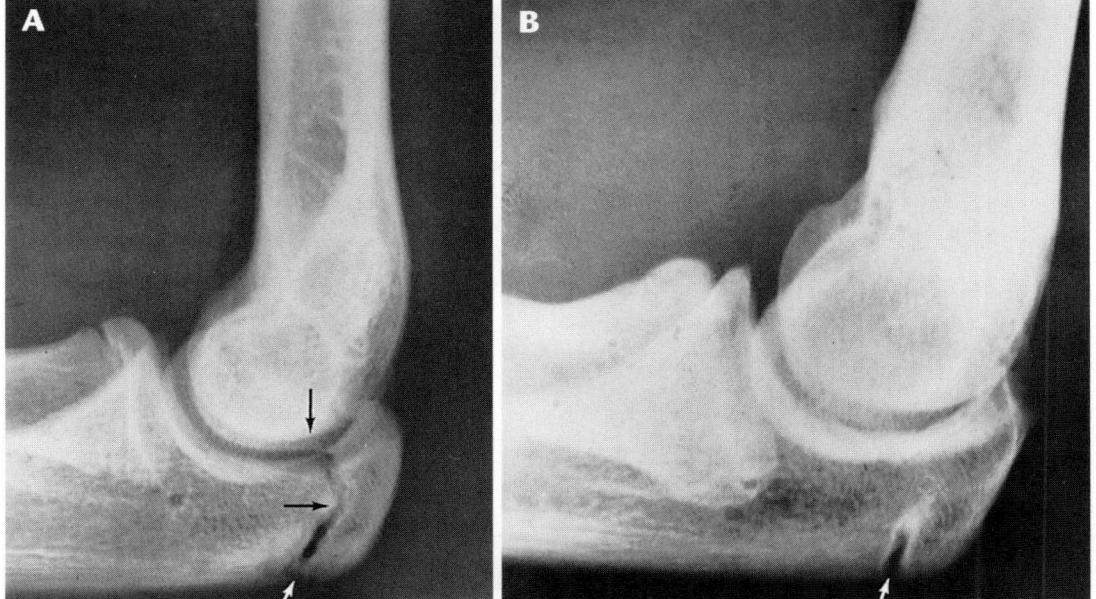

Figure 6–97. A, Normal appearance of the uniting olecranon ossification center in an adolescent. **B,** Incomplete union of the ossification center of the olecranon process—not a fracture—in an adult.

Figure 6–98. Persistent unfused apophyses of the olecranon in a middle-aged man.

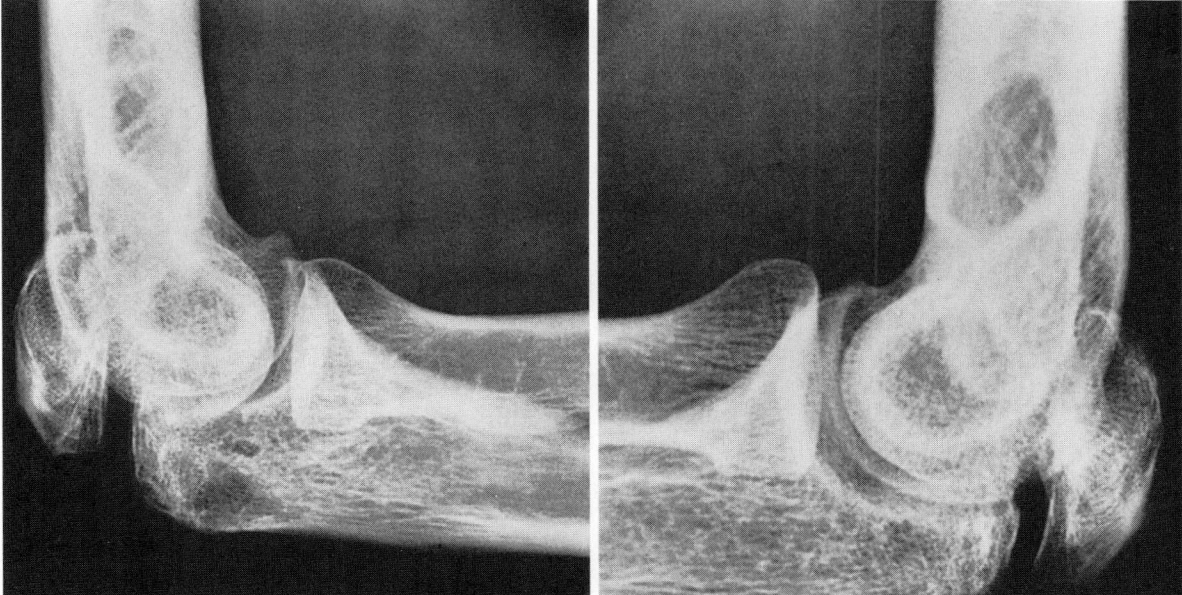

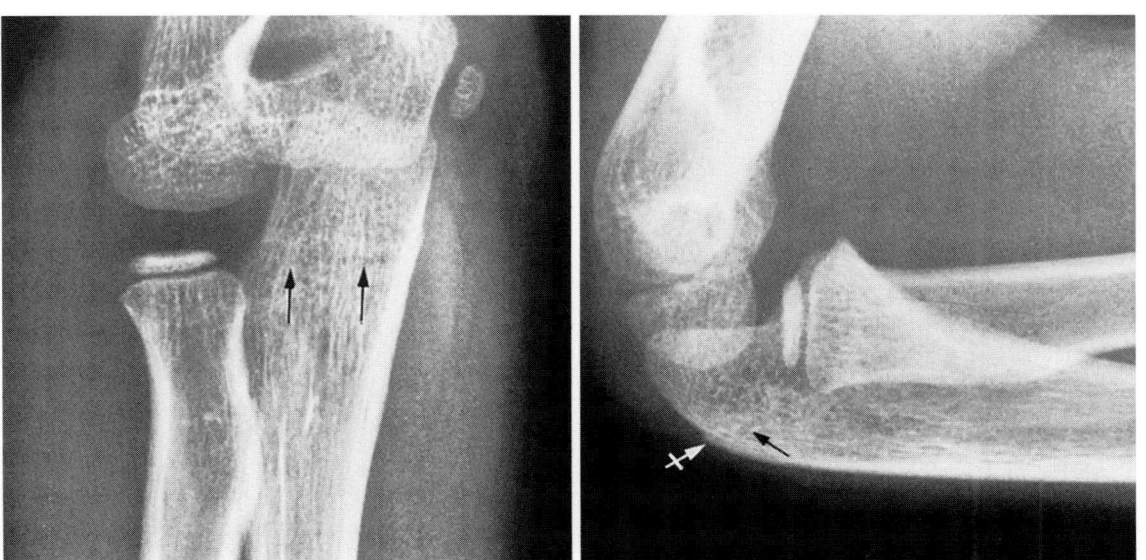

Figure 6–99. Simulated fracture of the ulna produced by trabeculations in the shaft (←) and a small excrescence in the cortex just below the location of the distal end of the unossified apophysis (↤).

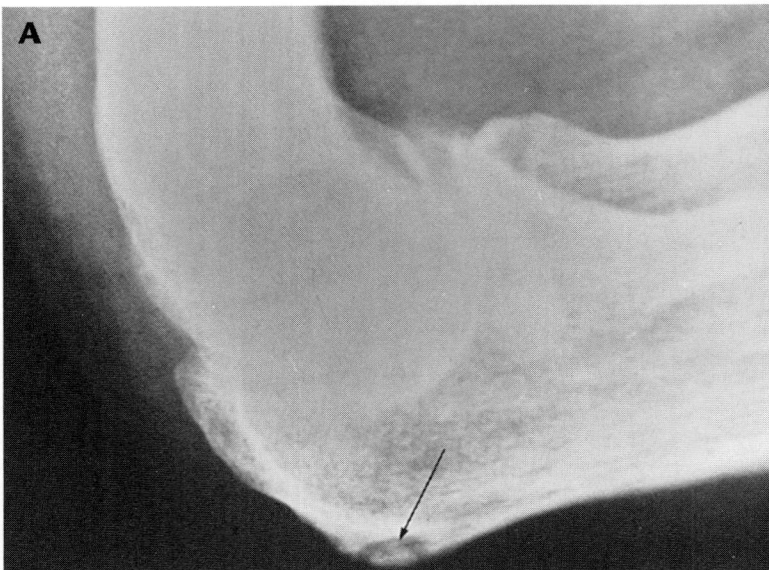

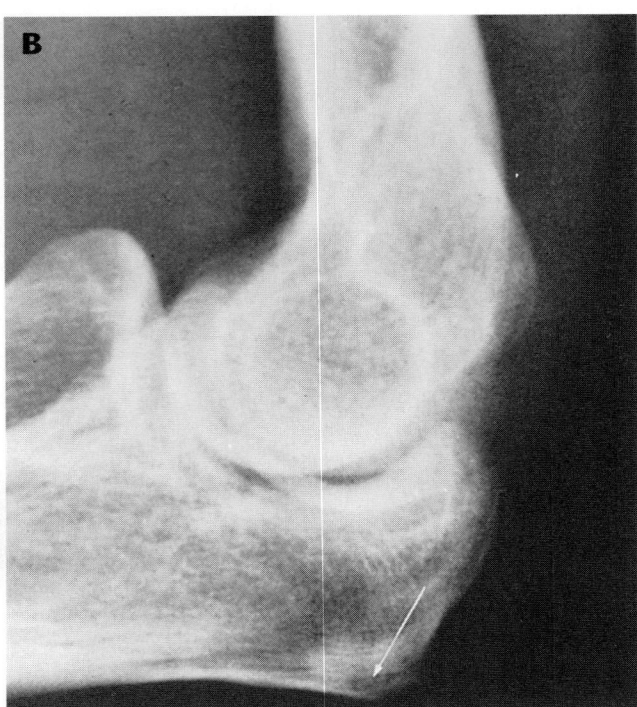

Figure 6–100. Unusual development of the olecranon in a single individual. **A,** Ossicle. **B,** Fossa.

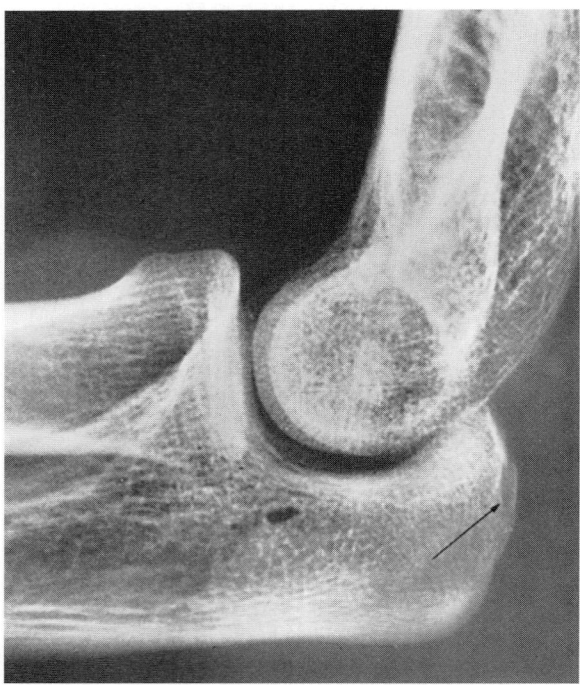

Figure 6–101. Residual irregularity of the olecranon after closure of the apophysis in a 19-year-old man.

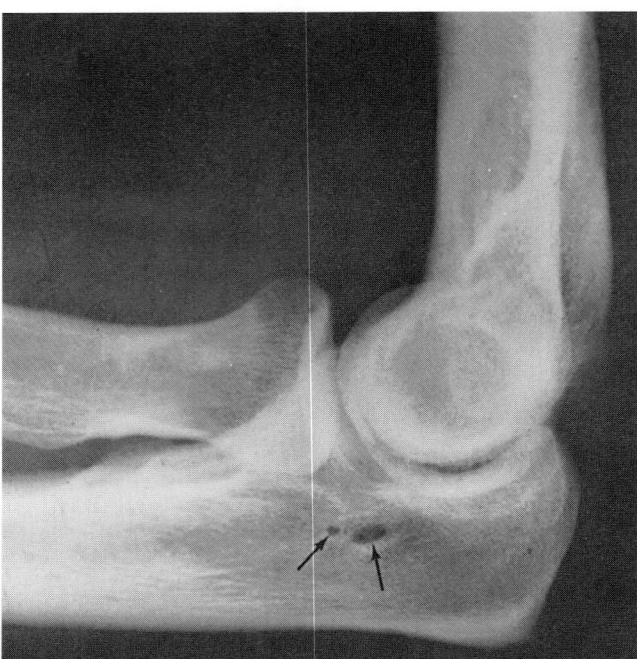

Figure 6–102. Normal foramina for nutrient vessels of the proximal ulna.

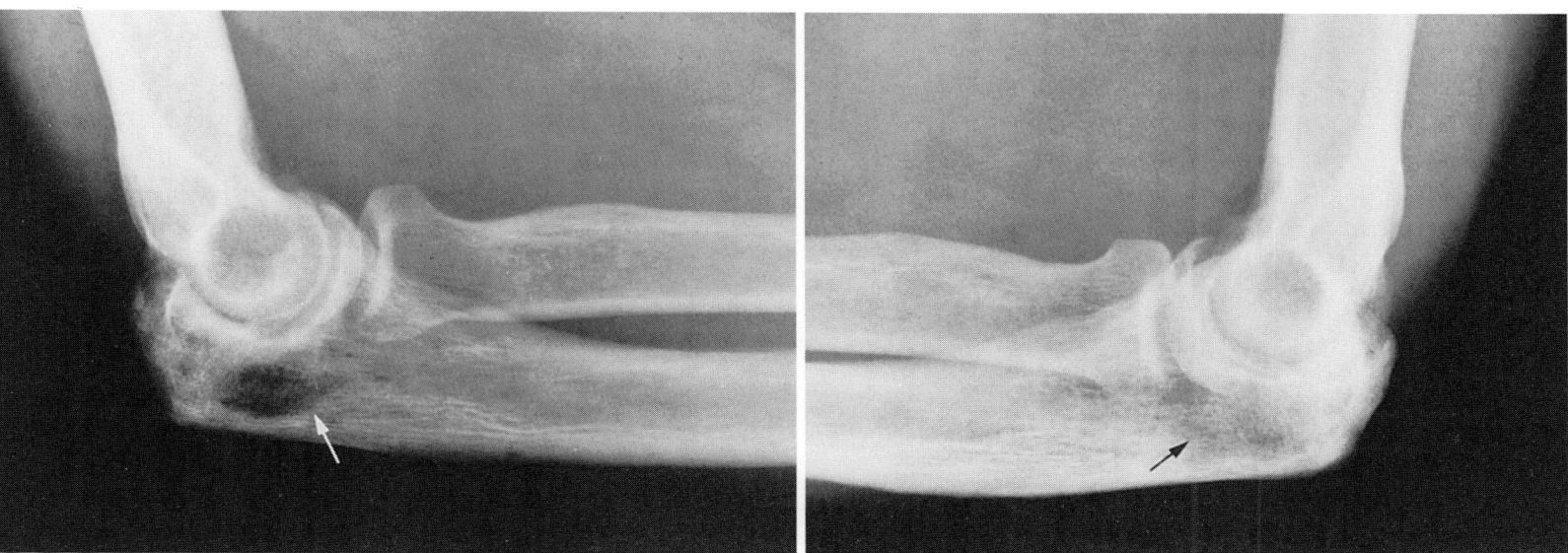

Figure 6–103. Cancellous bone of the proximal end of the ulnae, simulating destructive lesions in a 49-year-old man.

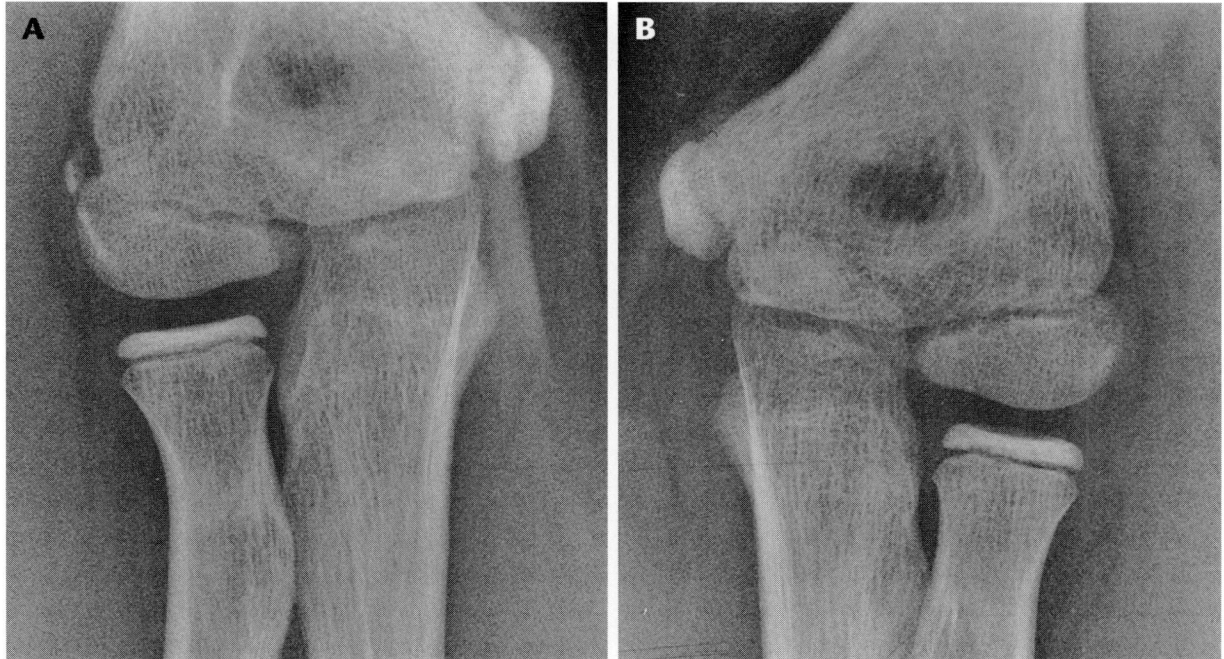

Figure 6–104. Normal sclerotic appearance of the epiphysis of the radial heads in an 11-year-old boy.

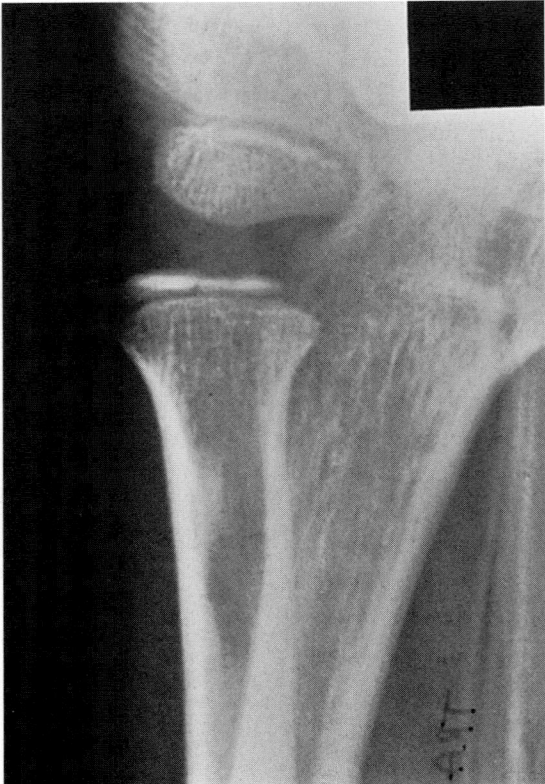

Figure 6–105. Cleft epiphysis of the radial head. (Ref: Harrison RB, Keats TE: Epiphyseal clefts. *Skeletal Radiol* 5:23, 1980.)

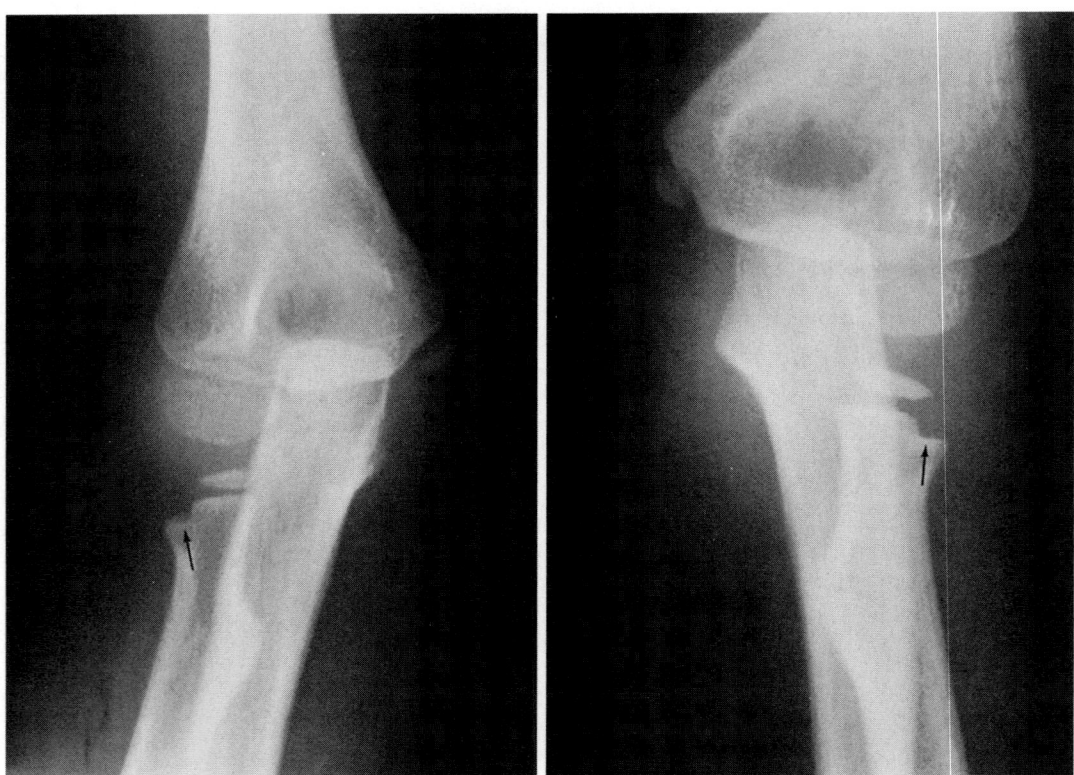

Figure 6–106. Notches on the lateral aspects of the radial metaphyses in a 6-year-old girl. These are filled in by further growth and disappear as the child matures (see following figure).

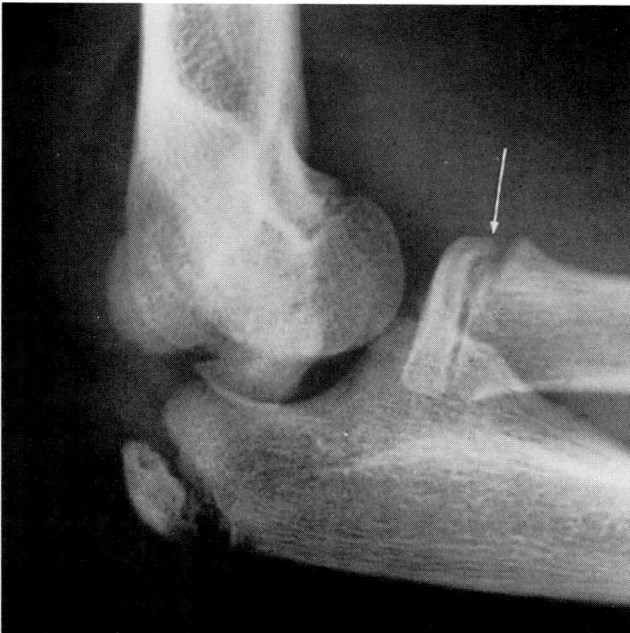

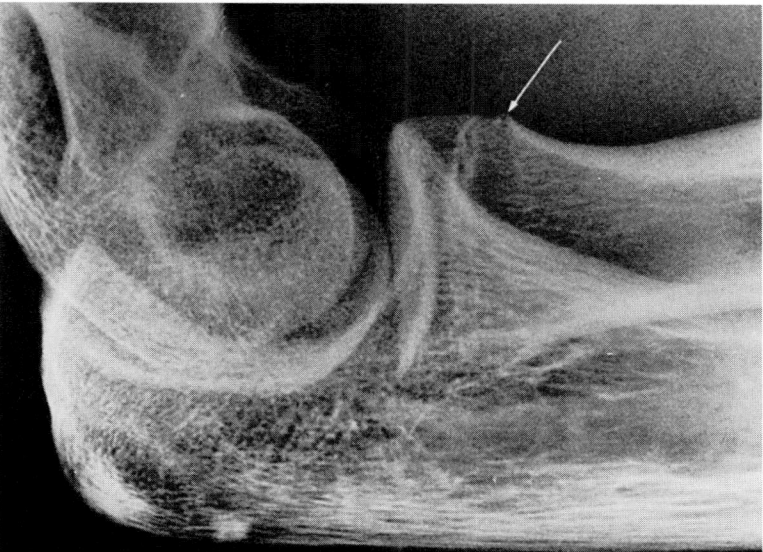

Figure 6–108. Small cleft in the radial metaphysis in a 16-year-old girl, which should not be mistaken for a fracture.

Figure 6–107. This patient illustrates the mechanism by which the notches seen in the preceding figure are obliterated. The fossa fills in by overgrowth of the epiphysis of the radial head. This is the same mechanism seen for completion of growth of the tibial tubercle. (Ref: McCarthy SM, Ogden JA: Radiology of postnatal skeletal development. IV. Elbow joint, proximal radius and ulna. *Skeletal Radiol* 9:17, 1982.)

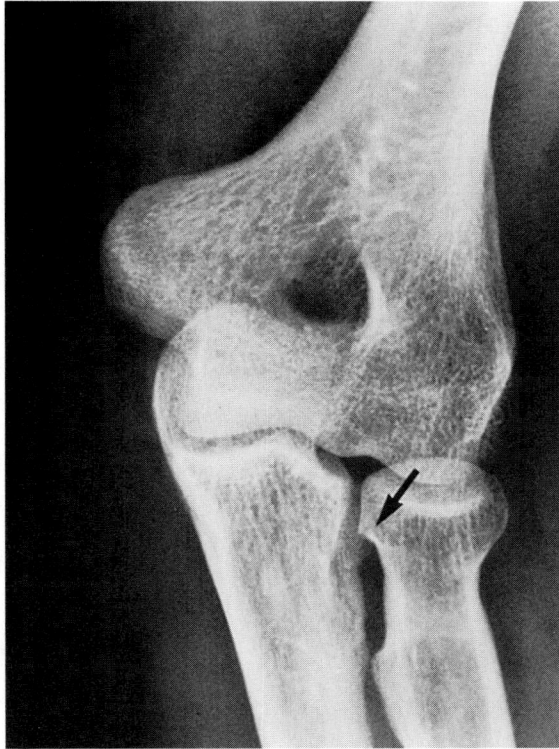

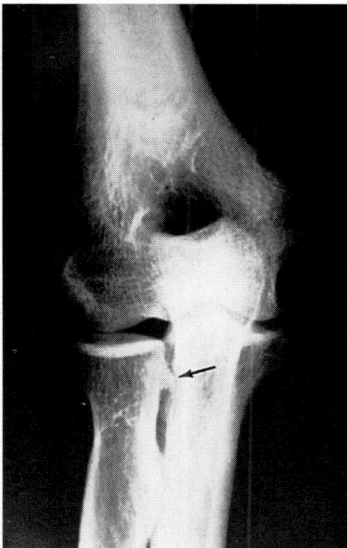

Figure 6–110. A small spur arising from the radial head.

Figure 6–109. Small cleft that might be mistaken for fracture in the medial aspect of the proximal radial metaphysis. There was no history of trauma.

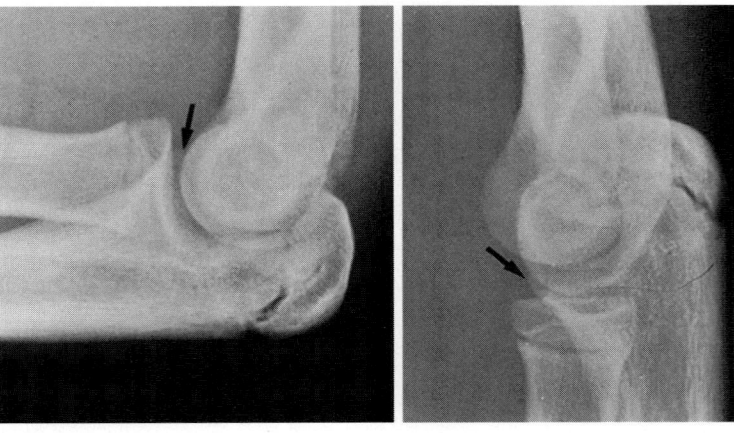

Figure 6–111. Ossification center at the tip of the coronoid process of the ulna (os cubiti anterius) in an adolescent.

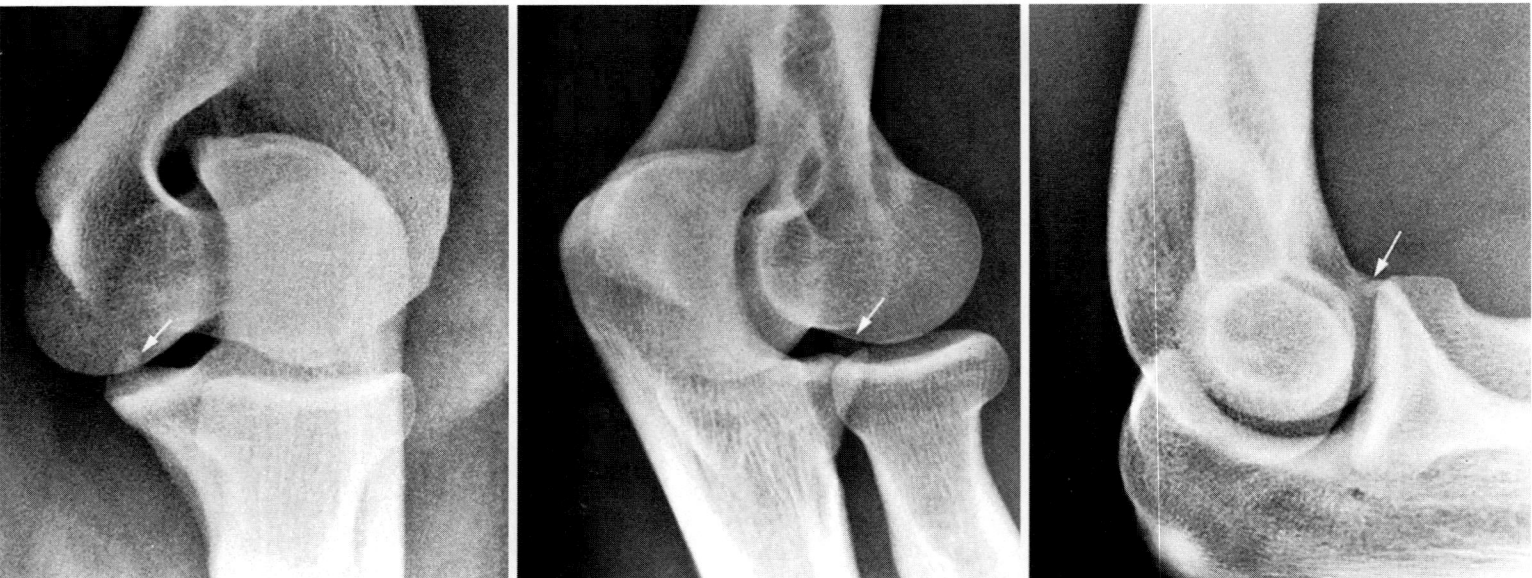

Figure 6–112. Accessory ossicle at the tip of the coronoid process. Old avulsion injuries may also manifest as ossicles of this type. (Ref: Glajchen N et al: Avulsion fracture of the sublime tubercle of the ulna. *Am J Roentgenol* 170:627, 1998.)

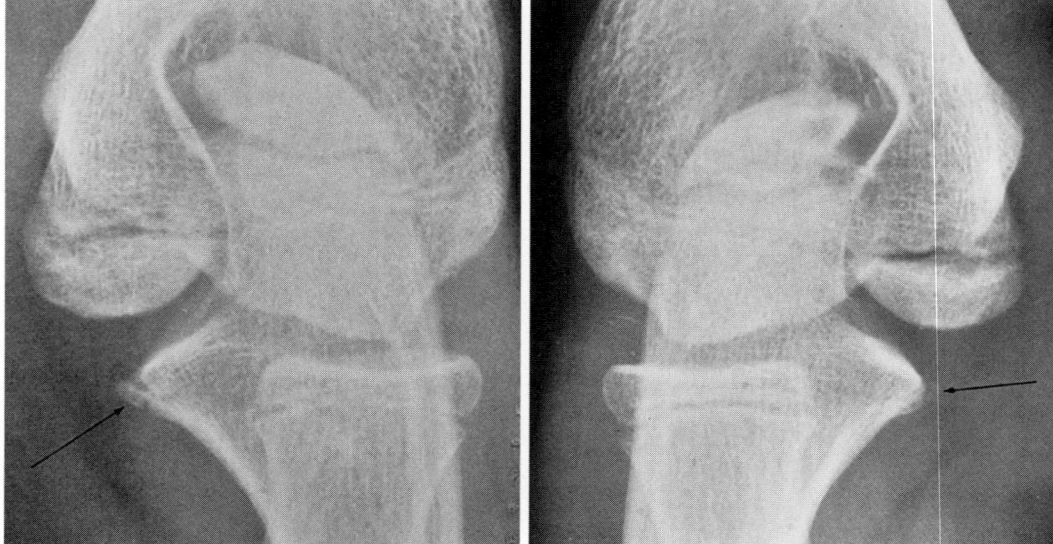

Figure 6–113. Accessory ossification centers for the tip of the coronoid process, which could be mistaken for a fracture.

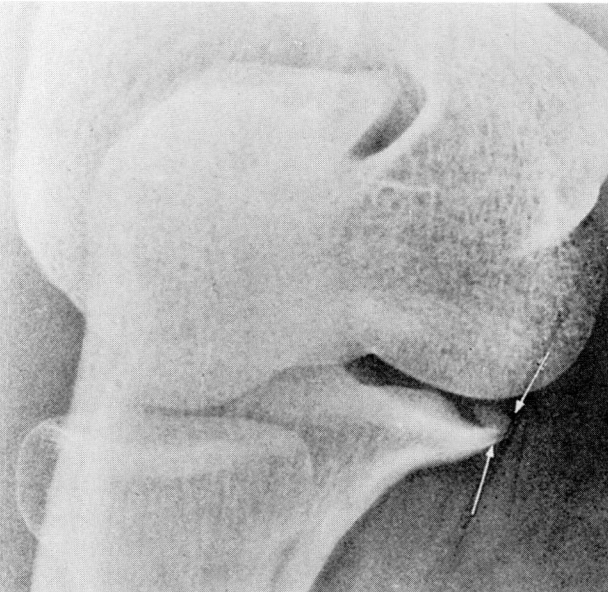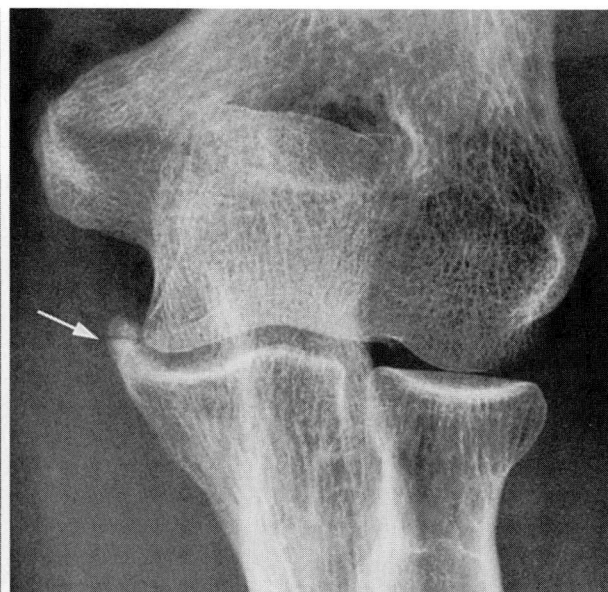

Figure 6–114. Persistent ossification center of the coronoid process of the ulna, which simulates a fracture.

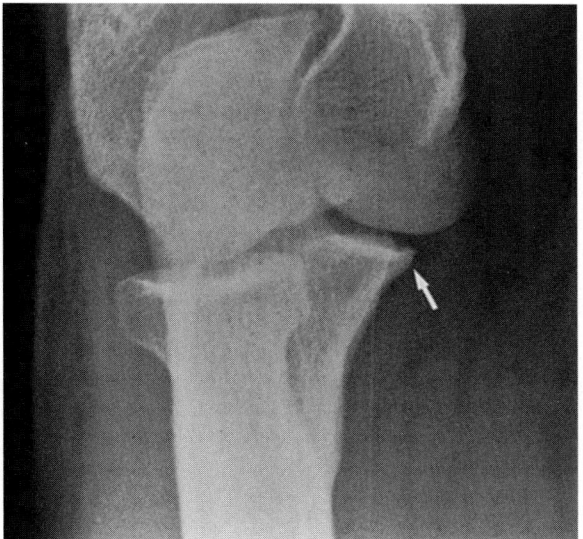

Figure 6–115. Partially fused ossicle at tip of the coronoid process of the ulna.

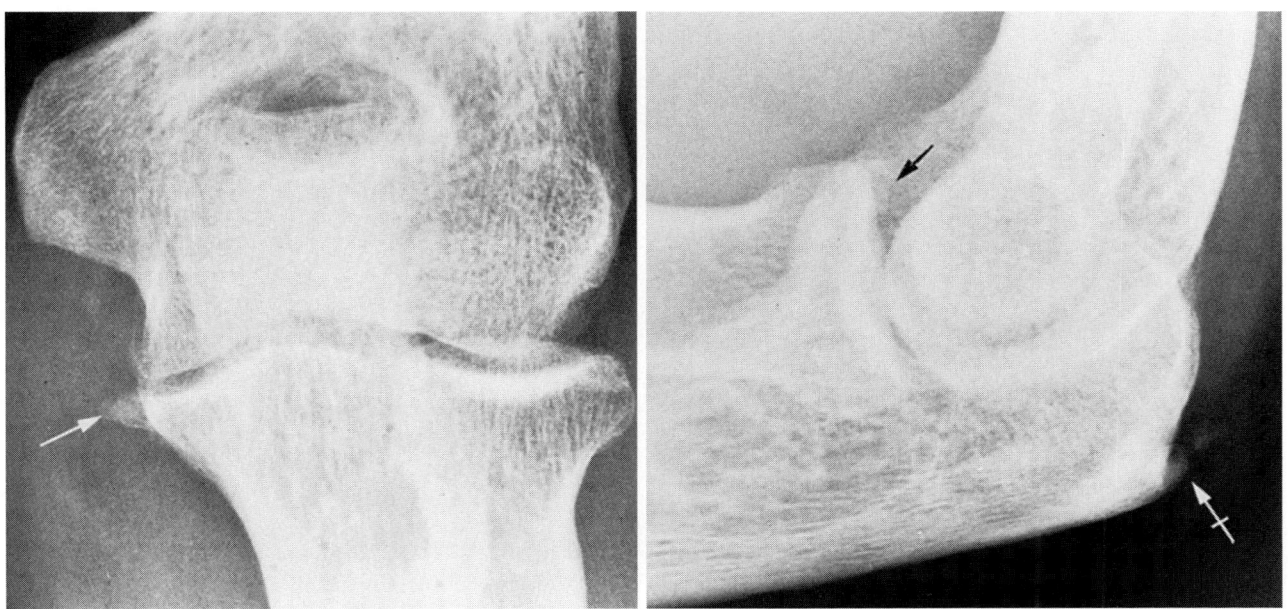

Figure 6–116. Tendinous calcification at the coronoid process (←) in the origins of the flexor digitorum superficiale and at the insertion of the triceps tendon (↔). These should not be mistaken for traumatic sequelae.

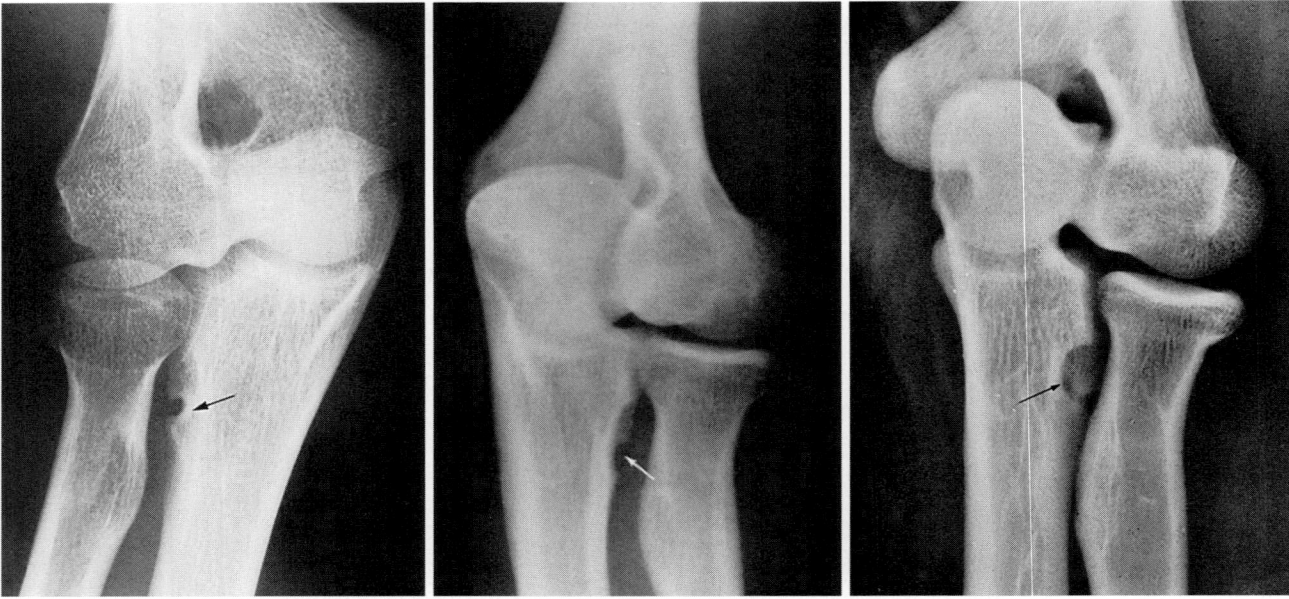

Figure 6–117. Examples of fossae in the ulna that represent the insertion point of the annular ligament. These should not be confused with a pathologic process. (Ref: Schoneich R: Tuberositas radii varietat "Bandgruber." *ROFO* 149:675, 1988.)

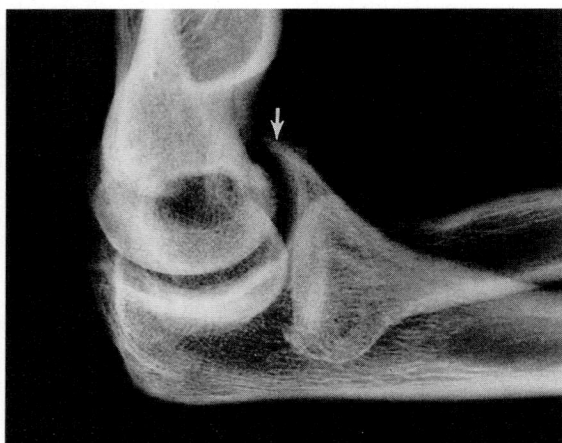

Figure 6–118. Unusually long coronoid process of the ulna, possibly related to stress.

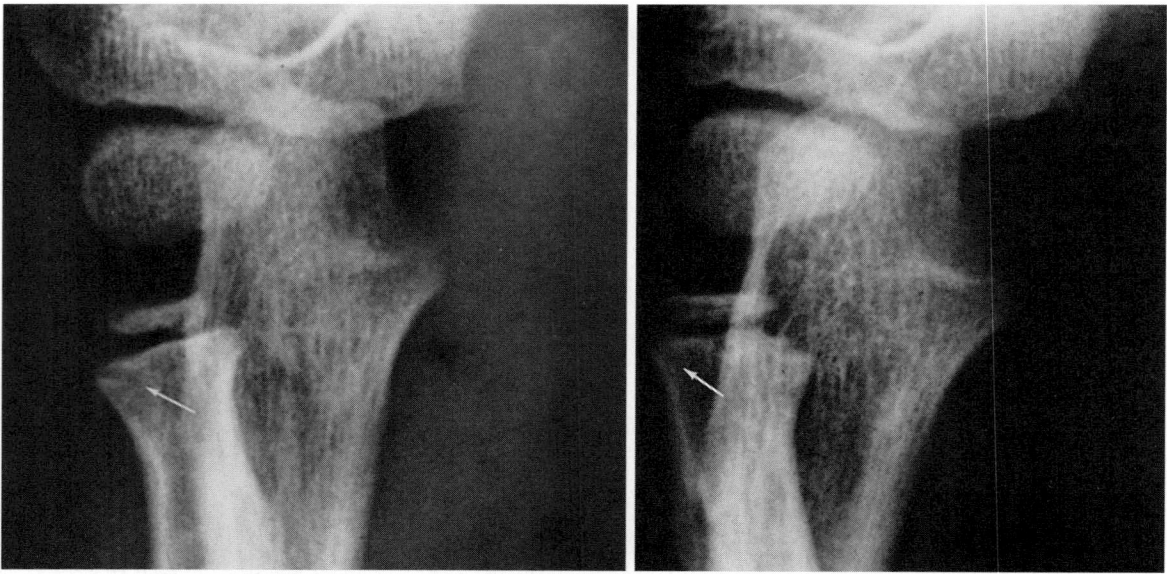

Figure 6–119. Oblique radiolucent clefts in proximal radial metaphysis in a young child. These oblique clefts are a common finding adjacent to the epiphyseal lines in young children and should not be mistaken for metaphyseal fractures. (Ref: Silberstein MJ et al: Some vagaries of the radial head and neck. *J Bone Joint Surg* 64A:1153, 1982.)

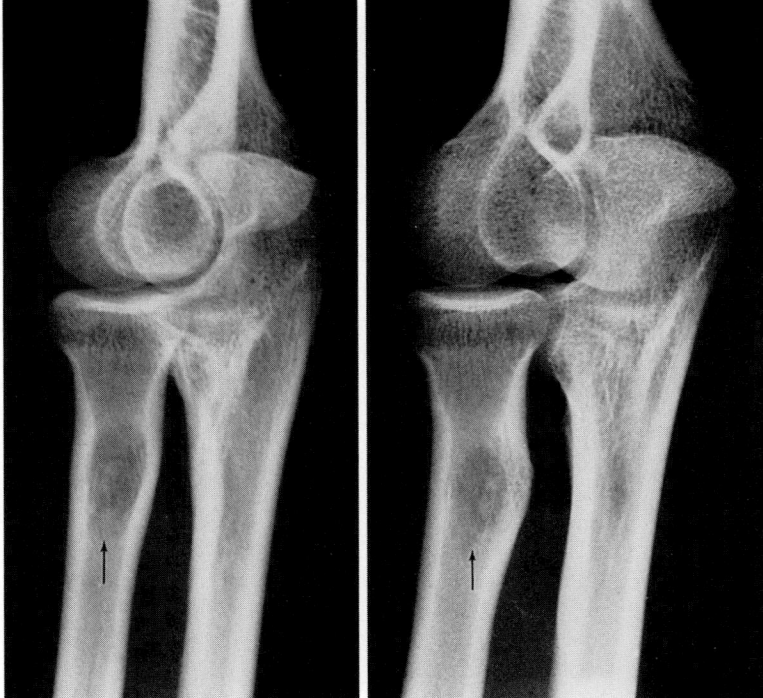

Figure 6–120. The radial tuberosity presents as a radiolucency and might be mistaken in both projections for an area of bone destruction.

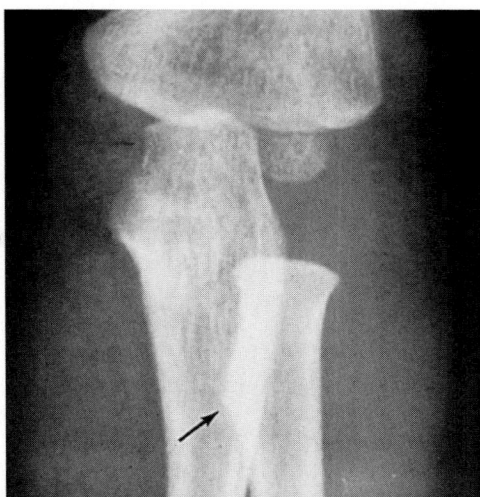

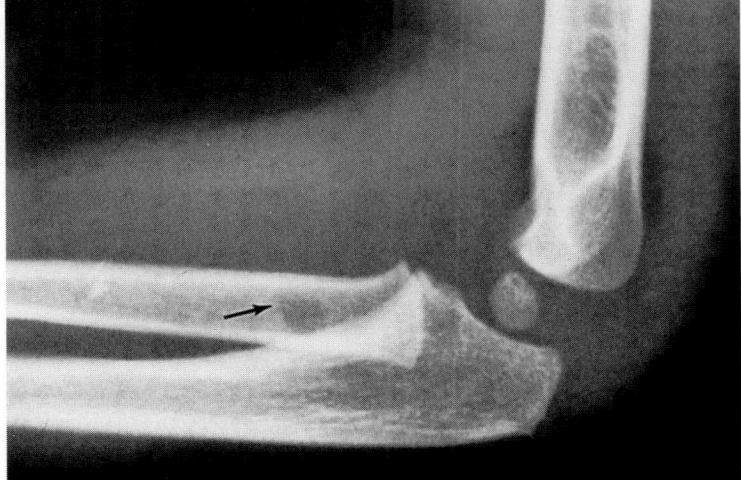

Figure 6–121. A radial tuberosity in a 4-year-old boy, simulating a focal destructive lesion only in the lateral projection.

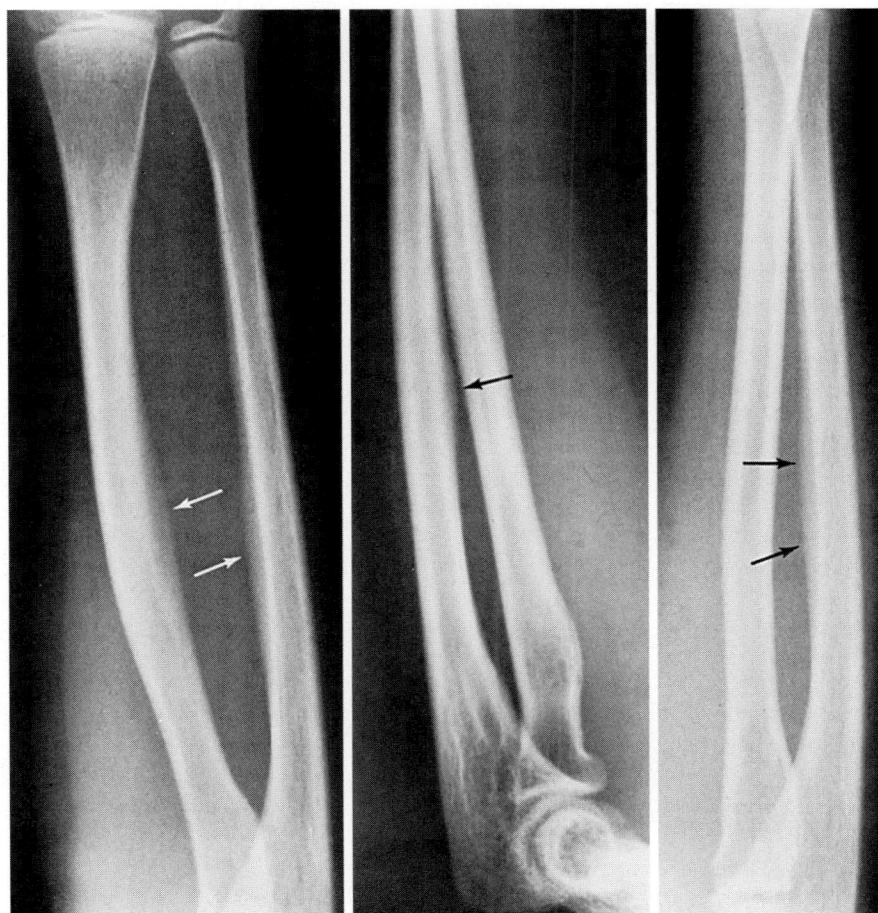

Figure 6–122. The interosseous ridges of the radius and ulna often cast shadows that may be mistaken for periostitis.

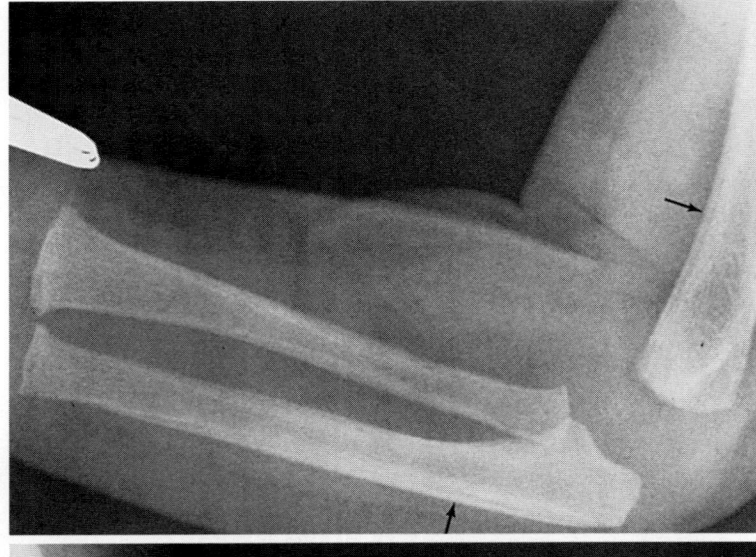

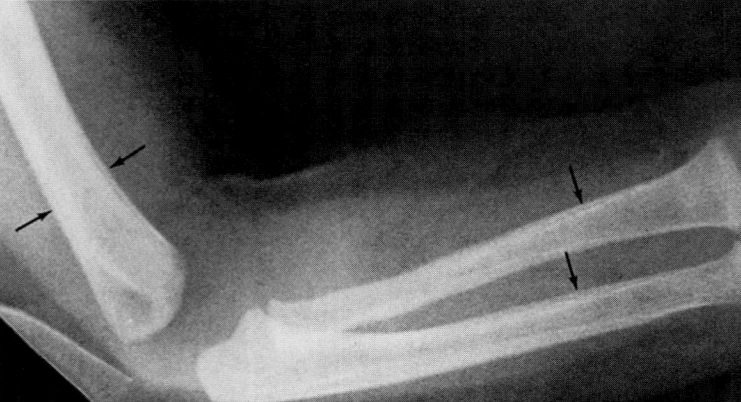

Figure 6–123. Physiologic "periostitis" of the newborn in a 2½-month-old infant. This is not seen before the age of 1 month, is symmetric in distribution although not necessarily concentric, and may be seen in only one view. (Ref: Shopfner CE: Periosteal bone growth in normal infants: A preliminary report. *Am J Roentgenol* 97:154, 1966.)

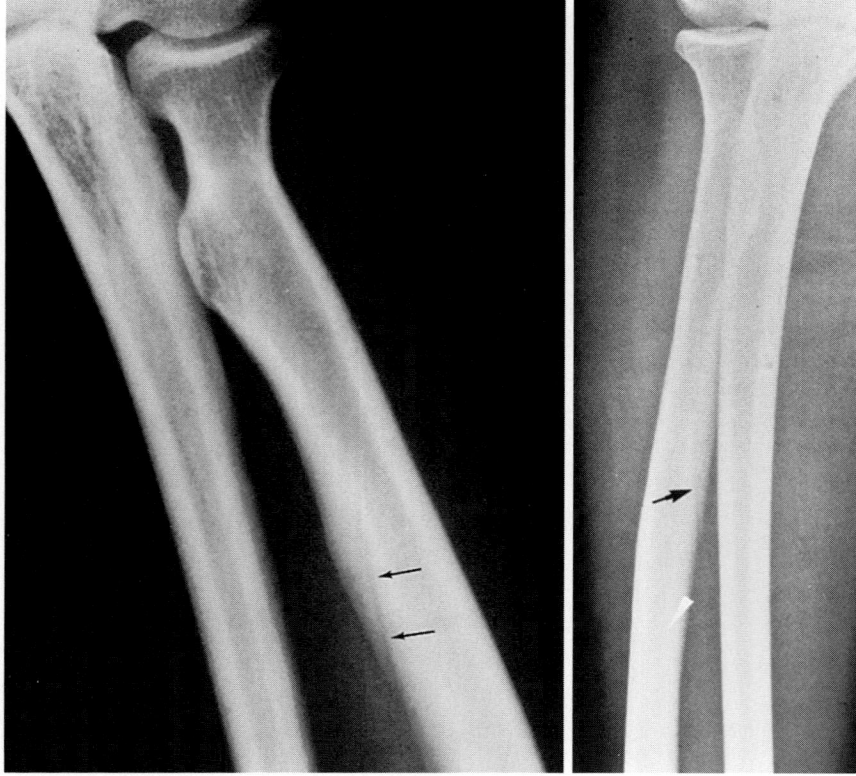

Figure 6–124. The nutrient channel of the radius.

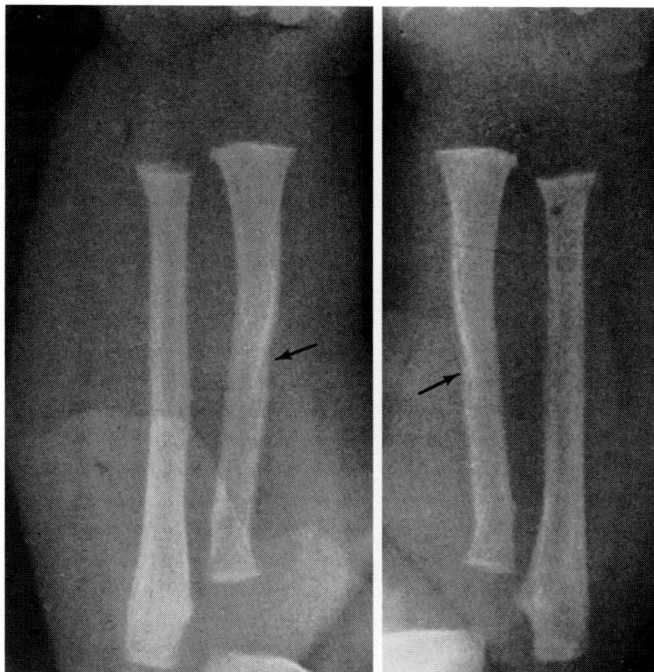

Figure 6–125. Normal undulations of the contour of the radii of the newborn. These disappear with increasing age.

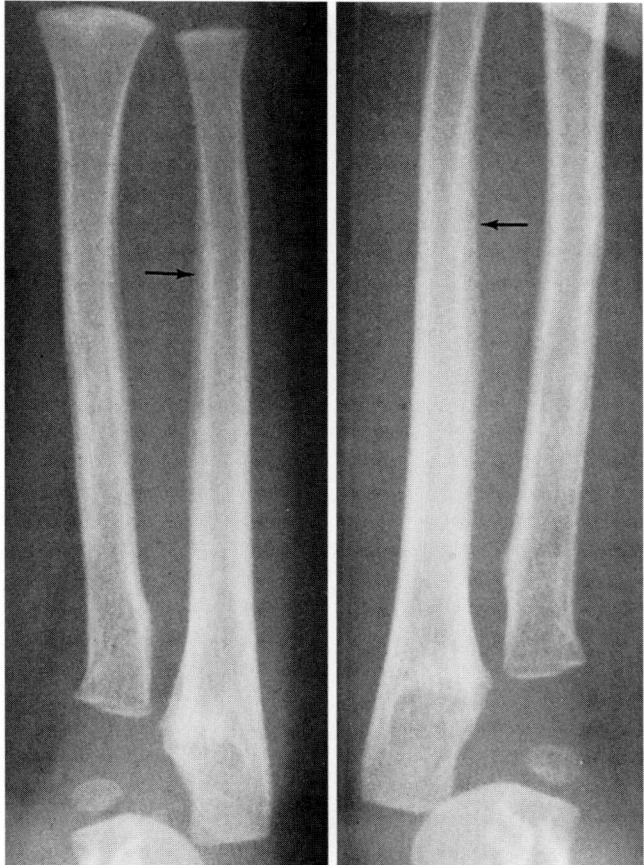

Figure 6–126. Cortical tunneling of the distal ulna may be seen in infants and older children and is of no clinical significance. (Ref: Weiss C: Normal roentgen variant: Cortical tunneling of the distal ulna. *Radiology* 136:294, 1980.)

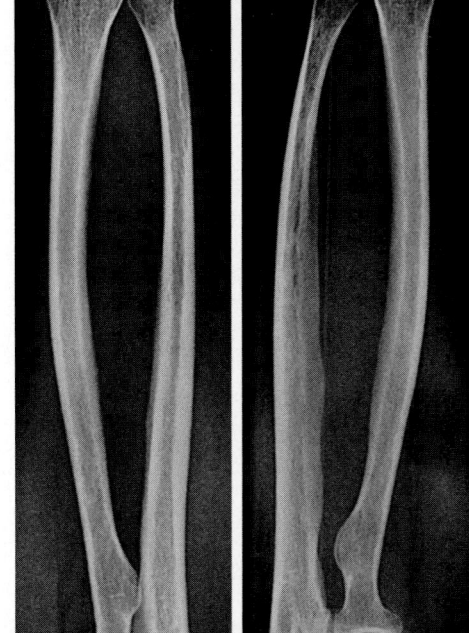

Figure 6–127. A, B, Bilateral physiologic bowing of both bones of the forearm seen in a patient with ulna minus variation.

The Distal Portion of the Forearm

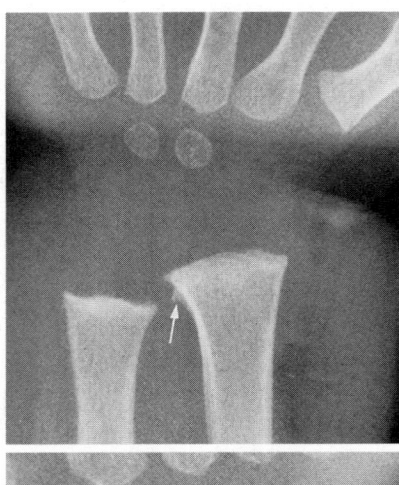

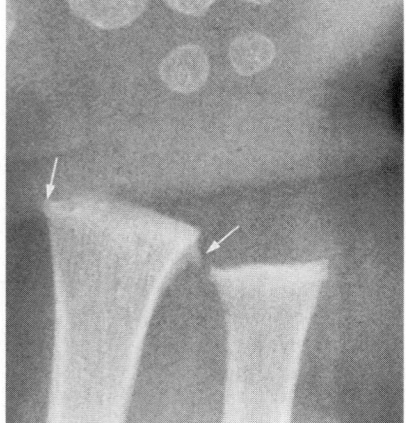

Figure 6–128. Small normal metaphyseal spurs of the distal radius in a healthy 1-year-old girl. (Ref: Kleinman PK et al: Normal metaphyseal radiologic variant, not to be confused with findings of infant abuse. *Am J Roentgenol* 156:781, 1991.)

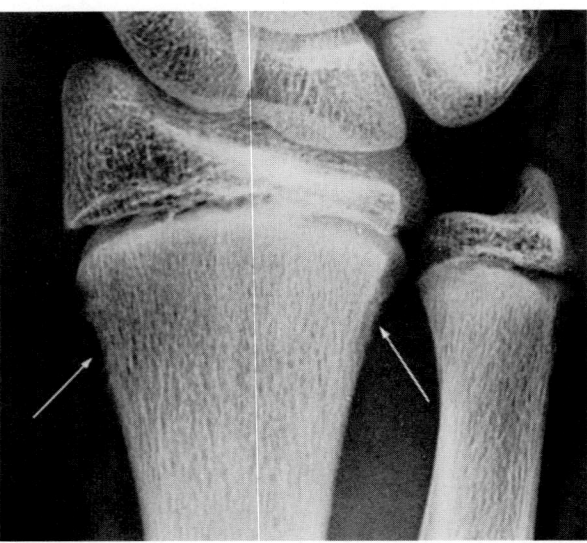

Figure 6–129. Normal metaphyseal irregularities of the radius in a 14-year-old boy. These changes were no longer present 1 year later.

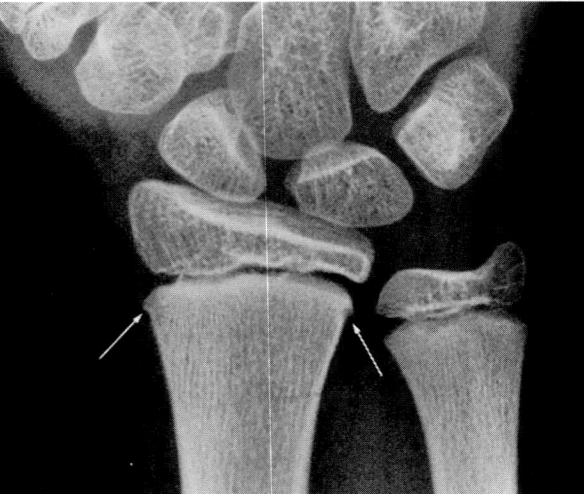

Figure 6–130. Small irregularities of the metaphysis in a 10-year-old girl (as in the preceding figure).

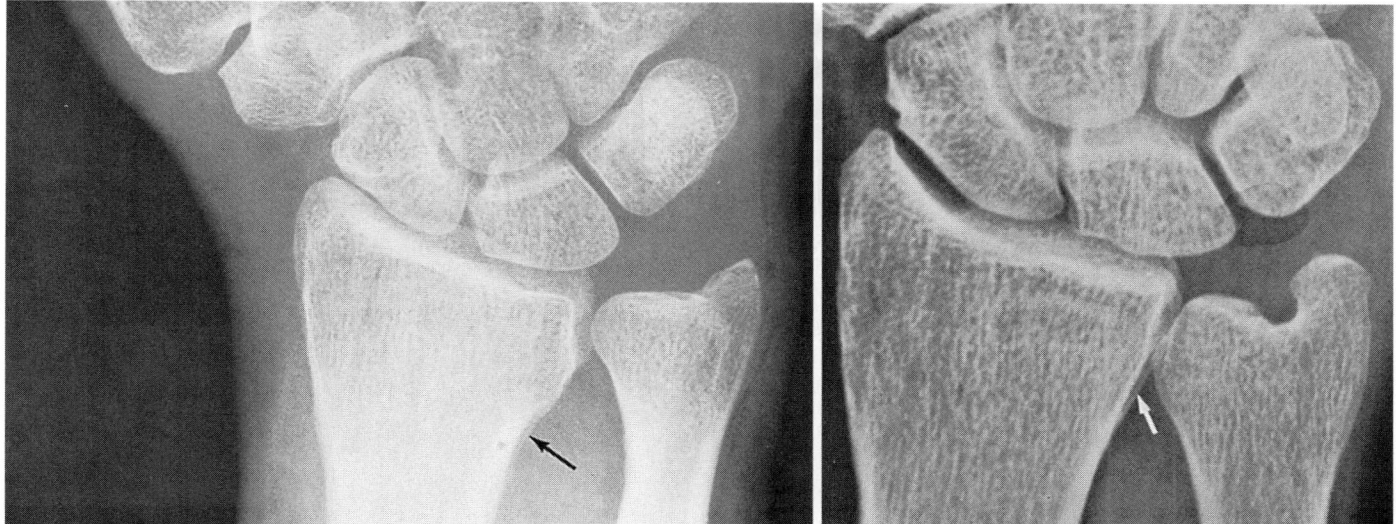

Figure 6–131. Two examples of thin flanges of bone simulating periostitis of the distal radius.

Figure 6–132. Examples of cortical irregularities at insertion of interosseous membrane simulating periostitis.

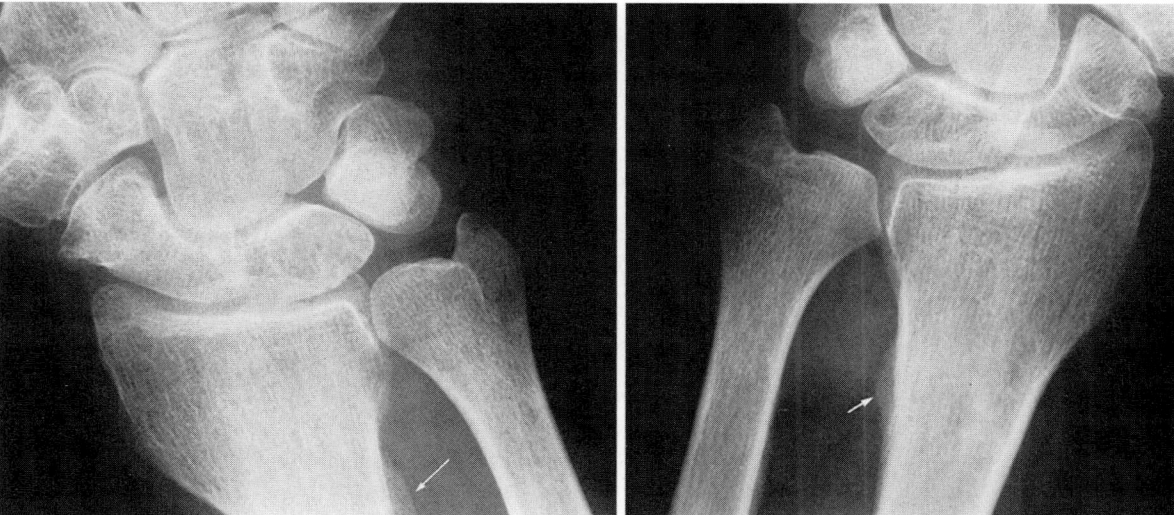

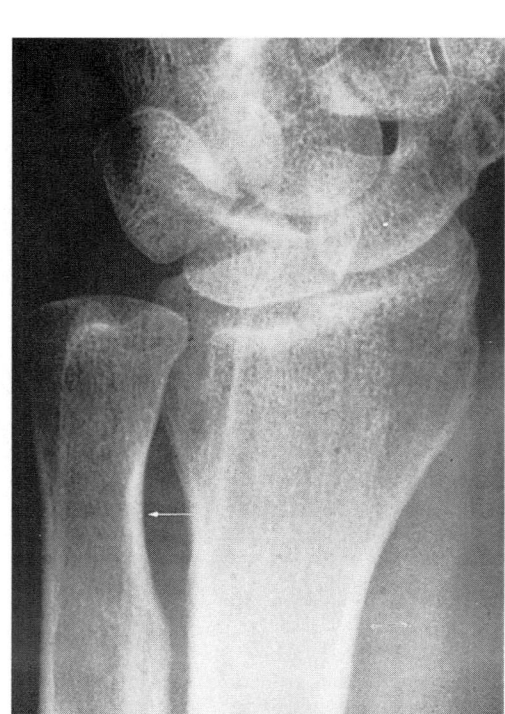

Figure 6–133. Developmental fossa in distal ulna.

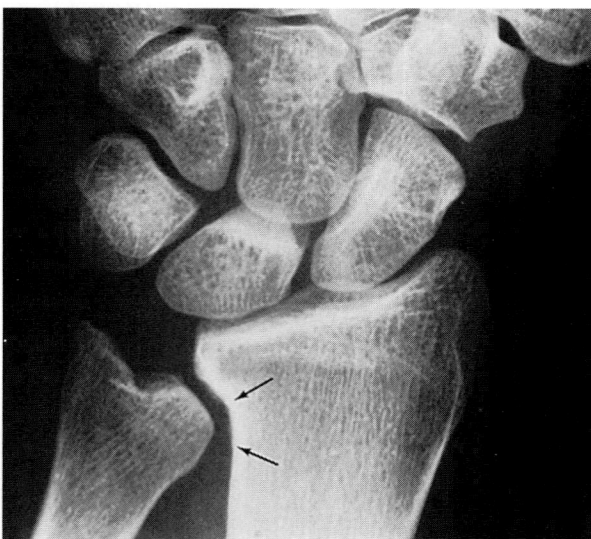
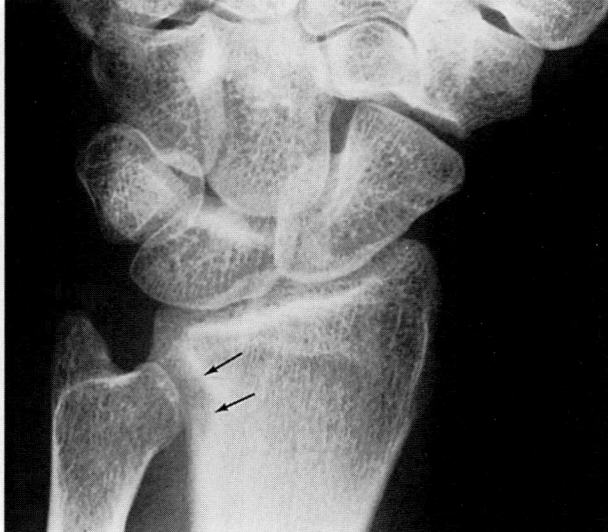

Figure 6–134. Short ulna (ulna minus variant) with a deep articulation with the radius, which resembles an erosive lesion. (Ref: Gelberman RH et al: Ulnar variance in Kienböck's disease. *J Bone Joint Surg* 57A:674, 1975.)

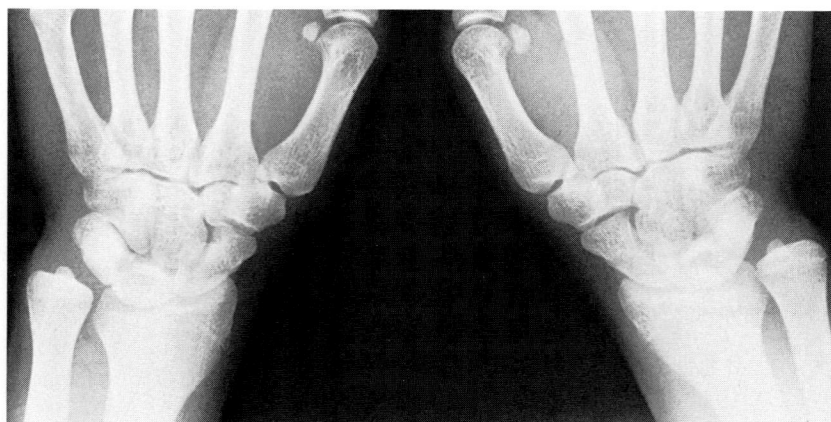
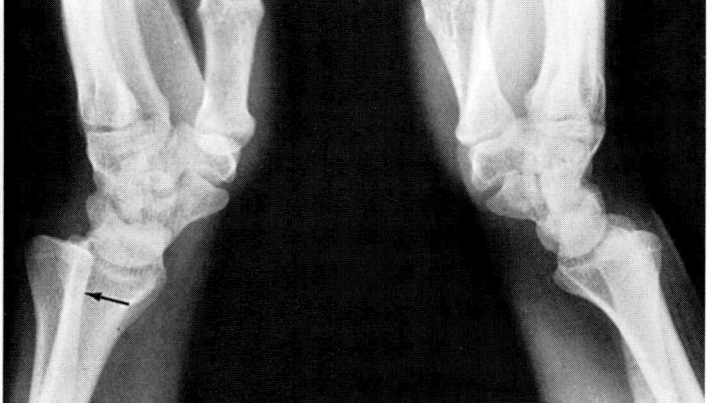

Figure 6–135. Unusually long ulnae (ulna plus variant), which may be mistaken for a dislocation of the distal radioulnar joint if the bilateral symmetry is not noted.

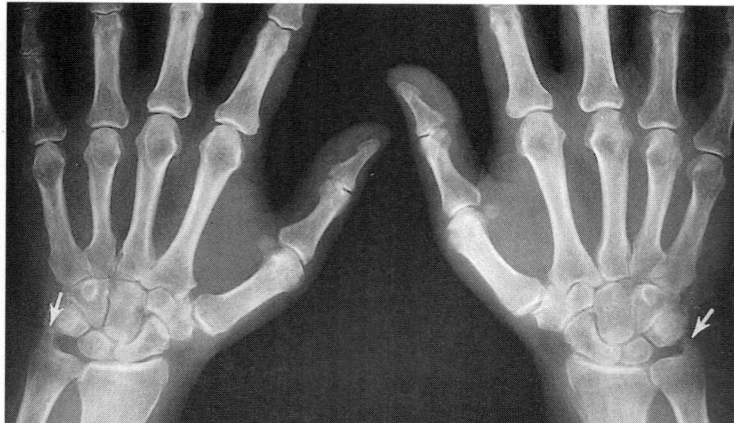

Figure 6–136. Ulna plus variant. Note close approximation of the ulnar styloid to the triquetrum bone. This variant may lead to ulnar impaction syndrome and injury to the triangular fibrocartilage. (Ref: Escobedo EM et al: MR imaging of ulnar impaction. *Skeletal Radiol* 24:85, 1995.)

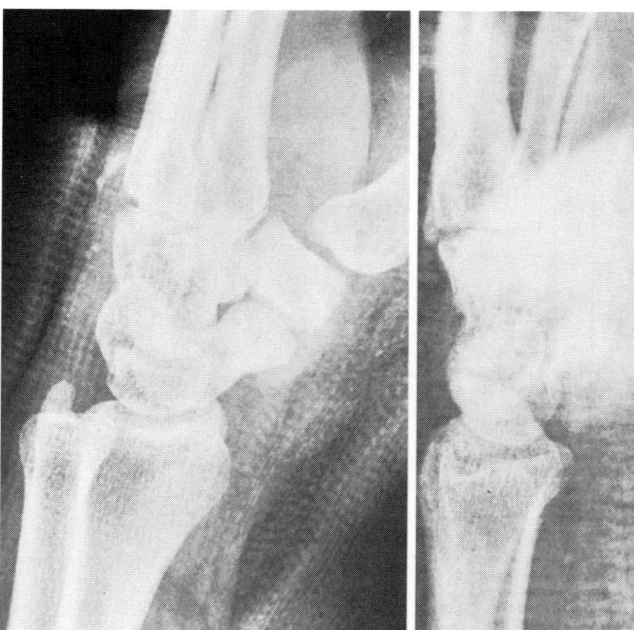

Figure 6–137. *Left,* Misdiagnosis of dislocation of the distal radioulnar joint by filming with wrist slightly rotated. *Right,* True lateral projection shows normal relationships.

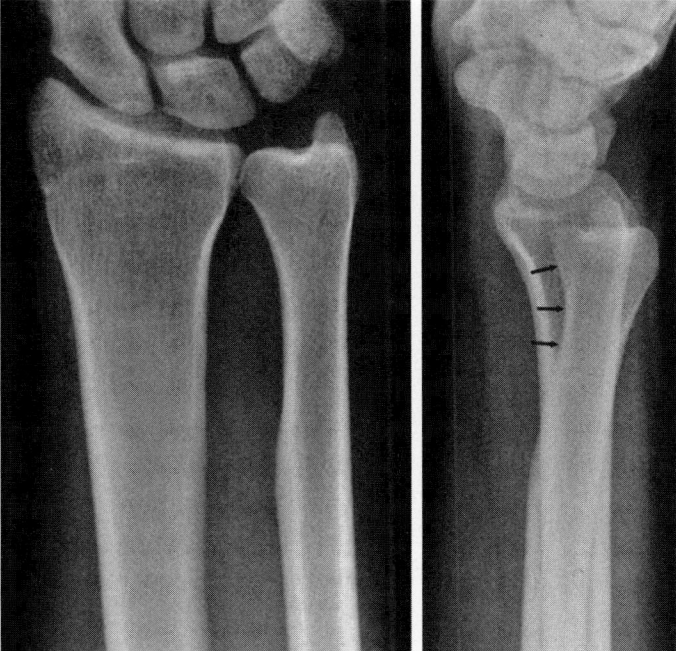

Figure 6–138. Apparent dorsal dislocation of the ulna caused by curvature of the shaft, seen in the lateral projection.

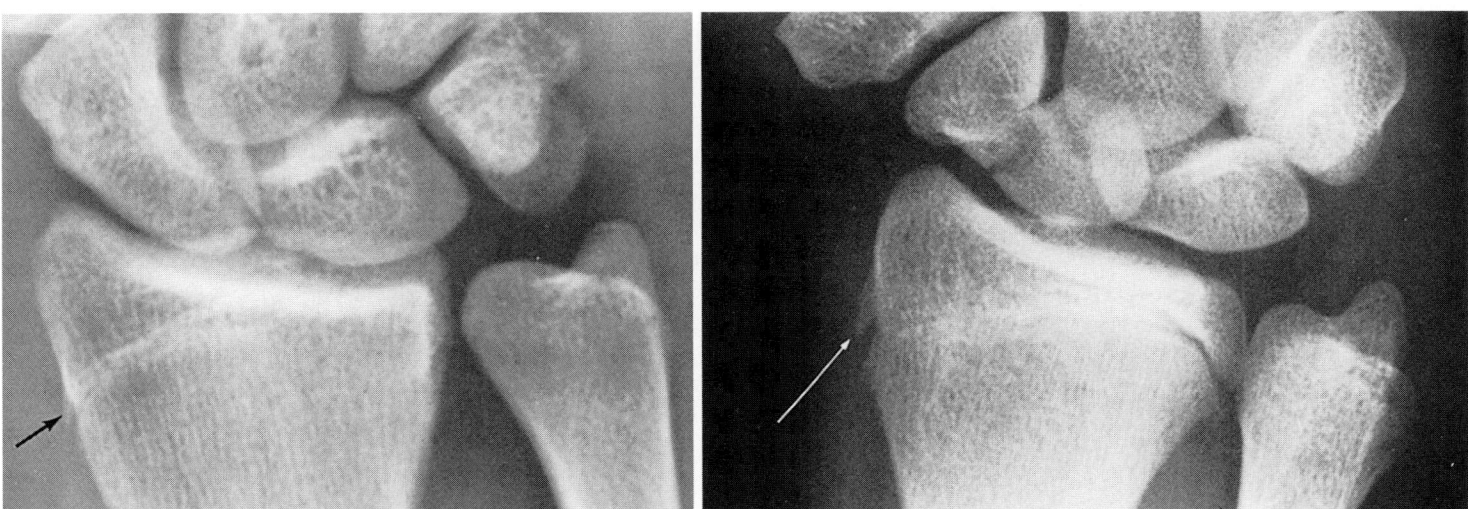

Figure 6–139. Normal spurlike projections of the epiphysis at the epiphyseal line, simulating avulsion injuries. (Ref: Keats TE, Harrison RB: The epiphyseal spur. *Skeletal Radiol* 5:175, 1980.)

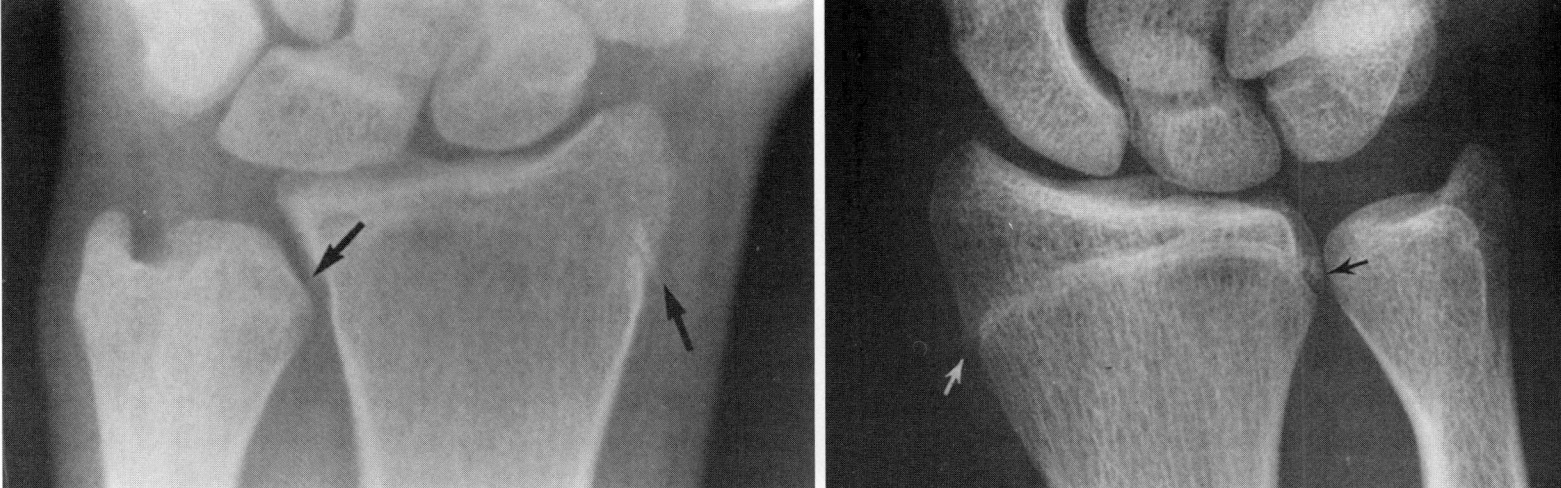

Figure 6–140. Two examples of epiphyseal spurs on medial and lateral aspects of the distal radius.

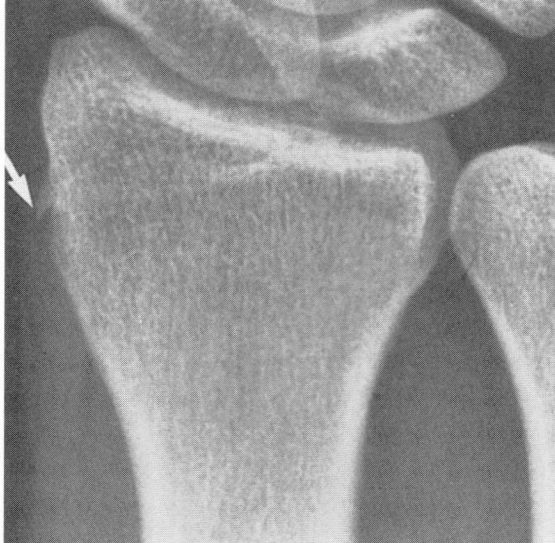

Figure 6–141. Residual epiphyseal spur after closure of the epiphyseal plate in a 20-year-old man.

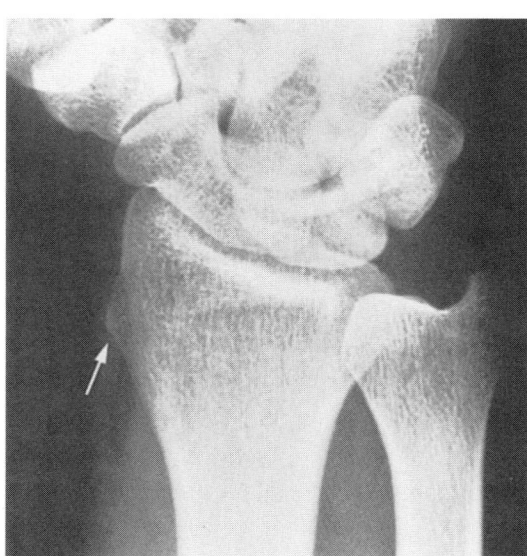

Figure 6–142. Closed epiphyseal spur at the edge of the closed physis mistaken for an avulsion fracture.

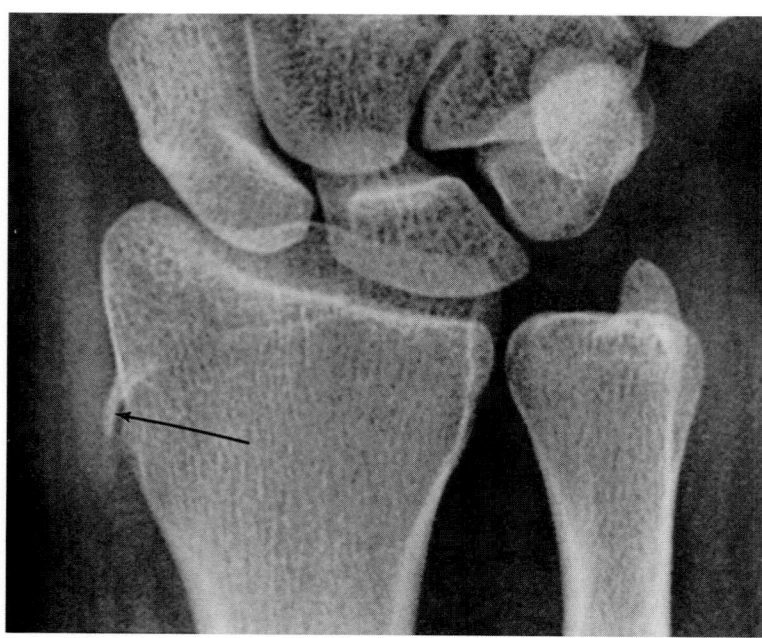

Figure 6–143. Large residual epiphyseal spur that might be mistaken for an avulsion.

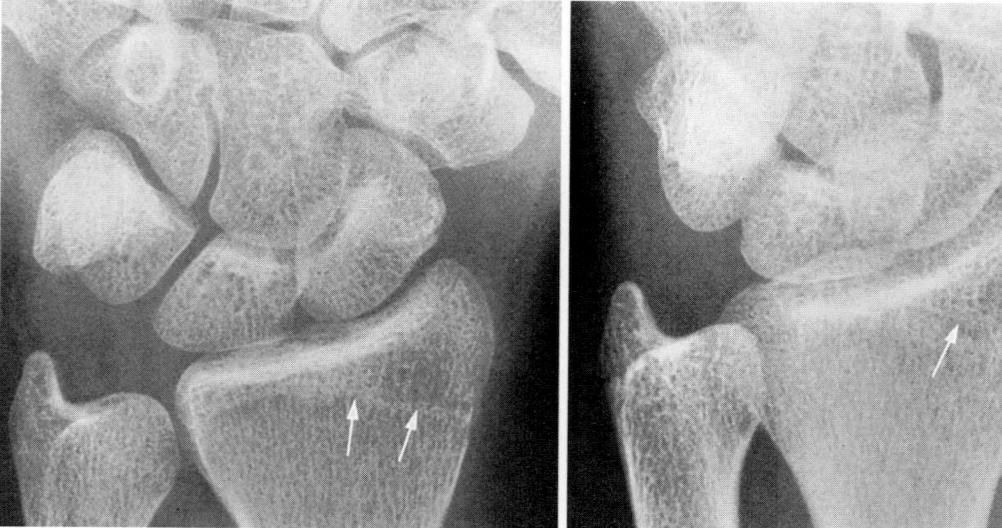

Figure 6–144. Remnants of the epiphyseal line simulating a fracture in an 18-year-old man.

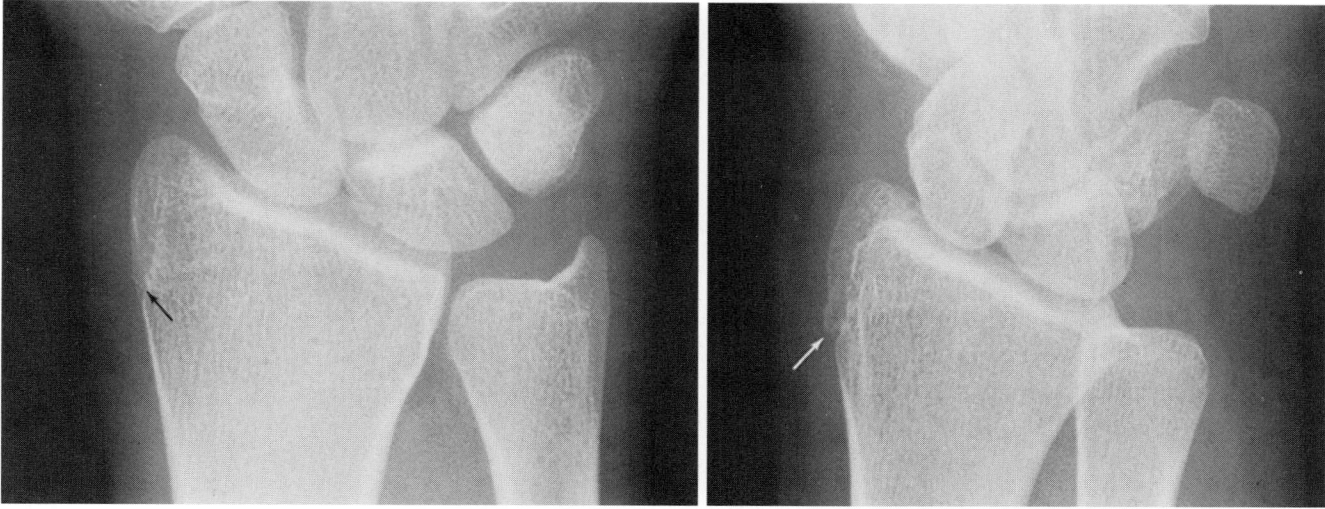

Figure 6–145. Remnants of the epiphyseal line in a 20-year-old man.

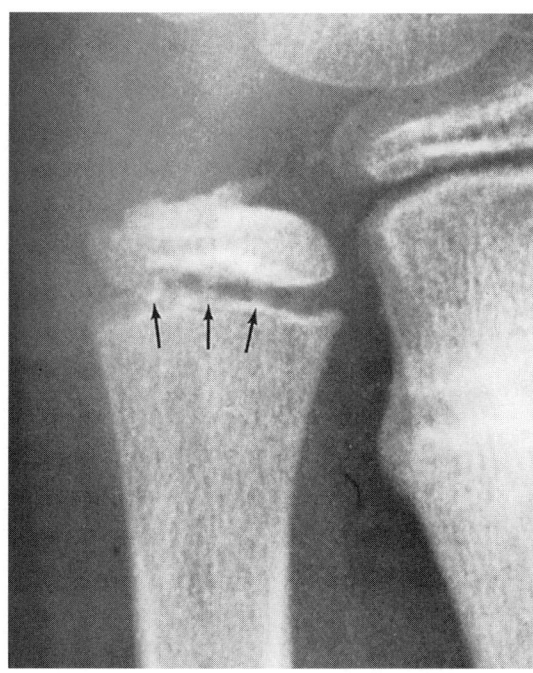

Figure 6–146. Small spicules in the epiphyseal cartilage of the ulna in a healthy 11-year-old girl. This is a normal finding of no significance.

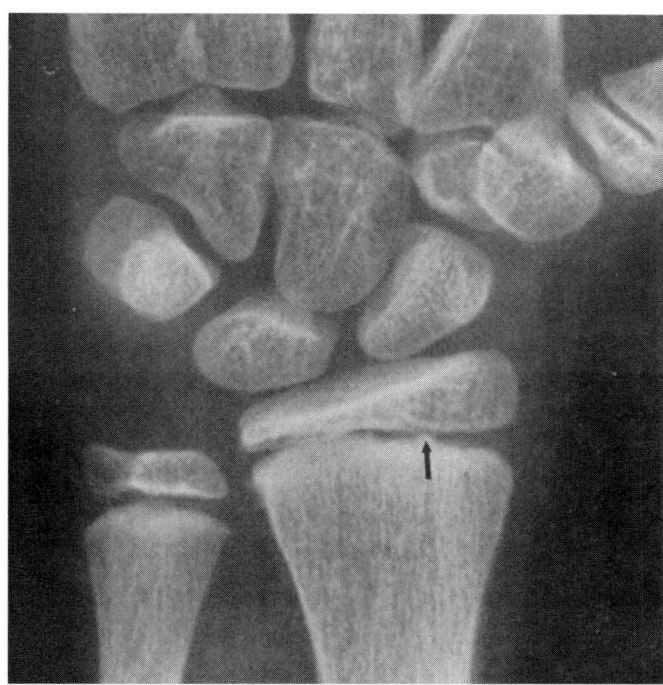

Figure 6–147. Spicule in the epiphyseal cartilage of the radius of a 12-year-old boy.

Figure 6–148. Spicules in the epiphyseal cartilage of the ulna in a 13-year-old boy.

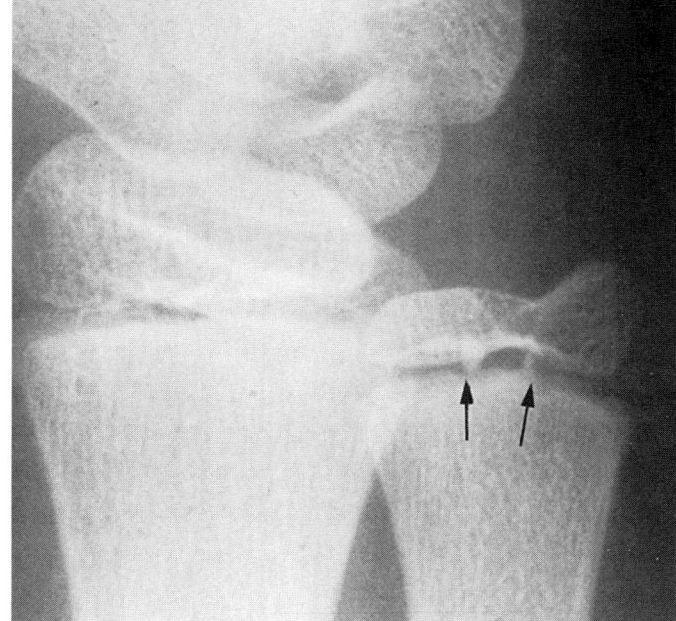

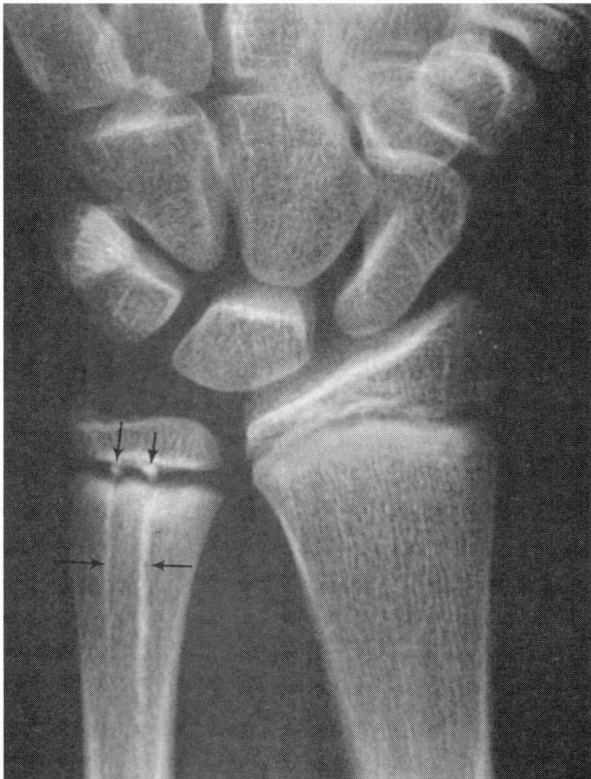

Figure 6–149. Spicules in the epiphyseal cartilage of the ulna with long streaks in the shaft in a healthy 12-year-old boy.

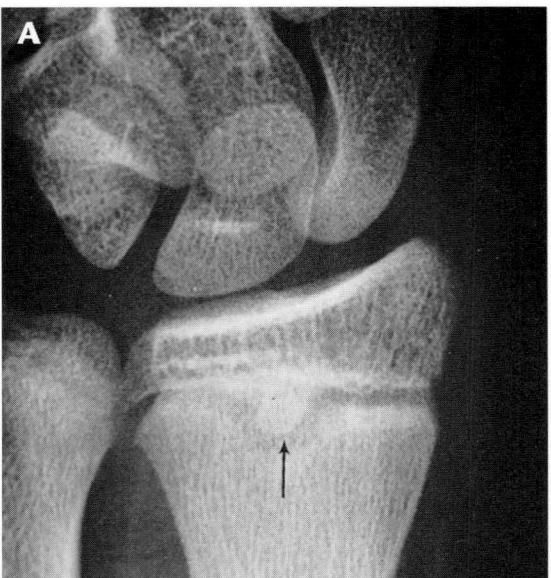

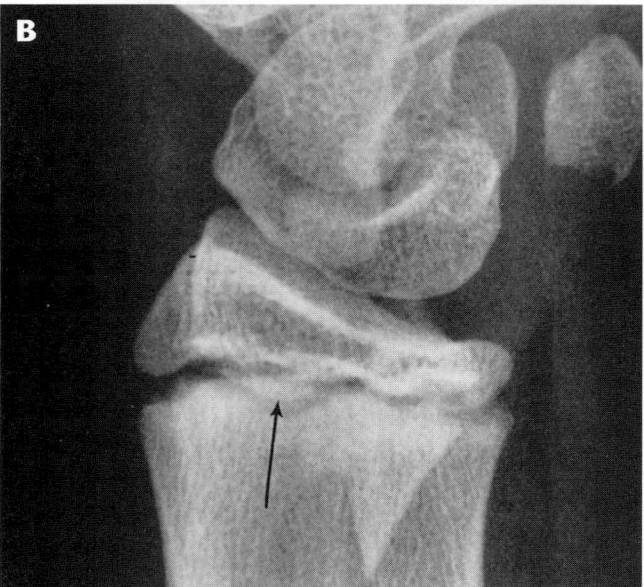

Figure 6–150. Reverse "tuck" in the physis of a 13-year-old boy. **A,** Frontal projection. **B,** Oblique projection.

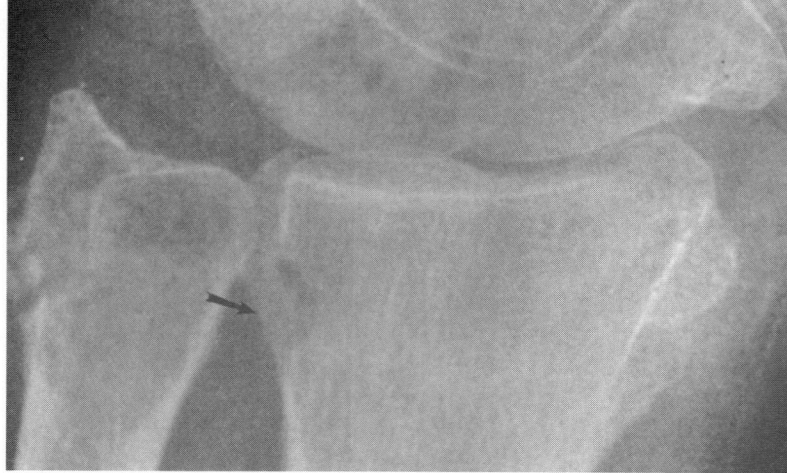

Figure 6–151. Deep symmetrical fossae below the radioulnar joint simulating erosions.

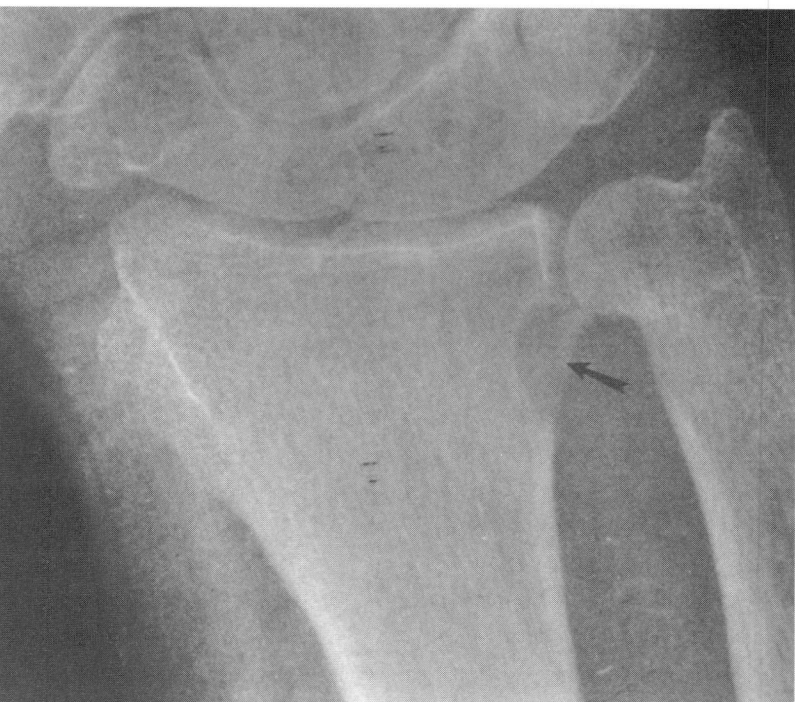

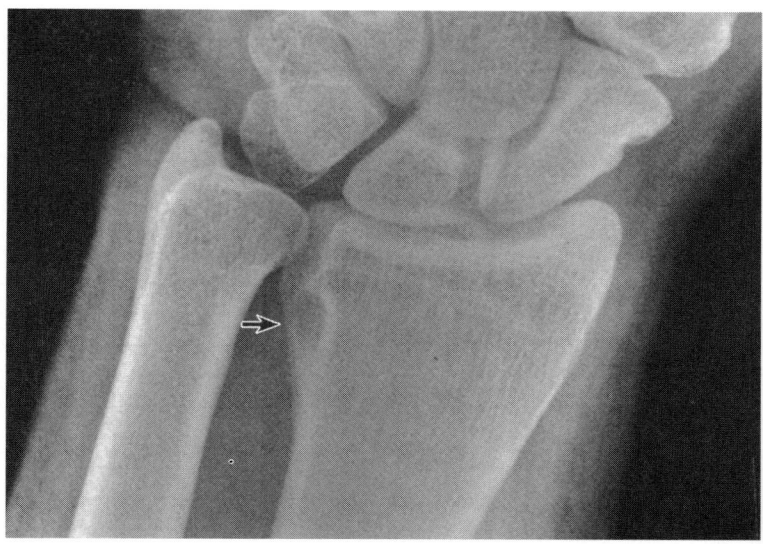

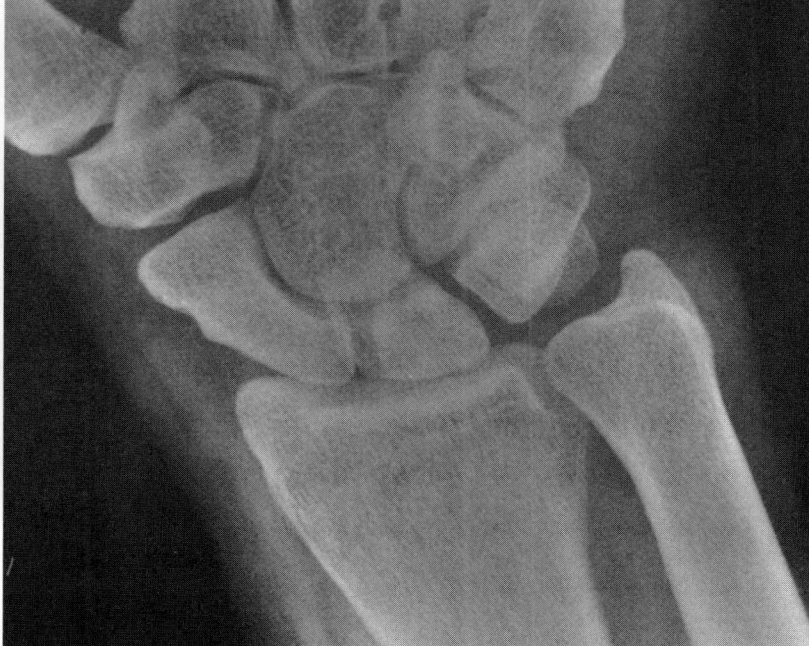

Figure 6–152. Deep asymmetric fossa on the left.

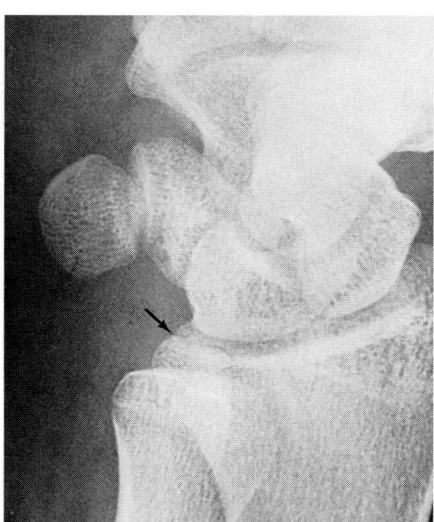

Figure 6–153. Closing distal radial epiphyseal line simulating a fracture. This situation prevails when the ulnar aspect of the distal radial epiphysis is thin, and the remnant of the epiphyseal line may be confused with an incomplete fracture. (From Teates CD: Distal radial growth plate remnant simulating fracture. *Am J Roentgenol* 110:578, 1970.)

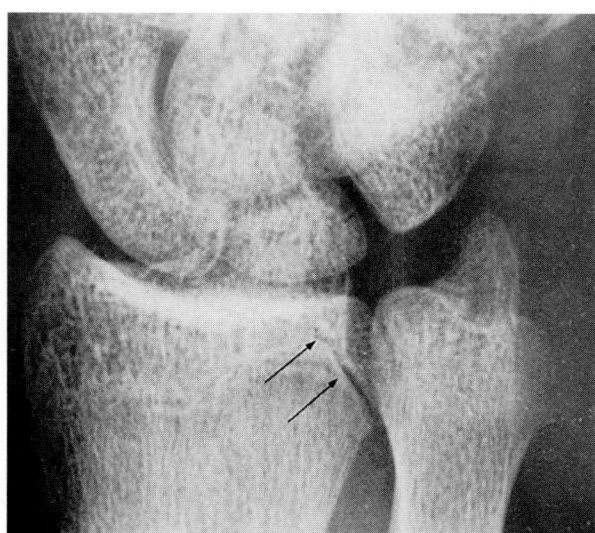

Figure 6–154. Simulated fracture of the radial epiphysis produced by superimposed projection of the epiphyseal plate at different levels.

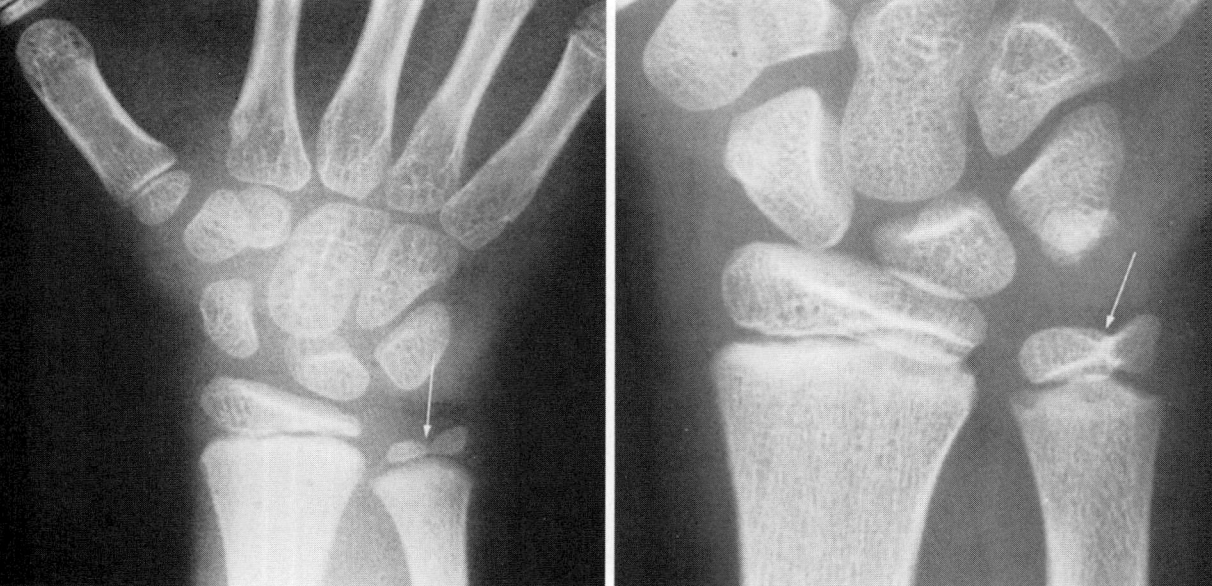

Figure 6–155. Examples of cleft distal ulnar epiphyses.

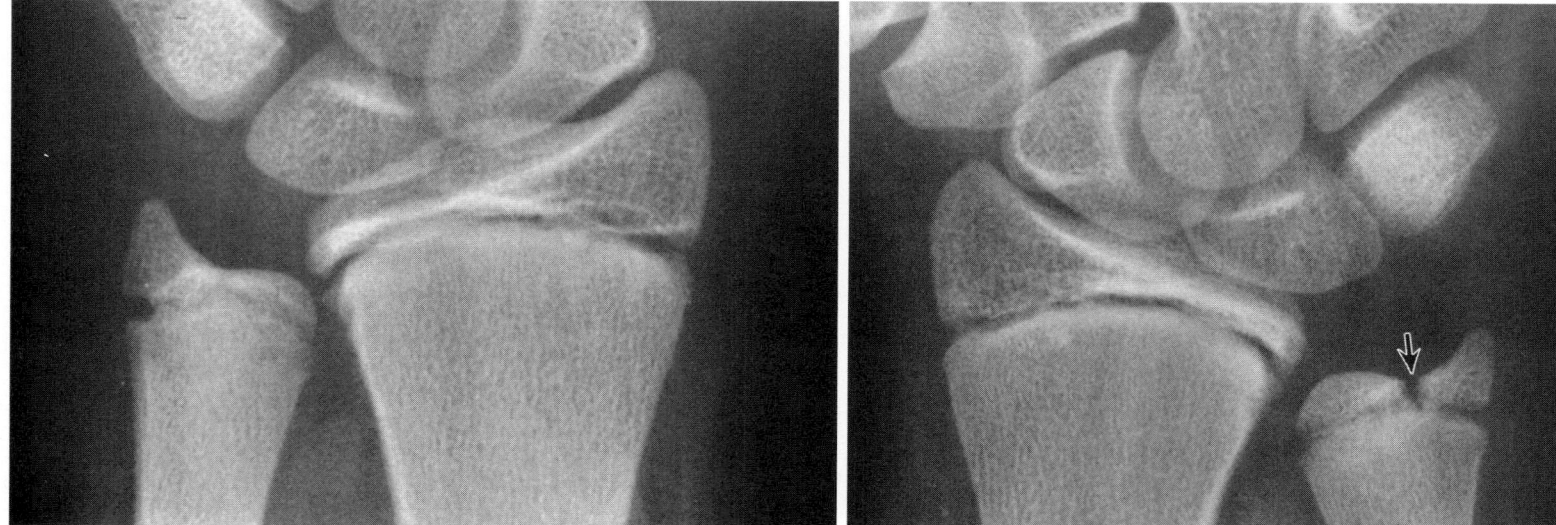

Figure 6–156. Unilateral cleft ulnar styloid epiphysis in a 14-year-old boy.

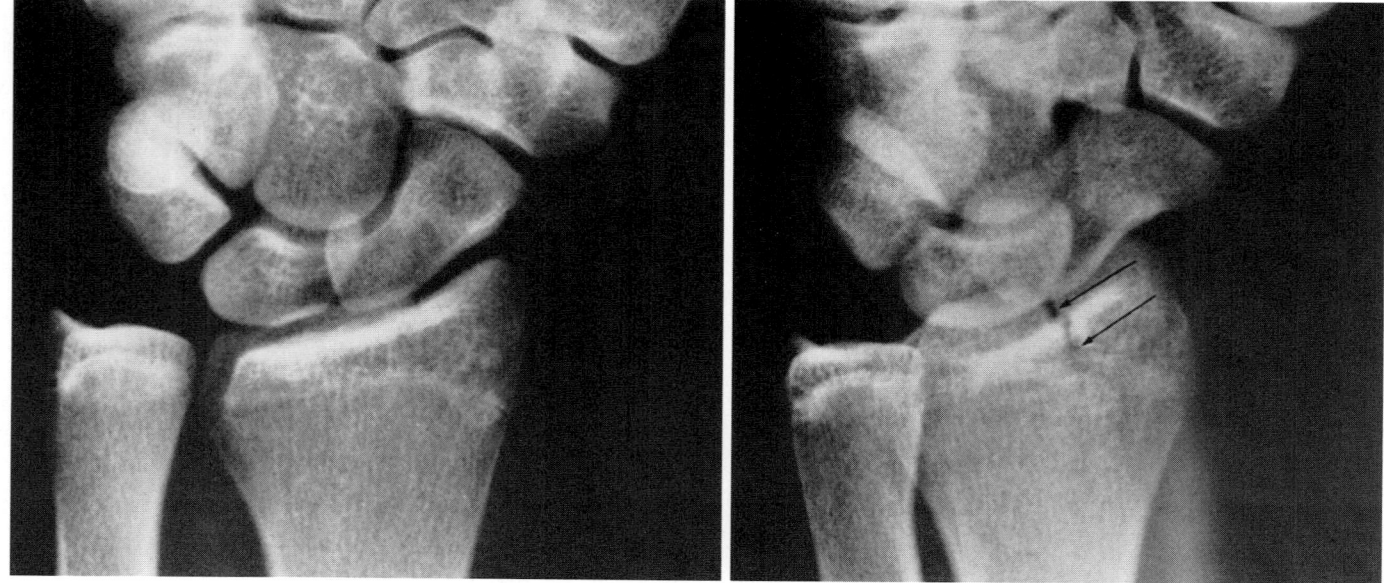

Figure 6–157. Cleft distal radial epiphysis seen only in the oblique projection. Any epiphysis or apophysis may develop from multiple centers. (Ref: Harrison RB, Keats TE: Epiphyseal clefts. *Skeletal Radiol* 5:23, 1980.)

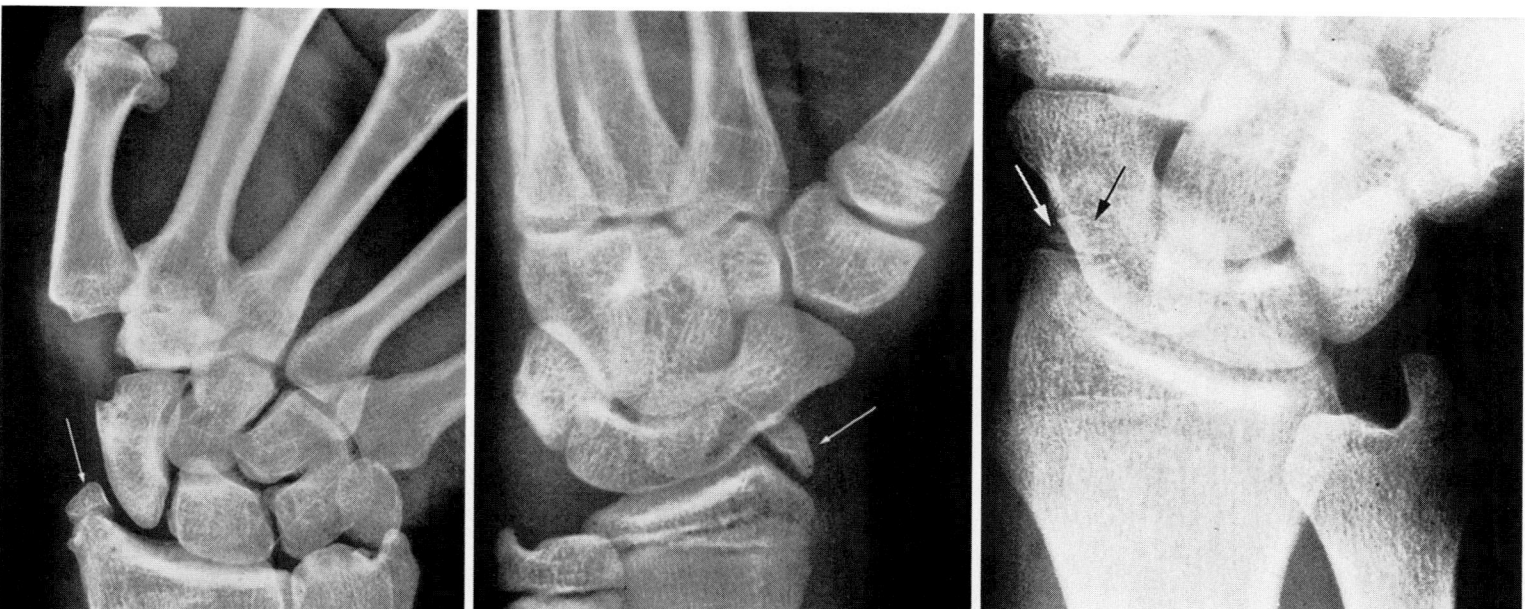

Figure 6–158. Separate ossification centers for the radial styloid process, which may persist into adult life and be mistaken for a fracture.

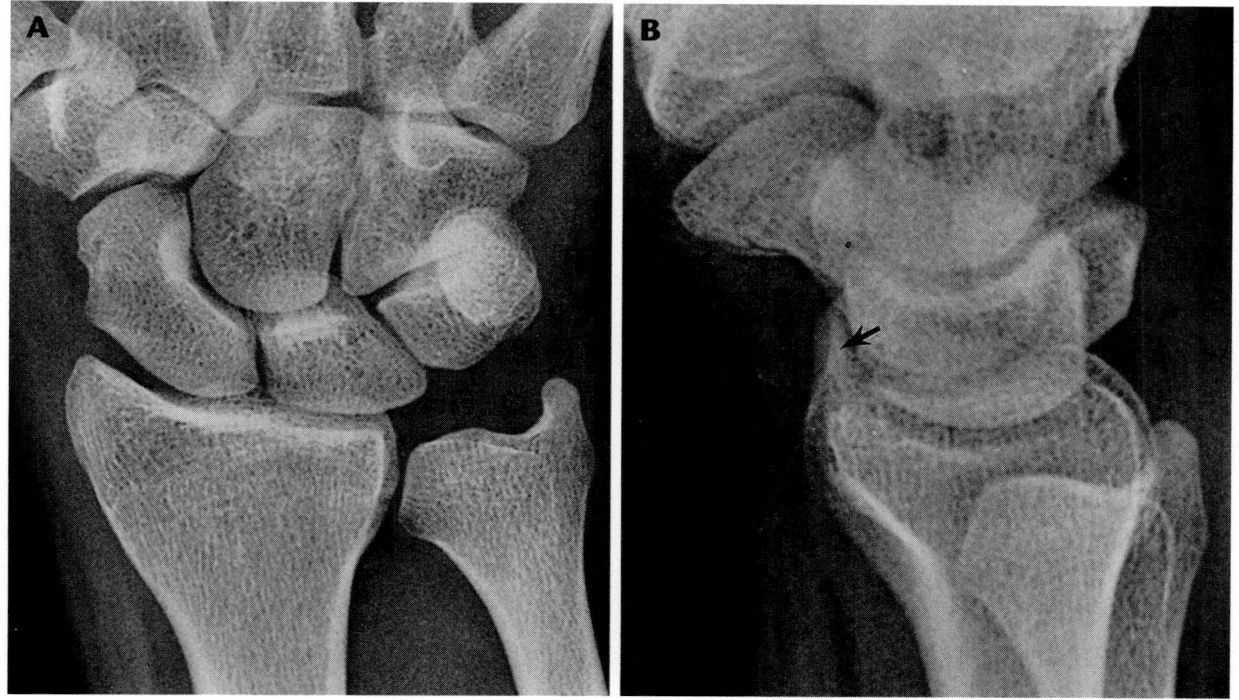

Figure 6–159. A, B, Unusually long distal extension of the radial styloid simulates a fracture fragment in the lateral projection (**B**) (*arrow*).

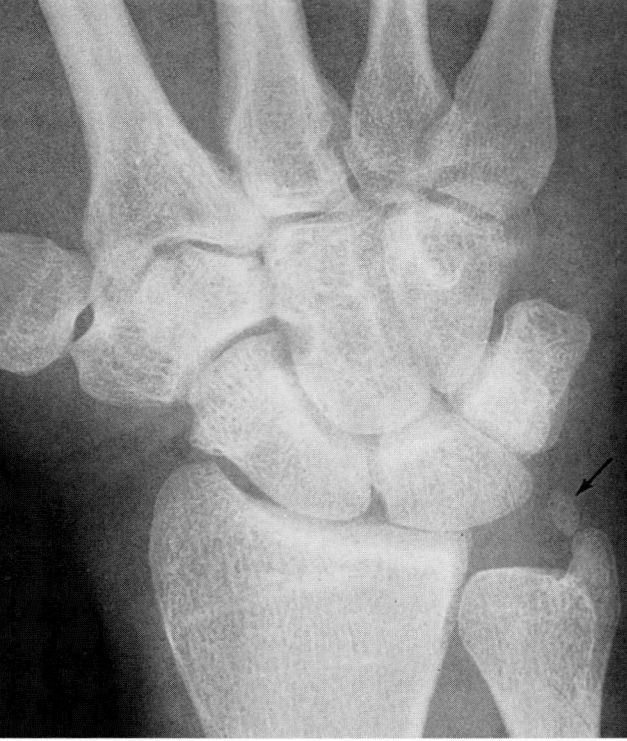

Figure 6–160. Accessory ossicle of the end of the ulnar styloid, which should not be mistaken for a fracture.

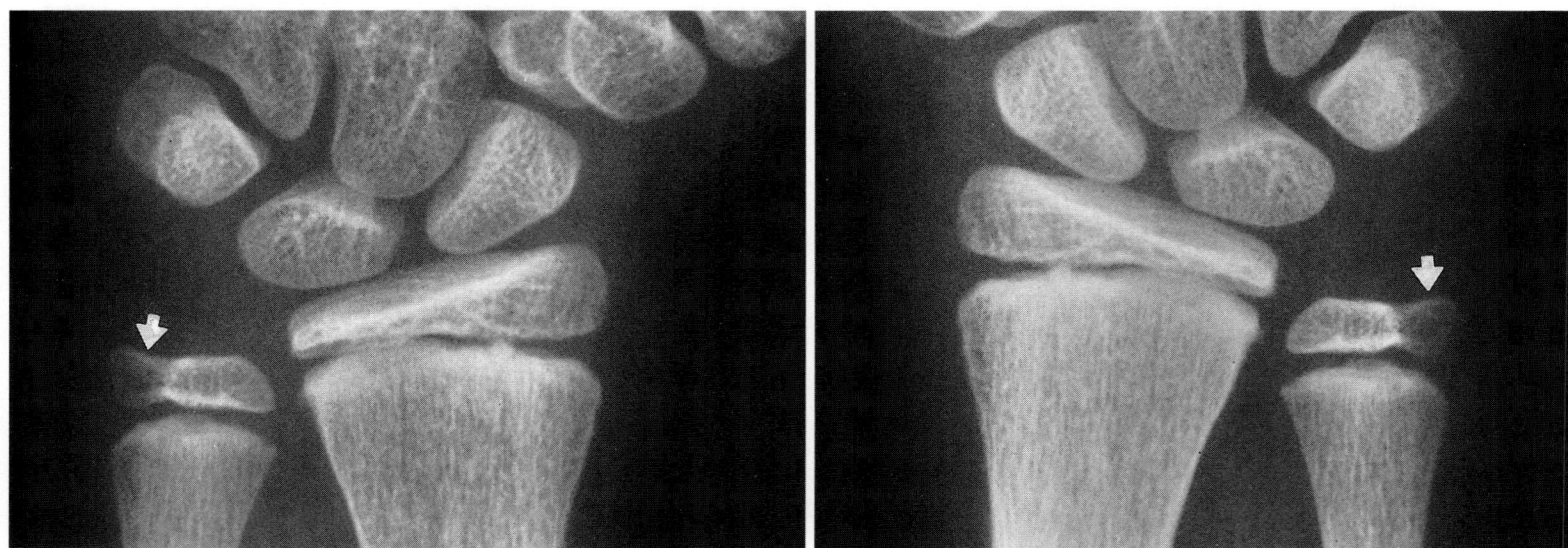

Figure 6–161. Unusual lucencies of the lateral aspects of the ulnar epiphyses.

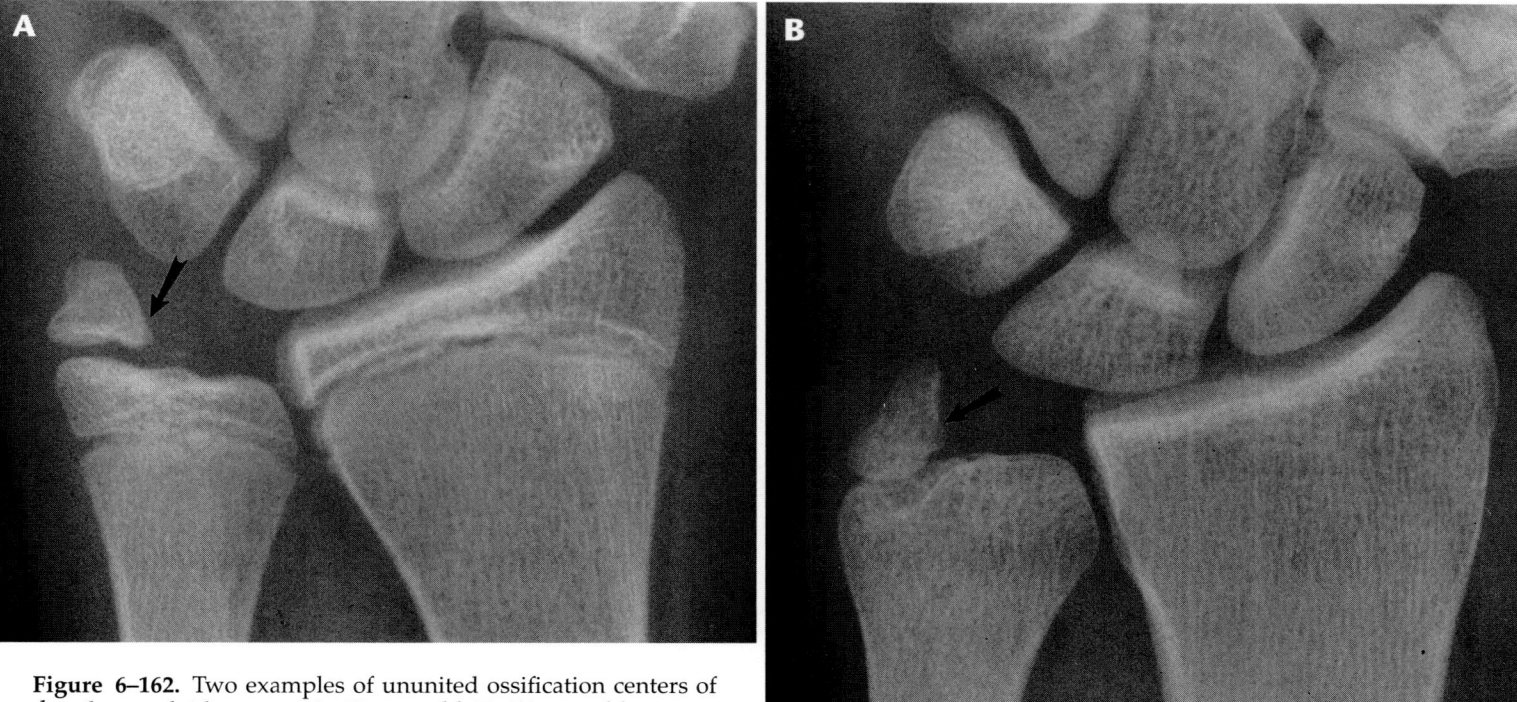

Figure 6–162. Two examples of ununited ossification centers of the ulnar styloid process. **A,** 15-year-old. **B,** 27-year-old.

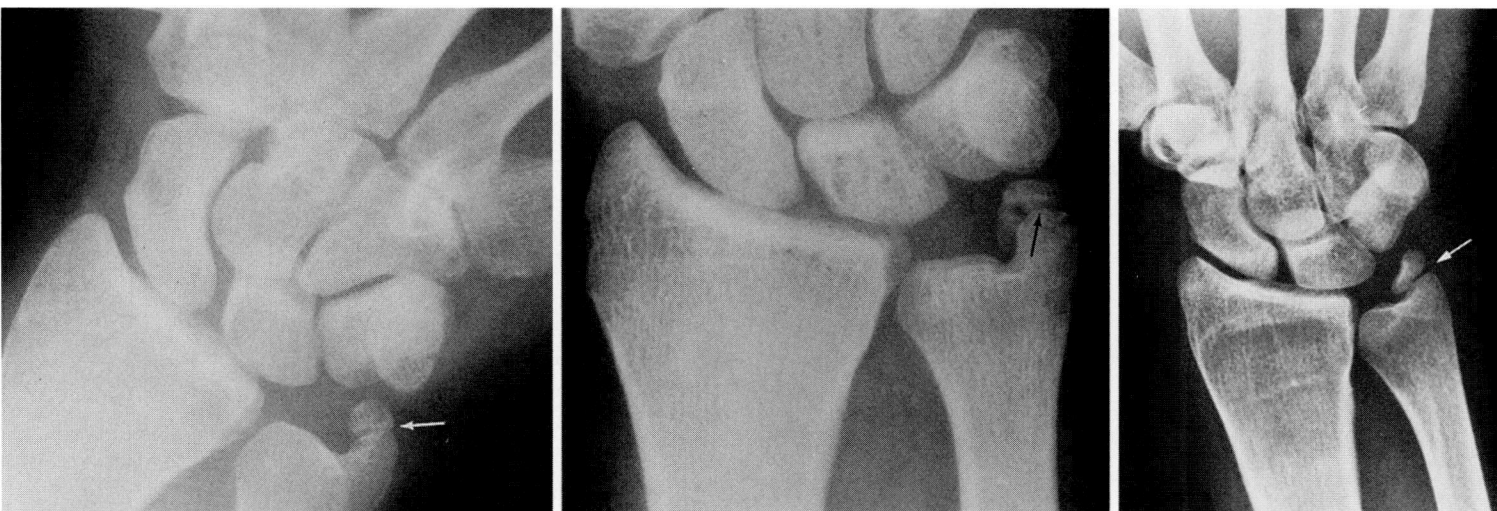

Figure 6–163. Accessory ossicles at the ulnar styloid, which articulate with the styloid process.

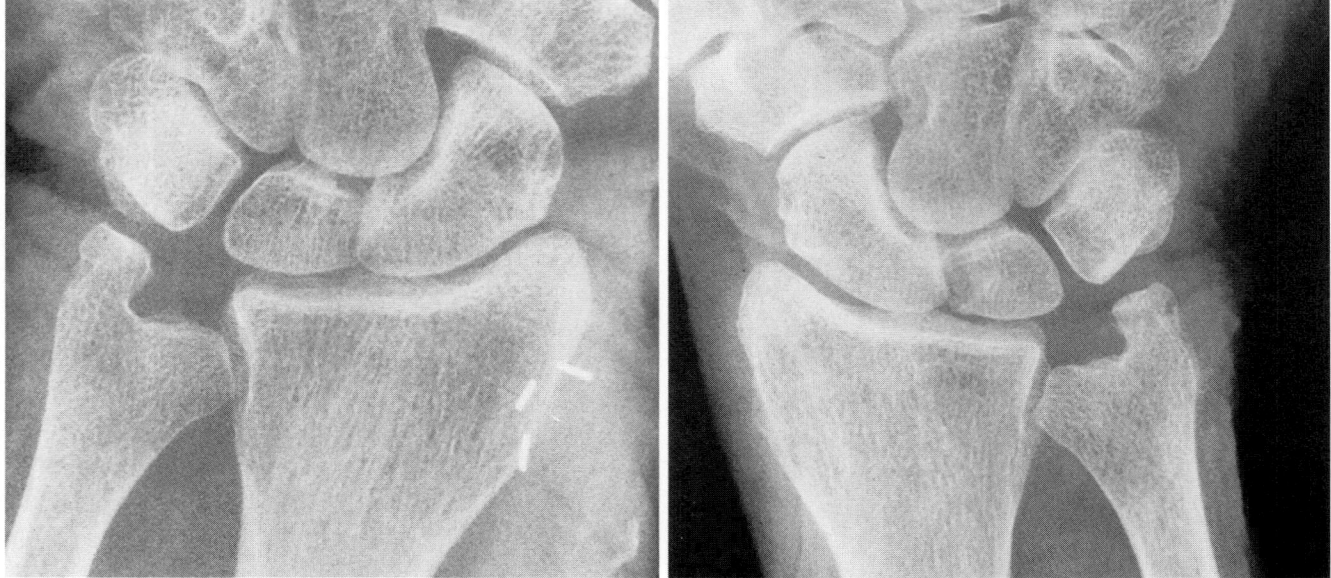

Figure 6–164. Unusual length and configuration of the ulnar styloid processes.

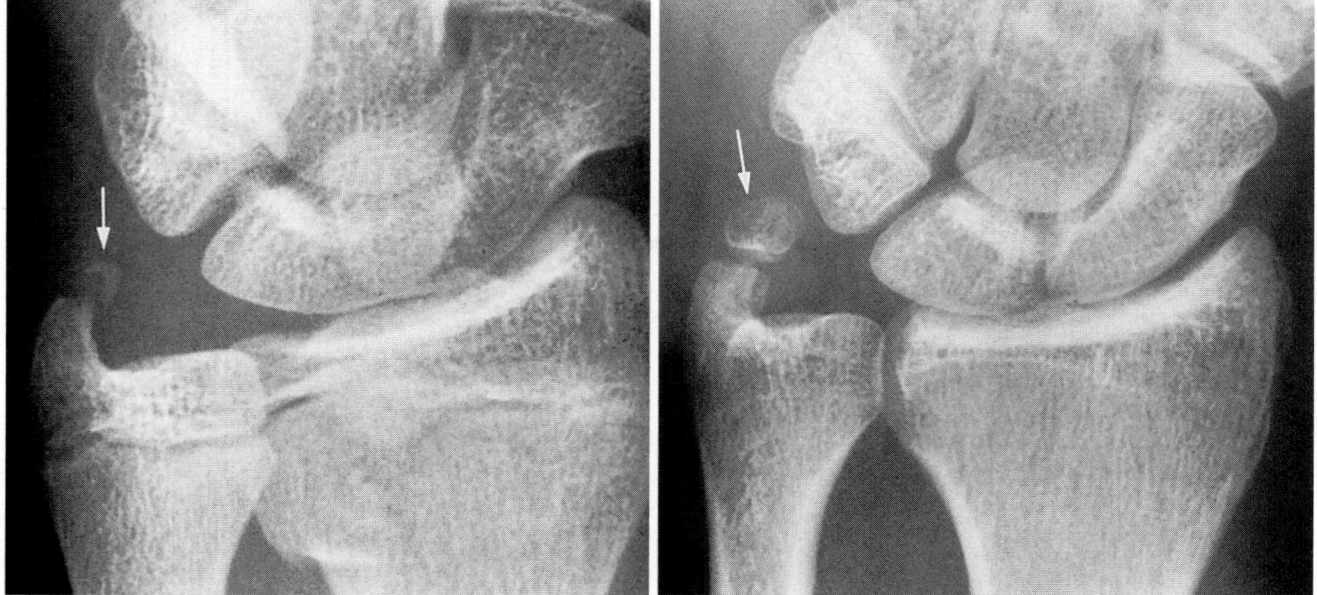

Figure 6–165. Not all styloid ossicles are developmental in origin; some may be of traumatic origin. *Left*, Fracture of the ulnar styloid in a 16-year-old. *Right*, At age 26 the fracture fragment has evolved into an ossicle.

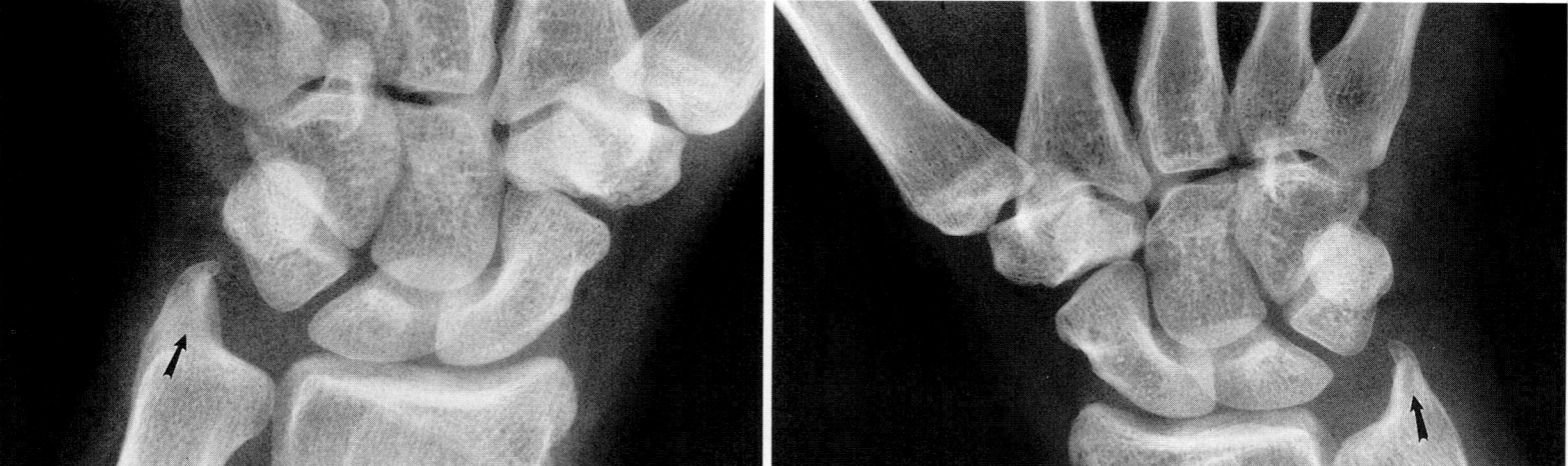

Figure 6–166. Unusual configuration of the ulnar styloids.

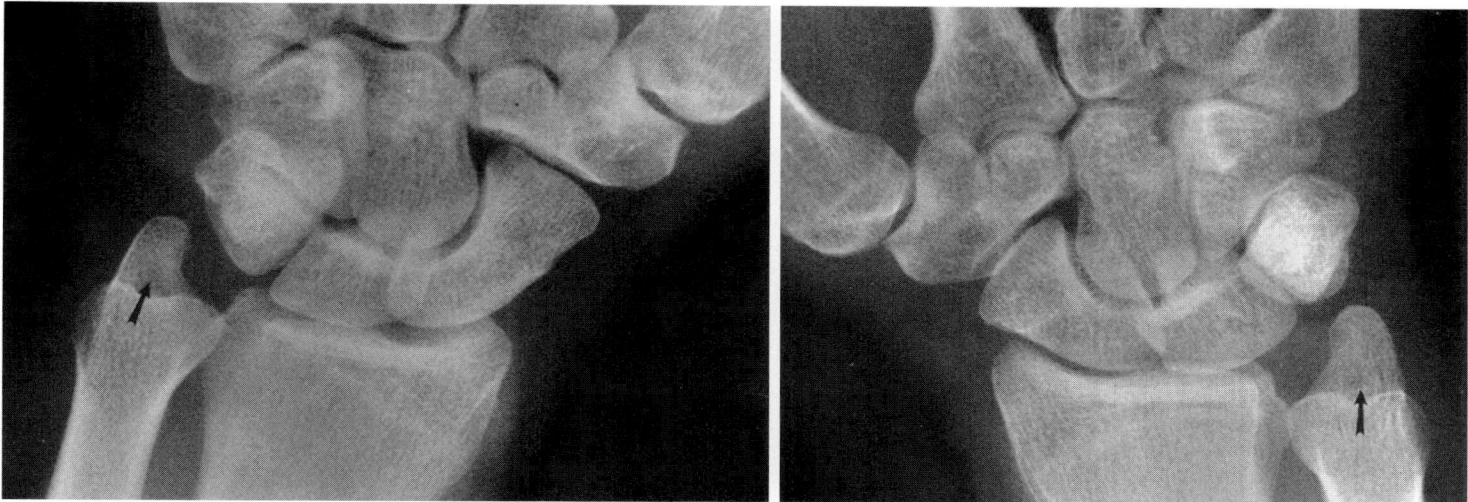

Figure 6–167. Huge ulnar styloid processes.

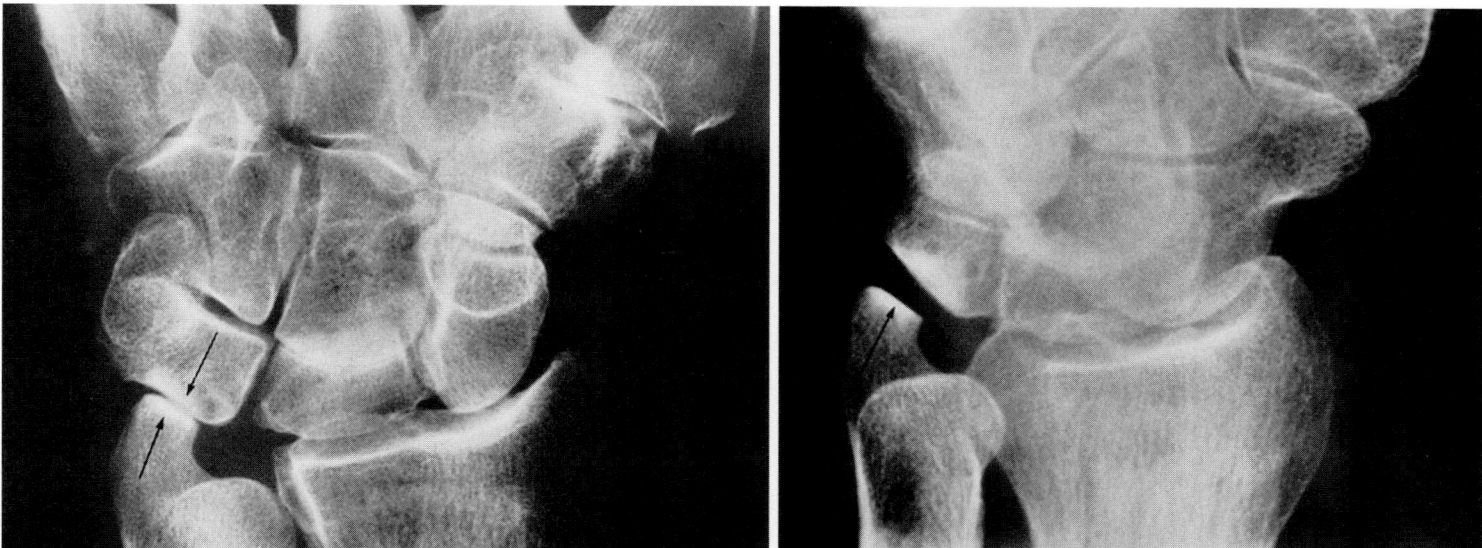

Figure 6–168. Unusually long ulnar styloid process, which articulates with the triquetrum.

Figure 6–169. Ring shadow on the ulnar styloid. This lesion is similar to other entities seen elsewhere in the wrist and hands that are probably fibrous in nature. They do not appear to be of clinical significance (see Figs. 6–268 and 6–304).

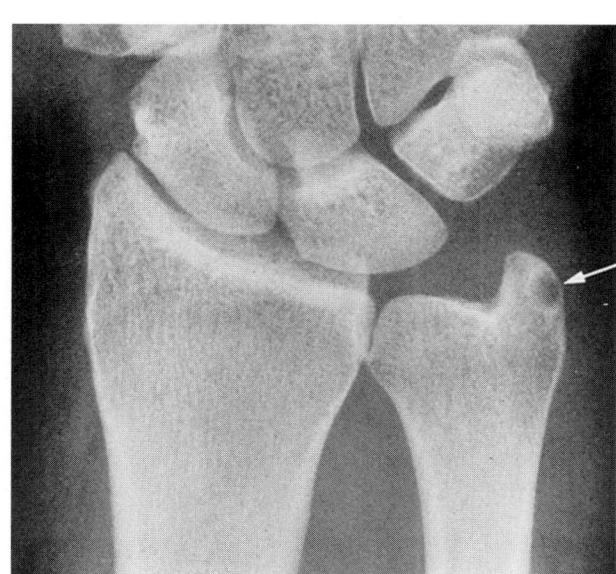

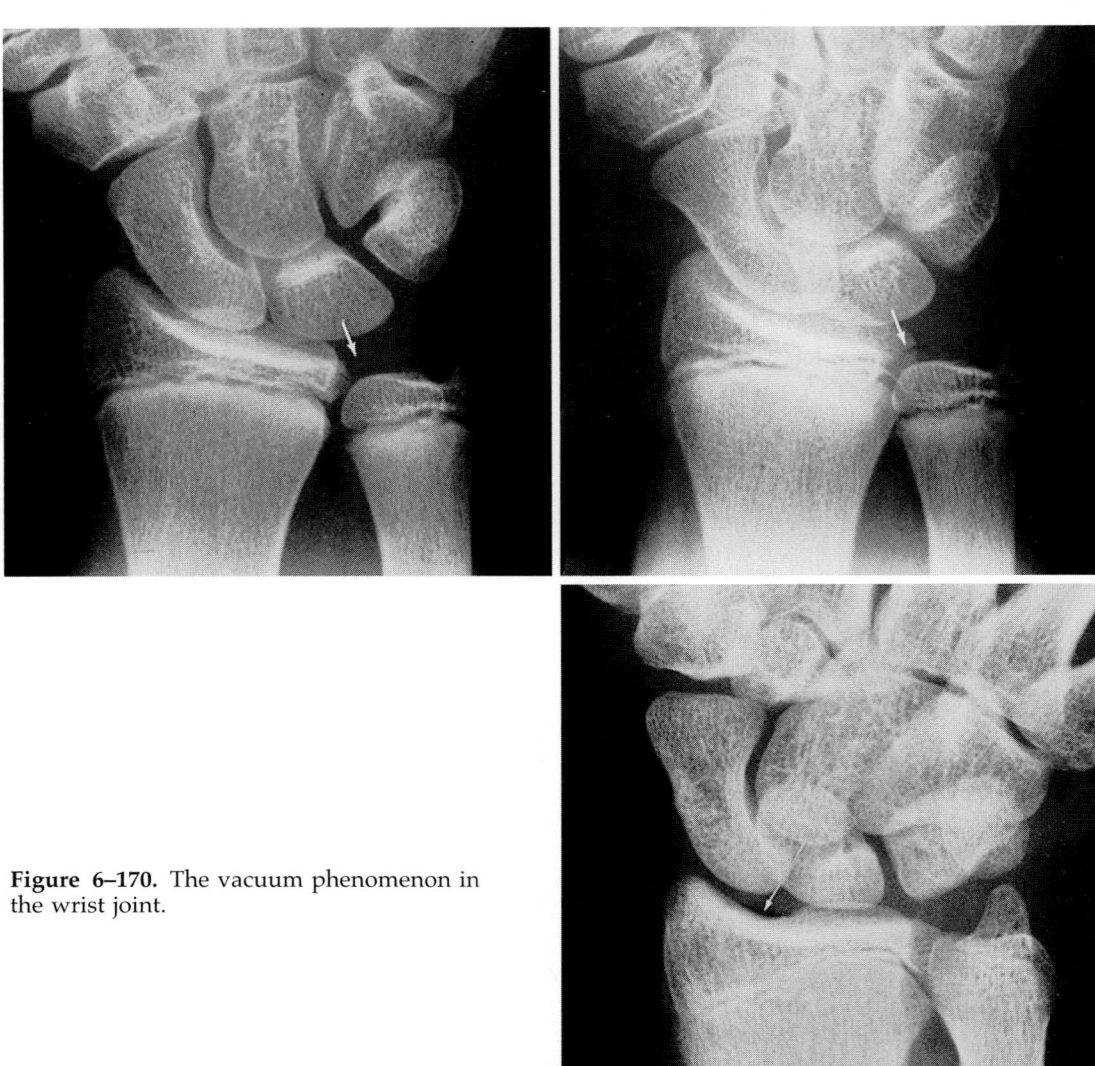

Figure 6–170. The vacuum phenomenon in the wrist joint.

The Hand

The Carpals

THE ACCESSORY OSSICLES

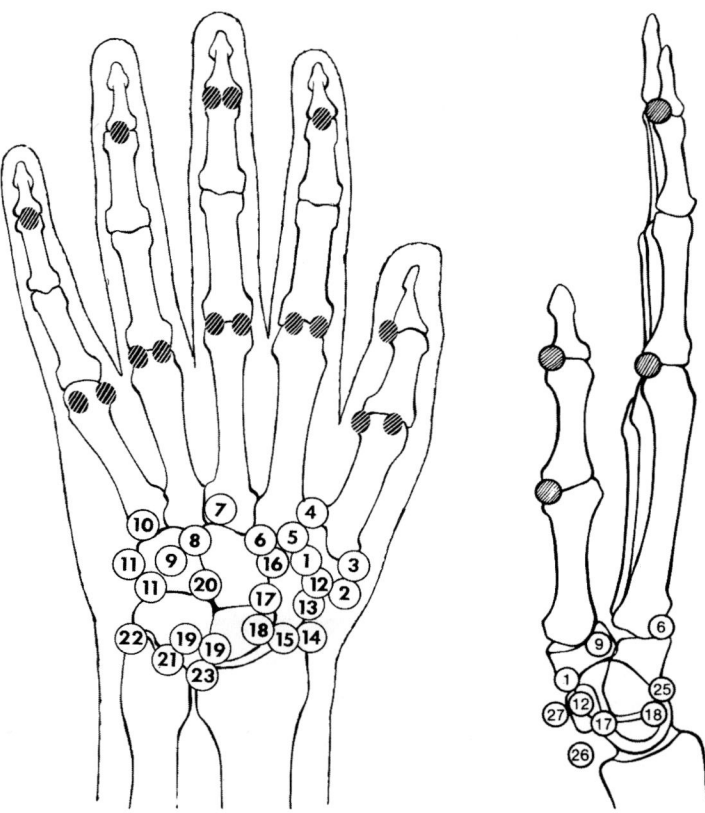

Figure 6–171. The accessory ossicles of the hand (after Kohler). The sesamoid bones are indicated by *shaded circles*. (Ref: Kohler A, Zimmer EA: *Borderlands of the normal and early pathologic findings in skeletal roentgenology,* 4th ed. New York, Thieme, 1993.) The MR appearances of these ossicles and other variants of the wrist are described by Timins. (Ref: Timins ME: Osseous anatomic variants of the wrist. Findings on MR Imaging. *Am J Roentgenol* 173:339, 1999.)

1. Epitrapezium
2. Calcification (bursa, flexor carpi radialis)
3. Paratrapezium (petrapezium)
4. Trapezium secundarium
5. Trapezoides secundarium
6. Os styloideum
7. Ossiculum Gruberi
8. Capitatum secundarium
9. Os hamuli proprium
10. Os vesalianum
11. Os ulnare externum (calcified bursa or tendon)
12. Os radiale externum
13. Fissure of traumatic origin
14. Persisting ossification center of the radial styloid process
15. Intercalary bone between the navicular and the radius (paranavicular)
16. Os carpi centrale
17. Hypolunatum
18. Epilunatum
19. Accessory bone between the lunate and the triangular bone
20. Epipyramis
21. So-called "os triangulare"
22. Persisting center of the ulnar styloid
23. Small ossicle at the level of the radioulnar joint
25. Avulsion from the triangular bone; no accessory ossicle
26. Tendon or bursal calcification
27. Calcification of the pisiform

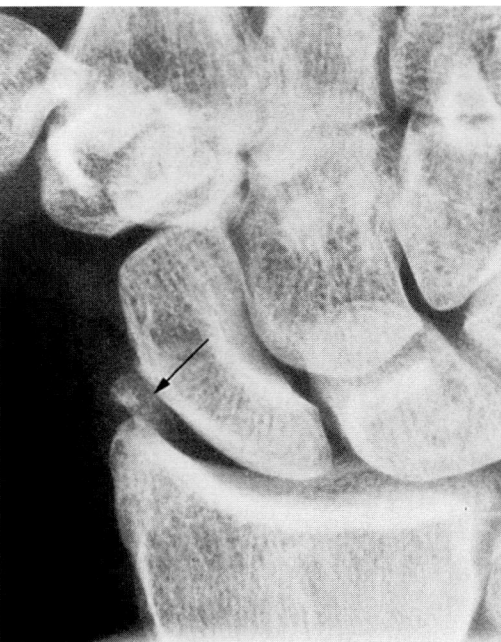

Figure 6–172. Accessory ossicle at the radial styloid process, representing a persistent ossification center.

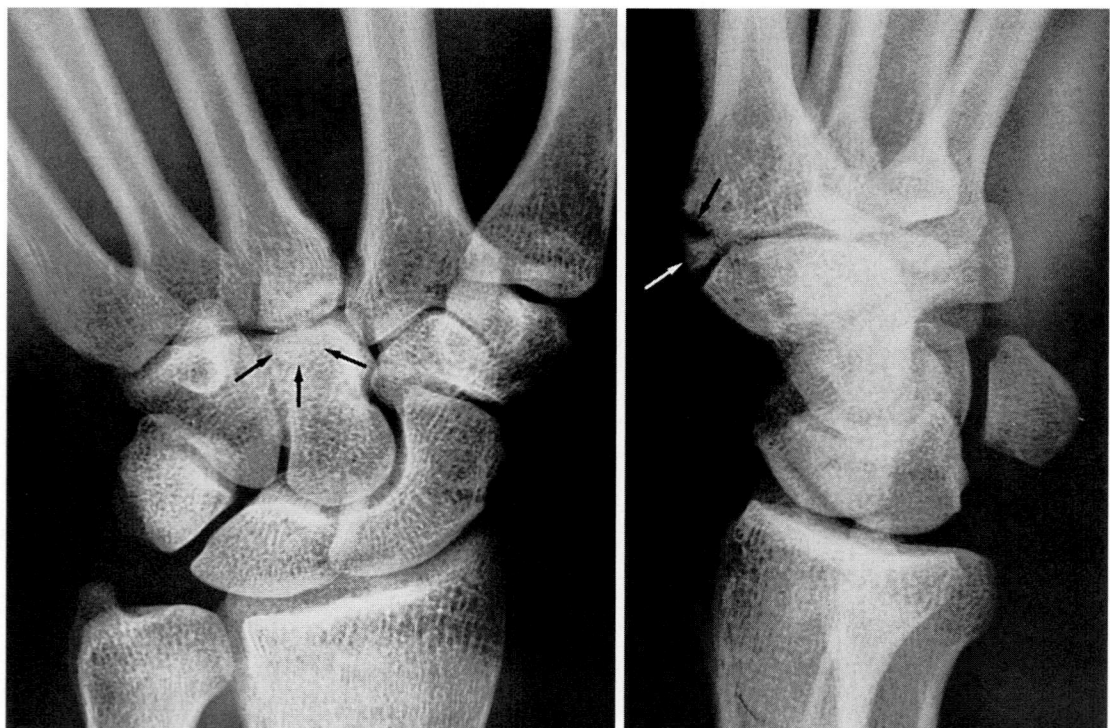

Figure 6–173. The os styloideum. This ossicle lies between the capitate and the base of the second and third metacarpals. It produces a small immovable protuberance on the dorsum of the hand and may give rise to symptoms. (Refs: Bassöe E, Bassöe H: The styloid bone and carpe bossu disease. *Am J Roentgenol* 74:886, 1955; Conway WE et al: The carpal boss: An overview of radiographic evaluation. *Radiology* 156:29, 1985.)

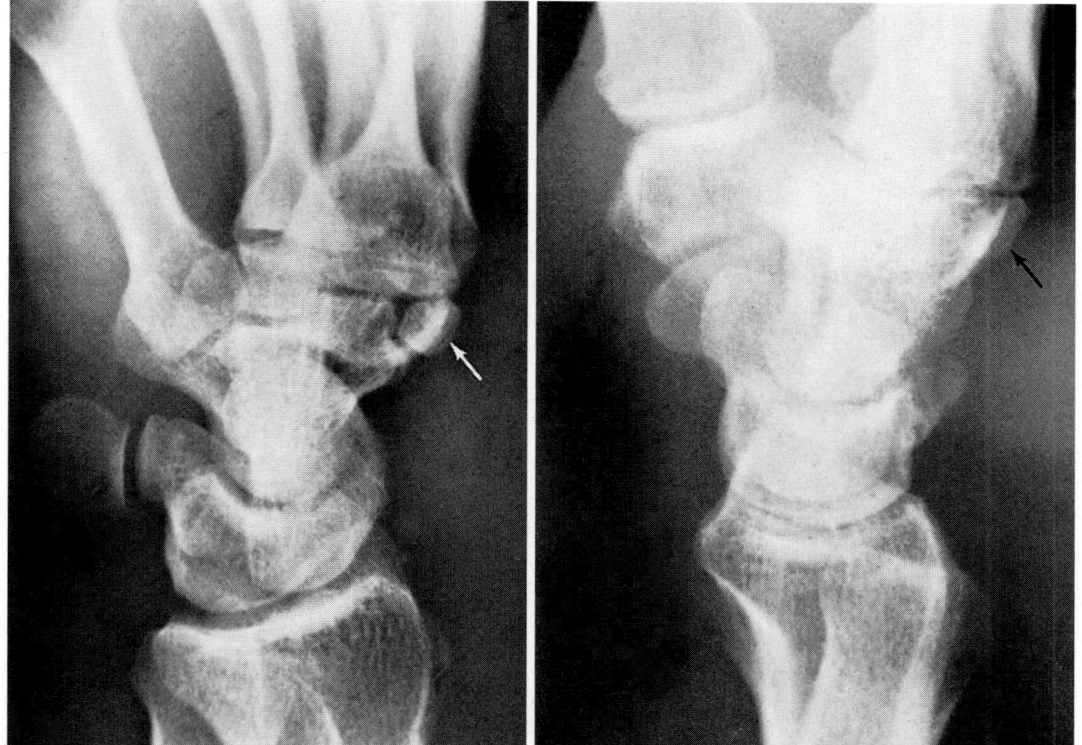

Figure 6–174. Two additional examples of the os styloideum.

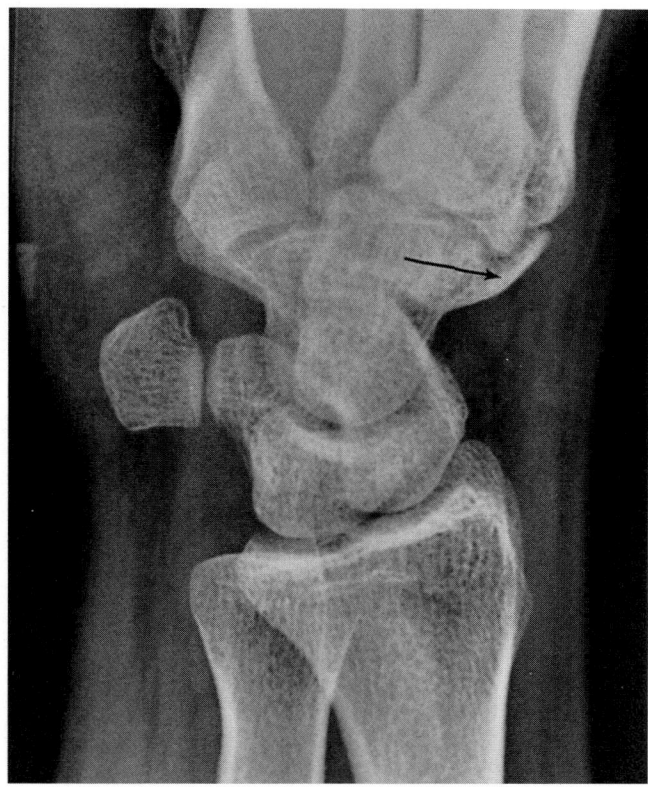

Figure 6–175. In the external oblique projection of the wrist, the dorsal aspect of the capitate is thrown into relief and simulates a fracture or an os styloideum.

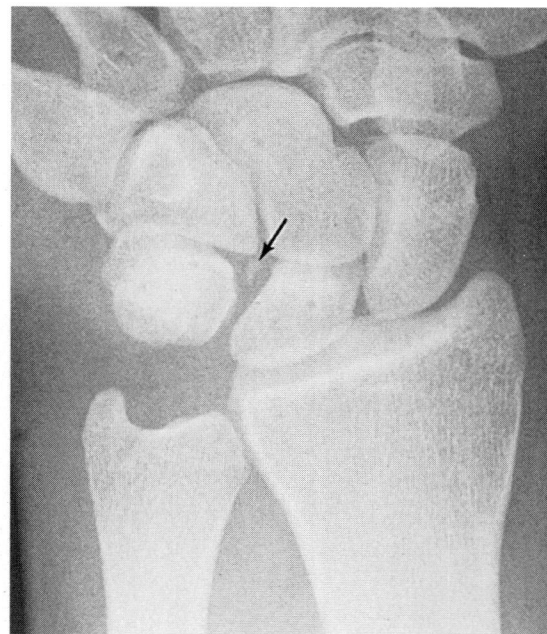

Figure 6–176. The os epitriquetrum (os epiphyramis). This ossicle is located on the dorsal and radial edge of the triquetrum and varies in size.

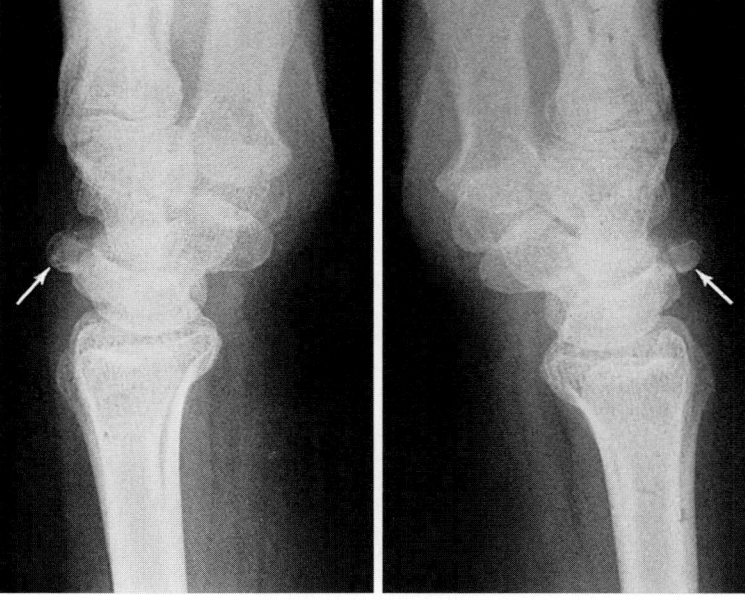

Figure 6–177. The os epilunatum.

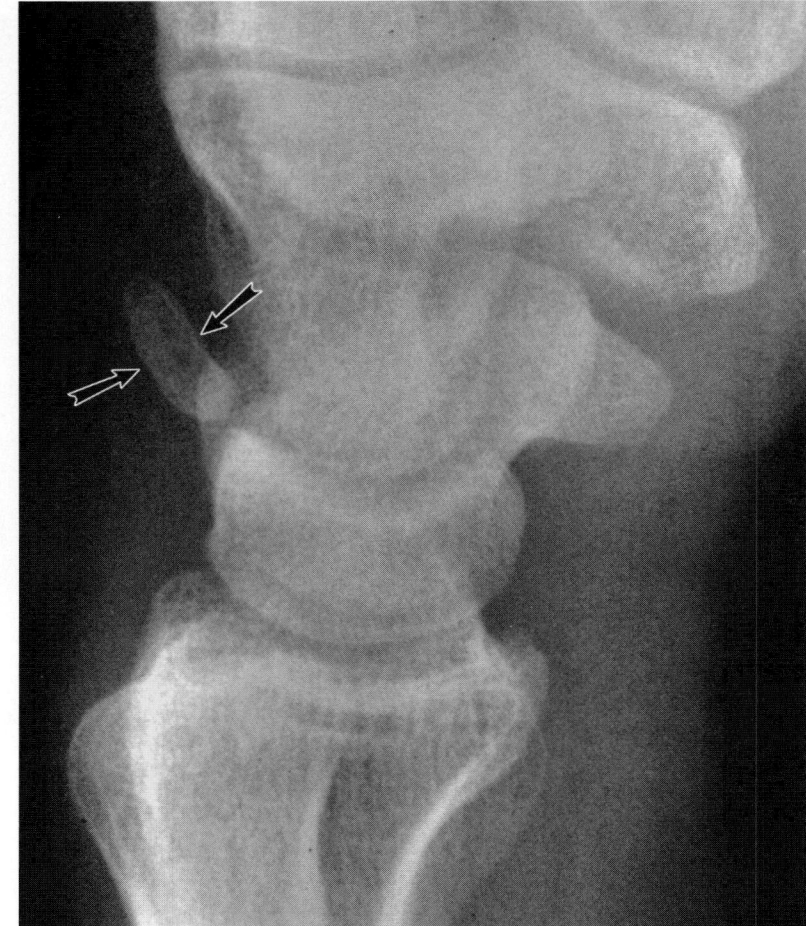

Figure 6–178. Large os epilunatum.

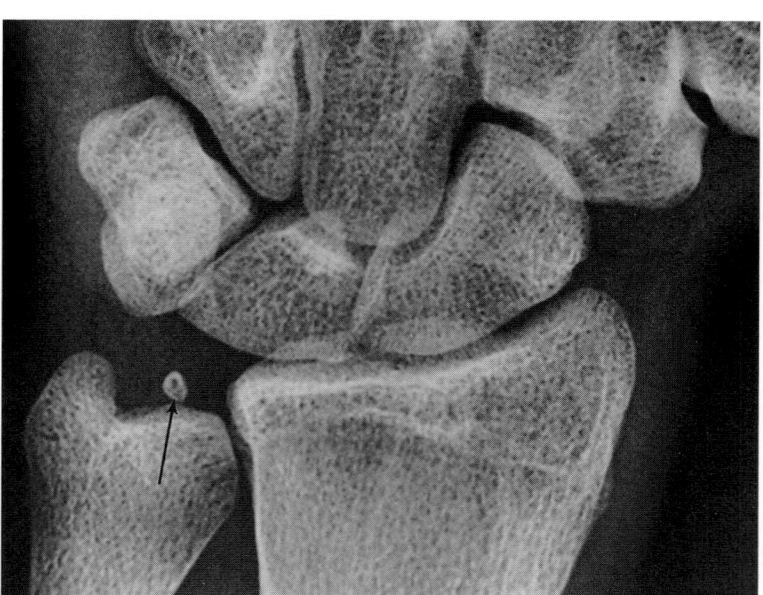

Figure 6–179. The os triangulare.

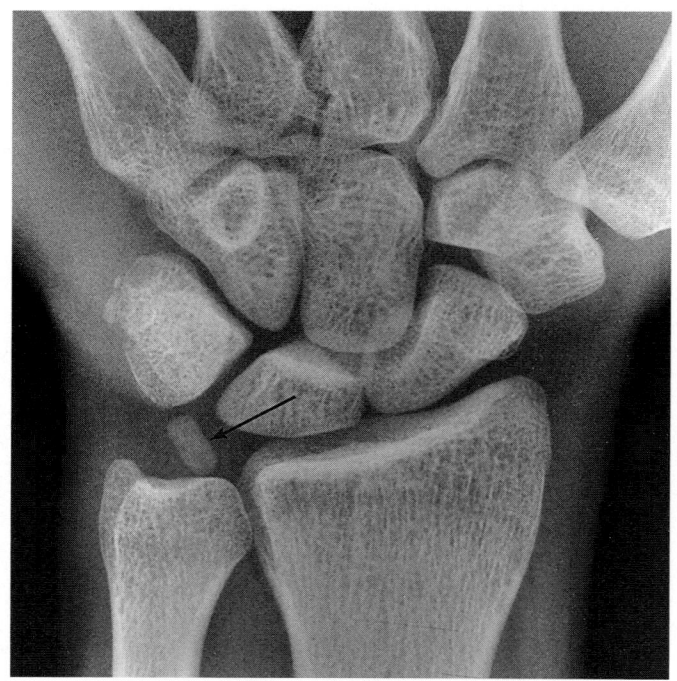

Figure 6–180. Large os triangulare.

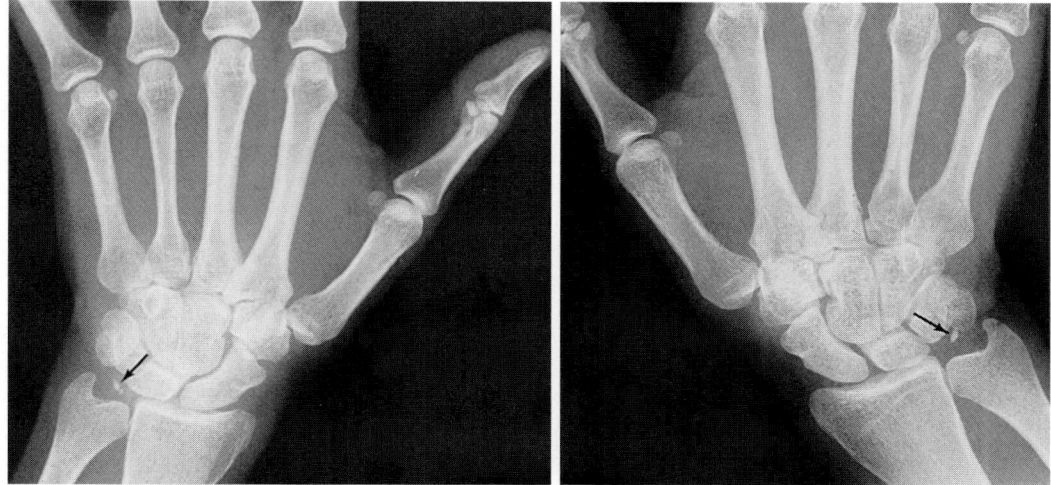

Figure 6–181. Bilateral os triangulare. Some osseous elements in this area may represent old avulsions of the styloid process. This is not true in this illustration, which is of a normal variation. (Ref: Kohler A, Zimmer EA: *Borderlands of the normal and early pathologic findings in skeletal roentgenology,* 4th ed. New York, Thieme, 1993, p. 130.)

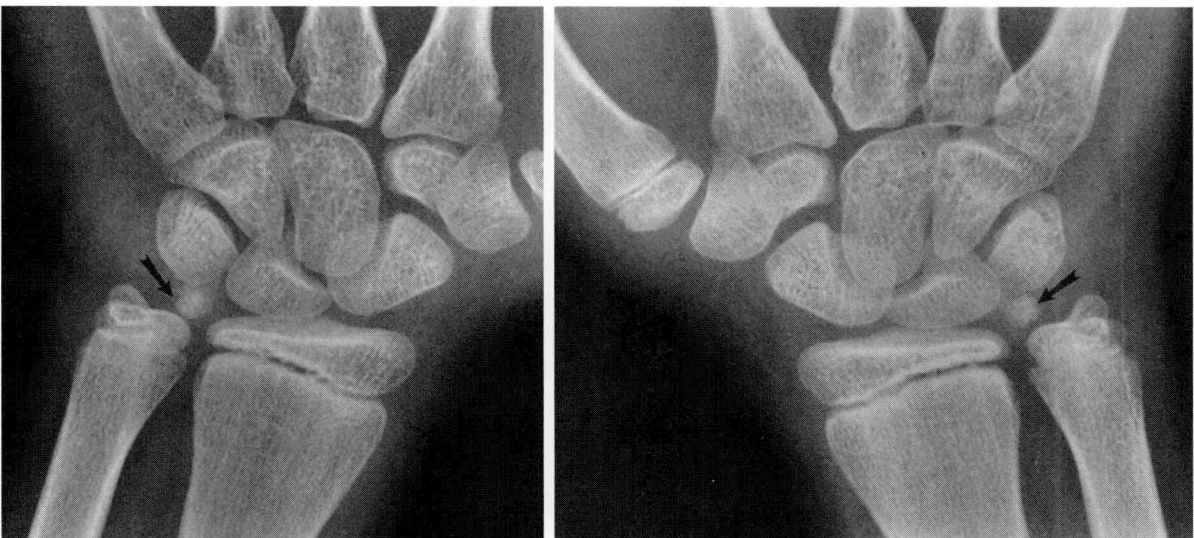

Figure 6–182. Large bilateral os triangulare.

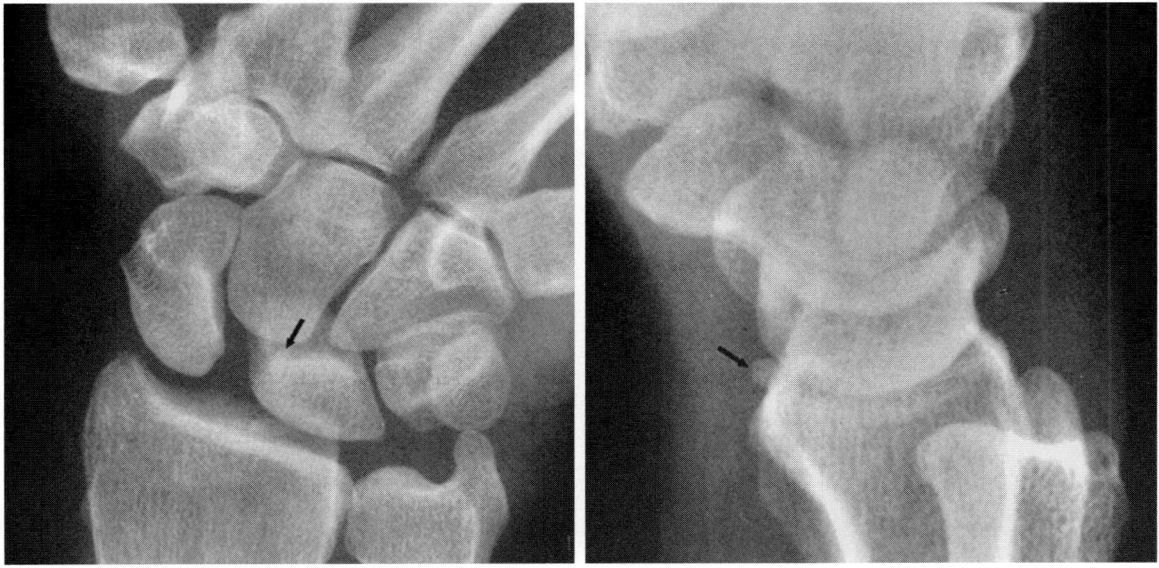

Figure 6–183. Accessory bone between the lunate and capitate bones.

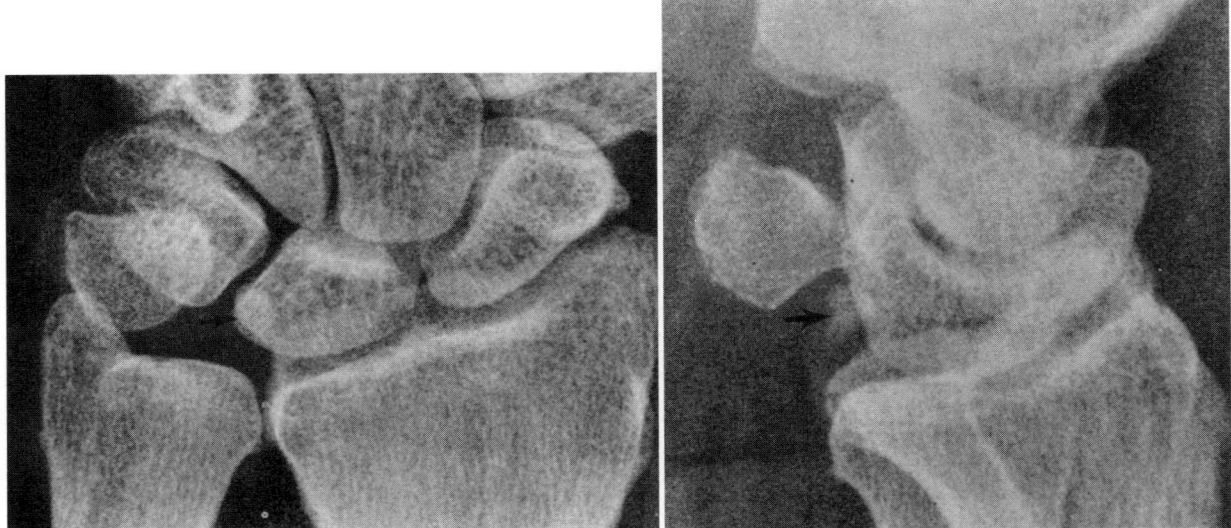

Figure 6–184. Another example of the ossicle between the lunate and triquetrum.

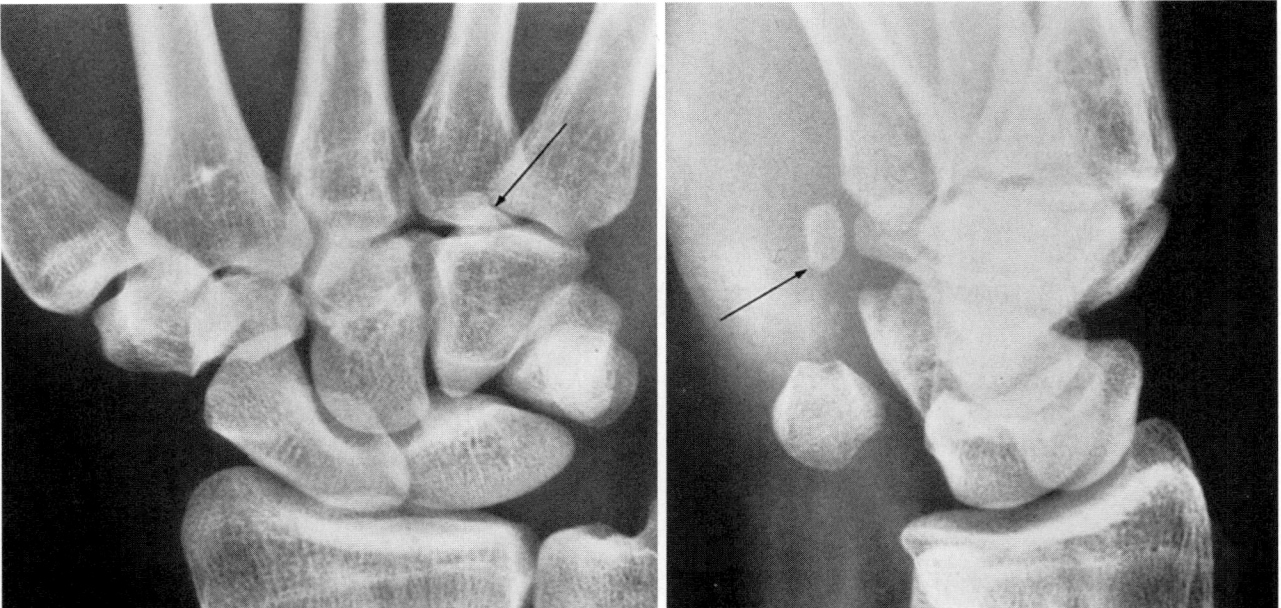

Figure 6–185. The os hamuli proprium.

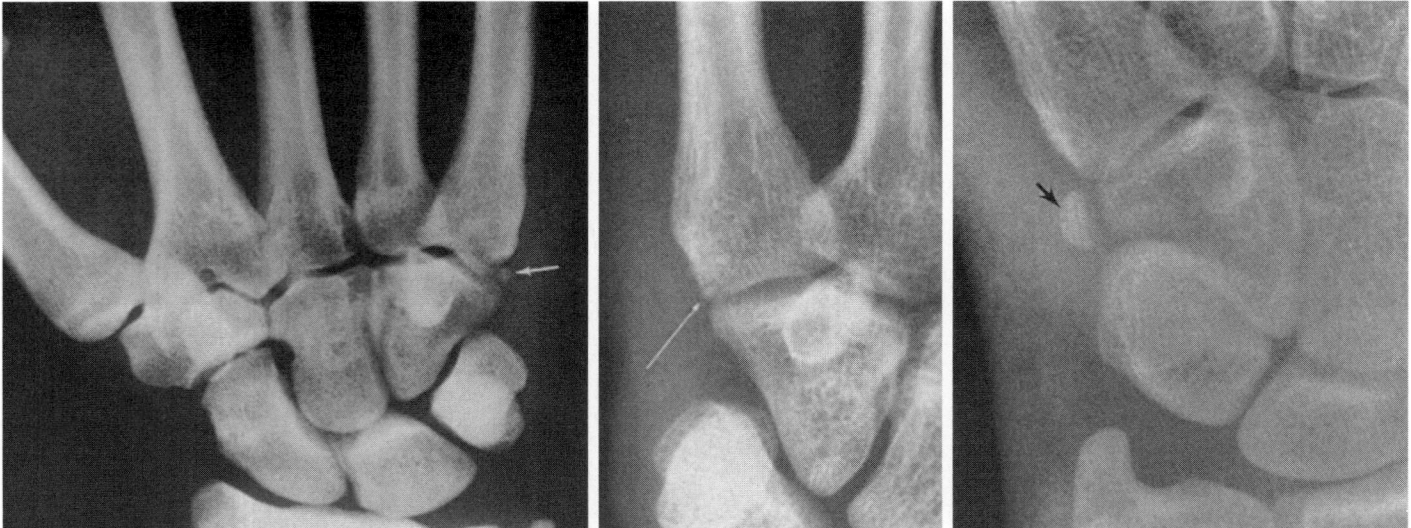

Figure 6–186. Examples of the os vesalianum.

The Carpals

THE CAPITATE AND LUNATE BONES

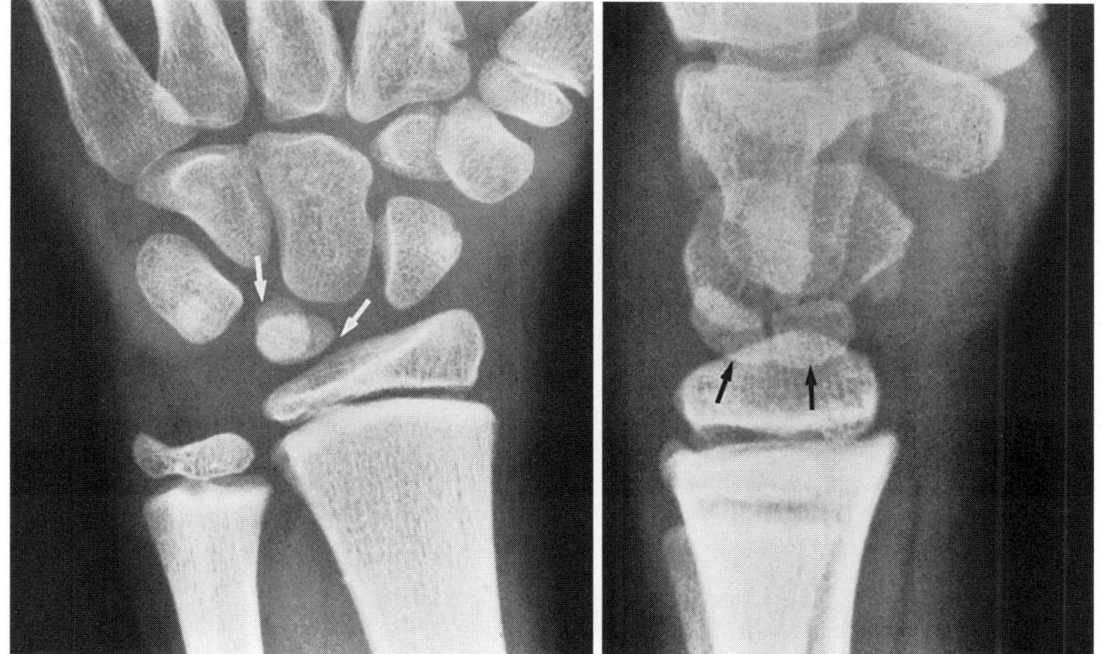

Figure 6–198. Bipartite lunate in a young child.

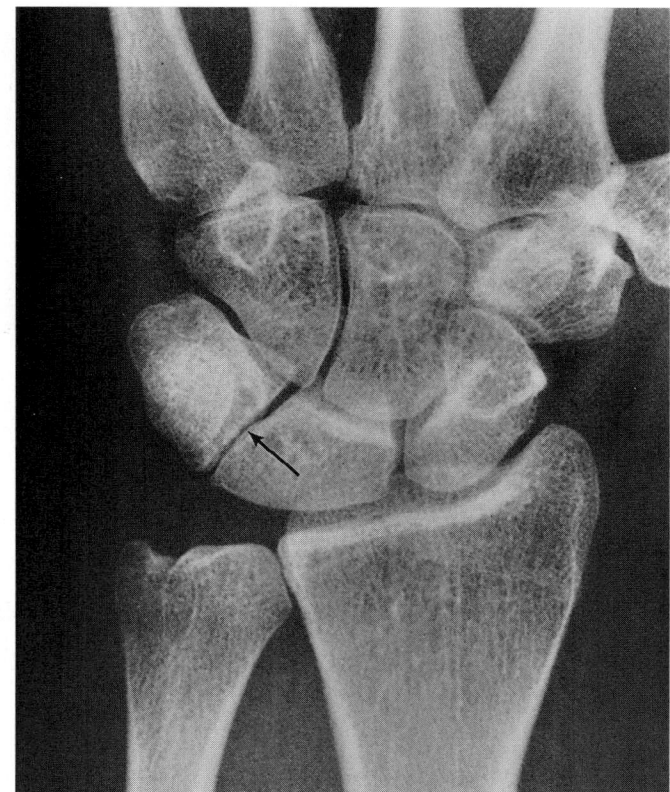

Figure 6–199. Abortive coalition between the lunate and triquetrum.

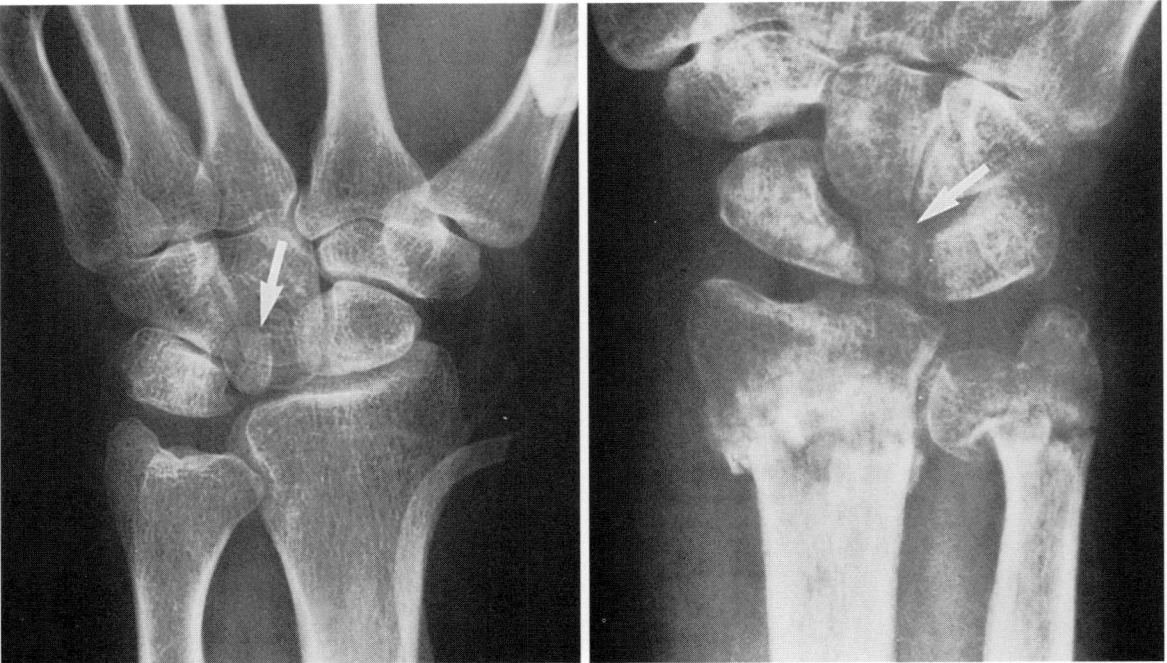

Figure 6–200. Bilateral hypoplastic lunates discovered as incidental findings after fracture of right wrist.

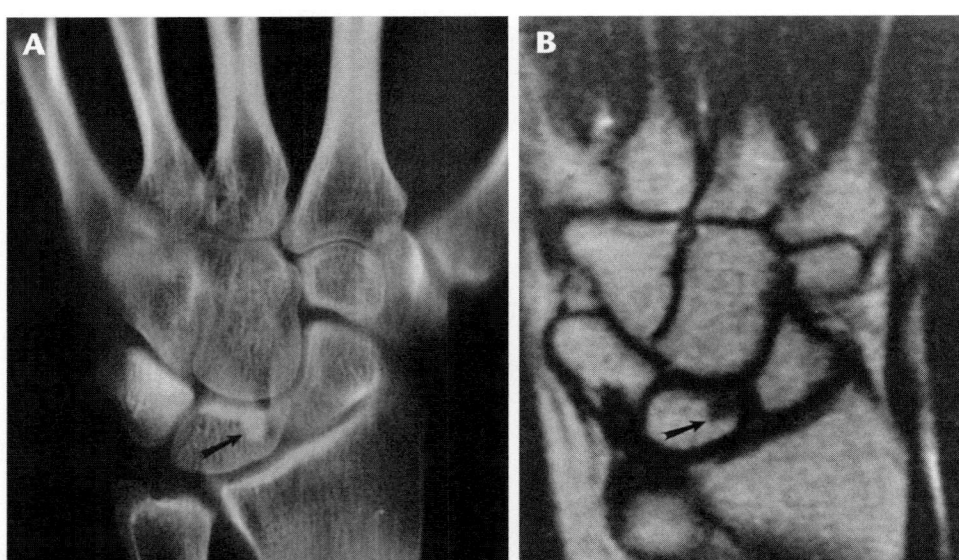

Figure 6–201. Bone island in the lunate. **A,** Plain film. **B,** Corresponding MRI.

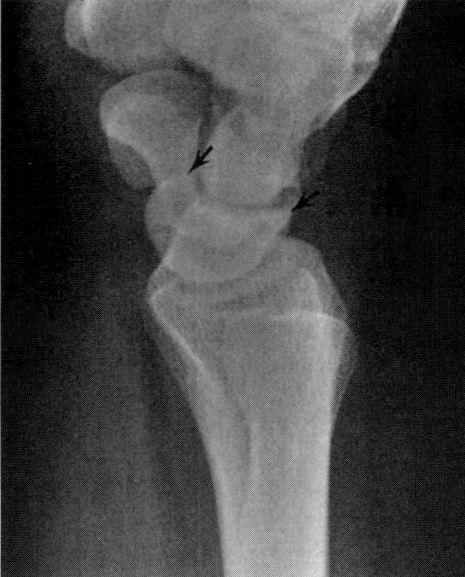

Figure 6–202. Dorsal flexion of the wrist in lateral projection can simulate dorsal instability of the lunate. Palmar flexion can similarly simulate volar instability of the lunate.

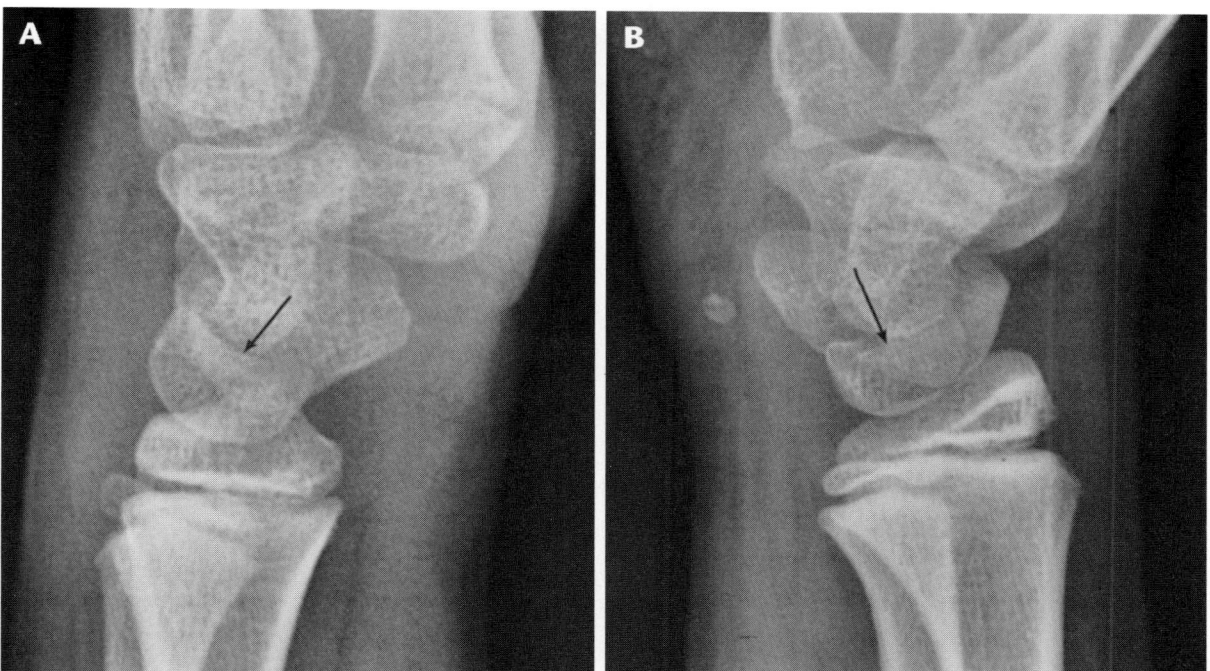

Figure 6–203. A, B, Unimportant bilateral volar tilt of the lunates in a 10-year-old boy. The right wrist was injured, and note that the lunate is tilted in a volar direction, despite the fact that the wrist is extended (**B**).

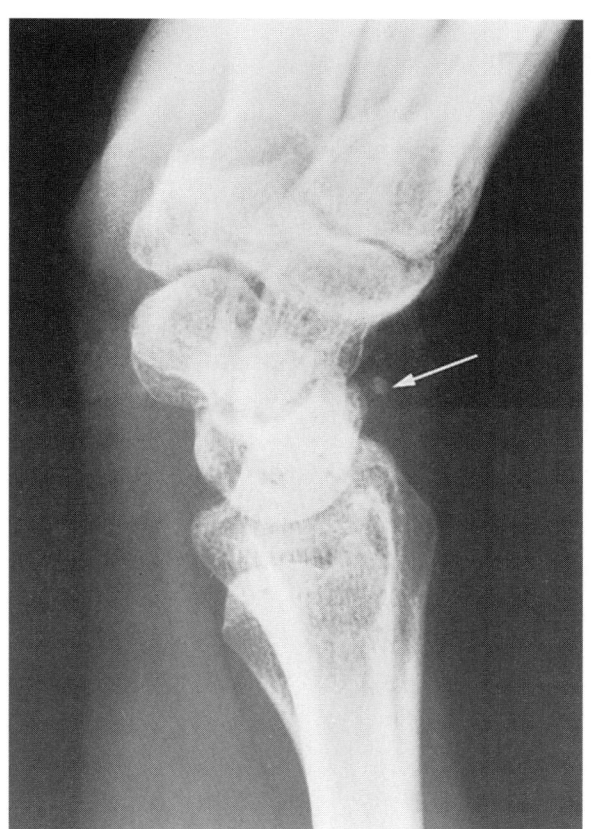

Figure 6–204. Small os epilunatum.

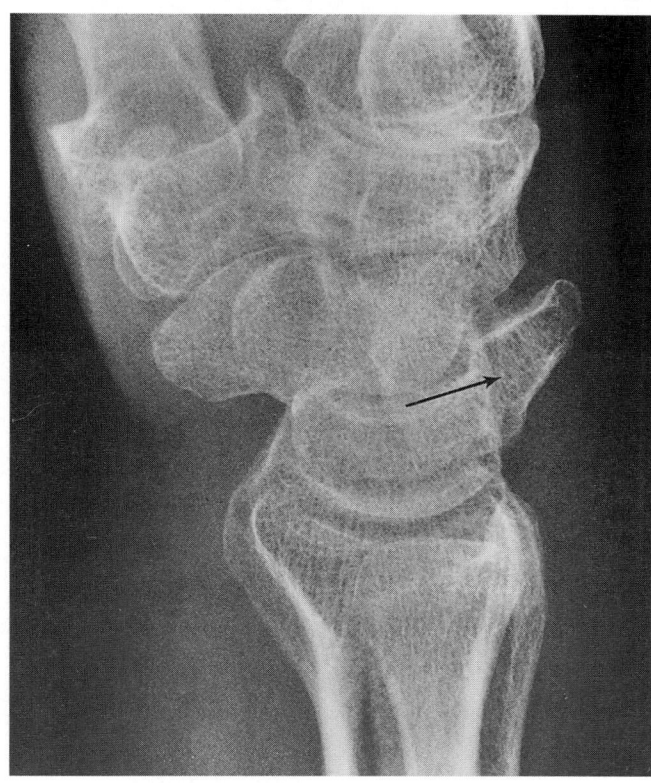

Figure 6–205. Huge os epilunatum.

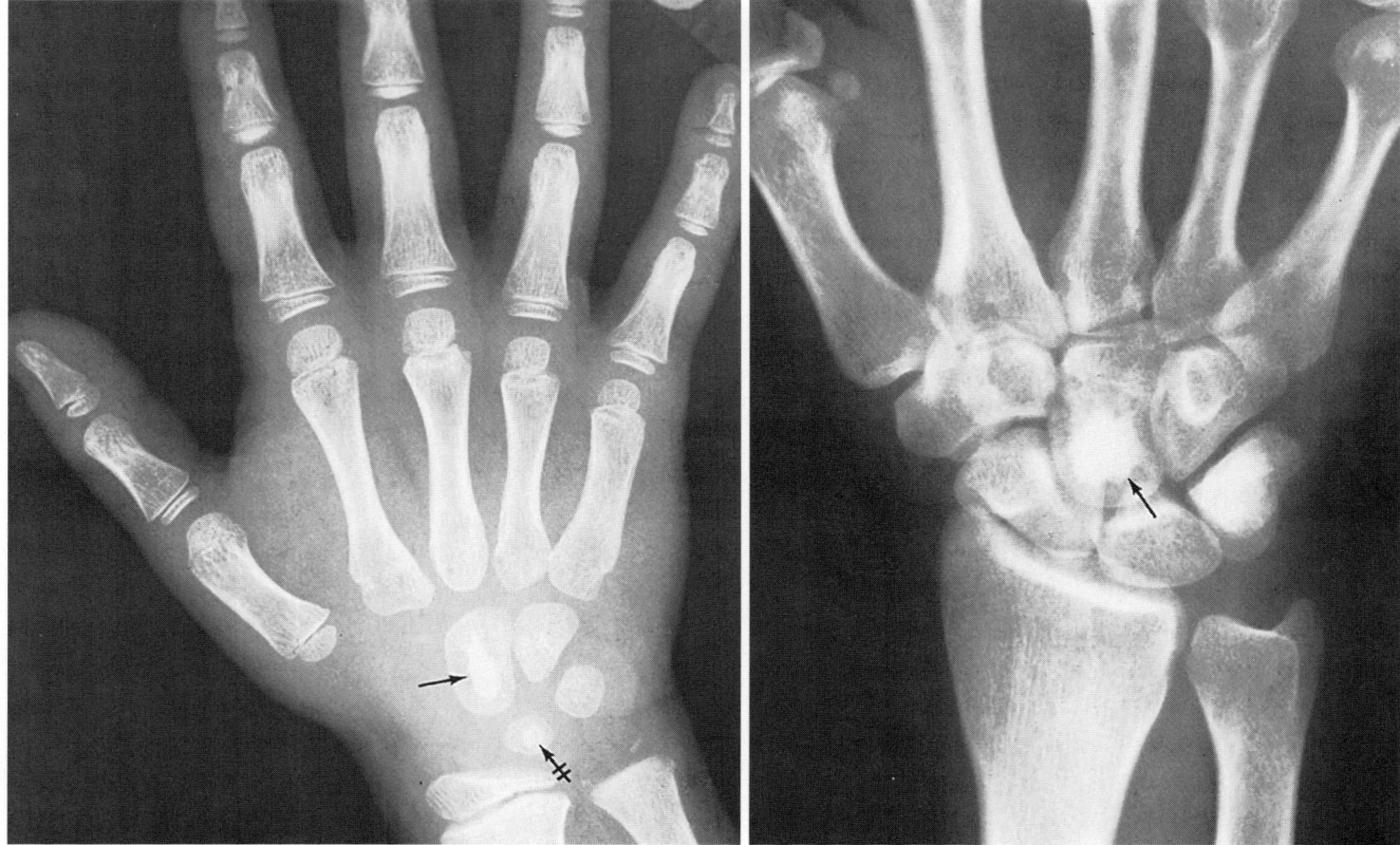

Figure 6–206. Two examples of asymptomatic and clinically unimportant bone islands in the capitate (←). A bone island also appears in the lunate in the first example (⇇).

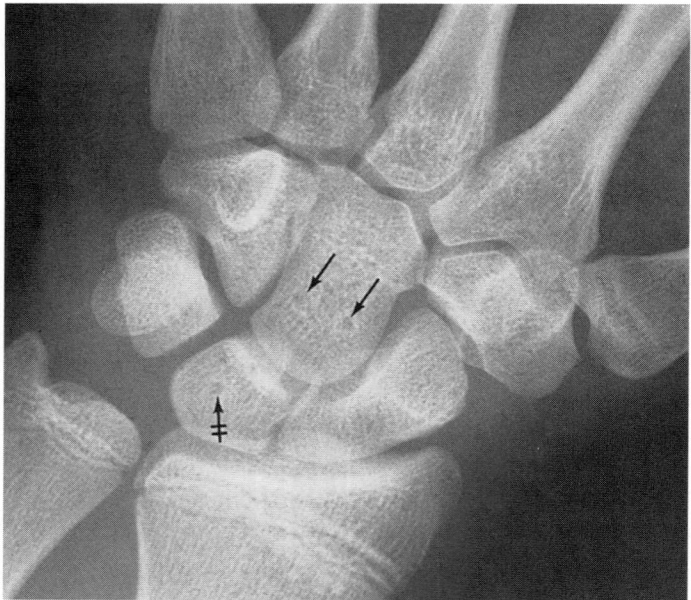

Figure 6–207. Vascular foramina in the capitate bone (←). A similar foramen is seen in the lunate (⇇).

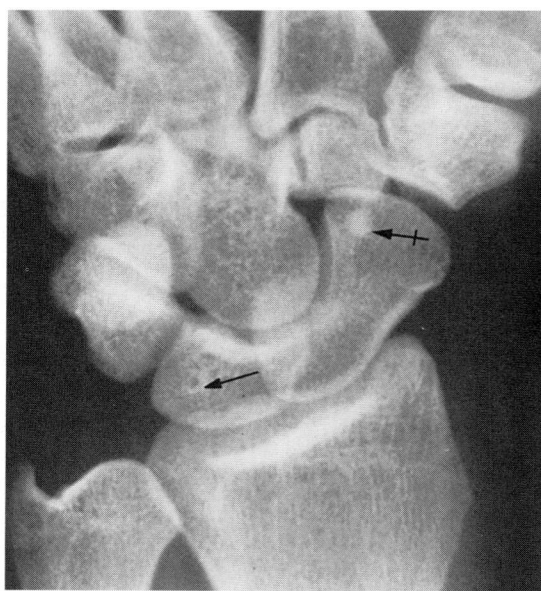

Figure 6–208. The vascular foramen of the lunate (←). A bone island is present in the navicular (↤).

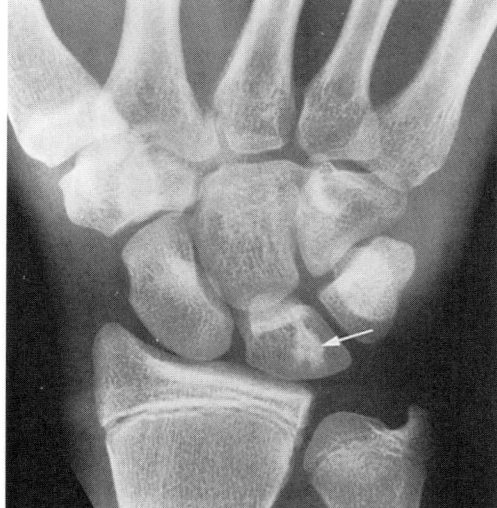

Figure 6–209. Bone island in the lunate in a 14-year-old boy.

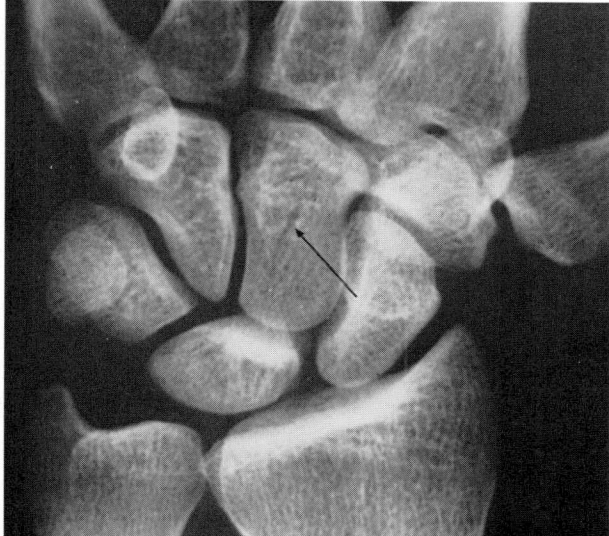

Figure 6–210. Lucent cleft in the capitate, simulating a fracture.

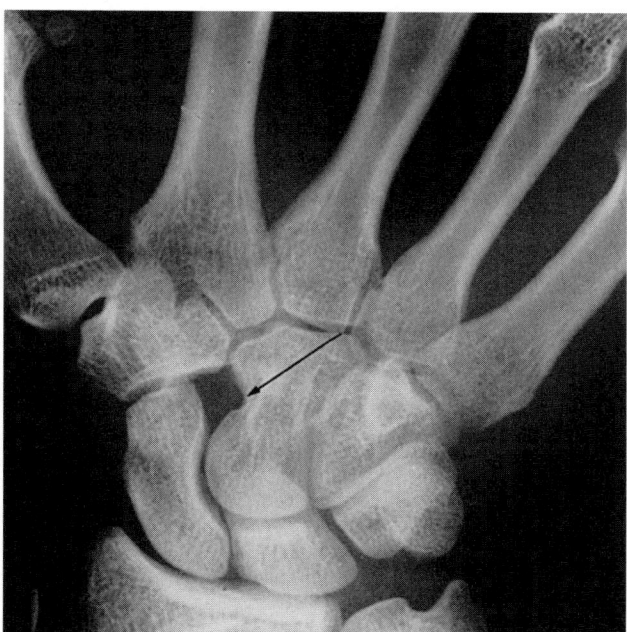

Figure 6–211. Deep fossa in the radial side of the capitate. The os carpi centrale may develop in this fossa (see Fig. 6–189).

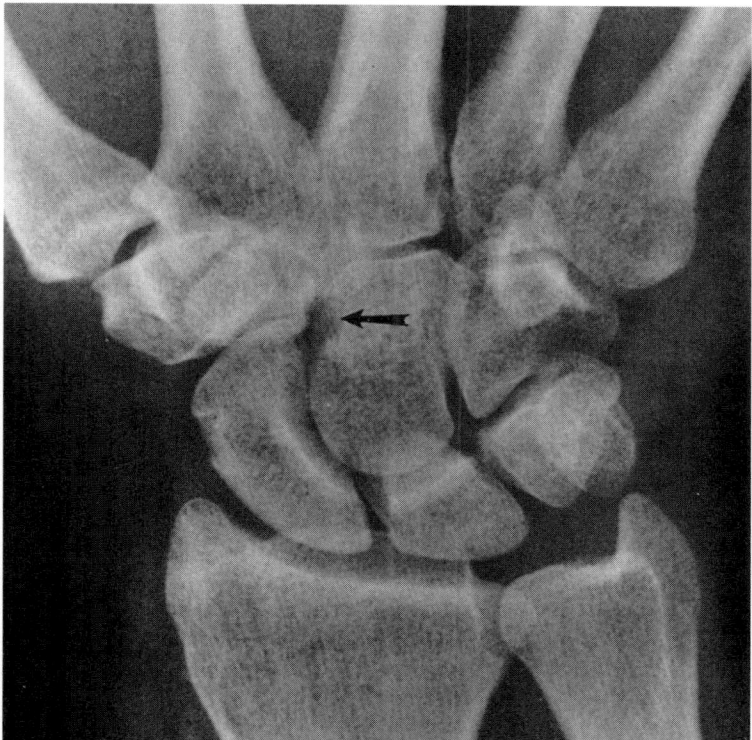

Figure 6–212. The capitate fossa may simulate an erosion.

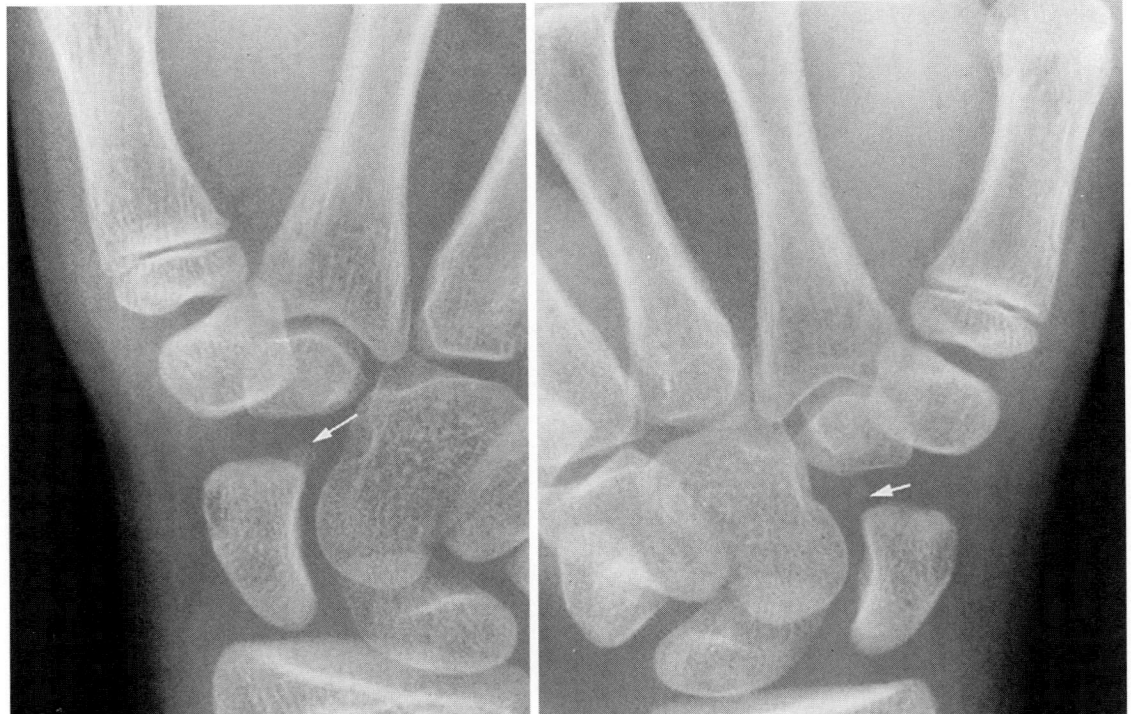

Figure 6–213. The os carpi centrale present bilaterally in a child.

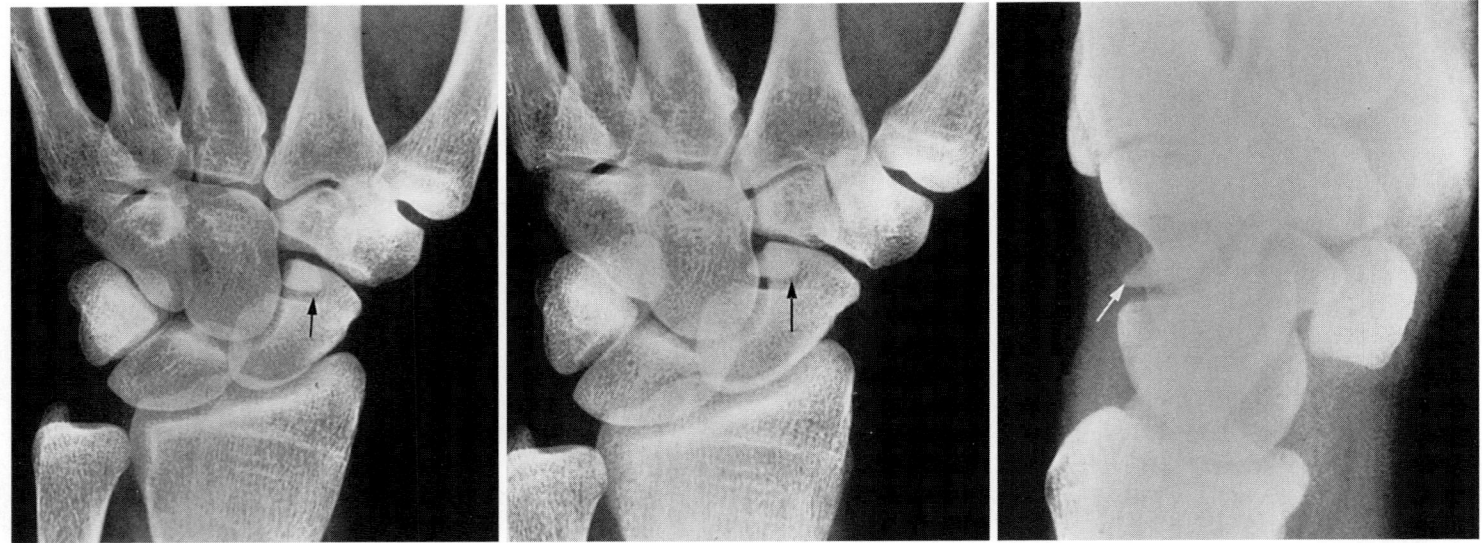

Figure 6–214. A large os carpi centrale in an adult. (Ref: Gersovich EO, Greenspan A: Case report 598. *Skeletal Radiol* 19:143, 1990.)

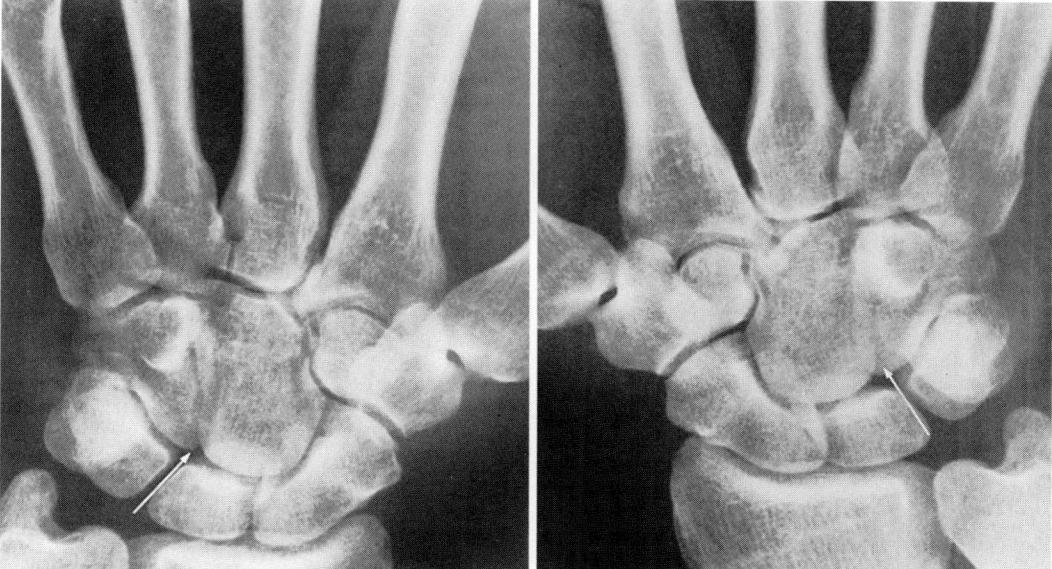

Figure 6–215. The joint between the capitate and hamate may be poorly visualized in normal individuals and should not be mistaken for the changes of an inflammatory arthritis.

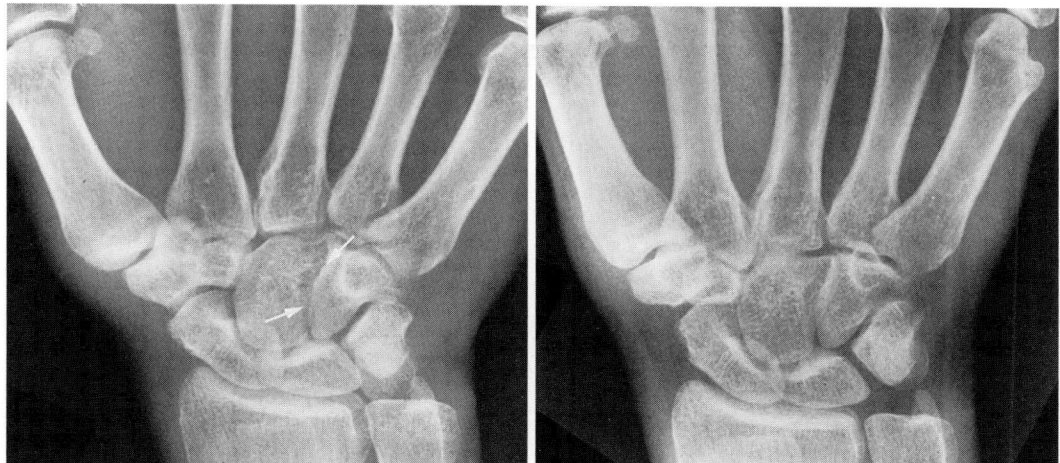

Figure 6–216. *Left,* Apparent loss of the joint space between the capitate and hamate produced by inability of the patient to flatten the hand. Note similar overlap of navicular and lunate. *Right,* Improved positioning shows normal relationships.

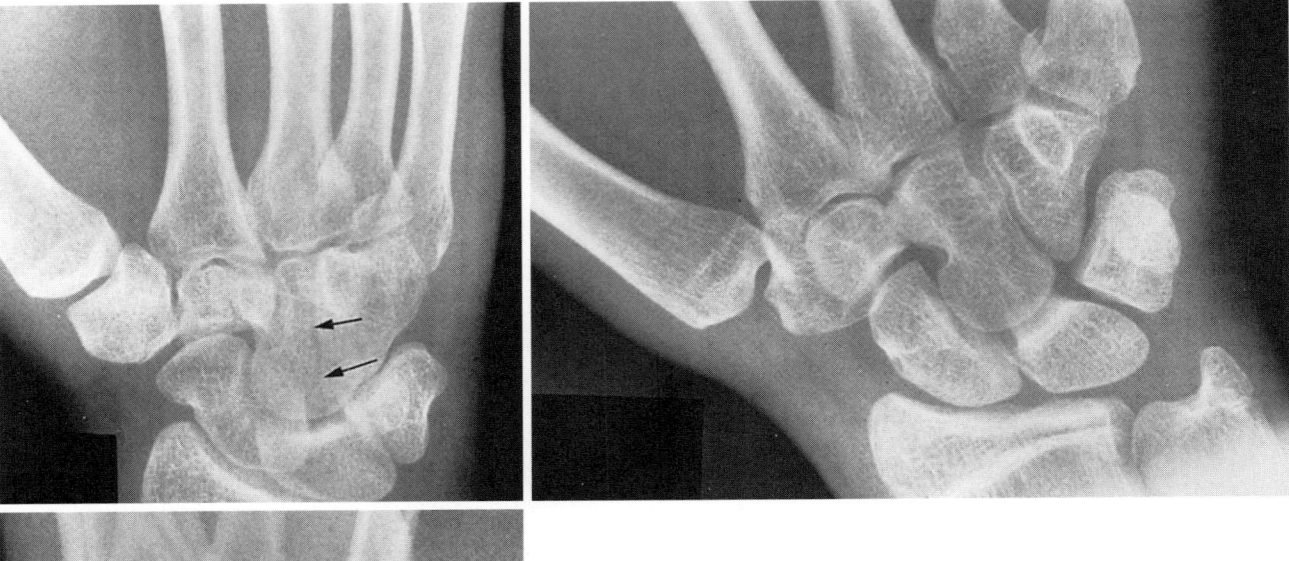

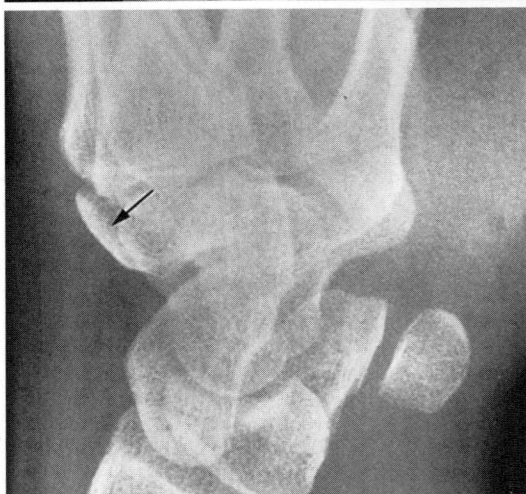

Figure 6–217. *Top left,* Poorly positioned PA view mistaken for fracture of the capitate as a result of overlap of the shadows of the capitate and hamate. *Top right,* Correct positioning shows no fracture. *Bottom left,* Off-lateral projection of wrist shows simulated fracture of the posterior aspect of the capitate.

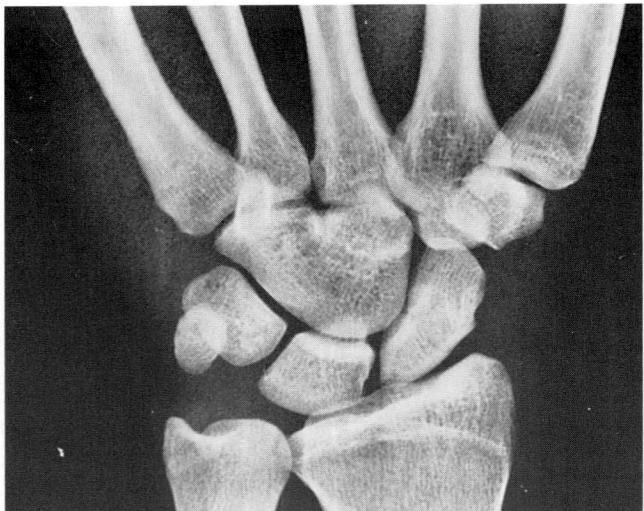

Figure 6–218. Congenital fusion of the capitate and hamate. Carpal fusions may occur as isolated anomalies or be associated with congenital malformation syndromes. The isolated fusions usually involve bones of the same row, such as triquetrum-lunate, capitate-hamate, or trapezium-trapezoid, while syndrome-related fusions often go across rows, such as, trapezium-scaphoid. (Ref: Poznanski AJ: *The hand in radiologic diagnosis,* 2nd ed. Philadelphia, WB Saunders, 1984, p. 201.)

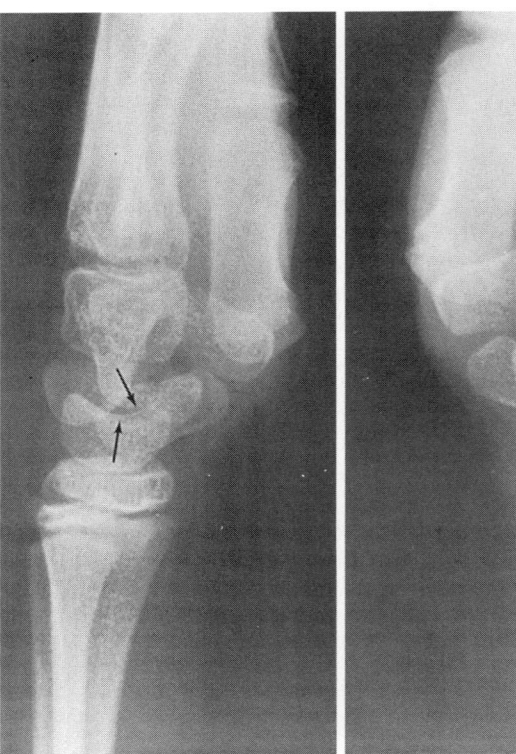

Figure 6–219. Variable relationships of capitate to lunate, depending on degree of flexion or extension of the hand.

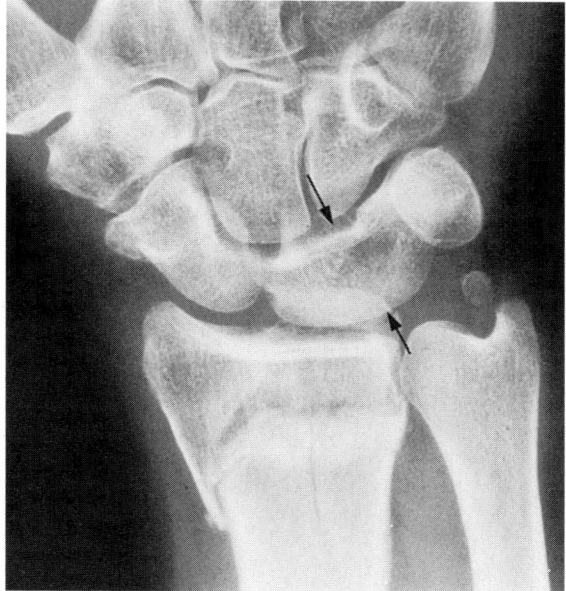

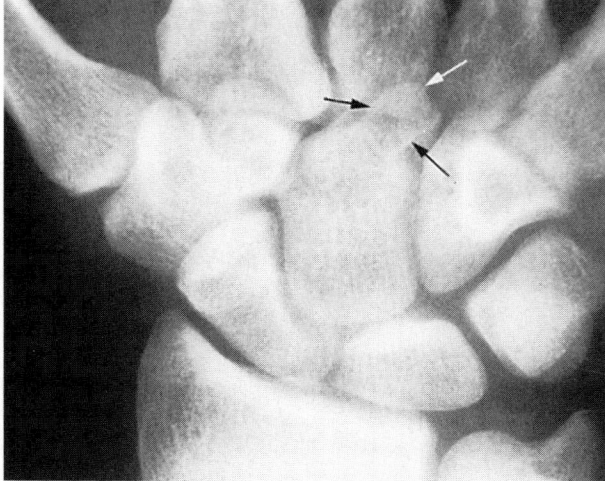

Figure 6–221. The os styloideum (see Figs. 6–173 and 6–174).

Figure 6–220. Congenital fusion of the lunate and triquetrum. Patients with this type of coalition may have a wide scapholunate space as a normal variation. (Ref: Metz VM et al: Wide scapholunate space in lunotriquetral coalition: A normal variant? *Radiology* 188:557, 1993.)

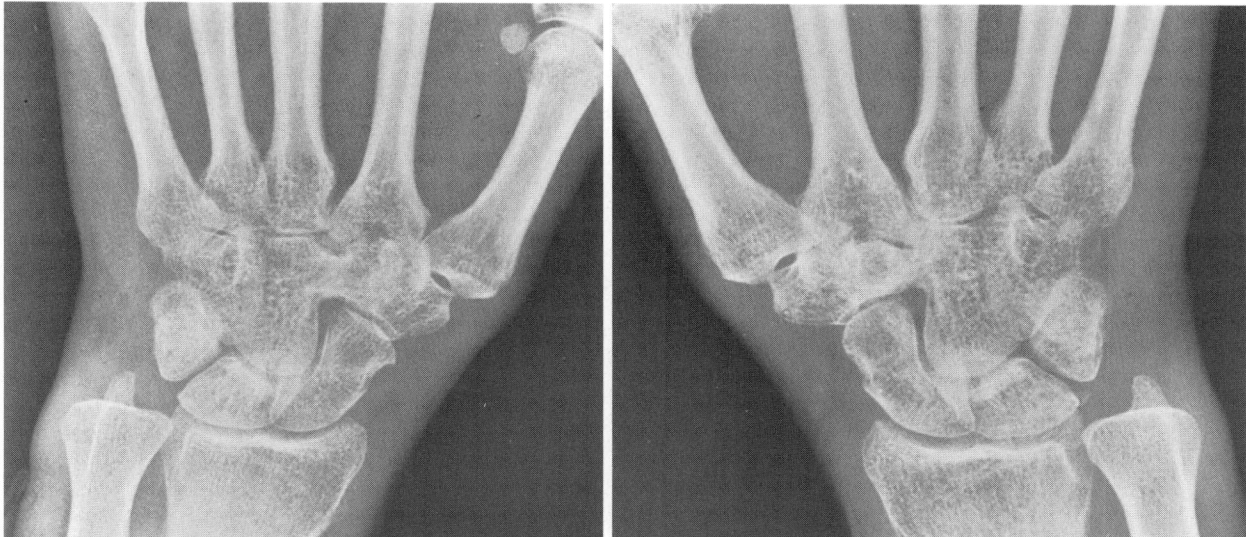

Figure 6–222. Bilateral congenital fusions of the capitate, hamate, trapezoid, and trapezium.

The Carpals

THE HAMATE BONE

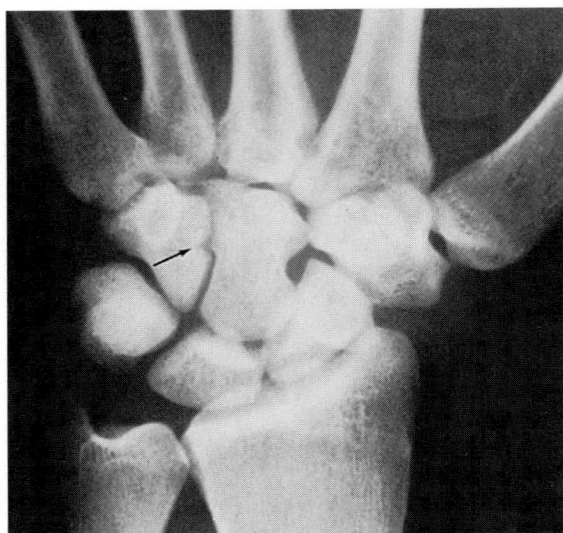

Figure 6–223. Developmental cleft in the lateral aspect of the hamate.

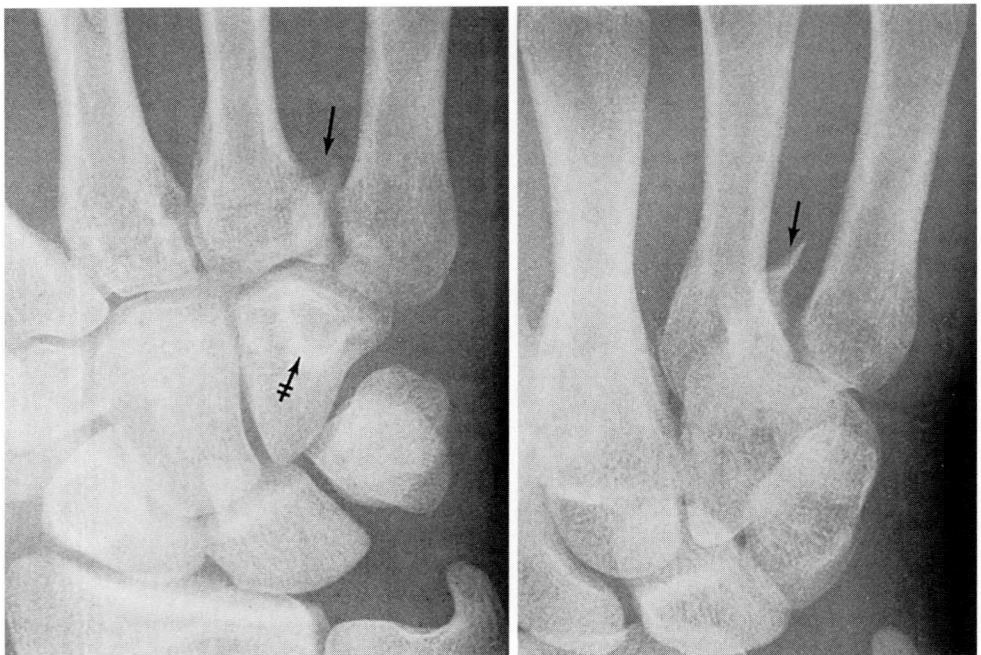

Figure 6–224. Elongated unciform process of the hamate, the origin of the flexor digiti quanti muscle (←). Note also the cystlike shadow produced by the base of the unciform process (↚).

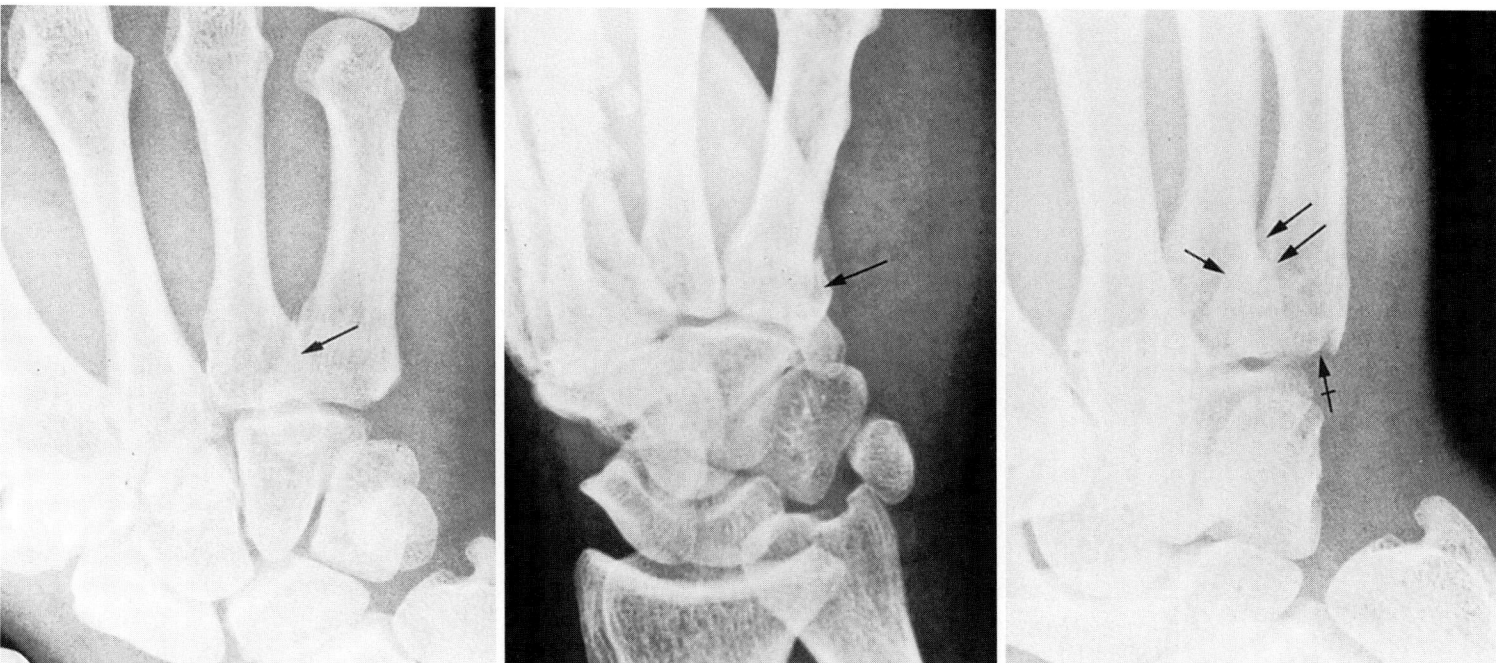

Figure 6–225. Elongated unciform process of the hamate misdiagnosed as a fracture (←). The cleft of the base of the fifth metacarpal is normal (↔).

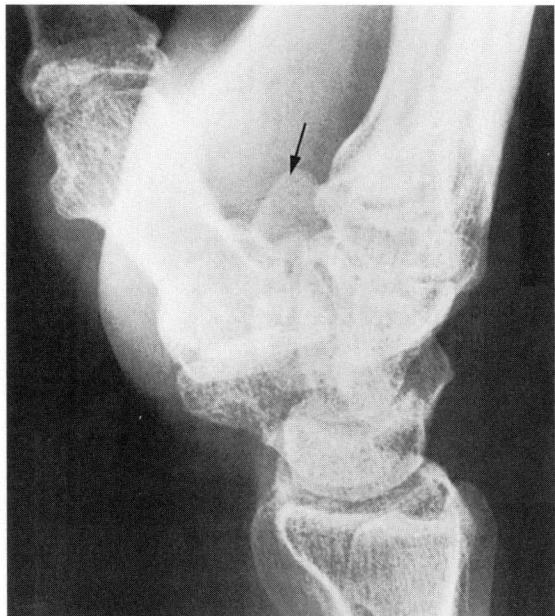

Figure 6–226. The hamulus of the hamate in lateral projection. This should not be mistaken for a trapezium secundarium.

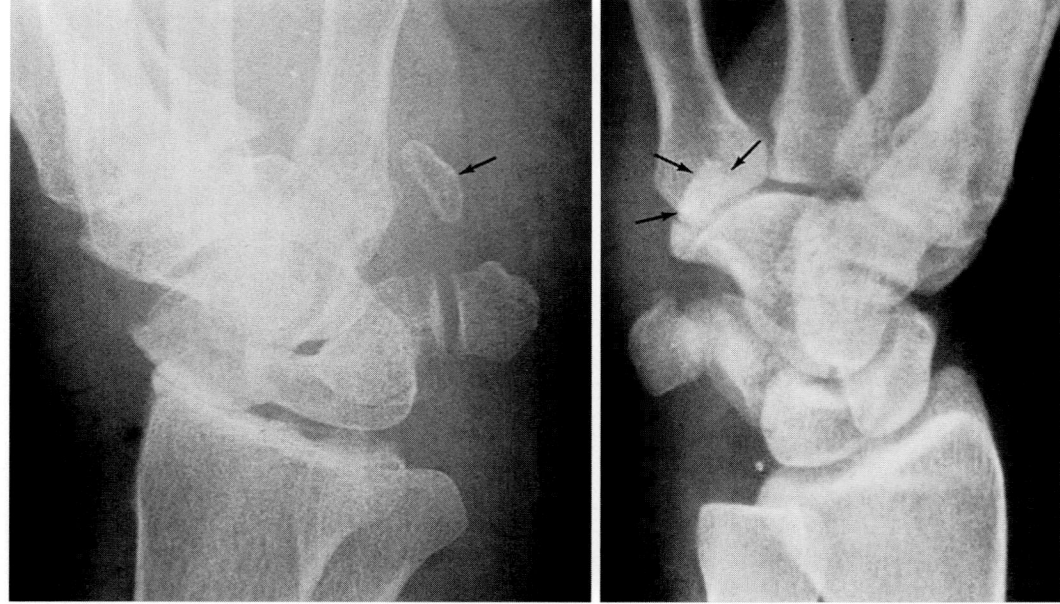

Figure 6–227. Two examples of the os hamuli proprium. The unciform process of the hamate may ossify independently and give the impression of an accessory bone or a fracture. (Ref: Kohler A, Zimmer EA: *Borderlands of the normal and early pathologic findings in skeletal roentgenology,* 4th ed. New York, Thieme, 1993, p. 95.)

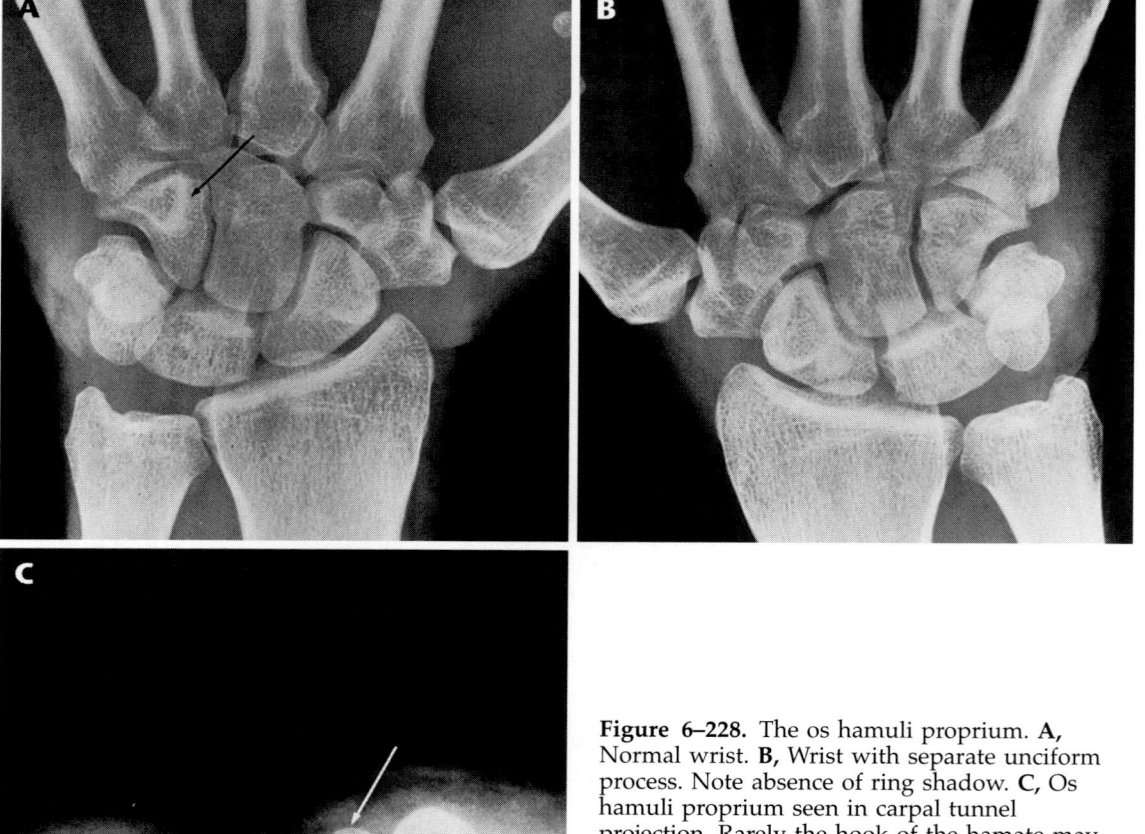

Figure 6–228. The os hamuli proprium. **A,** Normal wrist. **B,** Wrist with separate unciform process. Note absence of ring shadow. **C,** Os hamuli proprium seen in carpal tunnel projection. Rarely the hook of the hamate may be congenitally absent. (Ref: Seeger LL et al: Case report 464: Bilateral congenital absence of the hook of the hamate. *Skeletal Radiol* 17:85, 1988.)

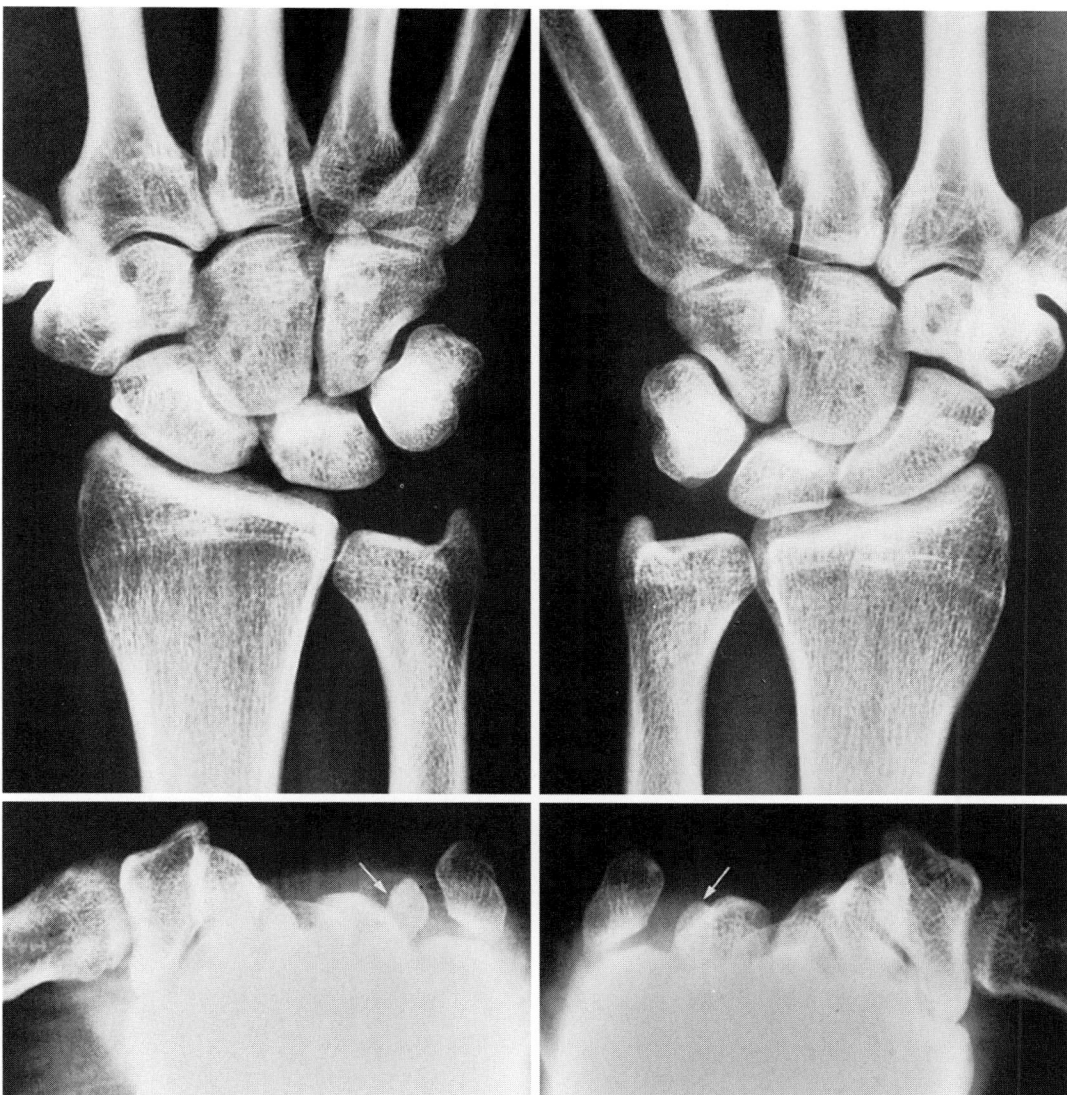

Figure 6–229. Bilateral os hamuli proprium. Note absence of ring shadows in the hamates in the frontal projections.

The Carpals

THE TRAPEZIUM AND TRAPEZOID BONES

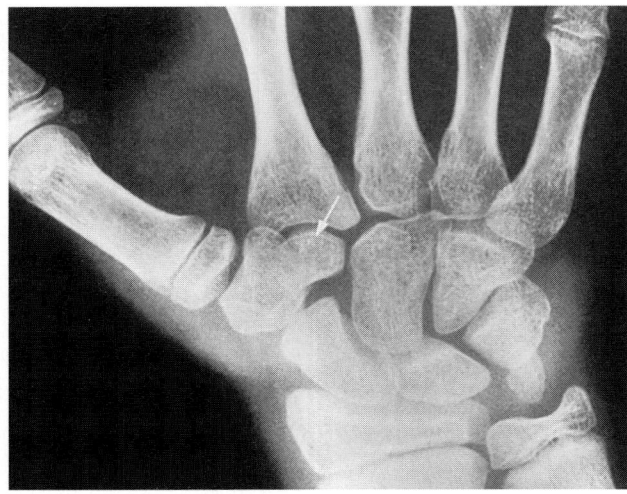

Figure 6–230. Hypoplasia of the trapezoid in a 13-year-old boy.

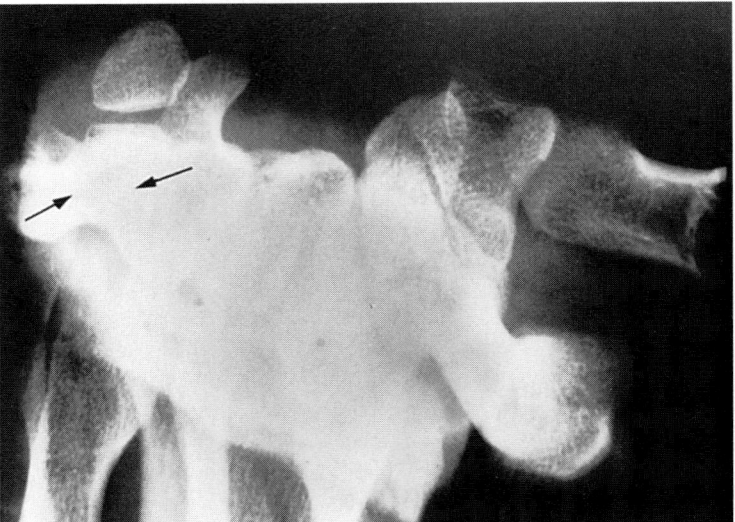

Figure 6–231. The carpal tunnel projection may produce an end-on view of the fifth metacarpal superimposed on the carpal bones. This may produce a ringlike radiolucency that should not be mistaken for a pathologic process. (Ref: Fodor T et al: Carpal tunnel ring artifact. *Am J Roentgenol* 144:765, 1985.)

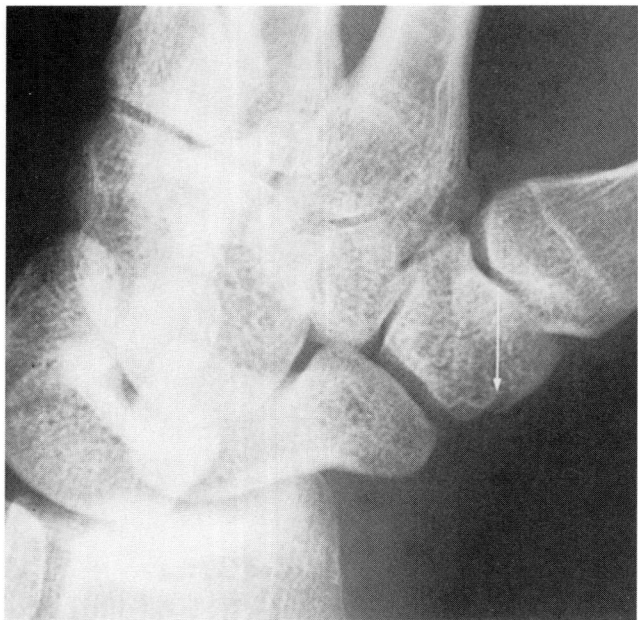

Figure 6–232. Irregularity of the radial aspect of the trapezium, simulating a fracture.

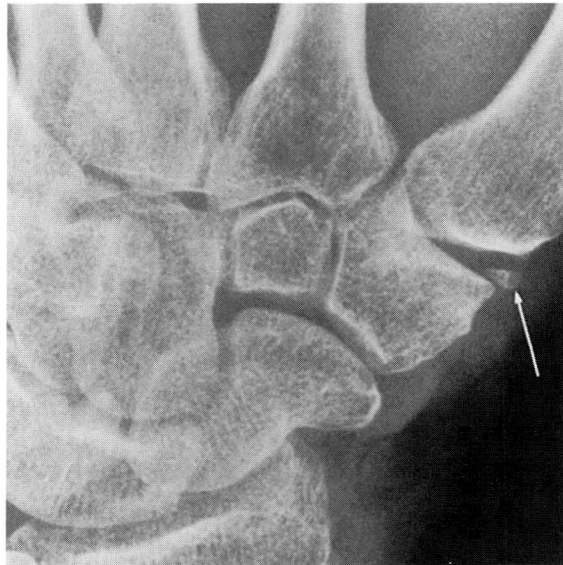

Figure 6–233. The os paratrapezium.

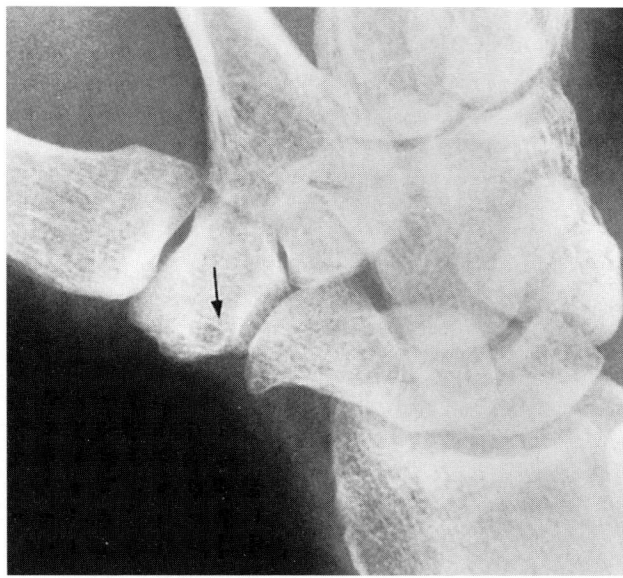

Figure 6–234. Ring lesion in the trapezium. These lesions are fibrous in nature and are seen elsewhere in the hand and wrist. They are apparently of no clinical significance (see Figs. 6–268 and 6–304.)

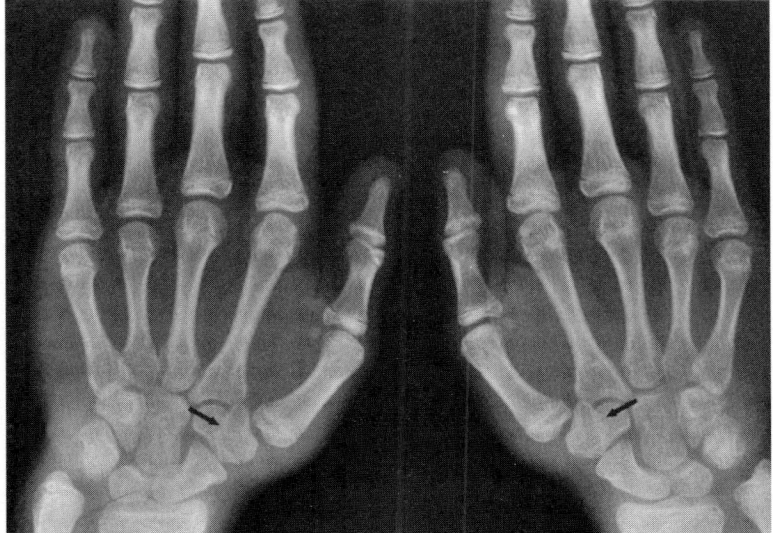

Figure 6–235. Bilateral coalition of the trapezium and trapezoid.

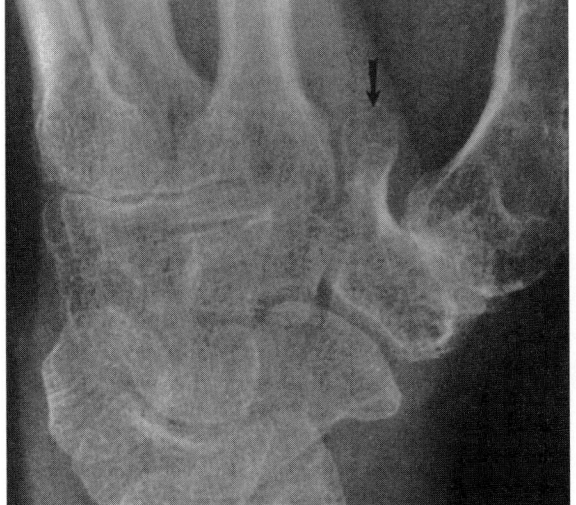

Figure 6–236. Osseous process arising from the trapezium (see the following figure).

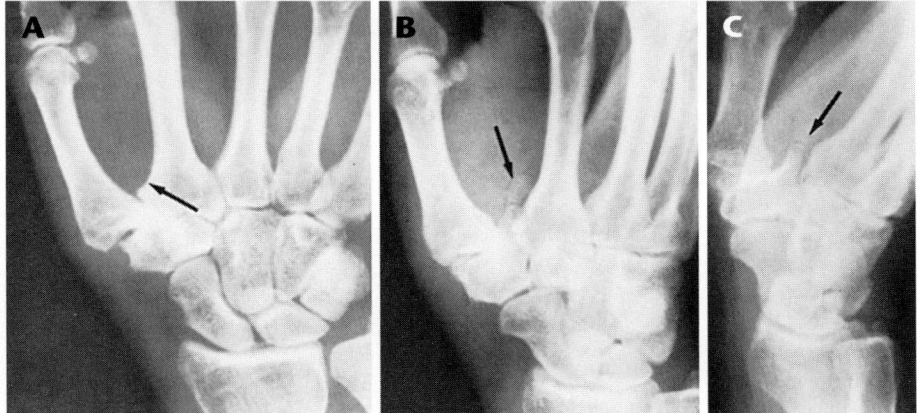

Figure 6–237. A, B, C, Attempted formation of an accessory metacarpal, seen best in **B,** arising from the trapezium.

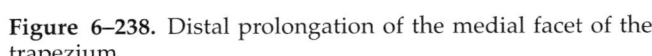

Figure 6–238. Distal prolongation of the medial facet of the trapezium.

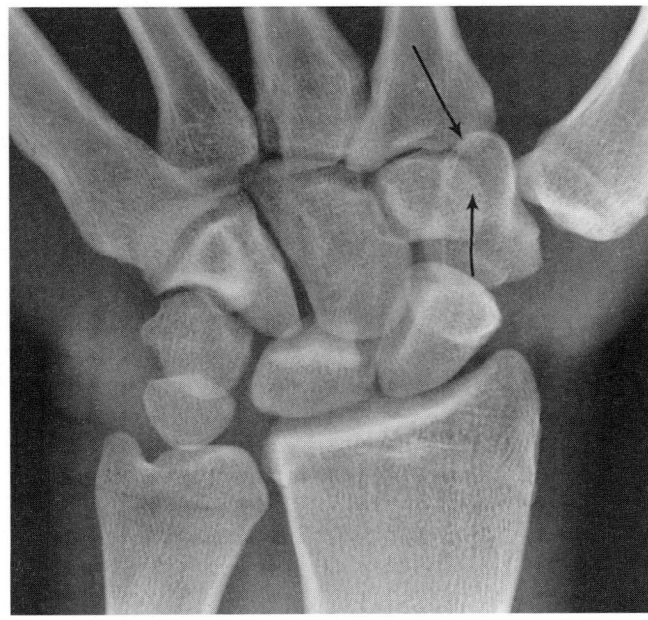

The Carpals

THE NAVICULAR BONE

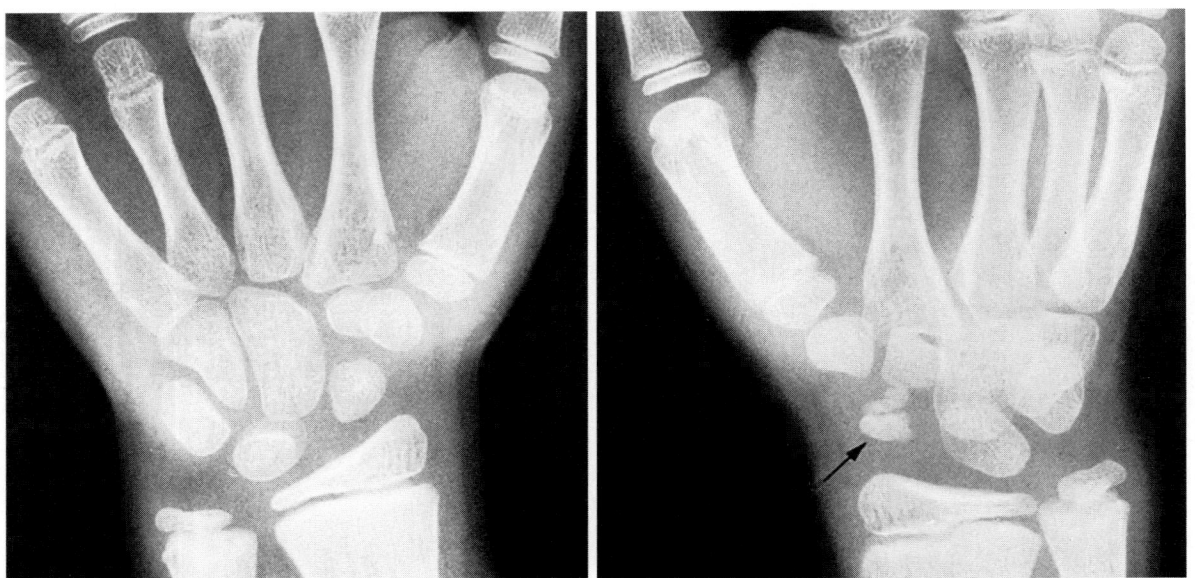

Figure 6–239. Unilateral development of the navicular from multiple foci in an 11-year-old boy.

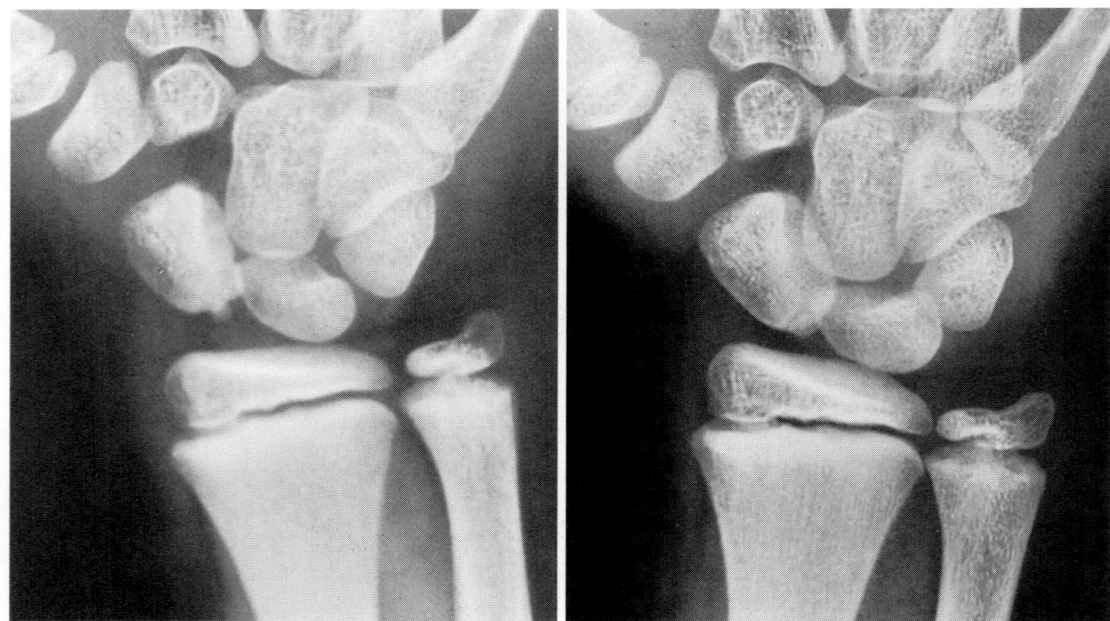

Figure 6–240. *Left*, Accessory ossification center for the navicular in a 10-year-old boy. *Right*, 5 months later, patient shows partial incorporation of the center.

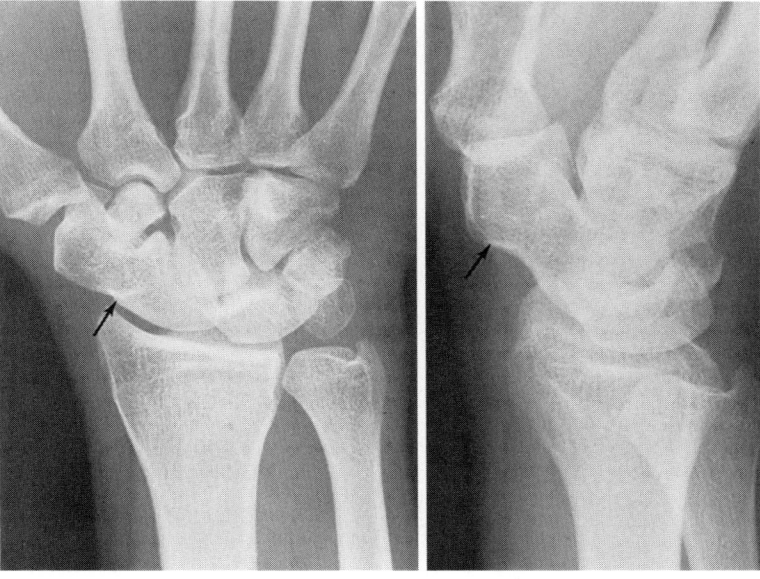

Figure 6–241. Congenital fusion of the navicular and trapezium. Such fusions are not uncommon and usually are of no significance. (Refs: O'Rahilly R: Survey of carpal and tarsal anomalies. *J Bone Joint Surg* 35A:626, 1953; Poznanski AJ: *The hand in radiologic diagnosis*, 2nd ed. Philadelphia, WB Saunders, 1984, p. 201.)

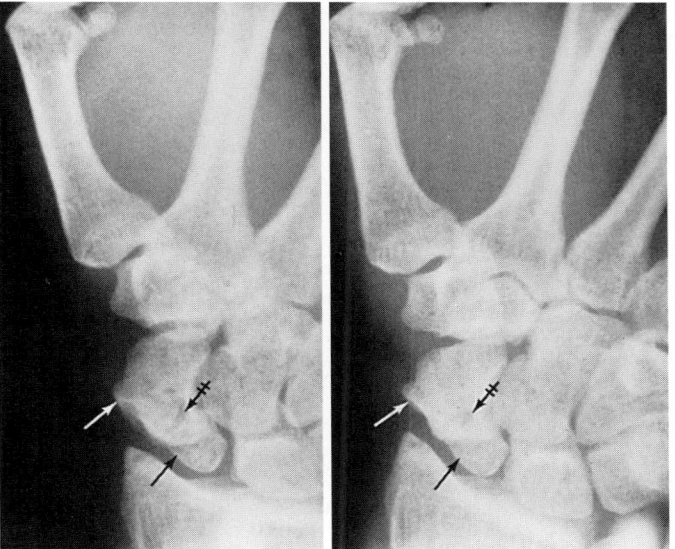

Figure 6–242. Two views of a bipartite navicular bone (←). Note the joint space, which is visible in both projections (◄#).

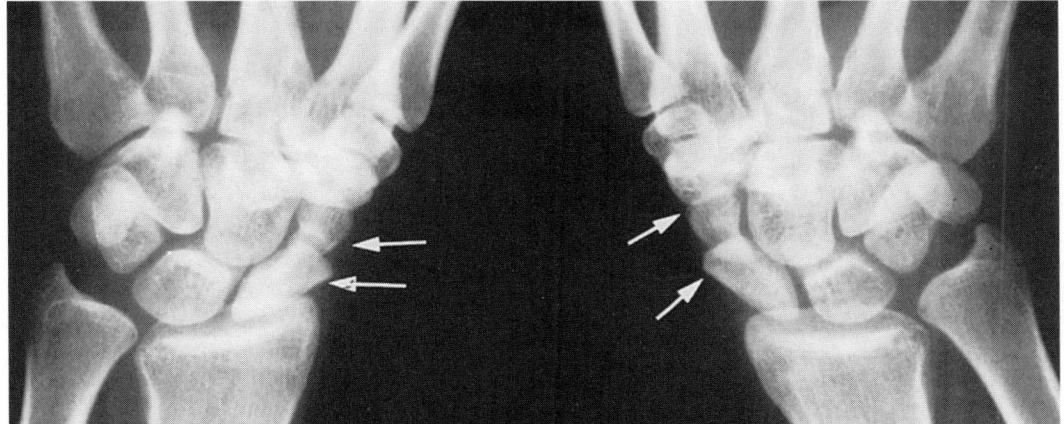

Figure 6–243. Bilateral bipartite navicular bones. (Ref: Waugh RL, Sullivan RF: Anomalies of the carpus with particular reference to the bipartite scaphoid (navicular). *J Bone Joint Surg* 32A:682, 1950.)

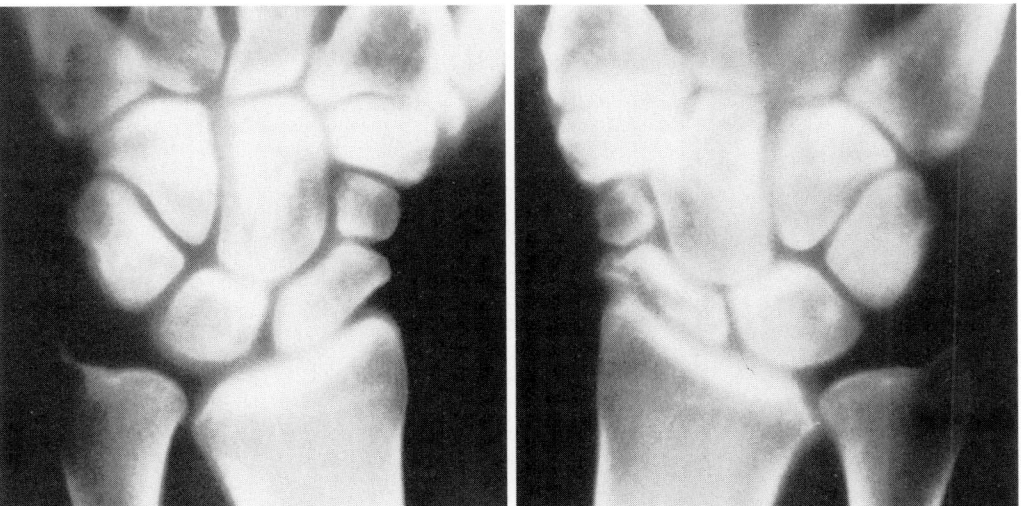

Figure 6–244. Bilateral bipartite navicular bone with aseptic necrosis of the proximal portion on the right.

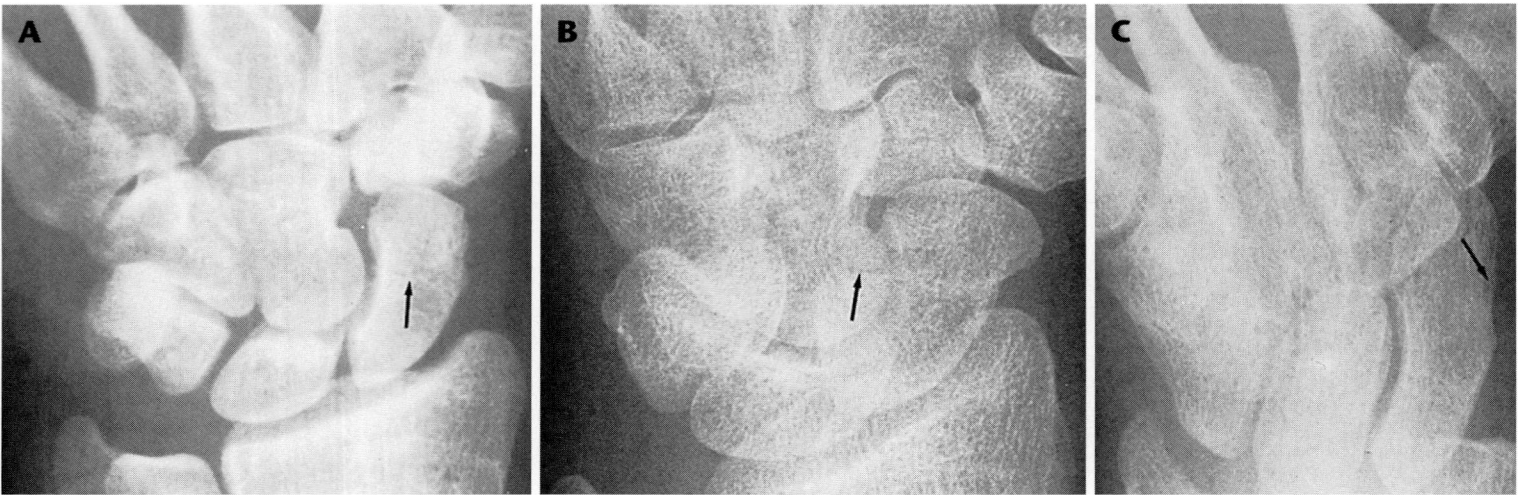

Figure 6–245. Partial division of the navicular bone, simulating a fracture. These clefts are best seen on the ulnar border (**A** and **B**) but may be seen on the radial border as well (**C**).

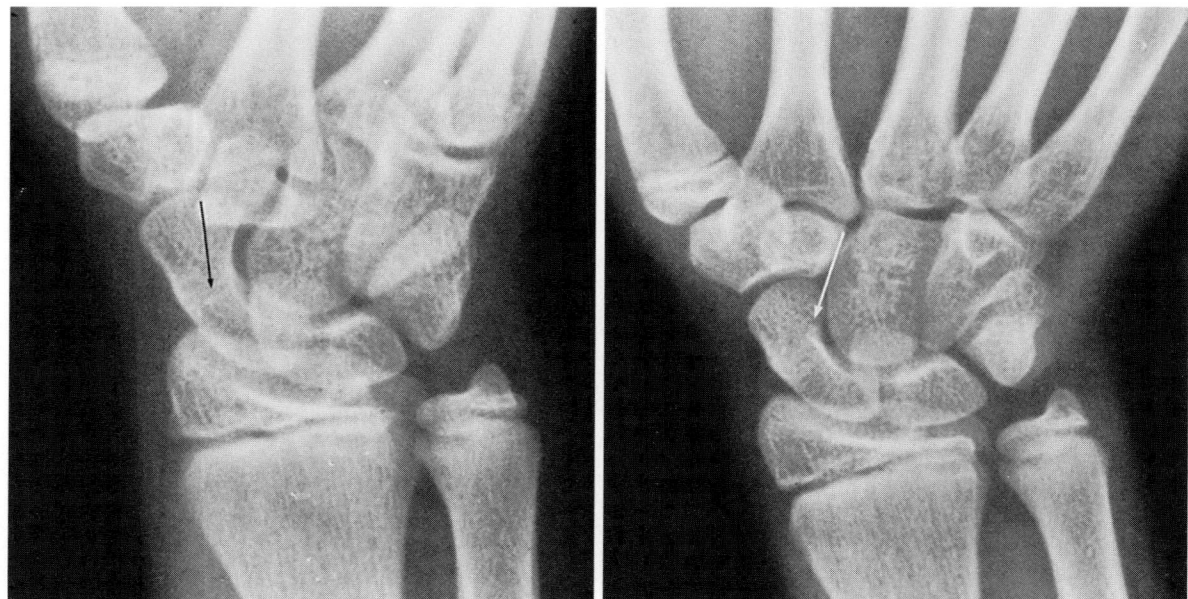

Figure 6–246. Incomplete cleft simulating a fracture in the navicular in a 10-year-old girl.

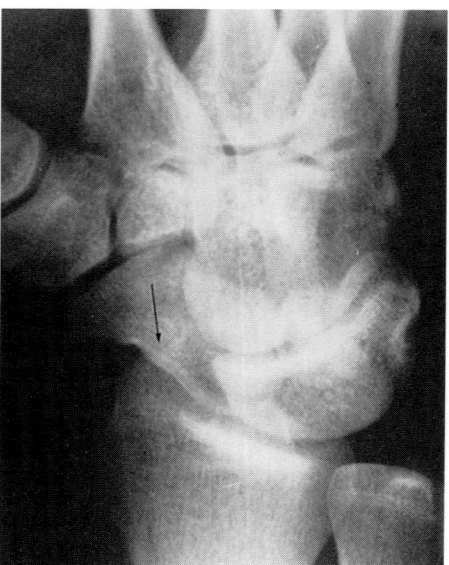

Figure 6–247. Simulated fracture of the navicular caused by Mach effect of underlying radial styloid.

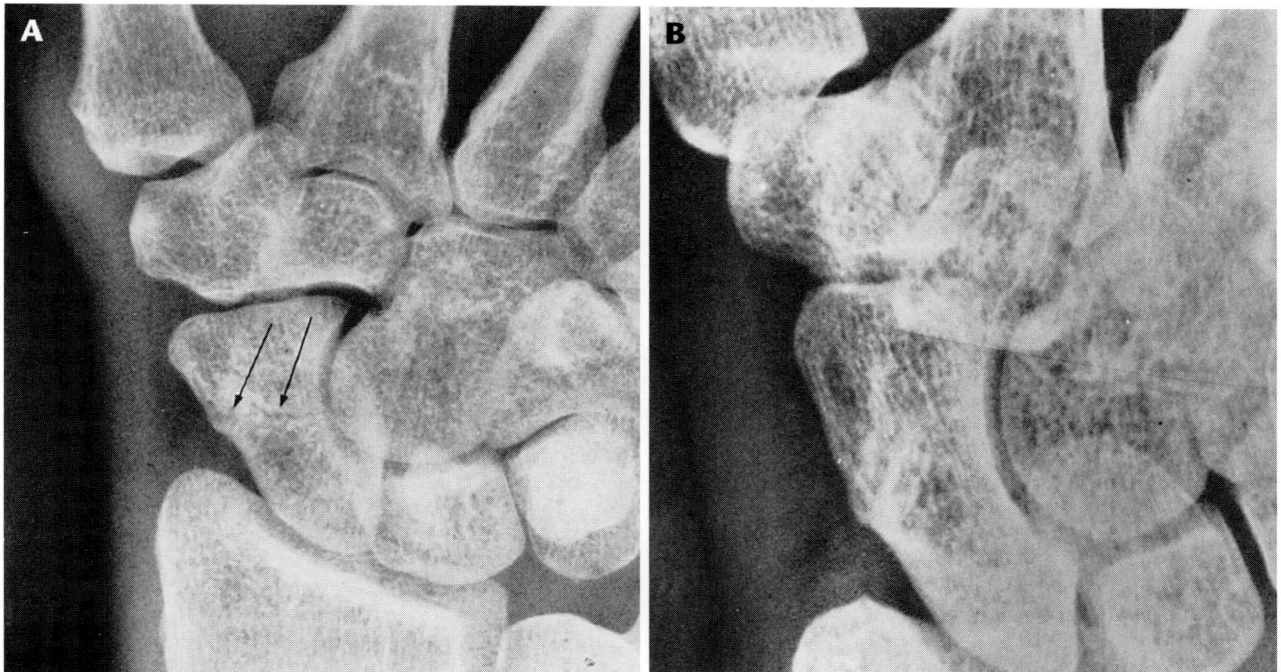

Figure 6–248. A, Simulated fracture of the navicular caused by trabecular pattern. **B,** Navicular view shows no fracture.

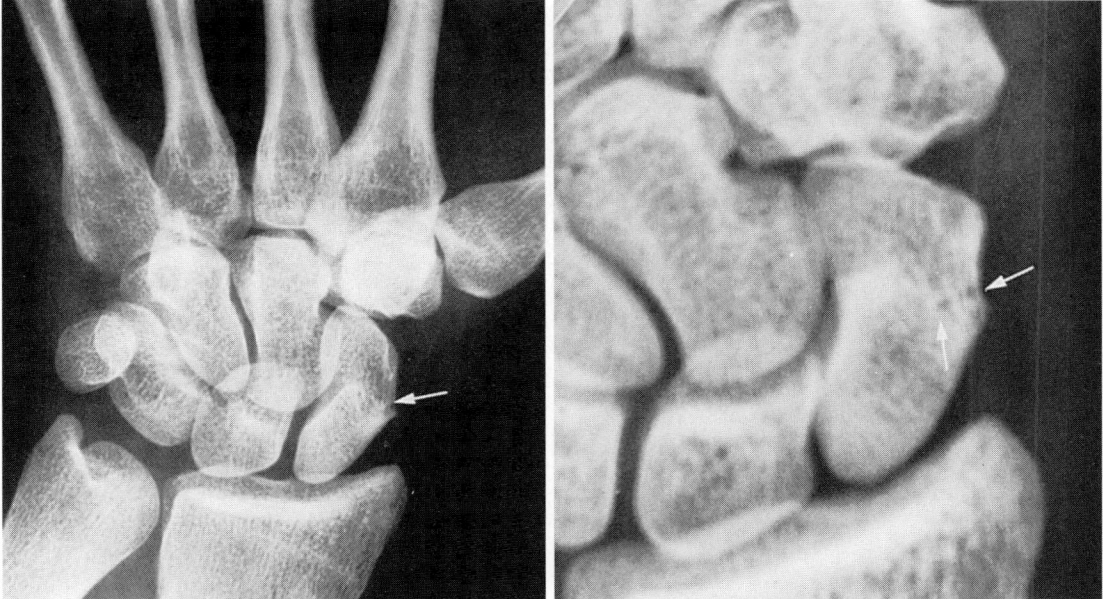

Figure 6–249. Simulated fracture of the navicular caused by trabecular pattern. *Left*, PA view. *Right*, Magnification view.

Figure 6–250. Trabecular pattern simulating a fracture of the navicular.

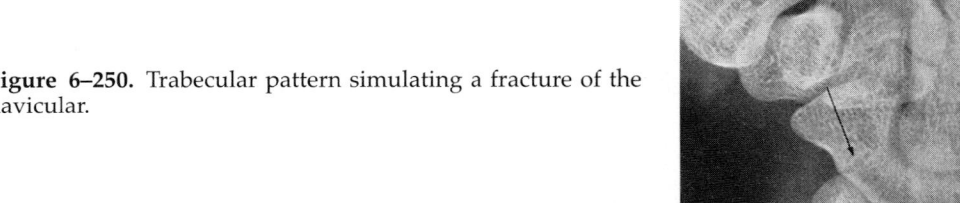

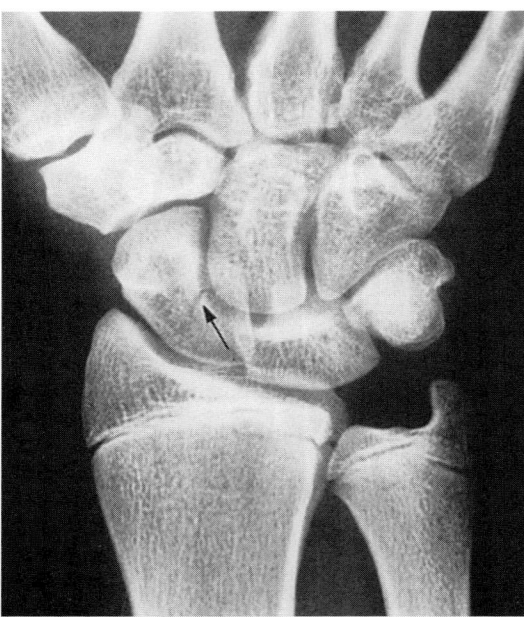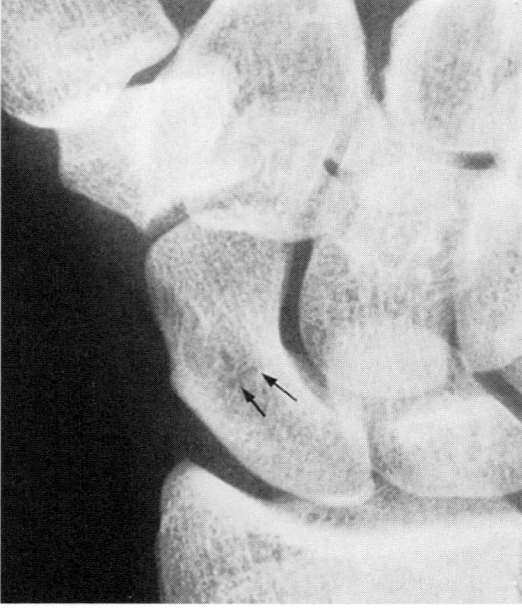

Figure 6–251. *Left,* Simulated fracture of the navicular caused by trabeculation. *Right,* navicular view shows no fracture but defines the trabecular nature of the pseudofracture.

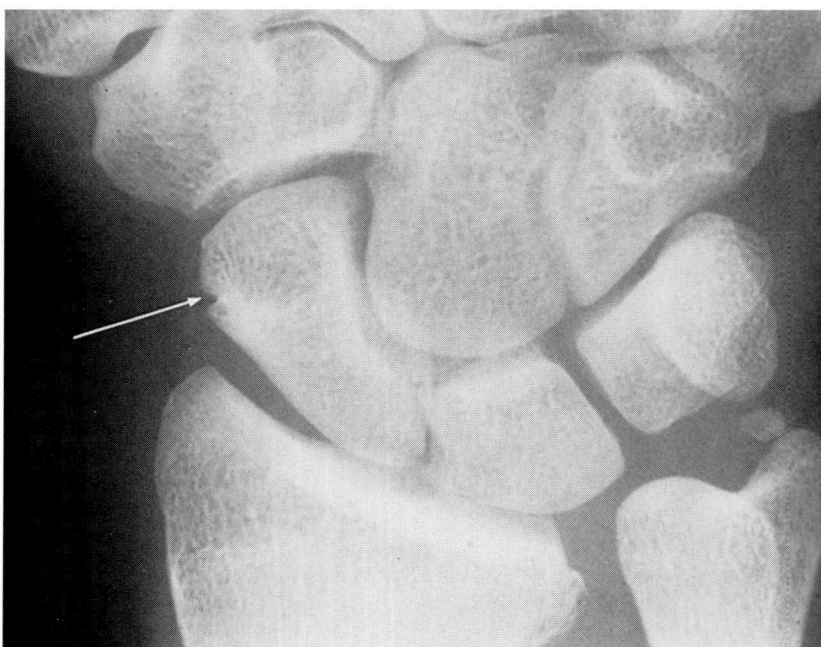

Figure 6–252. Developmental cleft on the radial border of the navicular.

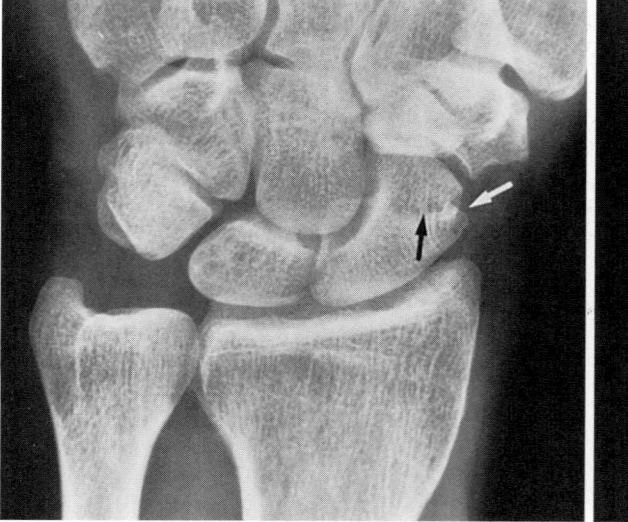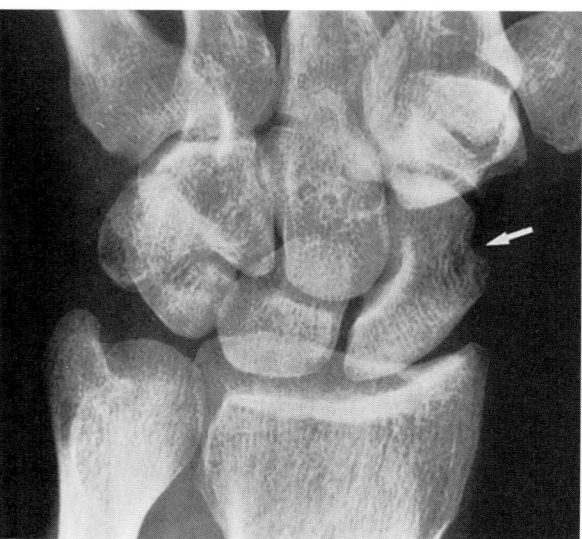

Figure 6–253. Simulated fracture of the navicular caused by a notch on lateral margin.

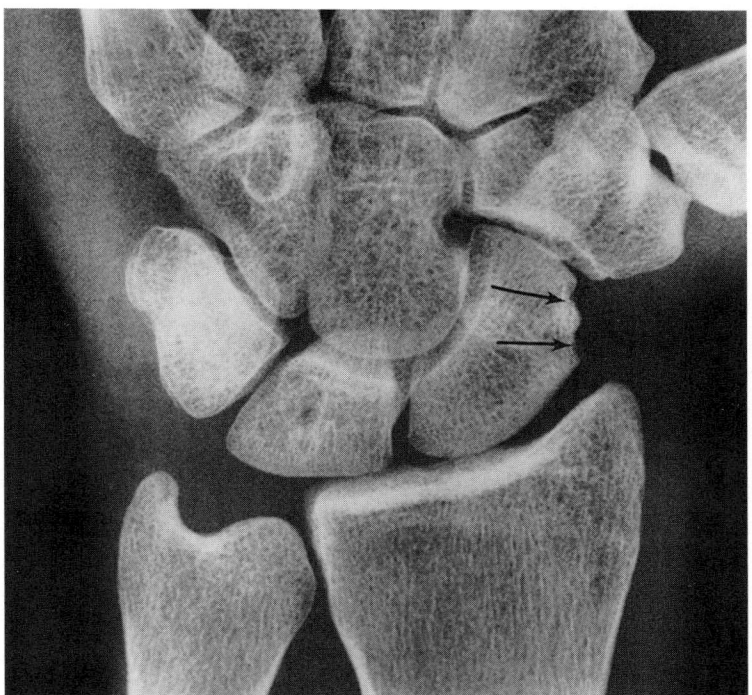

Figure 6–254. Normal undulations on the radial border of the navicular.

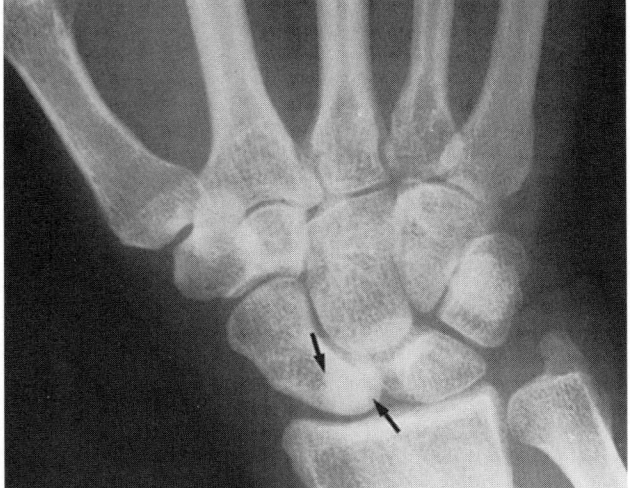

Figure 6–255. Bone island in the navicular.

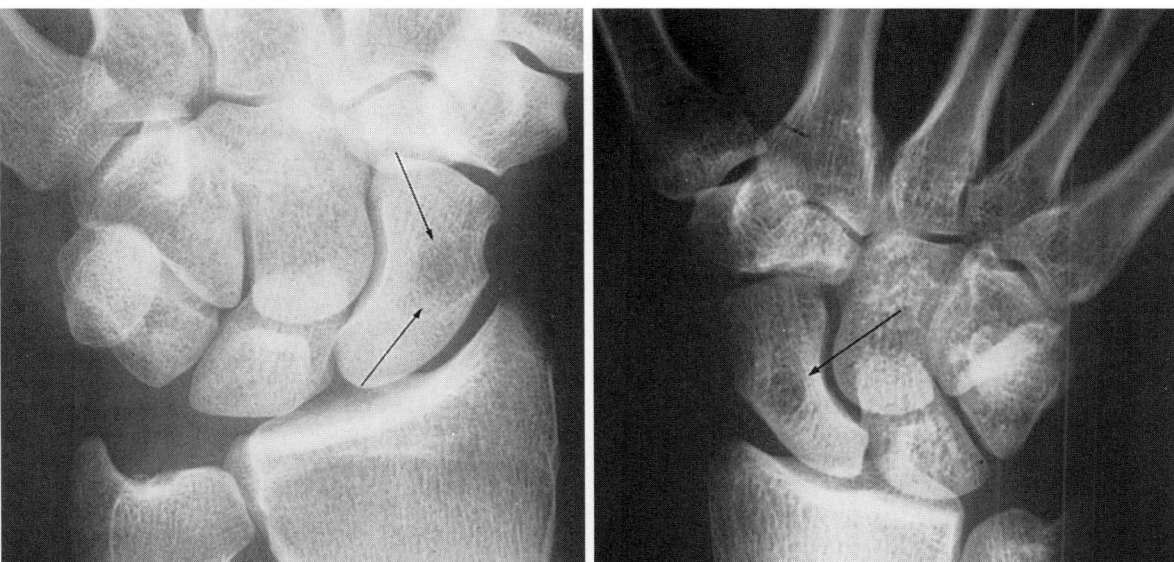

Figure 6–256. Simulated cysts of the navicular produced by trabecular pattern. Navicular views showed no abnormality.

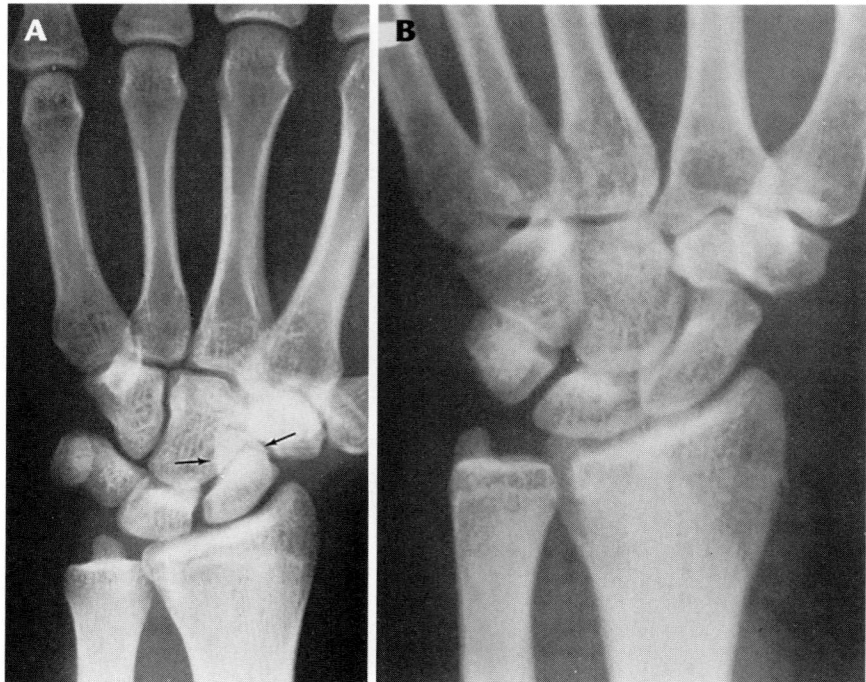

Figure 6–257. Rotary dislocation of the navicular may be simulated by faulty positioning of the wrist at the time of filming. **A,** Note position of the ulnar styloid, indicating rotation of the wrist. The foreshortened configuration of the navicular is similar to the appearance of rotary dislocation. **B,** Correct positioning of the wrist. Navicular assumes a normal configuration. (Ref: Hudson TM et al: Isolated rotary subluxation of the carpal navicular. *Am J Roentgenol* 126:601, 1976.)

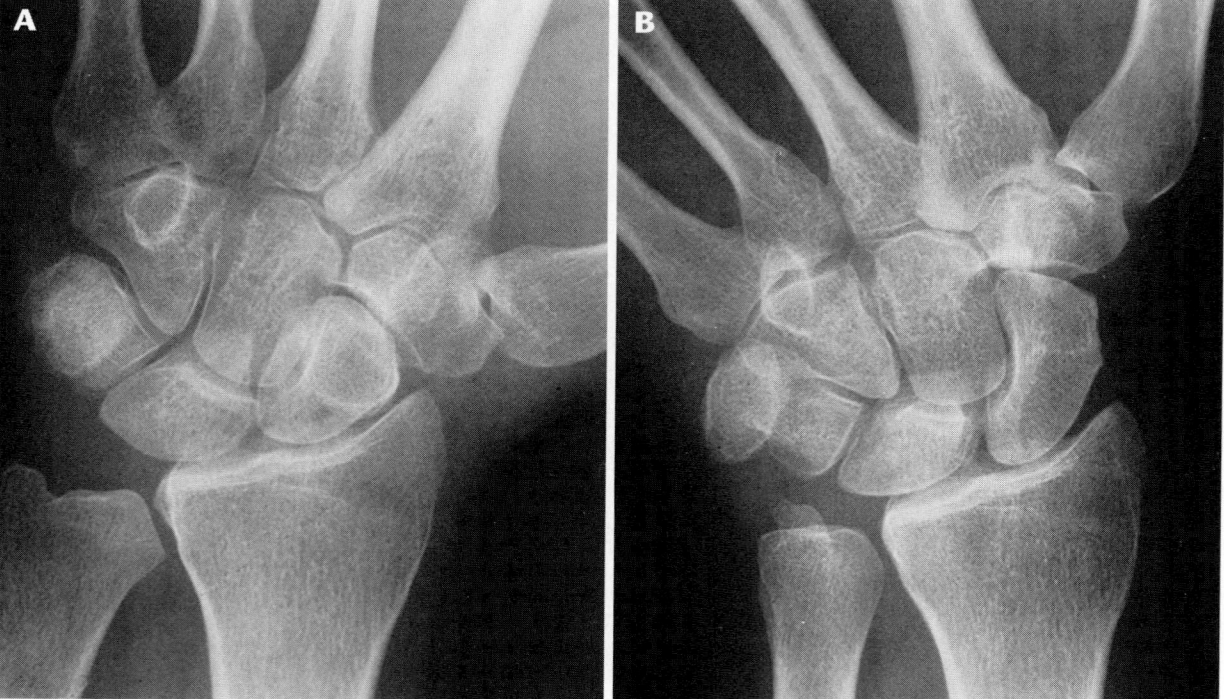

Figure 6–258. A, Simulated rotary dislocation of the navicular produced by filming in radial deviation of the wrist. **B,** Normal appearance of navicular with ulnar deviation.

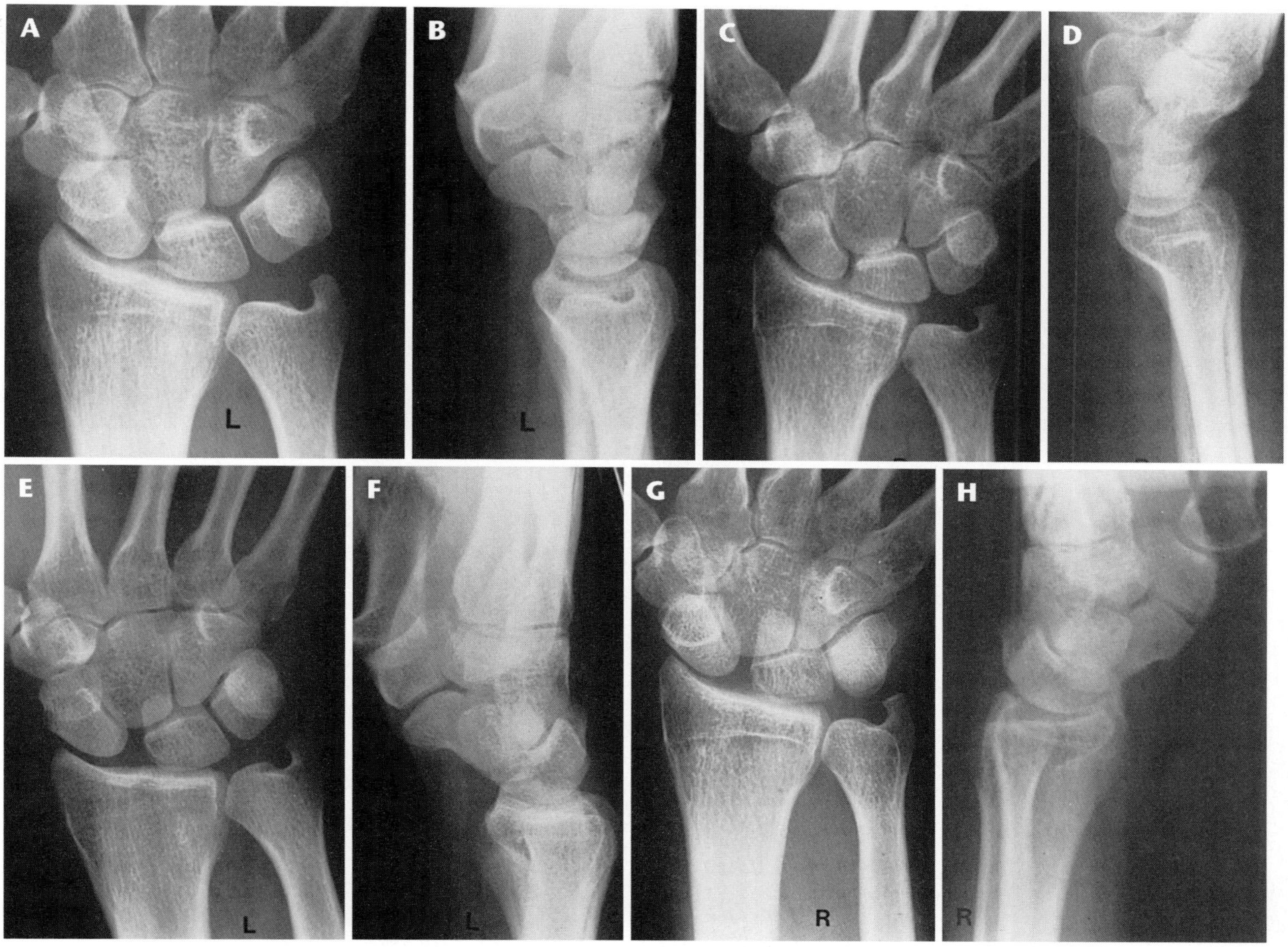

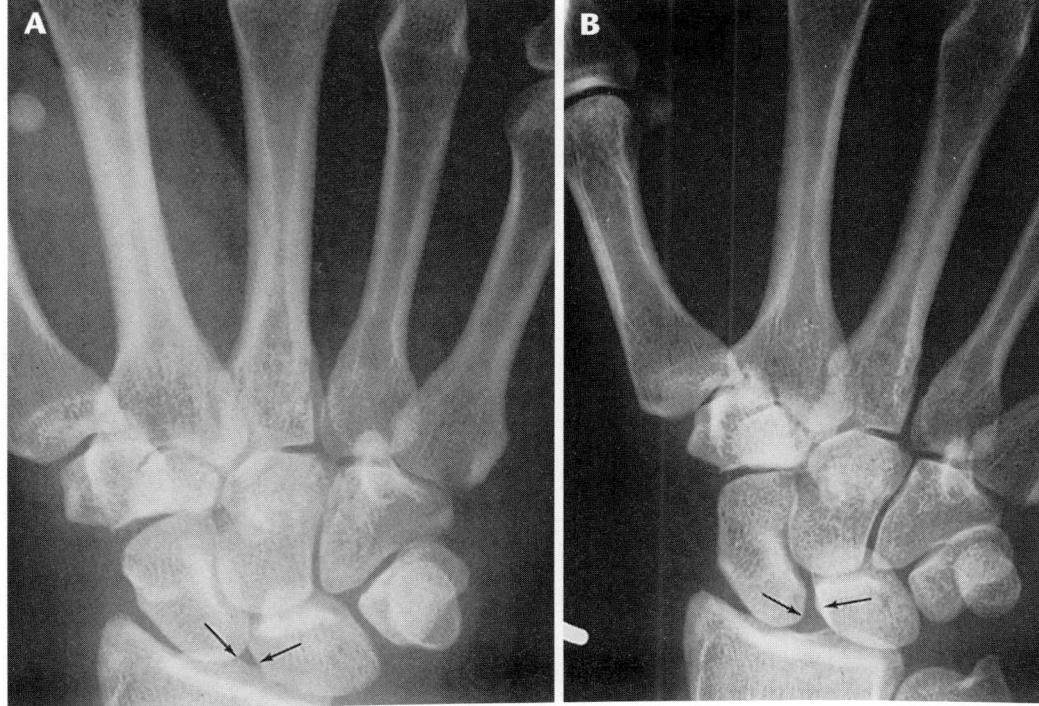

Figure 6–259. Voluntary bilateral painless subluxation of the naviculars in a 27-year-old man. **A–D,** Both wrists at rest. **E–H,** Both wrists with navicular subluxed at will.

Figure 6–260. The interval between the navicular and the lunate is not always a reliable indication of rotary dislocation of the navicular, since its width is dependent on the position of the thumb. Note change in interval between **A** and **B**.

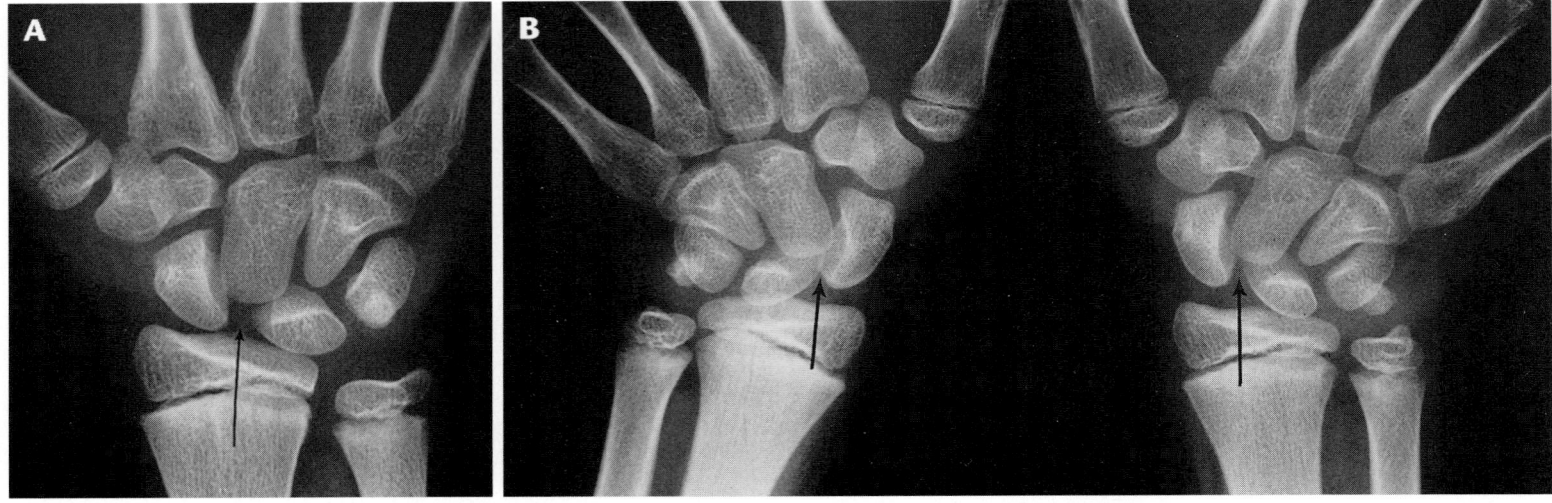

Figure 6–261. A, The navicular-lunate interval is normally wide in children and closes with subsequent growth. **B,** Note that the intervals close with ulnar deviation of the wrists.

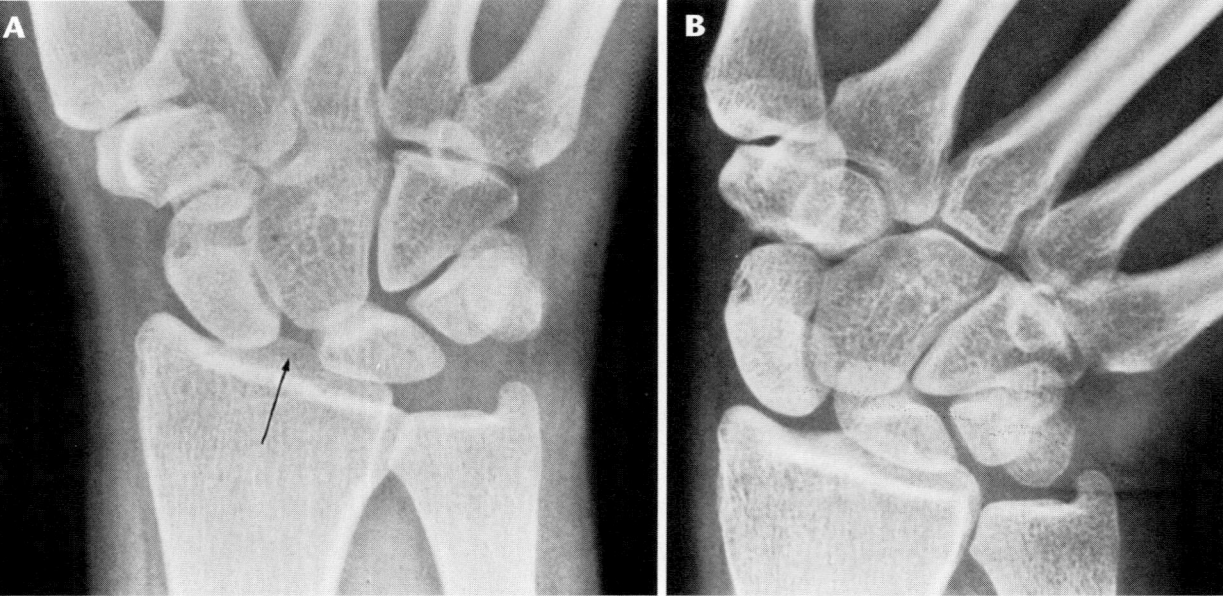

Figure 6–262. A, The navicular-lunate interval in normal individuals may be quite wide and is not an indication of traumatic dissociation in itself. **B,** Film made in ulnar deviation shows normal appearance of the navicular and decrease in the navicular-lunate interval.

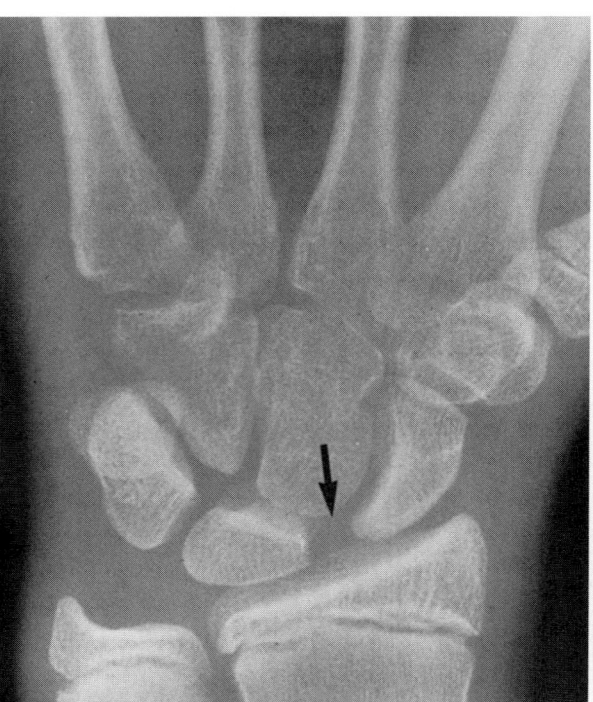
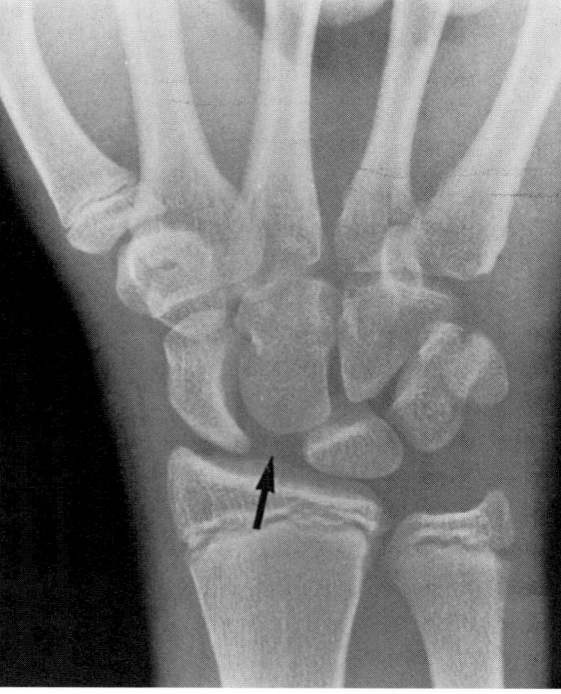

Figure 6–263. Wide navicular lunate interval in a 14-year-old boy. This appearance may be secondary to underdevelopment of the lunate, as in the preceding figure, or underdevelopment of the navicular, as in this case.

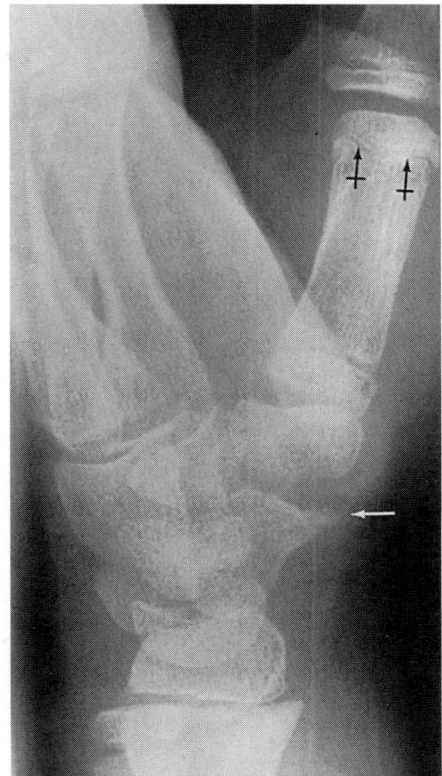

Figure 6–264. Accessory ossification center for the tubercle of the navicular in a 10-year-old girl (→). Note also accessory ossification center at the distal end of the first metacarpal (↠).

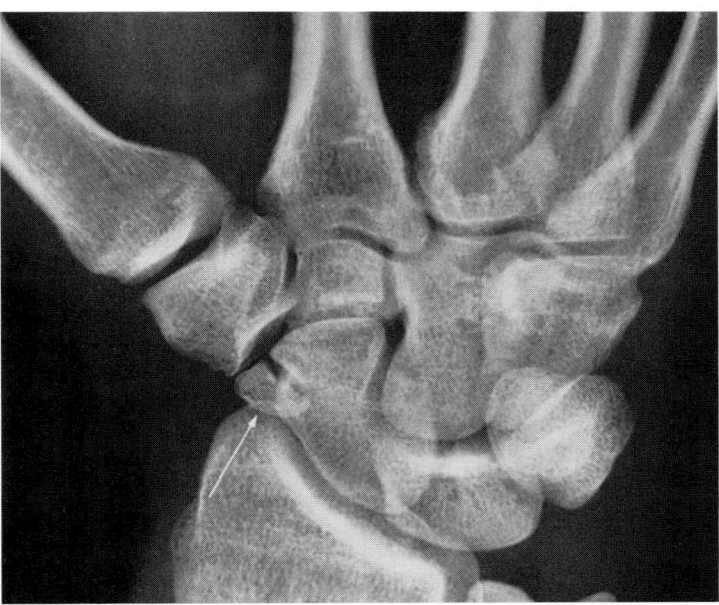
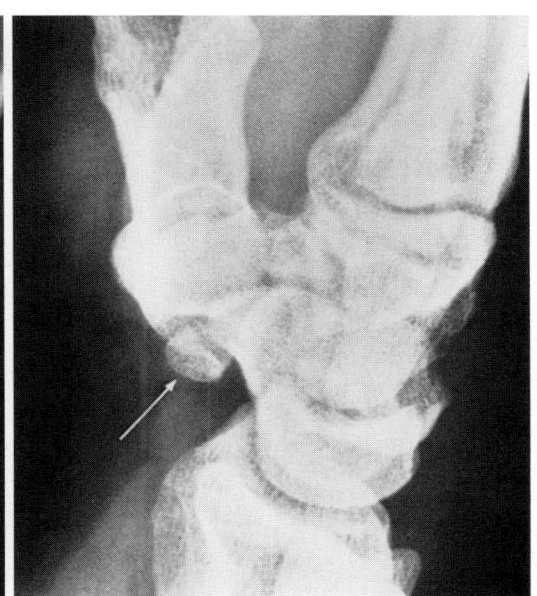

Figure 6–265. Accessory ossification center for the tubercle of the navicular, which failed to unite.

The Carpals

THE TRIQUETRUM BONE

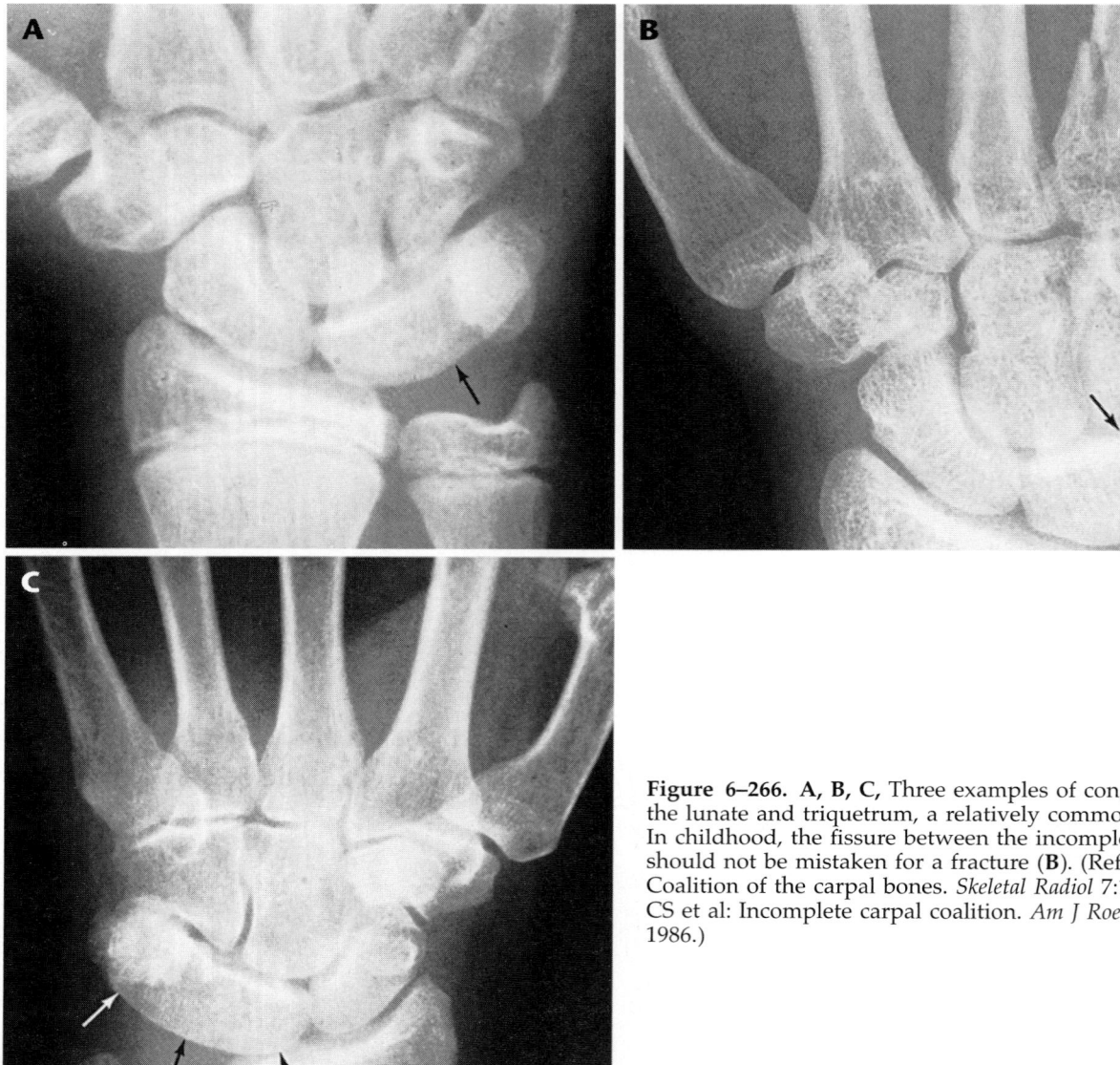

Figure 6–266. A, B, C, Three examples of congenital fusion of the lunate and triquetrum, a relatively common site of fusion. In childhood, the fissure between the incompletely fused bones should not be mistaken for a fracture (**B**). (Refs: Carlson DH: Coalition of the carpal bones. *Skeletal Radiol* 7:125, 1981; Resnik CS et al: Incomplete carpal coalition. *Am J Roentgenol* 147:301, 1986.)

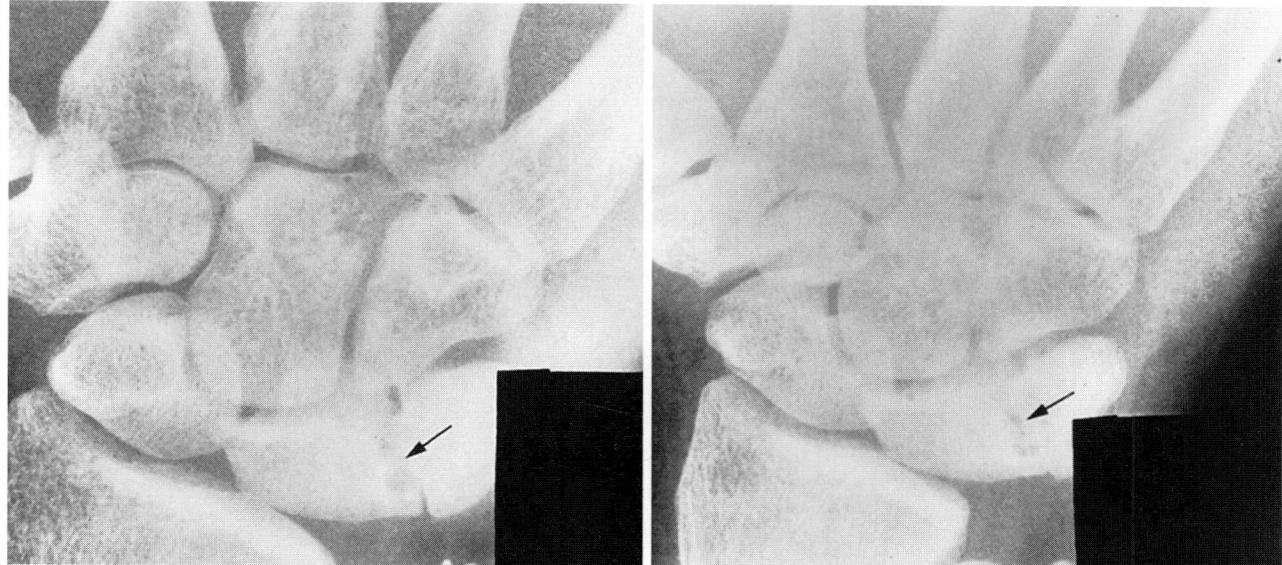

Figure 6–267. Incomplete coalition of the lunate and triquetrum bones.

Figure 6–268. Ring lesions in the triquetrum bone. These lesions are probably fibrous in nature and are seen elsewhere in the hand and wrist. They are apparently of no clinical significance and should be distinguished from traumatic cyst caused by occupational trauma (see Figs. 6–234 and 6–304).

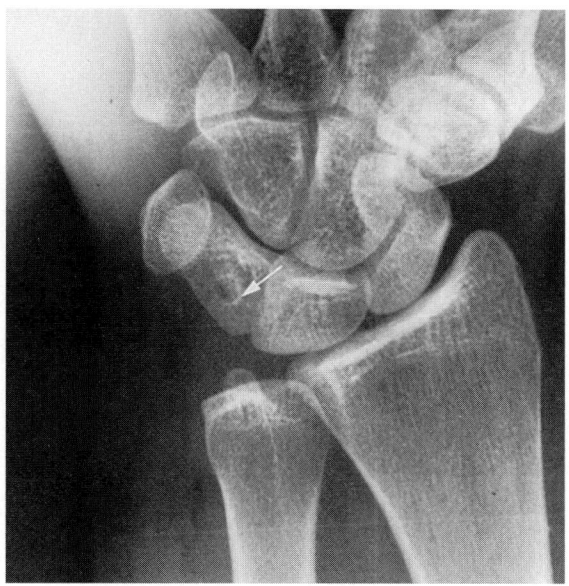

The Carpals
THE PISIFORM BONE

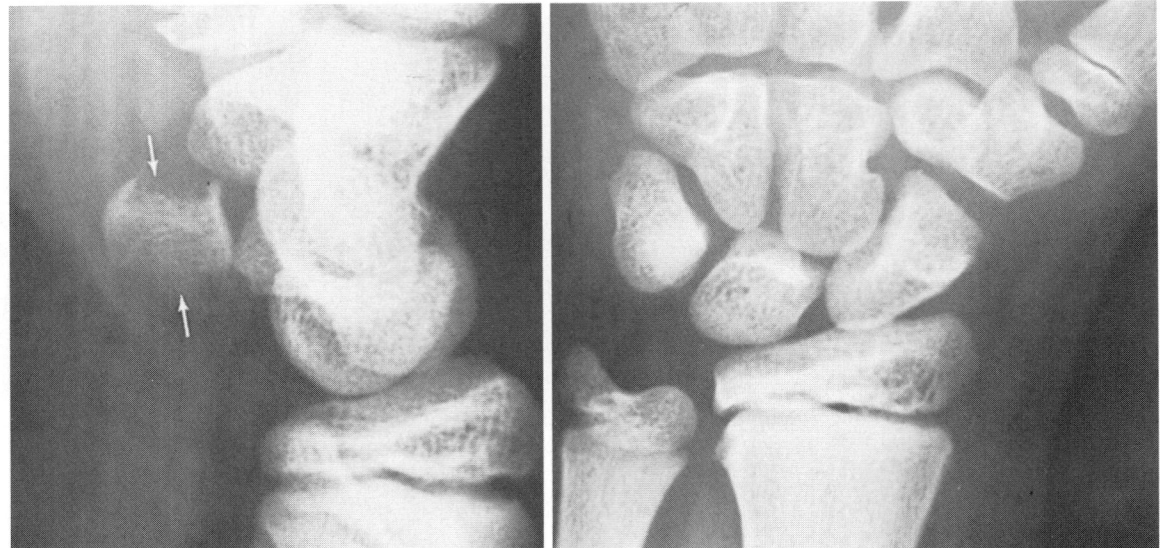

Figure 6–269. Normal irregularity of the pisiform in an 11-year-old boy. This irregularity is seen only in the lateral projection.

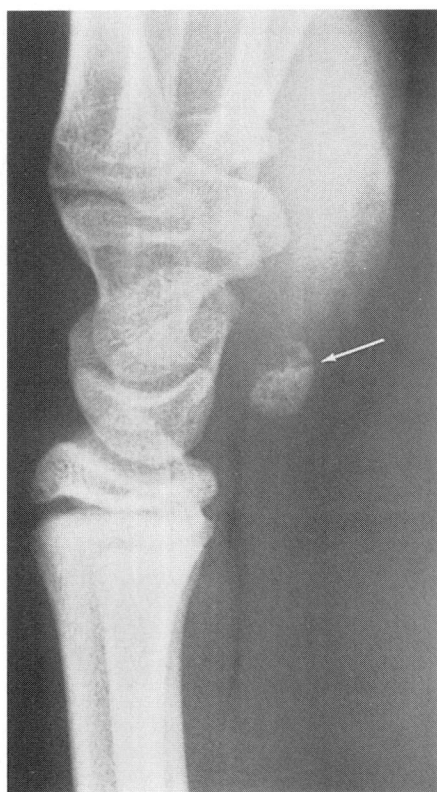

Figure 6–270. Developmental irregularity of the pisiform in an 11-year-old boy, simulating a fracture.

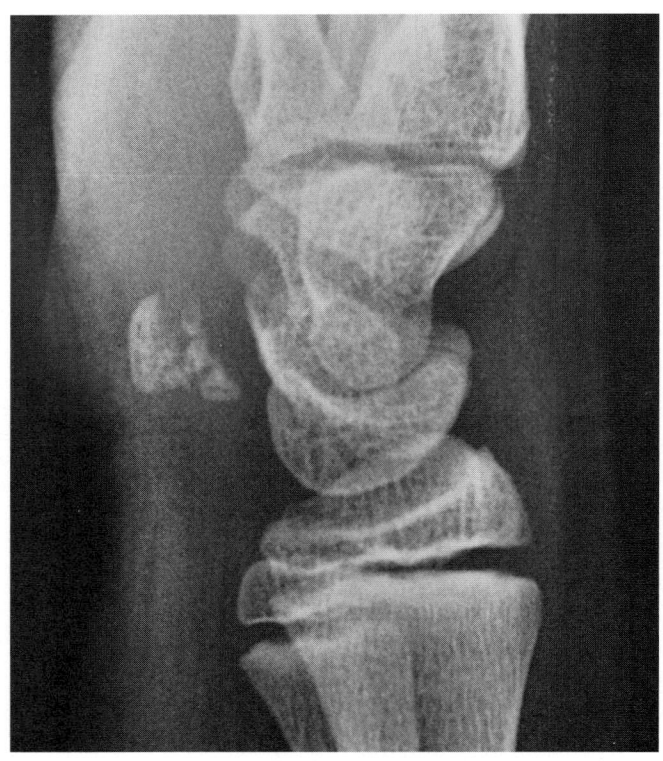

Figure 6–271. Multicentric pisiform in a 10-year-old girl.

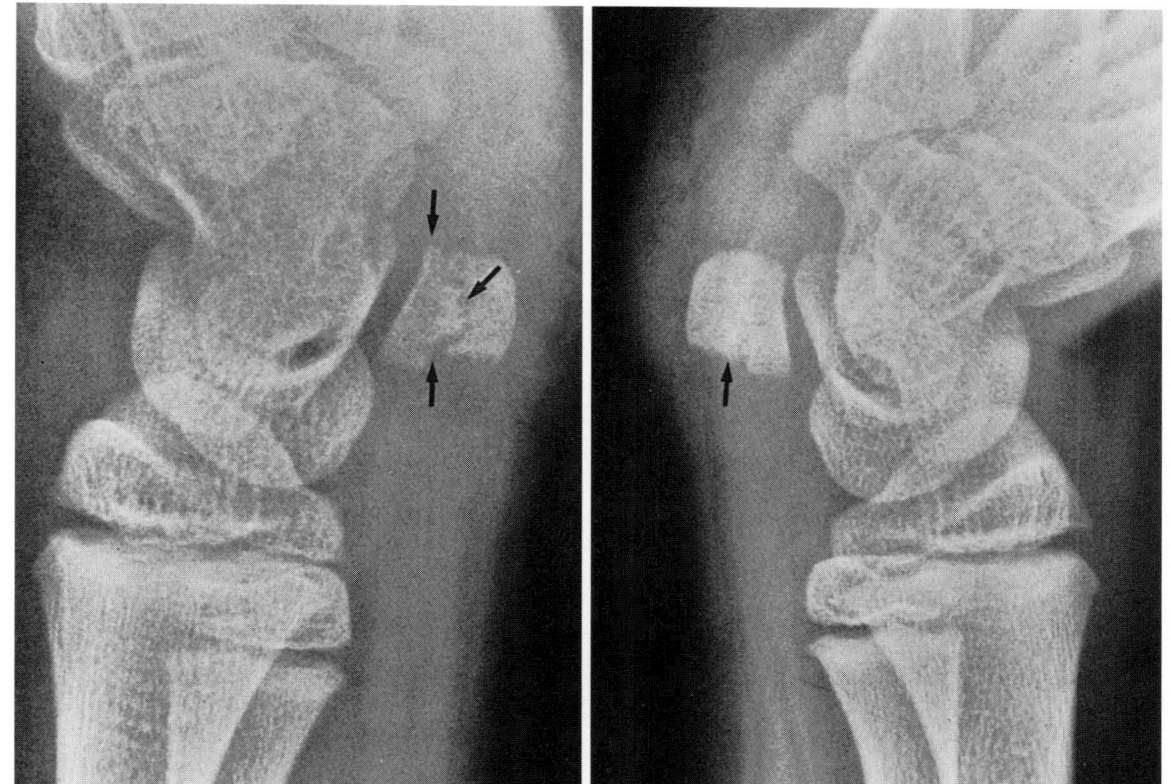

Figure 6–272. Bilateral irregularities in development of the pisiforms in a 12-year-old boy.

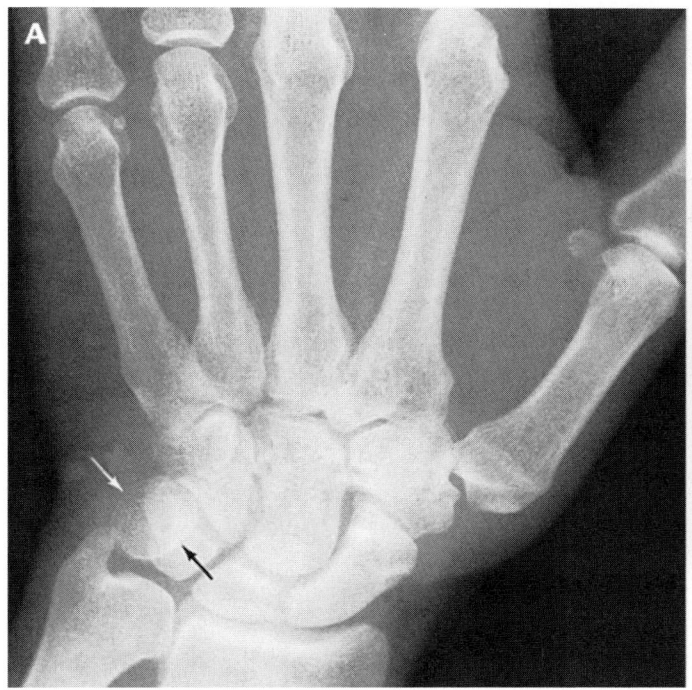

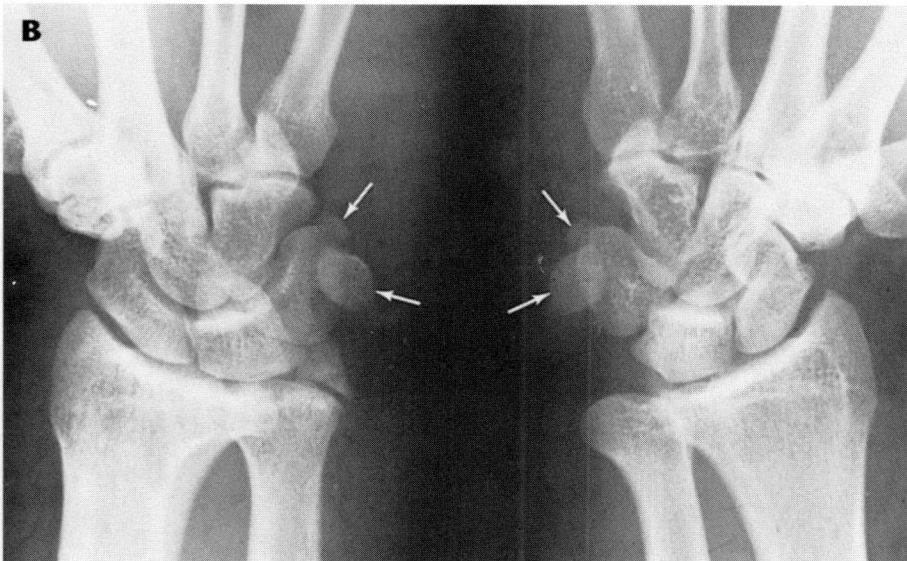

Figure 6–273. Variations in the pisiform bone. **A,** Normal but very large pisiform bone. **B,** Bipartite pisiform bones.

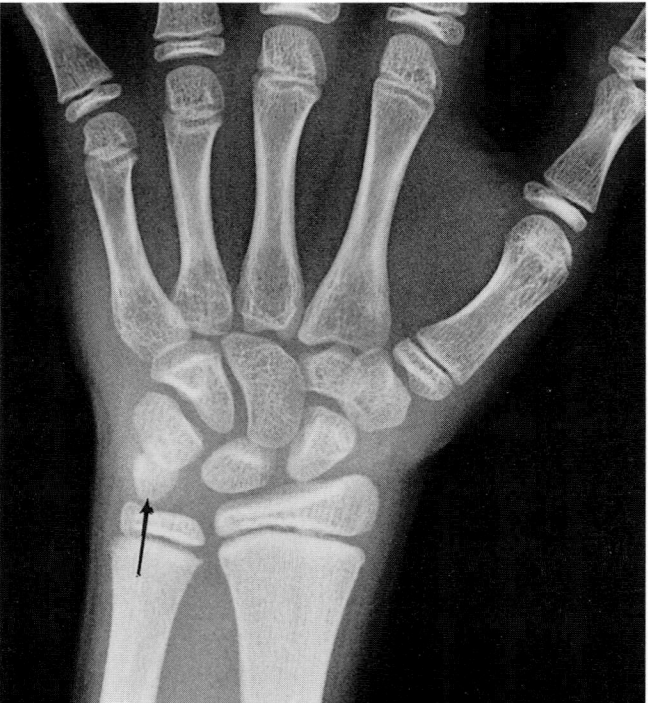

Figure 6–274. Unusually low position of the pisiform in a 12-year-old boy.

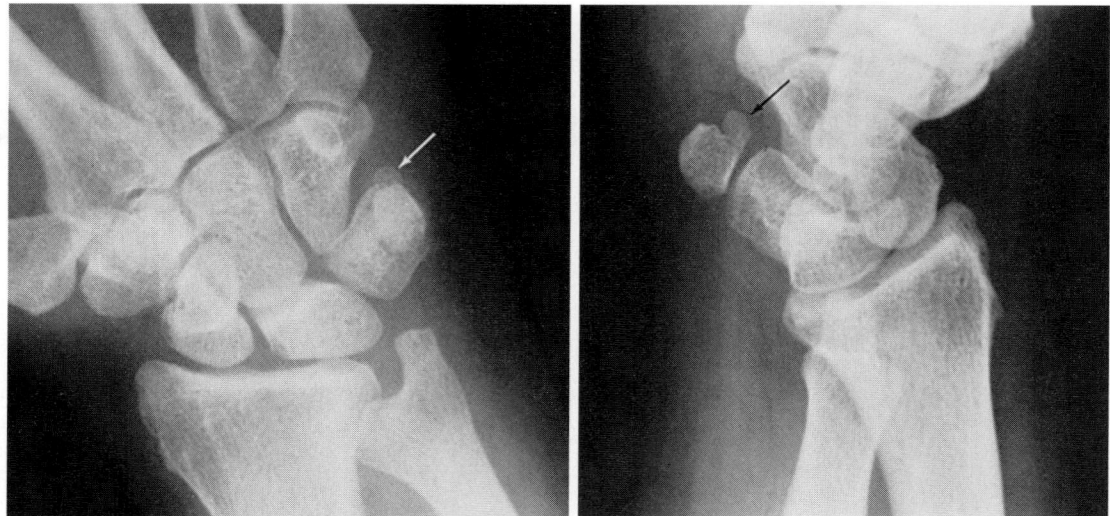

Figure 6–275. Bipartite pisiform bone.

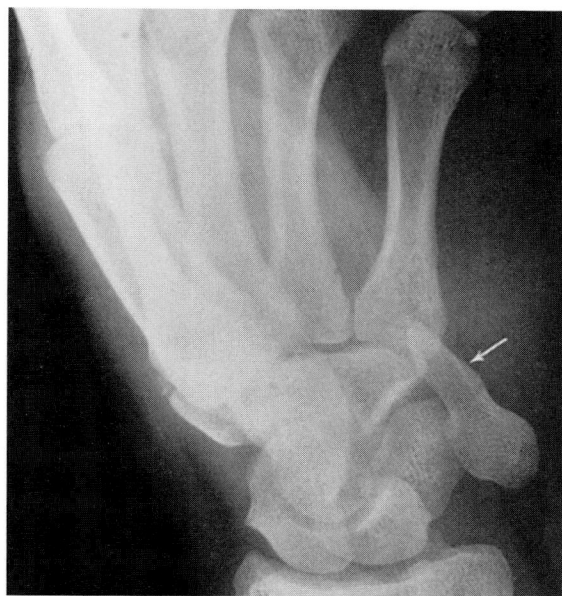

Figure 6–276. Exostosis-like process on the pisiform bone, a variation in development.

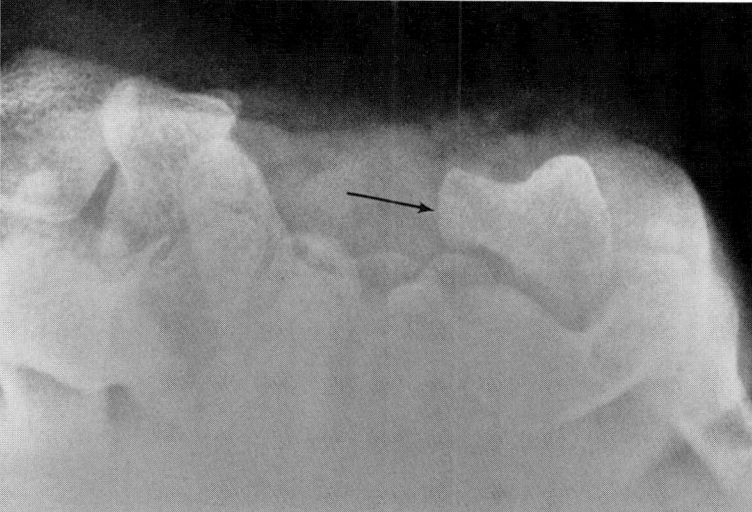

Figure 6–277. The exostosis-like process of the pisiform in the tunnel view.

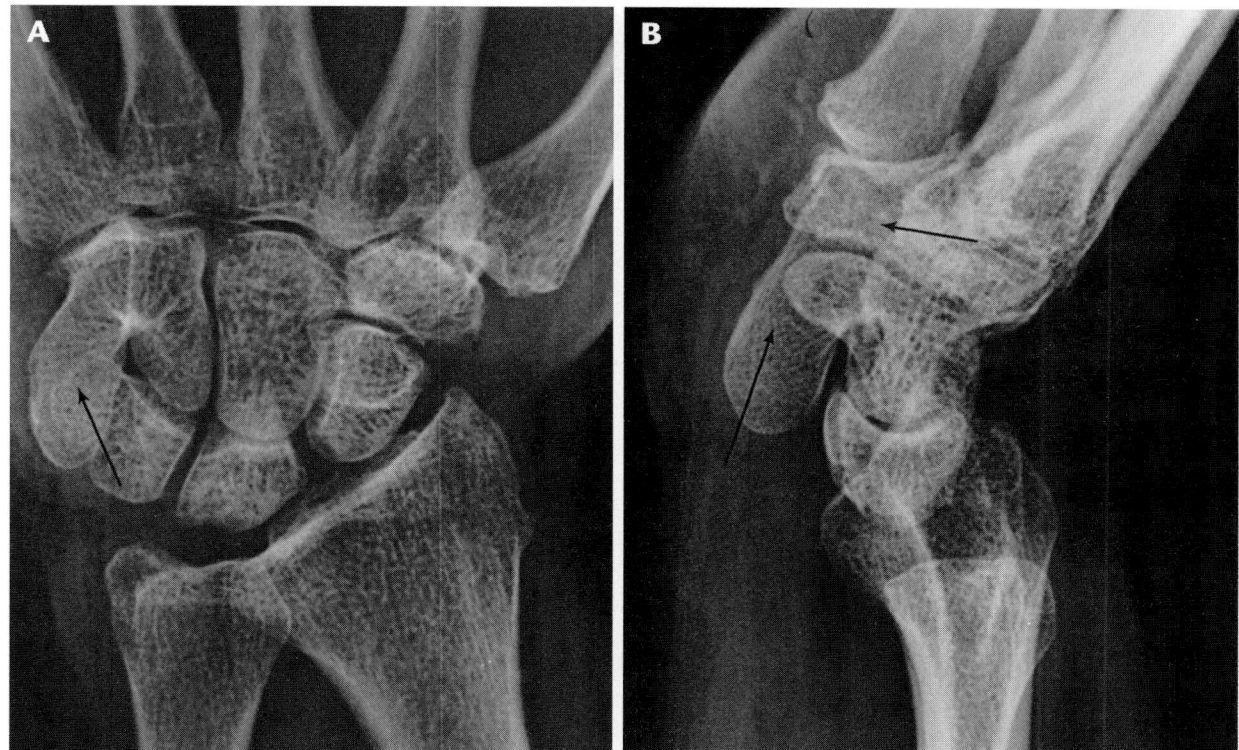

Figure 6–278. A, B, The exostosis of the pisiform with fusion to the hamate.

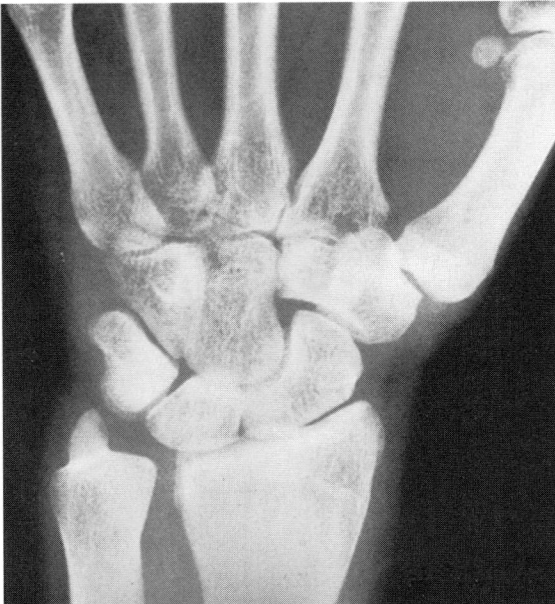

Figure 6–279. Congenital fusion of the triquetrum and pisiform bones.

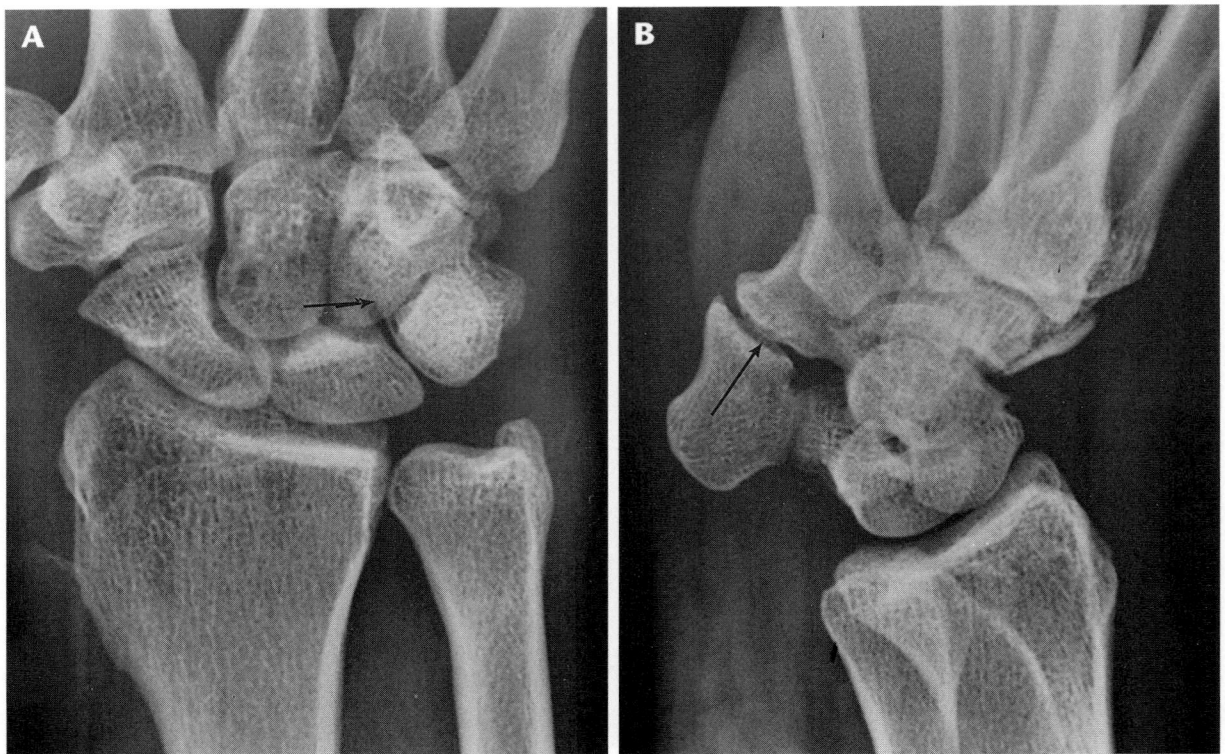

Figure 6–280. A, B, Congenital fusion of the triquetrum and pisiform bones with a pseudarthrosis between the pisiform and the hamate.

The Metacarpals

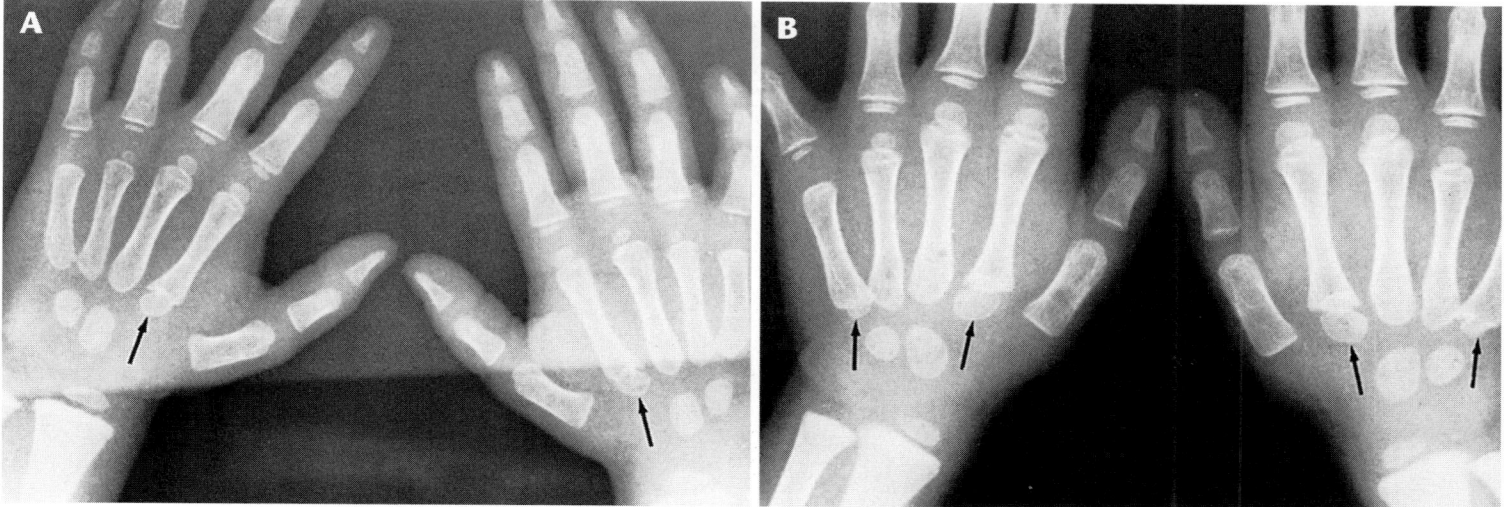

Figure 6–281. Two examples of accessory ossification centers at the bases of the metacarpals in 3-year-old (**A**) and 4-year-old (**B**) children. This finding is usually of no significance. (Ref: Ogden JD et al: Ossification and pseudoepiphysis formation in the "nonepiphyseal" end of bones of the hands and feet. *Skeletal Radiol* 23:3, 1994.)

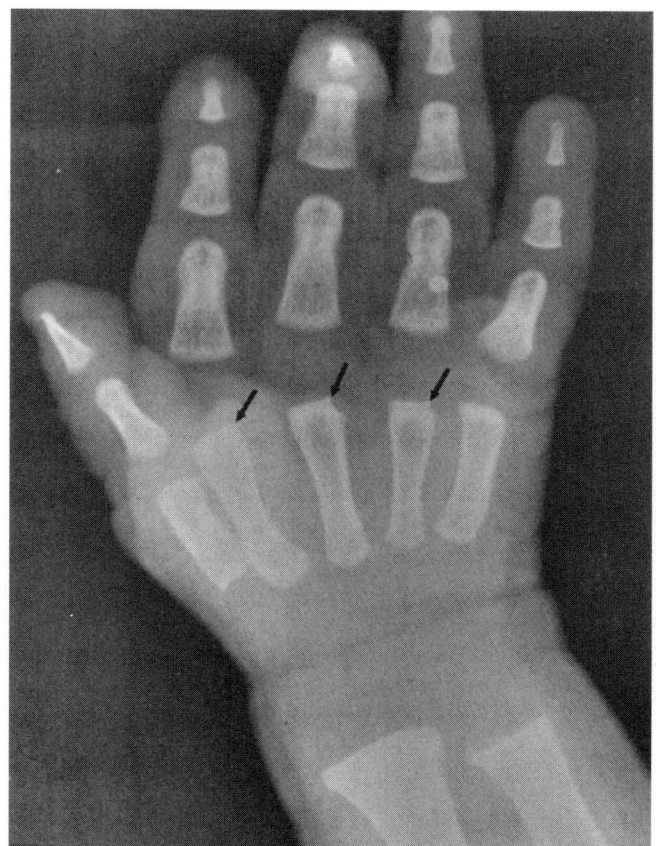

Figure 6–282. Spicules in the distal metaphyses of the metacarpals in a 3-month-old infant.

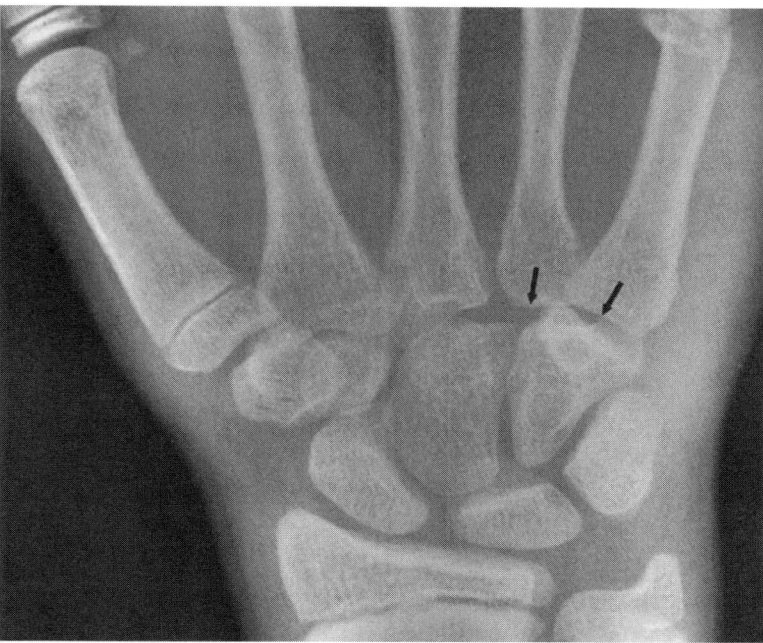

Figure 6–283. Striking clarity of the carpal-metacarpal joints in a 13-year-old boy simulating dislocation of the bases of the metacarpals.

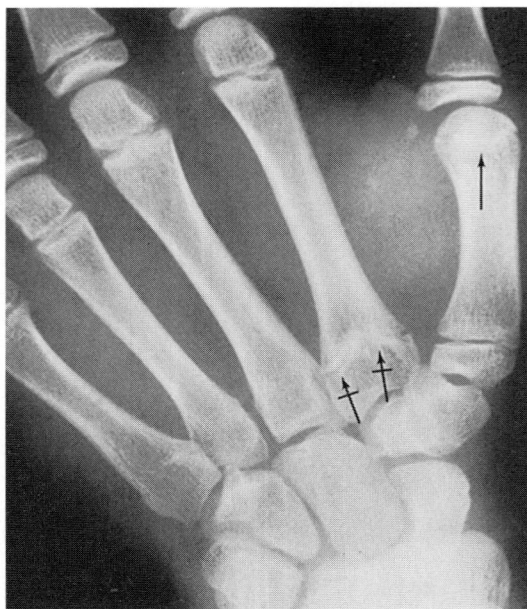

Figure 6–284. Accessory ossification center at distal end of the first metacarpal (→) and at the base of the second metacarpal (↦) in a 13-year-old boy.

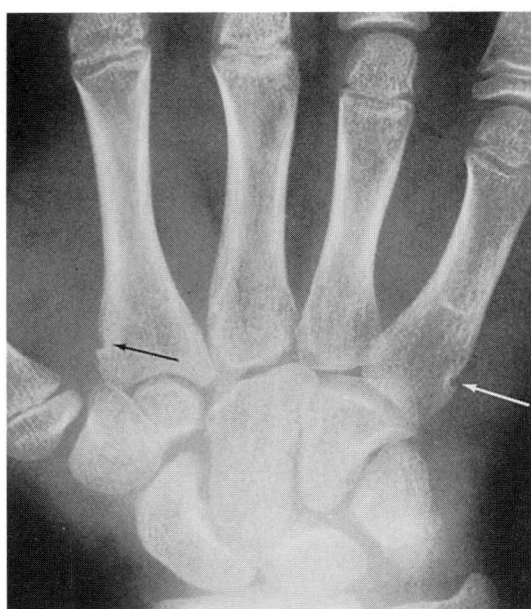

Figure 6–285. Remnants of closed secondary ossification centers in a 13-year-old boy.

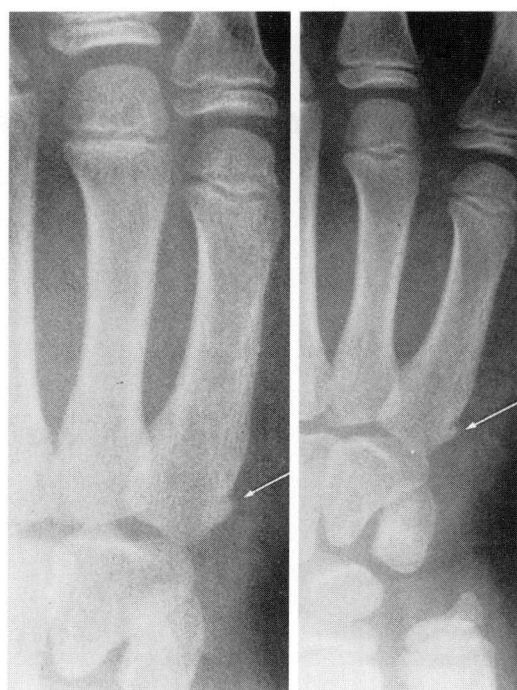

Figure 6–286. The clefts at the ulnar side of the base of the fifth metacarpal are particularly prone to misinterpretation as a fracture.

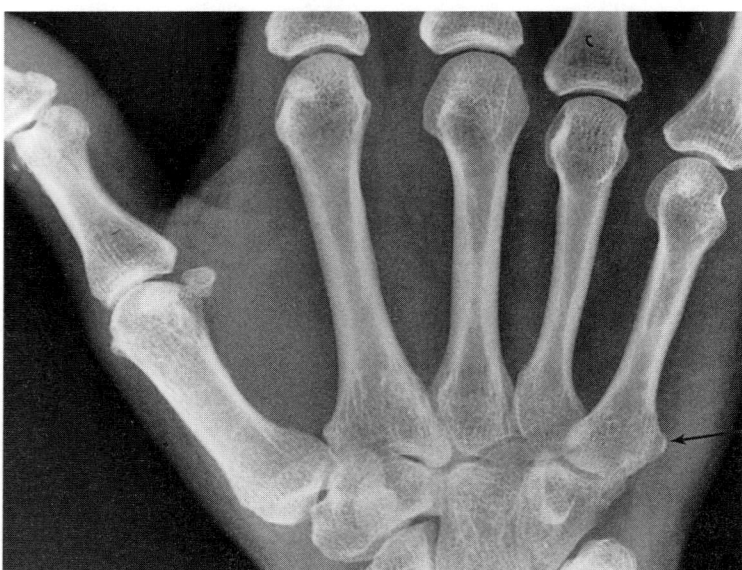

Figure 6–287. Developmental knob-like protuberance at the base of the fifth metacarpal.

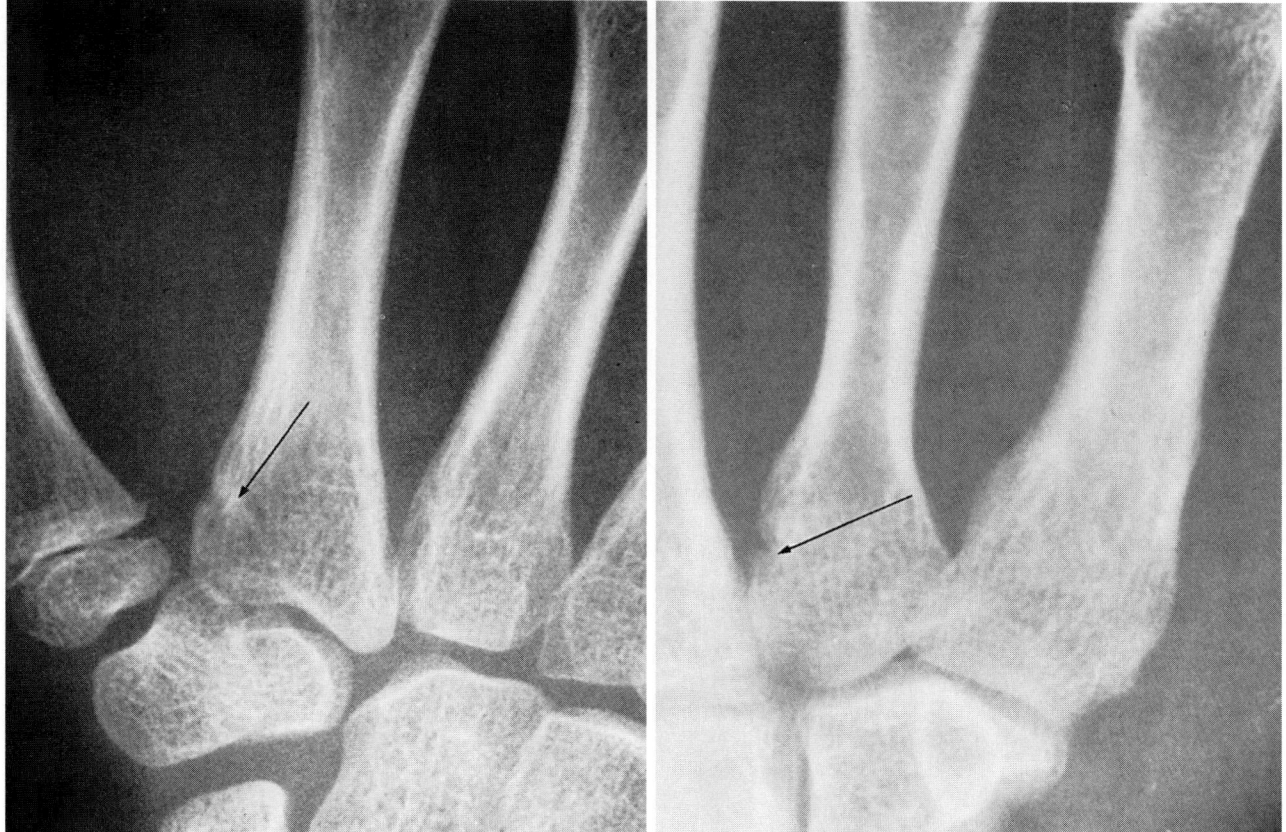

Figure 6–288. Clefts at the bases of the metacarpals may simulate fractures.

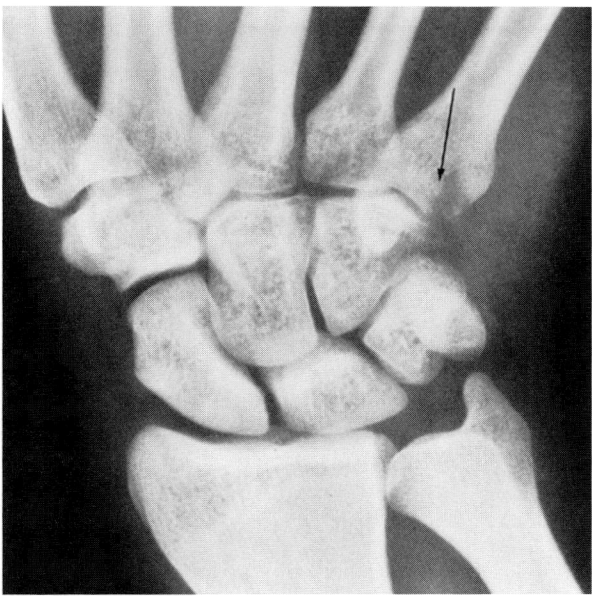

Figure 6–289. Fossa at the base of the fifth metacarpal may suggest abnormality.

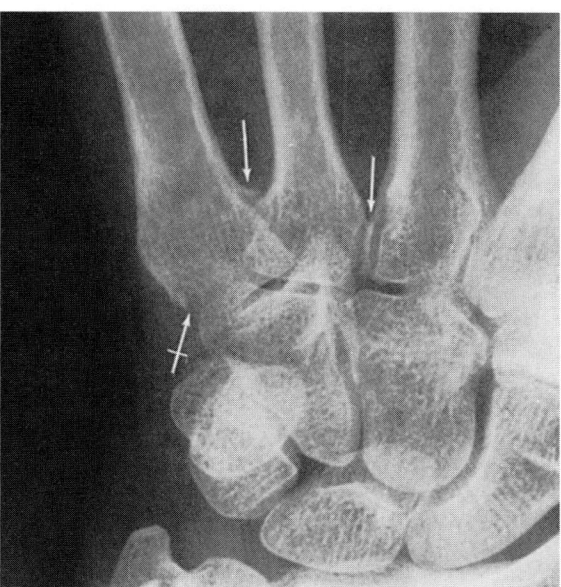

Figure 6–290. Normal shadows at the bases of the metacarpals that may be mistaken for fractures, produced by overlapping shadows of the osseous structures (→). Note also the normal fossa at the base of the fifth metacarpal (↦).

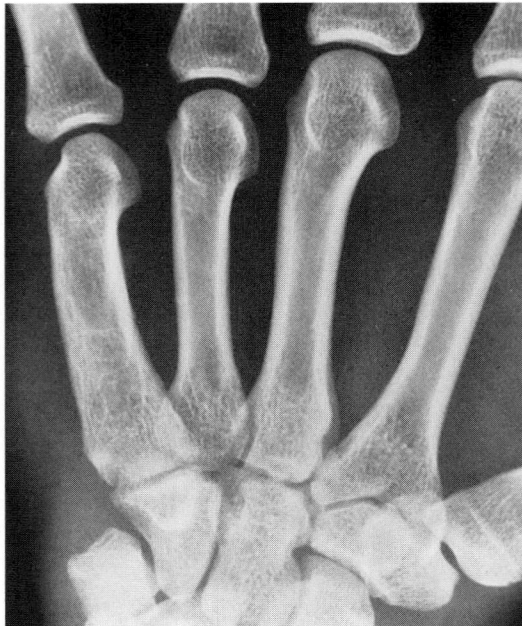

Figure 6–291. The fifth metacarpal may be broader than the others and may simulate abnormality.

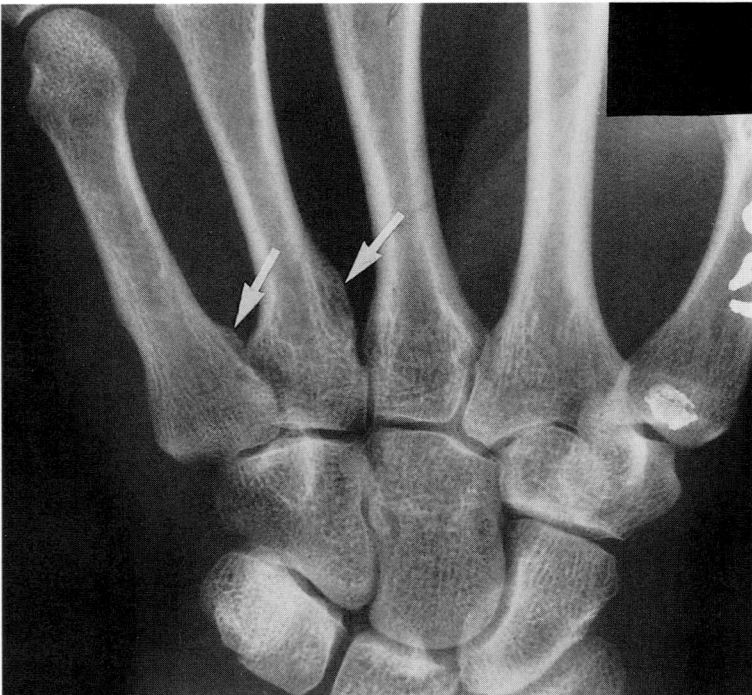

Figure 6–292. Bulges in the cortices at the bases of the fourth and fifth metacarpals.

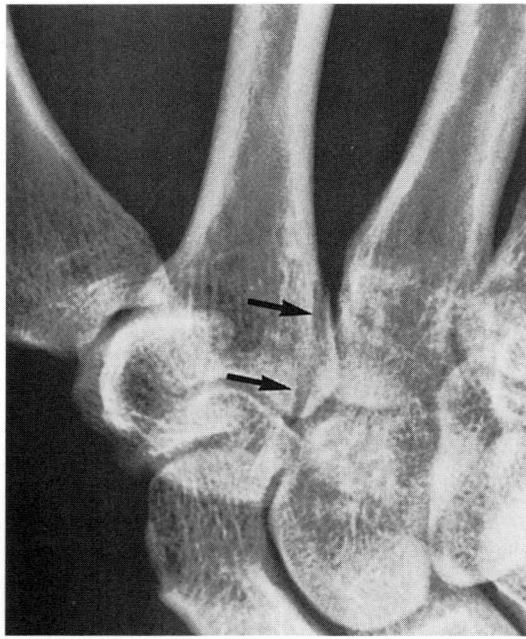

Figure 6–293. Overlapping shadows of the bases of the second and third metacarpals that simulate fracture.

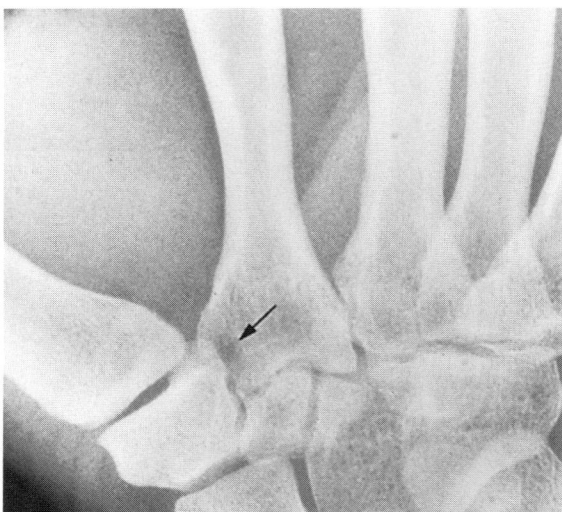

Figure 6–294. Normal lucency in the base of the second metacarpal simulating a cystlike lesion.

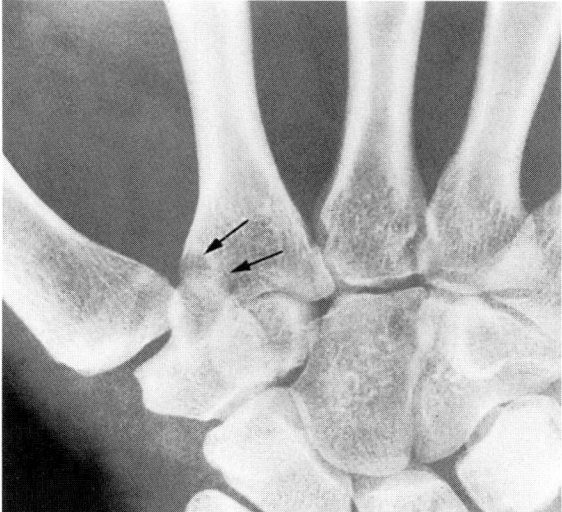

Figure 6–295. Another example of lesion shown in the preceding figure.

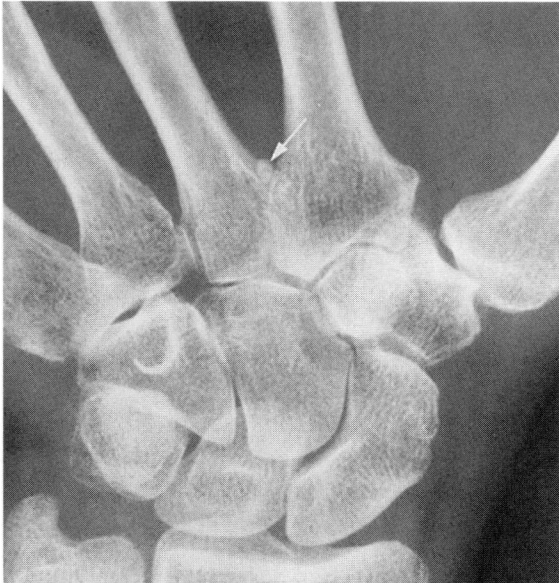

Figure 6–296. Ossicle between the bases of the second and third metacarpals.

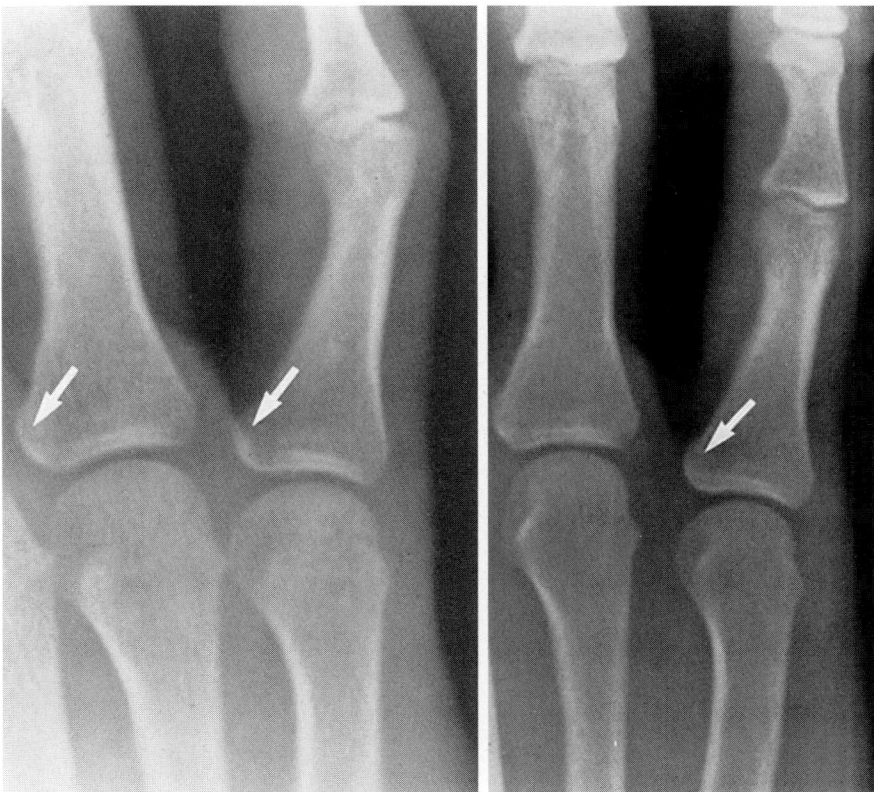

Figure 6–297. Simulated fractures of the bases of the phalanges of the fourth and fifth fingers.

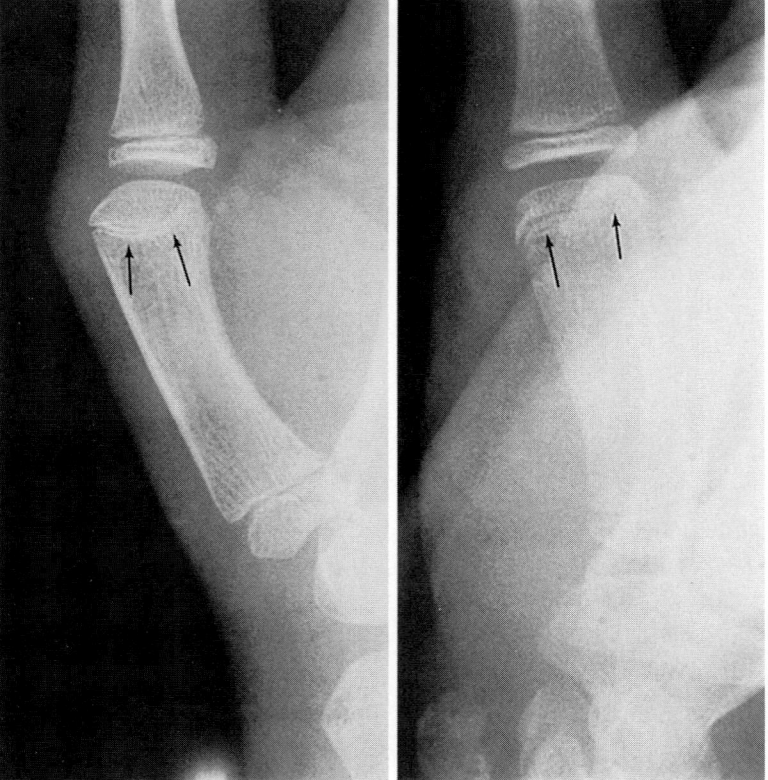

Figure 6–298. Accessory ossification center at the distal end of the first metacarpal, simulating a fracture.

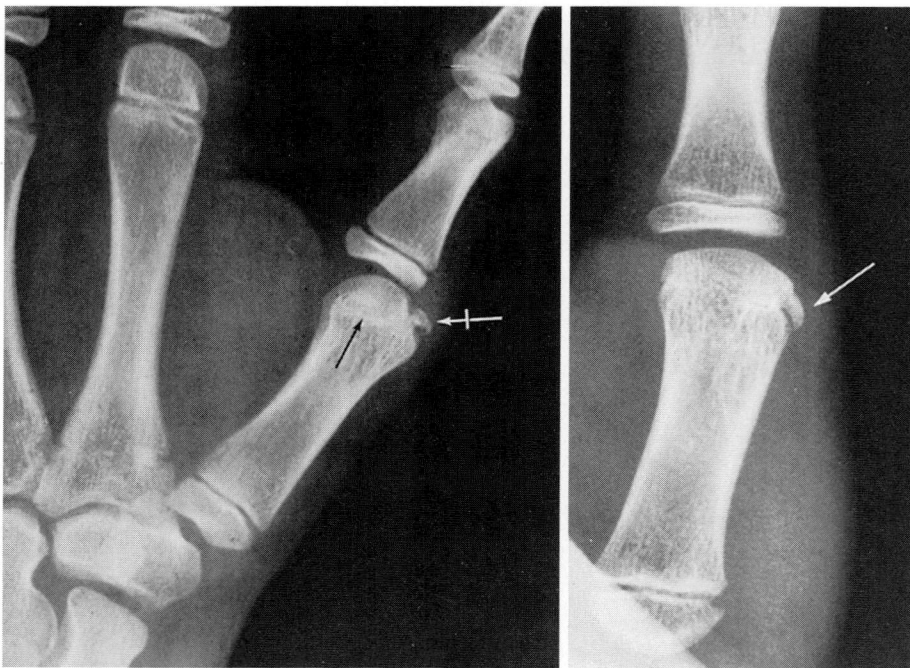

Figure 6–299. Two examples of accessory ossification centers at the distal end of the first metacarpal with spur at its medial margin. The epiphyseal spur is a normal variation.

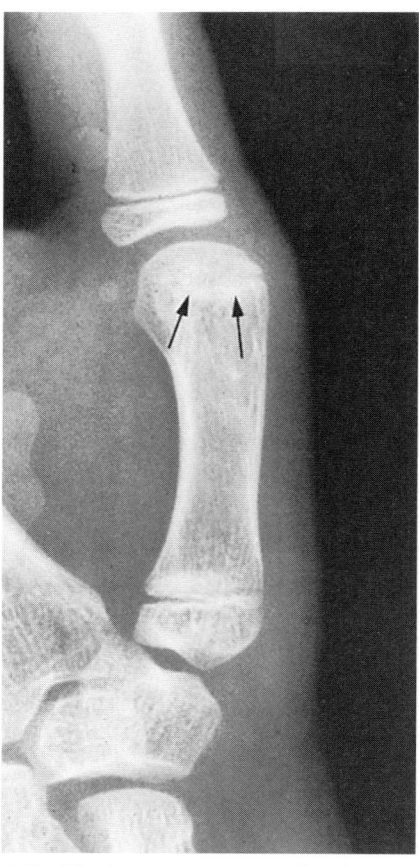

Figure 6–300. Closing accessory ossification center at the distal end of the first metacarpal in a 14-year-old boy.

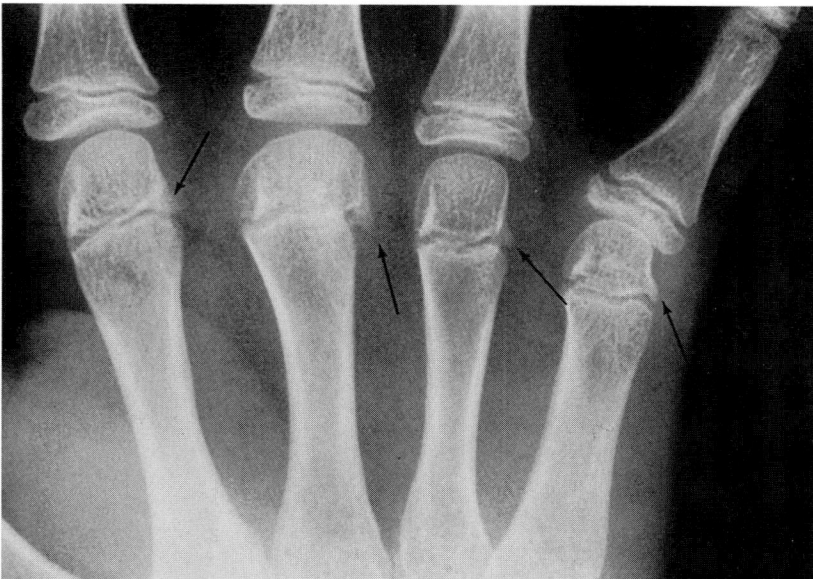

Figure 6–301. Spurring of the margins of ossification centers for the heads of the metacarpals in a 13-year-old boy. These spurs are transient events in the development of the epiphysis and are additional examples of the epiphyseal spur. (Ref: Keats TE, Harrison RB: The epiphyseal spur. *Skeletal Radiol* 5:175, 1980.)

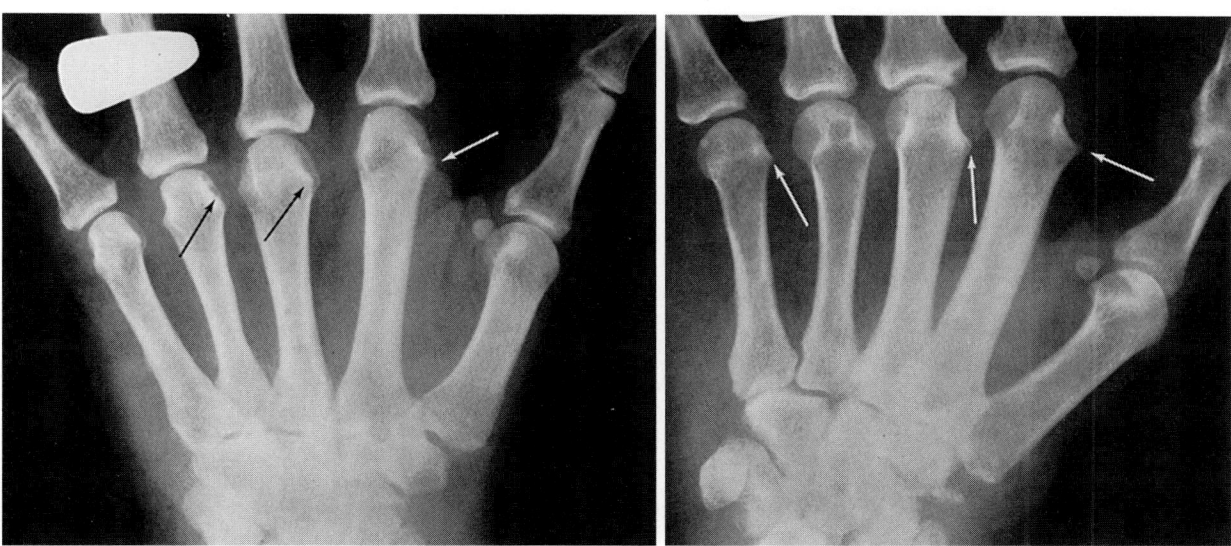

Figure 6–302. Prominent developmental spurlike protuberances at the radial sides of the distal metaphyses of the metacarpals.

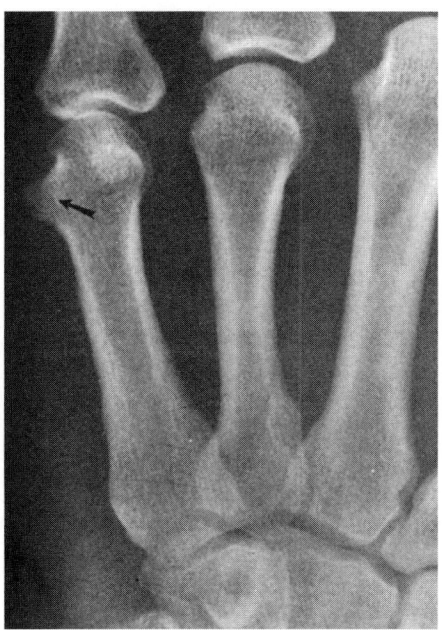

Figure 6–303. Exaggeration of the spurlike protuberance at the head of the fifth metacarpal.

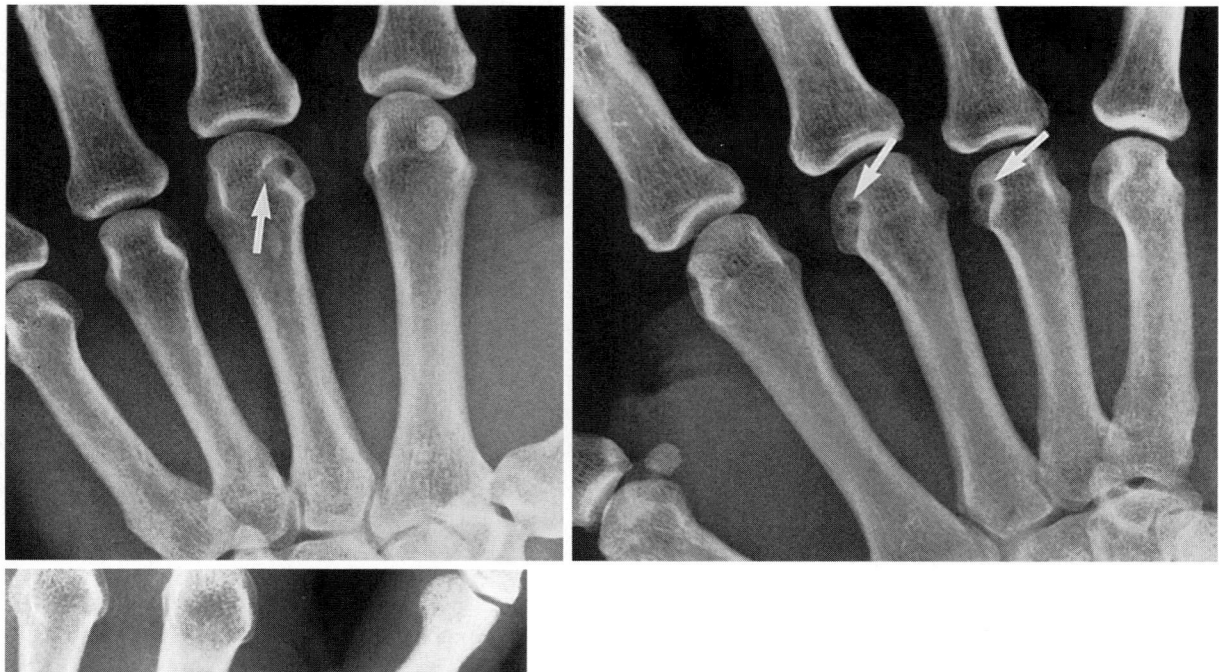

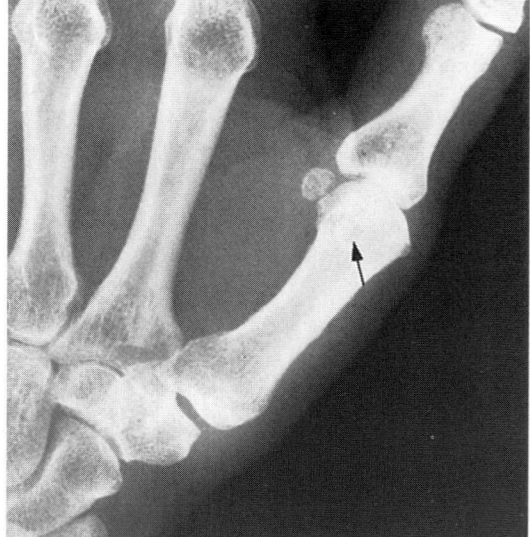

Figure 6–304. Ring lesions in the heads of the metacarpals. These are probably fibrous in nature and are apparently of no clinical significance (see Figs. 6–234 and 6–268).

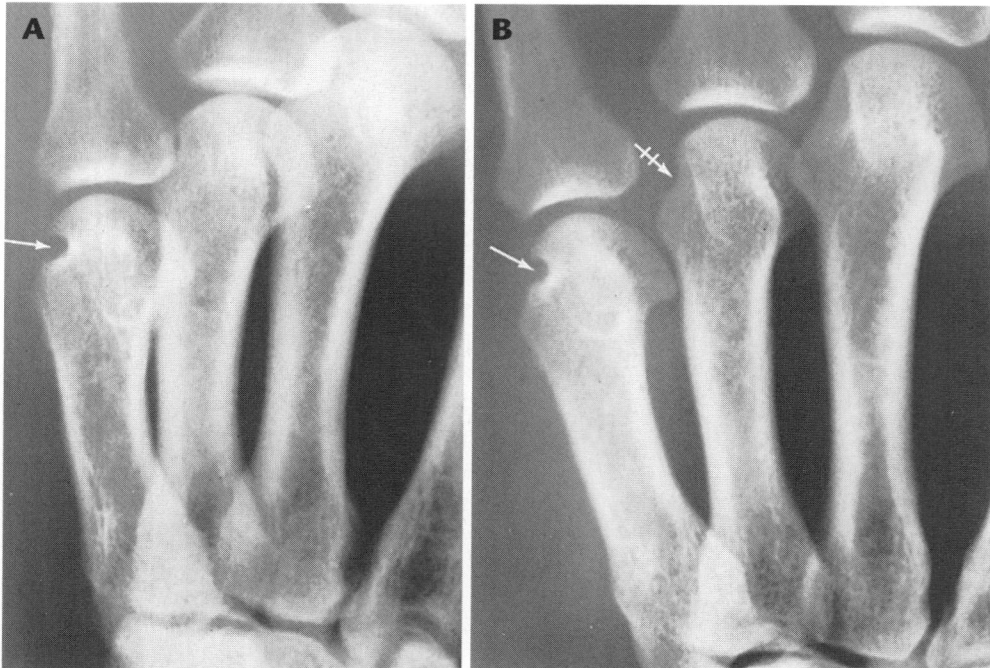

Figure 6–305. A, B, Normal exaggeration of the pitlike depression in the head of the fifth metacarpal (←). This does not represent an erosion. The more usual appearance is seen in the head of the fourth metacarpal in **B** (⇤).

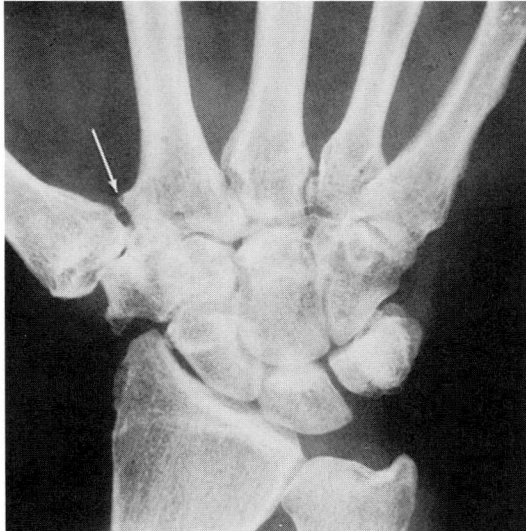

Figure 6–306. Developmental spurlike projection at the radial side of the base of the second metacarpal.

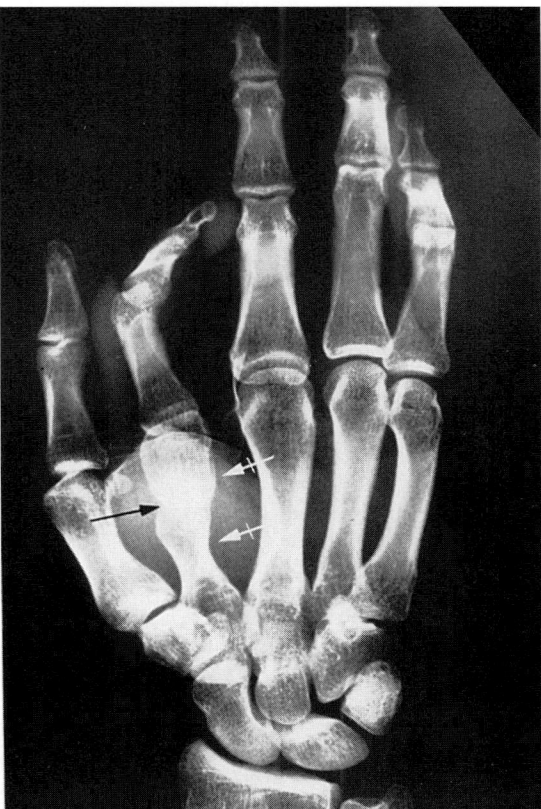

Figure 6–307. Duplication anomaly of the second metacarpal (↔) with an intervening articulation (←).

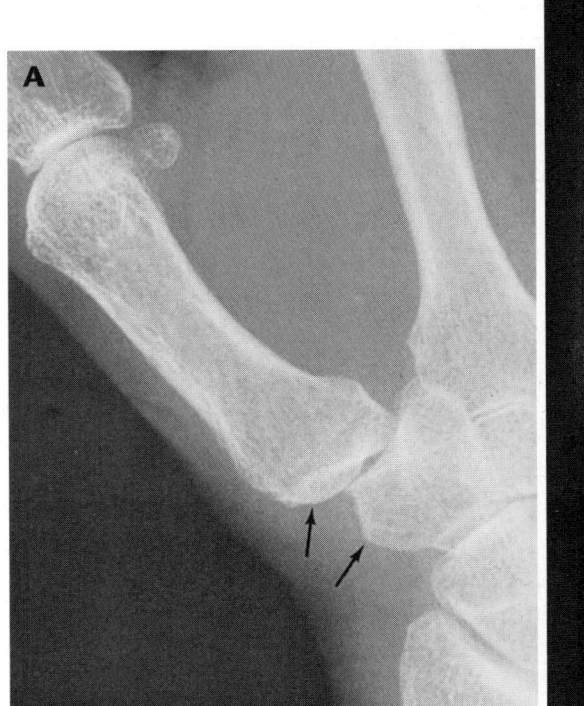

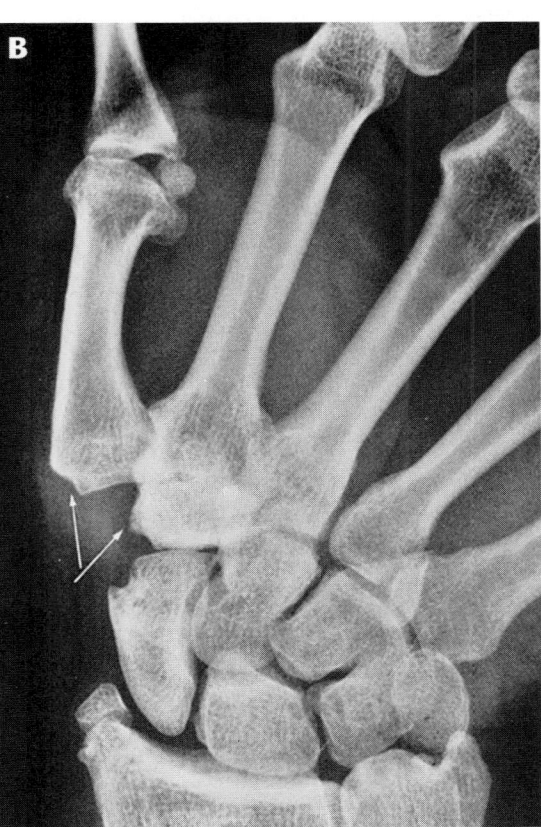

Figure 6–308. Normal relationships between the base of the first metacarpal and greater trapezium. This relationship is at times mistaken for a subluxation. **A,** Abduction of the thumb. **B,** Adduction of the thumb. (Ref: Lasserre C et al: Osteoarthritis of the trapeziometacarpal joint. *J Bone Joint Surg* 31B:534, 1949.)

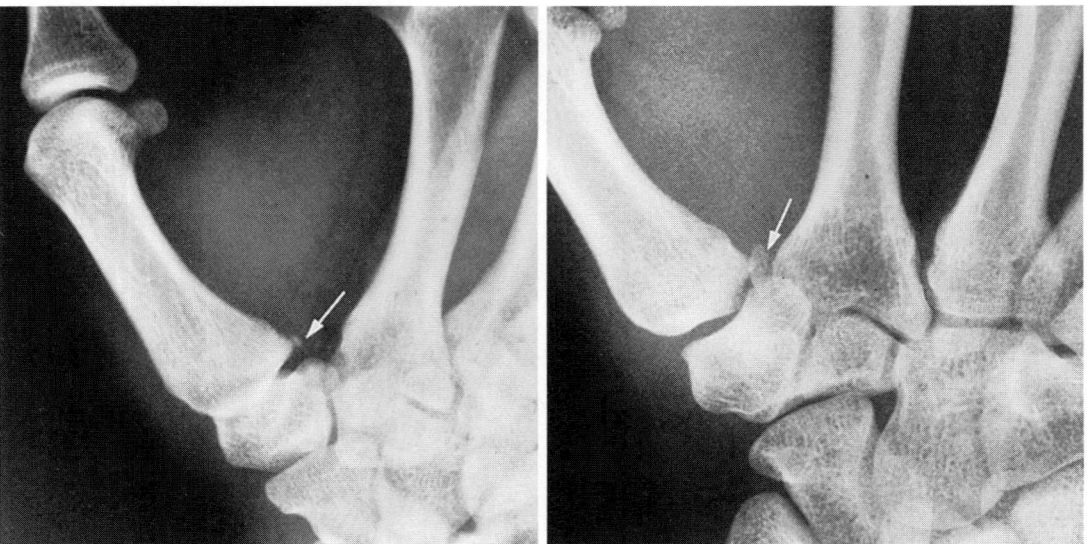

Figure 6–309. Two examples of the trapezium secundarium (see Fig. 6–193).

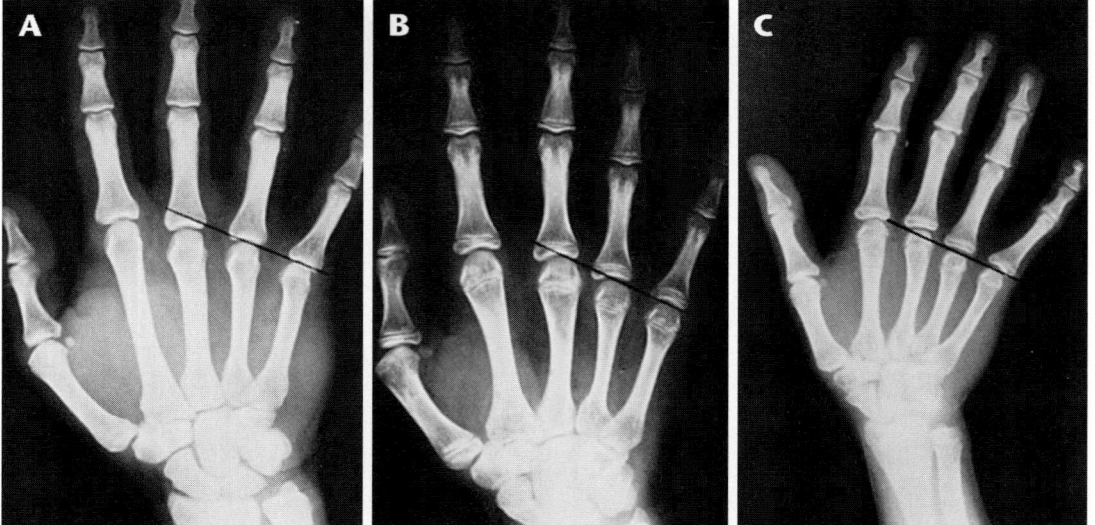

Figure 6–310. The metacarpal sign. A tangent drawn through the distal ends of the fourth and fifth metacarpals normally does not intersect the head of the third metacarpal. **A,** Normal. **B,** Borderline. **C,** Positive. A positive metacarpal sign is seen in some forms of gonadal dysgenesis but may also occur as a normal variant; its usefulness is therefore limited. (Ref: Bloom RA: The metacarpal sign. *Br J Radiol* 43:133, 1970.)

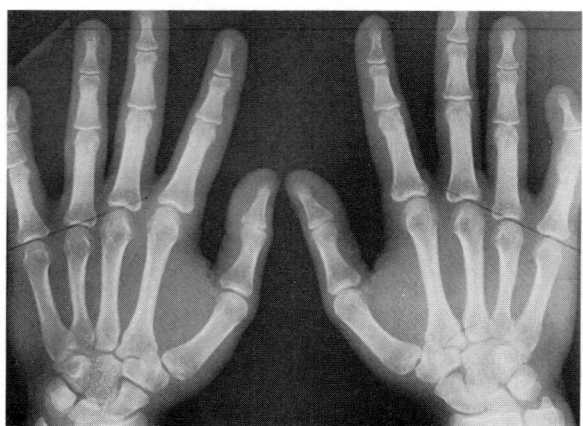

Figure 6–311. Short fourth metacarpals with positive metacarpal sign as a familial trait in a normal individual. Note the short middle phalanges of the fifth fingers, also a familial trait.

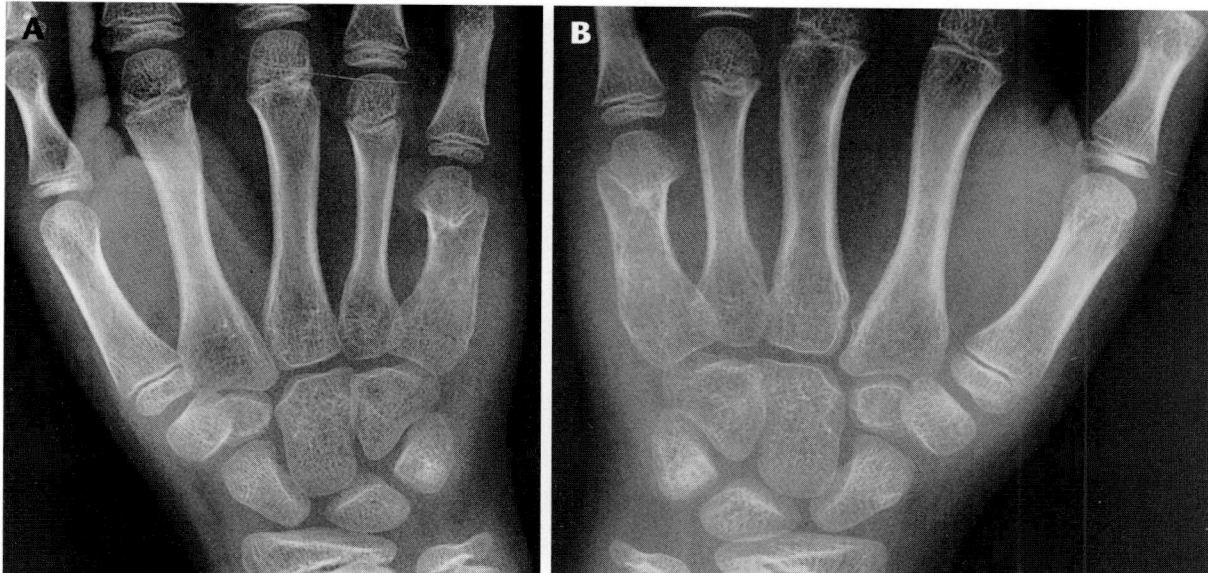

Figure 6–312. A, B, Bilateral short fifth metacarpals, usually a normal familial trait.

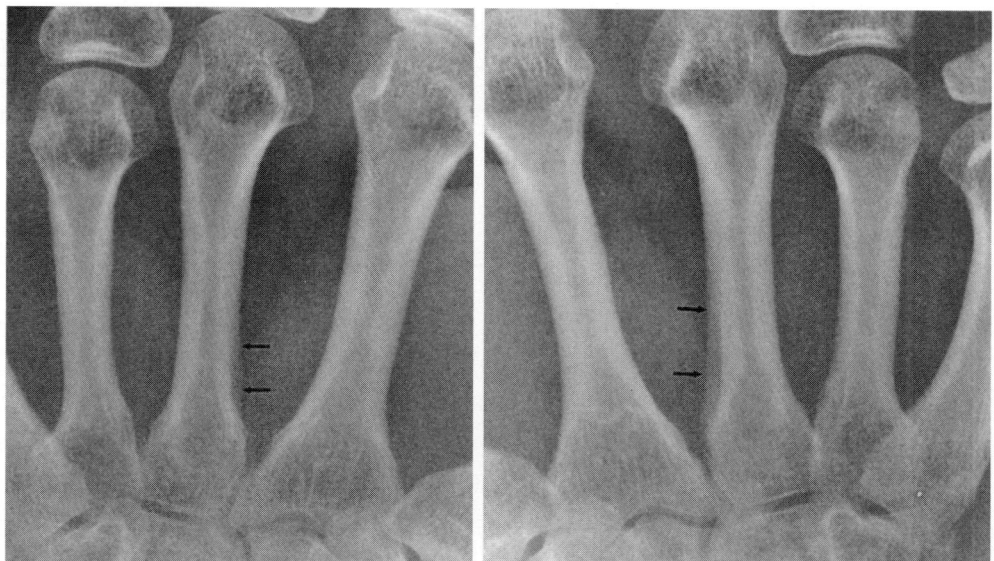

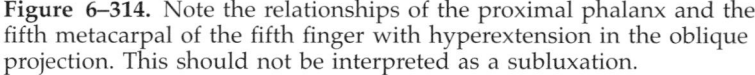

Figure 6–313. Osseous flanges on the metacarpal should not be mistaken for periostitis.

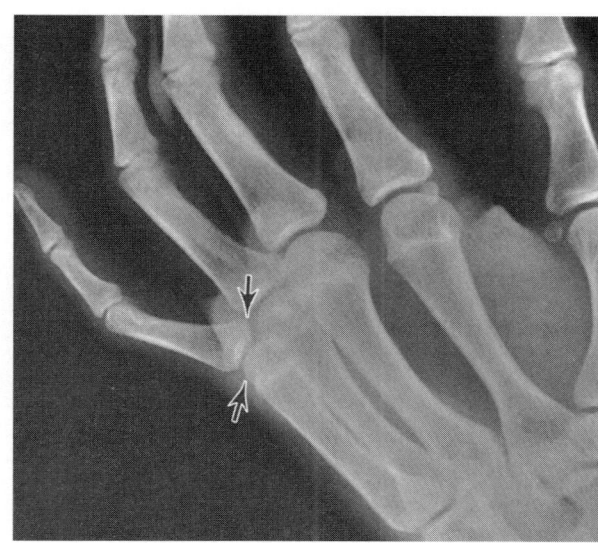

Figure 6–314. Note the relationships of the proximal phalanx and the fifth metacarpal of the fifth finger with hyperextension in the oblique projection. This should not be interpreted as a subluxation.

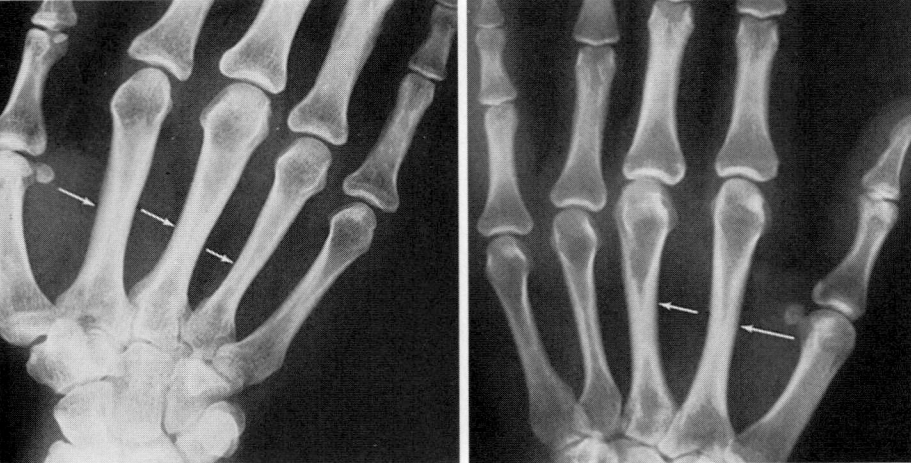

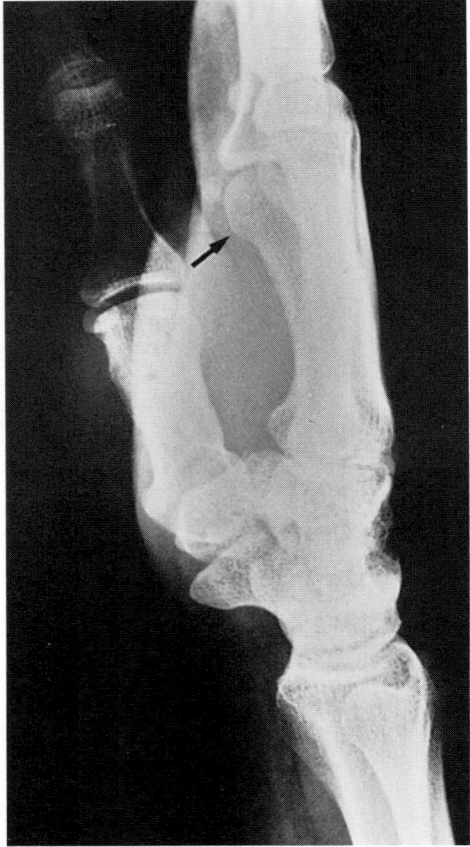

Figure 6–315. Examples of stenosis of the medullary cavities of the metacarpals, a finding of no clinical significance.

Figure 6–316. Normal palmar directed position of the head of the fifth metacarpal, not to be mistaken for displacement by trauma.

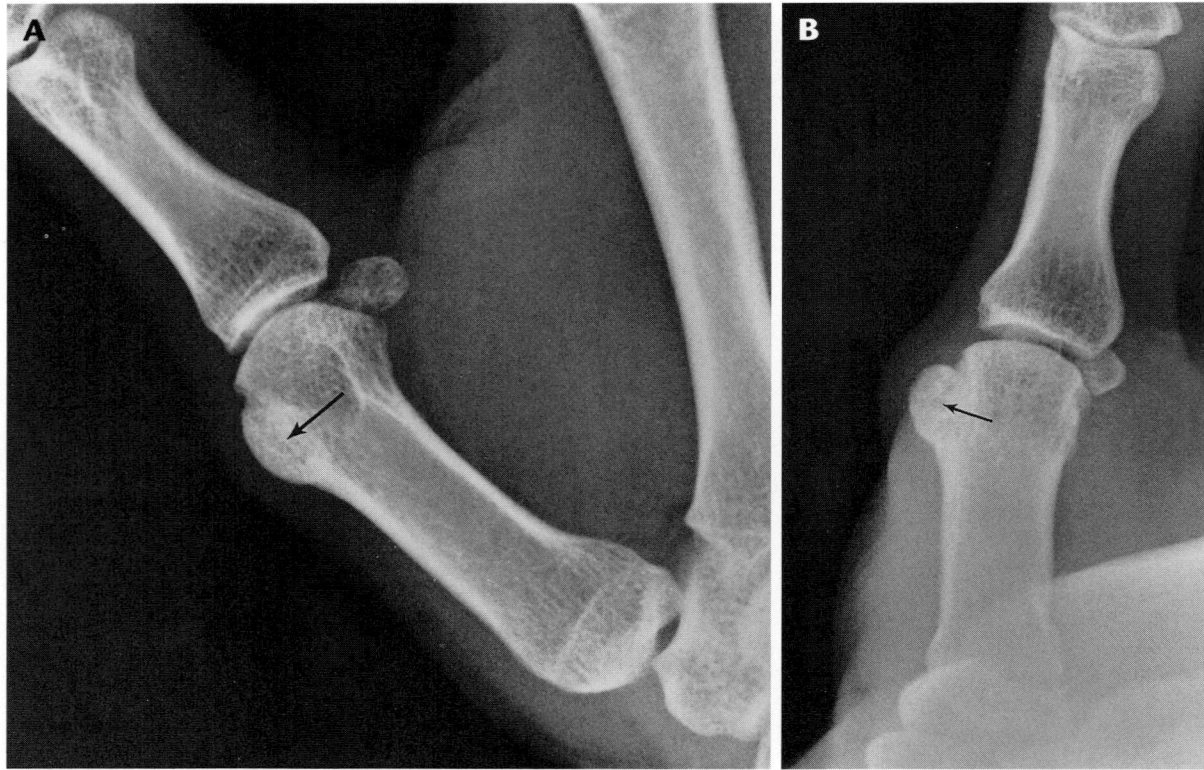

Figure 6–317. A, B, A knob-like developmental variation of the head of the first metacarpal that may be confused with sessile osteochondroma. There is no anatomic structure that can be implicated in its development. It may be seen on both medial and lateral aspects of bone. We have euphemistically termed it "The great knob of Keats."

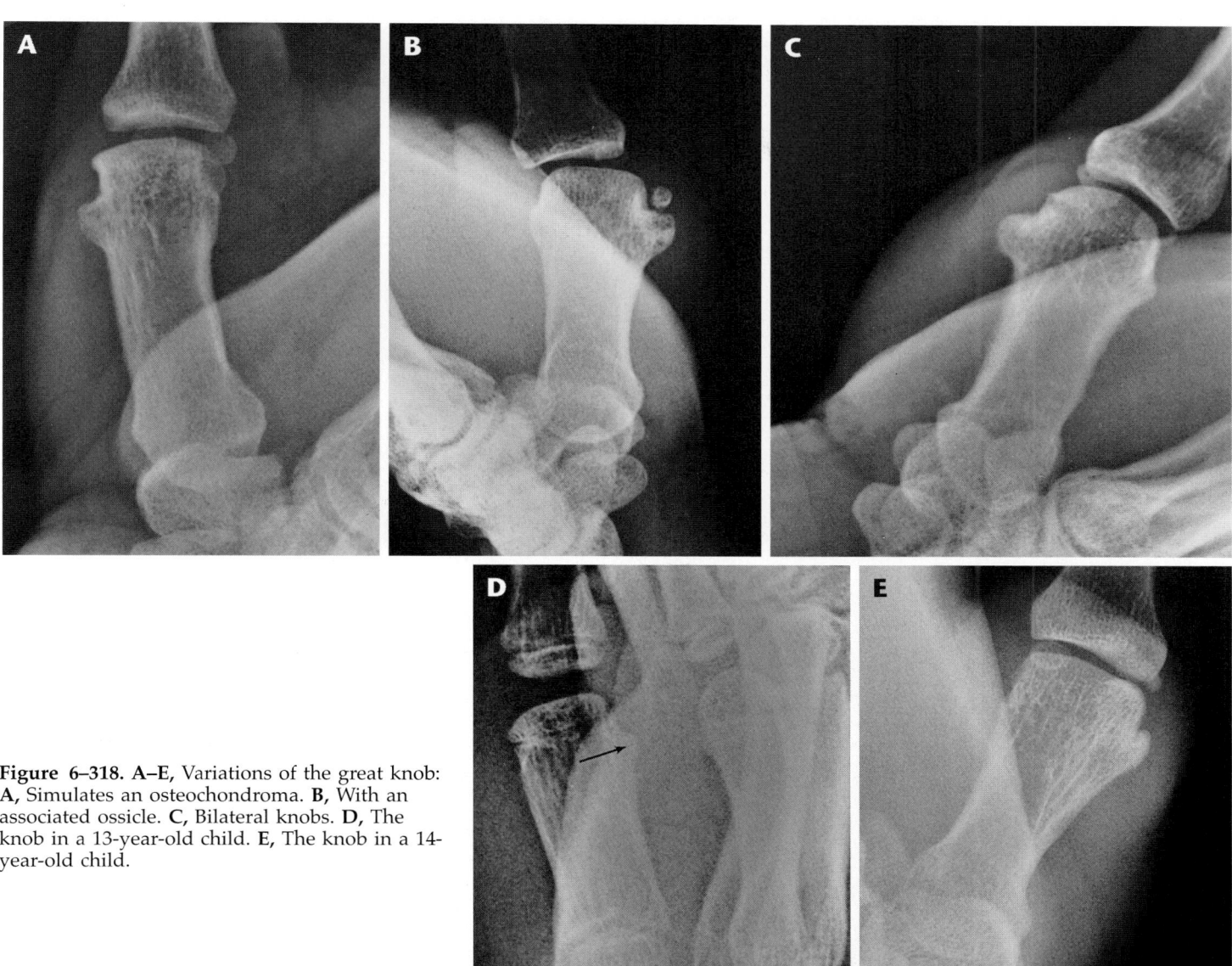

Figure 6–318. A–E, Variations of the great knob: **A,** Simulates an osteochondroma. **B,** With an associated ossicle. **C,** Bilateral knobs. **D,** The knob in a 13-year-old child. **E,** The knob in a 14-year-old child.

The Sesamoid Bones

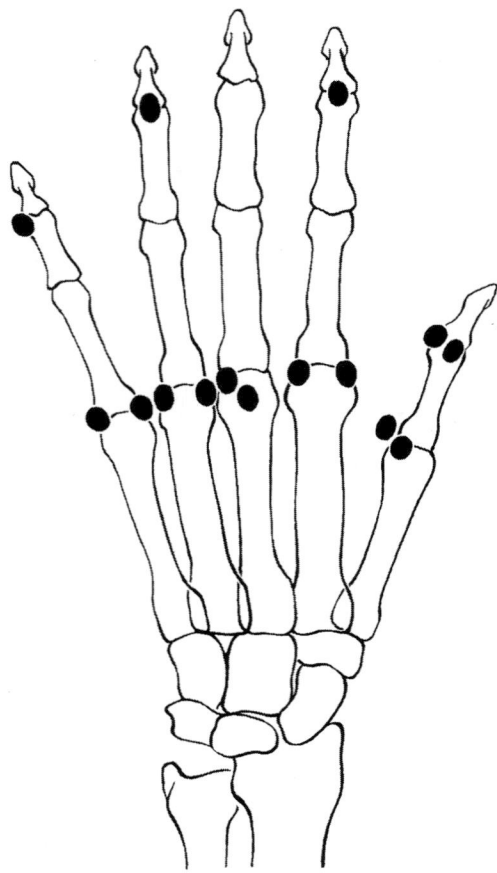

Figure 6–319. Diagram of all the recognized sesamoid bones of the hand (after Degen).

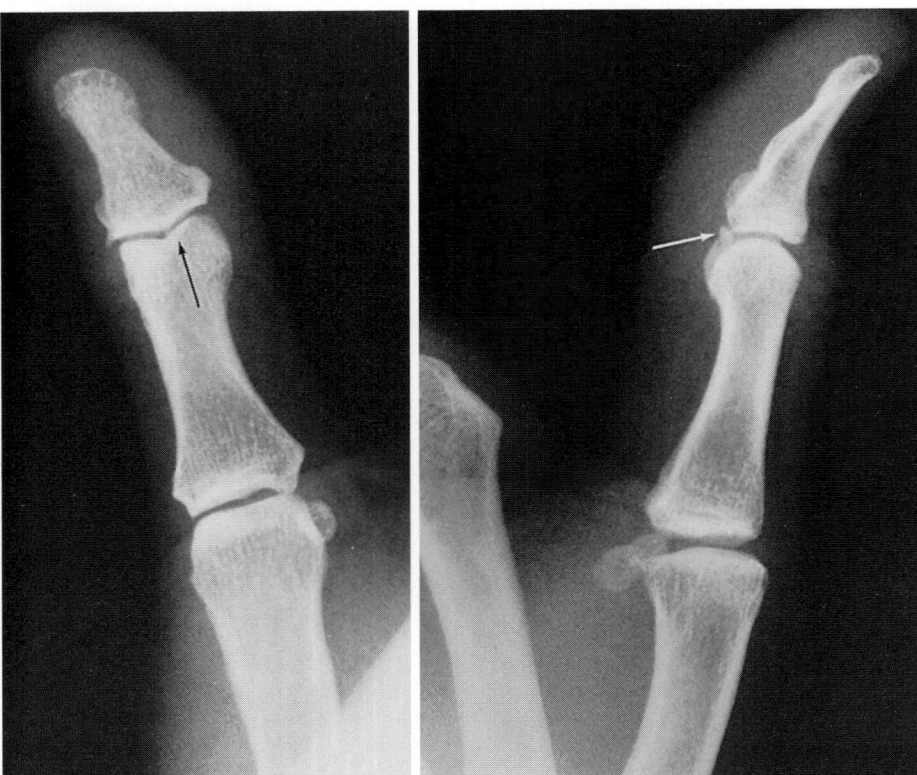

Figure 6–320. Sesamoid bone at the interphalangeal joint of the thumb.

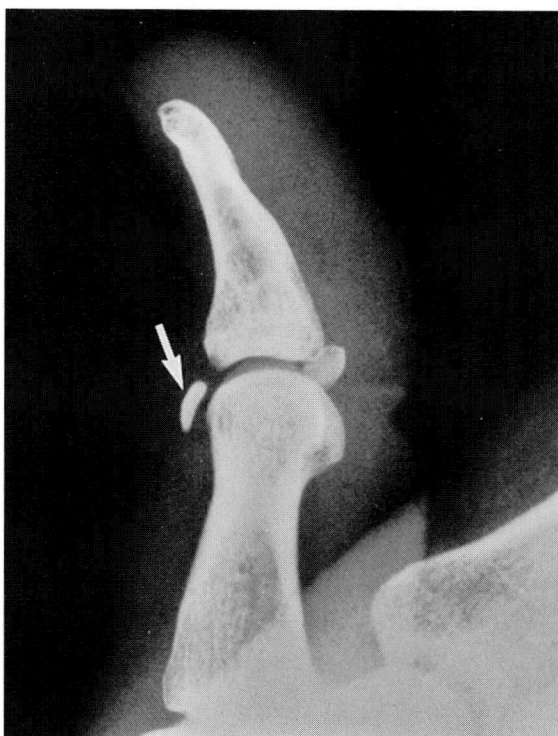

Figure 6–321. Unusual sesamoid in dorsal aspect of the interphalageal joint of the thumb.

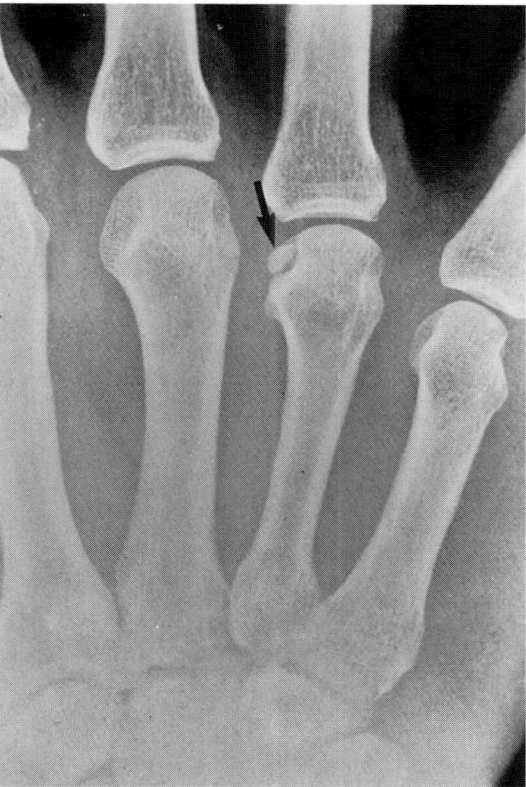

Figure 6–322. Solitary sesamoid bone at head of fourth metacarpal.

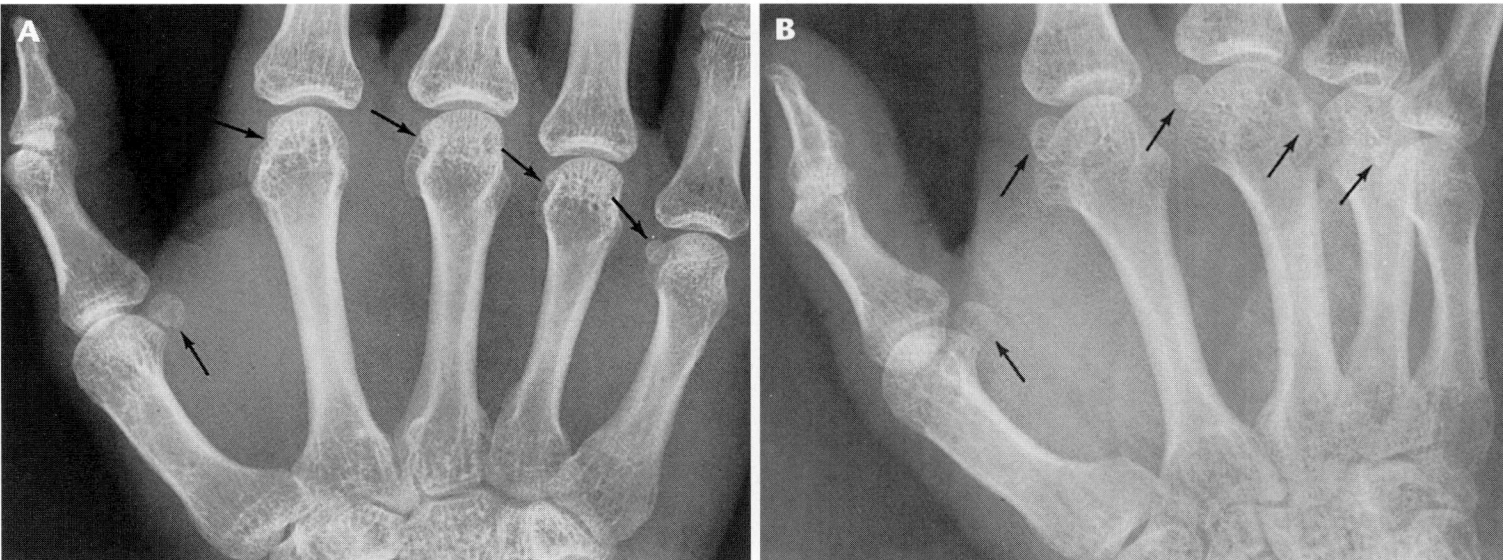

Figure 6–323. Sesamoid bones at each metacarpal head in frontal (**A**) and oblique (**B**) projections.

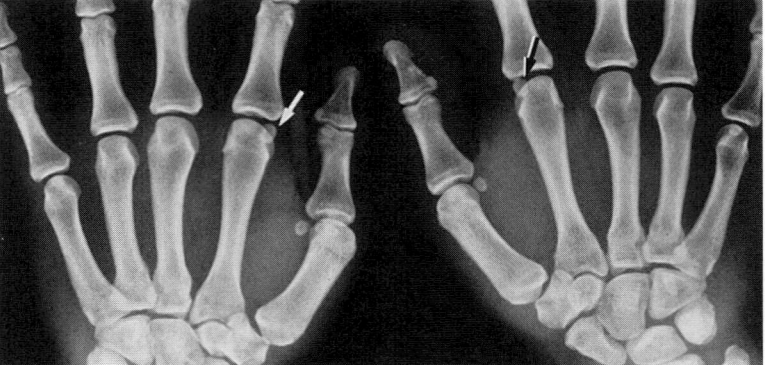

Figure 6–324. Solitary sesamoids at the heads of the second metacarpals.

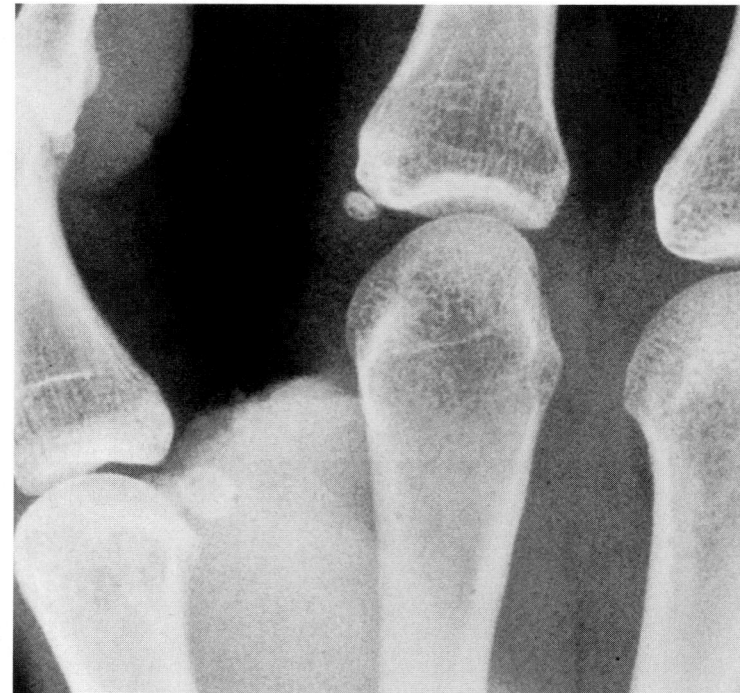

Figure 6–325. Ossicle at the base of the proximal phalanx of the index finger, possibly a sesamoid.

The Fingers

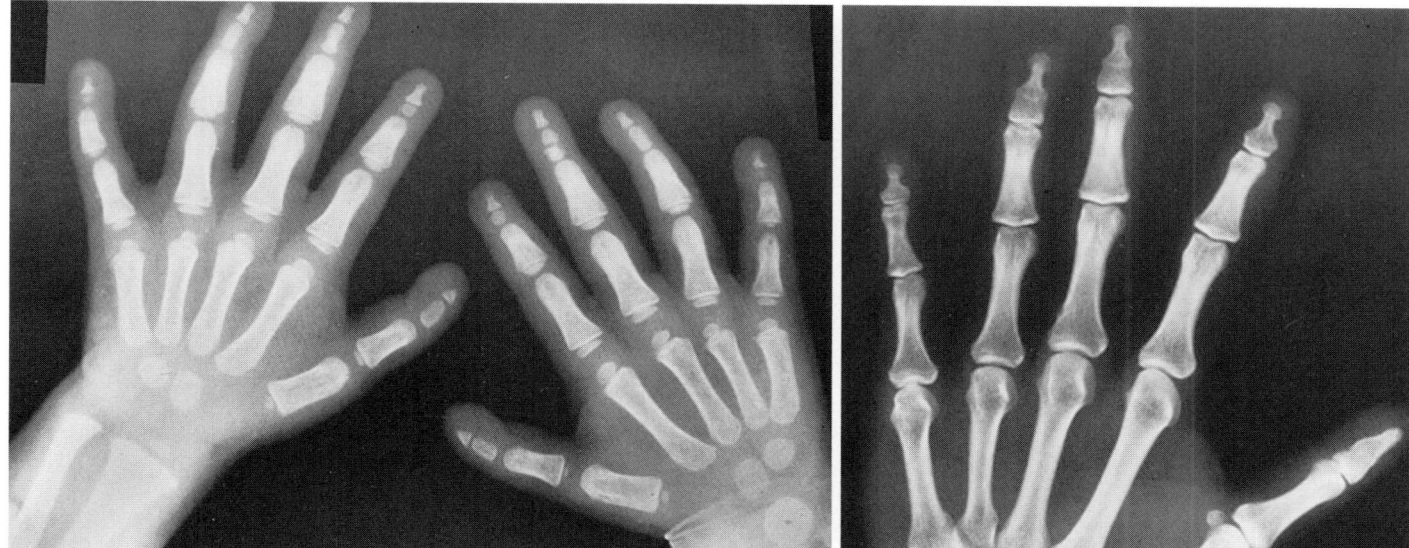

Figure 6–326. *Left,* Supernumerary phalanges in the distal digits of an otherwise healthy 10-month-old child. *Right,* Same patient at 19 years of age showing closing of the accessory centers of ossification. (Courtesy of Dr. N. Warn Courtney.)

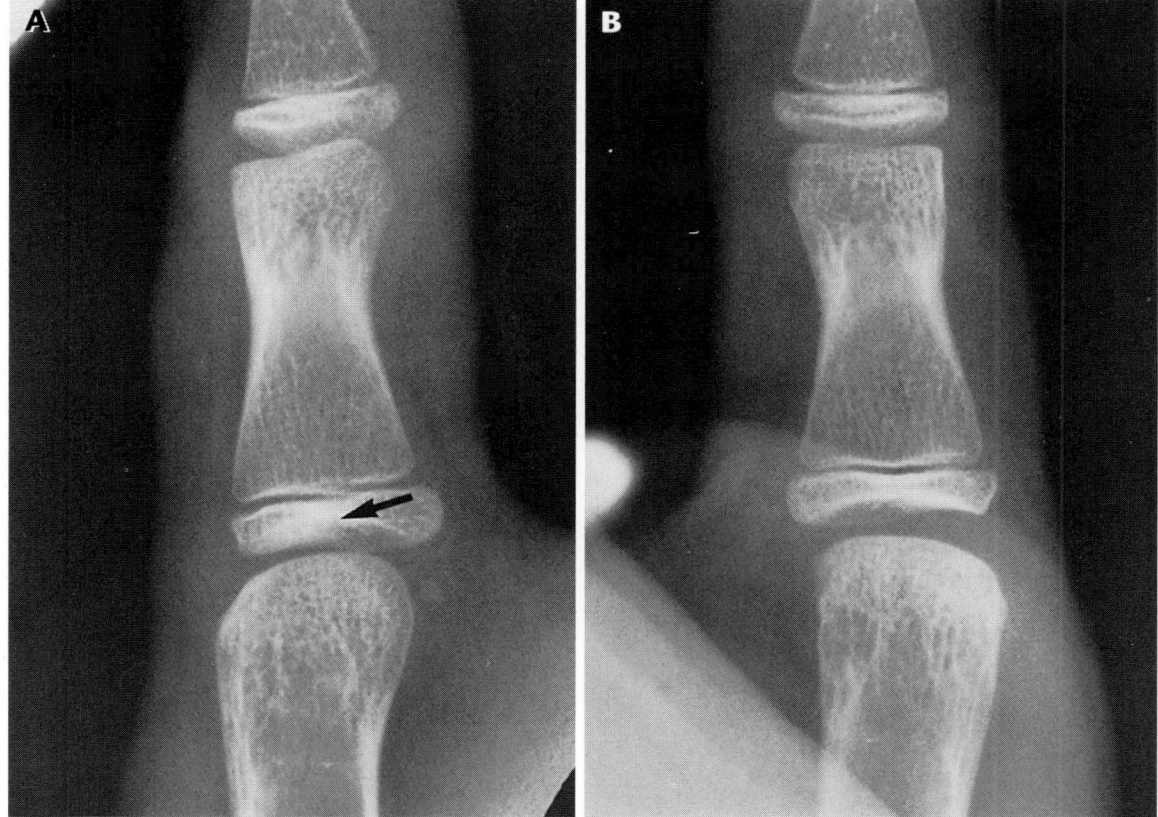

Figure 6–327. A, Cleft epiphysis of proximal phalanx of the thumb seen in the oblique projection. **B,** Cleft is not visible in frontal projection. (Ref: Harrison RB, Keats TE: Epiphyseal clefts. *Skeletal Radiol* 5:23, 1980.)

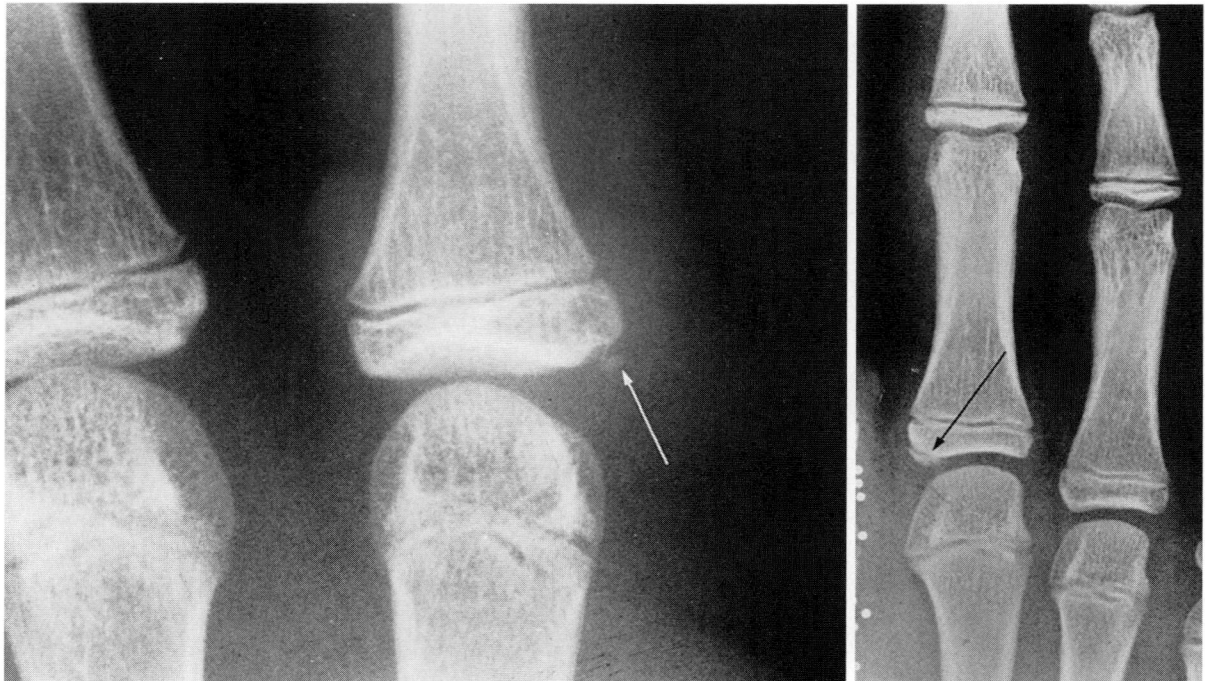

Figure 6–328. Accessory centers of ossification of the epiphyses of the proximal phalanges, simulating avulsion injuries.

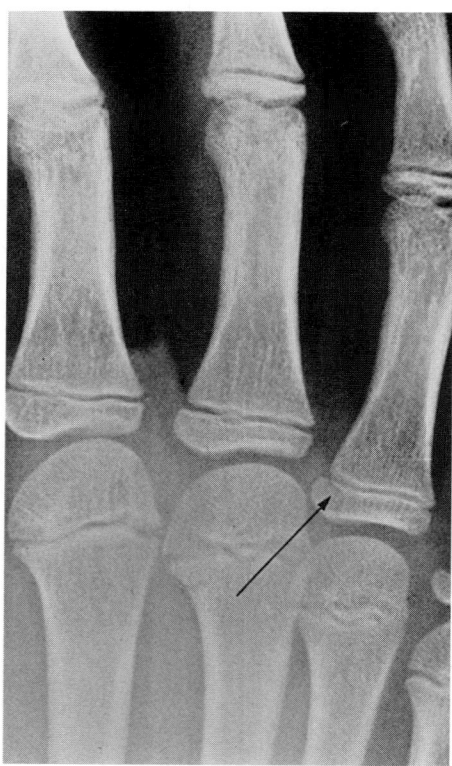

Figure 6–329. Mach effect of metaphysis superimposing on epiphysis, suggesting a fracture.

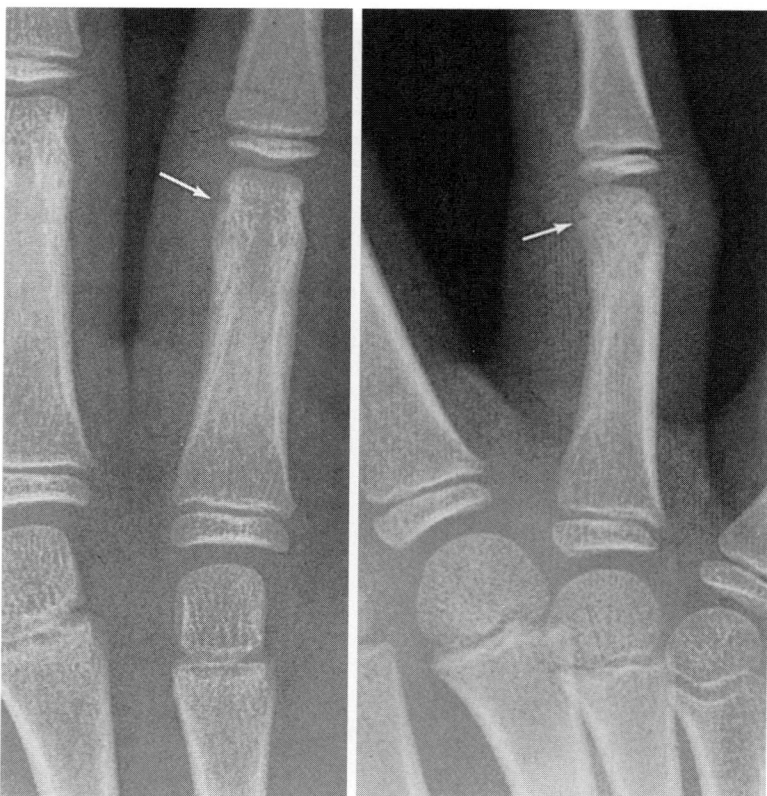

Figure 6–330. Attempt to form an accessory ossification center at the head of the proximal phalanx of the fourth finger in an 11-year-old boy. This might be mistaken for a fracture.

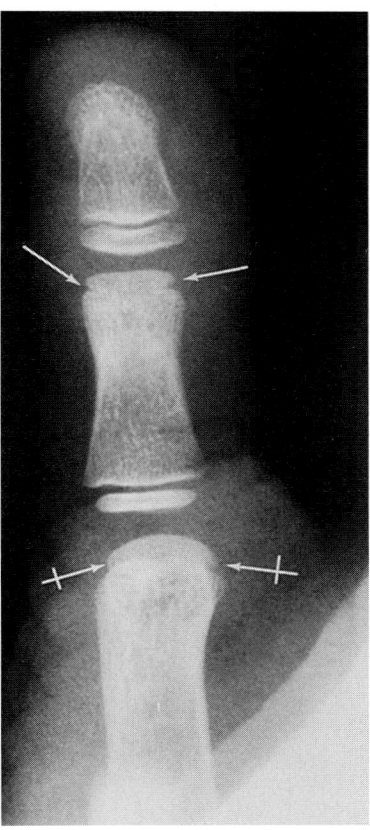

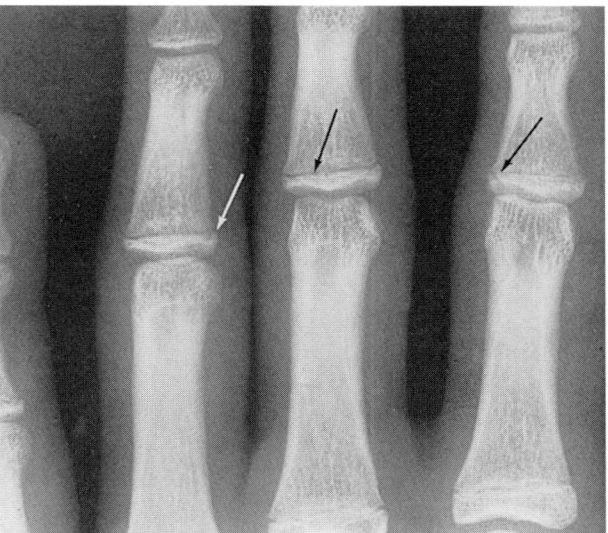

Figure 6–332. Normal lucent fissures in the epiphyses in a 14-year-old boy, which may be mistaken for fractures.

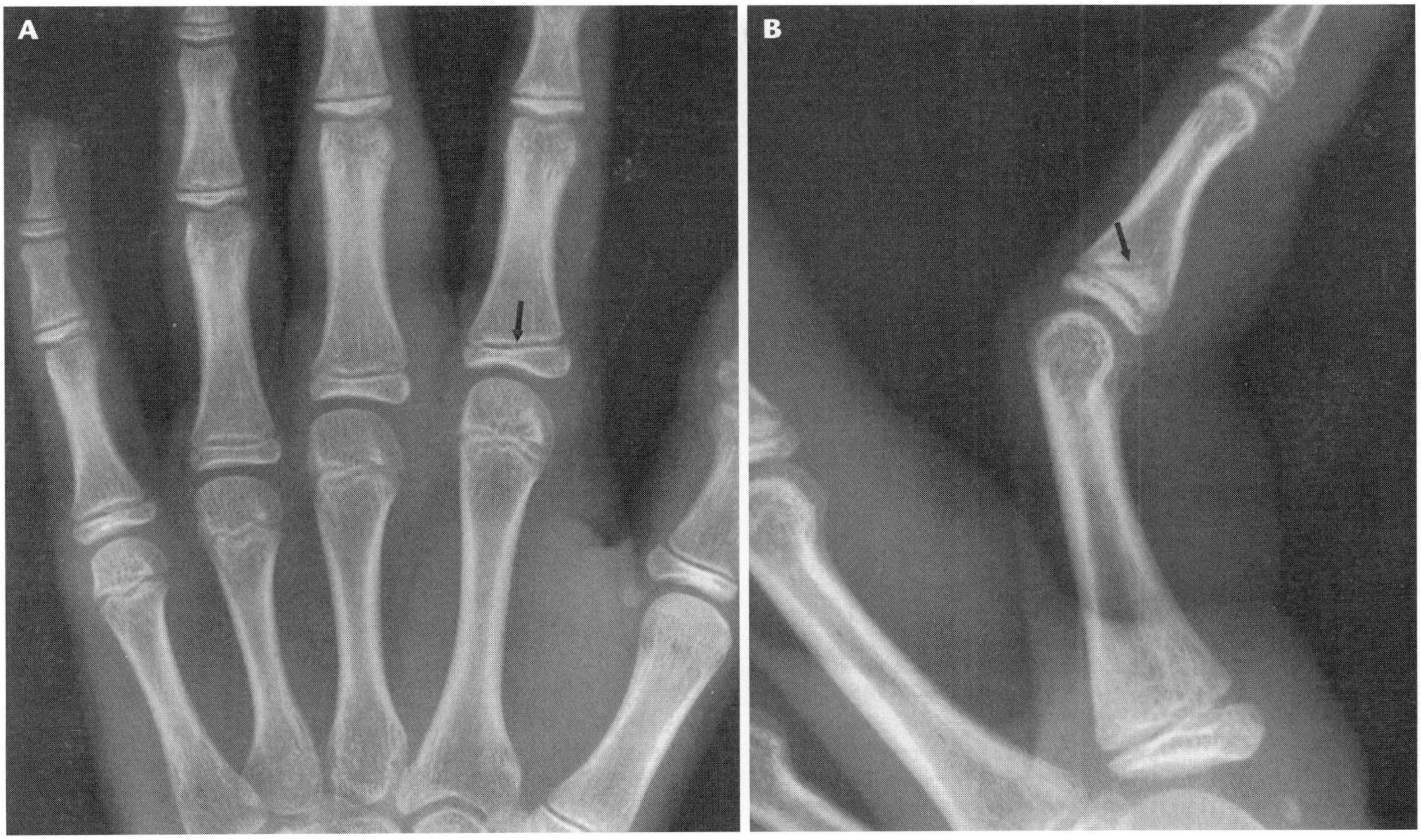

Figure 6–331. Attempt to form an accessory ossification center at the distal end of the proximal phalanx of the thumb in a 10-year-old boy (→). Note similar process at the end of the metacarpal (↦).

Figure 6–333. The epiphyseal line may simulate a fracture in the oblique projection. **A,** Frontal. **B,** Oblique.

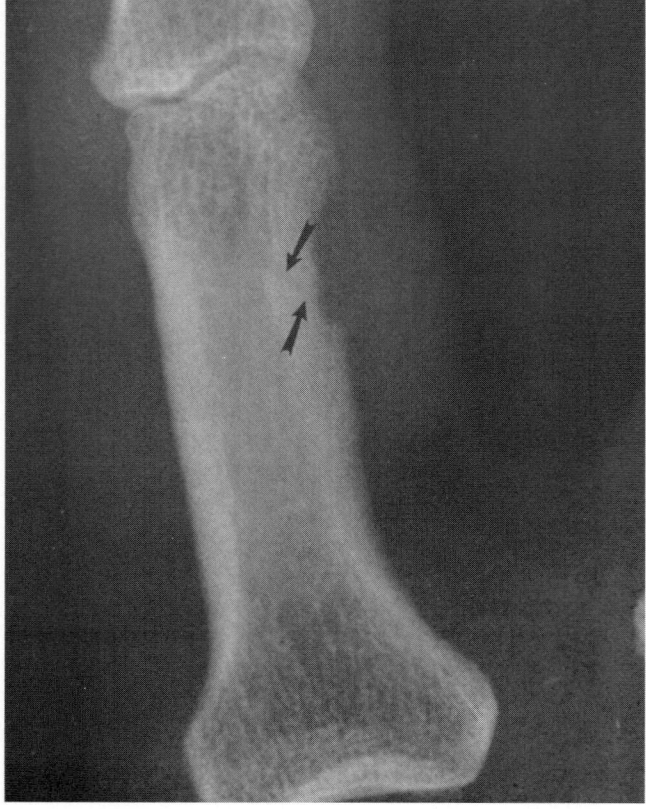

Figure 6–334. The nutrient foramen of the proximal phalanx.

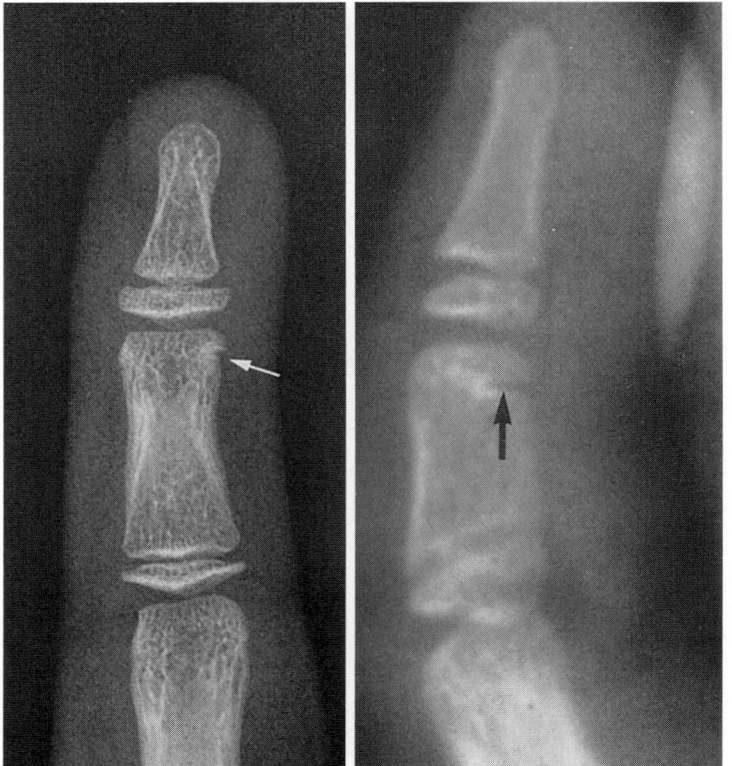

Figure 6–335. Developmental clefts in the middle phalanges. *Left,* 9-year-old child. *Right,* 10-year-old child.

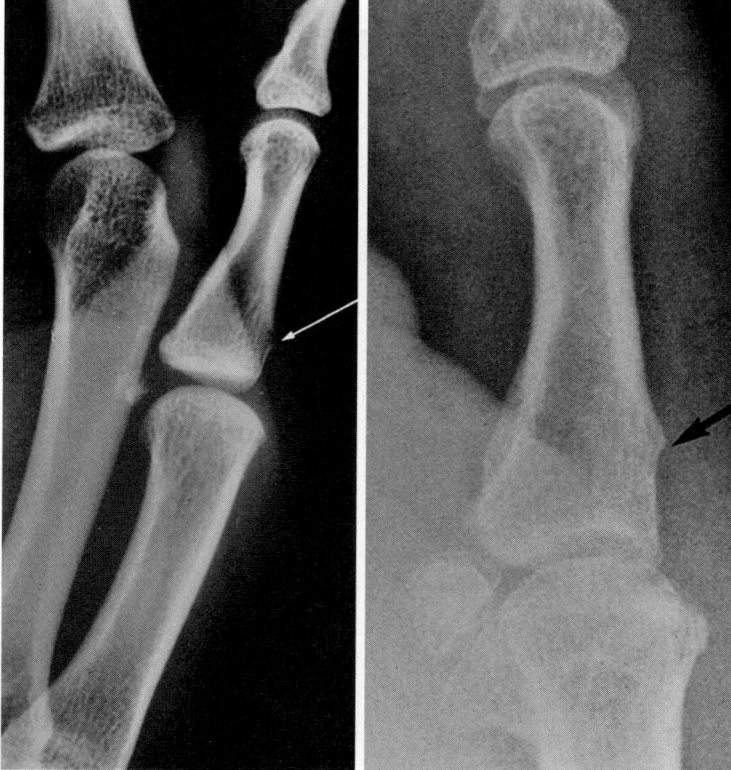

Figure 6–336. Two examples of a small spurlike excrescence in the cortex of the proximal phalanx of the thumb, which probably represents the insertion of the extensor pollicis brevis tendon.

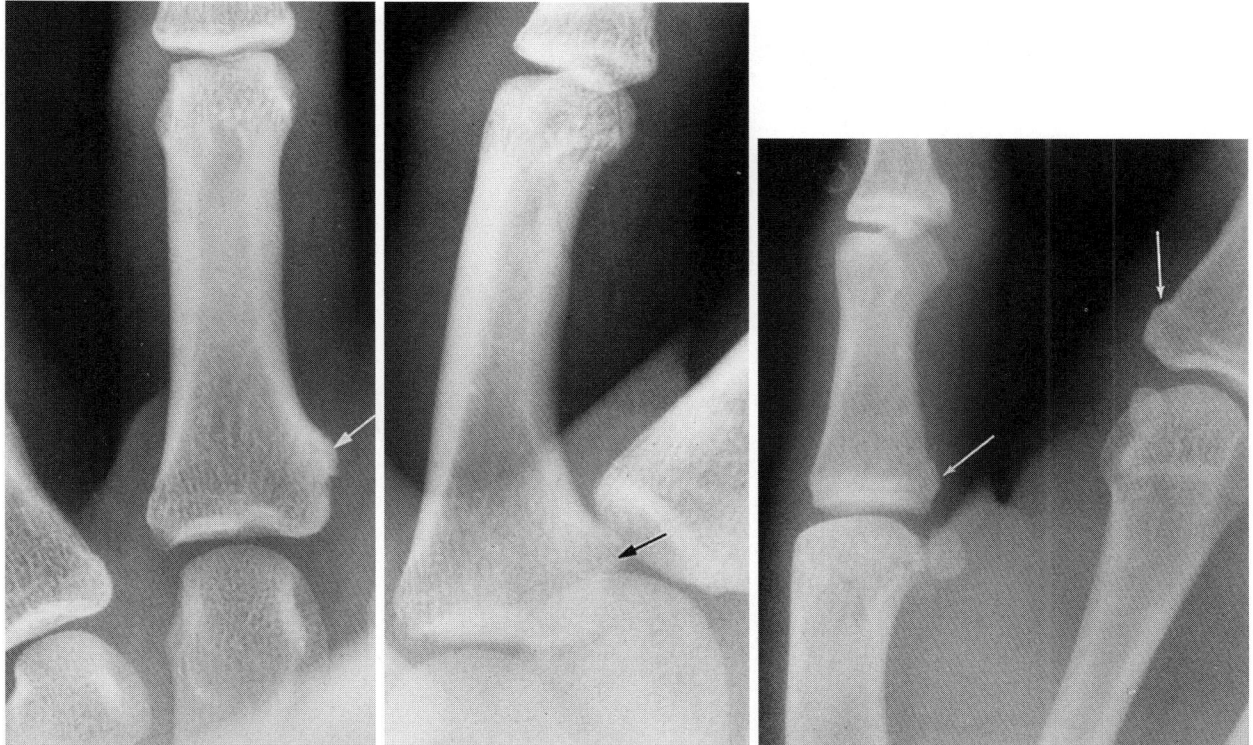

Figure 6–337. *Left* and *center*, Small, incidentally found excrescence at the base of the proximal phalanx of the fourth finger. *Right*, Normal tuberosities of the bases of the phalanges, not to be mistaken for torus fractures.

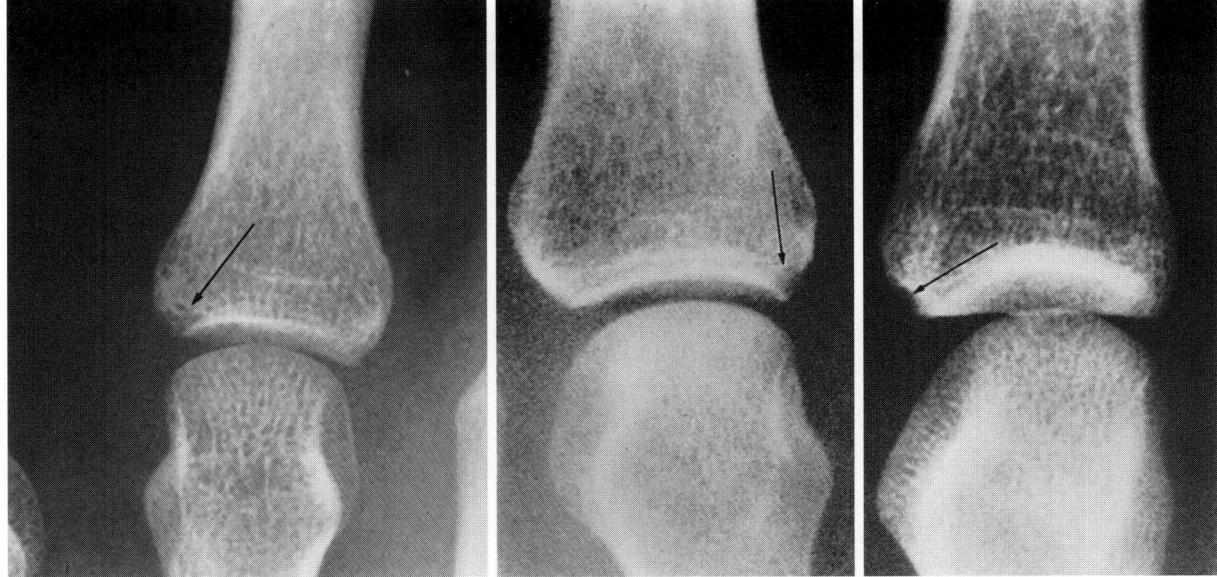

Figure 6–338. Small notches in the bases of the proximal phalanges should not be mistaken for the erosions of inflammatory arthritis, which should involve the heads of the metacarpals initially. (Ref: Stelling CB et al: Irregularities at the base of the proximal phalanges. *Am J Roentgenol* 138:695, 1982.)

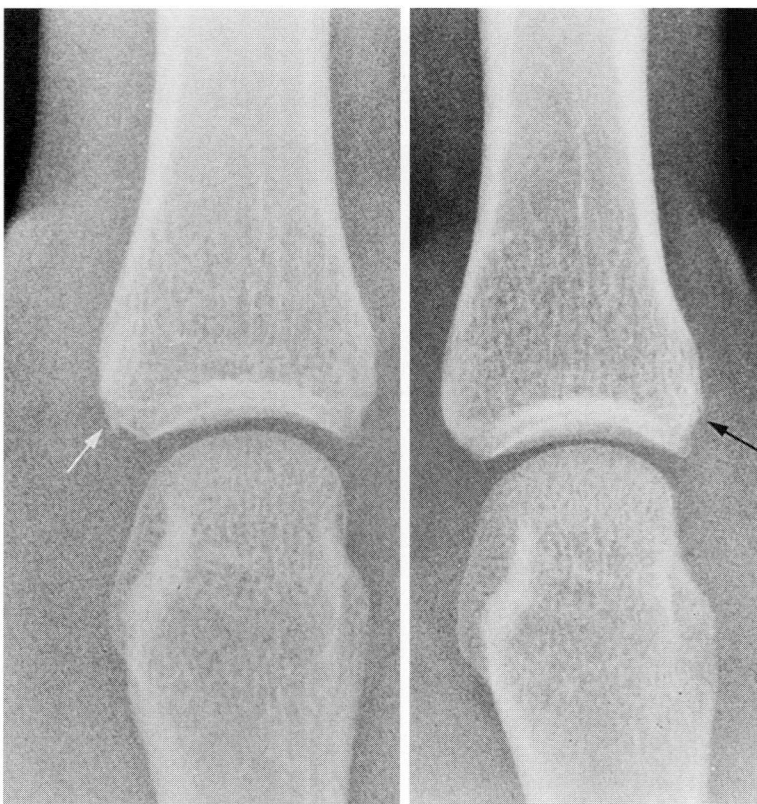

Figure 6–339. Bilateral, small spurlike projections from the bases of the proximal phalanges in a healthy 20-year-old woman.

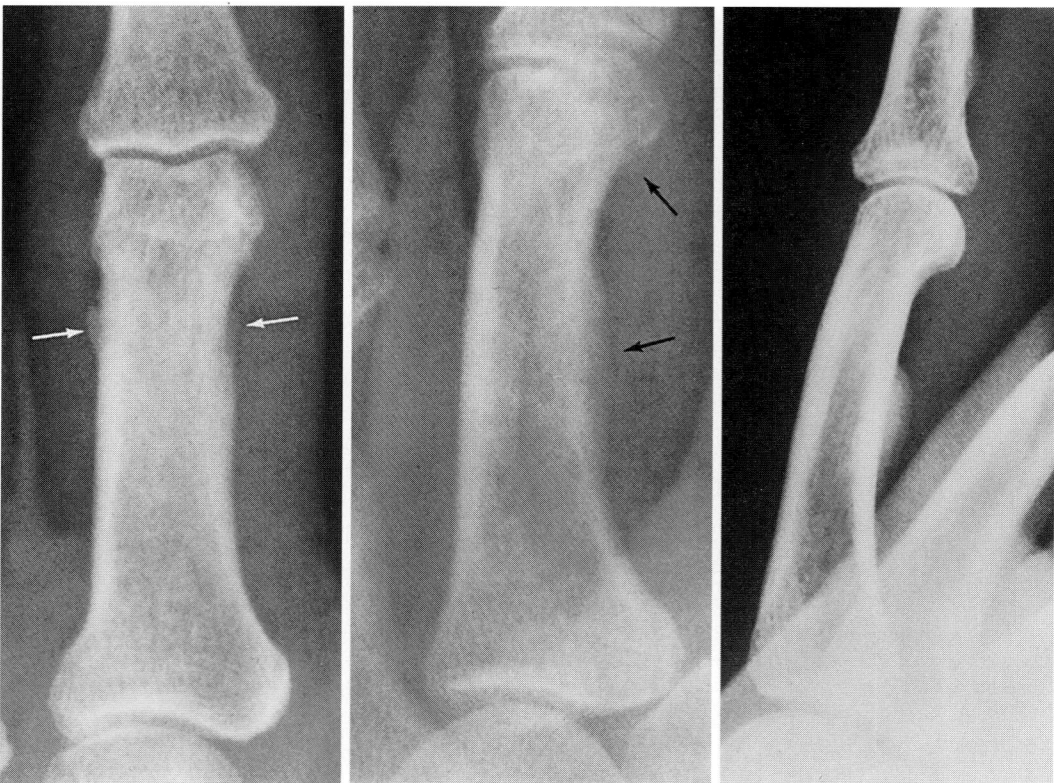

Figure 6–340. Normal ridges and projections of the proximal phalanx caused by tendon sheath attachments, which may simulate periostitis or calcifying hematoma.

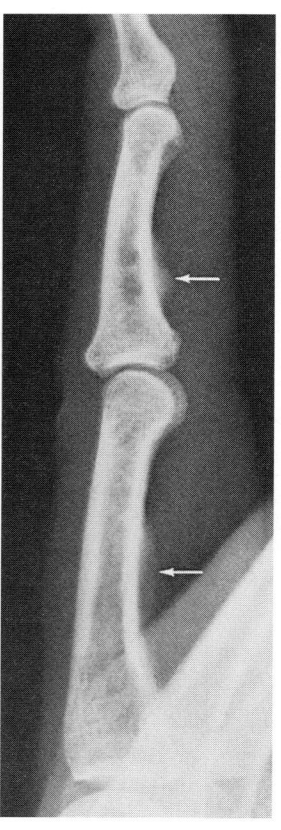

Figure 6–341. Normal irregularities of the palmar aspects of the proximal and middle phalanges of the index finger.

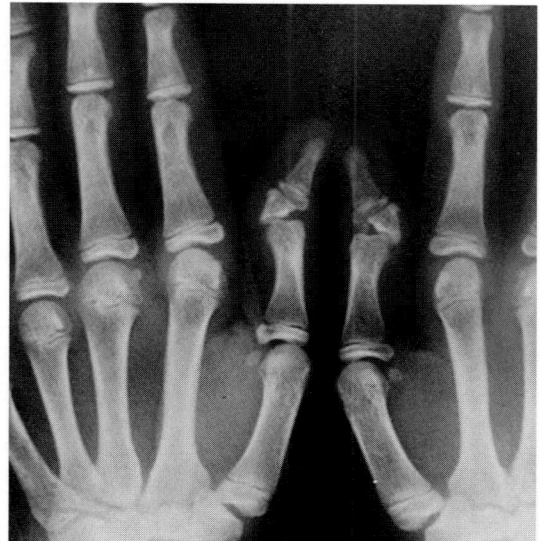

Figure 6–342. Abortive attempt to form triphalangeal thumbs. There were no associated anomalies in this patient.

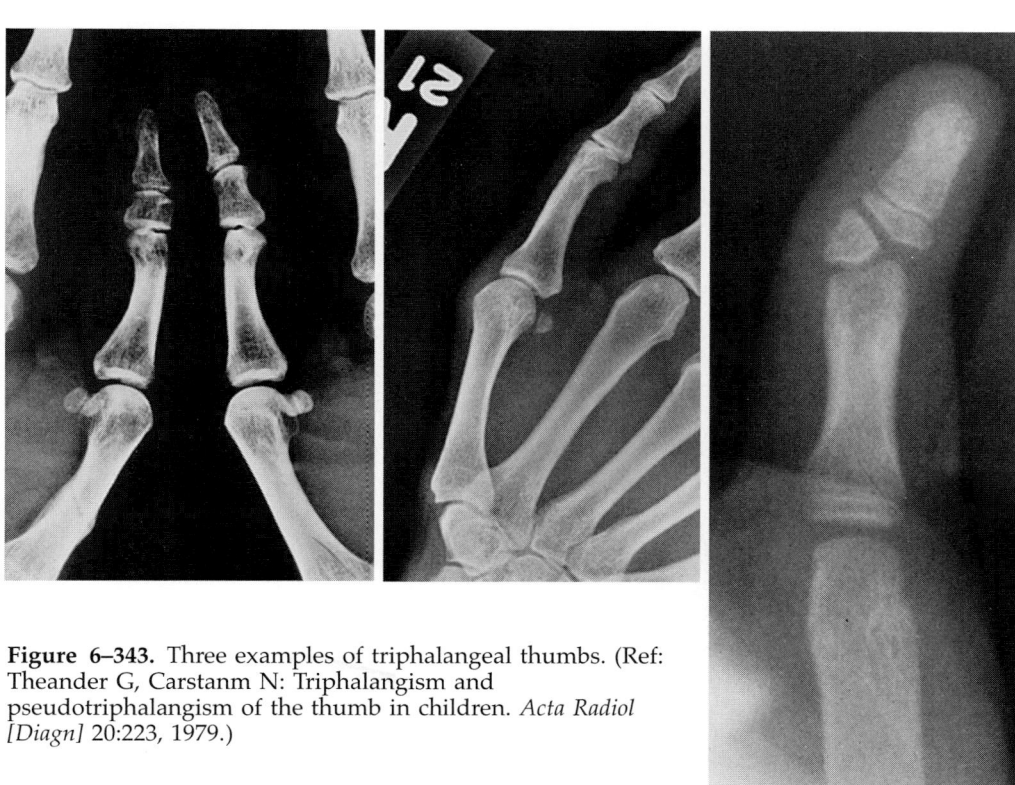

Figure 6–343. Three examples of triphalangeal thumbs. (Ref: Theander G, Carstanm N: Triphalangism and pseudotriphalangism of the thumb in children. *Acta Radiol [Diagn]* 20:223, 1979.)

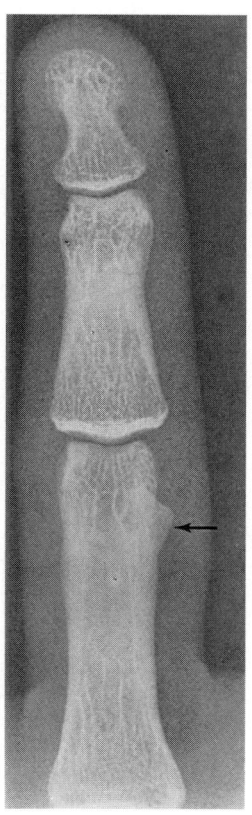

Figure 6–344. Exaggeration of normal irregularity of the head of the proximal phalanx of the third finger, not an exostosis.

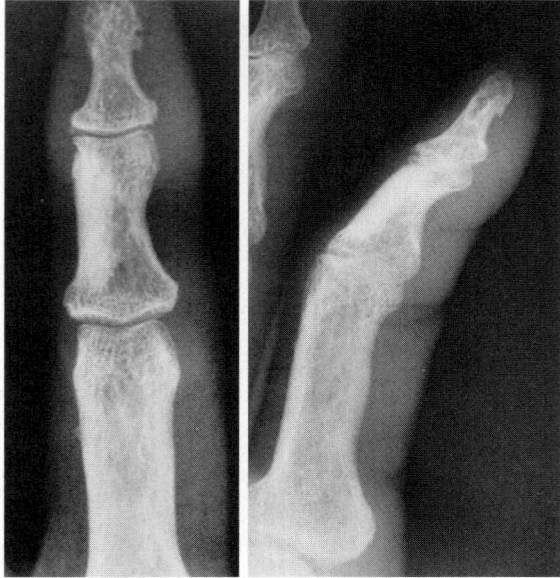

Figure 6–345. Osteosclerosis of the middle phalanx of the fifth finger.

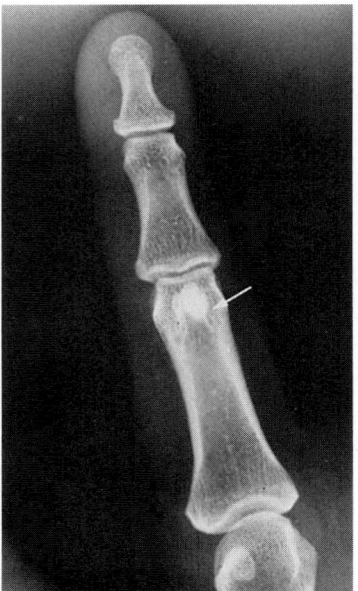

Figure 6–346. Bone island in the head of the proximal phalanx of the index finger.

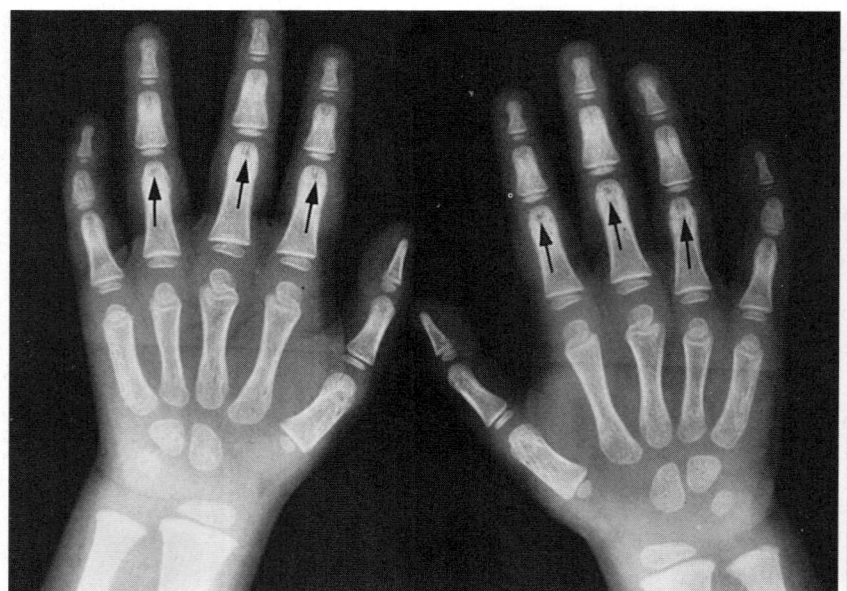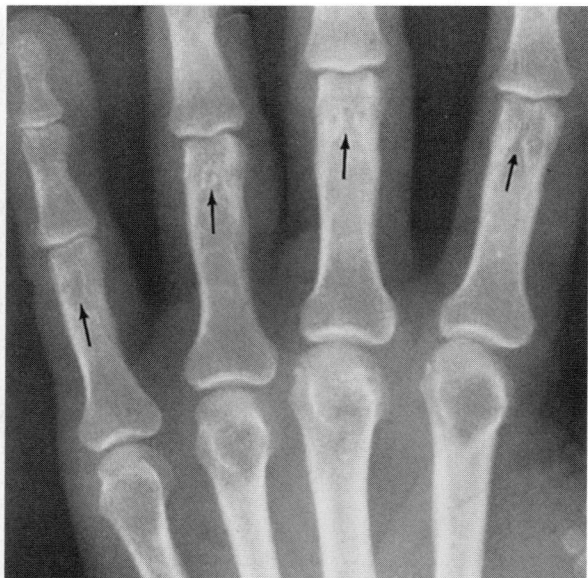

Figure 6–347. Nutrient foramina at the heads of the proximal phalanges. *Left*, 2-year-old child. *Right*, Adult.

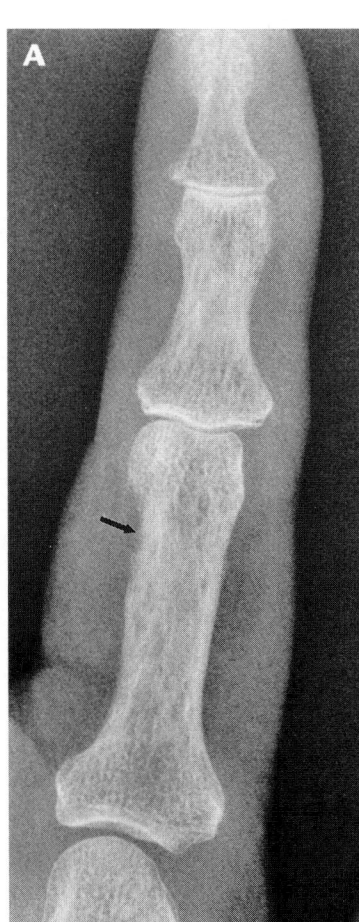

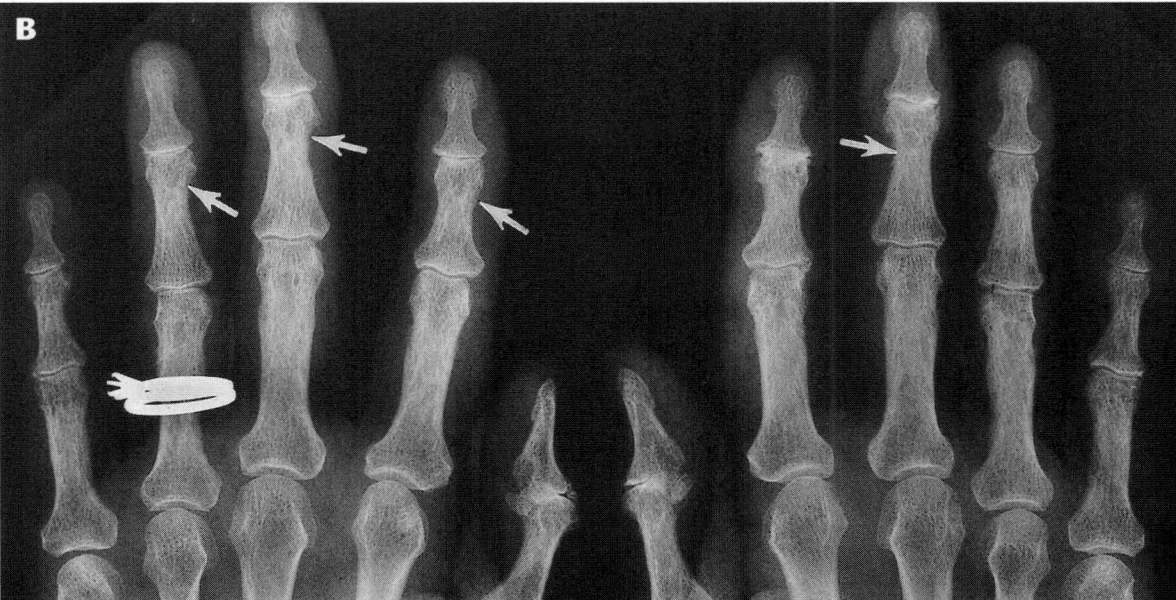

Figure 6–348. A, Cortical thinning of the lateral aspect of the shaft of the distal end of the proximal phalanx simulating bone destruction. This is seen in the presence of osteoporosis. **B,** Similar appearance in other fingers.

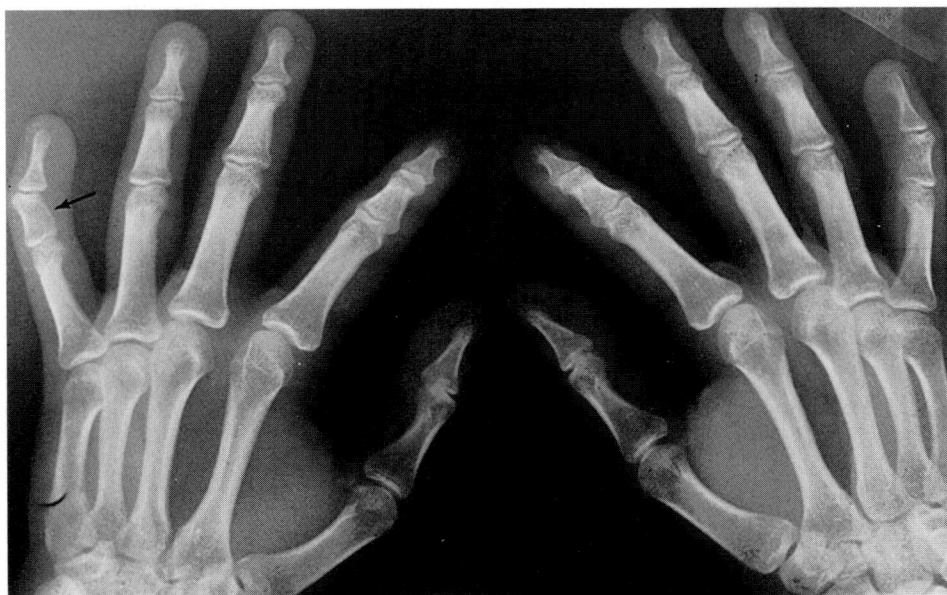

Figure 6–349. Short middle phalanges of the fifth fingers are associated with malformation syndromes, but may also be a normal familial trait, as in this 18-year-old woman. (Ref: Greulich WW: A comparison of the dysplastic middle phalanx of the fifth finger in mentally normal Caucasians, Mongoloids and Negroes with that of individuals of the same racial groups who have Down's syndrome. *Am J Roentgenol* 118:259, 1973.)

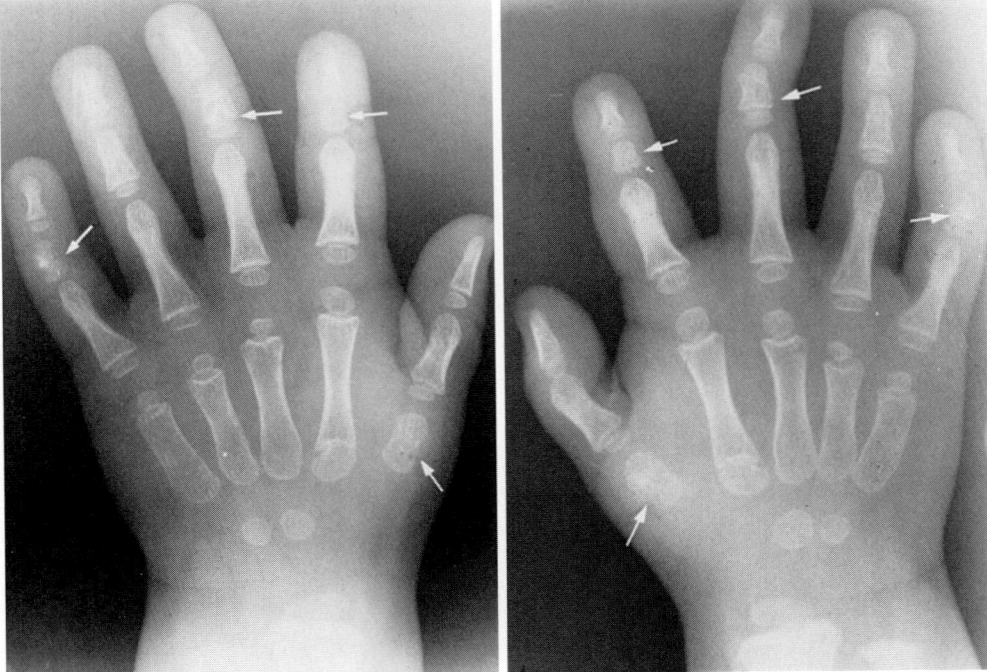

Figure 6–350. Anomalous development of the first metacarpals and the middle phalanges in a healthy 3-year-old child, representing a familial trait.

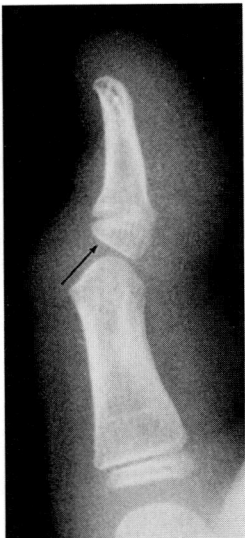

Figure 6–351. Normal relationships of the middle and distal phalanges of the thumb in a 9-year-old boy. Note wedged configuration of the epiphysis at the base of the distal phalanx.

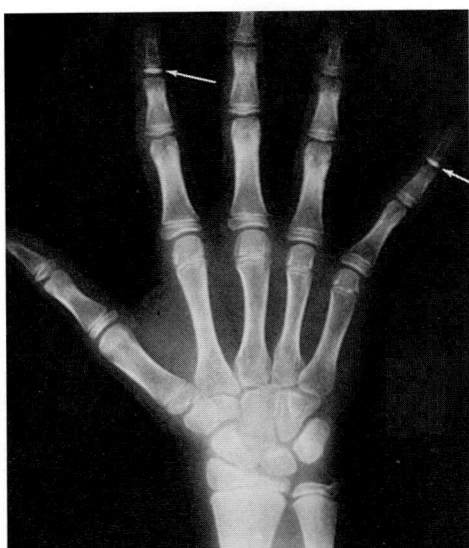

Figure 6–352. Ivory epiphyses in the hands of children may occur as isolated events without clinical significance. This is more common in children with retarded maturation. (Refs: Kuhns LR et al: Ivory epiphyses of the hands. *Radiology* 109:643, 1973; Van der Laan JG, Thijn CJ: Ivory and dense epiphyses of the hand. *Skeletal Radiol* 15:117, 1986.)

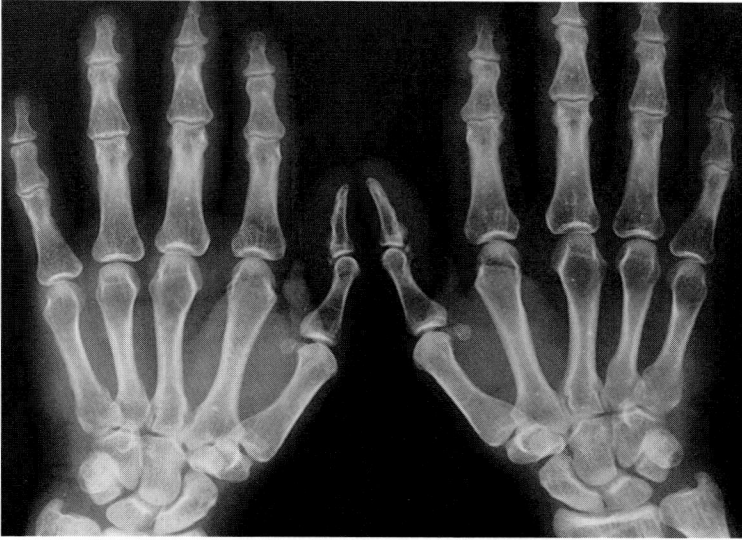

Figure 6–353. Speckled densities in the medullary cavities of the phalanges of both hands in a 58-year-old woman, probably representing prominent trabeculae in osteoporotic bone.

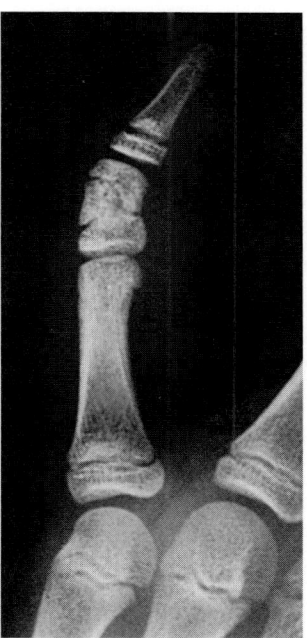

Figure 6–354. Unusual clinodactyly of the fifth finger in an otherwise normal 14-year-old boy.

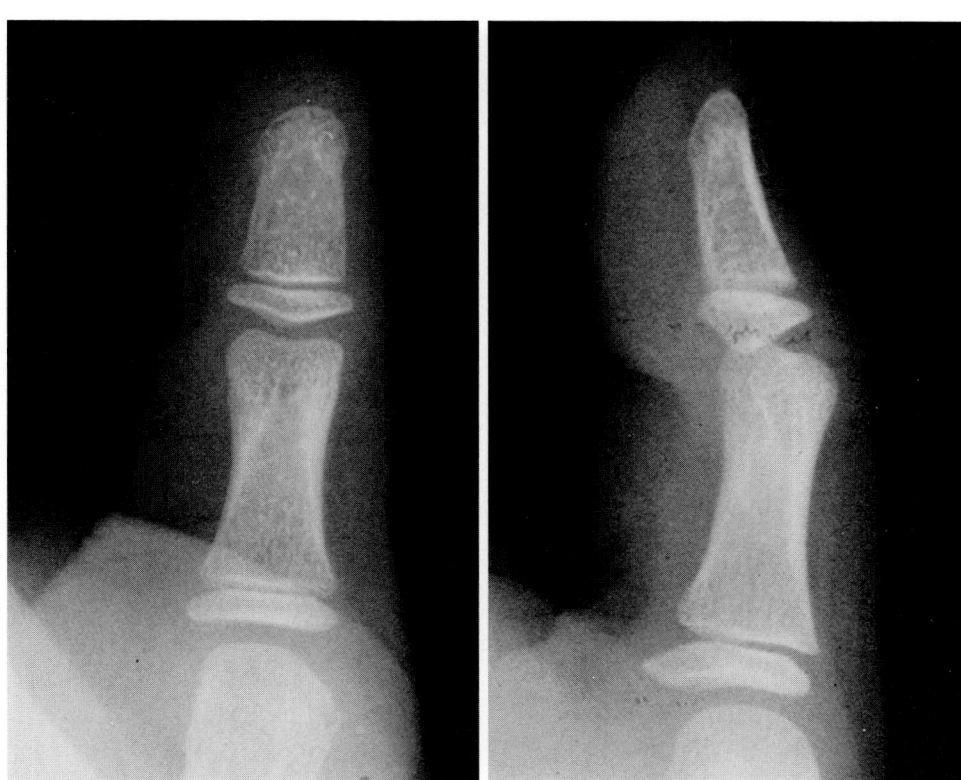

Figure 6–355. Unusually large epiphysis of the base of the thumb.

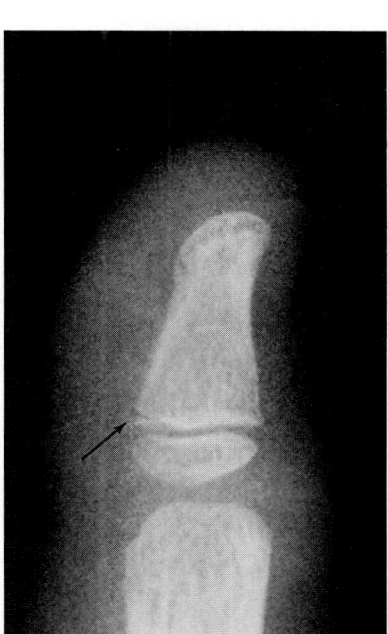

Figure 6–356. Horizontal fissure adjacent to the epiphyseal plate of the distal phalanx of the thumb in a 9-year-old child, not to be mistaken for a fracture.

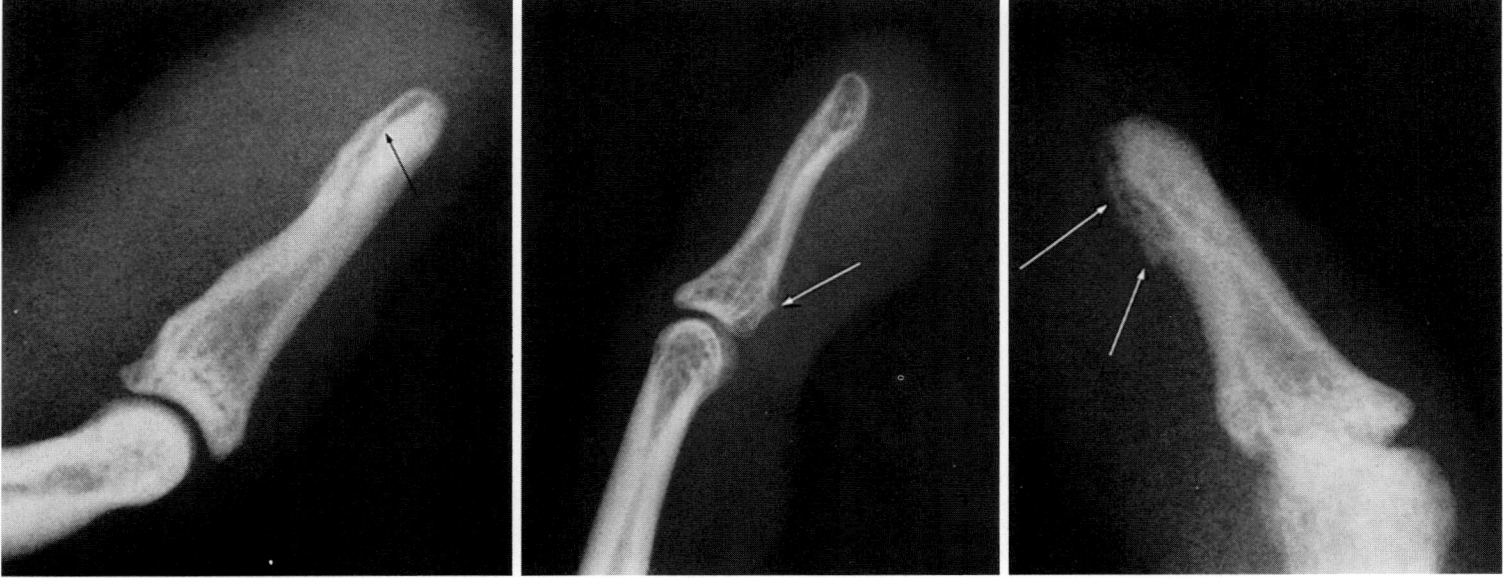

Figure 6–357. Normal configurations of the terminal phalanges, which should not be mistaken for the effects of trauma.

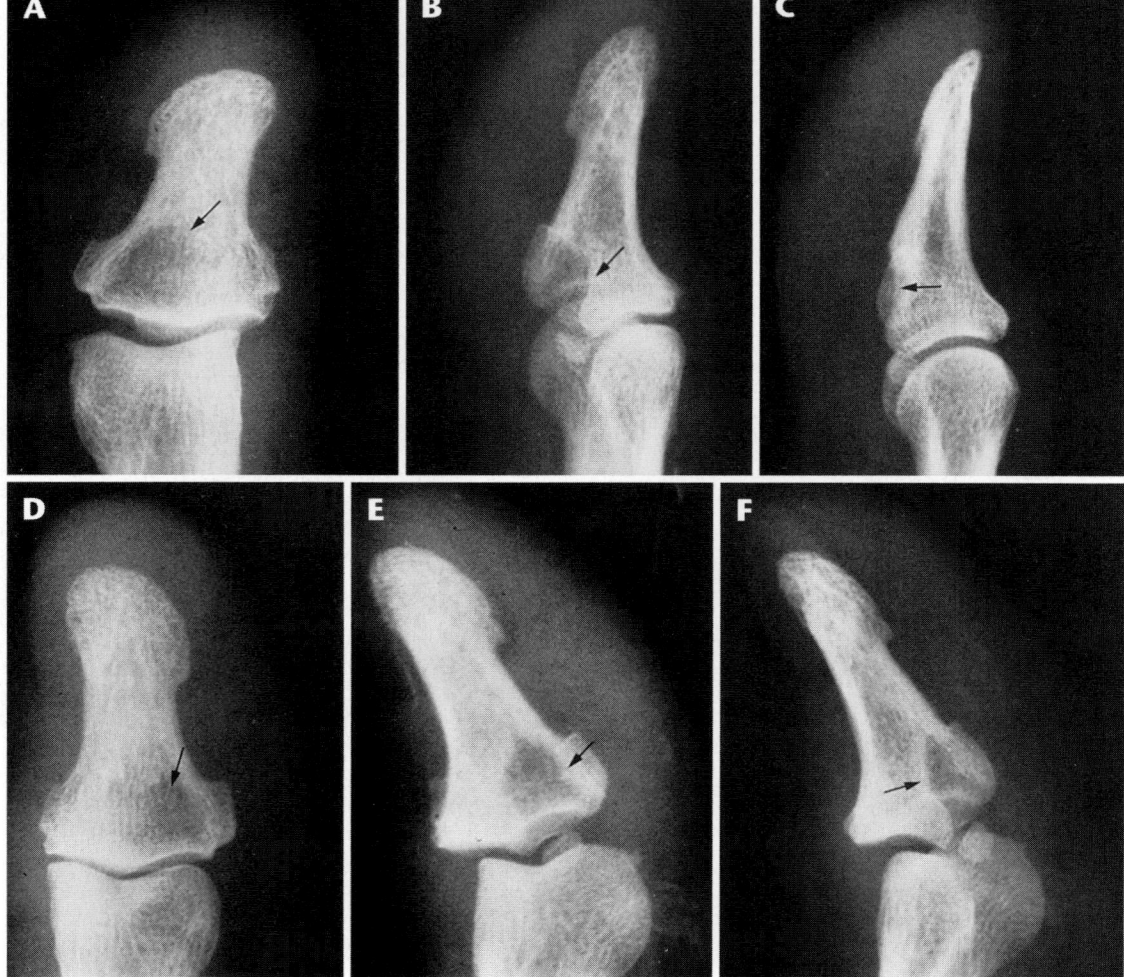

Figure 6–358. **A** and **B,** Fossa in the base of the distal phalanx of the thumb may simulate a destructive lesion. **C,** Lateral projection shows only the fossa. **D–F,** Similar appearance is seen on the opposite side.

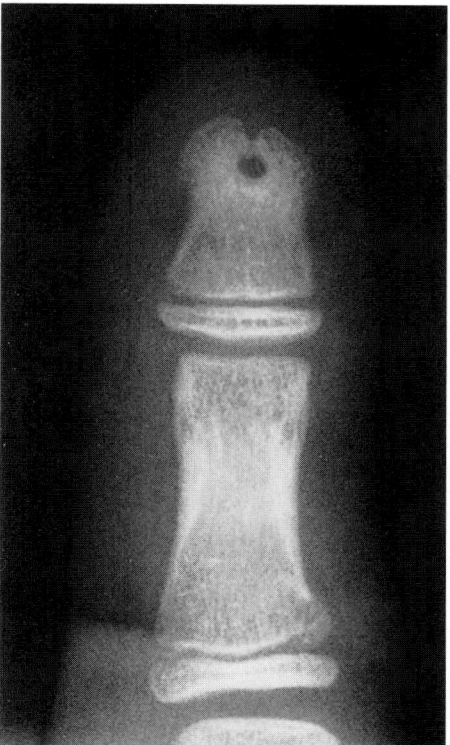

Figure 6–359. Attempted bifid distal phalanx.

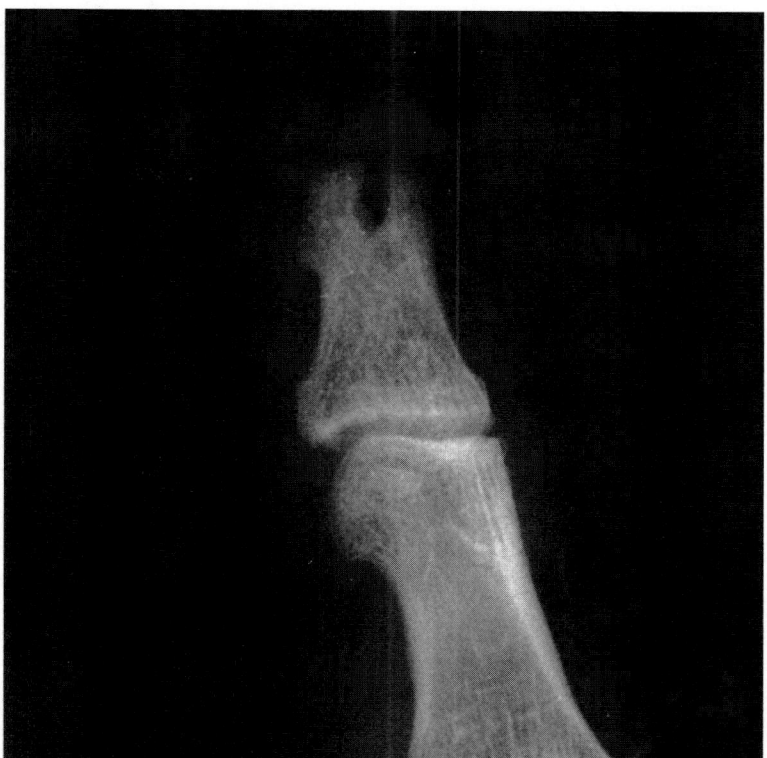

Figure 6–360. Bifid terminal digit of the thumb.

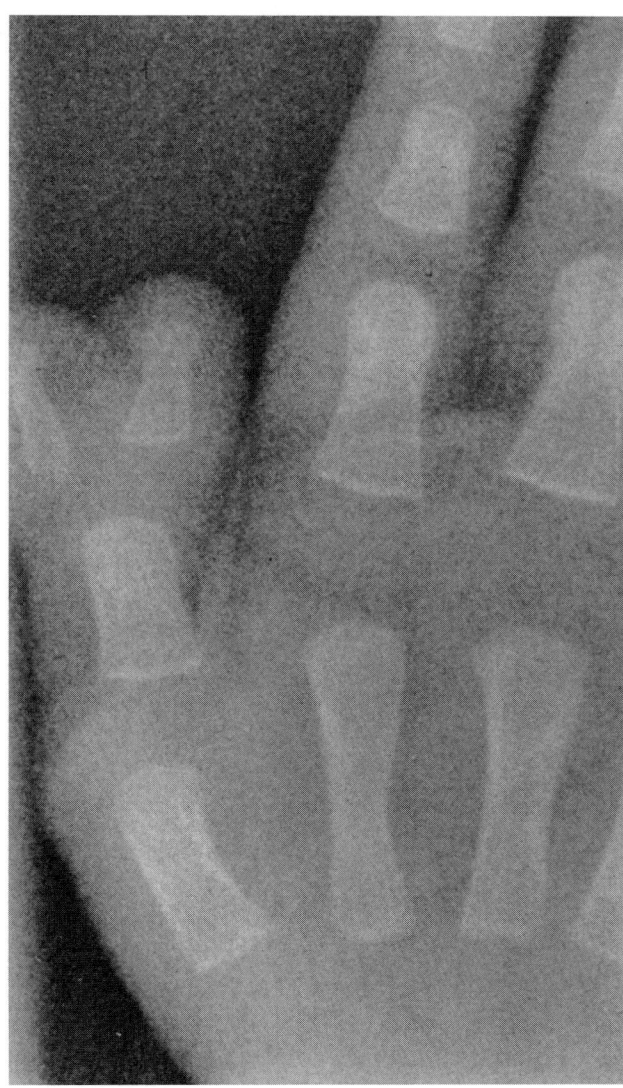

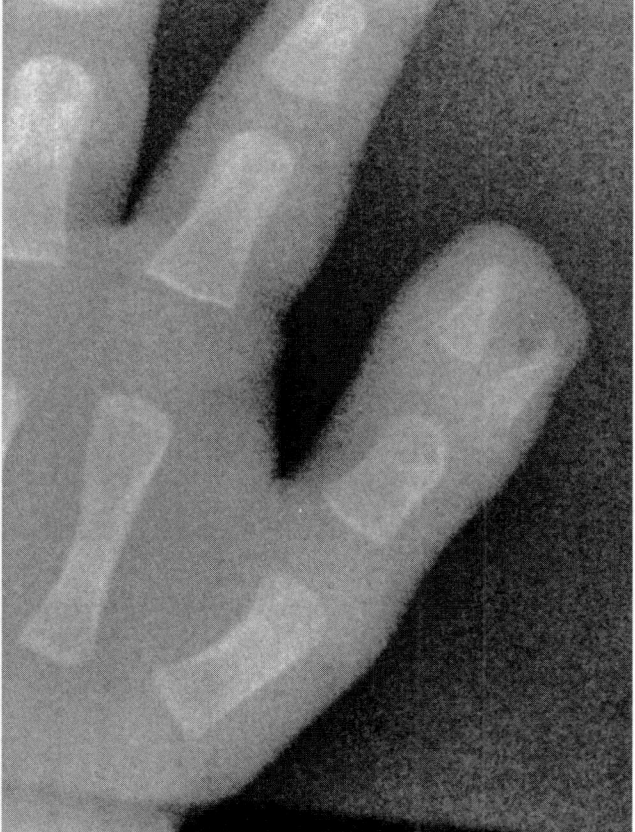

Figure 6–361. Duplication of the terminal phalanges of the thumbs.

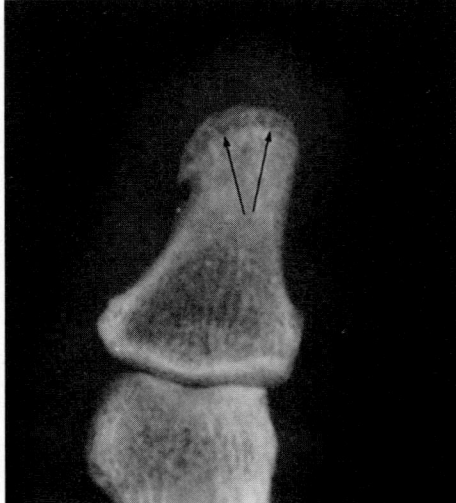

Figure 6–362. Soft tissue laceration simulating fracture of the ungual tuft.

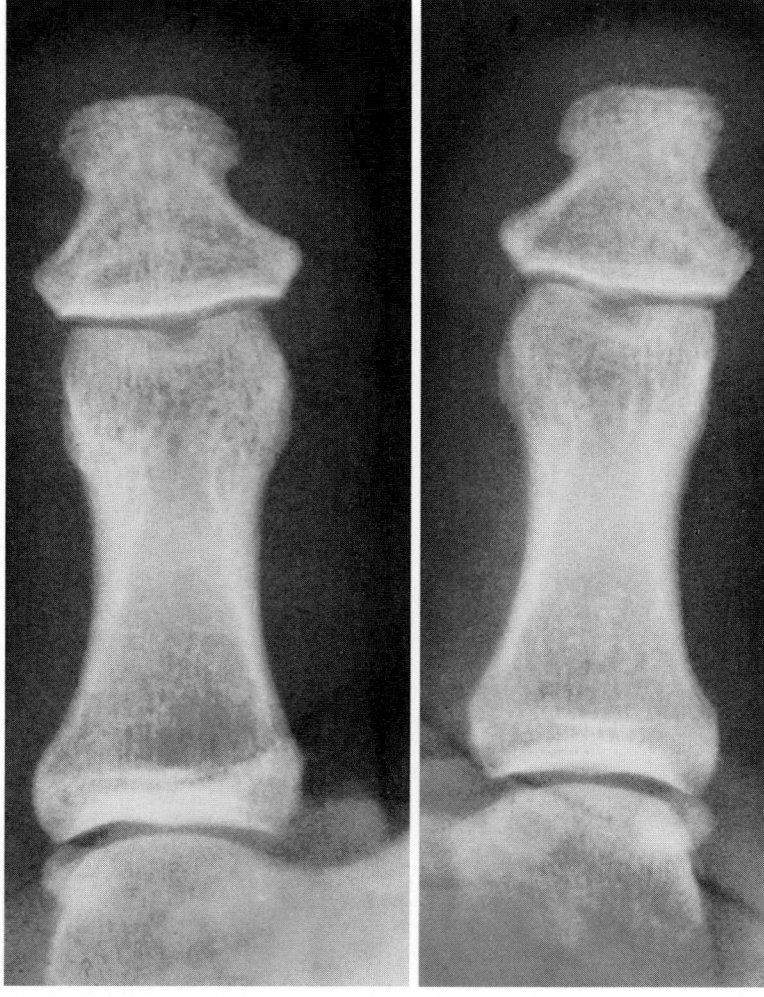

Figure 6–363. Familial broad thumbs. Short, broad, distal phalanges of the thumbs are often seen in malformation syndromes but may also occur as normal familial traits.

Figure 6–364. Sclerosis of the terminal phalanges is seen in the collagen diseases but may also occur in normal individuals, usually in females over 40 years of age. (Ref: Goodman N: The significance of terminal phalangeal osteosclerosis. *Radiology* 89:709, 1967.) The sclerosis begins early in adult life and regresses with old age. (Ref: Fischer E: Akroostiosklerose der finger, cine normale geschlects und altersabbangige endostale reaktion. *ROFO* 137:384, 1982.)

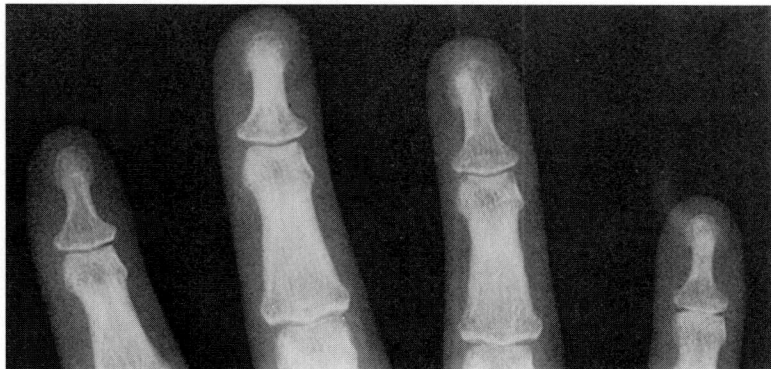

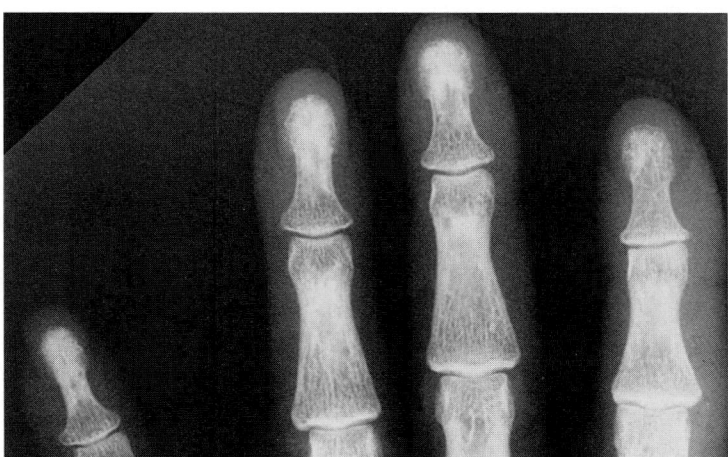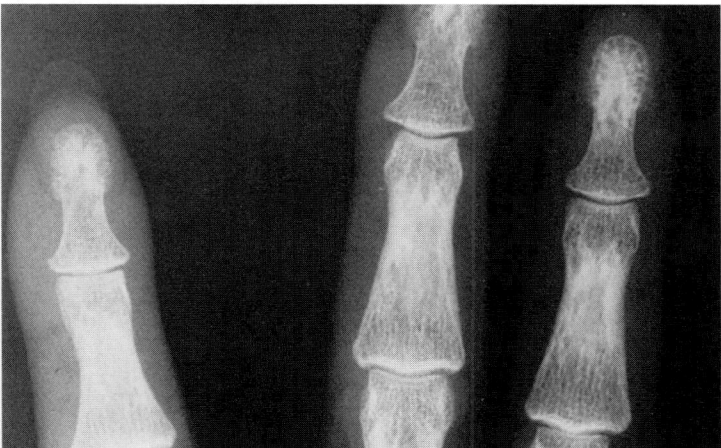

Figure 6–365. Bilateral terminal phalangeal sclerosis with varied degrees of involvement in a 60-year-old woman.

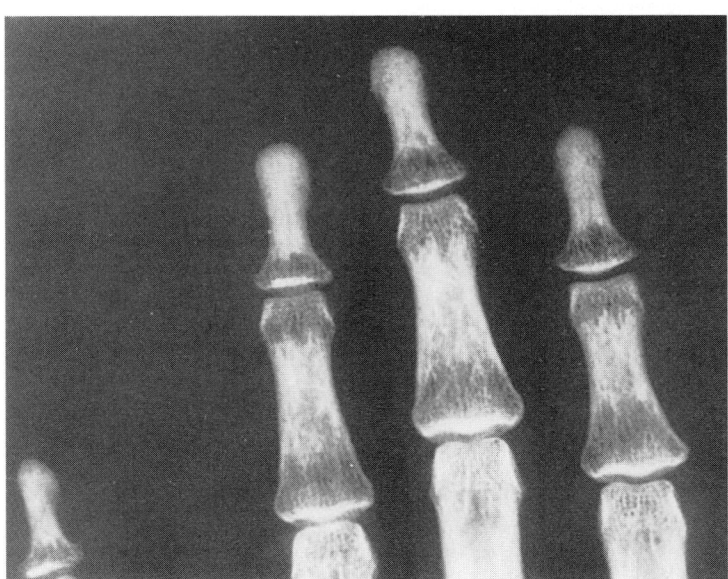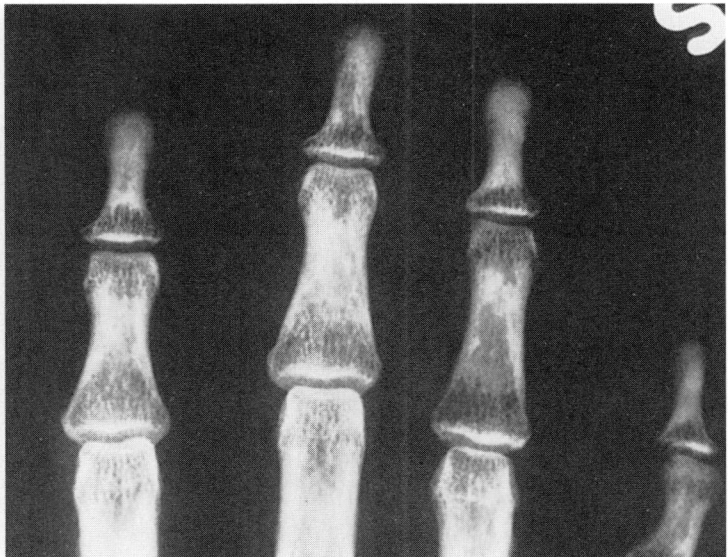

Figure 6–366. Persistence of terminal phalangeal sclerosis in an 80-year-old woman.

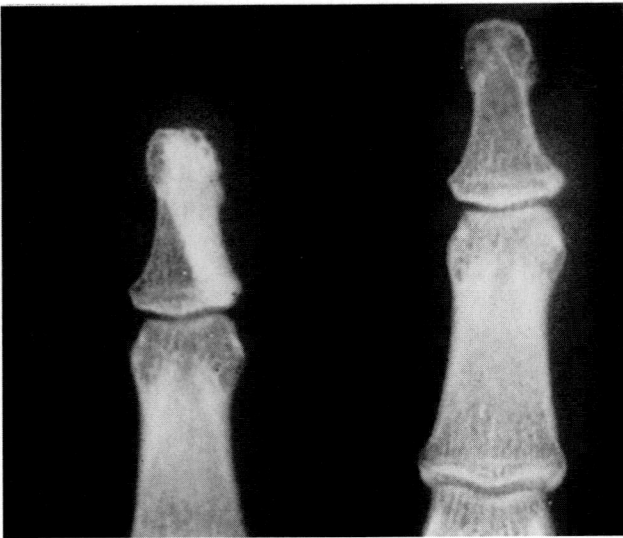

Figure 6–367. Terminal phalangeal sclerosis of a single digit.

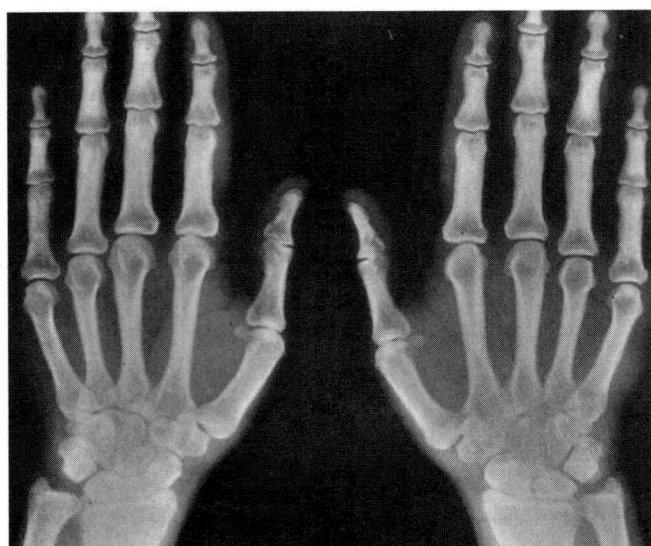

Figure 6–368. Sclerosis of all digits in a healthy 45-year-old woman.

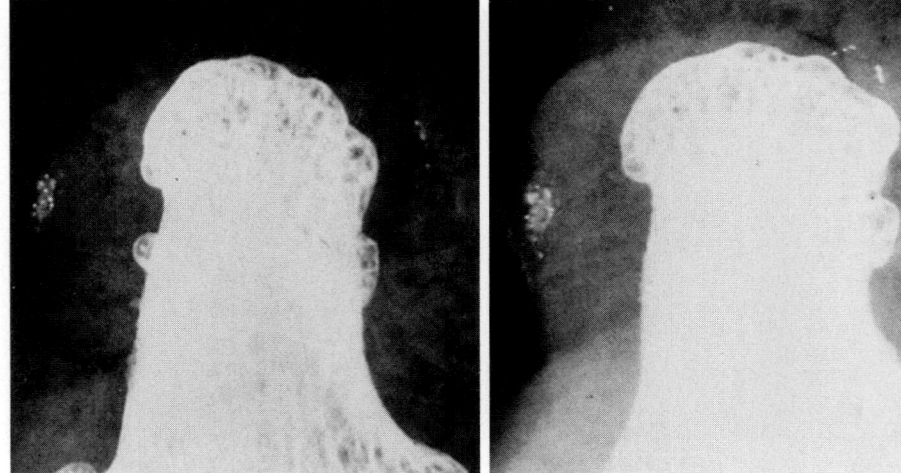

Figure 6–369. Soft-tissue calcification of the distal phalanges of the fingers, a finding of no clinical significance that may result from mechanical injury. (From Fischer E: Weichteilverkalkungen am rand der uberositas phalangis distalis der finger. *ROFO* 139:150, 1983.)

CHAPTER

7

The Lower Extremity

The Thigh

The Femoral Head and Hip Joint

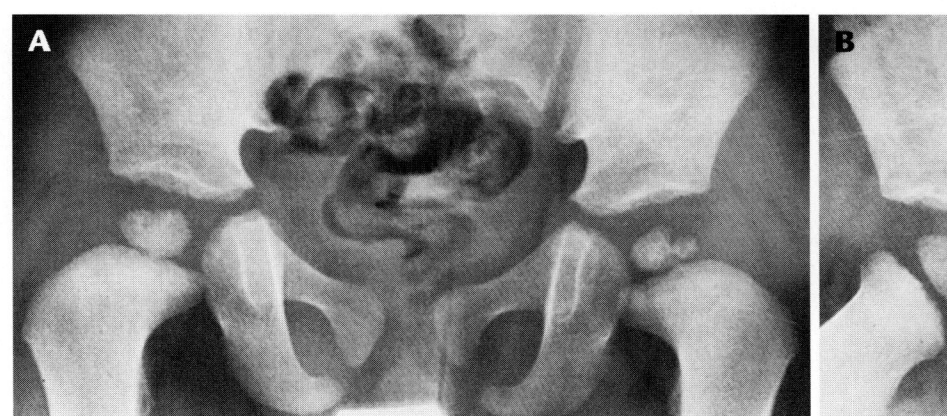
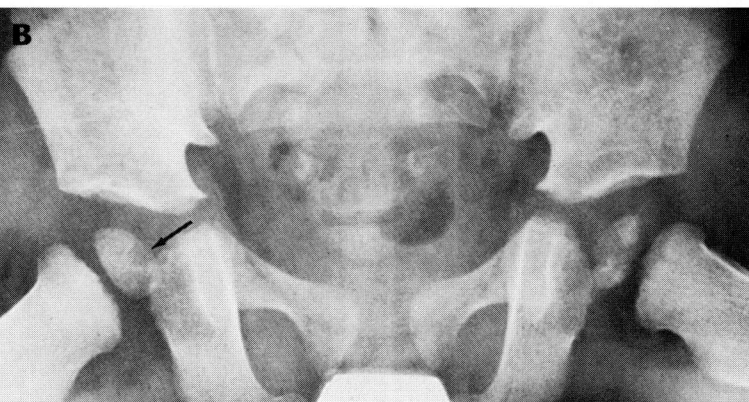

Figure 7–1. This 2-year-old infant has Perthes disease on his left side. However, the defect in the head of the right hip is a developmental variant, not incipient osteochondritis. **A,** Hips in neutral position. **B,** Hips in abduction. (Ref: Katz JF: "Abortive" Legg-Calvé-Perthes' disease or developmental variation in epiphysiogenesis of upper femur. *J Mount Sinai Hosp N Y* 132:651, 1965.)

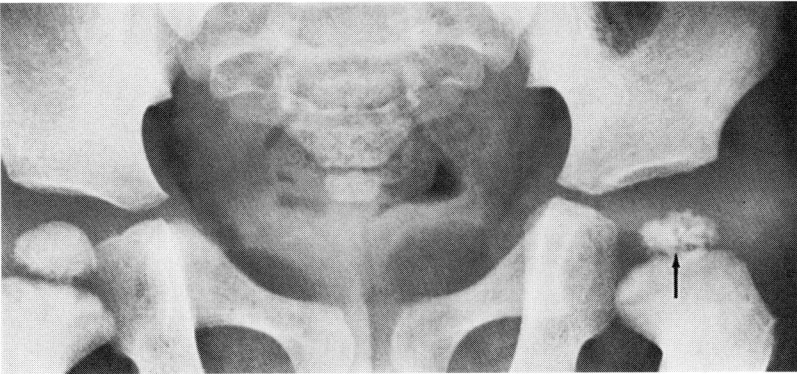

Figure 7–2. Normal irregular mineralization of the ossification center of one femoral head. This appearance in a single center in a young infant does not necessarily indicate disease. (Ref: Caffey J: *Pediatric x-ray diagnosis*, 9th ed. St. Louis, Mosby, 1993, p. 1497.)

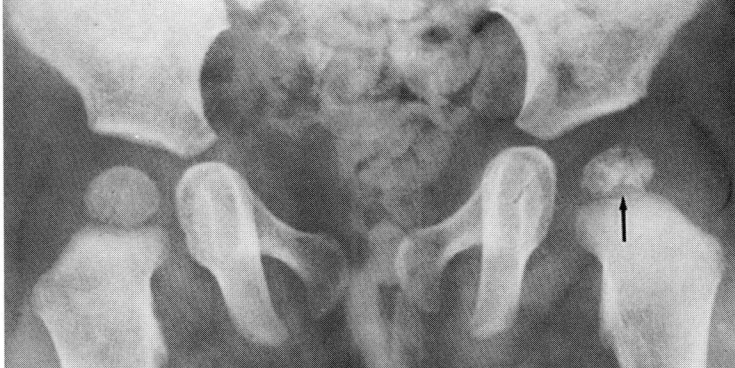

Figure 7–3. Normal stippled appearance of one ossification center in a 10-month-old infant. These centers evolve to normal contour with further growth. (Ref: Lemperg R et al: Asymmetry of the epiphyseal nucleus in the femoral head in stable and unstable hip joints. *Pediatr Radiol* 1:191, 1973.)

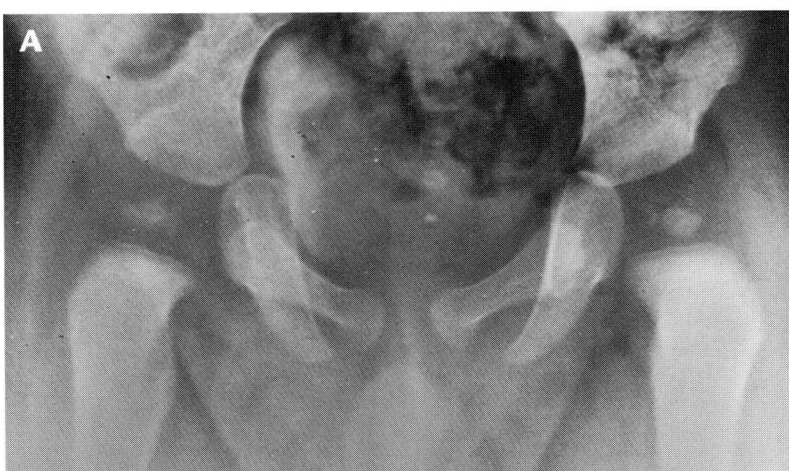
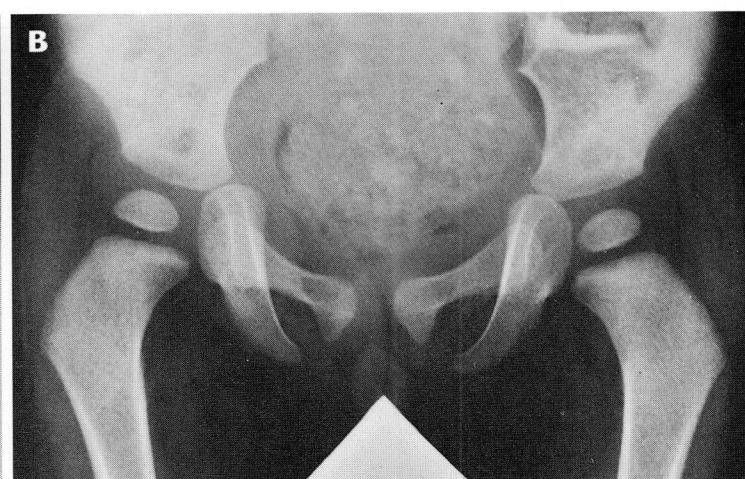

Figure 7–4. Bilateral stippled appearance of the capital femoral epiphyses with progression to normal appearance. **A,** 18 months of age. **B,** 30 months of age.

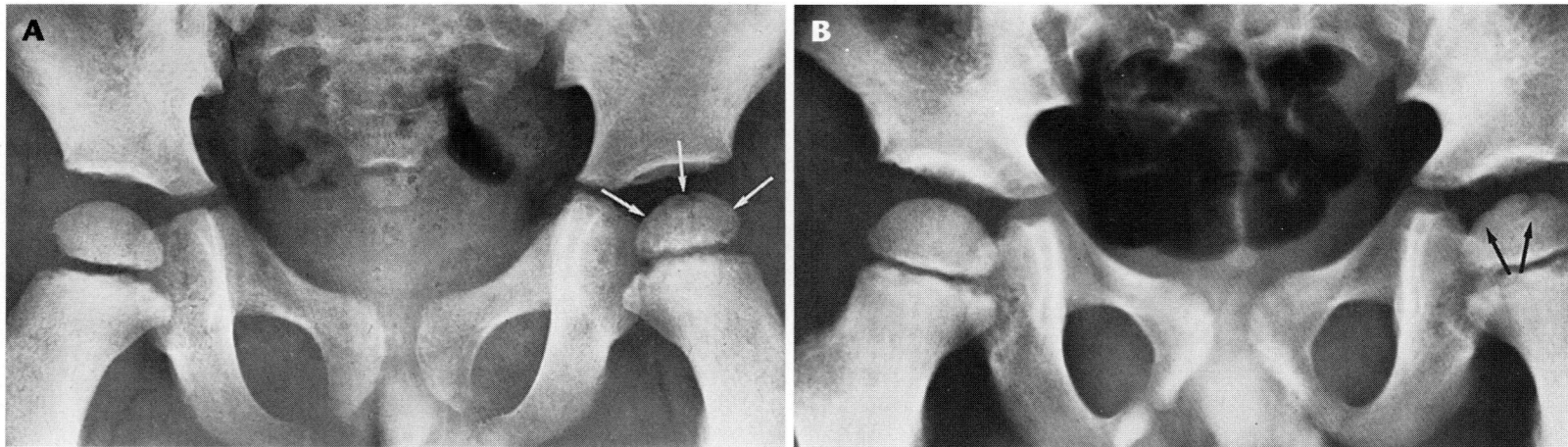

Figure 7–5. Two examples of normal developmental irregularity of the femoral heads in children without hip symptoms. **A,** 3-year-old boy. **B,** 4½-year-old boy.

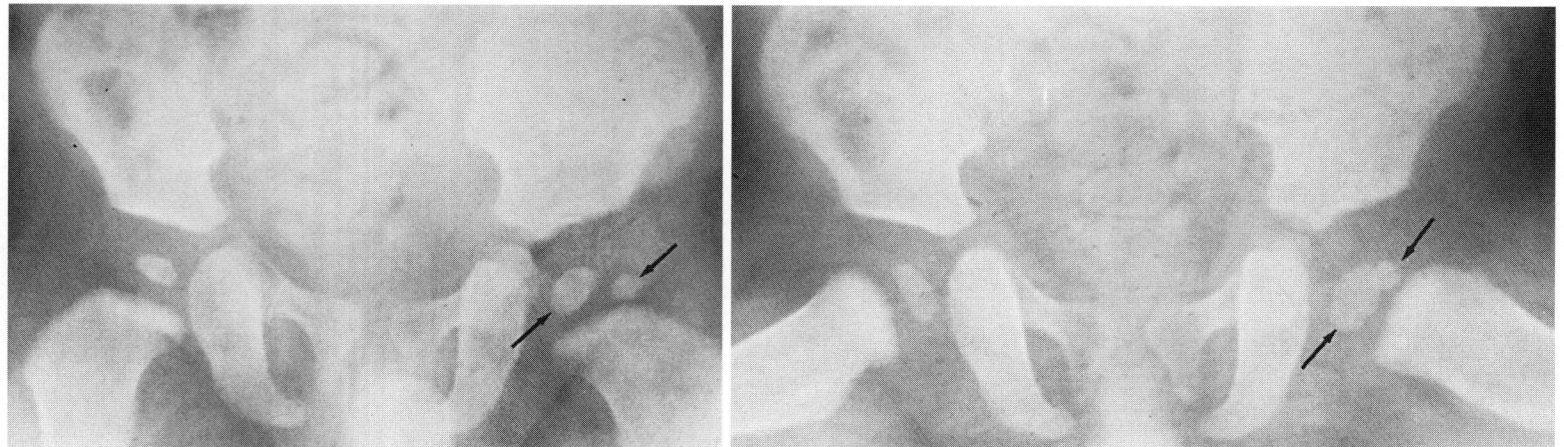

Figure 7–6. Double ossification centers for the capital femoral epiphysis. This is a normal variant, not an indication of disease.

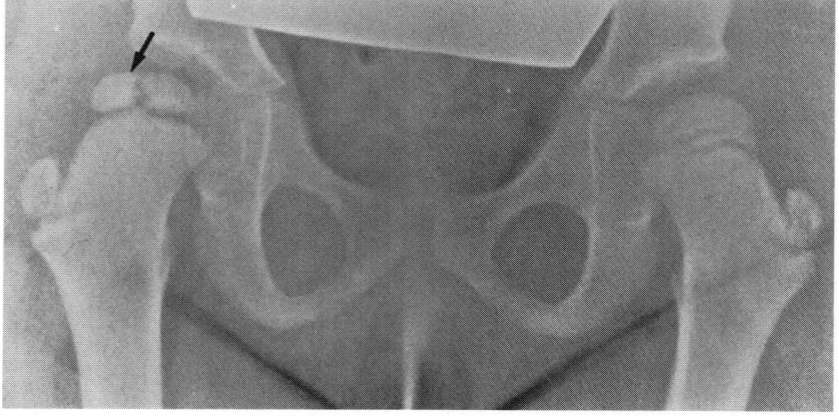

Figure 7–7. Cleft of the proximal femoral epiphysis in a 3-year-old girl.

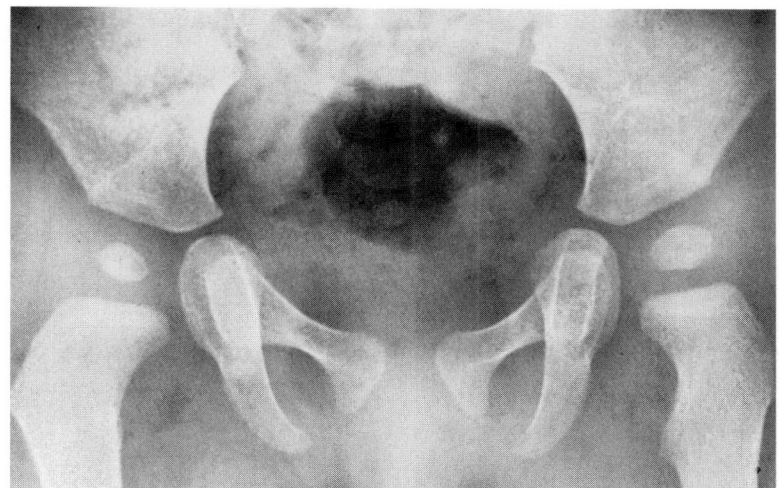

Figure 7–8. Normal asymmetry in size of the ossification centers of the femoral heads may be seen and is not necessarily indicative of congenital dislocation of the femoral head.

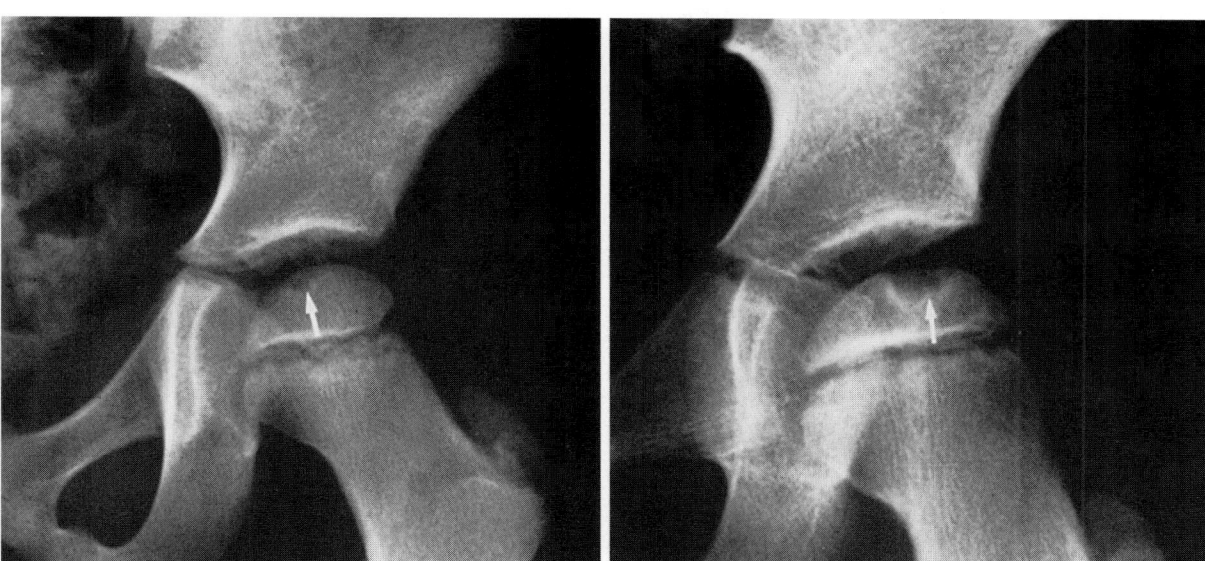

Figure 7–9. The femoral notch in two 9-year-old children. This defect is probably cartilaginous, since it does not communicate with the joint on arthrography. It may be seen as early as 4 years of age and disappears gradually over the course of months or years. (Ref: Ozonoff MB, Ziter FMH Jr: The femoral head notch. *Skeletal Radiol* 16:19, 1987.)

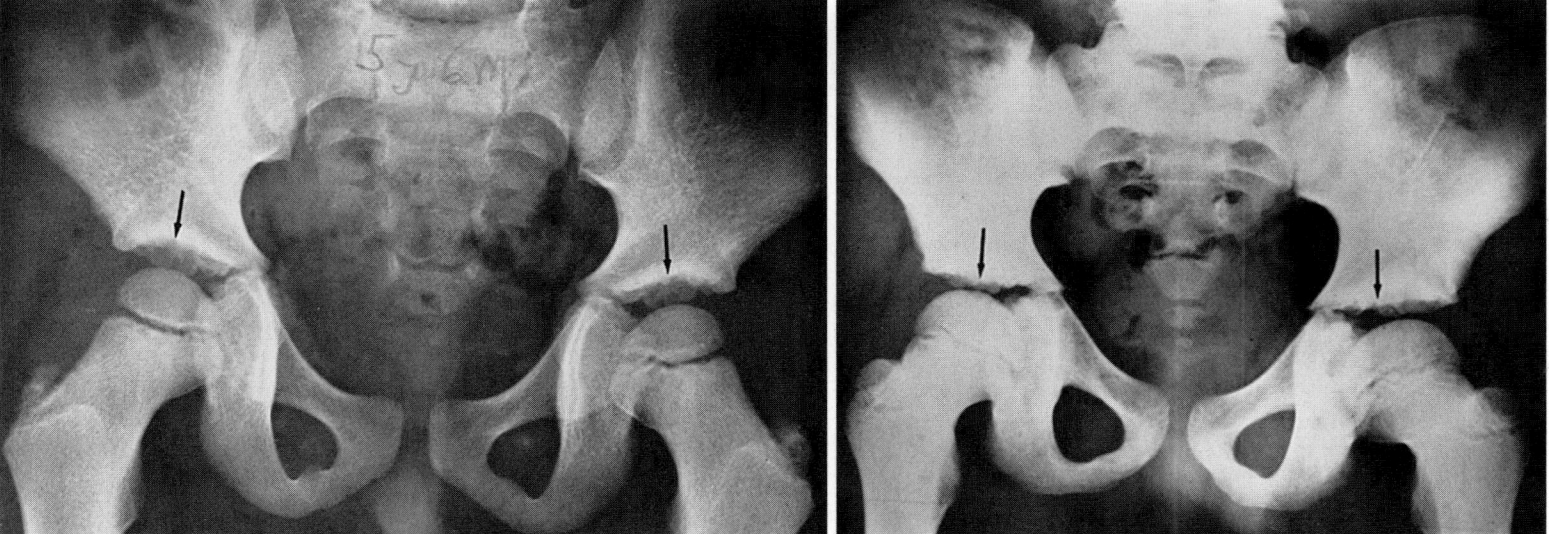

Figure 7–10. Two examples of the normal irregularity of the acetabular roofs in young children. This appearance is normal between the ages of 7 and 12 years.

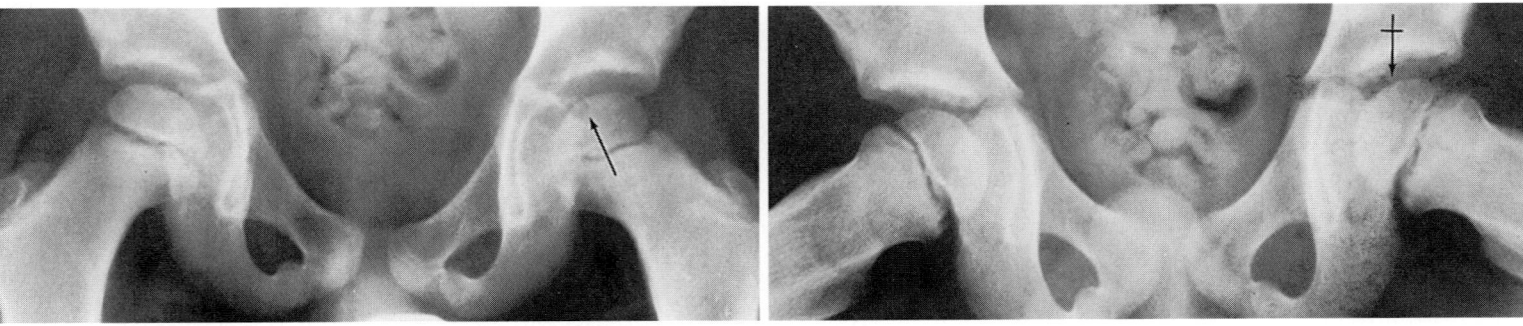

Figure 7–11. Apparent radiolucency of the femoral head in a 5-year-old boy (→) produced by superimposition of the normal irregularities of the acetabulum at this age (↦).

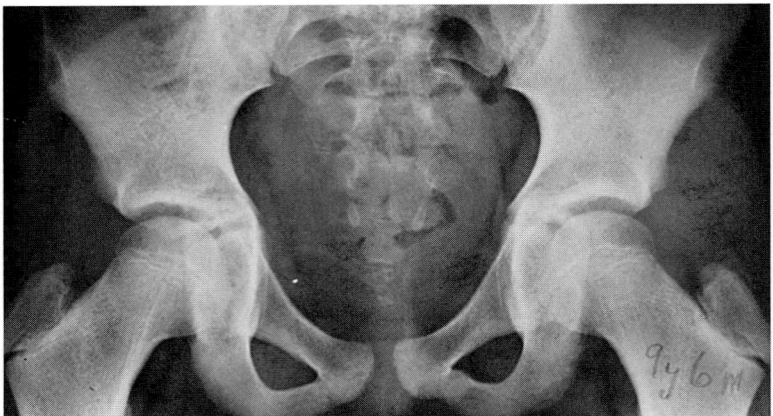

Figure 7–12. Normal intrapelvic protrusion of the acetabula. This is a normal phase of development between 4 and 12 years of age.

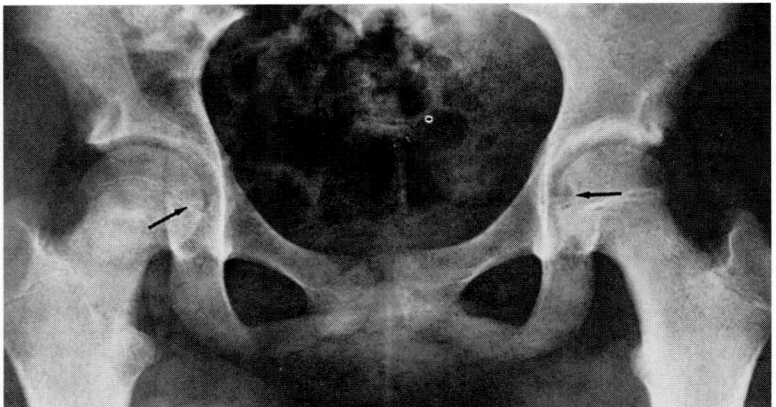

Figure 7–13. The fossa at the entry point of the acetabular nutrient vessels may simulate a destructive lesion of the femoral head.

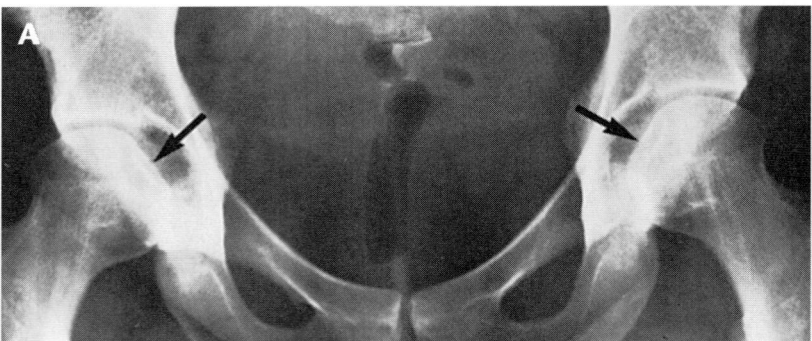

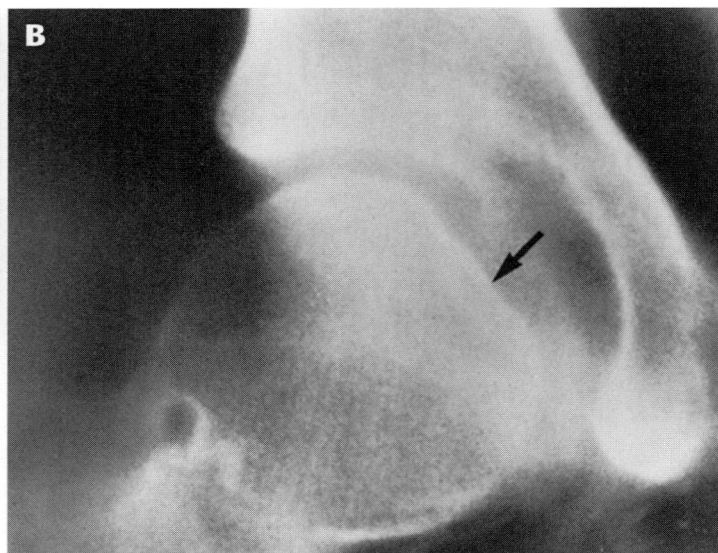

Figure 7–14. A, Unusually large bilateral fovea capitis, which may be mistaken for osteochondritis dissecans. **B,** Tomogram of right hip.

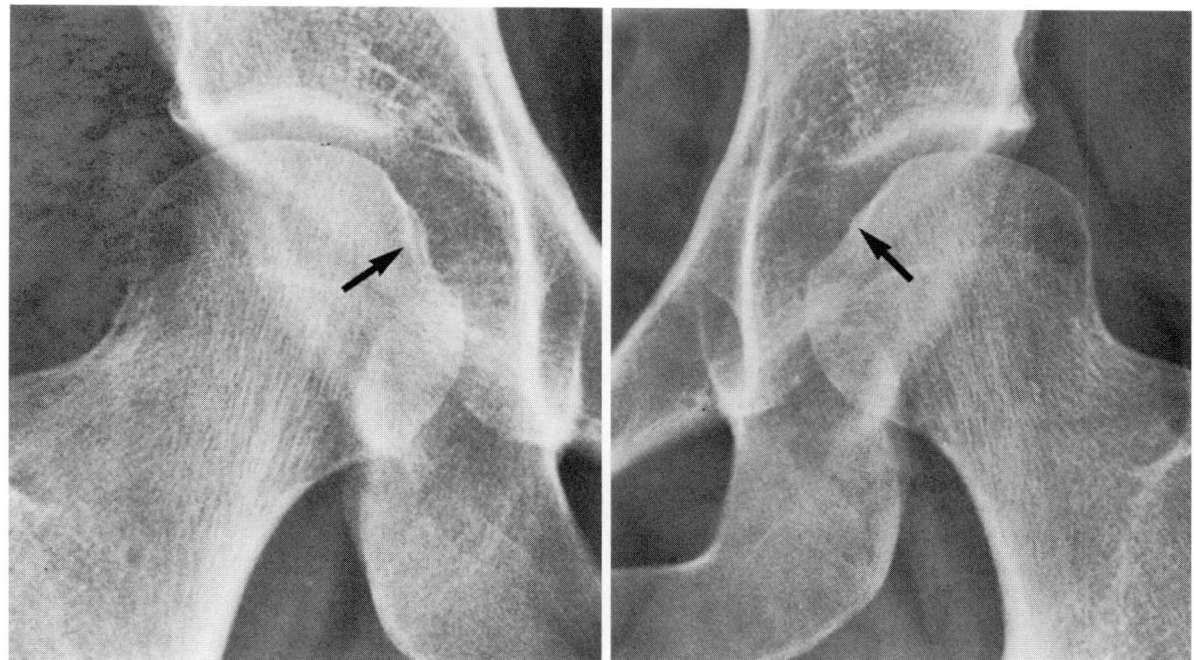

Figure 7–15. The same entity shown in Figure 7–14 in a 20-year-old man.

Figure 7–16. Large fovea capitis in a 26-year-old man.

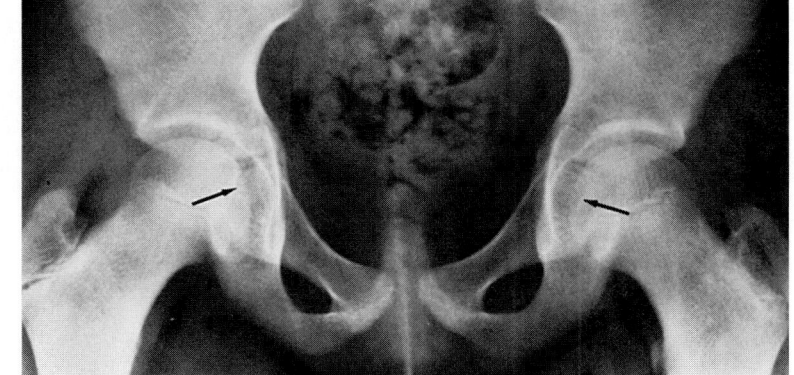

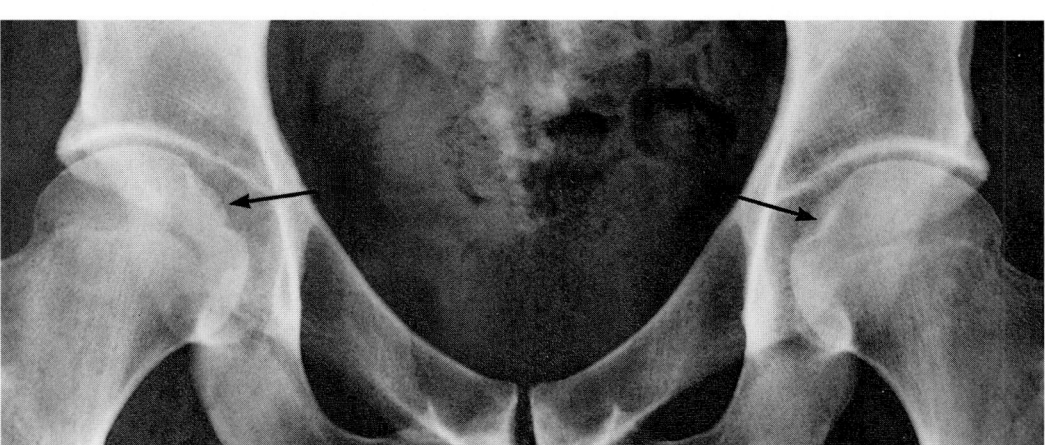

Figure 7–17. Normal asymmetry of the fovea capitis.

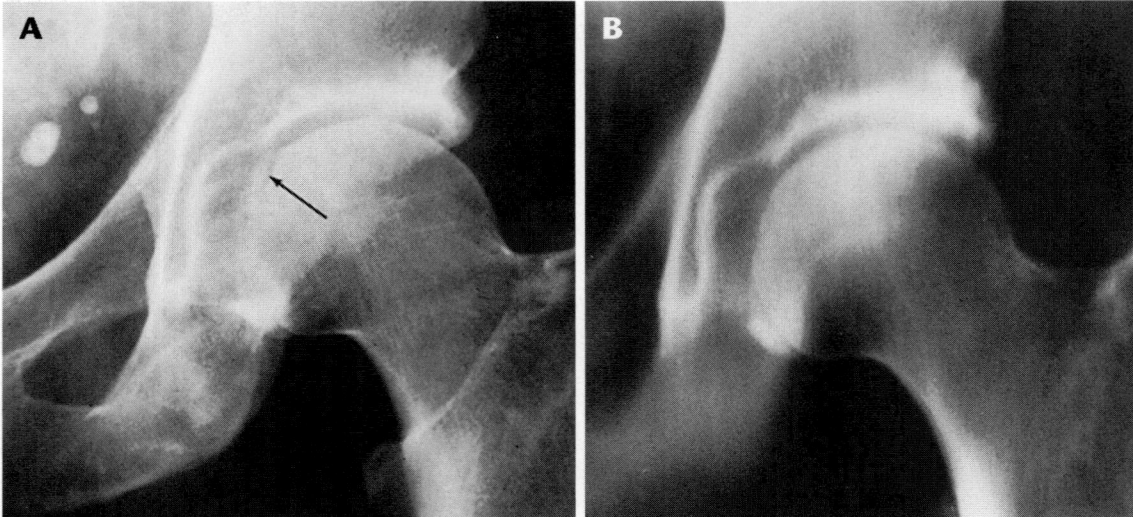

Figure 7–18. Simulated fracture or aseptic necrosis of the femoral head produced by the fovea capitis. **A,** Plain film. **B,** Tomogram. No fracture seen.

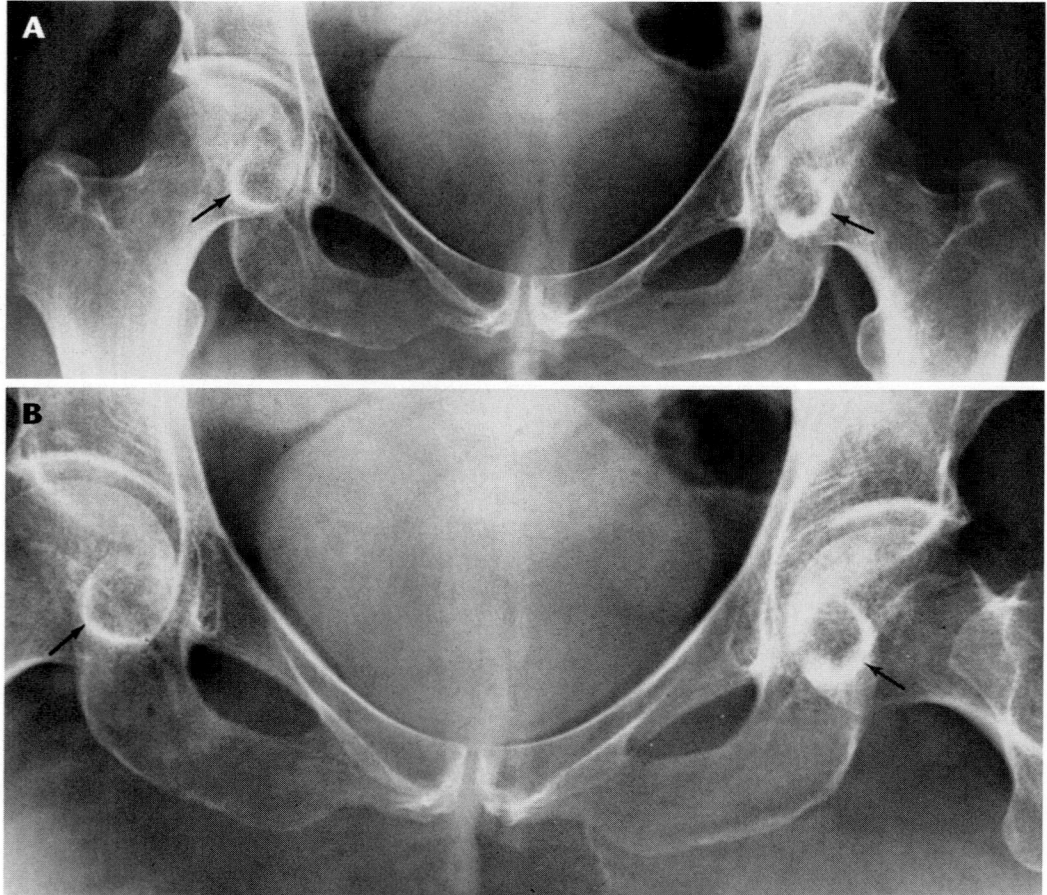

Figure 7–19. Simulated destructive lesions of the femoral heads produced by superimposition of the acetabular bone on the femoral head. **A,** Hips in neutral position. **B,** Hips in abduction.

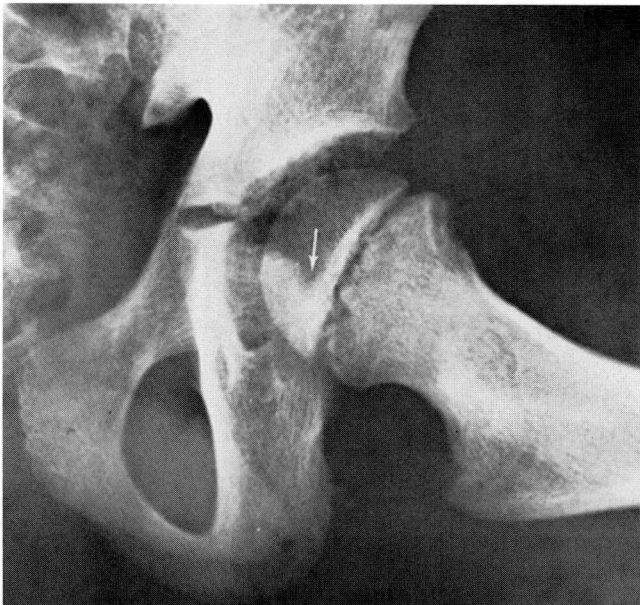

Figure 7–20. The shadow of the posterior acetabular margin superimposed on the femoral head may simulate the density of aseptic necrosis.

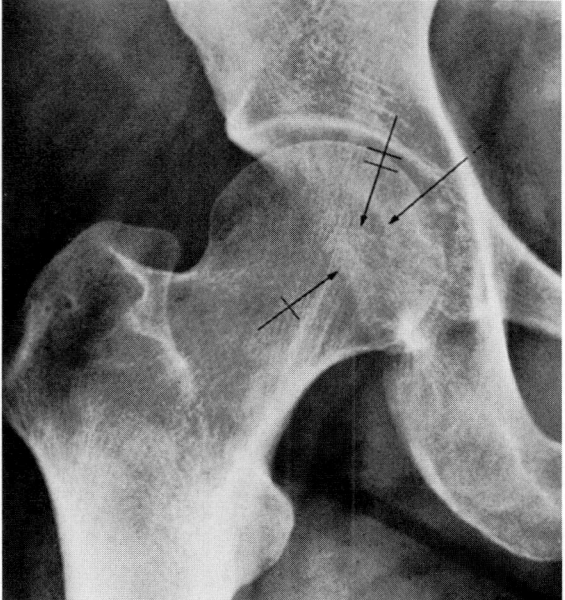

Figure 7–21. The lucent interval between the anterior (→) and the posterior lips of the acetabulum (↦) may simulate a lucent lesion of the femoral head (⊬).

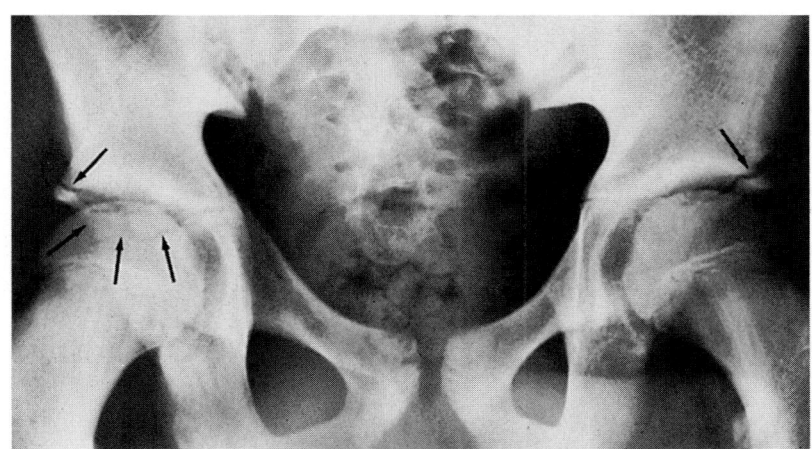

Figure 7–22. Ossification centers for the acetabulum, which may simulate fractures of the femoral head, in a 14-year-old boy.

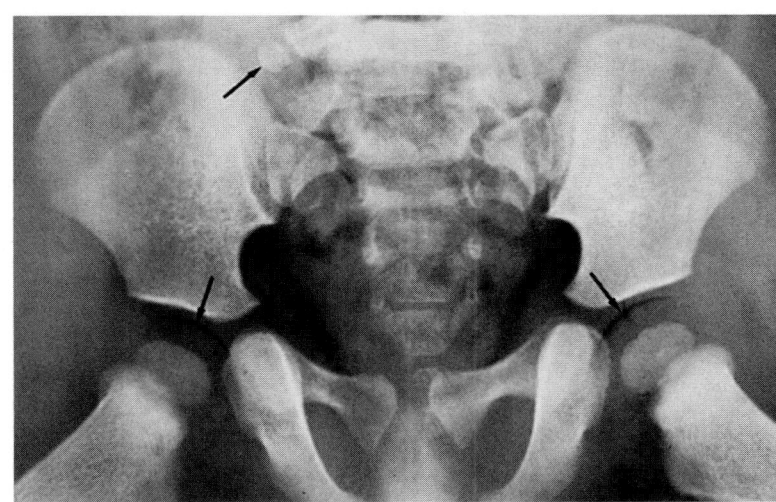

Figure 7–23. The "vacuum" phenomenon in normal hips of a 6-month-old child. The upper arrow indicates an accessory ossification center for the transverse process of L5.

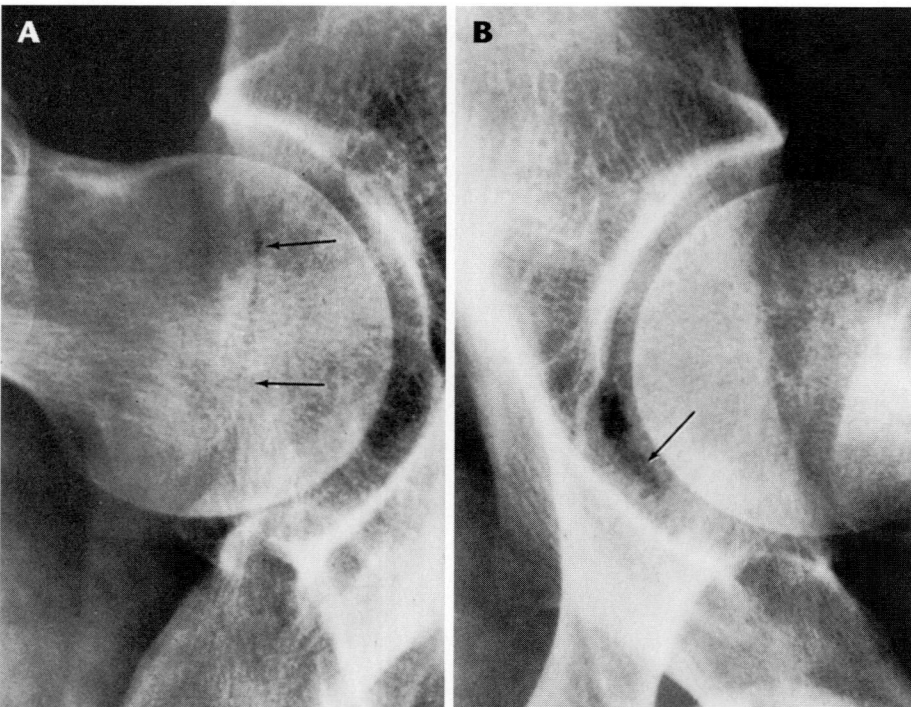

Figure 7–24. A, B, "Vacuum" phenomenon in the hips of an adult. Note how the radiolucency in **A** resembles a fracture line.

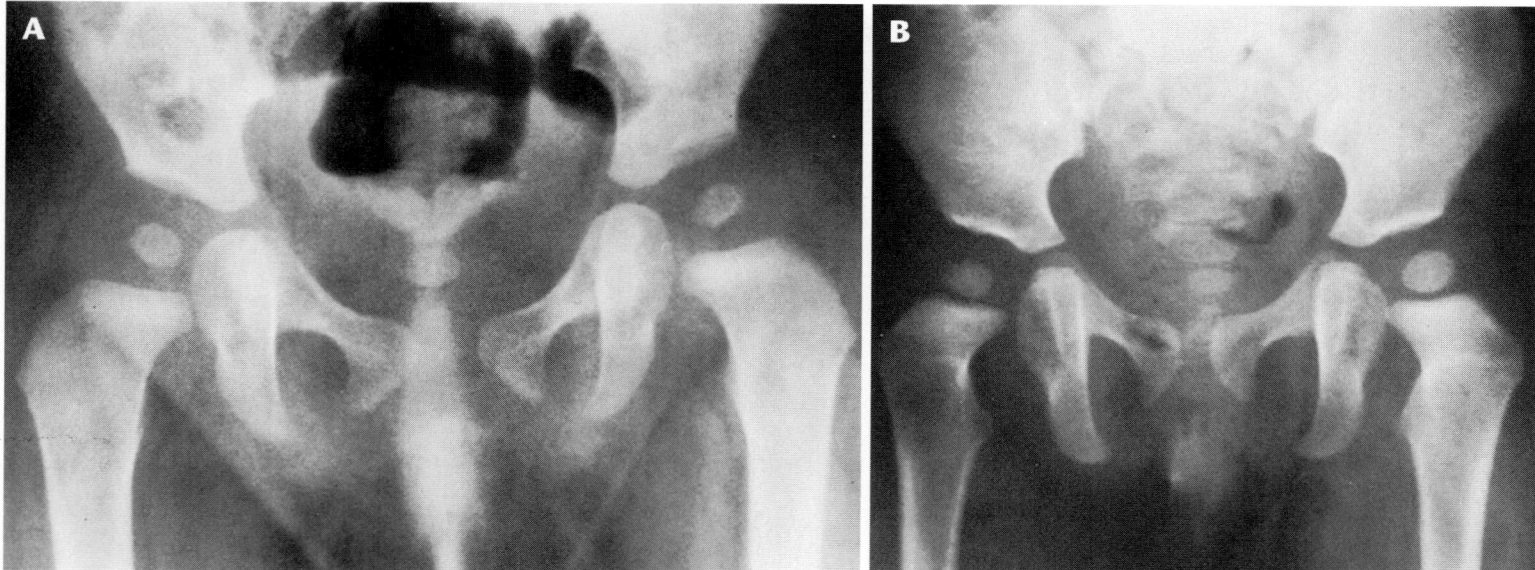

Figure 7–25. Two examples of the unreliability of Shenton's line after the newborn period. **A,** 5 month-old infant. **B,** 1-year-old child. Note particularly the asymmetry of the lines in **A.**

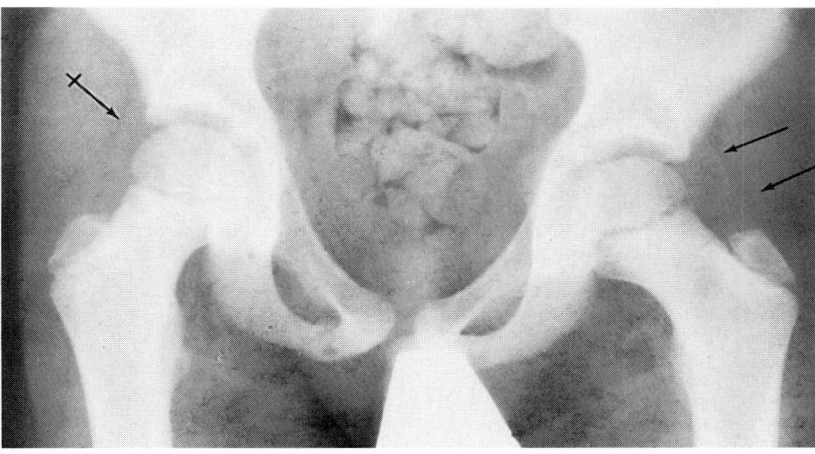

Figure 7–26. Apparent bulging of the hip "capsule," suggesting synovitis or hemarthrosis, may be produced by filming the hip in abduction and external rotation, as in this 6-year-old boy (→). Note normal fat lines on opposite side (↦). (Ref: Brown I: A study of the "capsular" shadow in disorders of the hip in children. *J Bone Joint Surg* 57B:175, 1975.)

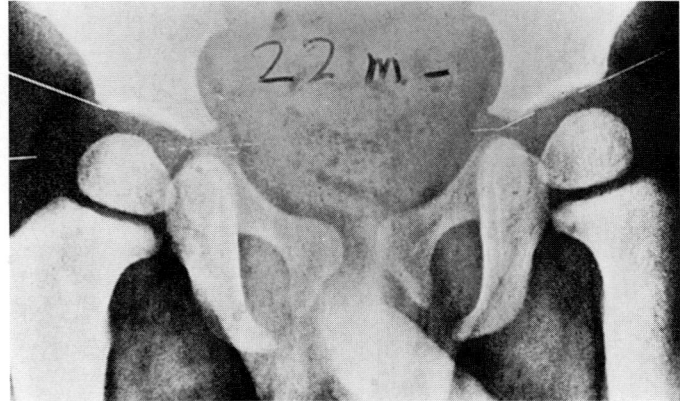

Figure 7–27. Plump femoral heads in a 22-month-old infant. (Courtesy of Dr. Clement Fauré.)

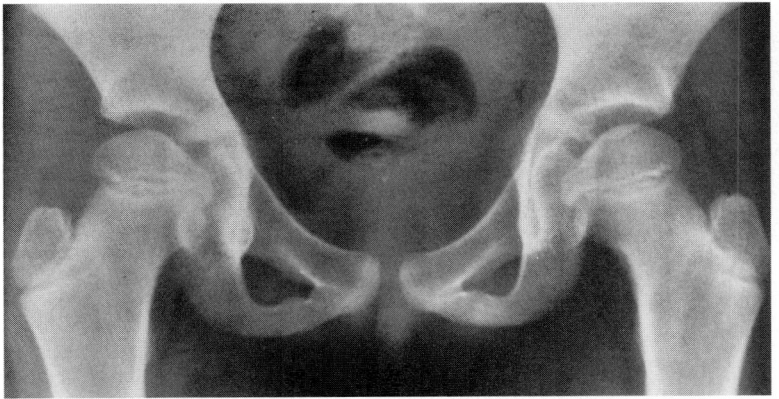

Figure 7–28. Variation in the configuration of the femoral heads in a 5-year-old child.

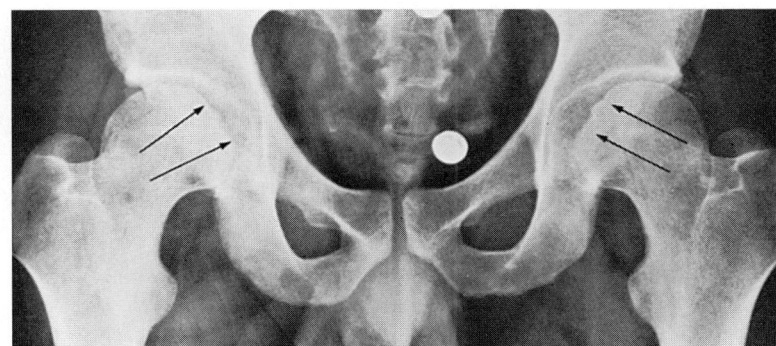

Figure 7–29. Unusual configuration of the femoral heads in a 26-year-old man, probably fovea capitis.

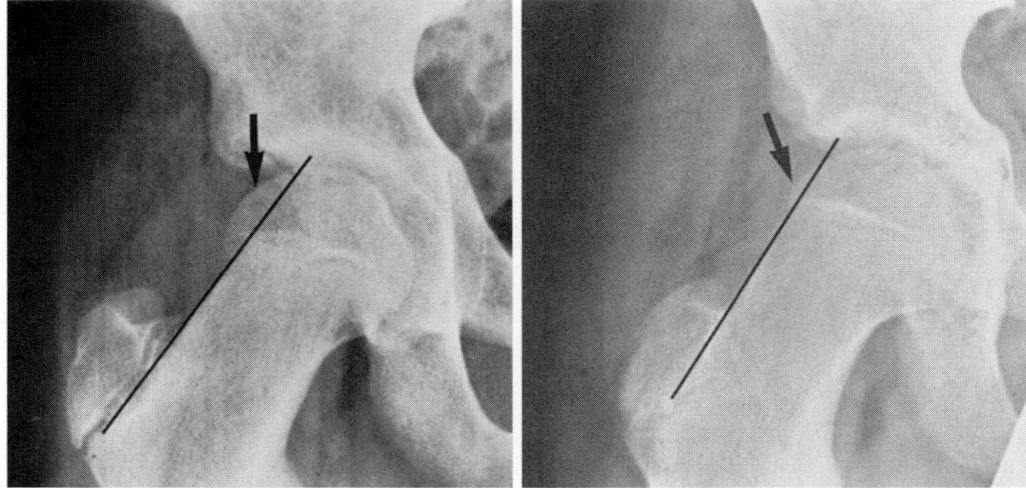

Figure 7–30. In using the line drawn along the femoral necks for the detection of slipped capital femoral epiphysis, note that there is great normal variability in the amount of femoral head that is intersected. This is illustrated in these two adolescent boys.

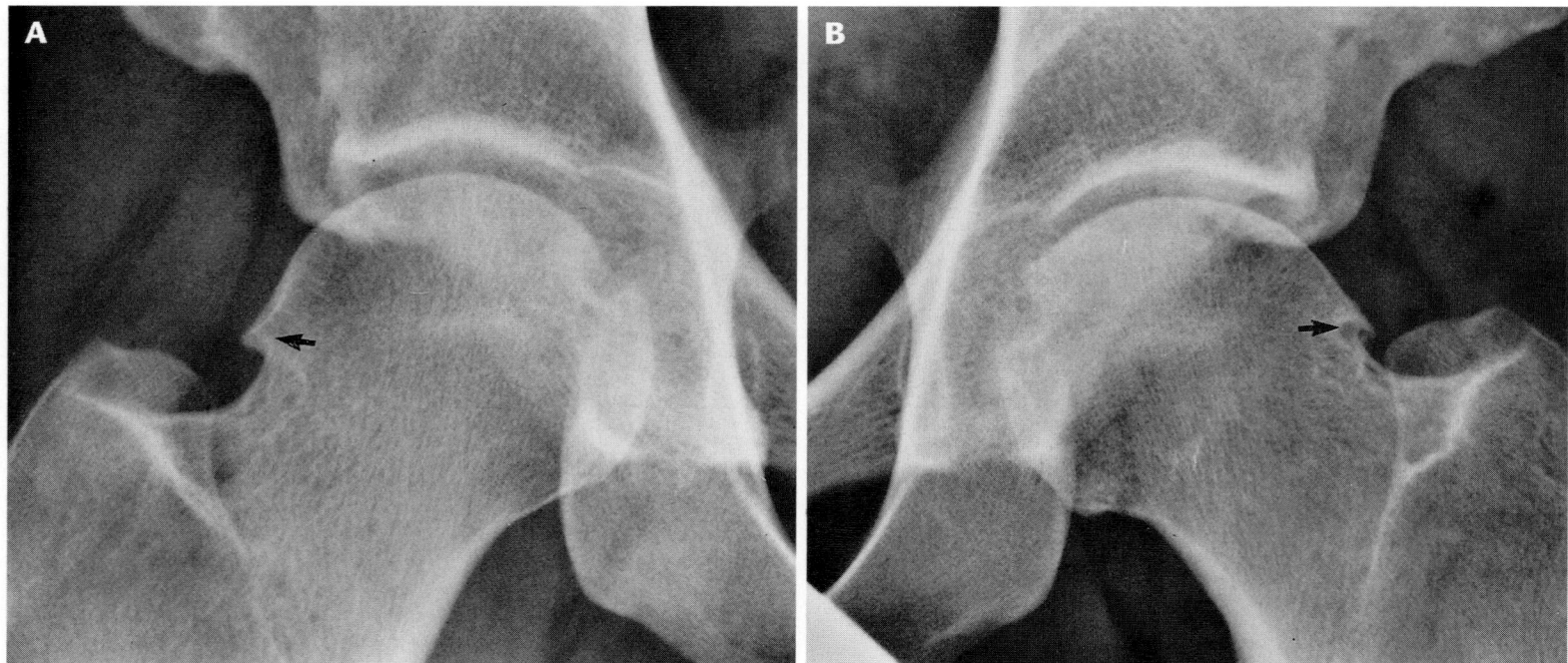

Figure 7–31. A, B, Bilateral developmental spurs at the edge of the closed physis in a 30-year-old man, possible remnants of epiphyseal spurs.

The Femoral Neck

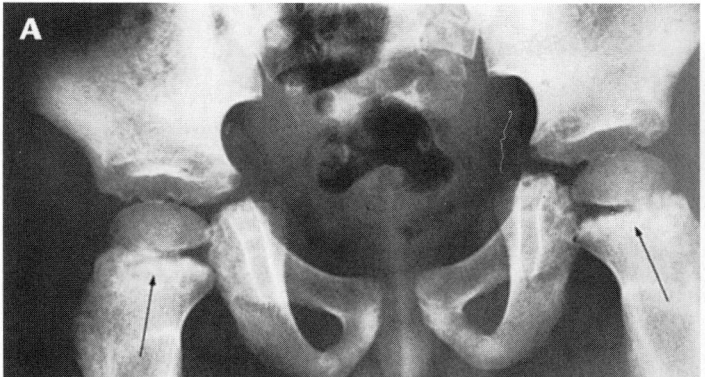
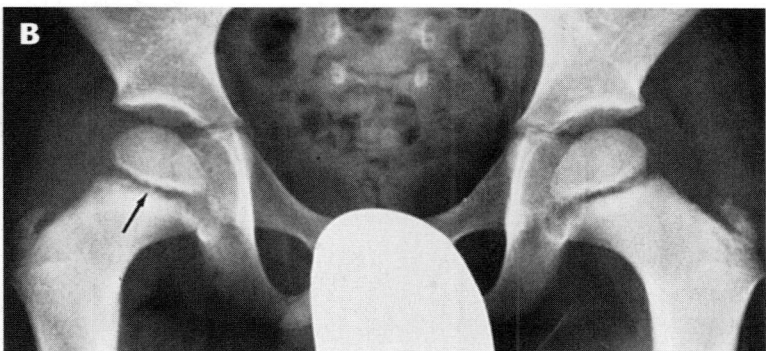

Figure 7–32. Normal irregularities of the metaphyseal bone at the epiphyseal line in early childhood. **A,** 4-year-old girl. **B,** 5-year-old boy.

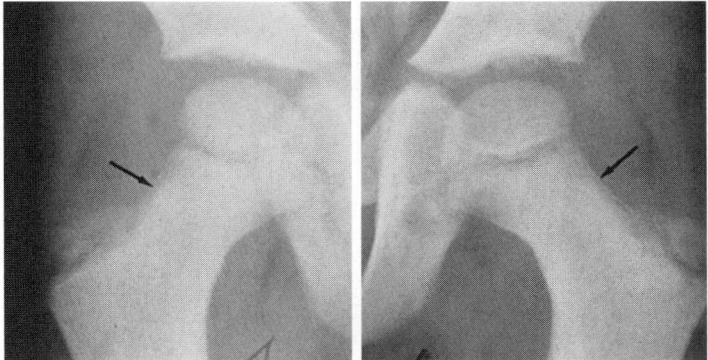

Figure 7–33. Normal double contour effect of cortex of superior aspect of the femoral neck in a 4-year-old boy. This is a common appearance in children of this age.

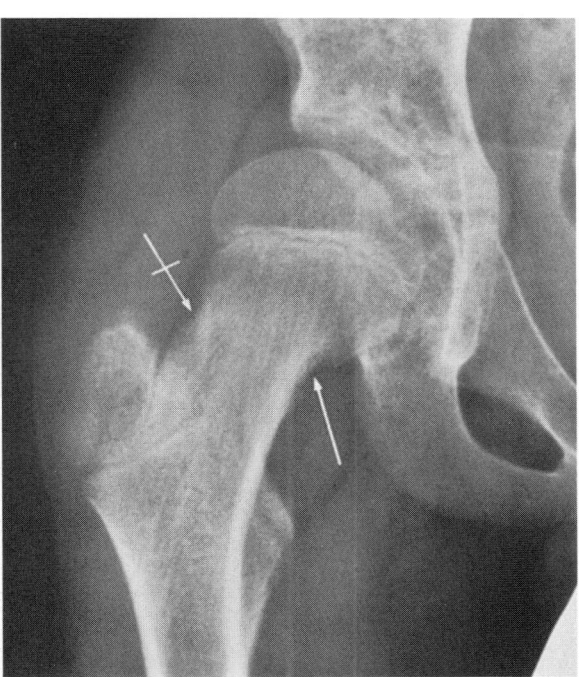

Figure 7–34. The upper femoral notch (←) in a 13-year-old boy. This is probably the same lesion seen in the humeral neck and other metaphyseal sites. The lesion disappears with growth and is of no significance. Note the poor definition of the upper margin of the femoral neck (↔), also a normal appearance at this age. (Ref: Ozonoff MB, Ziter FMH Jr: The upper femoral notch. *Skeletal Radiol* 14:198, 1985.)

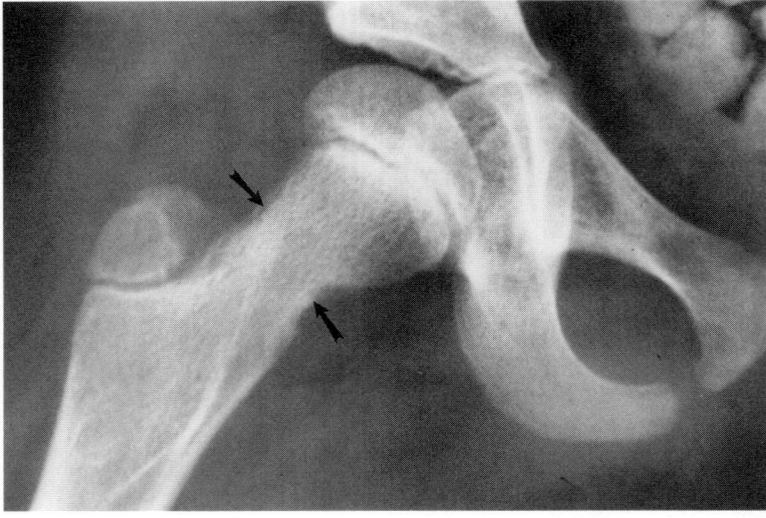
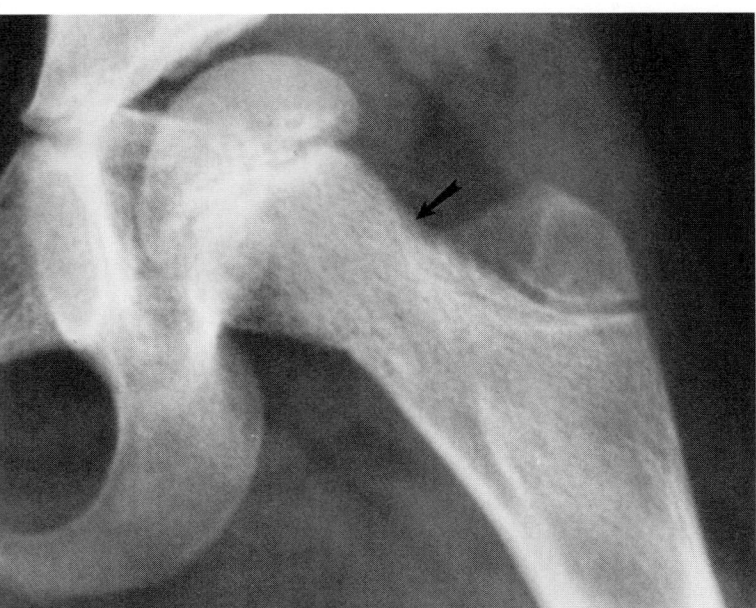

Figure 7–35. An additional example of the same entities described in Figure 7–34, seen bilaterally in a 12-year-old boy.

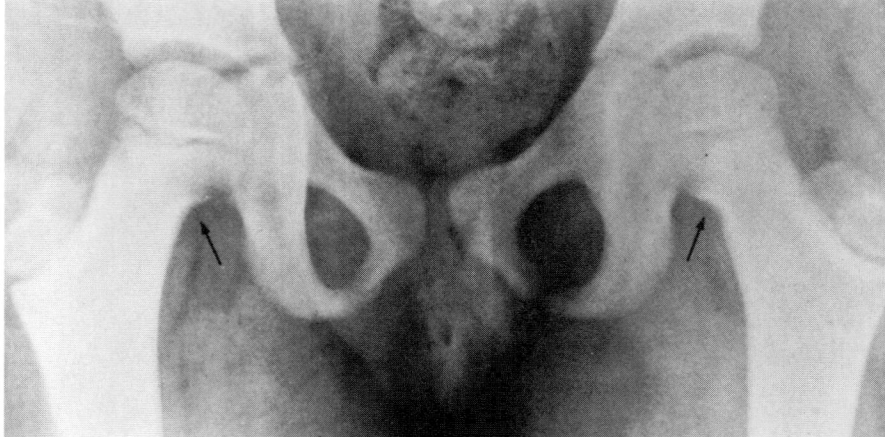
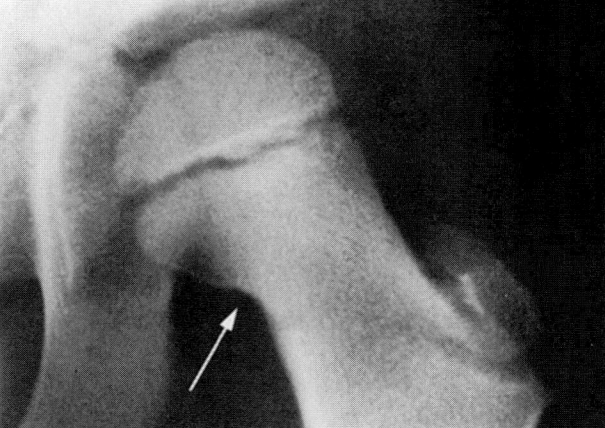

Figure 7–36. Two additional examples of the upper femoral notch.

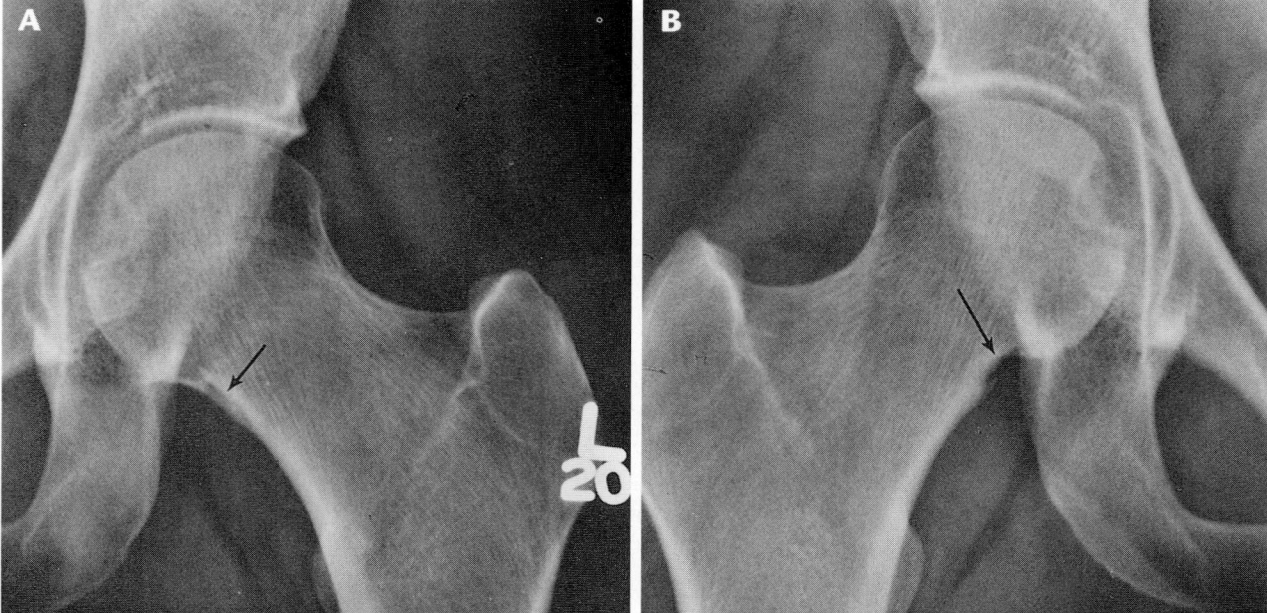

Figure 7–37. A, B, Probable residuals of the upper femoral notches in a 35-year-old woman.

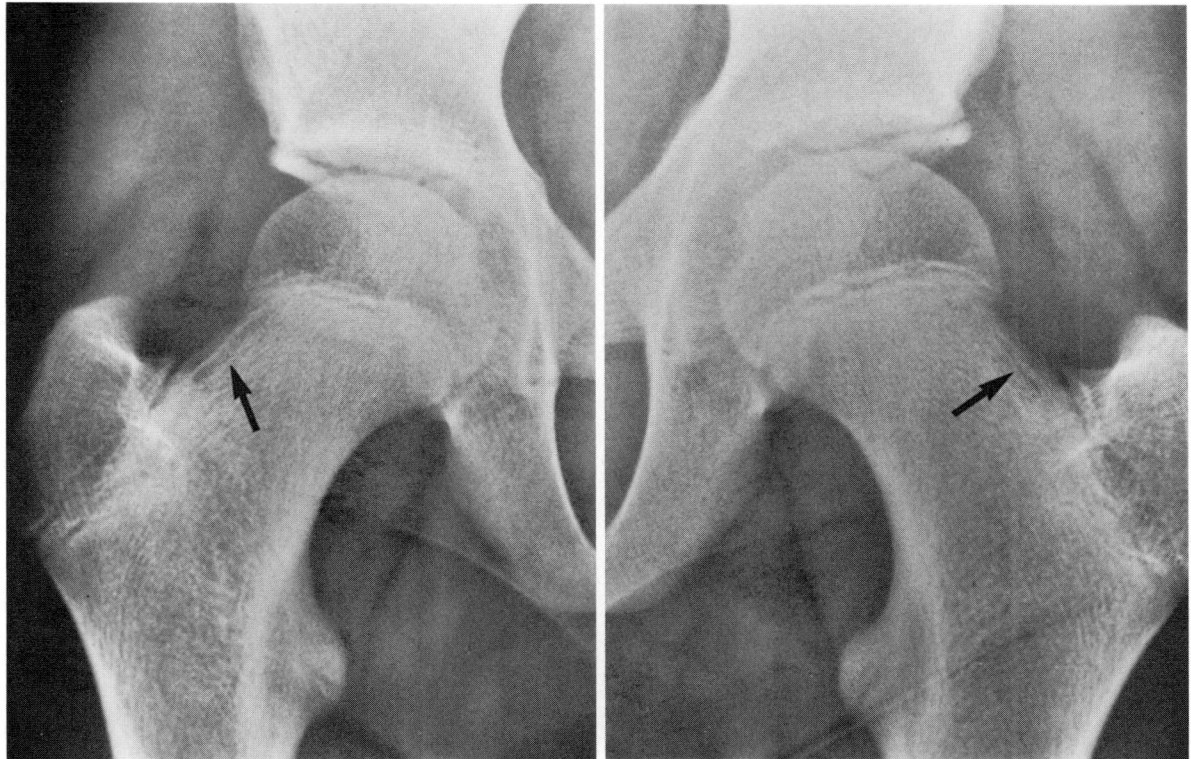

Figure 7–38. Normal irregularities and lucencies in the femoral necks of an 11-year-old boy.

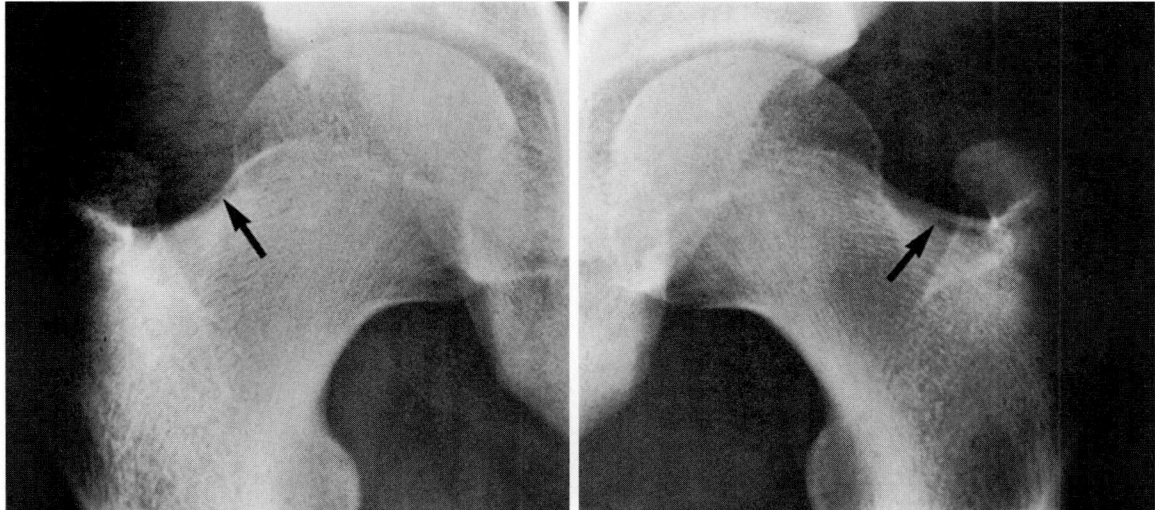

Figure 7–39. Normal lucencies in the femoral necks in a 16-year-old boy.

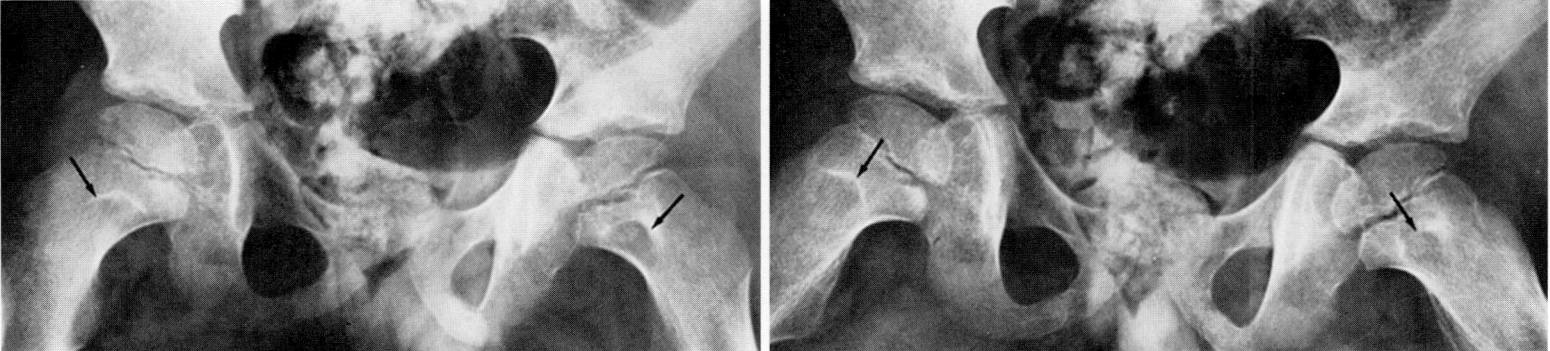

Figure 7–40. Normal lucencies in the necks of the femora (Ward's triangle) formed by the angle of the trabeculae in the neck of the femur.

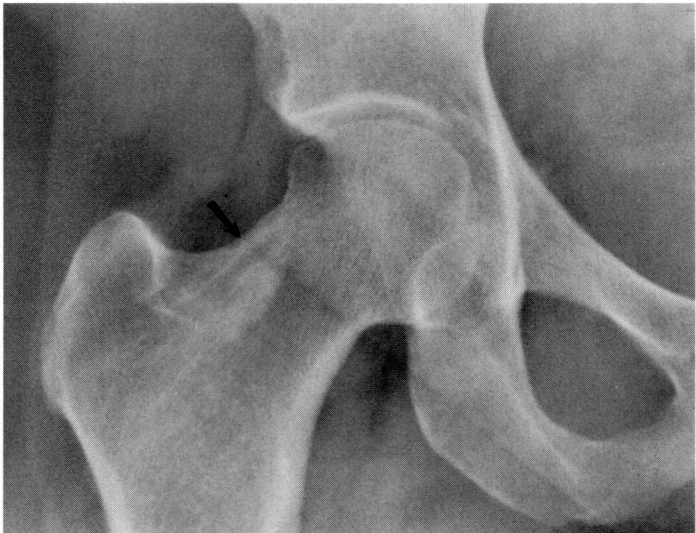

Figure 7–41. Simulated erosion of the right femoral neck in a 50-year-old man.

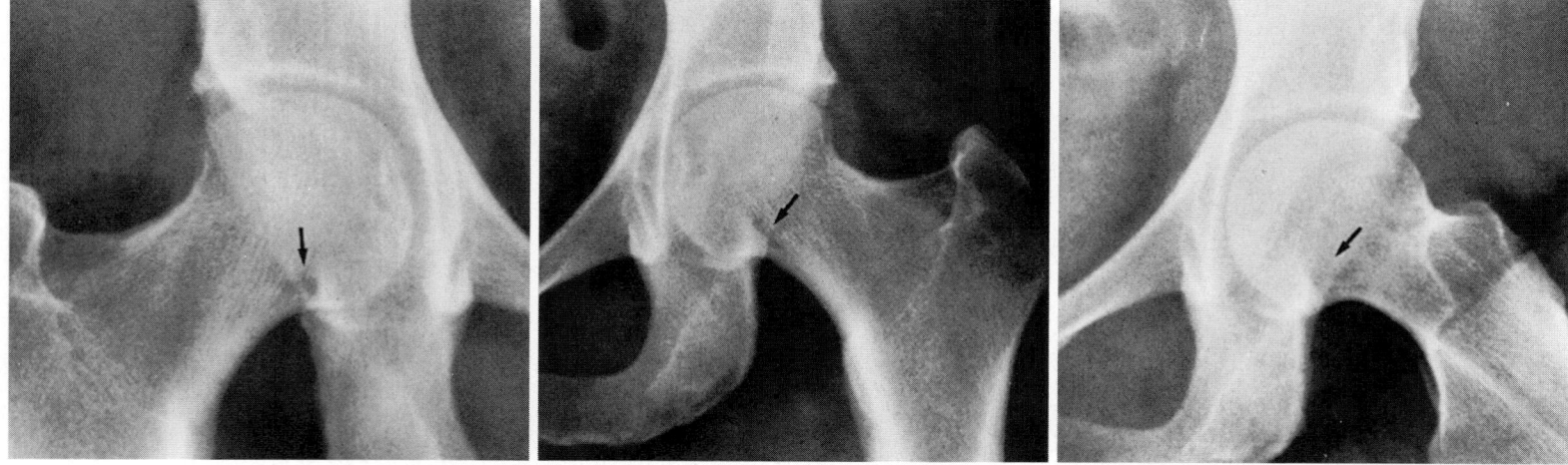

Figure 7–42. Bilateral localized trabecular radiolucencies in the femoral necks of a healthy 53-year-old woman.

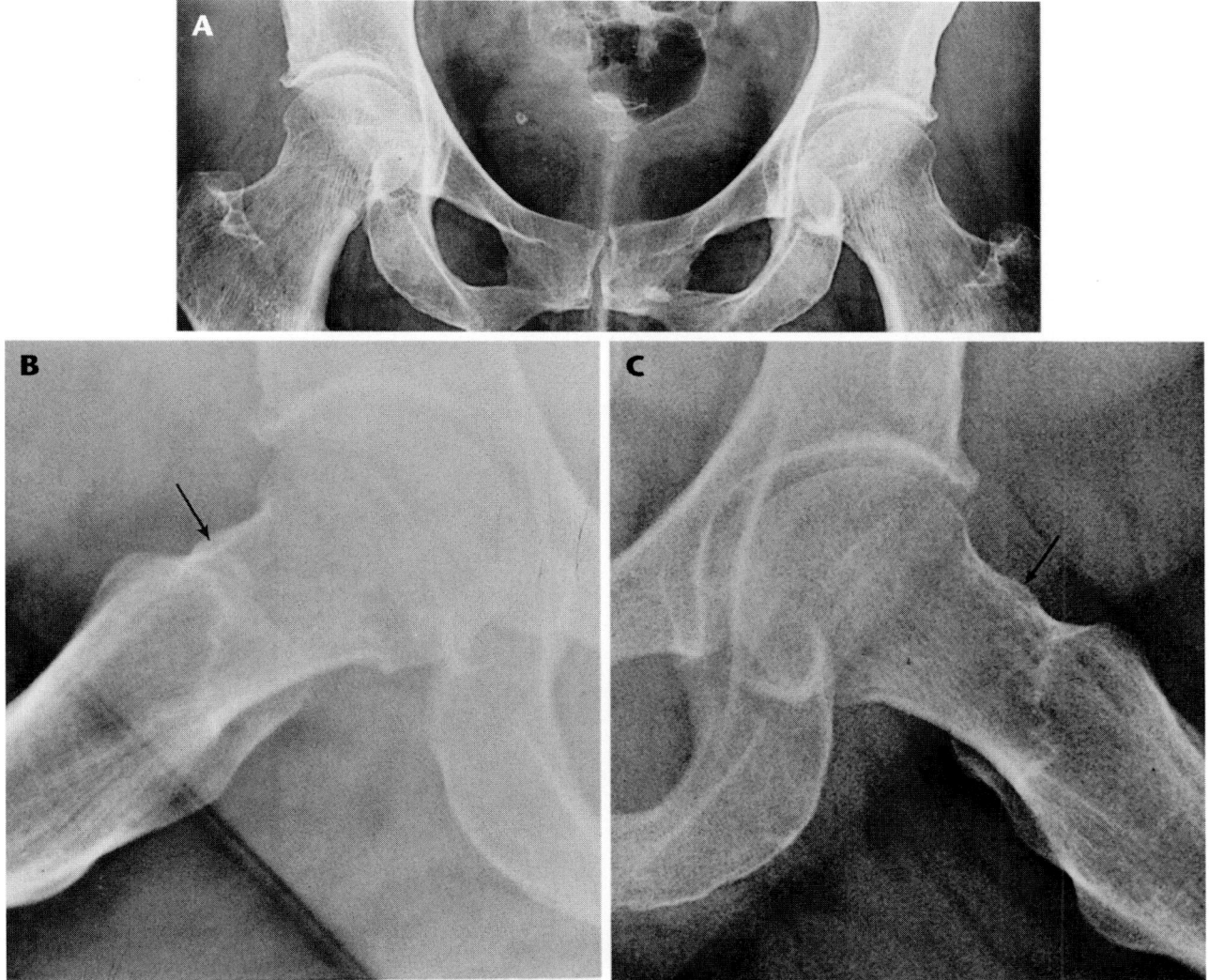

Figure 7–43. A–C, Normal irregularities of the femoral necks seen only in the frog-leg projection (**B** and **C**).

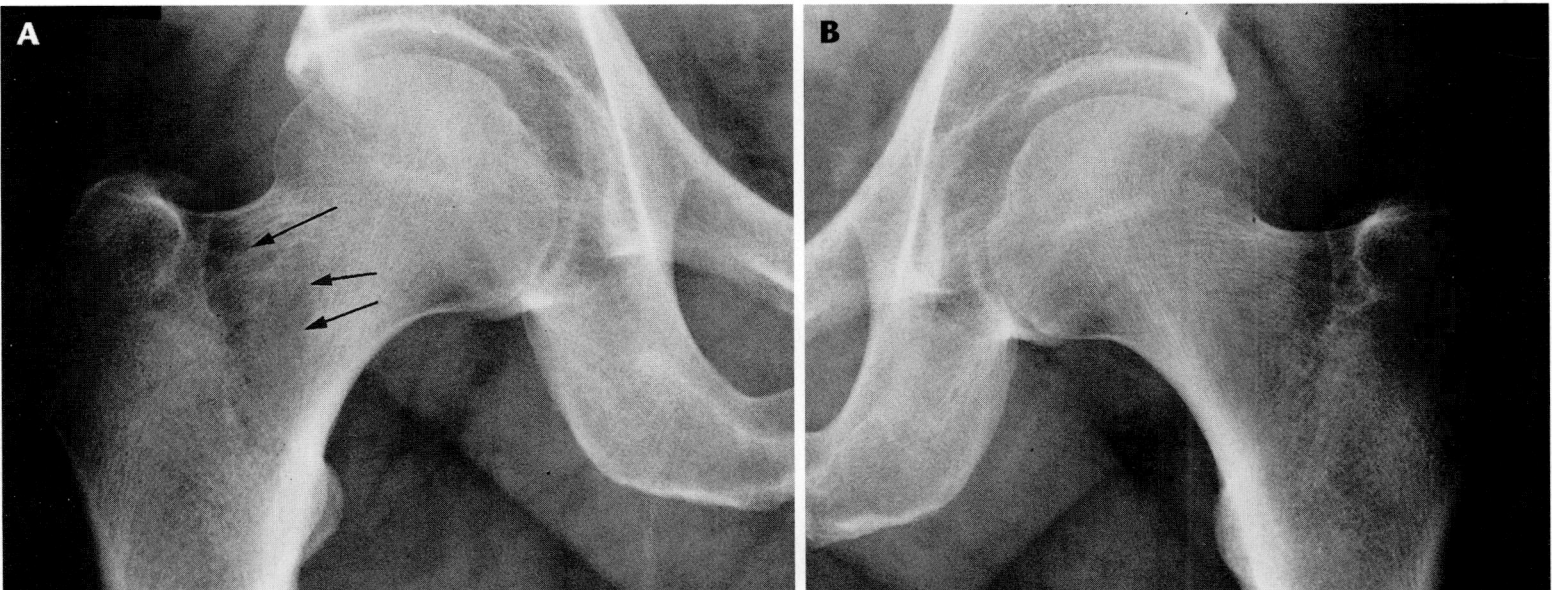

Figure 7–44. Asymmetric radiolucency of the right femoral neck (**A**), as compared to the left (**B**), probably due to asymmetry of position. MRI was normal.

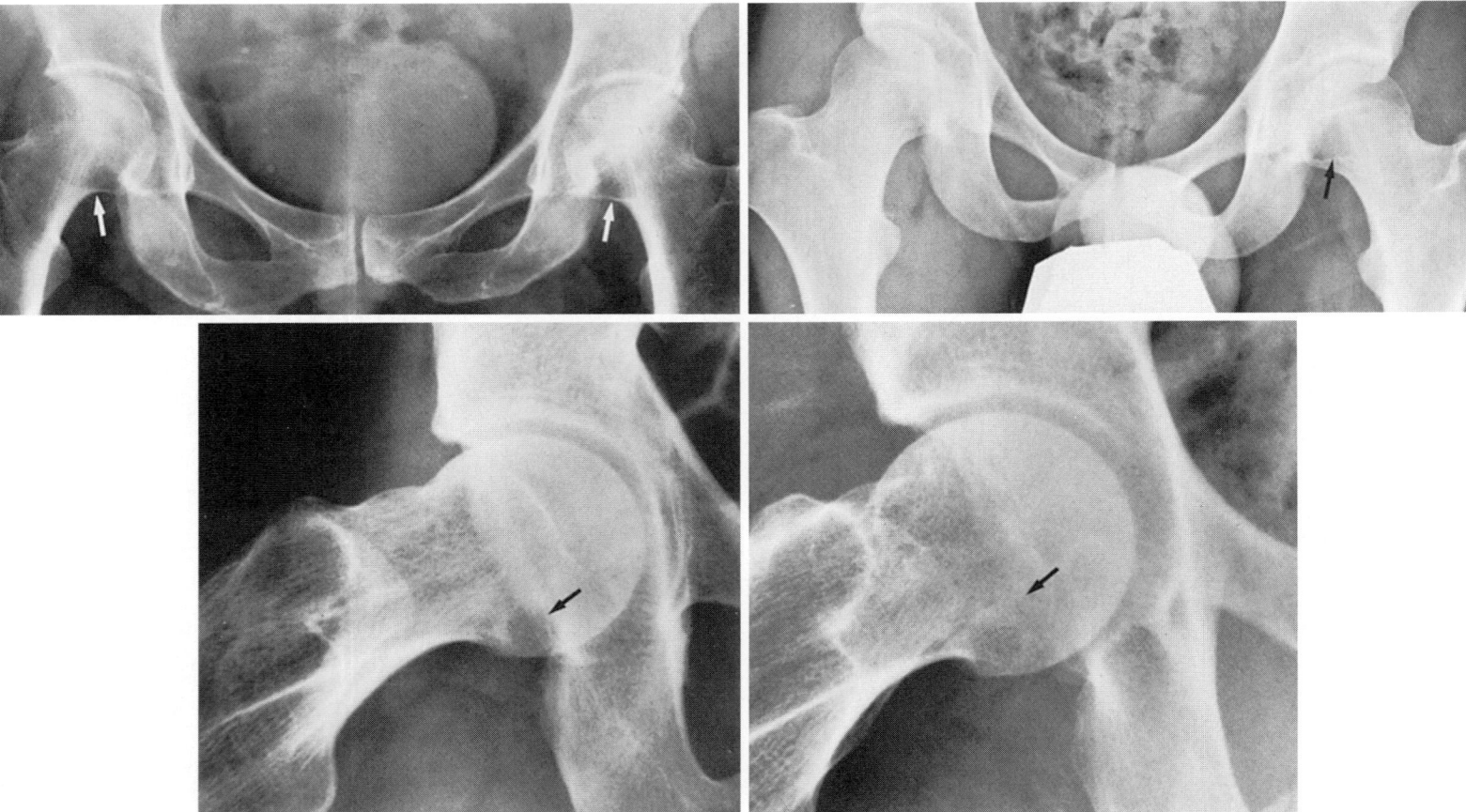

Figure 7–45. *Top left*, Normal triangular radiolucencies in the femoral necks produced by the heavy trabeculations in the center of the femoral neck and the overlap of the femoral head medially. *Top right*, This appearance may be asymmetric in its presentation. *Bottom left* and *right*, Similar radiolucencies may be seen in the frog-leg projection.

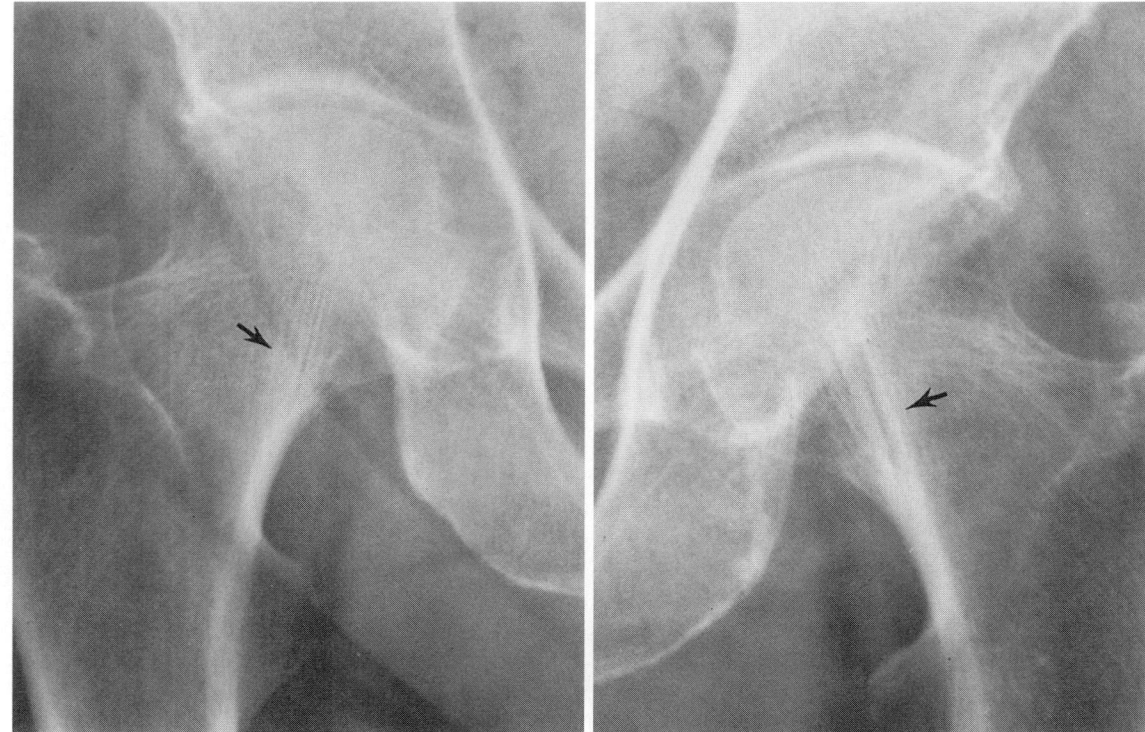

Figure 7–46. Trabecular reinforcement of the femoral necks secondary to osteoporosis. These alterations should not be confused with the trabecular changes of Paget's disease.

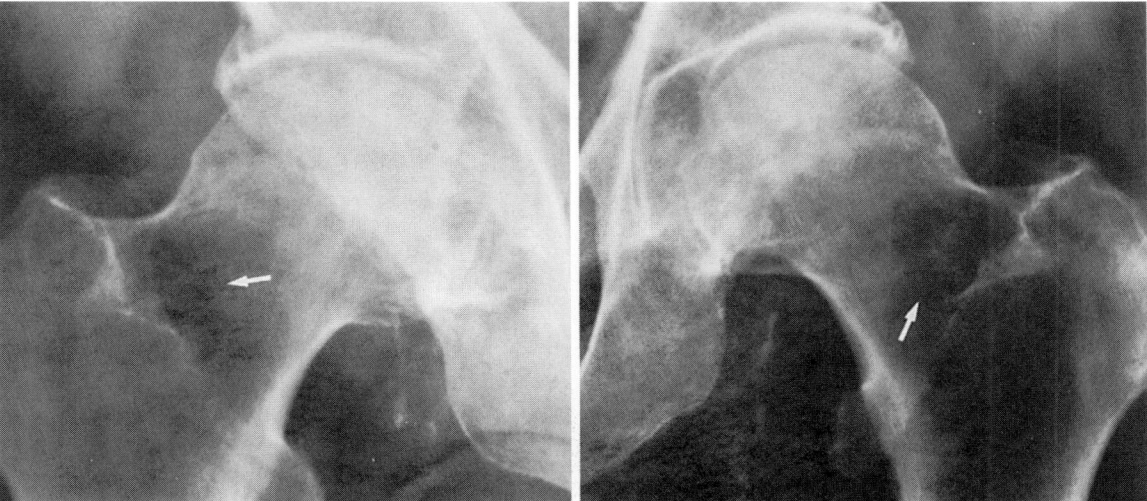

Figure 7–47. Relative radiolucencies in the femoral necks of an 85-year-old man, produced by the large trabeculations of the femoral neck inferior and medial to the edge of the greater trochanter.

Figure 7–48. Radiolucencies produced by overlap of the greater trochanter and the heavy trabeculation of the femoral neck in a 51-year-old man.

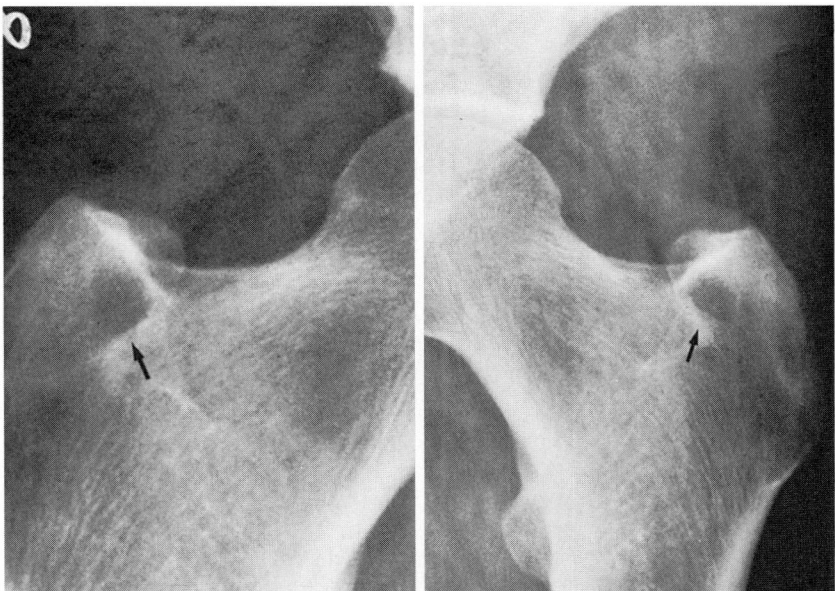

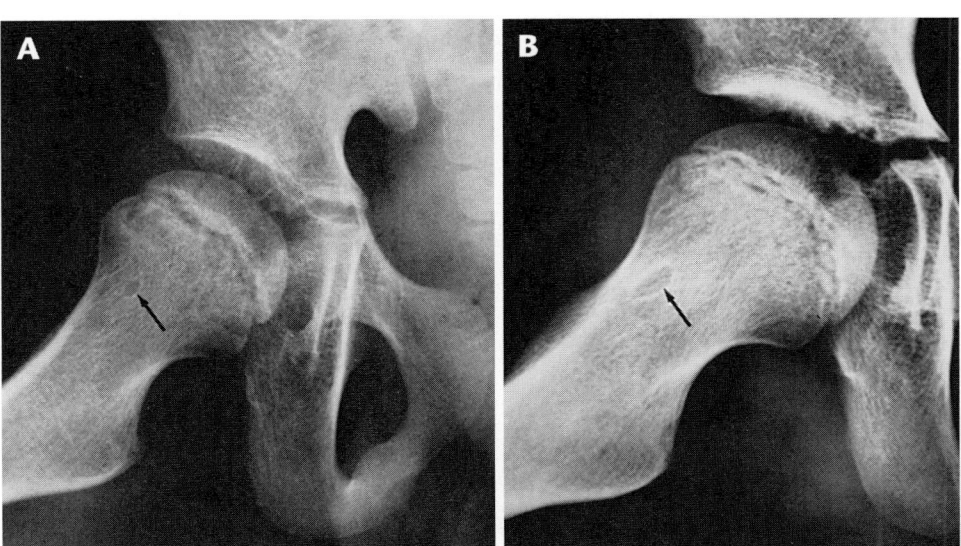

Figure 7–49. Typical juvenile benign cortical defects are occasionally seen in the femoral neck and are of no clinical significance. **A,** 7-year-old boy. **B,** Three years later, the lesion is slightly larger.

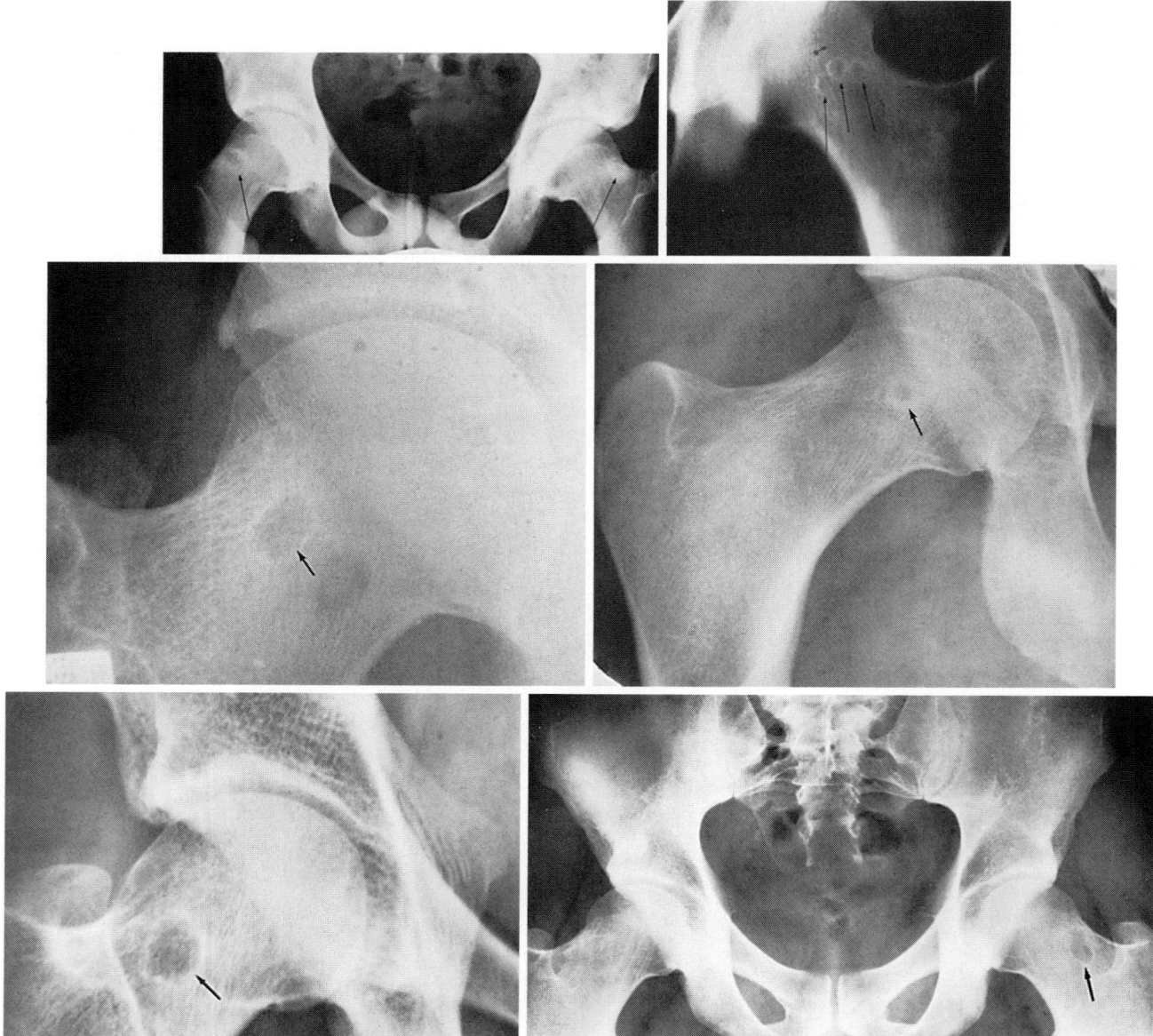

Figure 7–50. Examples of ringlike radiolucencies of the femoral necks with sclerotic borders. These are common lesions that are apparently of no clinical significance. There is evidence to suggest that they represent a subcortical pit formed by herniation of synovium through the cortical bone. (Ref: Pitt MJ et al: Herniation pit of the femoral neck. *Am J Roentgenol* 38:1115, 1982.) Rarely, these herniation pits may grow rapidly and suggest an aggressive lesion. In some cases these pits may enlarge, and the overlying cortex may fracture and become symptomatic. (Ref: Daenen B et al: Symptomatic herniation pits of the femoral neck. *Am J Roentgenol* 168:149, 1997.)

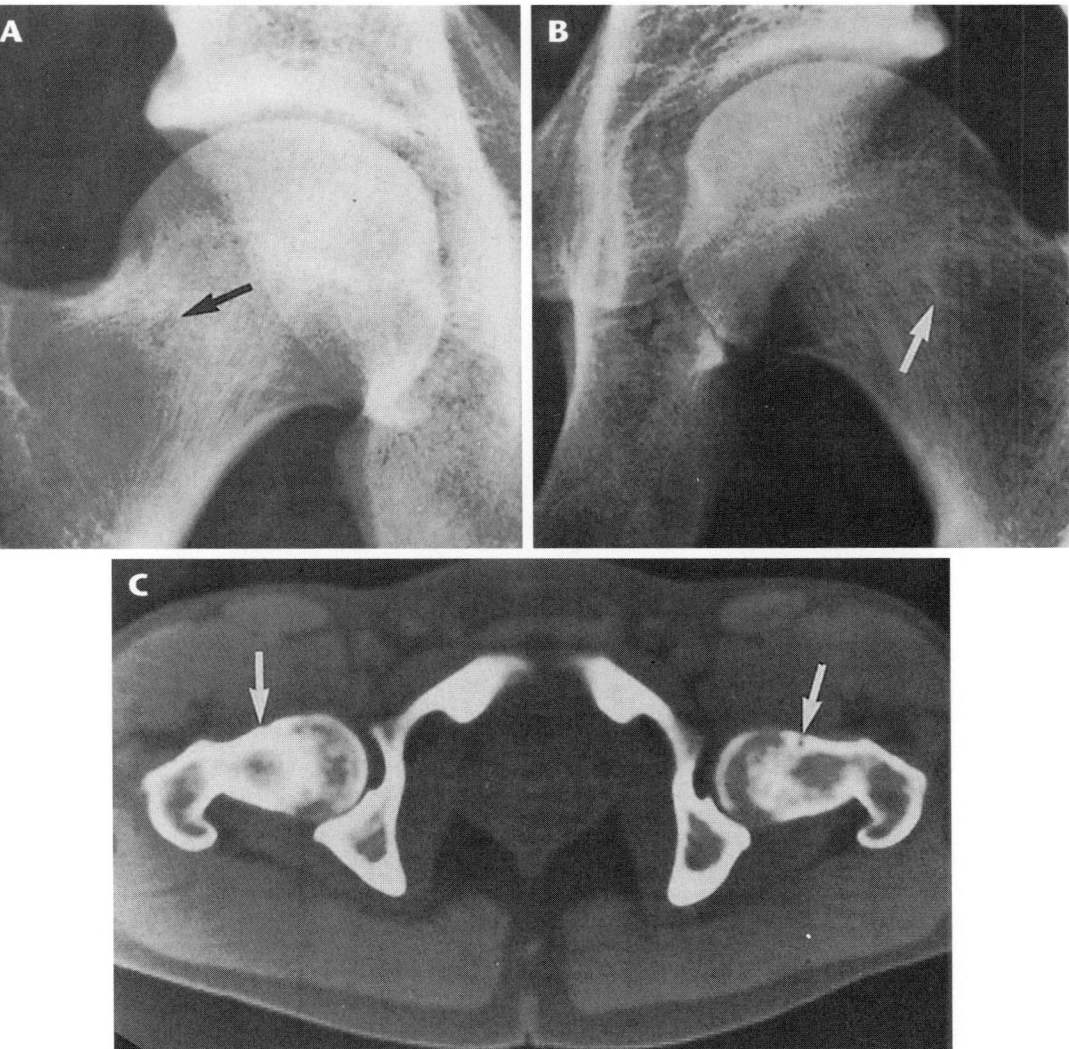

Figure 7–51. A and **B,** Bilateral herniation pits in a 25-year-old man. **C,** CT demonstration.

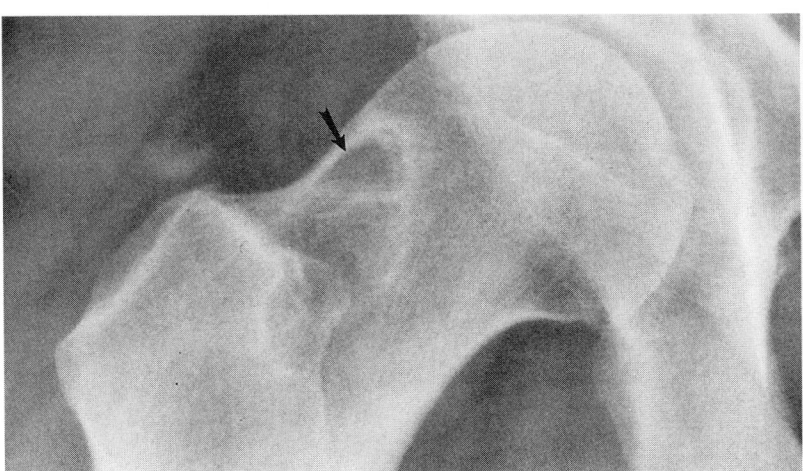

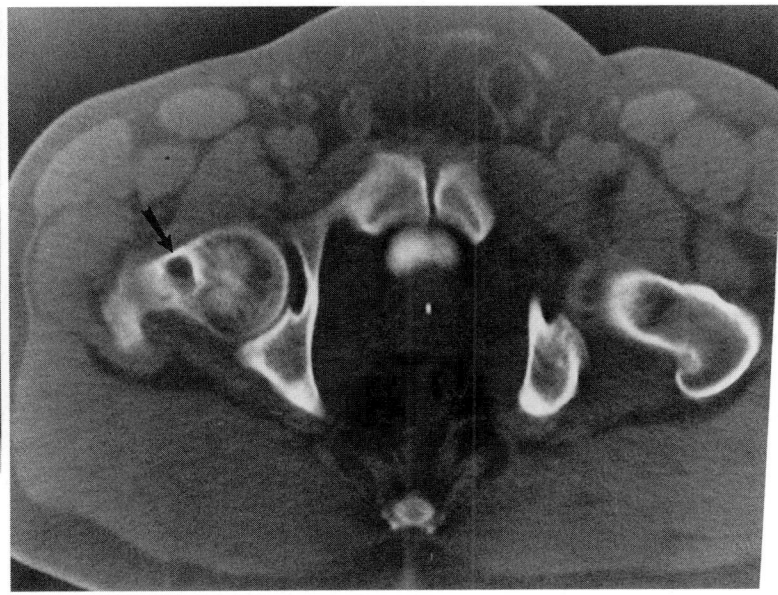

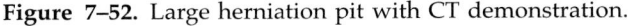

Figure 7–52. Large herniation pit with CT demonstration.

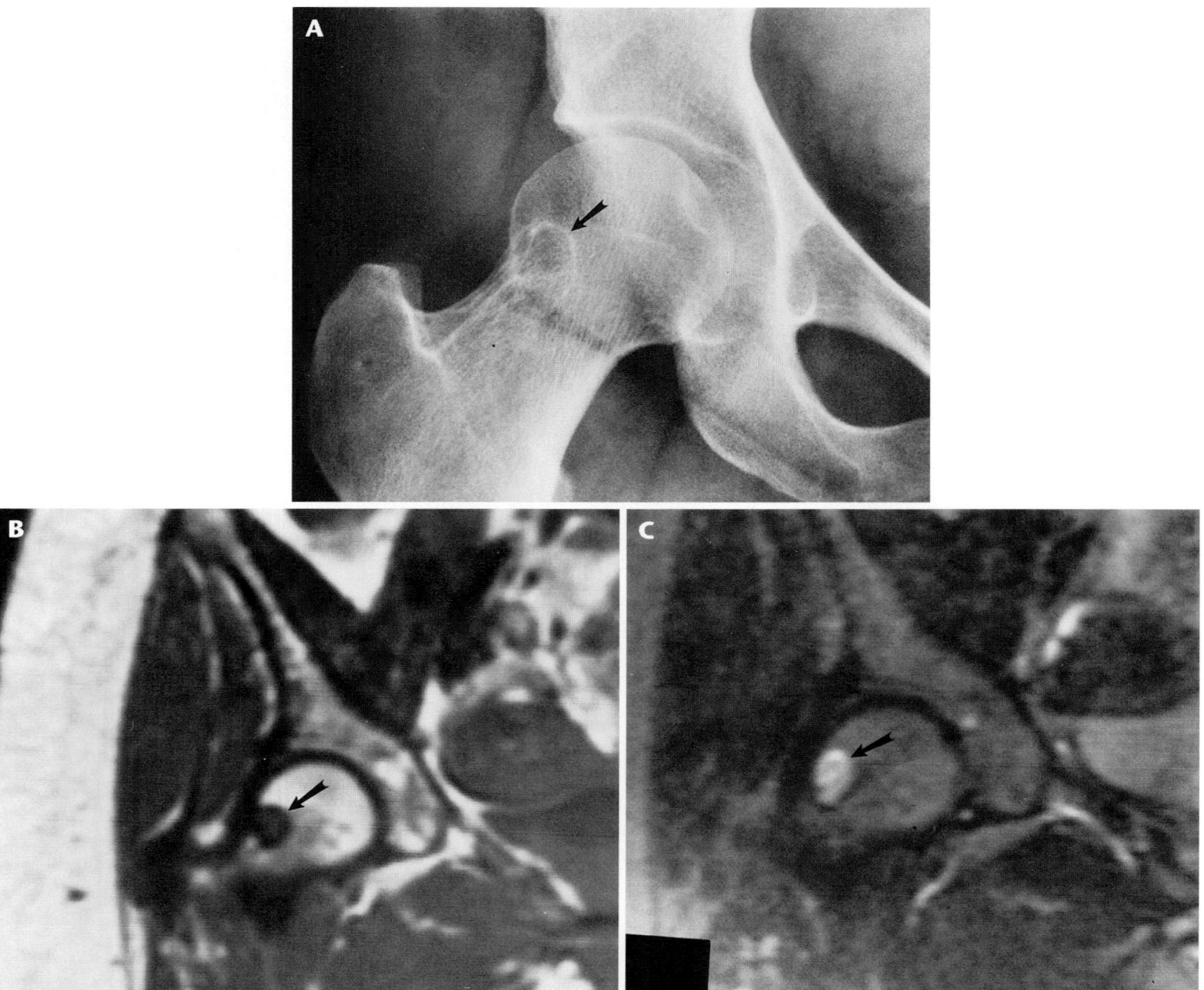

Figure 7–53. Large herniation pit. **A,** Plain film. **B,** T-1–weighted image. **C,** Fat-saturated image.

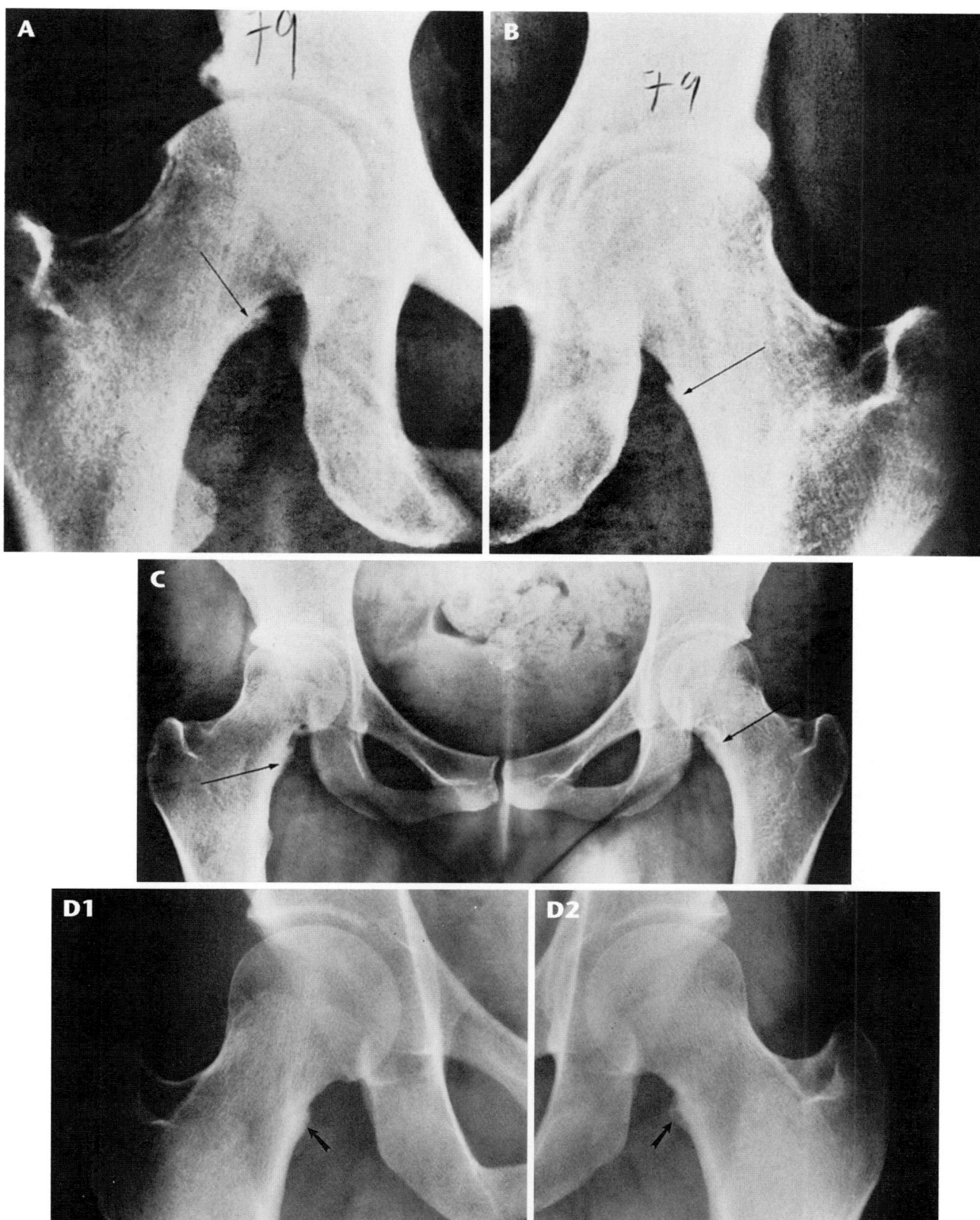

Figure 7–54. Examples of bony thickenings of the inferior aspect of the femoral necks, probably caused by ossification of the inferior retinaculum of the synovial capsule. (**A** and **B,** 34-year-old woman. **C, D1,** and **D2,** 25-year-old woman. (**A** and **B** courtesy of Dr. Clement Fauré.) (Ref: Fauré C et al: L'éperon pectineo-foveal du col fémoral. *J Radiol* 64:505, 1983.)

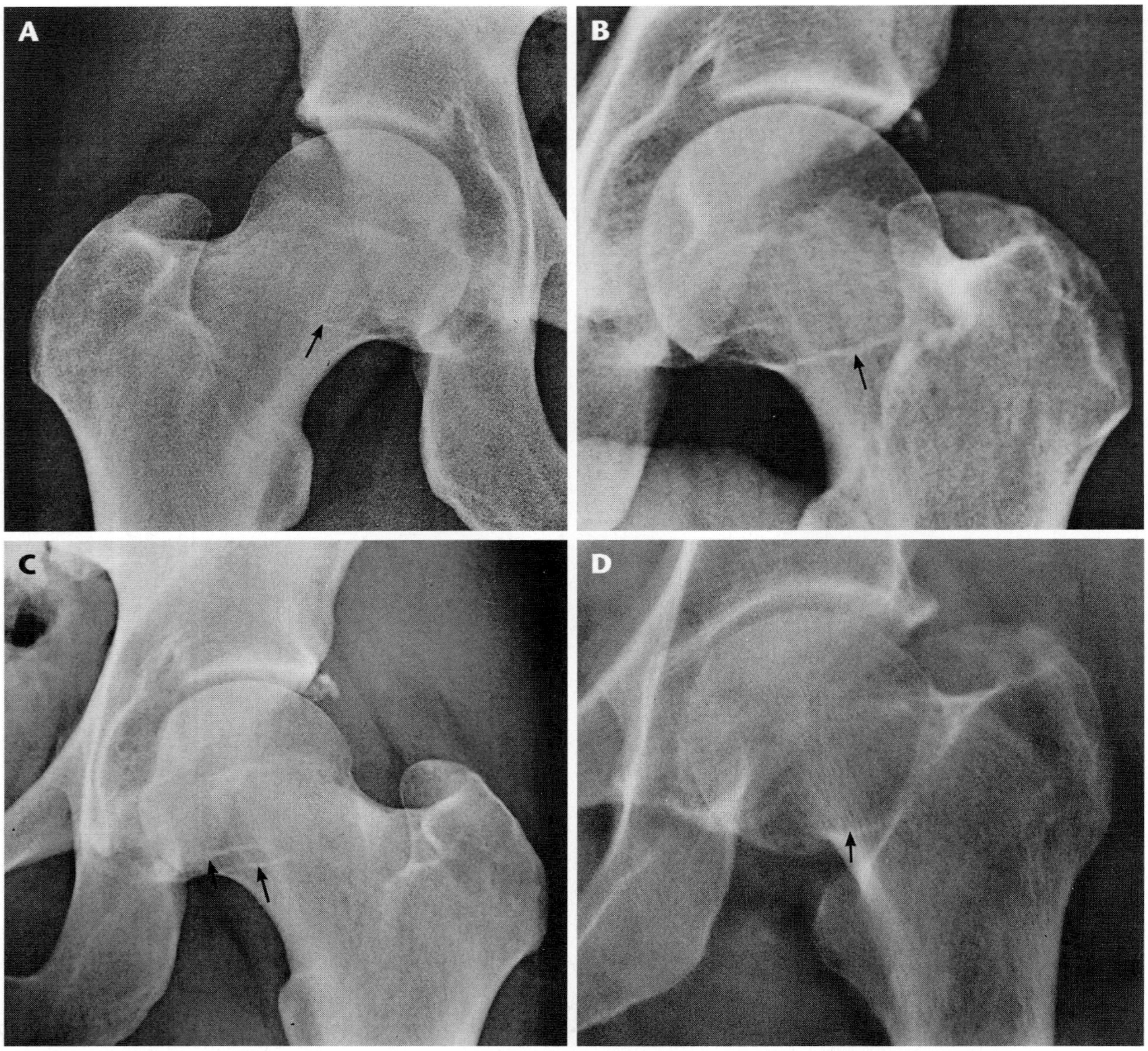

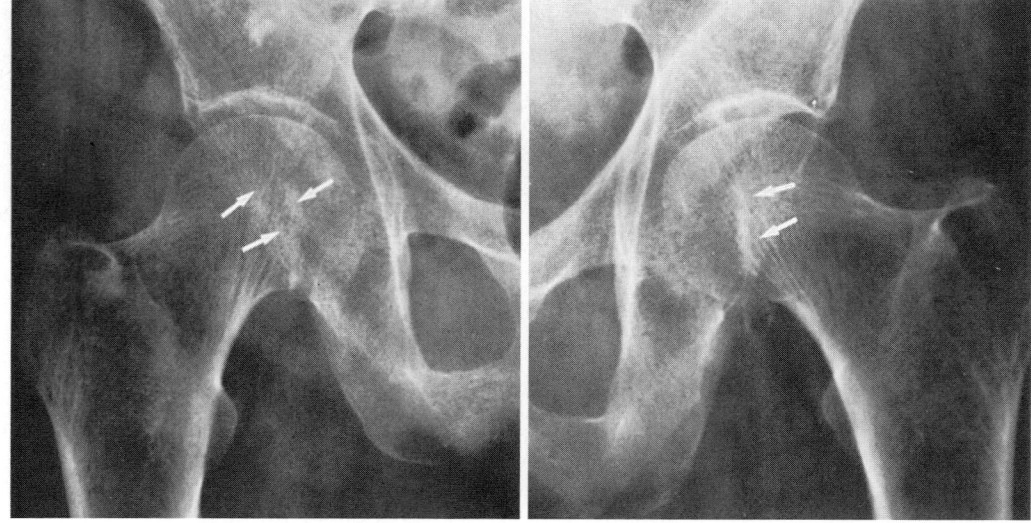

Figure 7–55. A–D, Four examples of the "white line" of the femoral neck, which probably represents the posterior insertion of the joint capsule. This may be confused with a fracture line.

Figure 7–56. Localized reinforcement of major trabeculae in a 75-year-old osteoporotic woman that might be mistaken for an insufficiency fracture.

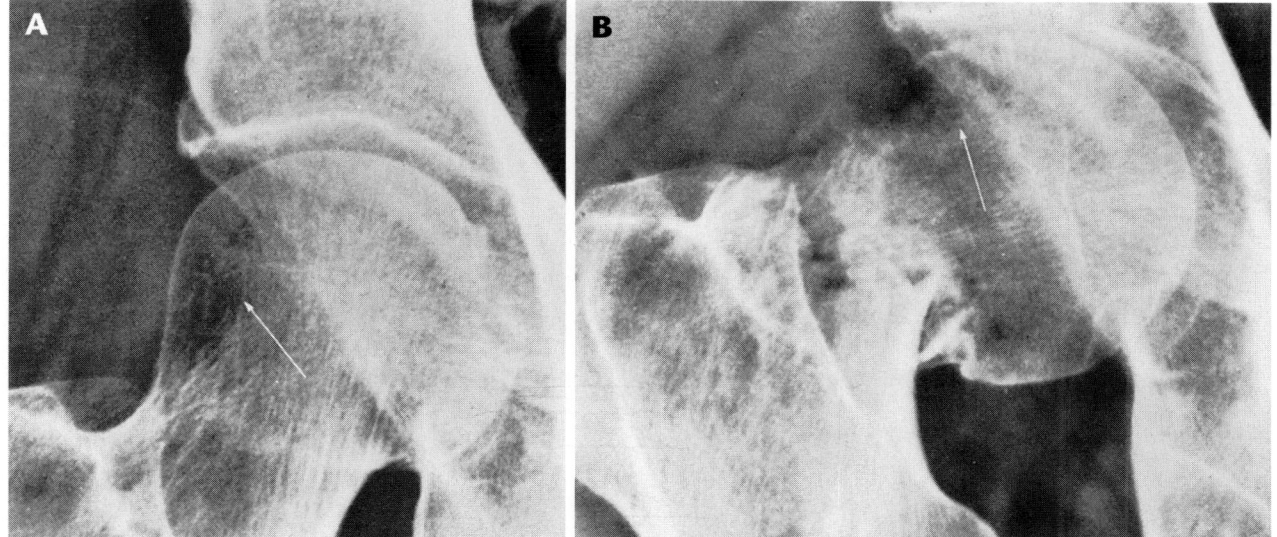

Figure 7–57. A, Normal area of radiolucency of the femoral neck, which becomes more marked in osteoporotic individuals. **B,** This area radiolucency simulates a pathologic fracture in patients with traumatic fracture of the femoral neck caused by rotation of the head. After reduction this appearance is no longer seen. (Ref: Pope TL Jr et al: Pseudopathologic fracture of the femoral neck. *Skeletal Radiol* 7:129, 1981.)

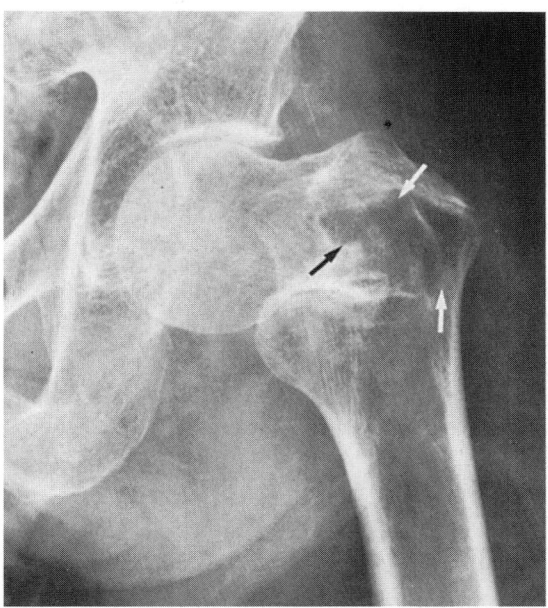

Figure 7–58. Additional example of a simulated destructive lesion following fracture of an osteoporotic femur.

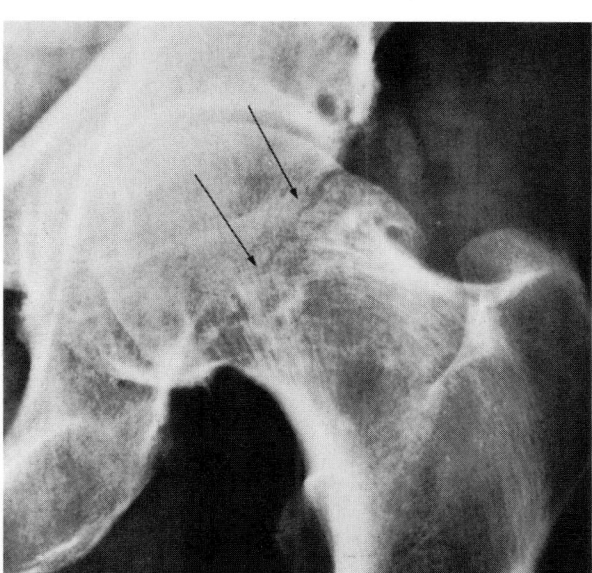

Figure 7–59. Hypertrophic changes at the femoral head may produce an appearance simulating a fracture of the femoral neck.

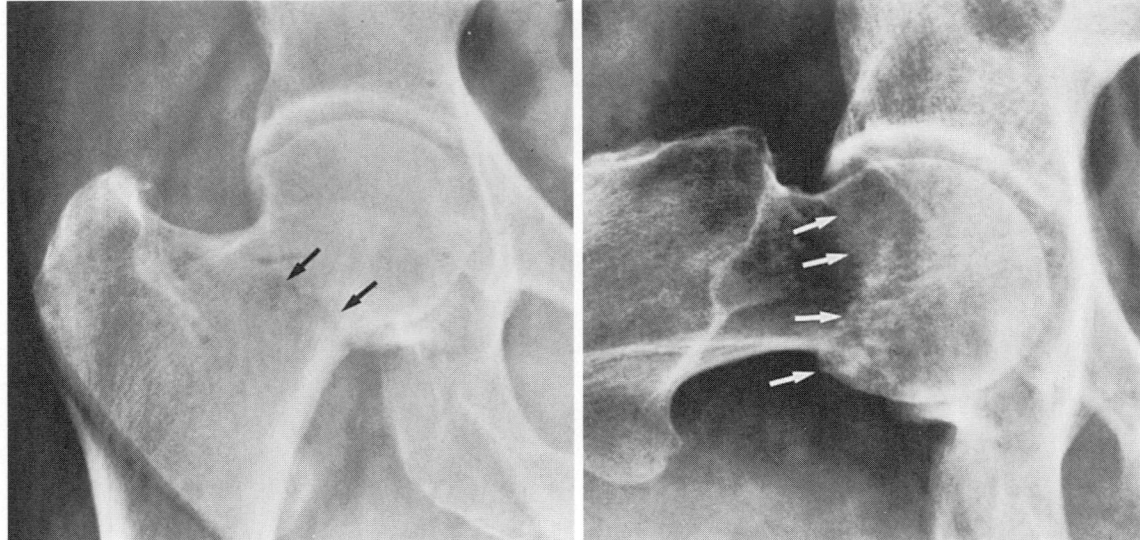

Figure 7–60. *Left*, Simulated fracture of the femoral neck in a 68-year-old woman, produced by hypertrophic lipping, best seen in the lateral projection (*right*).

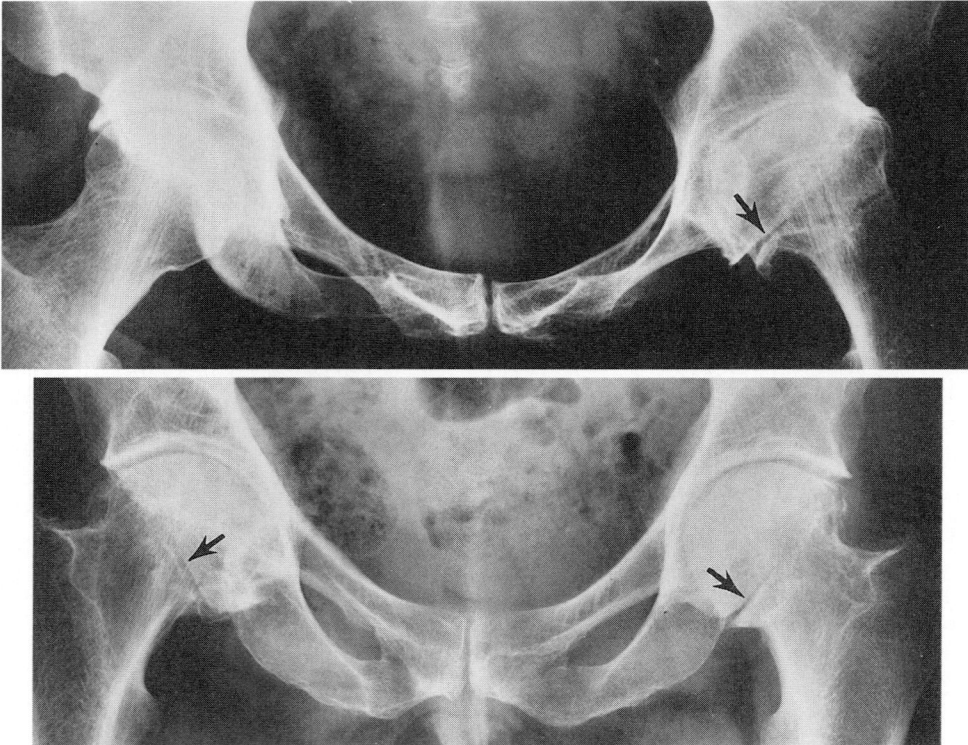

Figure 7–61. Simulated fractures of the femoral neck produced by hypertrophic lipping of the femoral head.

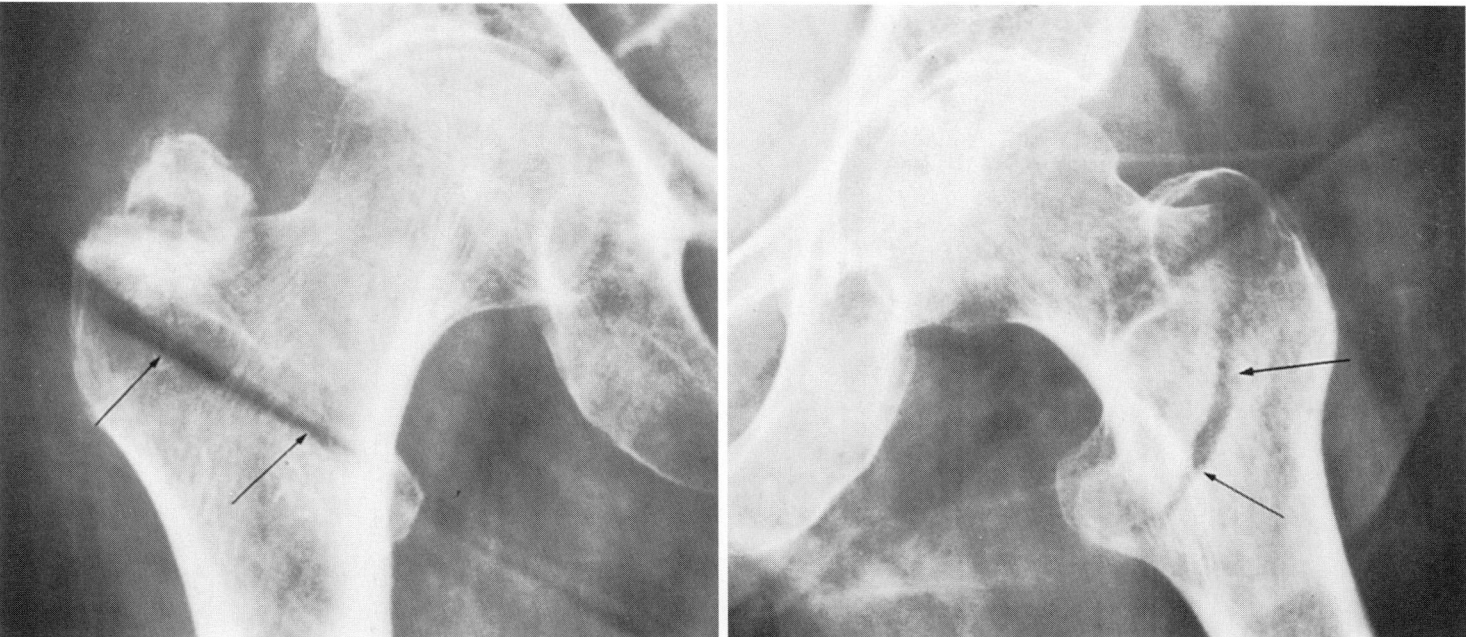

Figure 7–62. Two examples of skin folds simulating fractures of the femur.

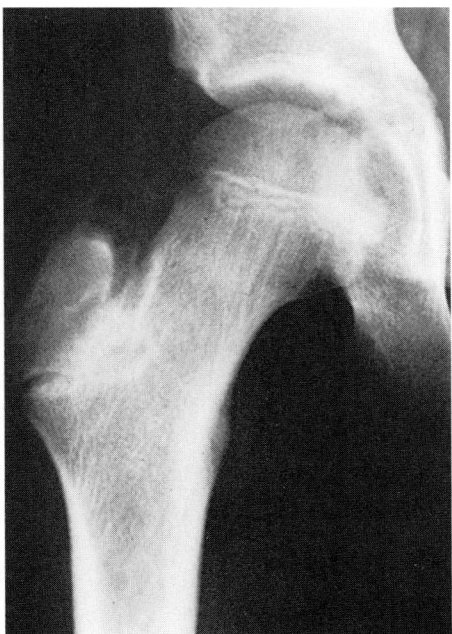

Figure 7–63. Prominent vertical striation of the bone of the femoral neck in a normal 12-year-old girl.

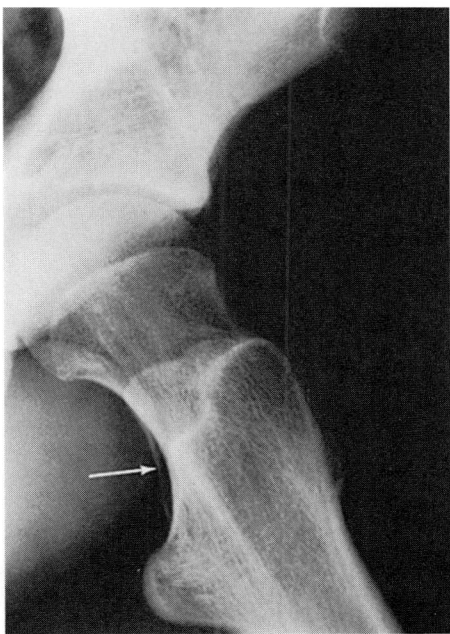

Figure 7–64. Simulated periostitis of the femoral neck, produced by the overlapping shadow of the greater trochanter.

The Trochanters

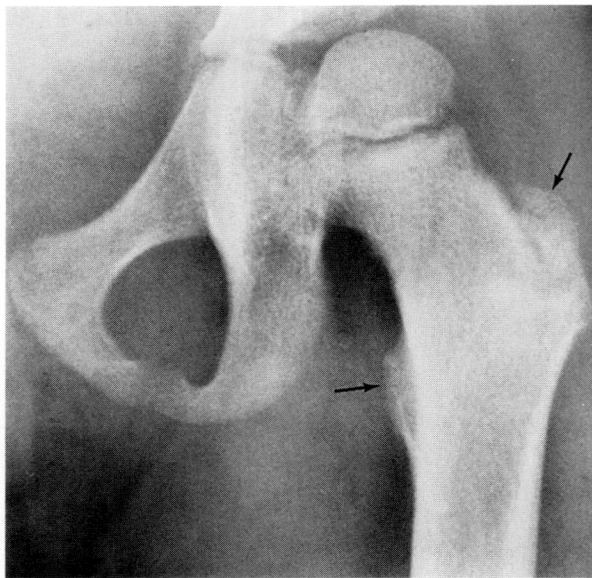

Figure 7–65. Normal irregularity of the ossification centers of the greater and lesser trochanters in a 3-year-old girl.

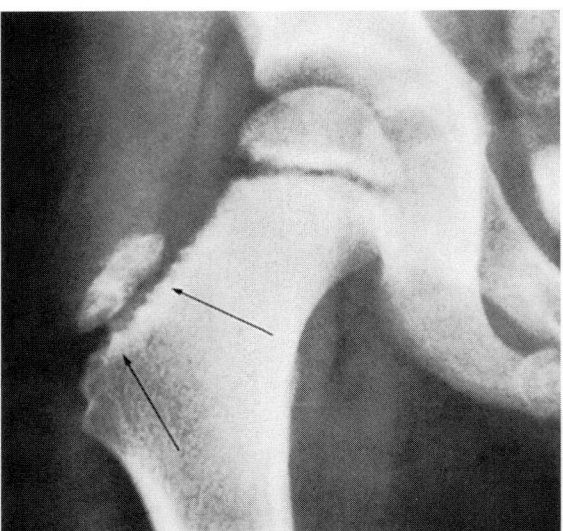

Figure 7–66. Normal irregularity of the trochanteric apophyseal line in a 7-year-old boy.

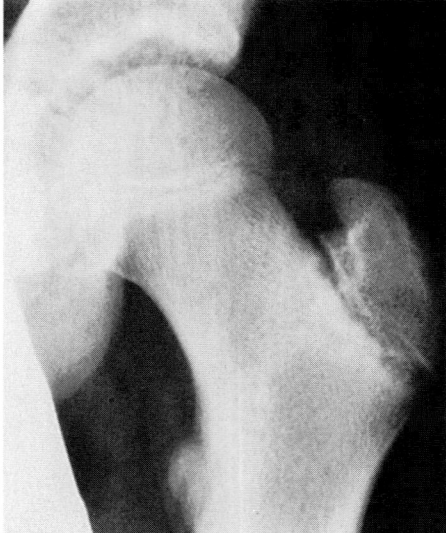

Figure 7–67. Normal irregularities of ossification of the greater trochanter in a 12-year-old boy.

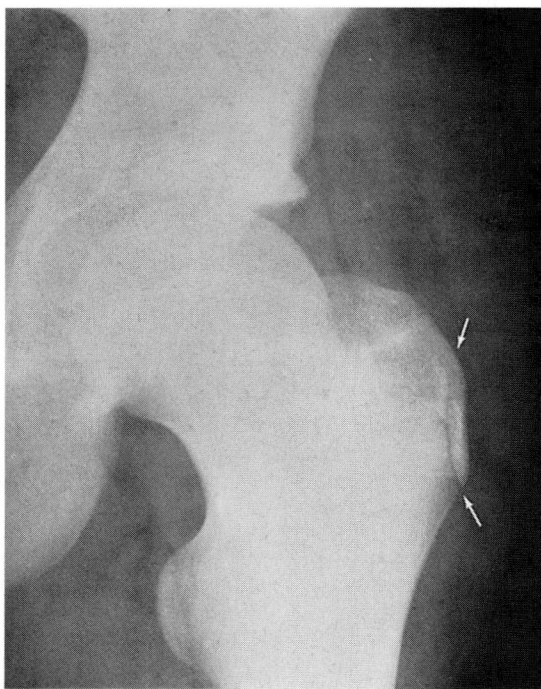

Figure 7–68. Ossification variant of the greater trochanter in a 15-year-old boy, simulating a fracture.

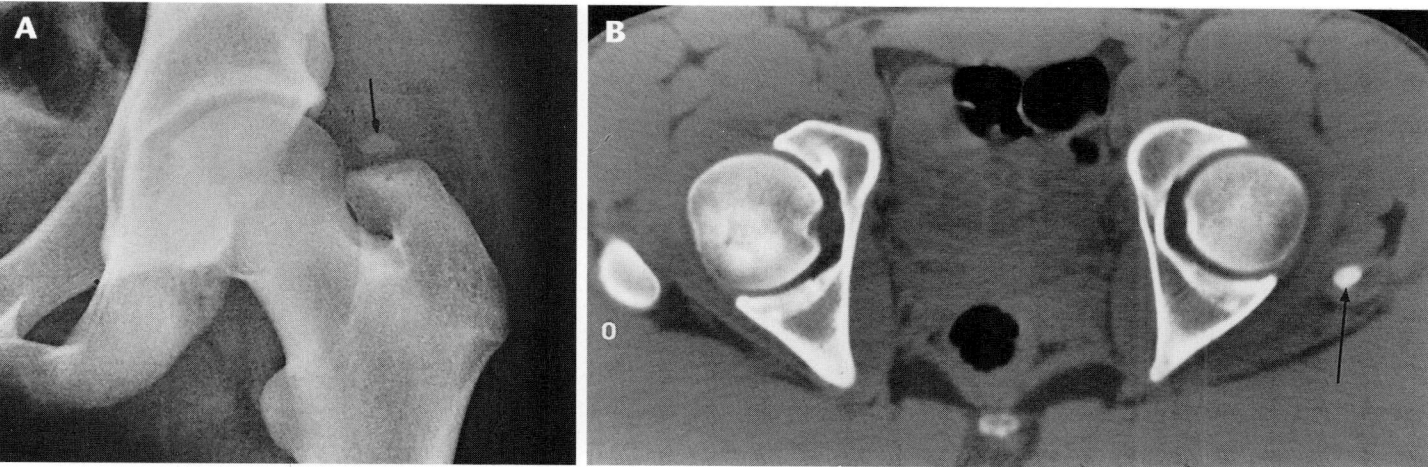

Figure 7–69. Accessory ossification center of the greater trochanter in a 16-year-old girl. **A,** Plain film. **B,** CT.

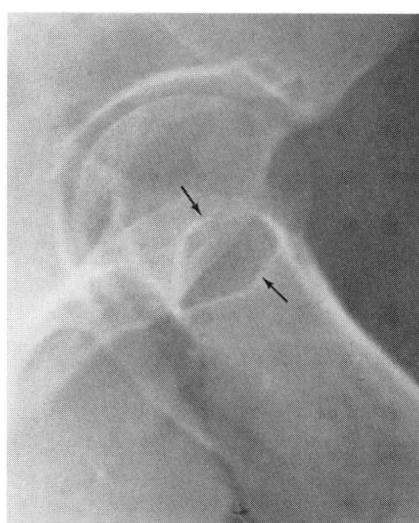

Figure 7–70. Simulated cyst of the femoral neck produced in abduction by the shadow of the greater trochanter.

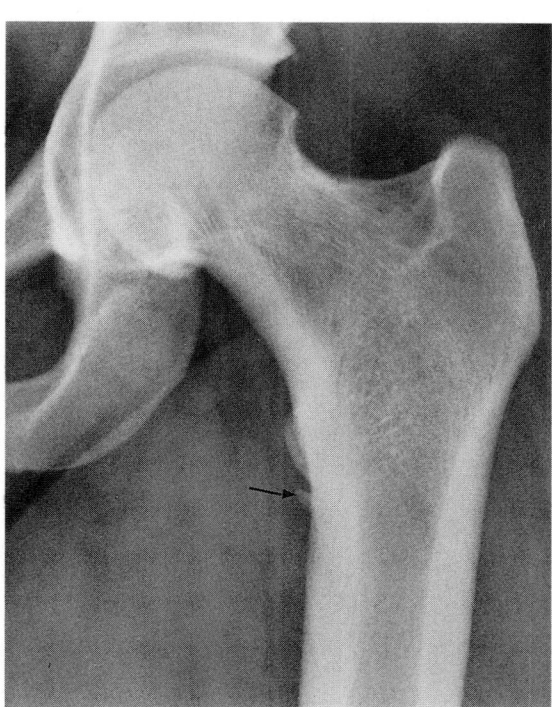

Figure 7–71. "Tug" lesion below lesser trochanter, an enthesopathy.

The Shaft of the Femur

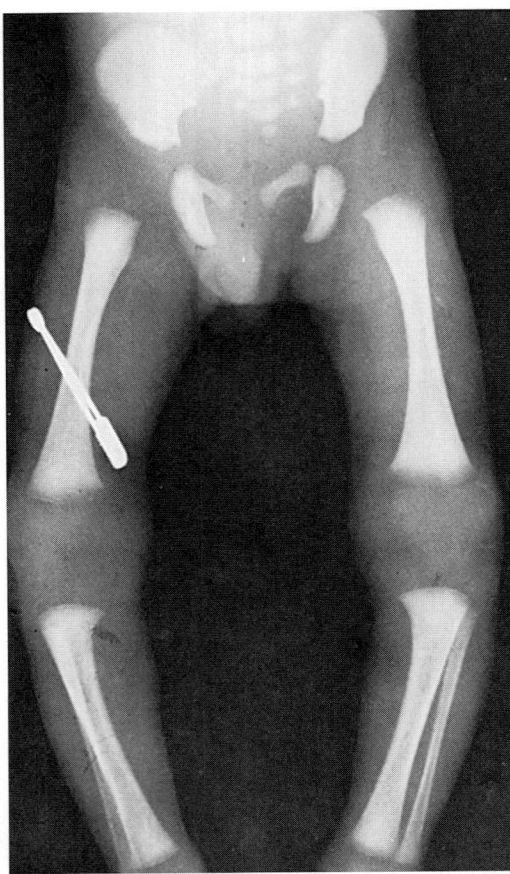

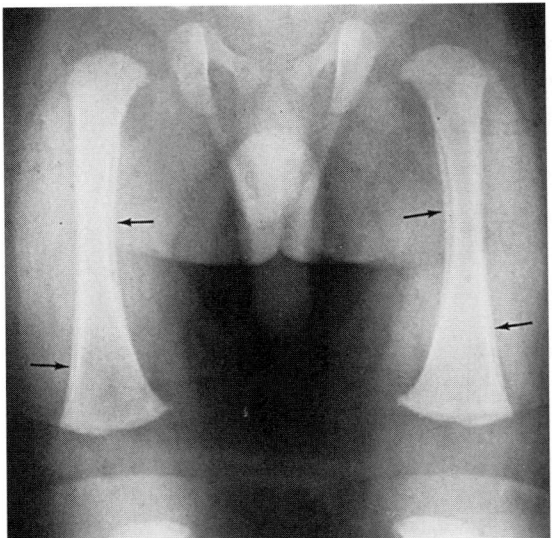

Figure 7–73. Physiologic "periostitis" of the newborn. This is not seen before the age of 1 month and is symmetric in distribution, although not necessarily concentric, and may be seen in only one view. (Ref: Shopfner CE: Periosteal bone growth in normal infants: A preliminary report. *Am J Roentgenol* 97:154, 1966.)

Figure 7–72. Normal osteosclerosis of the premature. This sclerosis is due to the proportionally thicker cortical bone and incomplete development of the medullary cavities. This appearance reverts to normal in the first weeks of life.

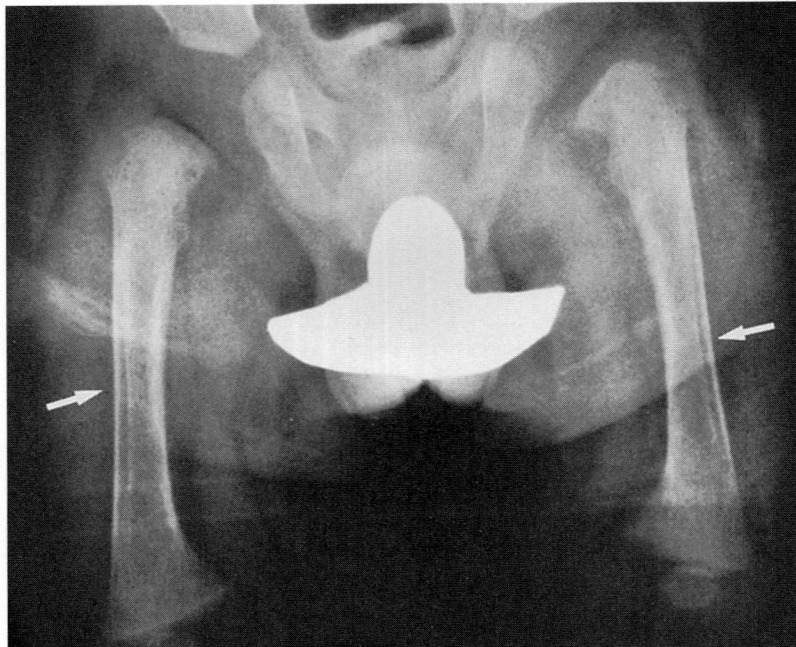

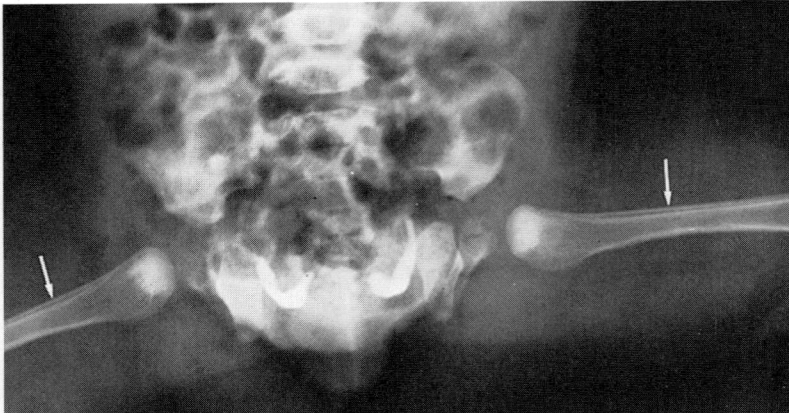

Figure 7–74. Additional examples of physiologic "periostitis" of the newborn, seen in two 4-month-old infants. Incorporation is evident and is essentially completed by 6 months of age.

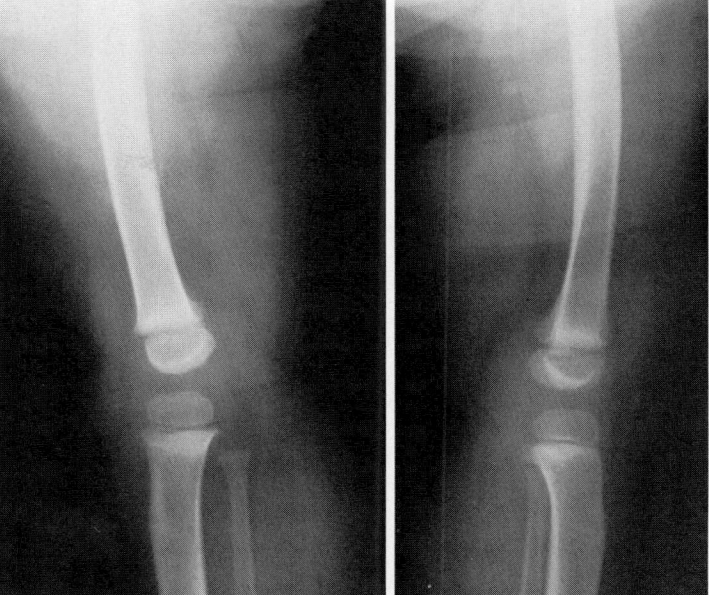

Figure 7–75. Physiologic anterior bowing of the femurs in a heavy 19-month-old girl. This is a self-limited phenomenon that disappears as the child matures.

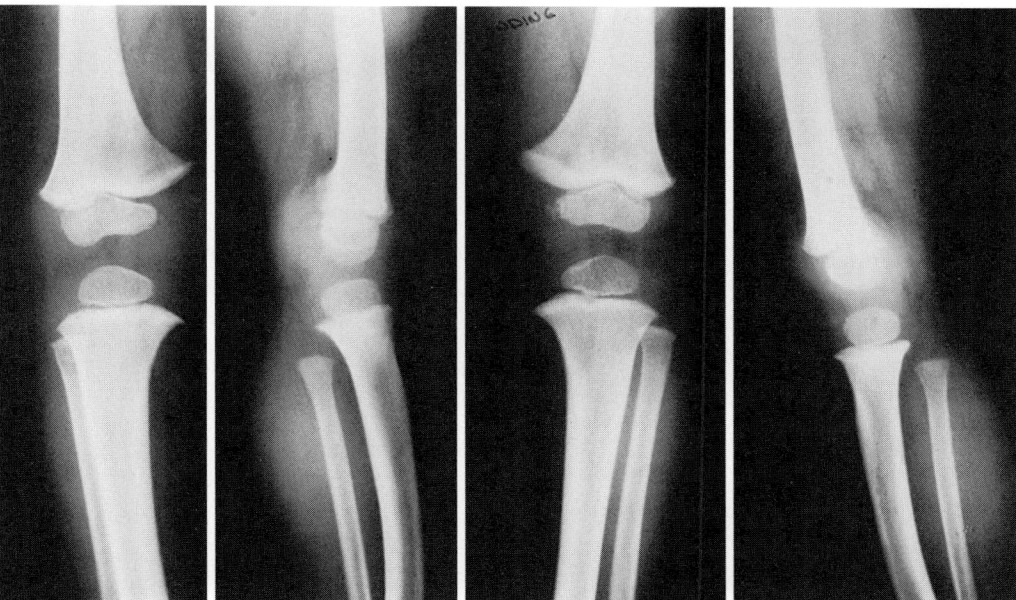

Figure 7–76. Combined anterior and lateral physiologic bowing of the tibias in a 12-month-old girl.

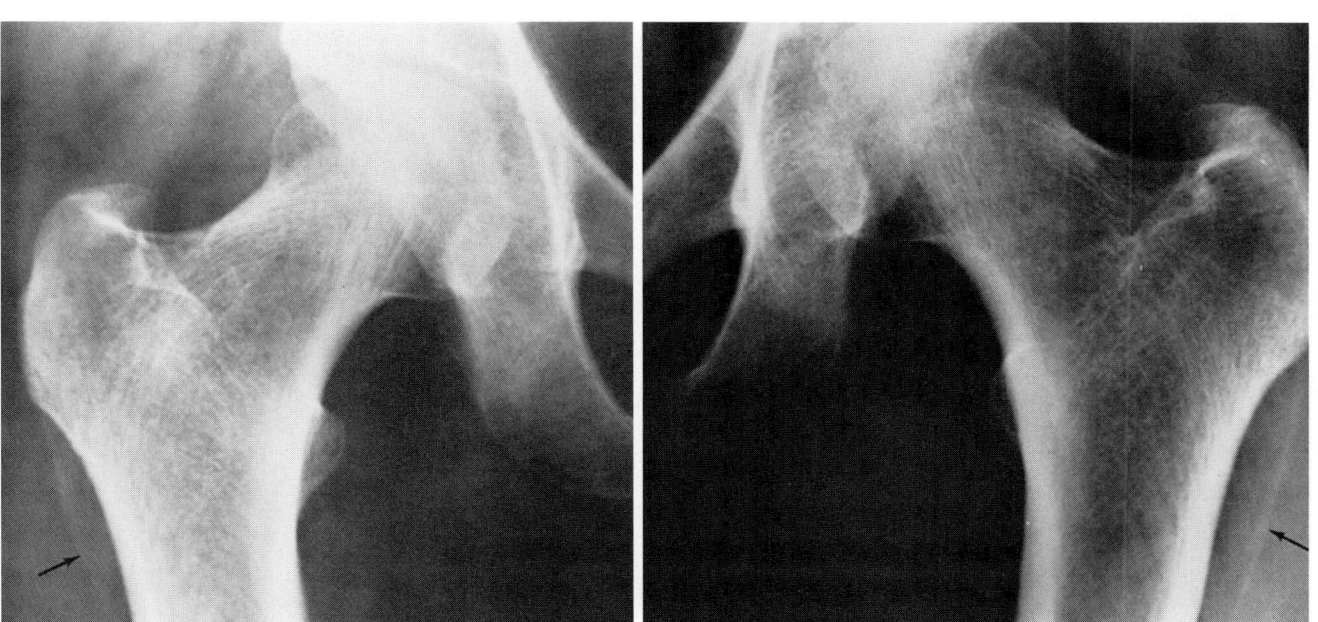

Figure 7–77. The shadow of the fascia lata, which may simulate new bone formation.

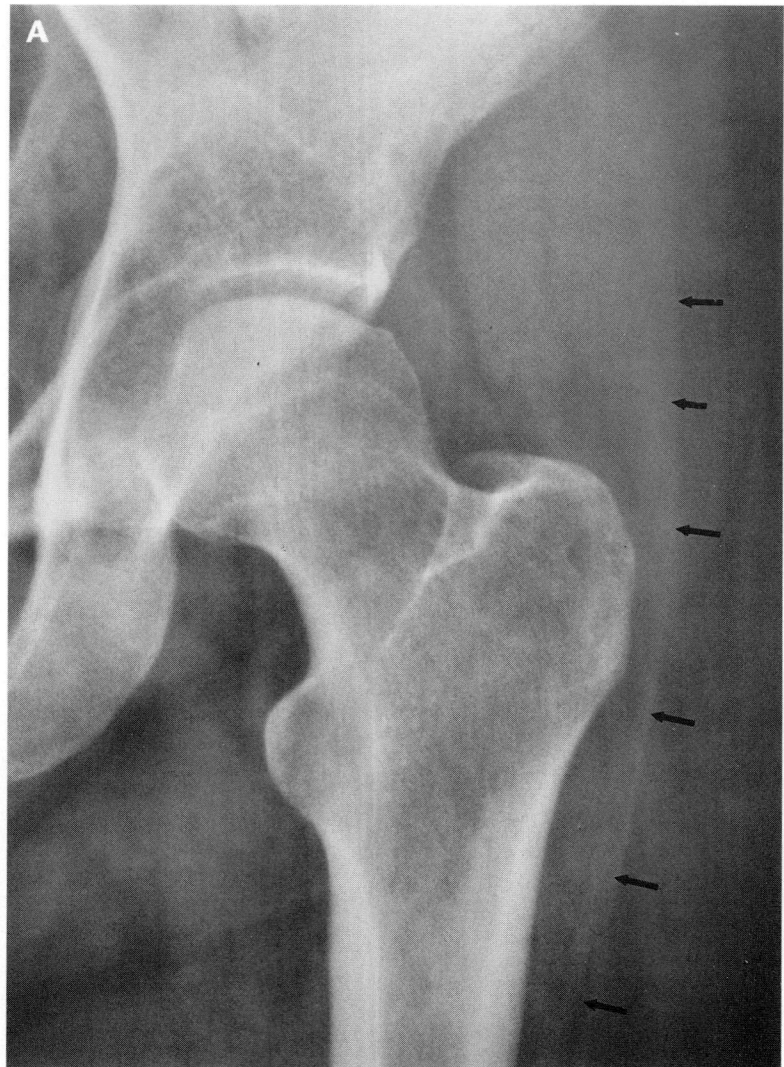

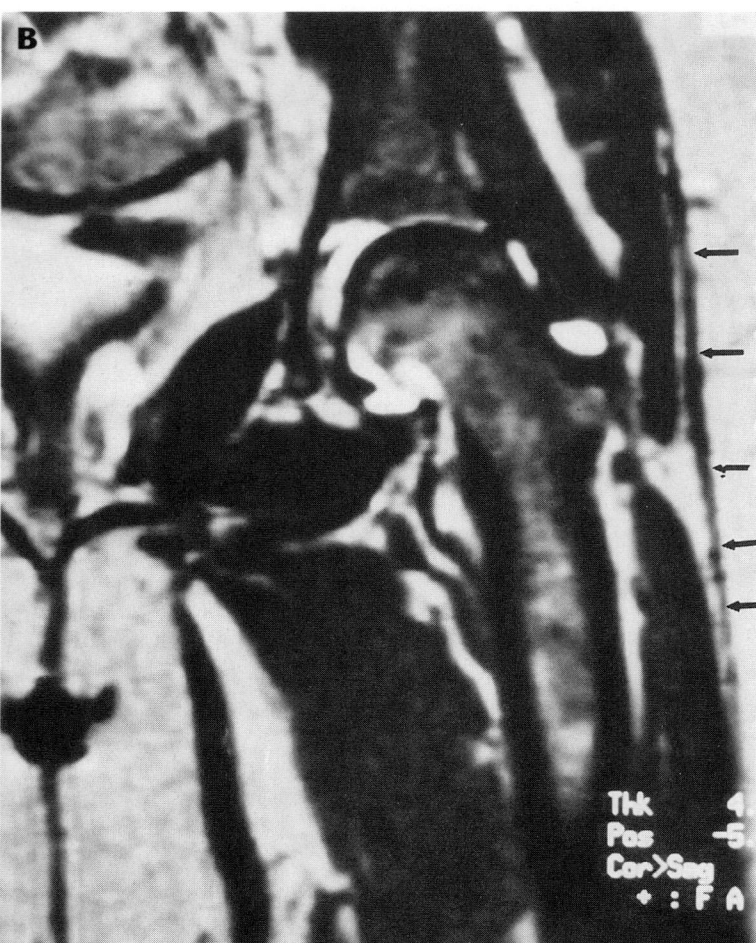

Figure 7–78. A, The shadow of the tensor fascia lata and iliotibial band by plain film. **B,** T-2–weighted MRI image.

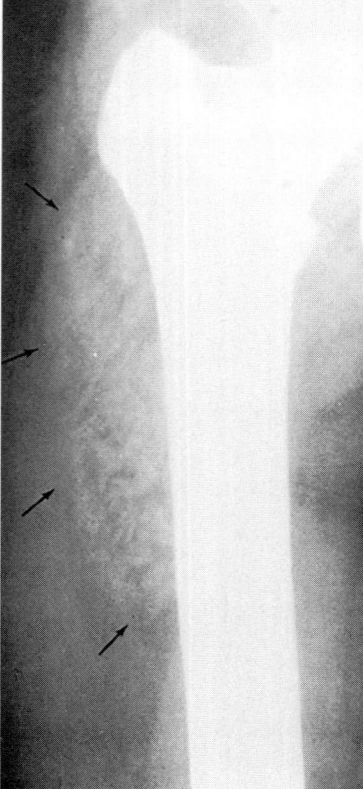

Figure 7–79. Muscle interleaved with fat may resemble a soft tissue mass, most commonly seen in women.

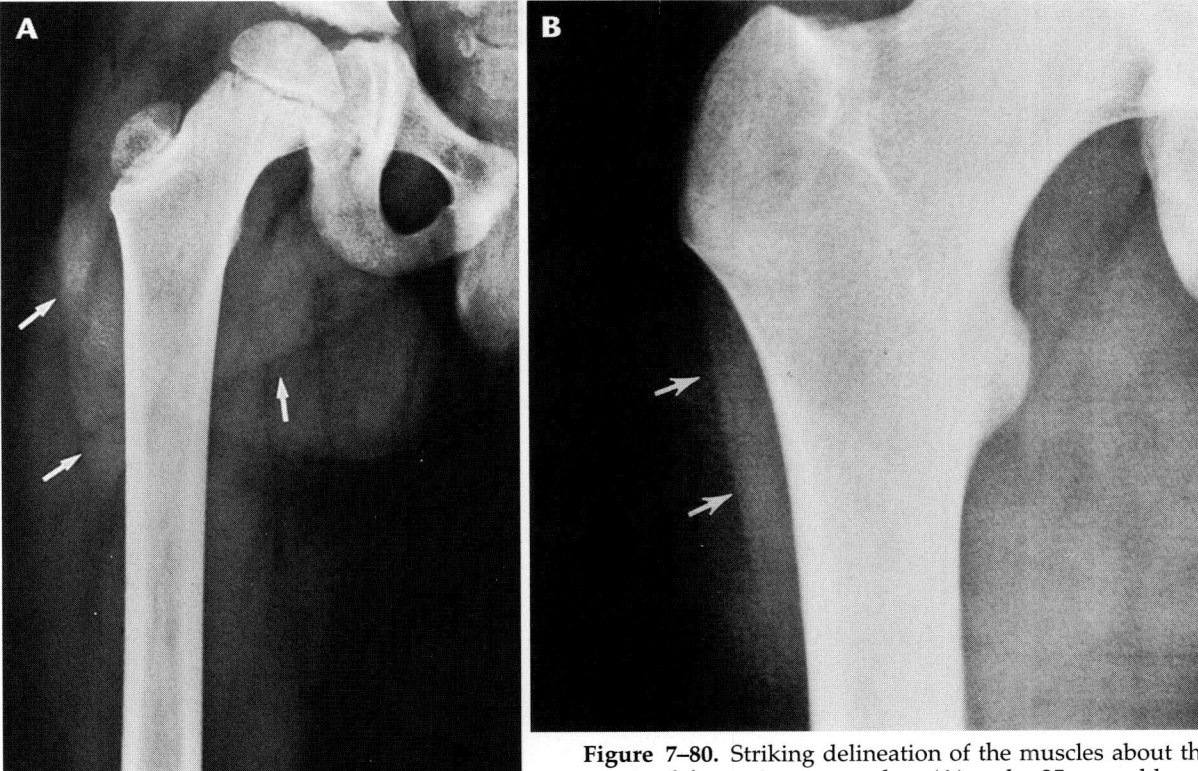

Figure 7–80. Striking delineation of the muscles about the proximal femur in a young boy (**A**) and a 25-year-old athlete (**B**).

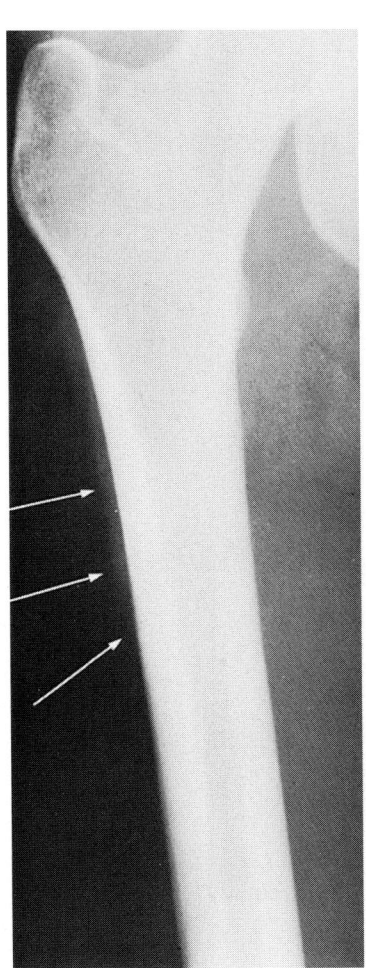

Figure 7–81. Soft tissue companion shadow of the femur.

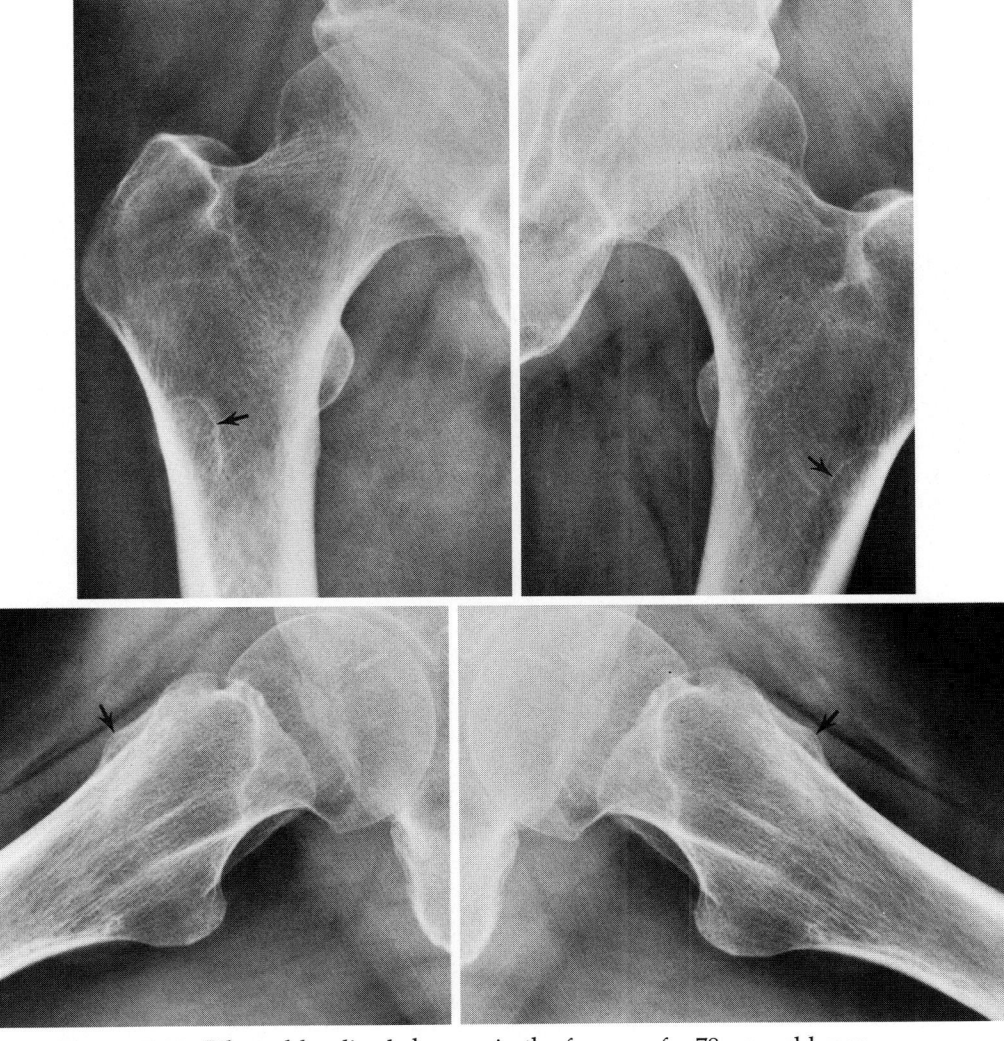

Figure 7–82. Bilateral localized changes in the femurs of a 78-year-old man, thought to represent the origin of the vastus lateralis muscles. (Courtesy of Dr. Ann Gabrielle Bergman.)

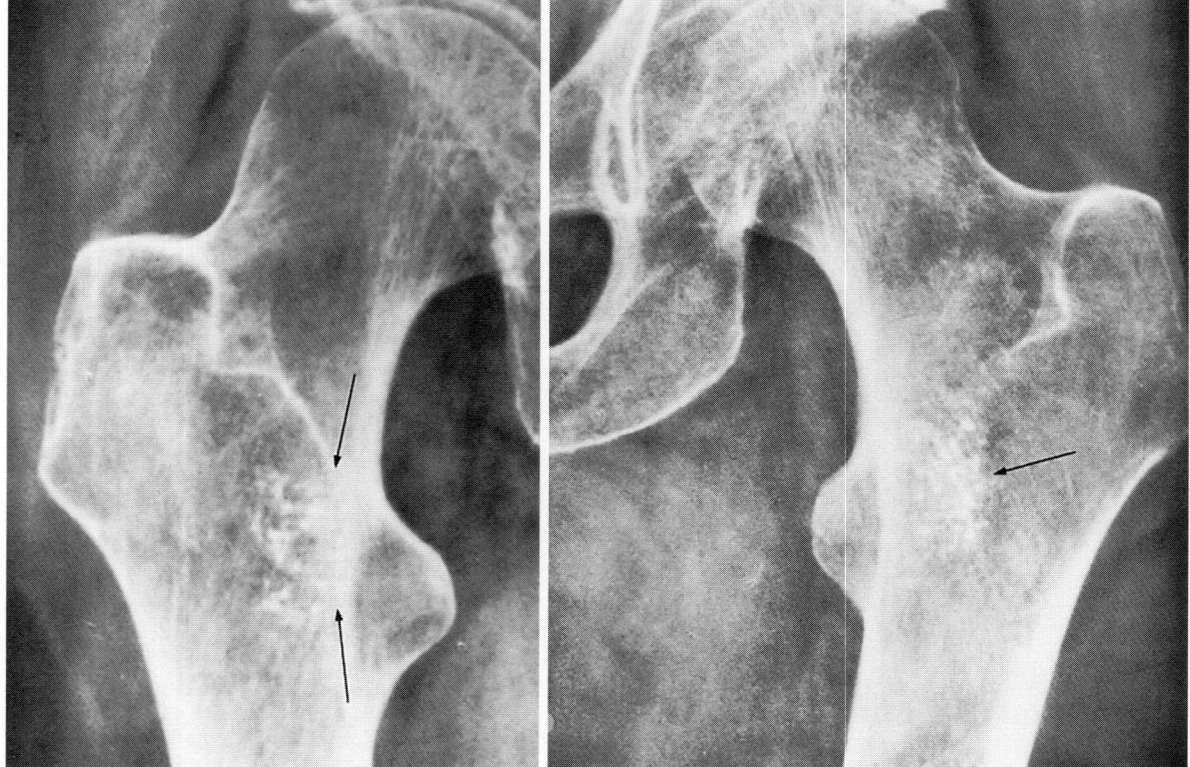

Figure 7–83. Speckled trabeculation of the intertrochanteric area, which should not be mistaken for cartilaginous tumor matrix or bone infarction. These are reinforced trabeculae seen in osteoporotic bone. (Ref: Kérr R et al: Computerized tomography of proximal femoral trabecular patterns. *J Orthop Res* 4:45, 1986.)

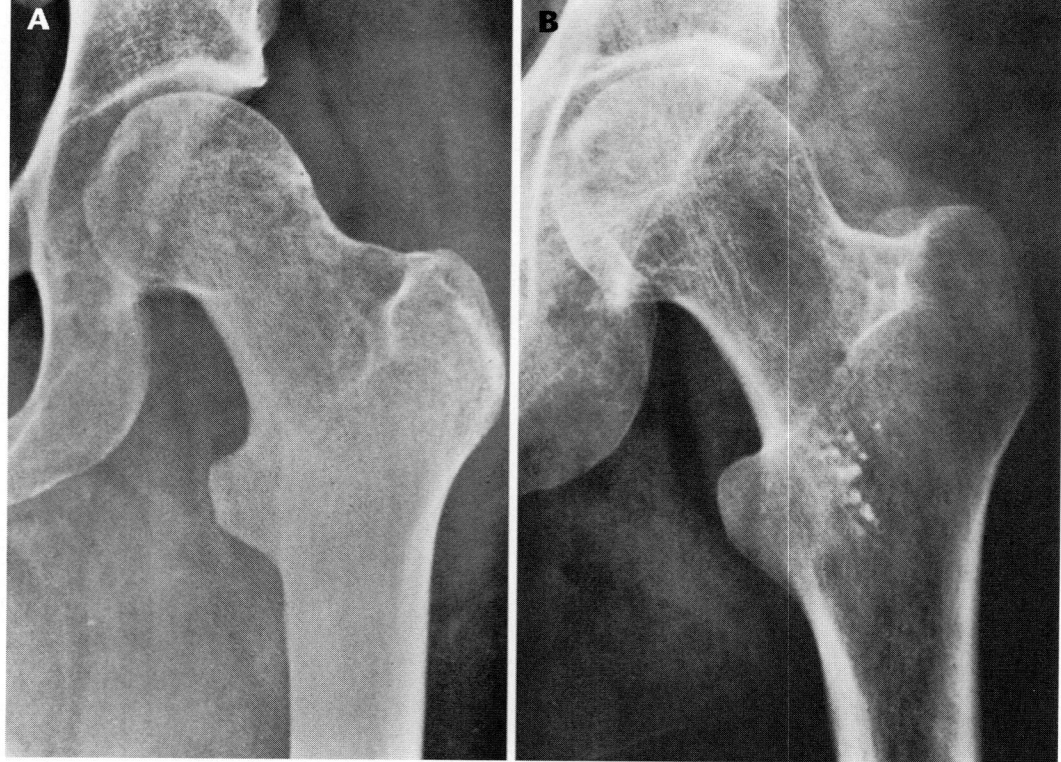

Figure 7–84. Development of the speckled pattern of the femur in a young woman immobilized after a stroke. **A,** Baseline. **B,** Four years later the bone has become osteopenic from disuse, and speckles have appeared.

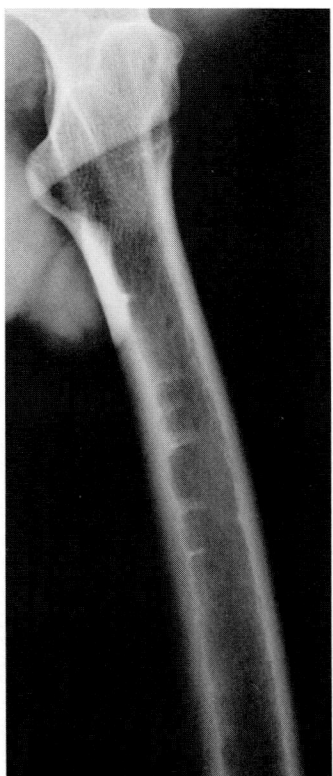

Figure 7–85. Multiple transverse lines in the femoral shaft in a healthy 35-year-old man. These were present bilaterally. Note the same phenomenon in the humerus (see Fig. 6–42).

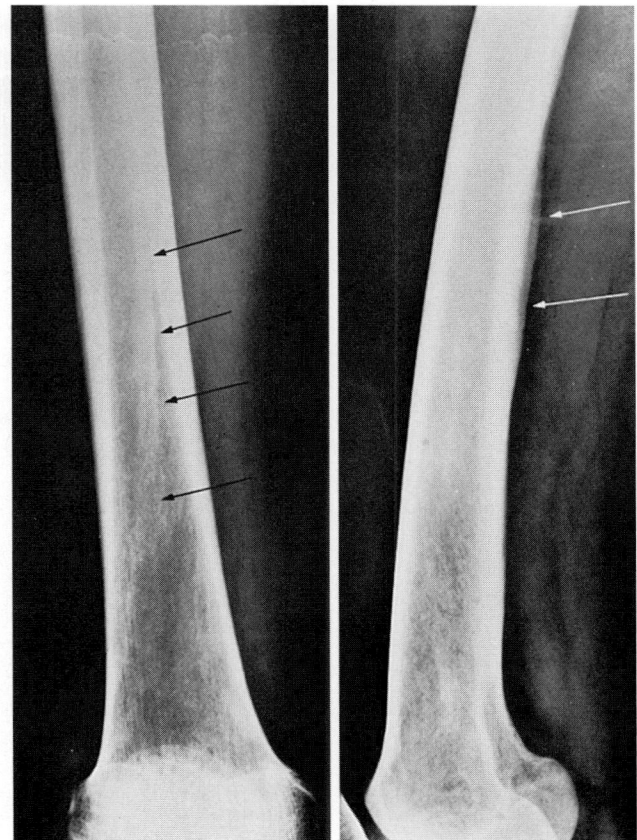

Figure 7–86. The femoral linea aspera-pilaster complex for the insertion of the adductor and extensor muscles. (Ref: Pitt MJ: Radiology of the femoral linea aspera-pilaster complex: The track sign. *Radiology* 142:66, 1982.)

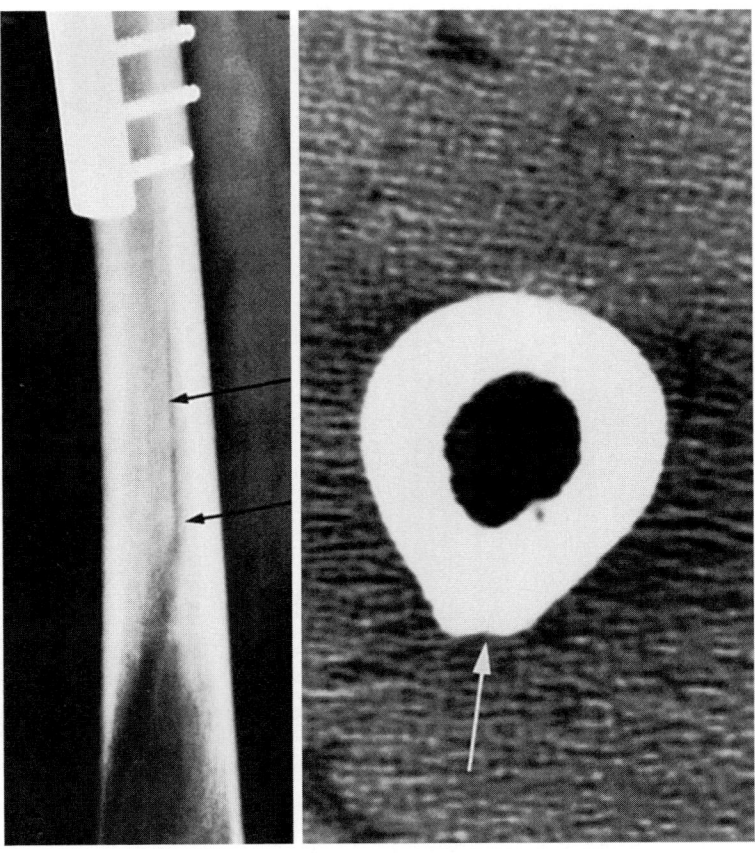

Figure 7–87. *Left,* The pilaster complex misdiagnosed as a fracture of the femur (*arrows*). *Right,* CT shows the cortical ridge (*arrow*) but no fracture.

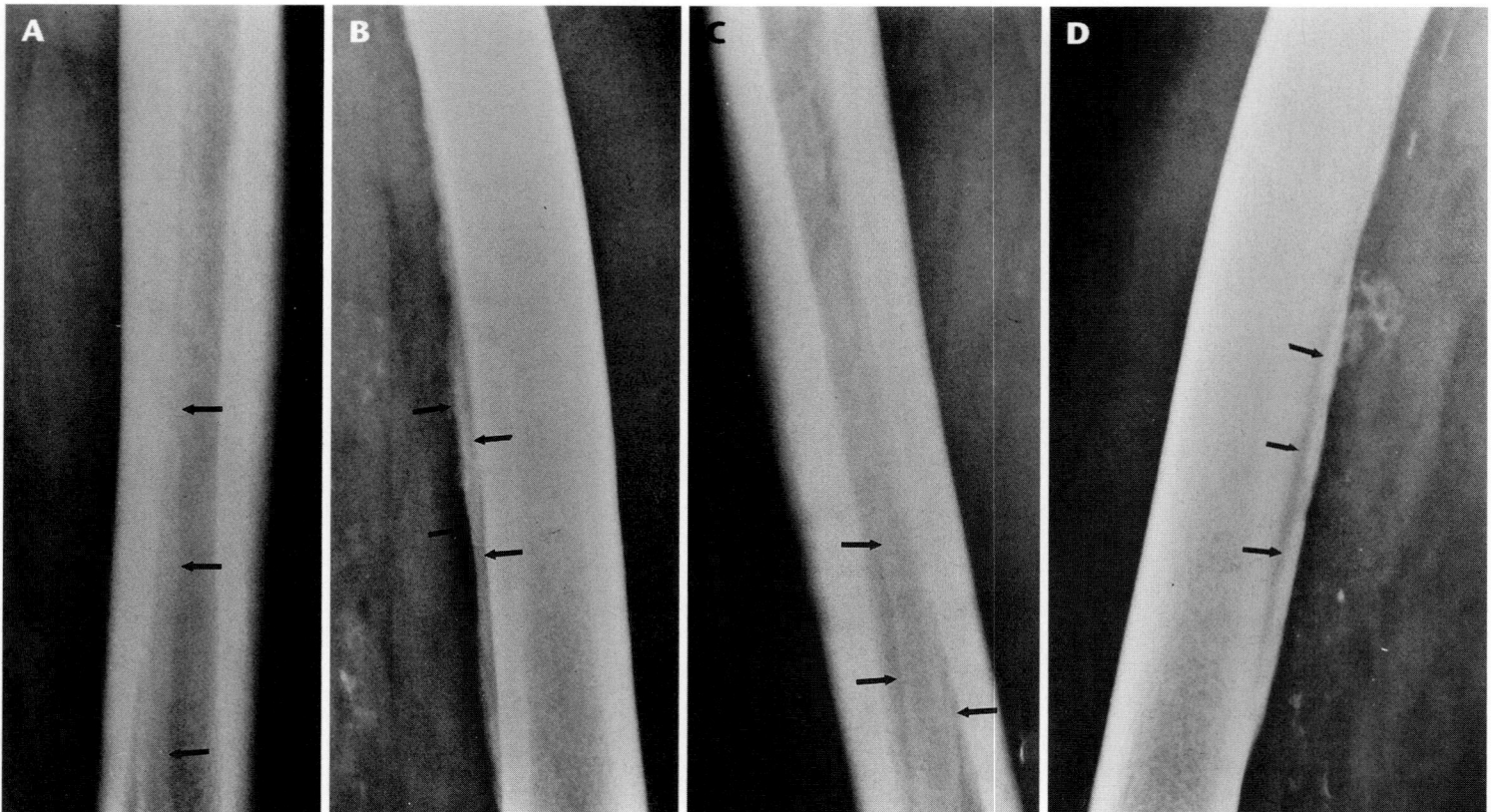

Figure 7–88. A–D, The same entity as Figure 7–87, seen bilaterally. Note the simulated periostitis in the lateral projections (**B** and **D**).

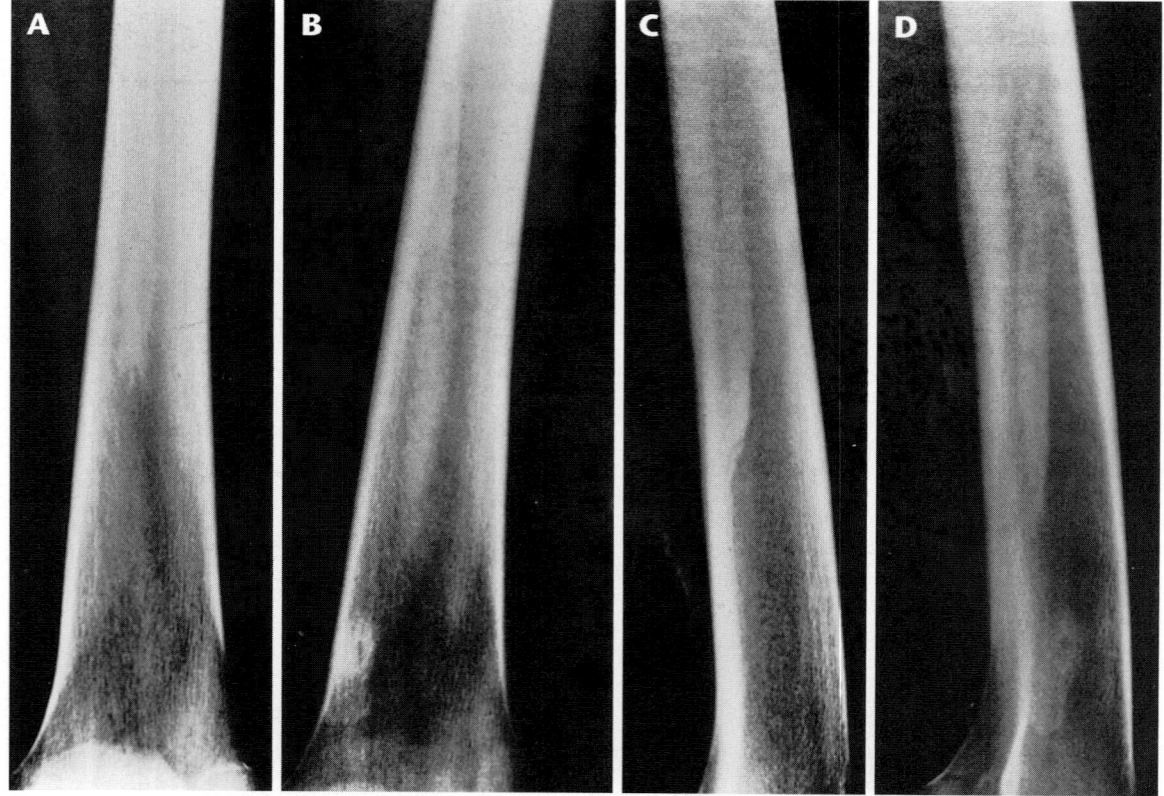

Figure 7–89. A–D, Bilateral linear intramedullary densities of the femurs in a 22-year-old woman. (Courtesy of Dr. J. C. Hoeffel.)

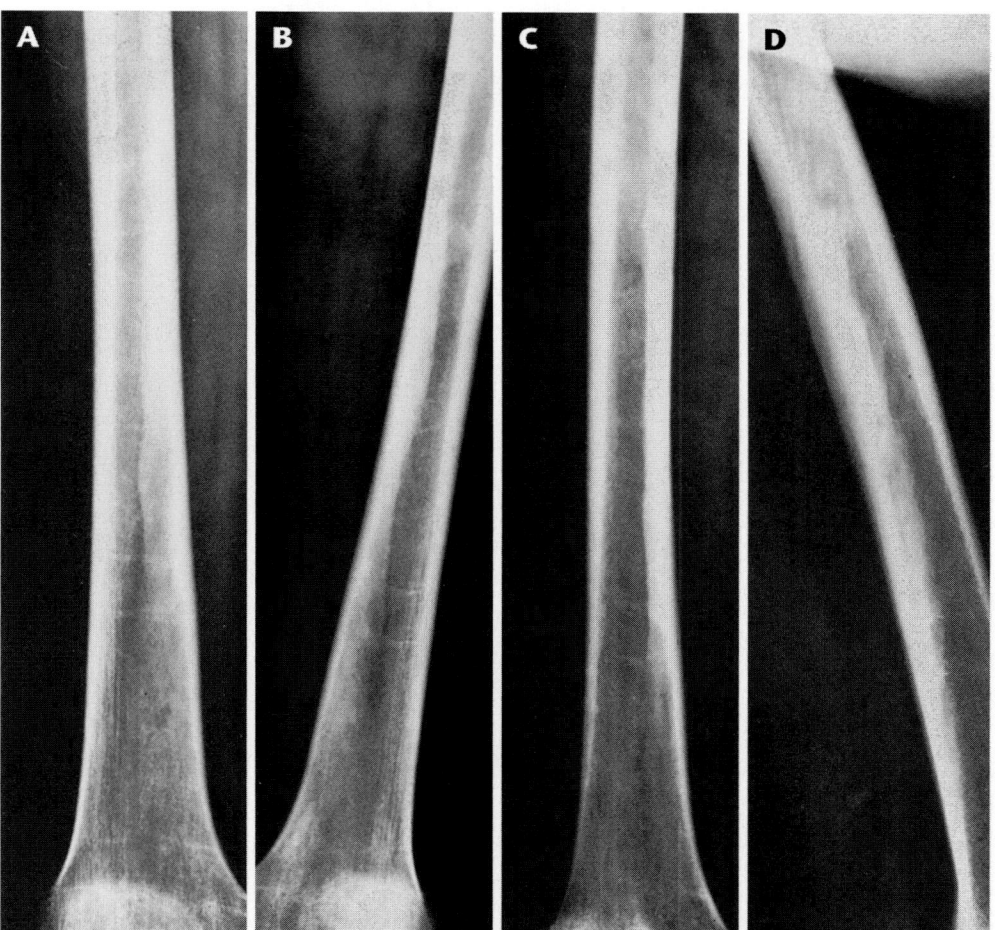

Figure 7–90. A–D, Bilateral linear intramedullary densities of the femurs in a 67-year-old woman. These are seen more frequently in elderly women without known disease and are apparently of no clinical significance.

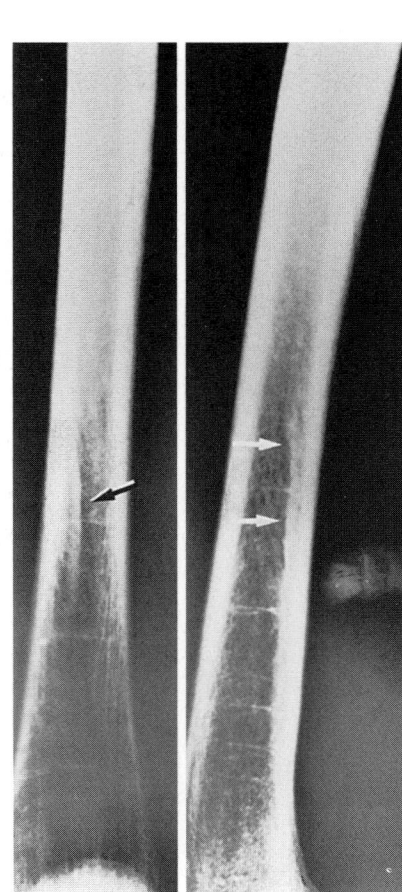

Figure 7–91. Same entity as shown in Figures 7–89 and 7–90 in a 70-year-old woman.

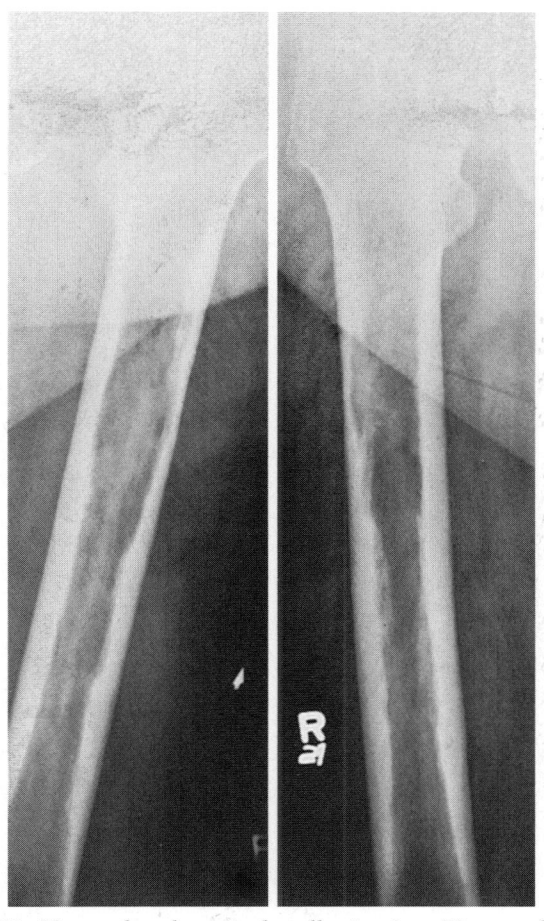

Figure 7–92. Unusual endocortical scalloping in a 70-year-old woman with no known disease, presumably representing a reflection of osteoporosis.

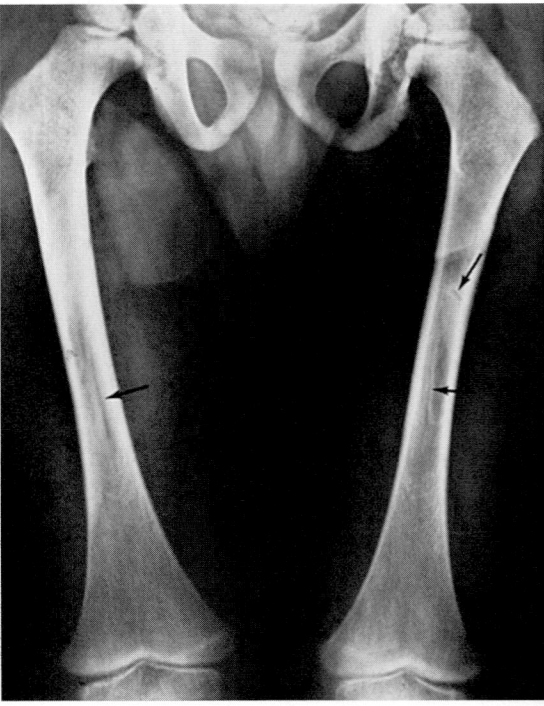
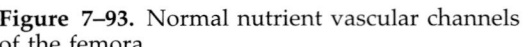
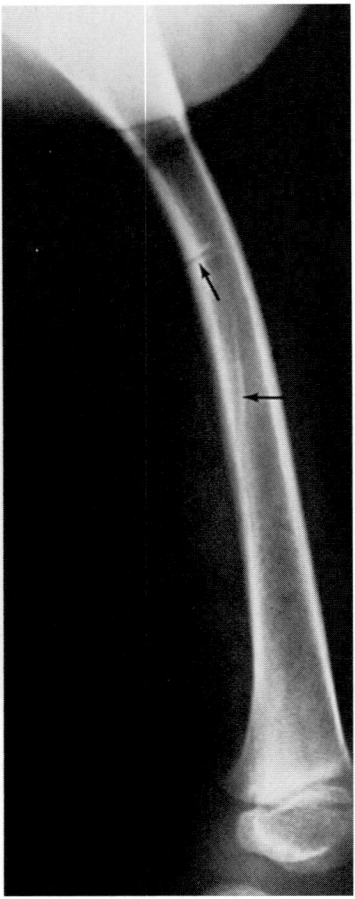

Figure 7–93. Normal nutrient vascular channels of the femora.

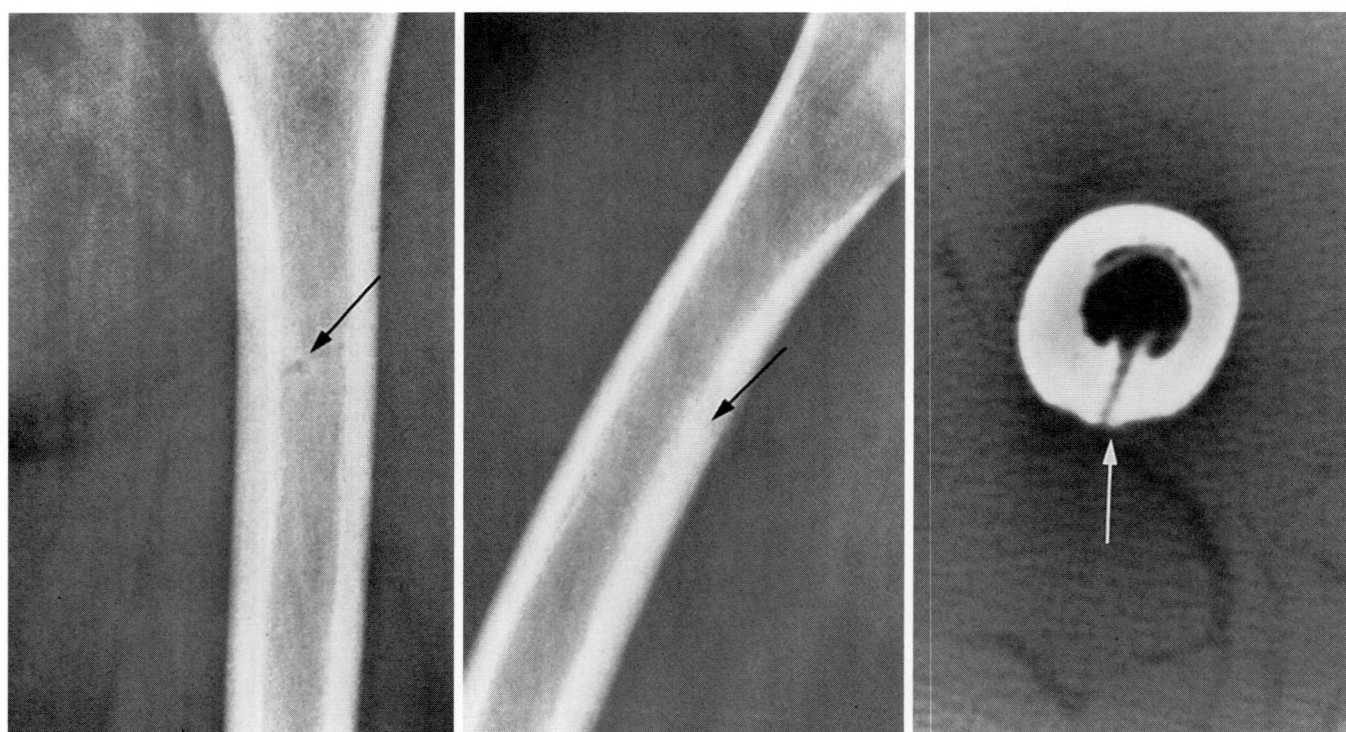

Figure 7–94. Nutrient foramen in a 7-year-old boy that, when added to the normal cortical thickening of the posterior aspect of the femur, was mistaken for an osteoid osteoma. *Left,* Frontal projection. *Center,* Lateral projection. *Right,* CT scan.

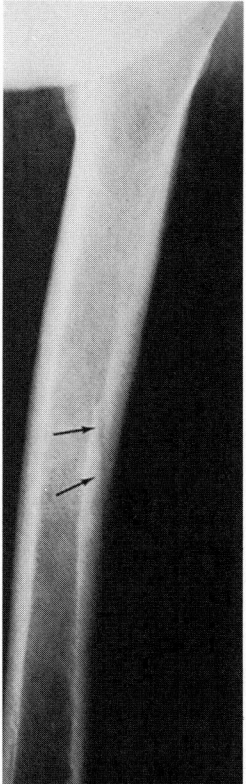

Figure 7–95. The nutrient channel of the femur.

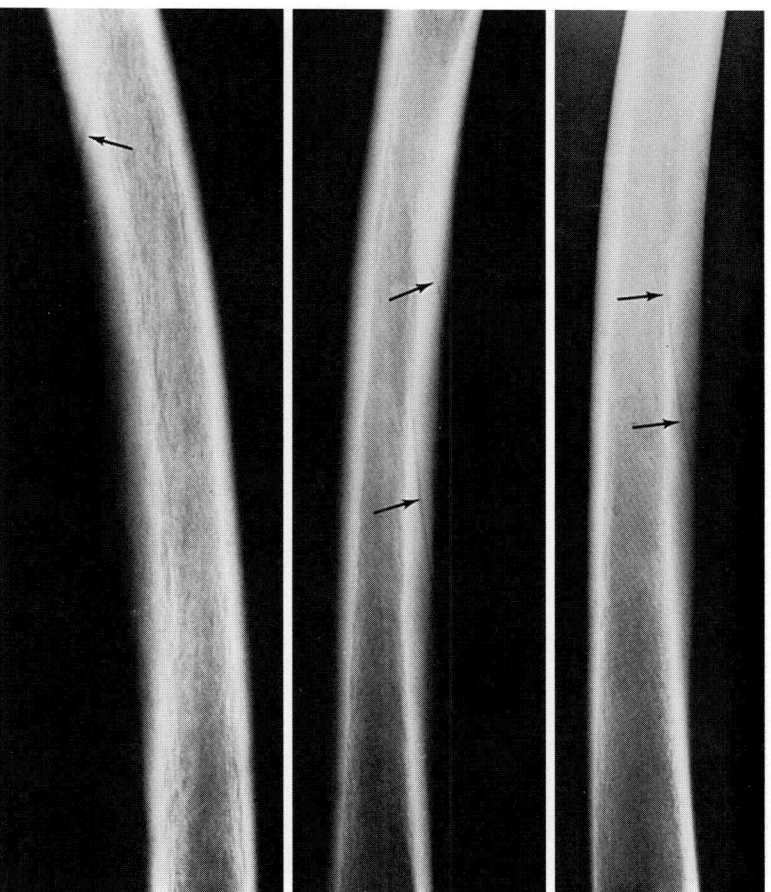

Figure 7–96. Three examples of lucent fissures in the posterior cortex of the femur, which might be mistaken for fracture lines.

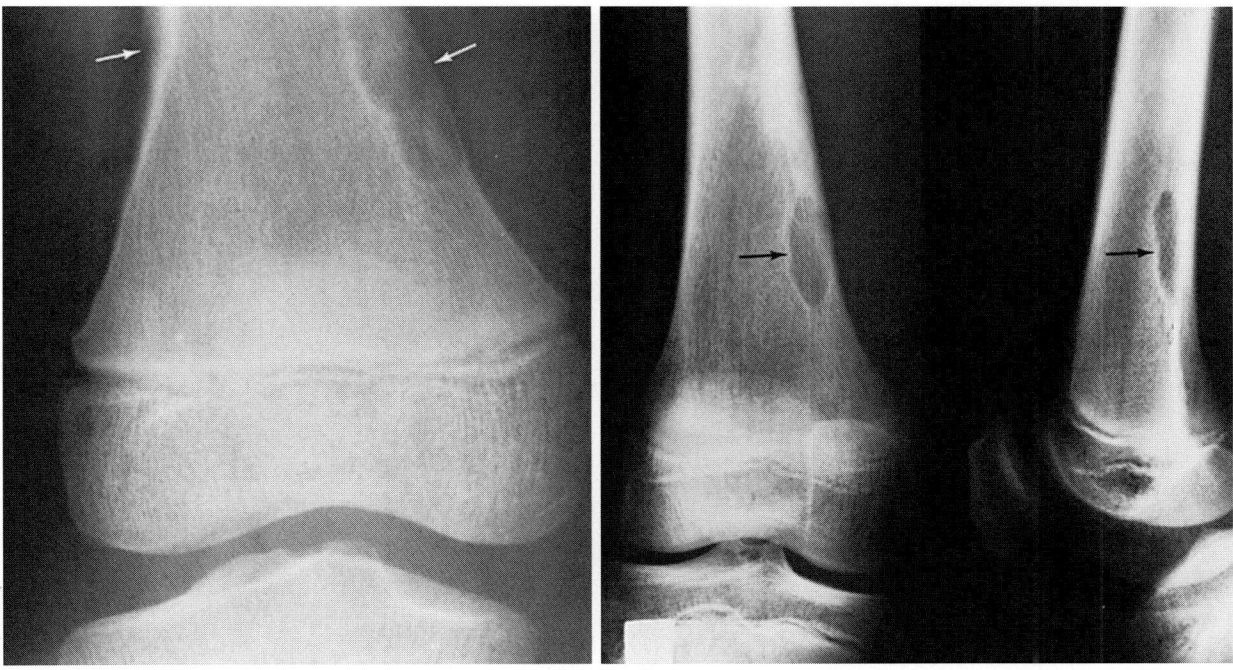

Figure 7–97. Typical juvenile benign cortical defects. These lesions are very common in the distal femur and are of no clinical significance. (Ref: Ritschl P et al: Fibrous metaphyseal defects: Determination of their origin and natural history using a radiomorphological study. *Skeletal Radiol* 17:8, 1988.)

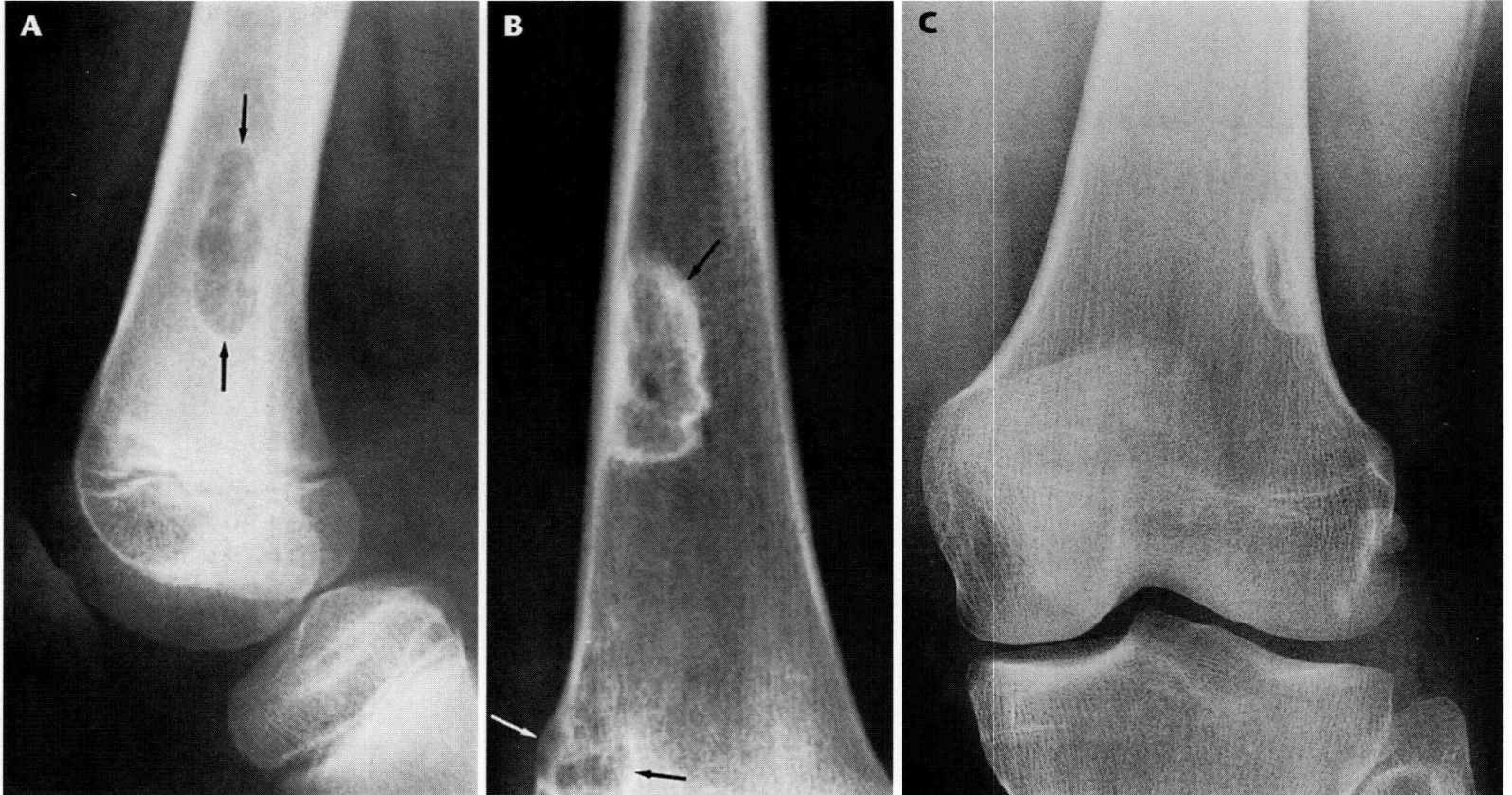

Figure 7–98. Additional examples of juvenile benign cortical defects. **A,** Multiloculate. **B,** Multiple lesions with thick sclerotic margins. **C,** Healing.

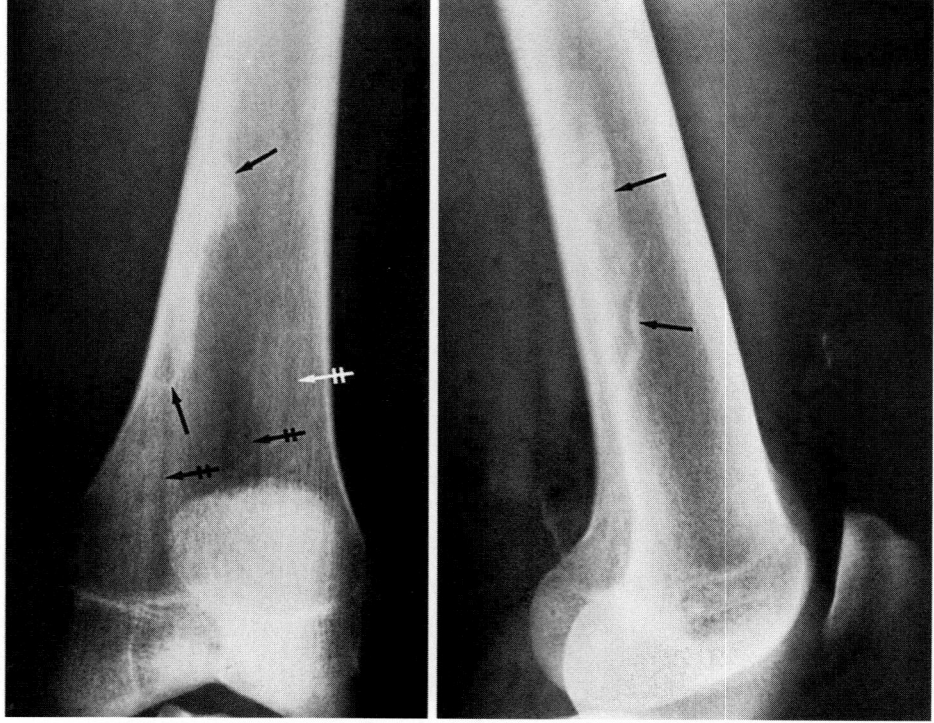

Figure 7–99. Healing juvenile benign cortical defect in a 17-year-old boy (←). Note mixed lucency and sclerosis. Note also longitudinal striations in the metaphysis, a common finding in young people (⊣⊦).

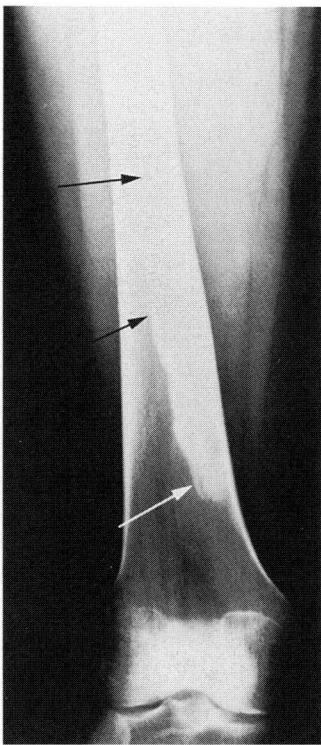

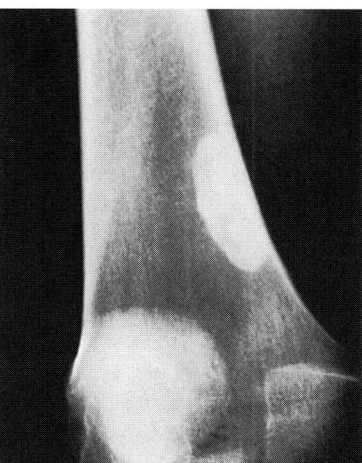

Figure 7–101. Very dense healed juvenile benign cortical defect in a 24-year-old woman.

Figure 7–100. Huge healed juvenile benign cortical defect in an 18-year-old woman.

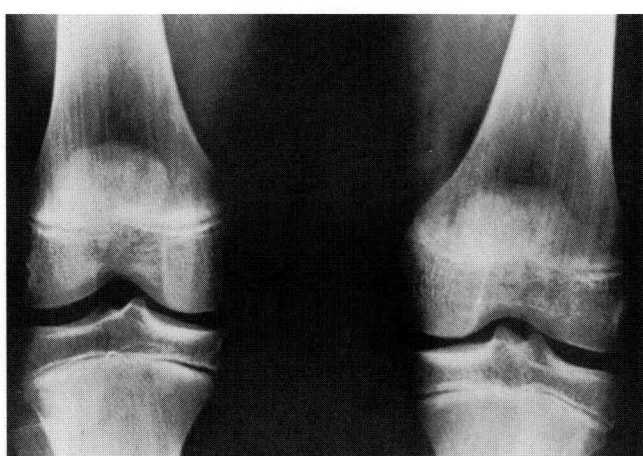

Figure 7–102. Prominent longitudinal striations of the bone in a normal 13-year-old girl.

The Distal End of the Femur

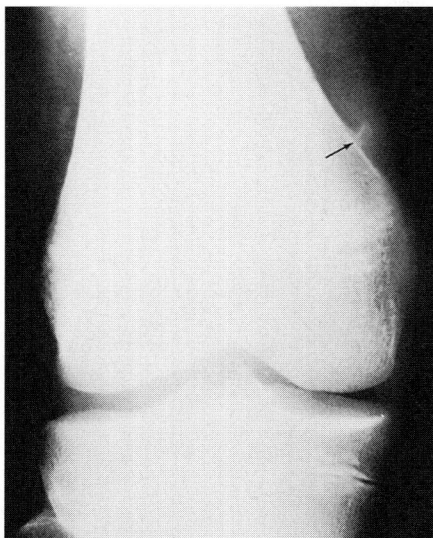

Figure 7–103. "Tug" lesion of the medial aspect of the distal femur in an adolescent, representing bone formation in the insertion of the adductor magnus muscle. (Ref: Barnes GR Jr, Gwinn JL: Distal irregularities of the femur simulating malignancy. *Am J Roentgenol* 122:180, 1974.)

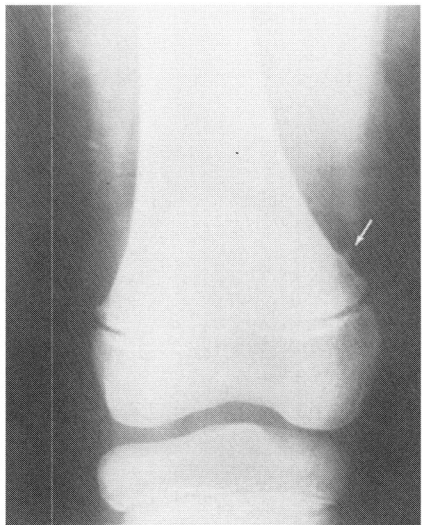

Figure 7–104. Small "tug" lesion in an 11-year-old girl.

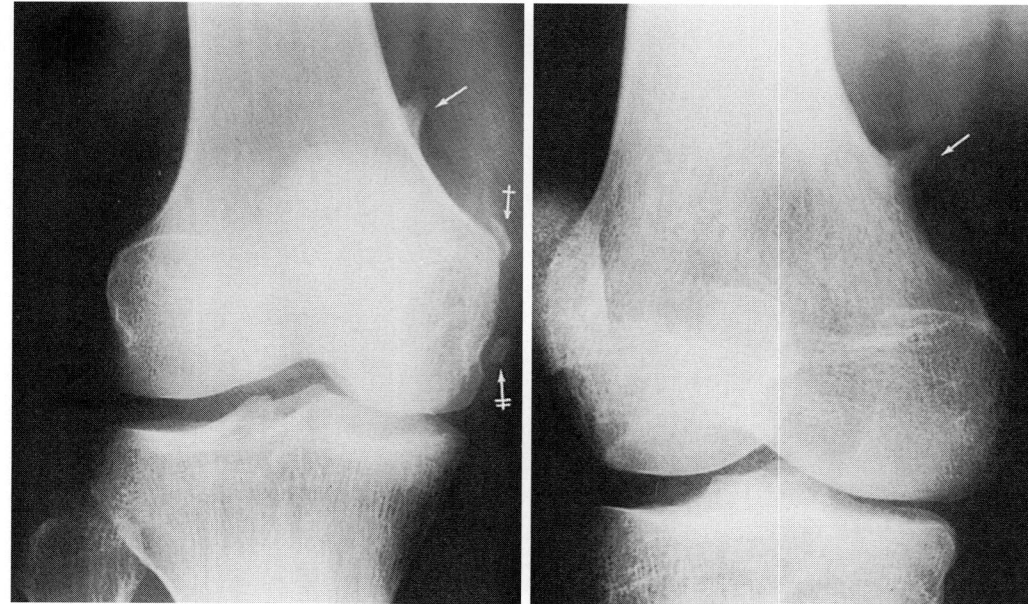

Figure 7–105. Additional example of the "tug" lesion of the femur in an adult (→). Note also calcification in the medial collateral ligament (↠) and an ossicle below of the same etiology (⇻).

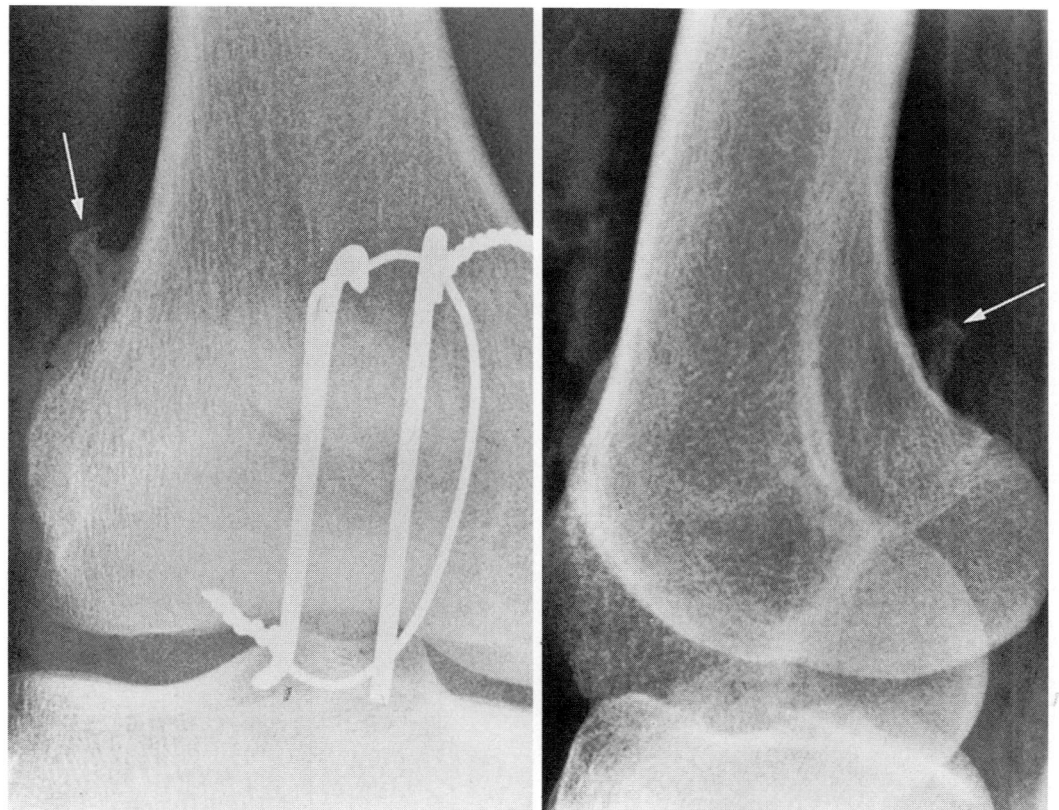

Figure 7–106. Very large "tug" lesion of the medial femoral metaphysis resembling an osteochondroma.

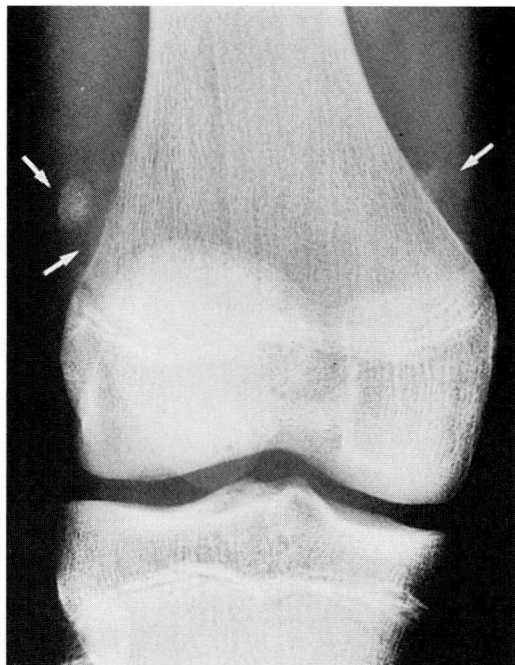

Figure 7–107. Bilateral "tug" lesions of the femur, probably secondary to a pull of the vastus lateralis and medialis.

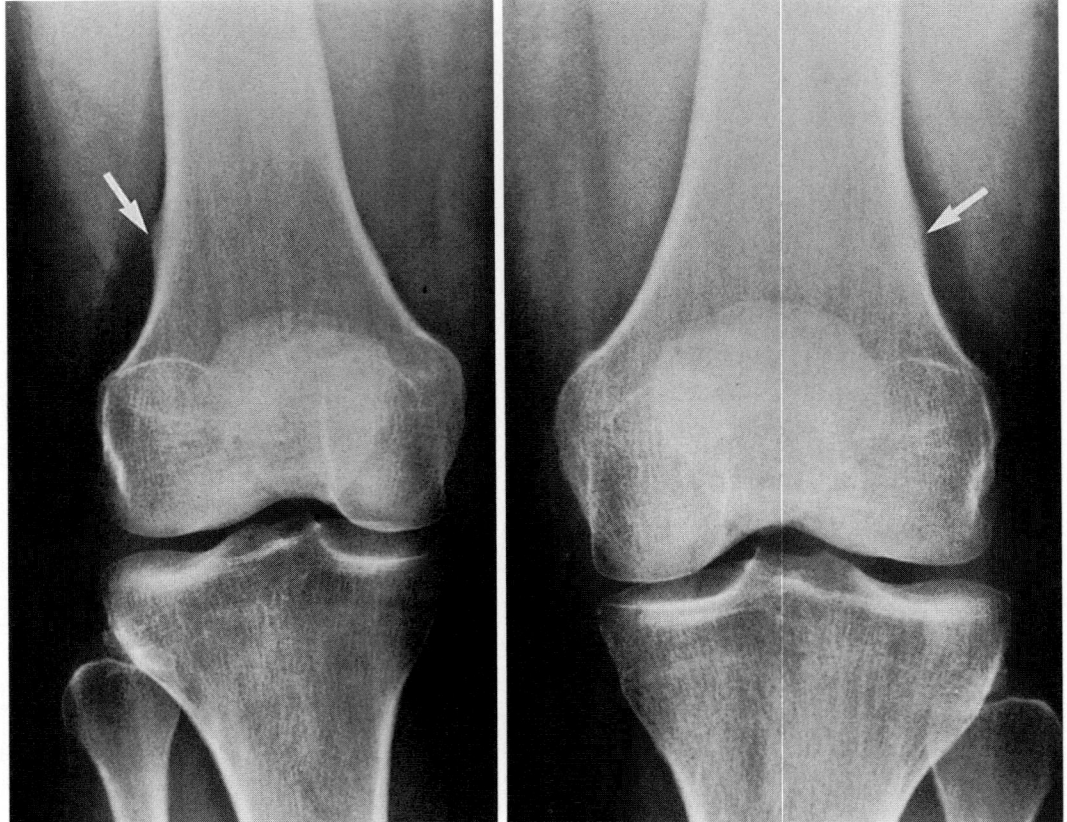

Figure 7–108. Bilateral cortical thickenings in a young man, related to insertion of the vastus lateralis muscle, a common radiologic finding.

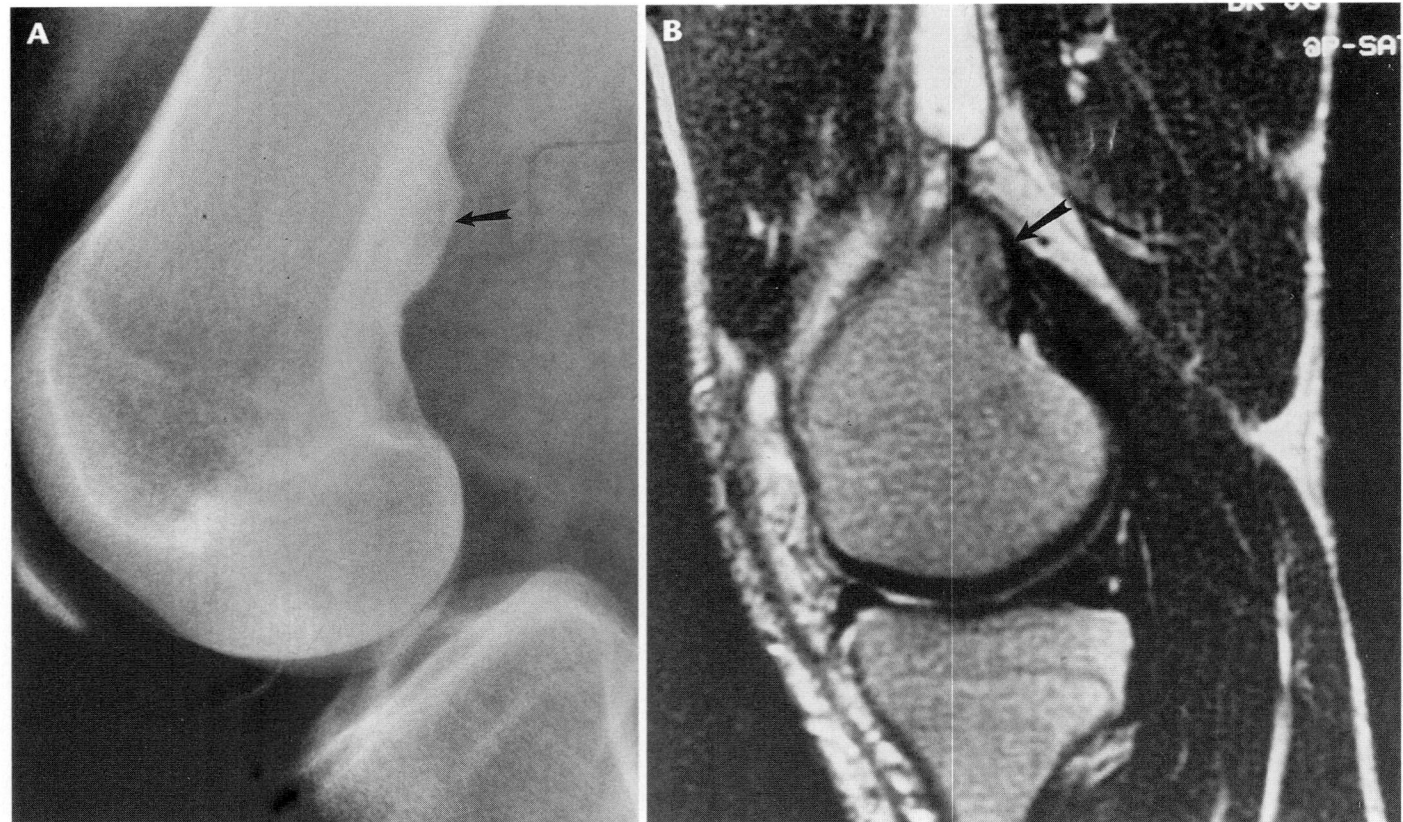

Figure 7–109. Prominent insertion of the medial head of the gastrocnemius. **A,** Plain film. **B,** T-2–weighted MR image.

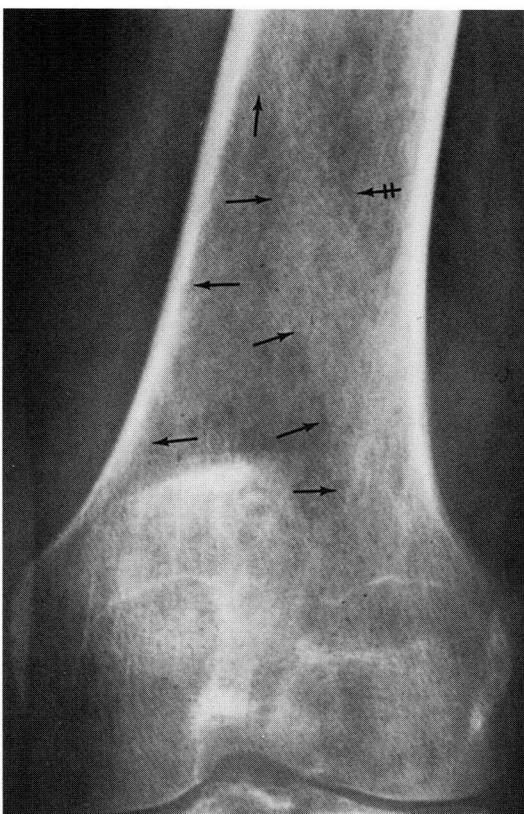

Figure 7–110. Normal triangular area of radiolucency seen in the metaphysis of the distal femur in an osteoporotic individual (←). The density in the midportion is related to the linea aspera (↤).

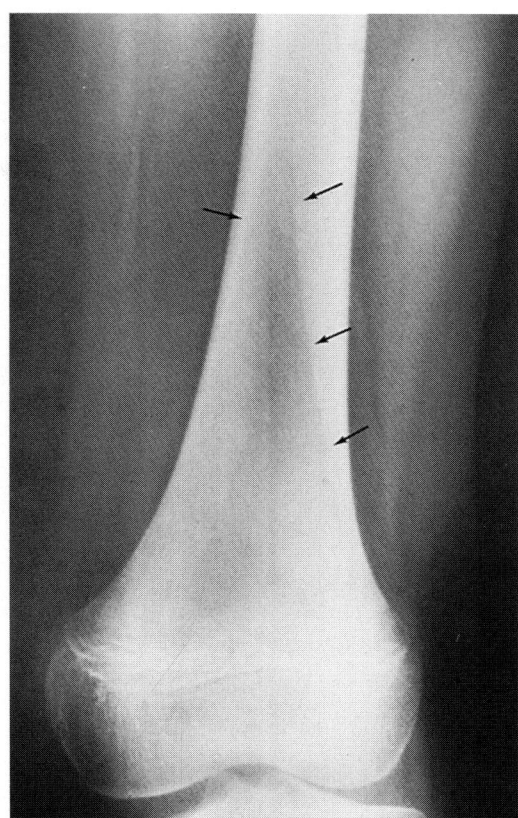

Figure 7–111. Triangular radiolucency in an 11-year-old girl.

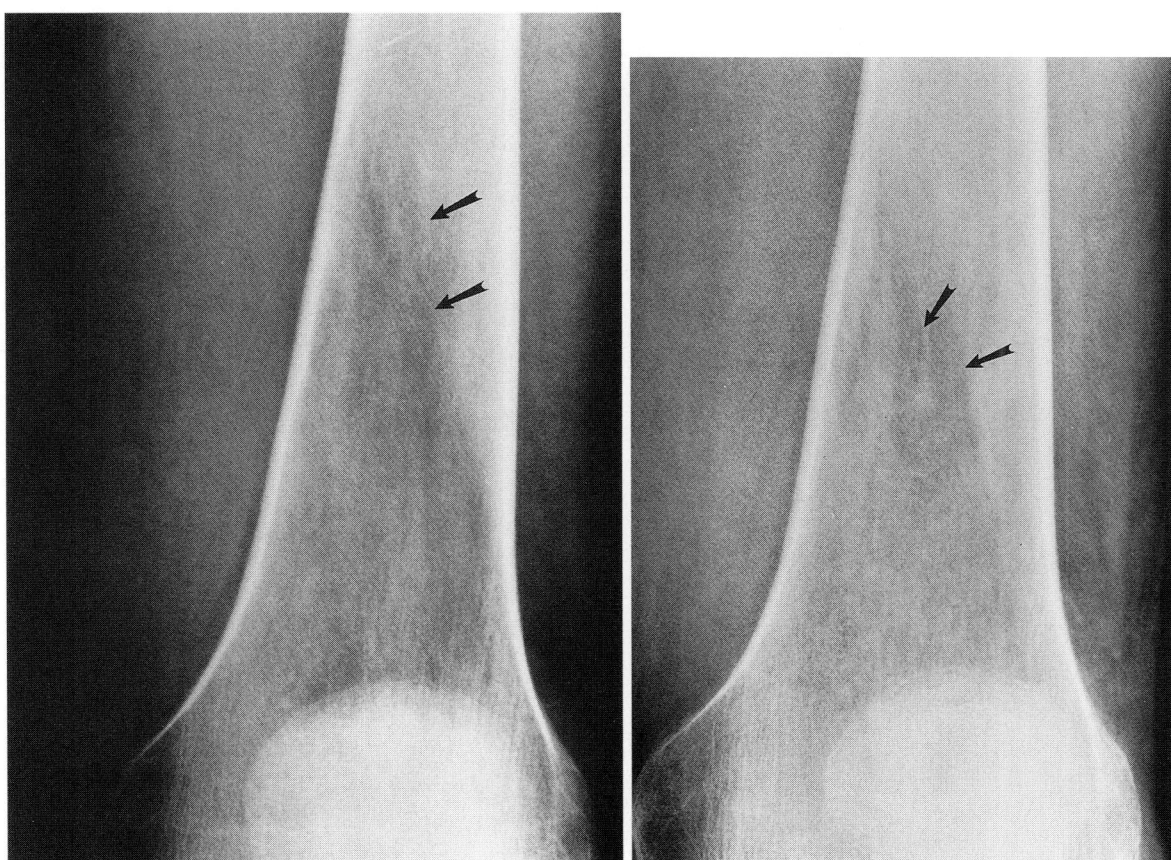

Figure 7–112. Normal lucencies in the distal femur mistaken for metastases in a patient with breast carcinoma. The lateral projections were normal.

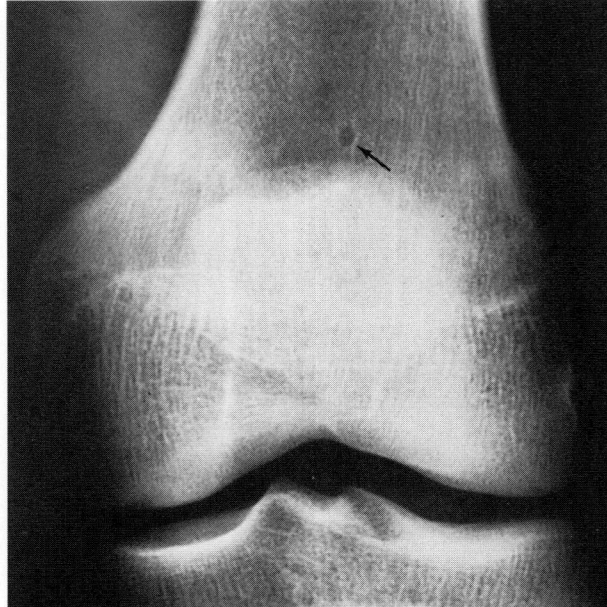

Figure 7–113. Nutrient foramen of the distal femur.

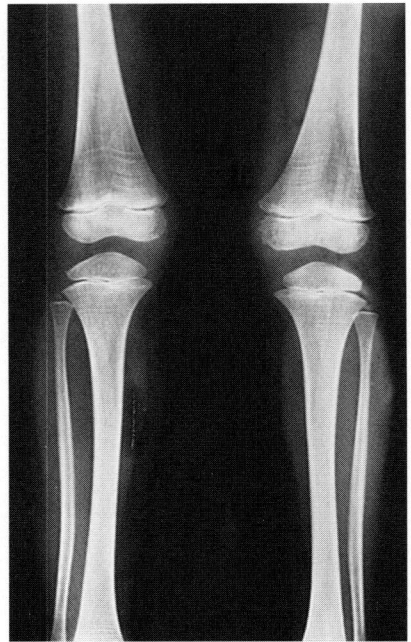

Figure 7–114. Examples of transverse ("growth") lines of the distal femoral metaphyses. Although frequently associated with disease states, these lines are often seen in patients without contributory history.

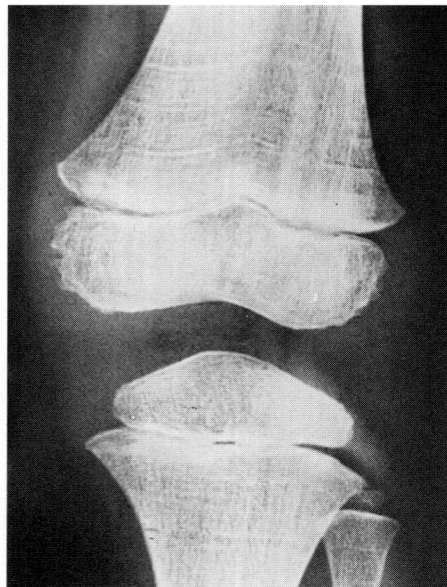

Figure 7–115. Detailed view of transverse lines of the distal femur in a younger child.

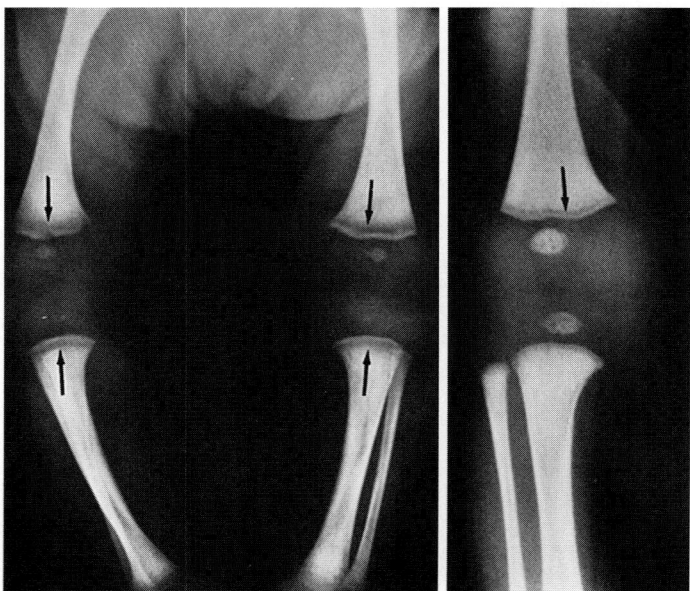

Figure 7–116. Two examples of normal metaphyseal radiolucencies, an accompanying feature of the osteosclerosis of the newborn (see Fig. 7–72). The new bone formed at the metaphysis is often more radiolucent, producing an appearance that might be mistaken for evidence of systemic disease. This finding is often the product of intrauterine stress.

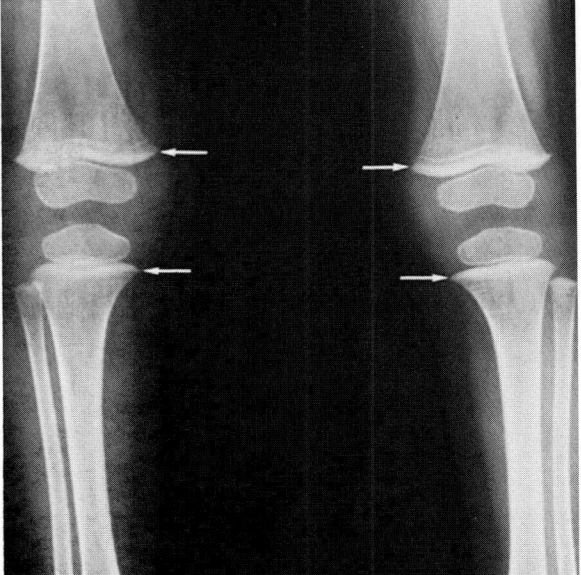

Figure 7–117. Dense zones of provisional calcification are often mistaken for the lines of heavy metal poisoning. These zones vary considerably in thickness in healthy children and in the same child at different ages. They tend to be proportionately thicker during the second to fifth years. (Ref: Caffey J: *Pediatric x-ray diagnosis*, 9th ed. Chicago, Mosby, 1993, p. 1465.)

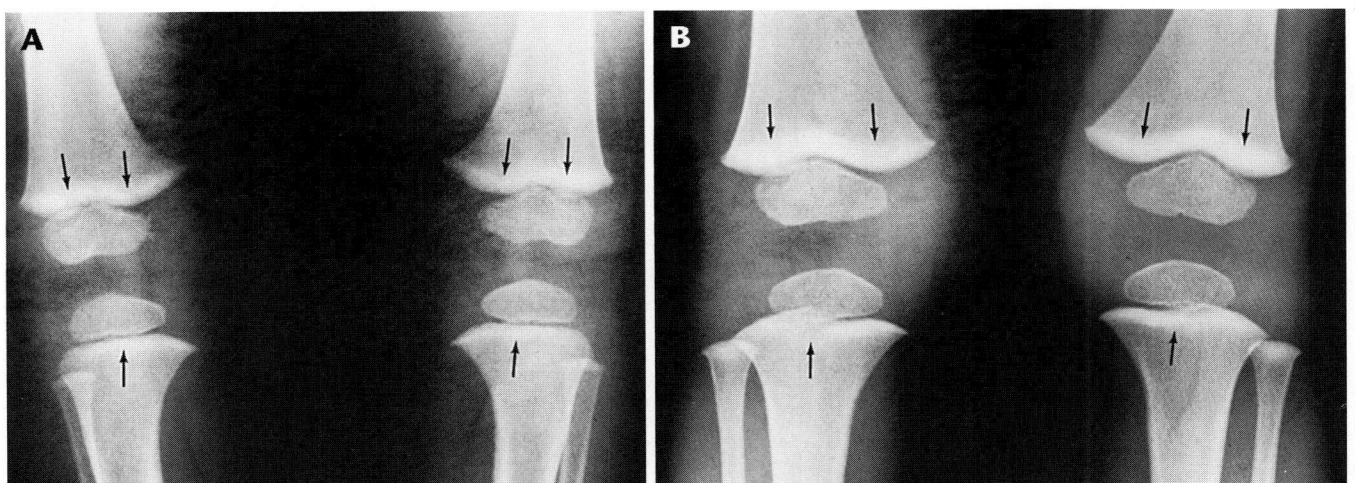

Figure 7–118. Additional examples of normal zones of provisional calcification. **A,** 14-month-old infant. **B,** 2-year-old infant.

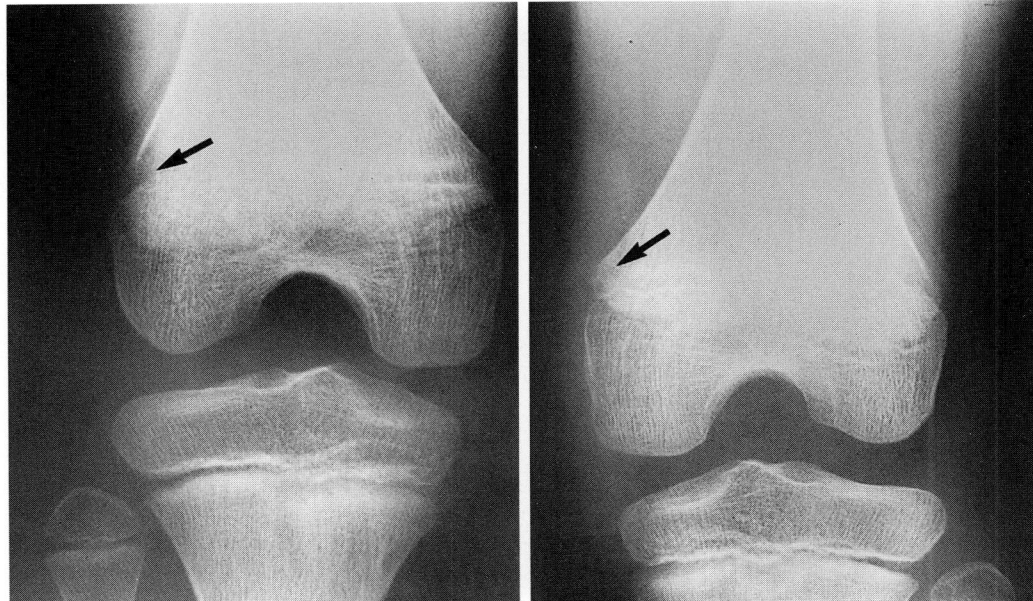

Figure 7–119. Simulated lesions of the femur produced by the edge of the growth plates in tunnel views in a 10-year-old boy.

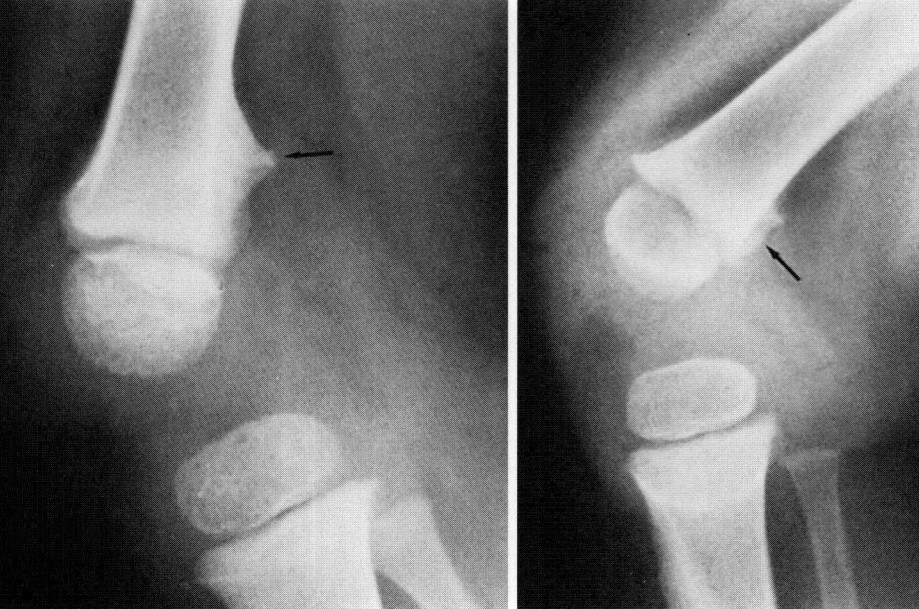

Figure 7–120. Two examples of normal irregularity in ossification of the posterior aspect of the distal femur in 2-year-old infants.

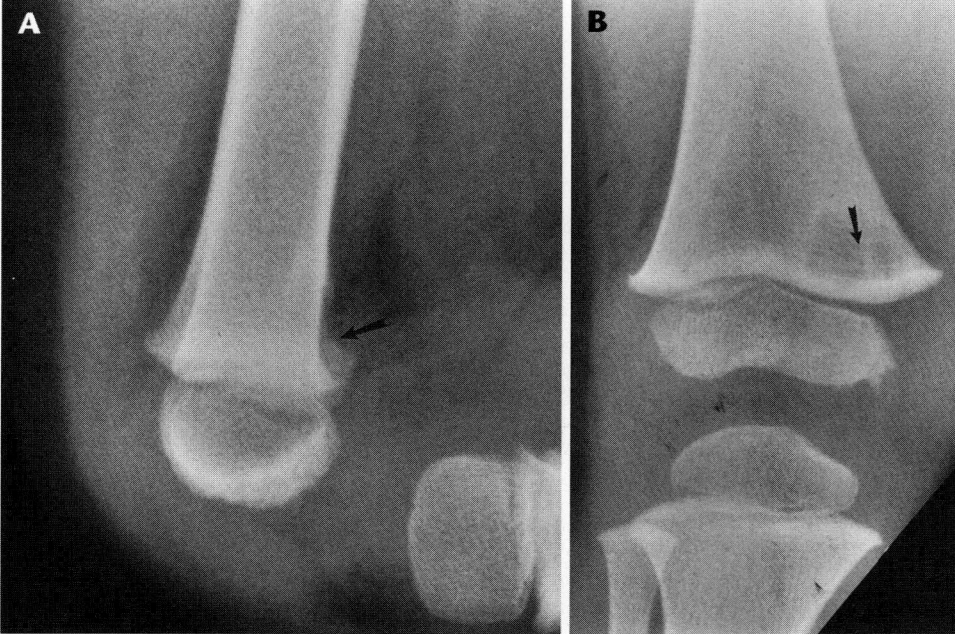

Figure 7–121. A, The posterior irregularity of the posterior aspect of the distal femur in a 2-year-old. **B,** Note the radiolucency in the medial aspect of the femoral metaphysis, which is probably the product of the posterior cortical irregularity.

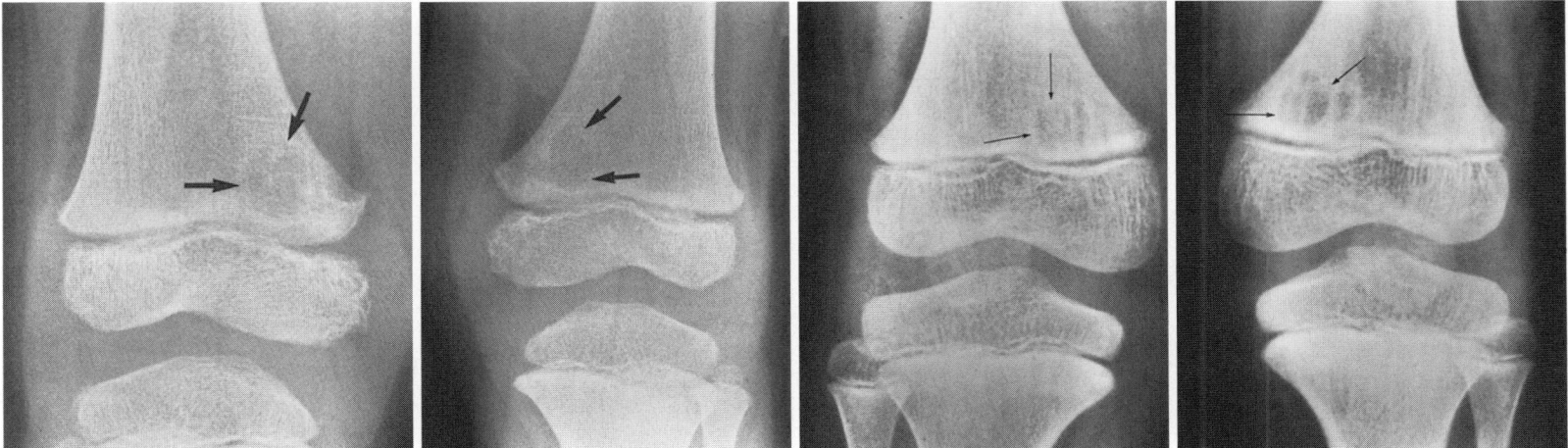

Figure 7–122. Four examples of the metaphyseal radiolucencies illustrated in the previous figure, seen in 5- and 6-year-old children.

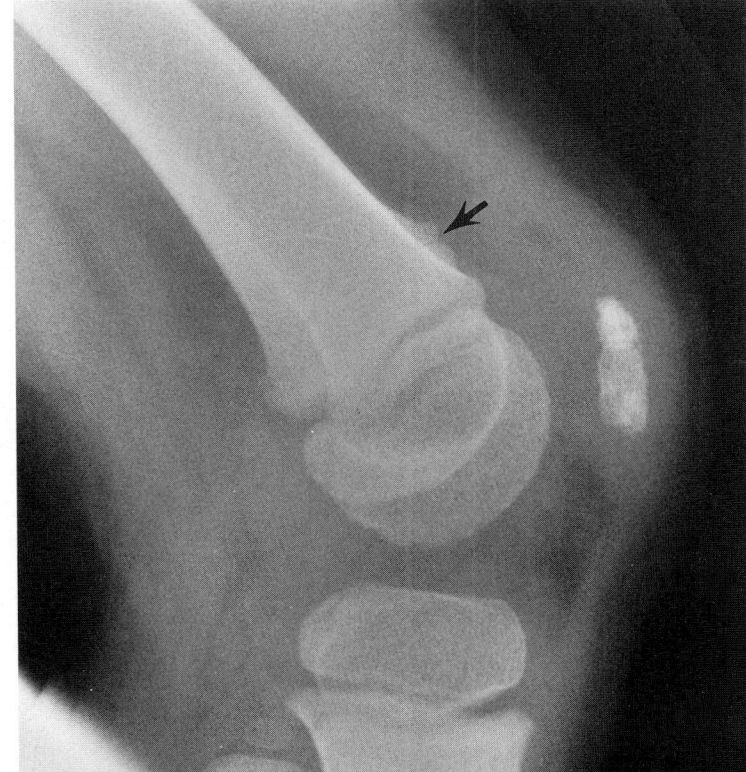

Figure 7–123. Irregularity of the anterior aspect of the femoral metaphysis in a 3-year-old boy, similar to that seen in Figures 7–120 and 7–127.

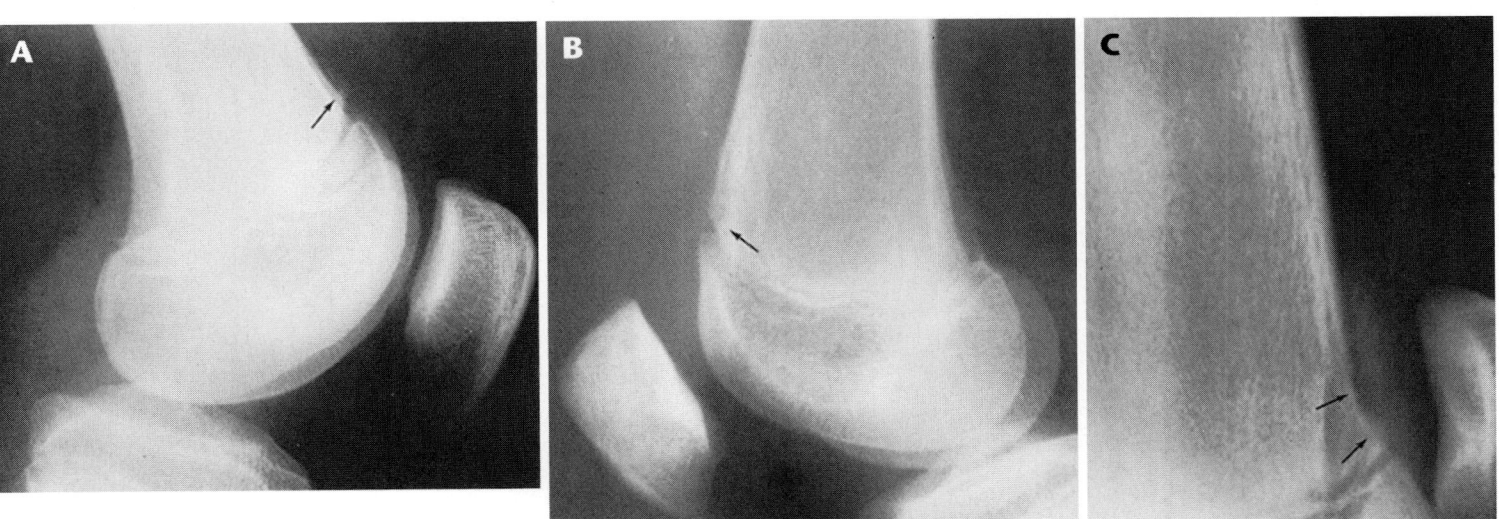

Figure 7–124. Three examples of irregularity of the cortex of the anterior aspect of the femur, immediately above the epiphyseal line. This entity is seen in adolescence and is a transient event. **A,** 11-year-old boy. **B,** 13-year-old boy. **C,** 15-year-old boy. (Ref: Keats TE: The distal anterior femoral metaphyseal defect: An anatomic variant that may simulate disease. *Am J Roentgenol* 121:101, 1974.)

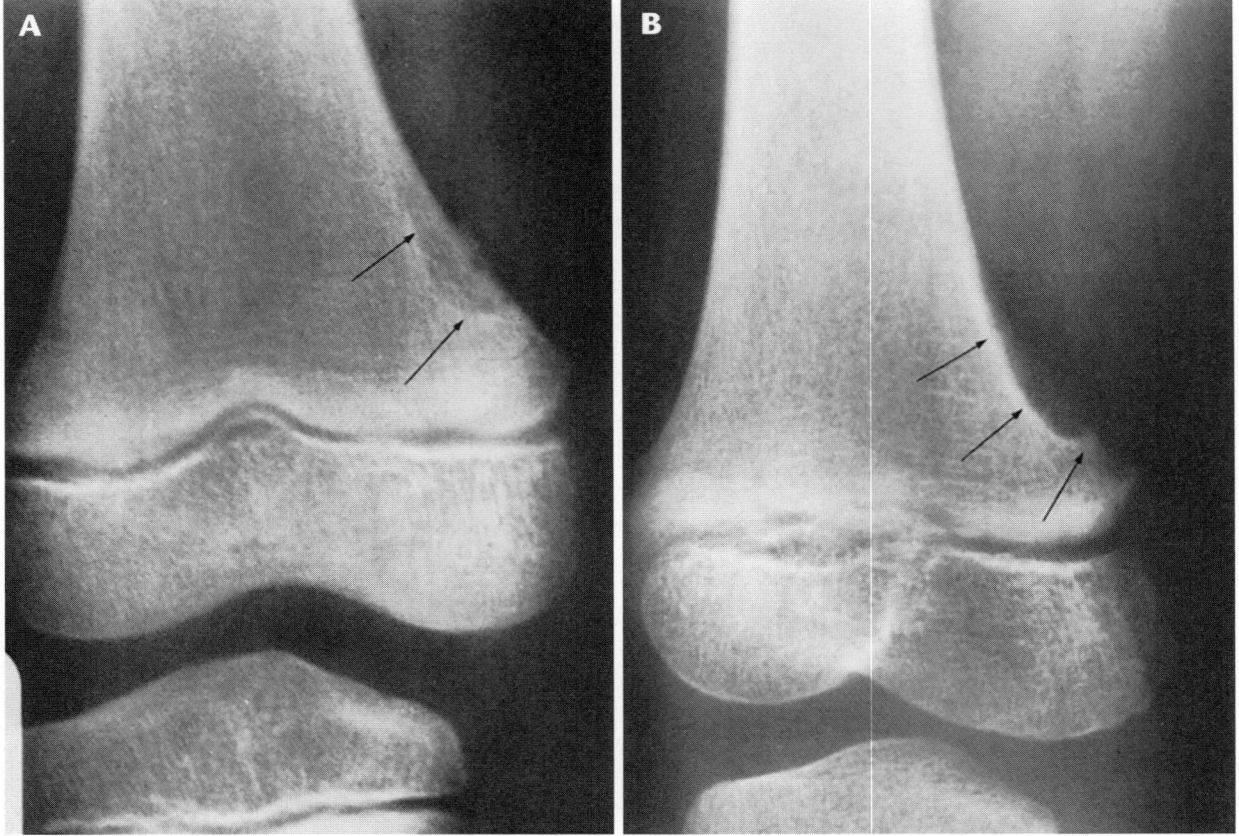

Figure 7–125. A, B, Irregular defect in the cortex of the medial posterior aspect of the distal femur is a common finding between the ages of 12 and 16 years. This is a fibrous lesion, which often demonstrates fine perpendicular spiculation of bone (**B**) and may be mistaken for a malignant bone tumor. It appears to be developmental in origin and disappears with advancing age. It seems to be similar in nature to other metaphyseal irregularities seen elsewhere in the body at the same age, and it is important to note that the metaphyseal irregularities in the medial posterior aspects of the distal end of the femur are cold on nuclear scanning, which would suggest that they are not avulsive in nature. (Refs: Brower AC et al: The histologic nature of the cortical irregularity of the medial posterior distal femoral metaphysis in children. *Radiology* 99:389, 1971; Burrows PE: The distal femoral defect: Technetium 99m pyrophosphate bone scan results. *J Can Assoc Radiol* 33:91, 1982.)

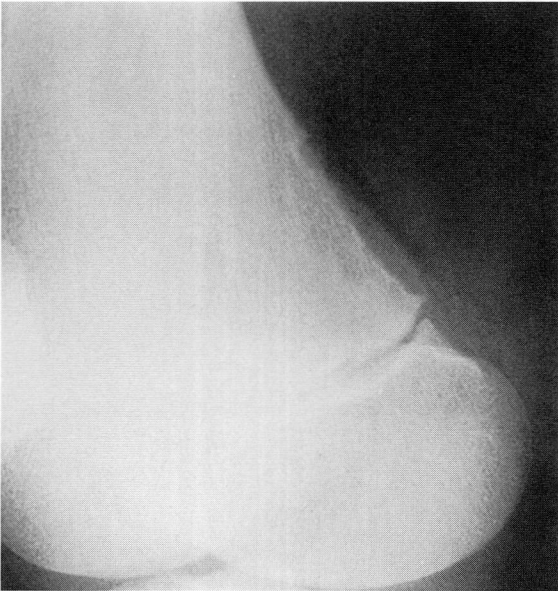

Figure 7–126. Good detail of the architecture of the medial femoral cortical irregularity in a 15-year-old boy.

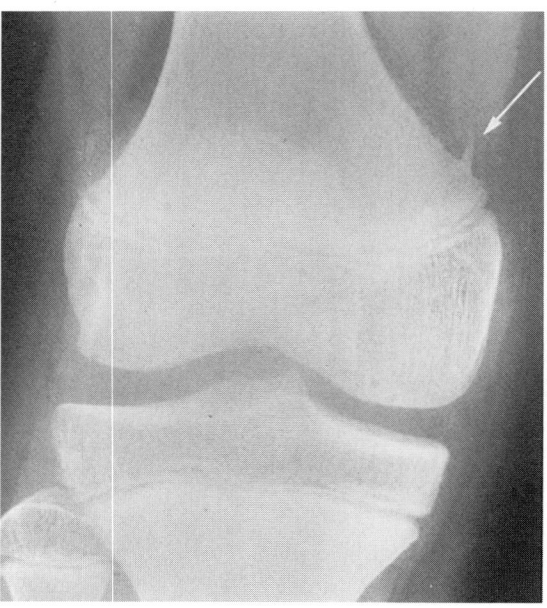

Figure 7–127. Medial femoral cortical irregularity in a 13-year-old boy with a large spur at the inferior margin of the lesion *(arrow).*

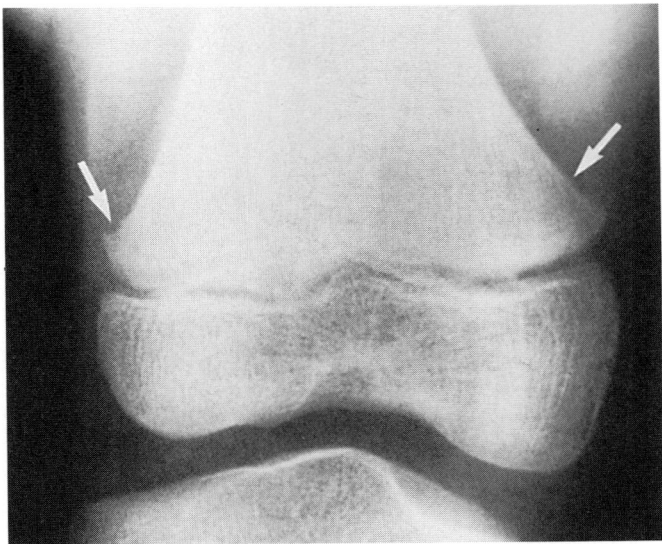

Figure 7–128. Distal femoral cortical irregularities on both sides in a 10-year-old boy.

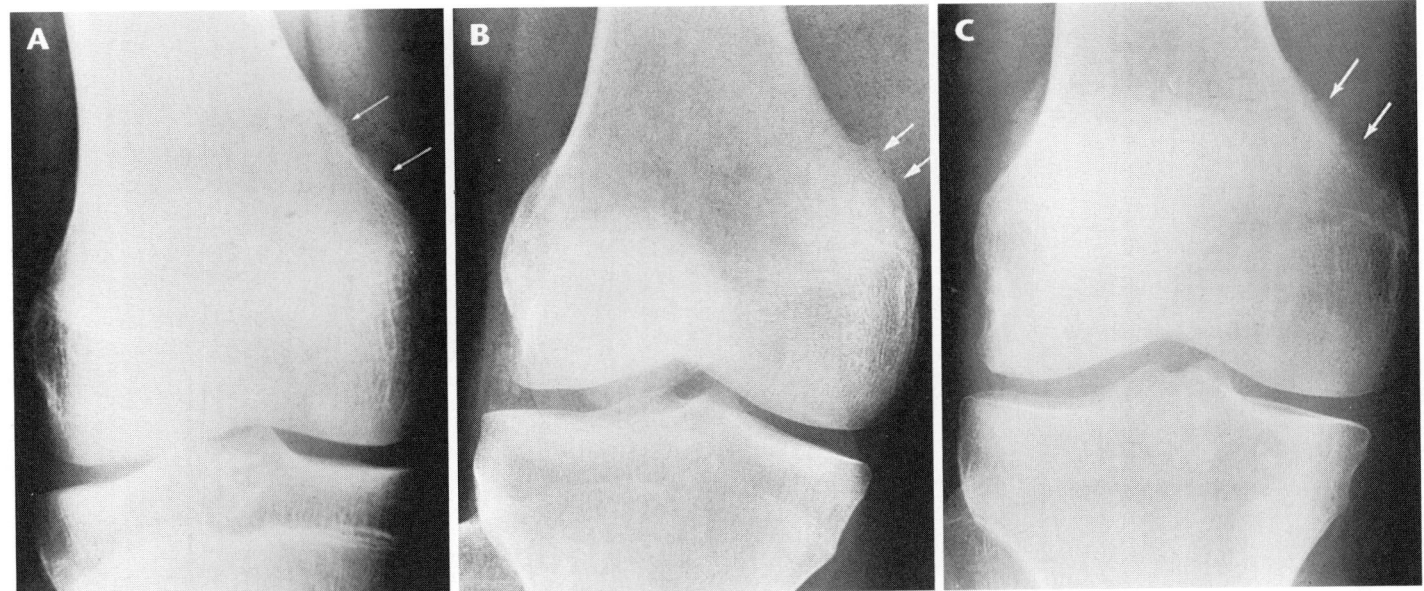

Figure 7–129. Residuals of the irregularity of the cortex in the area of the medial femoral defects described in Figures 7–127 and 7–128. **A,** 17-year-old boy. **B,** 23-year-old man. **C,** 35-year-old man.

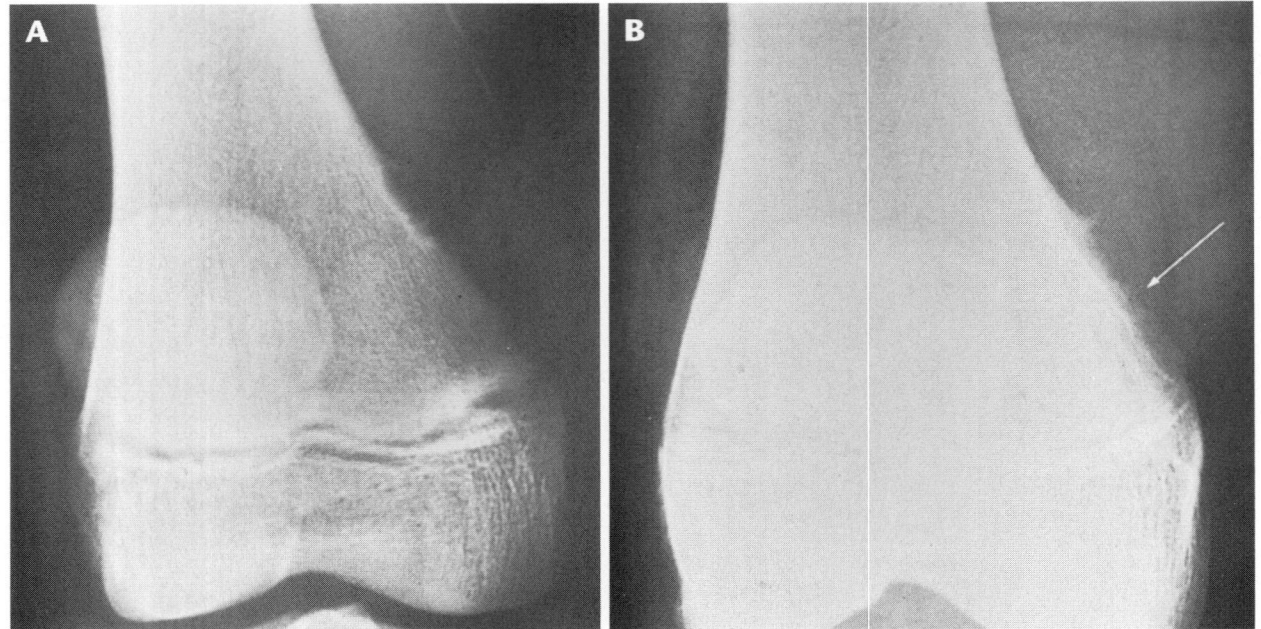

Figure 7–130. **A,** Typical benign cortical defect of the femur in a 12-year-old boy. **B,** Follow-up film made 3 years later shows the typical medial cortical irregularity. This evolution lends weight to the concept of the similar nature of these two entities.

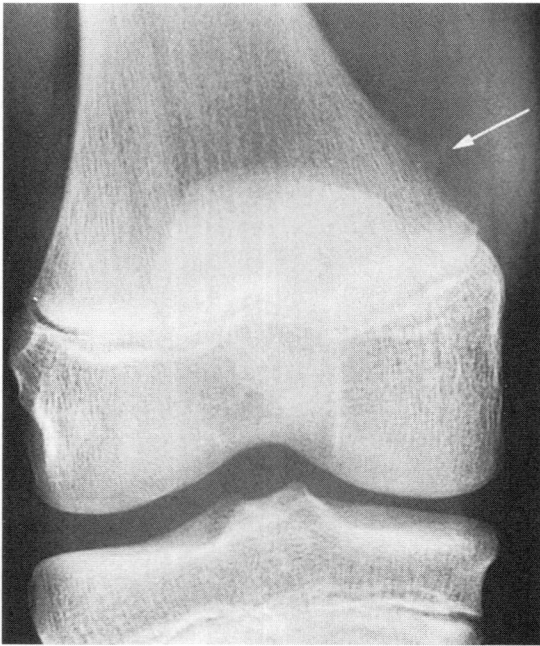

Figure 7–131. The medial distal femoral cortical irregularity in a 13-year-old boy. Note the spiculations of bone (*arrow*) and the absence of cortex. The nuclear scan was normal.

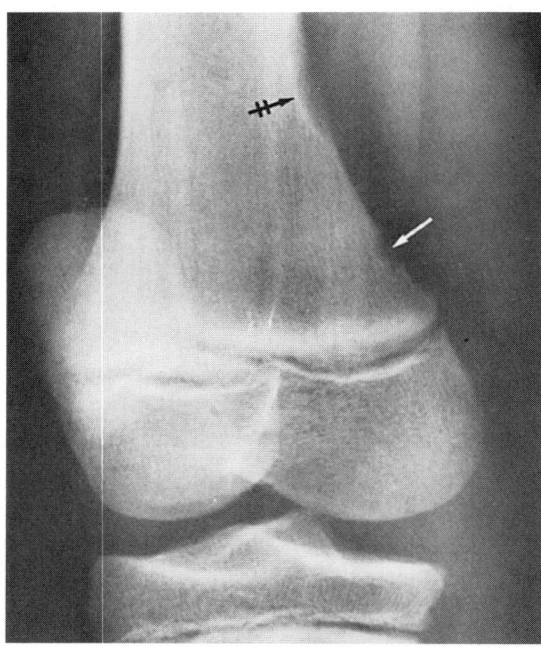

Figure 7–132. Coexistence of the medial posterior cortical defect (→) and a benign cortical defect (⊩→).

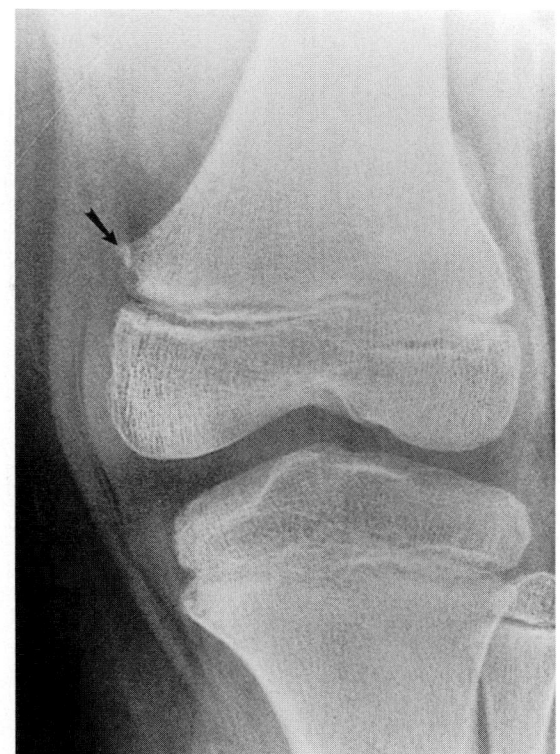

Figure 7–133. Unusual variation of the medial distal femoral irregularity in a 10-year-old boy.

Figure 7–134. Irregularity of the posterior aspect of the distal femur is a common finding in adolescents often mistaken for the new bone formation of a neoplasm. This lesion is apparently related to the medial cortical irregularity illustrated in Figure 7–125 and is of no clinical significance. It is cold on nuclear scanning, which suggests that it is not an avulsive injury and is more likely to be a reflection of growth. (Refs: Bufkin WJ: The avulsive cortical irregularity. *Am J Roentgenol* 112:487, 1971; Burrows PE et al: The distal femoral defect: Technetium 99m pyrophosphate bone scan results. *J Can Assoc Radiol* 33:91, 1982.)

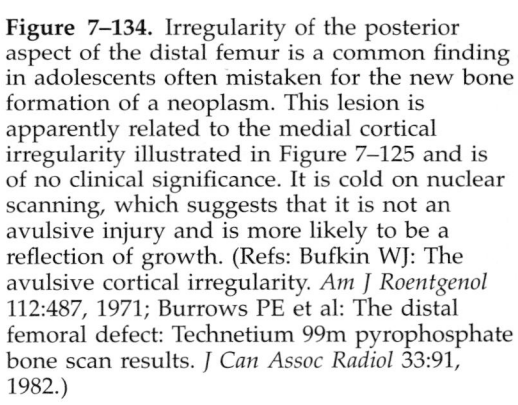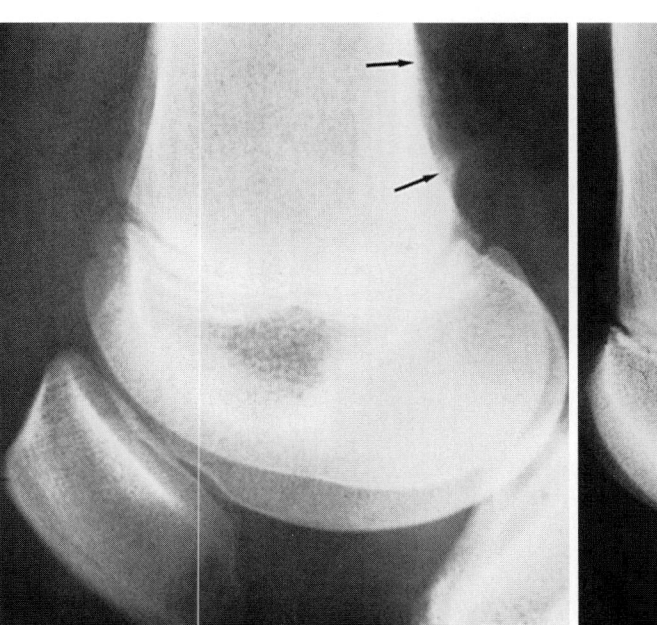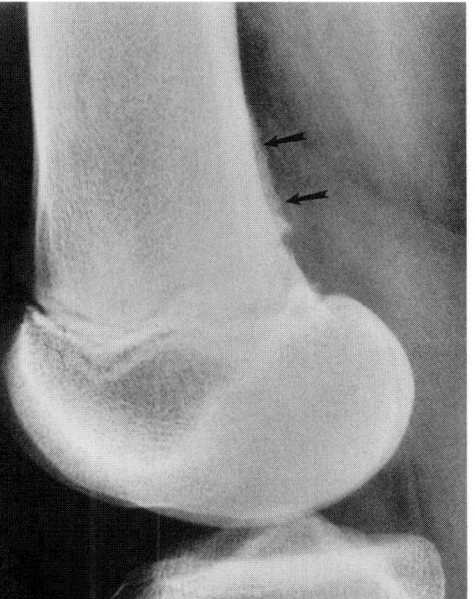

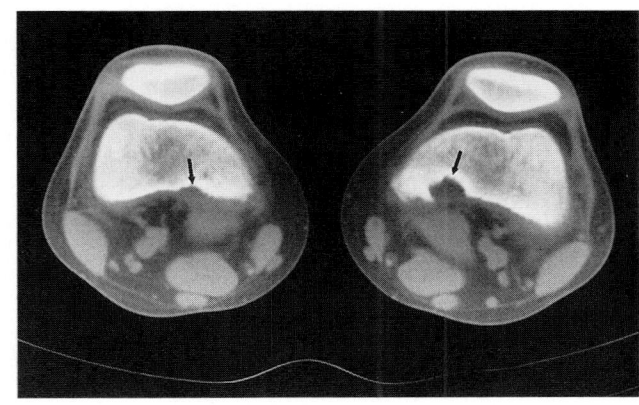

Figure 7–135. The posterior femoral cortical irregularities by CT.

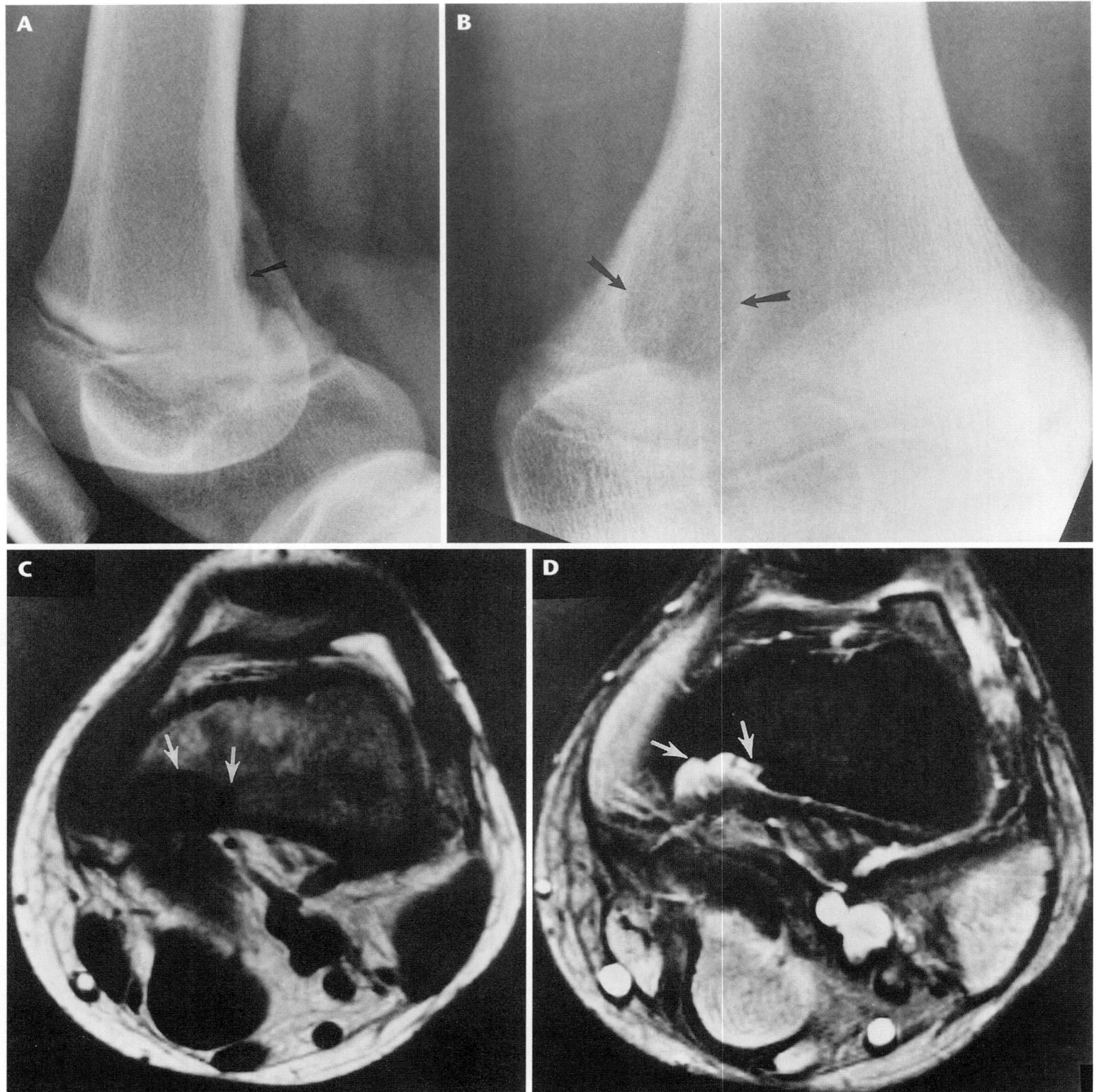

Figure 7–136. The posterior cortical irregularity of the femur in a 12-year-old boy. **A** and **B,** Plain films. **C,** T-1–weighted image shows area of low signal intensity in the cortex. **D,** T-2–weighted image shows an area of higher signal intensity. (Ref: Yamezaki T et al: MR findings of avulsive cortical irregularity of the distal femur. *Skeletal Radiol* 24:43, 1995.)

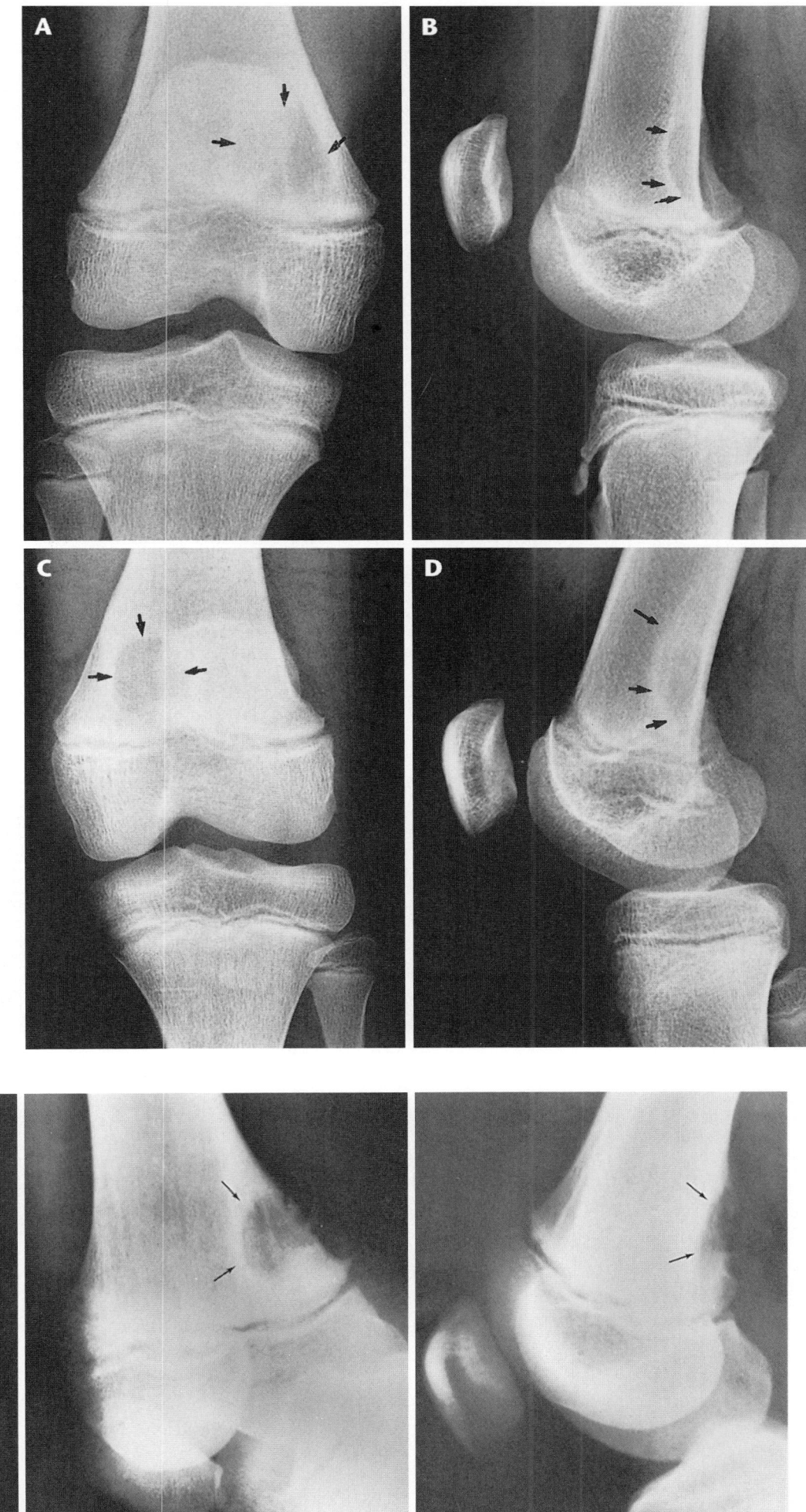

Figure 7–137. A–D, Huge symmetrical bilateral posterior cortical irregularities in a 10-year-old girl.

Figure 7–138. Large irregular posterior femoral defect in a 12-year-old girl, proved by biopsy to be fibrous in nature.

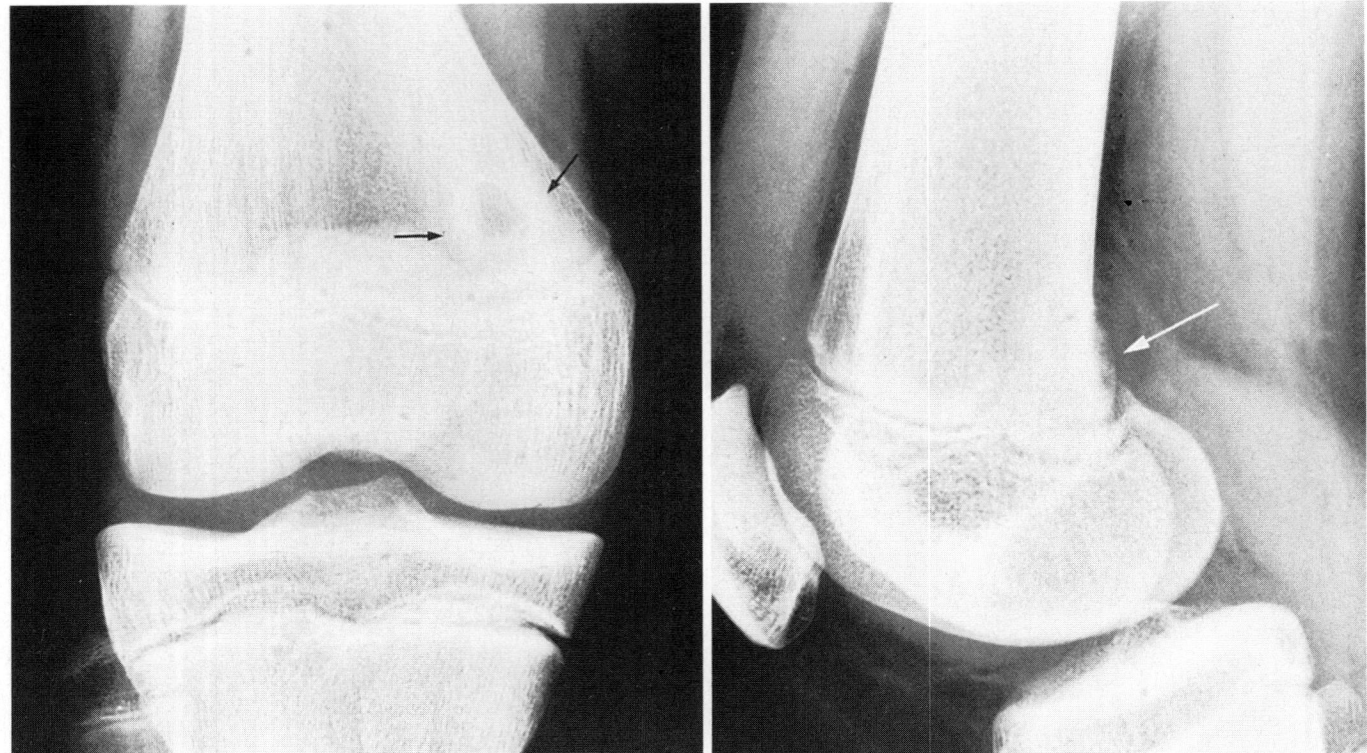

Figure 7–139. Well-defined posterior femoral defect in a 12-year-old girl.

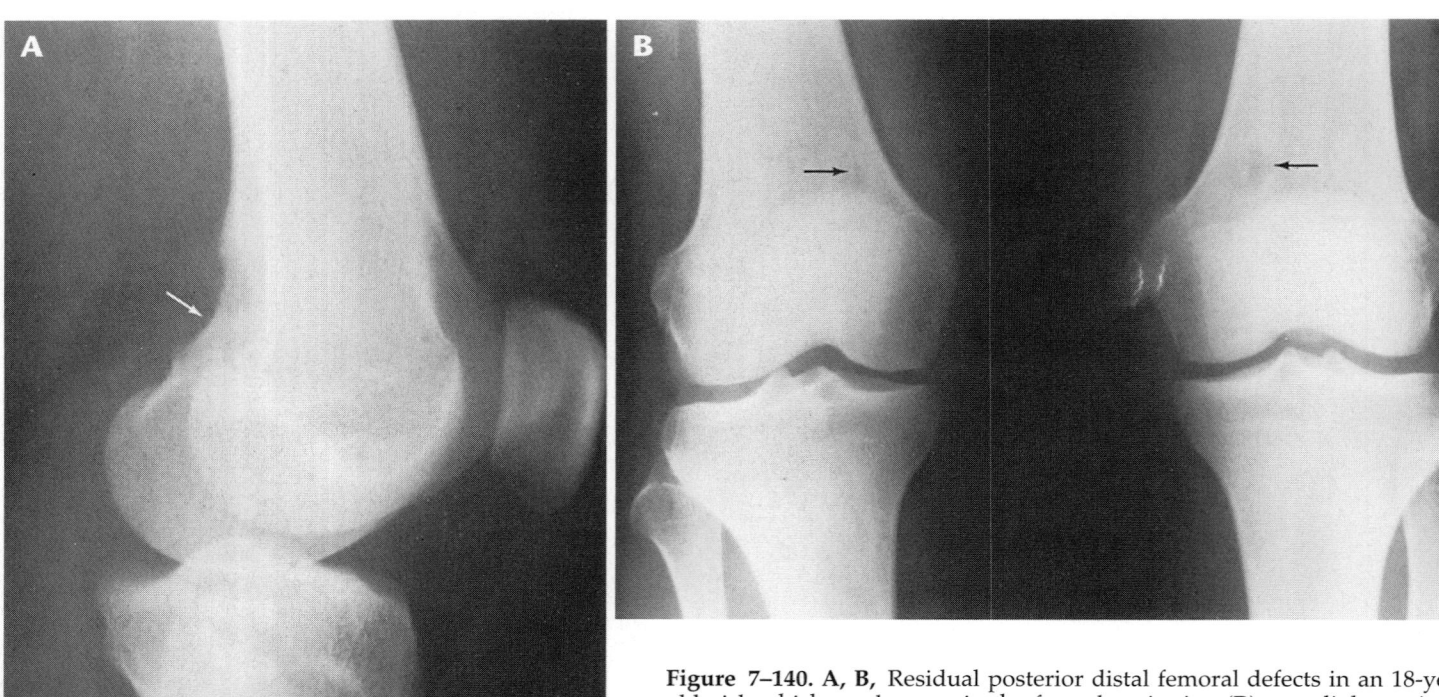

Figure 7–140. A, B, Residual posterior distal femoral defects in an 18-year-old girl, which can be seen in the frontal projection (**B**) as radiolucencies that might be mistaken for evidence of pathology.

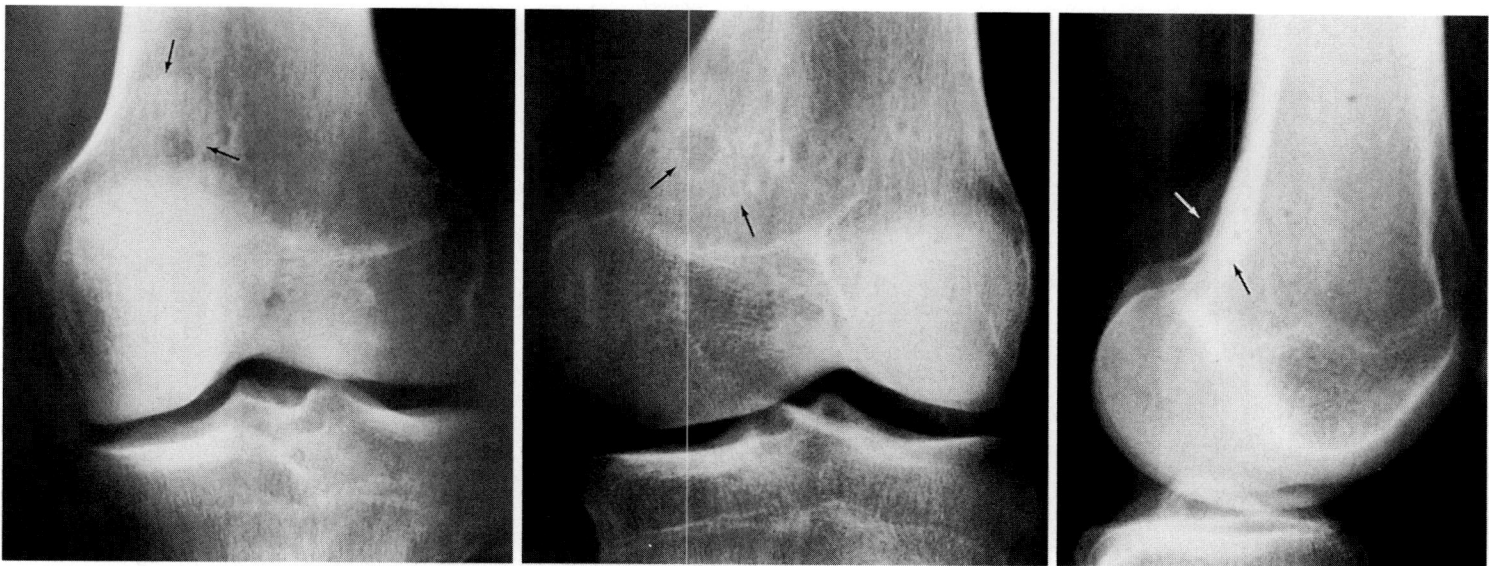

Figure 7–141. Residuals of the posterior femoral defect in a 30-year-old man.

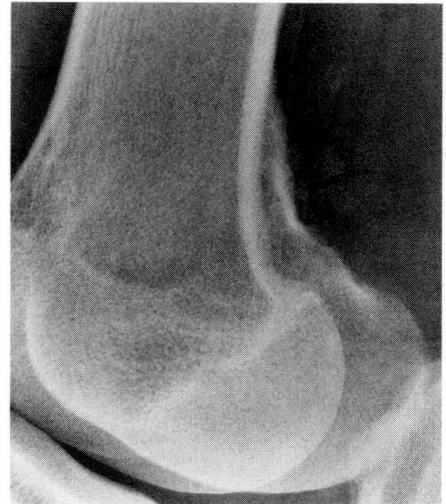

Figure 7–142. Residual of posterior femoral defect in a 46-year-old man, with a thin rim of bone.

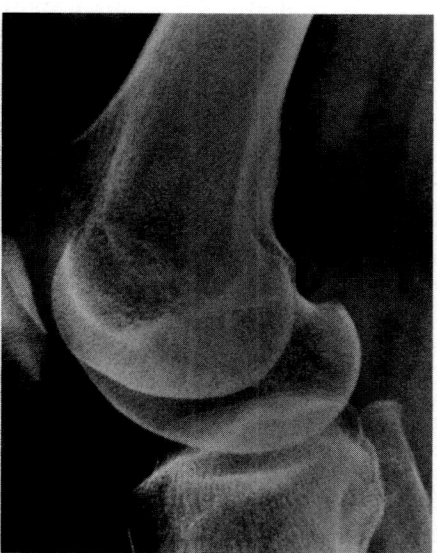

Figure 7–143. Developmental excavation on the posterior aspect of the medial femoral condyle.

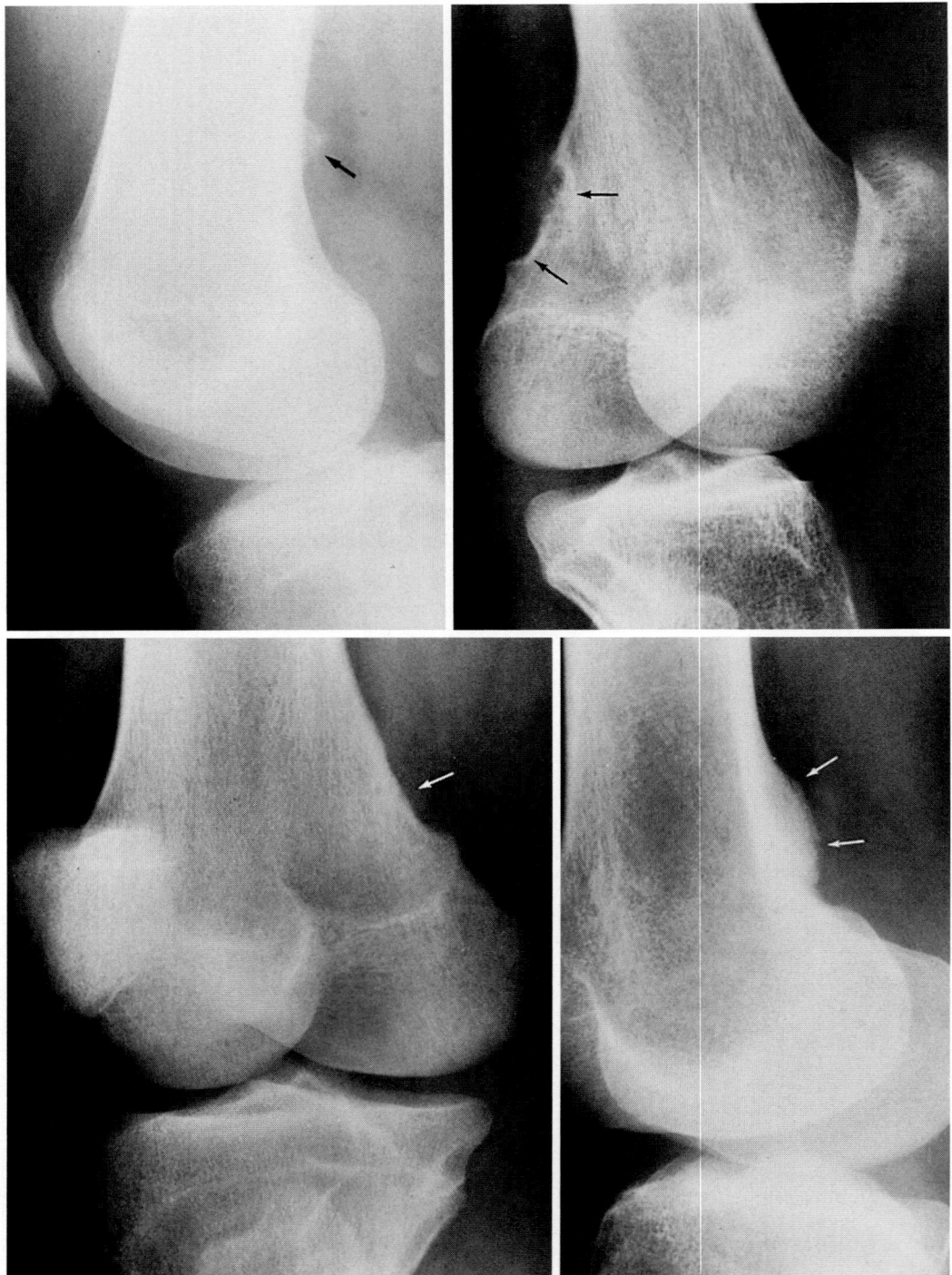

Figure 7–144. Four examples of cortical irregularities in the posterior cortex of the distal femur that have persisted into adult life, presumably the end product of the process shown in Figures 7–134 and 7–138. These defects are important only because they might be mistaken for significant lesions.

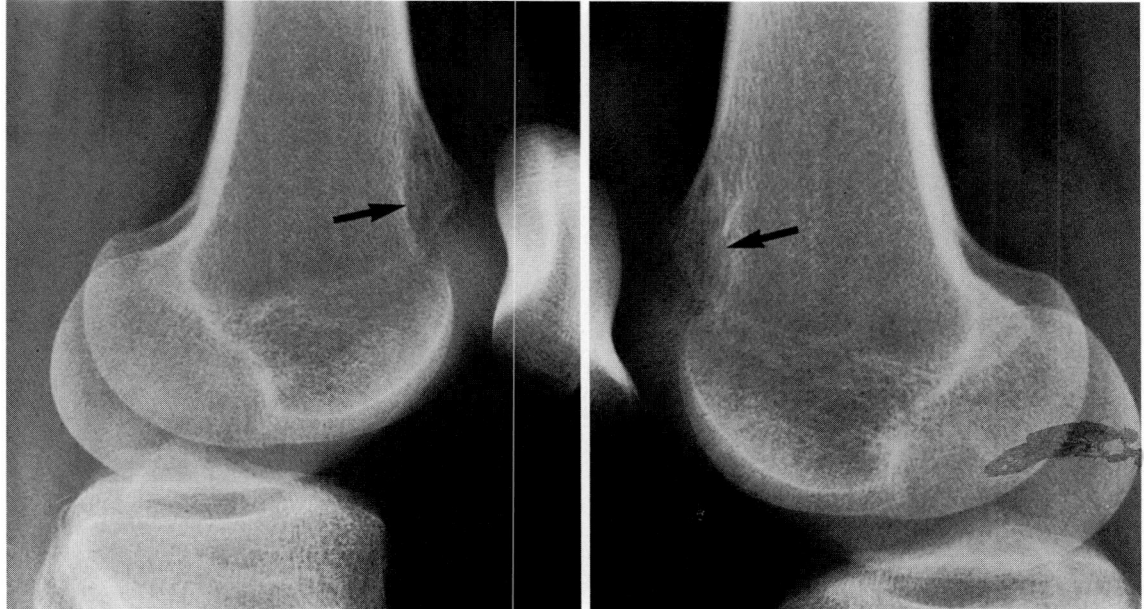

Figure 7–145. Simulated lesions of the anterior aspect of the distal femur, produced by rotation at the time of filming.

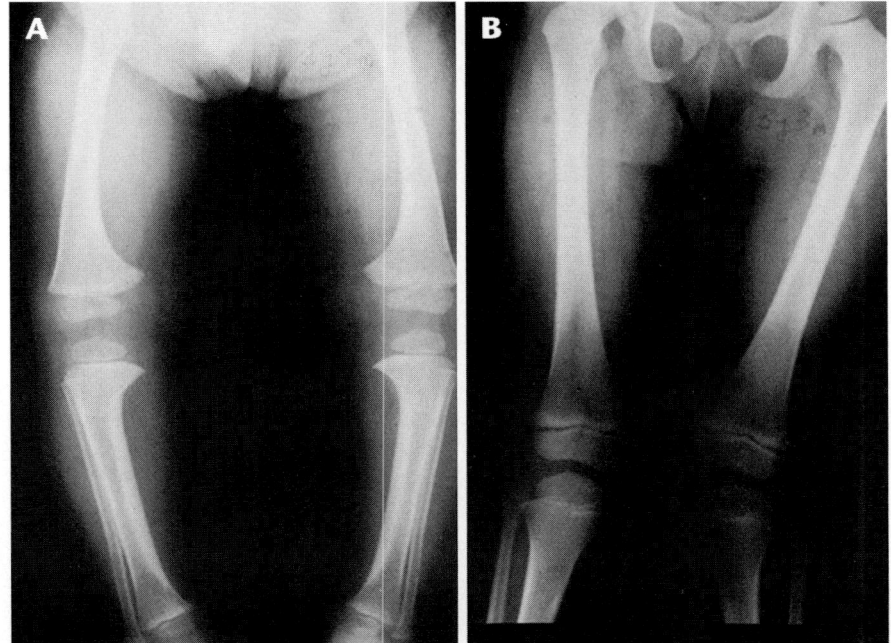

Figure 7–146. Physiologic bowing and knock-knee. **A,** Physiologic bowing in a 1½-year-old girl. **B,** Physiologic knock-knee in a 3½-year-old girl. In normal development, there is a varoid phase to the age of 2 years and a valgoid phase between 2 and 12 years of age. These are normal physiologic events that correct spontaneously. (Refs: Holt JF et al: Physiological bowing of the legs in young children. *JAMA* 154:390, 1954; Shopfner CE, Coin CG: Genu varus and valgus in children. *Radiology* 92:723, 1968.)

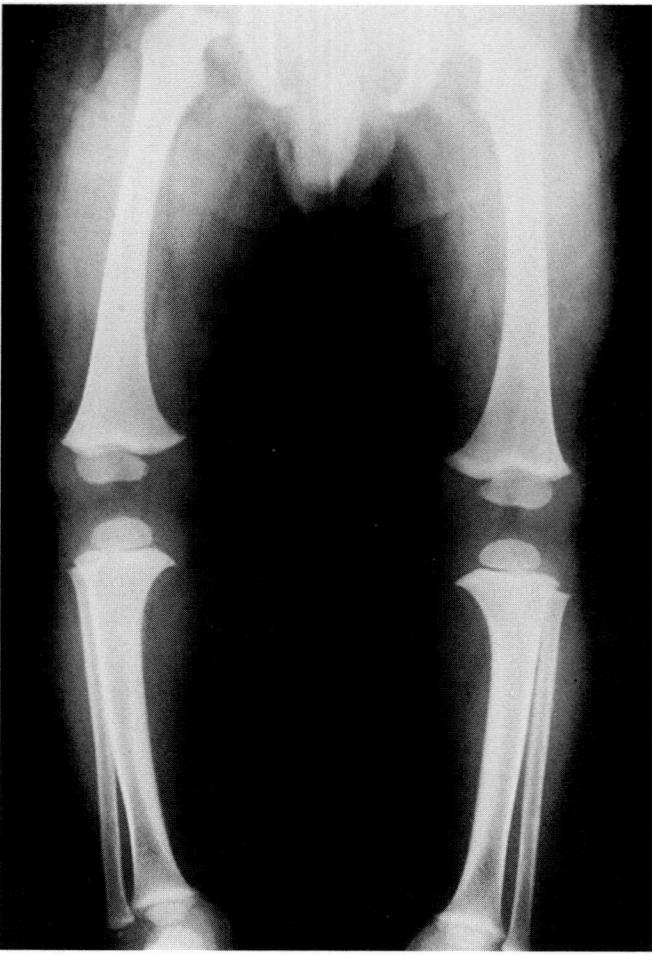

Figure 7–147. Physiologic bowing. Note the slight beaking of the medial tibial plateaus, the medial wedging of the ossification centers of the knees, and the thickening of the medial cortices of the tibias. These are all reflections of this physiologic state.

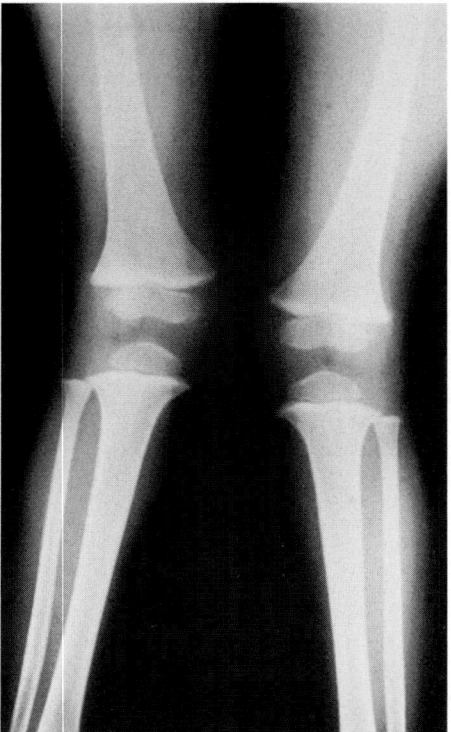

Figure 7–148. Physiologic knock-knees in a 3-year-old boy. Note lack of any architectural derangement.

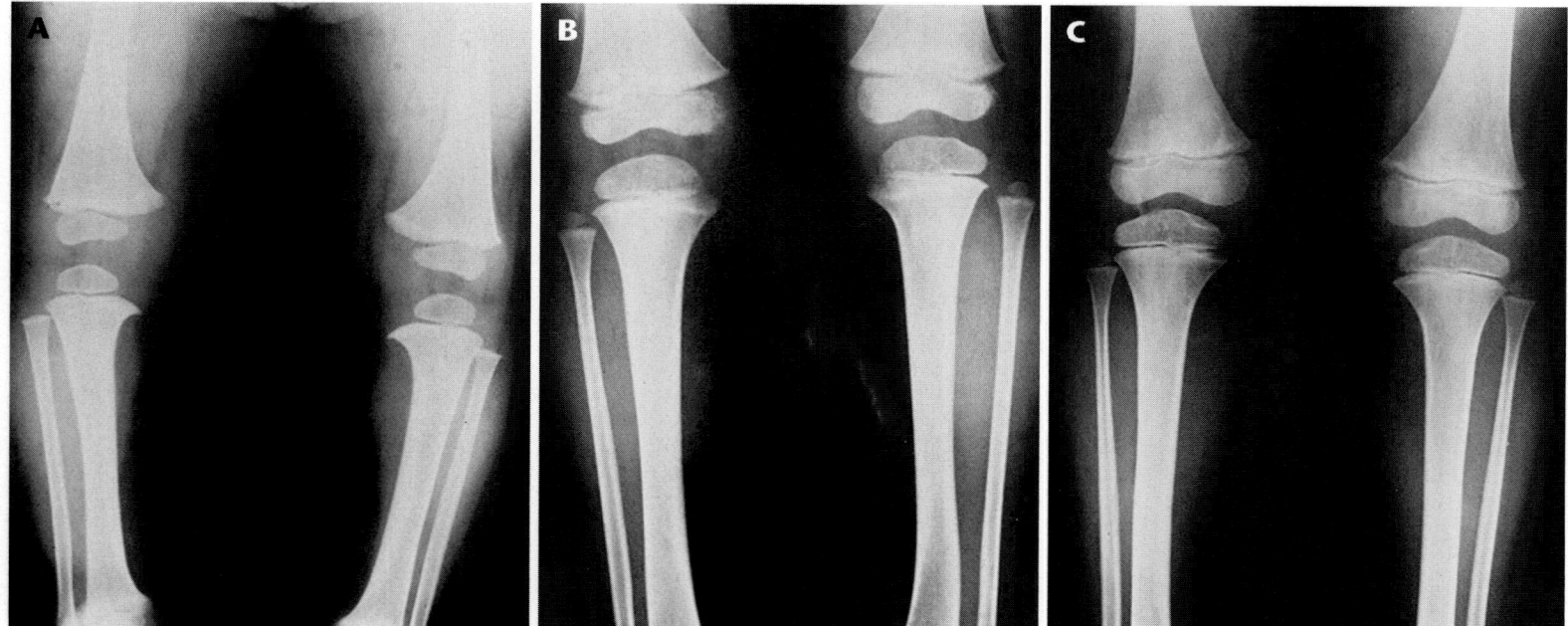

Figure 7–149. Evolution of physiologic bowing. **A,** 18-month-old. **B,** 2-year-old, showing spontaneous correction. **C,** 4-year-old. This appearance is normal.

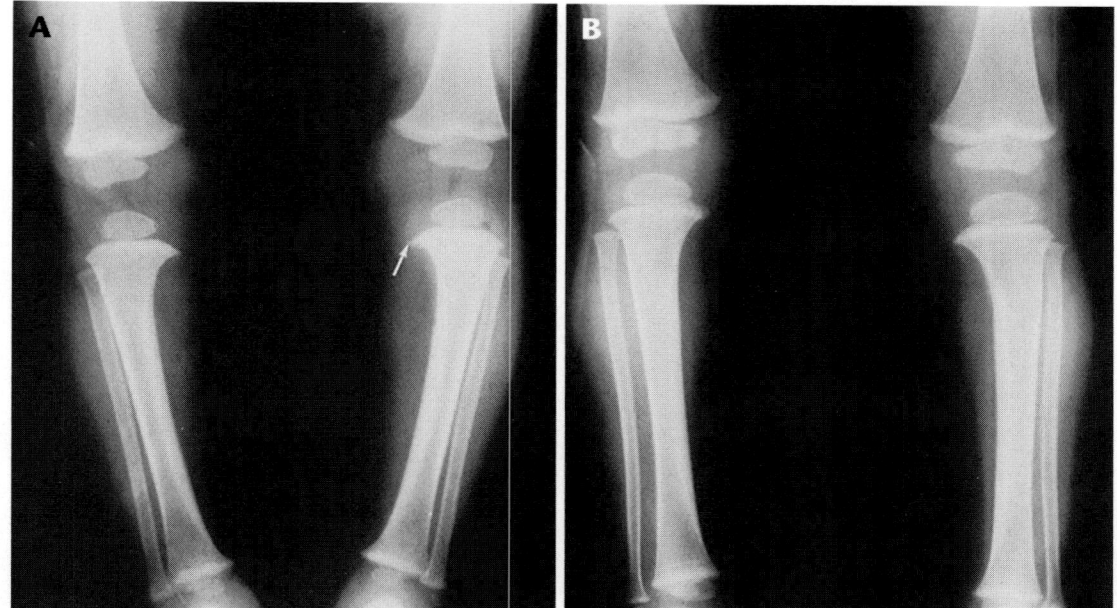

Figure 7–150. A, 1-year-old girl with physiologic bowing. Note the "fragmentation" of the medial aspect of the tibial metaphysis *(arrow)*. **B,** Same patient at age 2. Note conversion to mild knock-knee deformity and resolution of the changes of physiologic bowing.

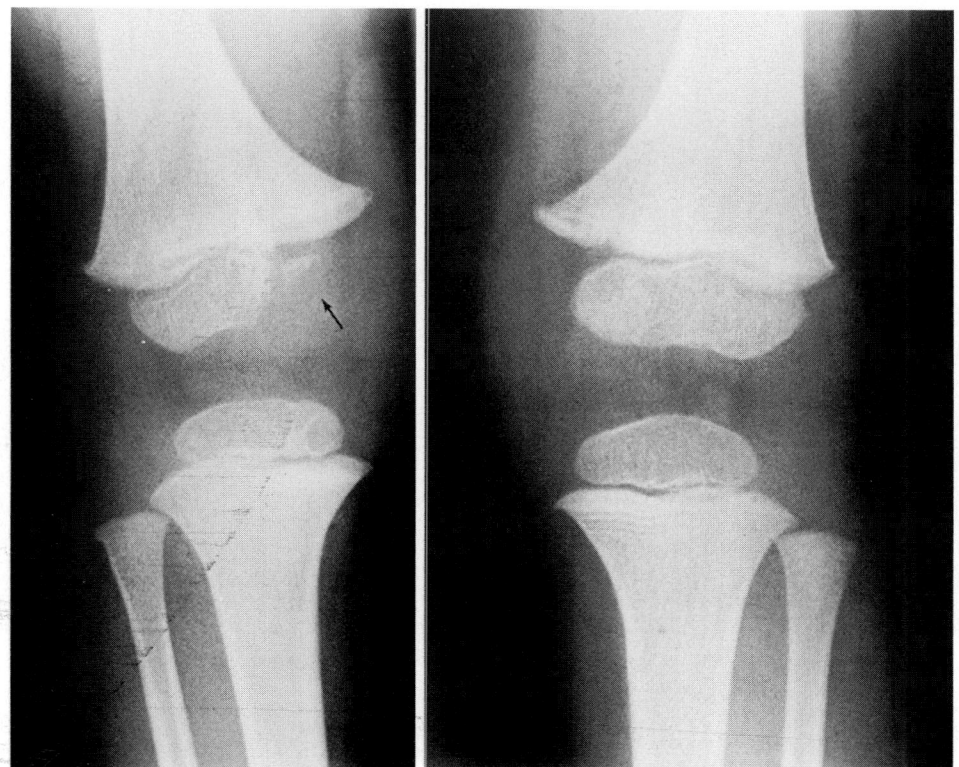

Figure 7–151. Asymmetric development of the distal femoral epiphysis in a 7-year-old boy with no symptoms referable to the knee joints.

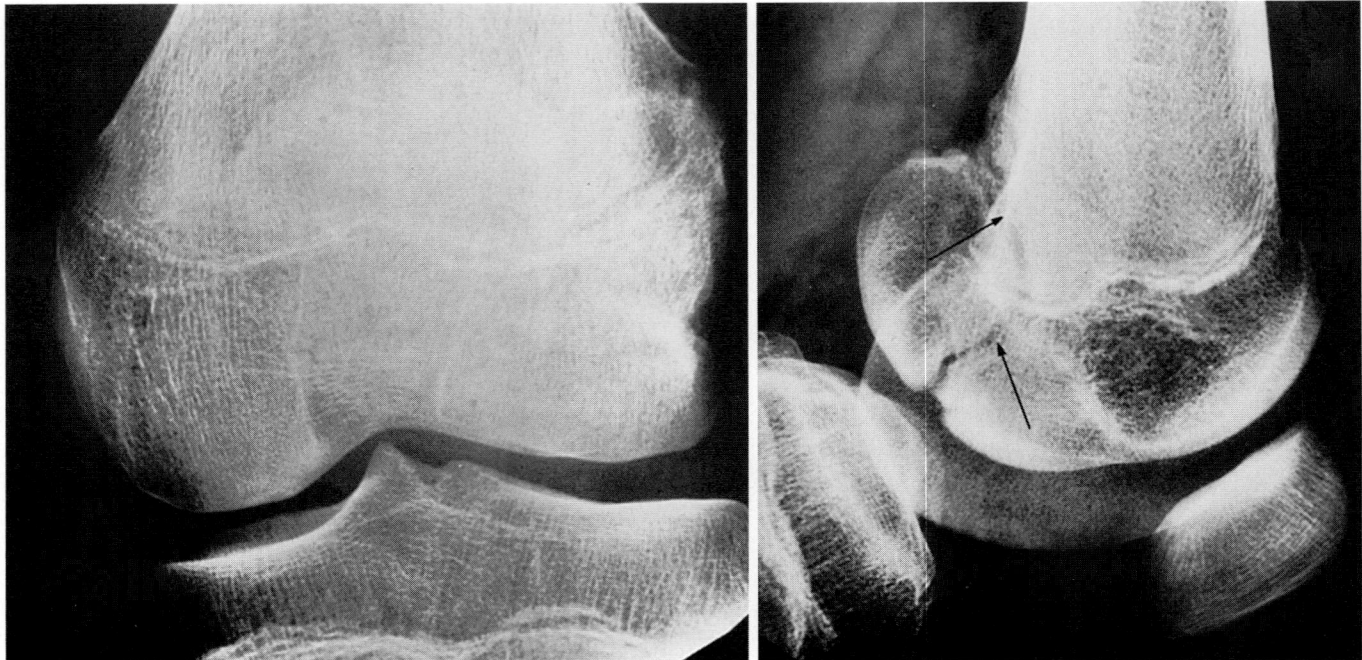

Figure 7–152. Cleft distal femoral epiphysis seen only in the lateral projection. Any epiphysis or apophysis may develop from multiple centers.

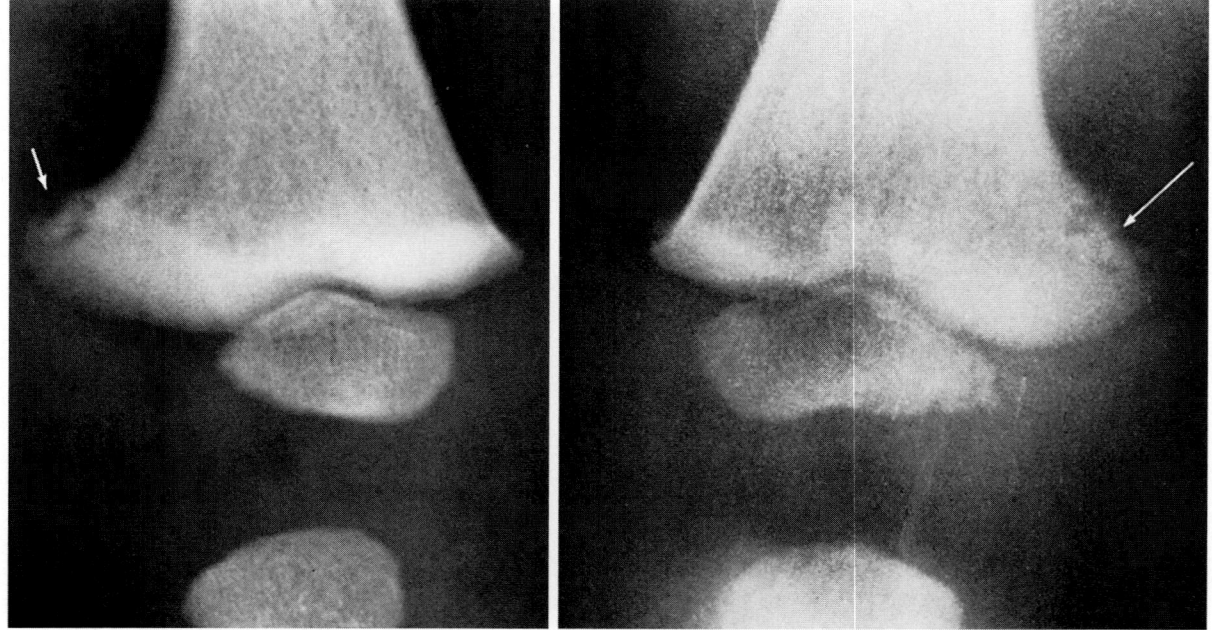

Figure 7–153. Normal irregularity of ossification of the medial femoral metaphyses in young children.

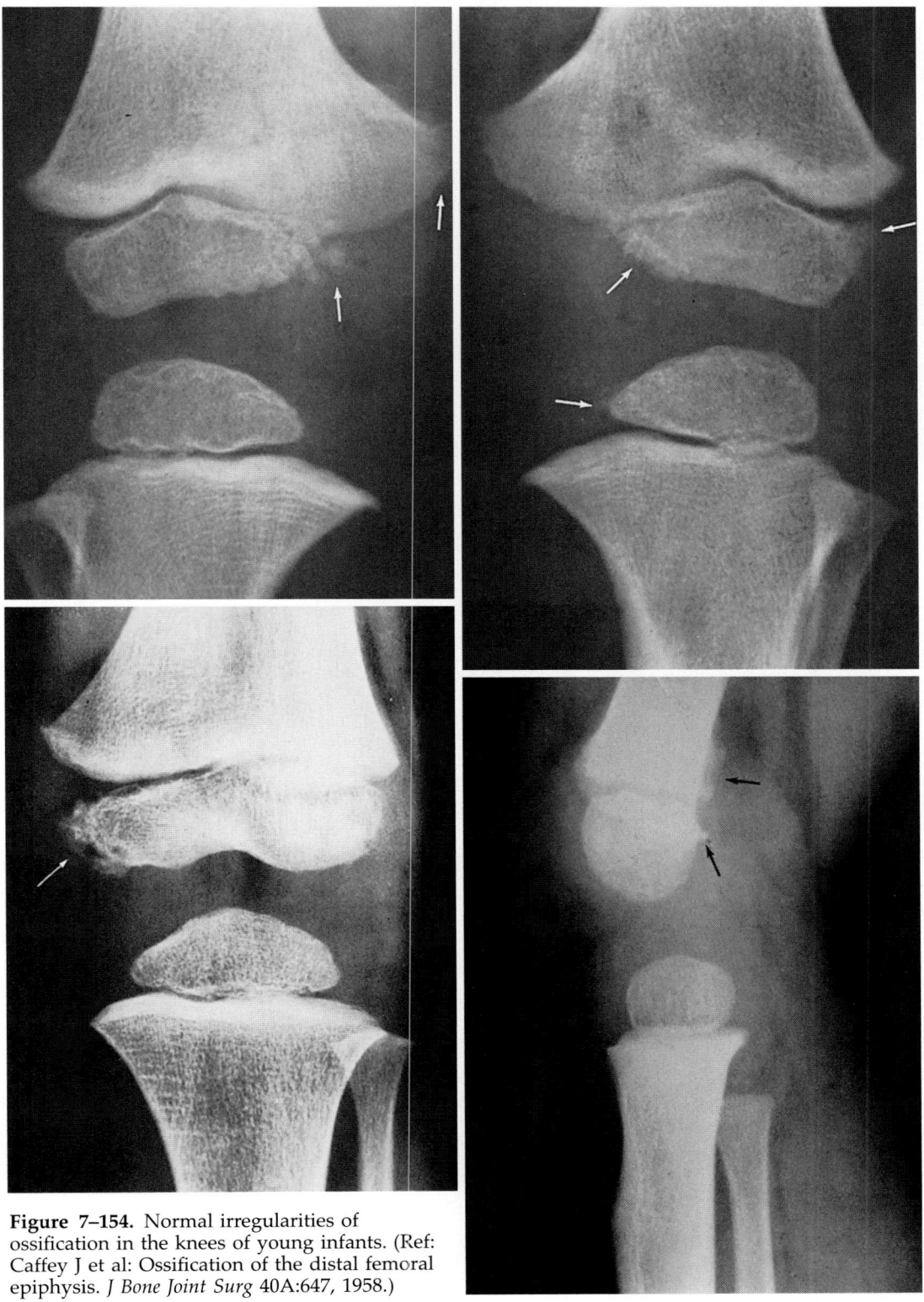

Figure 7–154. Normal irregularities of ossification in the knees of young infants. (Ref: Caffey J et al: Ossification of the distal femoral epiphysis. *J Bone Joint Surg* 40A:647, 1958.)

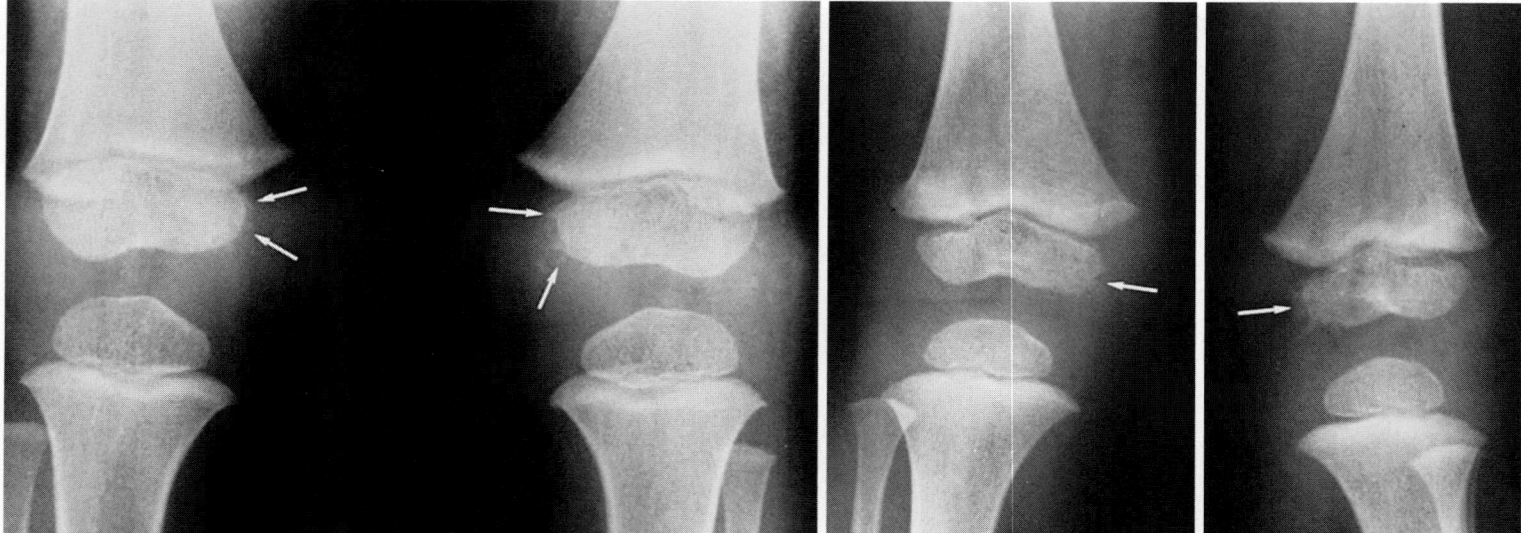

Figure 7–155. Additional examples of normal irregularities of the distal femoral epiphyses in 1-year-old children.

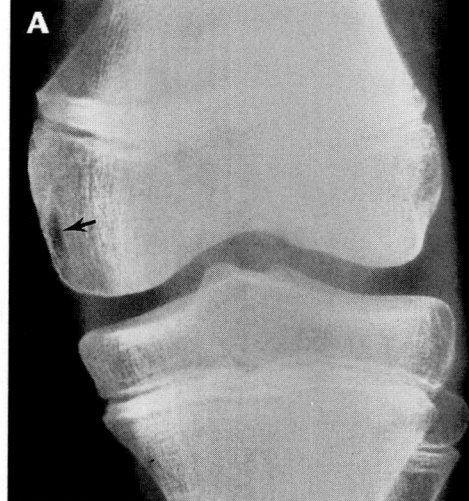

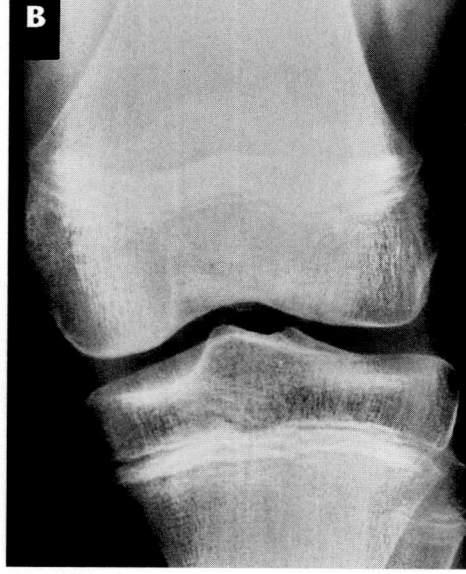

Figure 7–156. A, Apparent lucent lesion in the medial femoral condyle. **B,** Repositioned film shows no abnormality, the change being due to alteration in the beam direction.

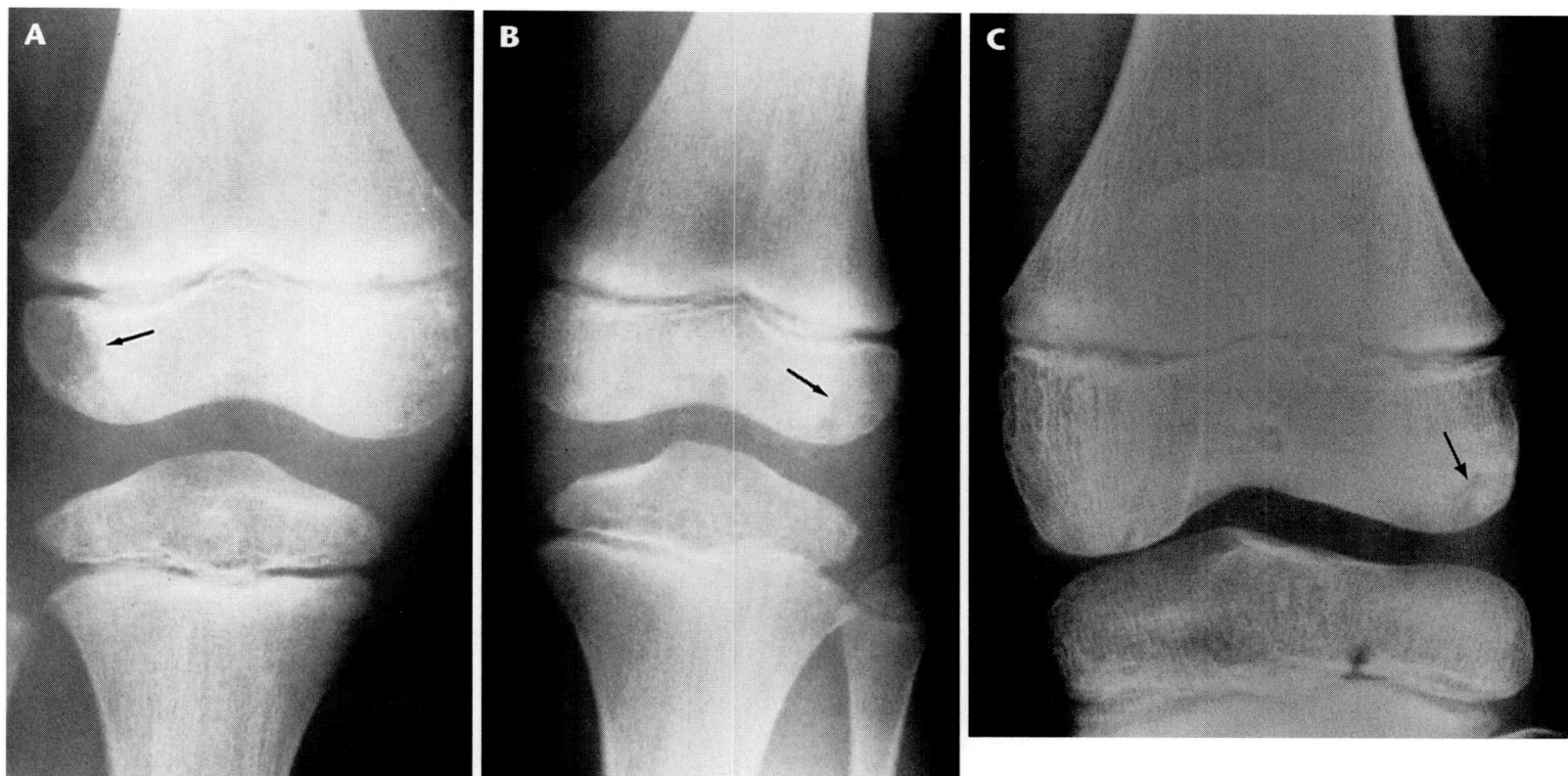

Figure 7–157. A, Normal developmental lucency of the lateral aspects of the distal femoral epiphysis, simulating a destructive lesion in a 6-year-old boy. **B,** Similar but less marked changes are present in the opposite limb. **C,** Similar changes in a 12-year-old boy.

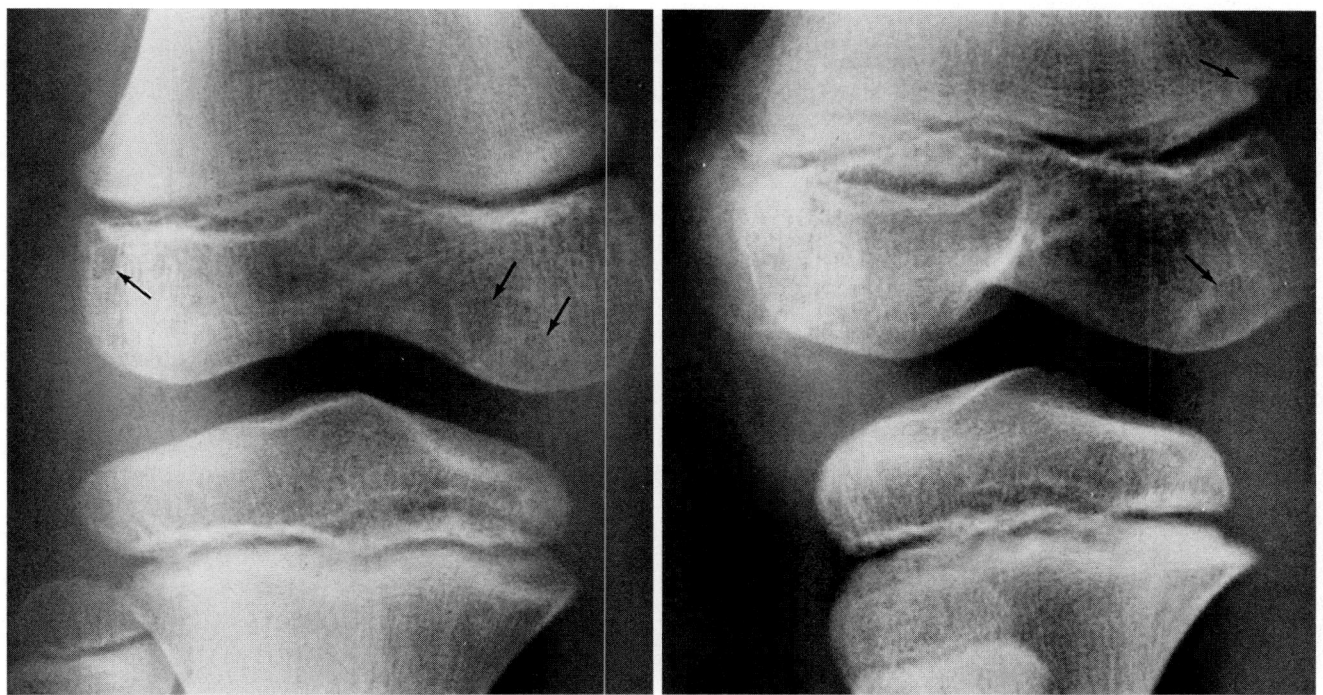

Figure 7–158. Normal developmental lucencies in the epiphyses and metaphyses of the distal femur in a 10-year-old boy.

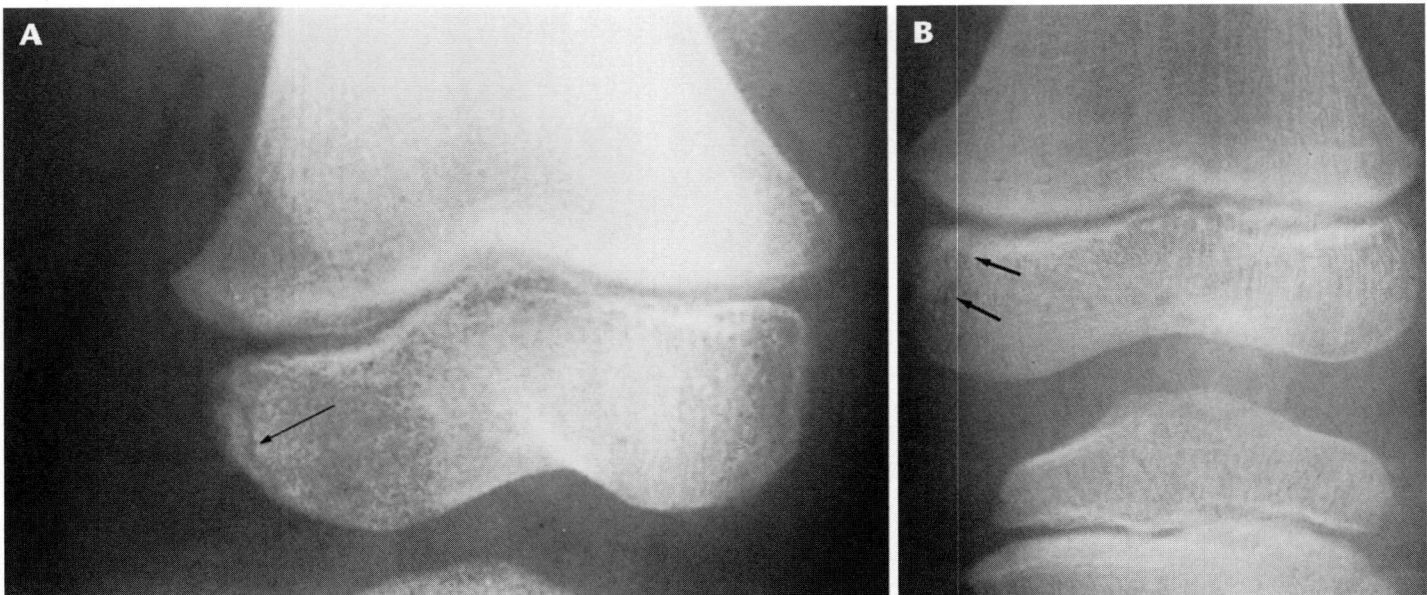

Figure 7–159. Developmental radiolucent stripes in the medial aspect of the distal femoral epiphysis, simulating a fracture. **A,** 5-year-old boy. **B,** 7-year-old boy.

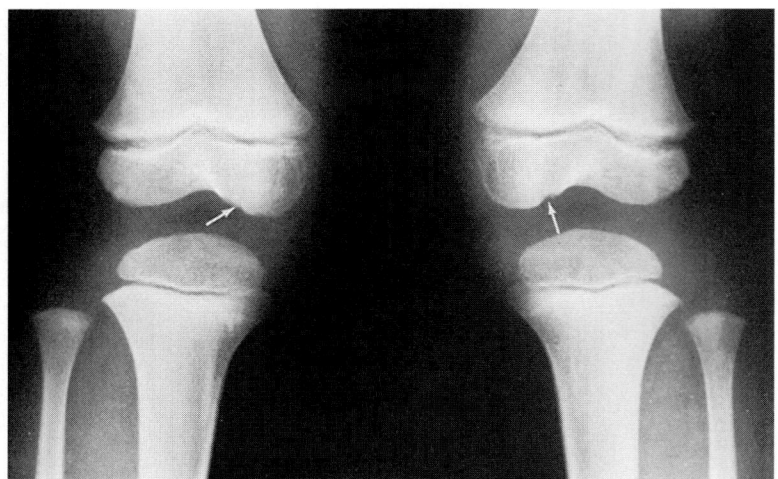

Figure 7–160. Normal irregular contours of the distal femoral epiphyses in a 4-year-old girl.

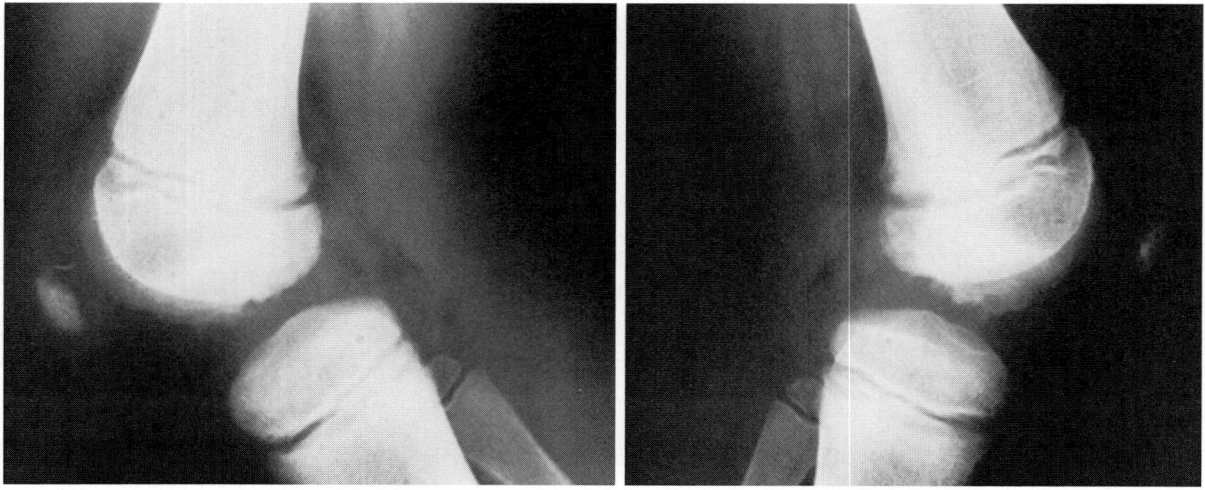

Figure 7–161. An excellent example of the normal irregularity of the distal femoral epiphyses in an 8-year-old, which explains the misleading shadows seen in the frontal projections of the knees of children of this age.

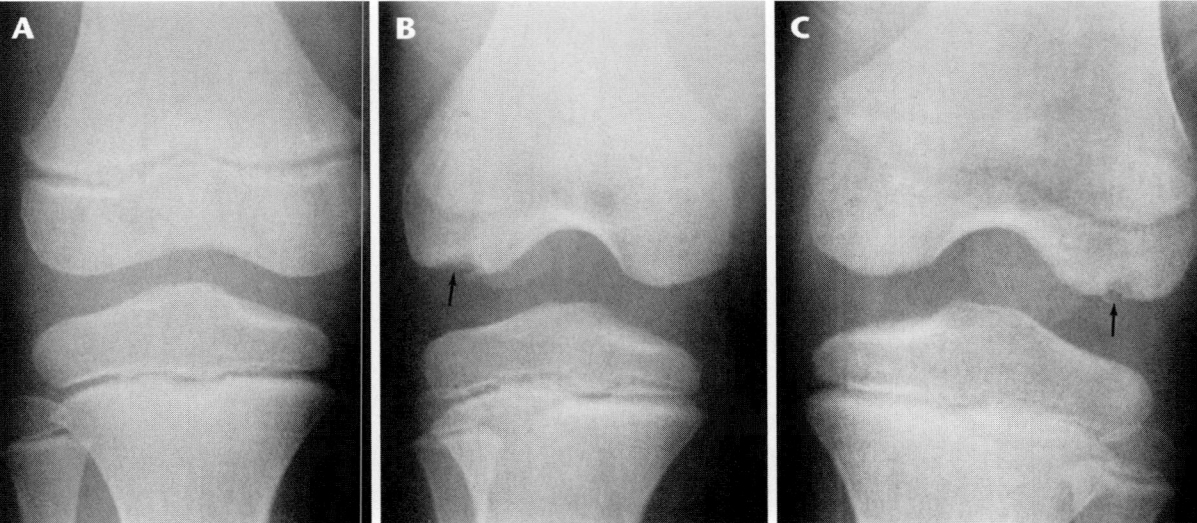

Figure 7–162. A–C, Normal irregularity of the lateral condyles of the femur in a 7-year-old boy. These irregularities are posteriorly located and are seen in the tunnel views of both knees (**B** and **C**) but not in the conventional anteroposterior projection (**A**). (Ref: Caffey J et al: Ossification of the distal femoral epiphysis. *J Bone Joint Surg* 140A:647, 1958.)

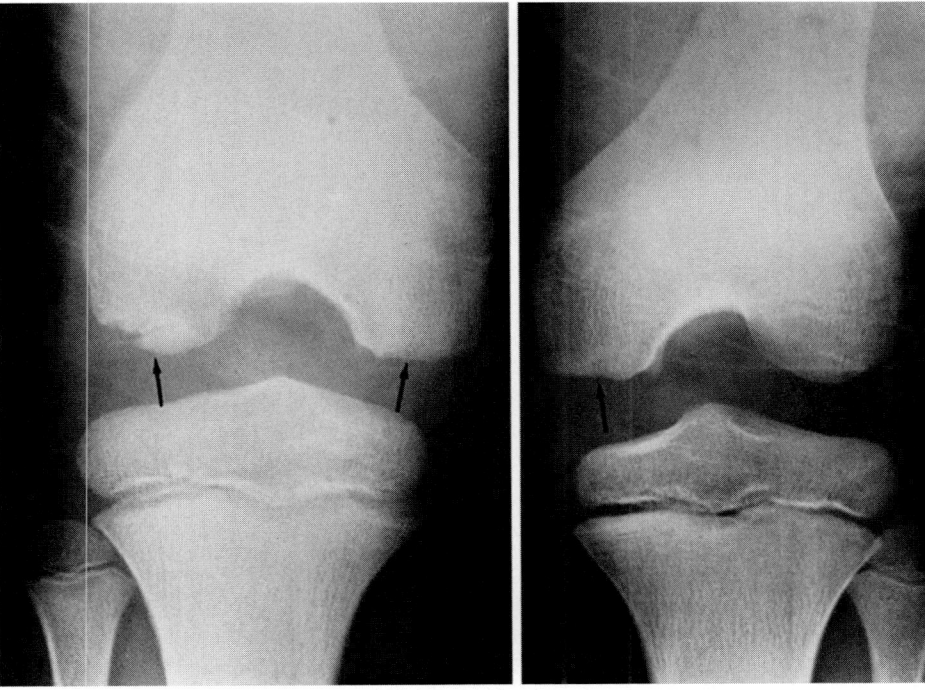

Figure 7–163. Medial and lateral femoral condylar irregularities seen in the tunnel views of both knees of a 10-year-old boy. These irregularities are often mistaken for evidence of osteochondritis.

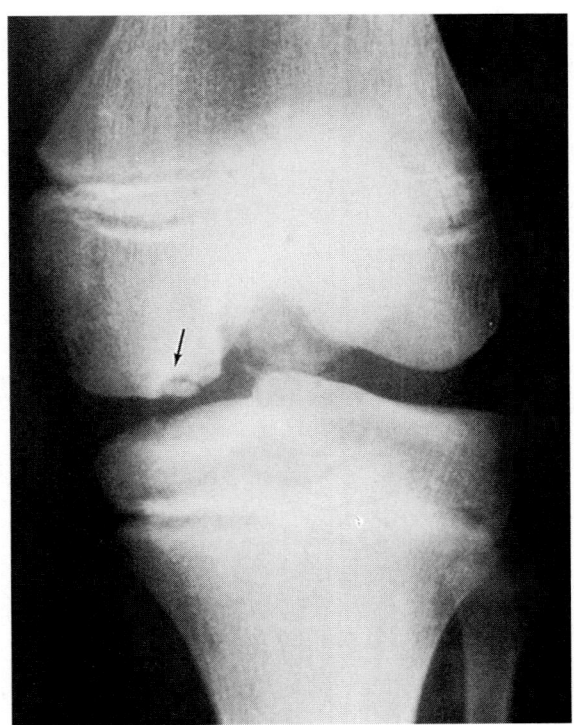

Figure 7–164. Simulated osteochondritis dissecans in a 6-year-old boy.

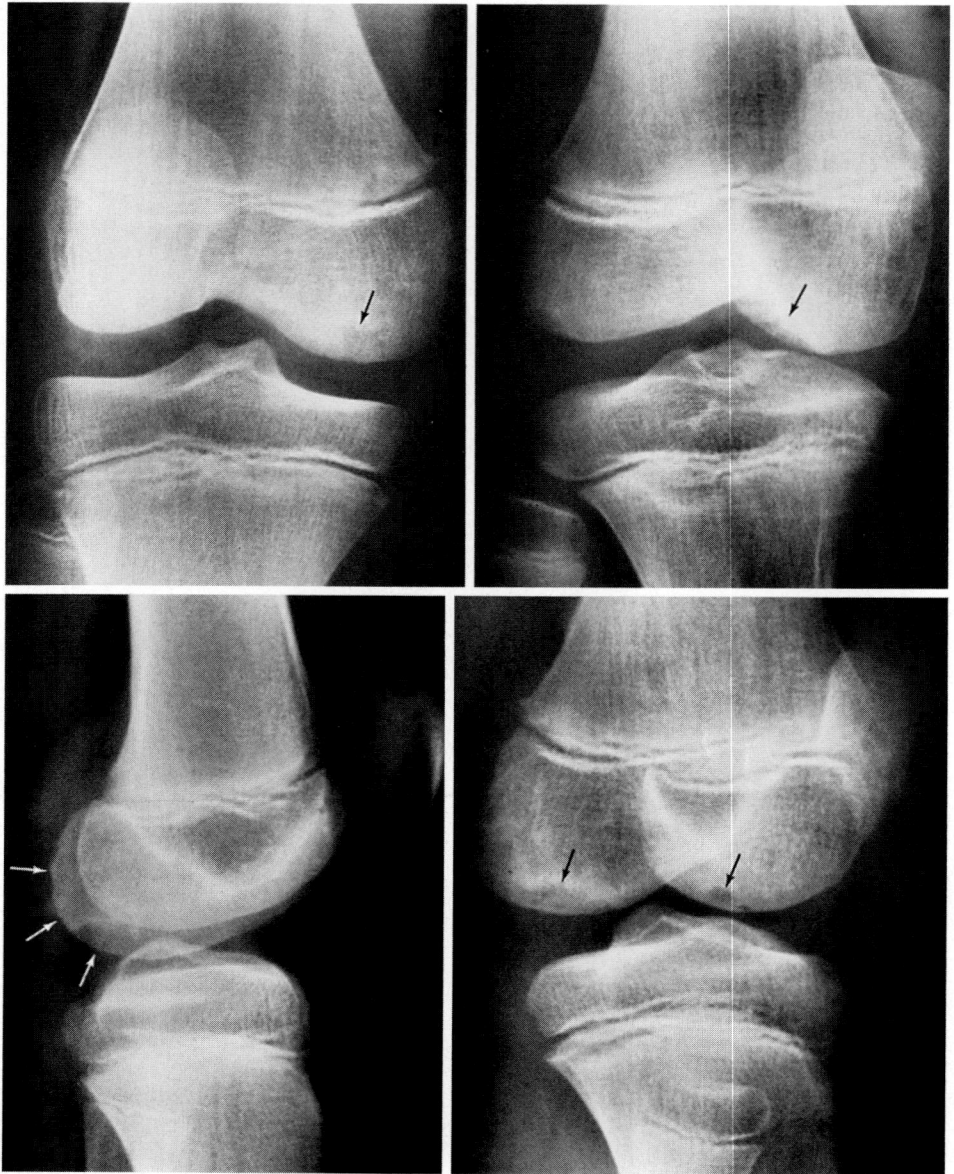

Figure 7–165. Normal developmental irregularities of the condyles in a 12-year-old boy, not to be mistaken for osteochondritis. (Ref: Caffey J: *Pediatric x-ray diagnosis.* 9th ed. St Louis, Mosby, 1993, p. 1504.)

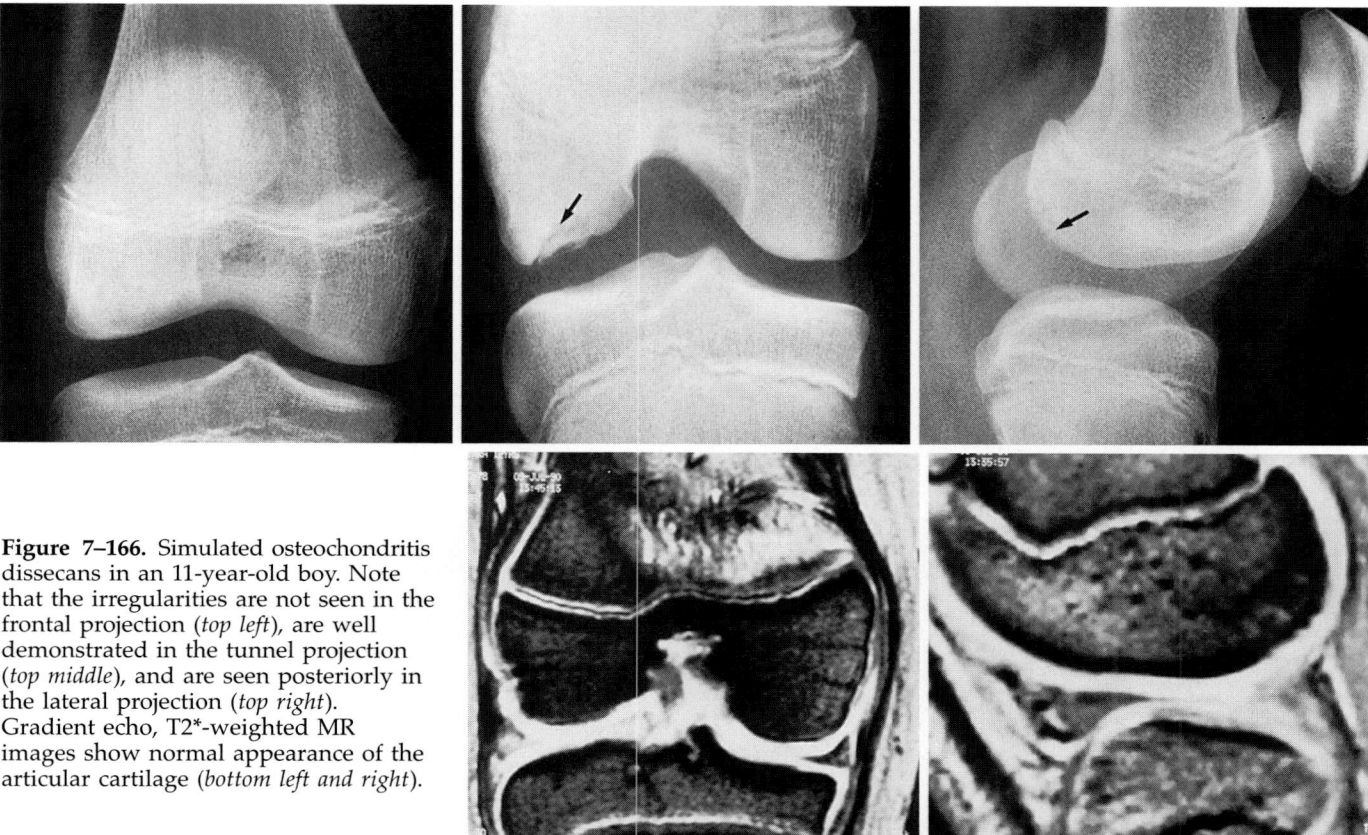

Figure 7–166. Simulated osteochondritis dissecans in an 11-year-old boy. Note that the irregularities are not seen in the frontal projection (*top left*), are well demonstrated in the tunnel projection (*top middle*), and are seen posteriorly in the lateral projection (*top right*). Gradient echo, T2*-weighted MR images show normal appearance of the articular cartilage (*bottom left and right*).

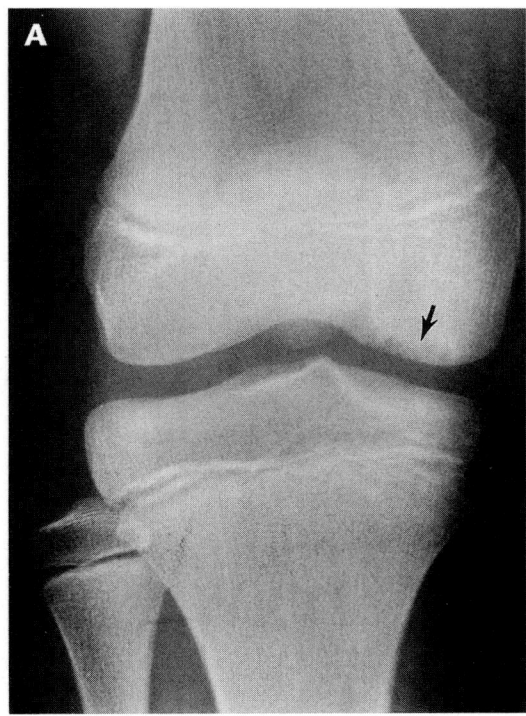

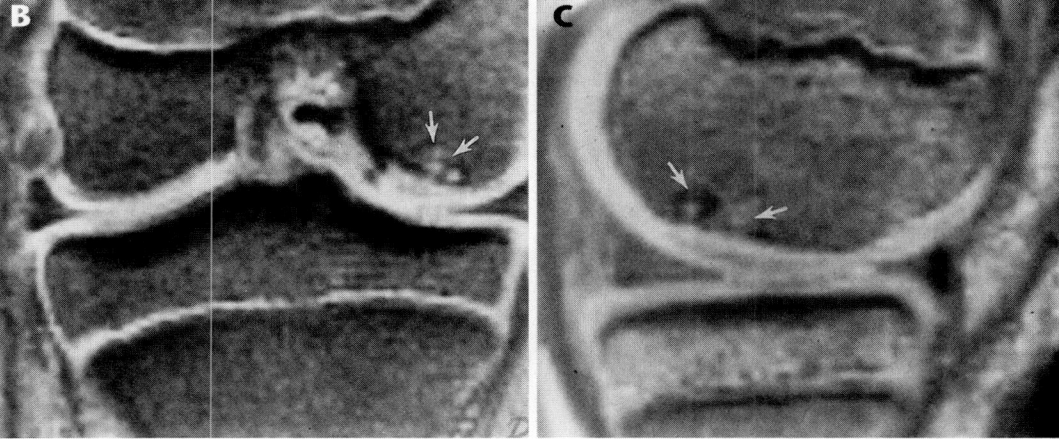

Figure 7–167. Normal irregularity in ossification of the medial femoral condyle in a 12-year-old boy, mistaken for osteochondritis dissecans. **A,** Plain film. **B** and **C,** Coronal and sagittal gradient echo, T2*-weighted images show typical ossification variant.

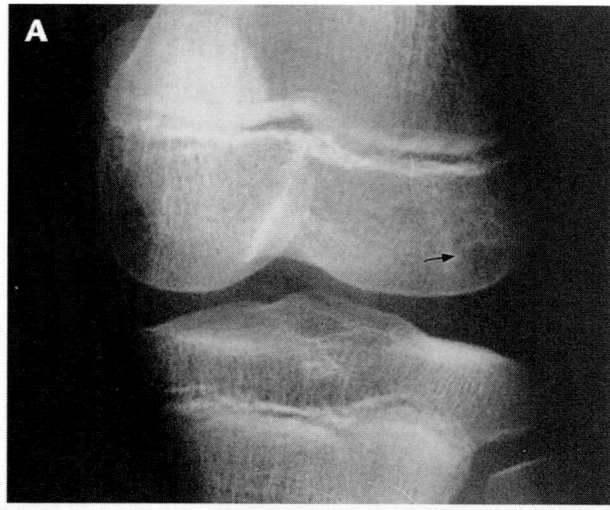

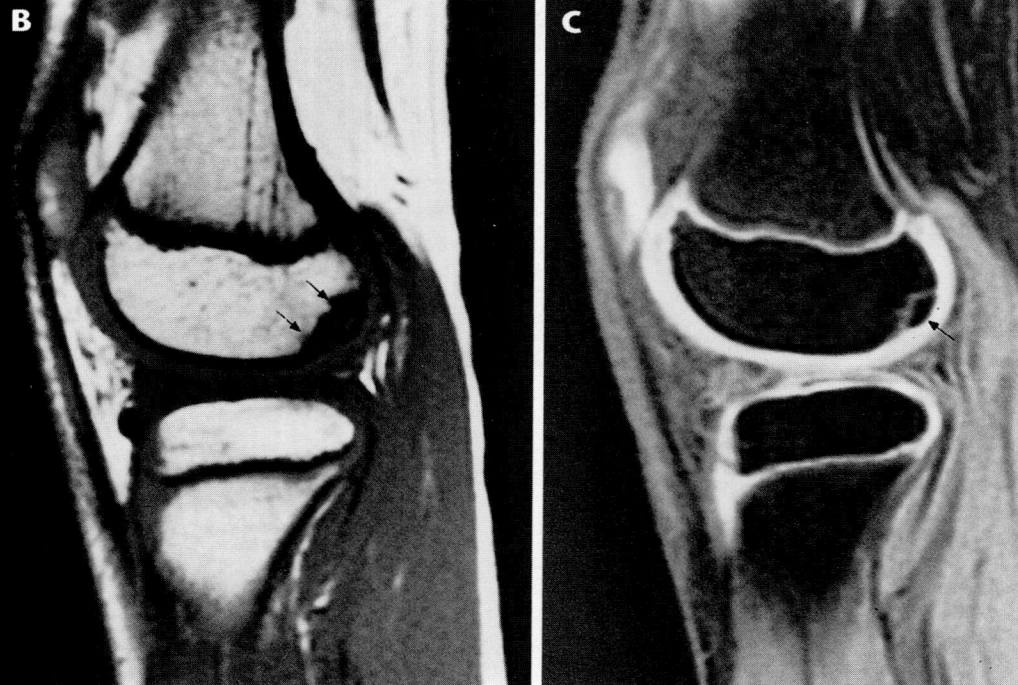

Figure 7–168. Normal irregularity in ossification of the medial femoral condyle in a 10-year-old girl simulating osteochondritis dissecans. **A,** Plain film. **B,** T-1–weighted, and **C,** Gradient echo, T-2–weighted MR images.

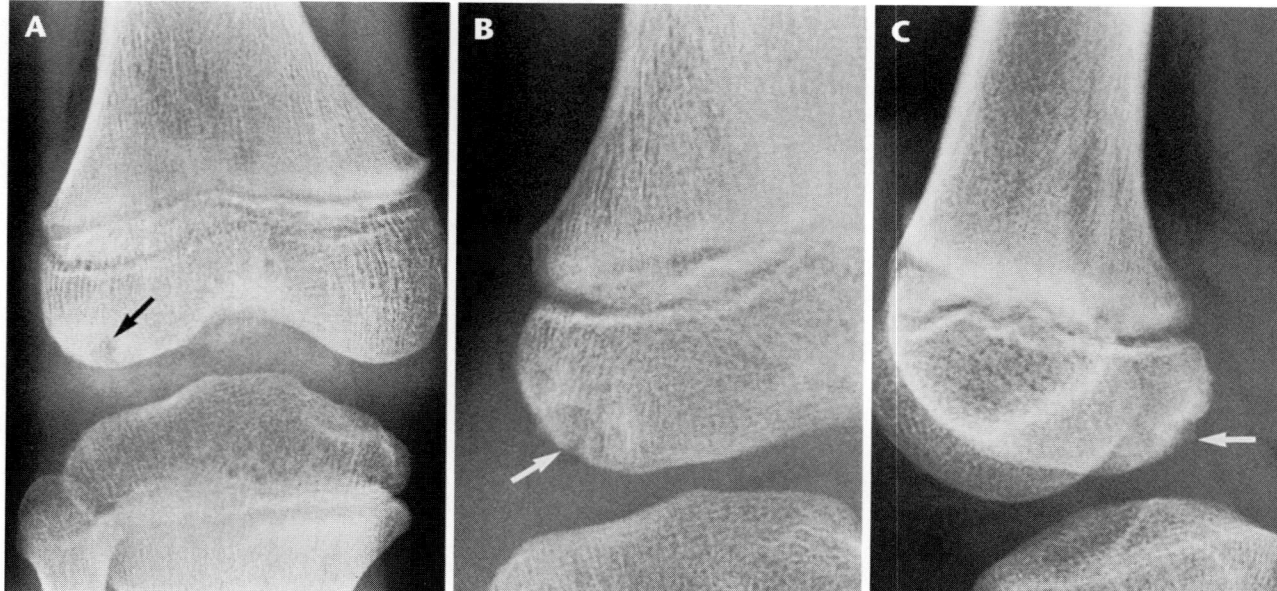

Figure 7–169. Normal irregularities in ossification of the lateral femoral condyle in an 8-year-old boy. **A,** Frontal projection. **B,** Oblique projection. **C,** Lateral projection.

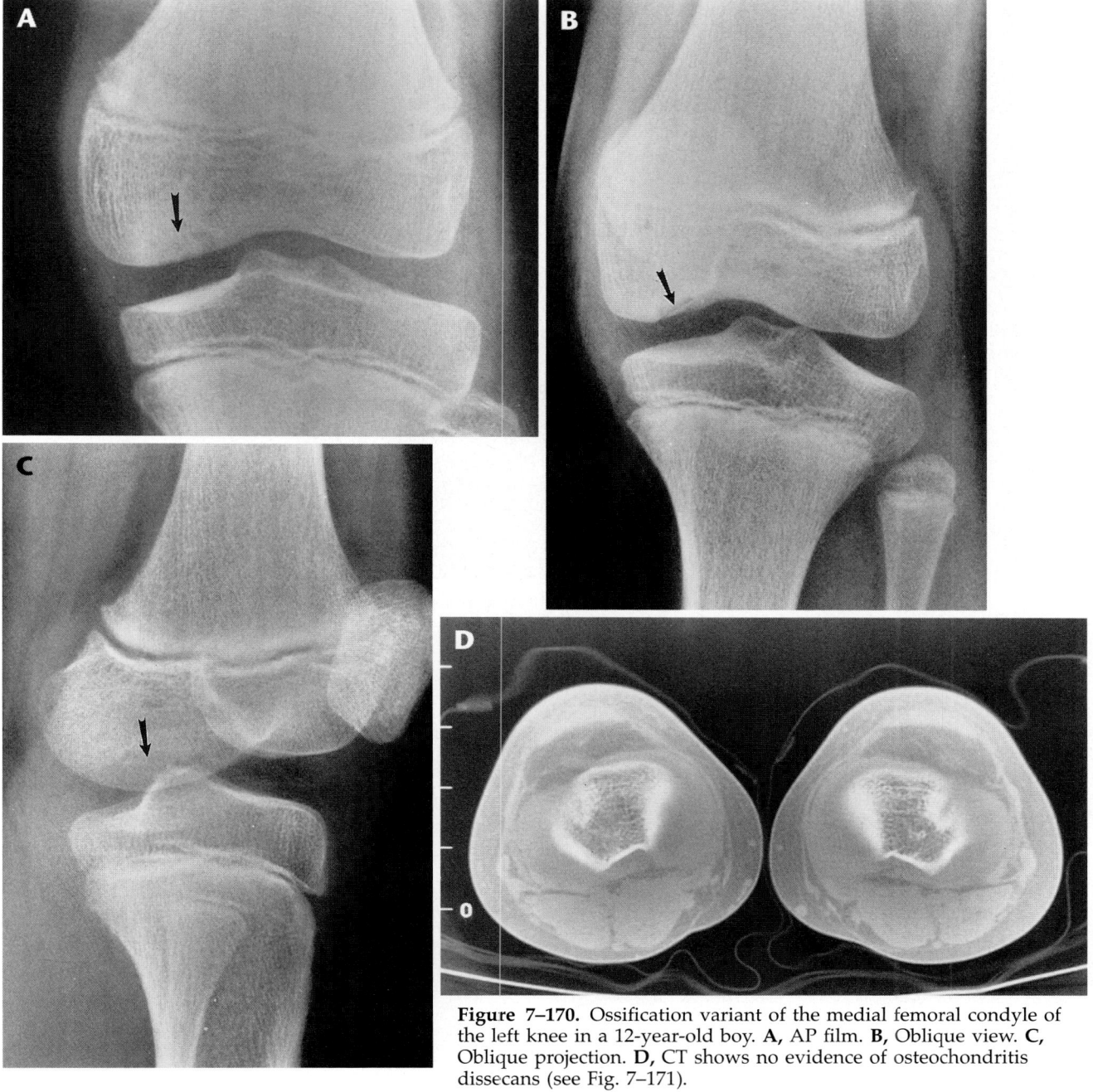

Figure 7–170. Ossification variant of the medial femoral condyle of the left knee in a 12-year-old boy. **A,** AP film. **B,** Oblique view. **C,** Oblique projection. **D,** CT shows no evidence of osteochondritis dissecans (see Fig. 7–171).

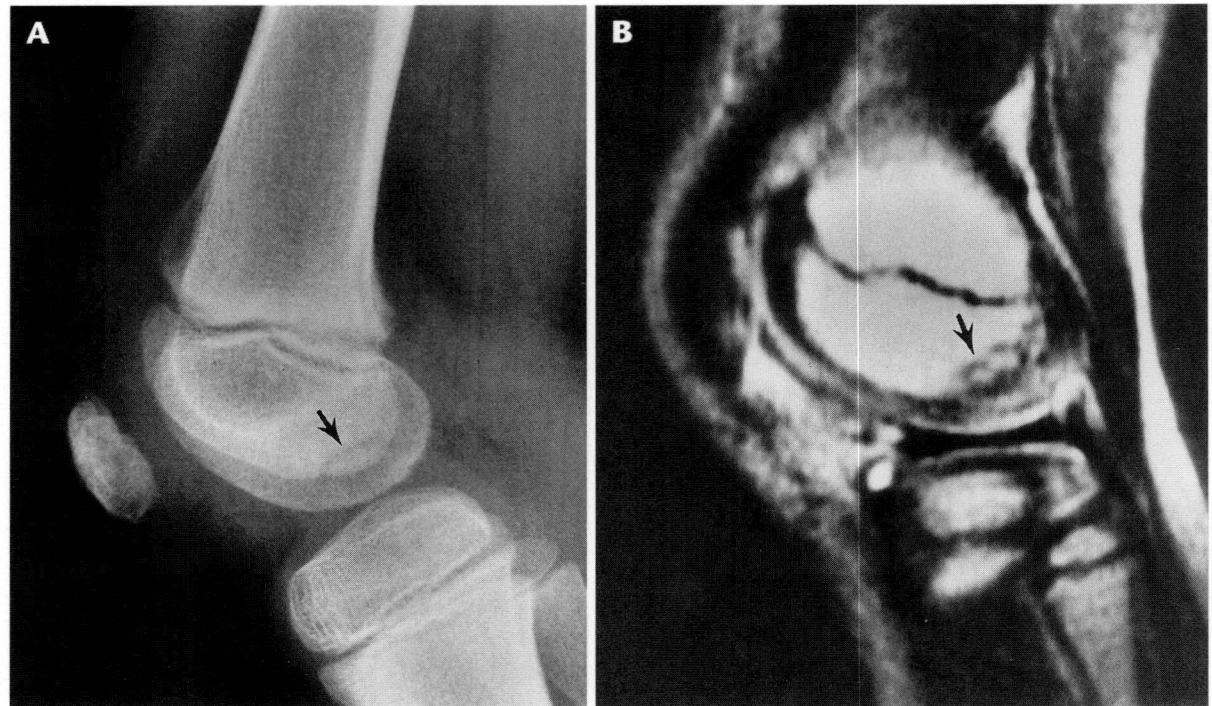

Figure 7–171. Simulated osteochondritis dissecans in a 10-year-old boy. **A,** Plain film. **B,** T-2–weighted image.

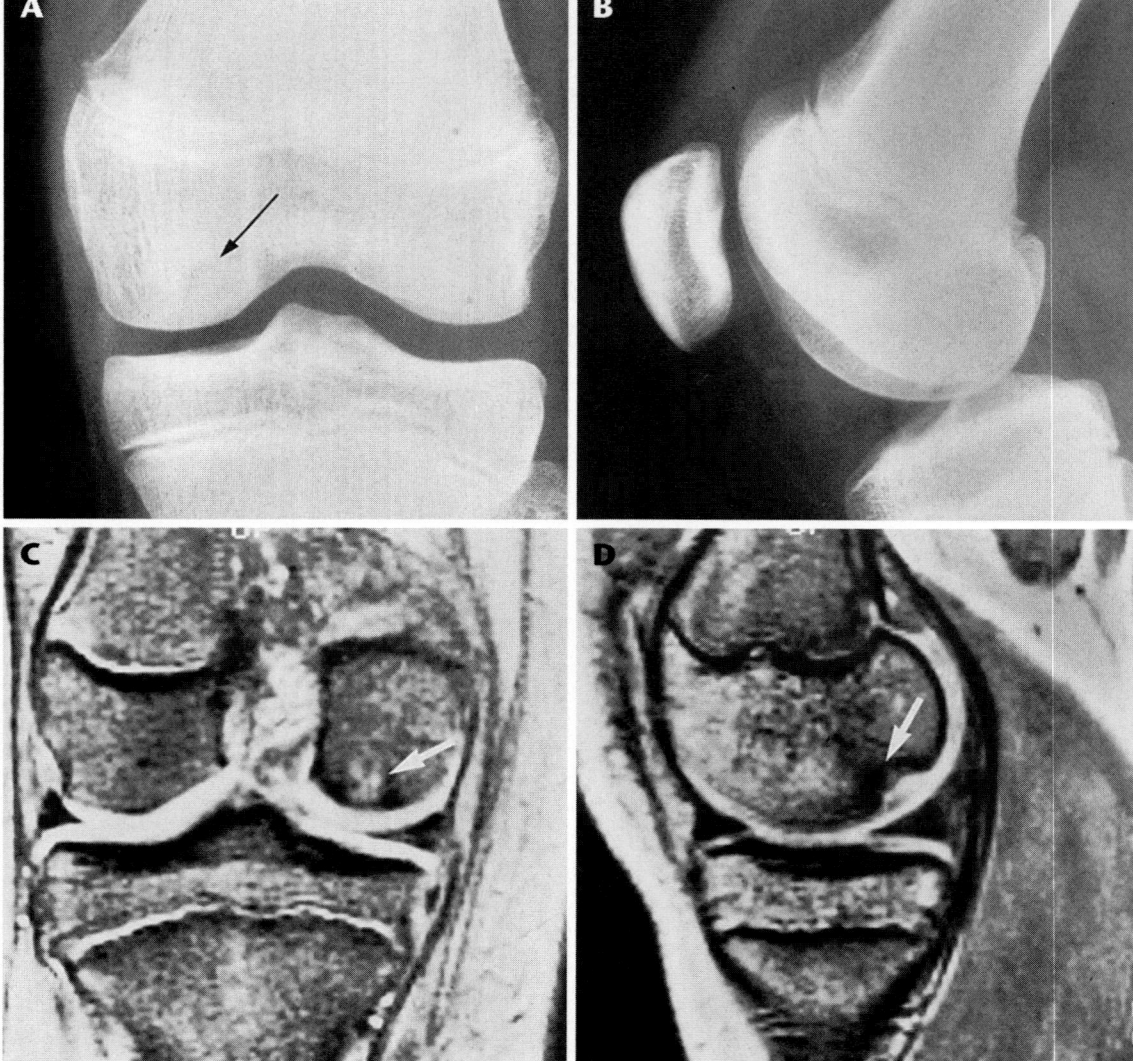

Figure 7–172. Apparent ossification variant of the medial femoral condyle in a 13-year-old boy. **A,** AP projection shows faint radiolucency. **B,** Lateral projection shows no abnormality. **C,** Coronal gradient echo, T2*-weighted MR image shows signal alteration in area of interest. **D,** Sagittal gradient echo T2*-weighted MR image shows a subchondral osseous defect. This entity bears a resemblance to the femoral head notch illustrated in Figure 7–9 and was not related to the patient's symptoms. (Ref: Nawata K et al: Anomalies of ossification in the posterior lateral femoral condyle: Assessment by MRI. *Pediatr Radiol* 29:781, 1999.)

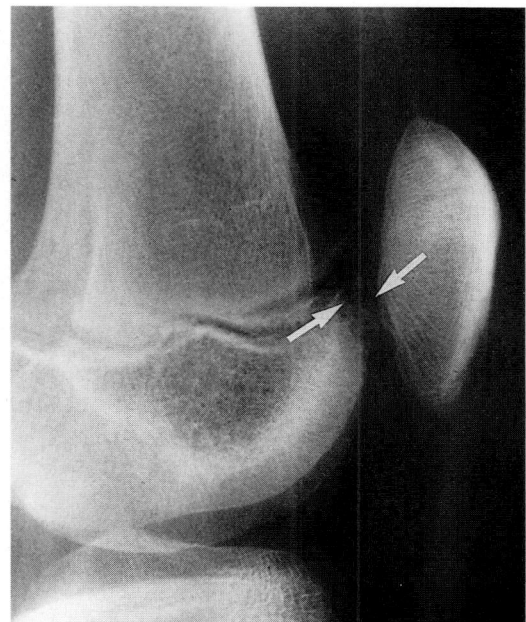

Figure 7–173. Accessory ossification center of the distal femoral epiphysis, seen in lateral projection.

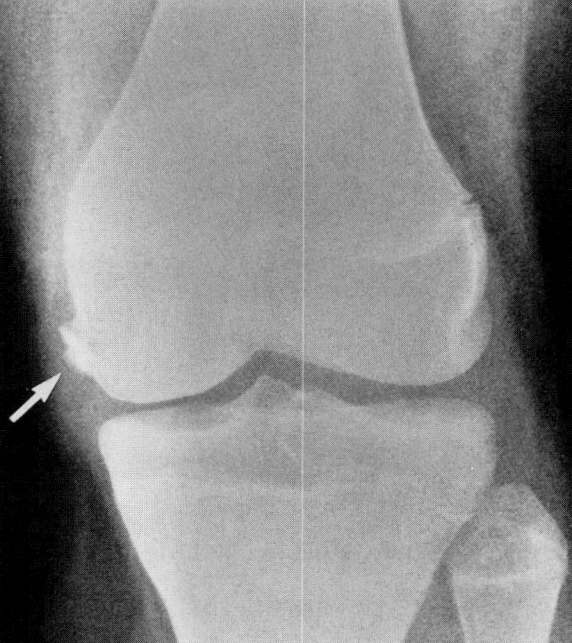
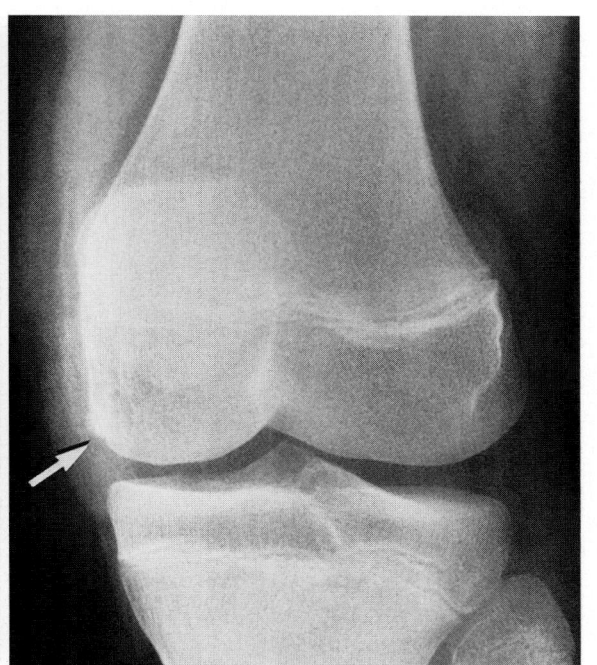

Figure 7–174. Spurlike configuration of the medial femoral epiphysis in a 12-year-old girl, not an epiphyseal osteochondroma. (Ref: Kohler A, Zimmer EA: *Borderlands of the normal and early pathologic findings in skeletal roentgenology,* 3rd ed. New York, Grune & Stratton, 1968, p. 415.)

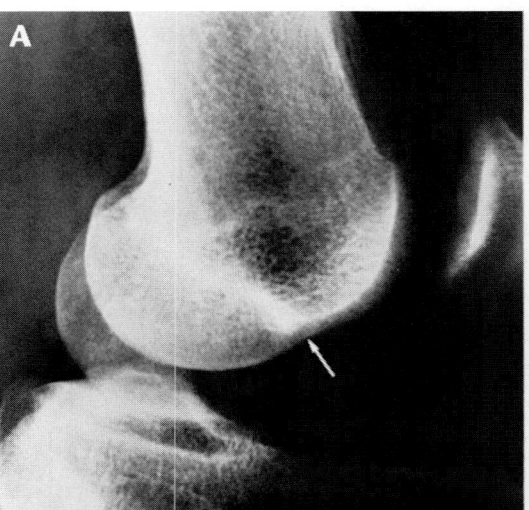
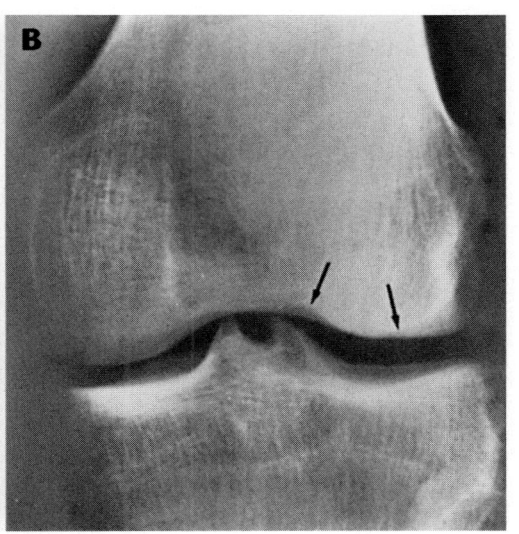

Figure 7–175. The terminal sulcus of the lateral condyle seen in the lateral projection (**A**) may reflect itself in the frontal plane (**B**) in a manner that suggests an abnormality.

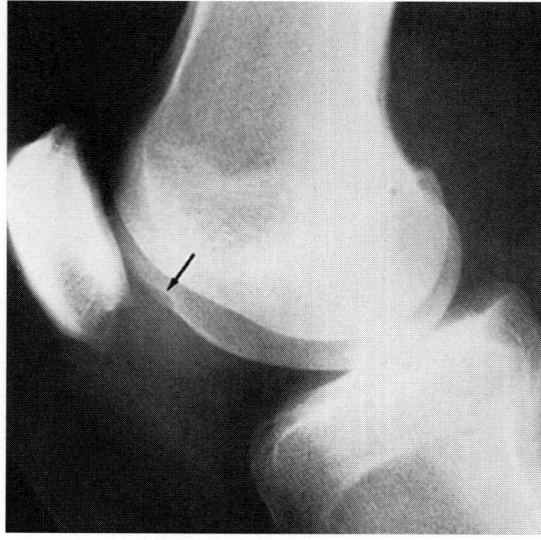
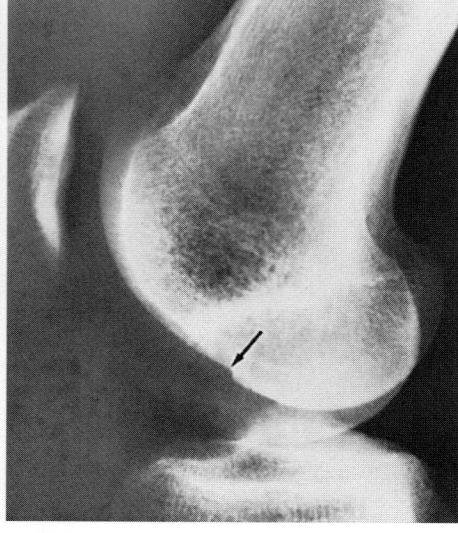

Figure 7–176. Two additional examples of normal contour irregularities of the condyles seen in lateral projection. This contour alteration may be seen in the patellar view as well (see Fig. 7–177.)

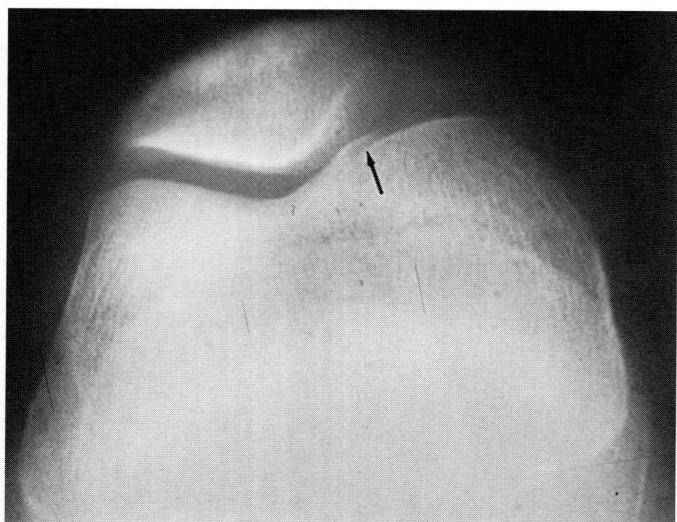

Figure 7–177. Normal contour alteration of the medial condyle seen in tangential projection.

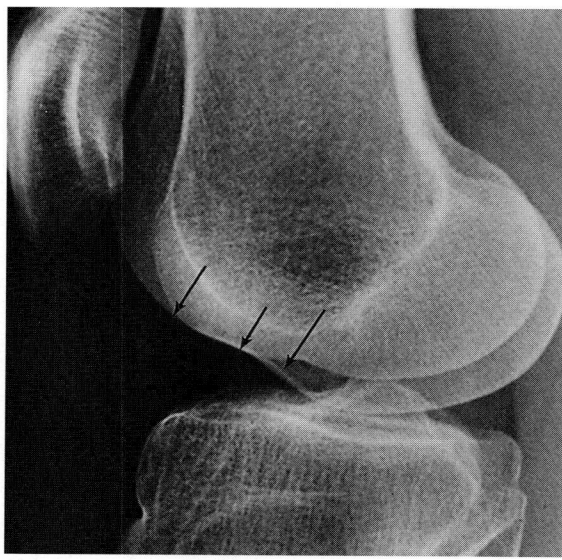

Figure 7–178. The lateral femoral condyle may normally appear flattened, not to be mistaken for evidence of an impaction fracture.

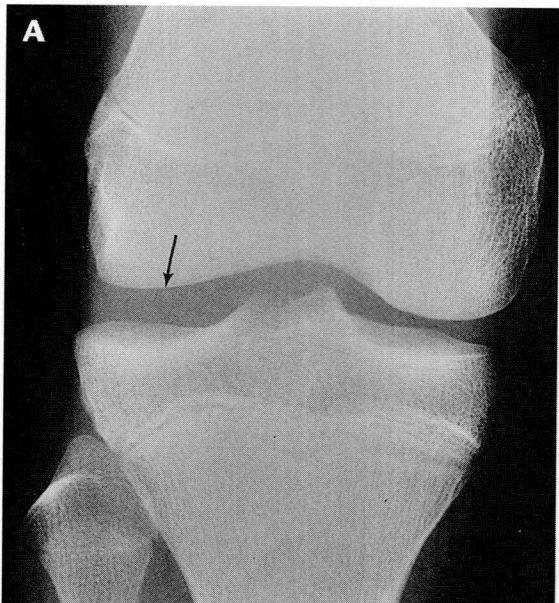
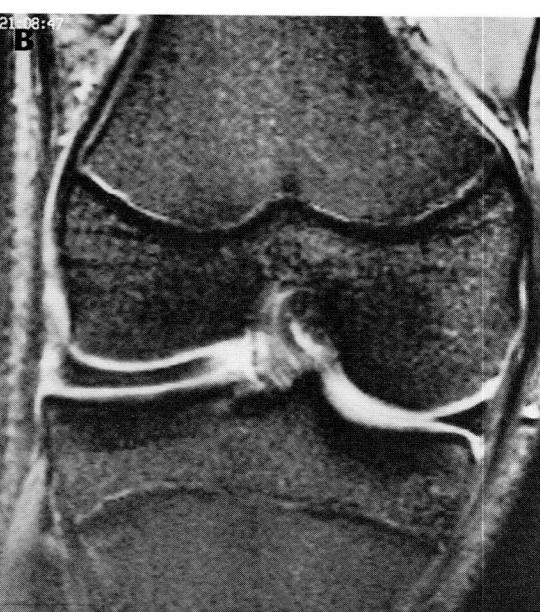

Figure 7–179. A, Flattening of the lateral femoral condyle may be associated with discoid lateral meniscus as documented by gradient echo, T2*-weighted coronal MR image (**B**).

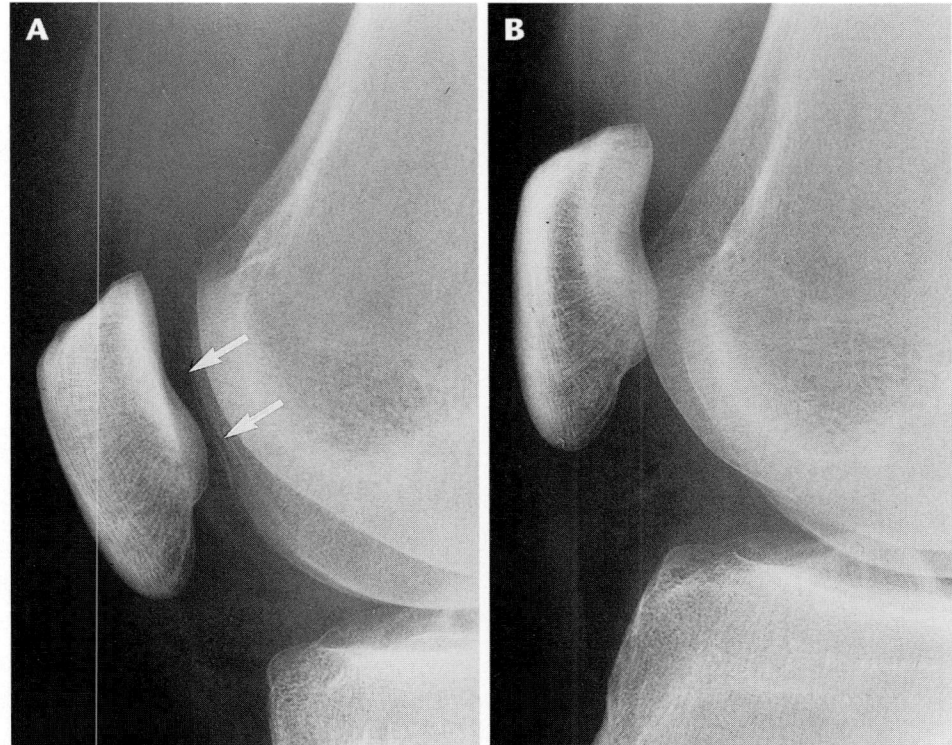

Figure 7–180. A, Simulated lesion of the anterior surface of the femoral condyle, produced by rotation. **B,** Normal appearance in repeat examination.

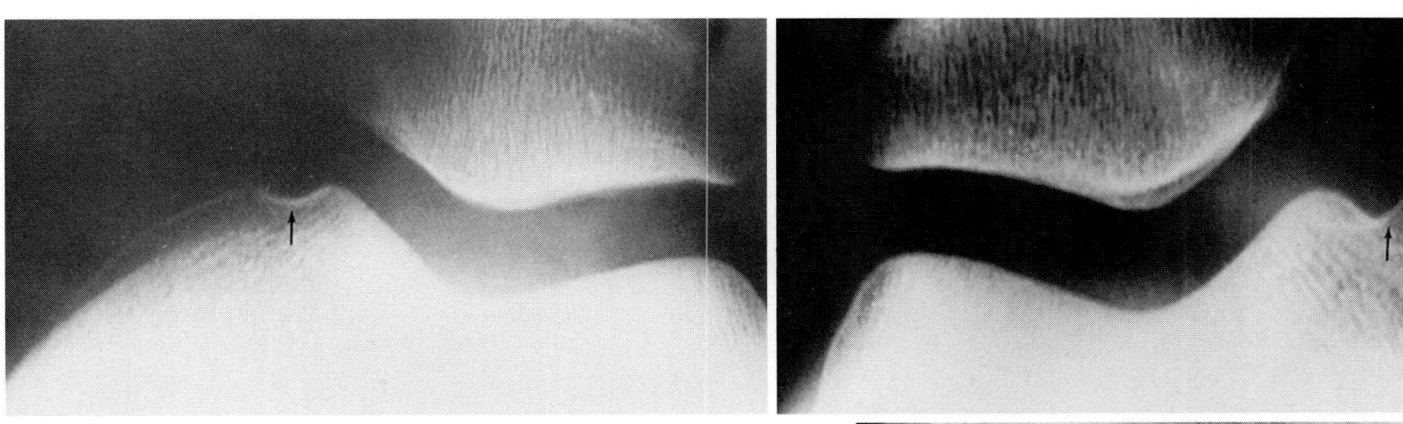

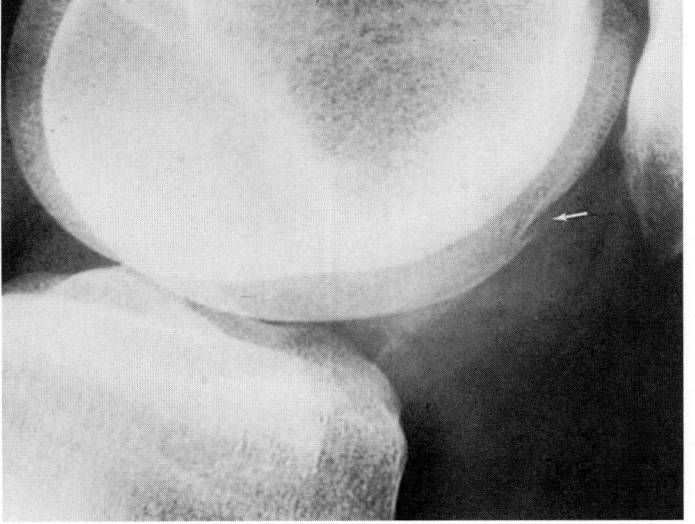

Figure 7–181. The grooves of the articular surface of the medial condyle of the femur represent a normal variant, which should not be confused with osteochondritis or a fracture. (Ref: Harrison RB et al: The grooves of the distal articular surface of the femur—A normal variant. *Am J Roentgenol* 126:751, 1976.)

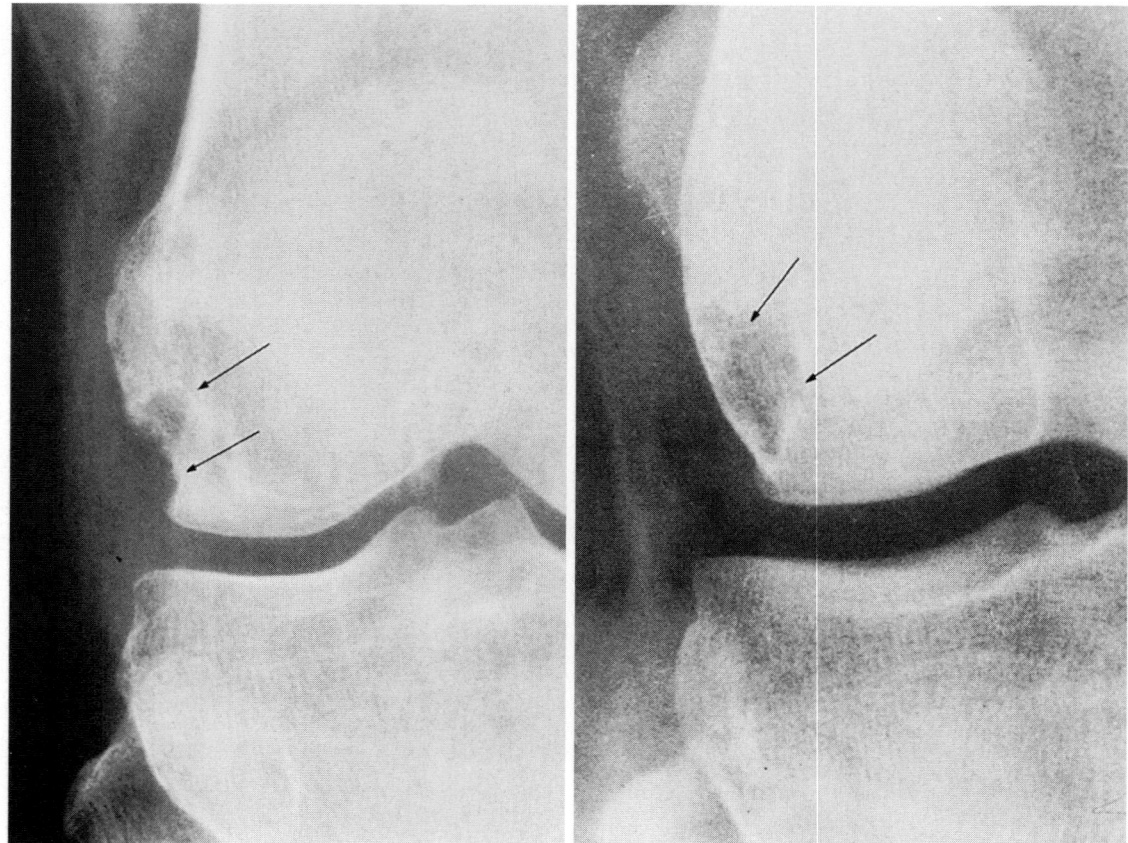

Figure 7–182. The groove for the popliteus tendon should not be mistaken for a pathologic process.

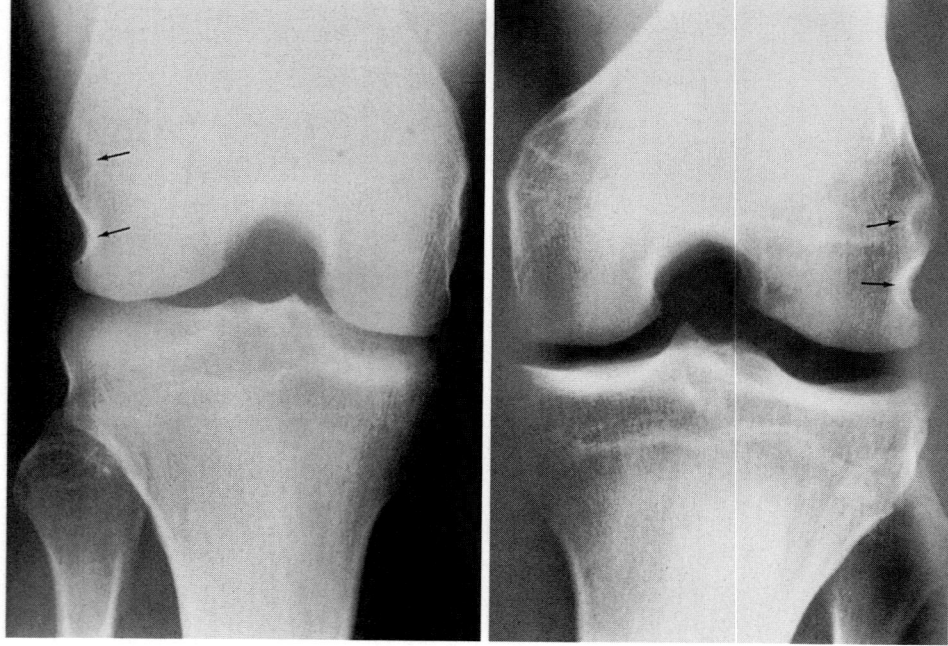

Figure 7–183. The grooves of the popliteus tendon seen in the tunnel view.

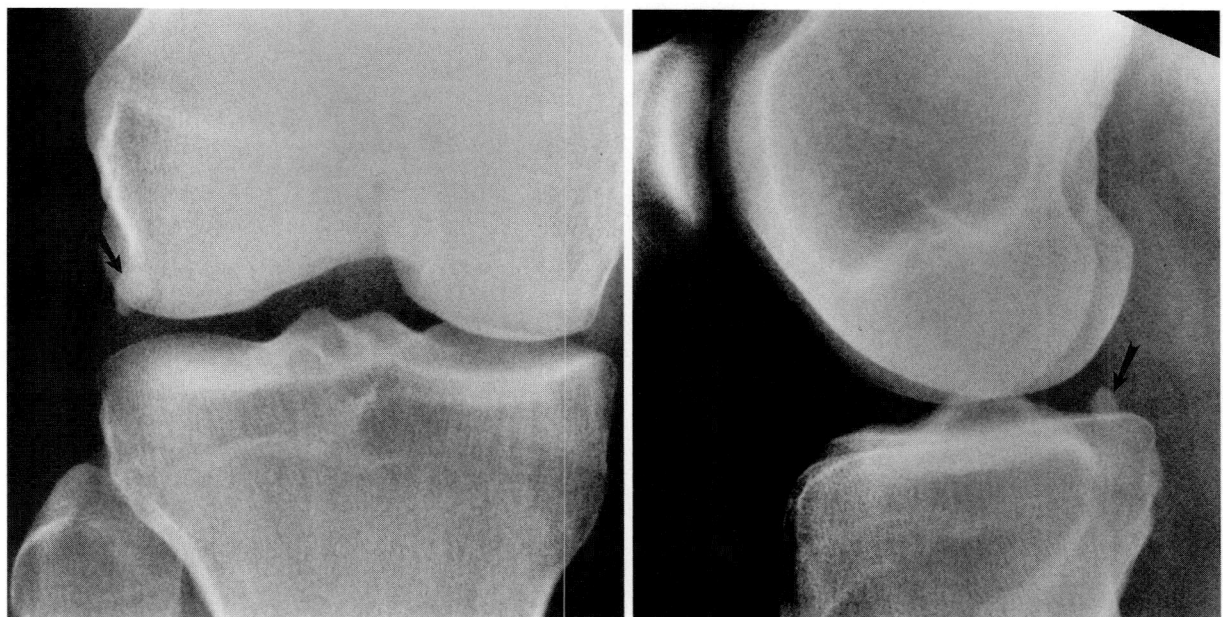

Figure 7–184. An ossicle in the popliteus groove. (Cyamella sesamoid in the popliteus tendon.)

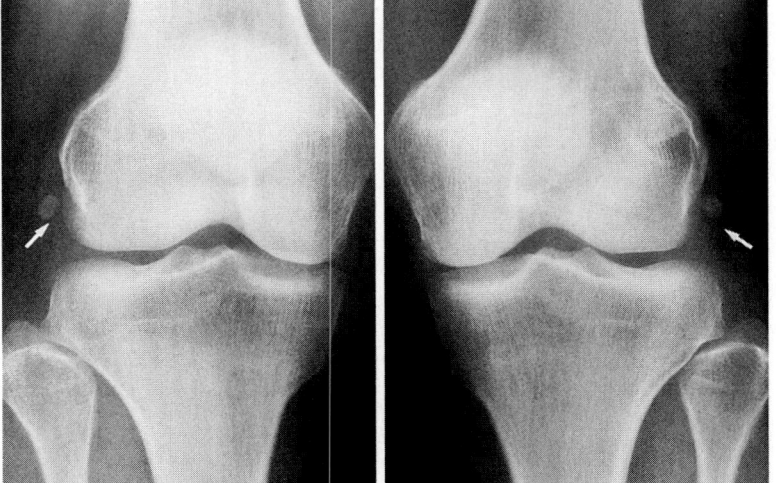

Figure 7–185. Bilateral cyamellae in shallow popliteus grooves.

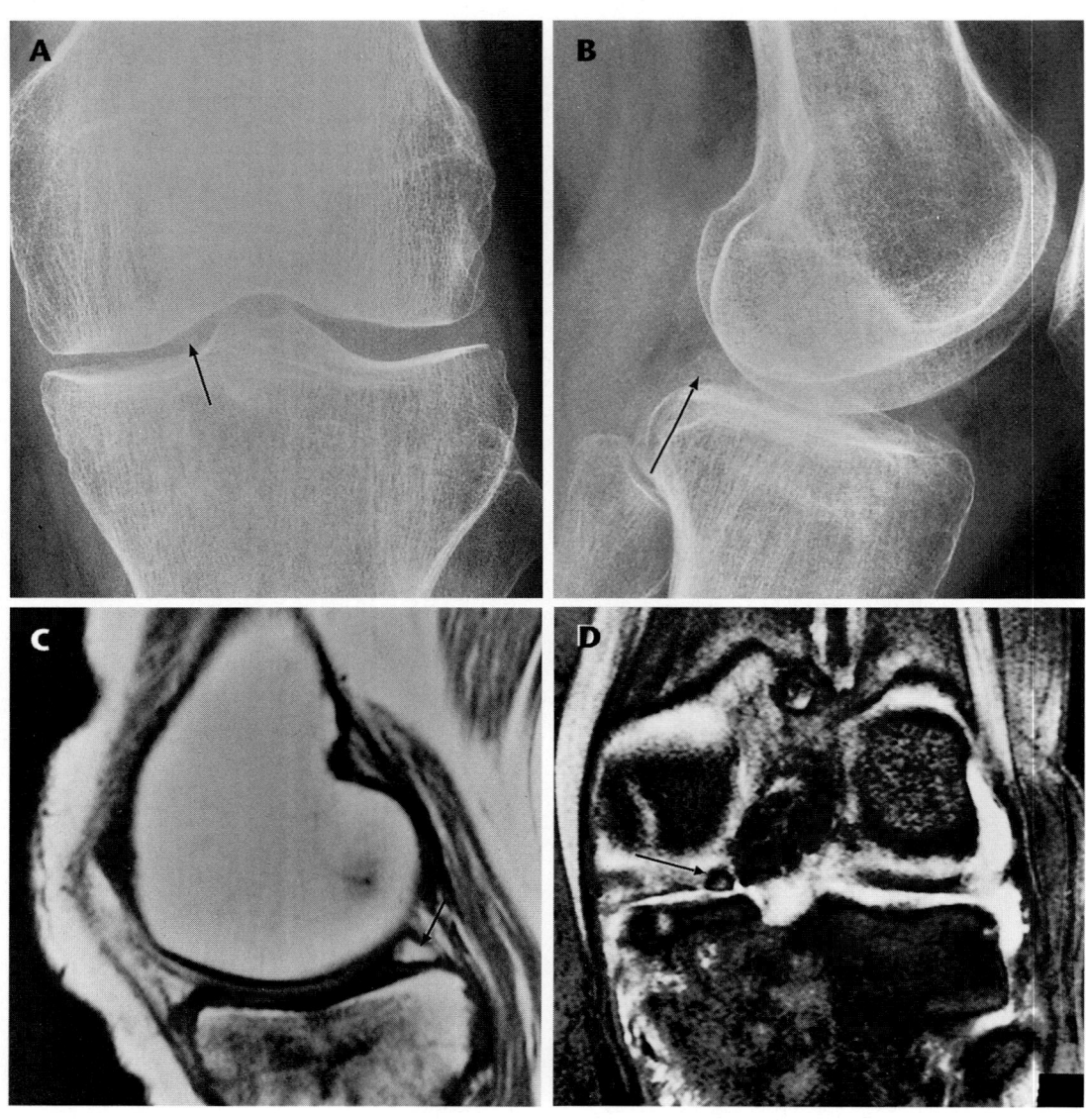

Figure 7–186. Meniscal ossicle of the medial meniscus. **A,** Anteroposterior projection. **B,** Lateral projection. **C,** Coronal STIR MR image. **D,** Sagittal T-1–weighted MR image. (Ref: Schwarkowski P, et al: Medial ossicle. *Radiology* 196:47, 1995.)

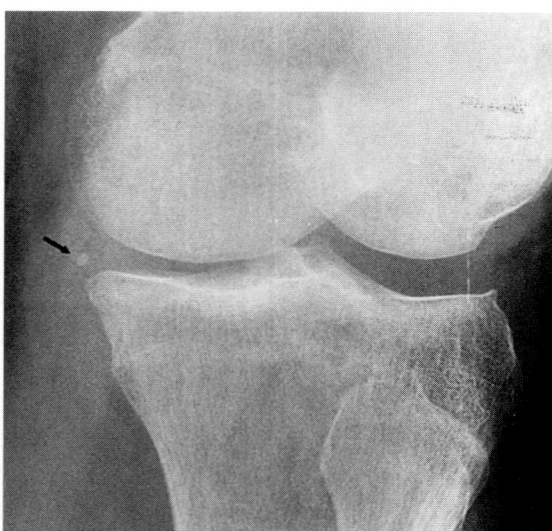

Figure 7–187. The meniscal ossicle in the posterior horn of the medial meniscus.

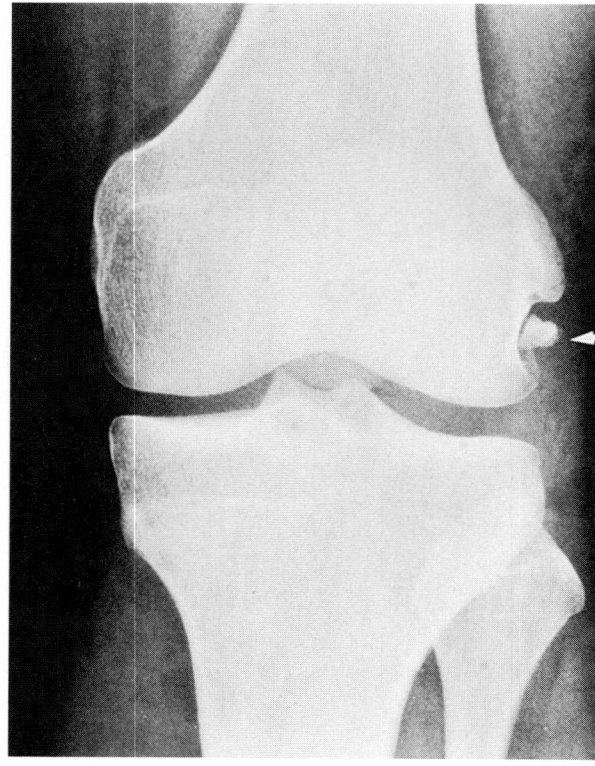

Figure 7–188. A large cyamella with overgrowth of the superior margin of the popliteus groove.

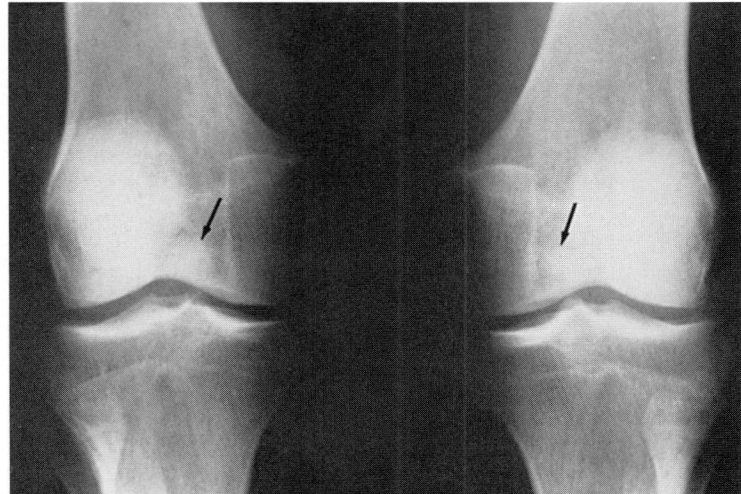

Figure 7–189. Normal areas of sclerosis of the intercondylar fossae in a 25-year-old man.

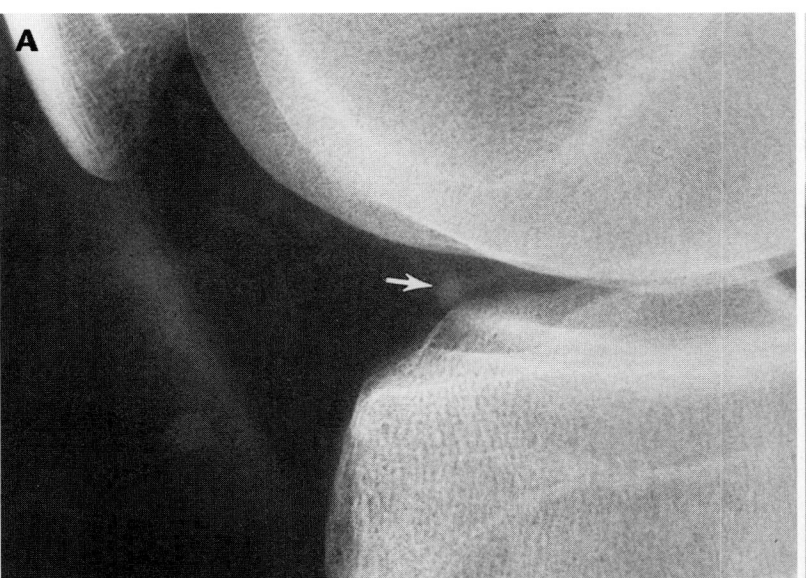

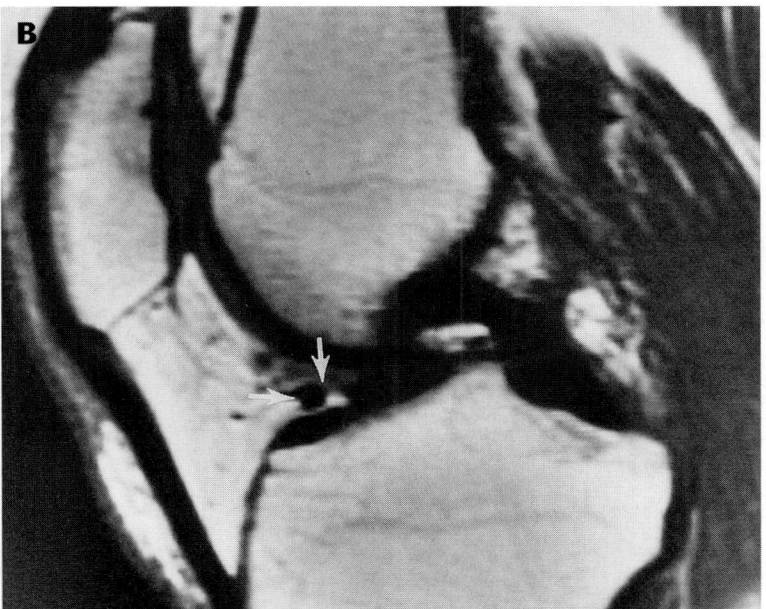

Figure 7–190. The transverse meniscal ligament. **A,** Plain film. **B,** T-1–weighted MR image. (Ref: Sintzoff SA et al: Transverse geniculate ligament of the knee: Appearance and frequency on plain radiographs. *Br J Radiol* 65:766, 1992.)

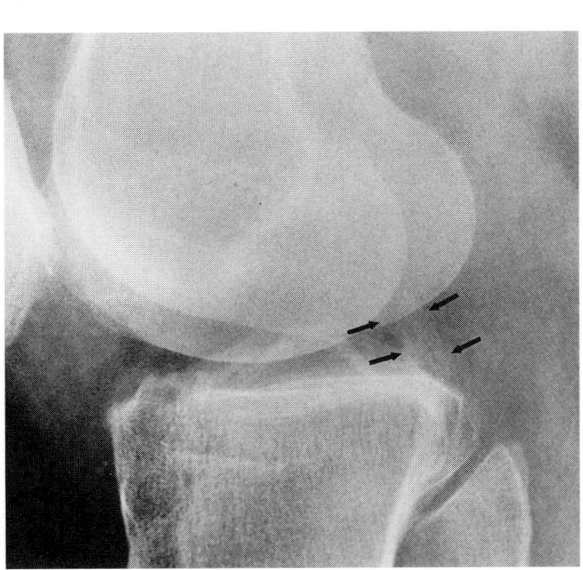

Figure 7–191. Calcification in the posterior cruciate ligament in a patient being examined for an acute injury.

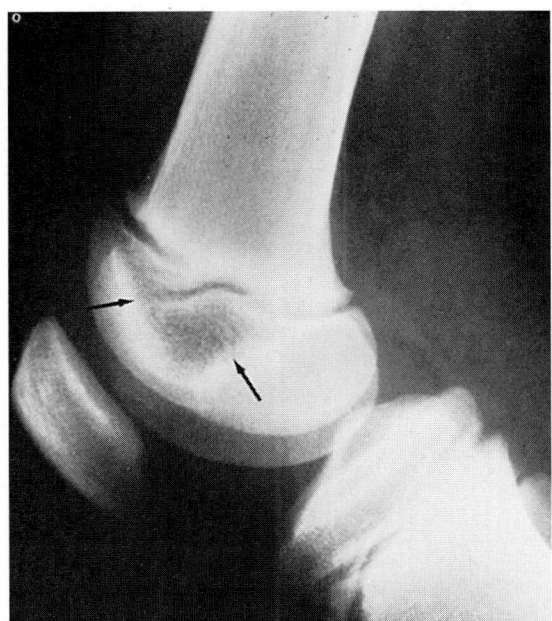

Figure 7–192. Normal radiolucent anterior segment of the distal femoral epiphysis in a 12-year-old boy, due to the fact that less bone is traversed anteriorly than posteriorly.

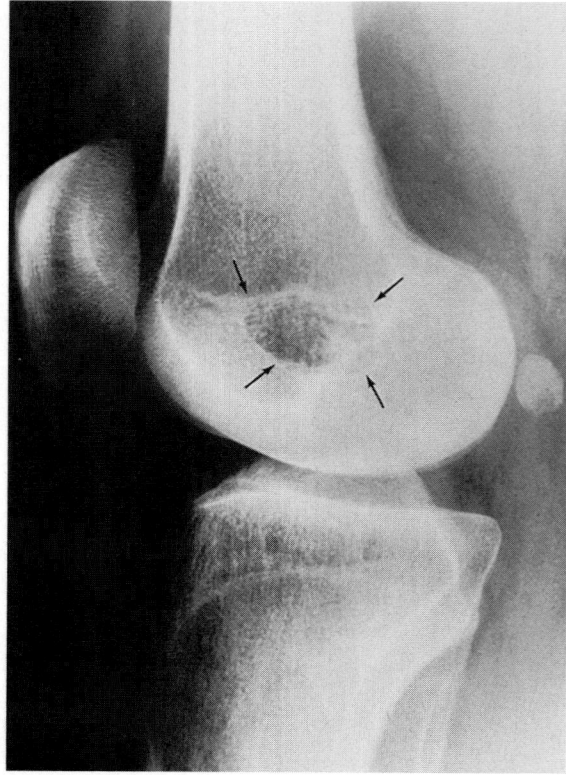

Figure 7–193. Normal radiolucency, simulating a cystic lesion.

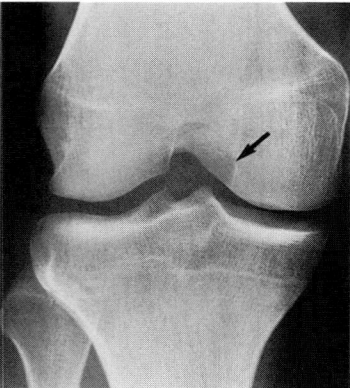

Figure 7–194. Triangular area of radiolucency, which may be confused with the defect of osteochondritis dissecans. (Ref: Weisman JC: The medial femoral triangle of radiolucency simulating osteochondrosis dissecans. *Am J Roentgenol* 58:166, 1947.)

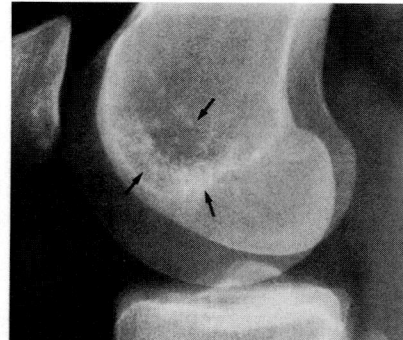

Figure 7–195. Stippled appearance of distal femur caused by the closing epiphyseal plate in a 13-year-old boy. This appearance should not be confused with chondroid matrix of a neoplasm.

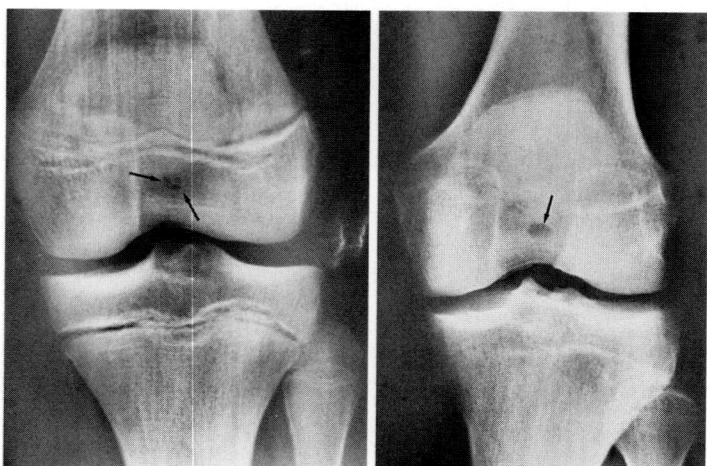

Figure 7–196. Two examples of the foramina for the nutrient vessels of the distal end of the femur.

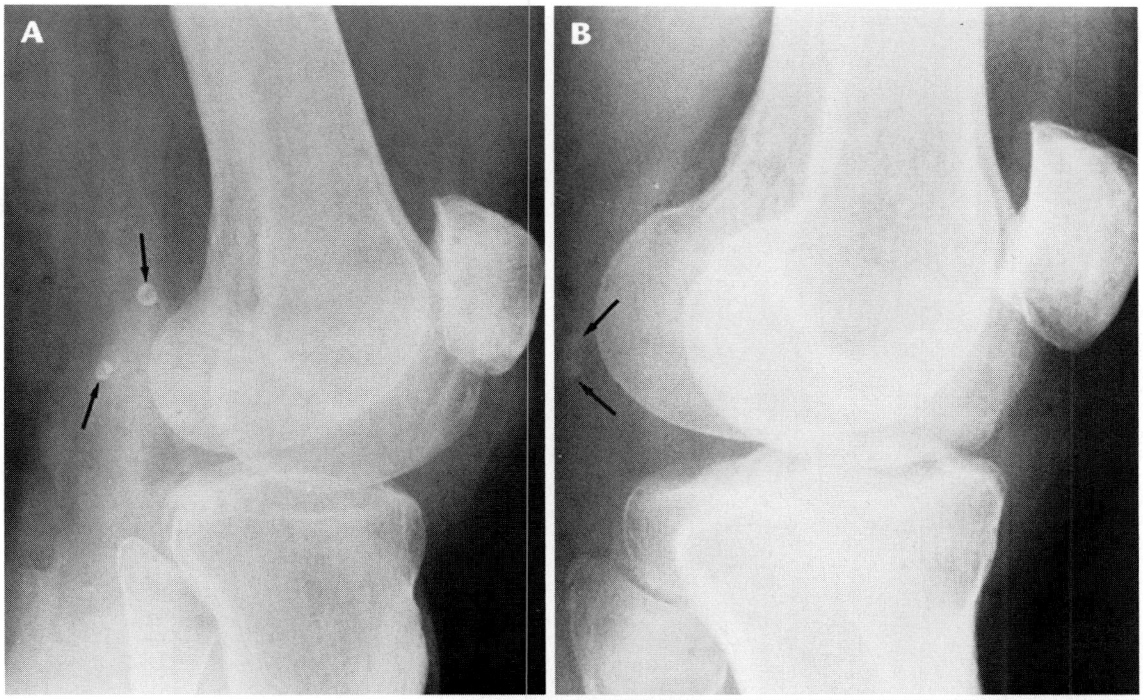

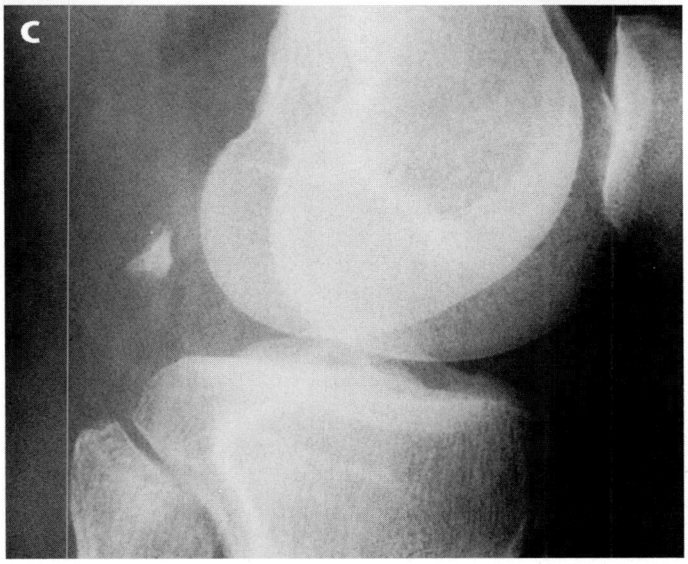

Figure 7–197. Variations in development of the fabella. **A,** Double fabella. **B,** Bifid fabella. **C,** Irregular fabella.

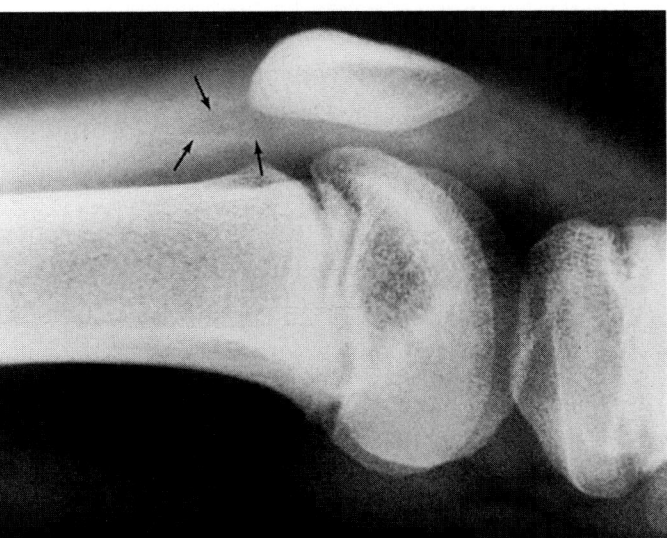

Figure 7–198. Fat pad between joint capsule and quadriceps tendon, which may be mistaken for a lipohemarthrosis. (Ref: Butt WP et al: Radiology of the suprapatellar region. *Clin Radiol* 34:511, 1983.)

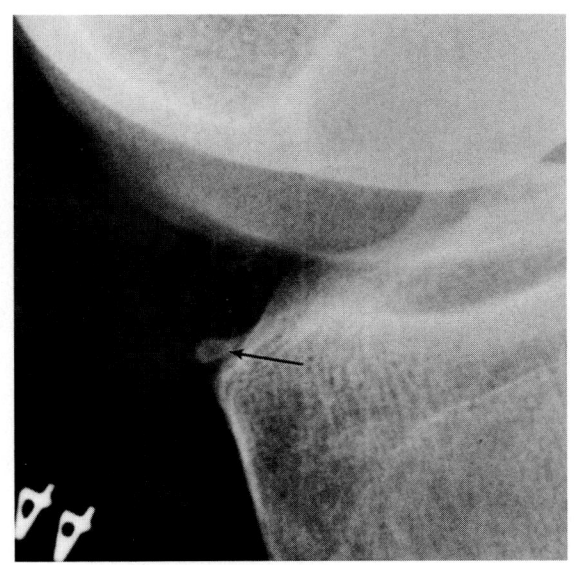

Figure 7–199. Ossicle in Hoffa's fat pad.

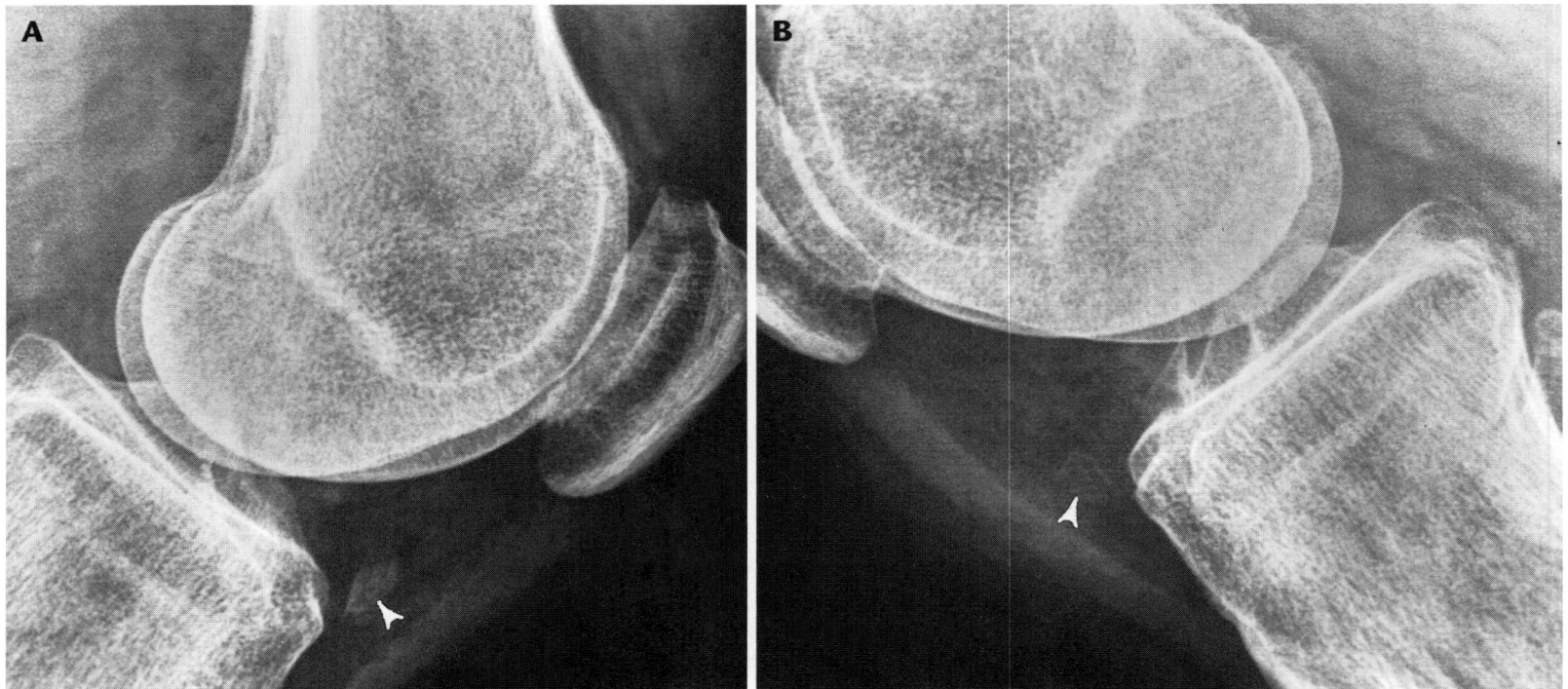

Figure 7–200. A, B, Bilateral ossification in Hoffa's fat pad.

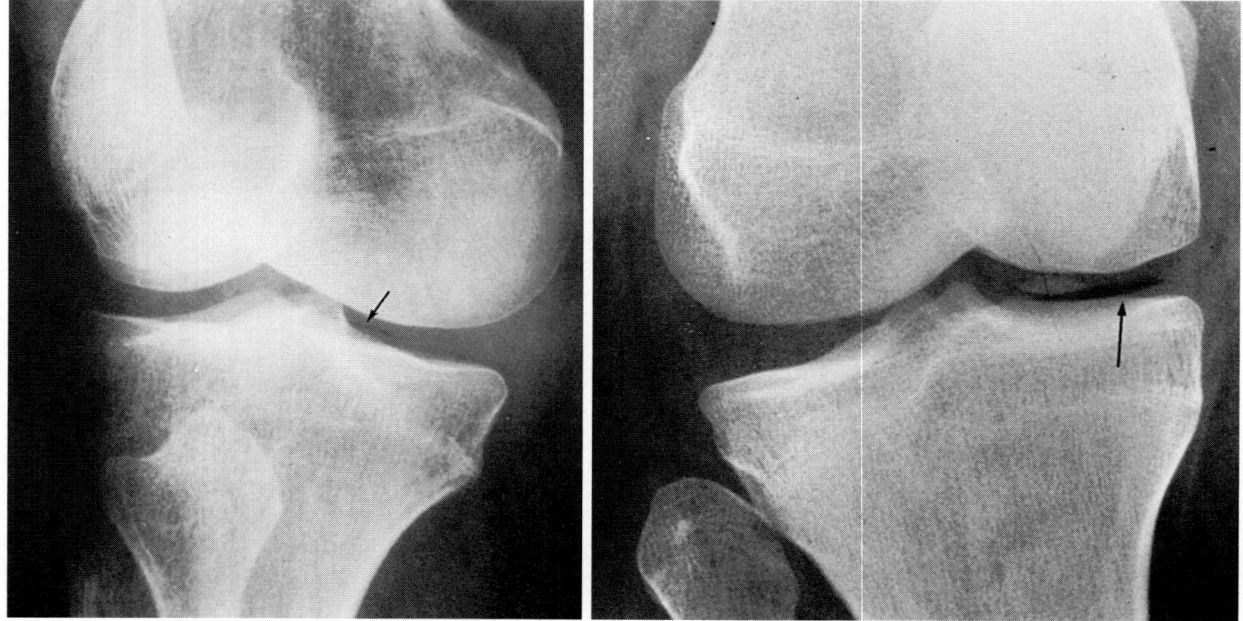

Figure 7–201. The vacuum phenomenon in the knee joint.

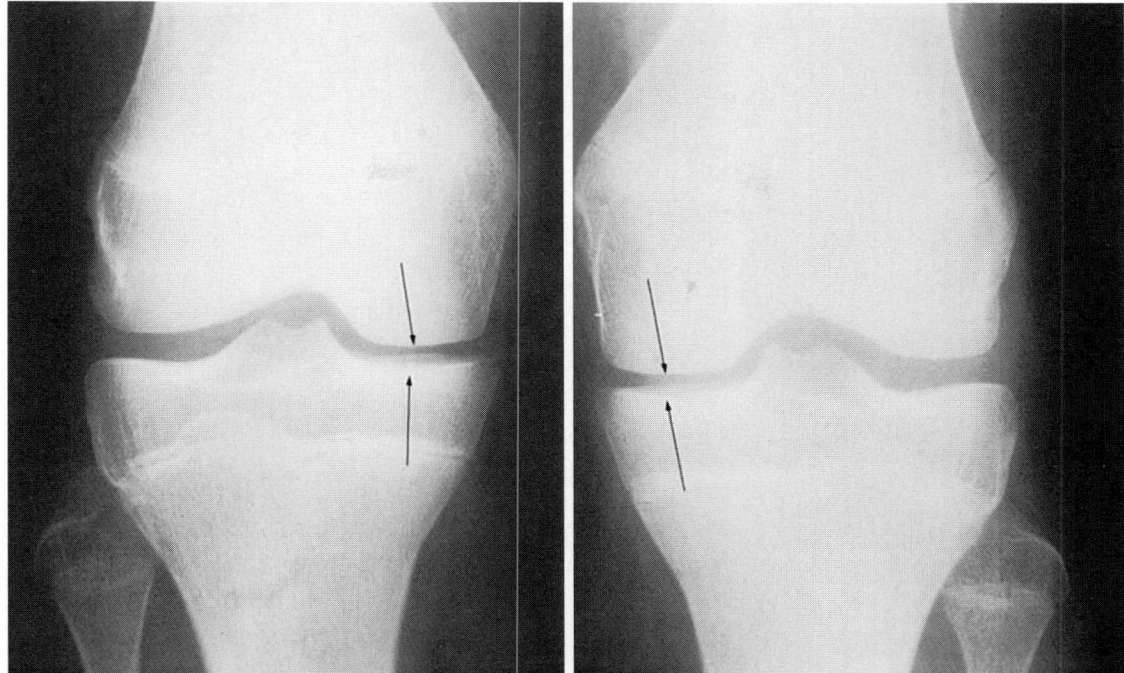

Figure 7–202. Simulated narrowing of the medial compartments of the knees in a 14-year-old girl. This misleading appearance is the result of the double contour of the medial tibial plateau. Measurements should be made from the articular surface of the distal femoral condyle to the most distal of the tibial articular margins (*arrows*). Measured in this fashion, the width of both compartments is equal. (Ref: Fife RS et al: Relationship between arthroscopic evidence of cartilage damage and radiographic evidence of joint space narrowing in early osteoarthritis of the knee. *Arthritis Rheum* 34:377, 1991.)

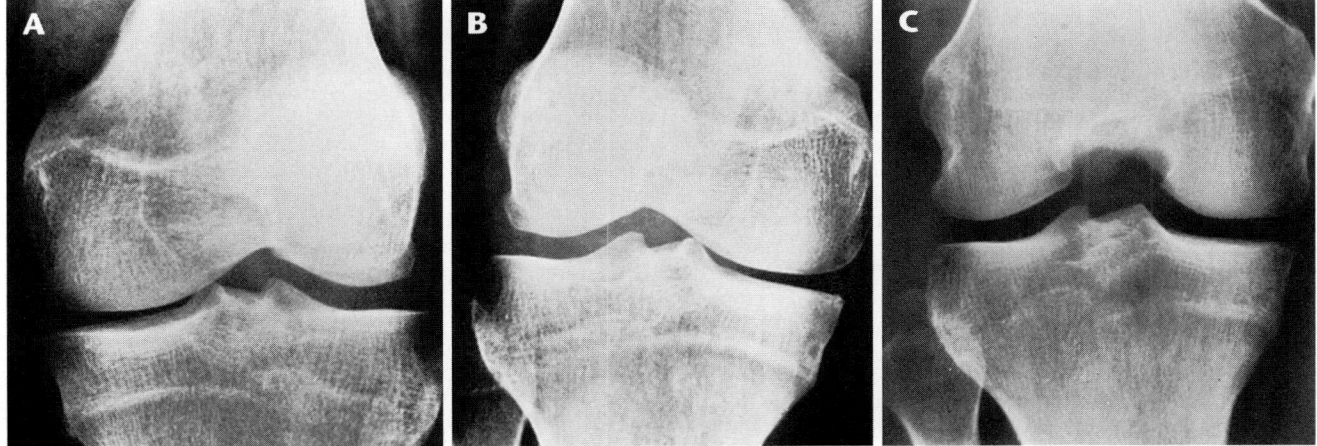

Figure 7–203. A and **B,** Simulated medial compartment narrowing on standing film on the same basis as Figure 7–202. This problem can also be resolved by tunnel projection (**C**), which demonstrates equality of measurement of both compartments.

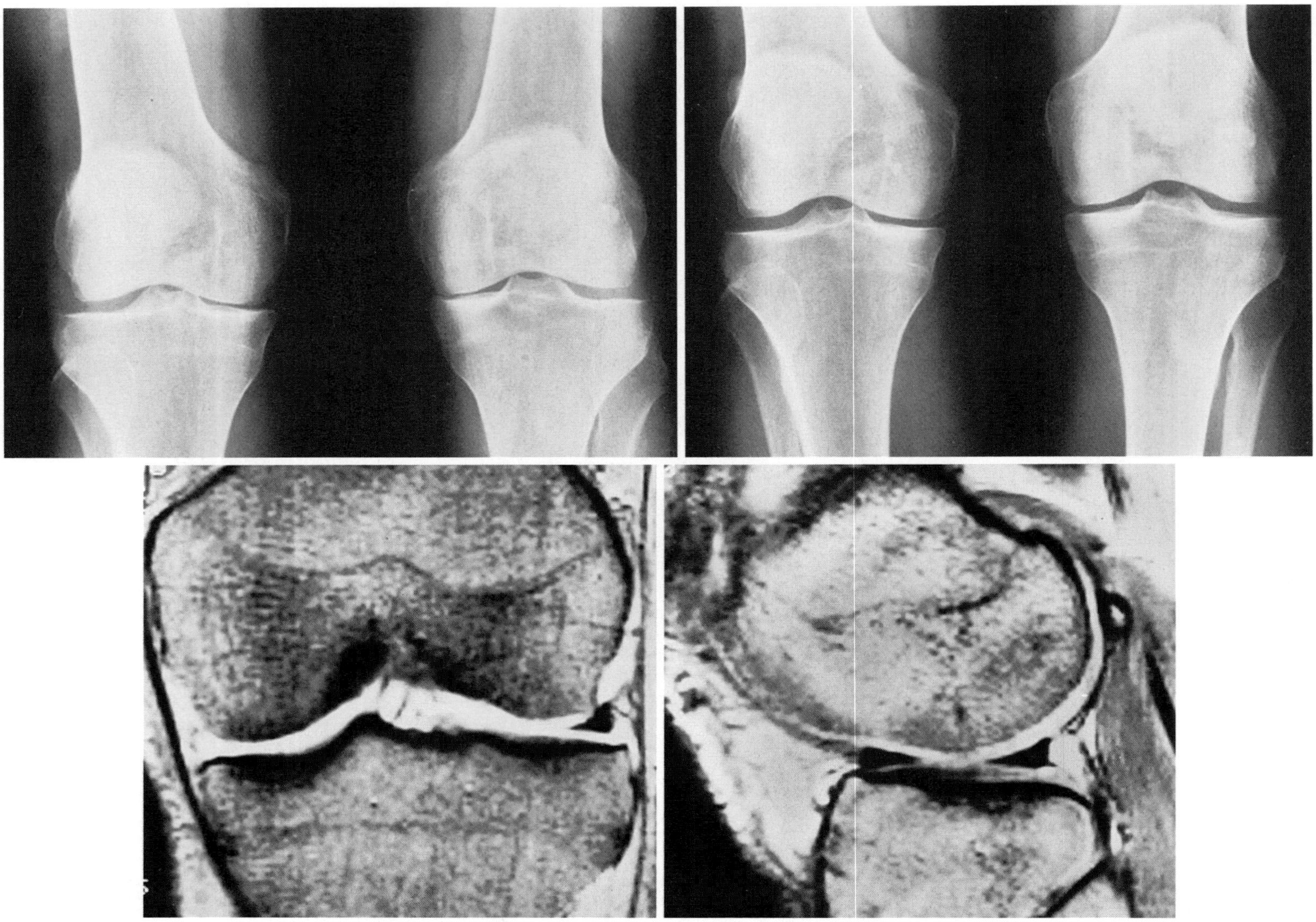

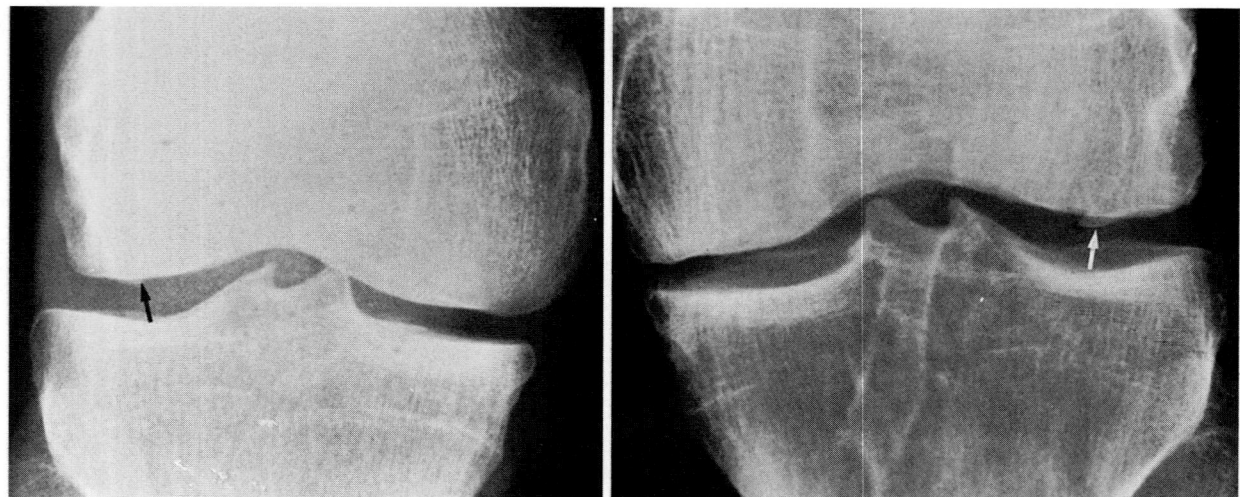

Figure 7–204. Some normal individuals show true asymmetry in the height of the medial and lateral compartments. *Top left*, 48-year-old male. Standing films show asymptomatic symmetrical narrowing of medial compartments. *Top right*, The same individual 10 years later shows no change in compartment height, and MR examination (coronal and sagittal gradient echo T2*-weighted images) at this time shows normal articular cartilage. These variations are probably related to known normal differences in thickness of articular cartilage in normal individuals. (Refs: Hall FM, Wyshak G: Thickness of articular cartilage in the normal knee. *J Bone Joint Surg* 62A:408, 1980; Fig. 7–162; Brandt KD et al: Radiographic grading of the severity of knee osteoarthritis. *Arthritis Rheum* 34:1381, 1991.)

Figure 7–205. Small excrescences on the articular surface of the femur.

The Patella

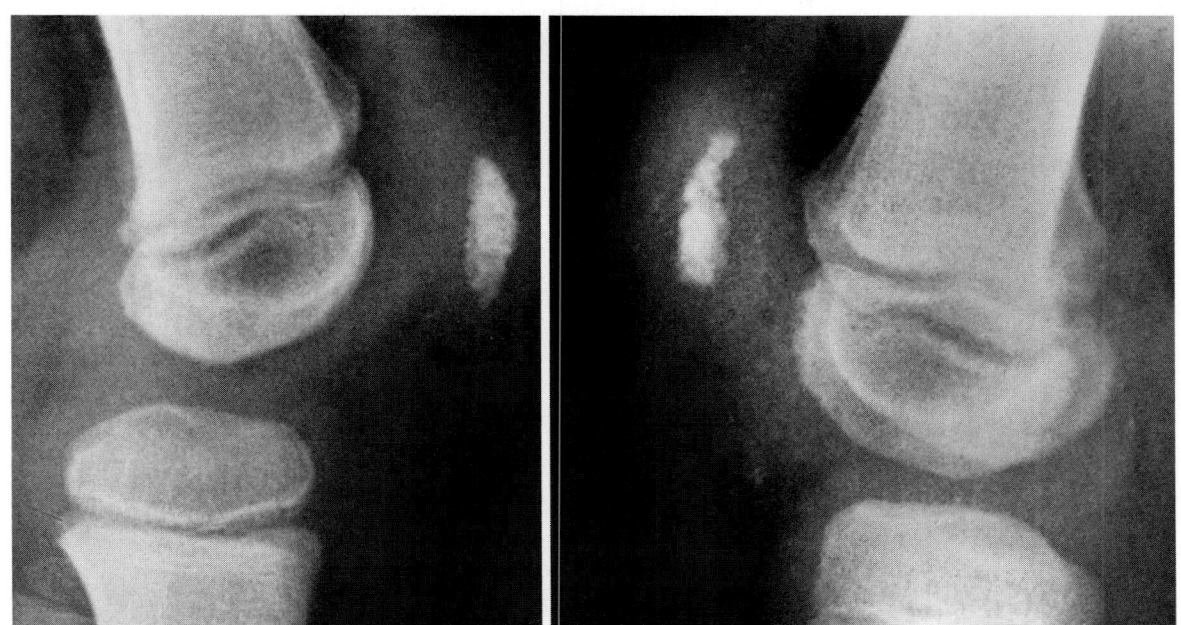

Figure 7–206. Normal irregularity of the growing patellae in a 7-year-old boy.

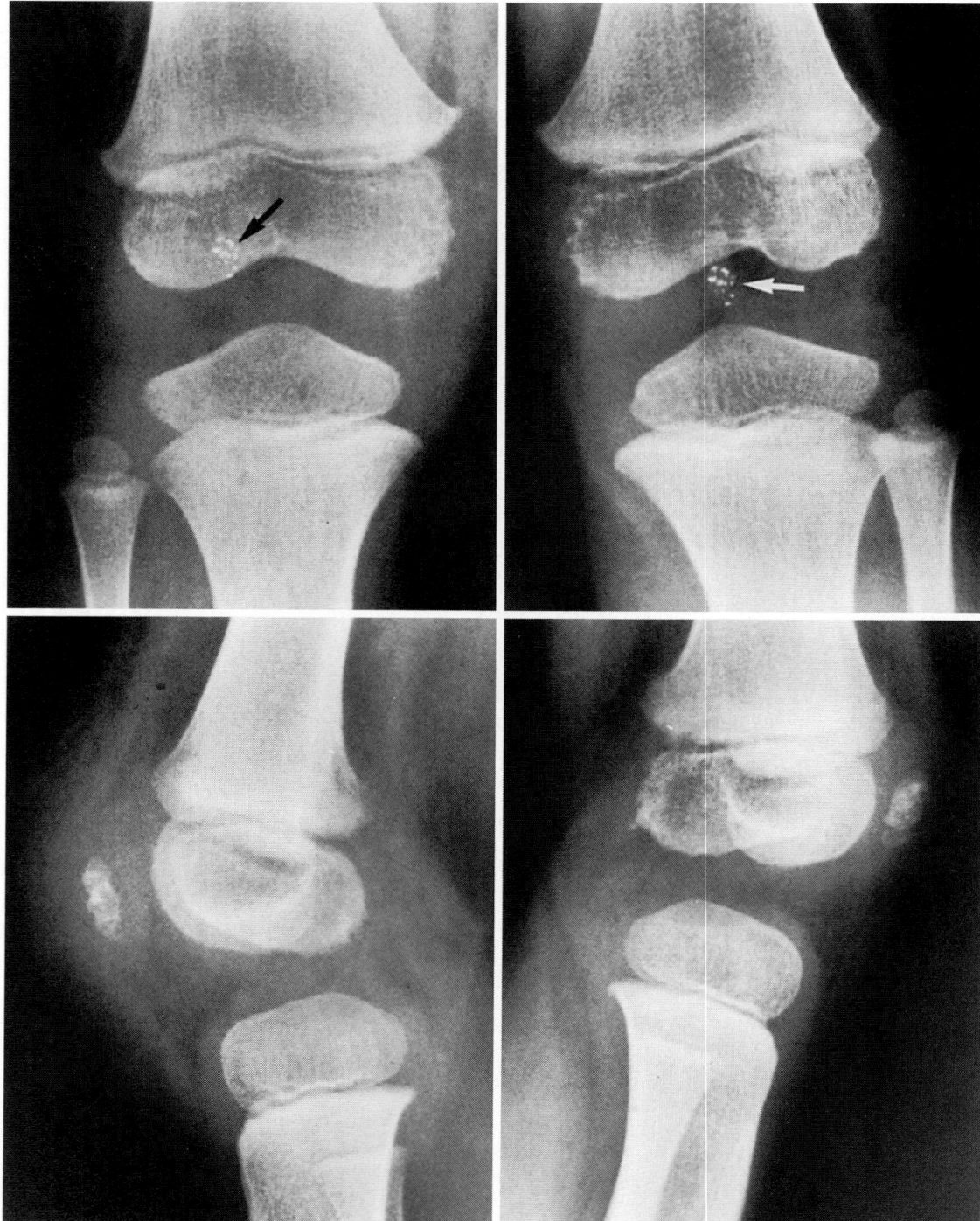

Figure 7–207. Unusual dense stippling of the patellae in a 2-year-old girl, best seen in the frontal projection. Note that the other epiphyses are normal.

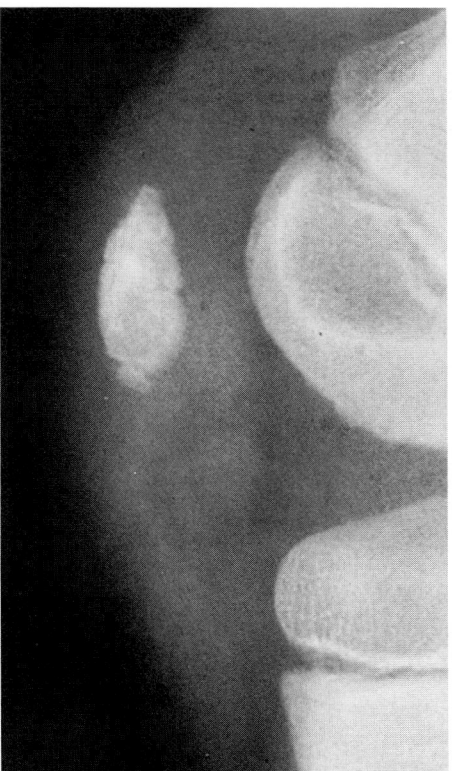

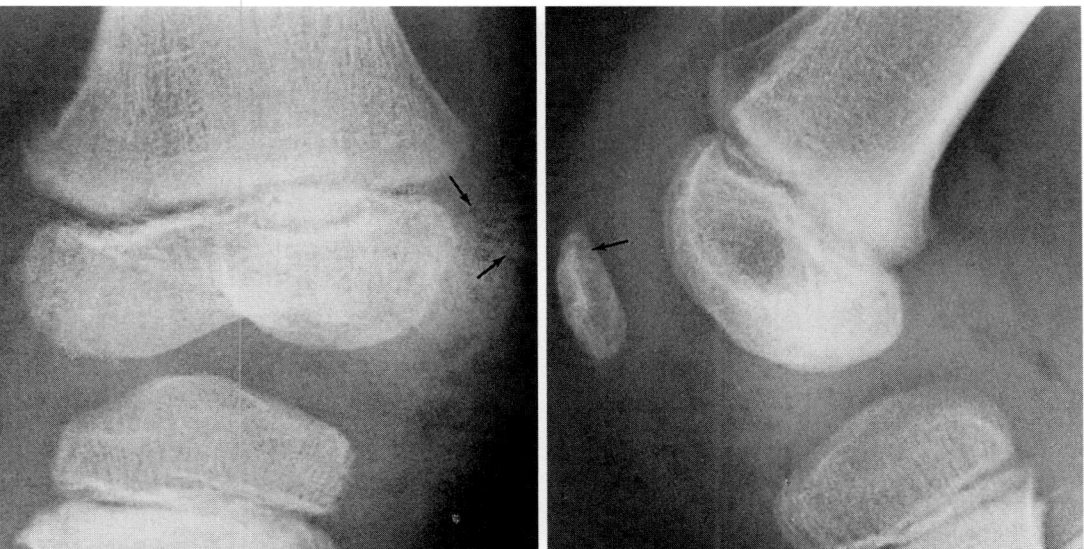

Figure 7–209. Normal variation in development of the patella in an 8-year-old boy, simulating a fracture.

Figure 7–208. Normal irregularity and clefts in the patella of a 6-year-old boy.

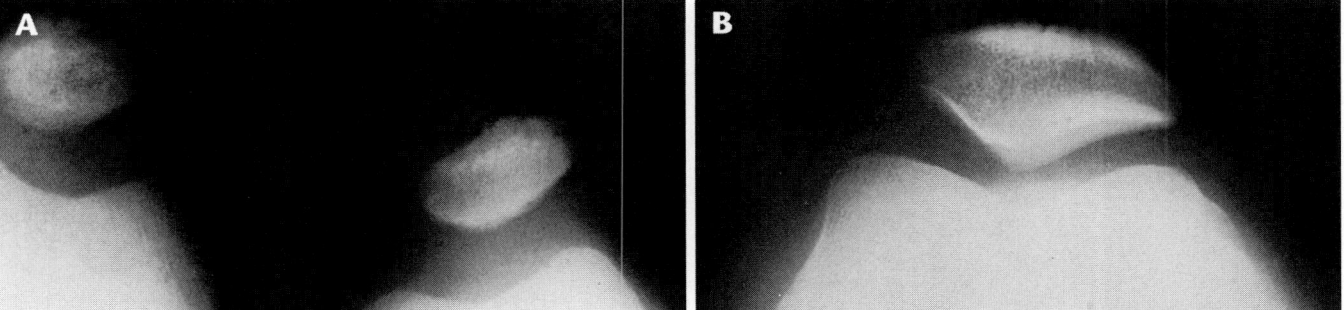

Figure 7–210. Normal developmental irregularities of the patellae, seen in the tangential projection. **A,** 7-year-old. **B,** 15-year-old.

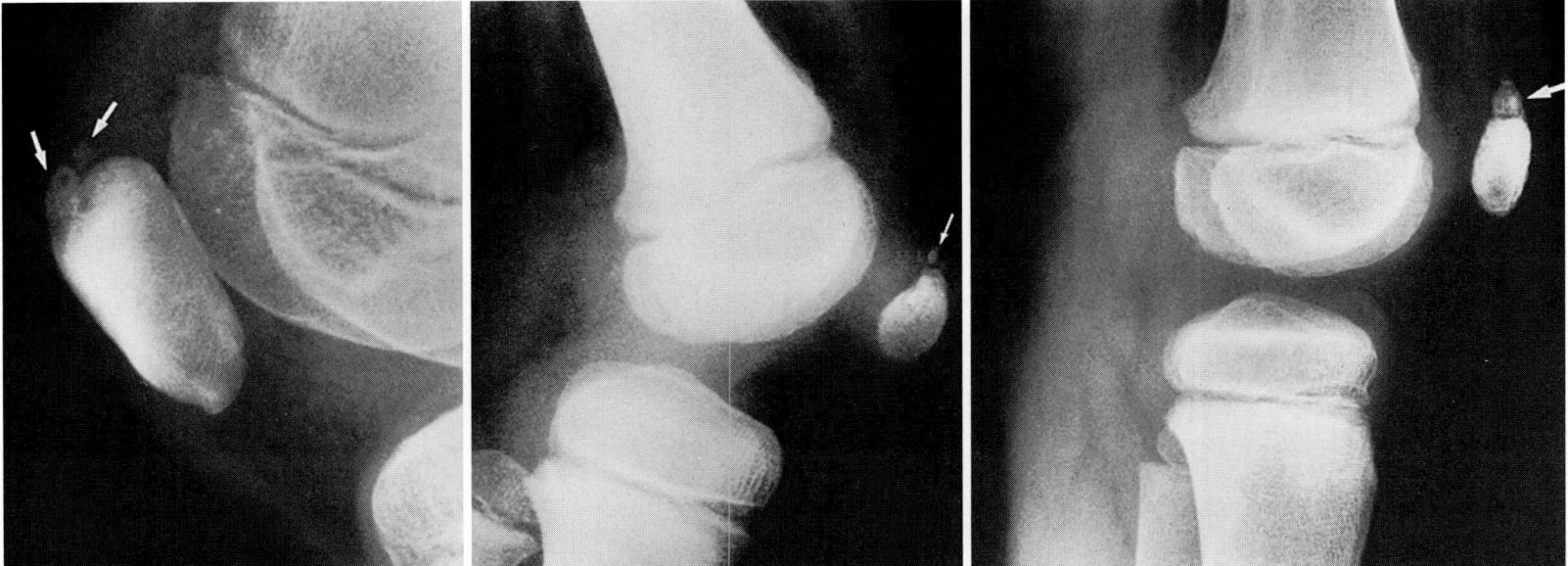

Figure 7–211. Three examples of accessory ossification centers at the superior pole of the patella.

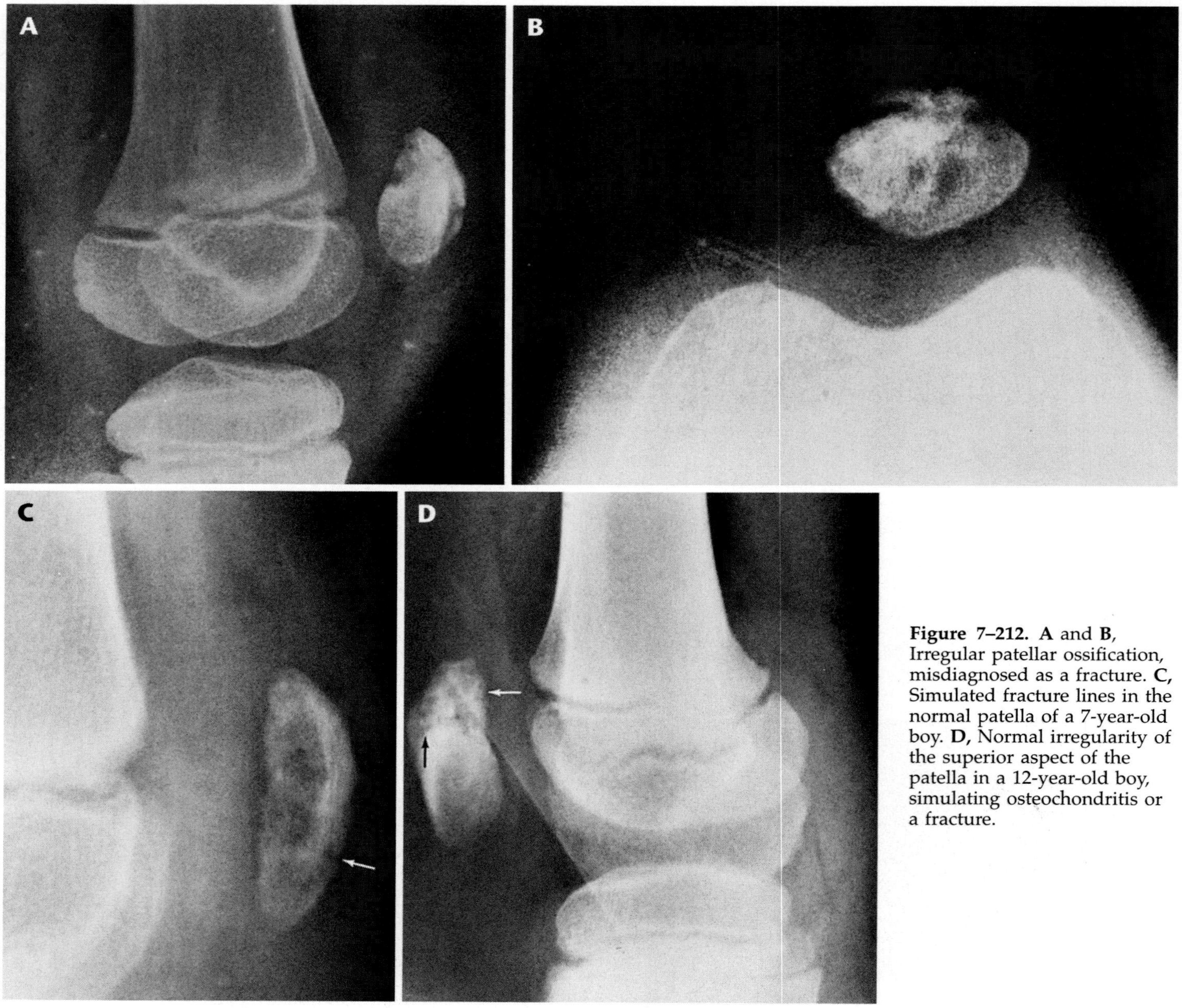

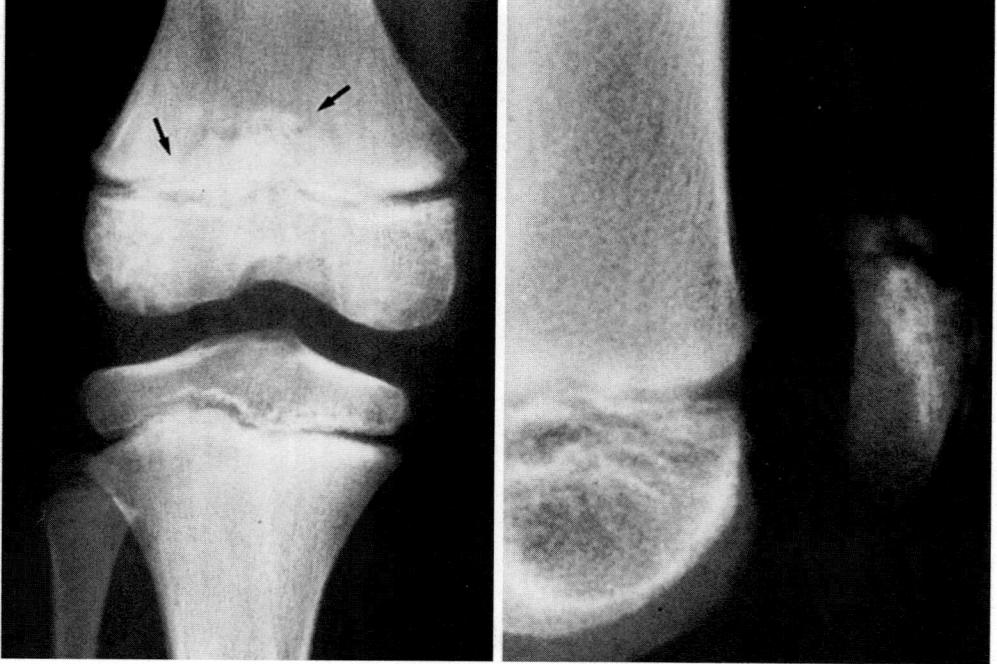

Figure 7–212. A and **B**, Irregular patellar ossification, misdiagnosed as a fracture. **C,** Simulated fracture lines in the normal patella of a 7-year-old boy. **D,** Normal irregularity of the superior aspect of the patella in a 12-year-old boy, simulating osteochondritis or a fracture.

Figure 7–213. Unusual patterns of ossification of the patella in a 6-year-old boy.

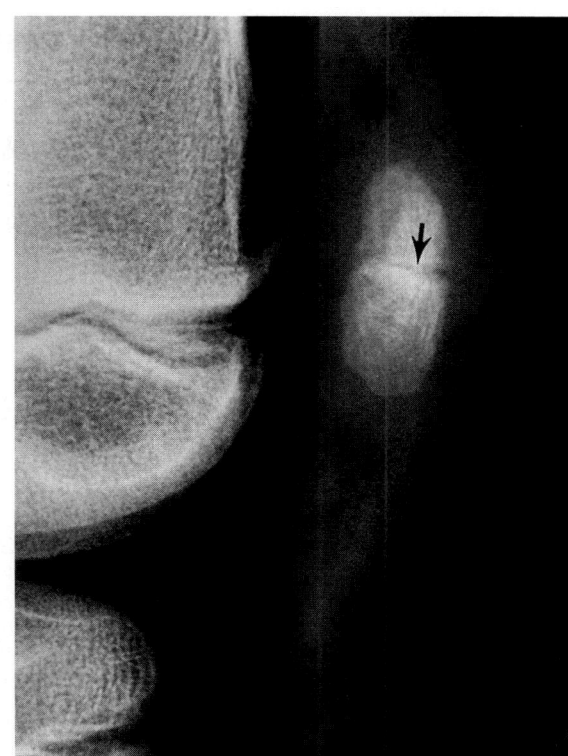

Figure 7–214. Variation in development of the patella in a 6-year-old, which might be mistaken for fracture.

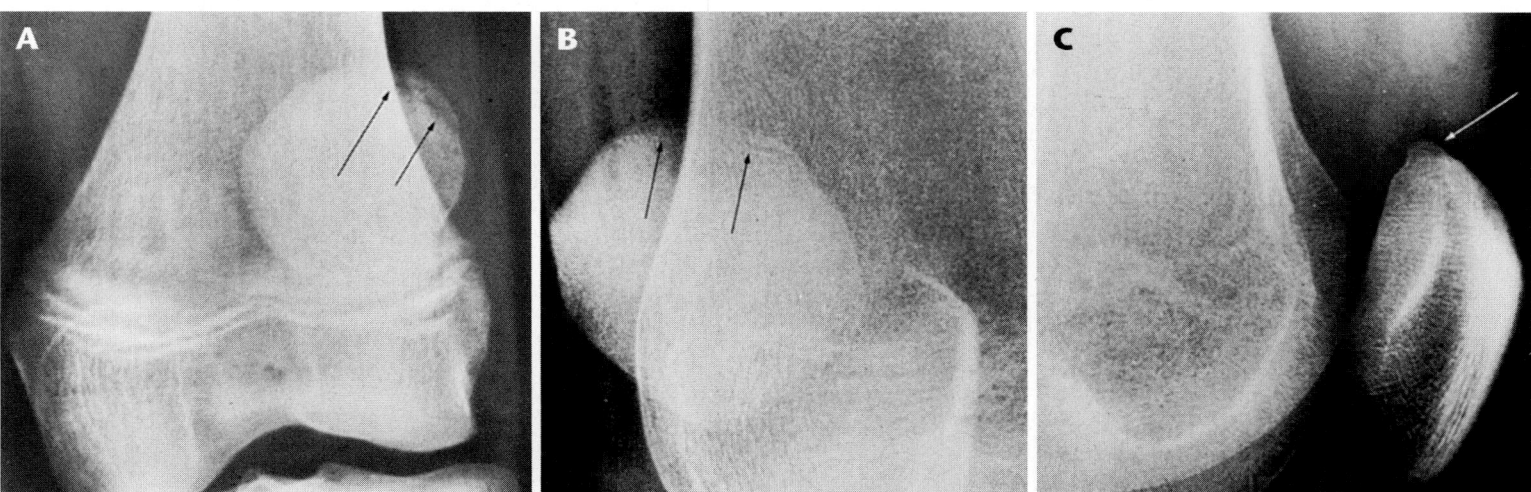

Figure 7–215. Apparent fracture of the superior aspect of the patella in a 14-year-old boy as a result of a secondary ossification center at the superior pole. (Ref: Ogden JA: Radiology of postnatal skeletal development. X. Patella and tibial tuberosity. *Skeletal Radiol* 11:246, 1984.)

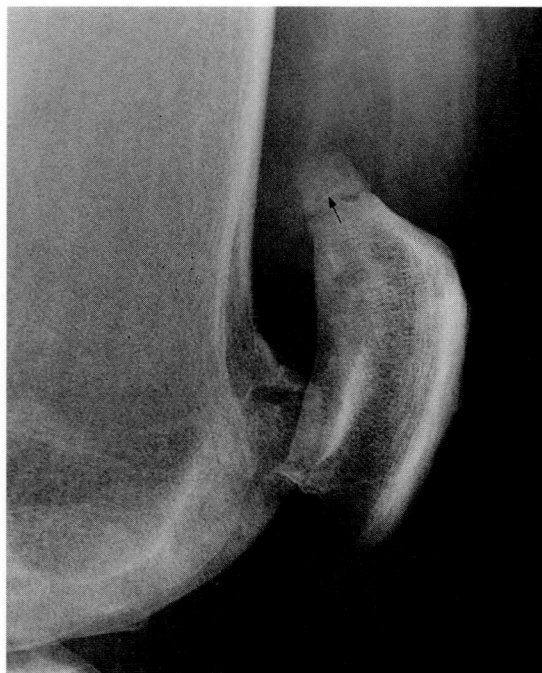

Figure 7–216. Unfused accessory ossification center at the upper pole of the patella in an 80-year-old man.

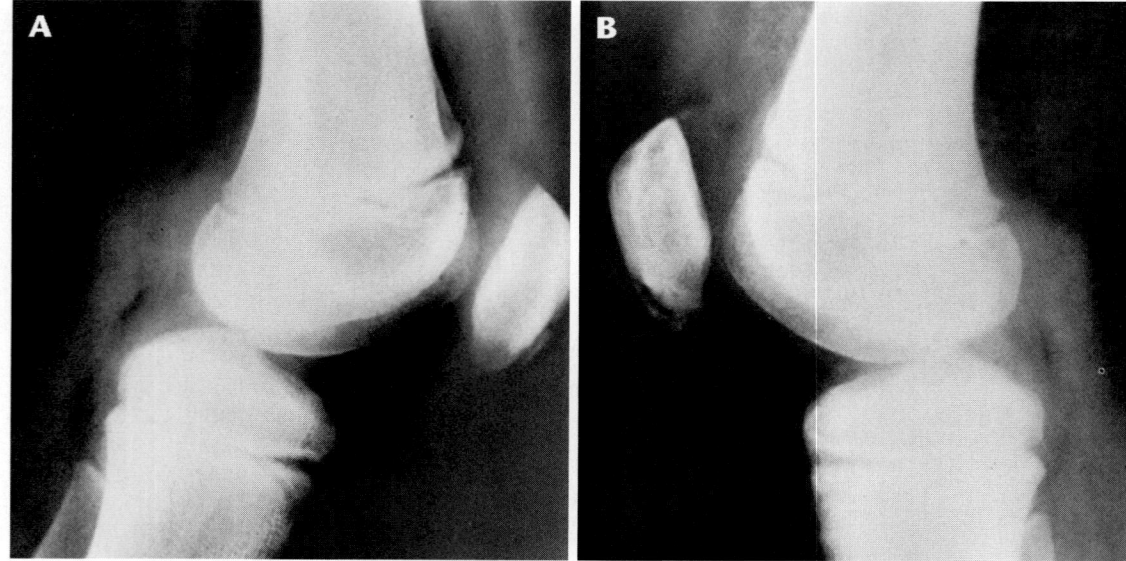

Figure 7–217. A, B, Normal asymmetric development of accessory ossification centers in a 9-year-old. Note apparent fragmentation of the lower pole of the patella in **B.**

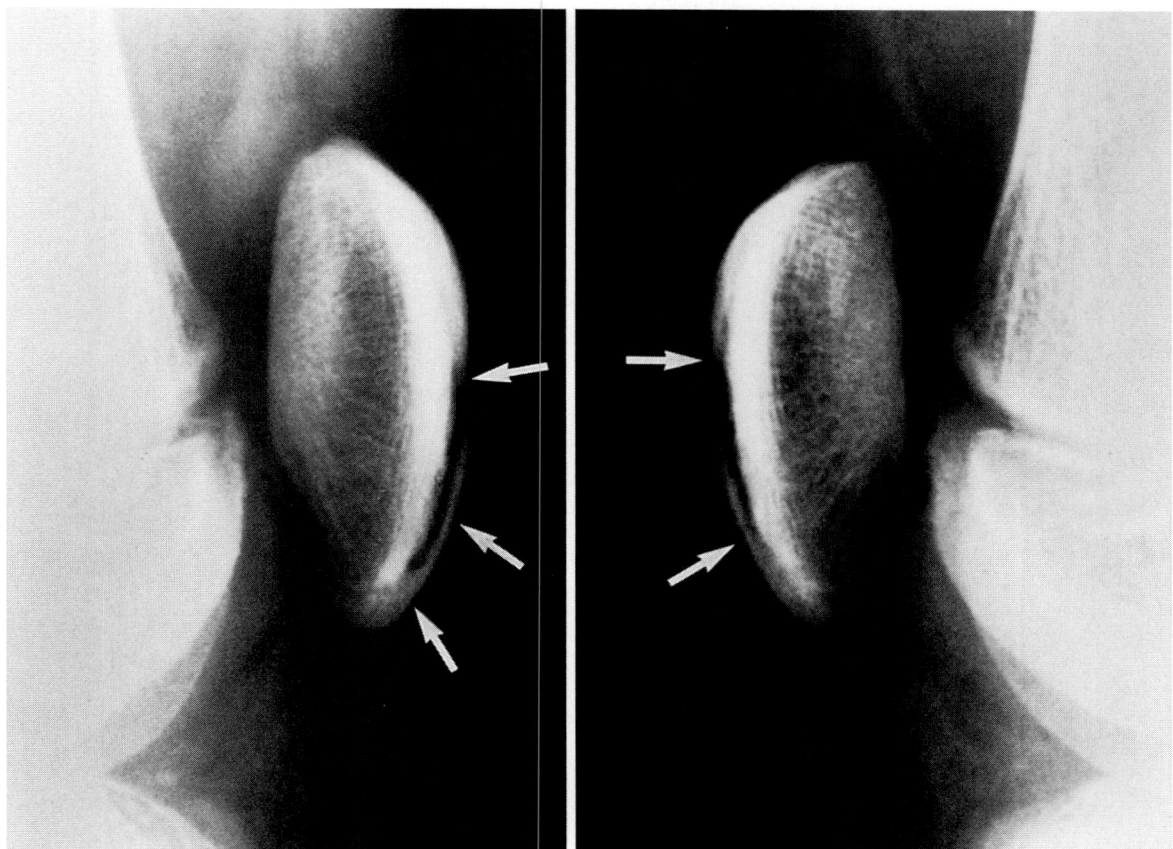

Figure 7–218. Long secondary apophysis of the anterior and inferior aspects of the patella in an 11-year-old boy.

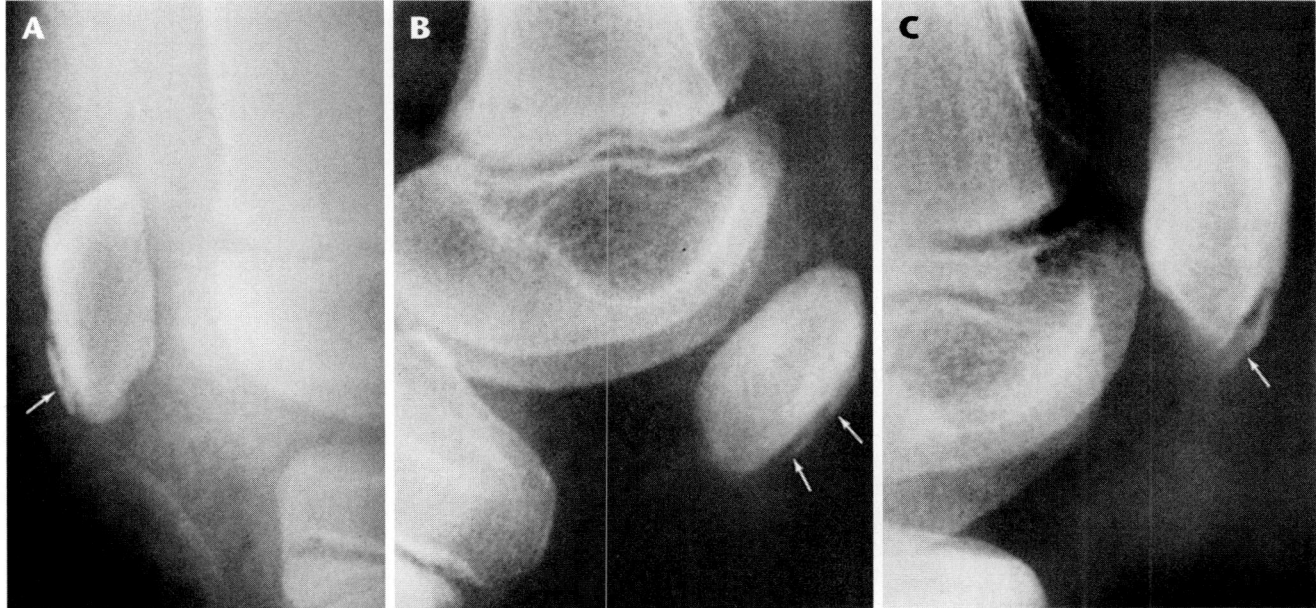

Figure 7–219. Three examples of accessory ossification centers simulating fractures. **A,** 7-year-old boy. **B,** 8-year-old boy. **C,** 12-year-old boy.

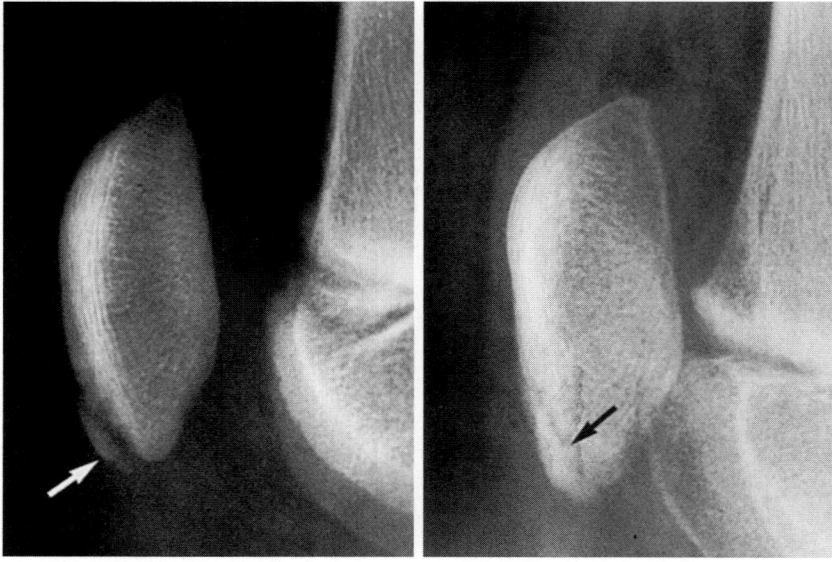

Figure 7–220. *Left,* Accessory ossification center in an 8-year-old boy diagnosed as a fracture. *Right,* Film made 1 month later with no treatment shows progressive closure of the secondary center.

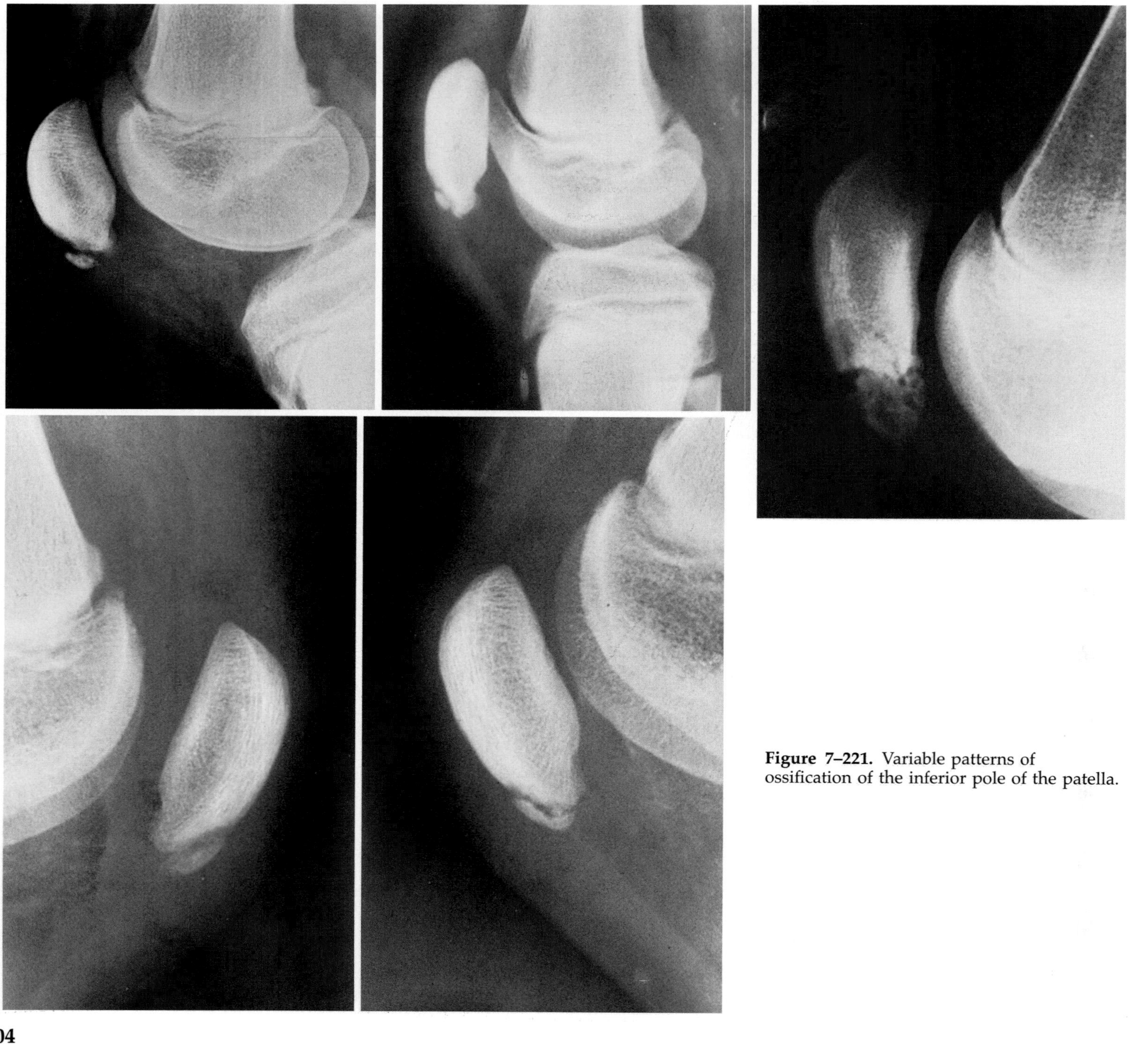

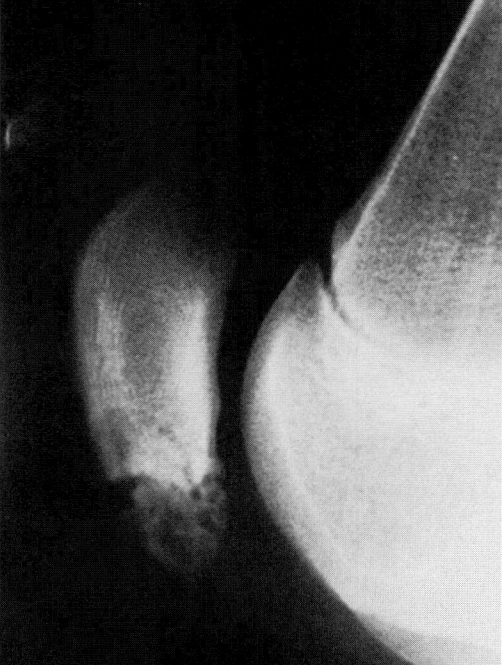

Figure 7–221. Variable patterns of ossification of the inferior pole of the patella.

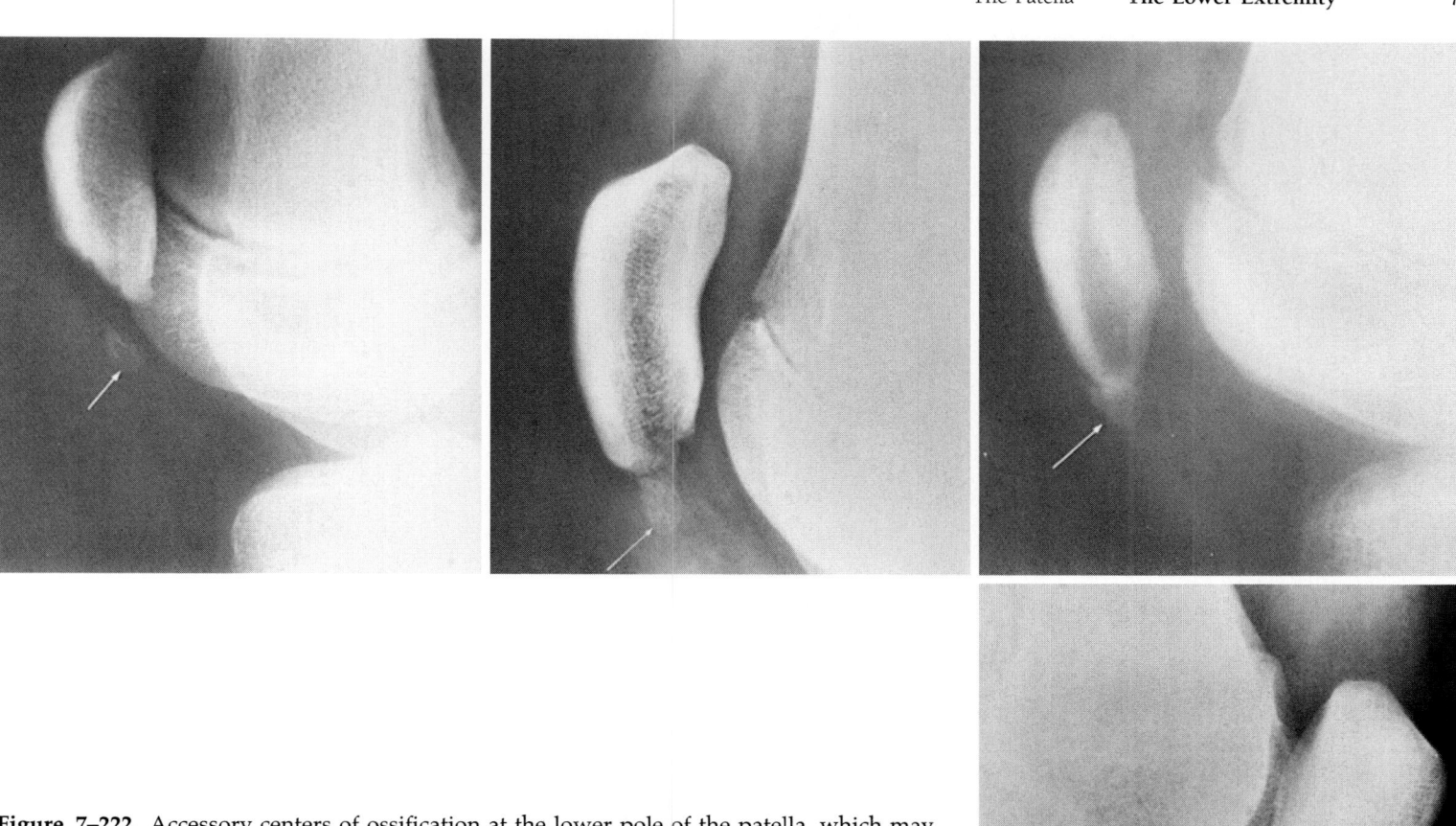

Figure 7–222. Accessory centers of ossification at the lower pole of the patella, which may be mistaken for a fracture.

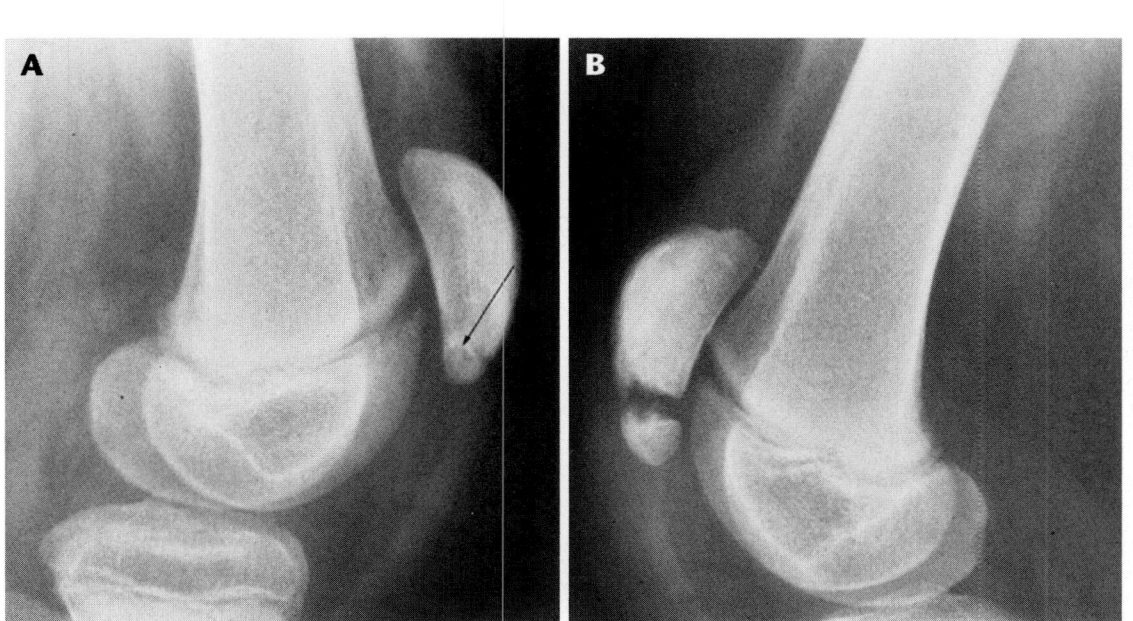

Figure 7–223. A, The closing accessory center at the inferior pole of the patella was suspected of being a fracture, and a comparison view was made of the opposite knee (**B**), showing an even more misleading appearance.

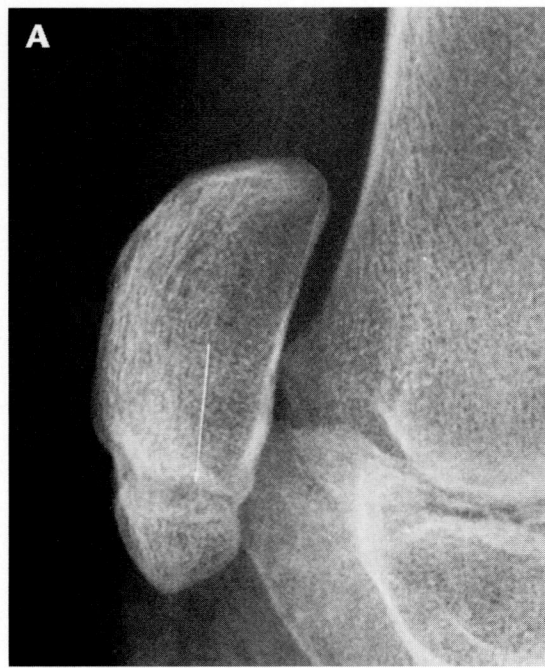
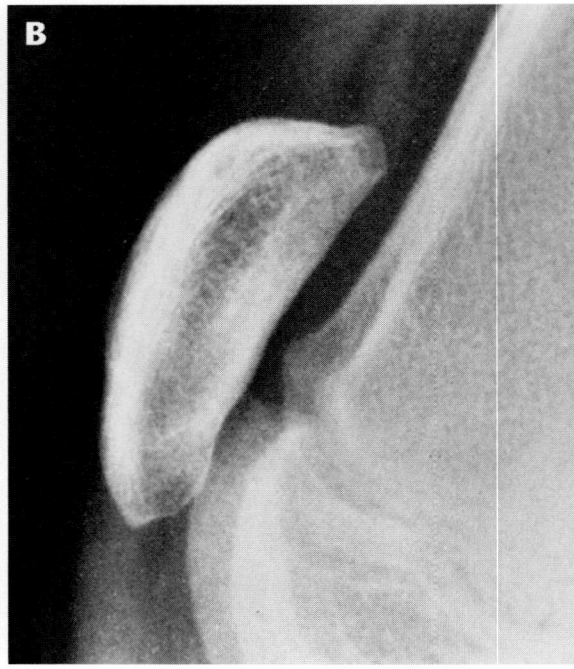

Figure 7–224. A, Fusing accessory centers of ossification at the inferior pole of the patella. **B,** After fusion is complete. Patellae with large accessory centers of this type often tend to attain the elongated configuration illustrated in **B.** They may be associated with patella alta.

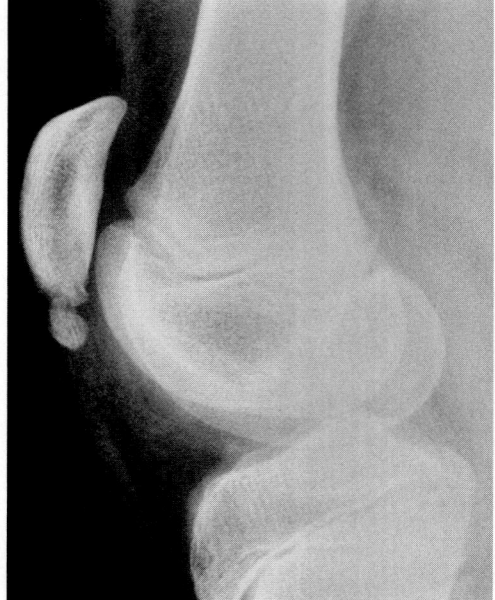
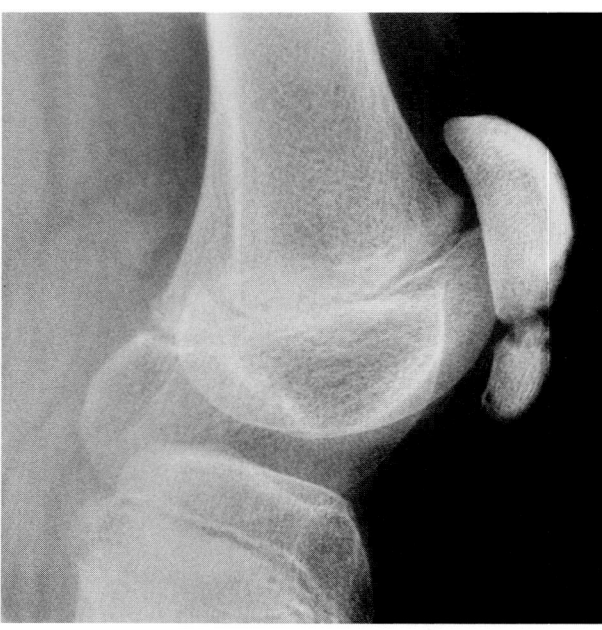

Figure 7–225. Variation in development of the patella in an 11-year-old child with cerebral palsy, possibly the result of traction by the quadriceps muscle and the patellar tendon. These centers often close, leaving an elongated patella.

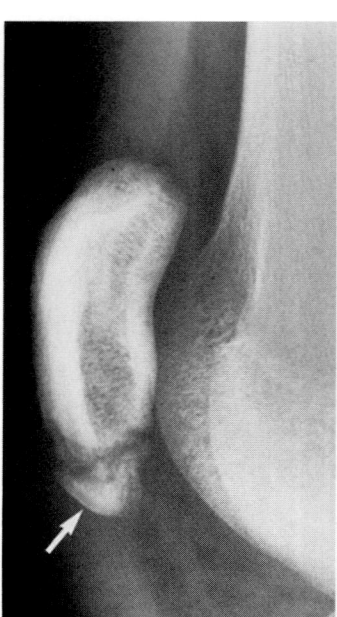
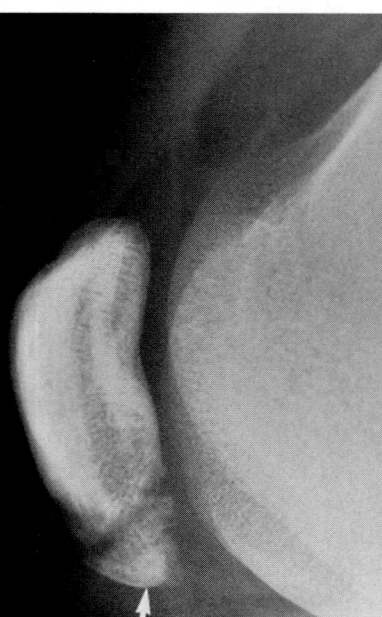
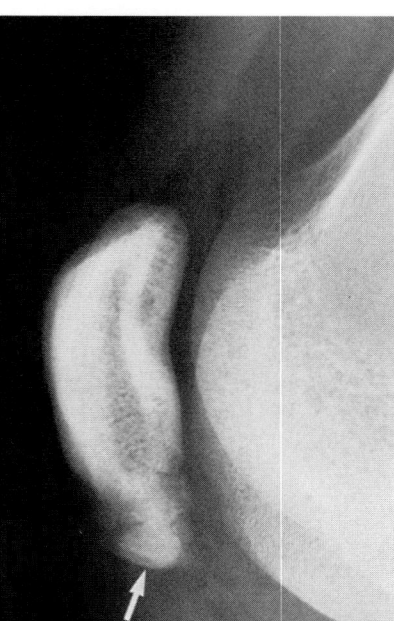

Figure 7–226. Unfused accessory ossification center at the inferior pole of the patella in a 19-year-old man, showing its closure over a 3-month period.

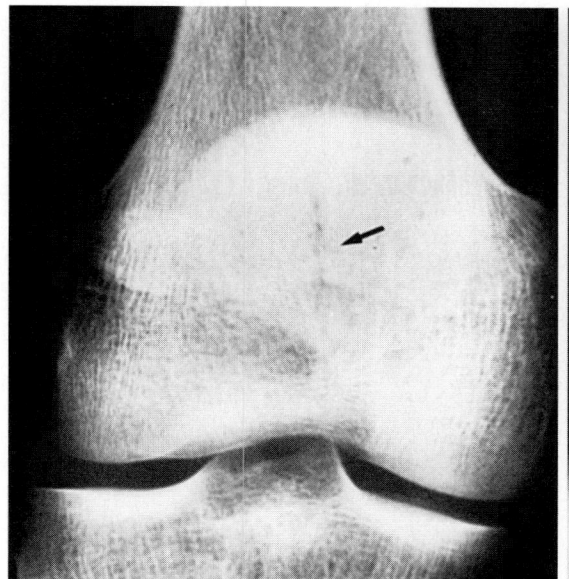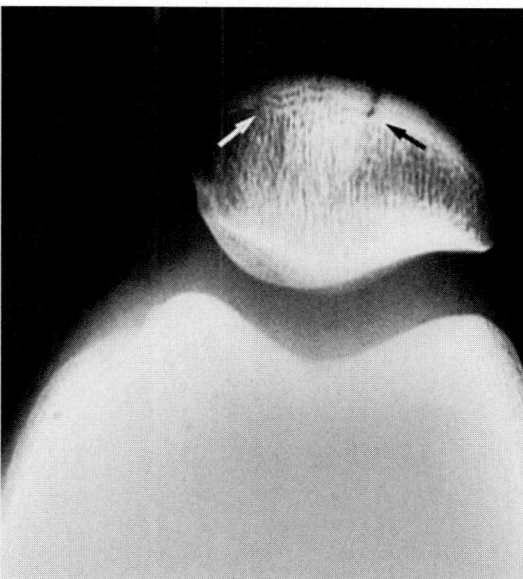

Figure 7–227. Developmental clefts in the patella of a 17-year-old boy.

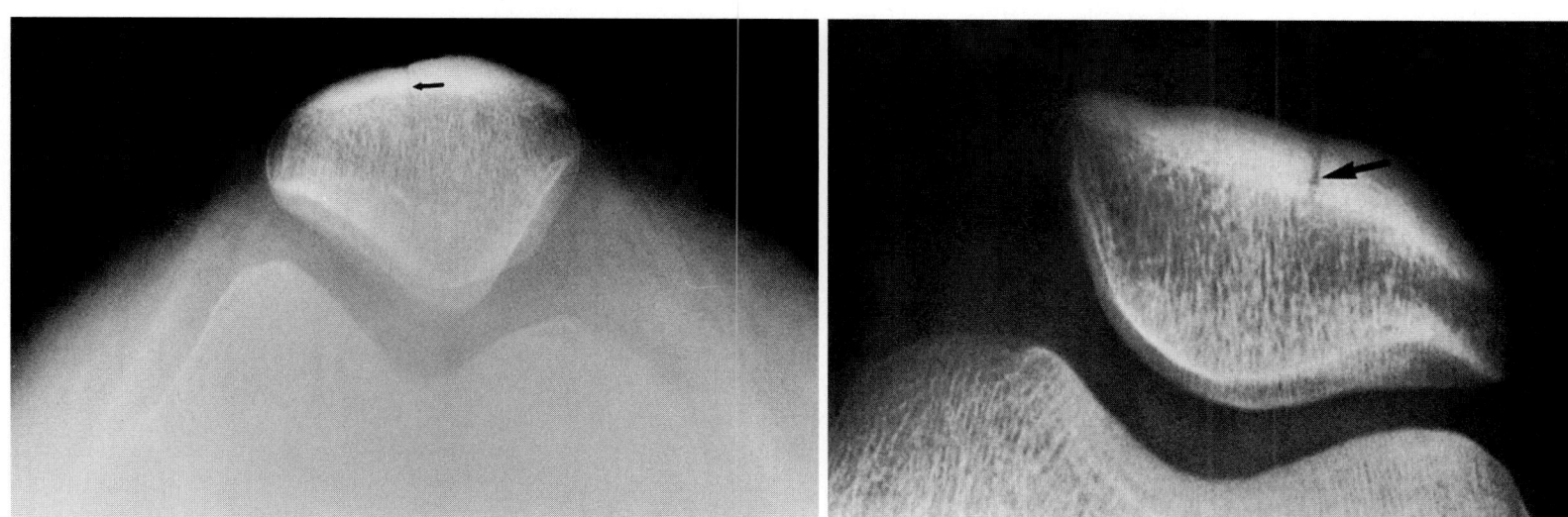

Figure 7–228. Patellar clefts.

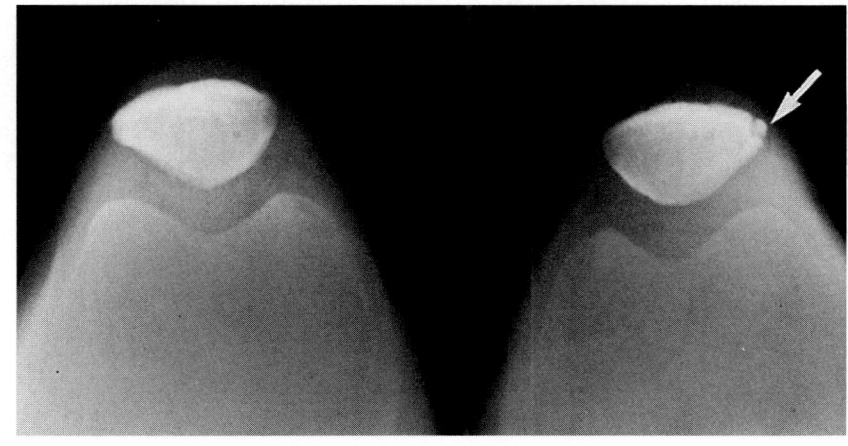

Figure 7–229. Accessory patellar ossification center, seen in tangential projection in a 2-year-old boy.

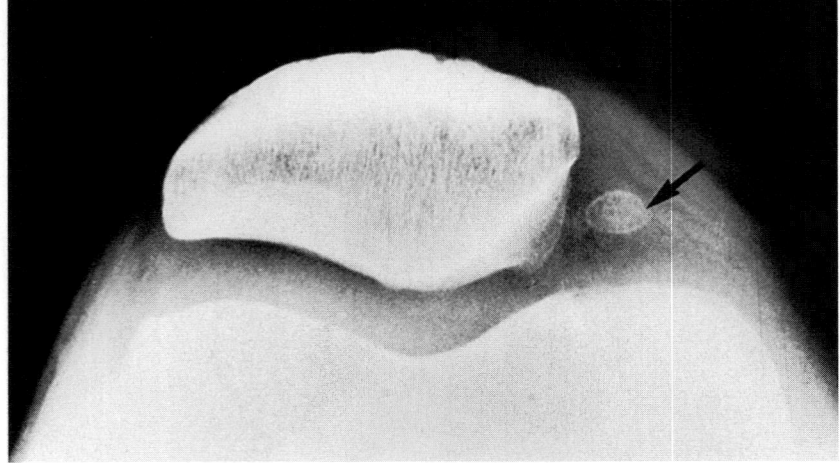

Figure 7–230. Accessory ossicle at the medial aspect of the patella.

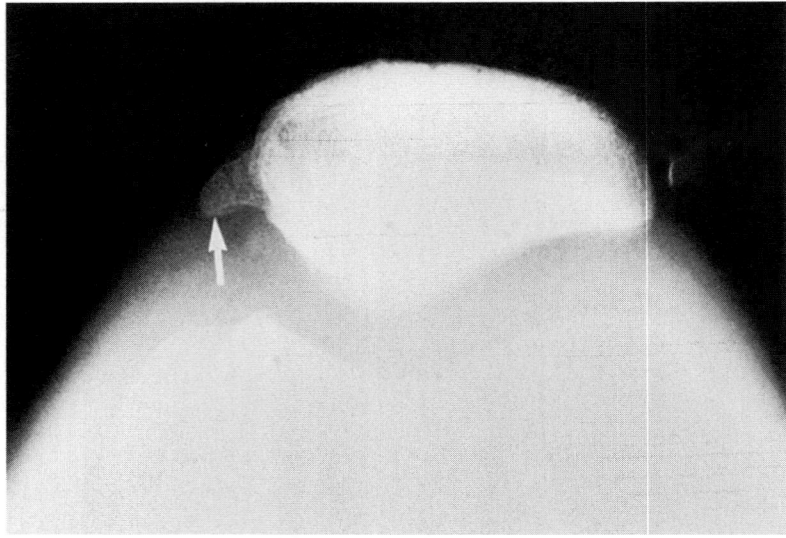

Figure 7–231. Unusual spurlike configuration of the medial aspect of the patella in a 20-year-old man.

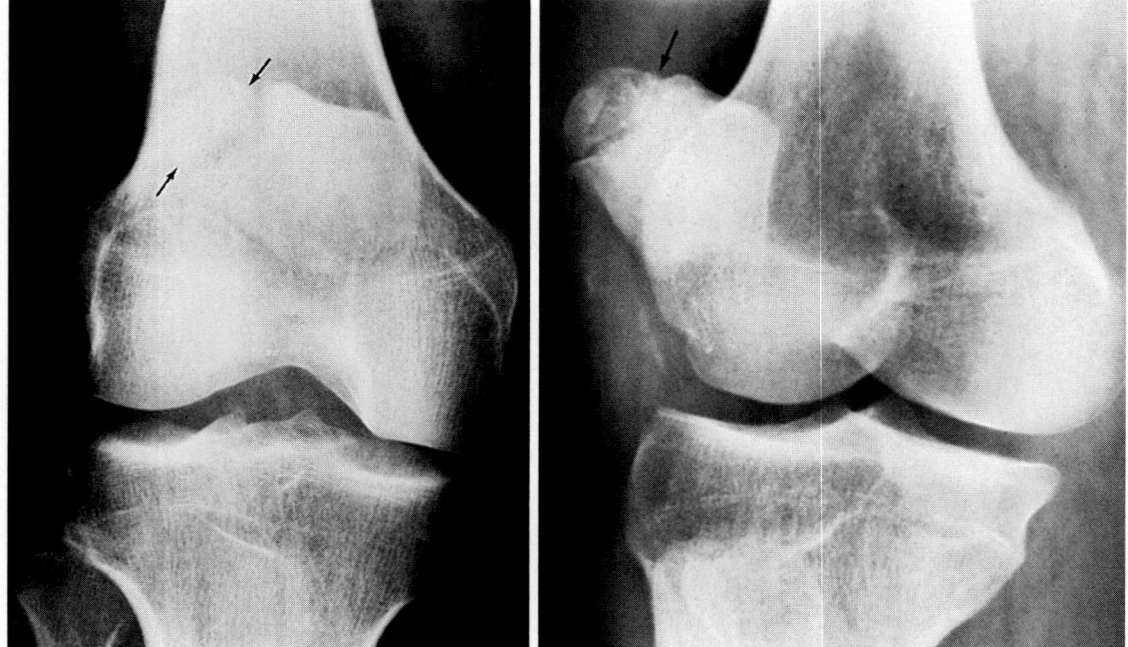

Figure 7–232. Bipartite patella, which may easily be mistaken for a fracture. Note the well-defined space between the major elements.

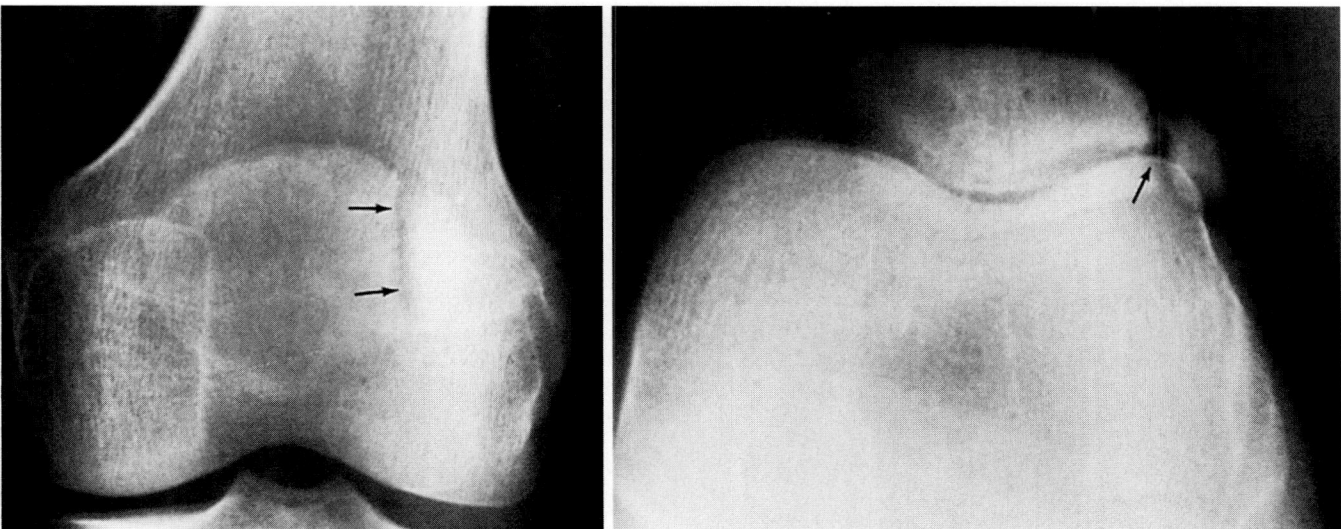

Figure 7–233. An additional example of a bipartite patella, which is well demonstrated in tangential projection. The rounded contour of the patellar elements seen in this projection is useful in the differentiation from fracture.

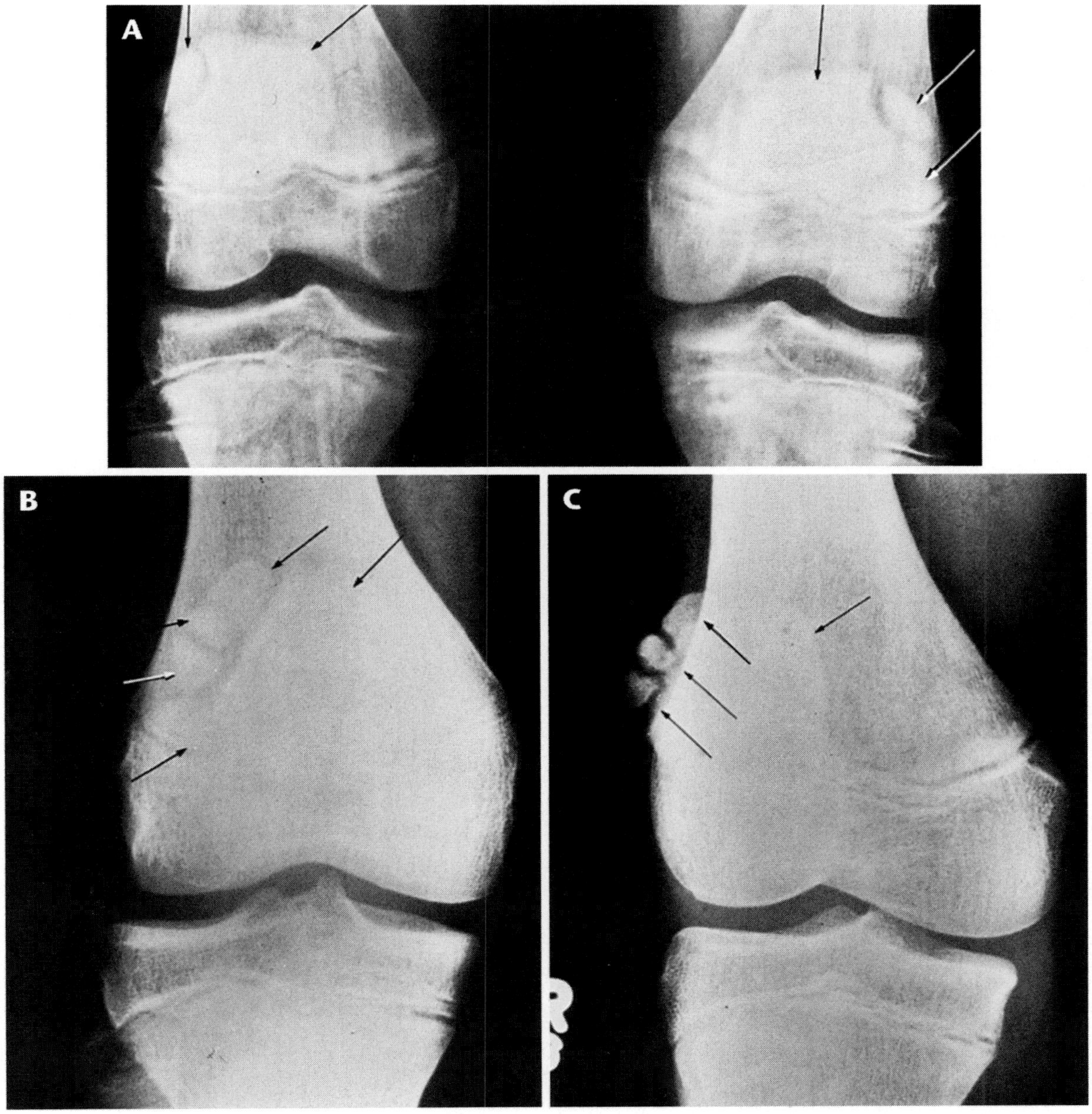

Figure 7–234. A, Segmented patellae with two pieces on patients right and three on the left. **B** and **C,** Segmented patella with four pieces.

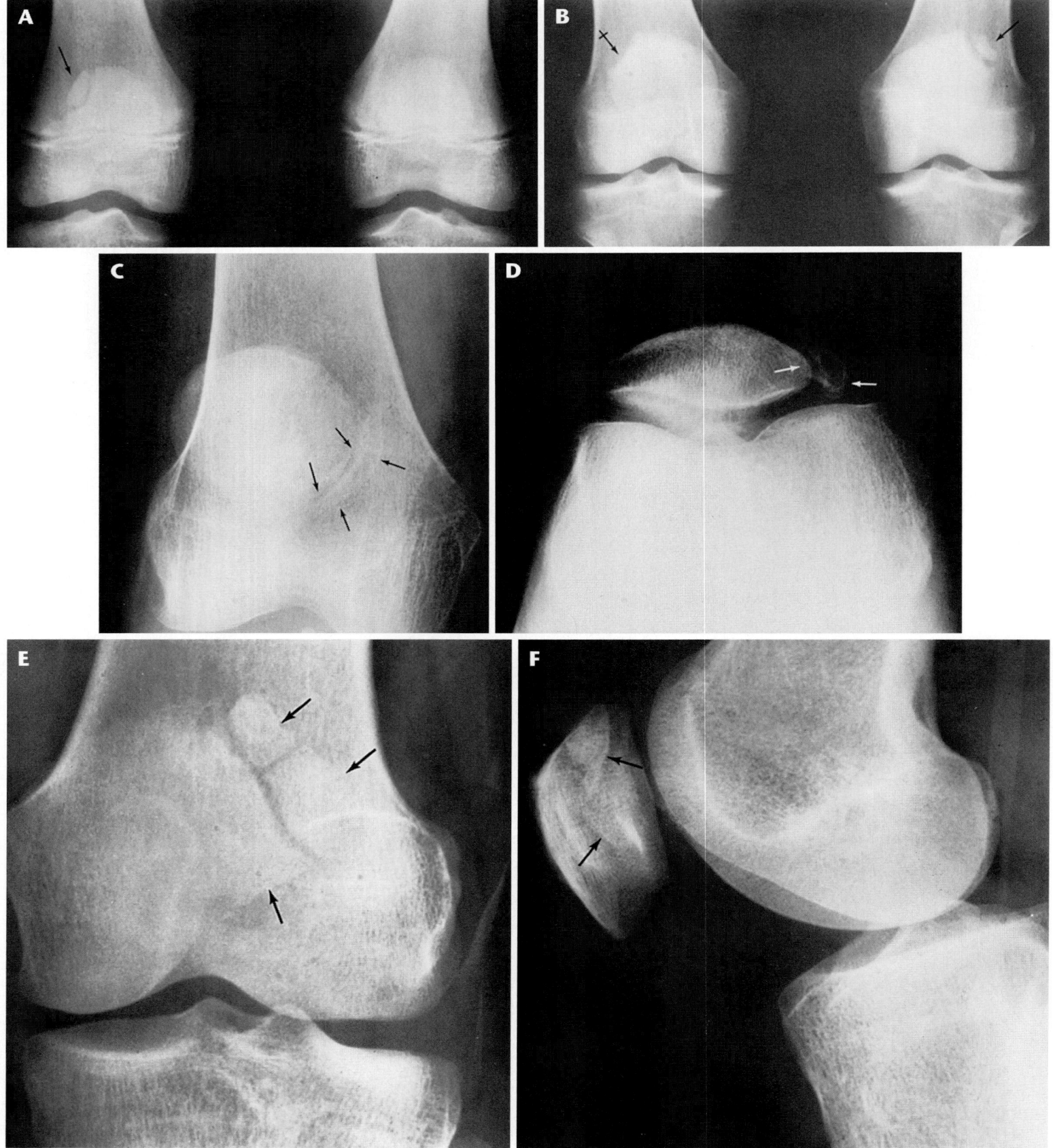

Figure 7–235. A, Unilateral bipartite patella. Note that the smaller elements in bipartite patellae often do not accurately correspond in size with the adjacent fossa. **B,** Unilateral bipartite patella (→) but with corresponding fossa on opposite side (↔). **C** and **D,** Bipartite patella on the medial side. The majority of bipartite patellae are located on the lateral side. **E, F,** Tripartite patella.

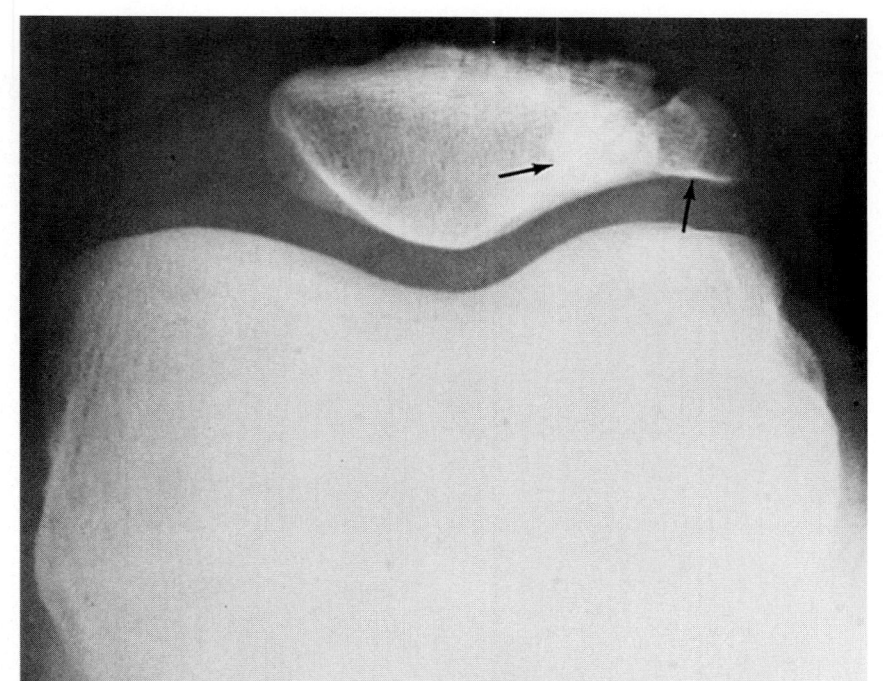

Figure 7–236. Tripartite patella. Note rounded contours in tangential projection.

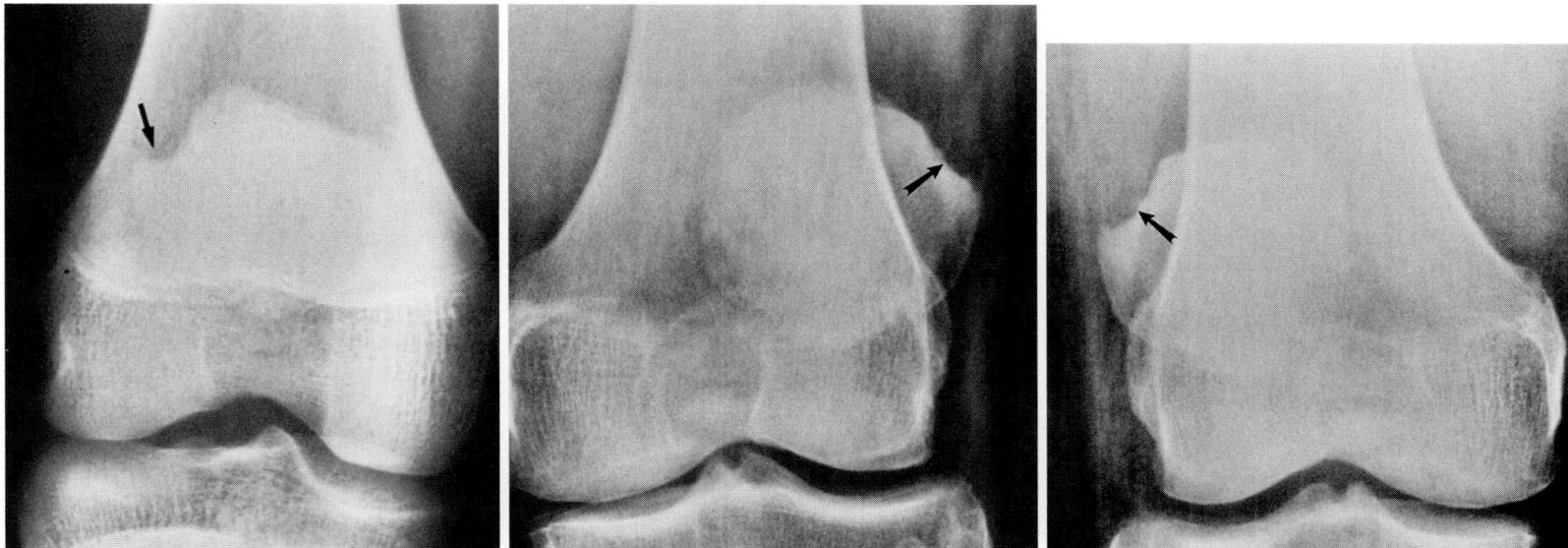

Figure 7–237. Three examples of forme fruste bipartite patella.

Figure 7–238. A, The smaller element of a bipartite patella is usually smaller than the fossa in the major portion. However, occasionally it is larger than the fossa (**B**).

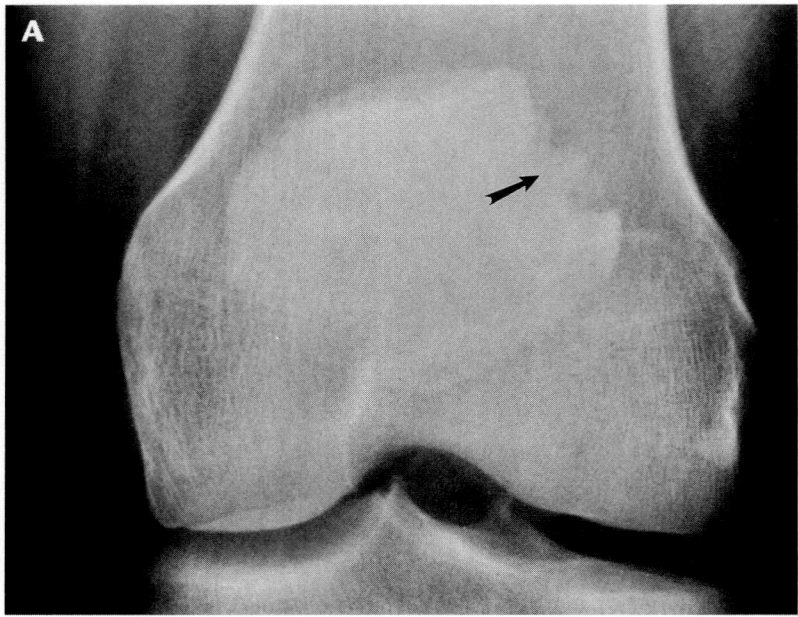 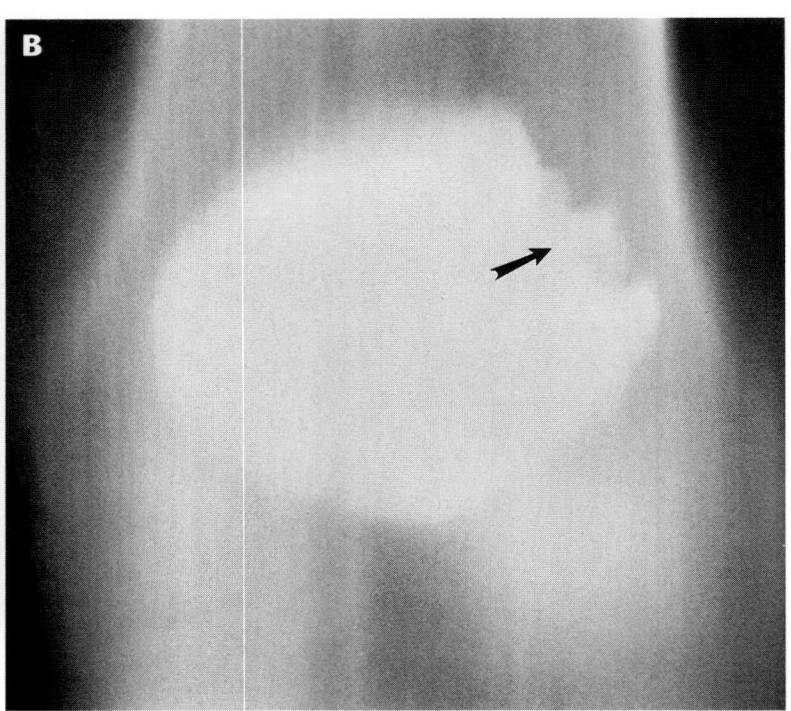

Figure 7–239. An unusual variety of partitioned patella. **A,** Plain film. **B,** Tomogram.

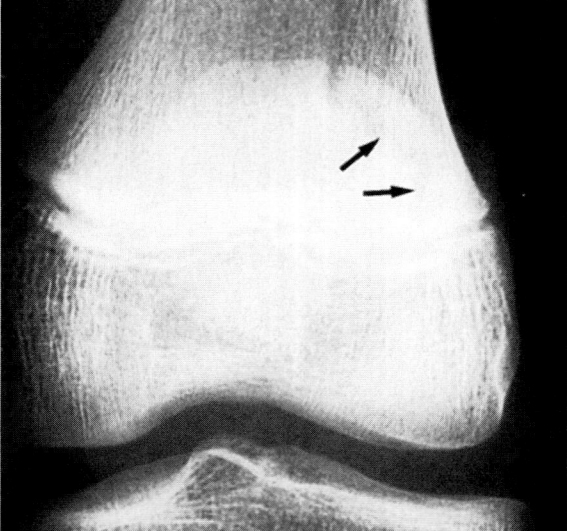 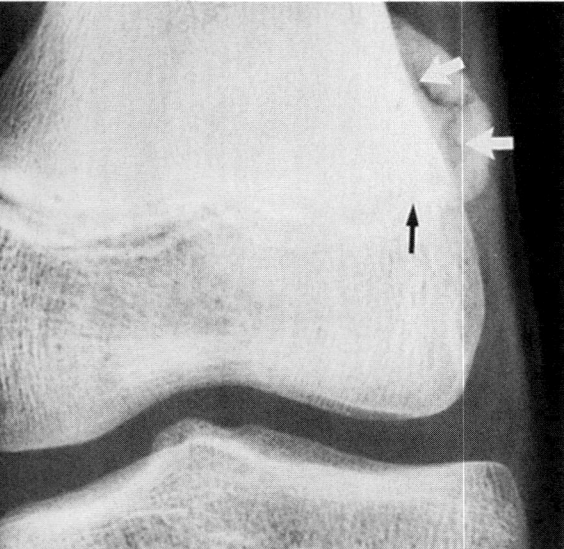

Figure 7–240. Segmented patella showing poor definition of septae in the oblique projection (*right*).

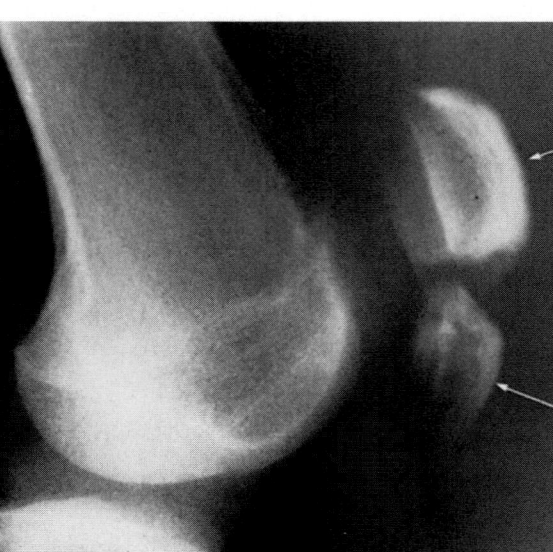 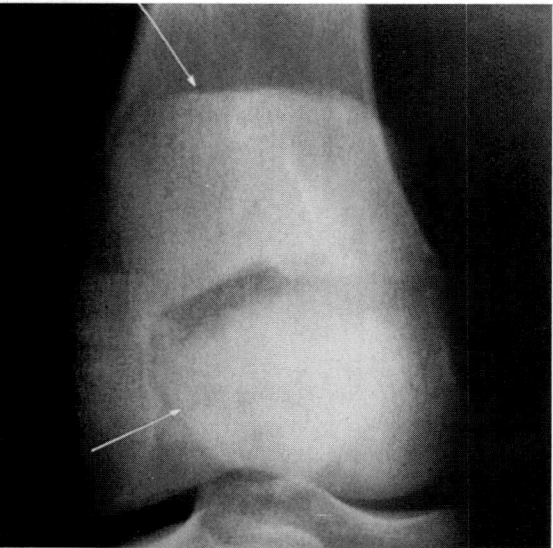

Figure 7–241. Horizontal bifid patella, a rare type of segmentation. (Ref: Weinberg S: Horizontal bifid patella. *Skeletal Radiol* 7:223, 1981.)

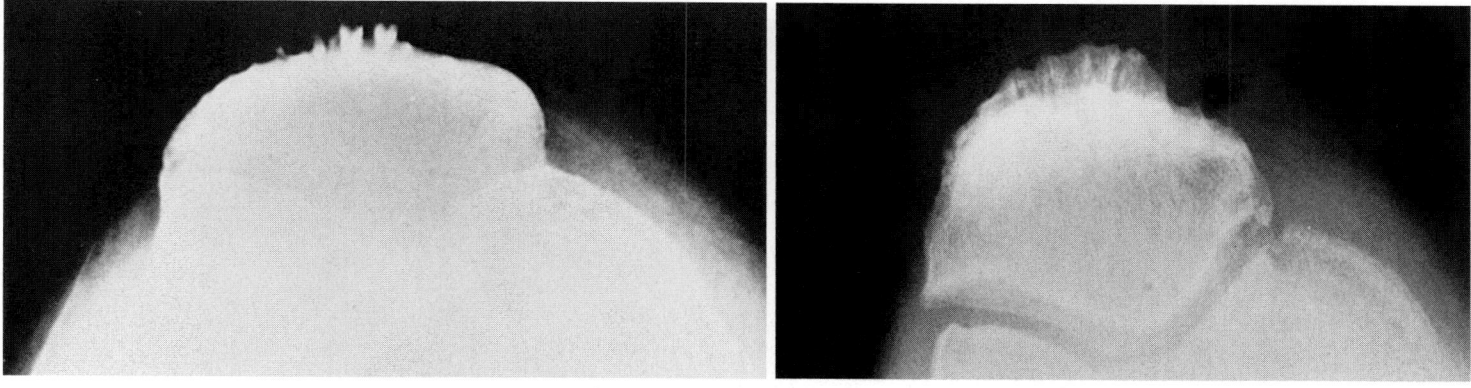

Figure 7–242. Patellar "teeth" caused by spurring of the tendon interdigitations. (Ref: Greenspan A et al: "Tooth" sign in patellar degenerative disease. *J Bone Joint Surg* 59A:483, 1977.)

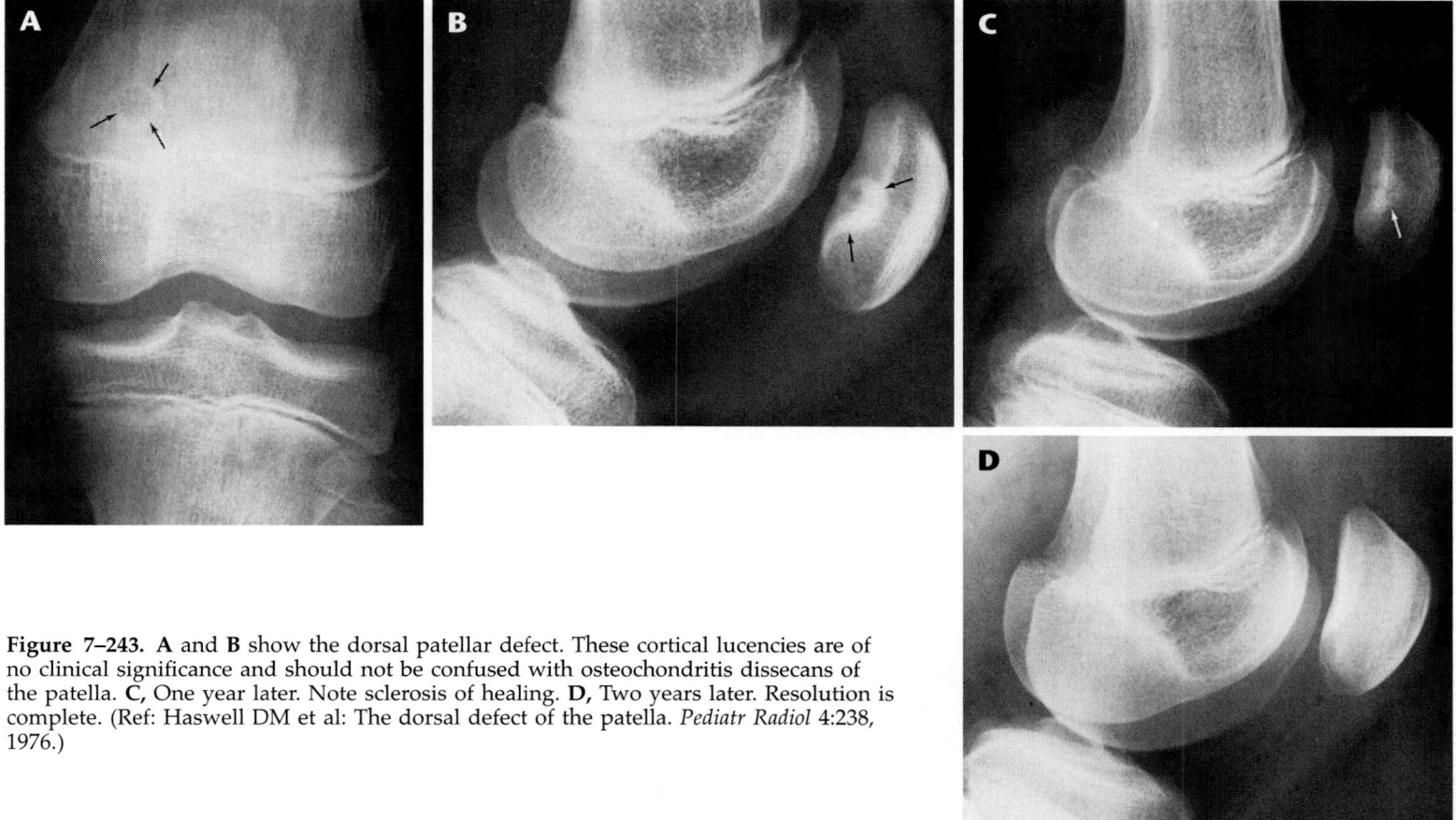

Figure 7–243. A and **B** show the dorsal patellar defect. These cortical lucencies are of no clinical significance and should not be confused with osteochondritis dissecans of the patella. **C,** One year later. Note sclerosis of healing. **D,** Two years later. Resolution is complete. (Ref: Haswell DM et al: The dorsal defect of the patella. *Pediatr Radiol* 4:238, 1976.)

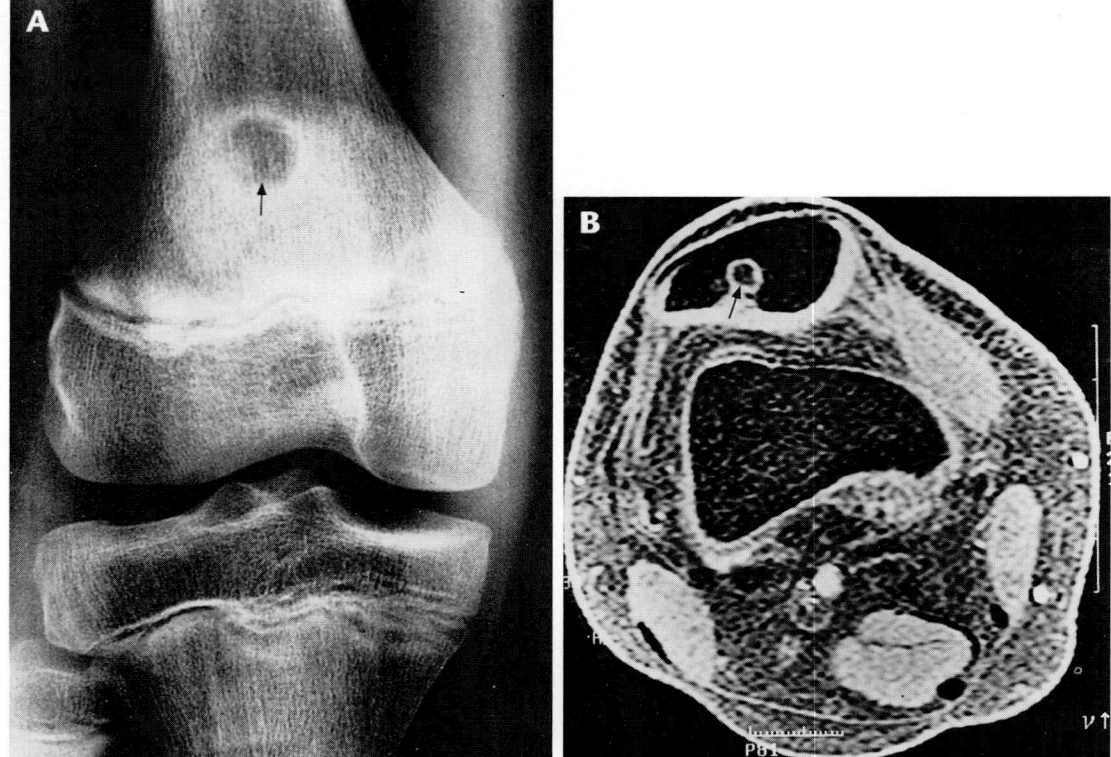

Figure 7–244. The dorsal patellar defect by plain film and MRI. **A,** Plain film. **B,** MRI gradient echo T2*-weighted image.

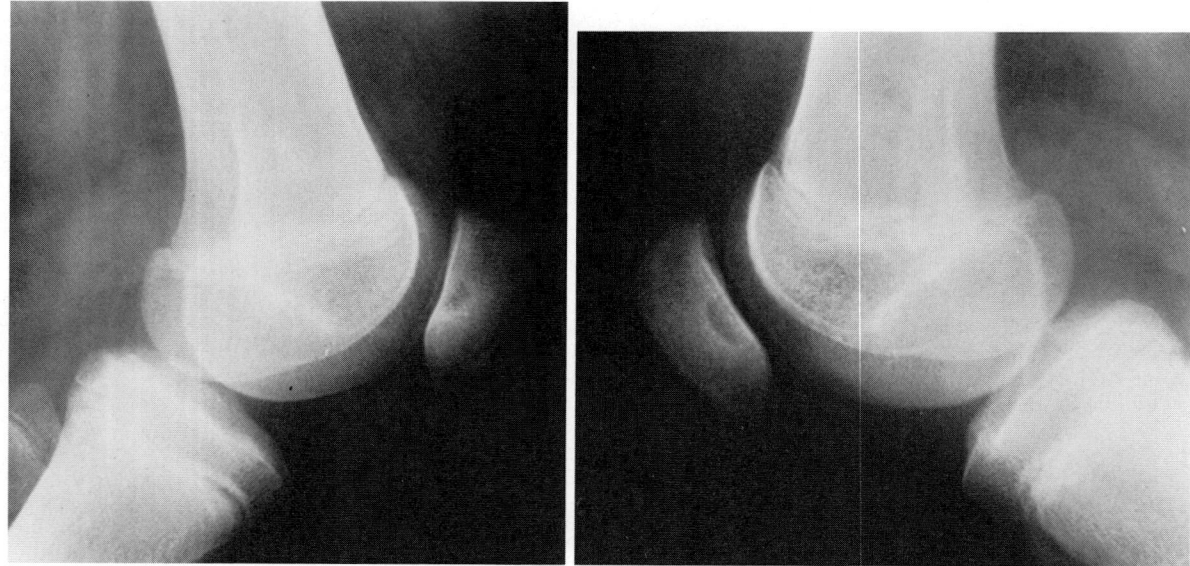

Figure 7–245. Bilateral dorsal patellar defects in a 13-year-old girl.

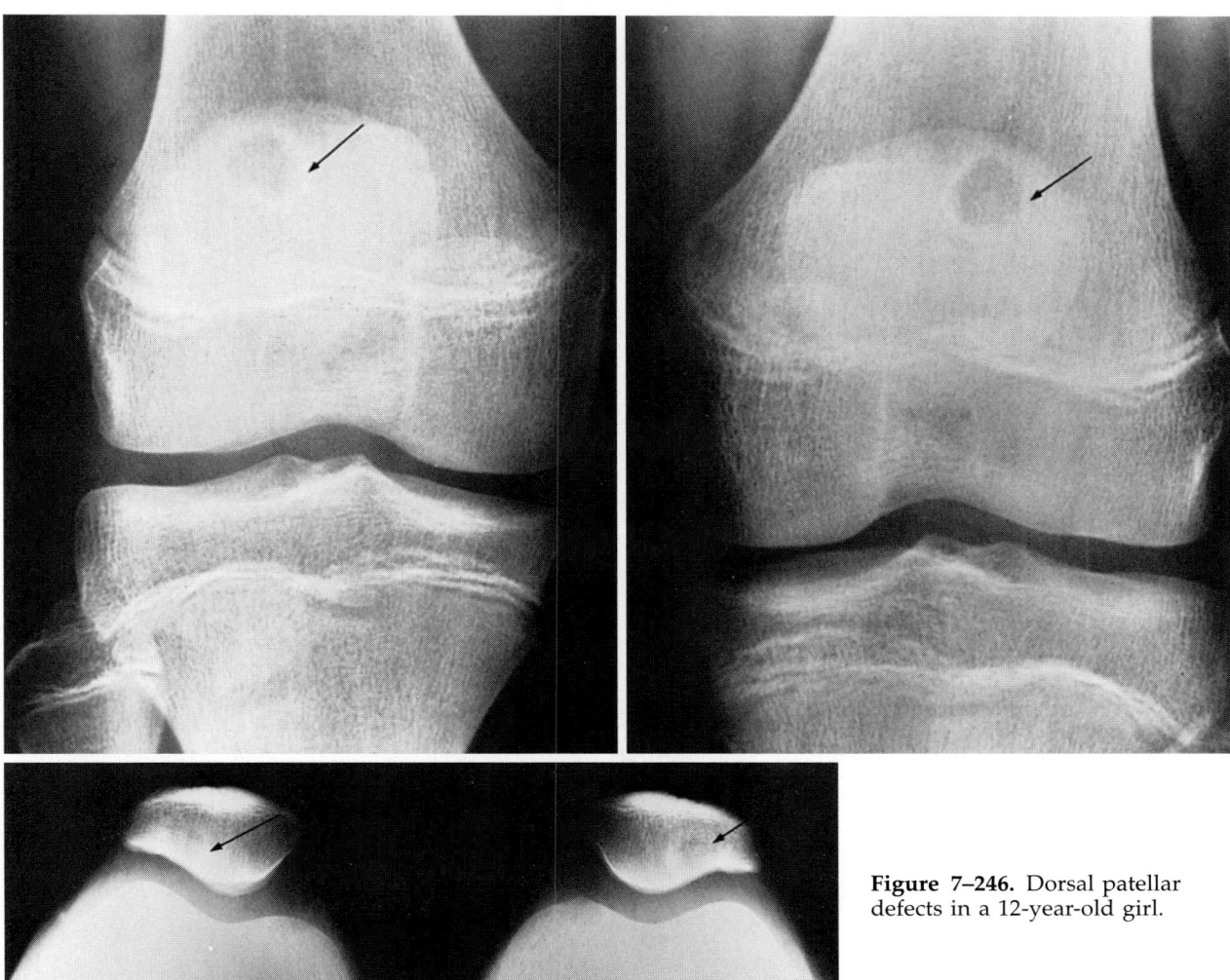

Figure 7–246. Dorsal patellar defects in a 12-year-old girl.

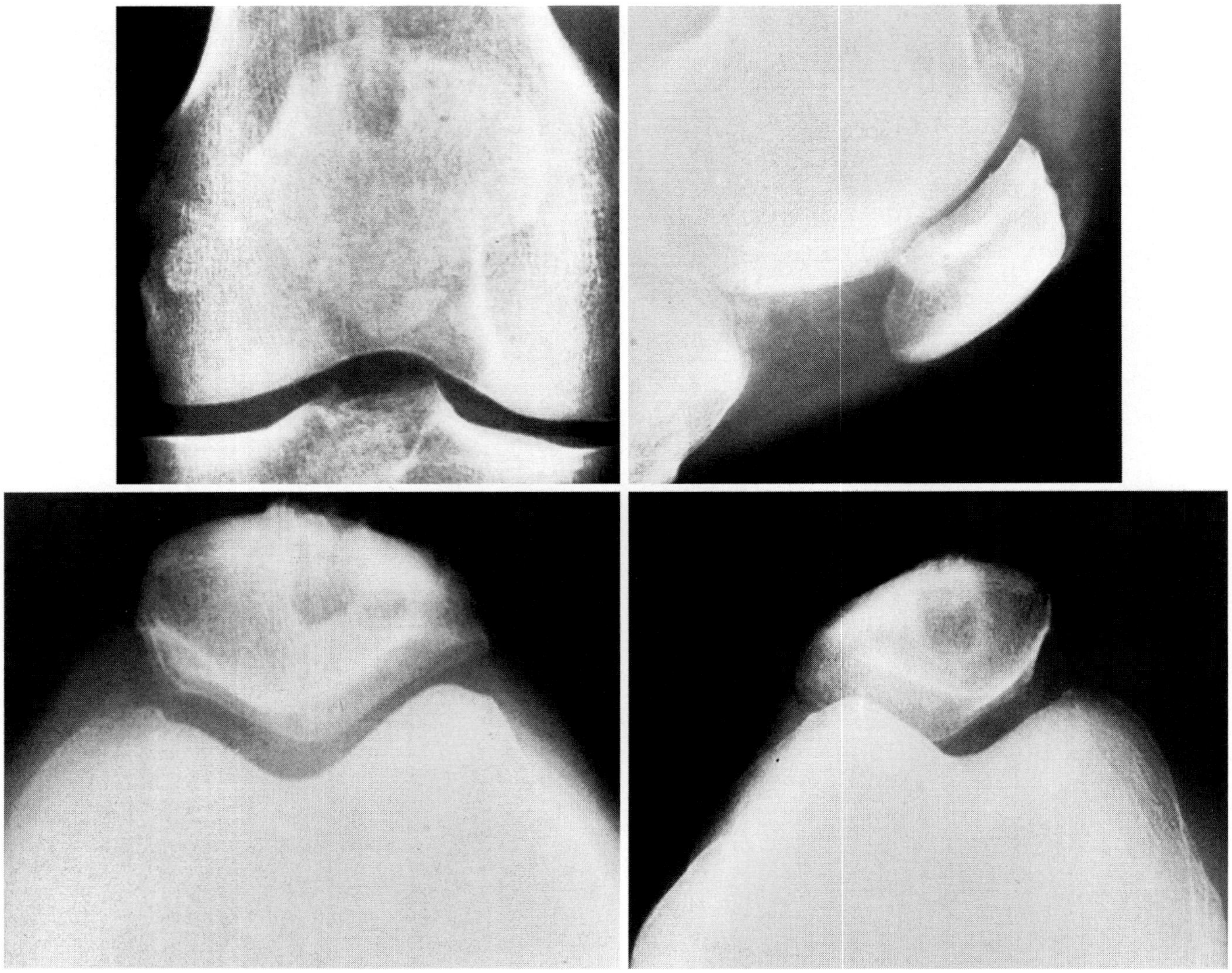

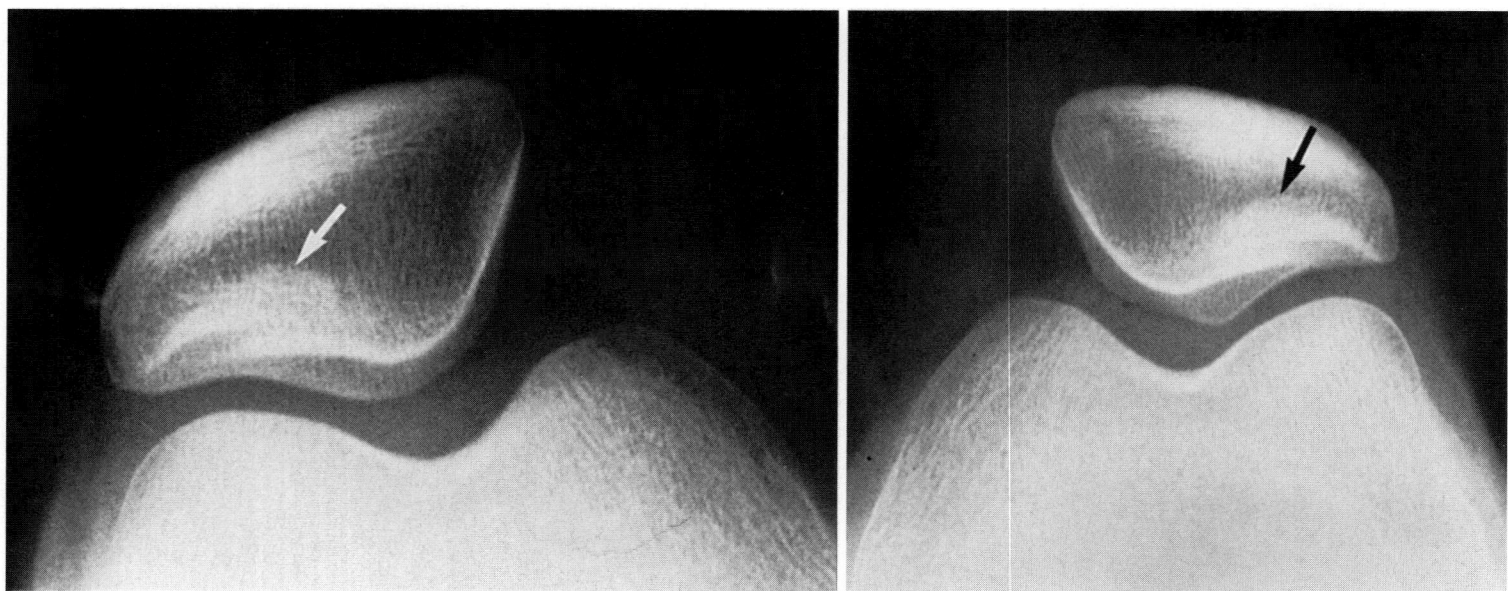

Figure 7–247. Dorsal defects in an elderly male. These defects are seen more commonly in young people but occasionally persist into later life. *Top left,* Frontal view. *Top right,* Lateral view. *Bottom,* Tangential views.

Figure 7–248. Bilateral areas of increased sclerosis in the posterior surfaces of the patellae in a 20-year-old woman.

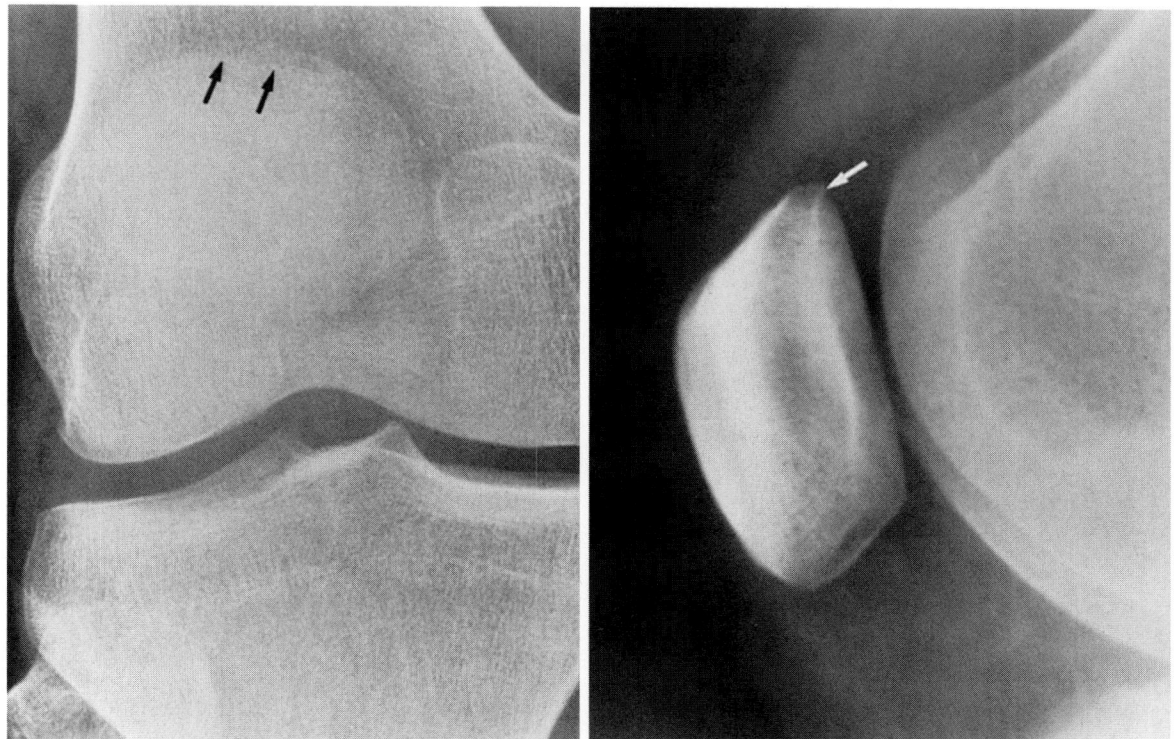

Figure 7–249. Simulated fracture of the upper pole of the patella, produced by a small flangelike projection, best seen in lateral projection.

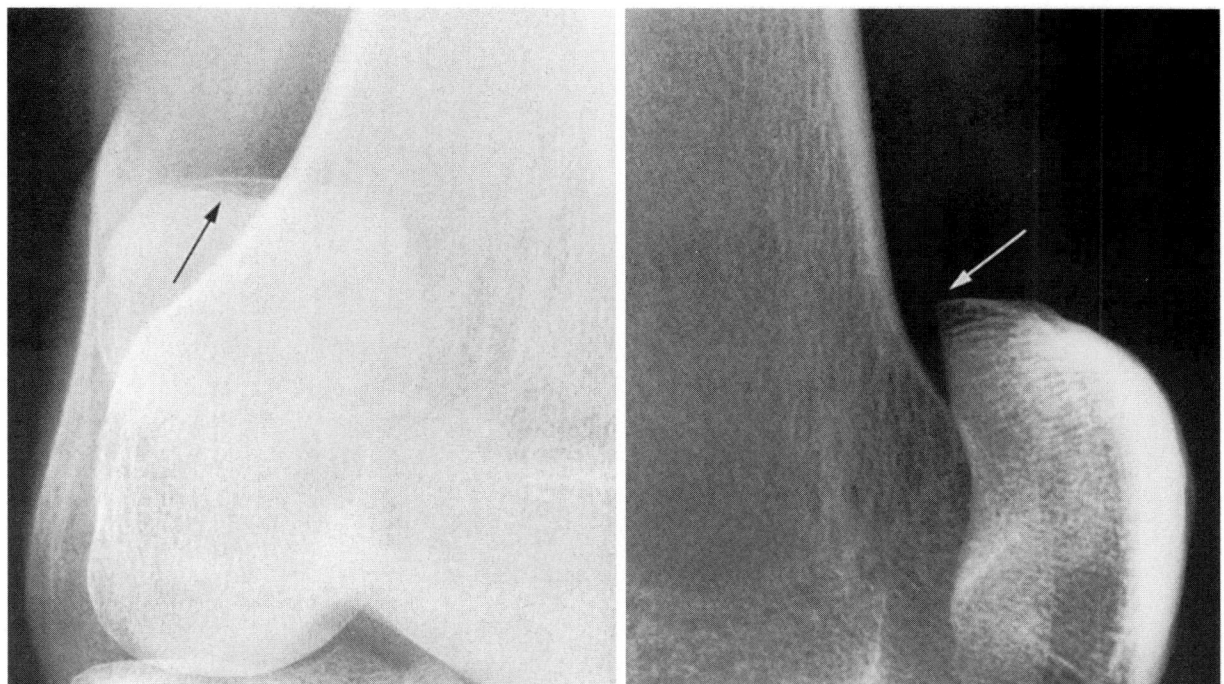

Figure 7–250. The lucency of the upper pole of the patella seen in Figure 7–249 is nicely demonstrated in this 33-year-old man.

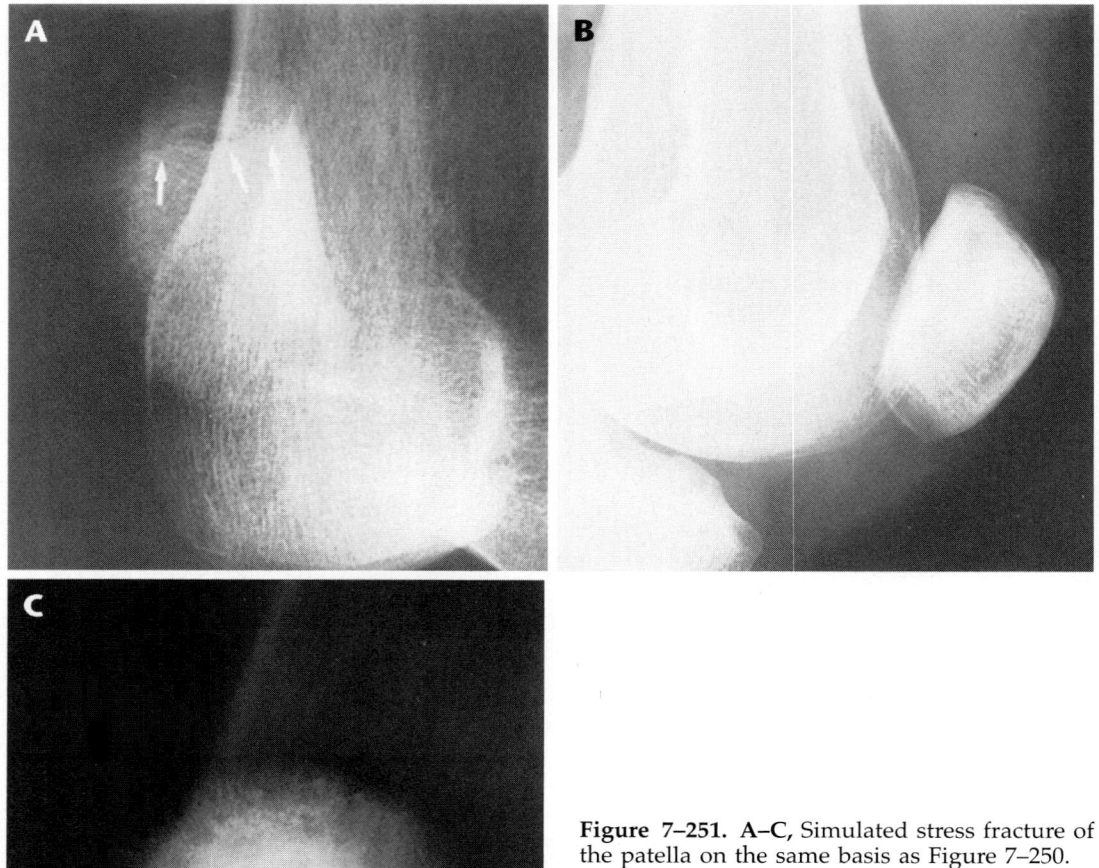

Figure 7–251. A–C, Simulated stress fracture of the patella on the same basis as Figure 7–250. Note that no discontinuity is seen in the lateral projection (**B**) or in the tomogram (**C**).

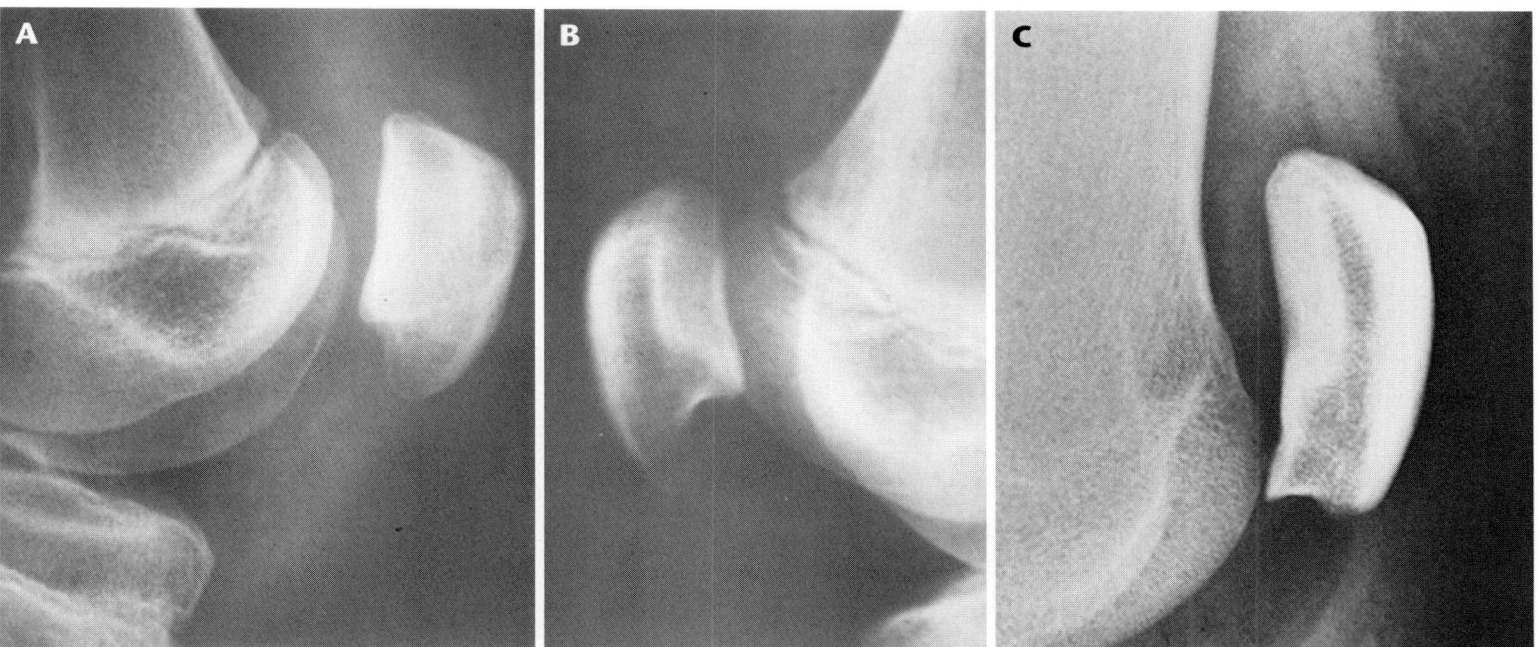

Figure 7–252. Unusual configurations of the lower poles of the patellae. **A** and **B,** 12-year-old. **C,** 14-year-old girl.

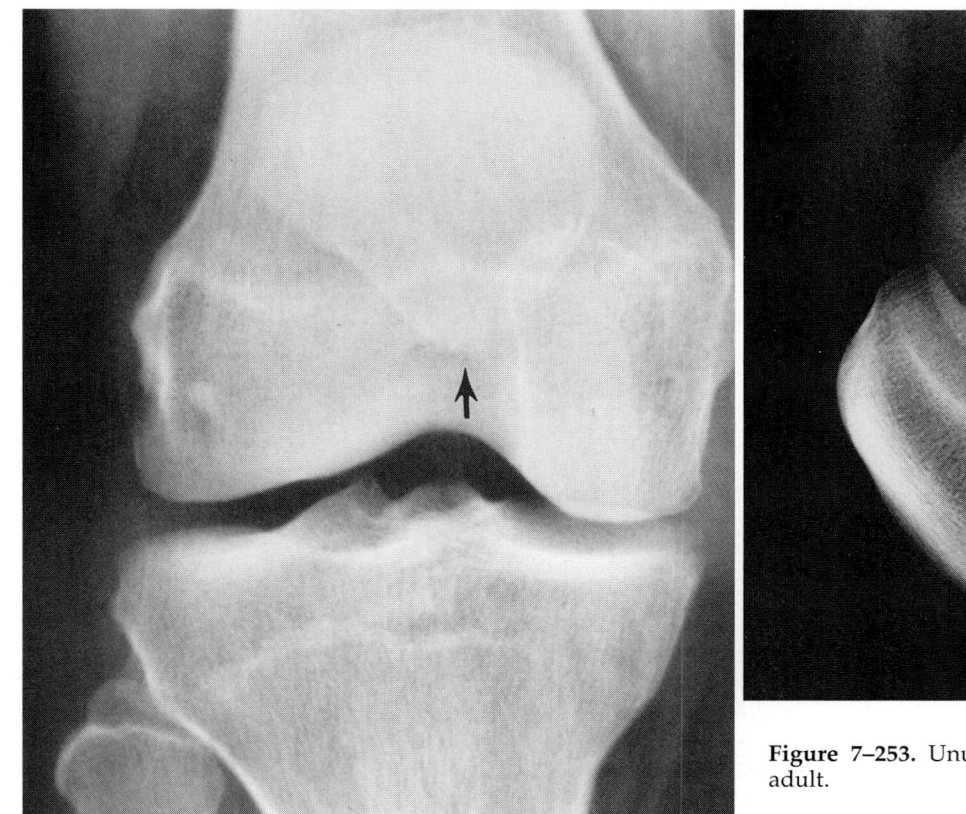

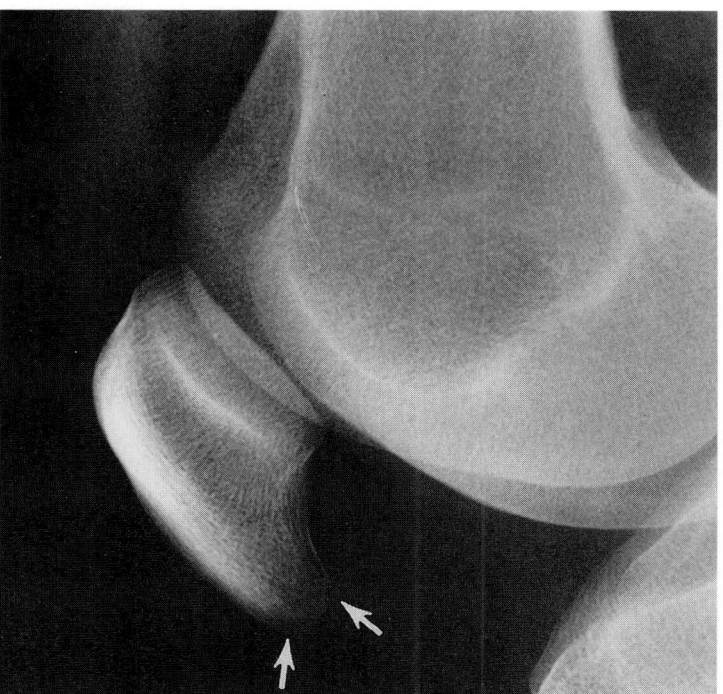

Figure 7–253. Unusual caudal extensions of the patella in an adult.

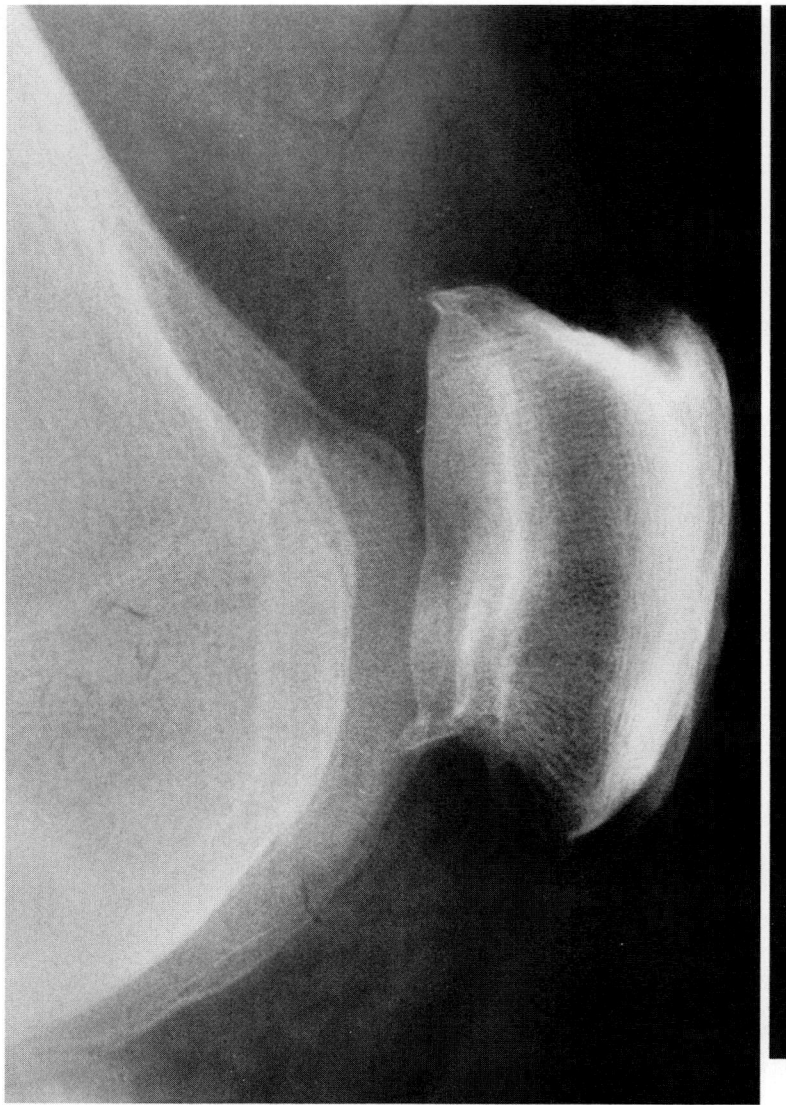
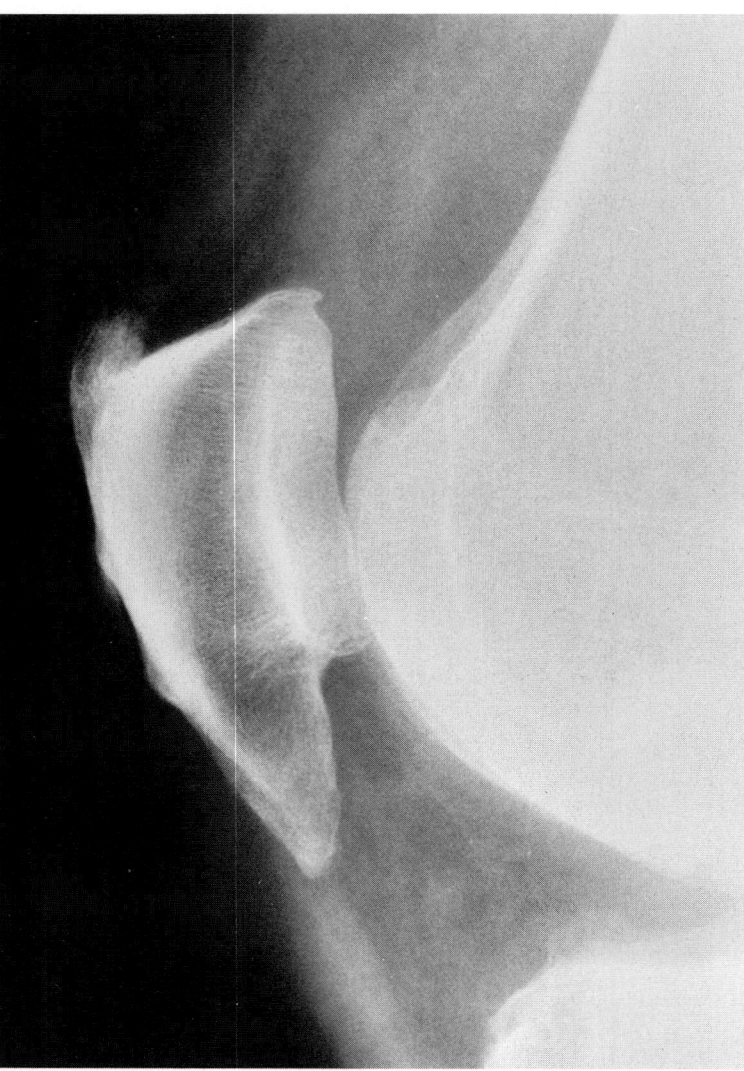

Figure 7–254. Unusual configurations of the patella resulting from enthesopathy.

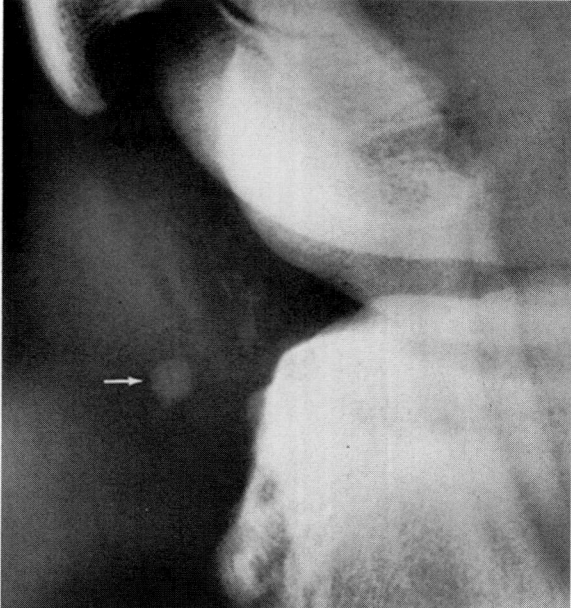
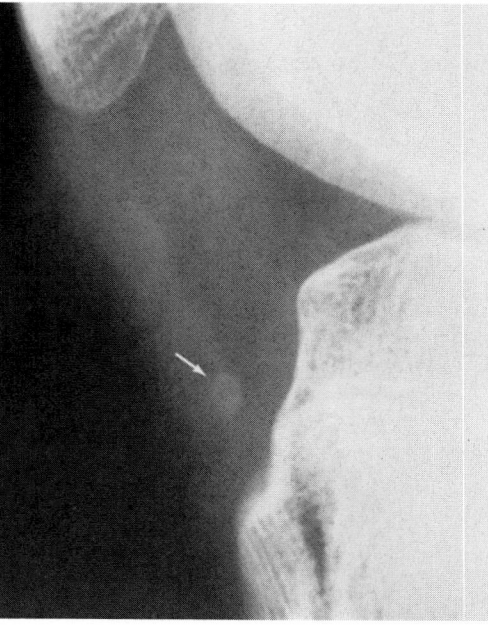

Figure 7–255. Two examples of ossicles or sesamoid bones in the patellar tendon.

The Leg

The Proximal Ends of the Tibia and Fibula

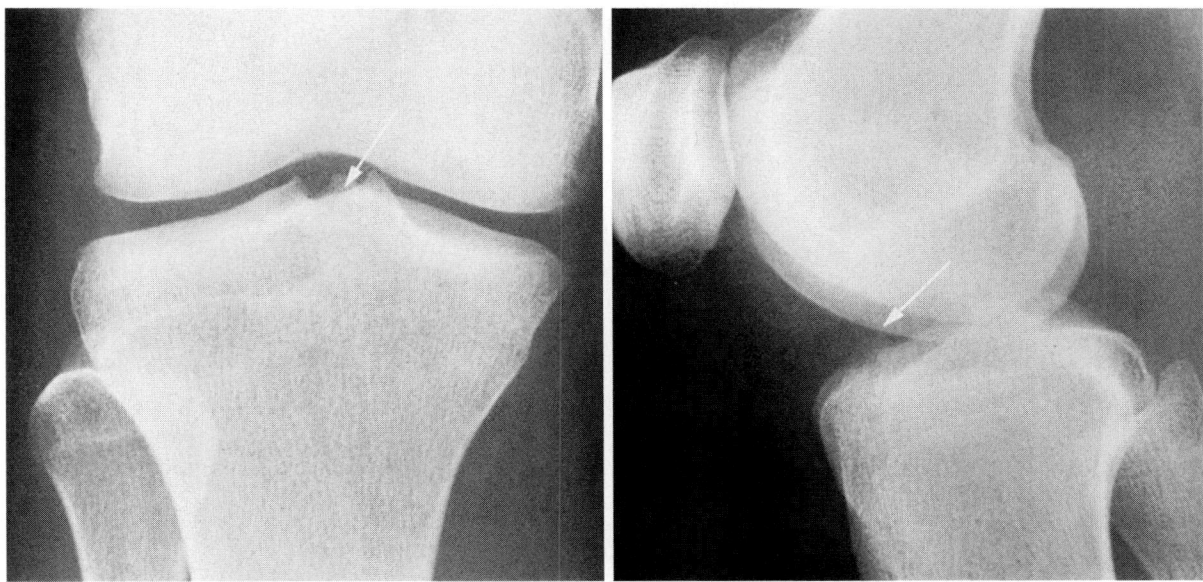

Figure 7–256. The third tibial spine is seen at the insertion of the anterior cruciate ligament in the anterior intercondylar area. (Ref: Kohler A, Zimmer EA: *Borderlands of the normal and early pathologic findings in skeletal roentgenology,* 4th ed. New York, Grune & Stratton, 1993, p. 742.)

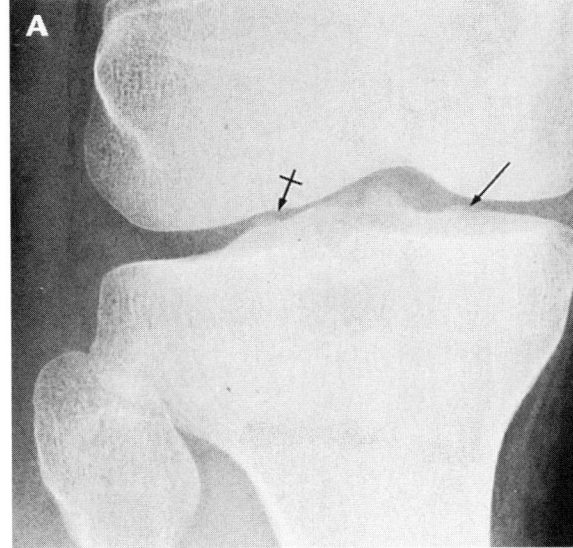

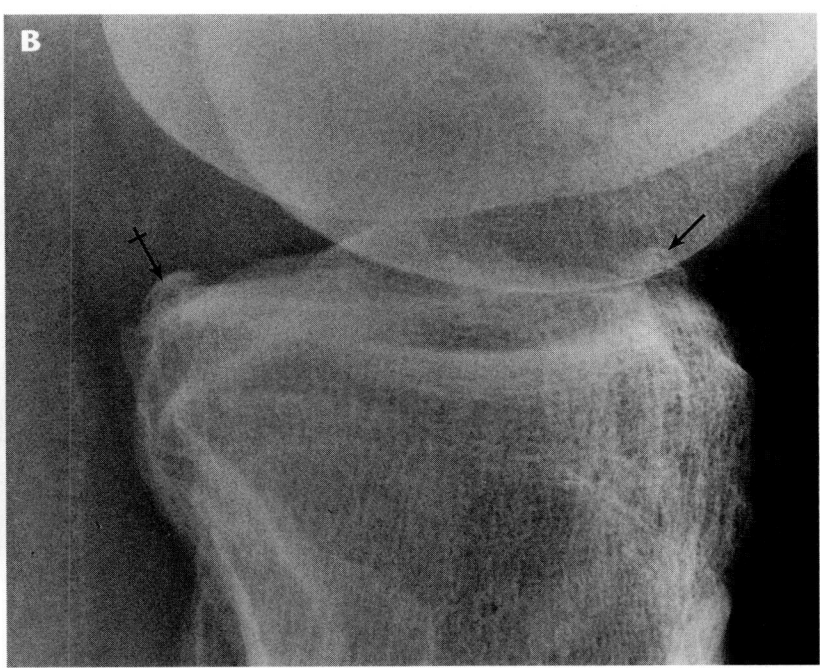

Figure 7–257. A, B, The third (←) and fourth (←+) tibial spines (see also Fig. 7–256). The fourth tibial spine is seen at the insertion by the posterior cruciate ligament in the posterior intercondylar area.

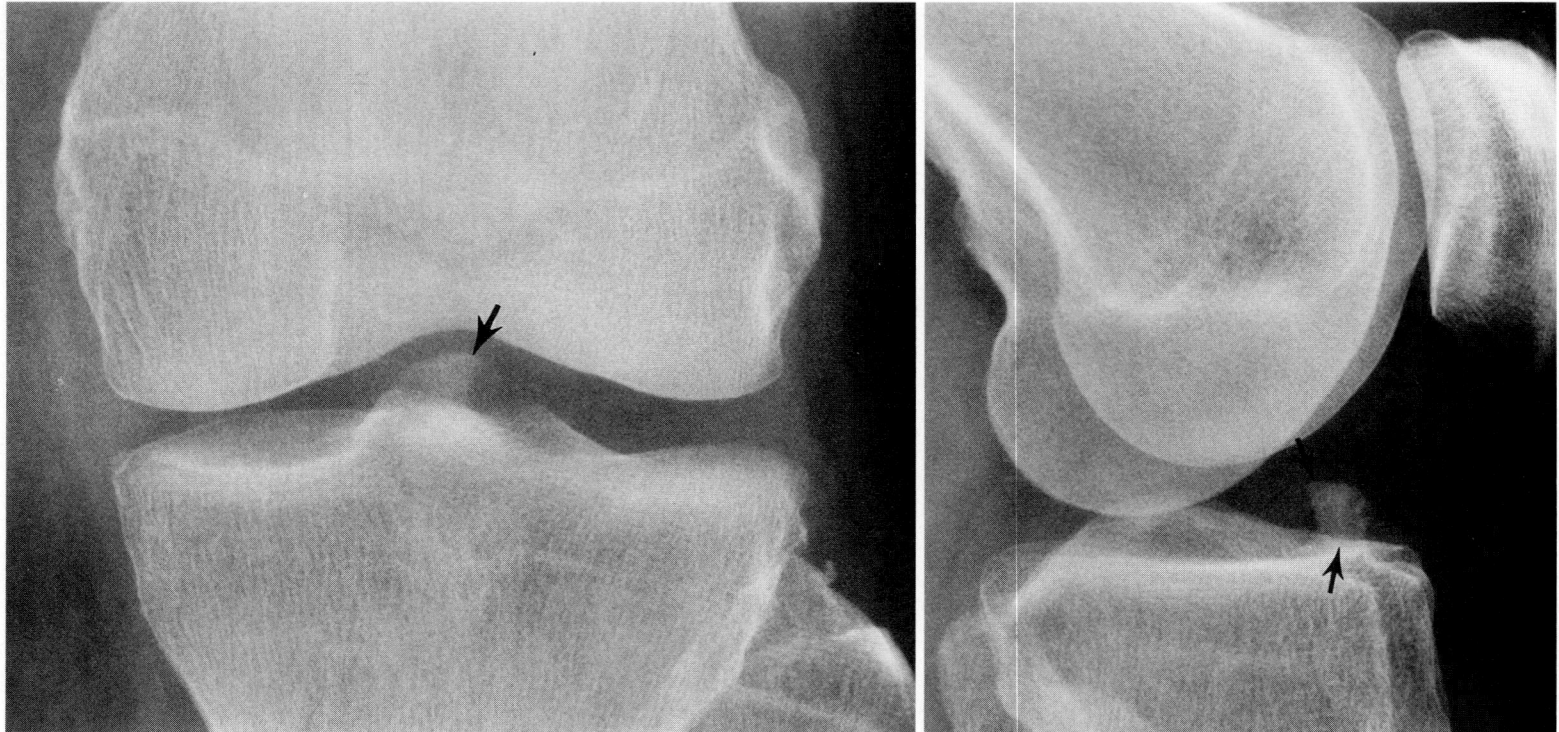

Figure 7–258. Spur on the tibial plateau in the absence of degenerative joint disease, possibly the origin of the anterior cruciate ligament. This entity is known as Parson's knob. Increasing size of the knob is said to be a reflection of enthesopathy. (Ref: Brossman J et al: Enlargement of the third intercondylar tubercle of Parson's as a sign of osteoarthritis of the knee. *Radiology* 198:845, 1996.)

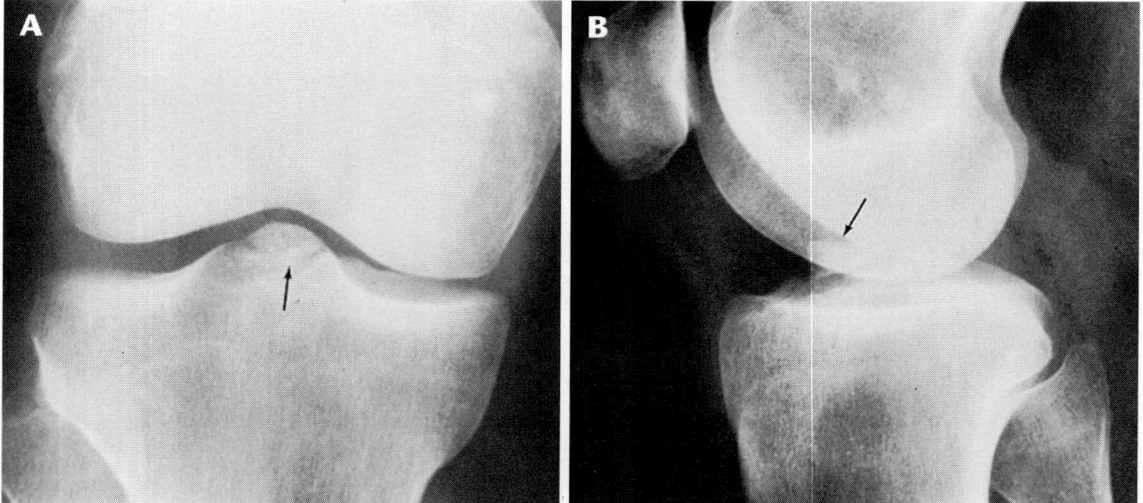

Figure 7–259. An ossicle in the intercondylar notch.

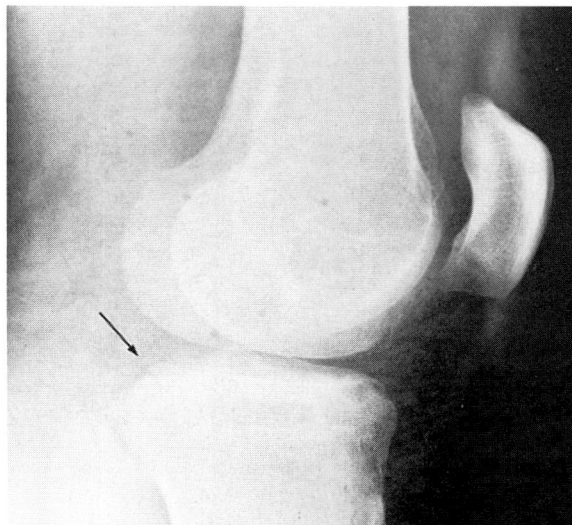

Figure 7–260. An ossicle at the fourth tubercle on the dorsal aspect of the proximal tibial surface. Note marked concavity of the posterior aspect of the patella. (Ref: Kohler A, Zimmer EA: *Borderlands of the normal and early pathologic findings in skeletal roentgenology,* 3rd ed. New York, Grune & Stratton, 1968, p. 441.)

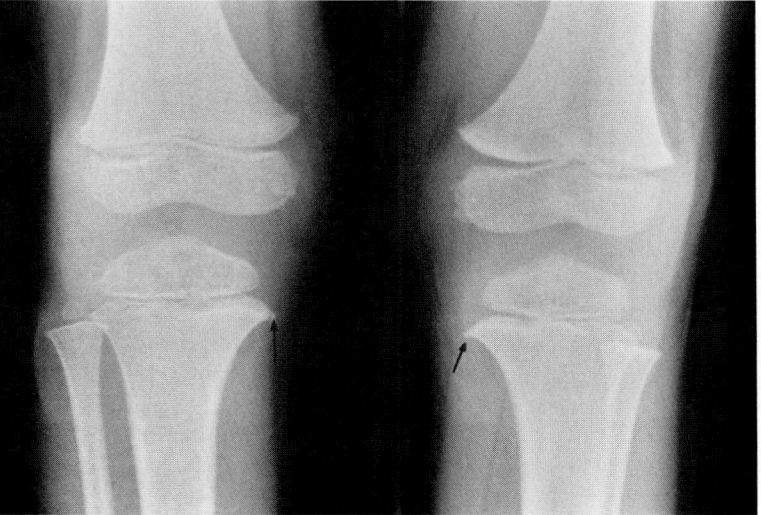

Figure 7–261. Bilateral accessory ossification centers at the medial edge of the proximal tibial metaphysis in a 7-year-old child.

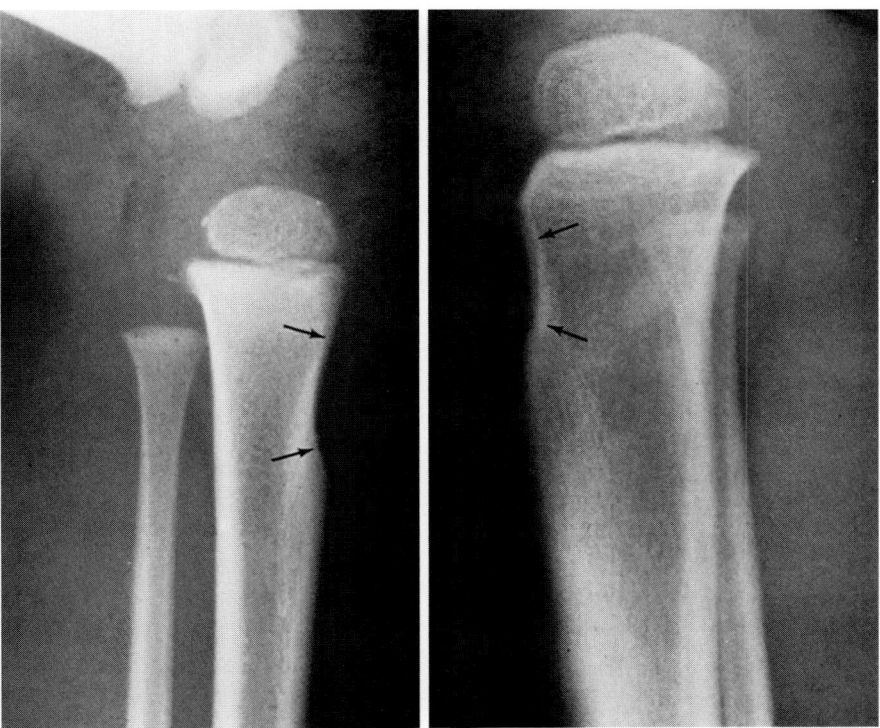

Figure 7–262. Normal depressions in the anterior tibia of a 4-year-old. These depressions disappear with the development of the ossification center for the tibial tubercle.

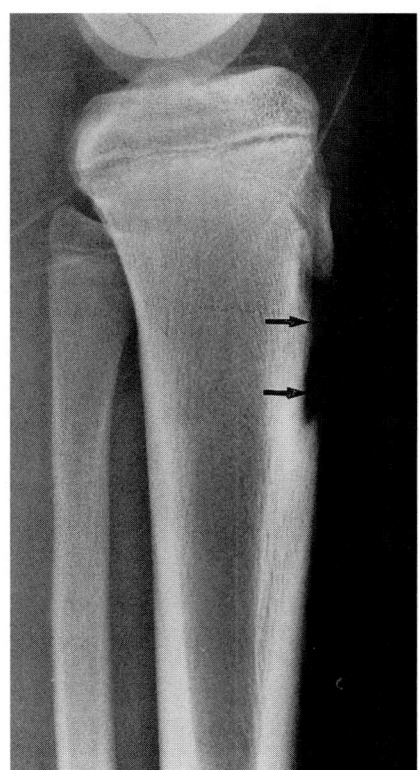

Figure 7–263. Unusually long anterior fossa for the developing tibial tubercle.

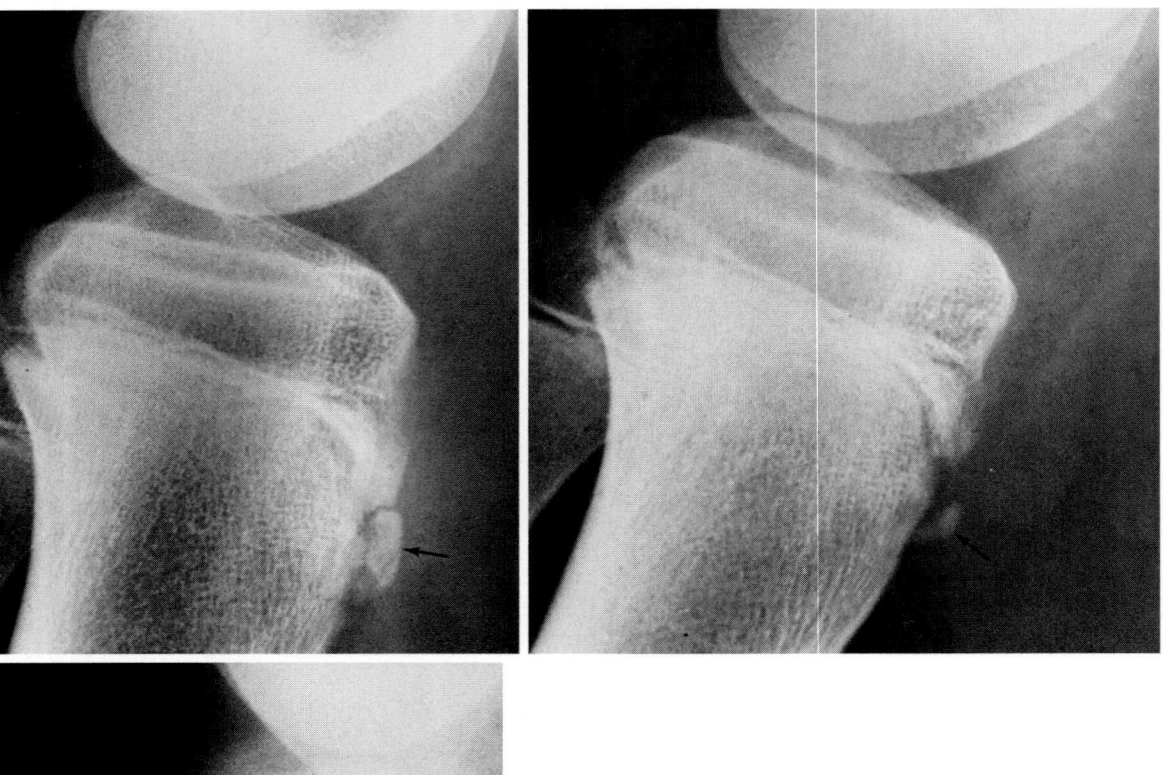

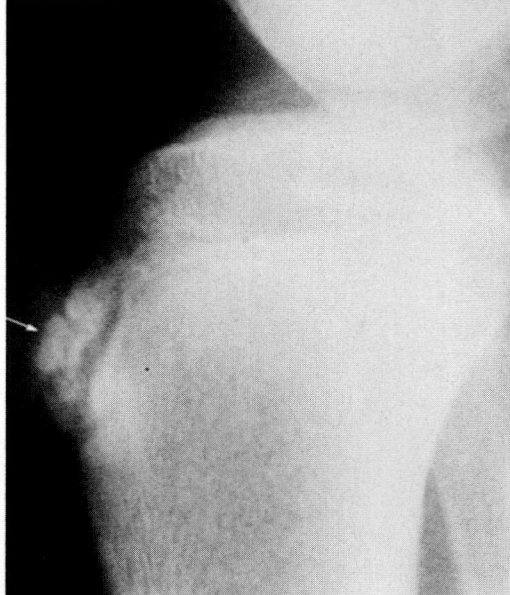

Figure 7–264. Normal variations in appearance of the apophysis of the tibial tubercle. None of these is necessarily indicative of Osgood-Schlatter disease.

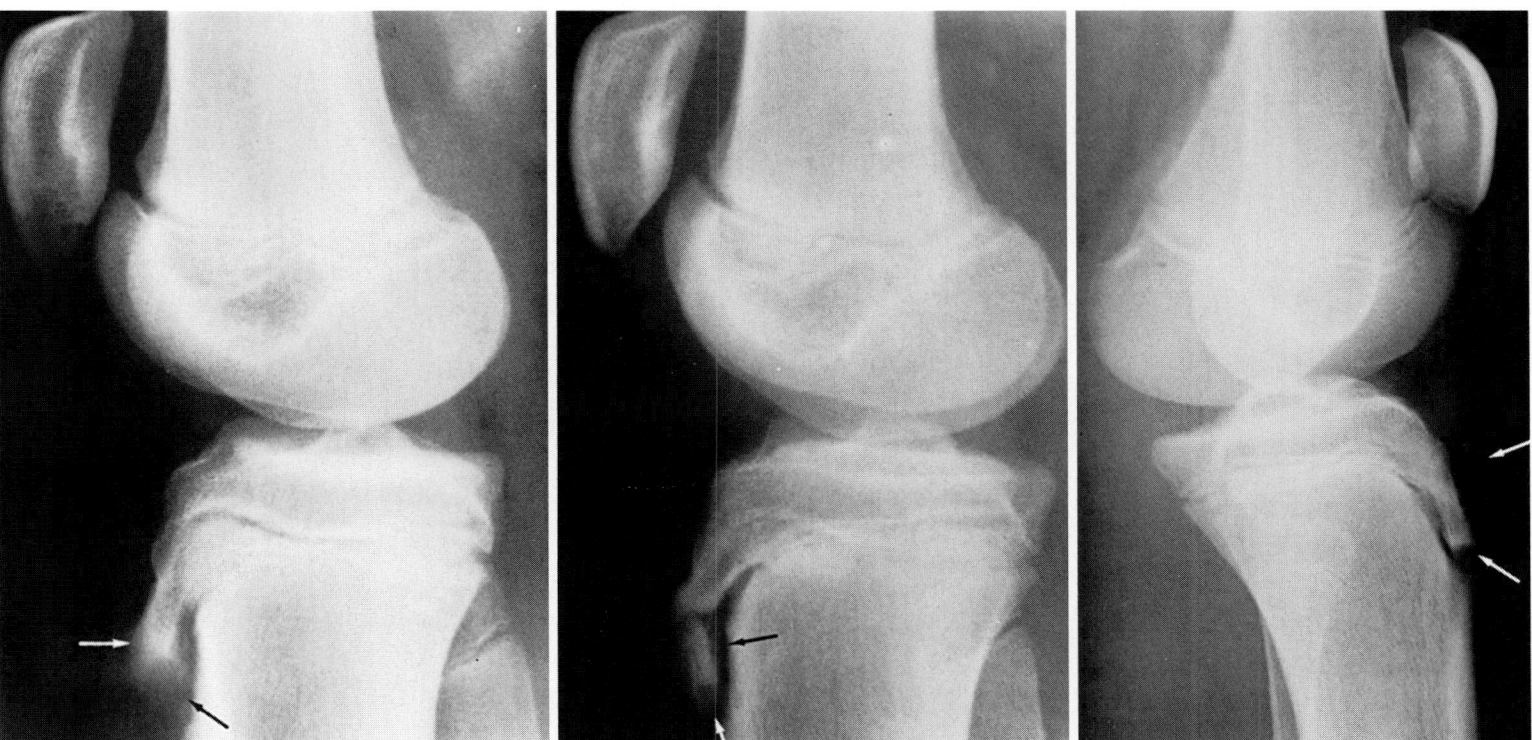

Figure 7–265. Three additional examples of normal variation in appearance of the ossification center of the tibial tubercle in adolescence.

Figure 7–266. A separate, ununited ossification center for the tibial tubercle in a young adult. This should not be confused with a fracture.

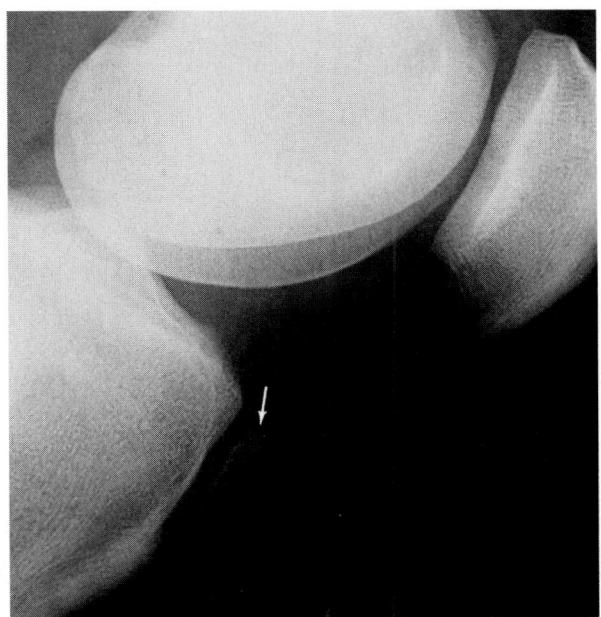

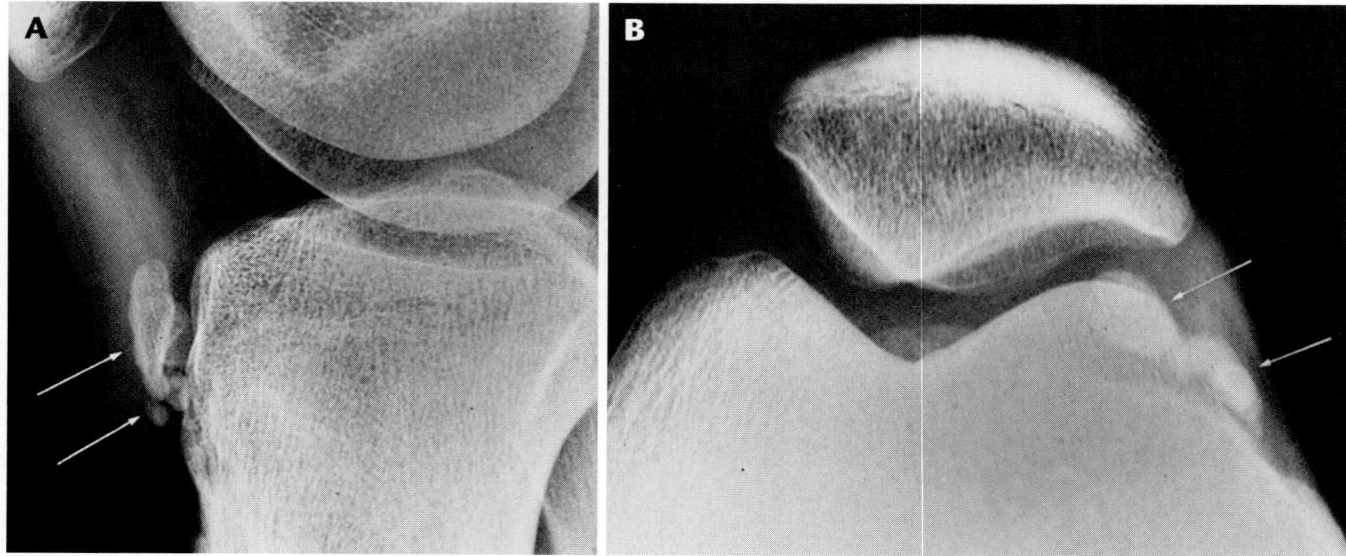

Figure 7–267. A, B, The unfused ossification centers for the tibial tubercle, seen in the tangential view (**B**). (Ref: Bloom R et al: Ossicles anterior to the proximal tibia. *Clin Imaging* 17:137, 1993.)

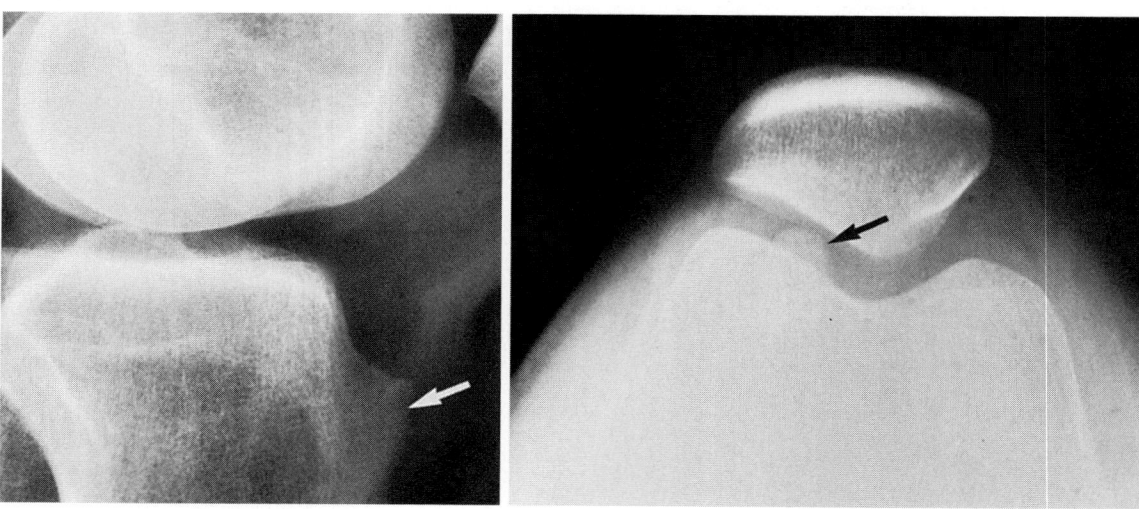

Figure 7–268. Large tibial tubercle simulating an intra-articular loose body on tangential projection (*arrow*).

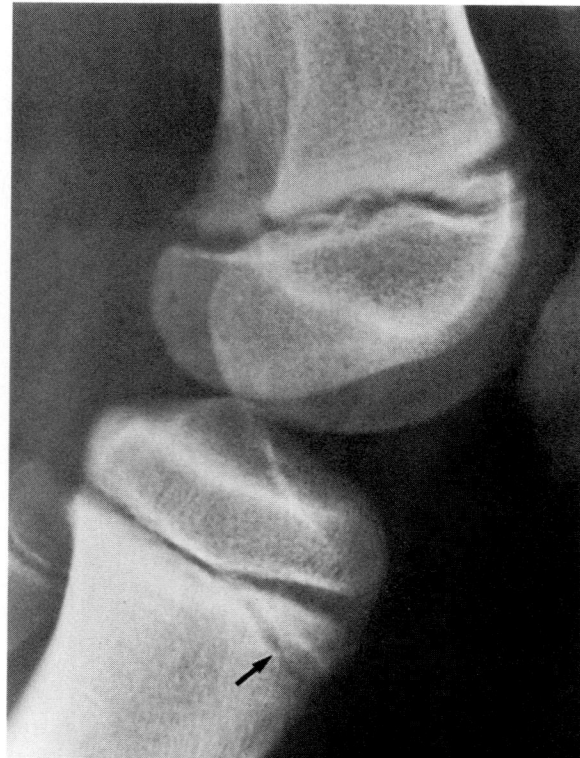

Figure 7–269. The edge of the proximal tibial epiphysis as seen in lateral projection may simulate a fracture.

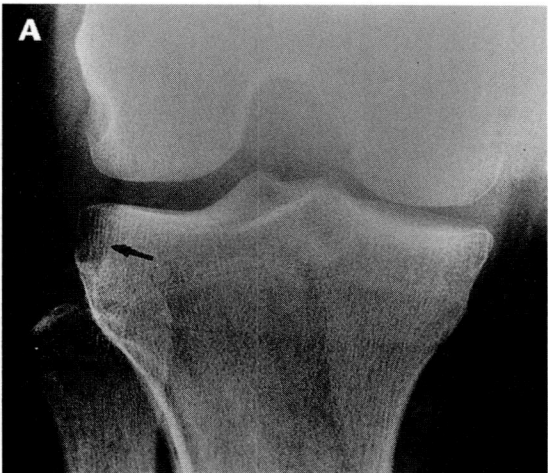
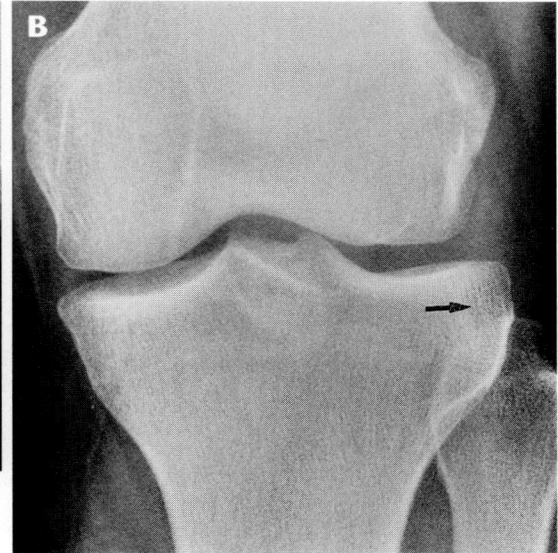

Figure 7–270. A, B, Bilateral factitious radiolucencies in the lateral aspects of the tibial plateaus in a 23-year-old man.

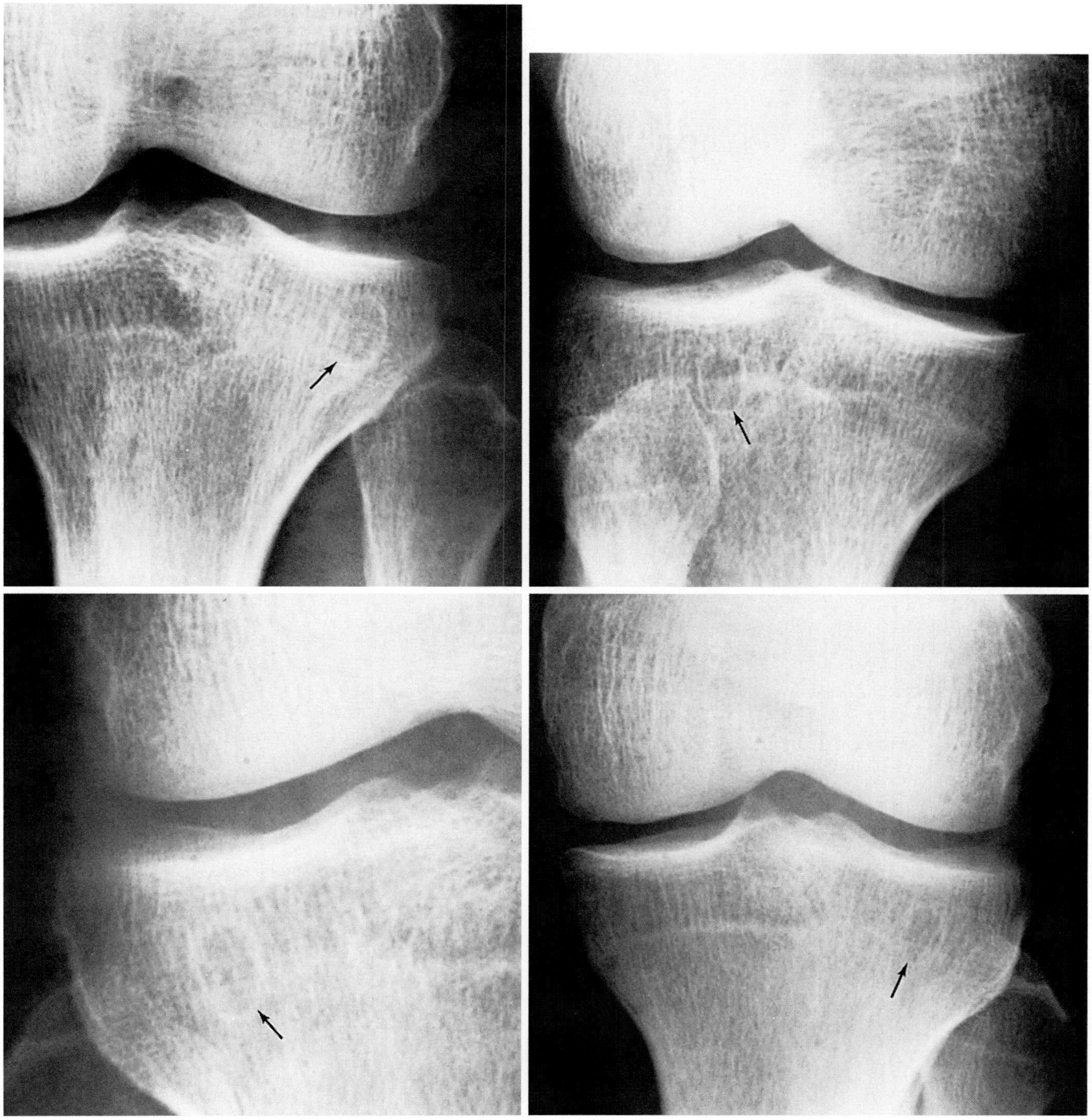

Figure 7–271. Ringlike lesions in the proximal tibia are of no clinical significance. They are probably fibrous in nature. Similar lesions are seen in the pelvis (see Fig. 4–35) and fibula (see Fig. 7–333).

727

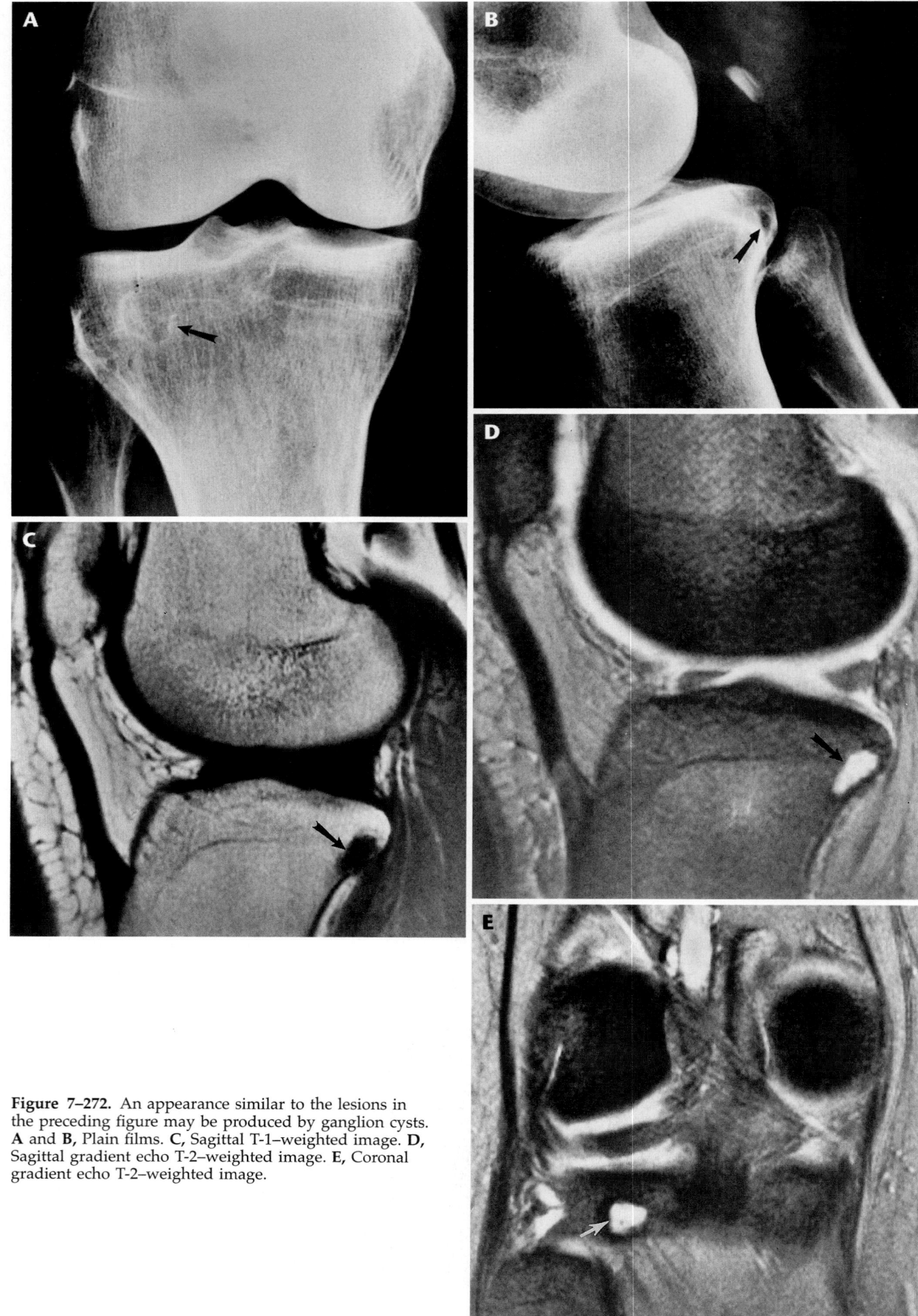

Figure 7–272. An appearance similar to the lesions in the preceding figure may be produced by ganglion cysts. **A** and **B**, Plain films. **C**, Sagittal T-1–weighted image. **D**, Sagittal gradient echo T-2–weighted image. **E**, Coronal gradient echo T-2–weighted image.

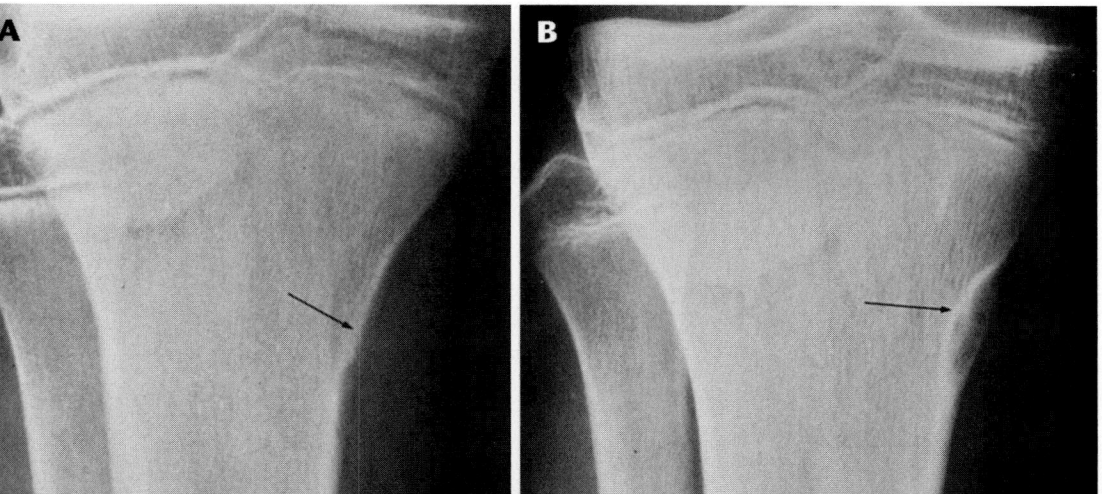

Figure 7–273. A, Medial metaphyseal cortical irregularity of the tibia in an adolescent. This is a developmental phenomenon similar to that seen in the humerus, the radius, and the femur. **B,** On follow-up, the irregularity was replaced by a typical benign cortical defect, suggesting the interrelationship of these lesions.

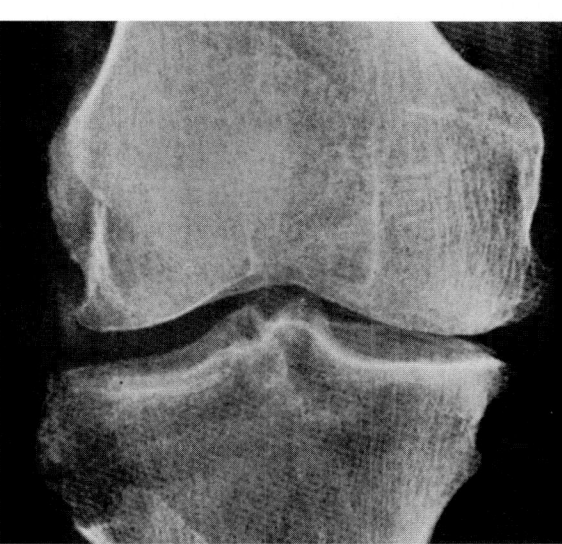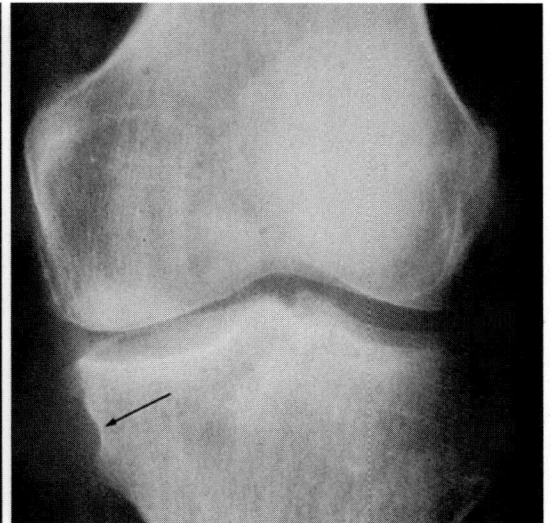

Figure 7–274. Normal fossae at the medial tibial metaphysis should not be mistaken for erosions. In the elderly they appear exaggerated because of spurring of the joint margin.

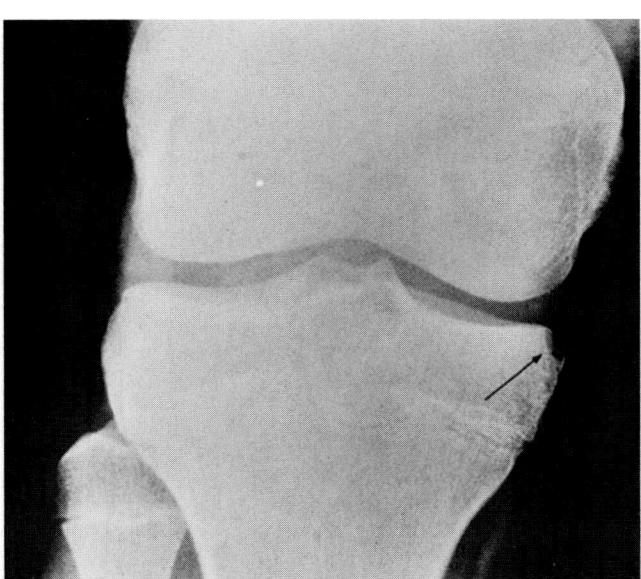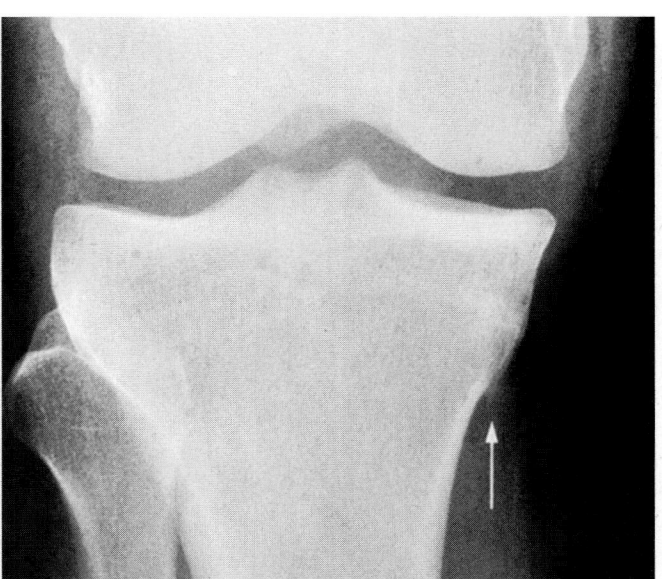

Figure 7–275. Developmental notch on the medial aspect of the tibial plateau in a 15-year-old boy.

Figure 7–276. Small spur at the medial tibial metaphysis, probably representing a "tug" lesion.

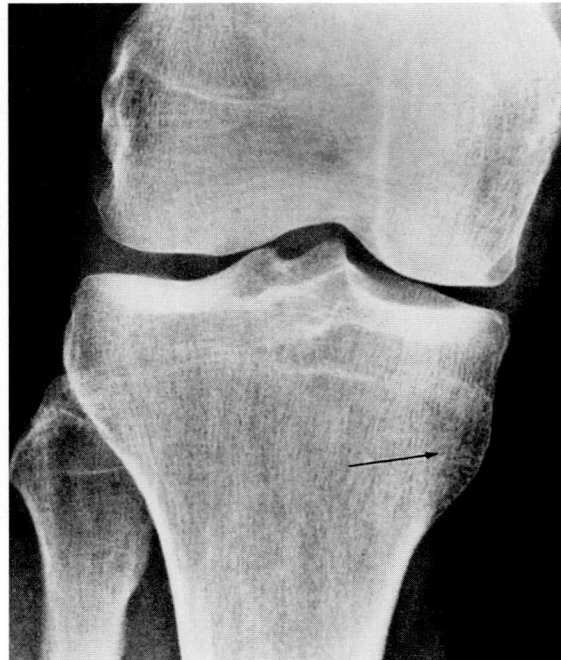

Figure 7–277. Developmental bulge of the medial tibial metaphysis.

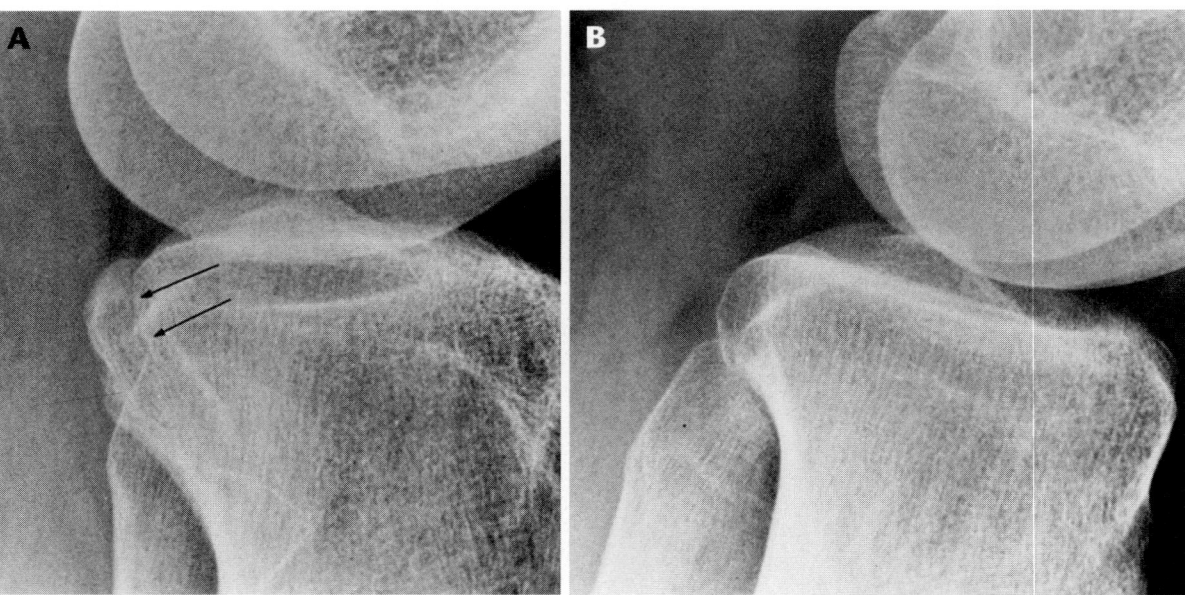

Figure 7–278. A, Simulated fracture of the proximal tibia caused by rotation at the time of filming. **B,** Correct position shows no fracture.

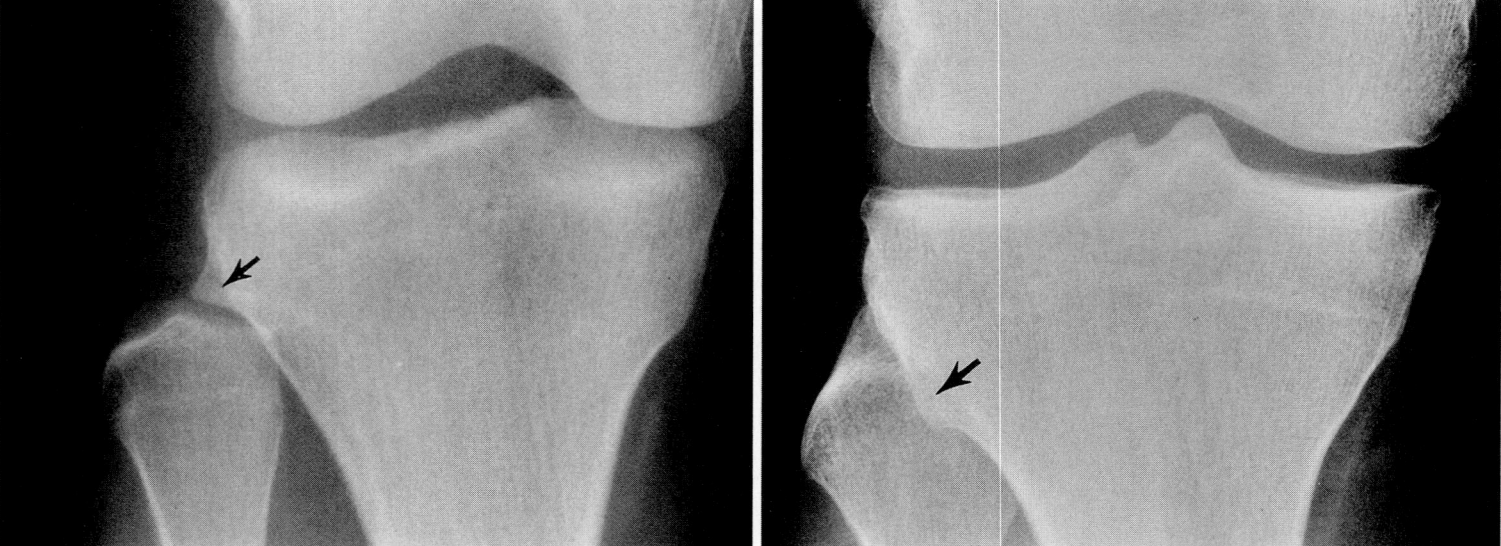

Figure 7–279. Spurlike extensions of the tibia in the tibial-fibular articulation.

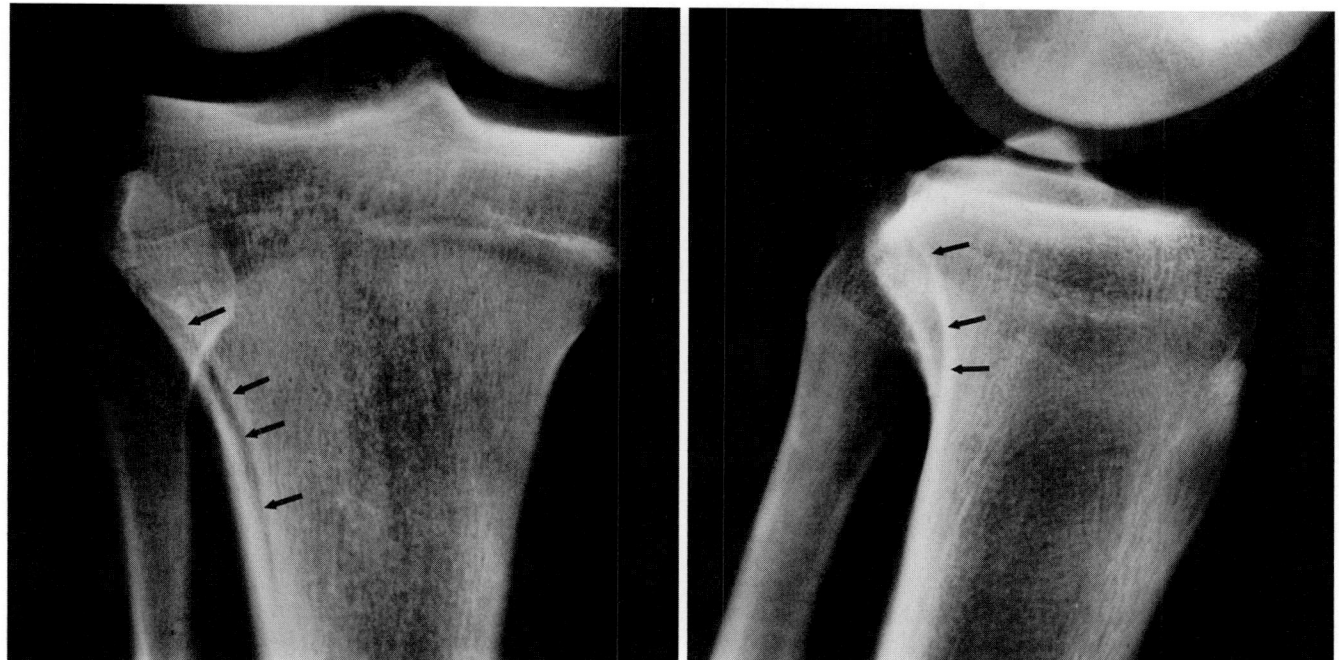

Figure 7–280. Prominent sulcus in the posterior lateral aspect of the tibia.

Figure 7–281. The open apophysis for the tibial tubercle, which should not be mistaken for a fracture.

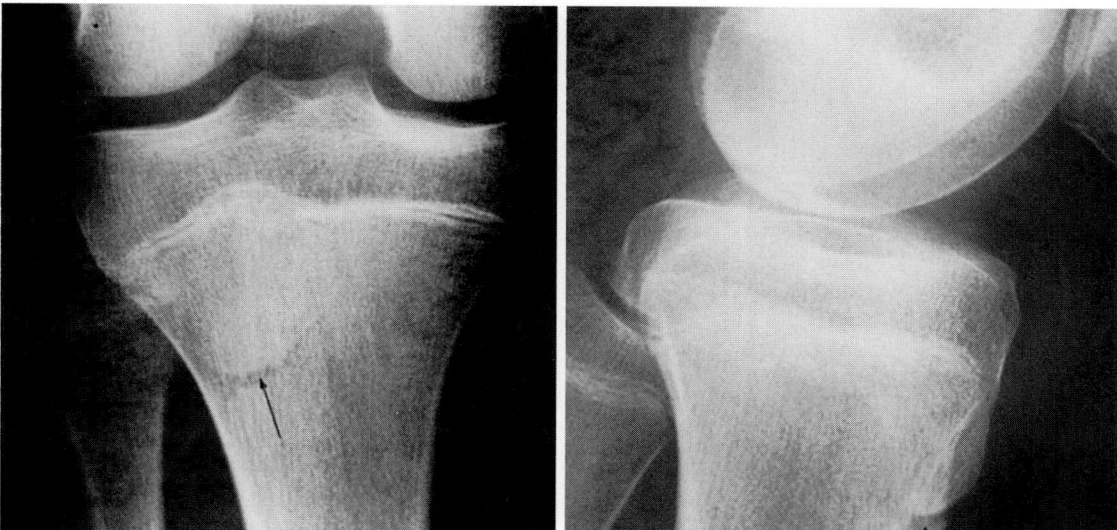

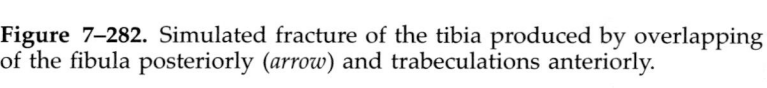

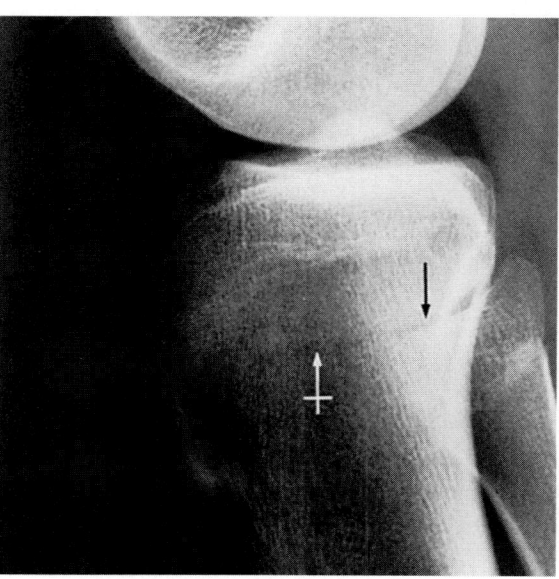

Figure 7–282. Simulated fracture of the tibia produced by overlapping of the fibula posteriorly (*arrow*) and trabeculations anteriorly.

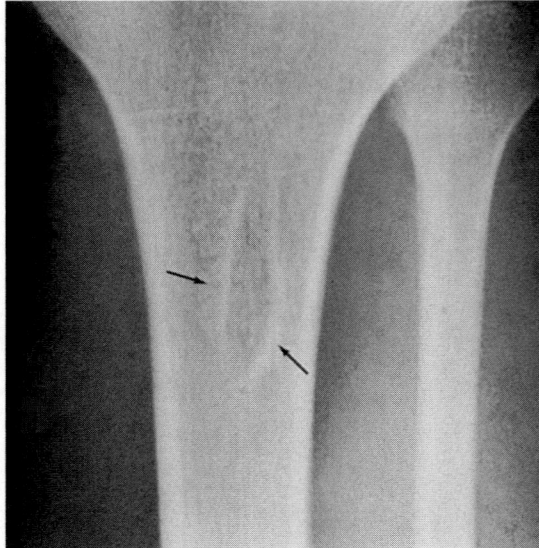

Figure 7–283. Radiolucency produced by the tibial tubercle en face.

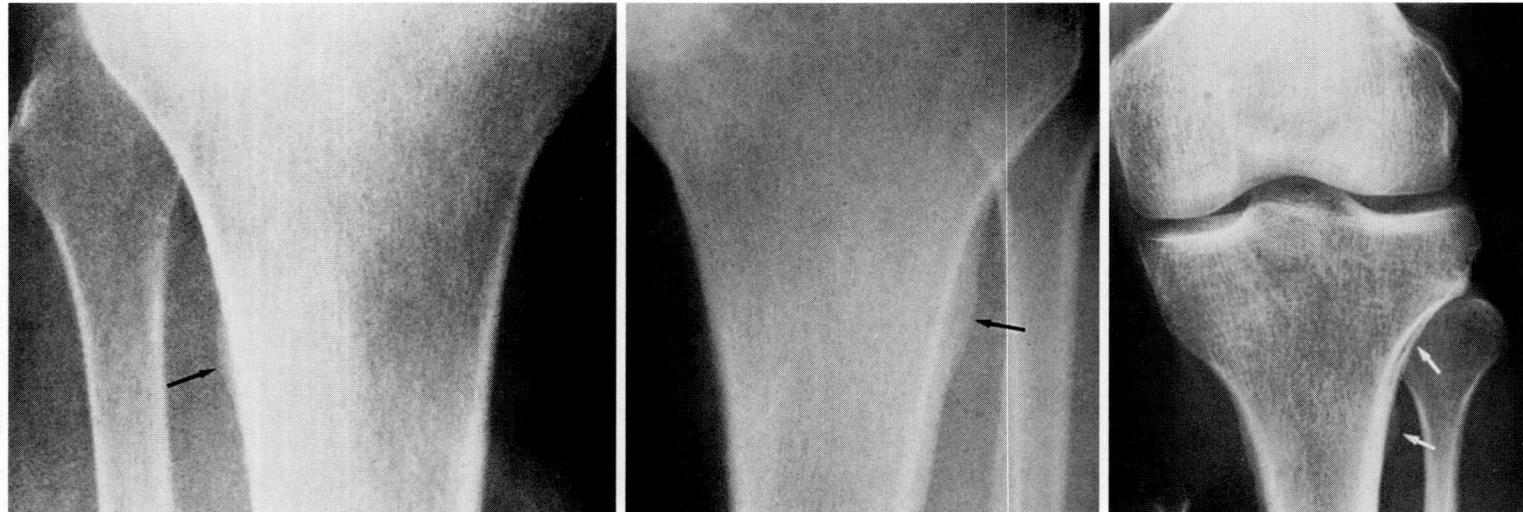

Figure 7–284. Three examples of pseudoperiostitis, simulated by the tibial tuberosity (*arrows*).

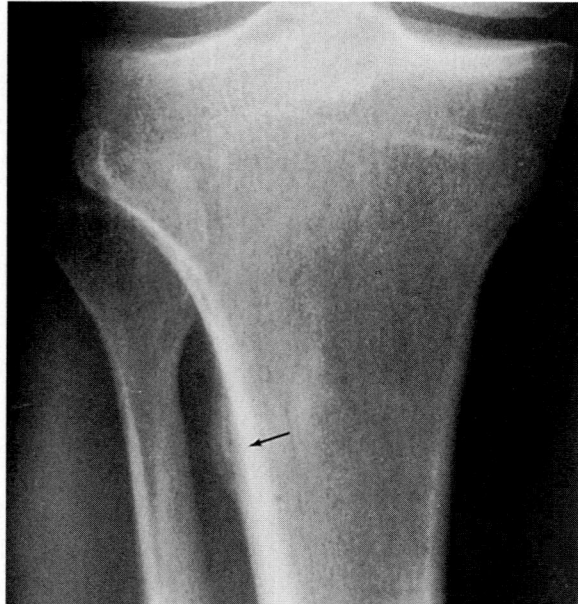

Figure 7–285. Laminated appearance of the tibial tubercle, not to be confused with periosteal new bone formation.

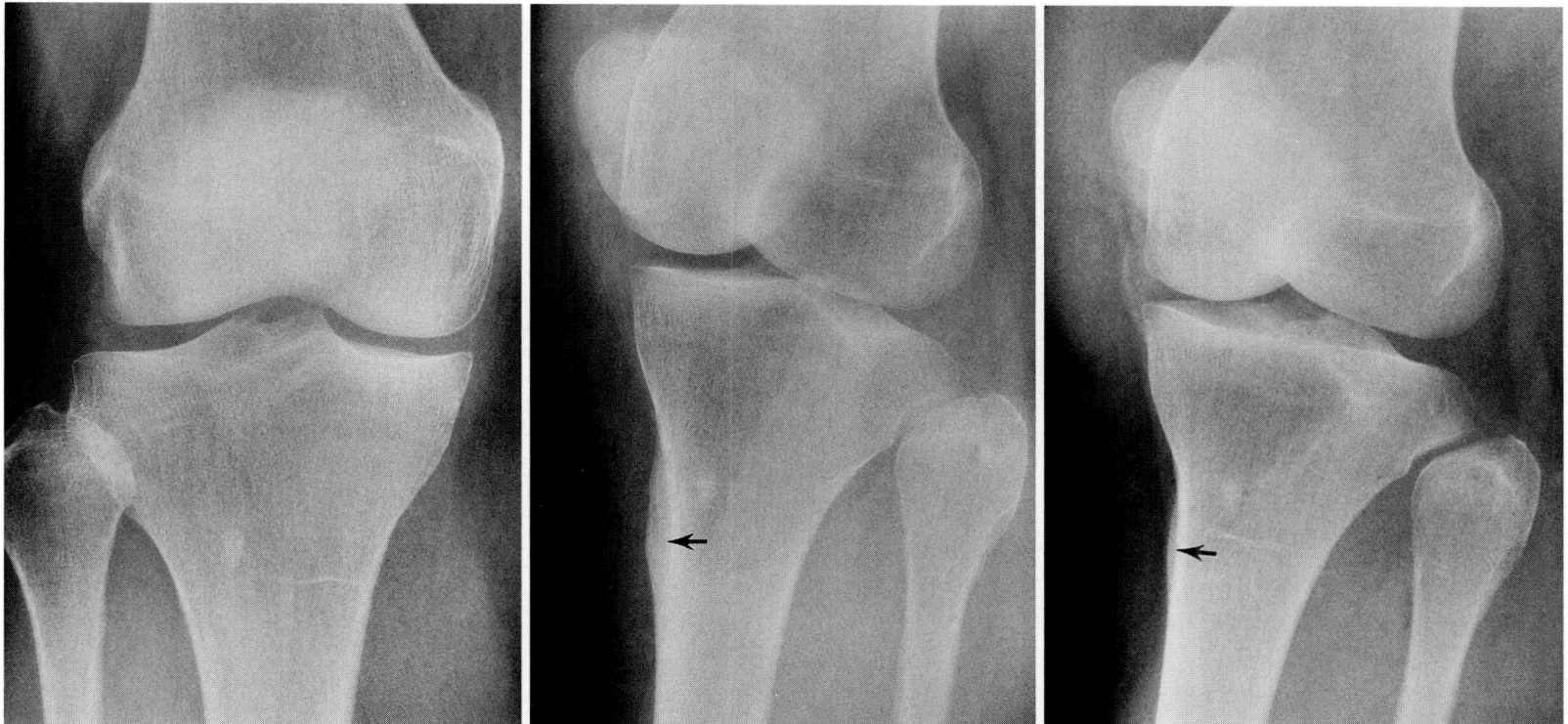

Figure 7–286. Note the varied prominence of the anterior tibial crest with various degrees of rotation. Note also the radiolucency that appears in the medial aspect of the tibial metaphysis with rotation.

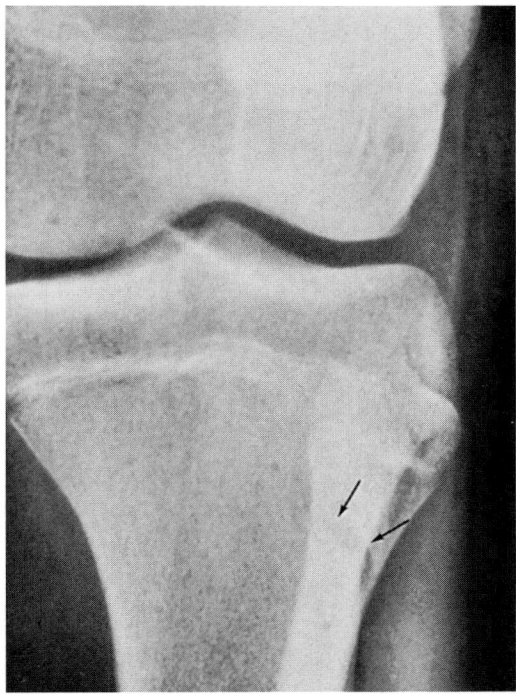

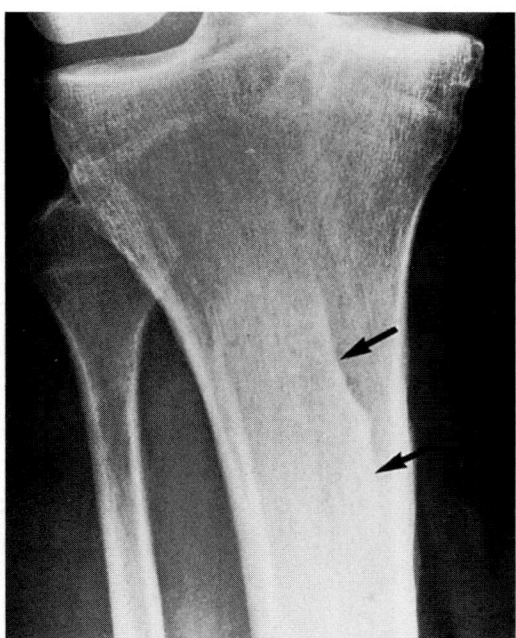

Figure 7–288. Thickening of the anterior cortex of the tibia, producing an unusual appearance in the frontal projection.

Figure 7–287. Apparent fracture of the neck of the fibula produced by rotation and overlap of the open apophysis of the tibial tubercle.

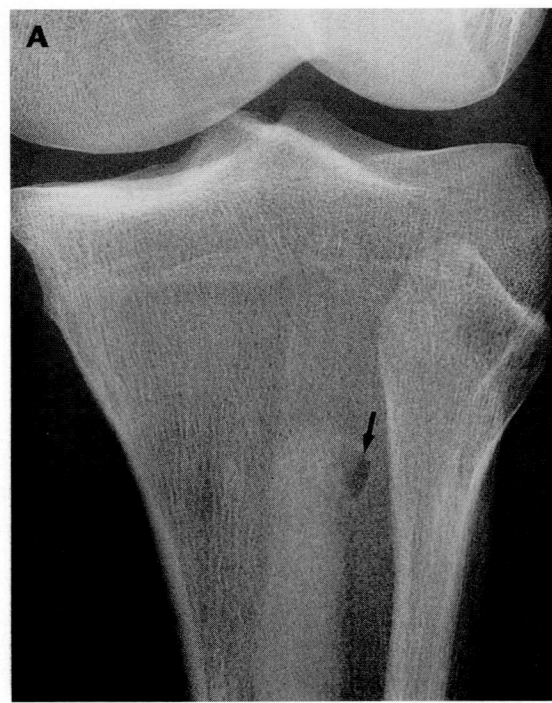
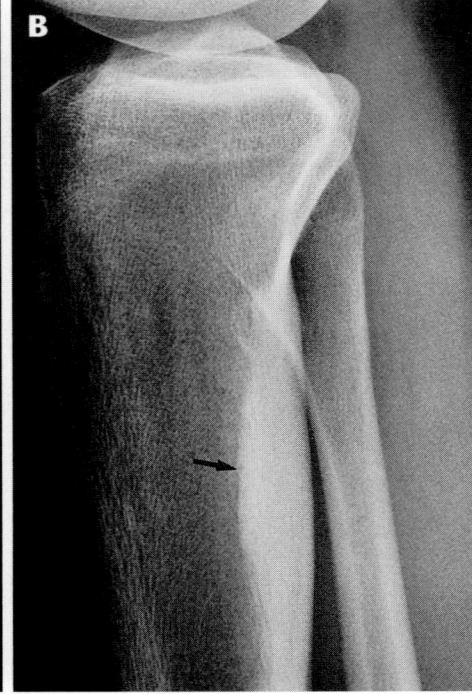

Figure 7–289. A, B, Healed benign cortical defect simulating the changes of a runner's stress fracture. Note remaining radiolucency in the proximal end of the lesion in **A.**

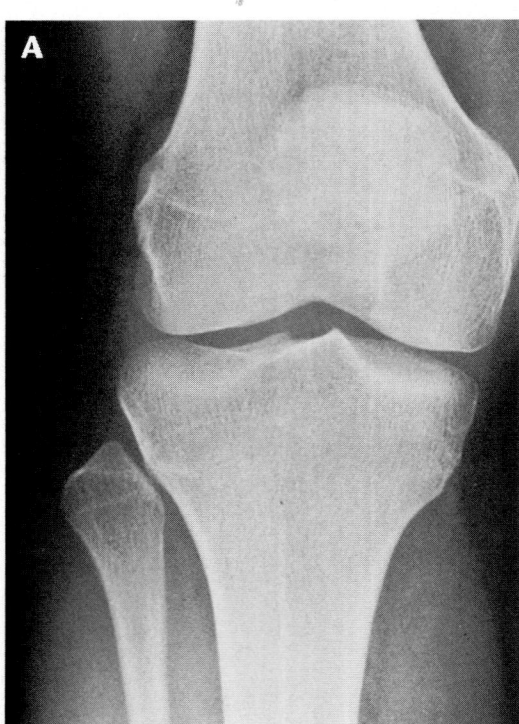
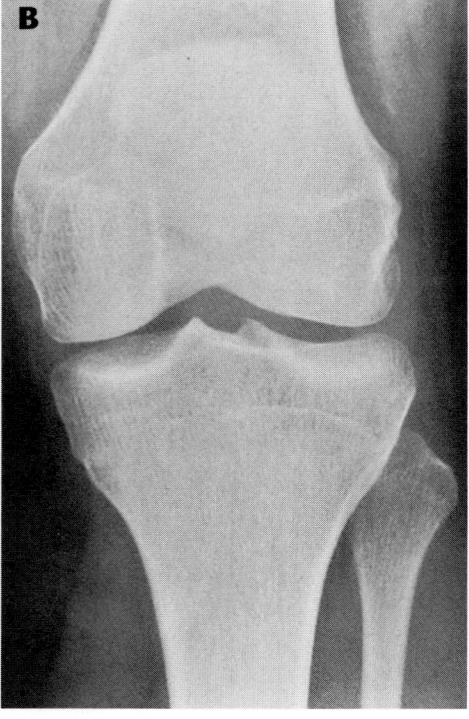

Figure 7–290. A, Simulated dislocation of the head of the fibula produced by filming in slight rotation. Note medial position of the patella. **B,** Opposite side showing proper positioning and normal relationships.

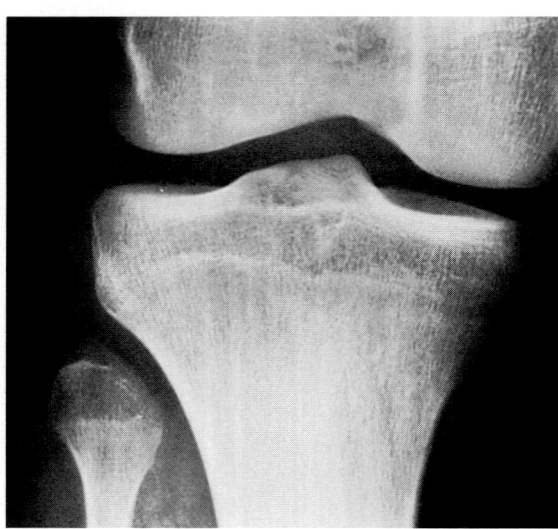
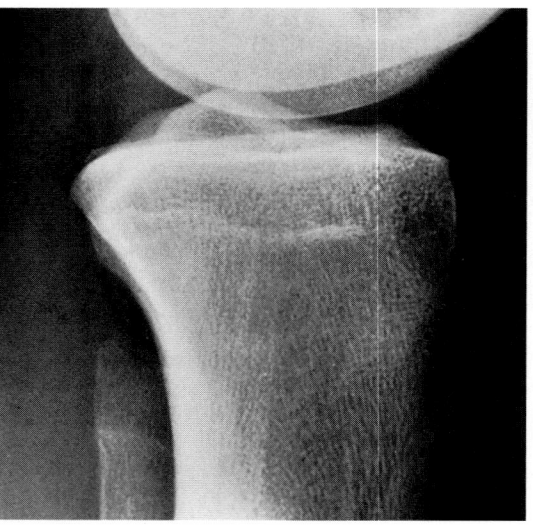

Figure 7–291. Short fibula.

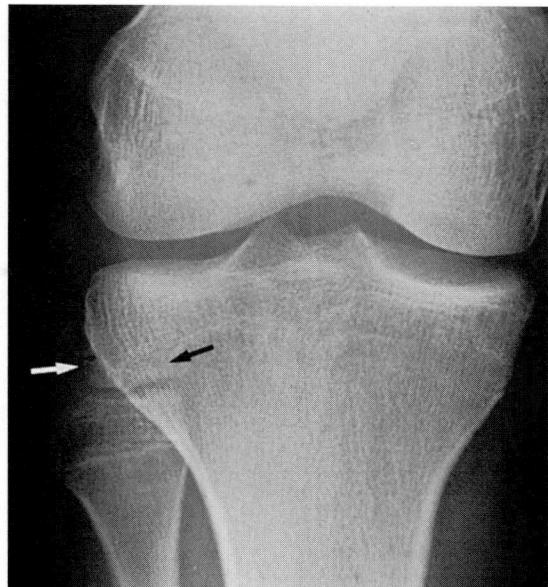

Figure 7–292. Accessory ossification center at the proximal end of the fibula.

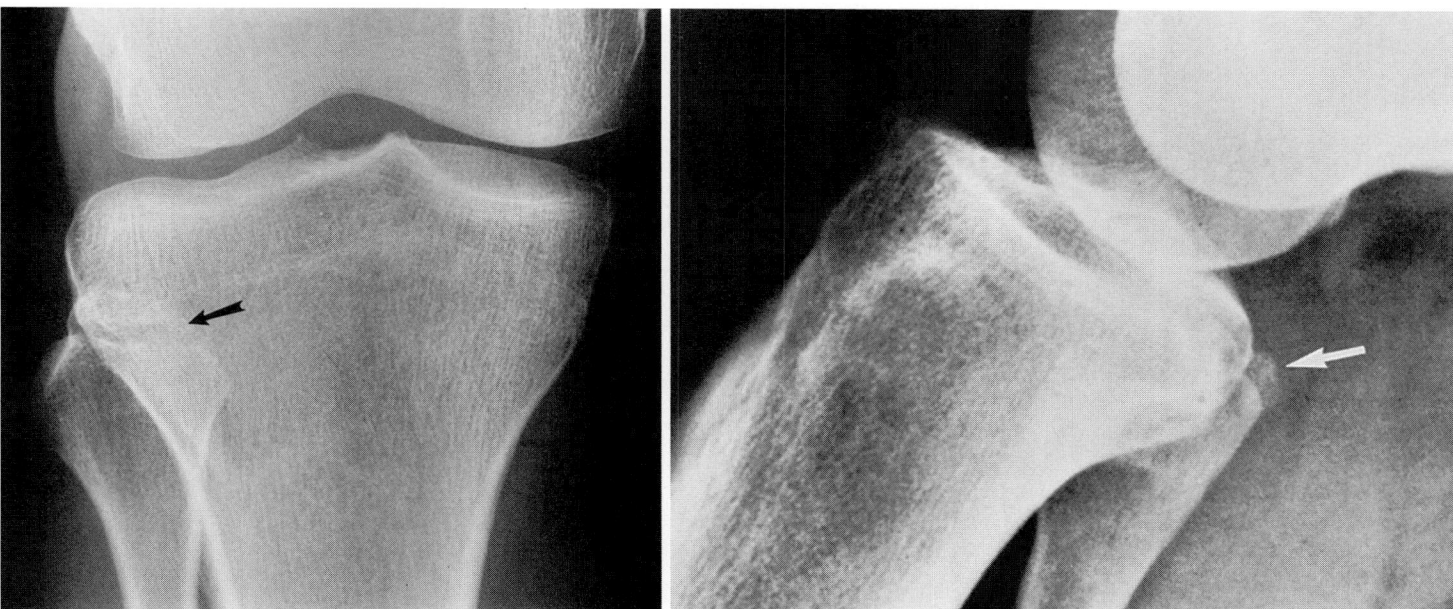

Figure 7–293. Accessory ossicle at the superior end of the fibula in a 44-year-old man.

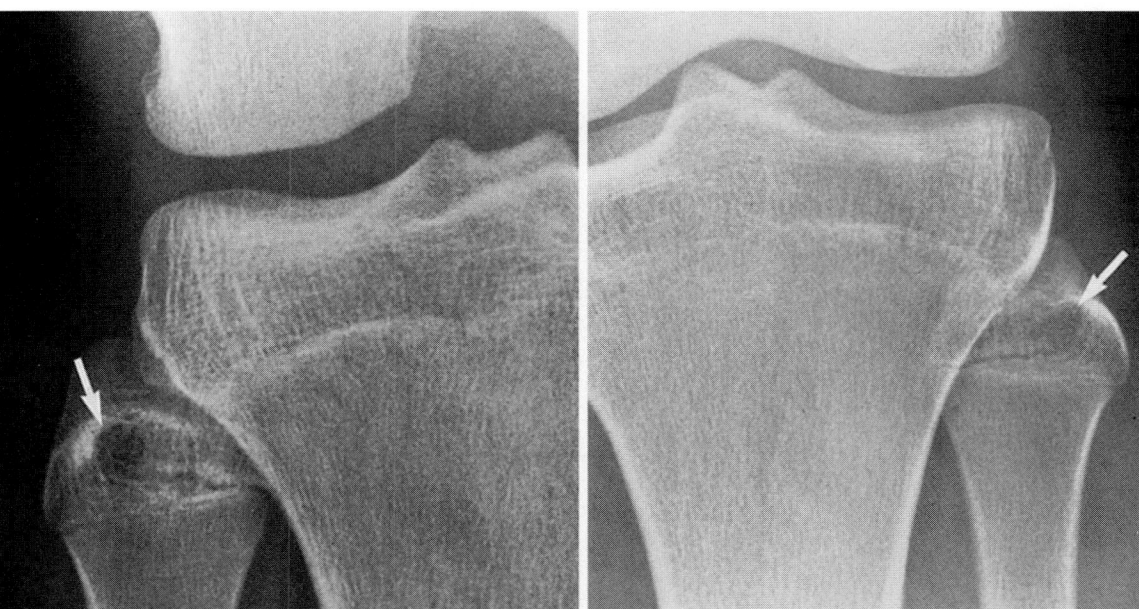

Figure 7–294. Normal lucency in the proximal fibular epiphyses in a 15-year-old girl.

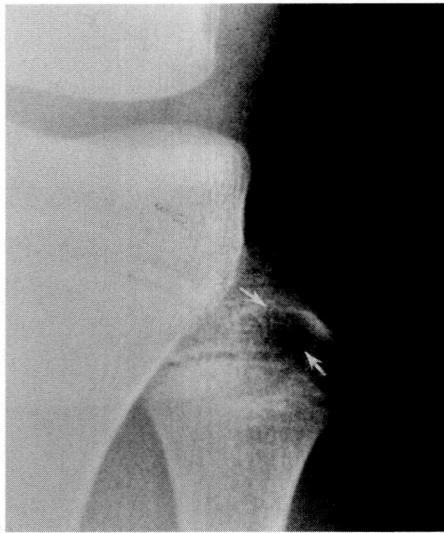

Figure 7–295. Normal lucency of the fibular head, simulating a cyst.

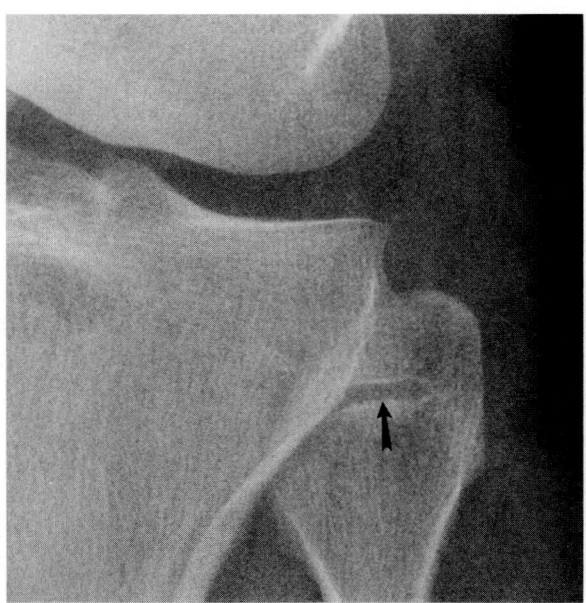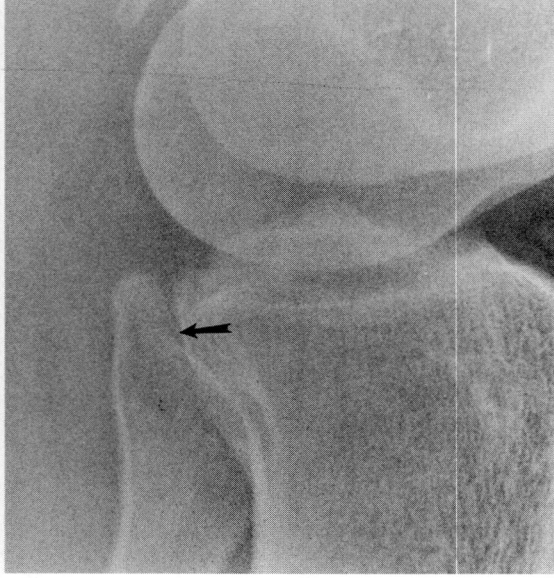

Figure 7–296. Simulated discontinuity of the head of the fibula produced by the elongated configuration of the proximal end of the fibular head.

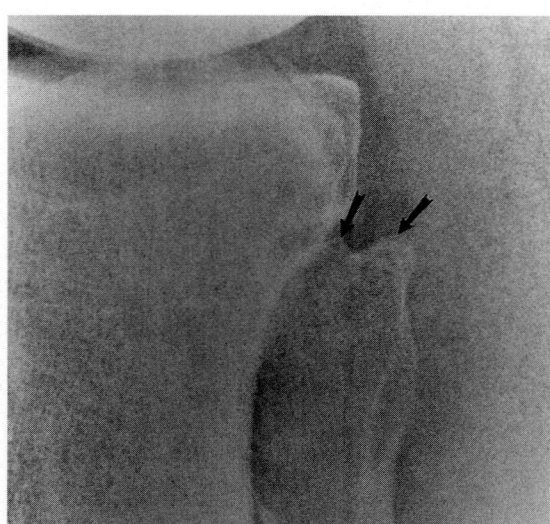

Figure 7–297. Unusual configuration of the proximal end of the fibula.

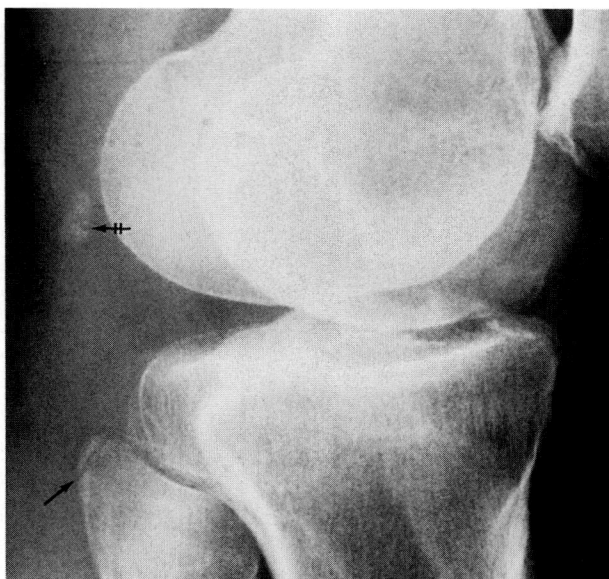

Figure 7–298. Ununited accessory ossification center at the head of the fibula, simulating a fracture (←). Note also the bifid fabella (⬿).

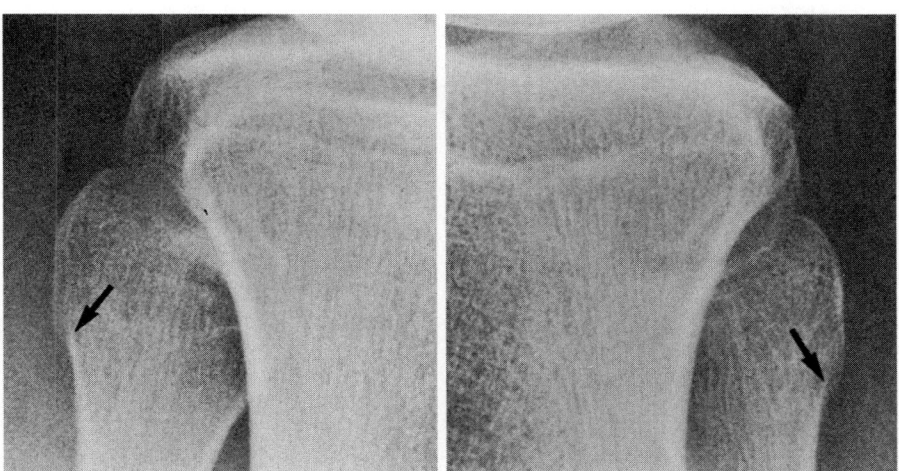

Figure 7–299. Two examples of simulated discontinuity of the cortex of the fibula in lateral projection, which may be mistaken for a fracture.

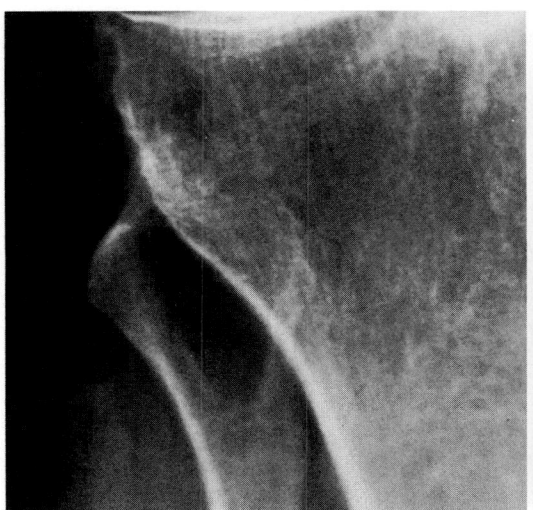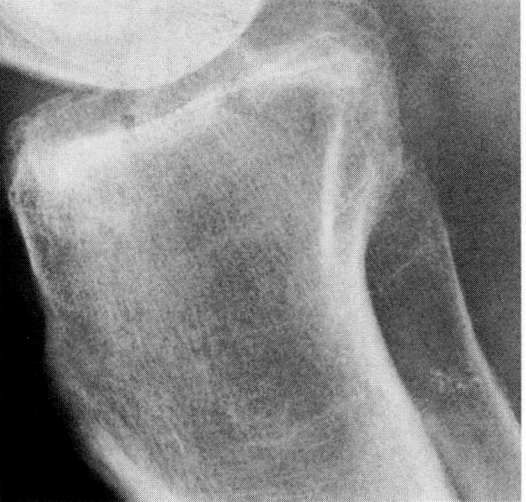

Figure 7–300. Simulated cyst of the head of the fibula as a result of the large amount of cancellous bone present in this area.

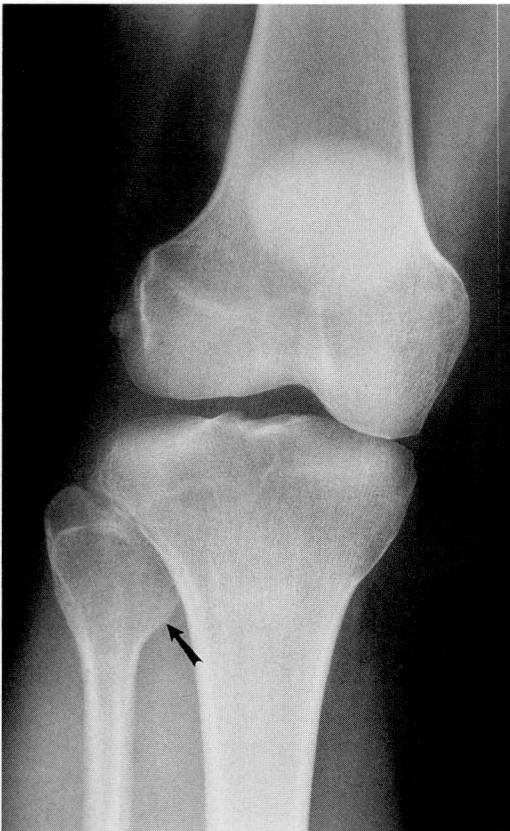

Figure 7–301. Unusual configuration of the proximal fibular metaphysis.

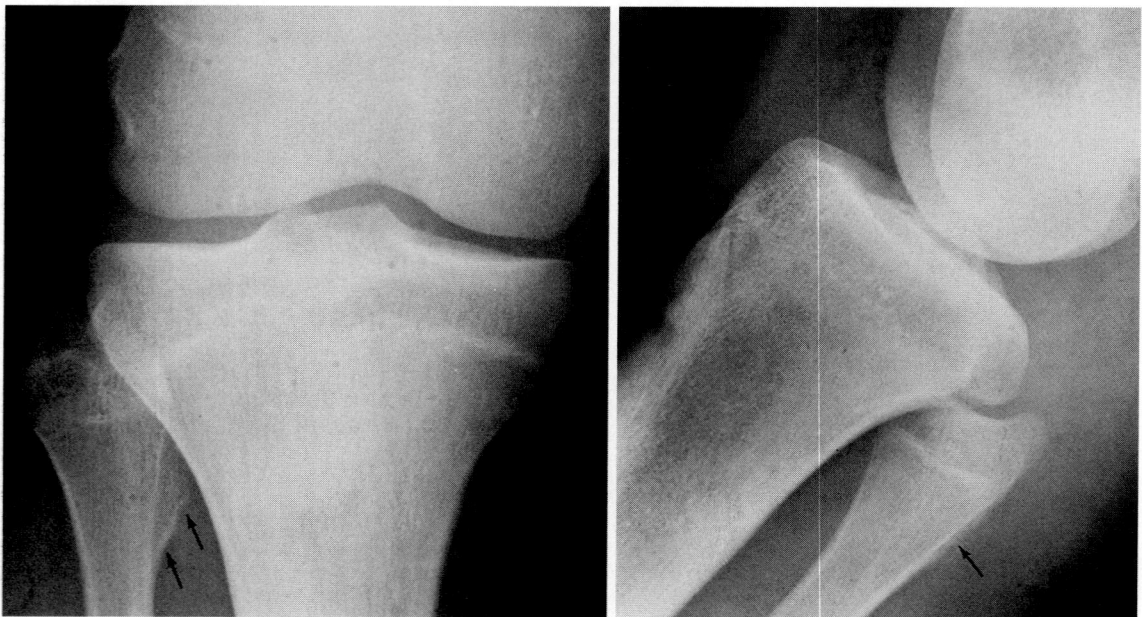

Figure 7–302. Developmental flangelike expansion of the neck of the fibula in a 15-year-old boy.

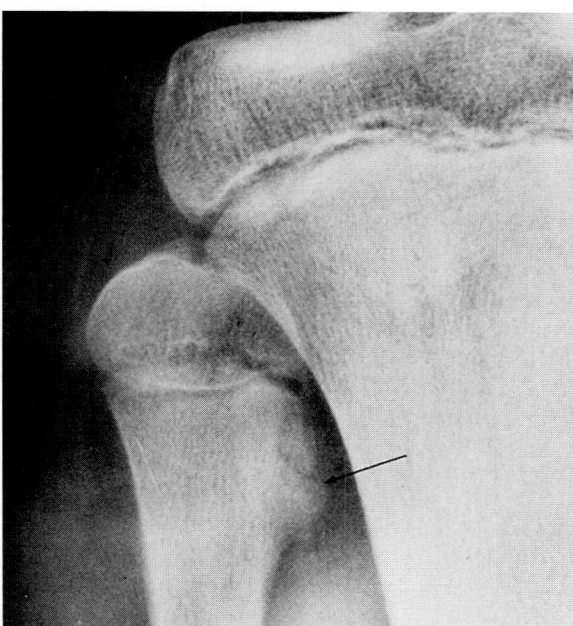

Figure 7–303. Metaphyseal irregularity of the medial aspect of the fibular metaphysis in a 13-year-old boy. This is probably a "tug" lesion in the origin of the soleus muscle.

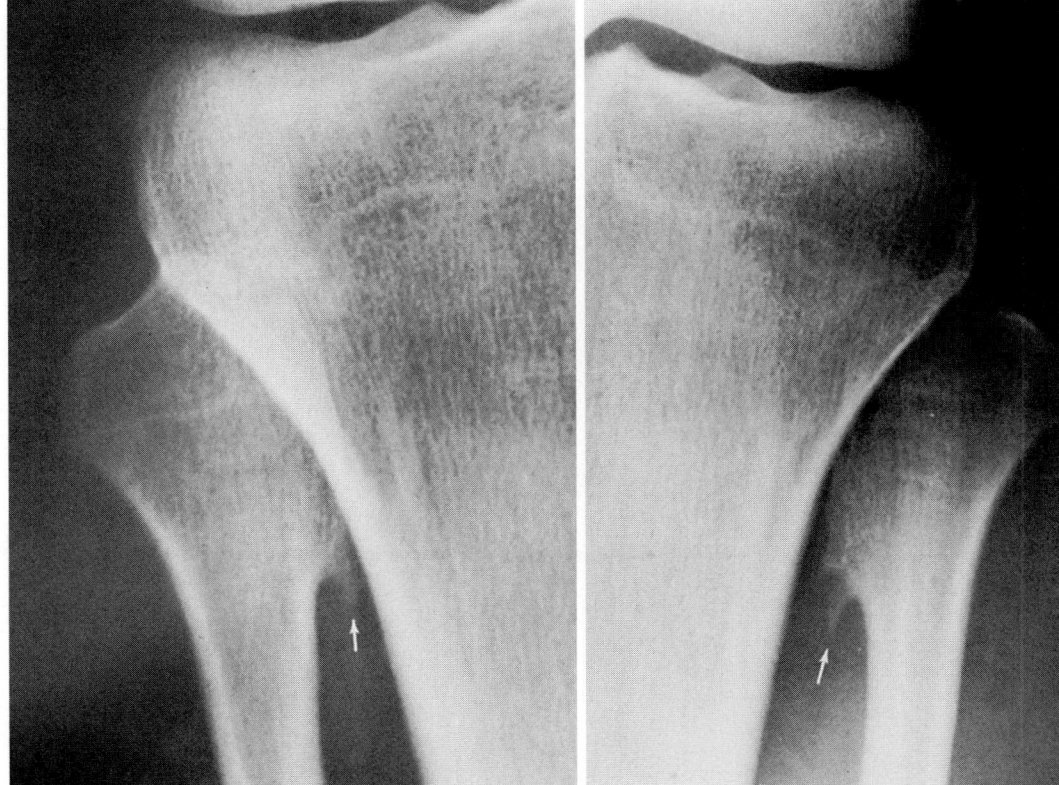

Figure 7–304. "Tug" lesions at the metaphysis of the proximal fibula at the origin of the soleus muscle, not to be mistaken for an osteochondroma.

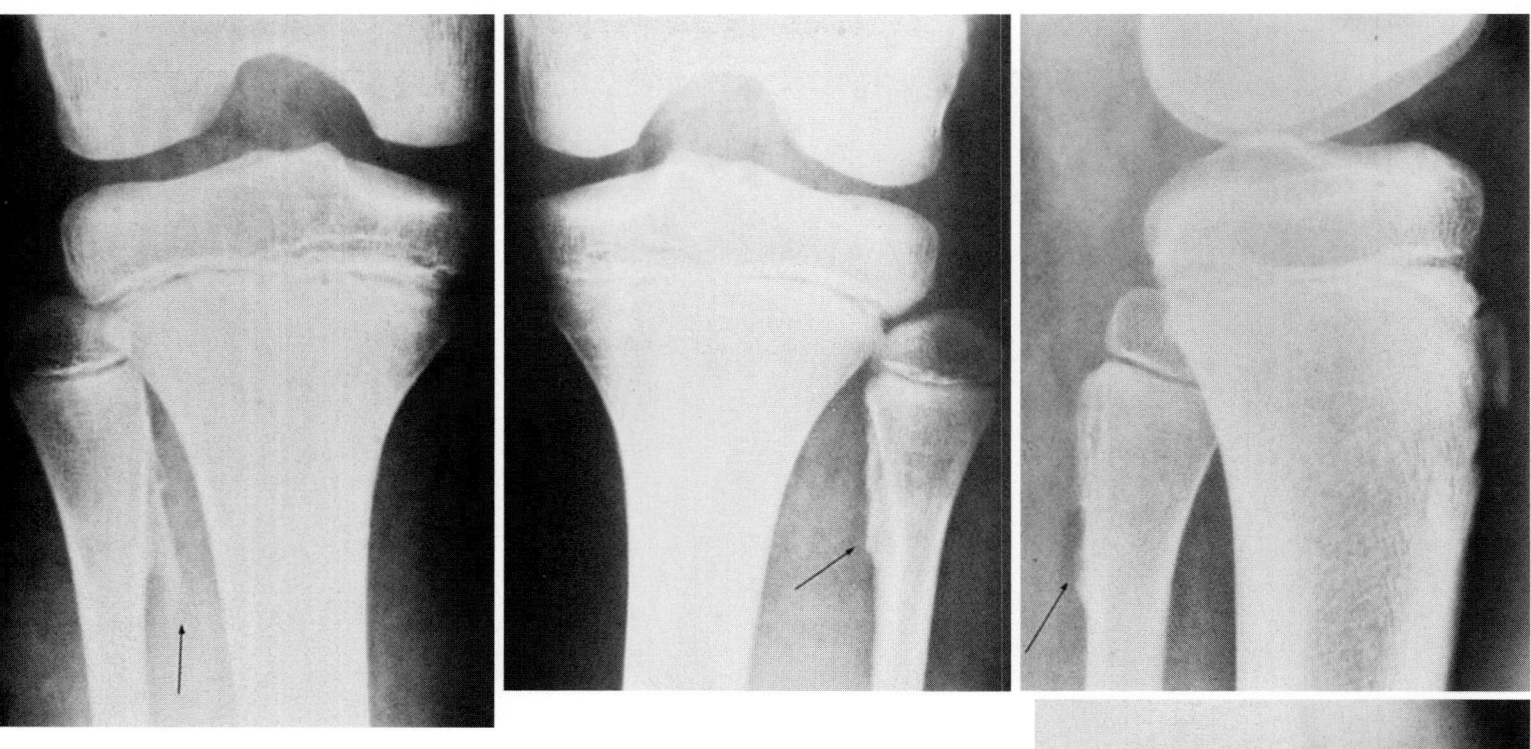

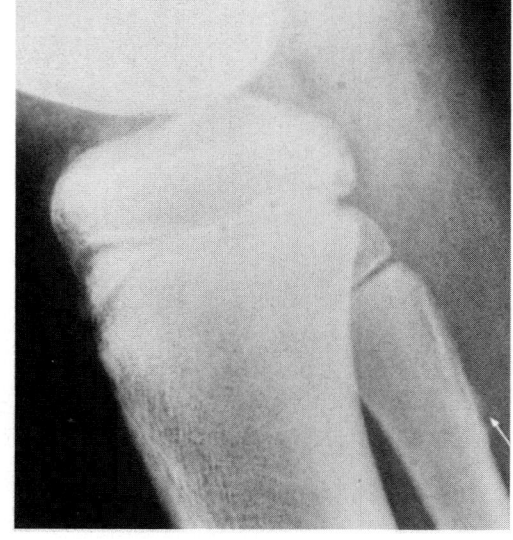

Figure 7–305. Example of marked "tug" lesions of the fibula in a 12-year-old long-distance swimmer. (Courtesy of Dr. John Earwaker.)

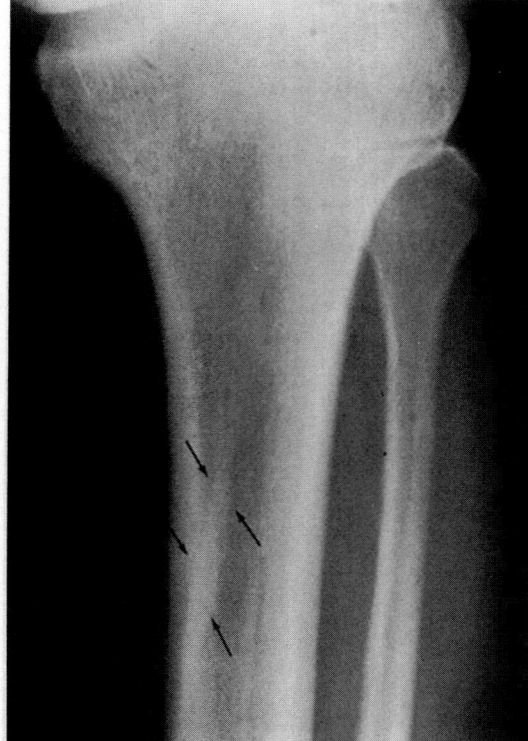

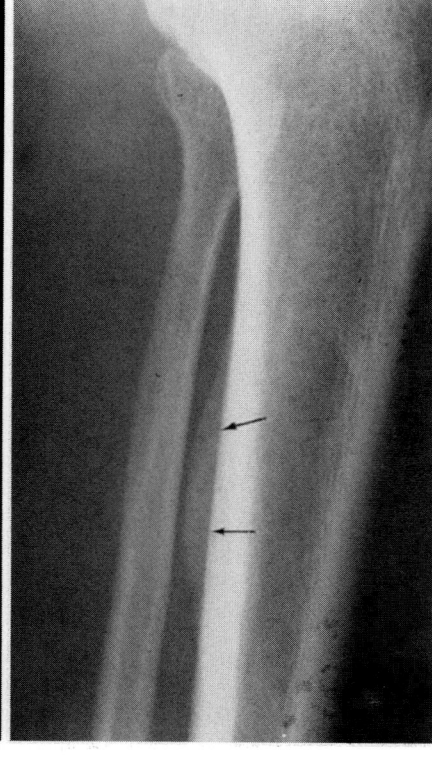

Figure 7–306. The soleal line represents a "tug" lesion at the origin of the soleus muscle. It should not be mistaken for periostitis. (Ref: Levine AH et al: The soleal line: A cause of tibial pseudoperiostitis. *Radiology* 119:79, 1976.)

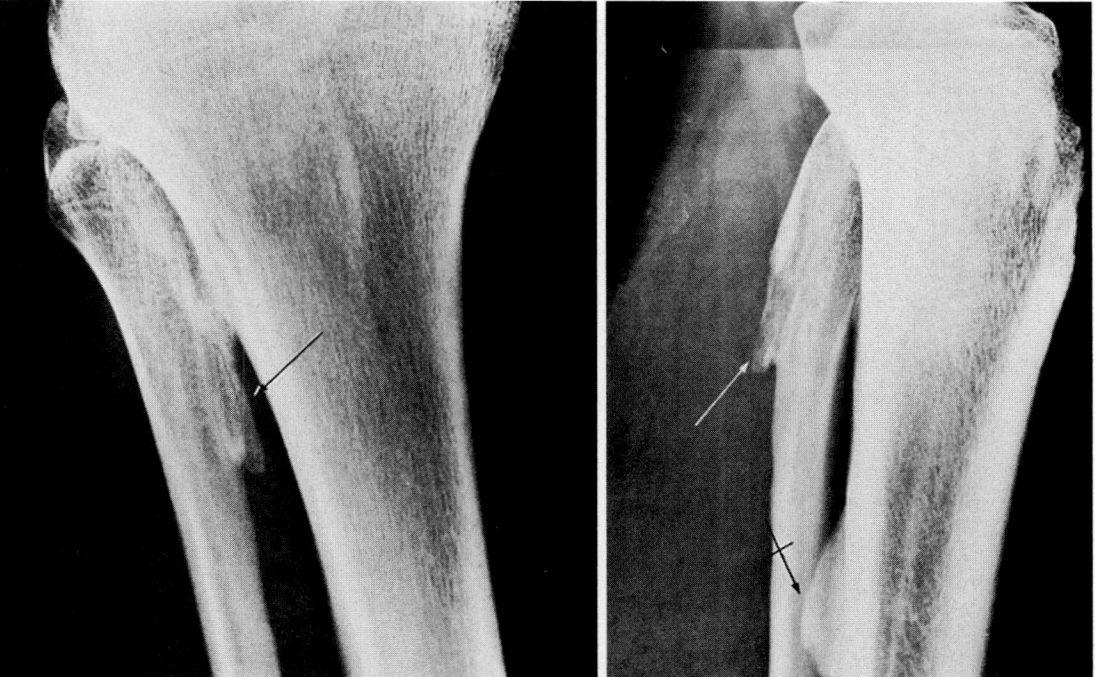

Figure 7–307. "Tug" lesions at both ends of the soleus muscle, producing a fibular spur (←) and the soleal line (↔).

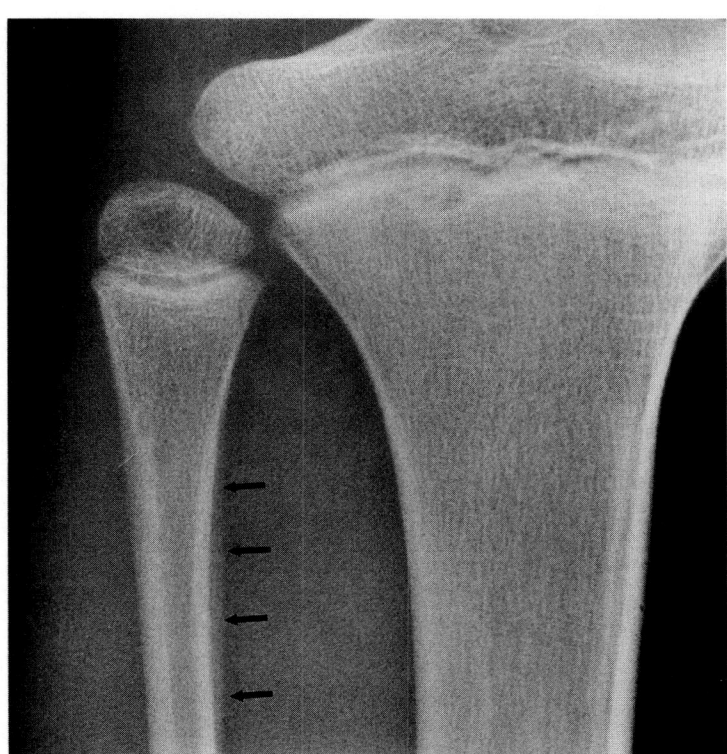

Figure 7–308. Prominence of the interosseous crest in the fibula, simulating periostitis.

The Shafts of the Tibia and Fibula

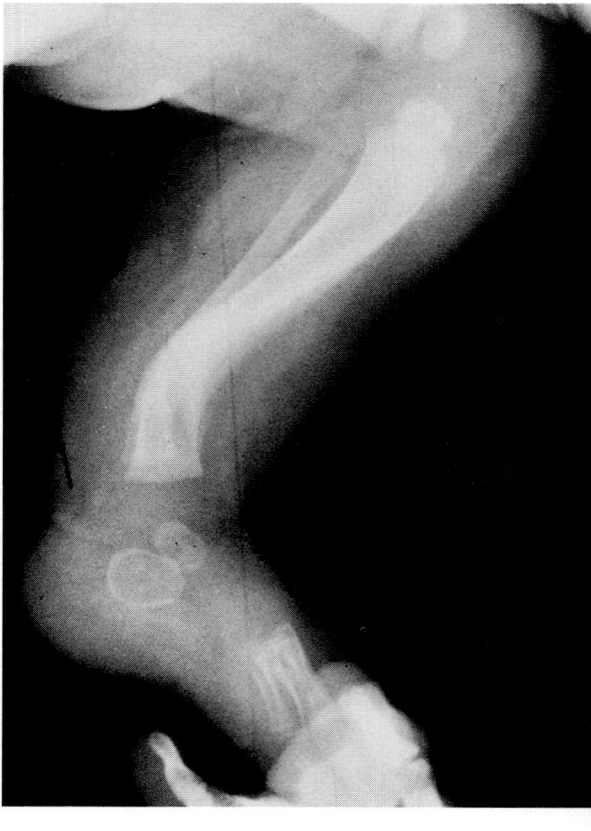

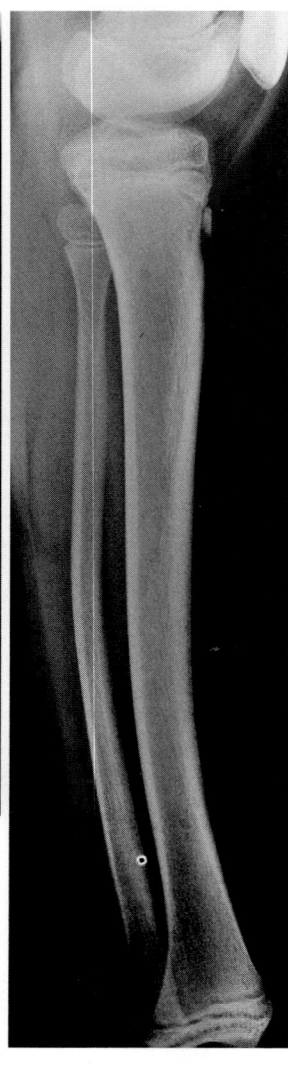

Figure 7–309. Two examples of prenatal posterior bowing of the tibia and fibula, probably relative to faulty fetal positions of the limbs in utero. (Ref: Silverman FN, Kuhn J: *Caffey's pediatric x-ray diagnosis*, 9th ed. St. Louis, Mosby, 1993, p. 1547.)

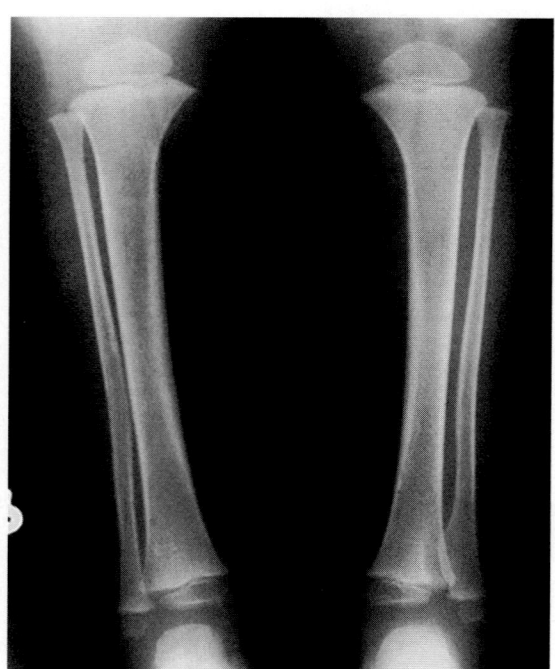

Figure 7–310. Physiologic bowing of the fibulae in a 19-month-old child, which should not be mistaken for plastic bowing fractures.

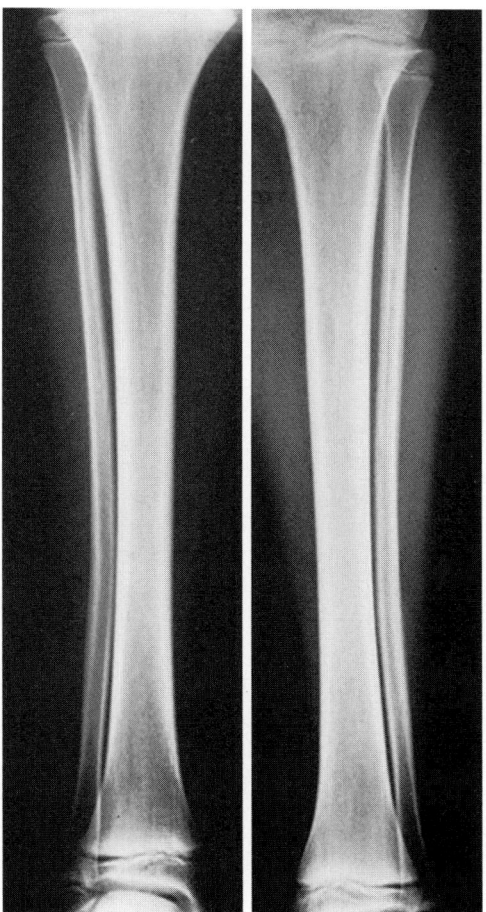

Figure 7–311. Physiologic bowing of the fibulae in an 11-year-old boy.

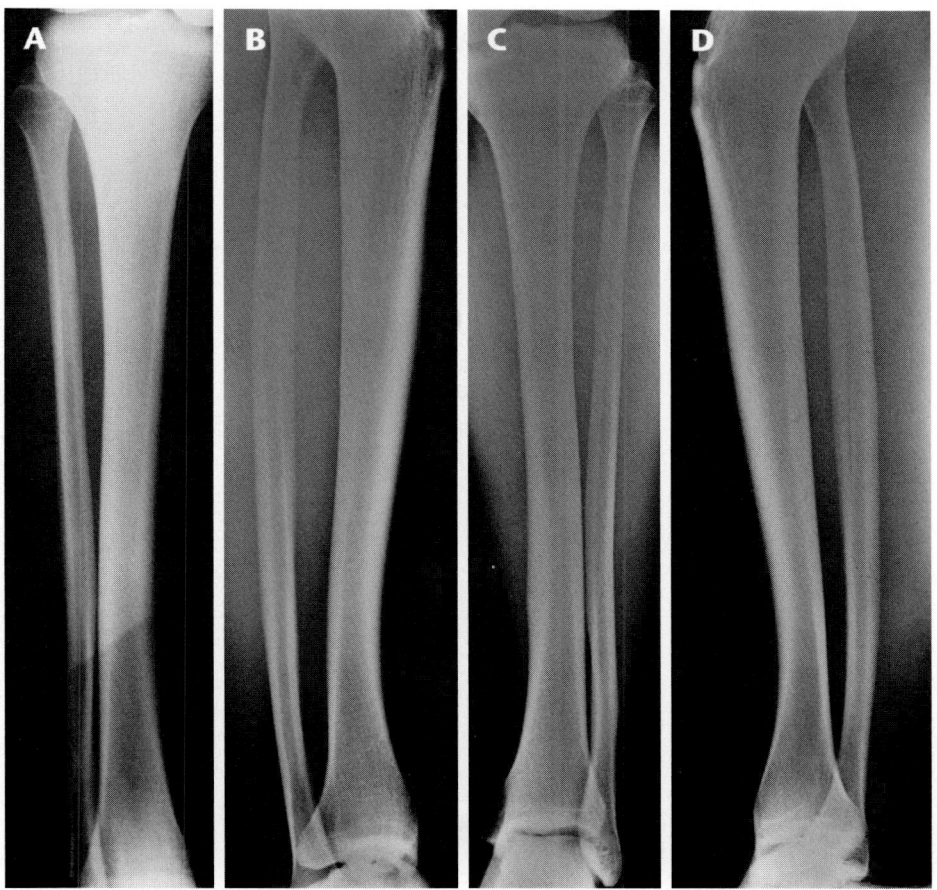

Figure 7–312. Physiologic bowing of the tibiae and fibulae in a 25-year-old man. **A** and **B,** Right leg. **C** and **D,** Left leg.

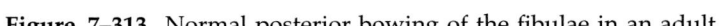
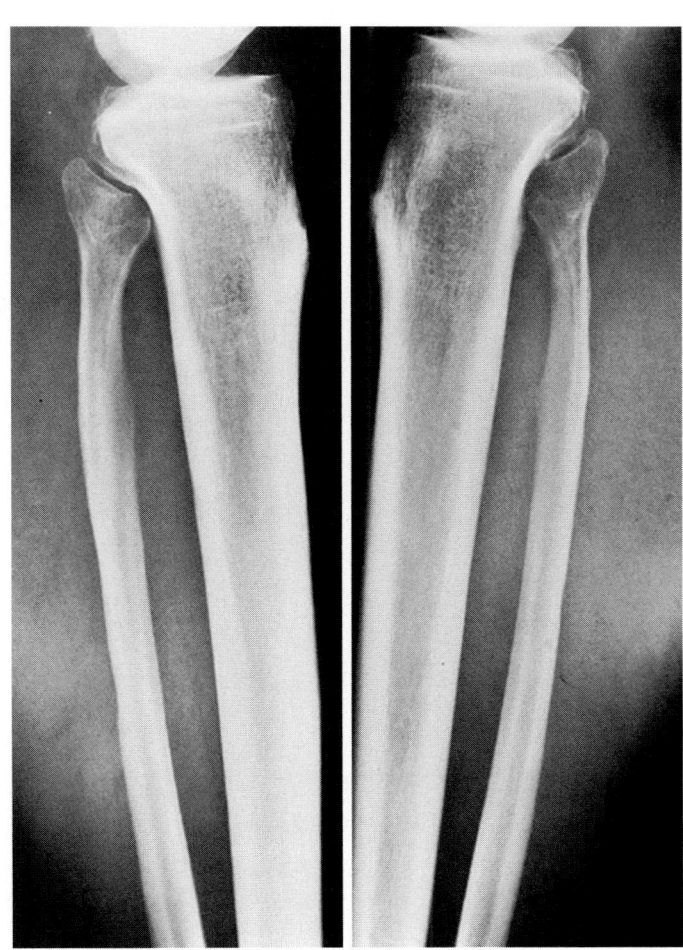

Figure 7–313. Normal posterior bowing of the fibulae in an adult.

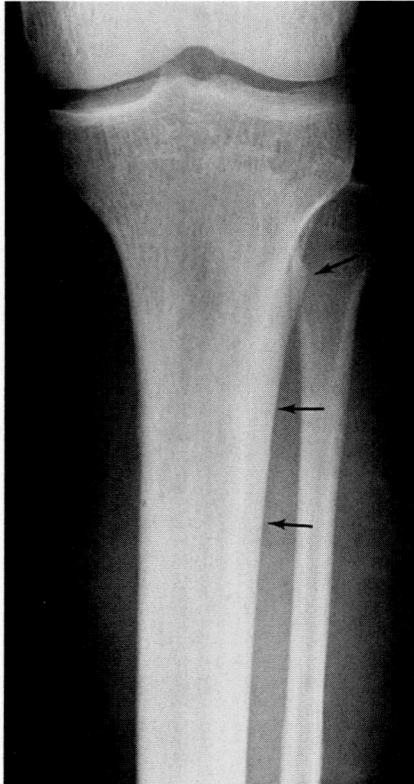

Figure 7–314. Spurious thickening of the lateral cortex of the tibia caused by slight external rotation of the leg. The density is due to the fact that the anterior tibial crest comes progressively more into profile. (Ref: Caffey J: *Pediatric x-ray diagnosis*, 9th ed. St Louis, Mosby, 1993, p. 1509.)

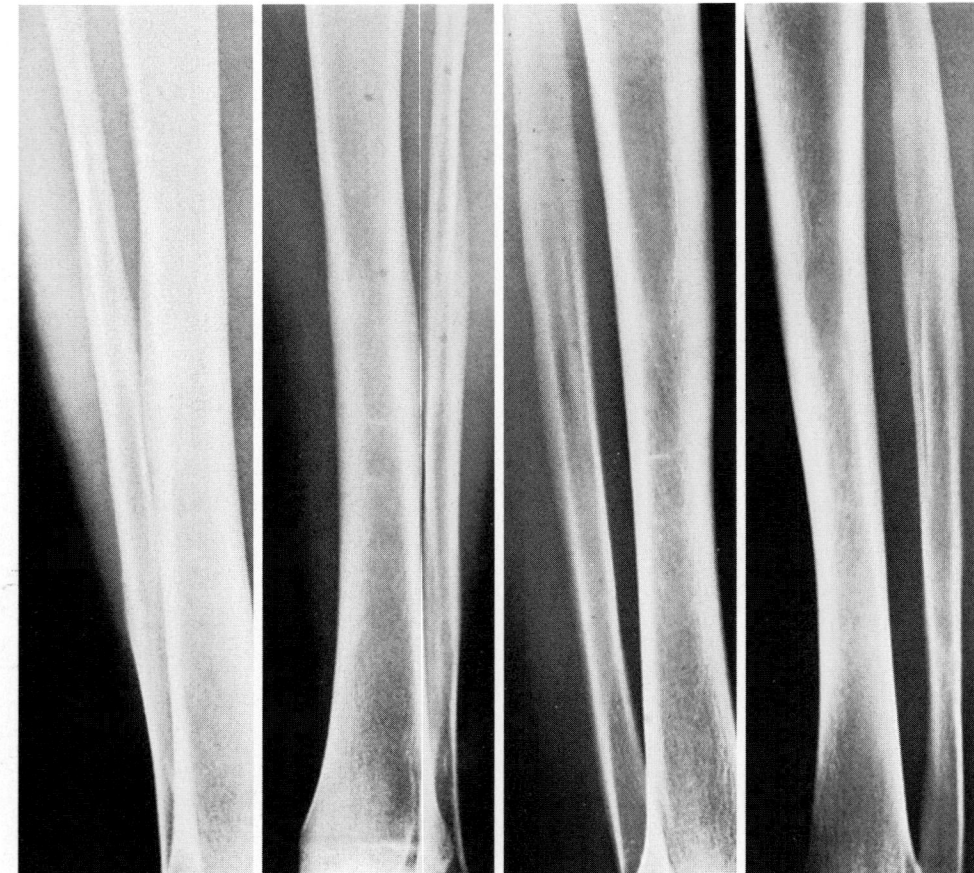

Figure 7–315. Normal cortical irregularities of the shafts of the fibulae. *Left,* Frontal projections. *Right,* Lateral projections.

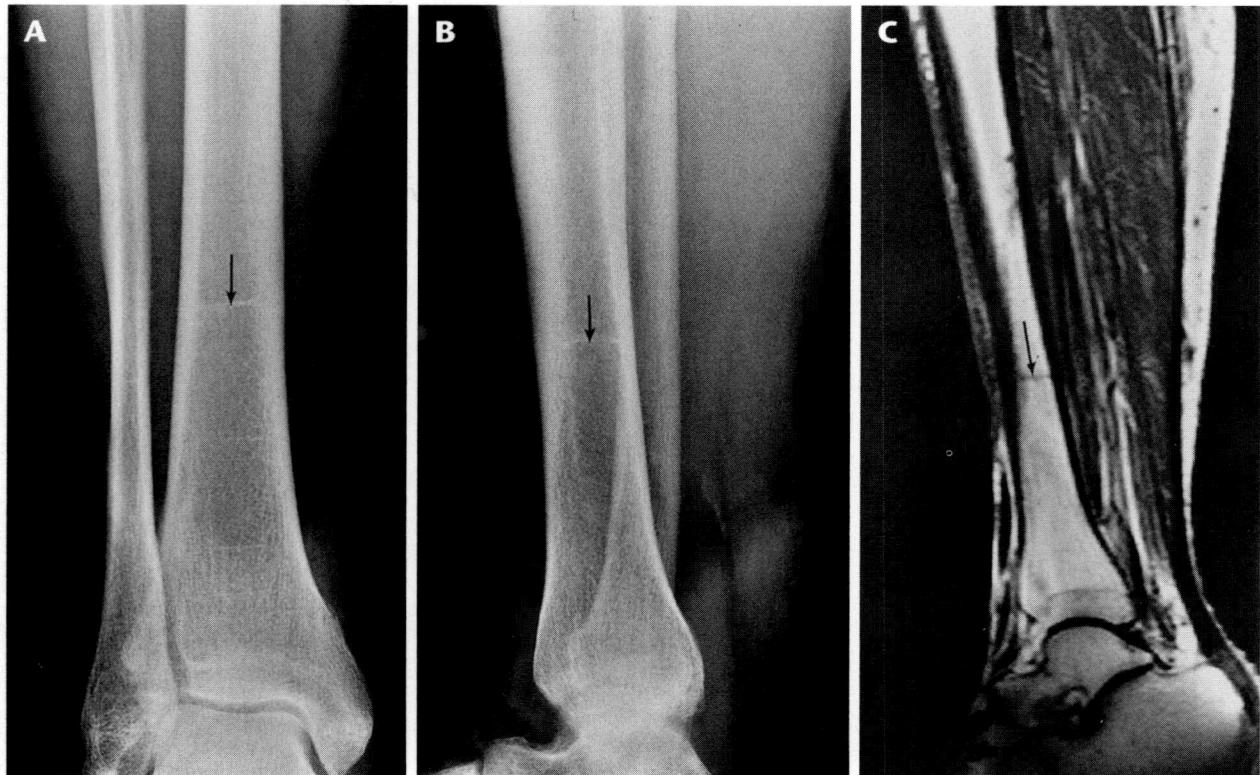

Figure 7–316. Transverse (growth arrest) line of the tibia. **A,** Frontal projection. **B,** Lateral projection. **C,** Sagittal T-1–weighted MR image.

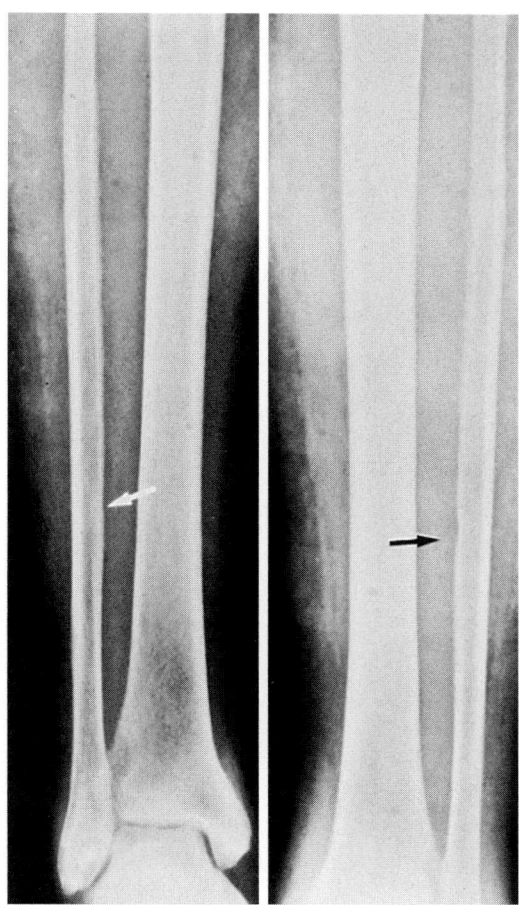

Figure 7–317. Localized bilateral symmetric undulations in the fibular cortex.

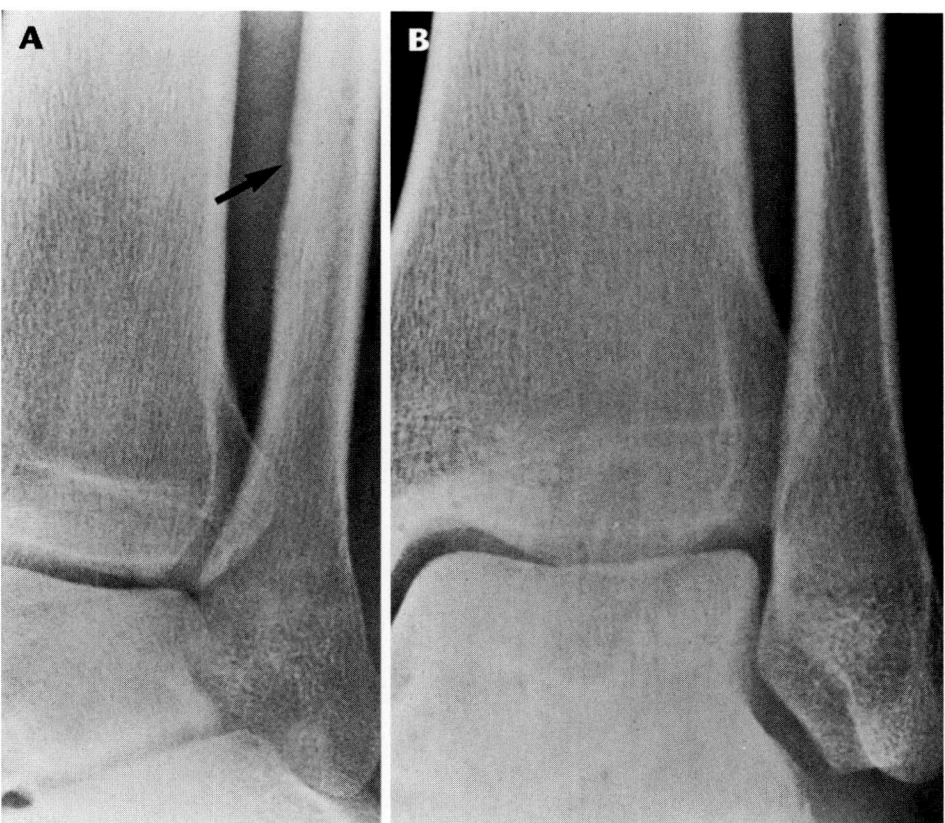

Figure 7–318. A, Notchlike lesion in distal fibula seen in the oblique projection. Note similarity to a notchlike defect in the humerus (Fig. 6–54). **B,** Lesion is not seen in the frontal projection.

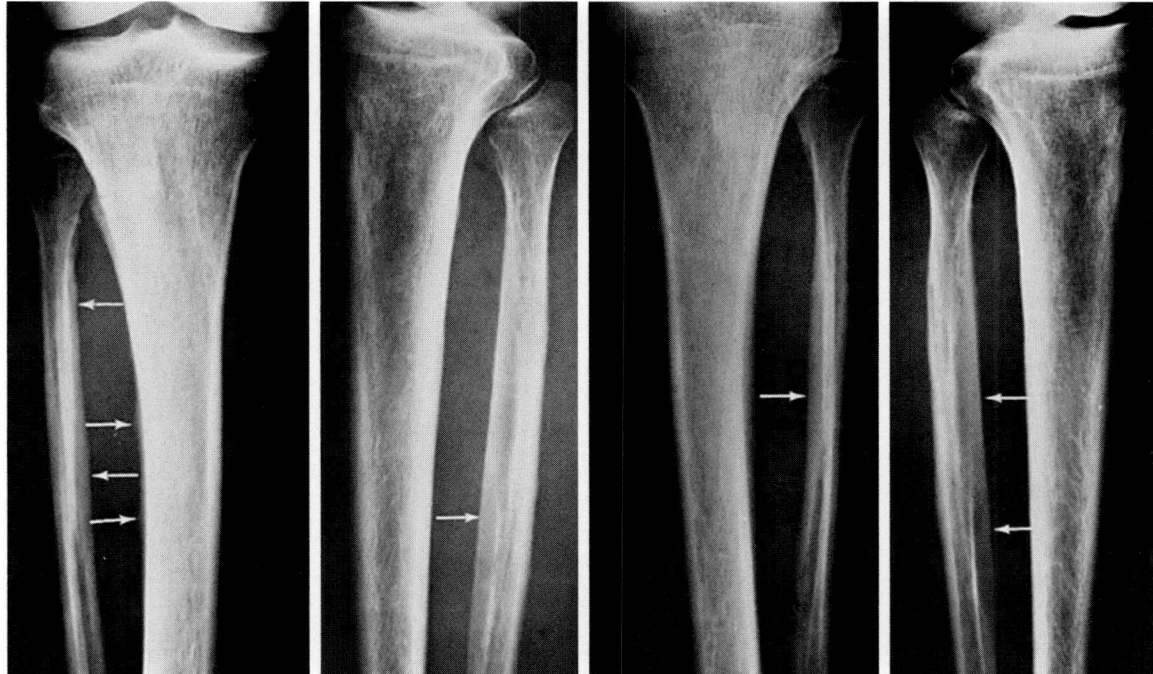

Figure 7–319. Normal irregularities of the cortices of the tibia and fibula caused by ossification of the interosseous membrane.

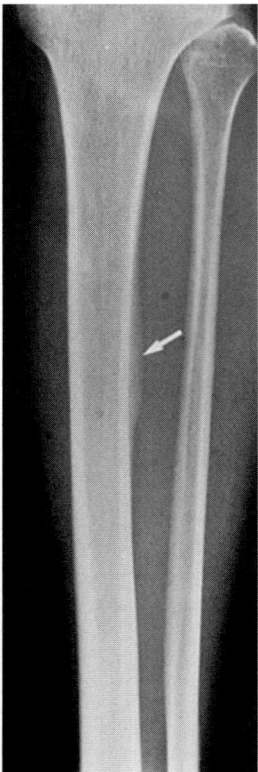

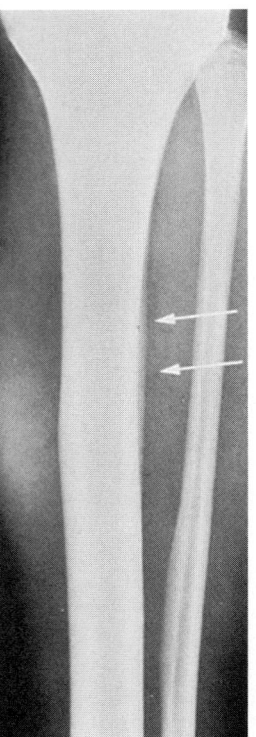

Figure 7–321. Localized ossification in the interosseous membrane.

Figure 7–320. Simulated isolated periostitis of the tibia as in Figure 7–319.

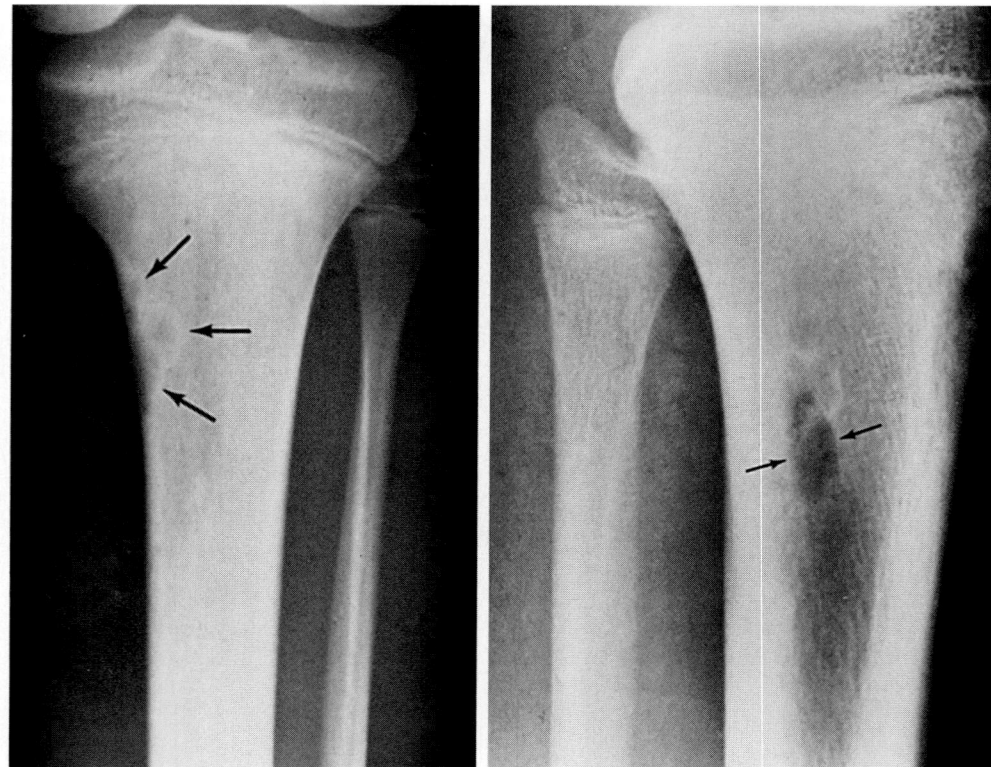

Figure 7–322. Two examples of juvenile benign cortical defects of the tibia. These lesions are common in the tibia and are of no clinical significance. (Ref: Caffey J: *Pediatric x-ray diagnosis*, 9th ed. St Louis, Mosby, 1993, p. 1499.)

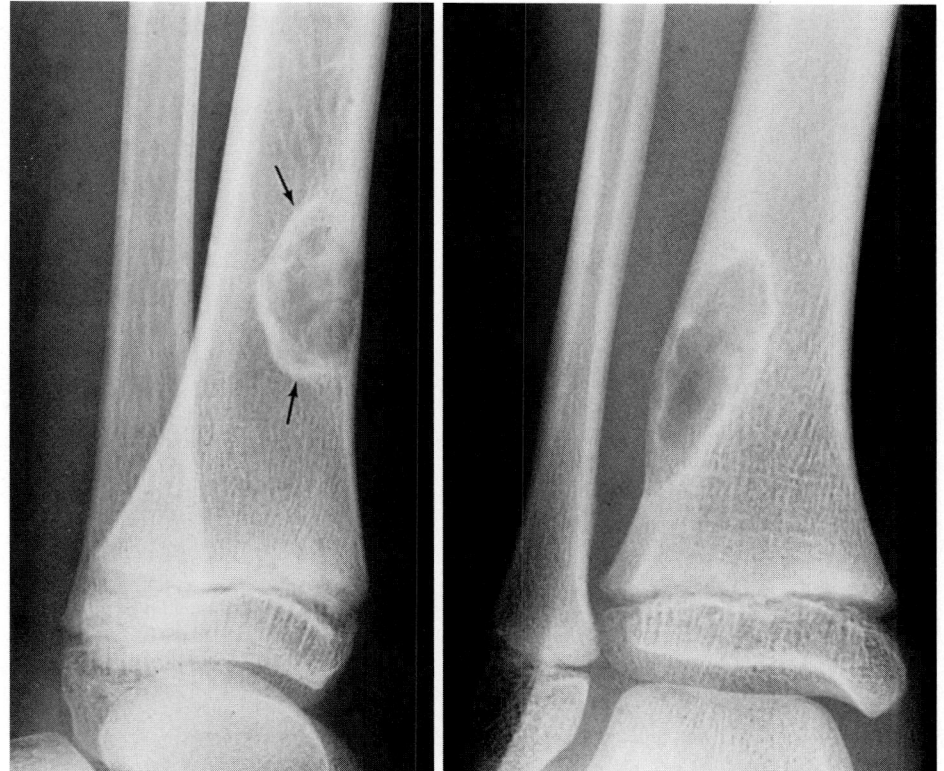

Figure 7–323. Two additional examples of benign cortical defects of the tibia.

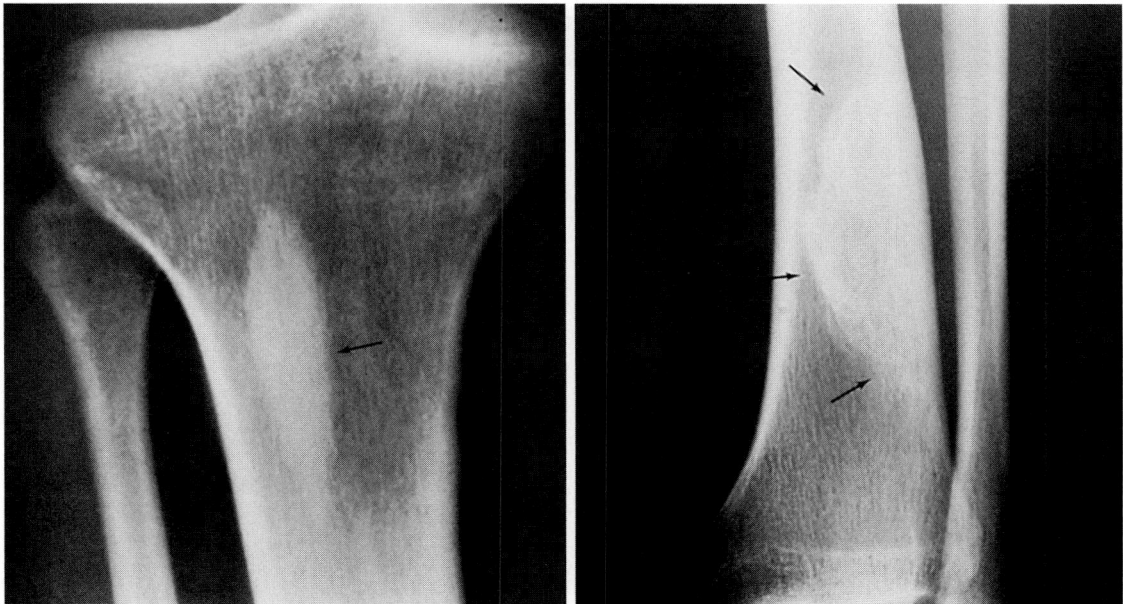

Figure 7–324. Two examples of healed juvenile benign cortical defects.

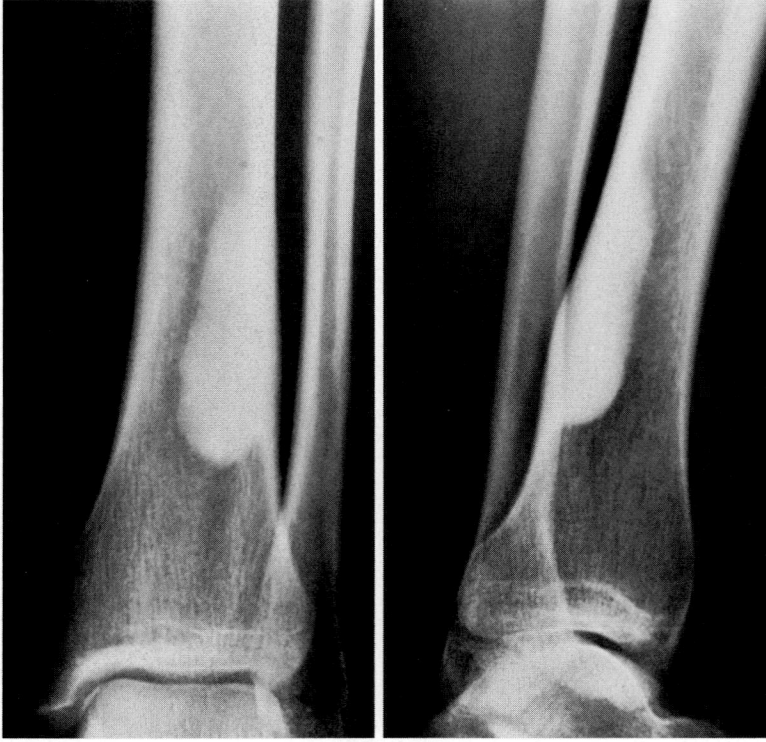

Figure 7–325. Very dense healed benign cortical defects.

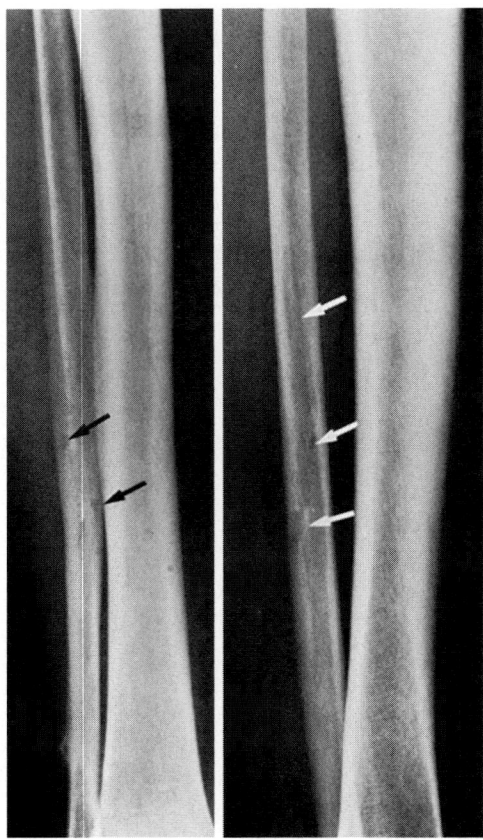

Figure 7–326. Nutrient vascular channels of the fibula.

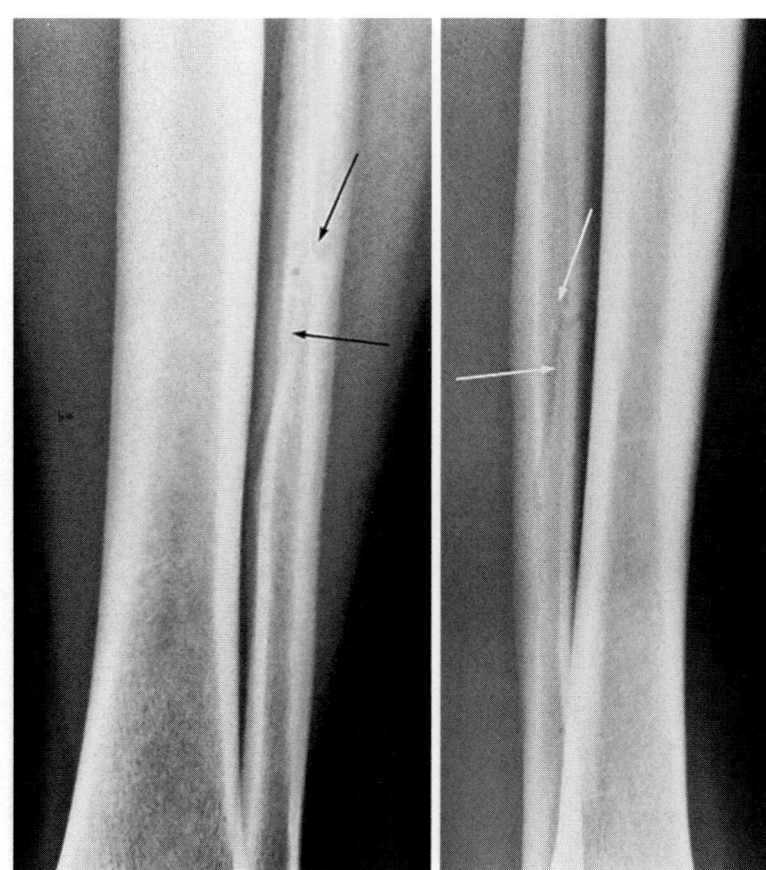

Figure 7–327. Nutrient channels of the fibula mistaken for fracture.

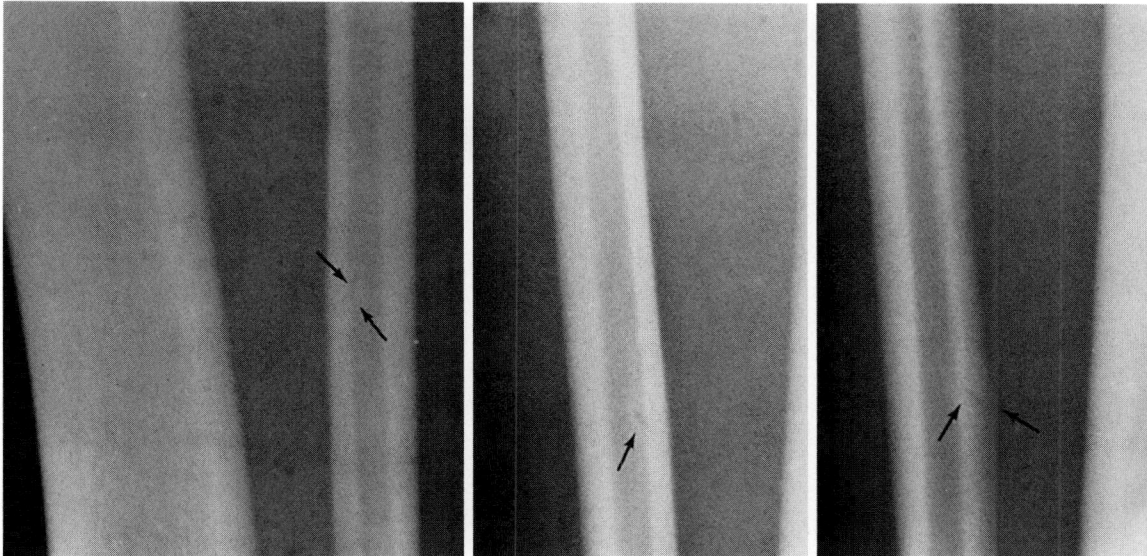

Figure 7–328. Three examples of nutrient foramina of the fibula that might be mistaken for fractures. (Ref: Lee J-H: Nutrient canal of the fibula. *Skeletal Radiol* 29:22, 2000.)

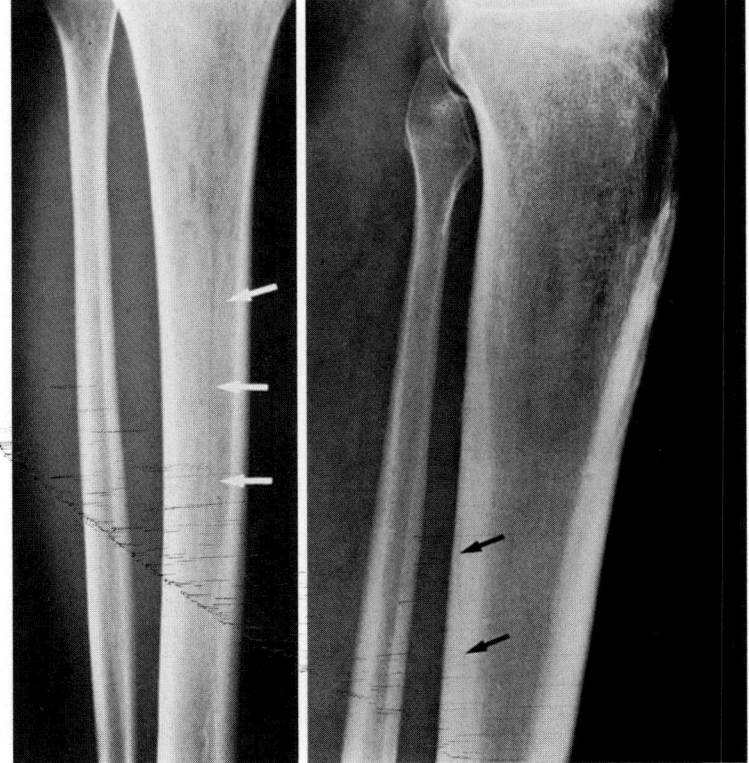

Figure 7–329. The nutrient channel of the tibia.

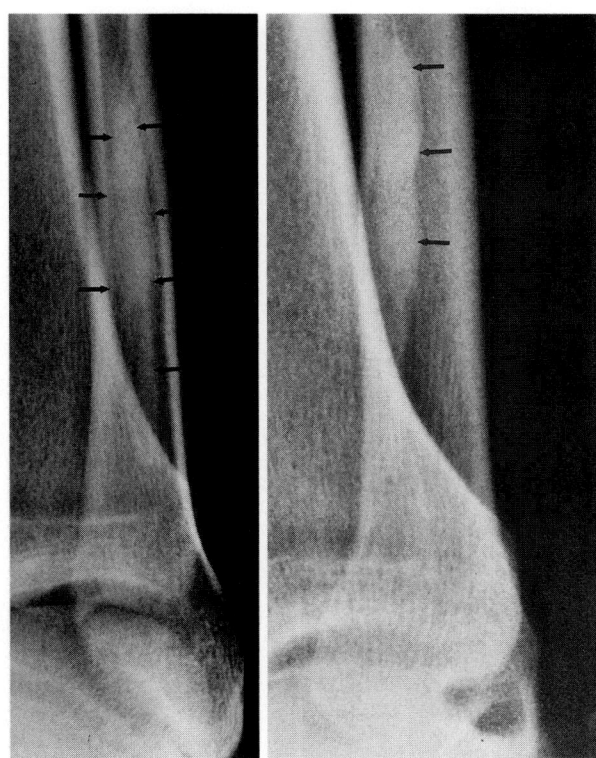

Figure 7–330. Large healed benign cortical defect of the fibula, an unusual site for this lesion.

The Distal Ends of the Tibia and Fibula

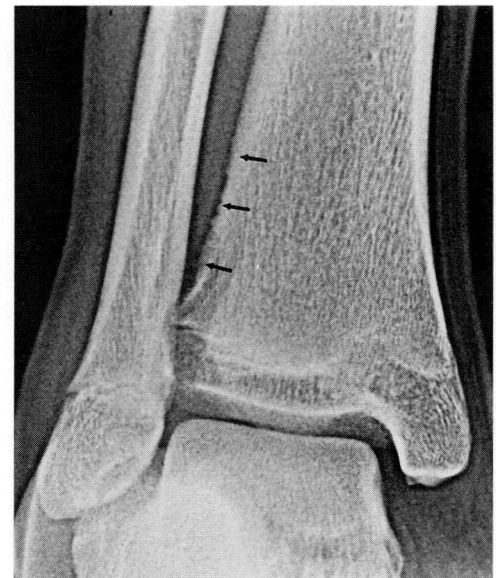

Figure 7–331. Normal metaphyseal irregularity of the tibia in a 14-year-old boy.

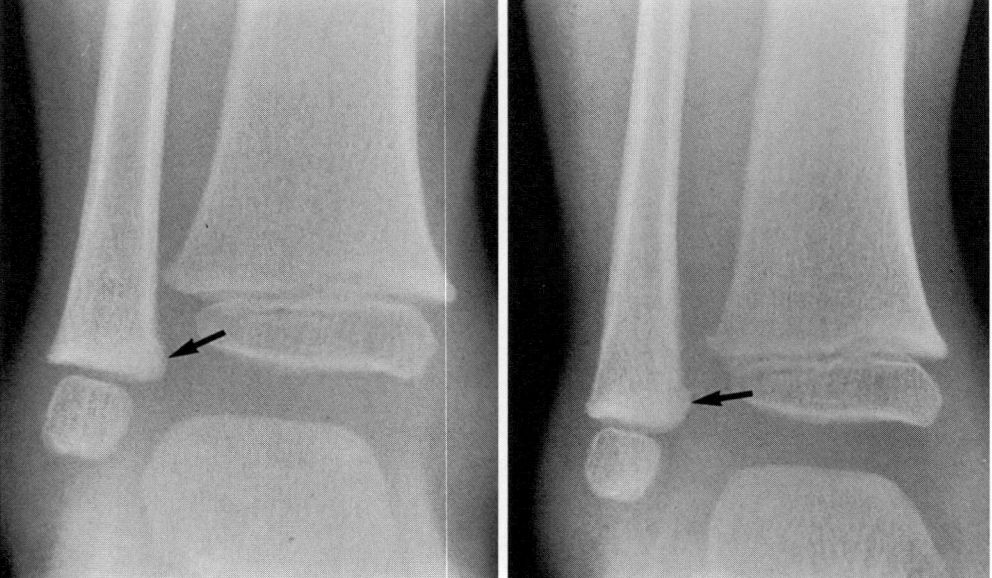

Figure 7–332. Normal bump in the medial cortex of the distal fibula of a 2-year-old child, which may simulate a torus fracture.

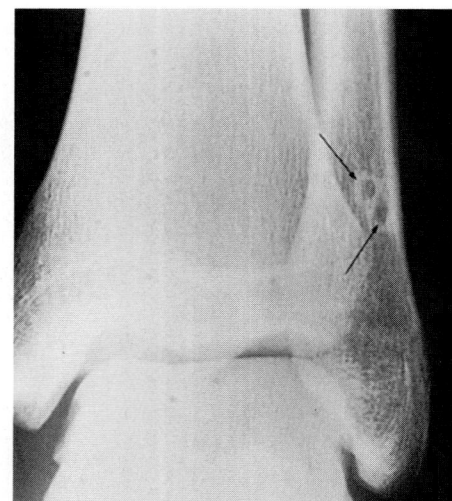

Figure 7–333. Ringlike lesions of the distal fibula. These are probably similar in nature to those seen in the proximal end of the tibia (Fig. 7–271) and are of no clinical significance.

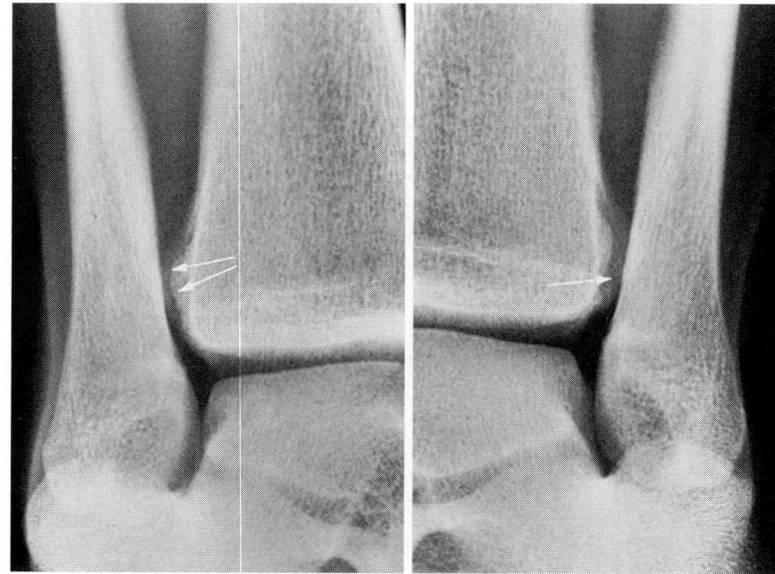

Figure 7–334. Tibial flange that might be mistaken for an avulsion fracture.

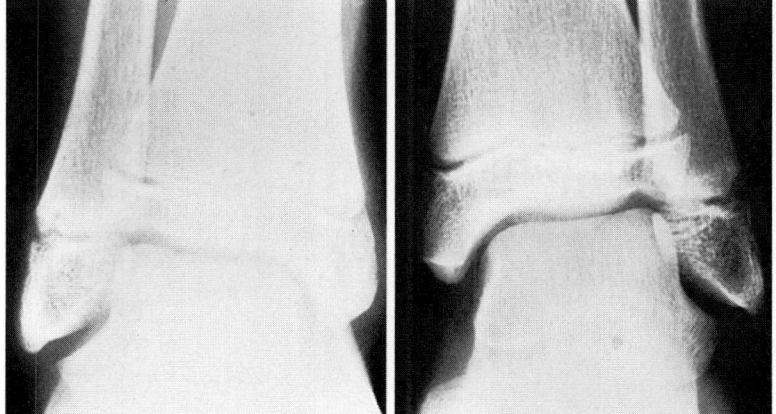

Figure 7–335. Normal radiolucencies in the distal fibular epiphyses.

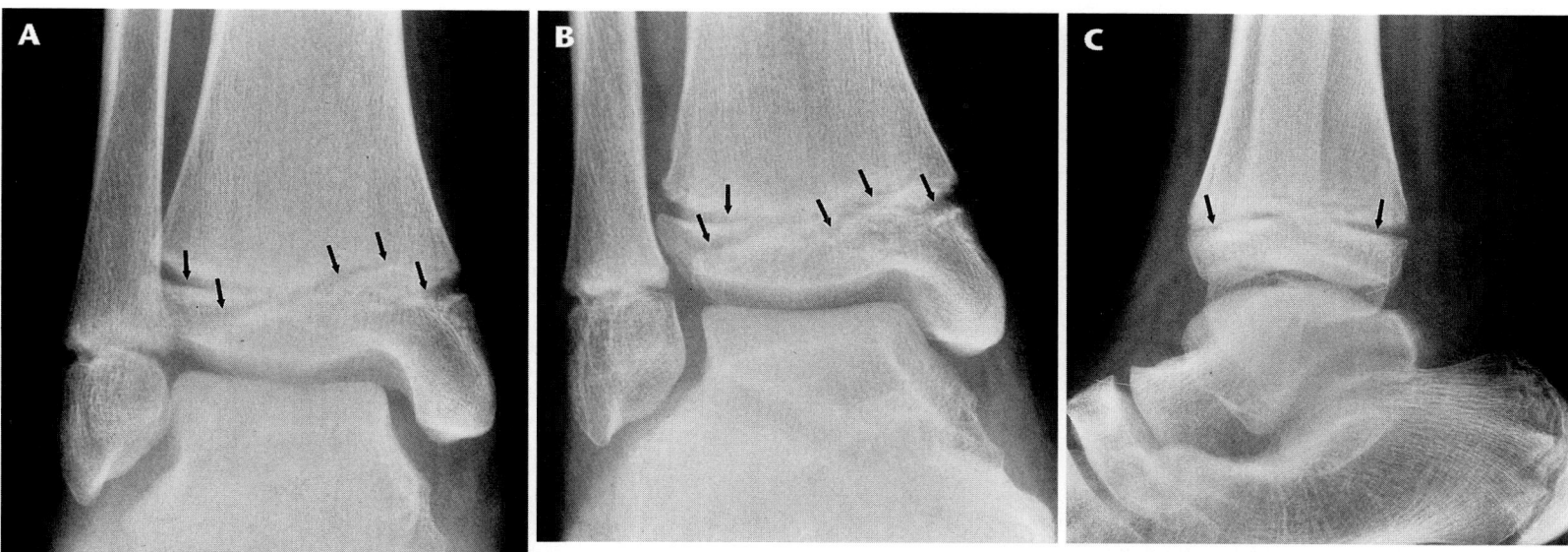

Figure 7–336. Normal 10-year-old. The physis may appear at different positions in the various projections and can be mistaken for evidence of an epiphyseal fracture. **A,** Anteroposterior projection. **B,** Oblique projection. **C,** Lateral projection. (Ref: Chung J, Jaramillo D: Normal maturing distal tibia and fibula: Changes with age at MR imaging. *Radiology* 194:227, 1995.)

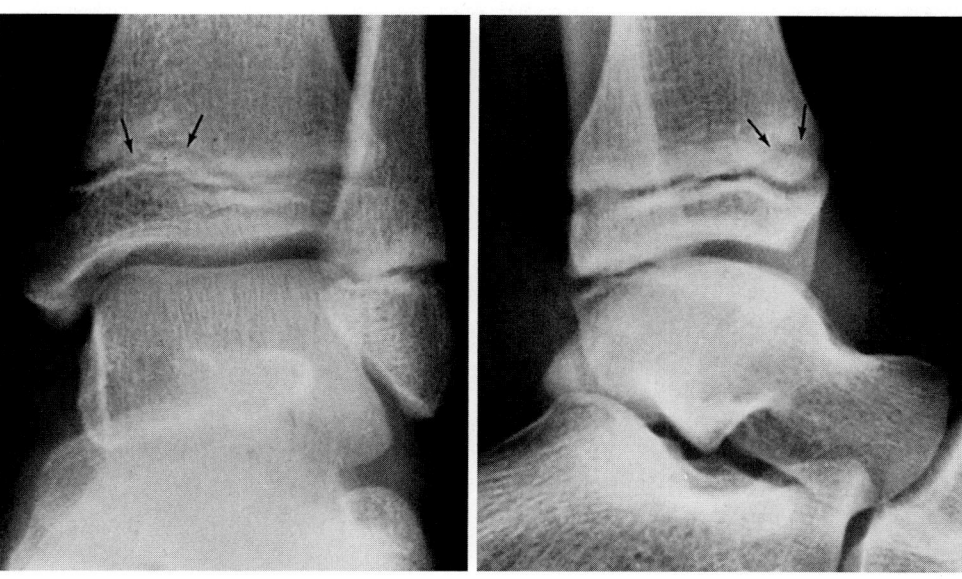

Figure 7–337. Normal localized angulation of the distal epiphyseal plate of the tibia in an 11-year-old boy (Kumphump). (Ref: Kump WL: Vertical fracture of the distal tibial epiphysis. *Am J Roentgenol* 97:676, 1966.)

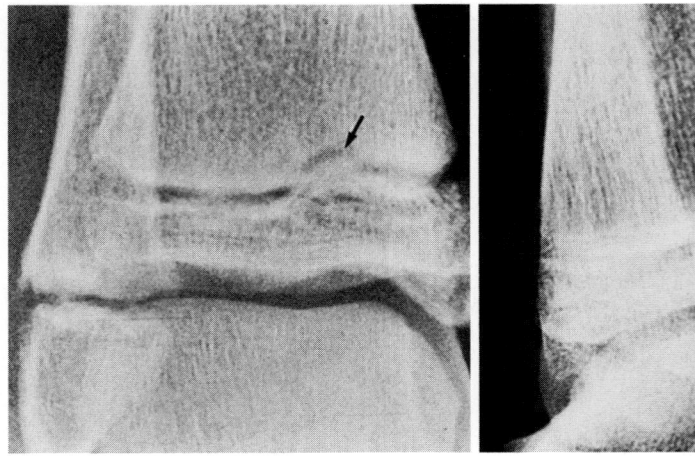

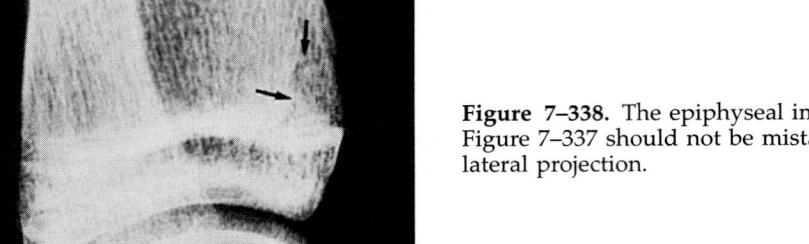

Figure 7–338. The epiphyseal impression illustrated in Figure 7–337 should not be mistaken for a fracture in the lateral projection.

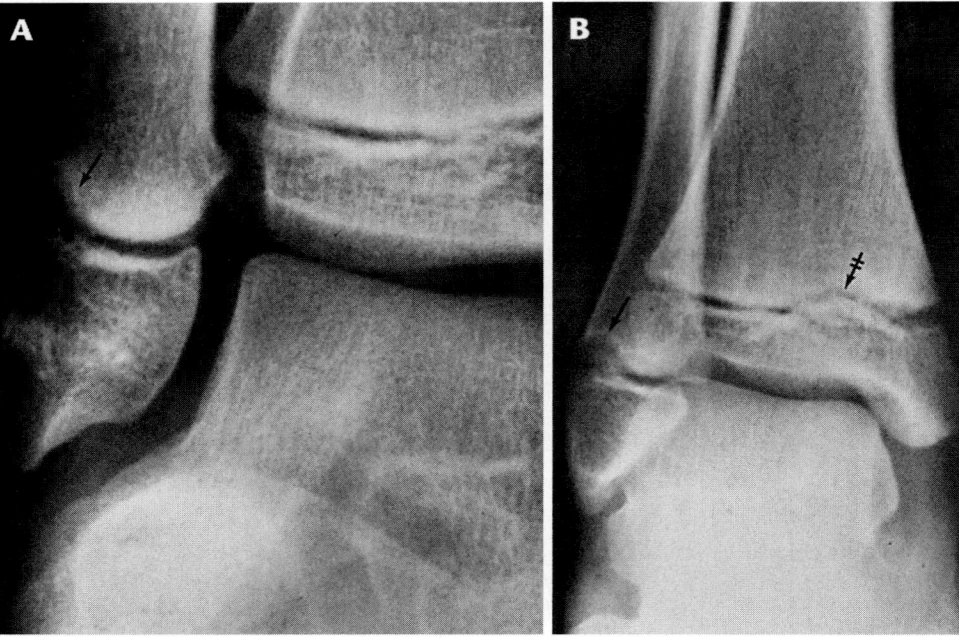

Figure 7–339. A, B, Two examples of normal localized depressions in the metaphyses of the distal fibula in 11-year-old boys (←). The angulation of the distal tibial epiphysis is also seen in **B** (⊬). (Ref: Ogden JA, McCarthy SM: Radiology of postnatal skeletal development. VIII. Distal tibia and fibula. *Skeletal Radiol* 10:209, 1983.)

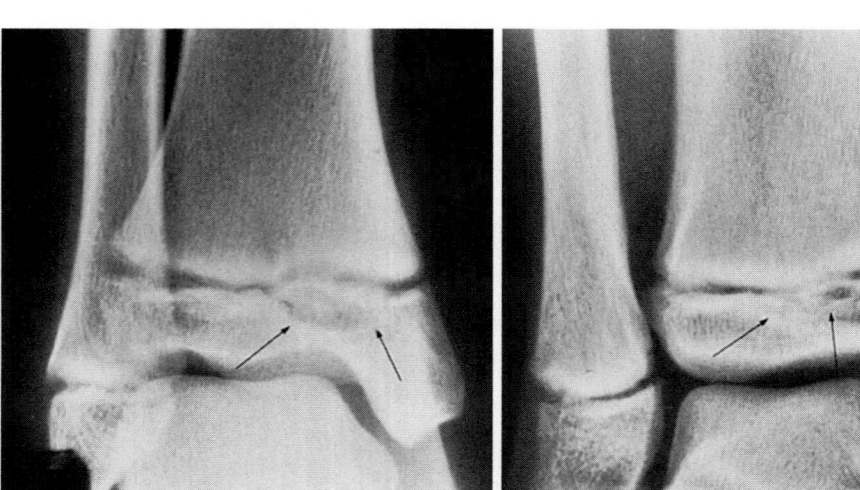

Figure 7–340. Occasionally the depression of the epiphyseal plate seen in Figures 7–337 and 7–339 may extend inferiorly into the epiphysis, rather than into the metaphysis.

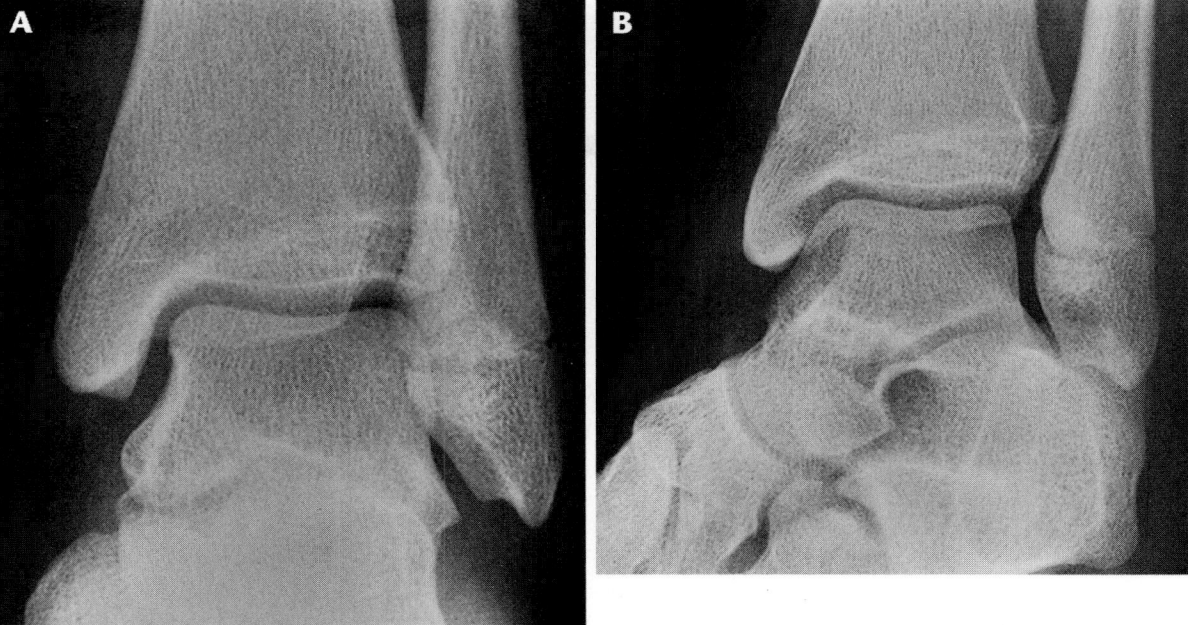

Figure 7–341. Discordant closure of the distal tibial and fibular physes in an 11-year-old girl. These closure rates cannot be reliably used to exclude a Salter-Harris Type I fracture of either bone. **A,** Frontal film. **B,** Oblique projection.

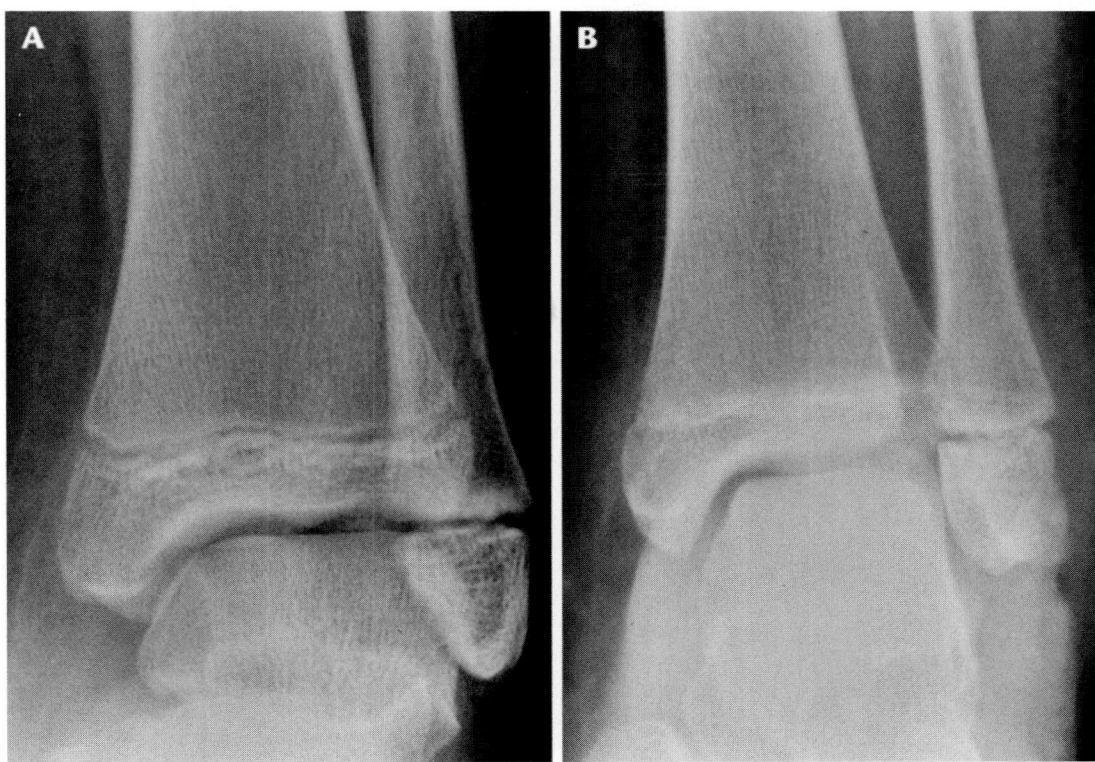

Figure 7–342. Another example of discordant maturation between the tibia and the fibula in the same subject. **A,** Age 9. **B,** Age 12.

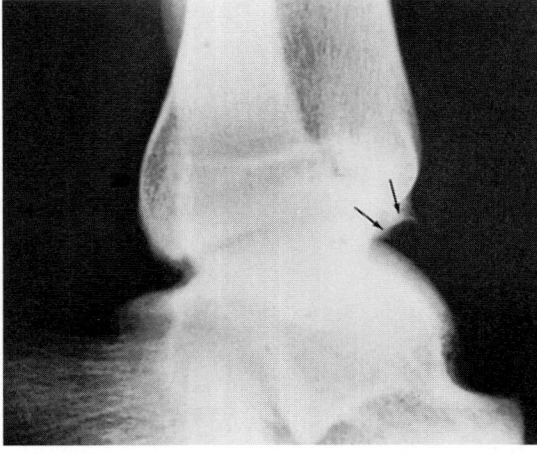

Figure 7–343. Exaggeration of the normal notch on the anterior surface of the distal portion of the tibia.

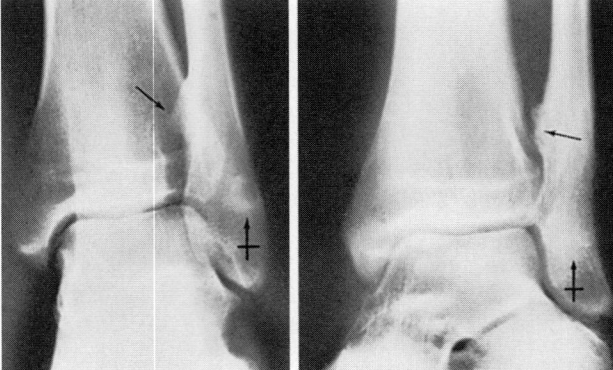

Figure 7–344. Calcification of the syndesmotic membrane (←). There is also an accessory bone at the lateral aspect of the distal fibula (↤).

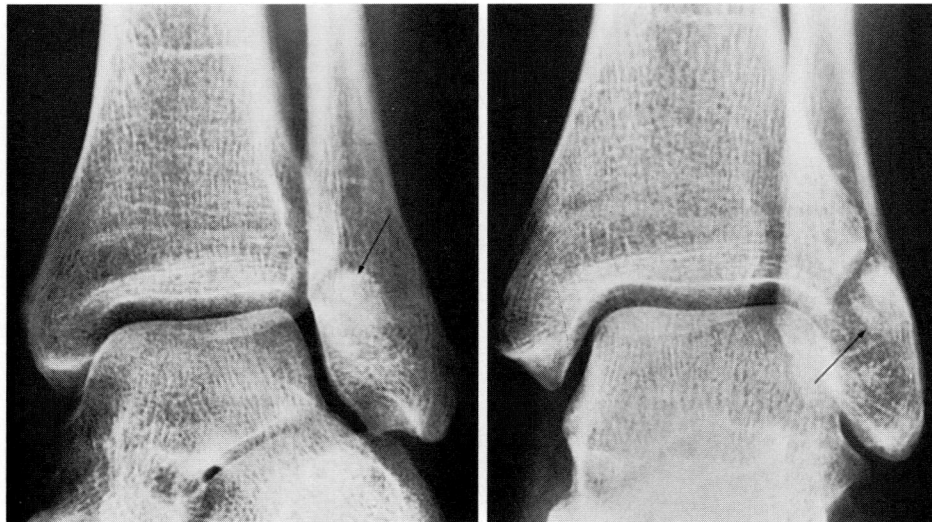

Figure 7–345. Another example of the accessory bone seen in Figure 7–344.

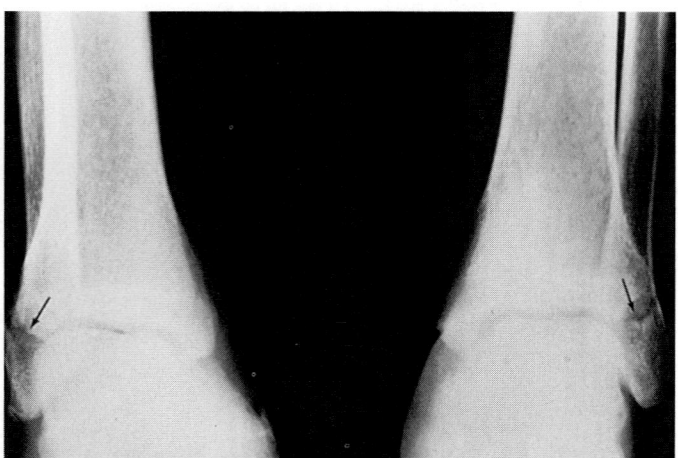

Figure 7–346. Overlapping of shadows of tibia and fibula, simulating fractures of the lateral malleoli.

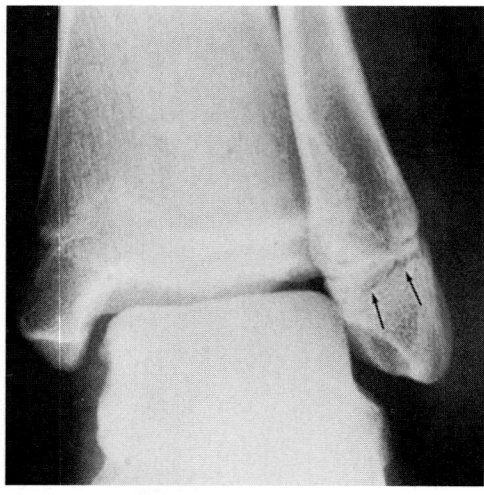

Figure 7–347. Simulated fracture of the lateral malleolus by the epiphyseal line.

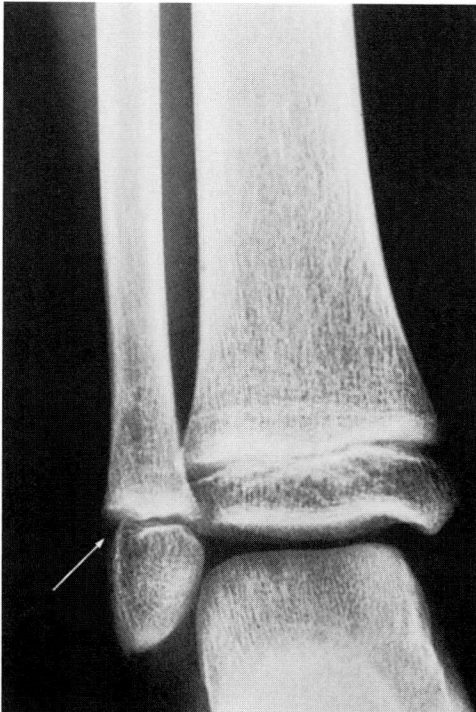

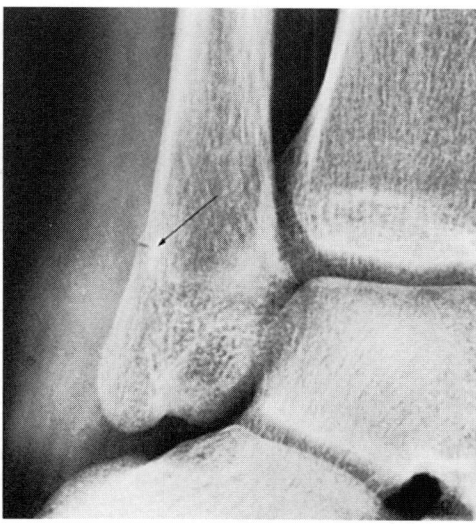

Figure 7–349. Closing epiphyseal line in a 13-year-old boy, misinterpreted as a fracture.

Figure 7–348. Normal offset of the distal fibular epiphysis, which might be mistaken for a fracture through the epiphyseal line.

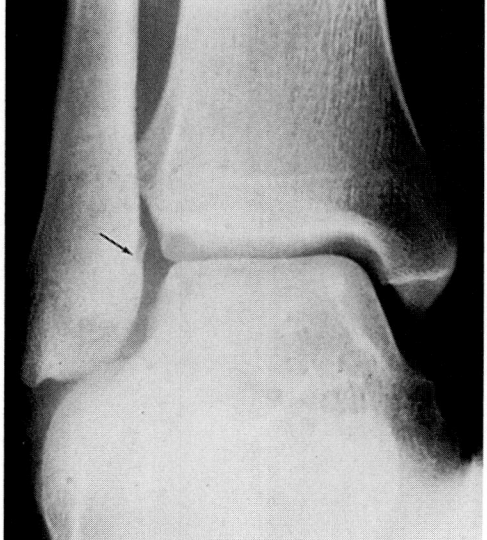

Figure 7–350. Residuals of the epiphyseal line of the fibula in an 18-year-old, not to be mistaken for fracture.

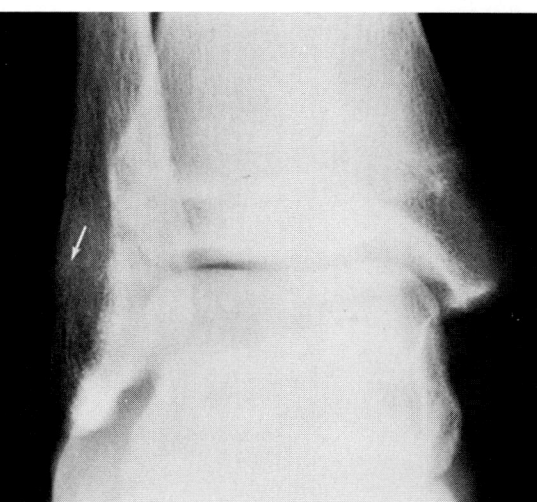
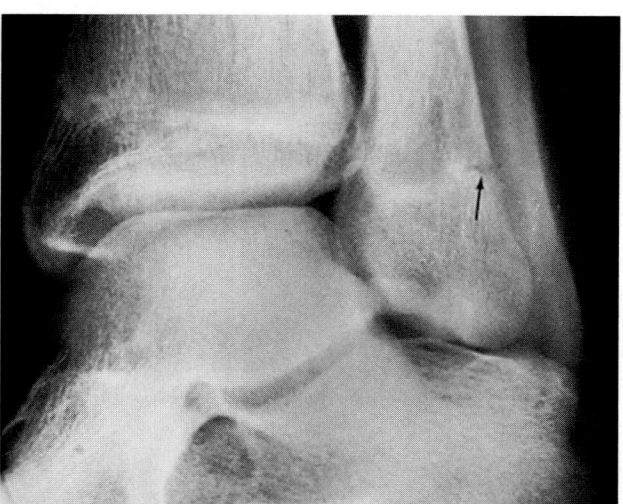

Figure 7–351. Residuals of the epiphyseal line of the fibula in a 19-year-old.

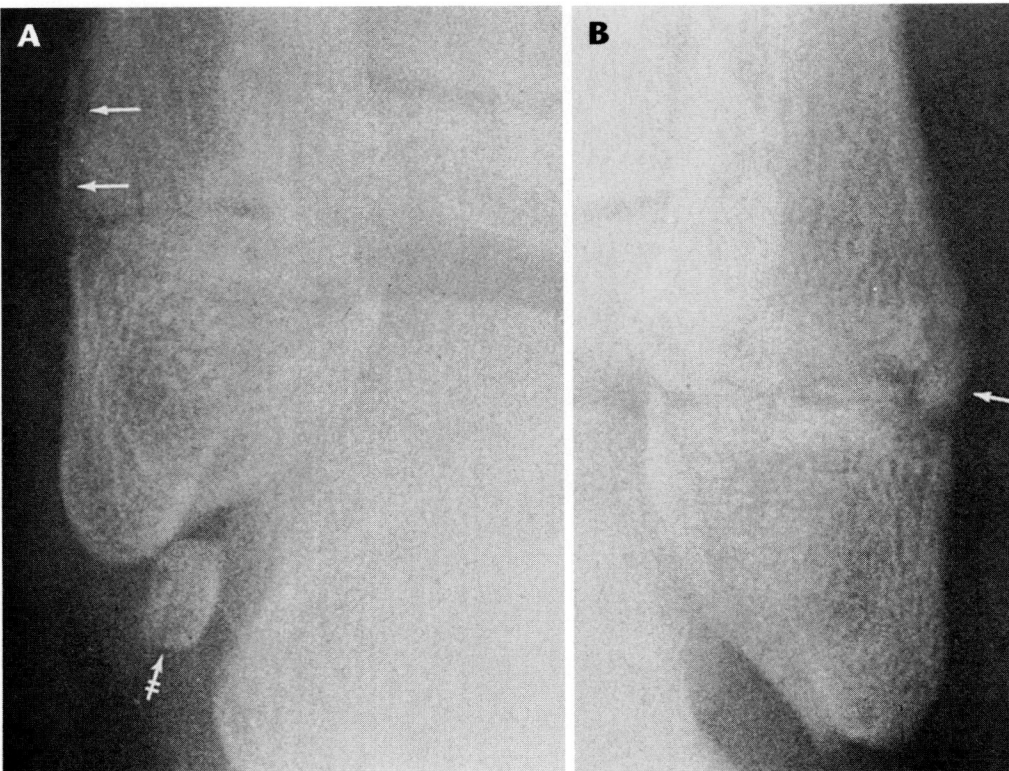

Figure 7–352. The fibular ossicle, a normal accessory ossification center, in a 12-year-old boy. In **A,** the ossicle is seen at the lateral aspect of the fibular metaphysis. In **B,** a large ossicle is visible at the lateral aspect of the epiphyseal line. These ossicles fuse after puberty and are often mistaken for fractures. A large os subfibulare is also present in **A** (⫬). (Ref: Caffey J: *Pediatric x-ray diagnosis*, 9th ed. St. Louis, Mosby, 1993, p. 1511.)

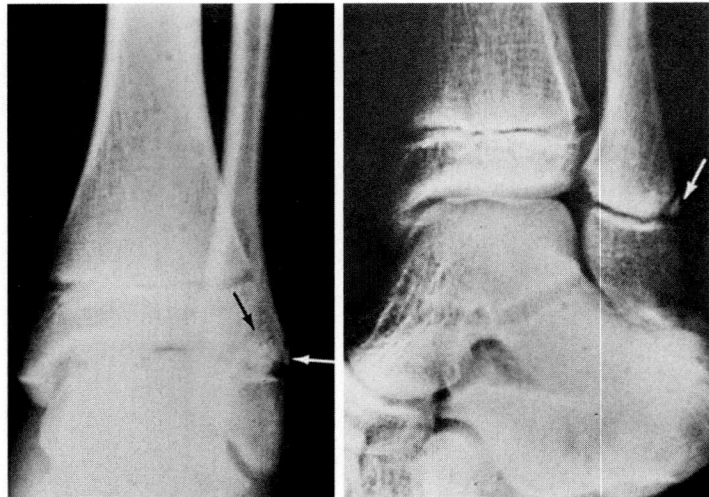

Figure 7–353. Another example of the fibular ossicle.

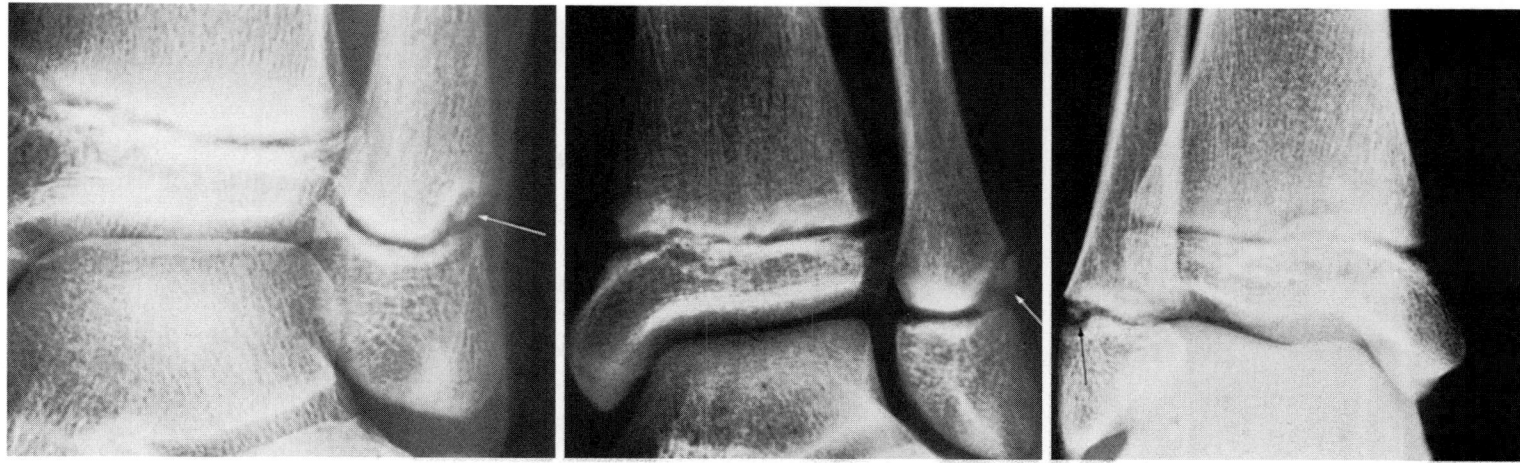

Figure 7–354. Three examples of fibular ossicles, all misinterpreted and treated as fractures.

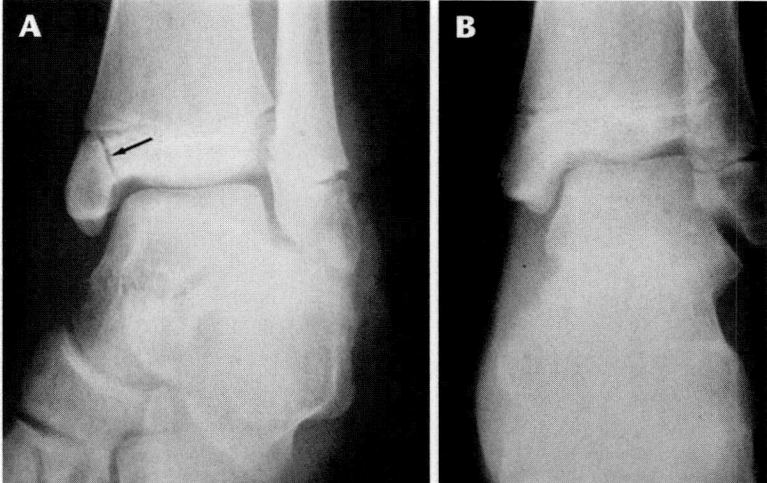

Figure 7–355. Cleft distal tibial epiphysis seen only in the oblique projection. Such clefting may be seen in many locations in late childhood.

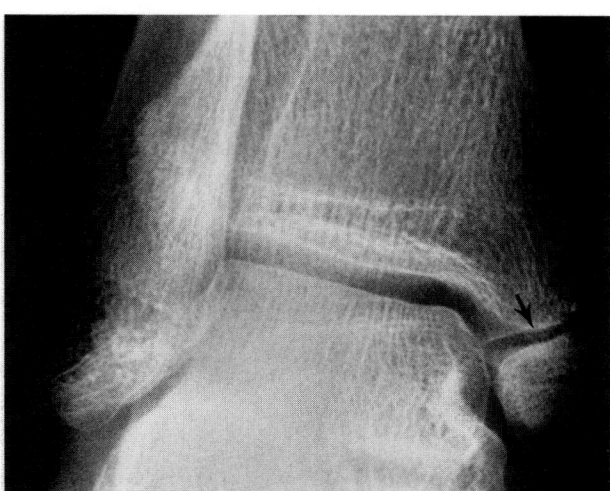

Figure 7–356. Failure of closure of the medial malleolus in an adult.

Figure 7–357. Cleft tibial epiphysis on the lateral side in a 16-year-old boy.

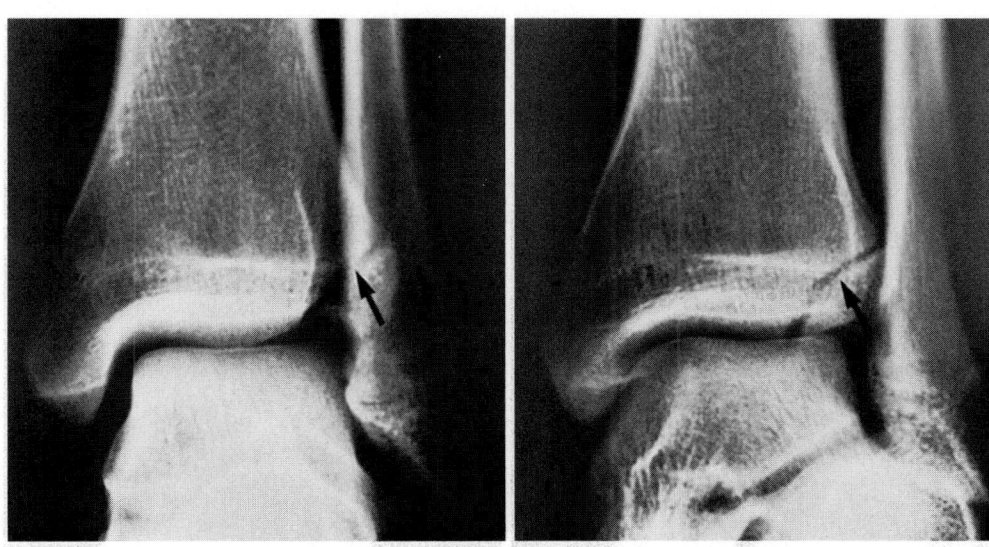

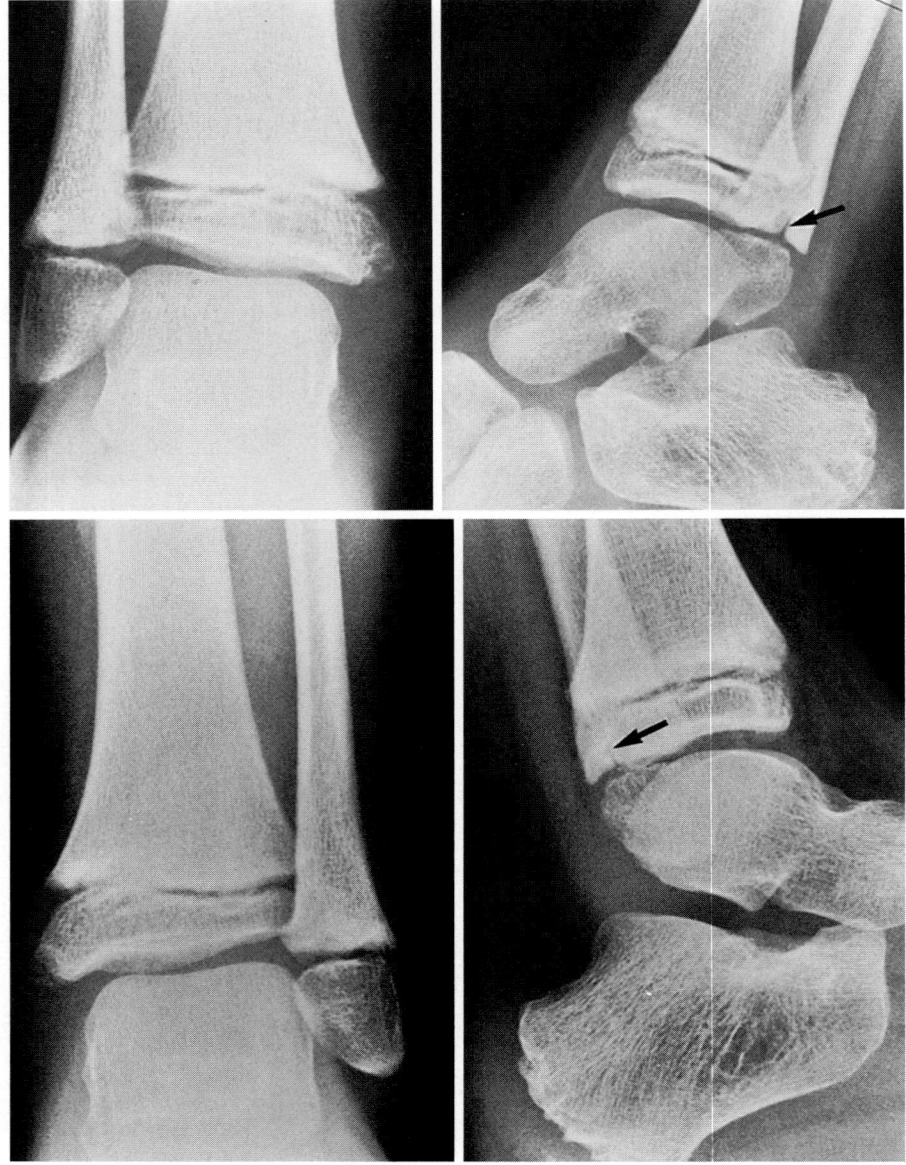

Figure 7–358. Cleft distal fibular metaphyses in a 7-year-old boy.

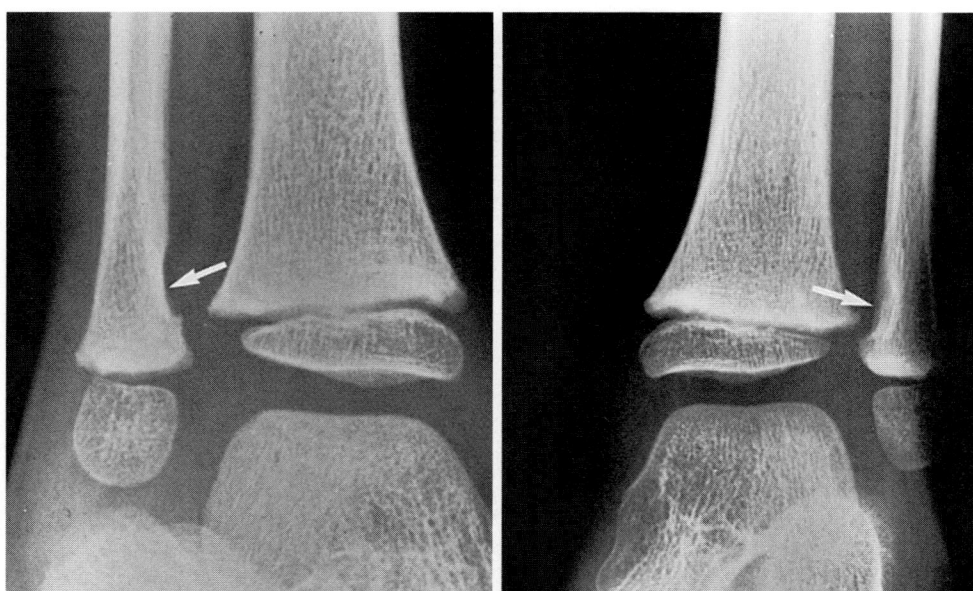

Figure 7–359. Bilateral metaphyseal defects in a 4-year-old boy, probably related to the metaphyseal defects seen in older children.

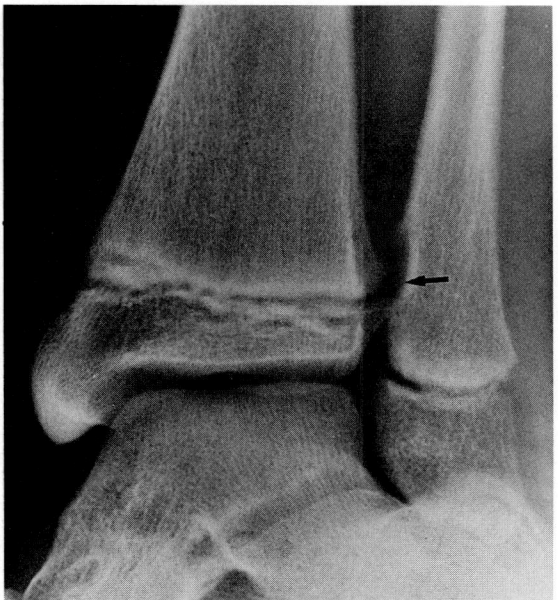

Figure 7–360. Same entity as noted in Figure 7–359 in a 10-year-old boy.

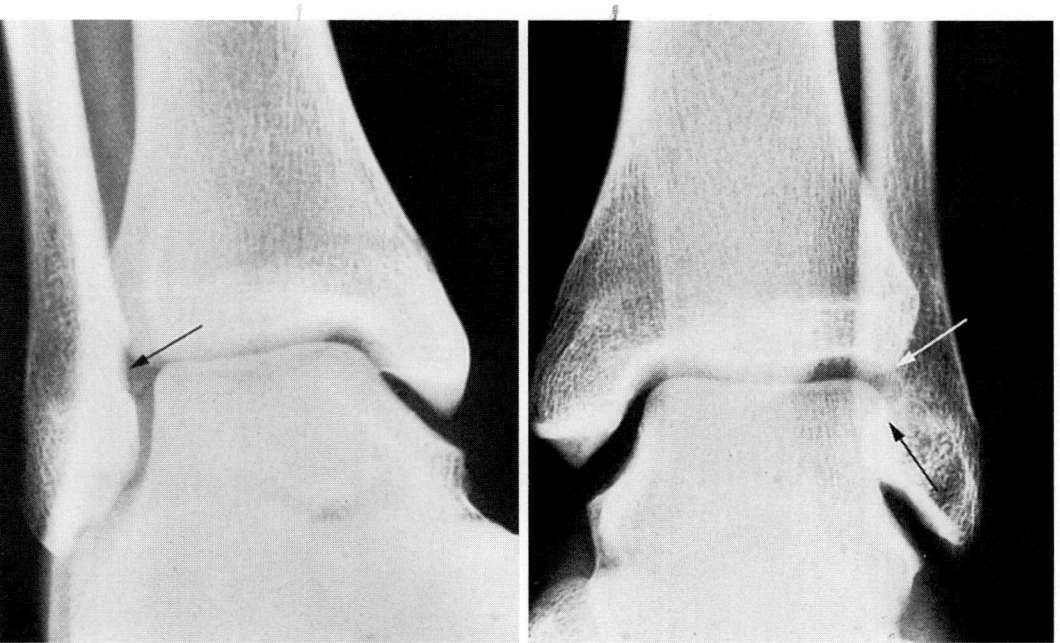

Figure 7–361. Developmental fossae or cortical defects in the medial aspects of the distal fibulae at the insertion of the anterior tibiofibular ligament are of no clinical significance. (Ref: Ehara S et al: Cortical defect of the distal fibula: Variant of ossification. *Radiology* 197:447, 1995.)

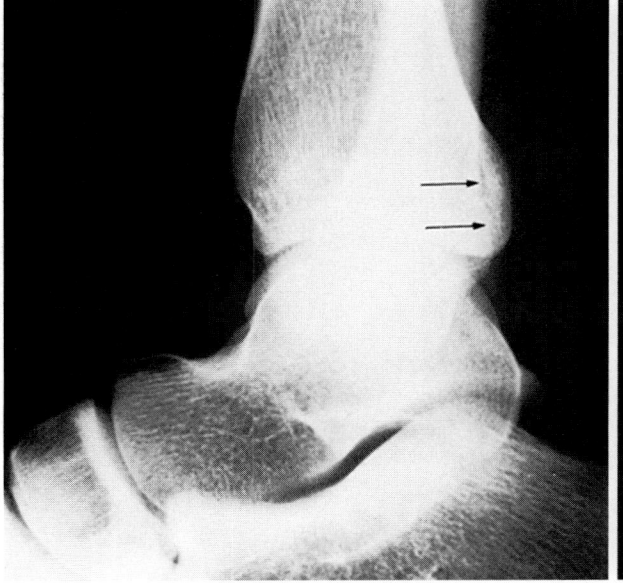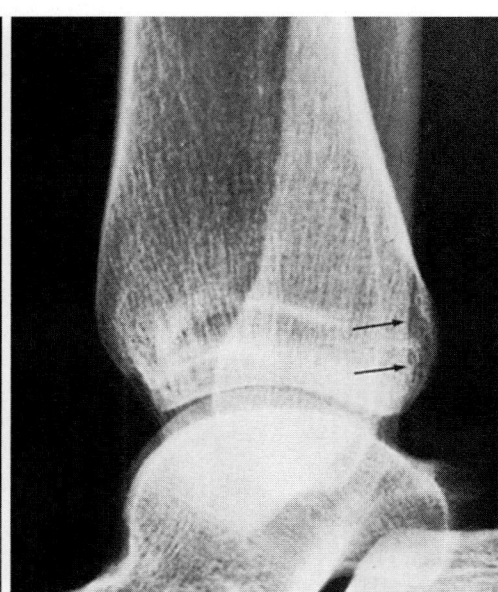

Figure 7–362. Simulated fractures of the posterior malleolus produced by Mach effect of overlap of the tibia and fibula.

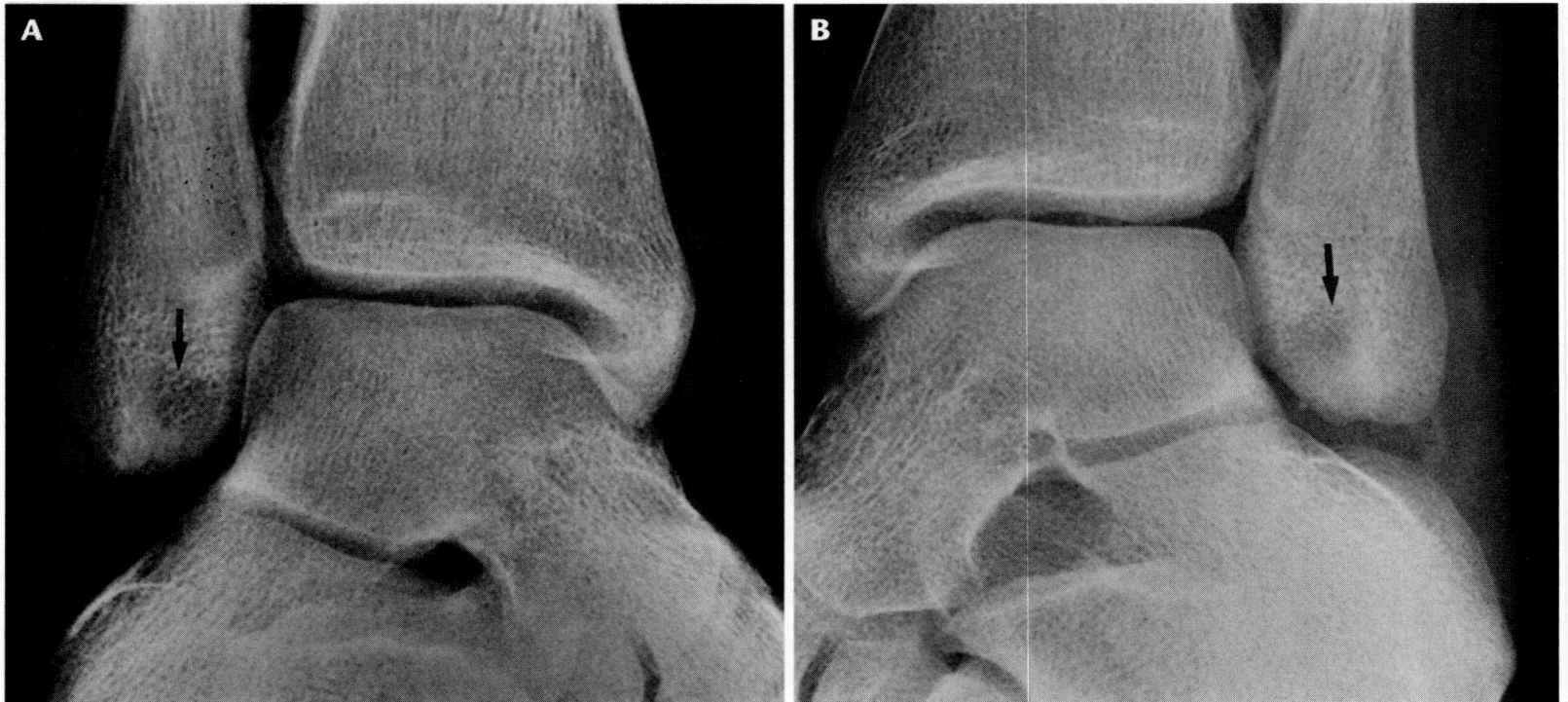

Figure 7–363. A, B, The normal fossae of the distal end of the fibulae.

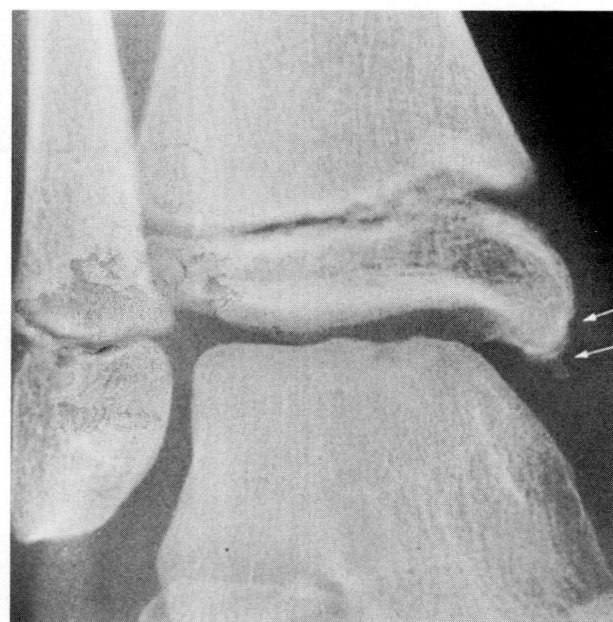

Figure 7–364. Irregularity of mineralization of the medial edge of the distal tibial epiphysis in an 8-year-old. This is similar to that seen in the distal femoral epiphysis.

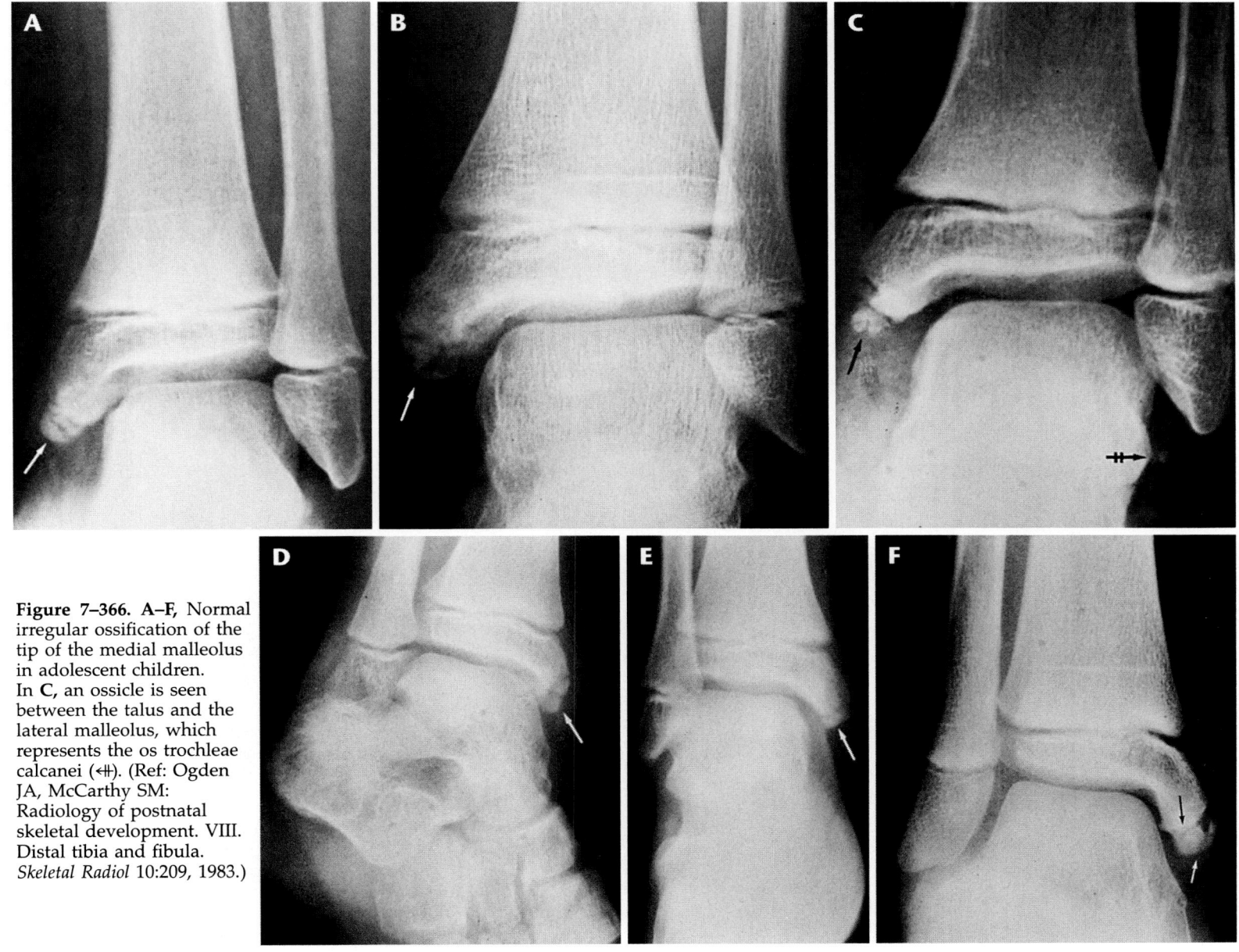

Figure 7–365. Bilateral separate secondary ossification centers for the medial malleoli in an 8-year-old boy, which may be mistaken for fractures.

Figure 7–366. A–F, Normal irregular ossification of the tip of the medial malleolus in adolescent children. In **C,** an ossicle is seen between the talus and the lateral malleolus, which represents the os trochleae calcanei (⊬). (Ref: Ogden JA, McCarthy SM: Radiology of postnatal skeletal development. VIII. Distal tibia and fibula. *Skeletal Radiol* 10:209, 1983.)

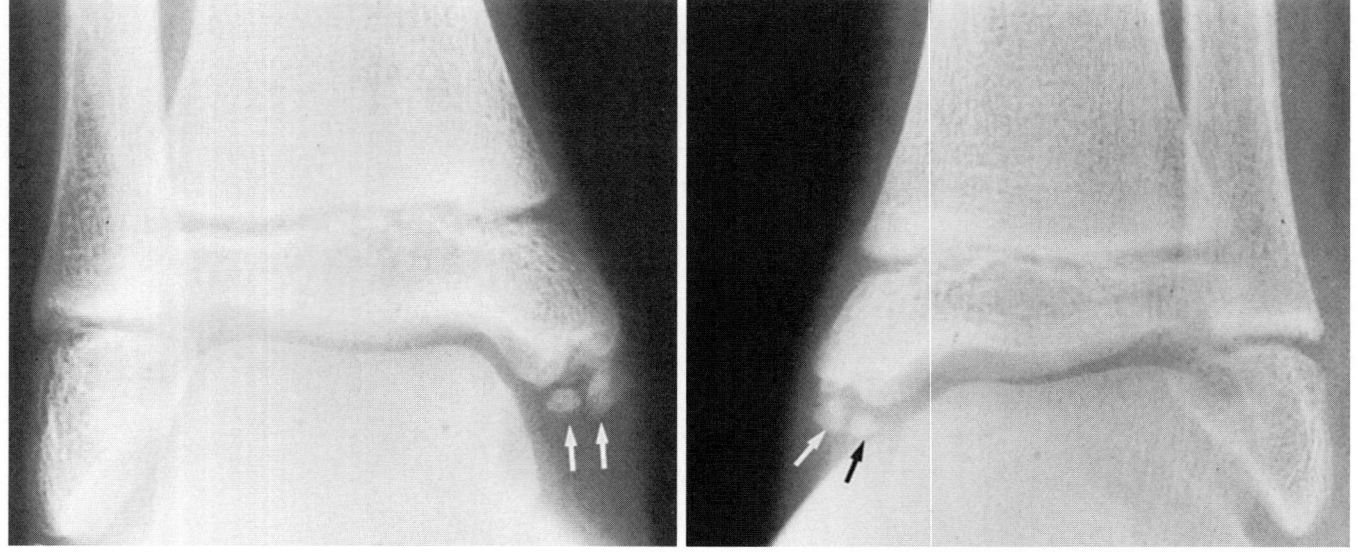

Figure 7–367. Bilateral multicentric ossification of the medial malleolus in a 9-year-old girl.

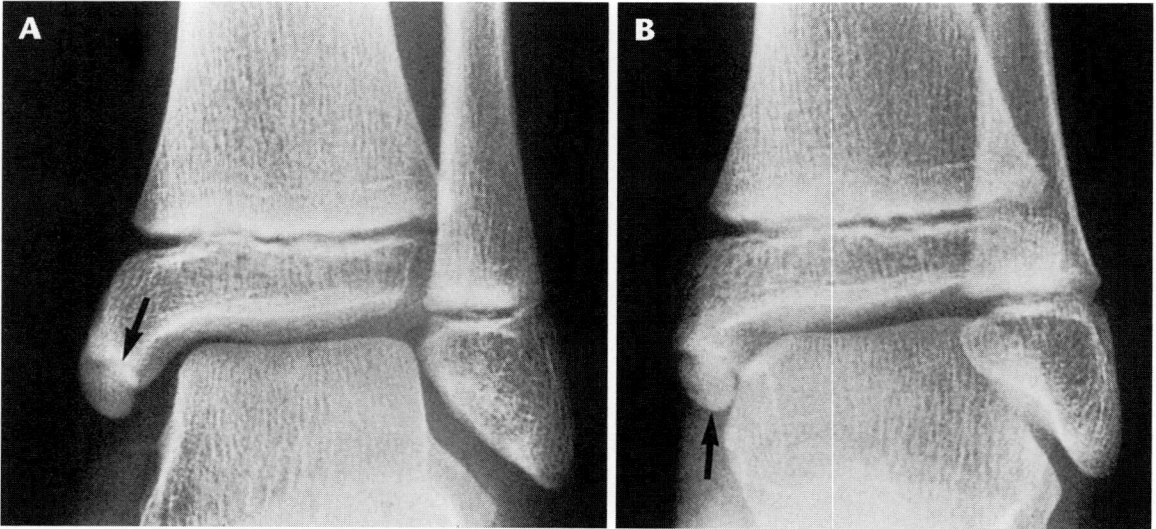

Figure 7–368. A, Medial malleolar ossicle simulating a fracture in frontal projection. **B,** Oblique projection shows cortication of the ossicle.

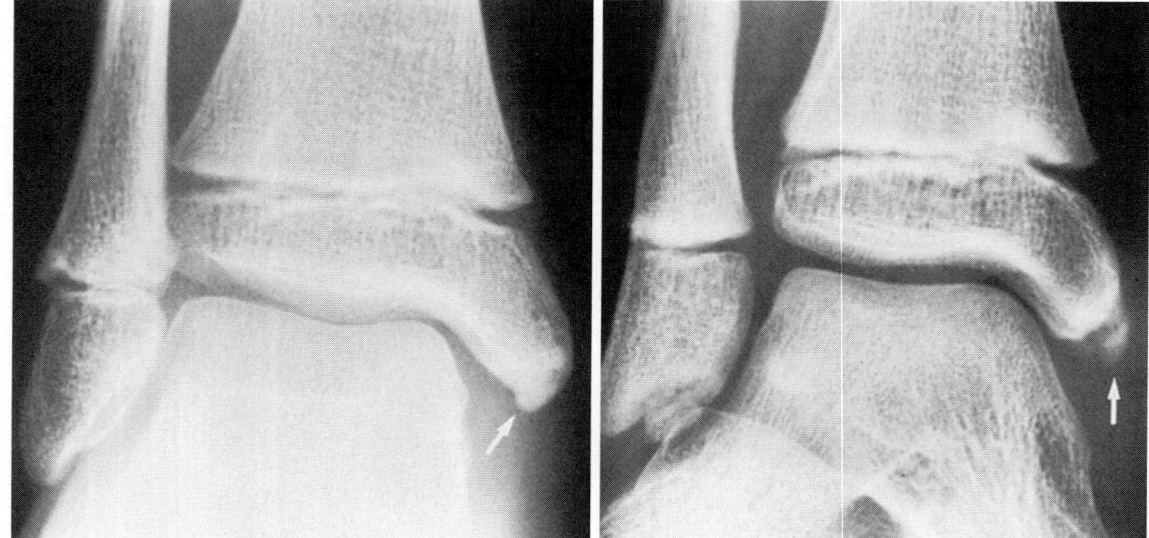

Figure 7–369. Closing accessory ossification center for the medial malleolus in an 8-year-old boy.

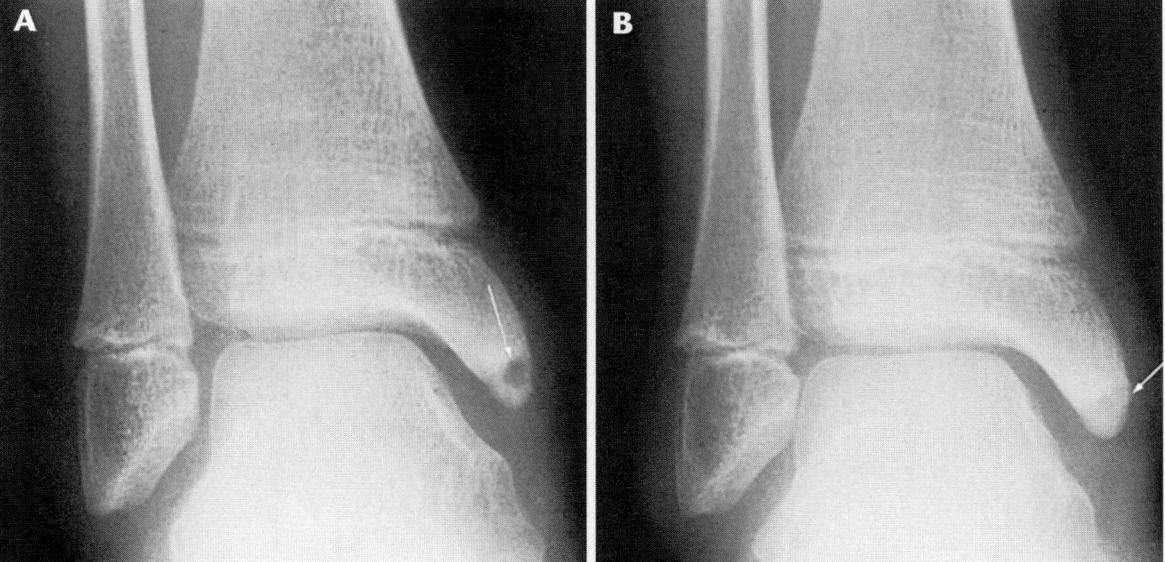

Figure 7–370. A, Developmental radiolucency in the medial malleolus in a 9-year-old boy secondary to the presence of a secondary ossification center. **B,** Follow-up 4 months later shows closing of secondary ossification center.

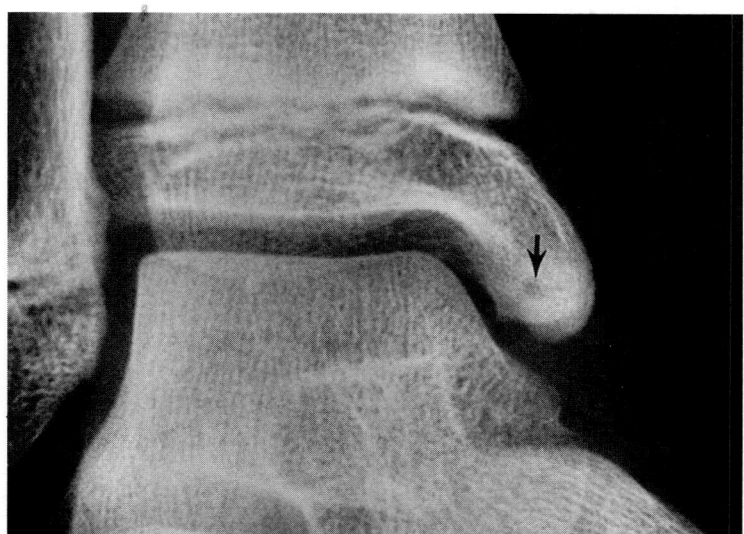

Figure 7–371. Developmental lucency in the medial malleolus in a 10-year-old boy similar to that seen in Figure 7–370.

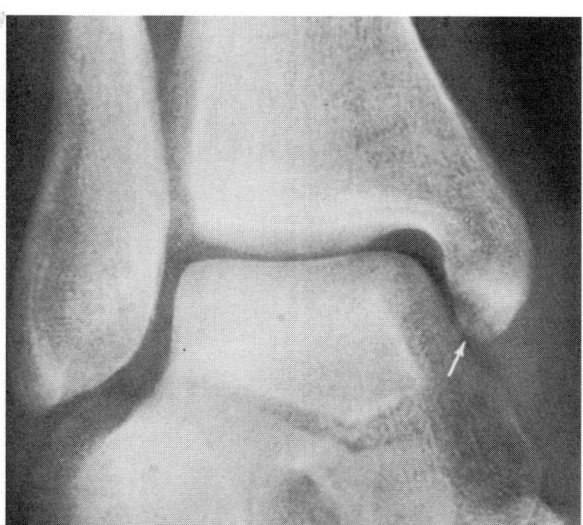

Figure 7–372. Persistent irregular ossification of the medial malleolus in an adult.

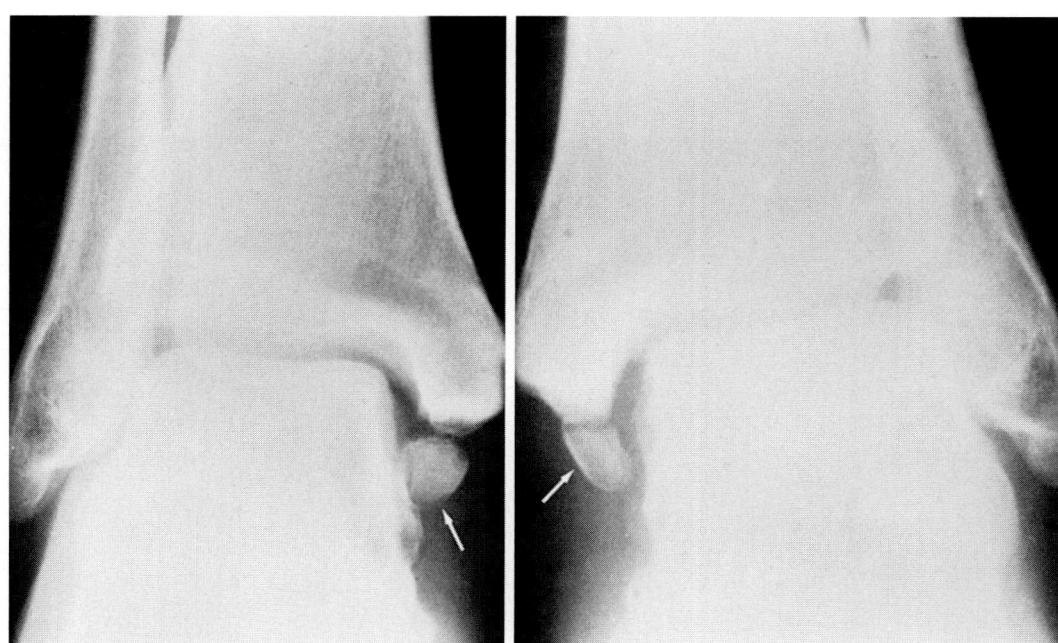

Figure 7–373. Large bilateral os subtibiale, accessory ossification centers that have persisted into adult life and are frequently mistaken for fractures.

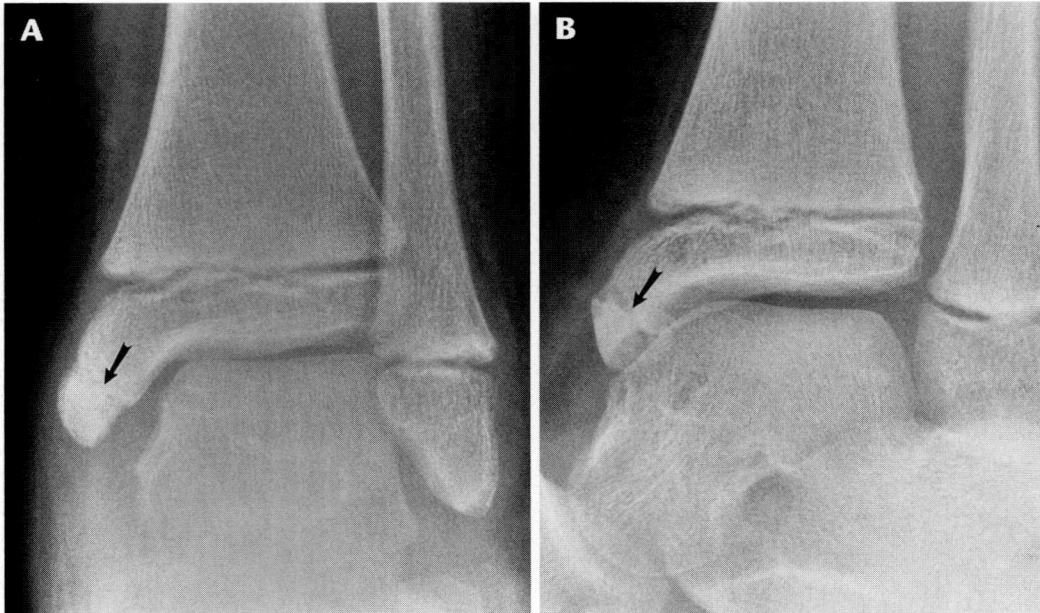

Figure 7–374. Large separate ossification center of the medial malleolus in a 14-year-old boy misdiagnosed as a fracture. **A,** Anteroposterior projection. **B,** Oblique projection.

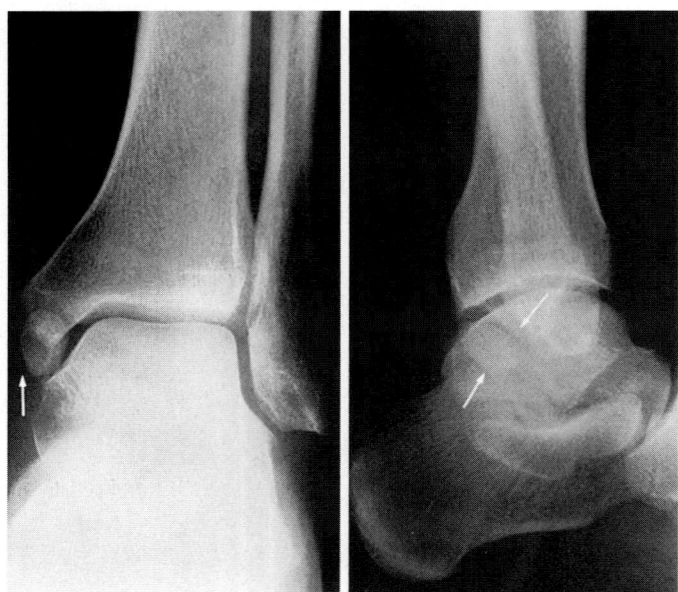

Figure 7–375. The os subtibiale. This is a rare accessory bone related to the posterior colliculus of the medial malleolus, as opposed to the more common os subtibiale, which is related to the anterior colliculus that forms the tip of the malleolus. (Coral A: The radiology of skeletal elements in the subtibial region: Incidence and significance. *Skeletal Radiol* 16:298, 1987.)

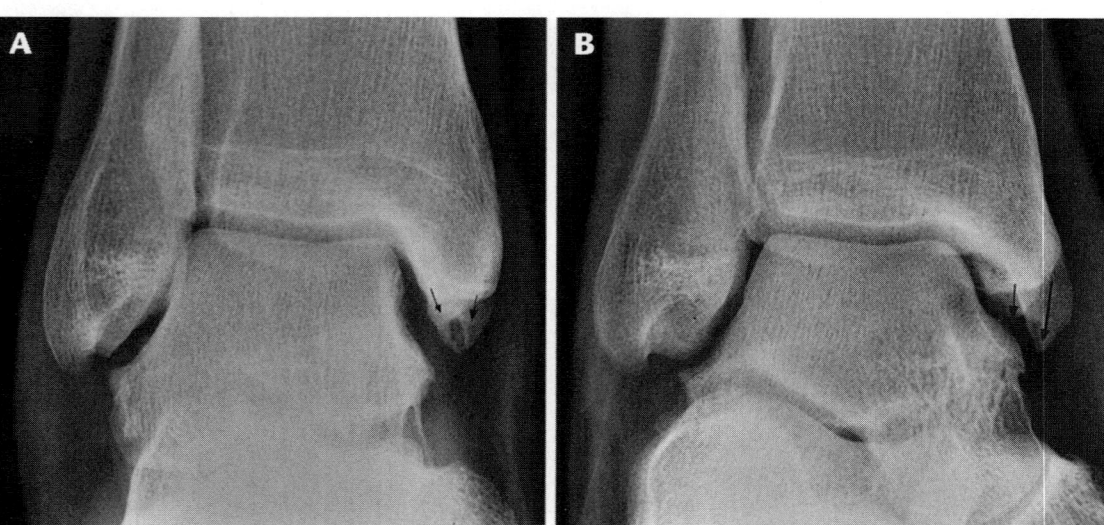

Figure 7–376. Bifid medial malleolus, representing the anterior and posterior colliculi. **A,** Frontal projection. **B,** Oblique projection.

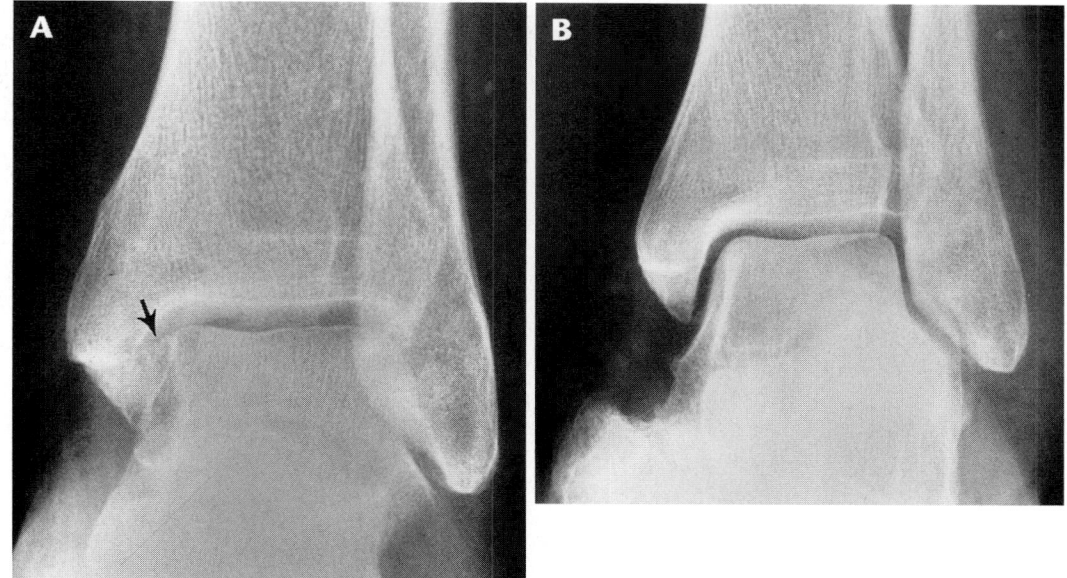

Figure 7–377. A, Simulated fracture of the medial malleolus secondary to rotation produced by poor positioning. **B,** Correct anteroposterior projection shows no fracture.

Figure 7–378. Unfused accessory ossification center of the distal tibia, producing unusual appearance of the upper margin of the talus. **A,** Frontal projection. **B,** Oblique projection. **C,** Tomogram.

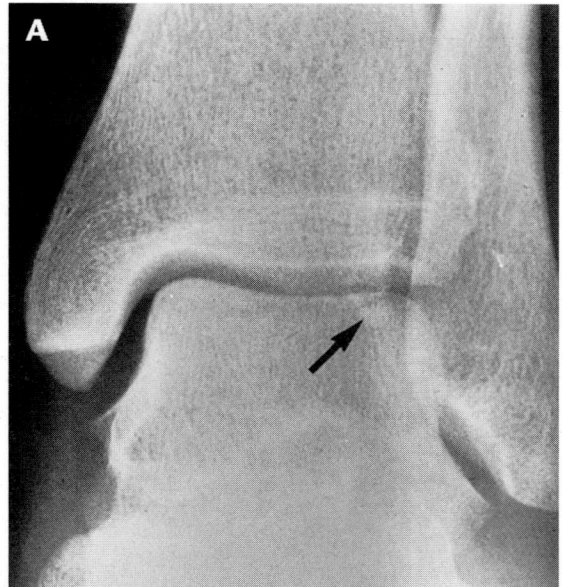

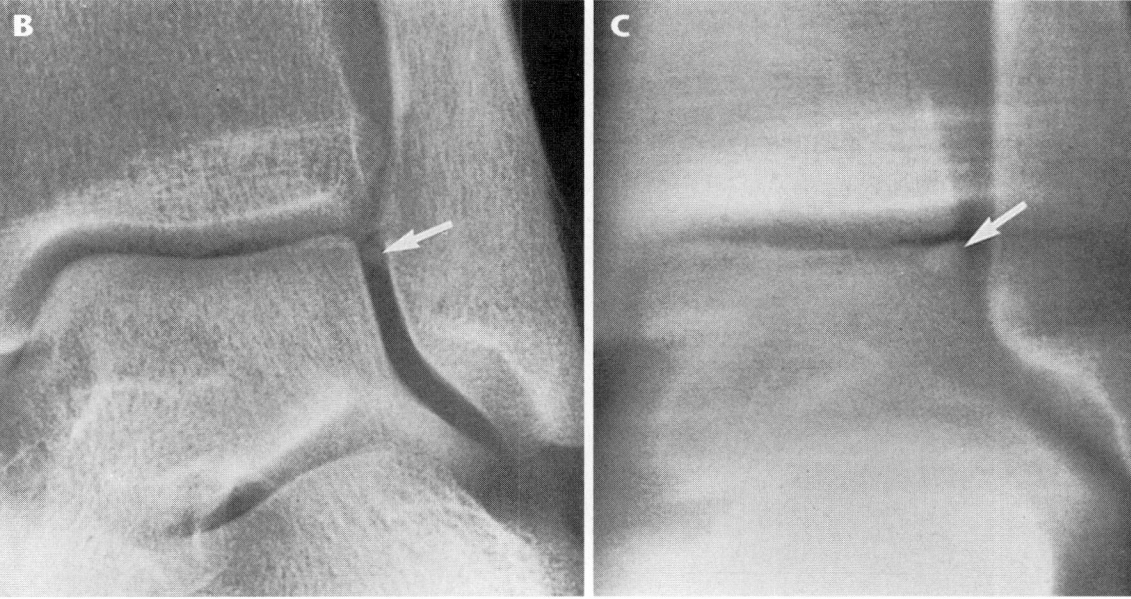

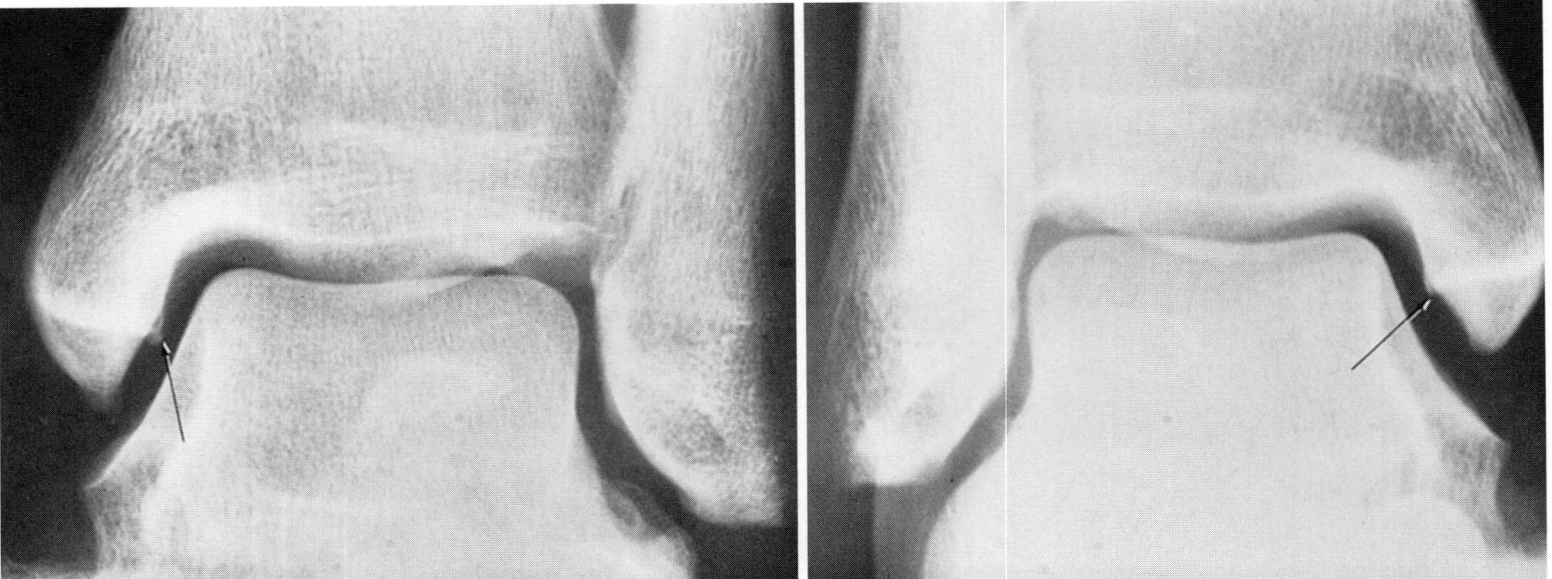

Figure 7–379. Bony flanges on the lateral aspects of the medial malleoli, which should not be mistaken for avulsion injuries.

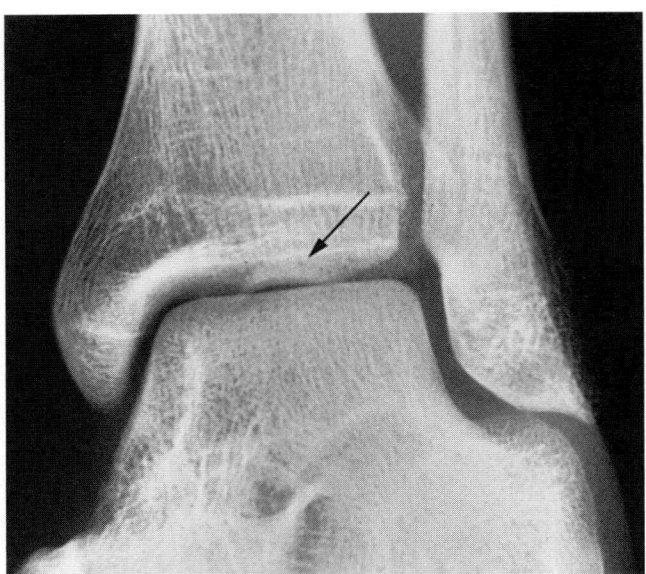

Figure 7–380. Normal band of density in the articular surface of the posterior malleolus.

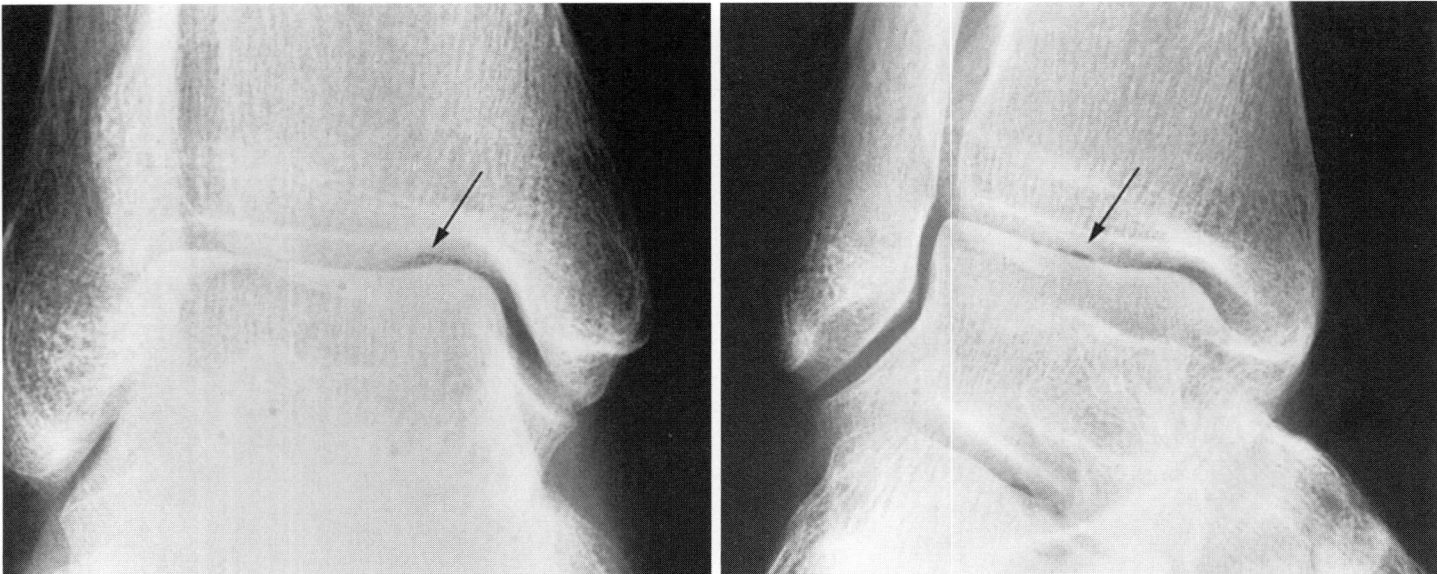

Figure 7–381. Small fossa on the articular surface of the posterior malleolus of no clinical significance.

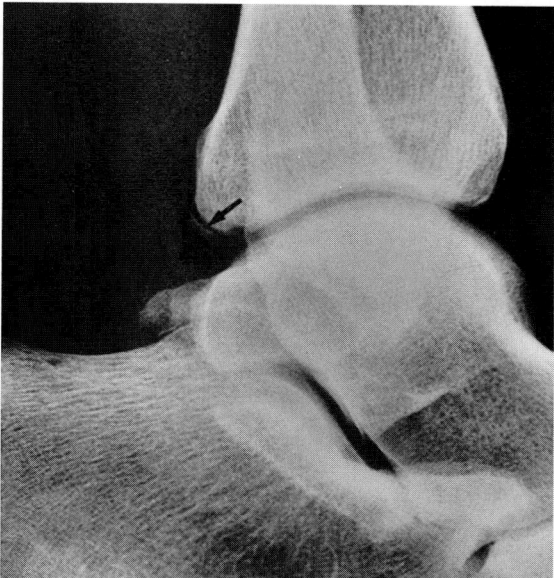

Figure 7–382. Persistent accessory ossification center of the posterior malleolus.

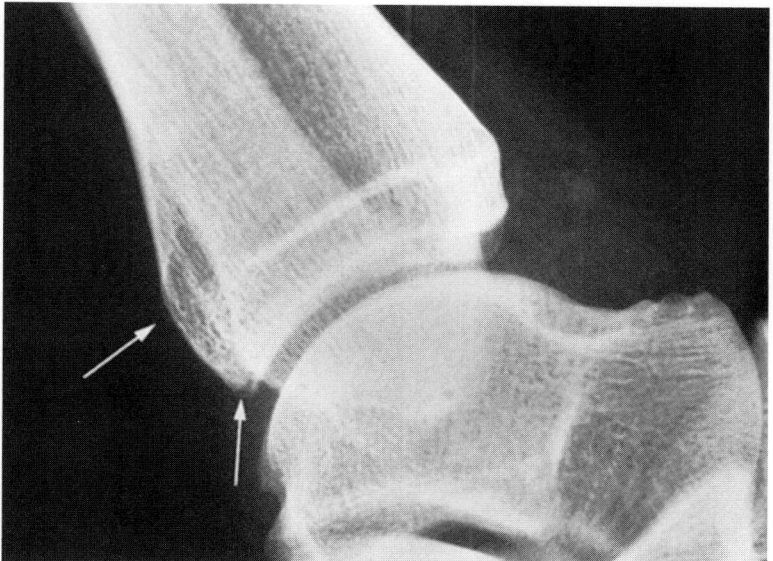

Figure 7–383. Normal undulations of the cortex of the posterior malleolus.

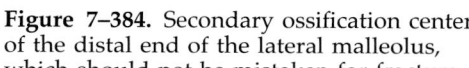

Figure 7–384. Secondary ossification center of the distal end of the lateral malleolus, which should not be mistaken for fracture.

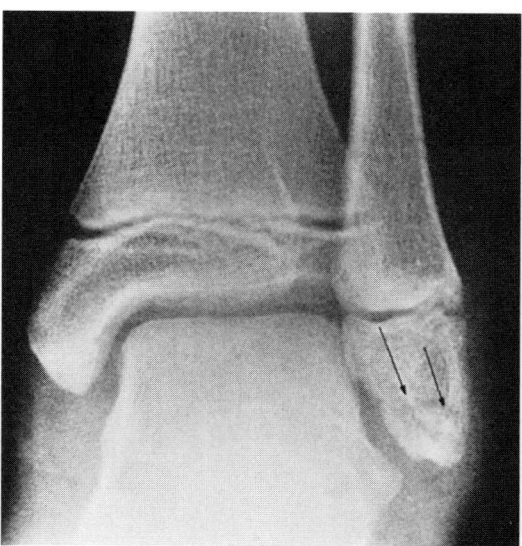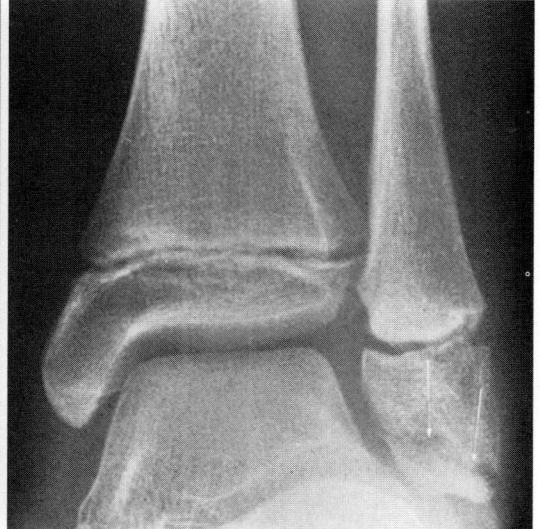

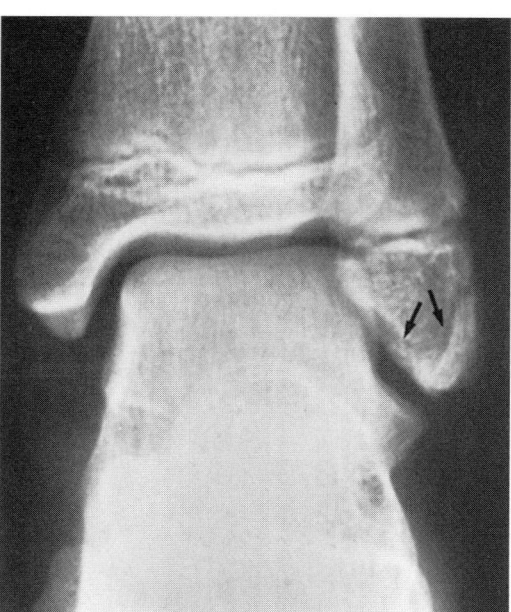

Figure 7–385. Secondary ossification center of the lateral aspect and distal end of the lateral malleolus in a 12-year-old girl.

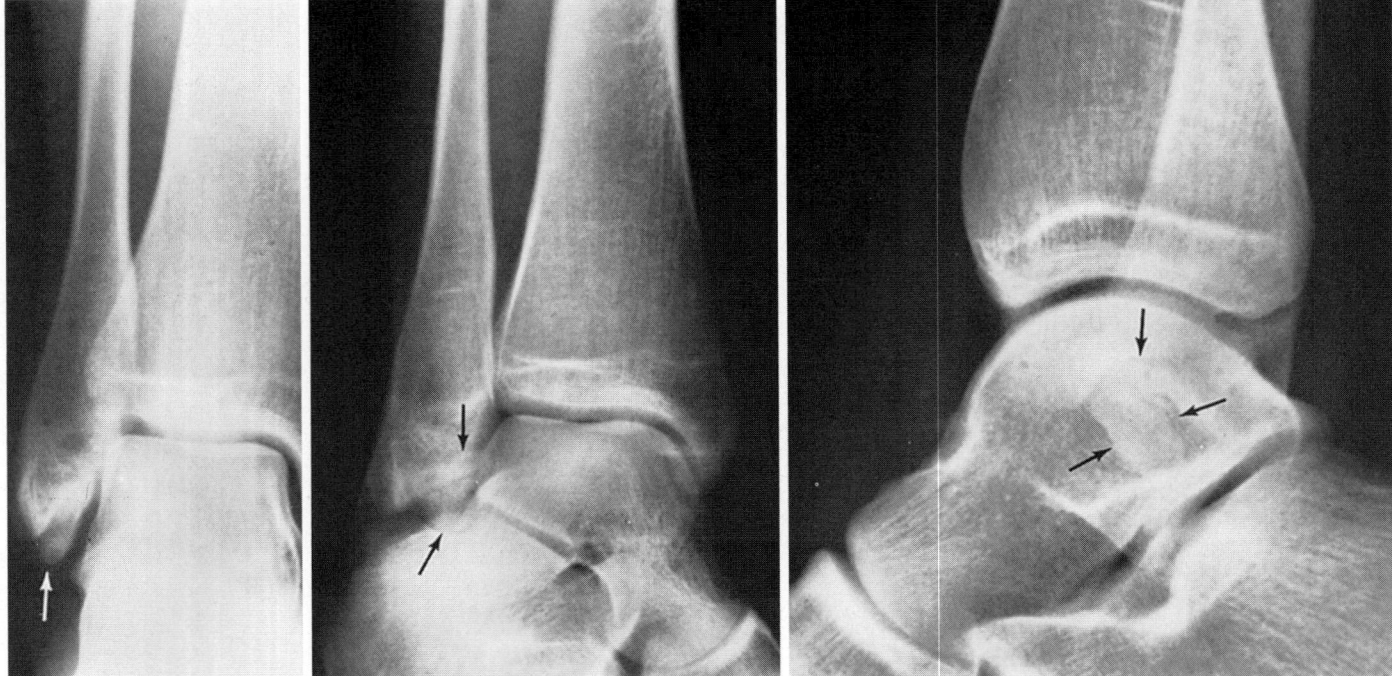

Figure 7–386. Large os subfibulare at the tip of the lateral malleolus with inset into the adjacent malleolus.

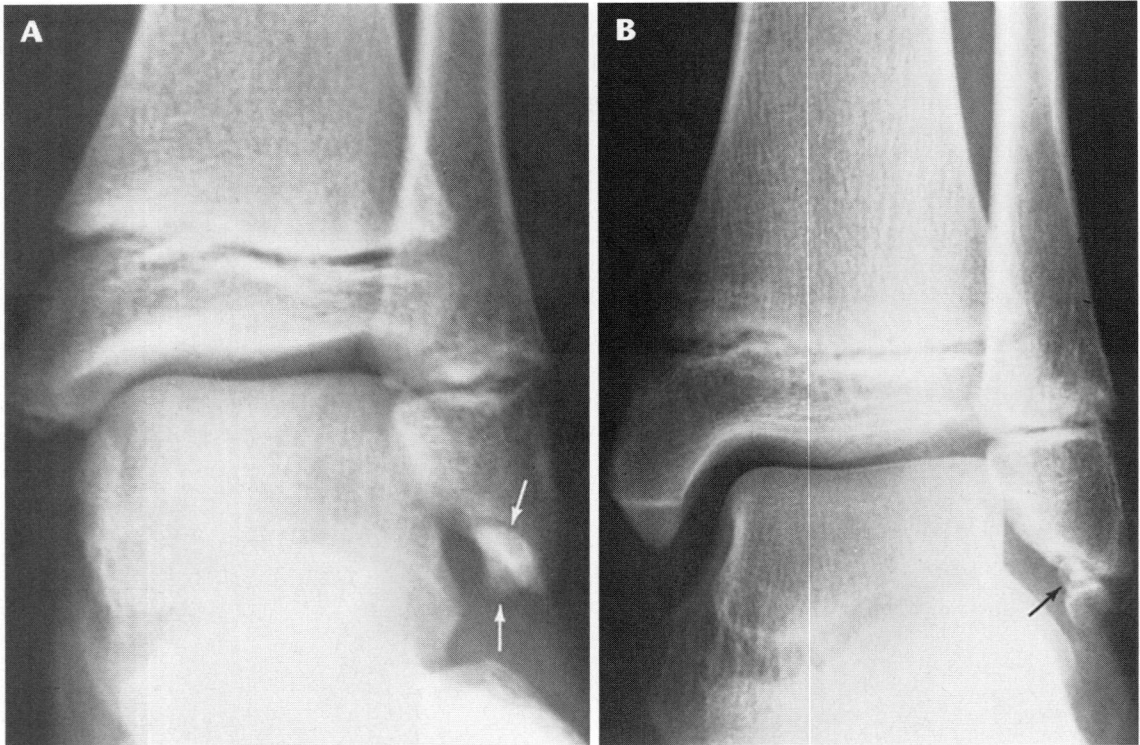

Figure 7–387. Large os subfibulare. **A,** 11-year-old boy. **B,** 14-year-old boy. Ossicles in this location may be symptomatic in children. (Ref: Griffiths JD, Menelaus MB: Symptomatic ossicles of the lateral malleolus in children. *J Bone Joint Surg* 69B:317, 1987.)

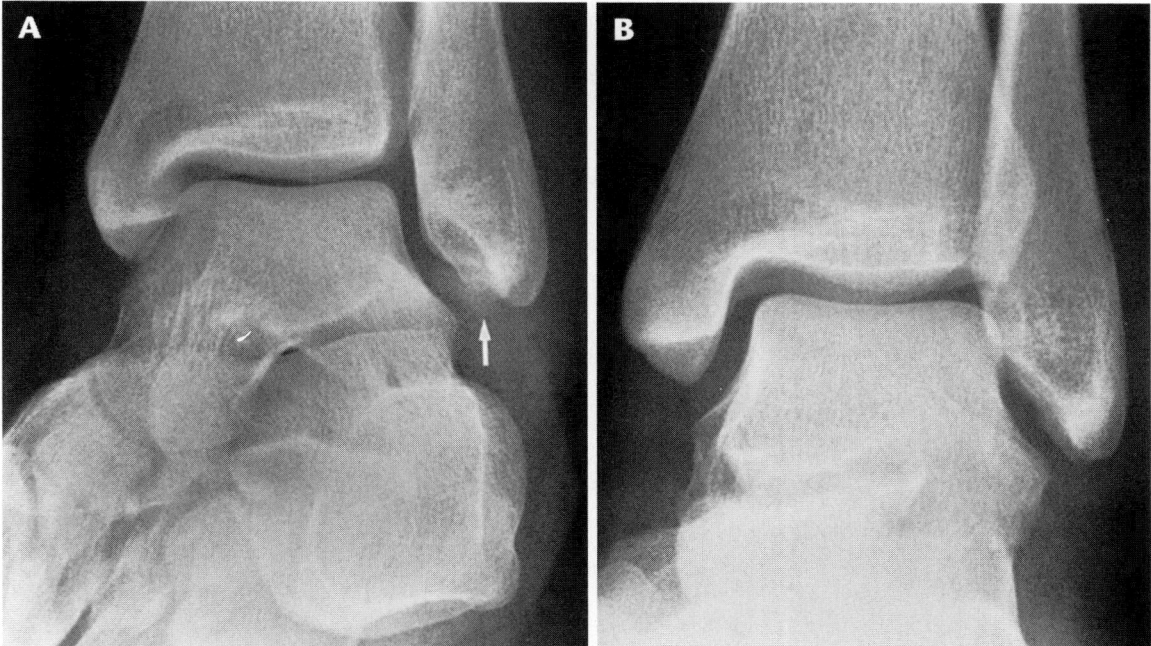

Figure 7–388. A, Os subfibulare seen only in oblique projection. **B,** Frontal projection.

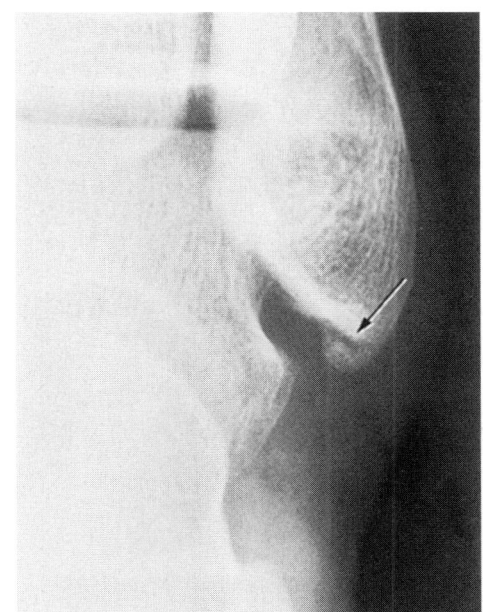

Figure 7–389. Simulated fracture of the tip of the lateral malleolus caused by trabeculations. Note that the cortical margins are intact.

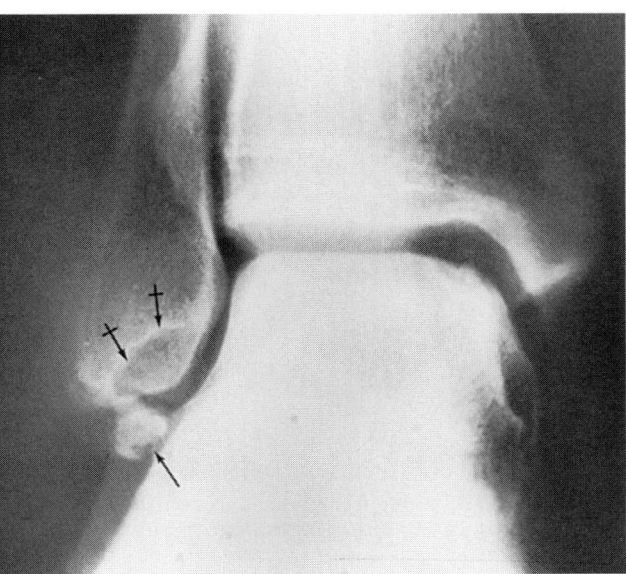
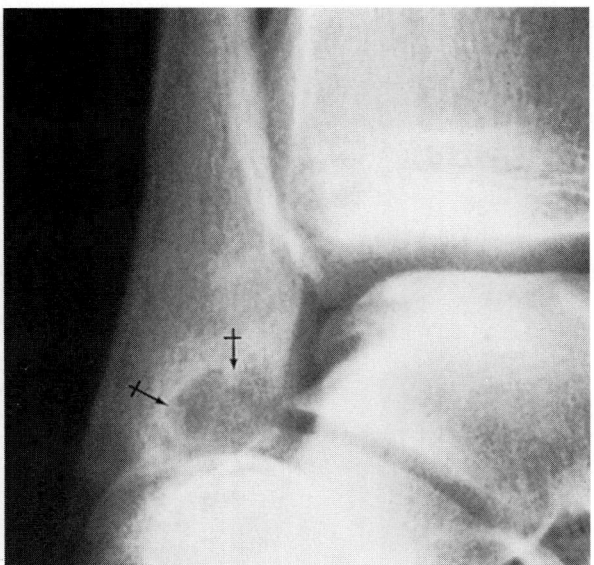

Figure 7–390. Os subfibulare (→) with deep fossa in distal end of the fibula (↠).

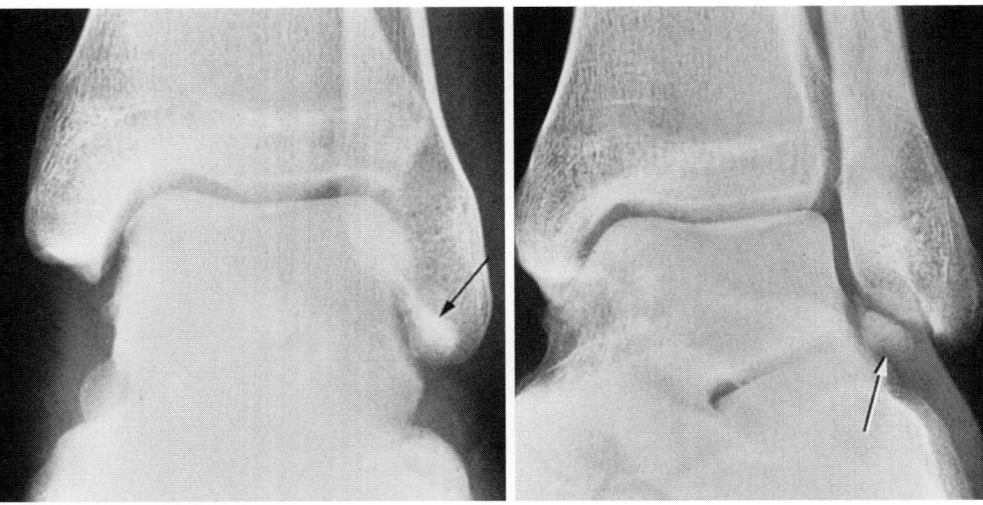

Figure 7–391. Large os subfibulare mistaken for a fracture. This ossicle can sometimes be differentiated from a fracture by mentally subtracting the ossicle from the fibula and determining whether the architecture of the fibula is correct without the additional osseous element.

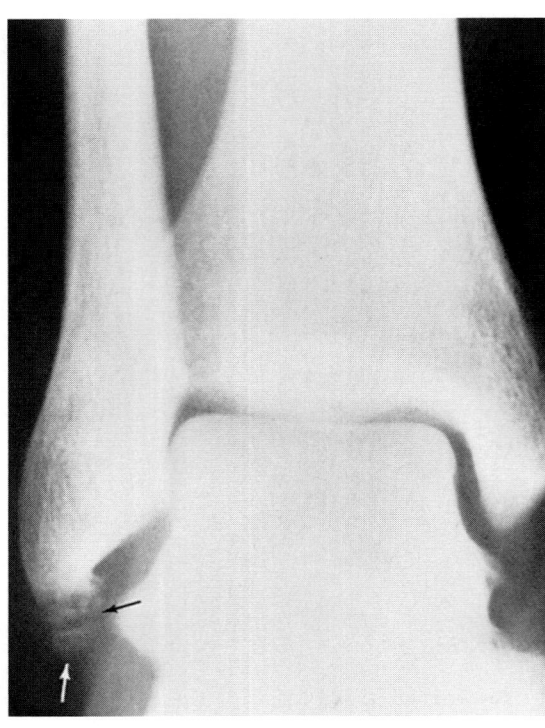

Figure 7–392. An example of the os subfibulare. Multiple irregular fragments have persisted into adult life in a 19-year-old man.

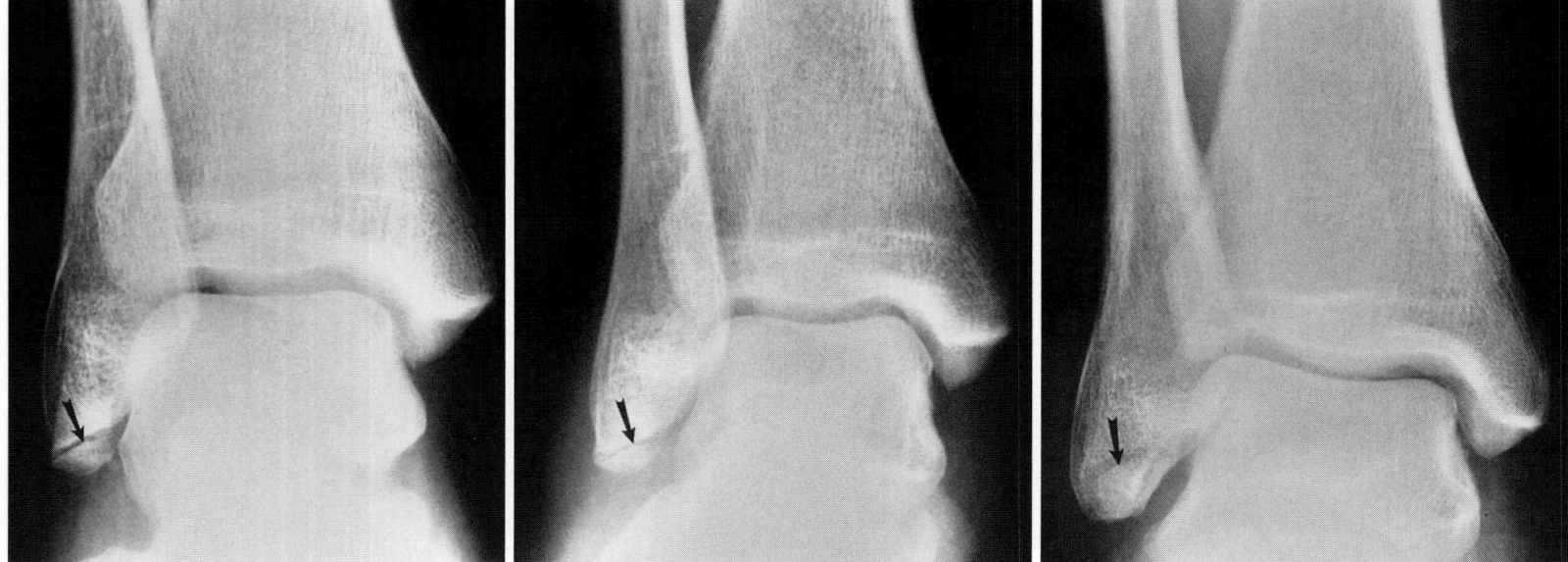

Figure 7–393. Os subfibulare, which resemble fractures. Such ossicles are occasionally a source of pain. (Ref: Berg EE: The symptomatic os subfibulare. *J Bone Joint Surg* 173A:1251, 1991.)

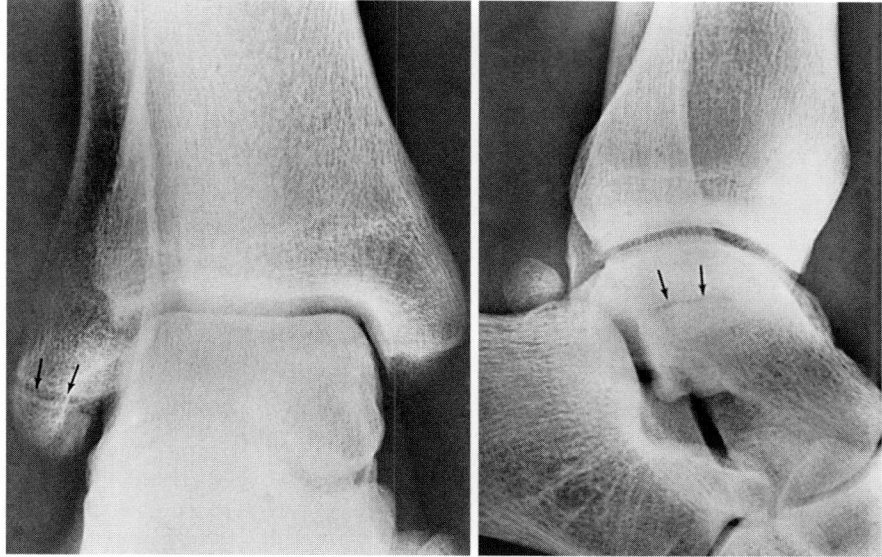

Figure 7–394. Incomplete fusion of the ossification center for the lateral malleolus in an adult, simulating a fracture.

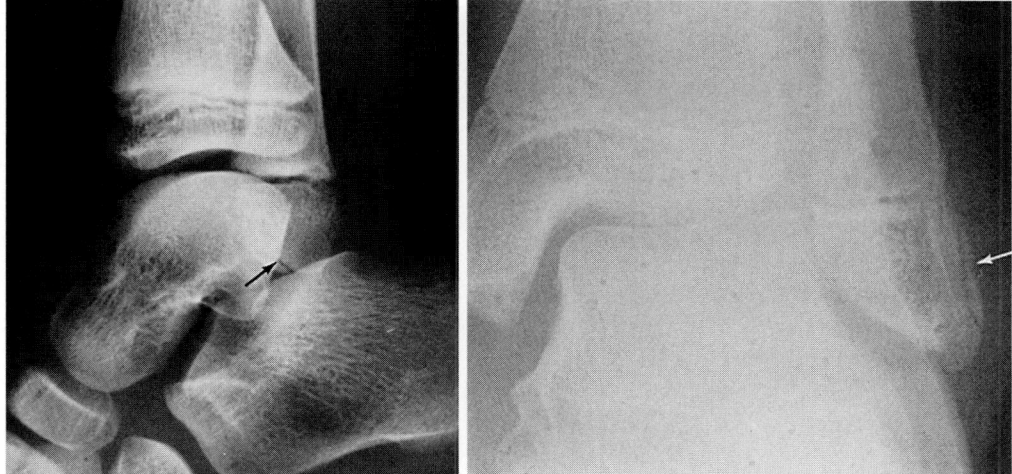

Figure 7–395. Scalelike secondary ossification centers that resemble fractures.

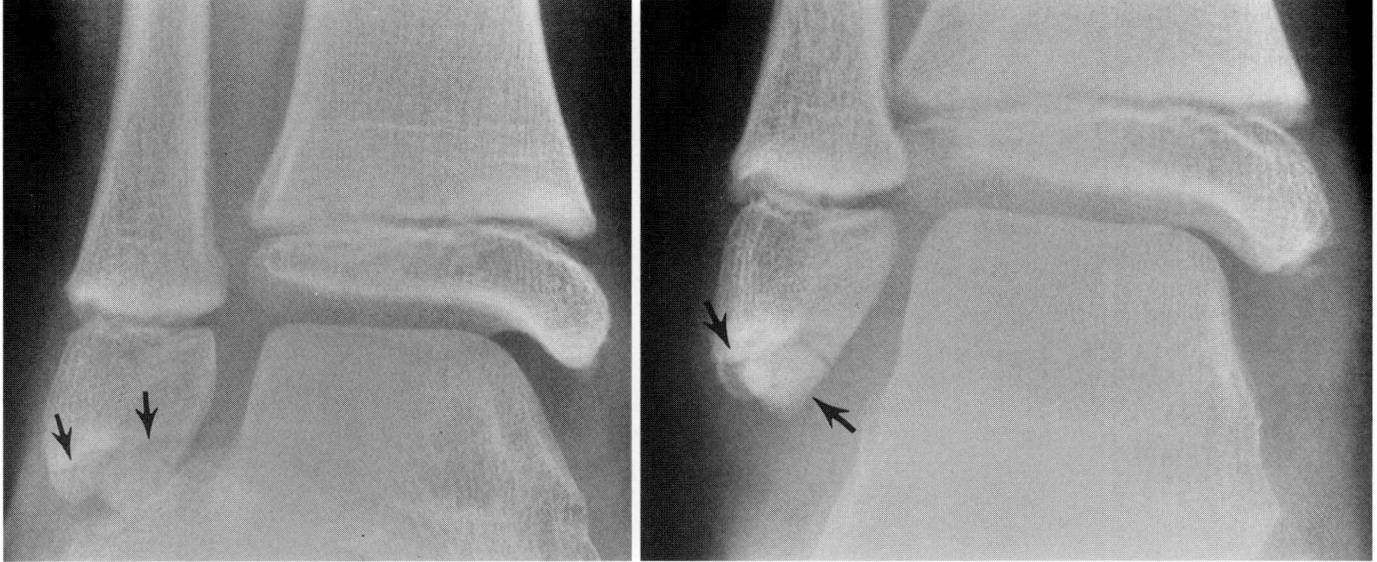

Figure 7–396. Accessory ossification centers of the lateral malleolus in a 10-year-old boy, treated as a fracture for 6 months.

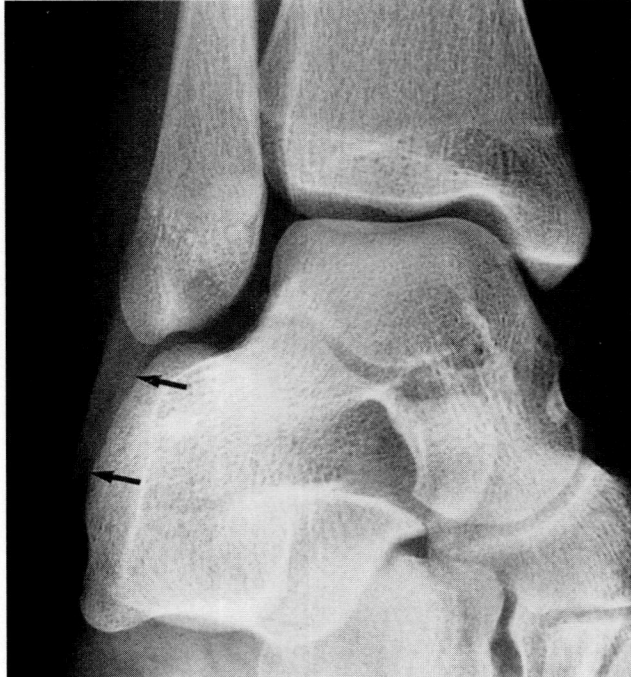

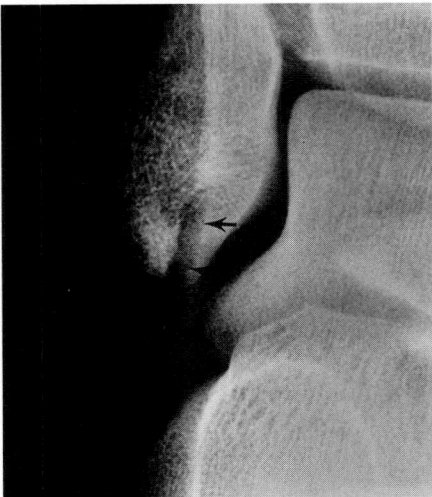

Figure 7–398. Simulated fracture of the lateral malleolus produced by overlying soft tissue shadow of the Achilles tendon.

Figure 7–397. The shadow of the Achilles tendon in the oblique projection.

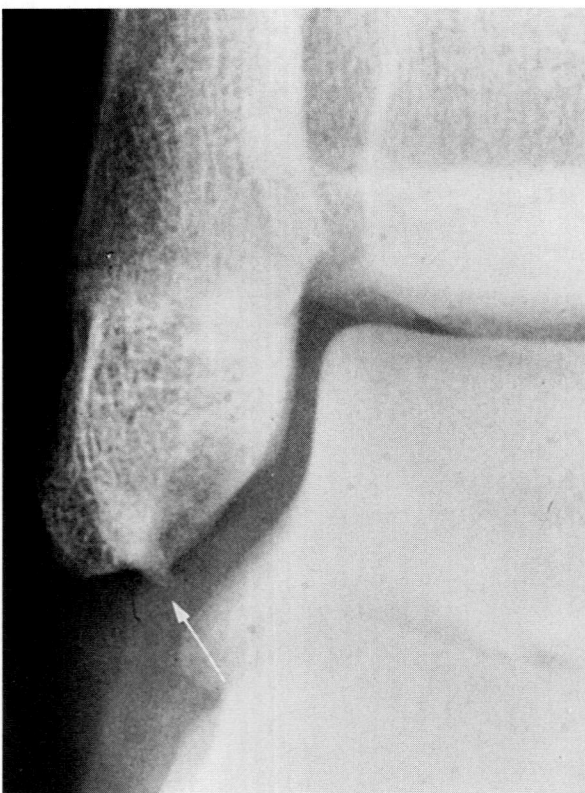

Figure 7–399. Spurlike extension of the distal end of the lateral mallelous.

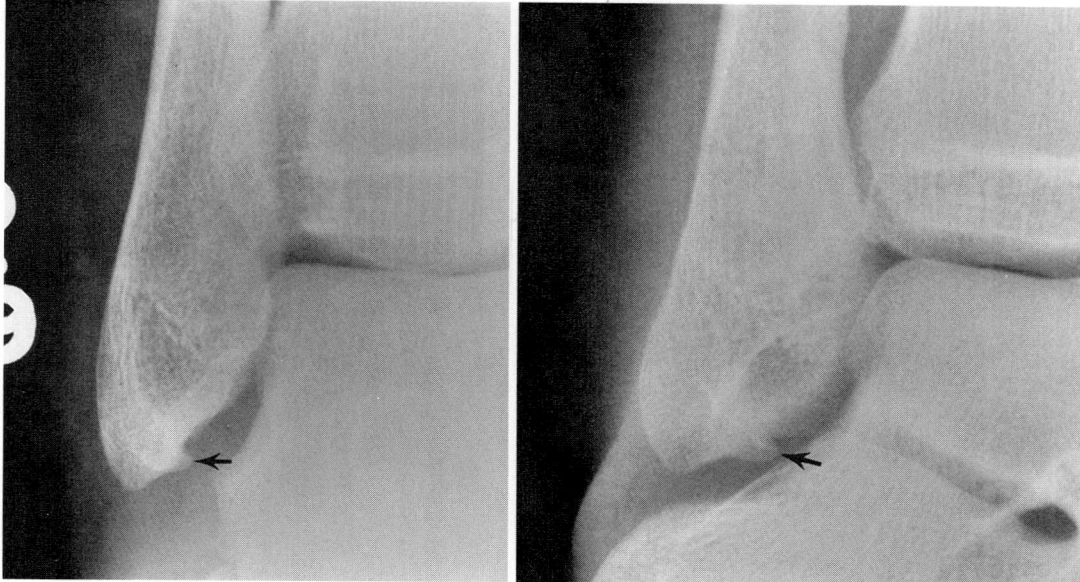

Figure 7–400. Another example of the entity illustrated in Figure 7–399.

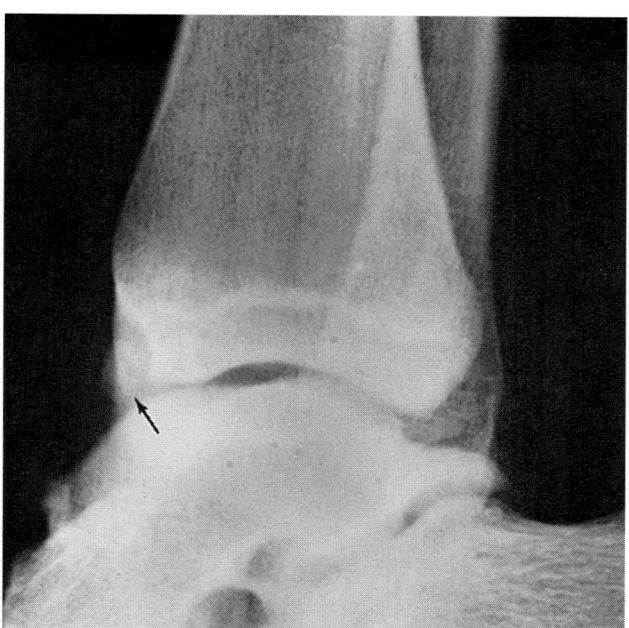

Figure 7–401. The os talotibiale, an accessory ossicle.

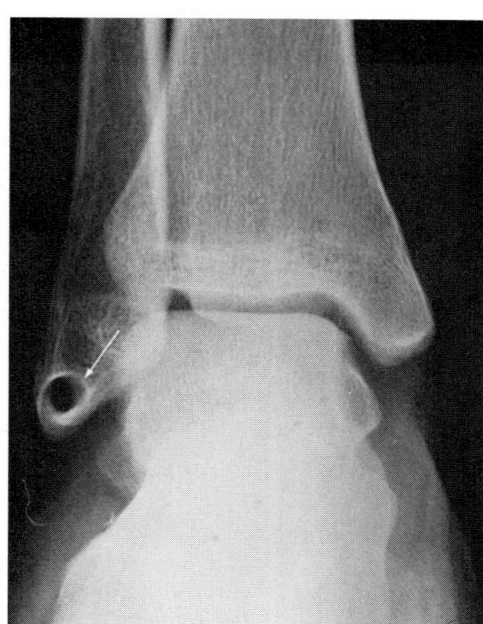

Figure 7–402. "Foramen" in the lateral malleolus, detected as an incidental finding.

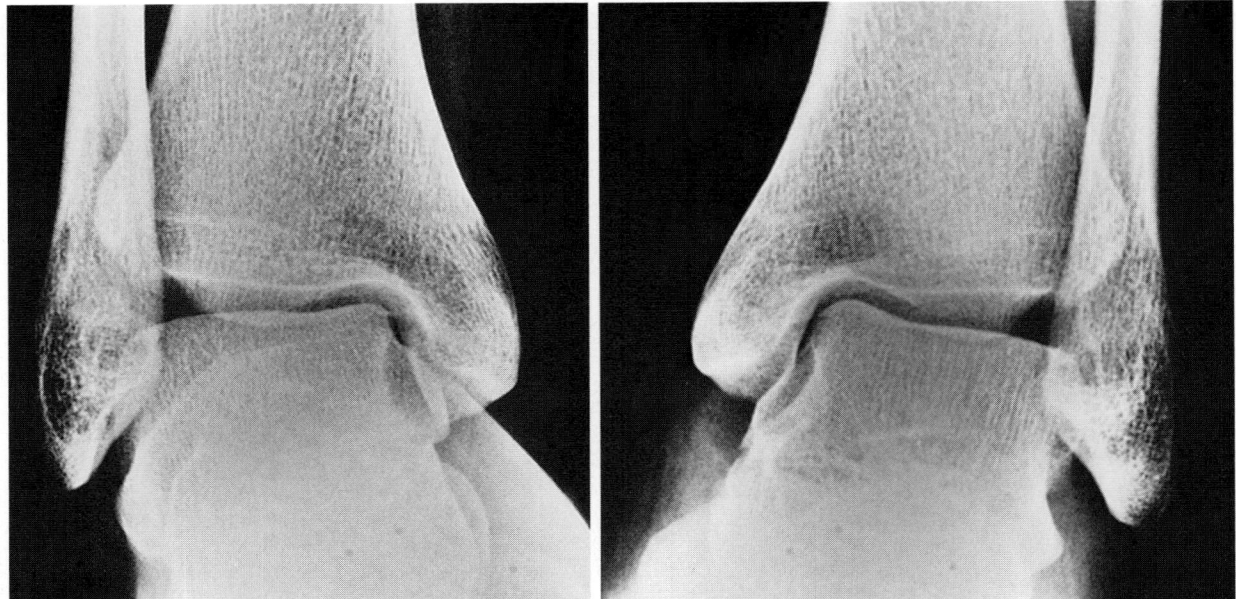

Figure 7–403. Stress views of a normal ankle demonstrate the degree of joint widening. This is subject to great variability and illustrates the need for comparison views of the opposite side.

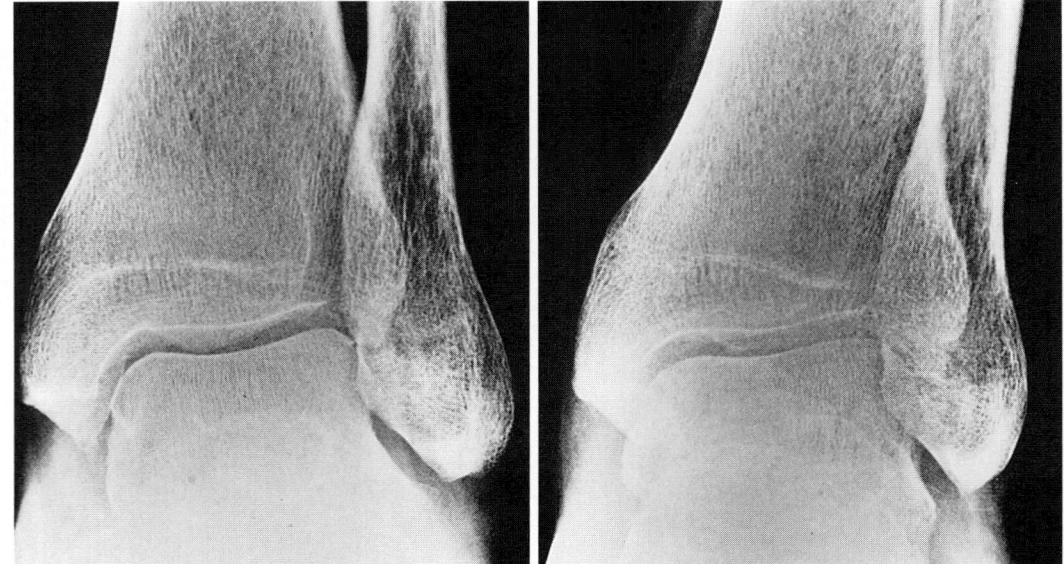

Figure 7–404. Pseudotalar tilt produced by improper positioning of the foot at the time of filming. (Ref: Bigongiari LR: Pseudotibiotalar slant: A positioning artifact. *Radiology* 122:669, 1977.)

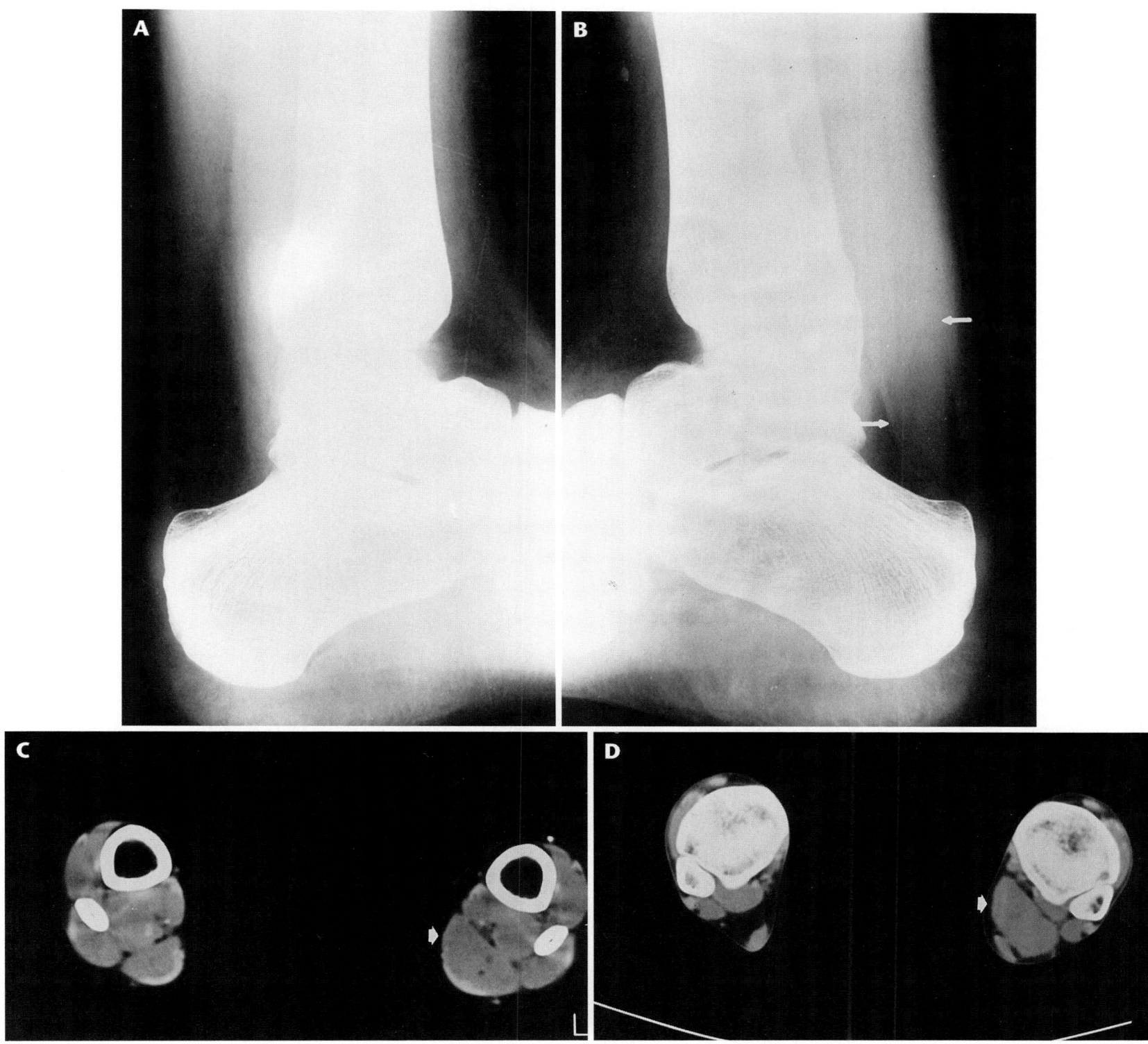

Figure 7–405. The accessory soleus muscle. **A,** No abnormality of posterior soft tissues of right ankle. **B,** Soft tissue mass in posterior soft tissues of left ankle. **C,** CT images of each calf show a mass with the density of muscle in the left calf (*arrows*). The right calf is normal. **D,** CT images of both ankles show a well-defined mass between the tibia and the Achilles tendon on the left (*arrow*). (Ref: Apple JS et al: Case report 376. *Skeletal Radiol* 15:398, 1986; Yu JS, Resnick D: MR imaging of the accessory soleus muscle appearance in 6 patients and a review of the literature. *Skeletal Radiol* 25:525, 1994.)

The Foot

The Tarsals

THE ACCESSORY OSSICLES

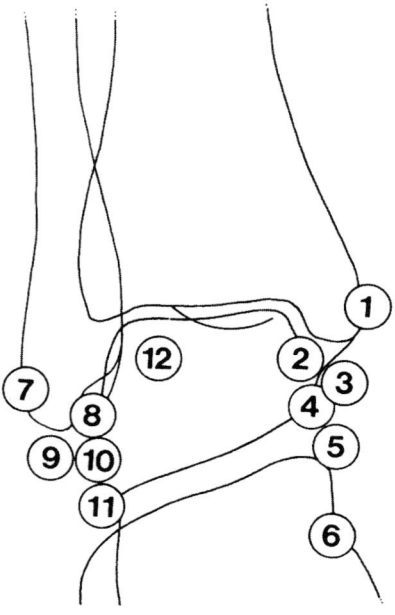

Figure 7–406. Accessory skeletal elements as seen on an anteroposterior radiograph of the ankle joint. (Ref: Kohler A, Zimmer EA: *Borderlands of the normal and early pathologic findings in skeletal roentgenology,* 3rd ed. New York, Grune & Stratton, 1968.)
1. Accompanying shadow on the internal malleolus (patella malleoli)
2. Intercalary bone (or sesamoid) between the internal malleolus and the talus
3. Os subtibiale
4. Talus accessorius
5. Os sustentaculi
6. Os tibiale externum
7. Os retinaculi
8. Intercalary bone (or sesamoid) between the external malleolus and the talus
9. Os secundarius
10. Talus secundarius
11. Os trochleare calcanei
12. Os trigonum

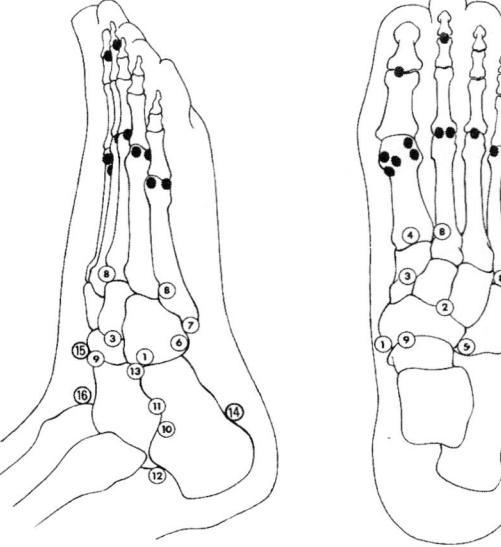

Figure 7–407. The accessory bones of the foot (after Kohler). (Ref: Kohler A, Zimmer EA: *Borderlands of the normal and early pathologic findings in skeletal roentgenology,* 3rd ed. New York, Grune & Stratton, 1968.) The sesamoid bones are indicated by *shaded circles.* These ossicles are usually of no clinical significance, but their recognition is important in the differential diagnosis of fracture. (Ref: Zatzkin HR: Trauma of the foot. *Semin Roentgenol* 5:419, 1970.)
1. Os tibiale externum
2. Processus uncinatus
3. Os intercuneiforme
4. Pars peronea metatarsalia
5. Cuboides secundarium
6. Os peroneum
7. Os vesalianum
8. Os intermetatarseum
9. Os supratalare
10. Talus accessorius
11. Os sustentaculum
12. Os trigonum
13. Calcaneus secundarius
14. Os subcalcis
15. Os supranaviculare
16. Os talotibiale

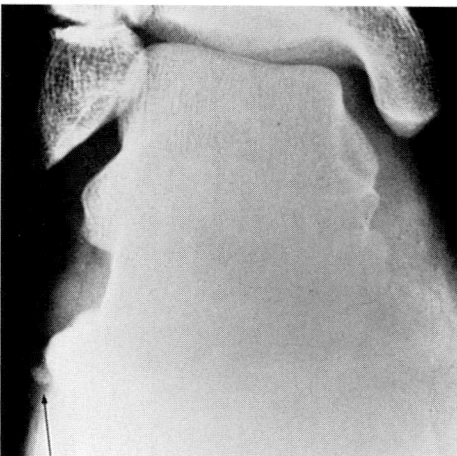

Figure 7–408. The os talocalcanei. (Ref: Kohler A, Zimmer EA: *Borderlands of the normal and early pathologic findings in skeletal roentgenology,* 3rd ed. New York, Grune & Stratton, 1968, p. 488.)

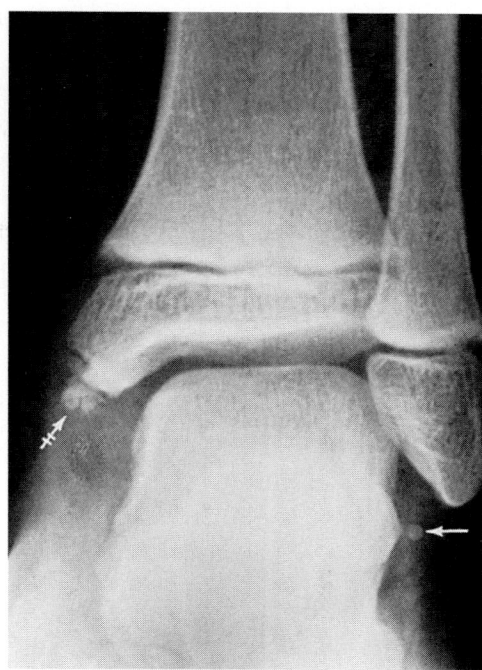

Figure 7–409. The talus secundarius (←). Secondary ossification centers are seen at the medial malleolus (⟻).

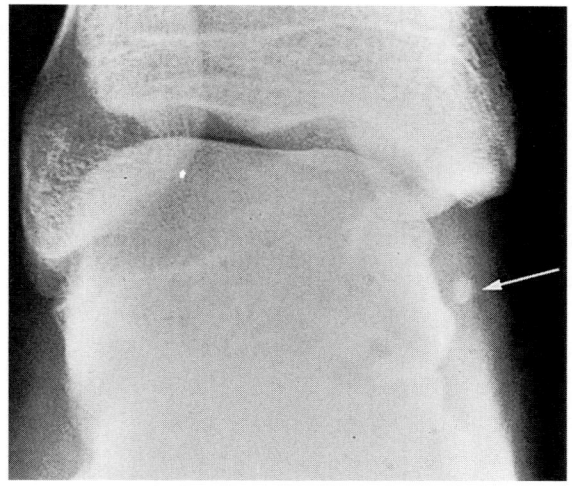

Figure 7–410. The talus accessorius.

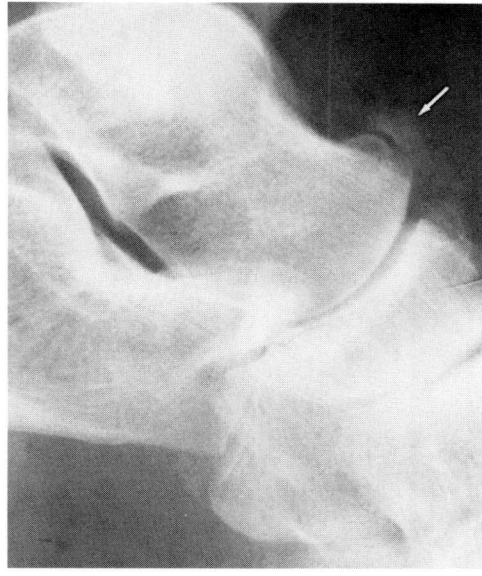

Figure 7–411. The os supratalare.

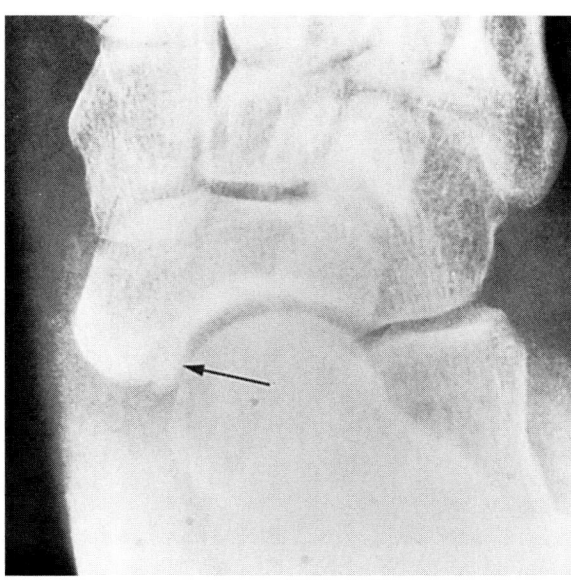

Figure 7–412. The os supratalare.

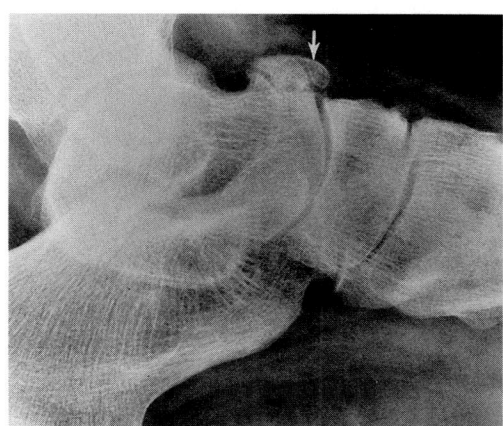

Figure 7–413. Large os supratalare.

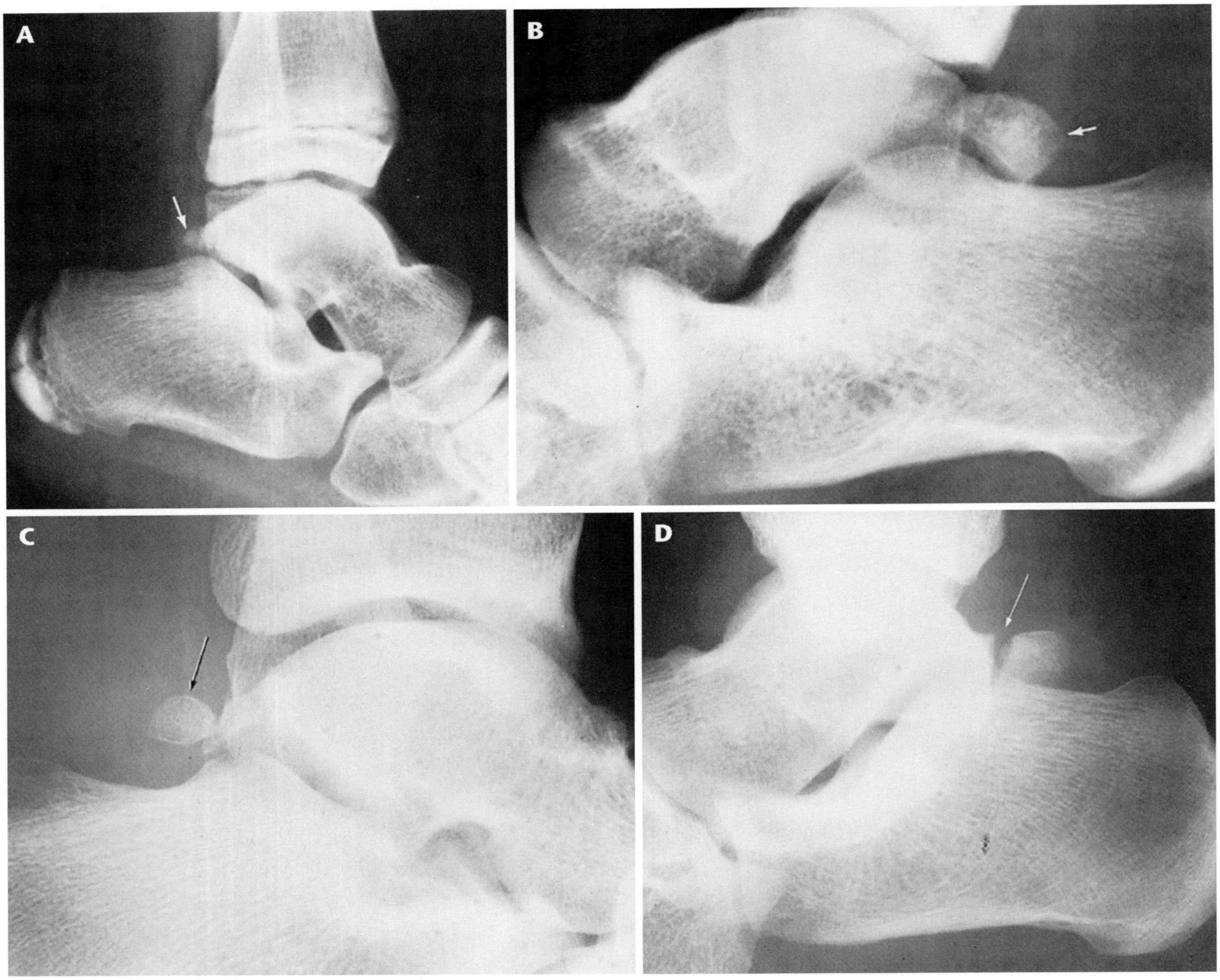

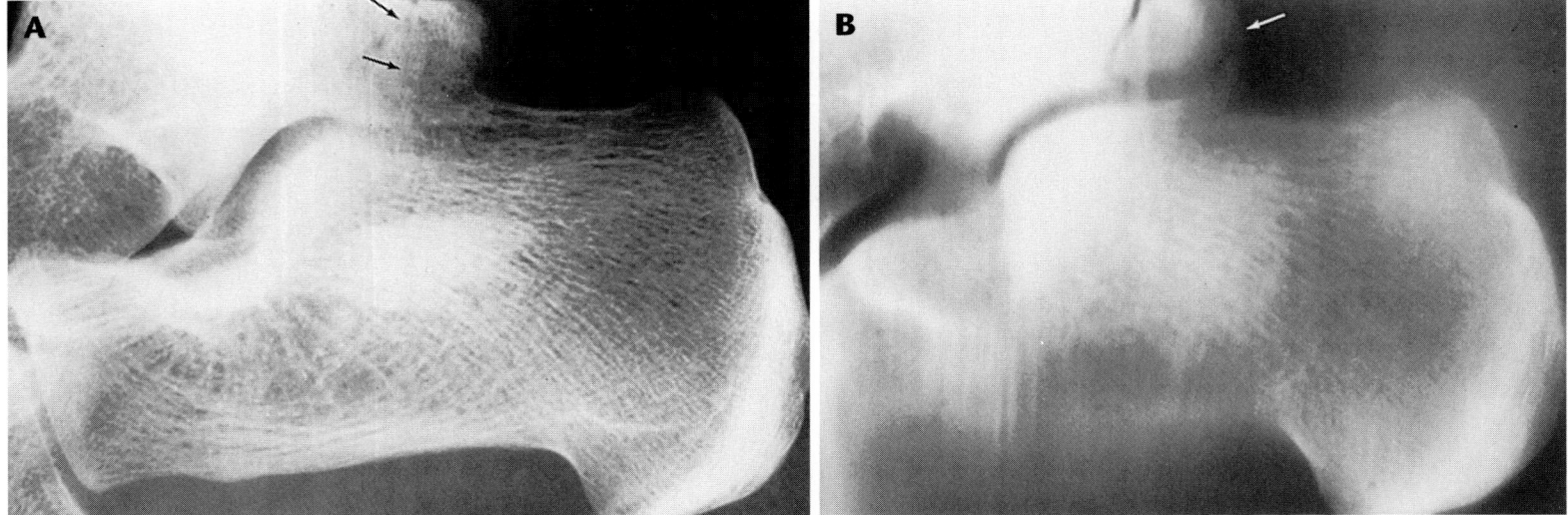

Figure 7–414. A–D, Variable appearance of the os trigonum. The multicentric appearance in **A** might be mistaken for a fracture.

Figure 7–415. A, The os trigonum may closely simulate a fracture of the posterior process of the talus. **B,** It may also require tomography for resolution.

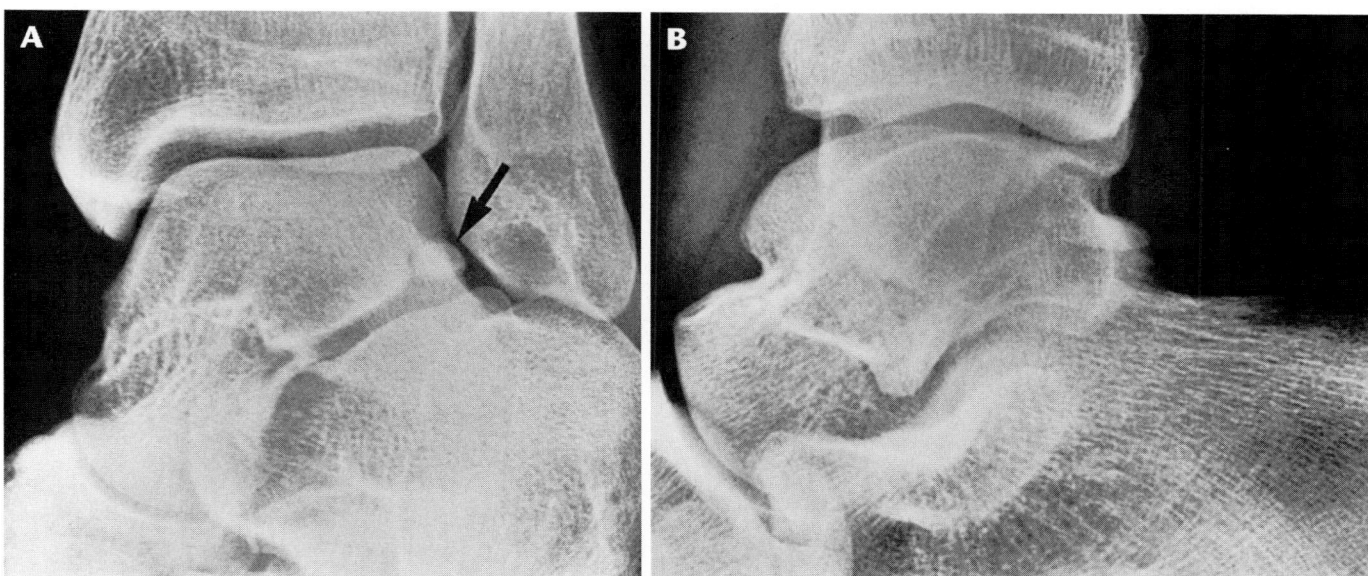

Figure 7–416. A, Os trigonum in the oblique projection may not be seen as an isolated entity in the lateral projection (**B**).

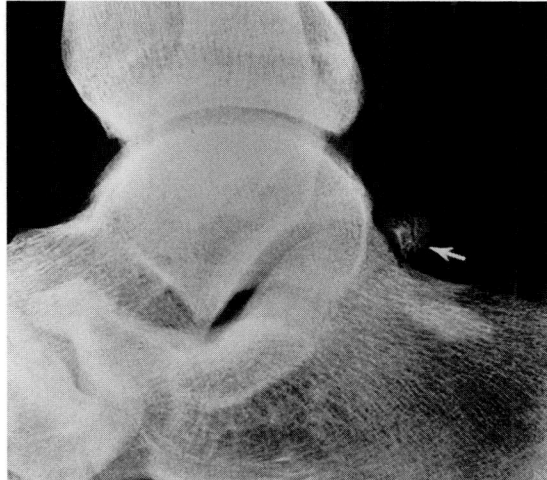

Figure 7–417. Low position of the os trigonum.

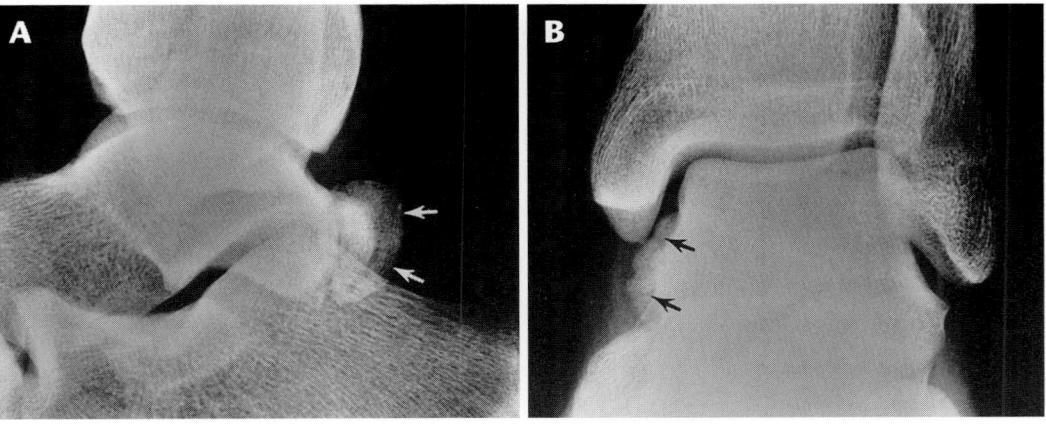

Figure 7–418. A–B, Unusual configuration of the os trigonum that can also be seen in the anteroposterior projection (**B**).

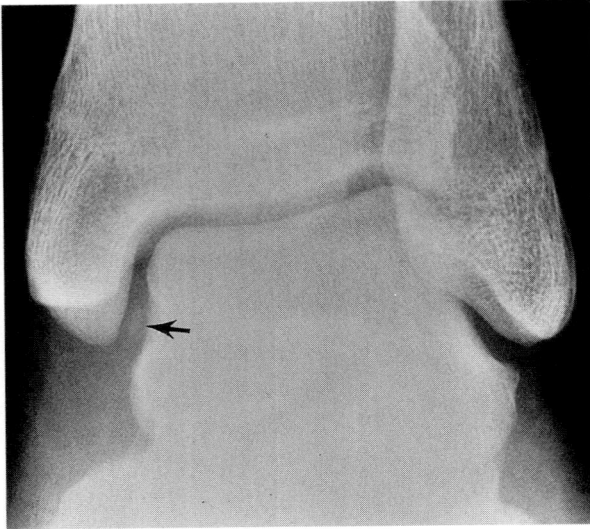

Figure 7–419. Intercalary bone (or sesamoid) between the medial malleolus and the talus.

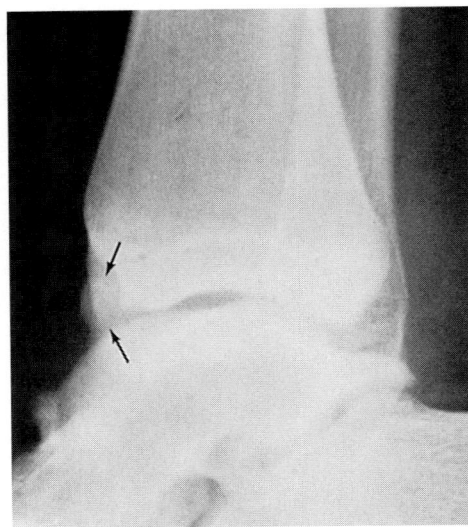

Figure 7–420. The os talotibiale.

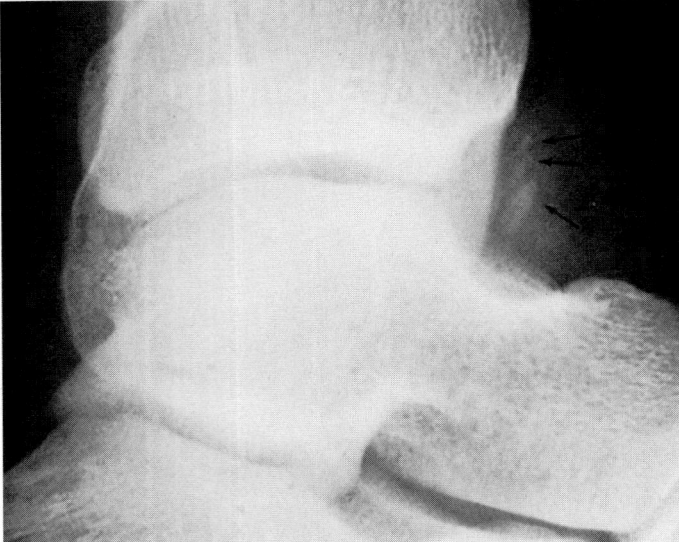

Figure 7–421. A multicentric os talotibiale.

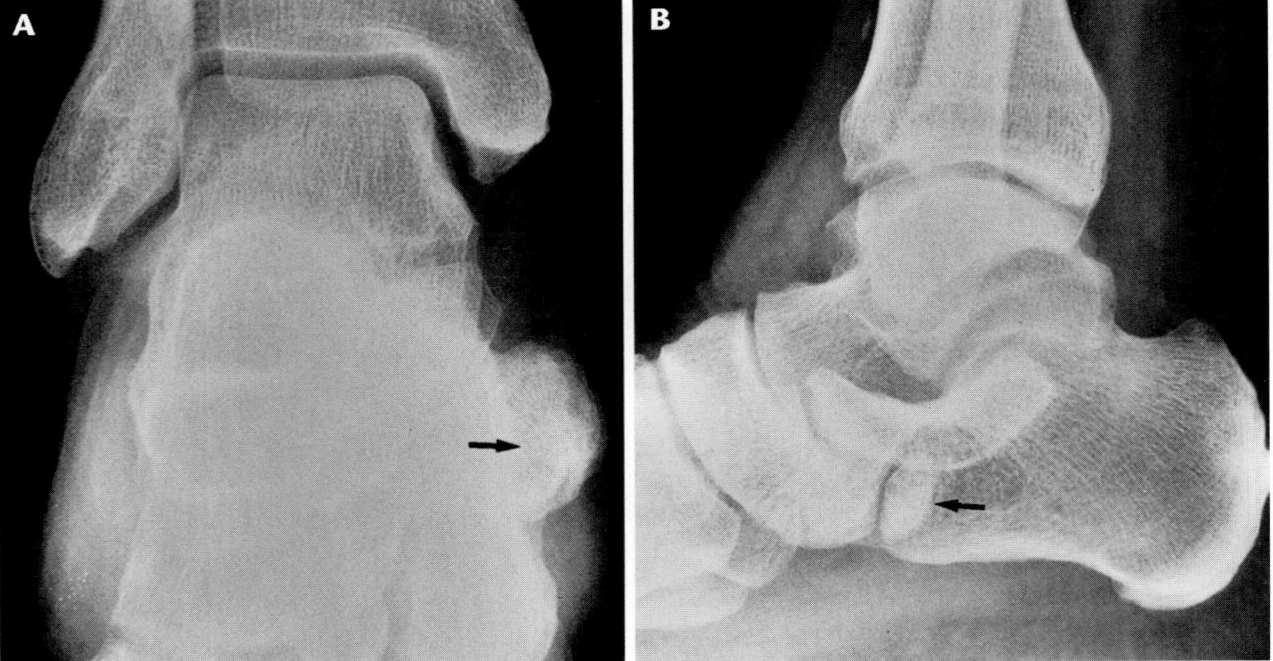

Figure 7–422. A, B, The os sustentaculum. (Ref: Kohler A, Zimmer EA: *Borderlands of the normal and early pathologic findings in skeletal roentgenology,* 4th ed. New York, Grune & Stratton, 1993, p. 802.) See also Figure 7–476.

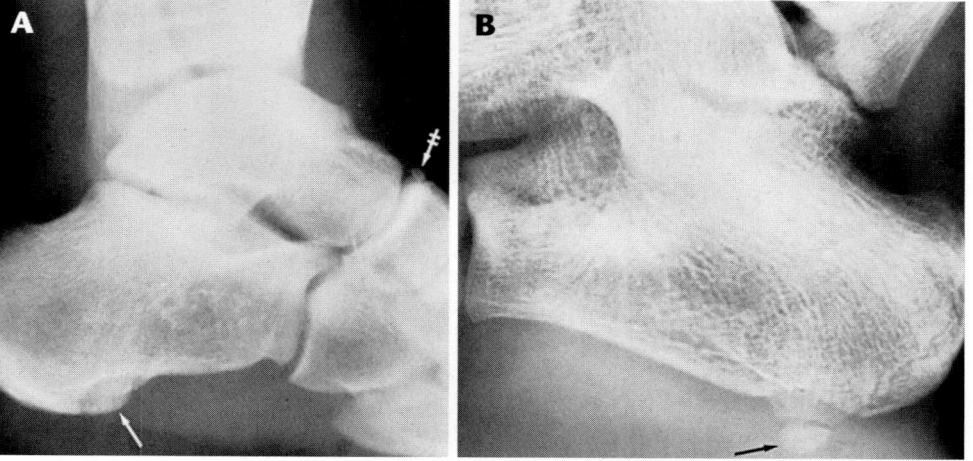

Figure 7–423. Two accessory bones of the calcaneal tuberosity. **A,** Os subcalcus (←). An os supranaviculare is also present (⊬). (Ref: Kohler A, Zimmer EA: *Borderlands of the normal and early pathologic findings in skeletal roentgenology,* 3rd ed. New York, Grune & Stratton, 1968, p. 486.) **B,** Accessory bone arising from the tip of the trochlear process on the lateral wall of the calcaneus, seen in oblique projection. (Ref: Caffey J: *Pediatric x-ray diagnosis,* 9th ed. St. Louis, Mosby, 1993, p. 1515.)

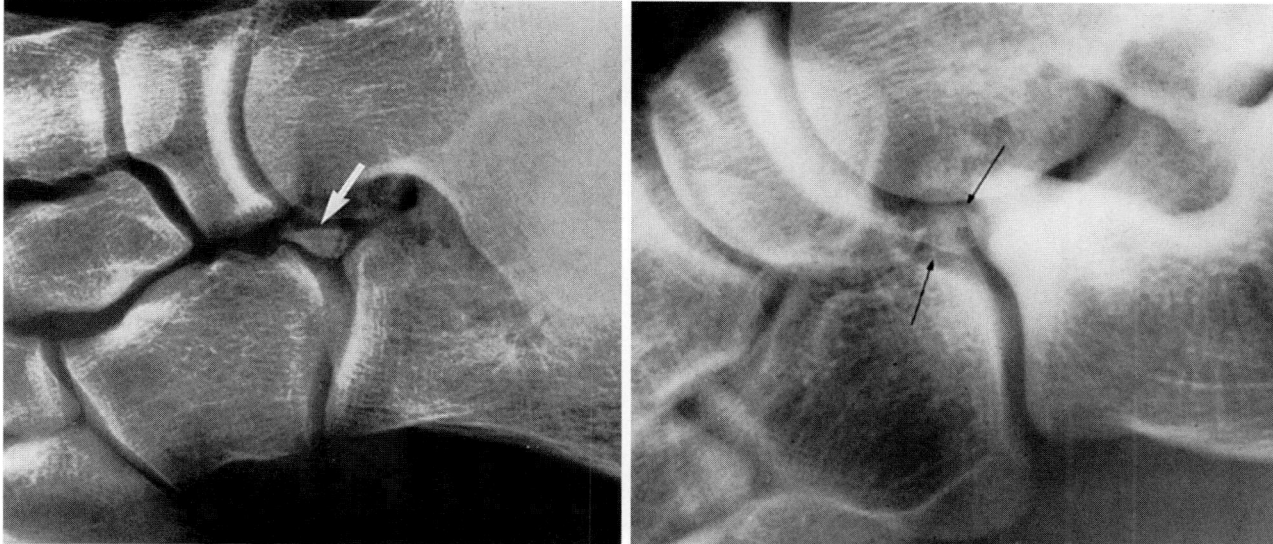

Figure 7–424. The calcaneus secundarius.

Figure 7–425. A small os peroneum.

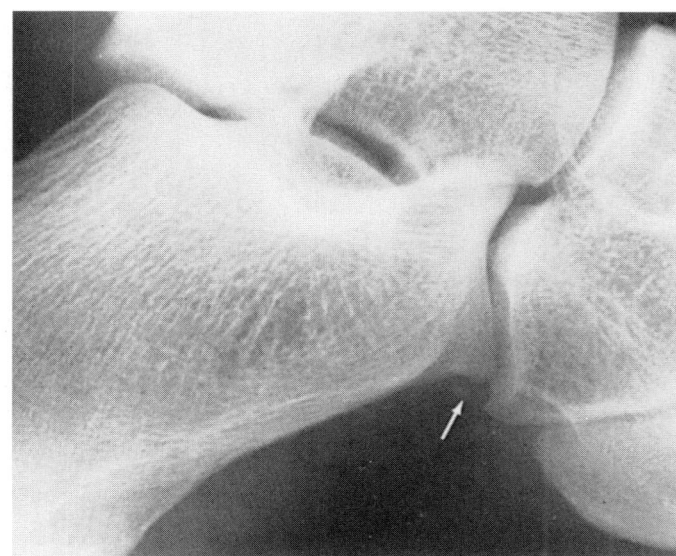

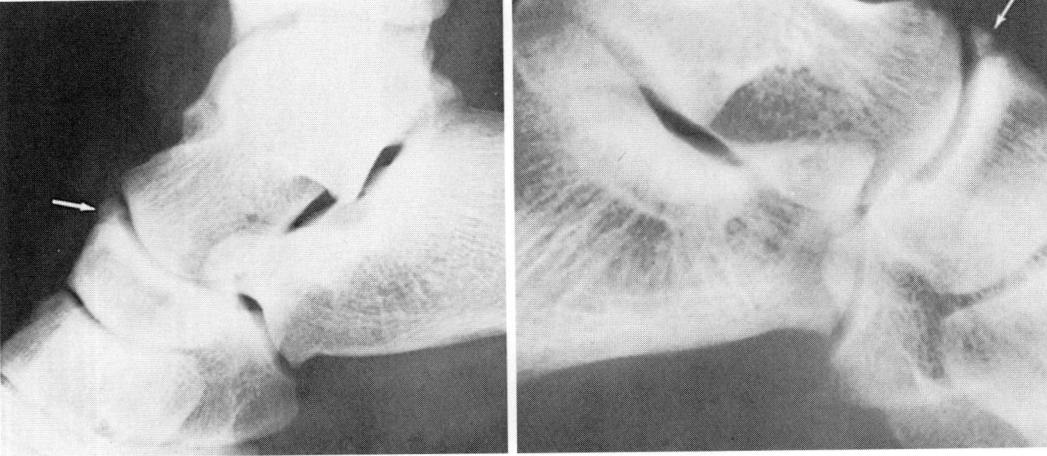

Figure 7–426. Two examples of the os supranaviculare. This ossicle is often confused with an avulsion fracture.

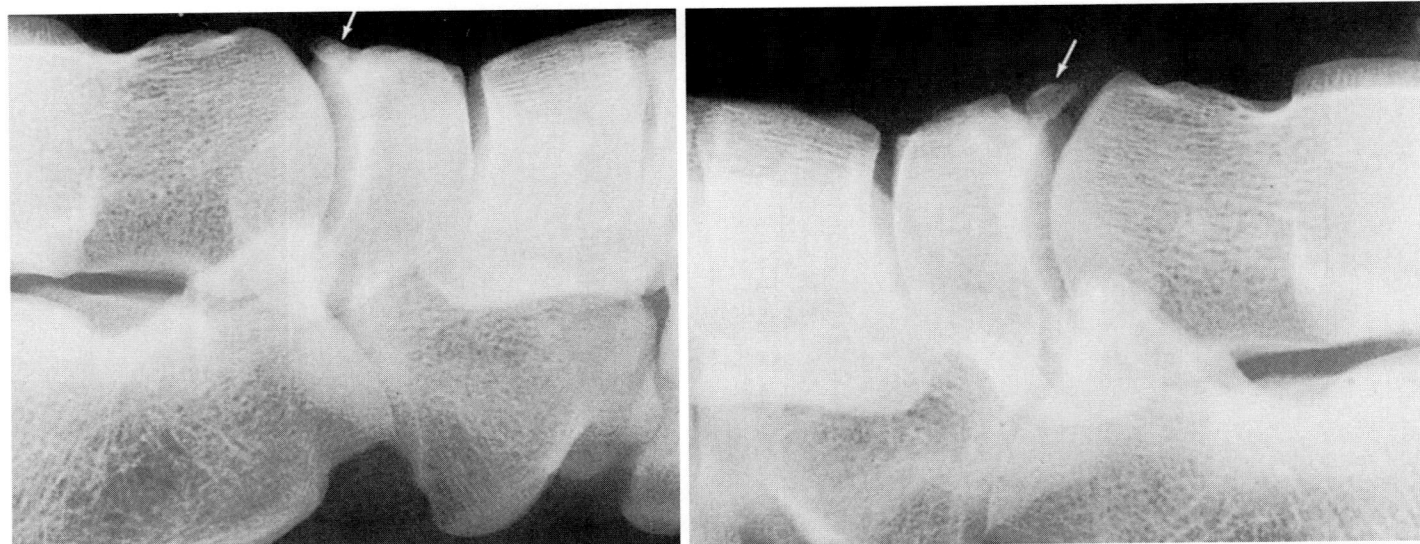

Figure 7–427. Bilateral os supranaviculare.

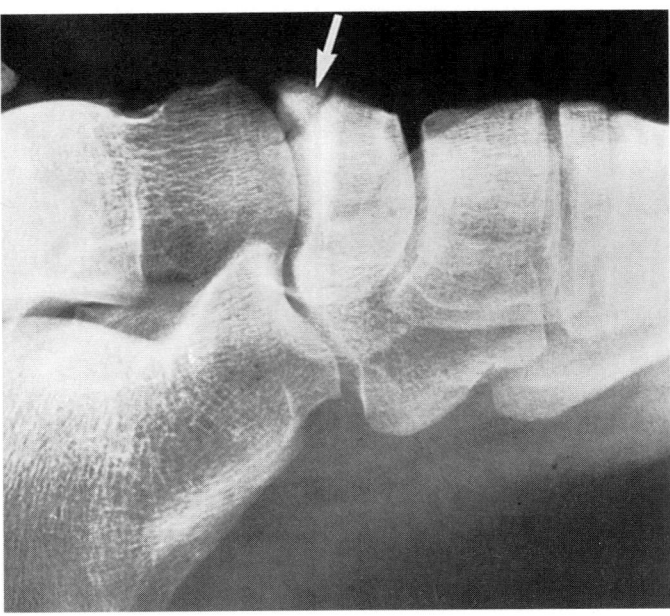

Figure 7–428. Large os supranaviculare.

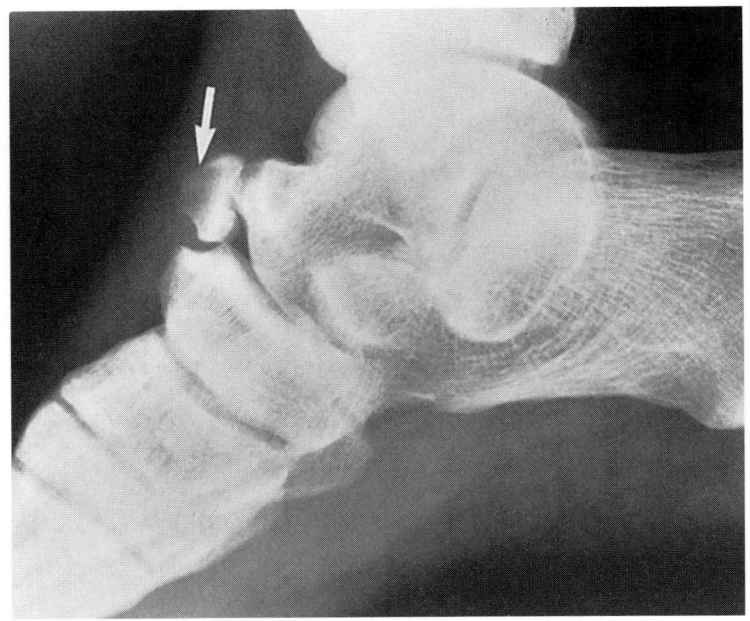

Figure 7–429. Huge os supranaviculare with articulations with both the talus and navicular.

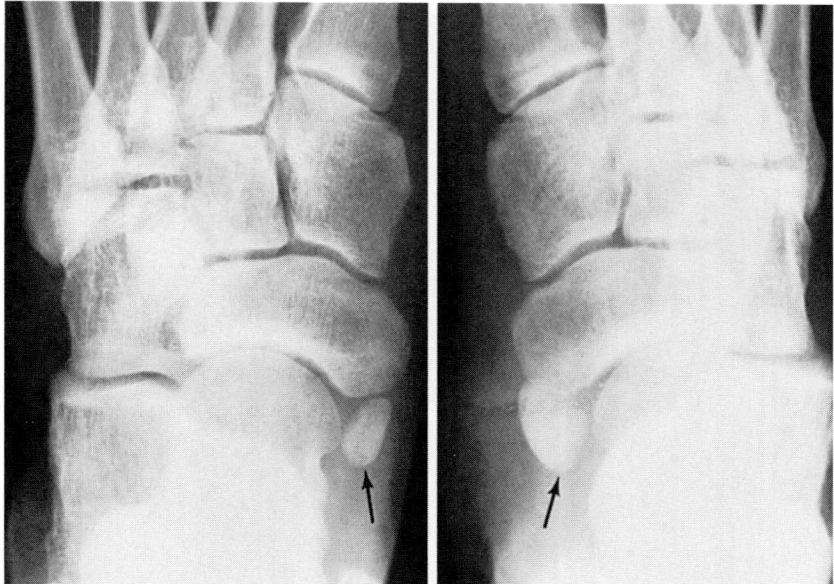

Figure 7–430. Large, bilateral os tibiale externum.

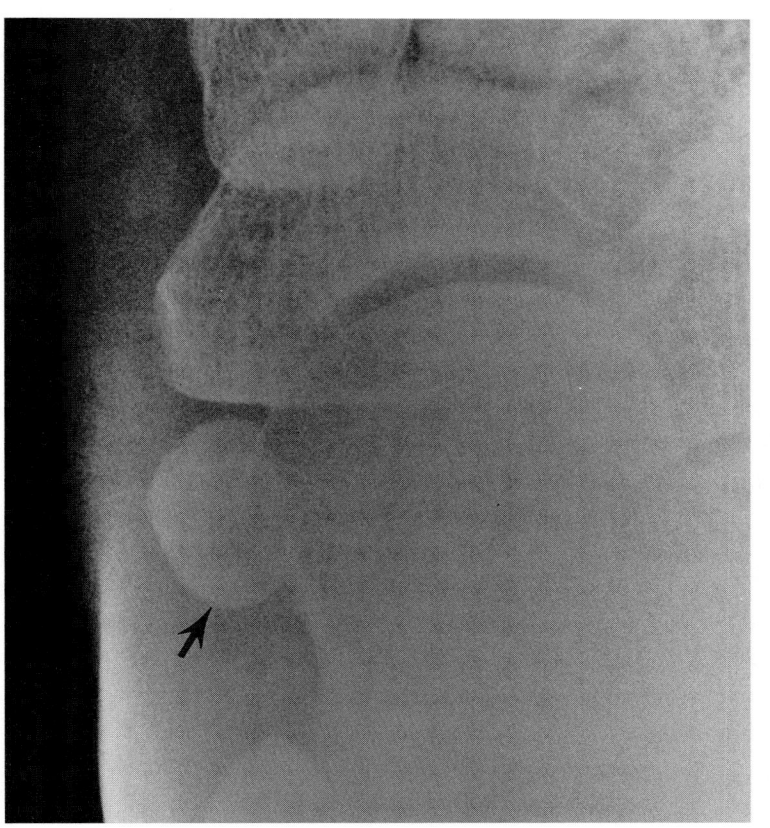

Figure 7–431. Huge os tibiale externum.

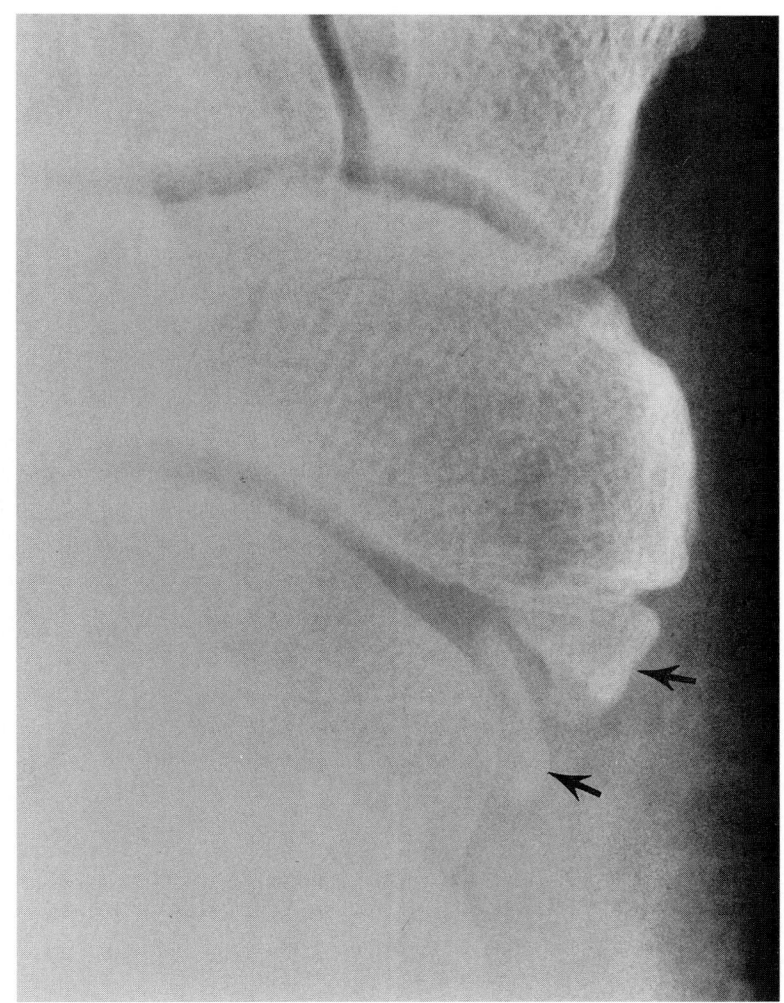

Figure 7–432. Bipartite os tibiale externum.

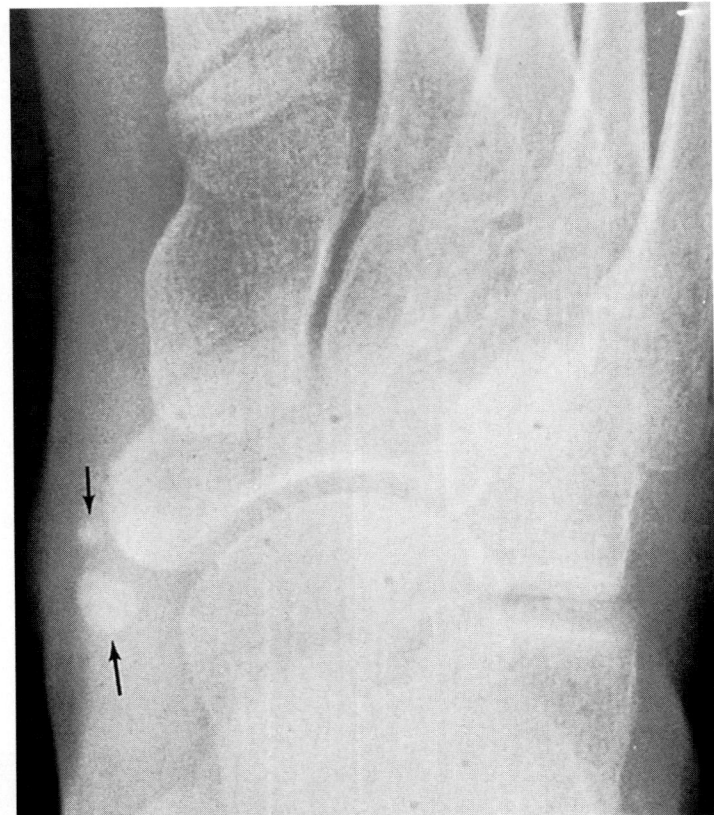

Figure 7–433. Bipartite os tibiale externum.

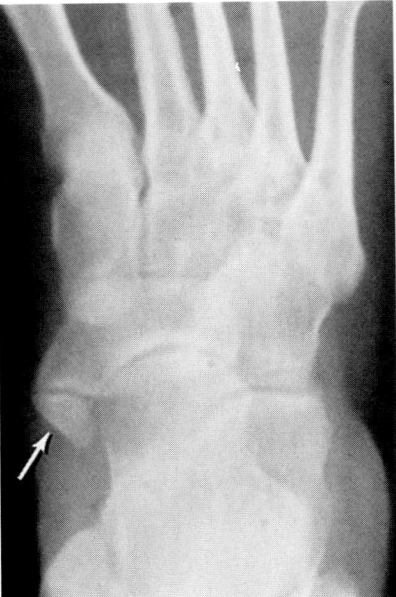

Figure 7–434. Partially fused os tibiale externum (accessory navicular).

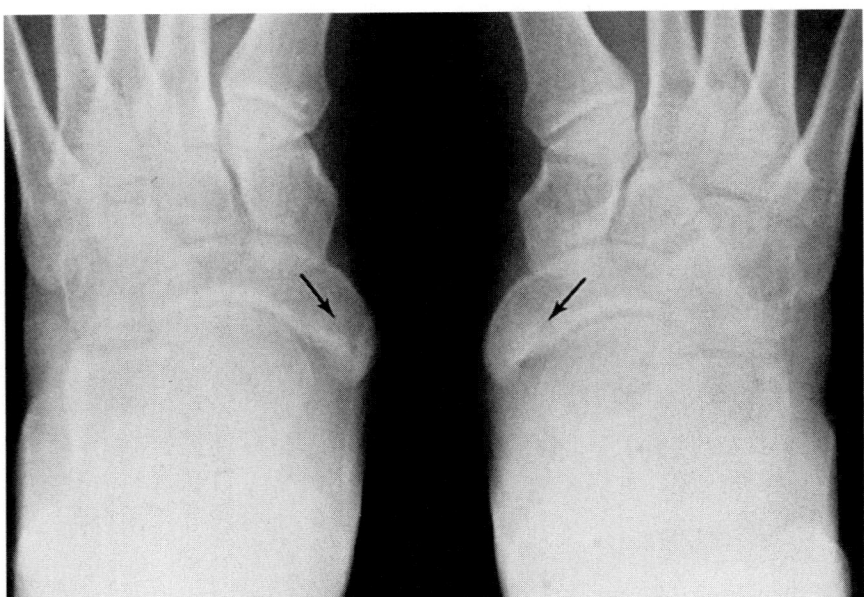

Figure 7–435. Virtually complete fusion of the os tibiale externum to the navicular bone (cornuate navicular).

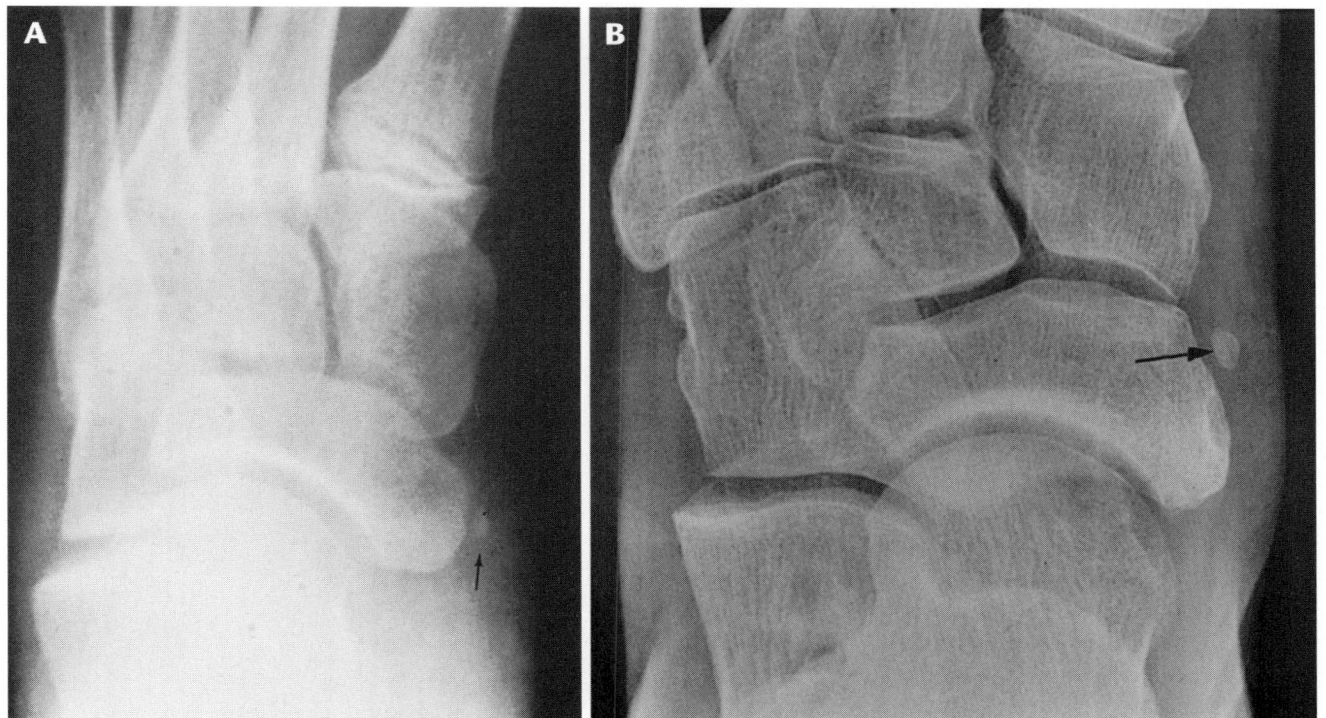

Figure 7–436. A, B, Two examples of an unnamed ossicle adjacent to the navicular.

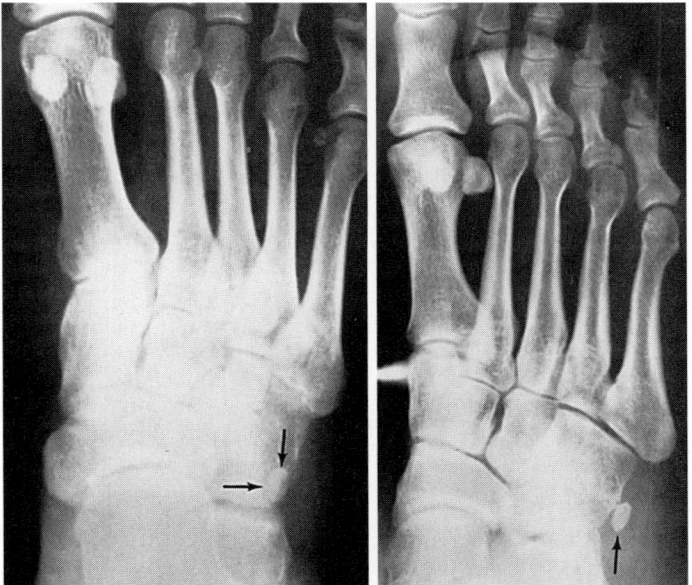

Figure 7–437. The os peroneum.

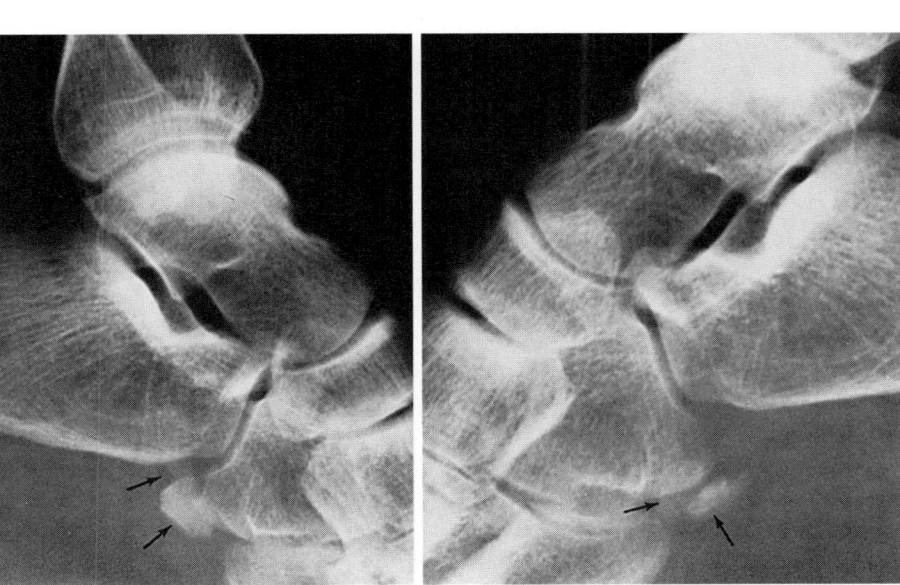

Figure 7–438. Large, multicentric os peroneum.

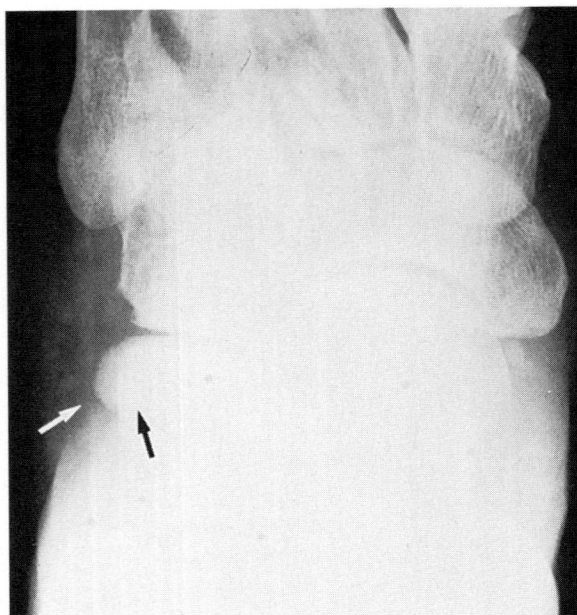

Figure 7–439. The os peroneum in frontal projection.

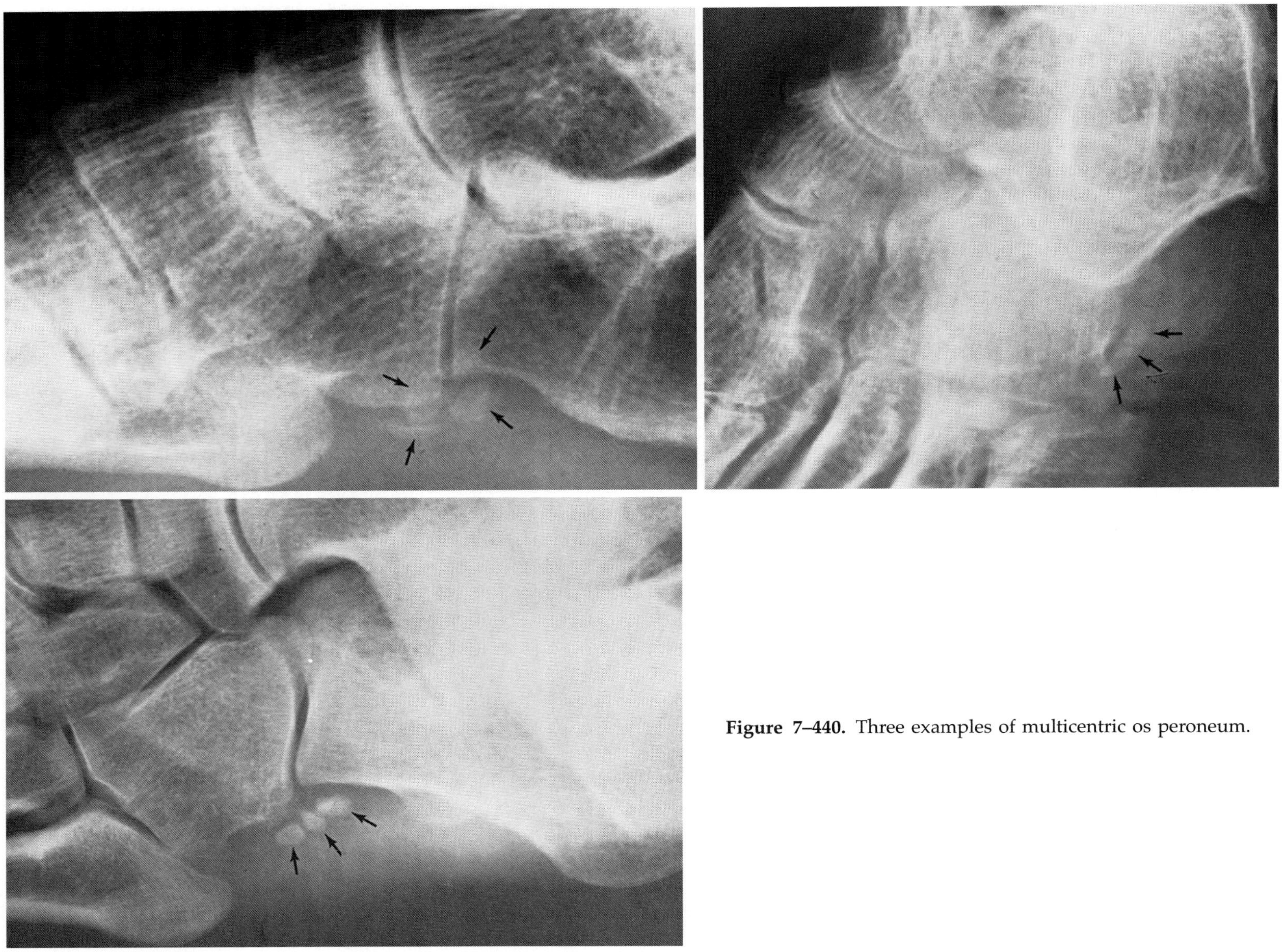

Figure 7–440. Three examples of multicentric os peroneum.

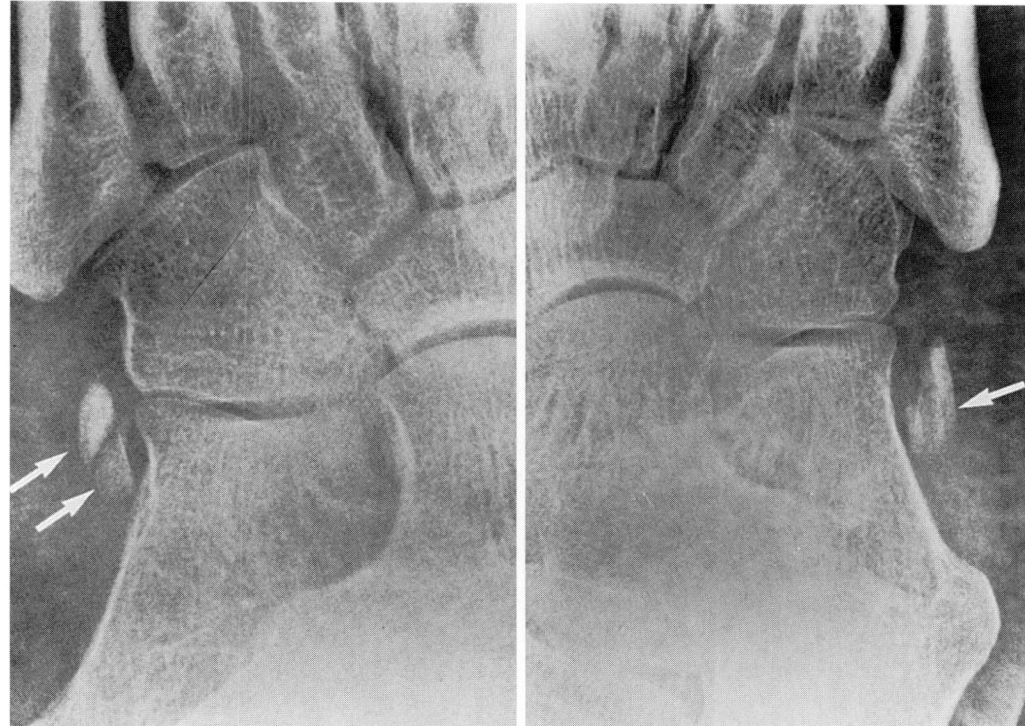

Figure 7–441. Unusual os peroneum.

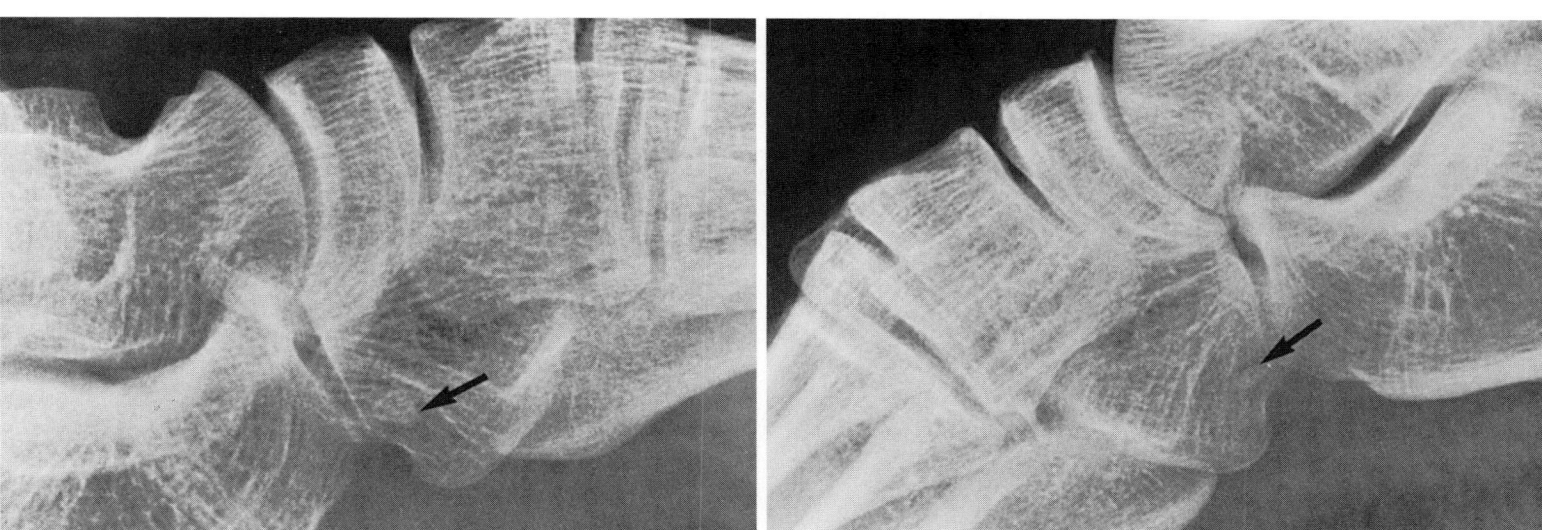

Figure 7–442. Os peroneum may be high in position and superimposed on the cuboid.

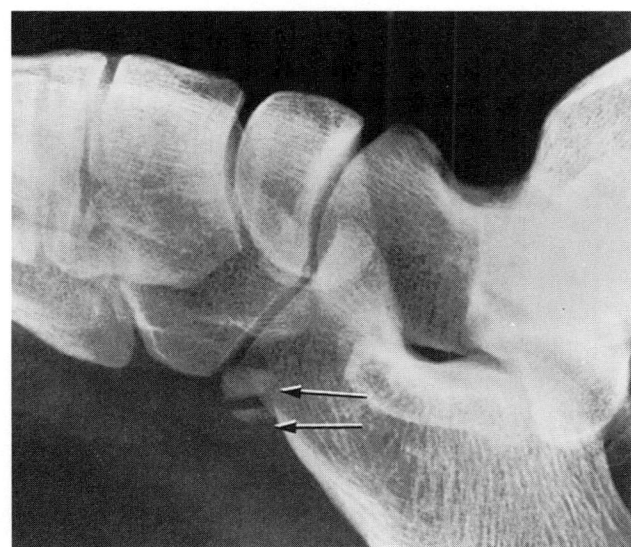

Figure 7–443. Bipartite os peroneum simulating a fracture.

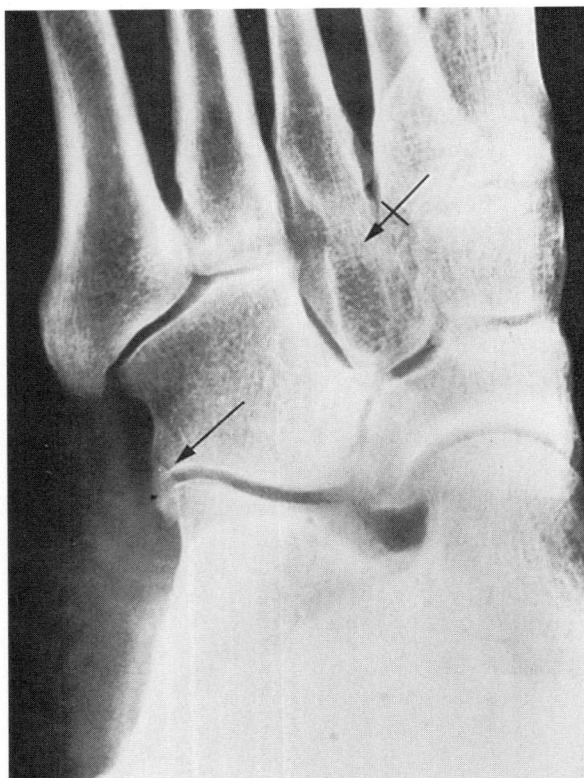

Figure 7–444. Os peroneum simulating partial coalition of the cuboid and calcaneus (←). Note the simulated fusion between the lateral cuneiform and third metatarsal.

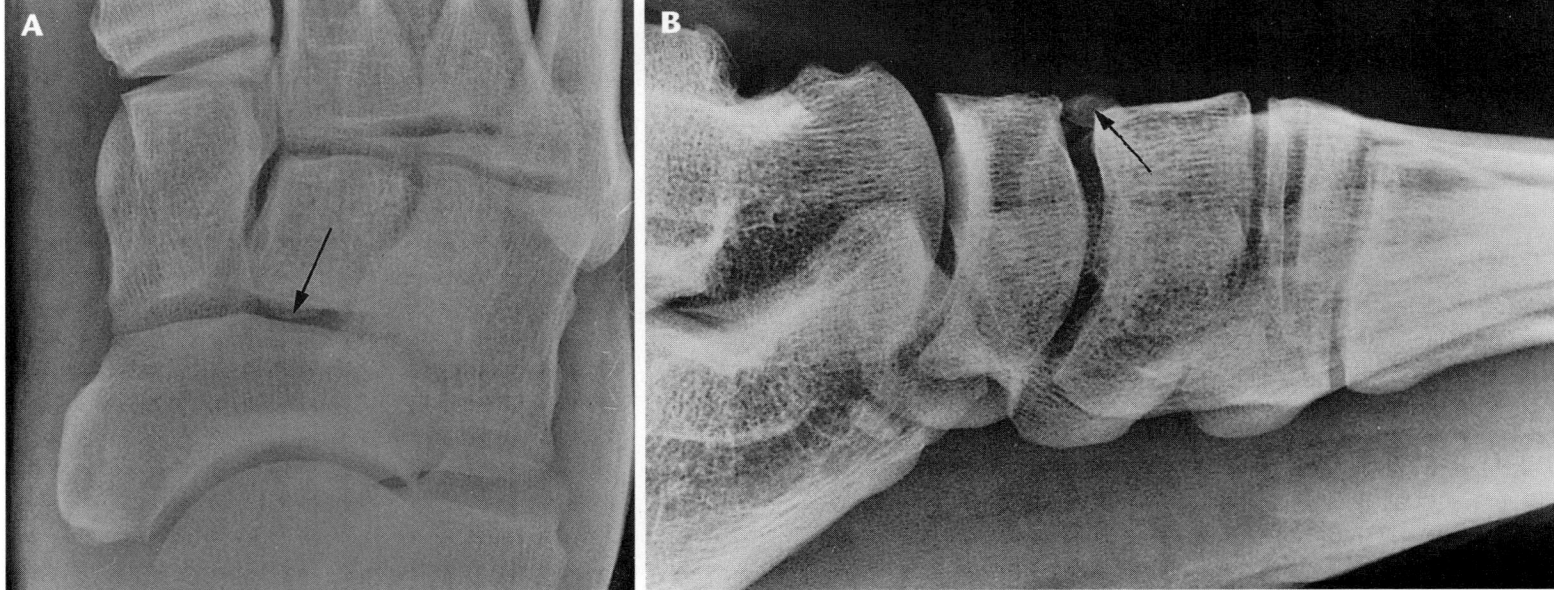

Figure 7–445. A, B, The os intercuneiform.

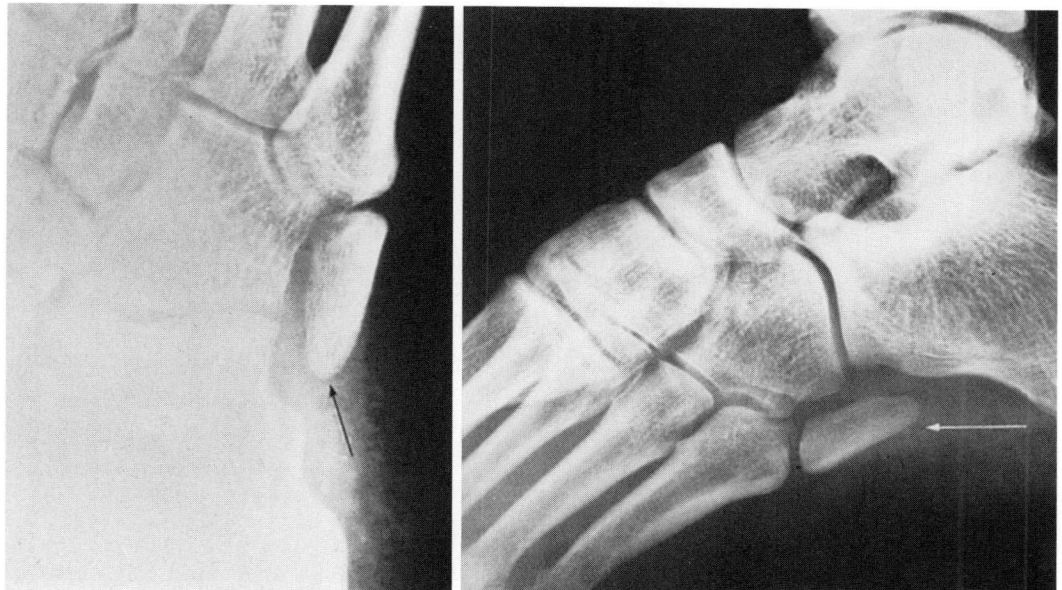

Figure 7–446. Huge os vesalianum (see Fig. 7–589).

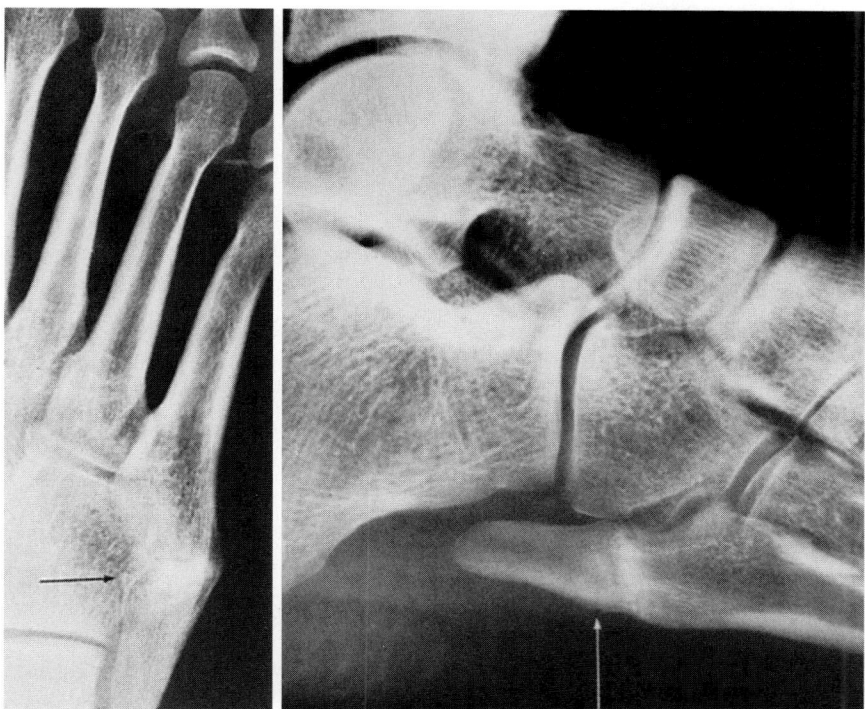

Figure 7–447. Huge os vesalianum fused to the base of the fifth metatarsal.

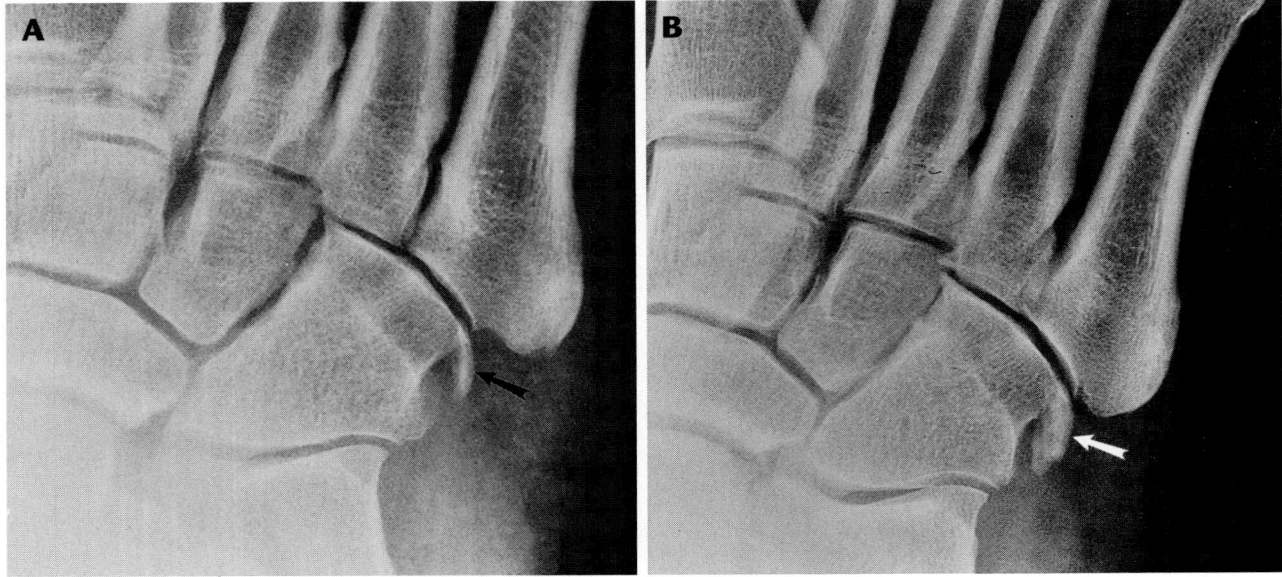

Figure 7–448. A, B, Two examples of an unnamed element, probably in the peroneus longus tendon.

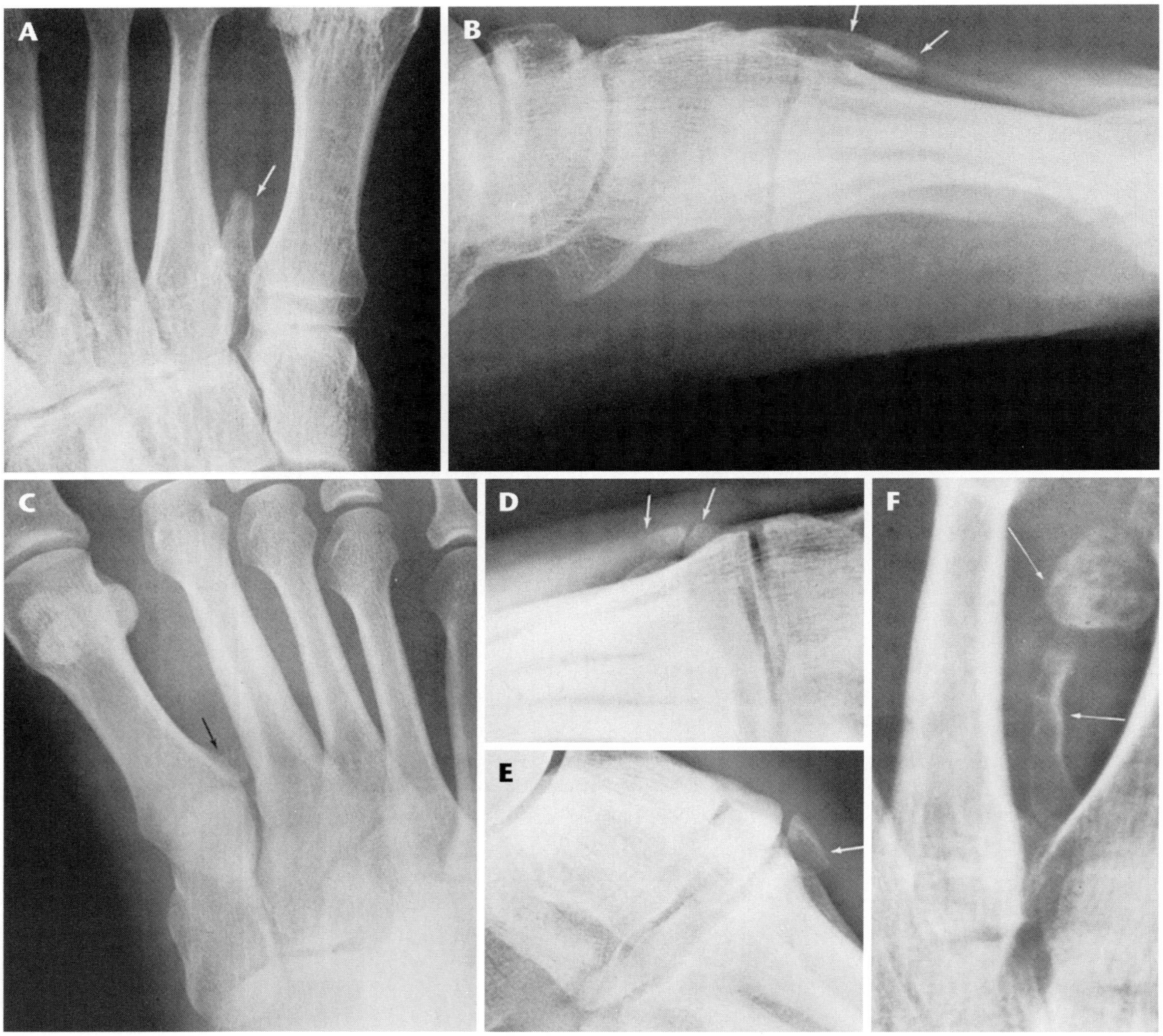

Figure 7–449. A–F, Six examples of the variable appearance of the os intermetatarseum. Note the accessory ossicle at the distal end in **F.**

The Tarsals

THE TALUS

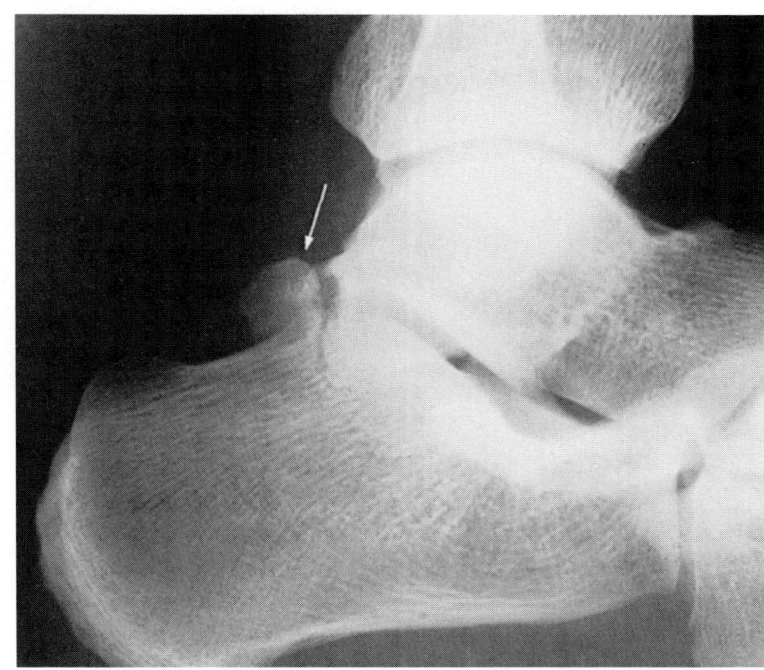

Figure 7–450. Os trigonum, which should not be mistaken for fracture of the posterior process of the talus. Symptoms related to the os trigonum are best delineated by MRI. (Ref: Karasick D, Schweitzer ME: The os trigonum syndrome. *Am J Roentgenol* 166:125, 1996.)

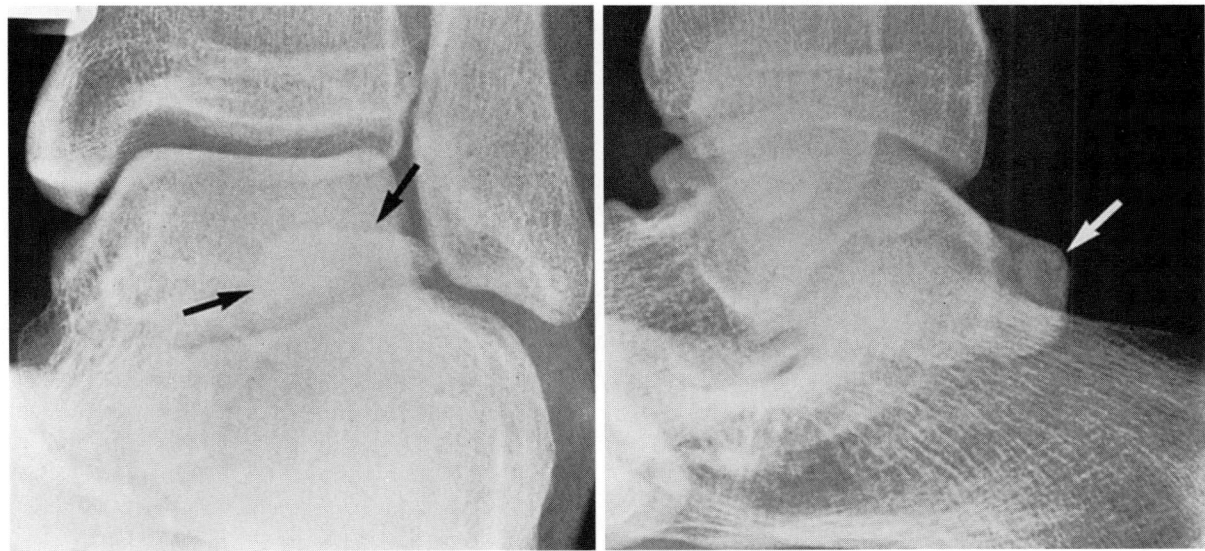

Figure 7–451. Huge posterior process of the talus.

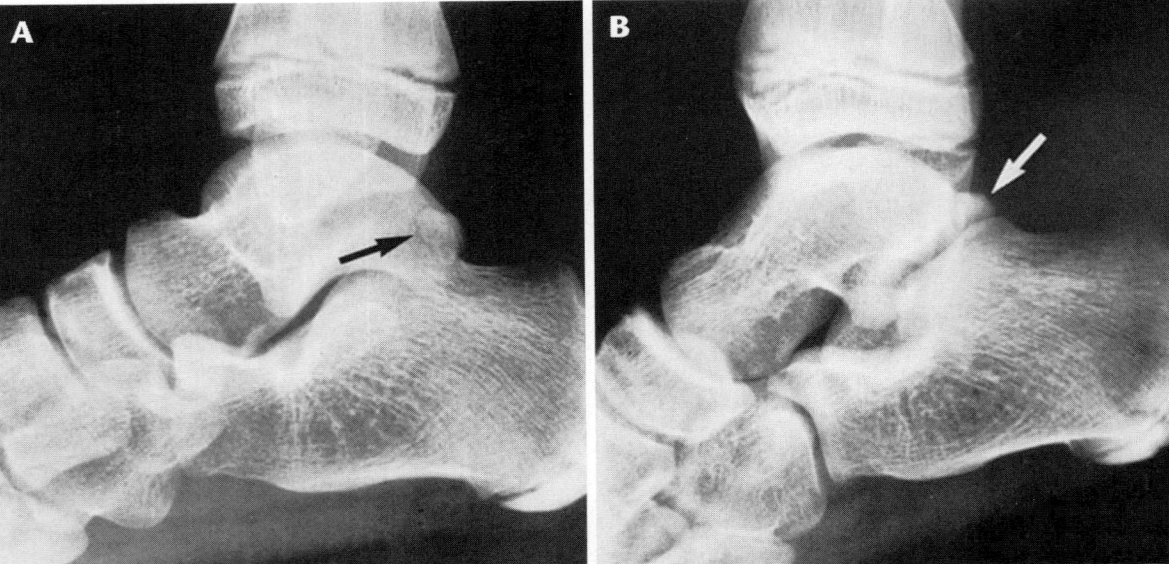

Figure 7–452. A, Os trigonum may be projected onto the talus and simulate a fracture. **B,** True lateral projection shows usual appearance of the os trigonum.

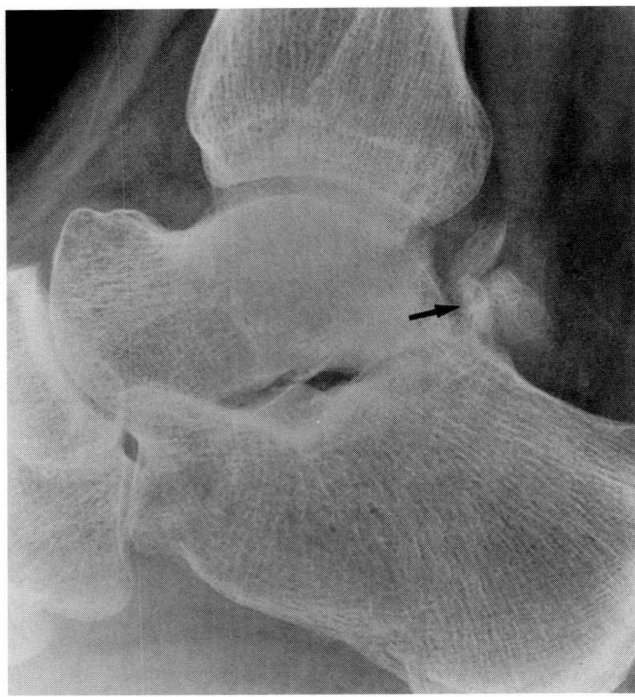

Figure 7–453. Multicentric os trigonum.

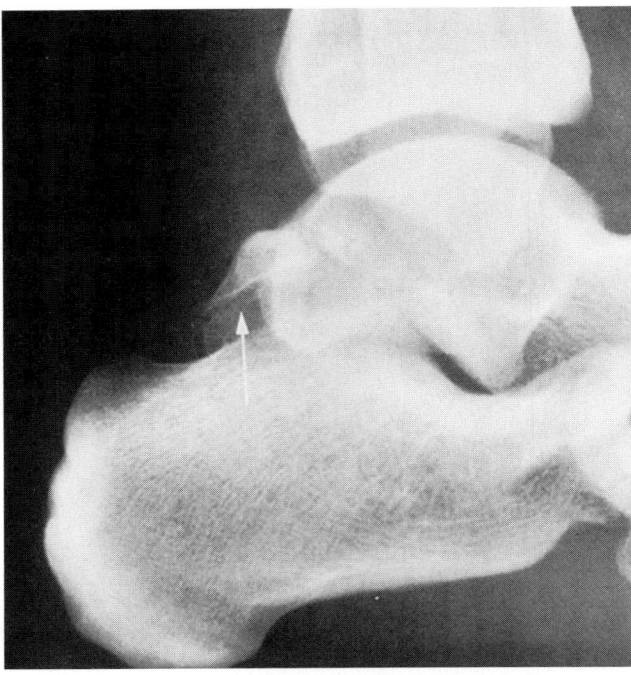

Figure 7–454. An unusual os trigonum that articulates with the posterior process of the talus (*arrow*).

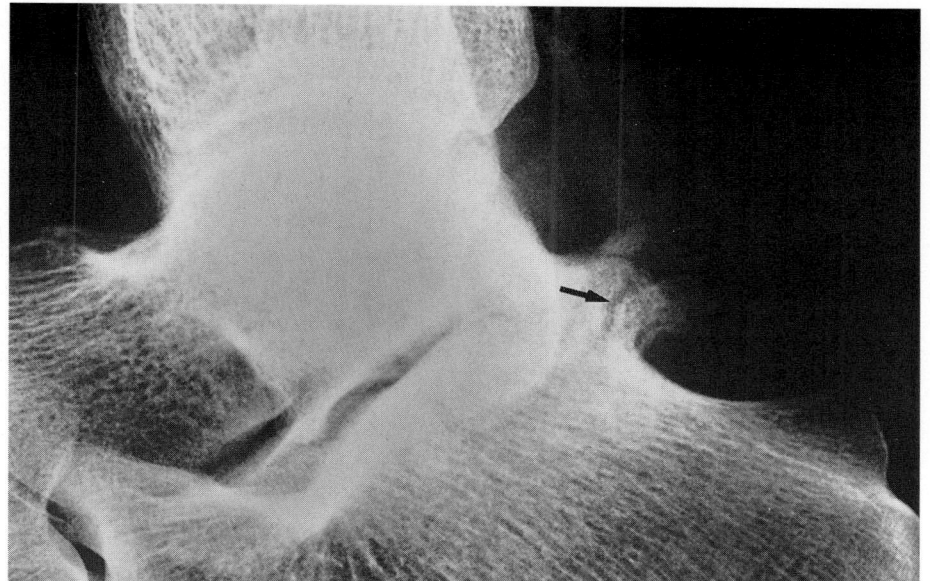

Figure 7–455. Unusual posterior process of the talus and os trigonum with articulation with the calcaneus.

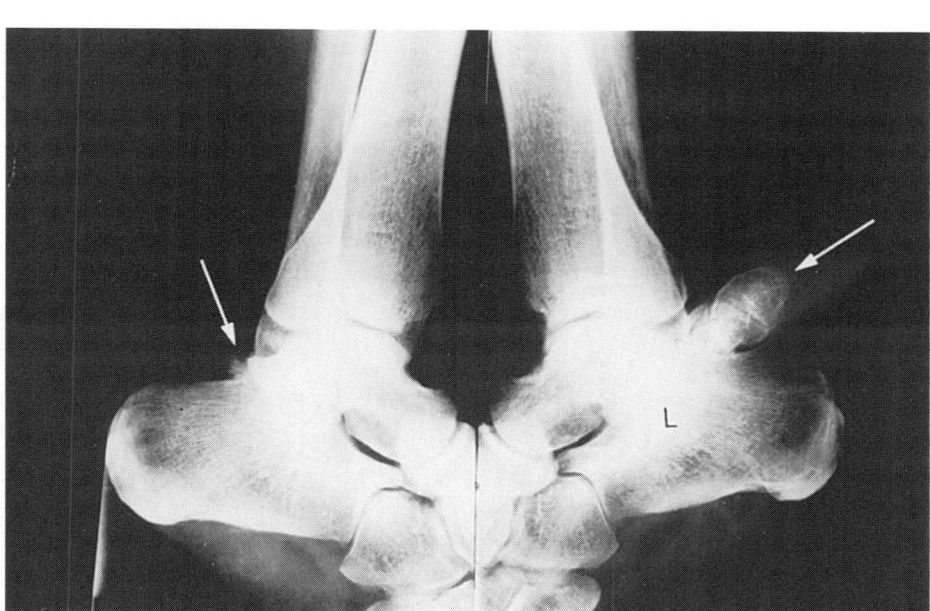

Figure 7–456. Os accessorium supracalcaneum seen prominently on the left and minimally on the right (*arrows*). This ossicle is separate from the posterior process of the talus and articulates with the posterosuperior margin of the calcaneus. (From Milgrom C et al: Open-quiz solutions: Case report 341. *Skeletal Radiol* 15:150, 1986.)

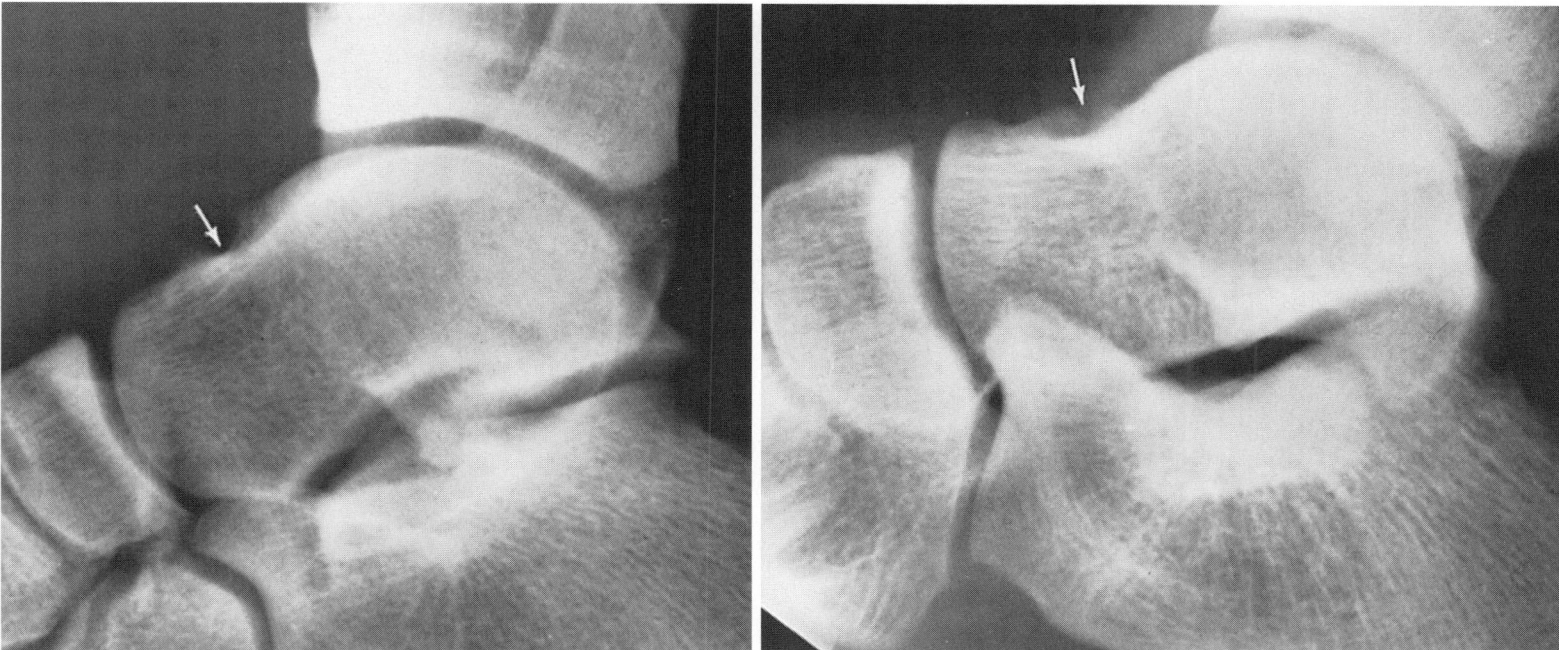

Figure 7–457. Two examples of normal saucerlike depressions on the superior aspect of the talus. (Ref: Resnick D: Talar ridges, osteophytes and beaks: A radiologic commentary. *Radiology* 151:329, 1984.)

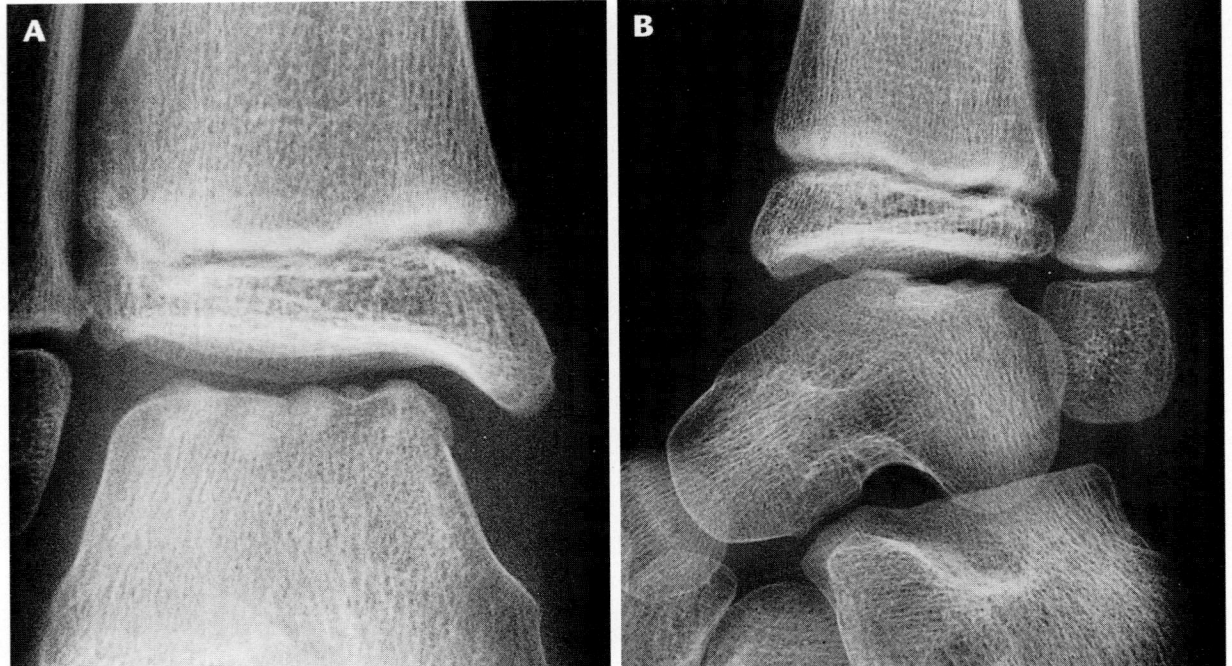

Figure 7–458. A, B, Irregular ossification of the dome of the talus in a 6-year-old child with no symptoms referable to the ankle.

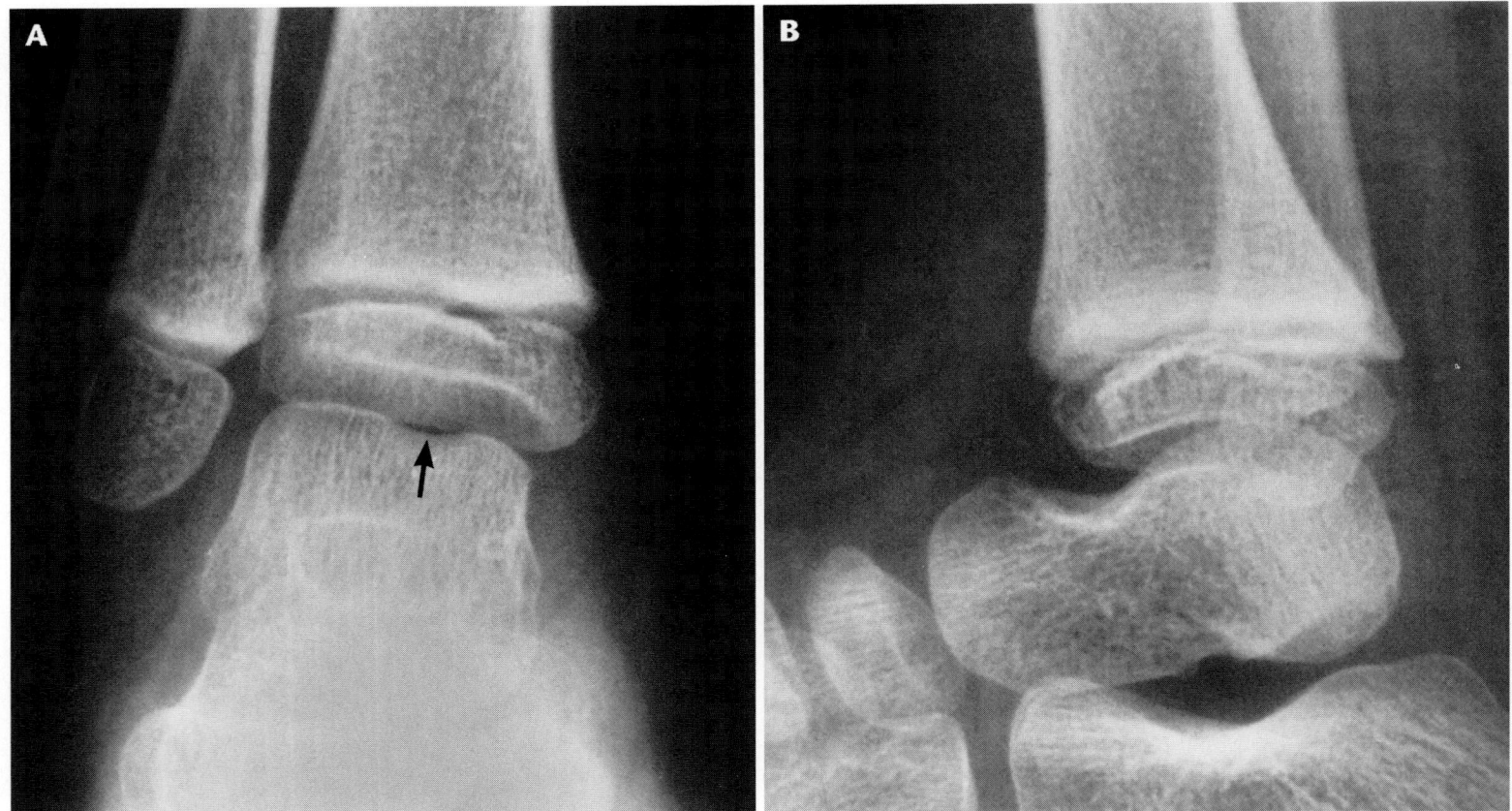

Figure 7–459. A, B, Forme fruste of bipartate talus (see Fig. 7–481). (Ref: Kohler A: *Borderlands of the normal and early pathologic findings in skeletal radiography,* 4th ed. New York, Thieme, 1993, p. 793.)

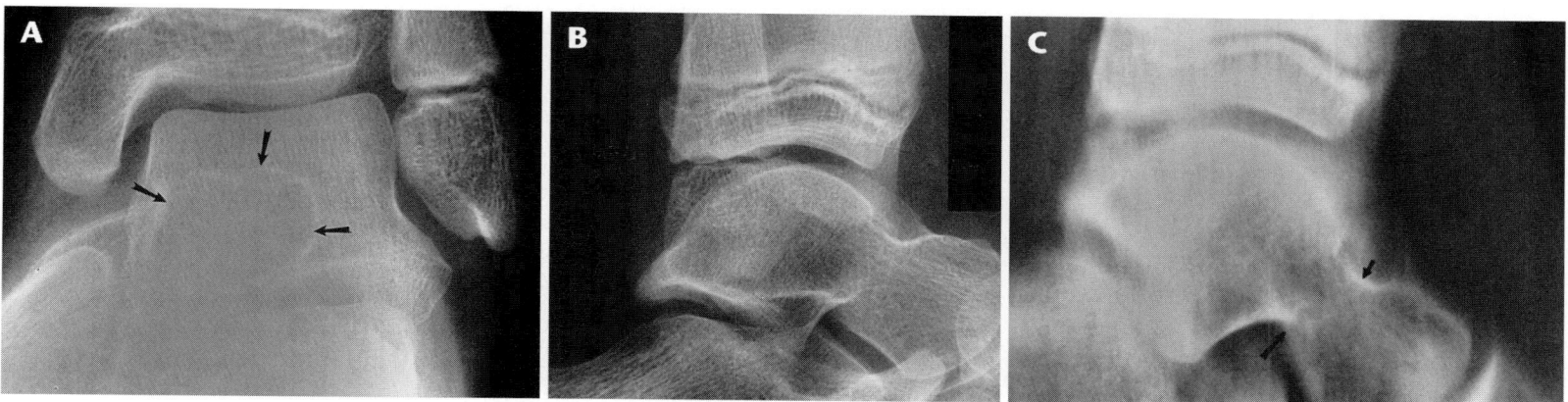

Figure 7–460. Simulated cyst of the talus produced by through projection of the narrow waist of the bone. **A** and **B**, Plain films. **C**, Tomogram.

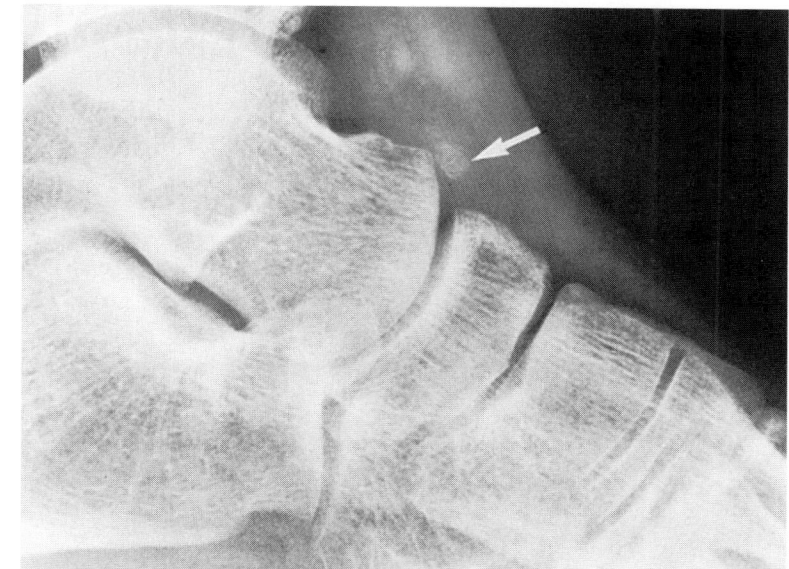

Figure 7–461. Os supratalare.

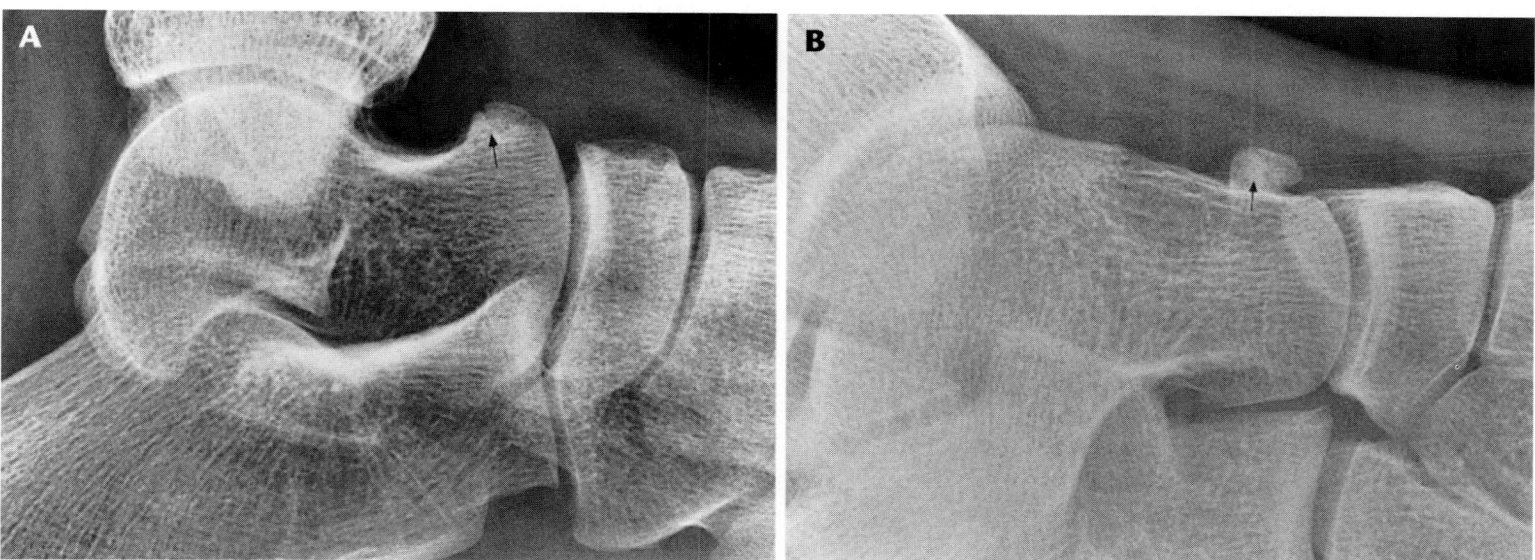

Figure 7–462. A, B, Large os supratalare.

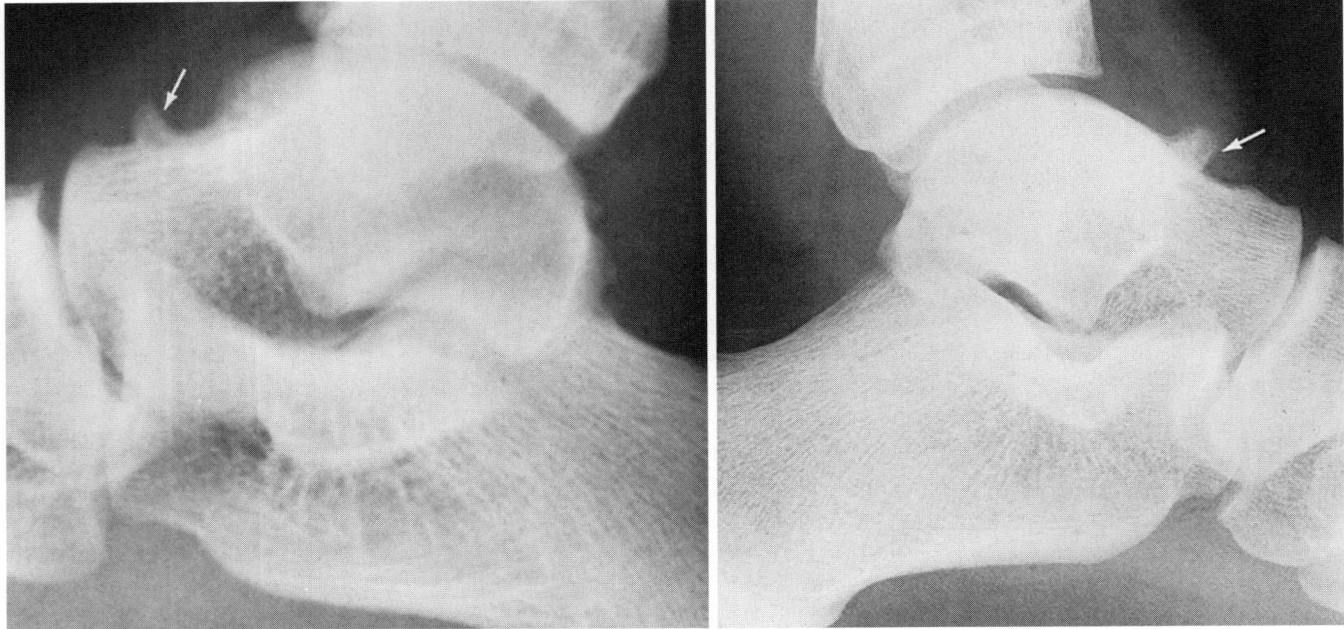

Figure 7–463. Two examples of the talar beak, illustrating its varied appearance. This structure is a developmental variant that should not be confused with hypertrophic spurring seen adjacent to the talonavicular joint.

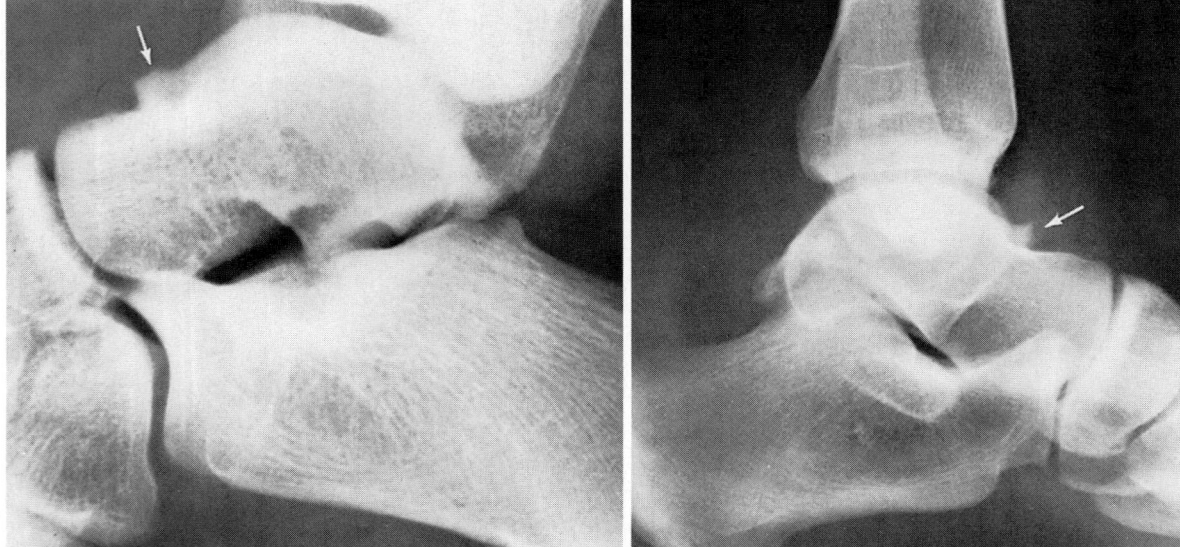

Figure 7–464. Two additional examples of the talar beak.

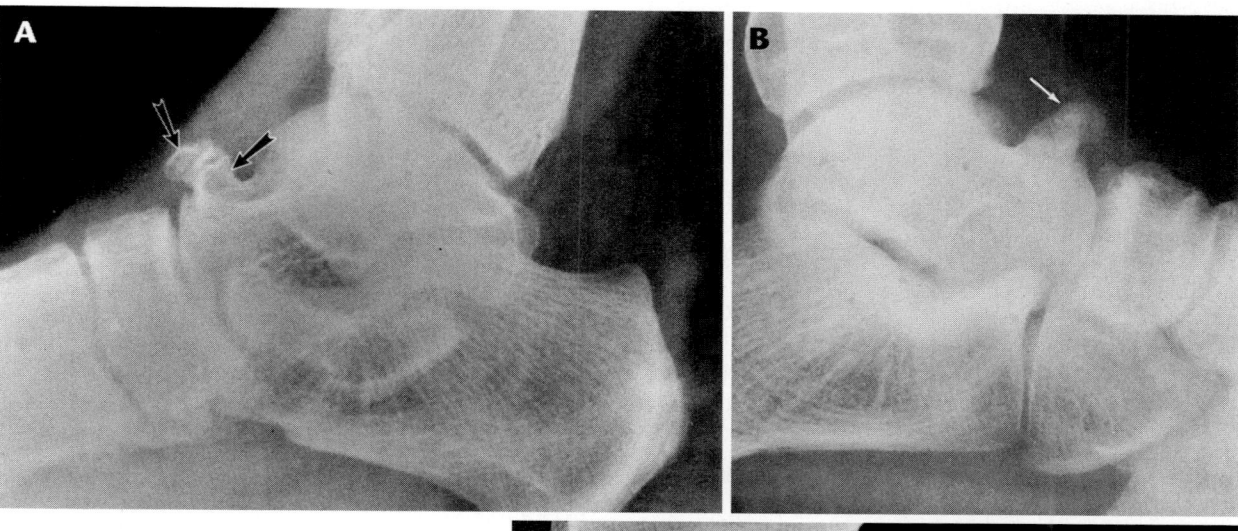

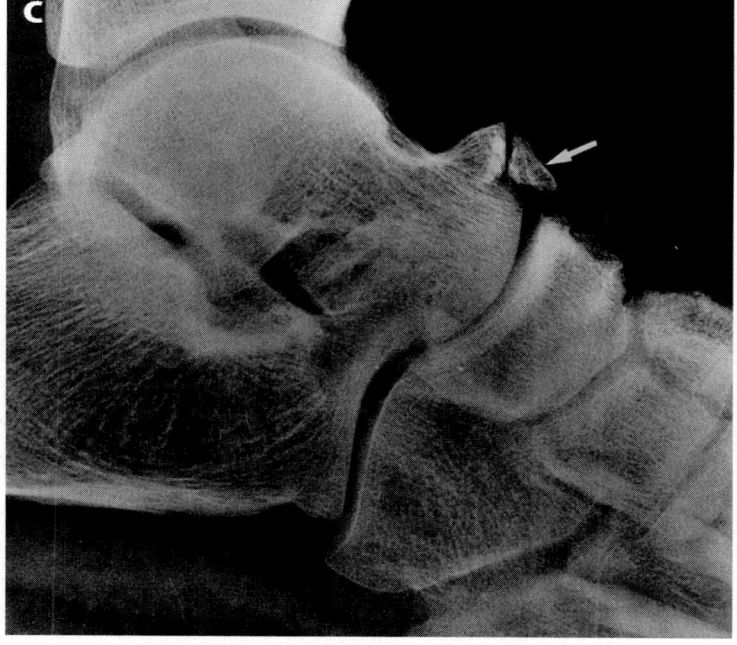

Figure 7–465. A–C, Examples of large talar beaks with ossicles at the tip. (Ref: Keats TE: Hypertrophy of the talar beak. *Skeletal Radiol* 4:37, 1979.)

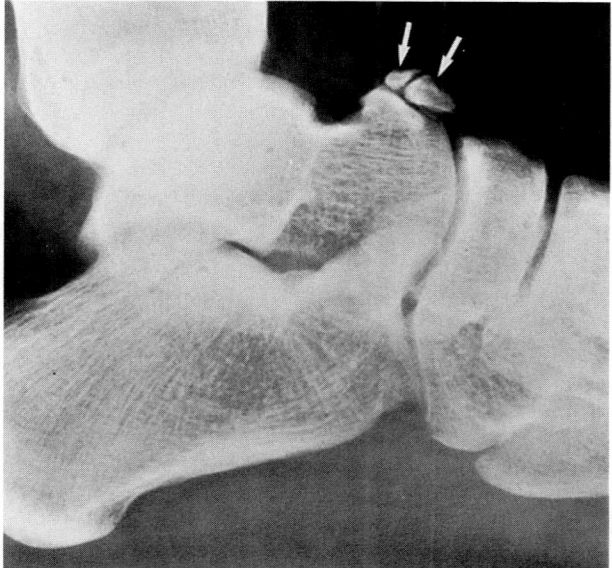

Figure 7–466. Talar beak with two large articulating ossicles.

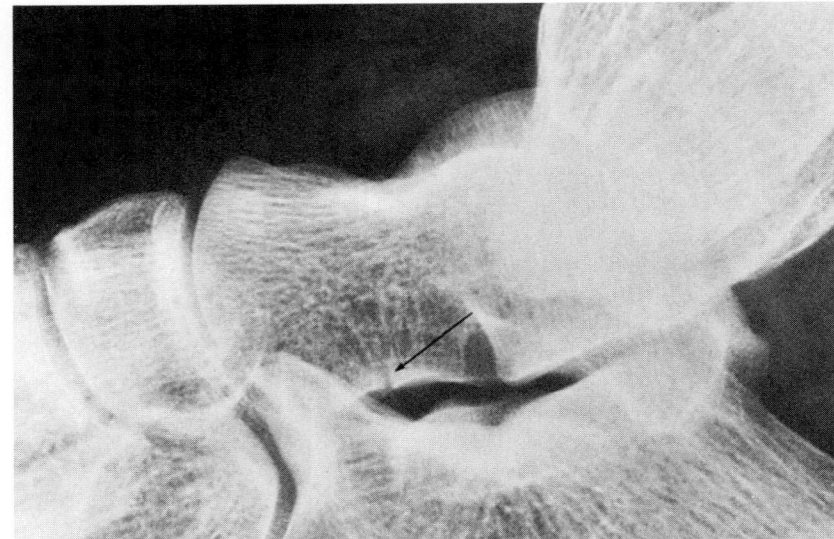

Figure 7–467. Prominent trabecular pattern simulating fracture of the talus.

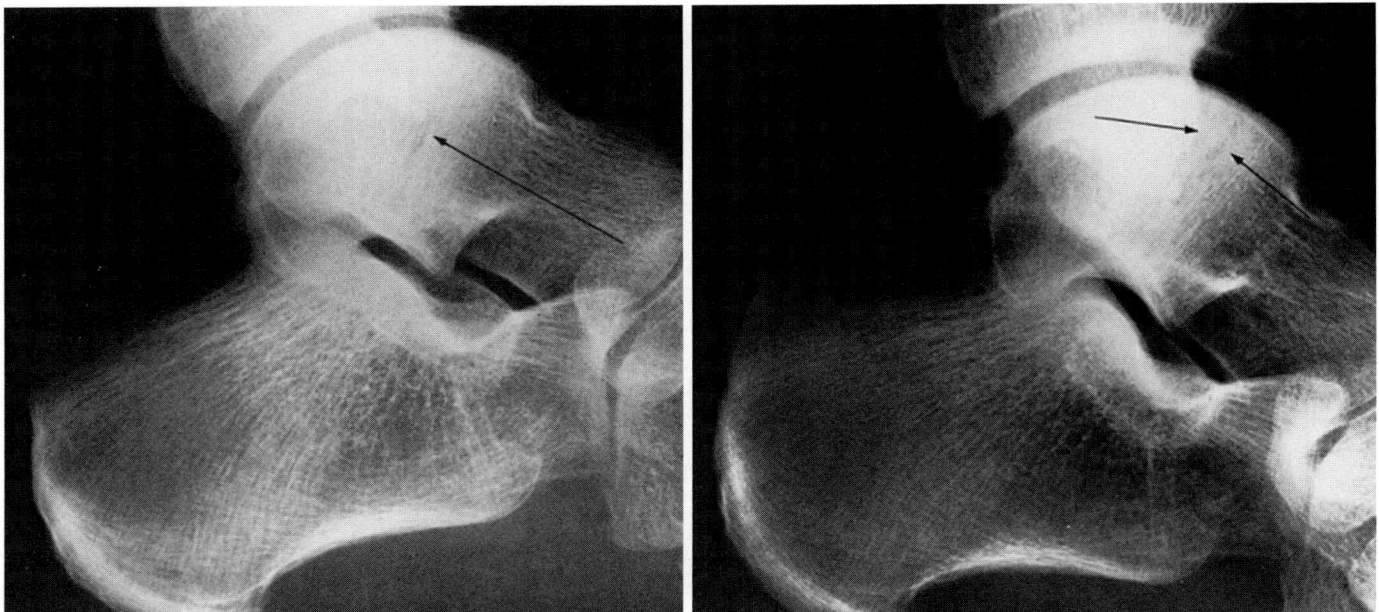

Figure 7–468. Simulated fractures of the talus produced by prominent trabeculae.

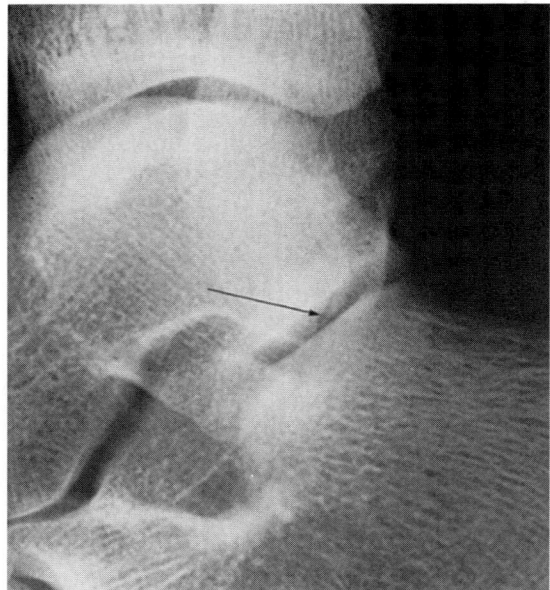

Figure 7–469. Simulated fracture of the talus produced by overlapping of the lateral malleolus and posterior process of the talus.

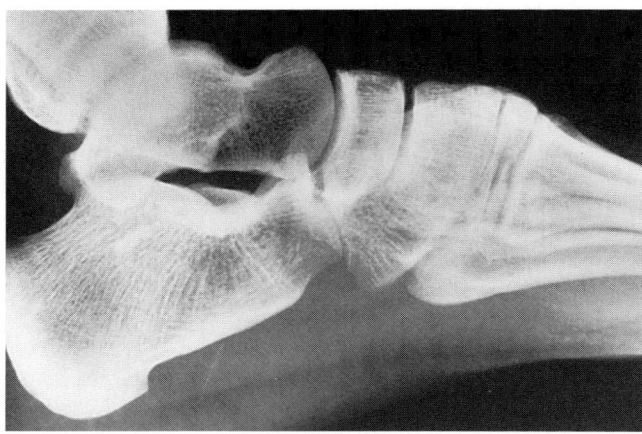

Figure 7–470. Unusual width of the subtalar joint simulating talocalcaneal dislocation produced by poor positioning for the lateral projection. Note the foreshortening of the talus in the vertical plane.

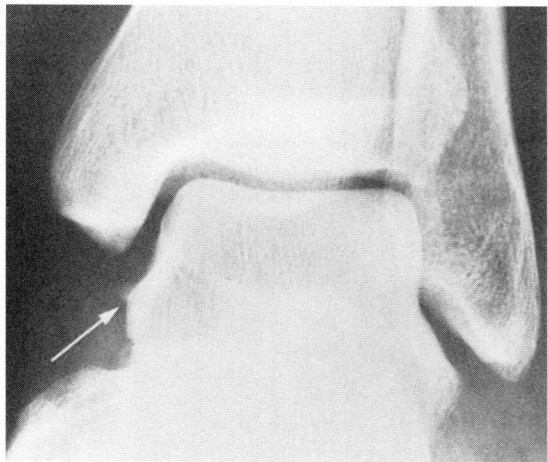

Figure 7–471. The talus accessorius.

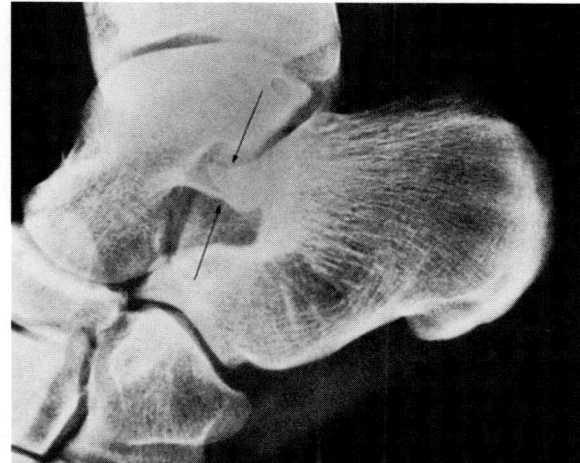

Figure 7–472. Simulated talocalcaneal coalition produced by improper positioning during filming. (Ref: Shaffer HA, Harrison RB: Tarsal pseudocoalition: A positional artifact. *J Can Assoc Radiol* 31:236, 1980.)

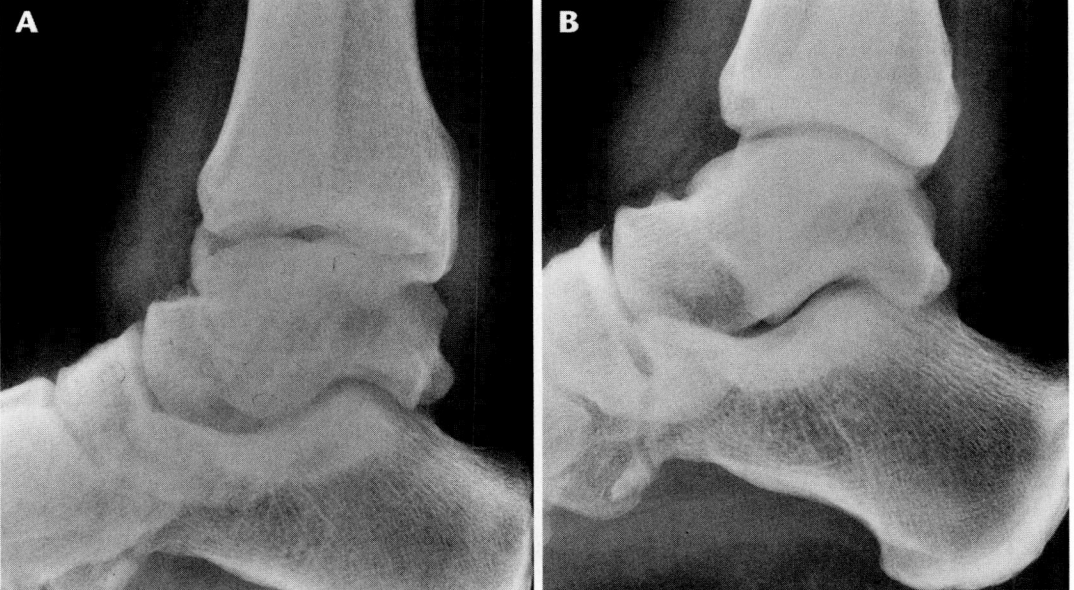

Figure 7–473. A, Simulated talar dislocation produced by rotation. **B,** True lateral projection shows normal relationships.

Figure 7–474. Partially fused talus secundarius.

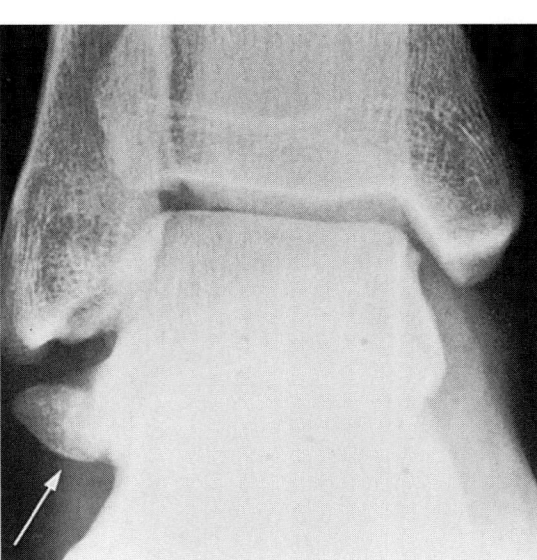

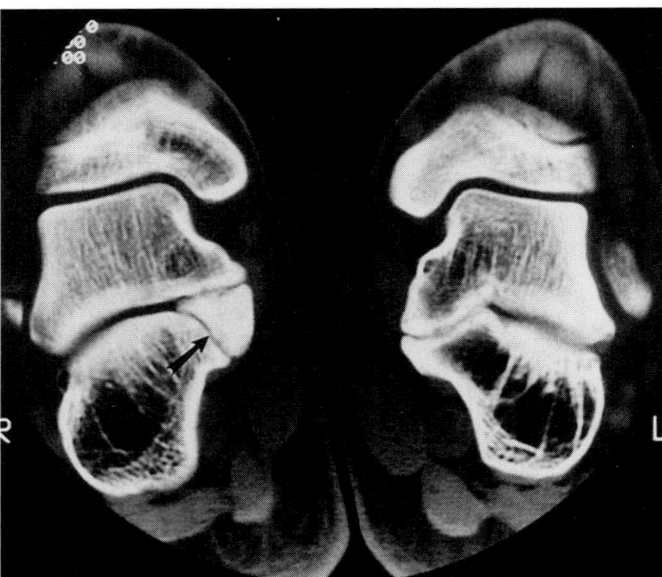

Figure 7–475. Os sustentaculum tali by CT. Note coalition on the left. The sustentaculi are accessory bones lodged at the posterior end of the sustentaculum tali, slightly to its superior side. (Ref: March HC, London RI: The os sustentaculi. *Am J Roentgenol* 76:1114, 1956.) This anomaly may be incorporated in an accessory joint between the sustentaculum tali and the talus. (Ref: Bloom RA et al: The assimilated os sustentaculi. *Skeletal Radiol* 15:455, 1986.)

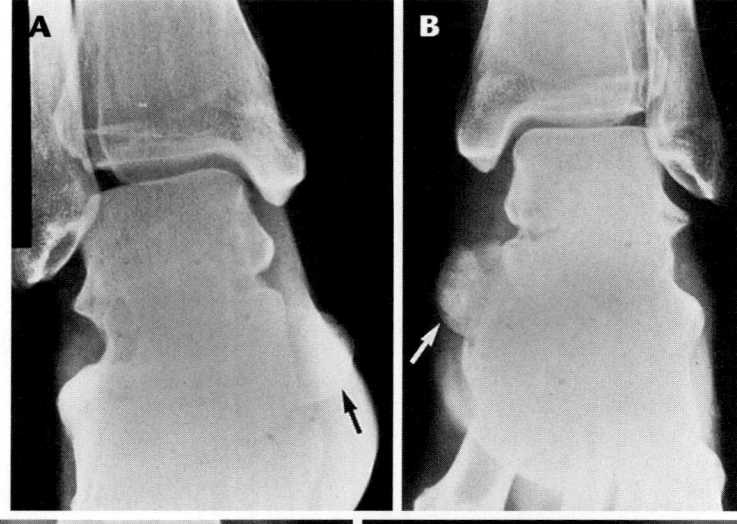

Figure 7–476. Large os tibiale externa may be confused with os sustentaculi. The latter are lower in position. **A** and **B,** Frontal projections. **C** and **D,** Lateral projections. **E** and **F,** Axial projections of the calcaneus.

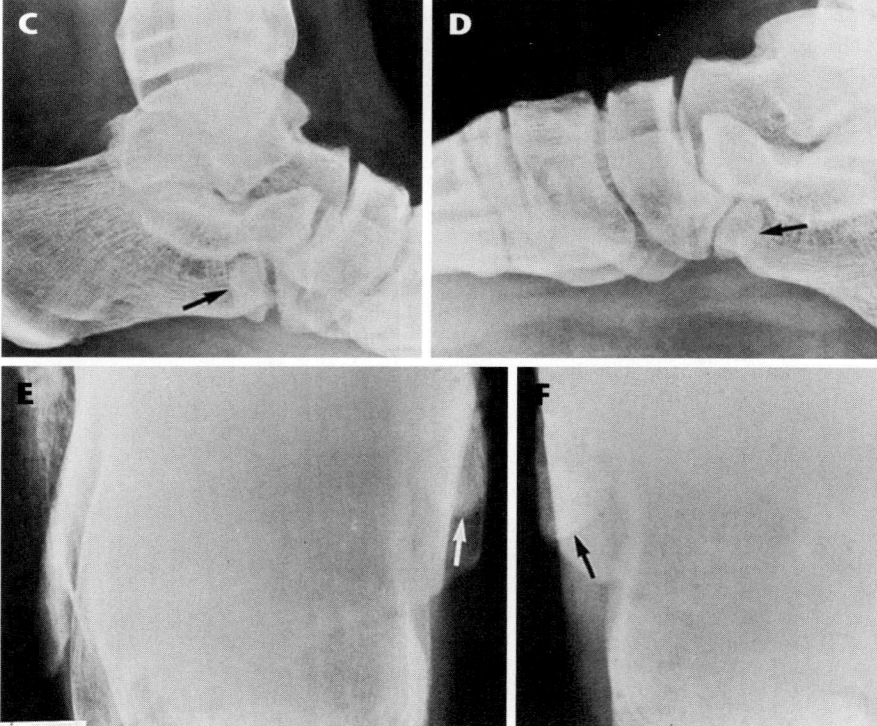

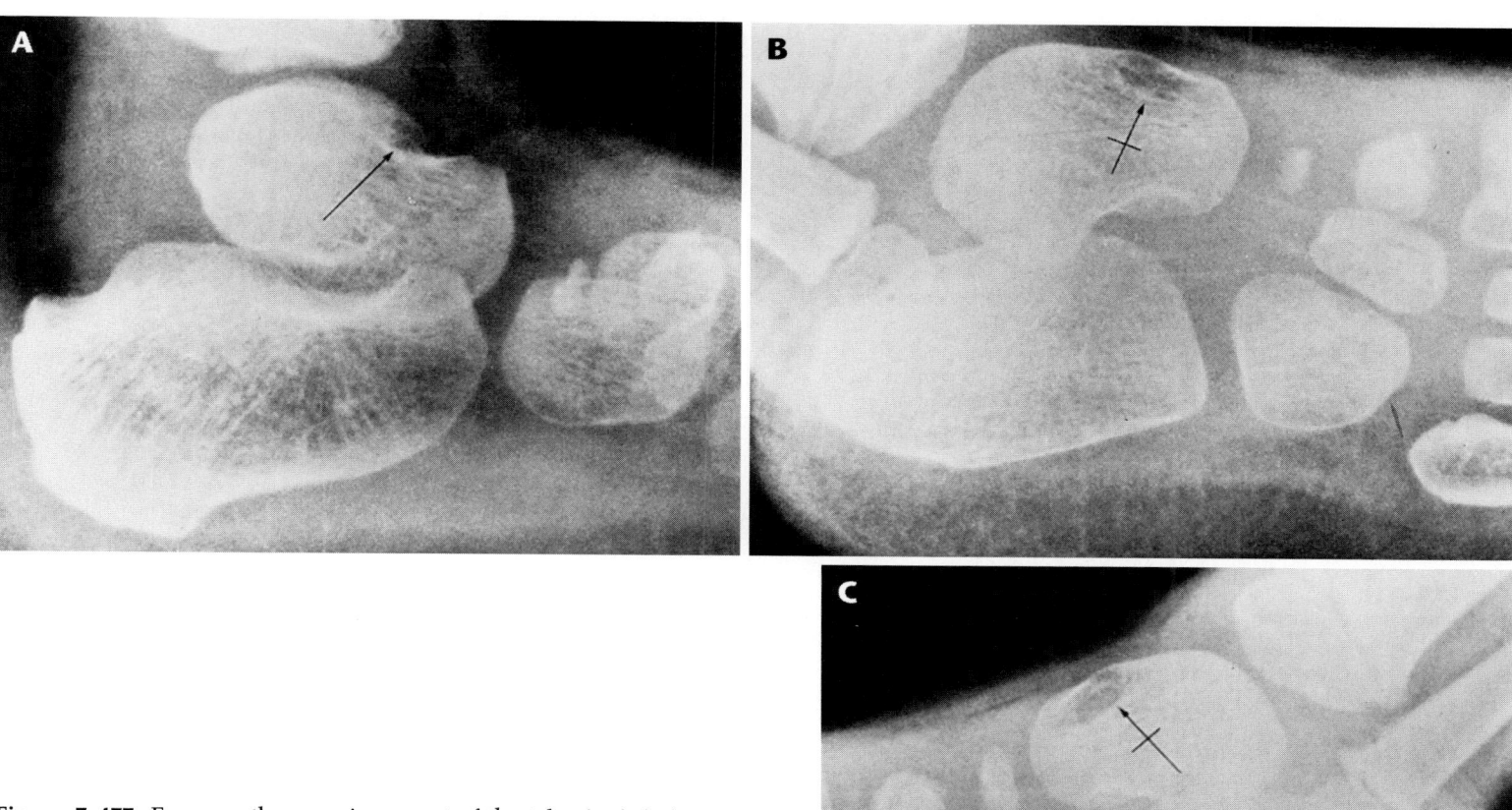

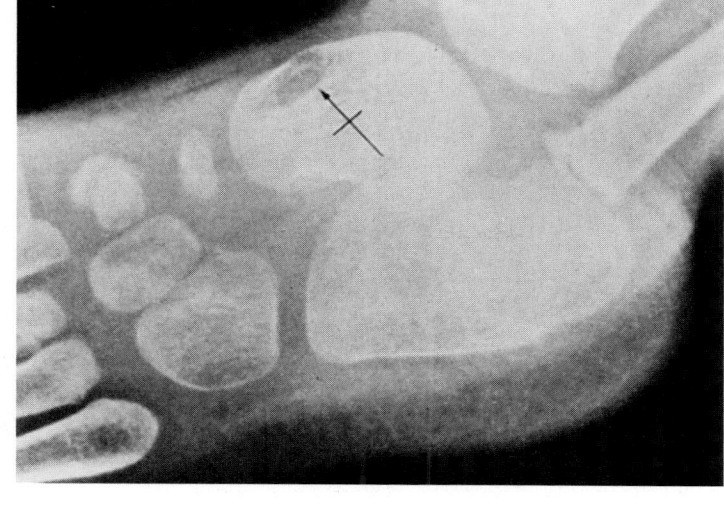

Figure 7–477. Fossa on the superior aspect of the talus in **A** (→) may produce apparent abnormalities in the oblique projections (**B** and **C**, ↦).

Figure 7–478. Nutrient foramen of the talus.

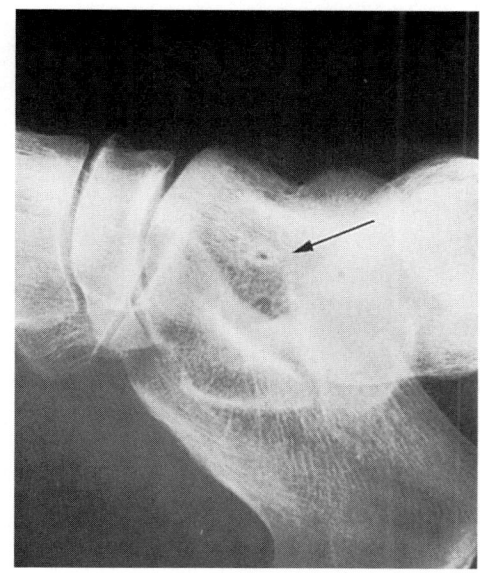

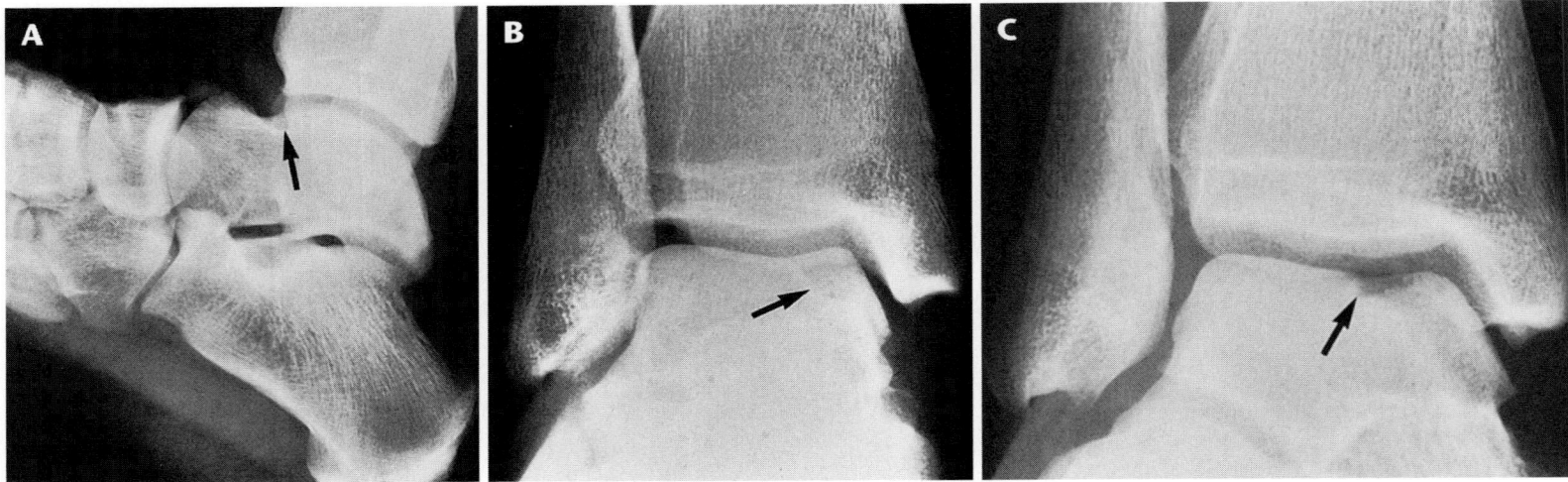

Figure 7–479. A, Deep fossa on the superior aspect of the talus in an adult, producing apparent abnormalities in the frontal and oblique projections (**B** and **C**).

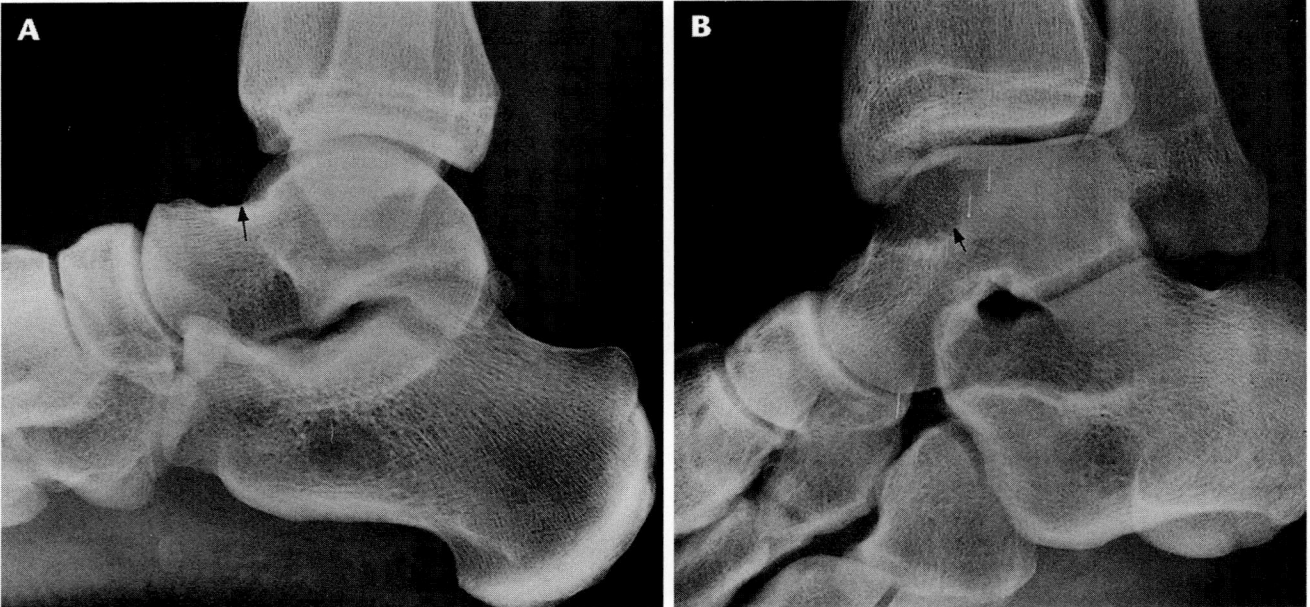

Figure 7–480. The fossae described, in Figure 7–479, if deep, may simulate a destructive lesion in the oblique projection. **A,** Lateral projection. **B,** Oblique projection.

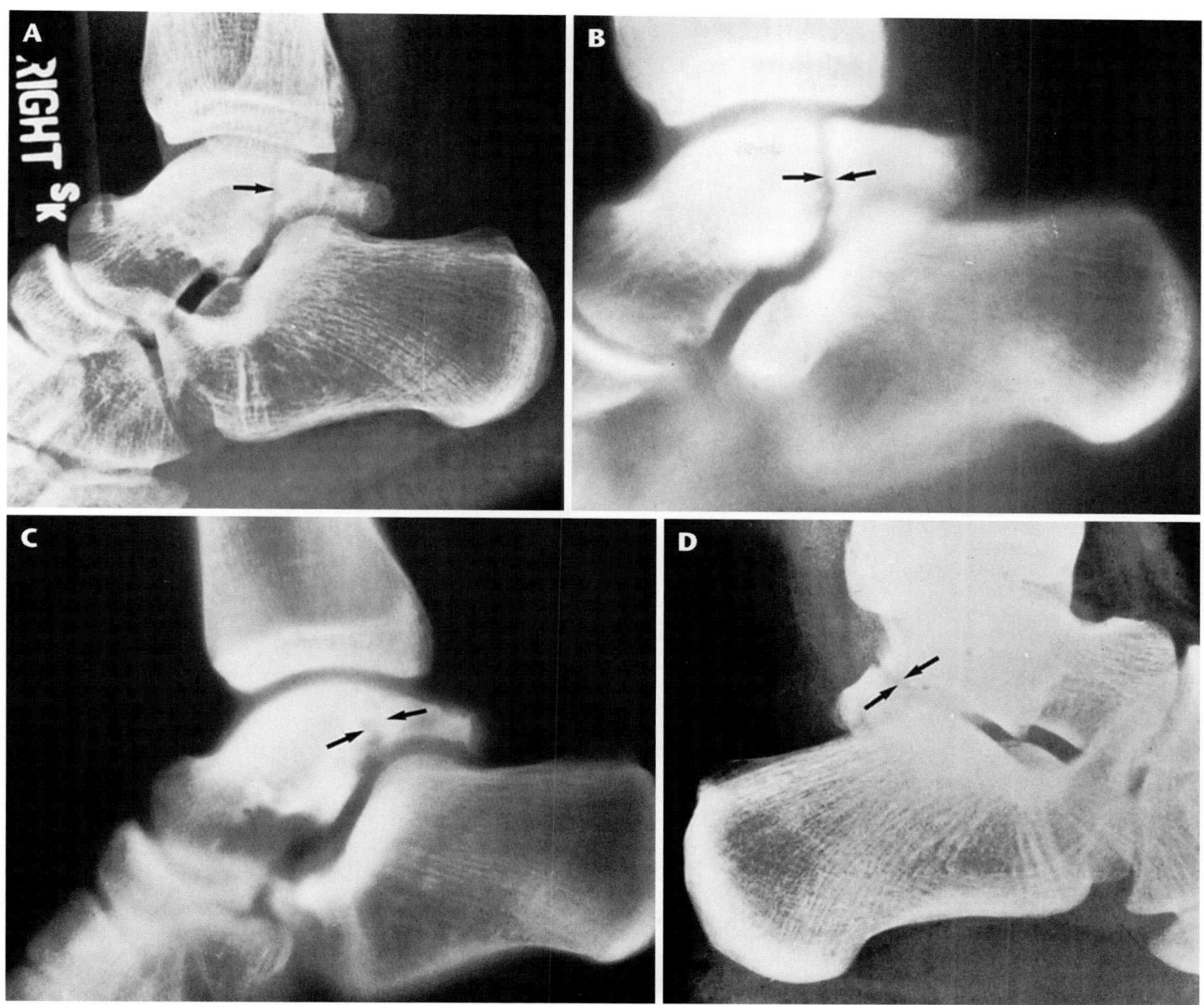

Figure 7–481. Talus partitus, an unusual developmental anomaly in which the talus is partitioned. **A,** Right ankle, plain film. **B** and **C,** Right ankle tomograms. **D,** Similar but less marked appearance of the left talus. (Ref: Schreiber A et al: Talus partitus. *J Bone Joint Surg* 67B:430, 1985.) (Courtesy of Dr. L. W. Bassett.)

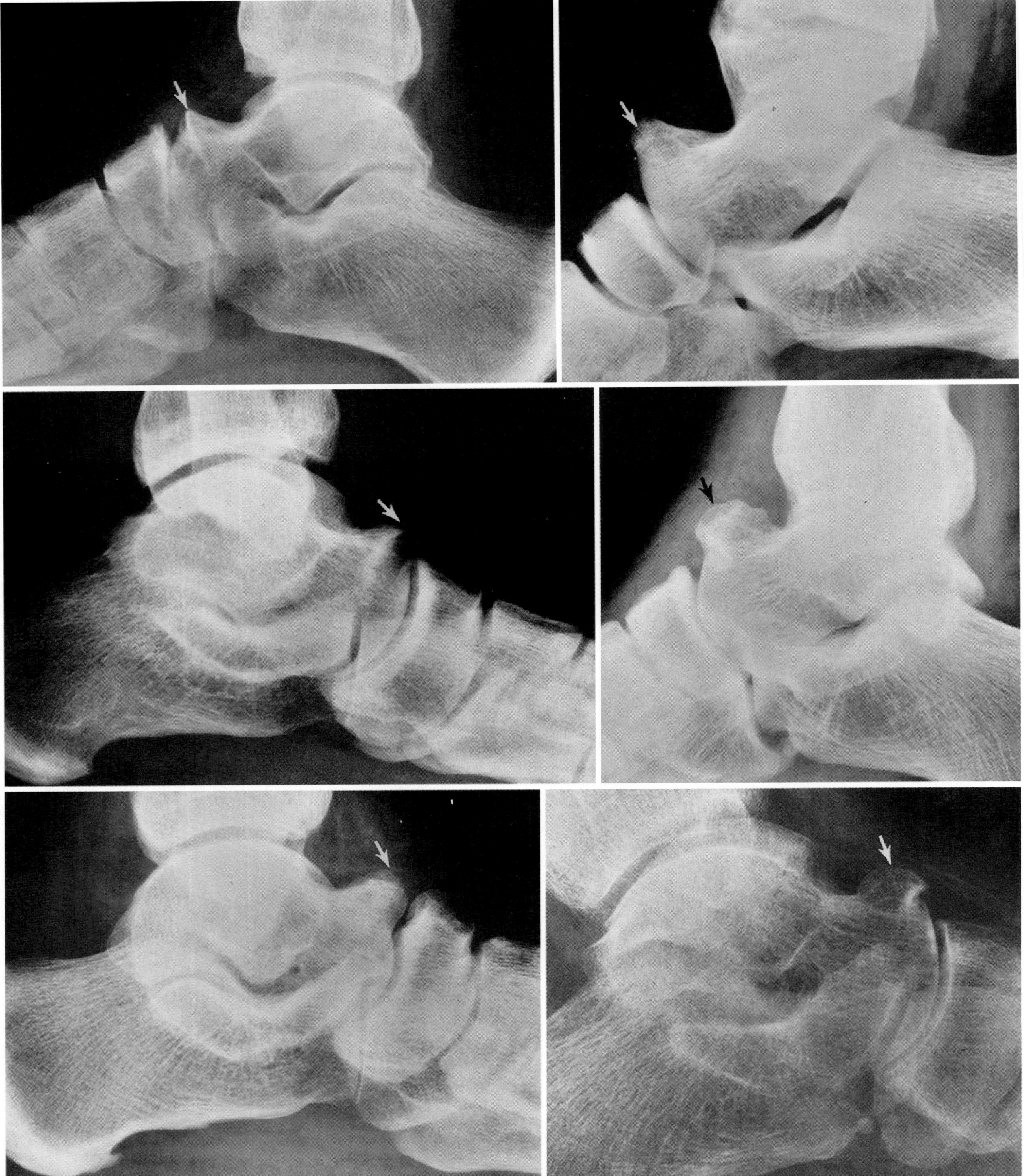

Figure 7–482. Some unusually prominent anterior processes of the talus, which should not be confused with the degenerative spurs that develop at the articulation secondary to tarsal coalition.

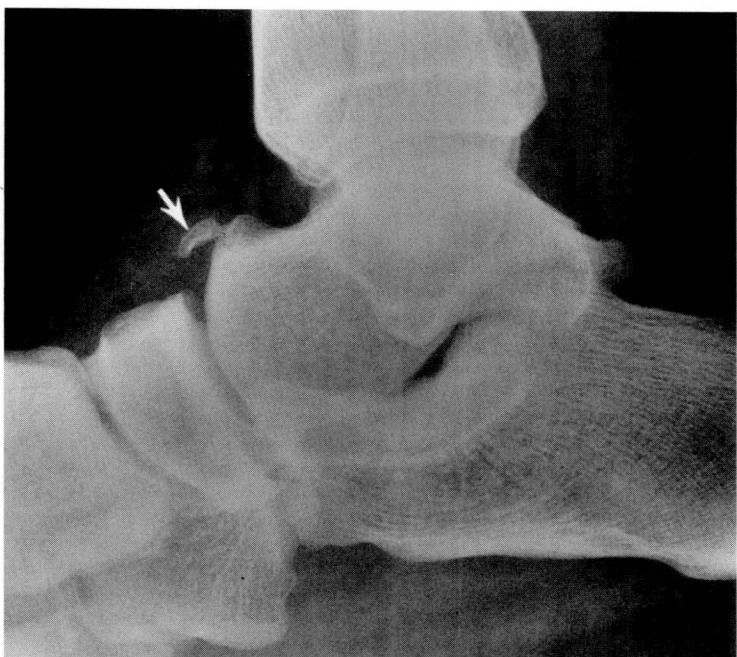

Figure 7–483. Unusual configuration of the distal end of the talus, with an accessory ossicle at its distal end.

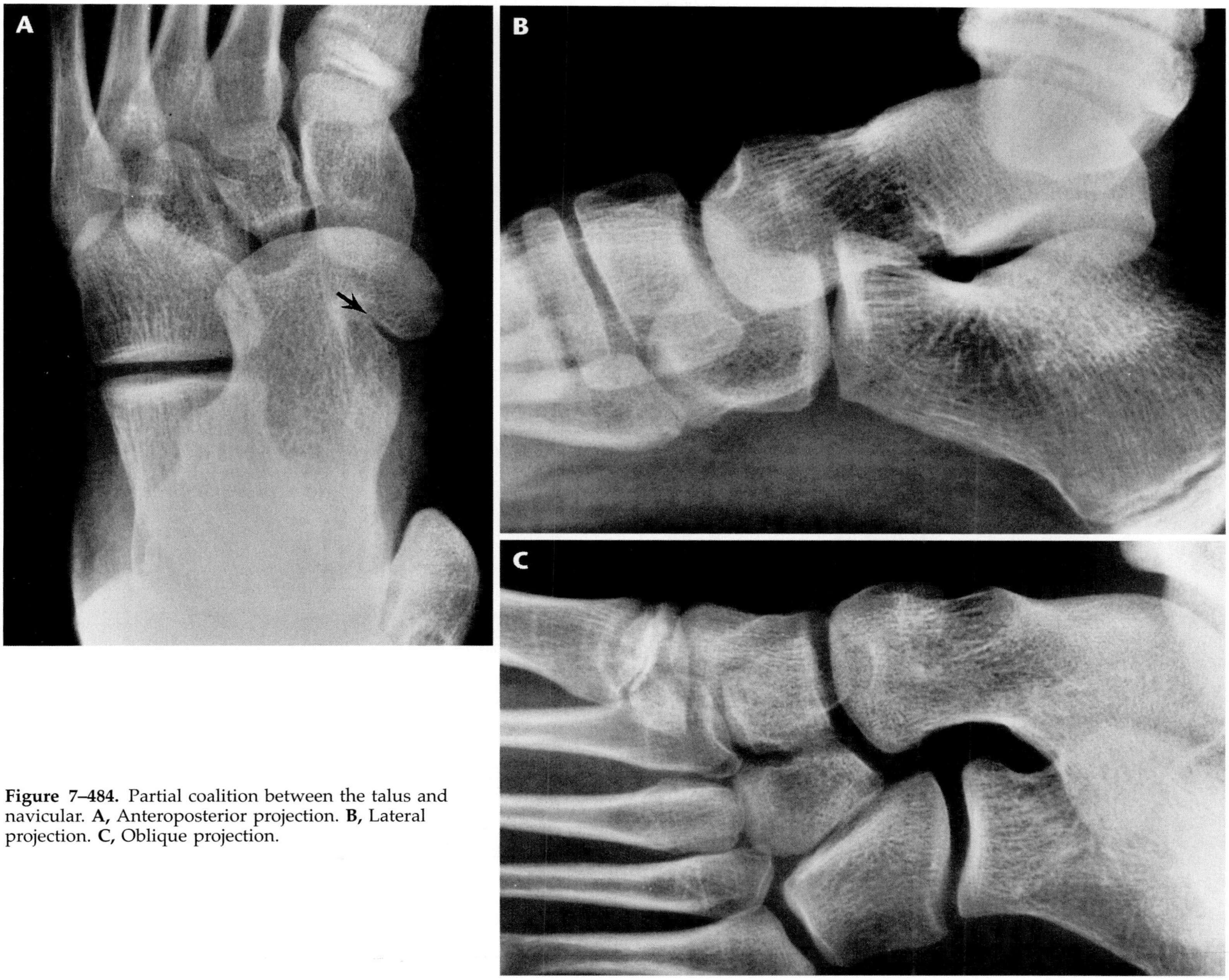

Figure 7–484. Partial coalition between the talus and navicular. **A,** Anteroposterior projection. **B,** Lateral projection. **C,** Oblique projection.

THE CALCANEUS

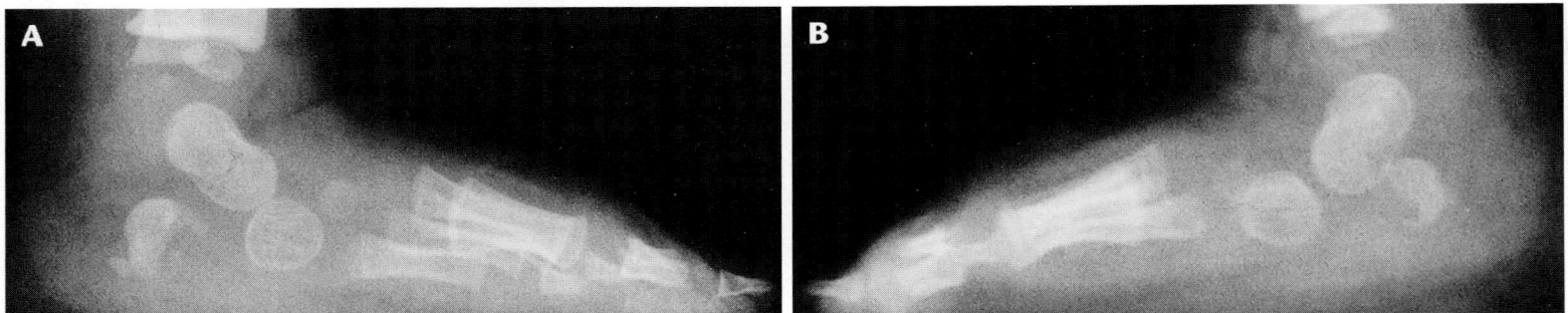

Figure 7–485. A, B, Bilateral calcaneal hypoplasia in a 1½-year-old child.

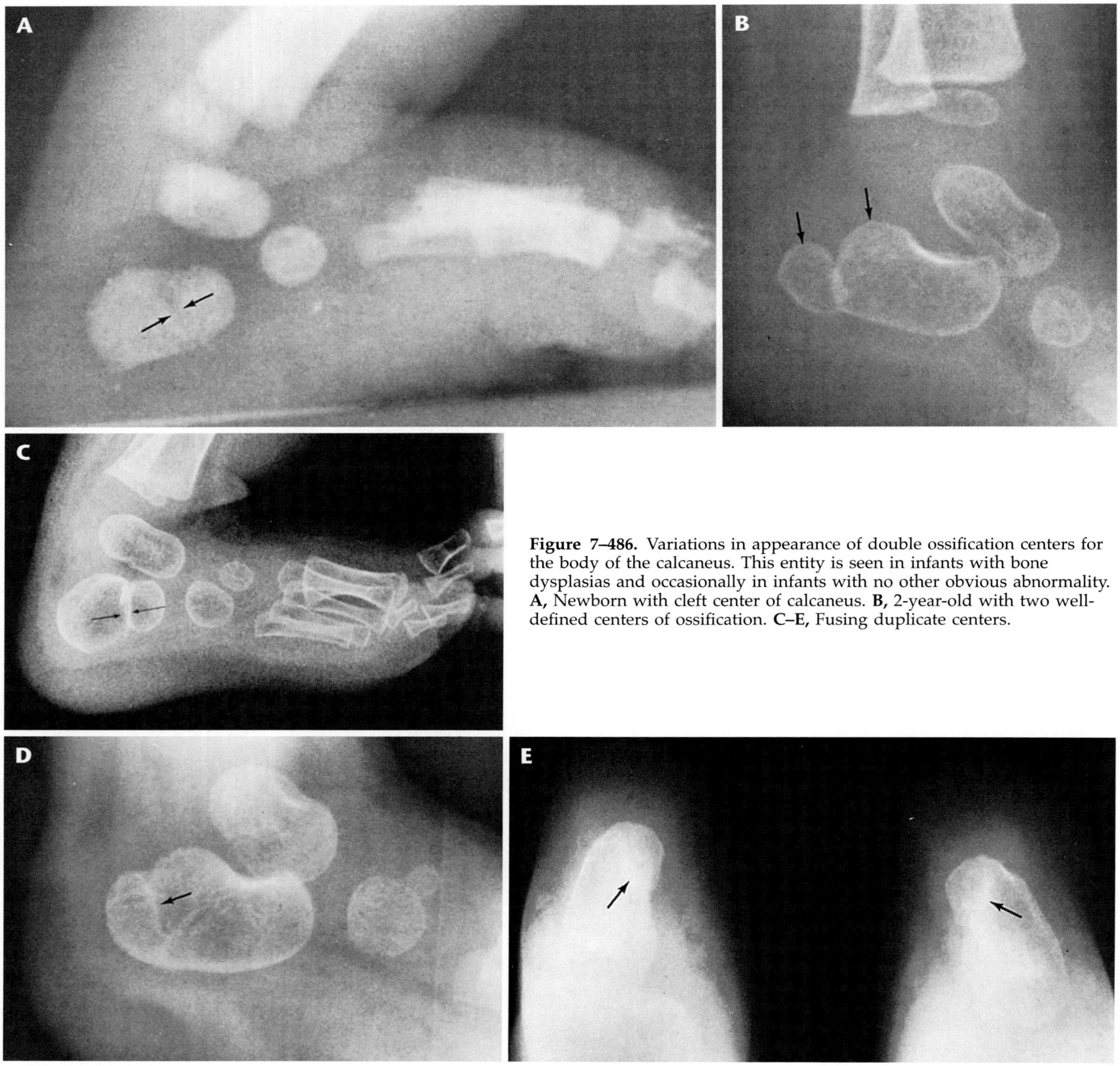

Figure 7–486. Variations in appearance of double ossification centers for the body of the calcaneus. This entity is seen in infants with bone dysplasias and occasionally in infants with no other obvious abnormality. **A,** Newborn with cleft center of calcaneus. **B,** 2-year-old with two well-defined centers of ossification. **C–E,** Fusing duplicate centers.

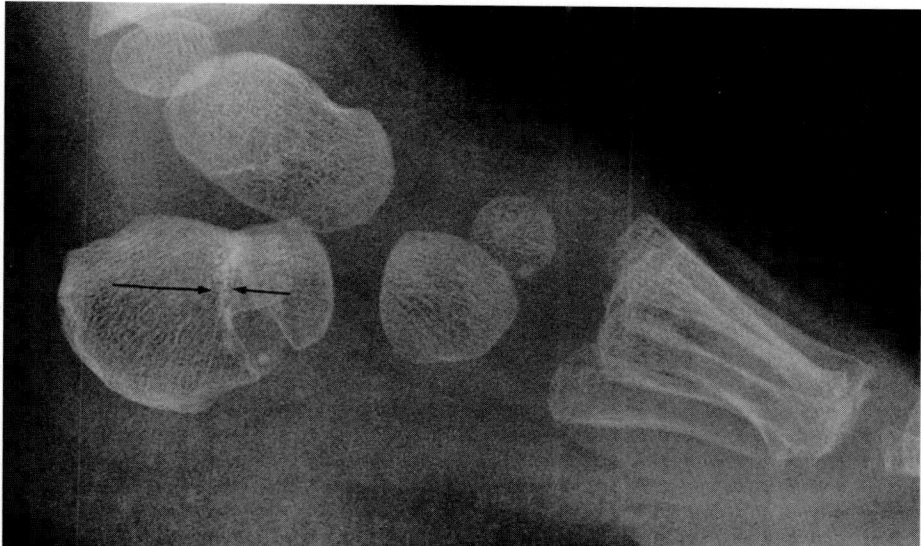

Figure 7–487. Double ossification centers for the calcaneus with irregular mineralization.

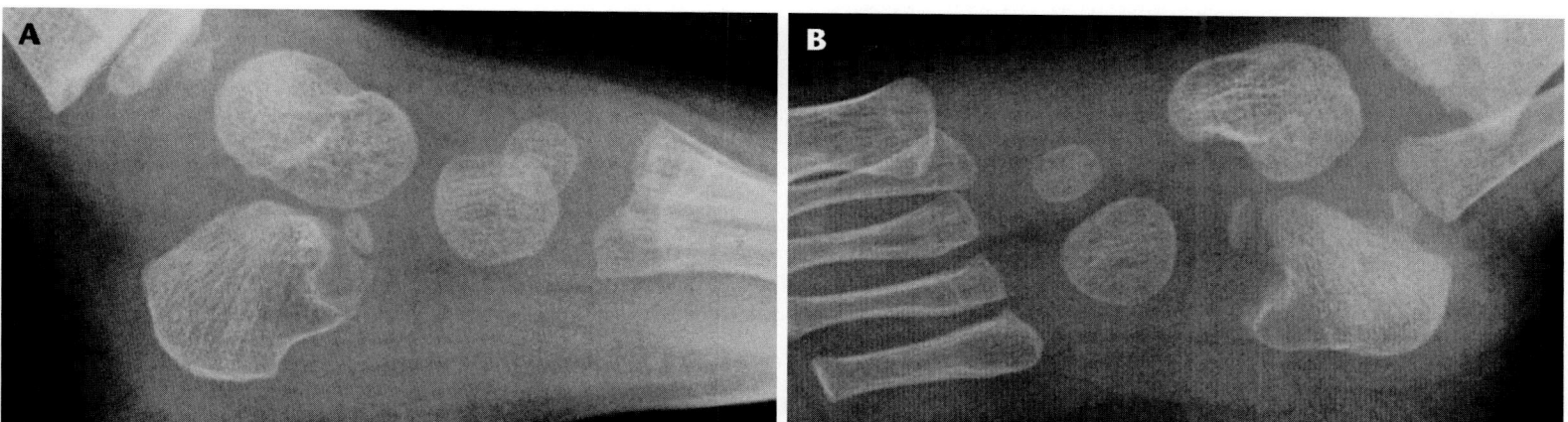

Figure 7–488. A, B, Striking irregular patterns of ossification of the calcaneus seen bilaterally in a 2-year-old child.

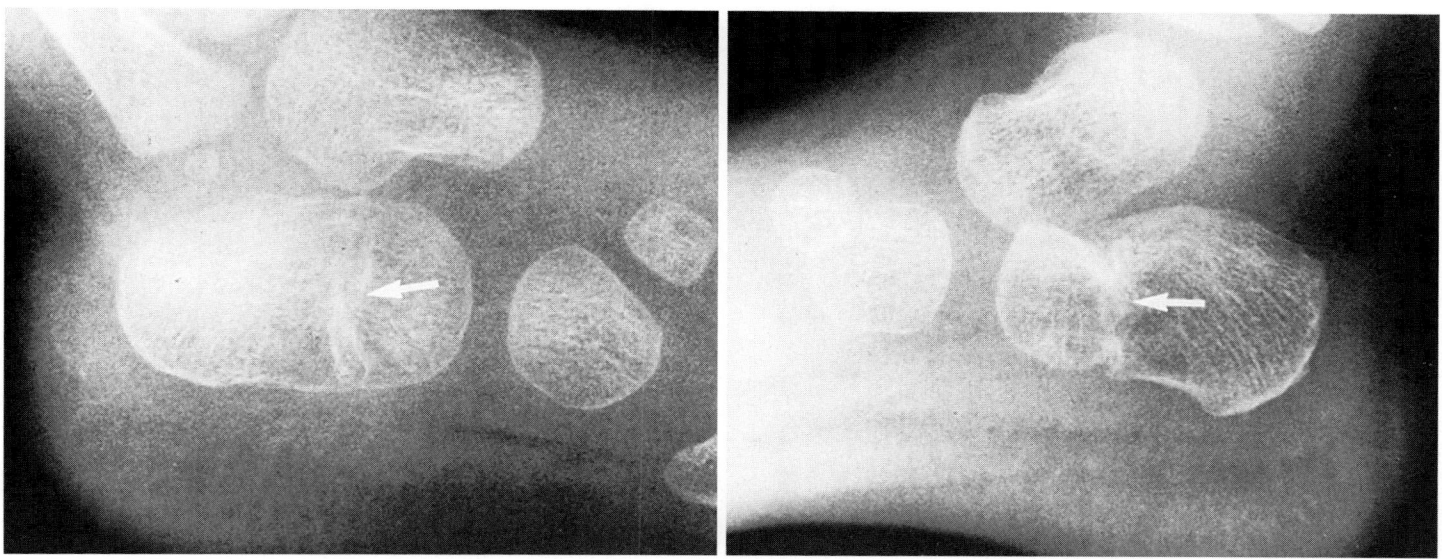

Figure 7–489. Closing bilateral duplicate ossification centers of the calcaneus.

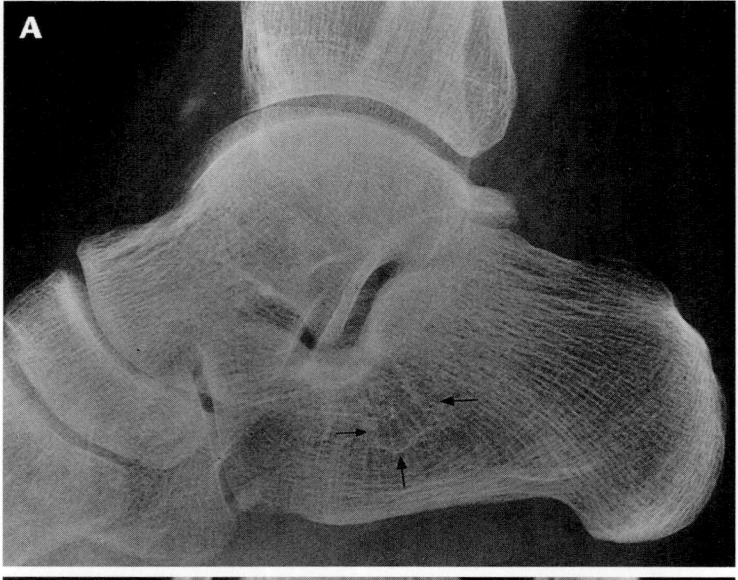

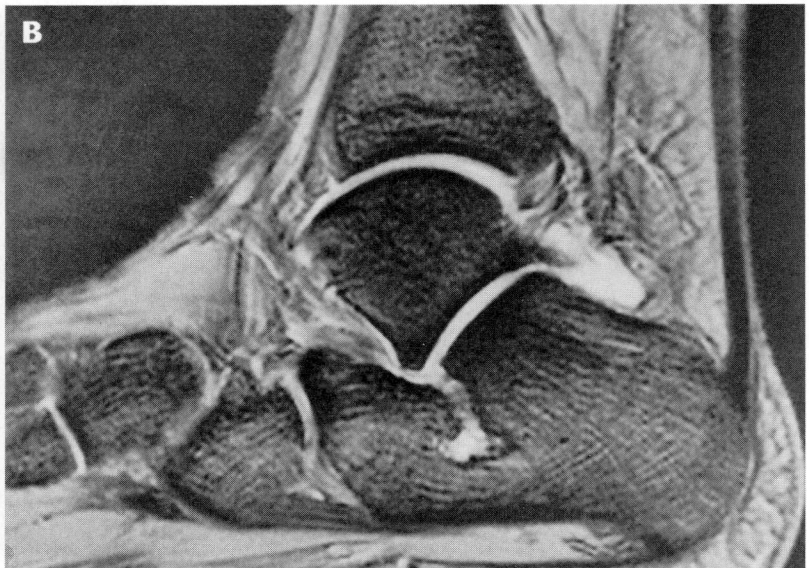

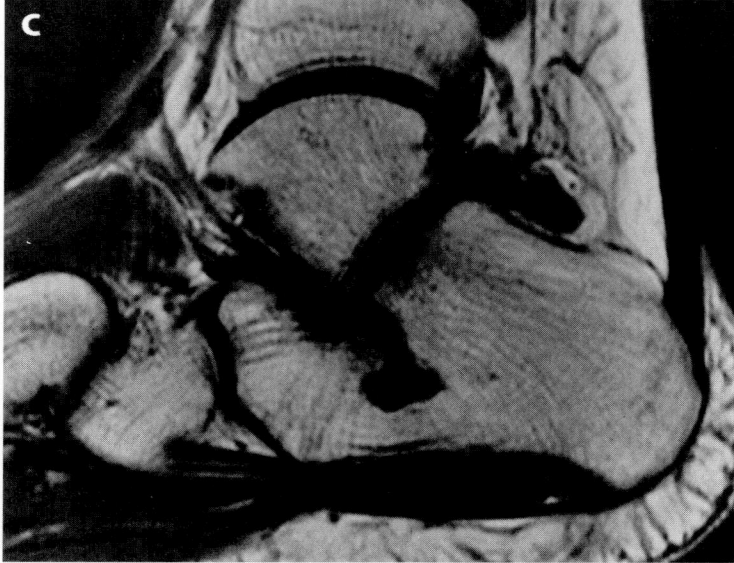

Figure 7–490. A, Irregular lucency in mid-portion of calcaneus. **B** and **C,** MR images show signal pattern of cartilage. **B,** Gradient echo T-2–weighted; **C,** T-1–weighted. The lesion probably represents a remnant of the divided ossification centers of early life.

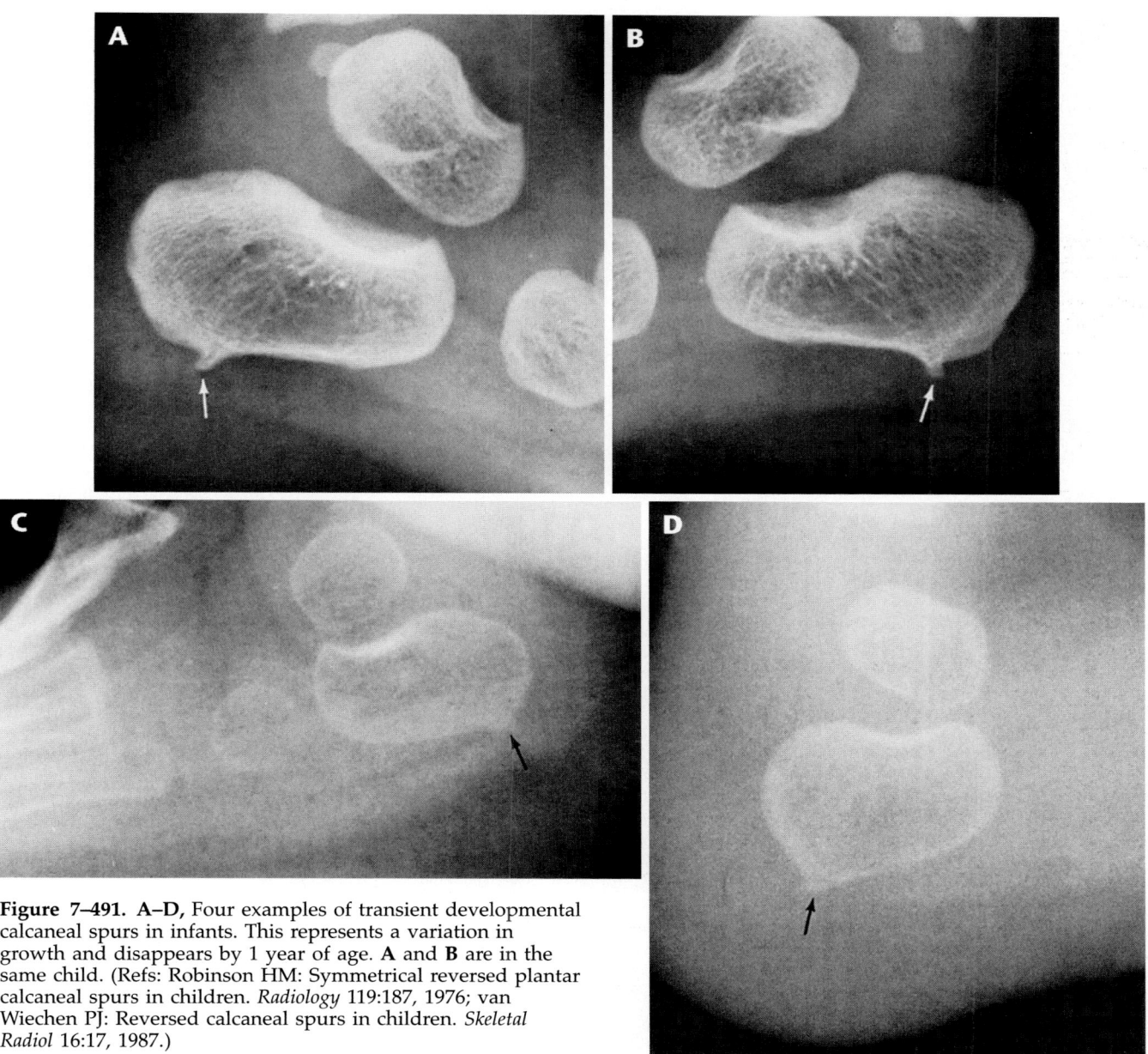

Figure 7–491. A–D, Four examples of transient developmental calcaneal spurs in infants. This represents a variation in growth and disappears by 1 year of age. **A** and **B** are in the same child. (Refs: Robinson HM: Symmetrical reversed plantar calcaneal spurs in children. *Radiology* 119:187, 1976; van Wiechen PJ: Reversed calcaneal spurs in children. *Skeletal Radiol* 16:17, 1987.)

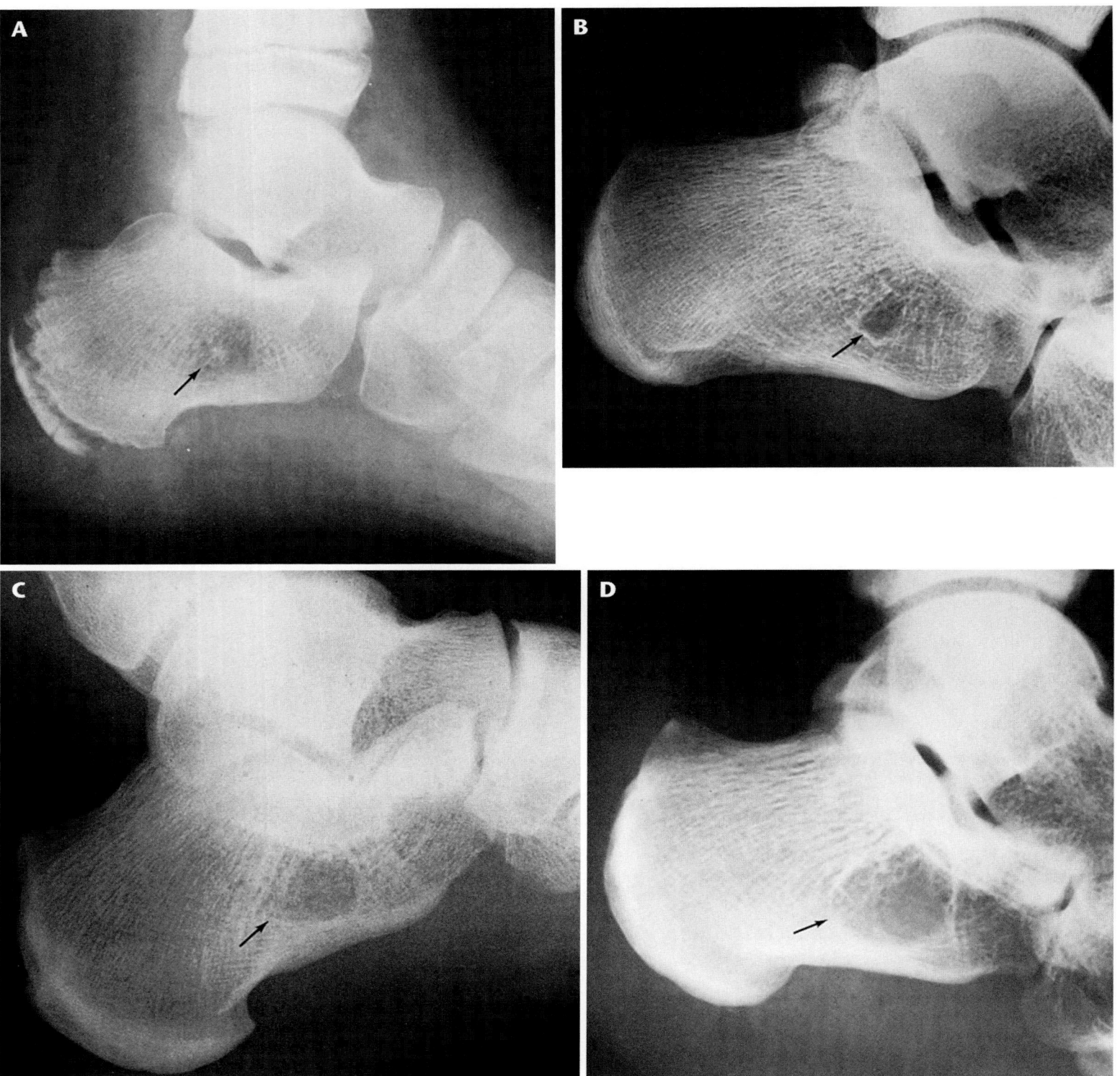

Figure 7–492. A–D, Four examples of simulated calcaneal cyst caused by the normal arrangement of the trabecular pattern in this area. The presence of the nutrient channel within the cyst, as in **A,** is useful in identifying the area of radiolucency as a pseudocyst. This variant is confused with true cyst of the calcaneus. (Ref: Keats TE: The calcaneal nutrient canal. *Skeletal Radiol* 3:329, 1979.)

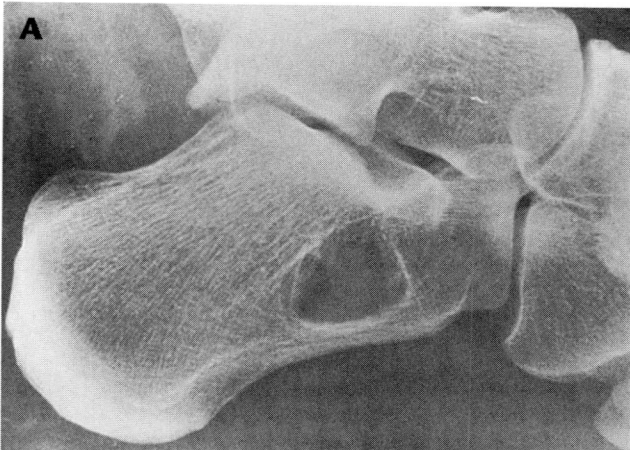

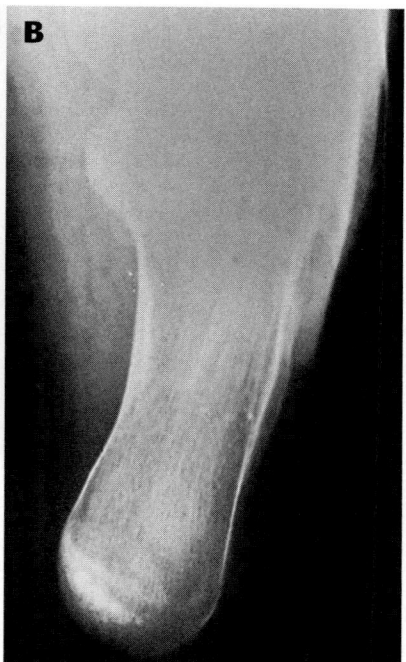

Figure 7–493. Calcaneal pseudocyst. The problem of distinguishing the pseudocyst (**A**) from a true cyst is most simply solved by using the axial projection of the calcaneus on which the pseudocyst will not be apparent (**B**).

Figure 7–494. The calcaneal pseudocyst seen in axial CT projection.

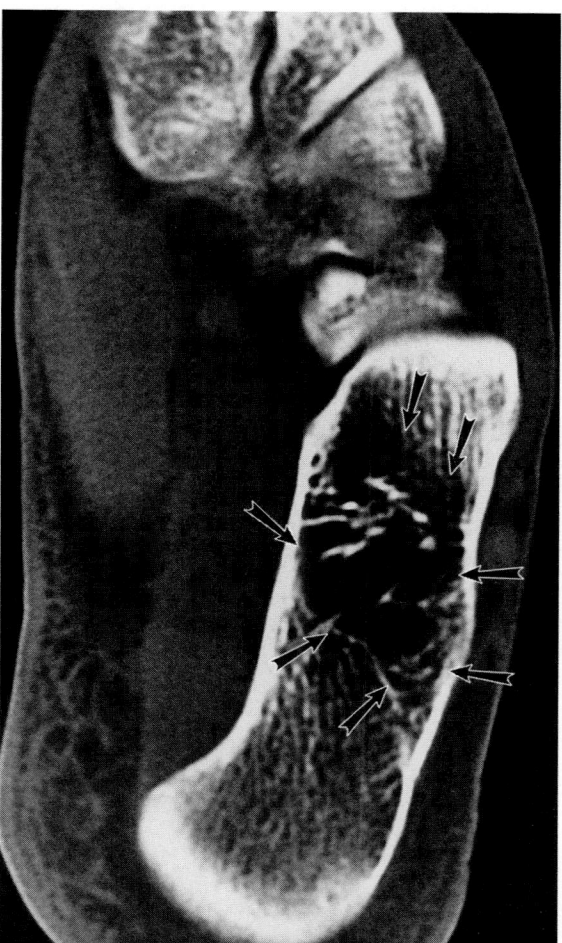

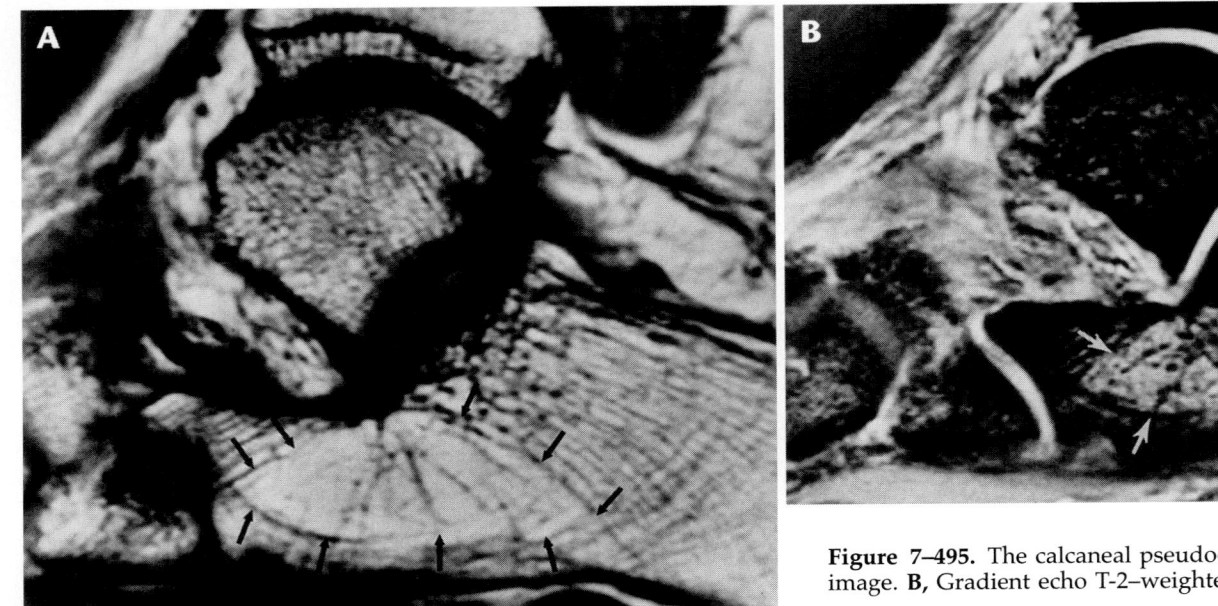

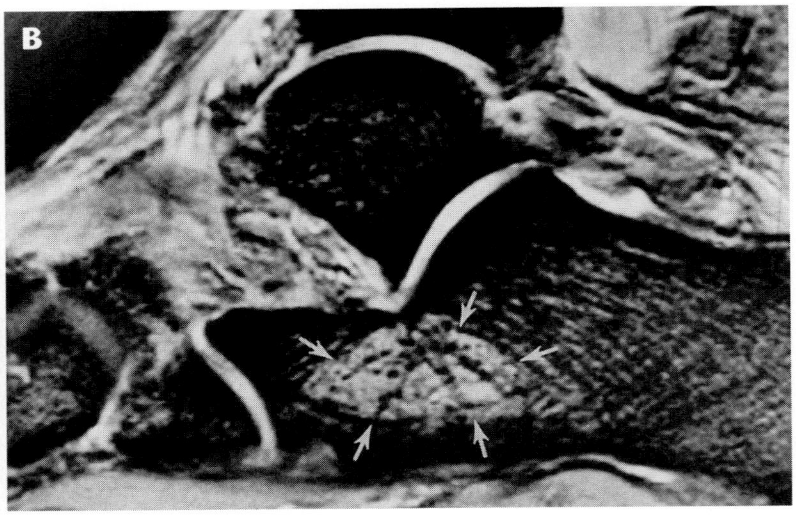

Figure 7–495. The calcaneal pseudocyst by MRI. **A,** T-1–weighted image. **B,** Gradient echo T-2–weighted image.

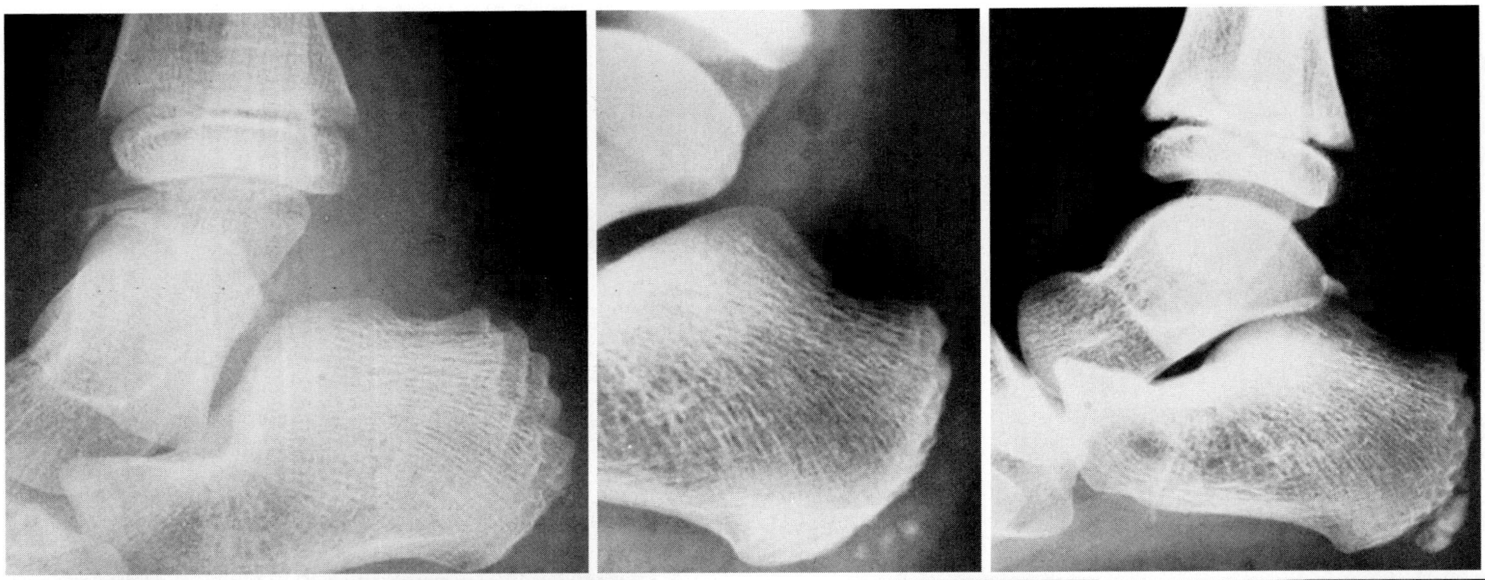

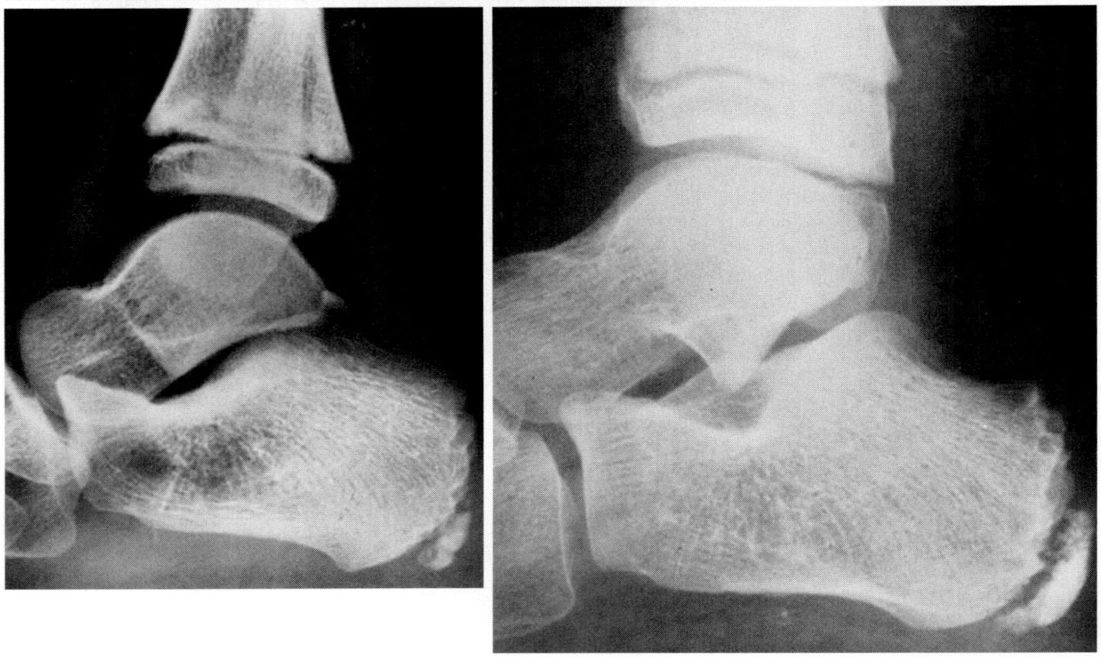

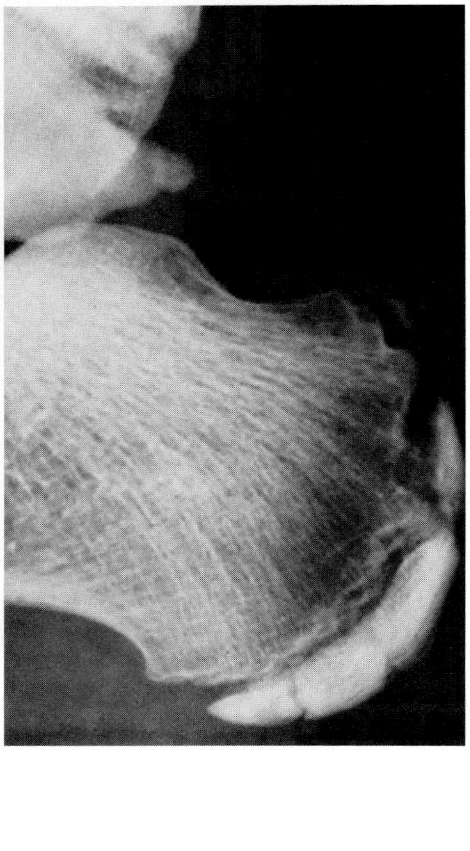

Figure 7–496. Normal variations in appearance of the growing calcaneus in adolescence. The irregularity of the calcaneal tuberosity before fusion of the secondary ossification center, as well as the density and fragmentation of the secondary ossification center, are normal manifestations of growth.

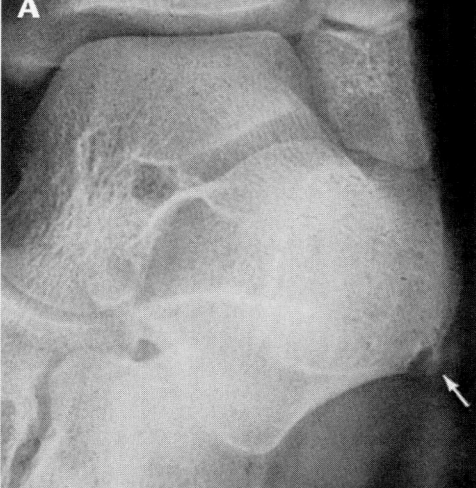

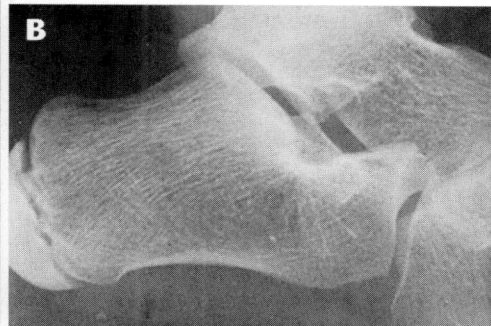

Figure 7–497. Simulated fracture of the calcaneal tuberosity by the apophysis in the oblique projection of the foot. This is seen before the calcaneal apophysis is closed and is produced by projection of the caudal tip of the apophysis into the soft tissues, as illustrated in the oblique view (**A**). This appearance is not seen in the lateral projection (**B**). (From Keats TE: Four normal anatomic variations of importance to radiologists. *Am J Roentgenol* 78:89, 1957.)

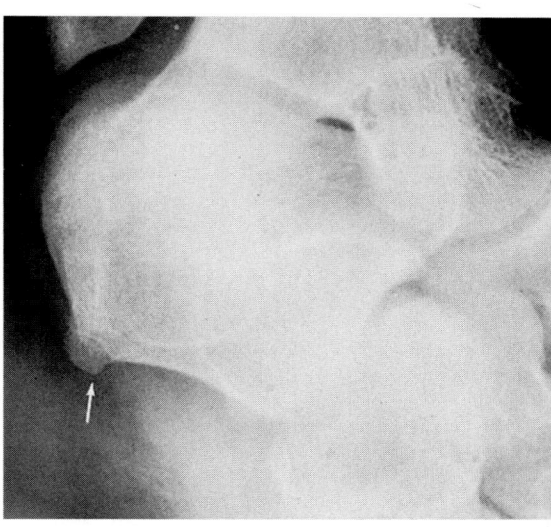

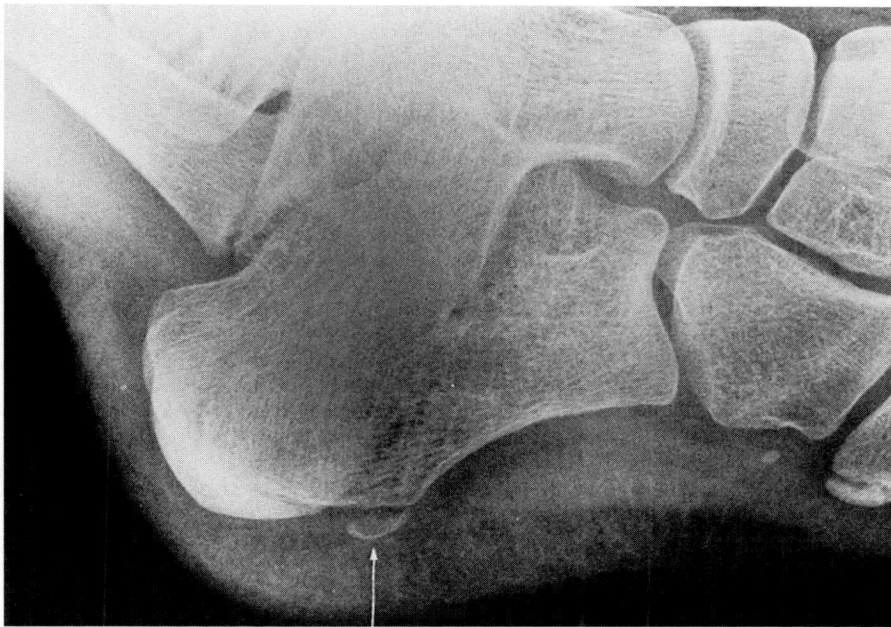

Figure 7–498. Two more examples of the tip of the ossification center of the calcaneal tuberosity, seen in oblique projection.

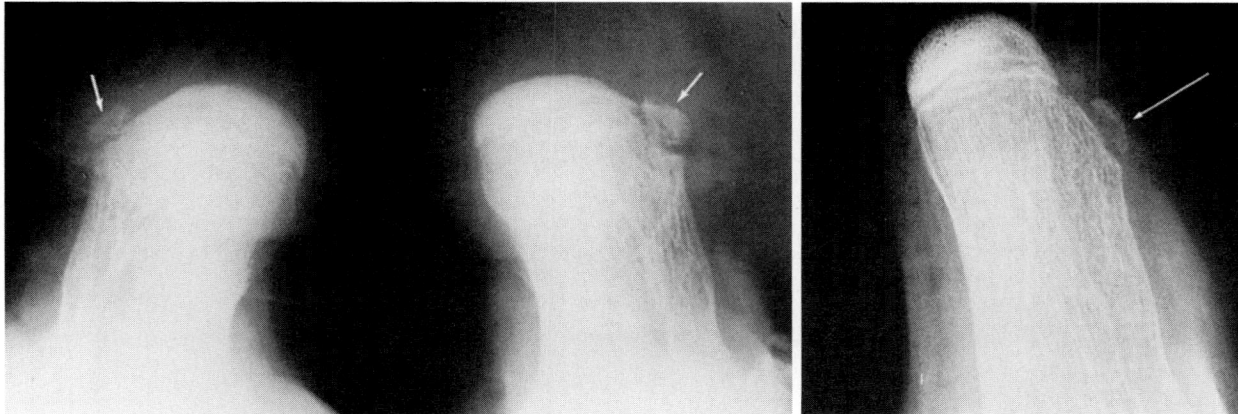

Figure 7–499. Appearance of the calcaneal apophyses in an adolescent. This projection may show centers of ossification that are not visible in the lateral projection.

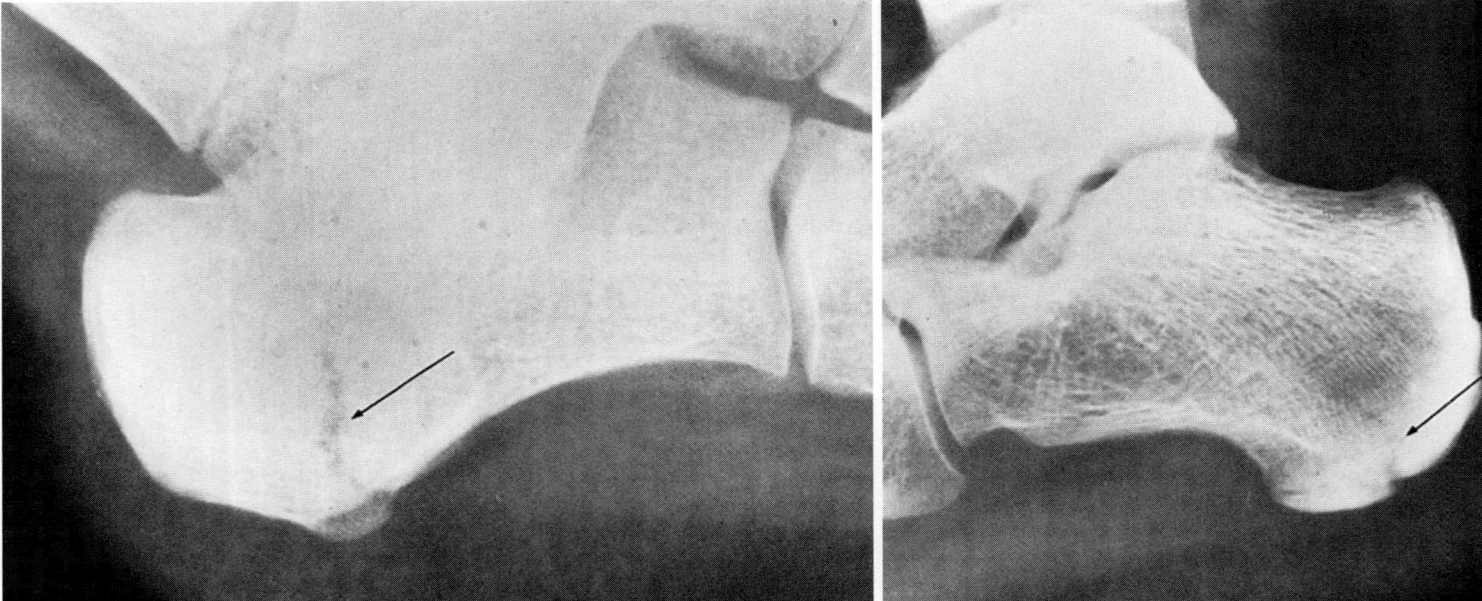

Figure 7–500. Simulated fractures of the calcaneus produced by the unfused secondary ossification center for the calcaneal tuberosity.

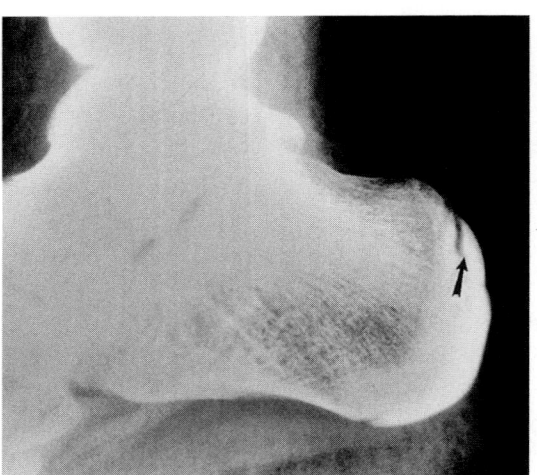

Figure 7–501. Proximal end of the closing calcaneal apophysis, which should not be mistaken for fracture.

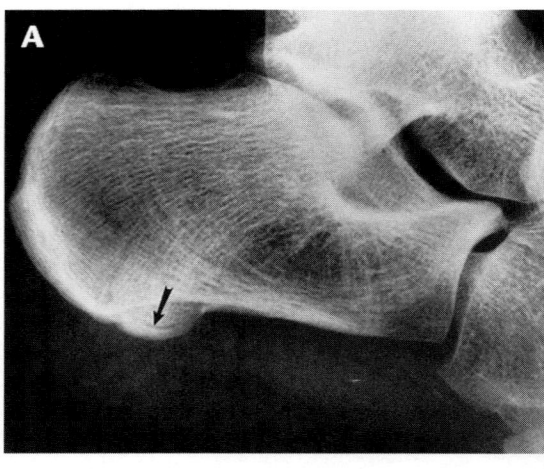 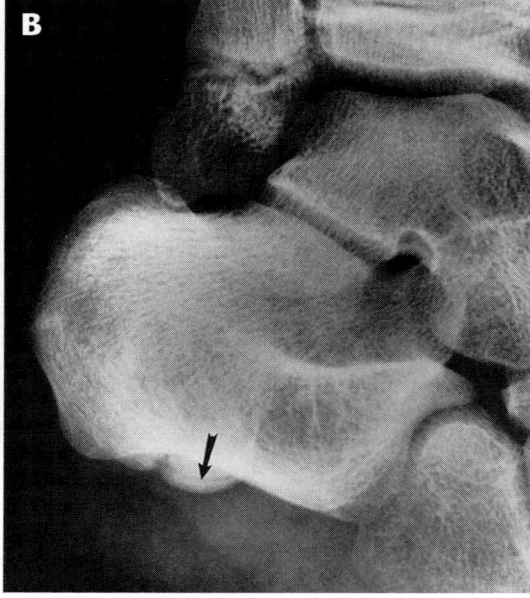

Figure 7–502. Closing calcaneal apophysis in a 13-year-old boy. **A,** Lateral projection. **B,** Oblique projection.

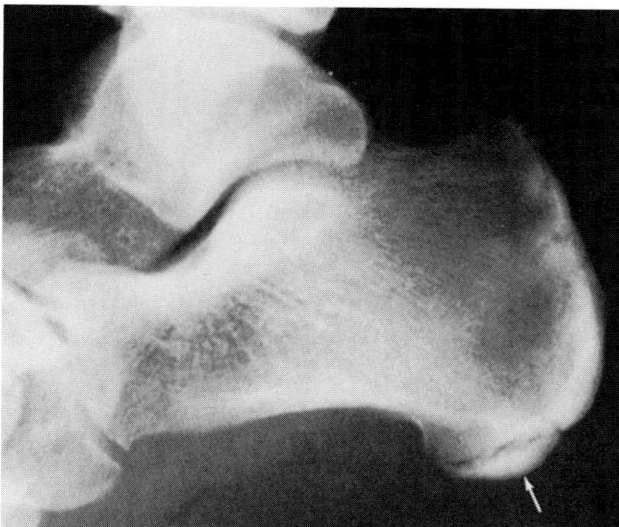

Figure 7–503. Incomplete closure of the distal portion of the calcaneal apophysis in a 15-year-old boy.

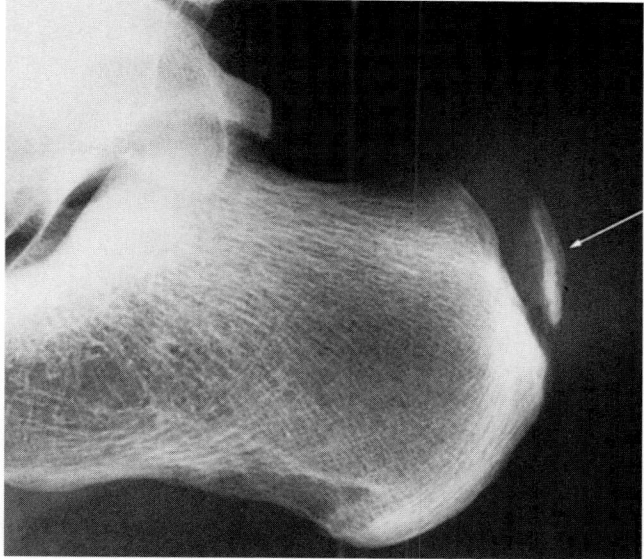

Figure 7–504. Failure of union of a portion of the calcaneal apophysis in an adult.

Figure 7–505. Shelflike configuration of the superior aspect of the calcaneus, not to be mistaken for an erosion.

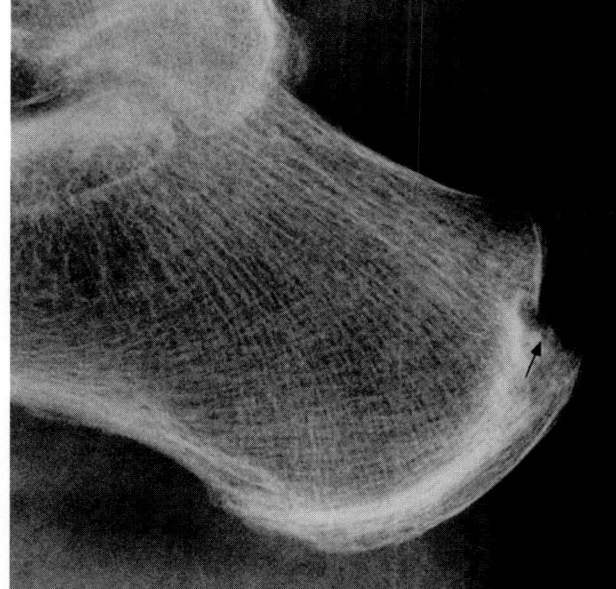

Figure 7–506. A, B, Secondary ossification center at the tip of the trochlear process on the lateral wall of the calcaneus, but seen well only in the oblique projection (←). **B,** The trochlear process may be so prominent, as in this case, as to suggest an exostosis (⊪).

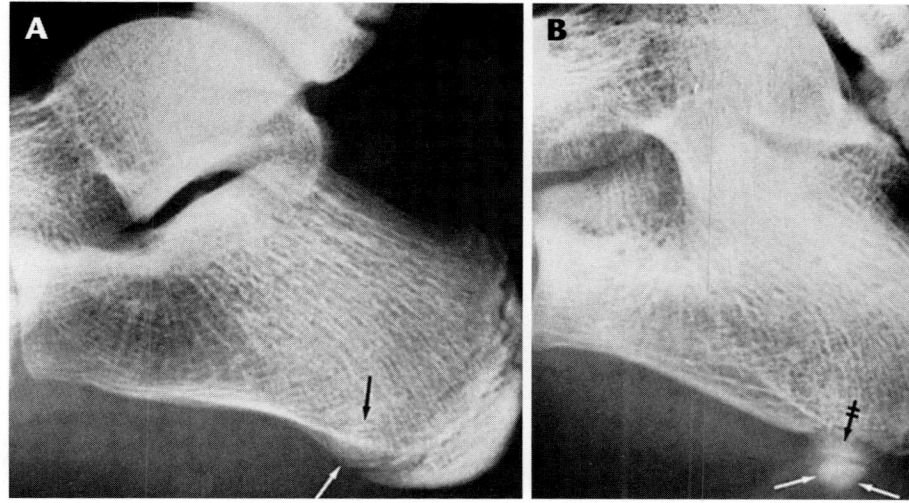

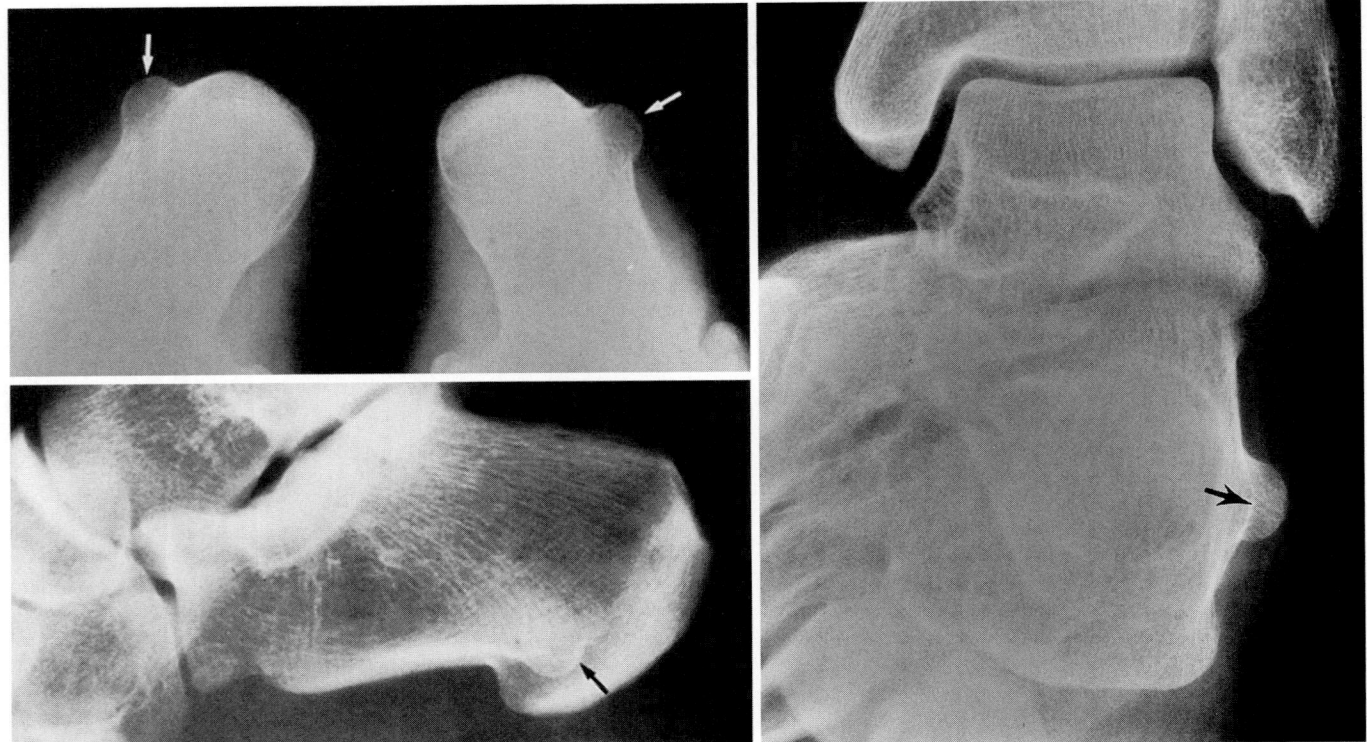

Figure 7–507. The trochlear process of the calcaneus, not to be mistaken for an exostosis.

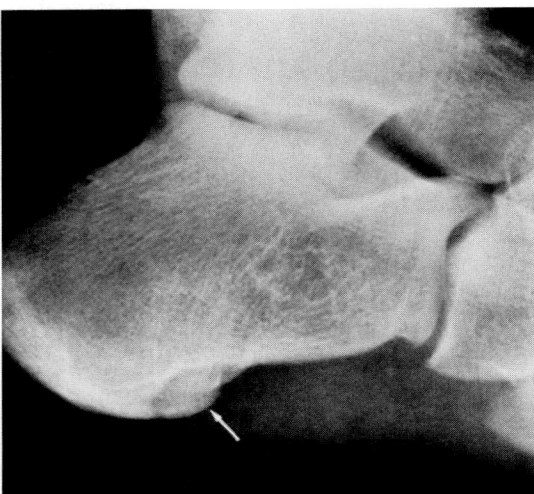

Figure 7–508. Os subcalcis, not an avulsion fracture.

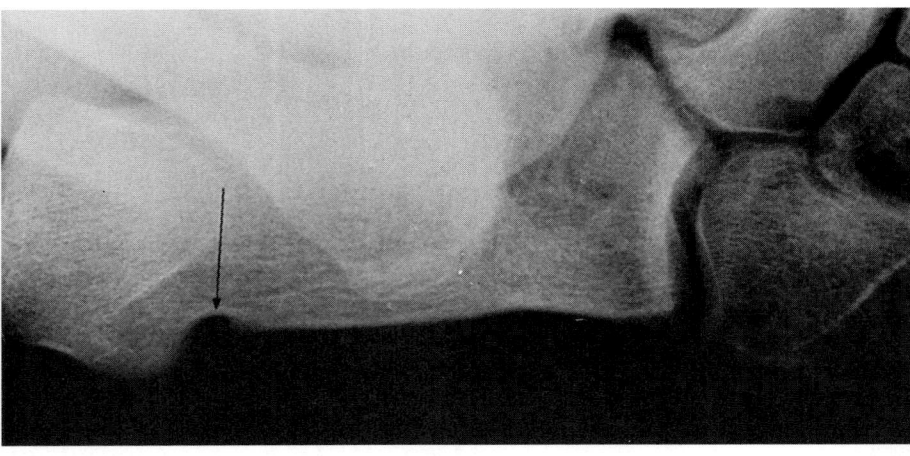

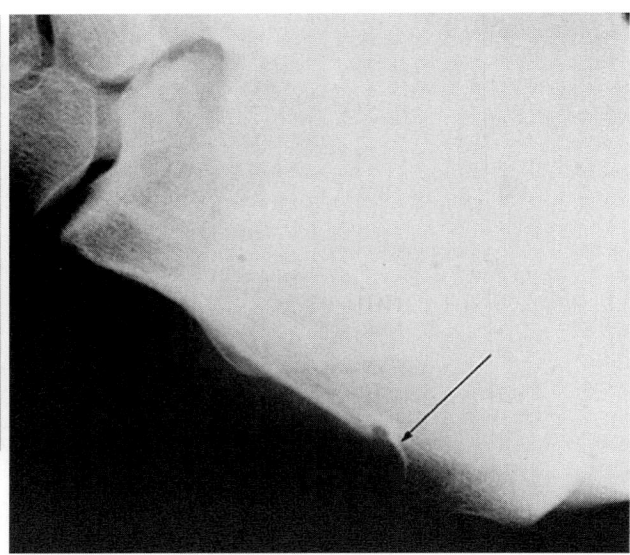

Figure 7–509. Developmental fossae in the calcaneal tuberosity, seen in oblique projection.

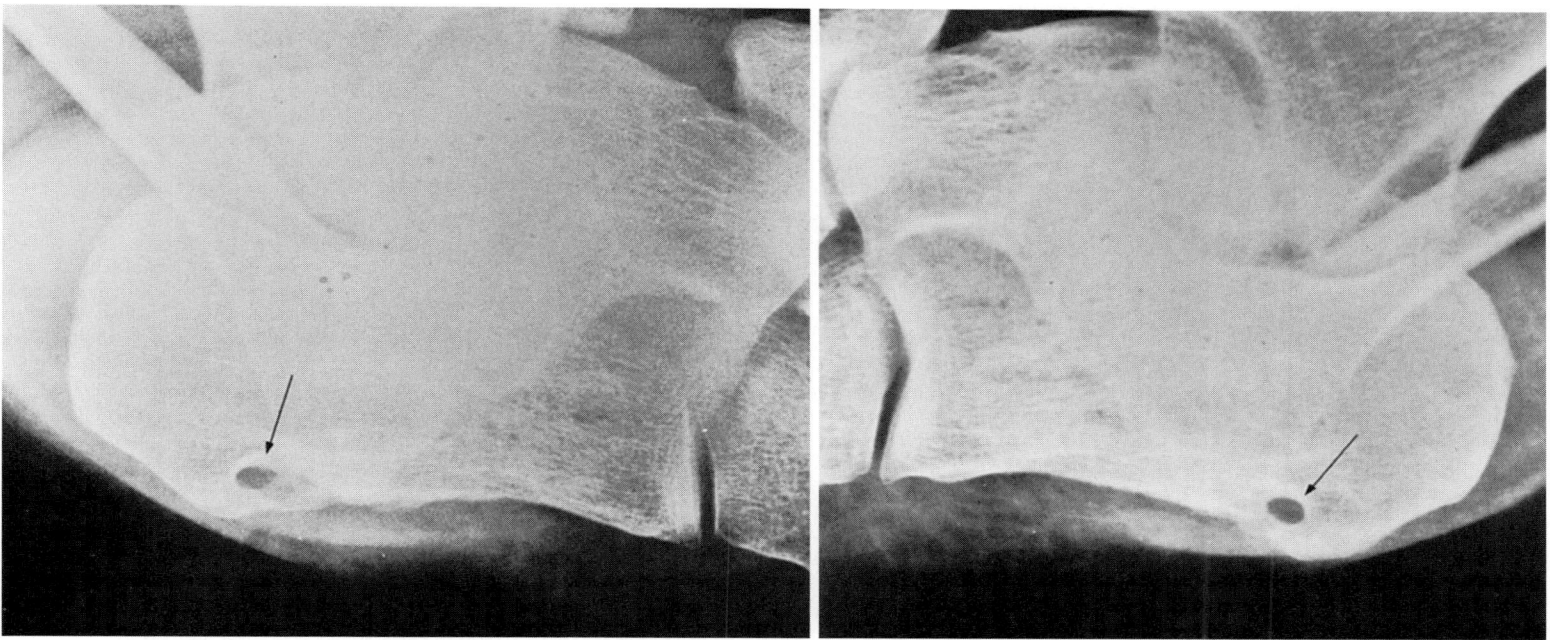

Figure 7–510. Developmental foramina in the calcaneal tuberosities, seen in oblique projection. This entity is probably related to the one in Figure 7–509.

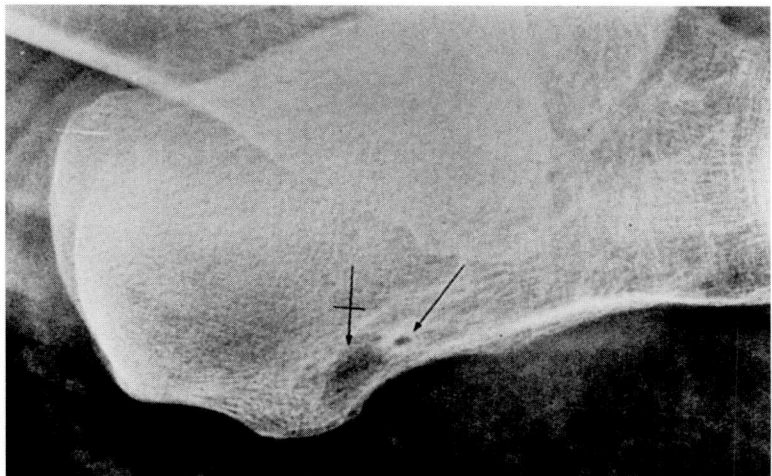

Figure 7–511. Nutrient channel of the calcaneus (→) and a fossa (↠), which might be mistaken for an abnormality.

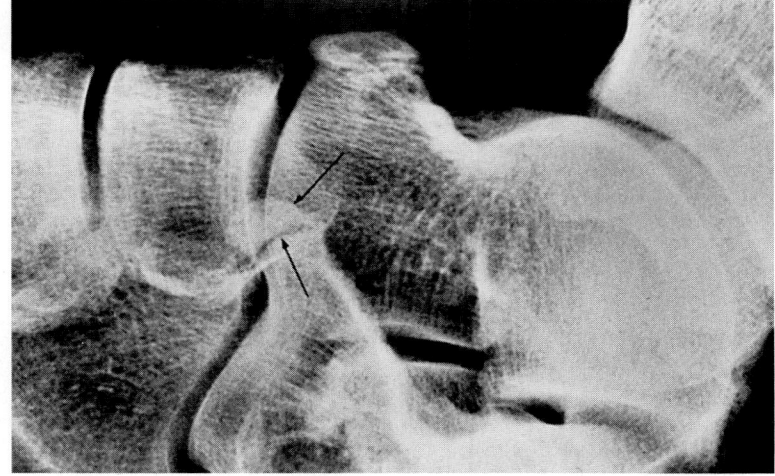

Figure 7–512. Calcanus secundarius should not be mistaken for a fracture of the anterior process of the calcaneus.

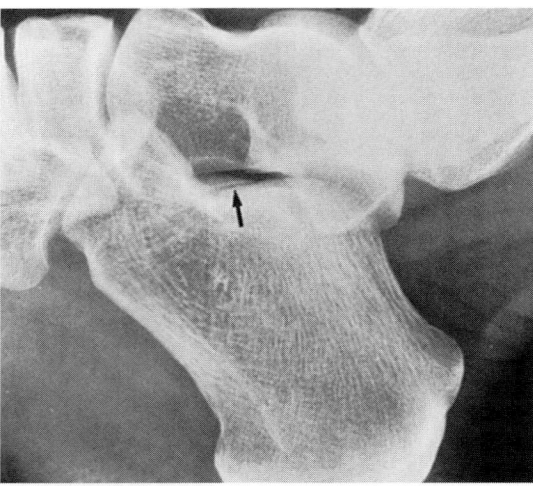

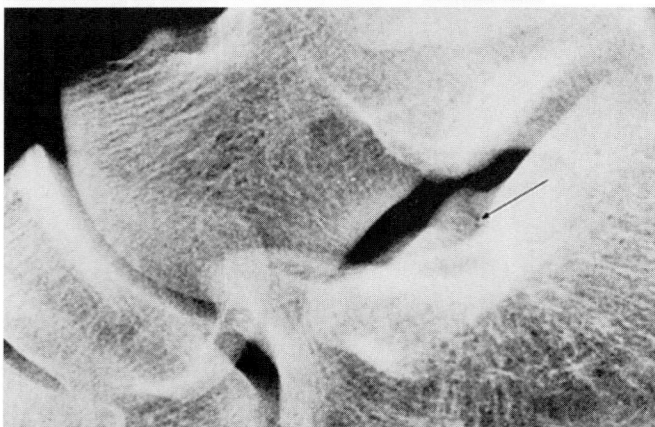

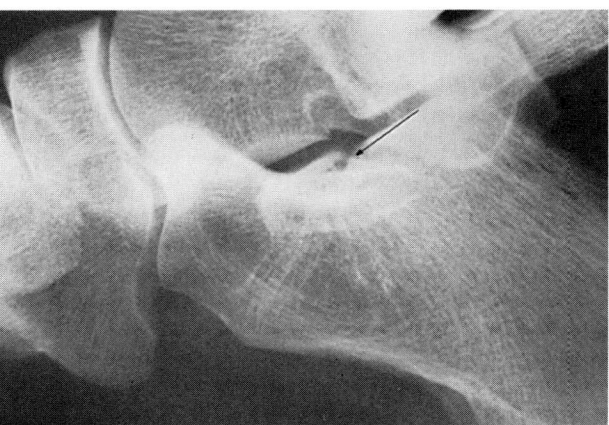

Figure 7–513. Three examples of simulated fractures of the superior margin of the calcaneus produced by the sustentaculum tali.

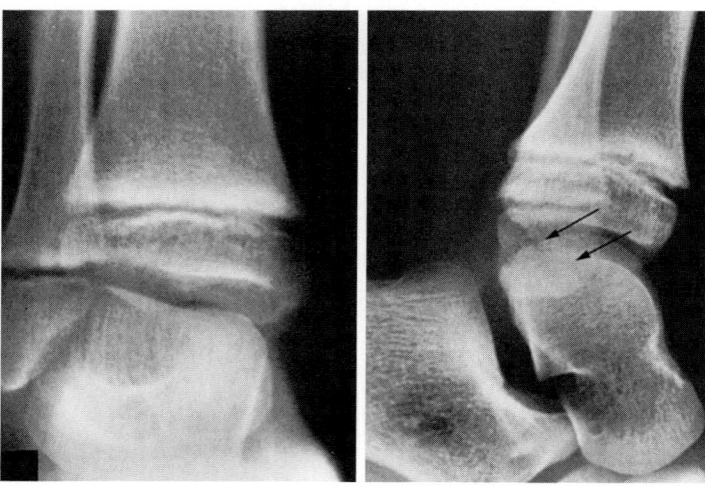

Figure 7–514. Simulated fracture of the talus in lateral projection, produced by overlapping shadow of the distal fibular epiphysis in an 8-year-old girl.

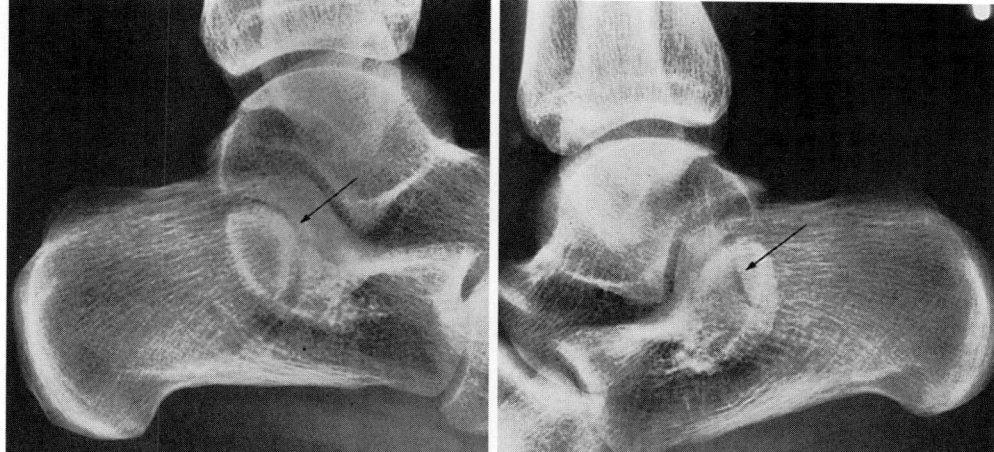

Figure 7–515. Simulated fractures produced by the sustentaculum tali.

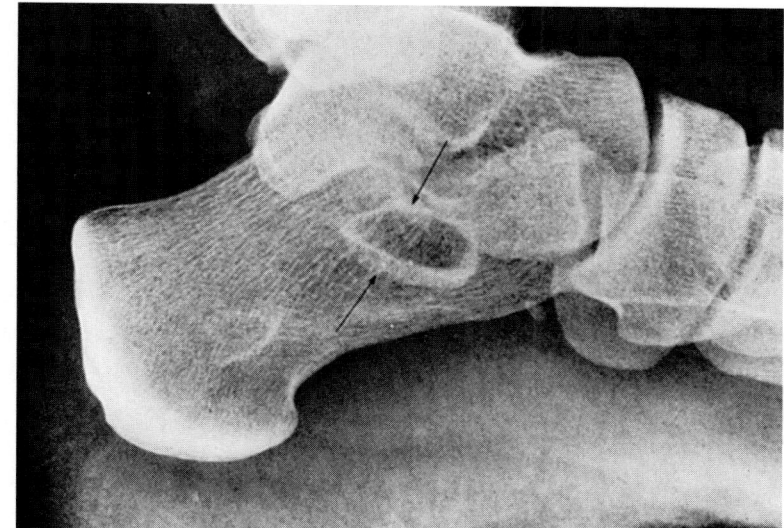

Figure 7–516. Simulated cyst produced by the sustentaculum tali.

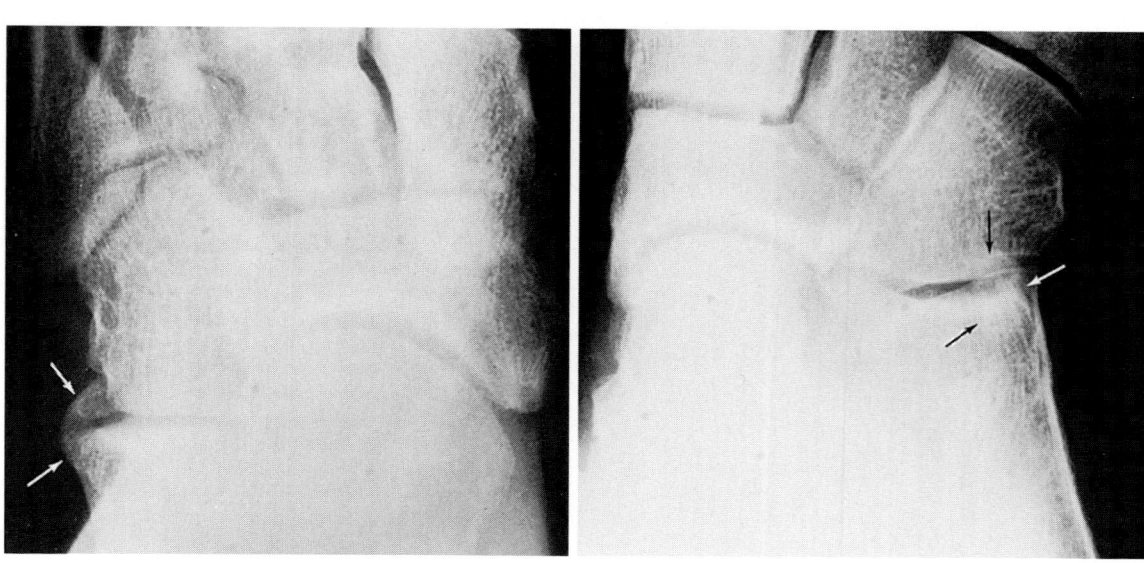

Figure 7–517. Incomplete osseous bridge between the calcaneus and the cuboid.

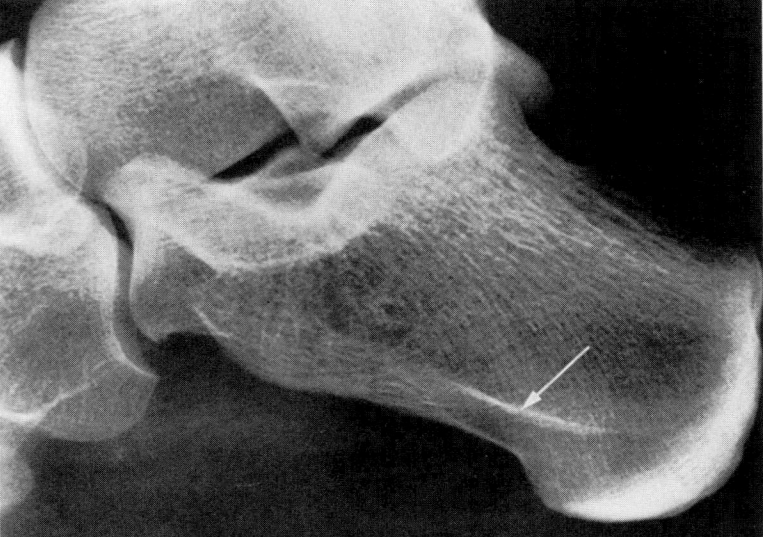

Figure 7–518. Prominent trabeculation in the calcaneus, mistaken for a stress fracture. This is a rather common finding.

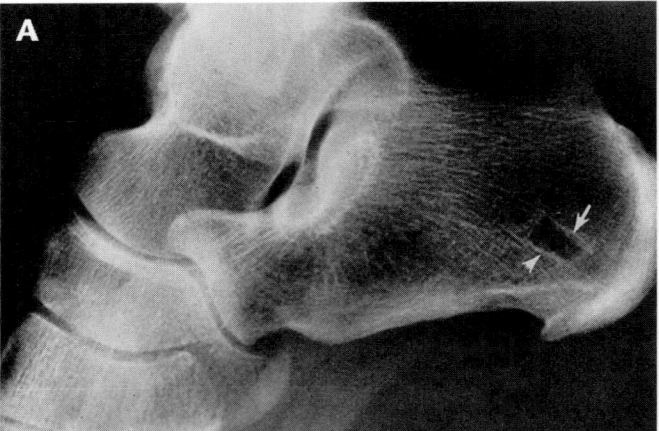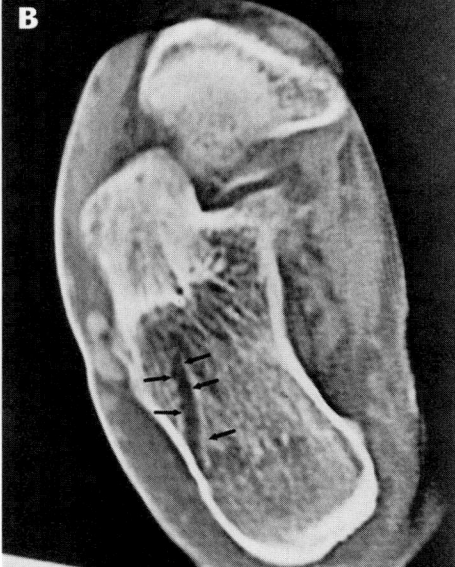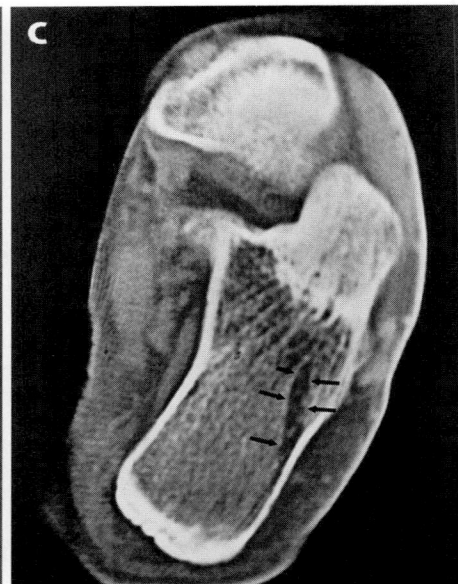

Figure 7–519. A, Simulated lesion in the calcaneus produced by prominent trabeculation, seen in axial CT bilaterally (**B** and **C**).

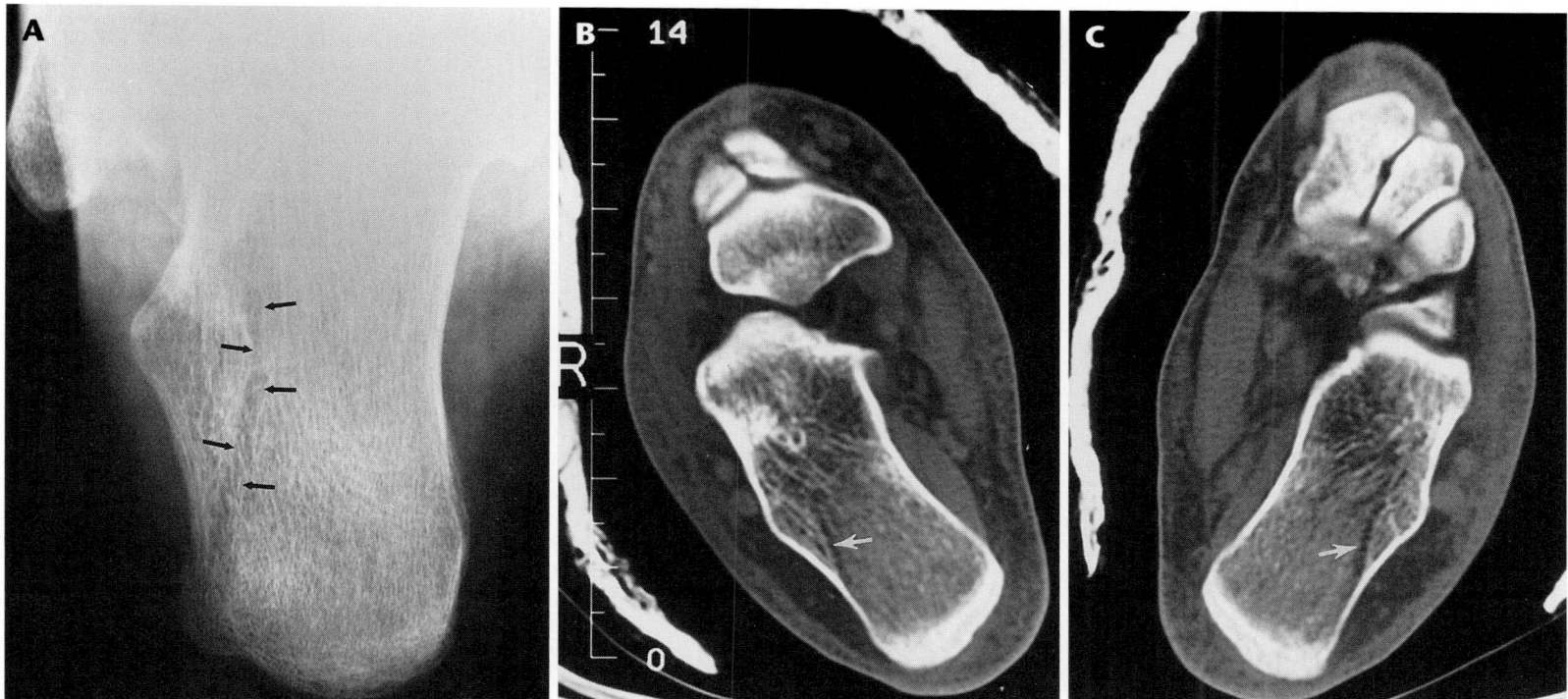

Figure 7–520. **A,** Simulated fracture in axial projection of the calcaneus, produced by the same mechanism as the preceding case. Demonstrated by axial CT in both calcanei (**B** and **C**).

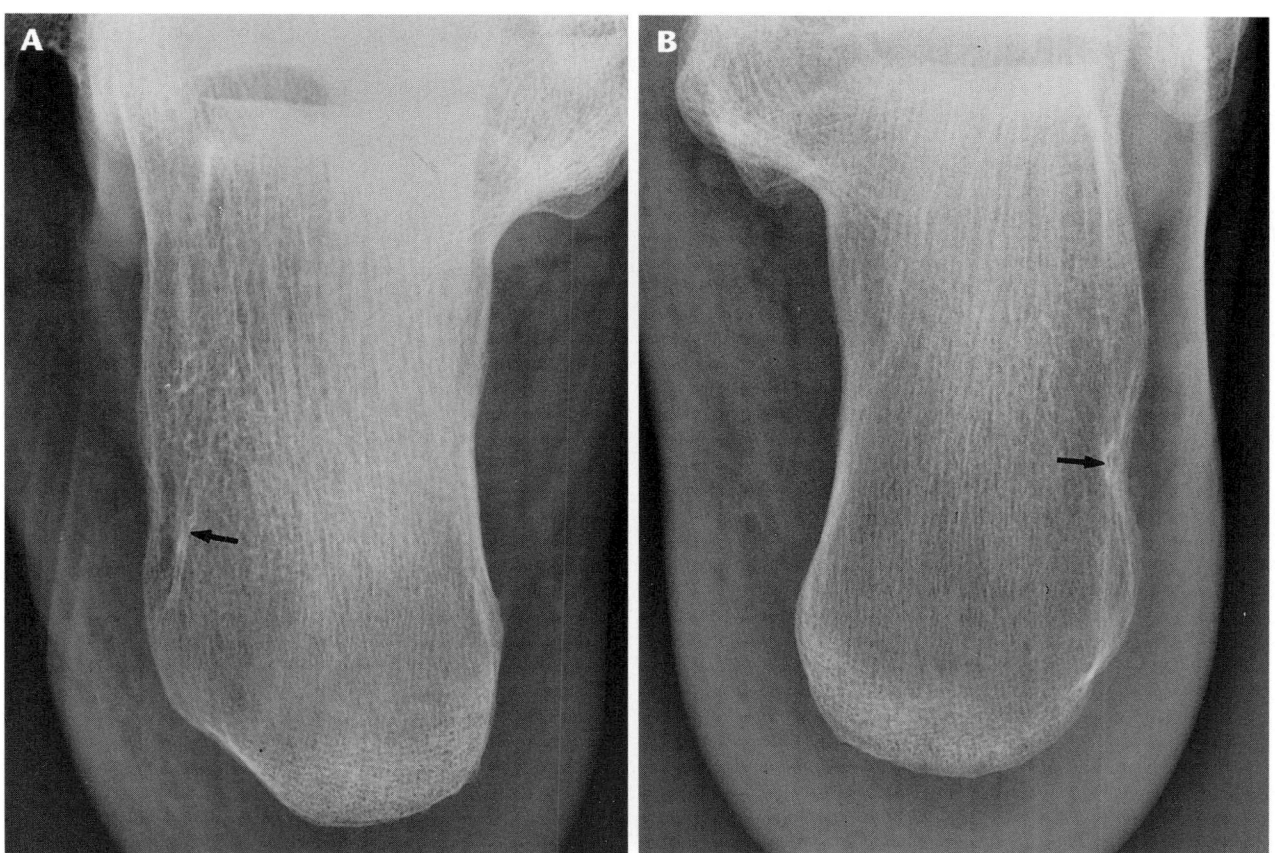

Figure 7–521. **A, B,** Normal contour alterations seen in the axial projection of the calcanei, which should not be mistaken for fractures.

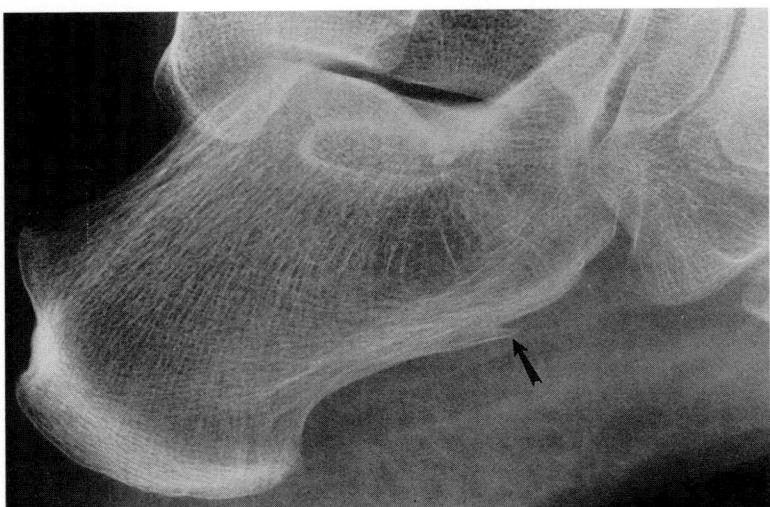

Figure 7–522. Secondary attachment site of the plantar fascia, not to be confused with a spur or exostosis.

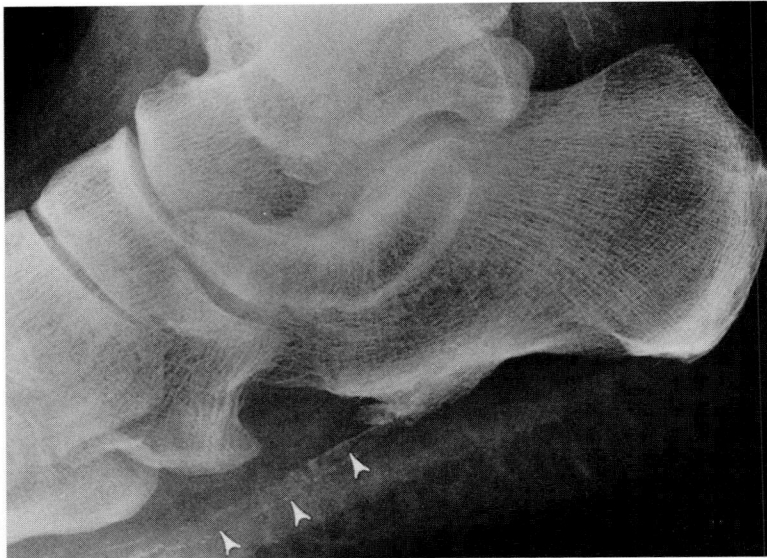

Figure 7–523. Calcification in the plantar fascia in a healthy 24-year-old man, a finding of no clinical significance.

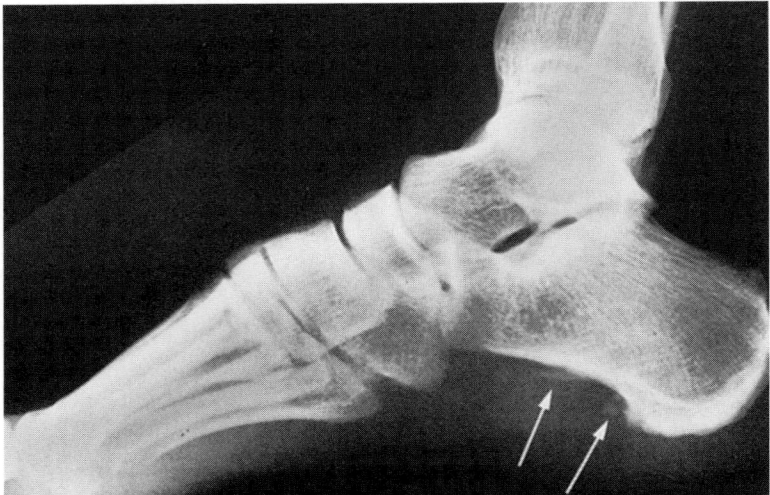

Figure 7–524. Vascular calcification in the plantar soft tissues and exostosis-like protrusion from the plantar surface of the calcaneus.

The Tarsals

THE TARSAL NAVICULAR

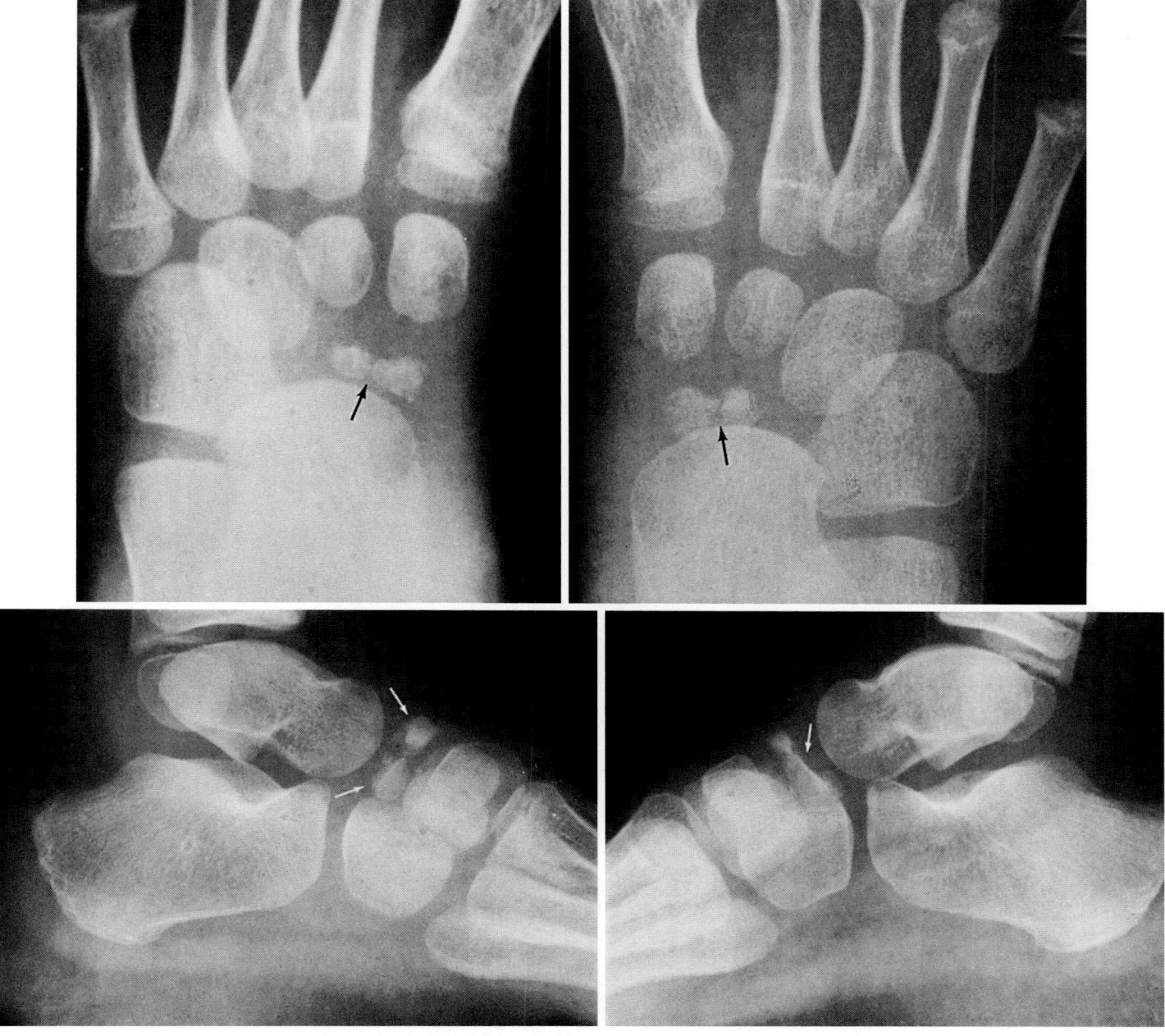

Figure 7–525. Normal ossification of the navicular from duplicate irregular centers in a 6-year-old.

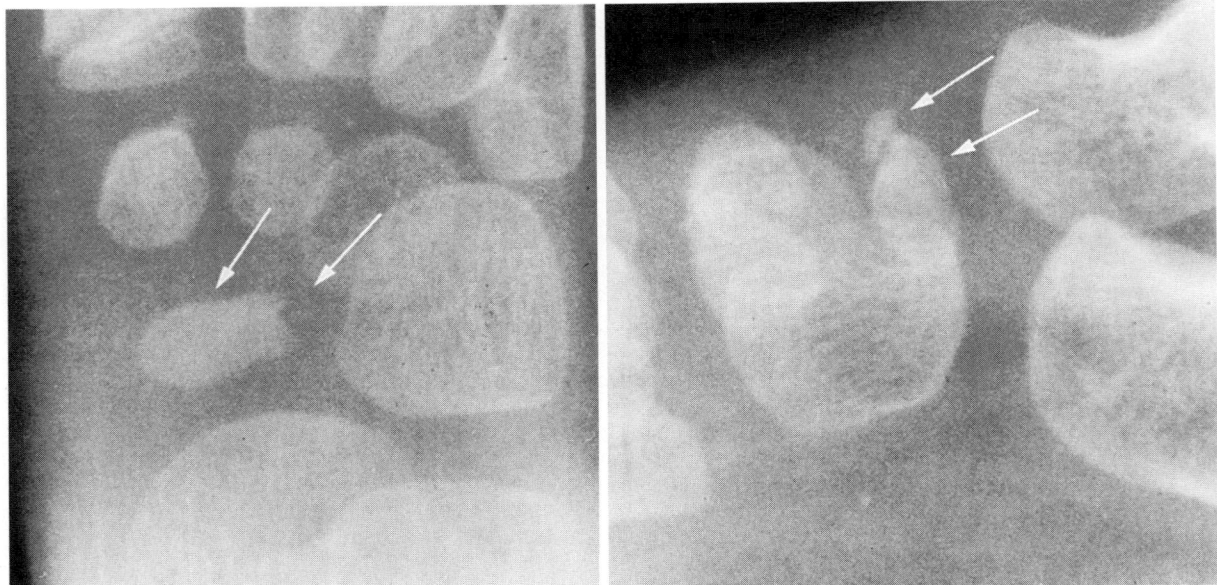

Figure 7–526. Duplicate ossification centers of the navicular of different sizes.

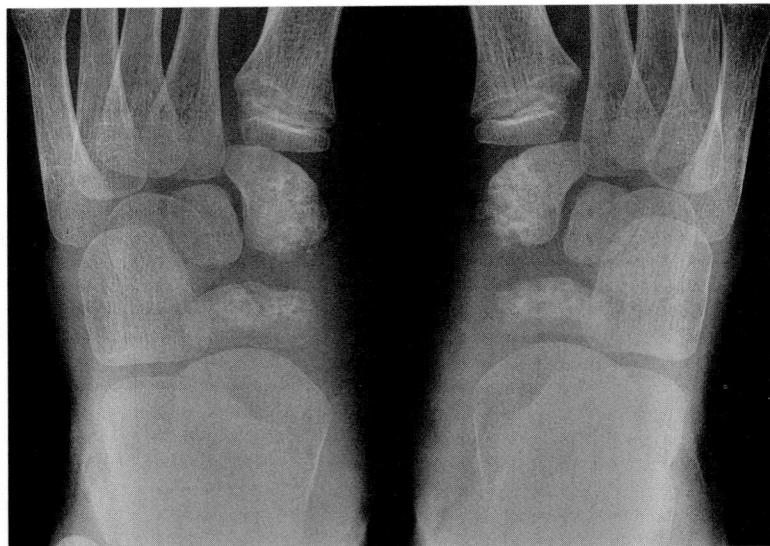

Figure 7–527. Normal irregular ossification of the naviculars and first cuneiforms in an 8-year-old child.

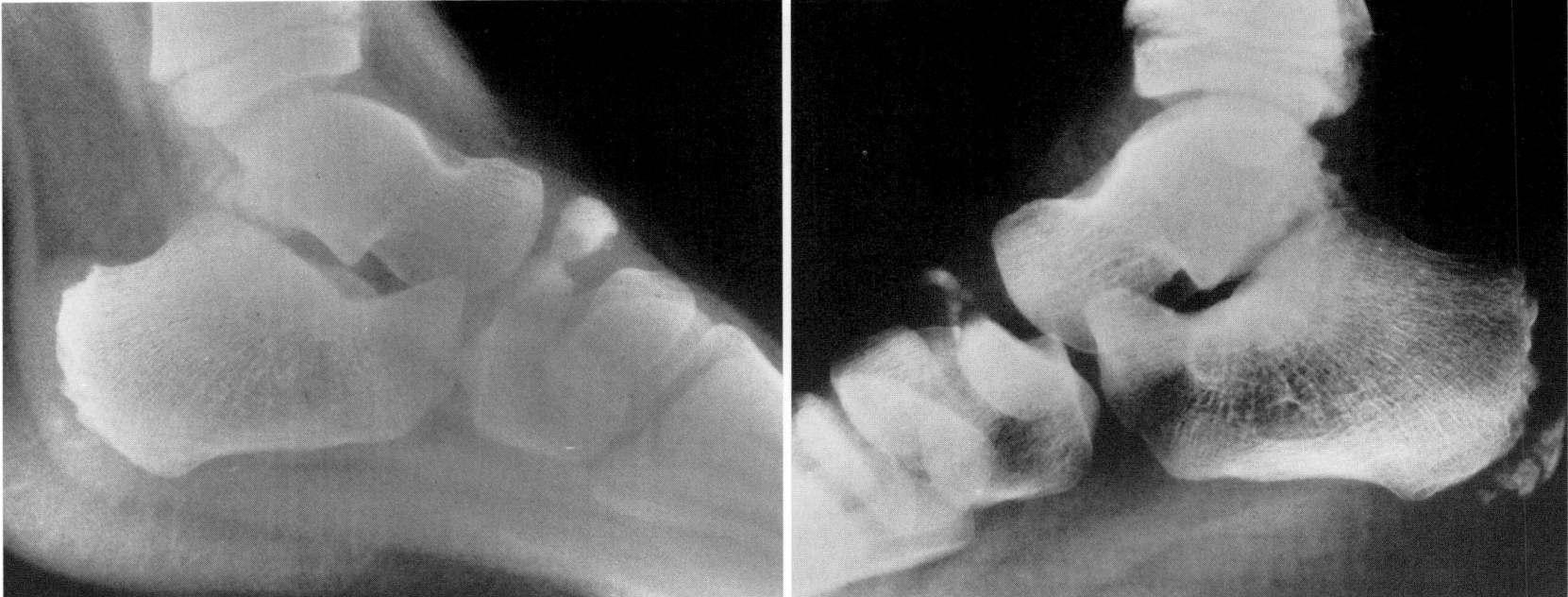

Figure 7–528. Bilateral irregular ossification of the tarsal naviculars in an 8-year-old boy. Note also the asymmetric appearance of the calcaneal apophyses.

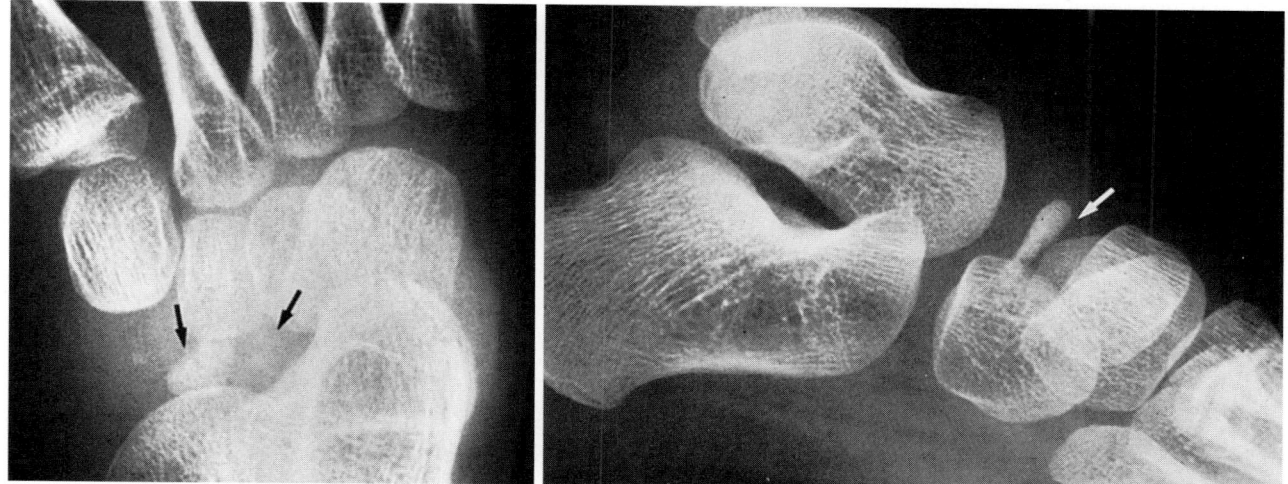

Figure 7–529. Irregular ossification of the tarsal navicular, mistaken for Köhler's disease in a 5-year-old boy.

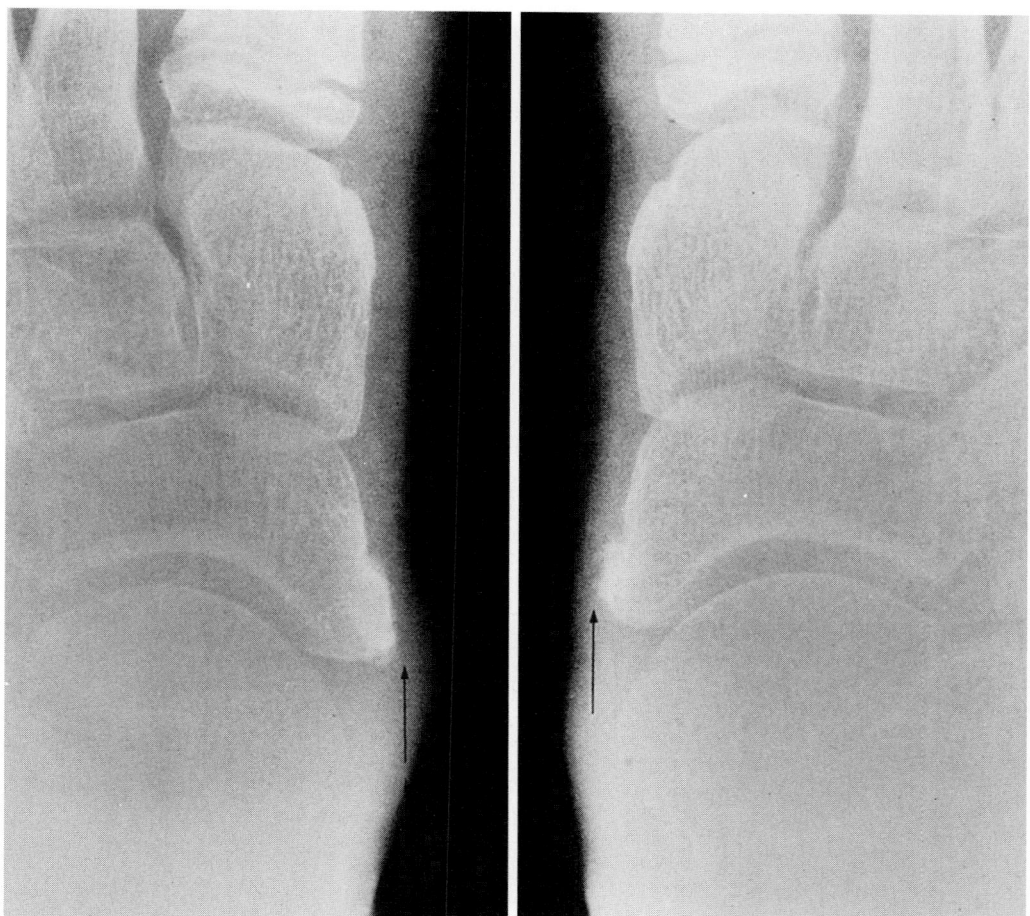

Figure 7–530. Developmental irregularity of the medial aspect of the naviculars in a 12-year-old boy.

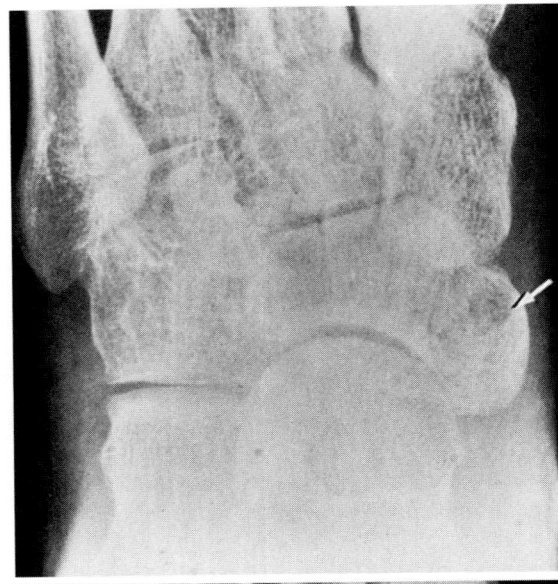

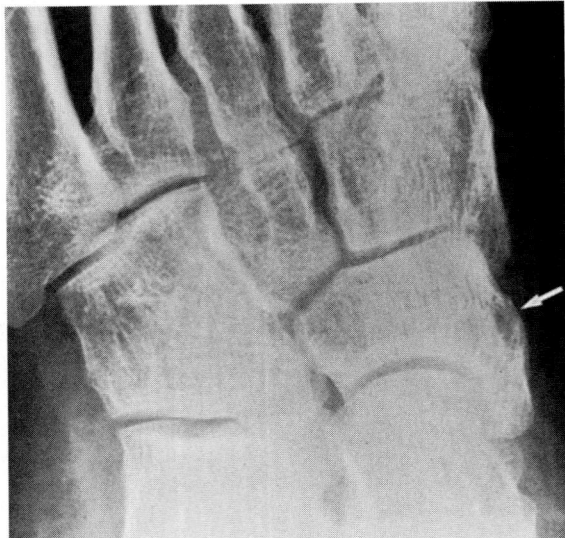

Figure 7–531. Simulated cyst of the navicular, produced by configuration of upper cortical margin.

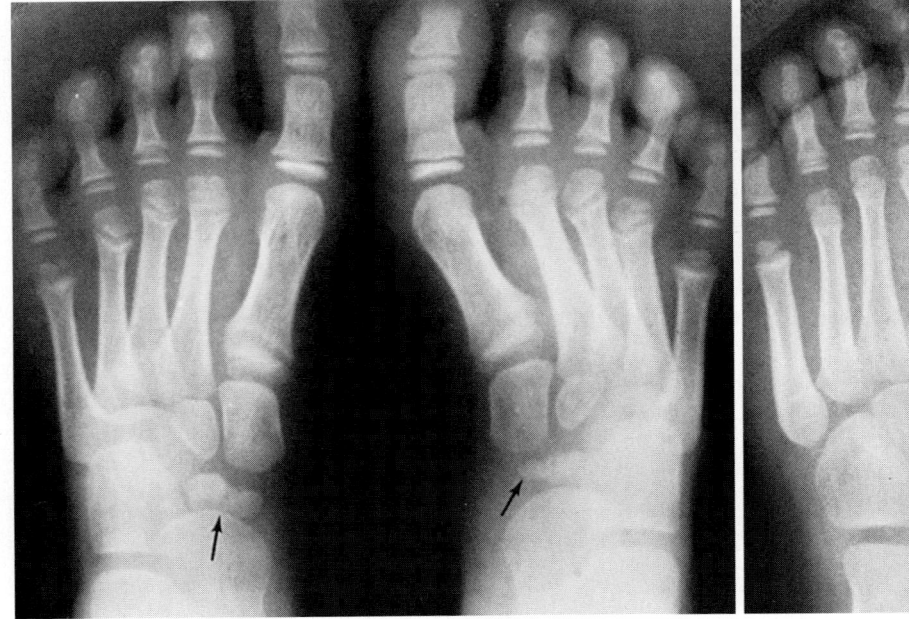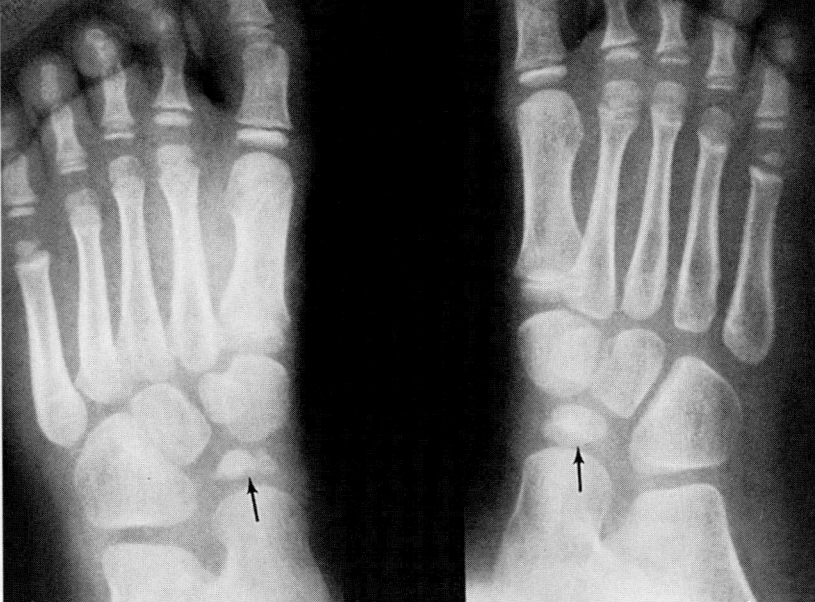

Figure 7–532. Normal ossification of the navicular from multiple centers in an 8-year-old boy. This appearance may be confused with osteochondritis or a fracture.

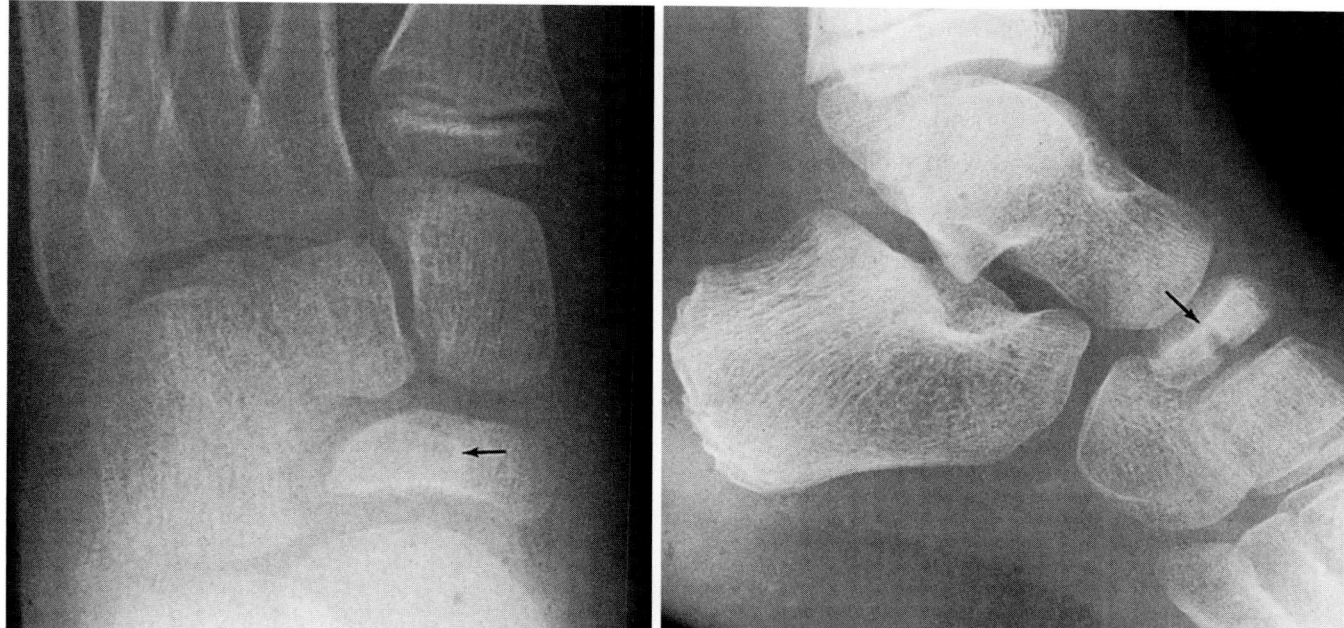

Figure 7–533. Incomplete fusion of duplicate ossification centers for the navicular in an 8-year-old boy, simulating a fracture.

Figure 7–534. Bilateral bipartite tarsal naviculars in an adult. Note the unusual configuration of the bone in the frontal projections. (Refs: Kohler A, Zimmer EA: *Borderlands of normal and early pathologic findings in skeletal radiography,* 4th ed. New York, Thieme, 1993, p. 817; Shawdon A et al: The bipartite tarsal navicular bone: Radiographic and computed tomography findings. *Australas Radiol* 39:192, 1995.)

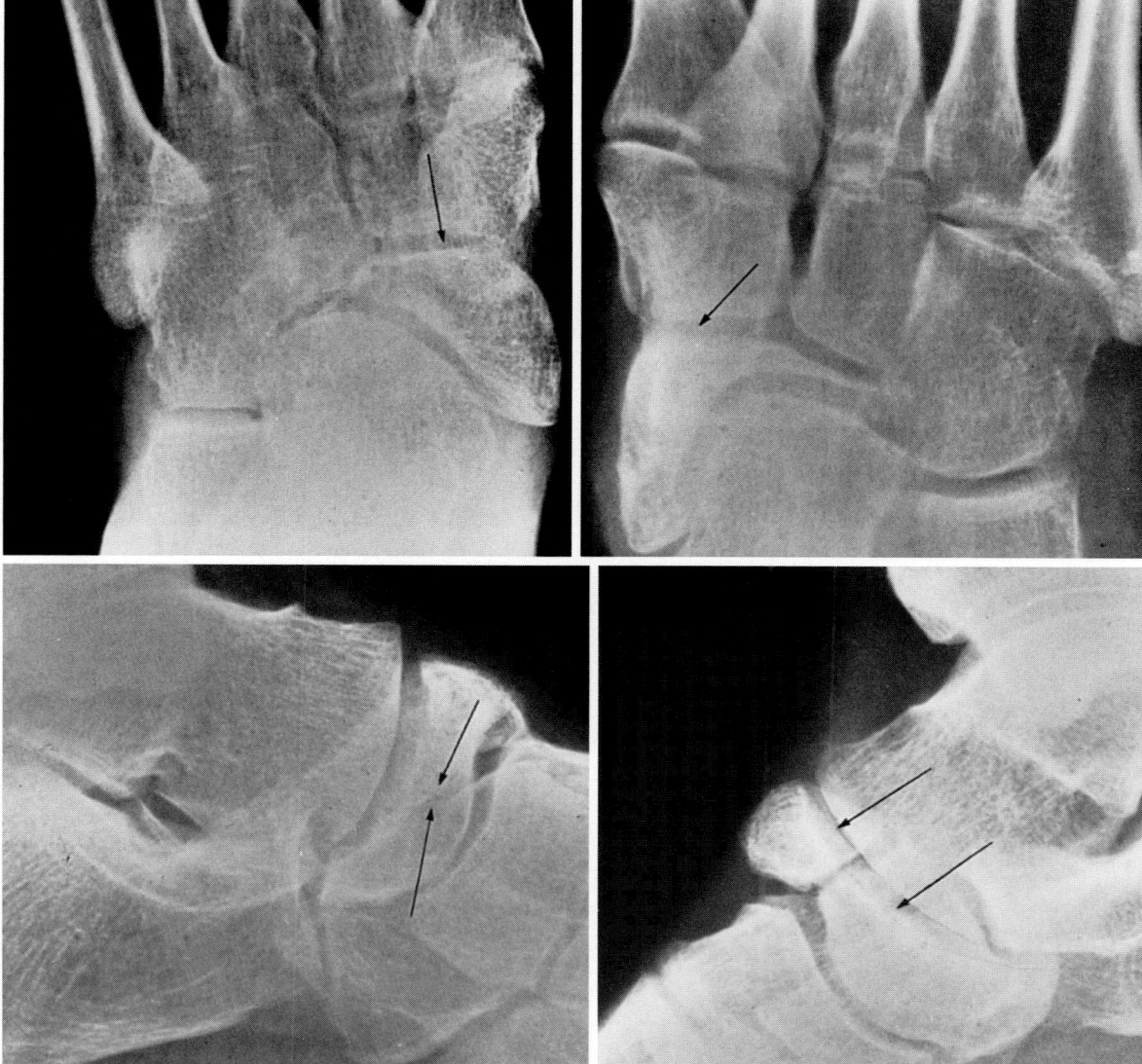

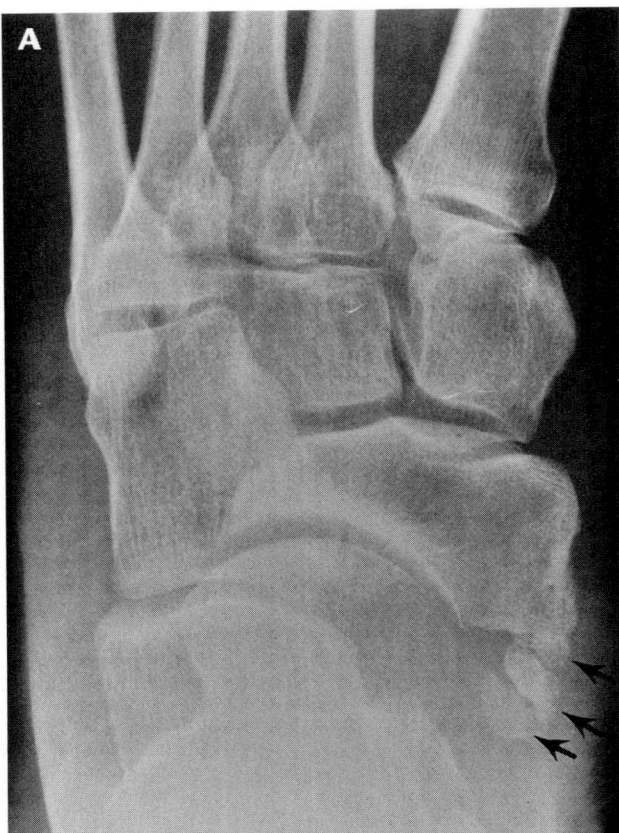

Figure 7–535. Abortive bipartite navicular. Note similarity of configuration of the navicular in comparison with Figure 7–534. **A,** Anteroposterior projection. Note multicentric os tibiale externum (*arrow*). **B,** Lateral projection. **C,** Oblique projection. See Figure 7–536.

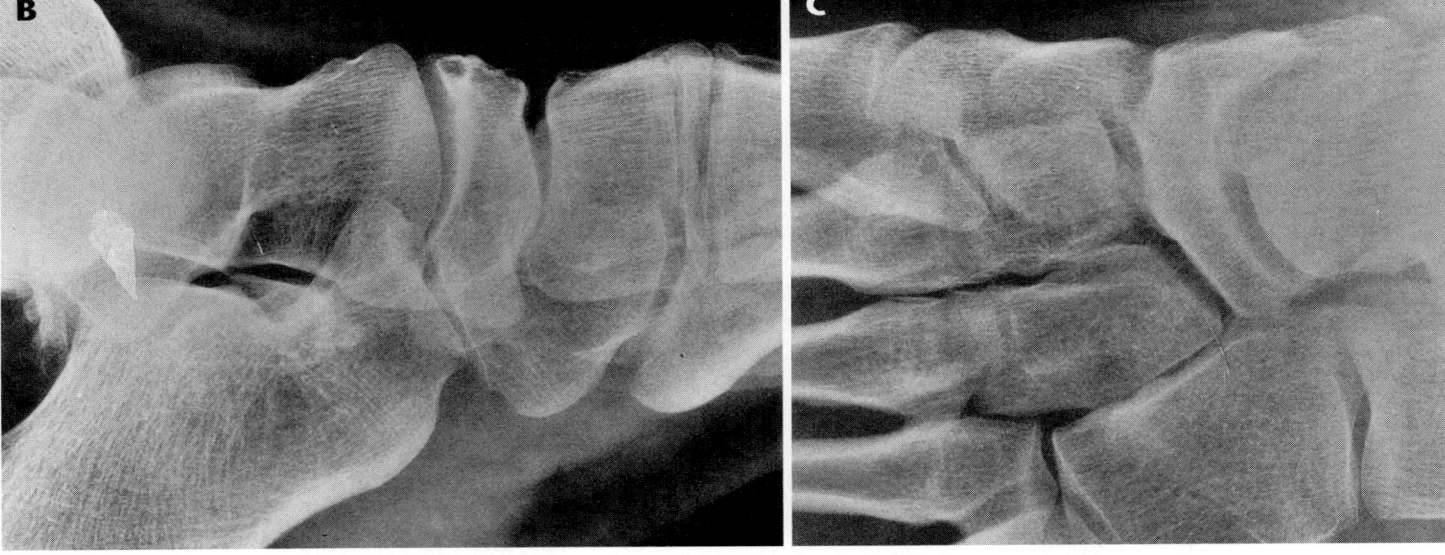

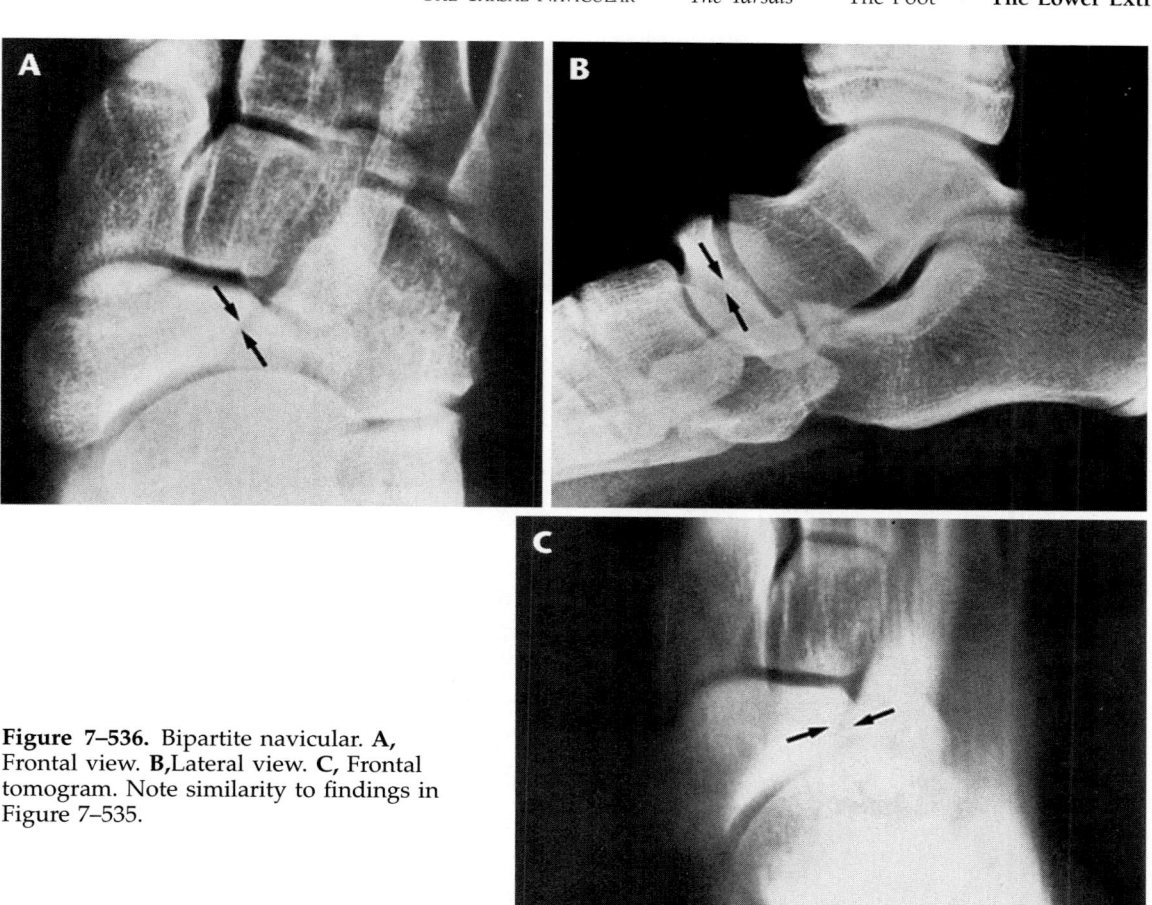

Figure 7–536. Bipartite navicular. **A,** Frontal view. **B,** Lateral view. **C,** Frontal tomogram. Note similarity to findings in Figure 7–535.

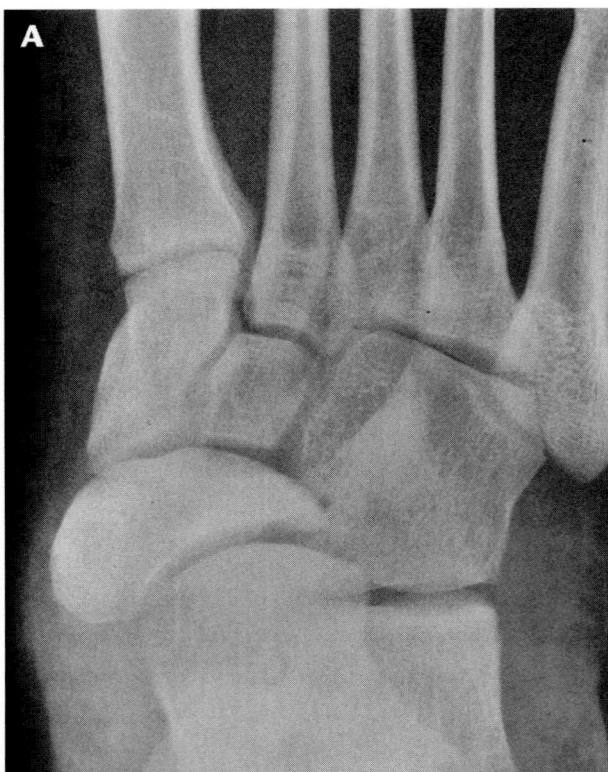

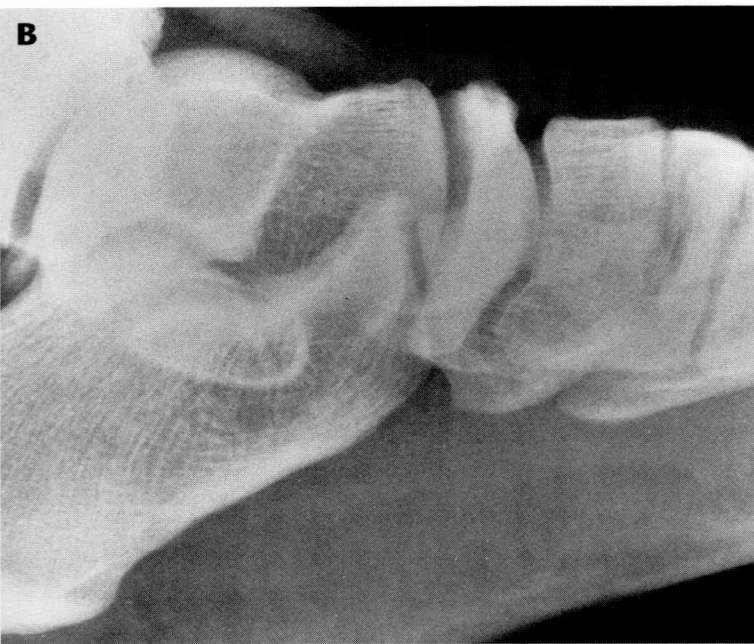

Figure 7–537. The same entity as illustrated in Figure 7–536 without division. Note the similarity in appearance of the navicular as compared with the fully developed bipartite navicular. **A,** Anteroposterior projection. **B,** Lateral projection. **C,** Oblique projection.

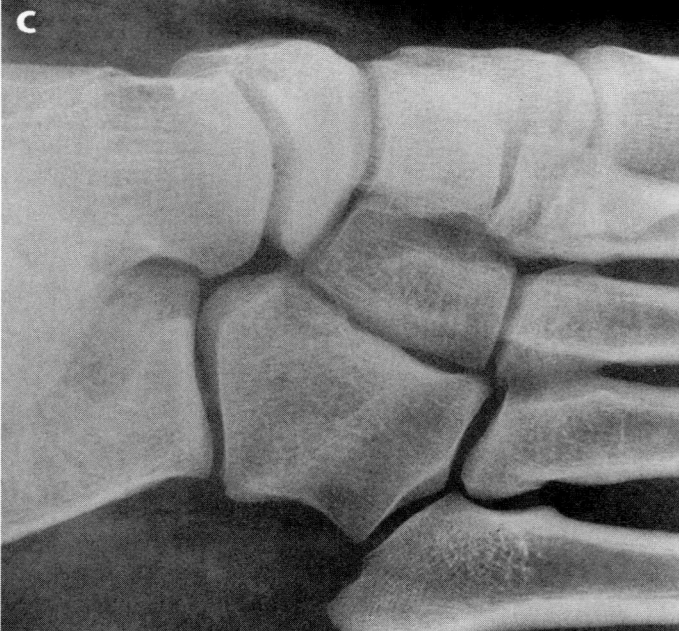

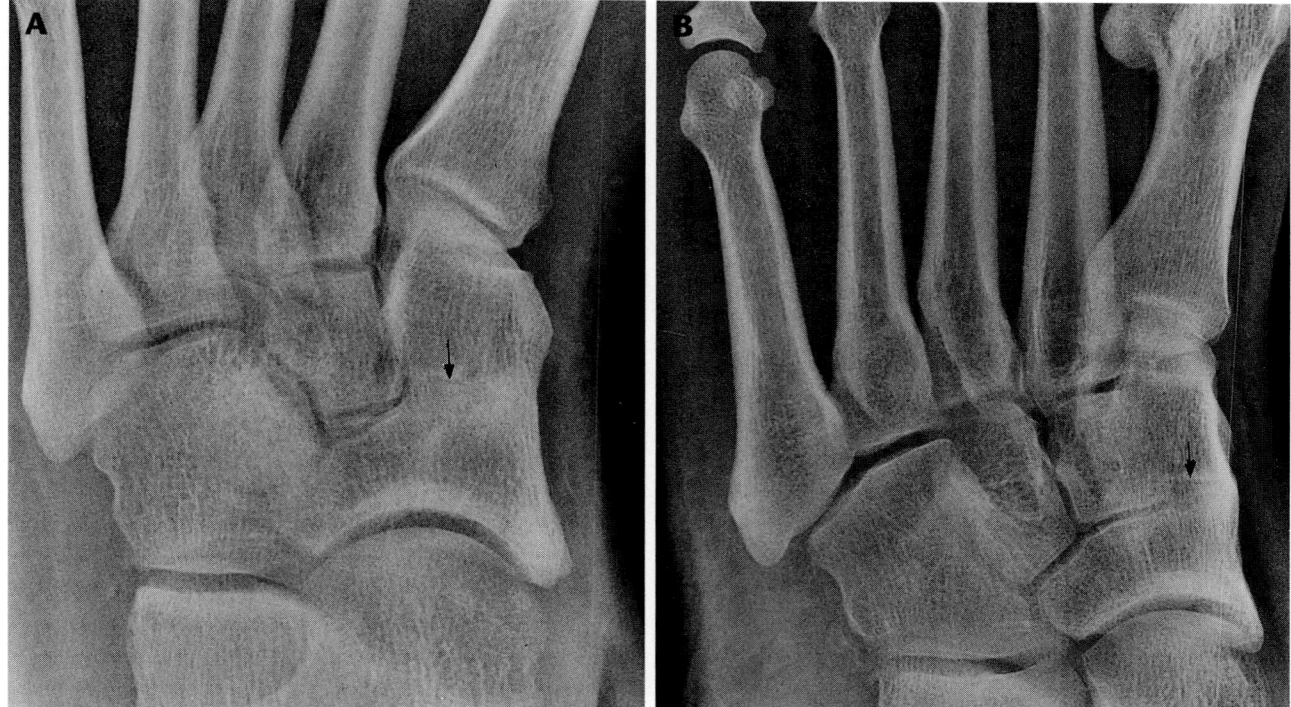

Figure 7–538. A, B, Partial coalition of the navicular and the first cuneiform.

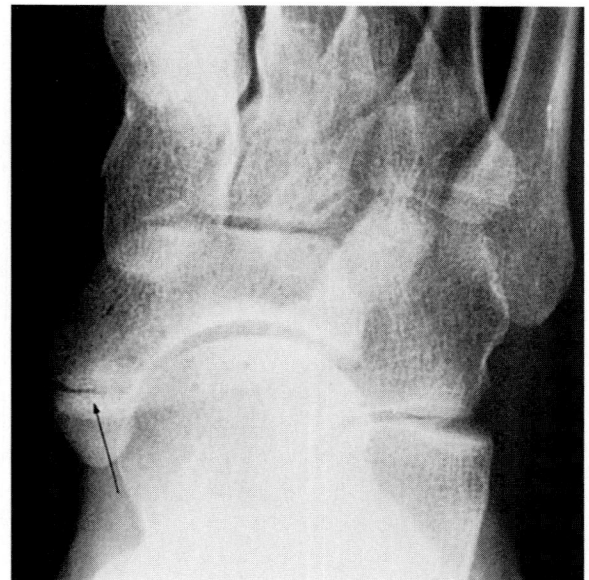

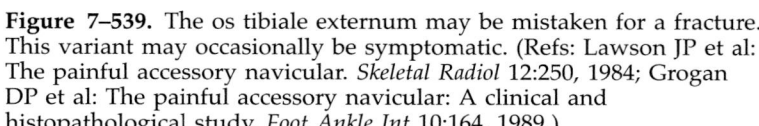
Figure 7–539. The os tibiale externum may be mistaken for a fracture. This variant may occasionally be symptomatic. (Refs: Lawson JP et al: The painful accessory navicular. *Skeletal Radiol* 12:250, 1984; Grogan DP et al: The painful accessory navicular: A clinical and histopathological study. *Foot Ankle Int* 10:164, 1989.)

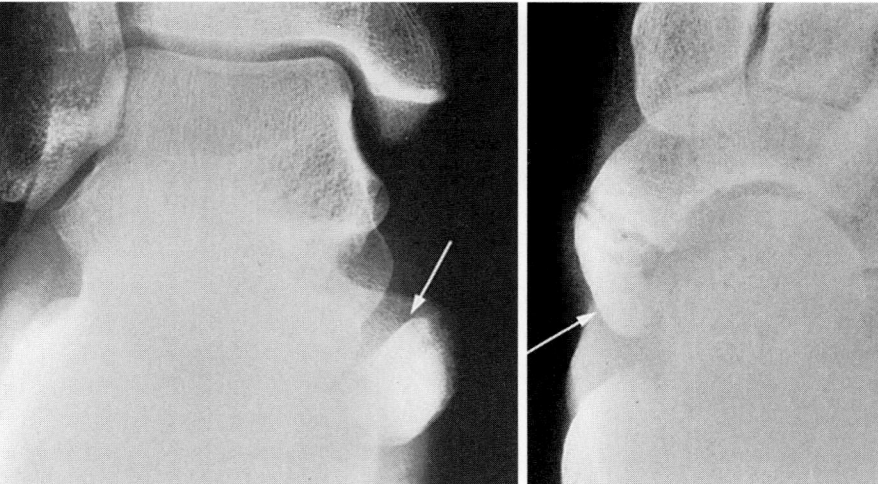

Figure 7–540. Huge os tibiale externum.

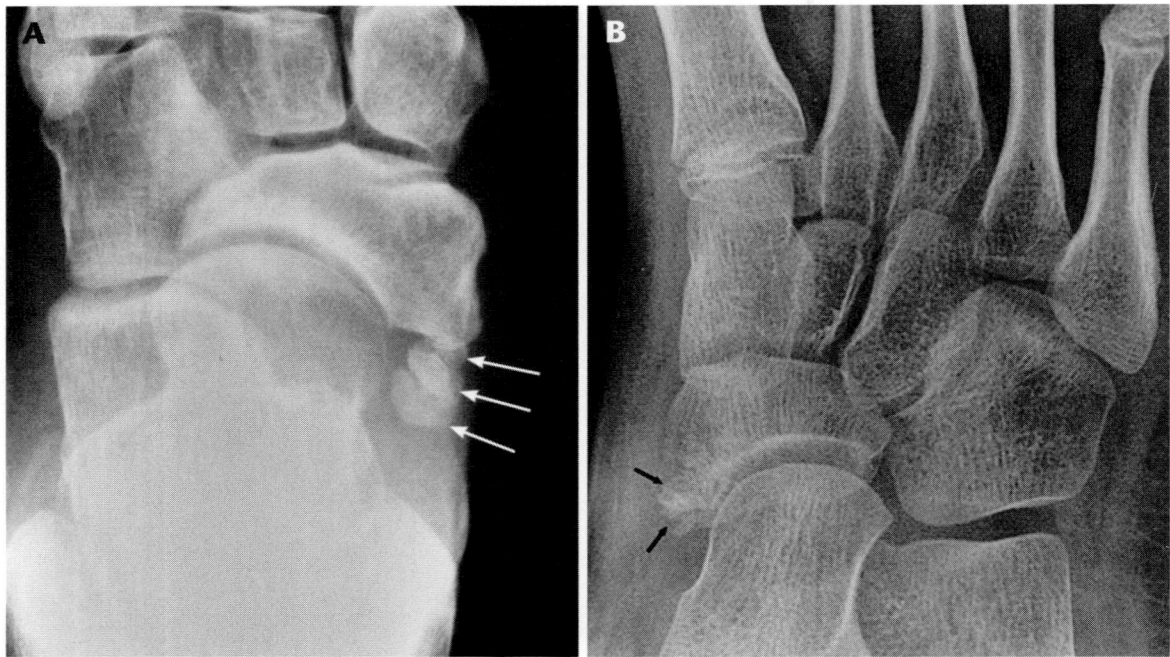

Figure 7–541. A, B, Two examples of multicentric ossification of the os tibiale externum.

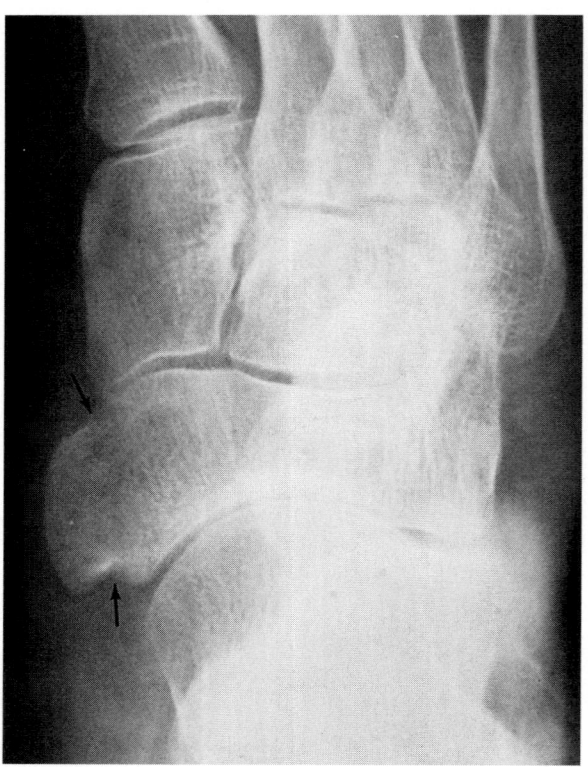

Figure 7–542. Fusion of an os tibiale externum to the navicular.

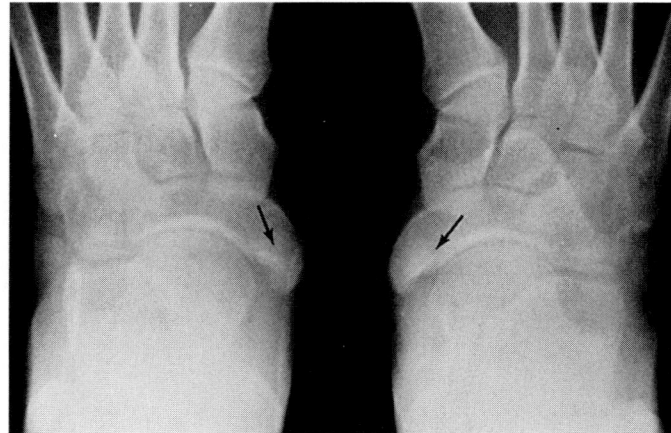

Figure 7–543. Bilateral partial fusion of the os tibiale externum to the navicular. The *arrows* point to the remnants of the line of fusion.

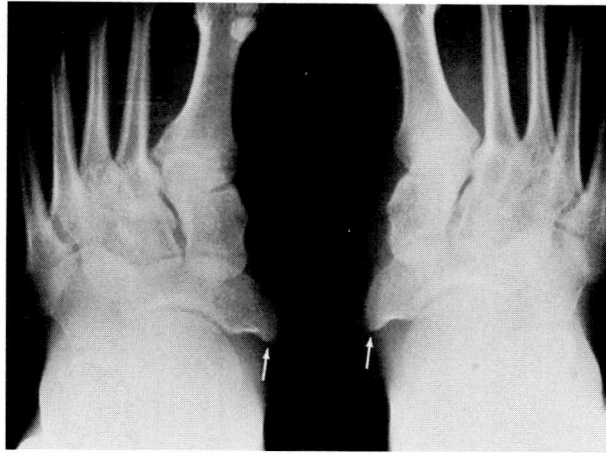

Figure 7–544. Configuration of the naviculars, suggesting complete incorporation of the os tibiale externum (cornuate navicular).

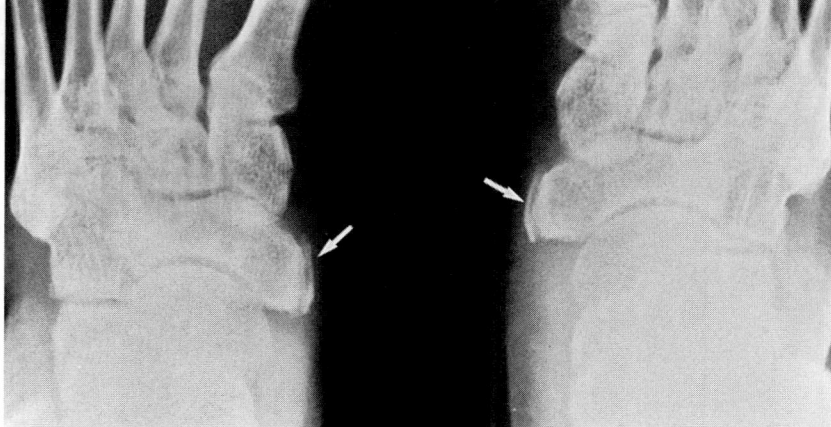

Figure 7–545. Unusual bilateral os tibiale externum.

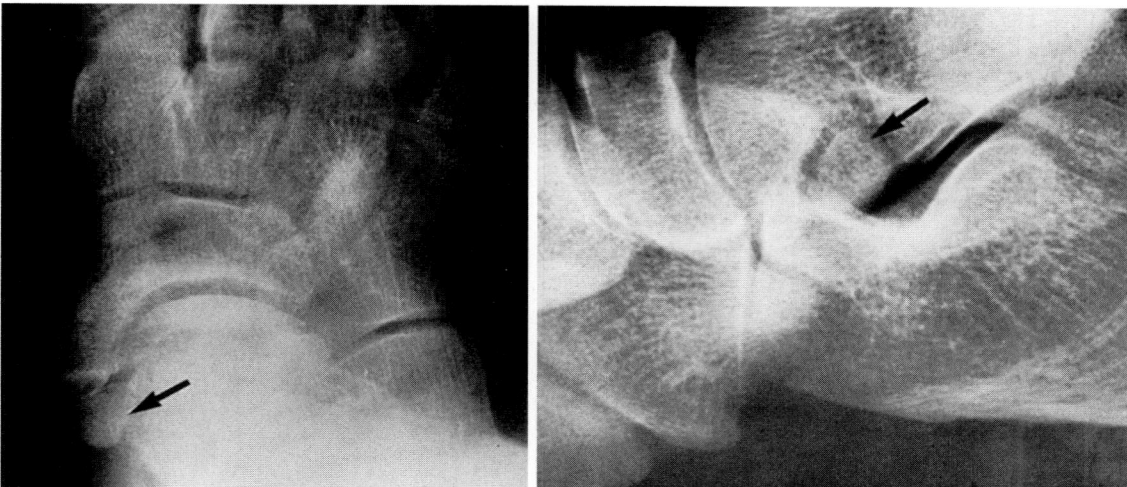

Figure 7–546. The os tibiale externum in frontal (*left*) and lateral (*right*) projection.

Figure 7–547. Os tibiale externum in lateral projection simulating a fracture of the cuboid.

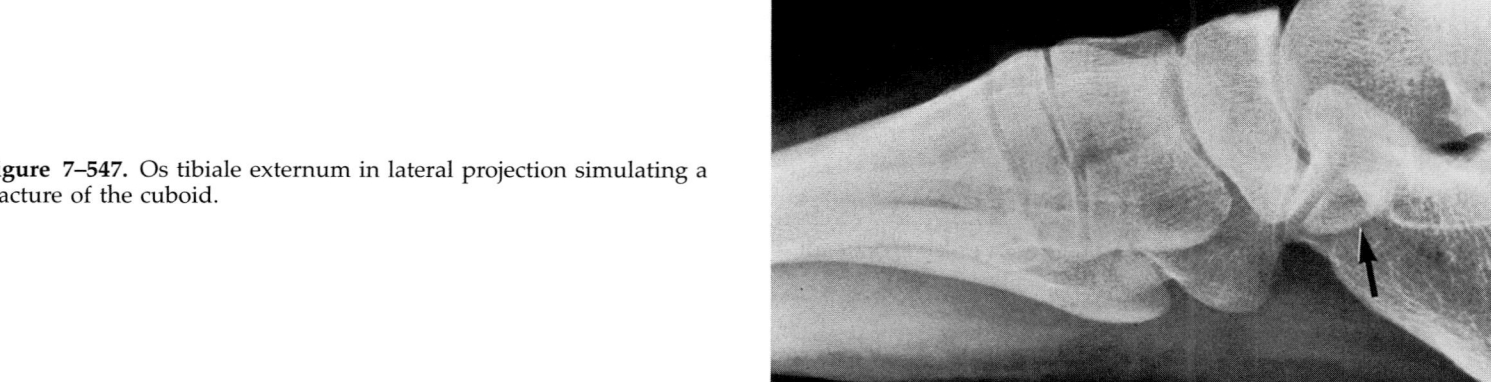

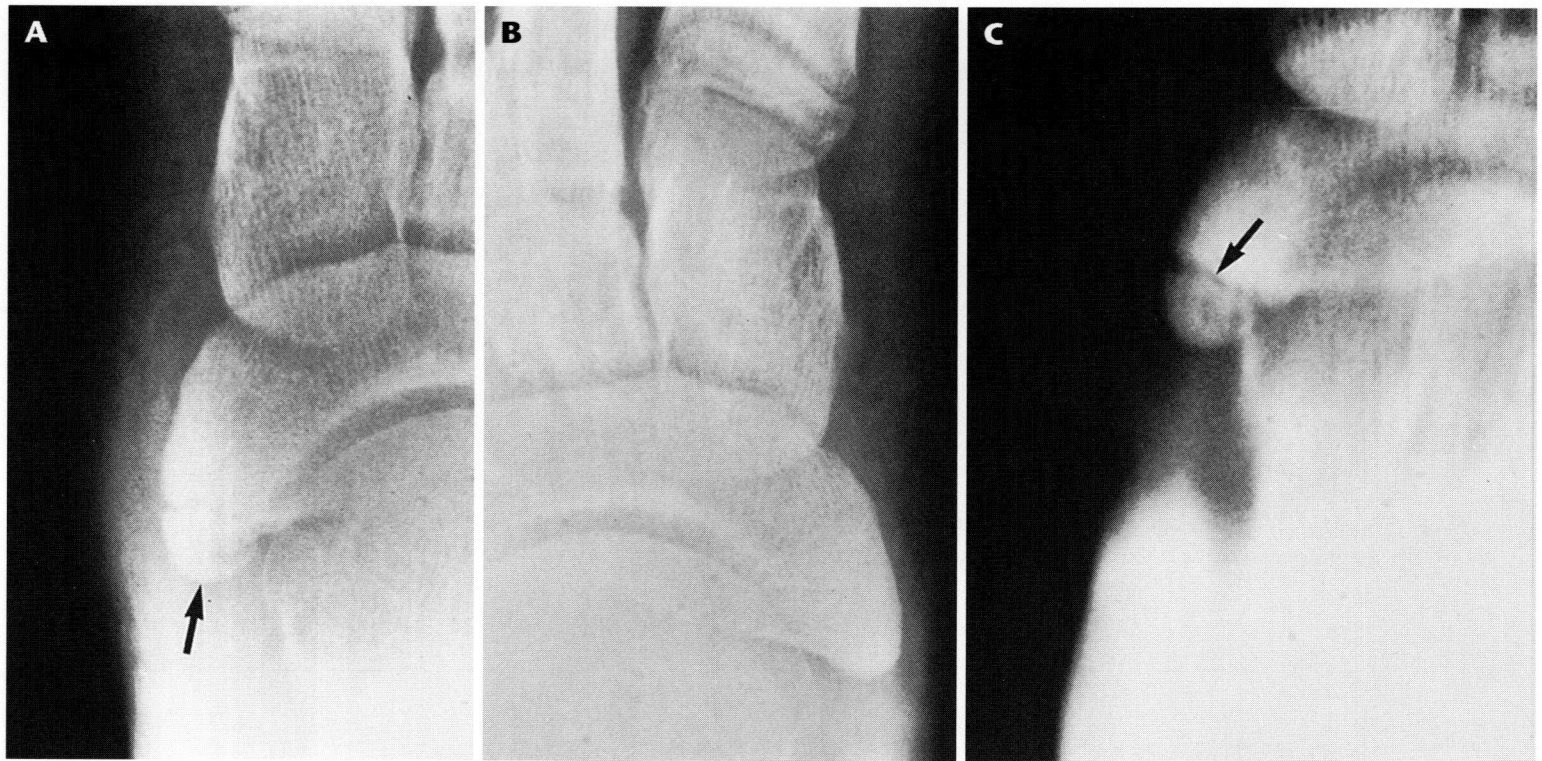

Figure 7–548. **A** and **B,** Os tibiale externum originally diagnosed as a fracture because of its presence on one side only. **C,** Tomogram confirming nonfracture.

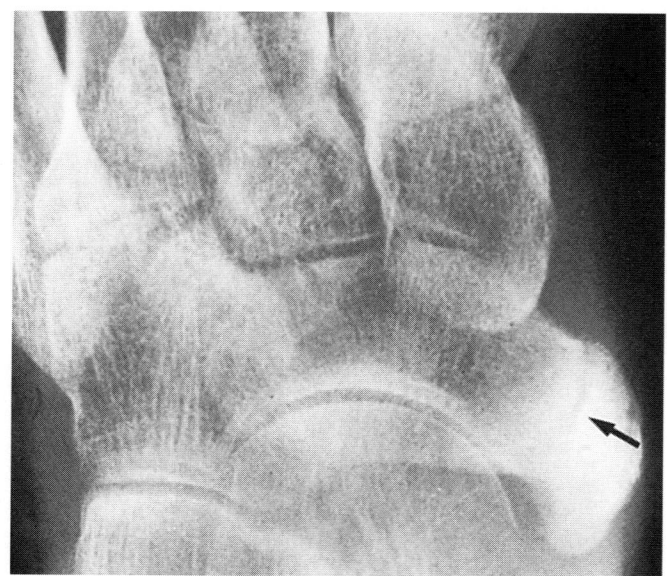

Figure 7–549. Partial fusion of the os tibiale externum, which was mistaken for a fracture.

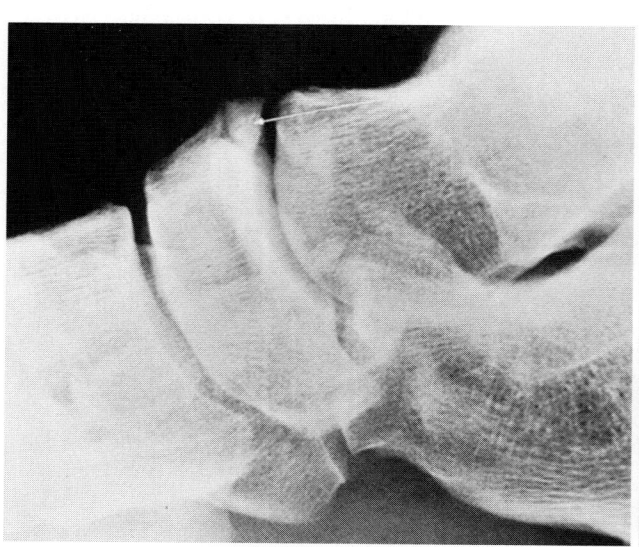
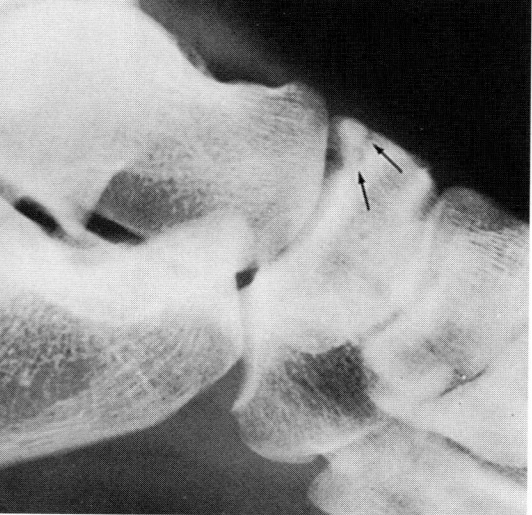

Figure 7–550. Partial incorporation of the os supranaviculare, which might be mistaken for an avulsion fracture.

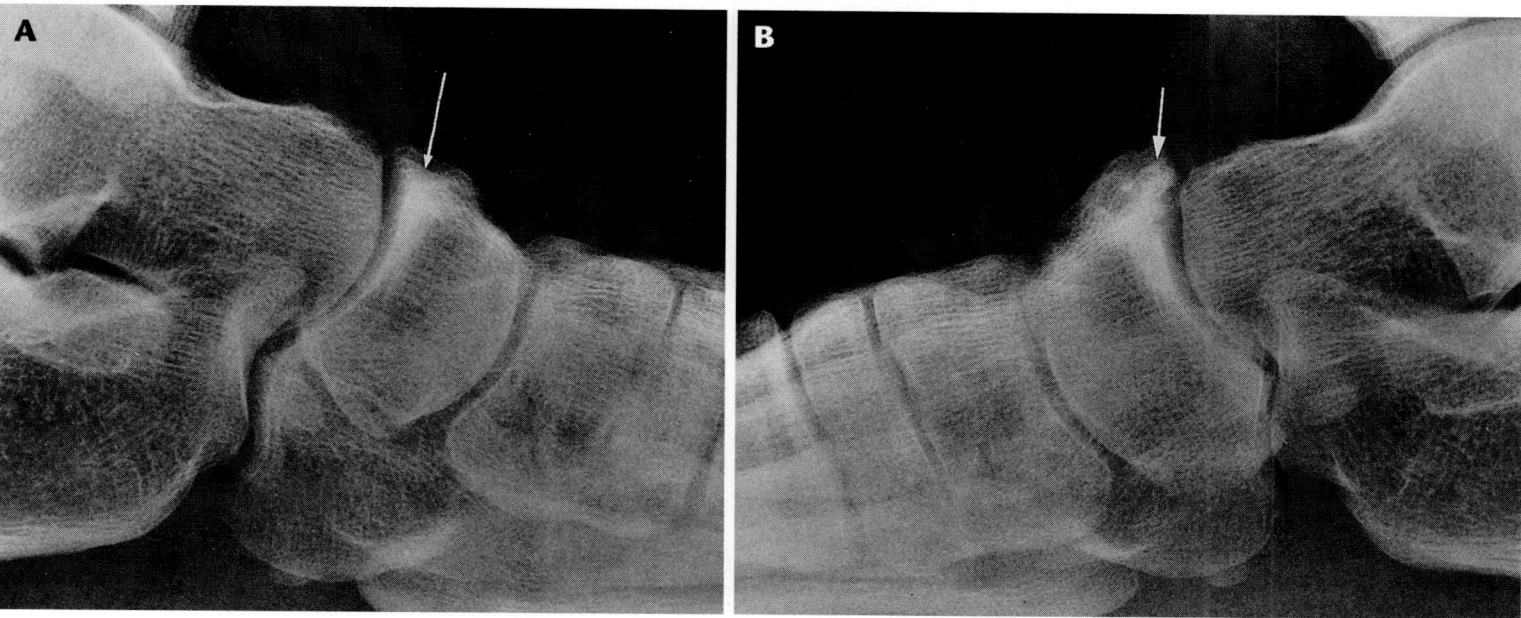

Figure 7–551. A, B, Bilateral total incorporation of the os supranaviculare.

Figure 7–552. Normal irregularity of the joint margins of the navicular and cuboid in oblique projection. This entity should not be mistaken for a manifestation of arthritis.

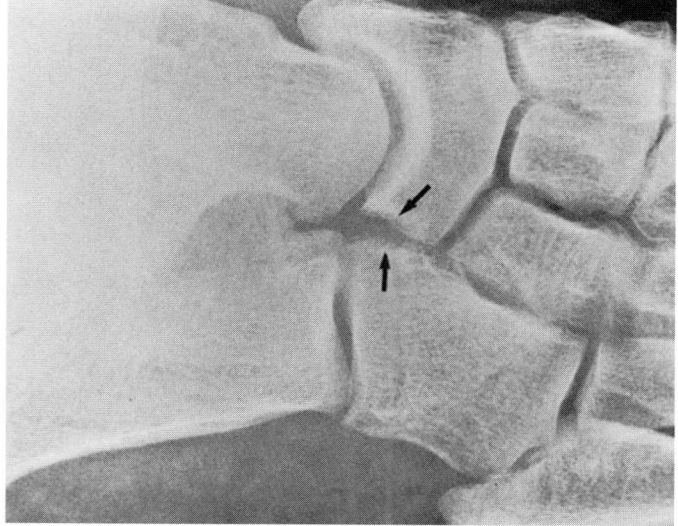

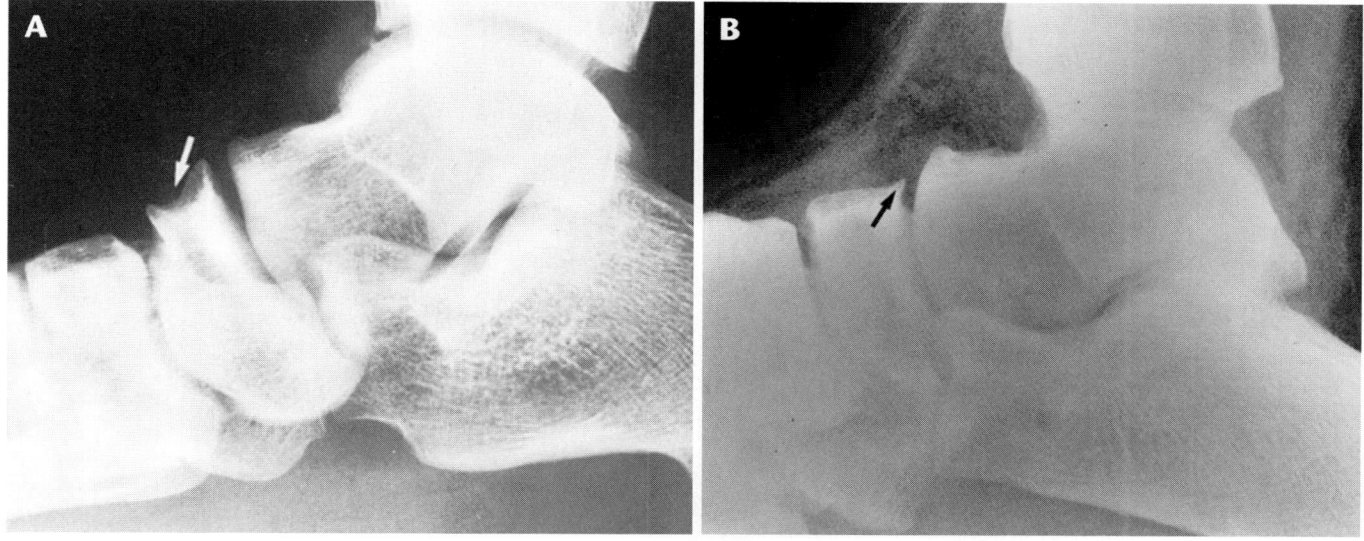

Figure 7–553. A, B, Unusual configuration of the superior aspect of the navicular in young subjects.

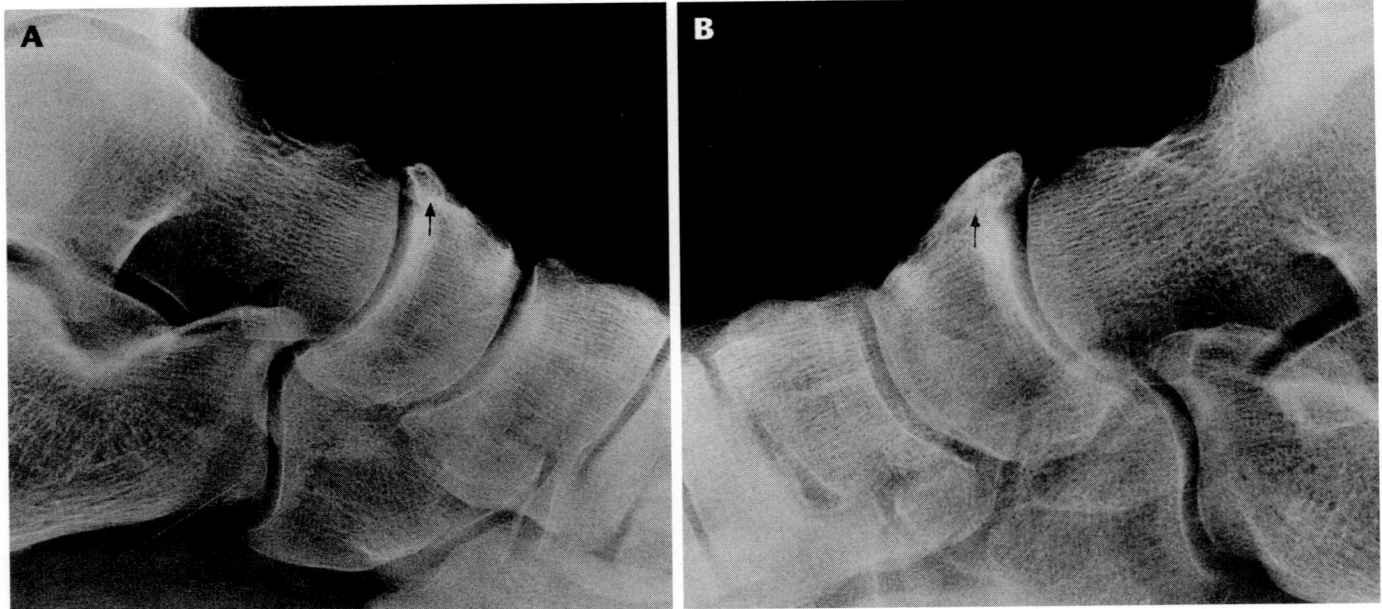

Figure 7–554. A, B, Bilateral incorporated os supranaviculare.

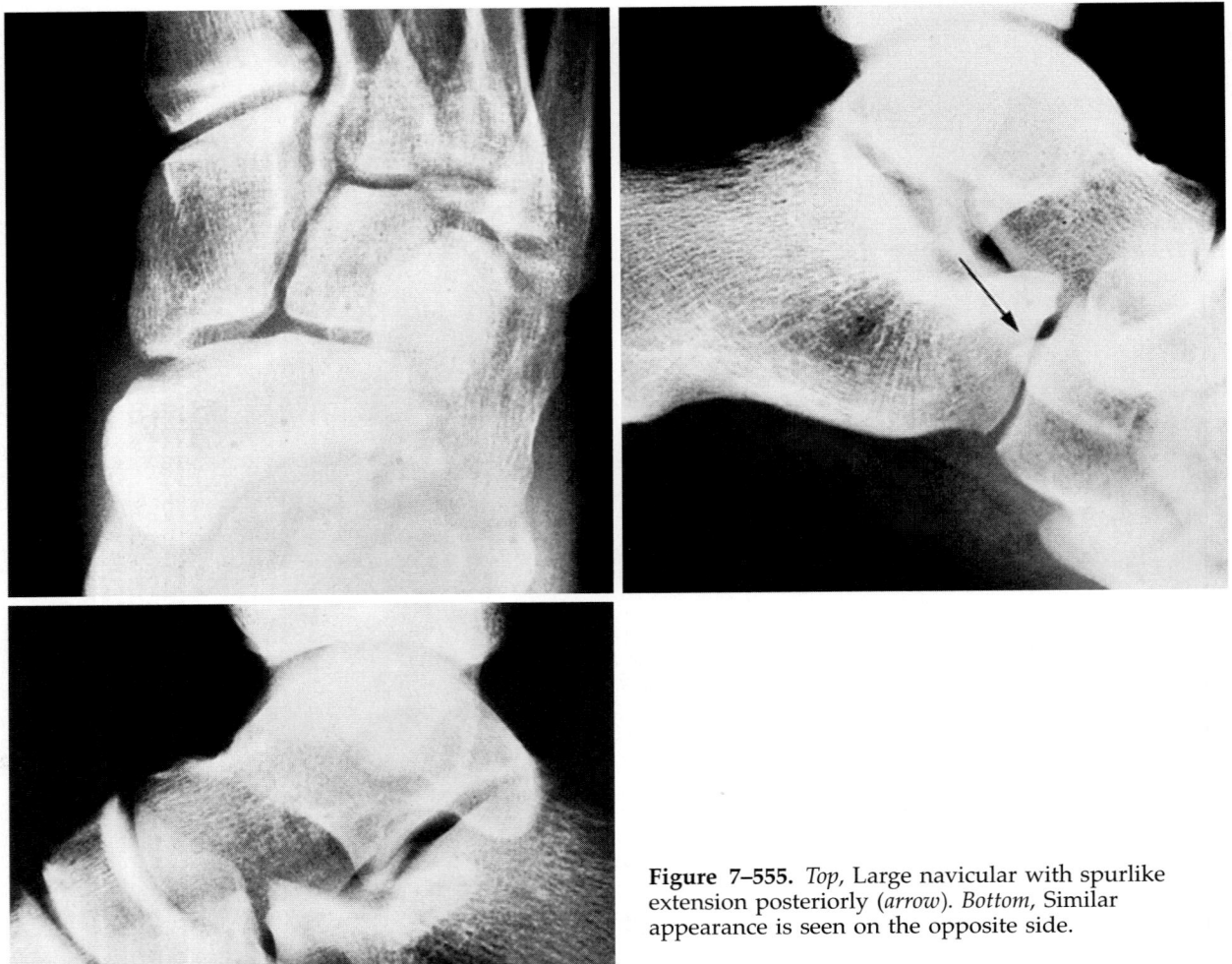

Figure 7–555. *Top,* Large navicular with spurlike extension posteriorly (*arrow*). *Bottom,* Similar appearance is seen on the opposite side.

The Tarsals

THE CUNEIFORMS

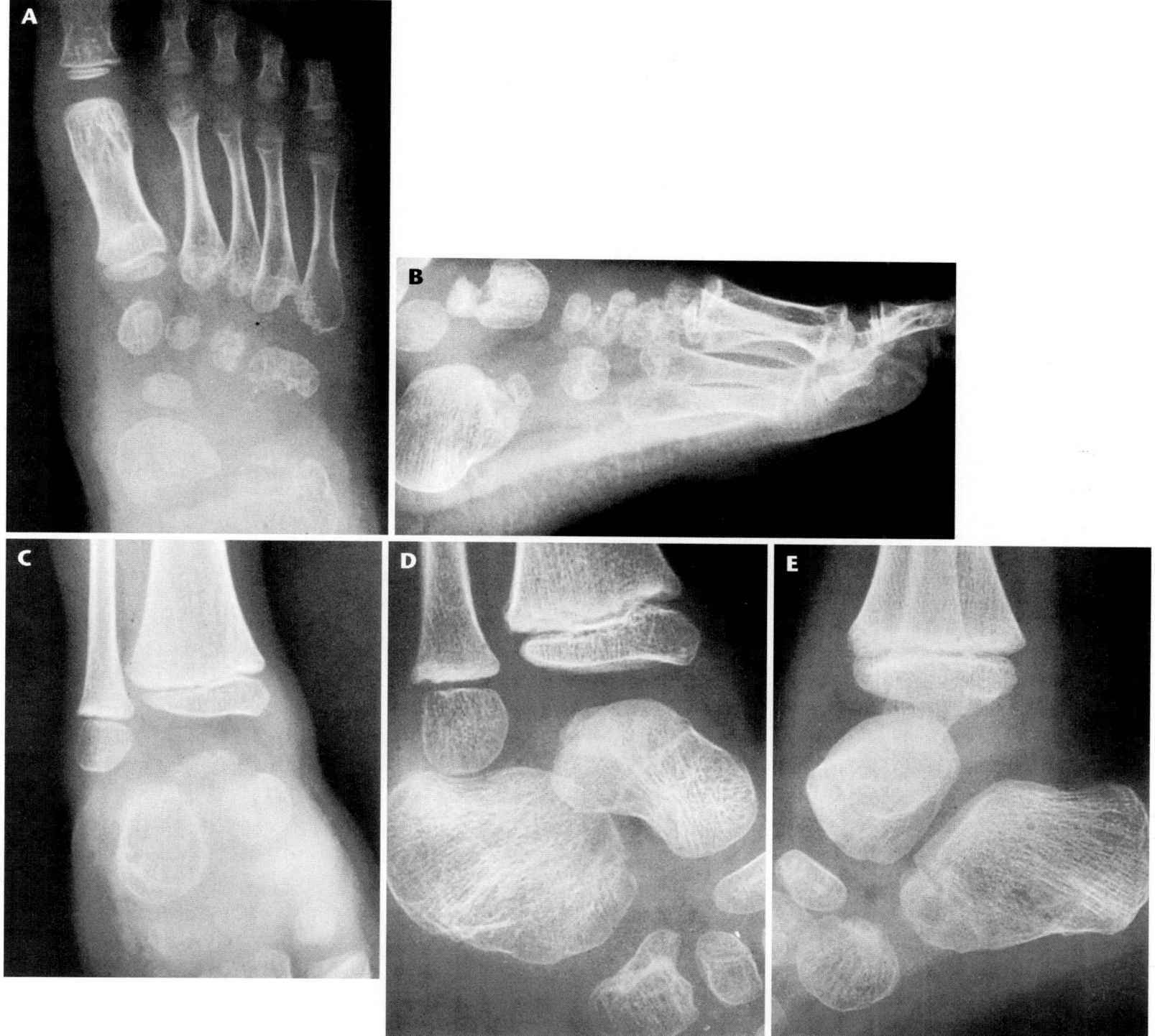

Figure 7–556. Normal irregular ossification of the tarsal bones of the right foot in a 4-year-old child (**A–C**). Note bipartite ossification of calcaneus and talus as well as the irregularity of the cuneiforms. **D,** Right foot at age 6. Note residual irregularities in the posterior aspect of the talus. **E,** Left foot at age 6. Note some persistence of the bifid calcaneus.

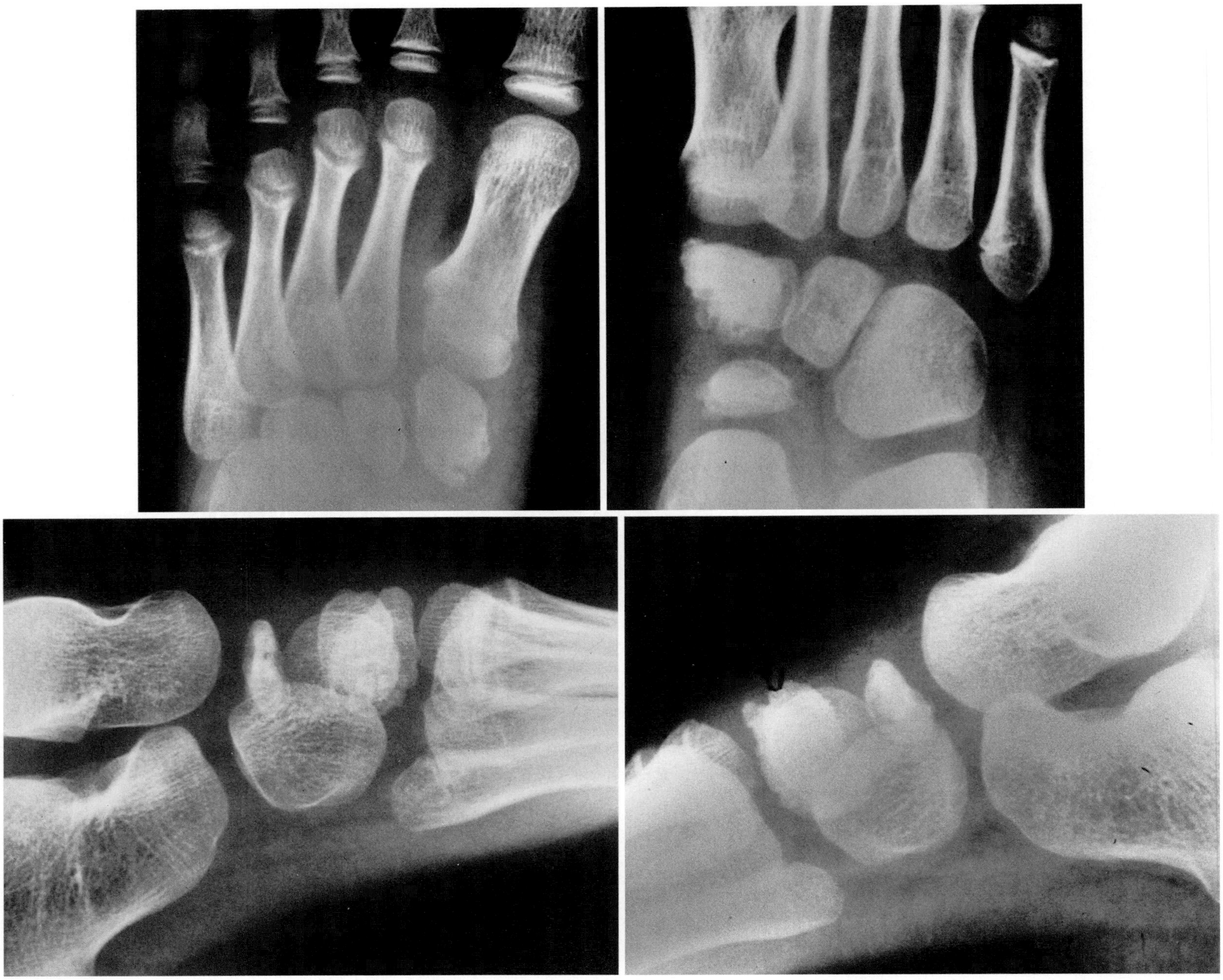

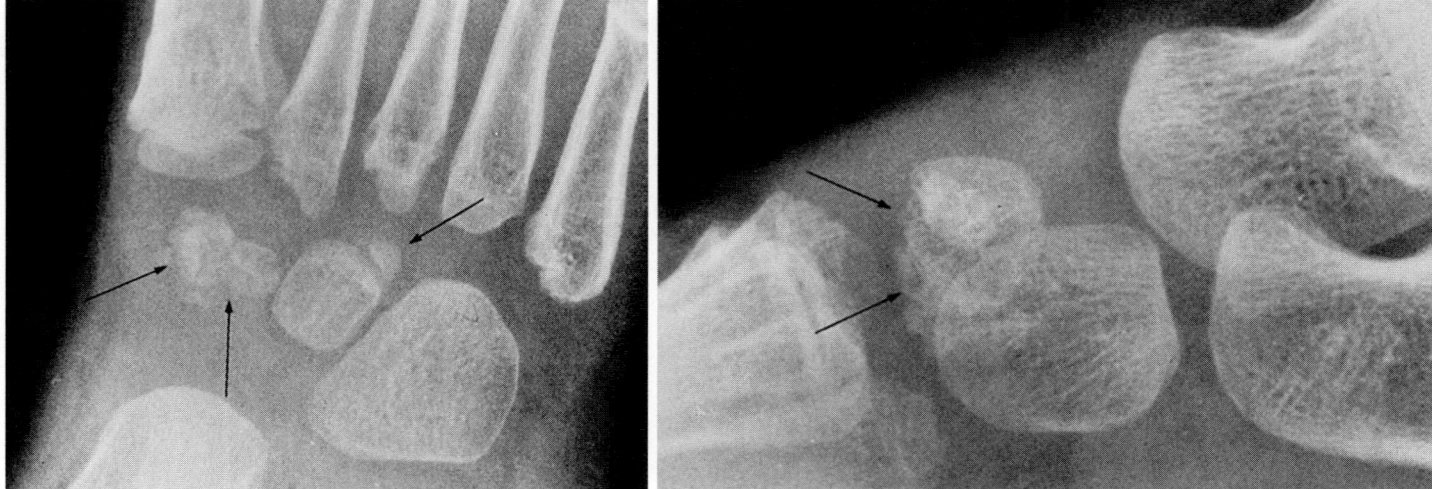

Figure 7–557. Bilateral developmental tarsal irregularity in a 6-year-old boy. These irregularities disappear with growth.

Figure 7–558. Irregular ossification of the cuneiforms in a 4-year-old boy.

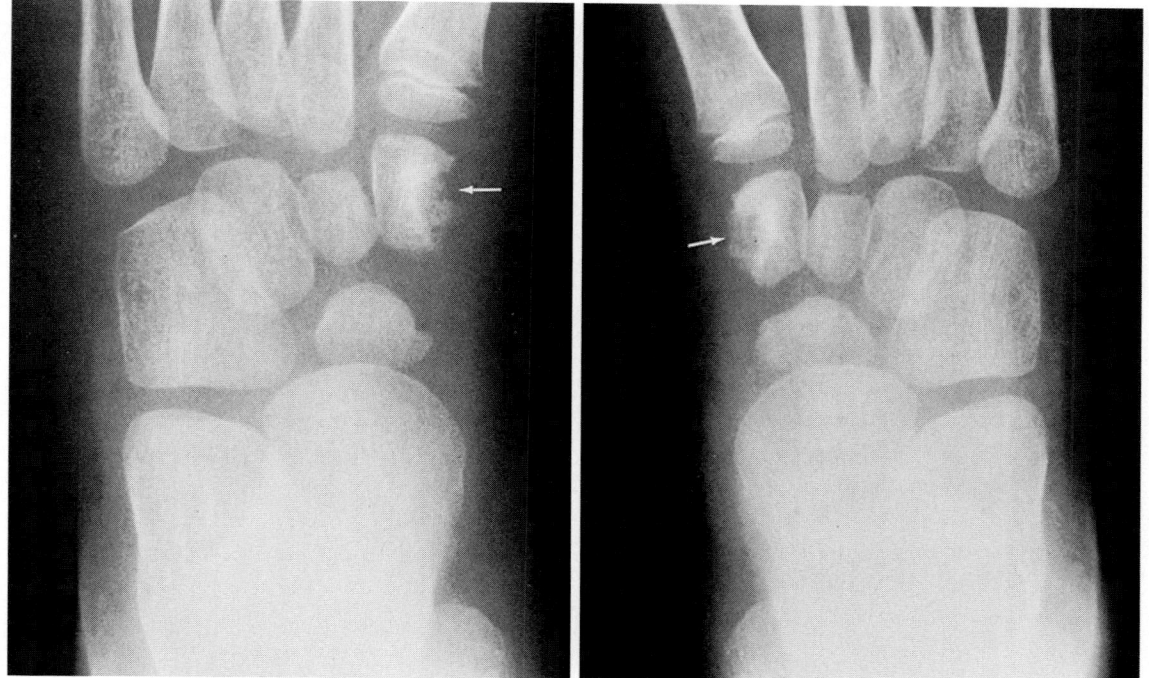

Figure 7–559. Irregular ossification of the first cuneiforms in a 6-year-old boy.

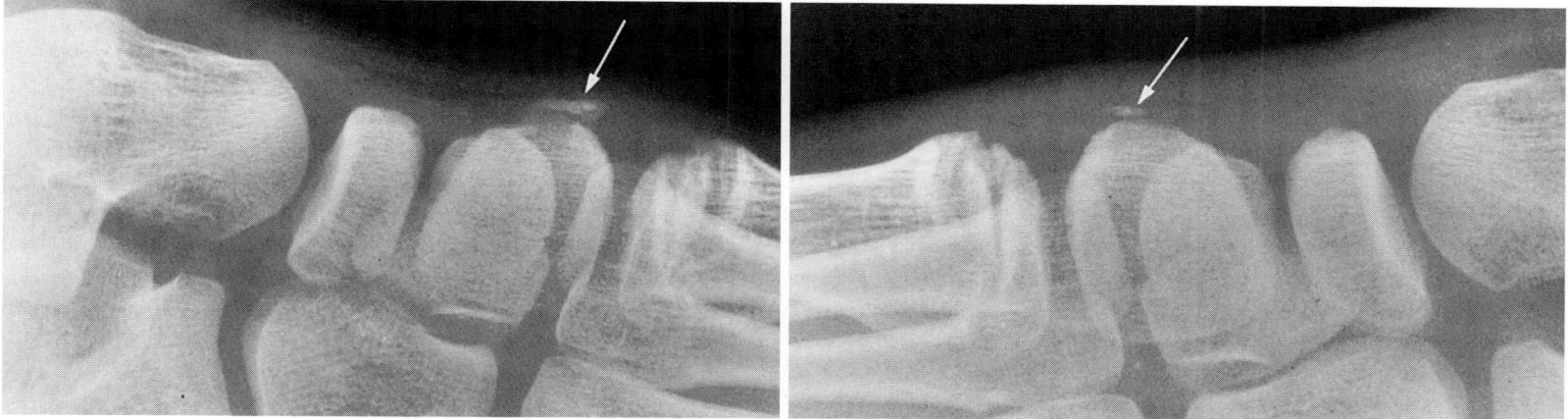

Figure 7–560. Bilateral accessory ossification centers at the tip of the first cuneiform in a 9-year-old boy.

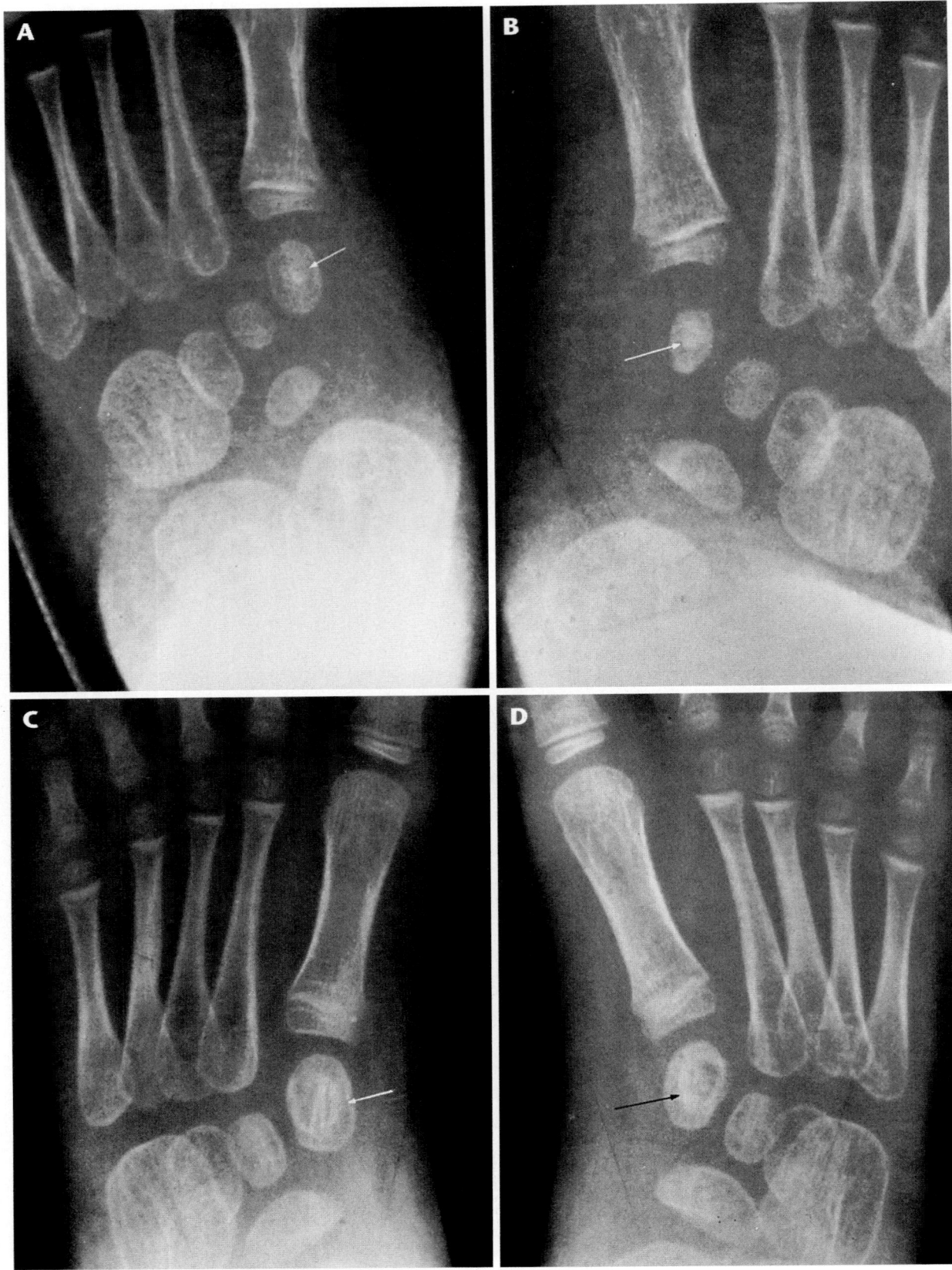

Figure 7–561. A and **B,** Central densities within the first cuneiform of a 3-year-old boy. **C** and **D,** one year later.

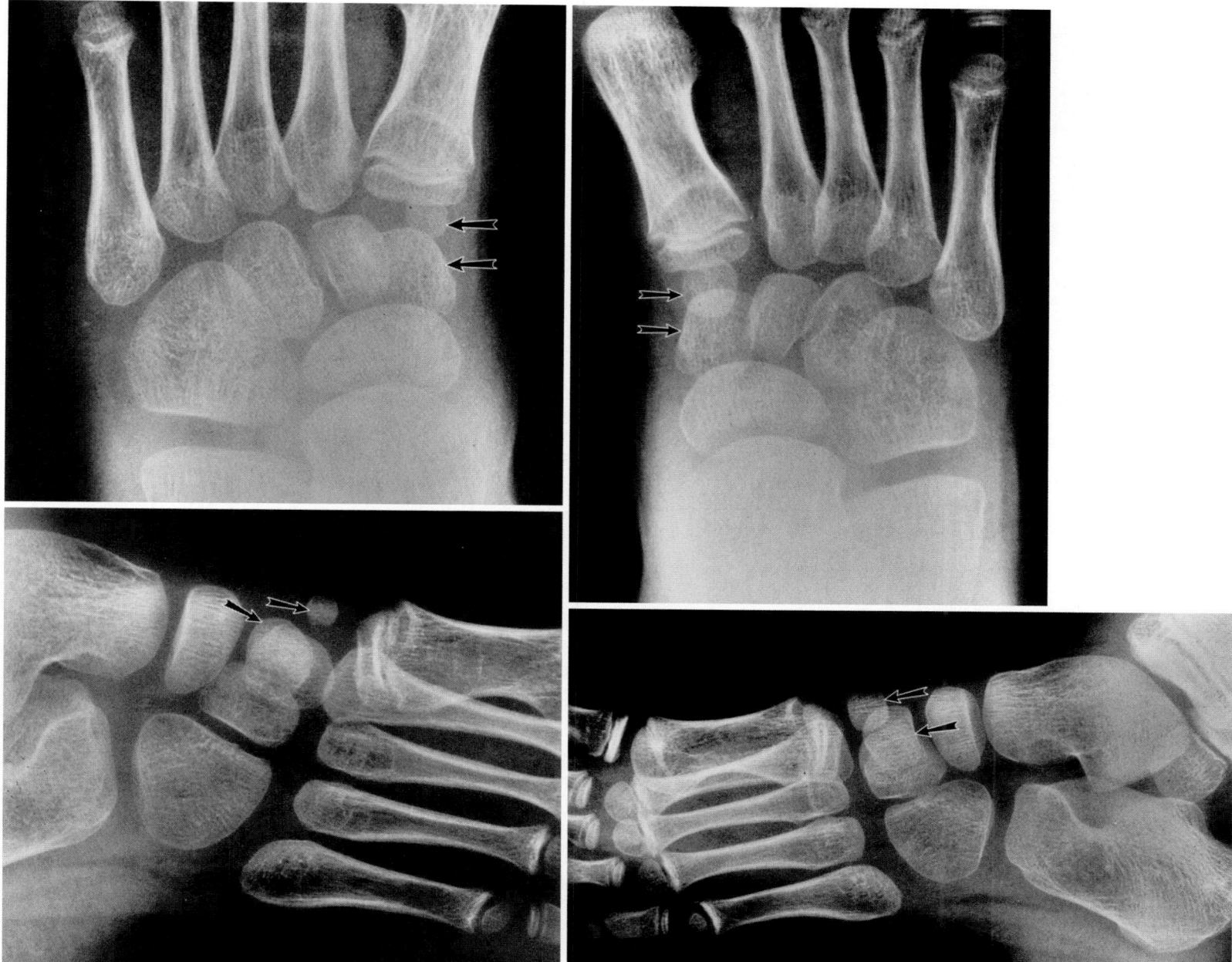

Figure 7–562. Bilateral bipartate first cuneiforms in a 6-year-old boy. (Ref: Kohler A, Zimmer EA: *Borderlands of the normal and early pathologic findings in skeletal roentgenology,* 4th ed. New York, Thieme, 1993, p. 832.)

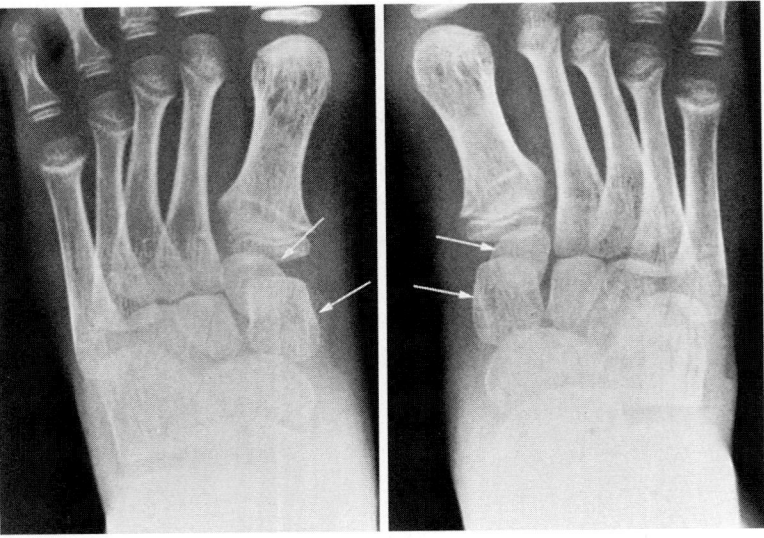

Figure 7–563. Bilateral bipartite first cuneiforms in a 6-year-old.

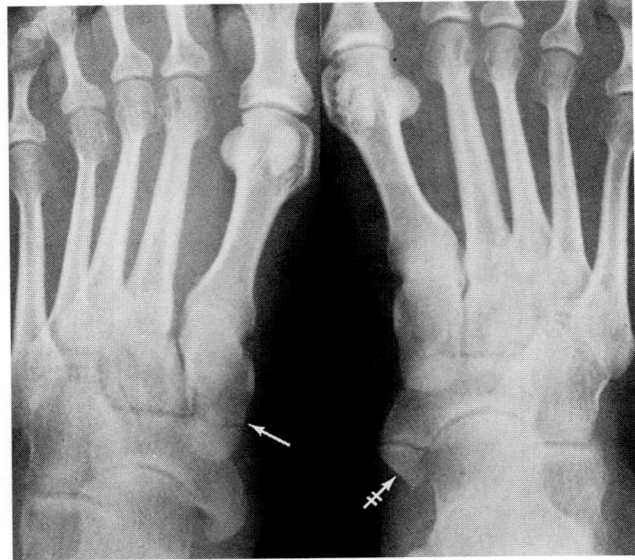

Figure 7–564. Bipartite first cuneiform on the patient's left foot (←). The right foot shows an os tibiale externum (⊬). The bipartite first cuneiform is more commonly divided into dorsal and plantar segments. (Ref: Kohler A, Zimmer EA: *Borderlands of the normal and early pathologic findings in skeletal roentgenology,* 4th ed. New York, Theime, 1993, p. 832.)

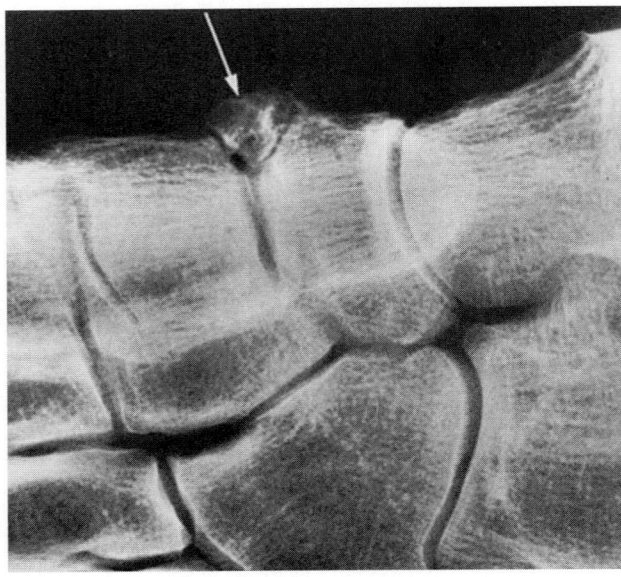

Figure 7–565. The os intercuneiform.

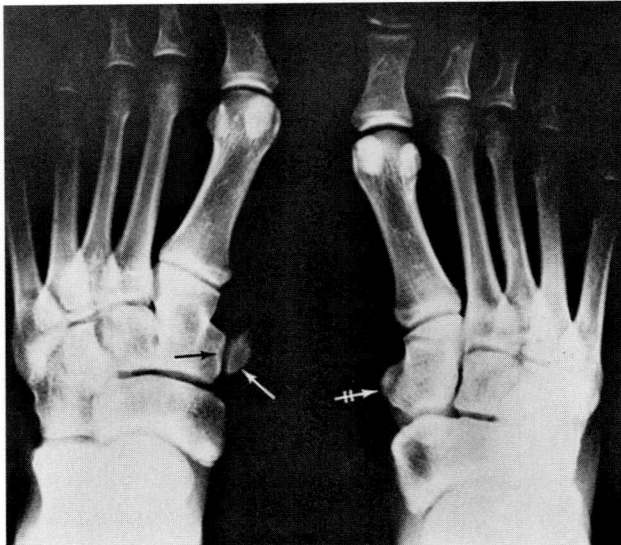

Figure 7–566. Supernumerary bone arising from the left first cuneiform (←). On the right foot, it is represented by an osseous protuberance (⊬). (Ref: Rao B: Supernumerary toe arising from the medial cuneiform. *J Bone Joint Surg* 61A:308, 1979.)

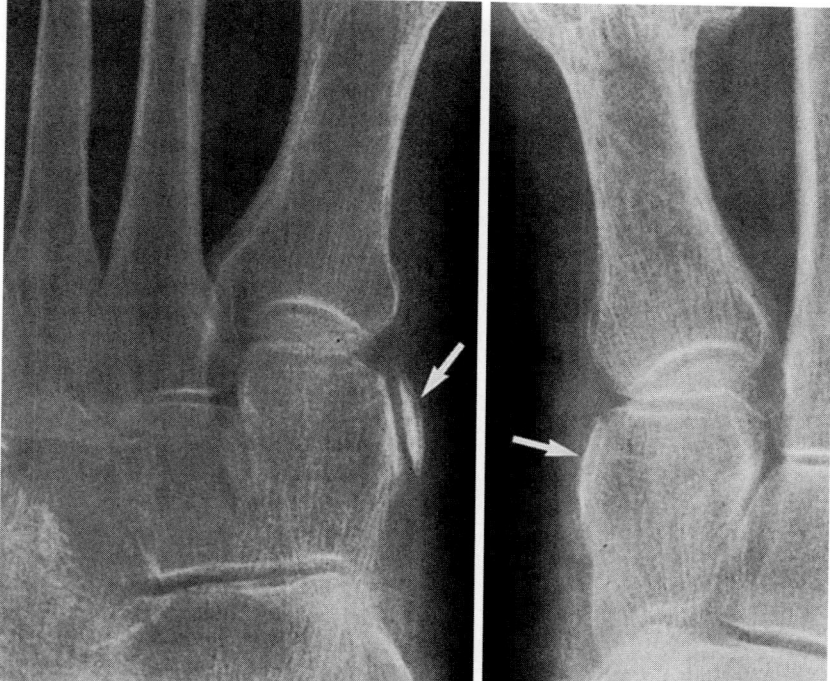

Figure 7–567. Supernumerary bones arising from the first cuneiform.

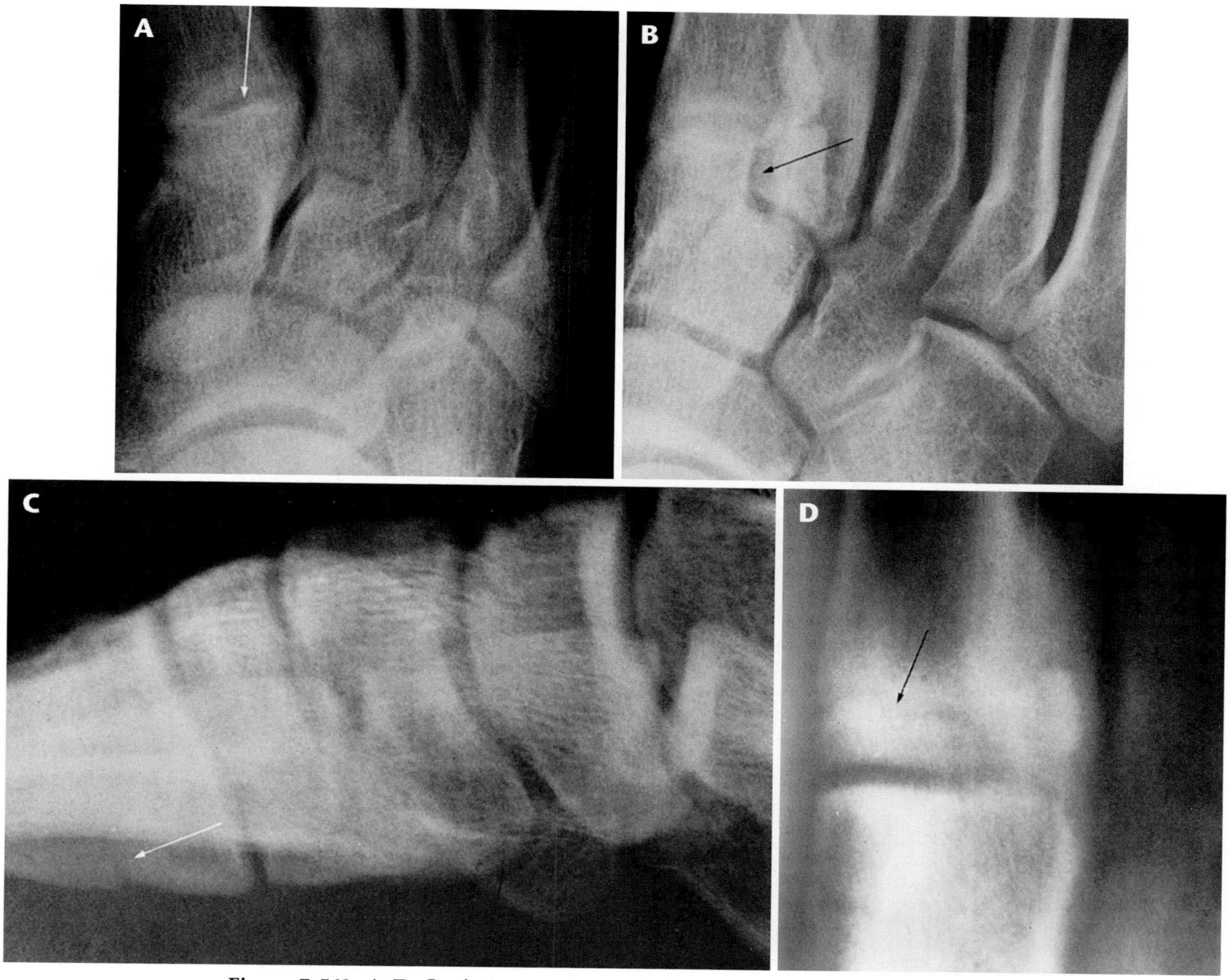

Figure 7–568. A–D, Confusing appearance at base of first metatarsal, simulating a fracture in a 15-year-old boy, produced by overlapping shadows of the first cuneiform and the epiphysis of the base of the first metatarsal. The epiphyseal line at the base of the metatarsal is seen in **C** and demonstrated by tomography in **D**.

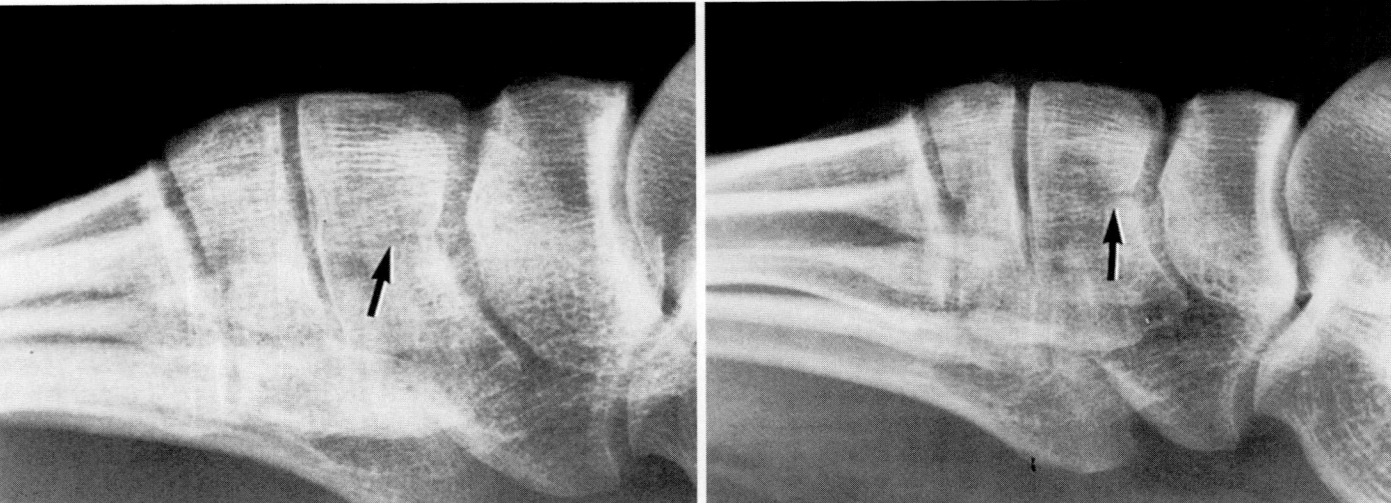

Figure 7–569. Simulated fractures produced by overlapping shadows of the cuneiforms.

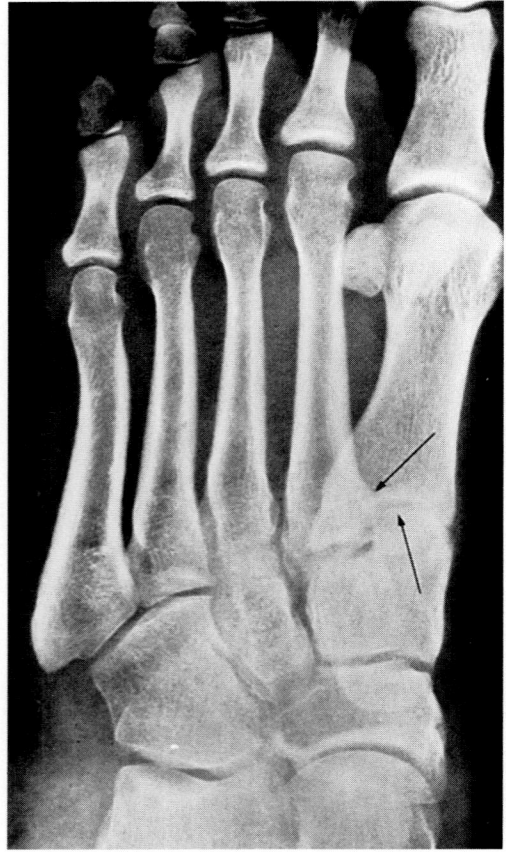

Figure 7–570. The overlapping relationships illustrated in Figure 7–569 are better defined in the adult.

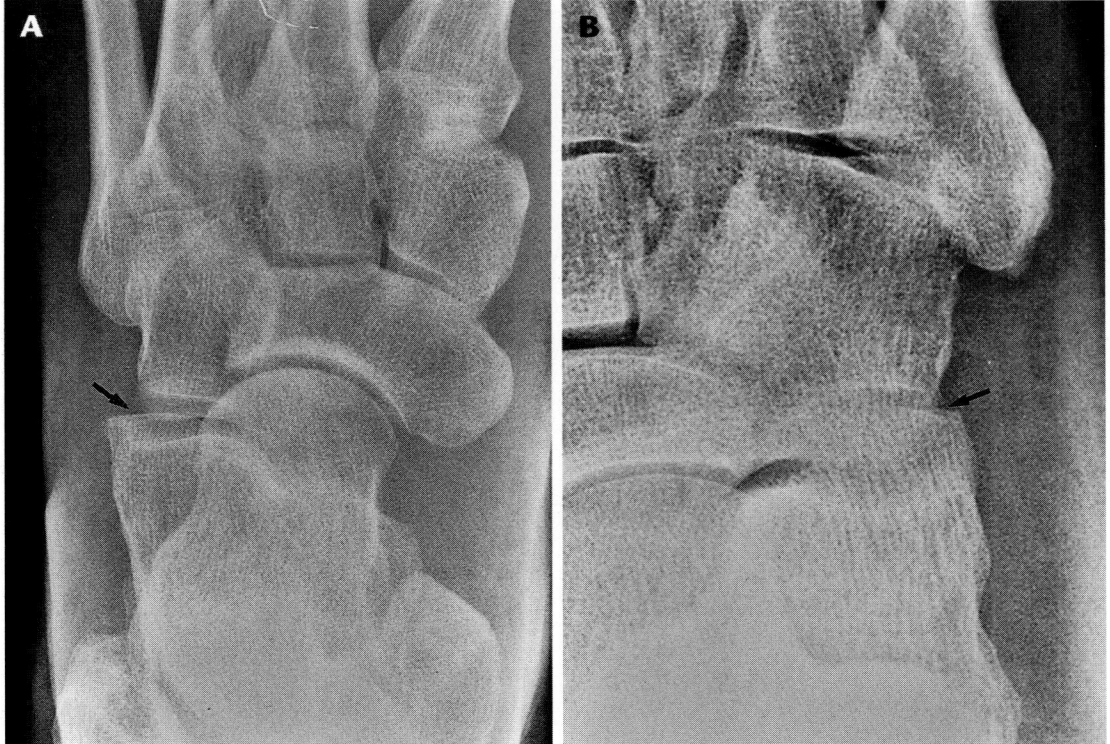

Figure 7–571. A, B, Two examples of simulated subluxation of the cuneiforms from the cuboid resulting from foot positioning. Cases proved normal by CT.

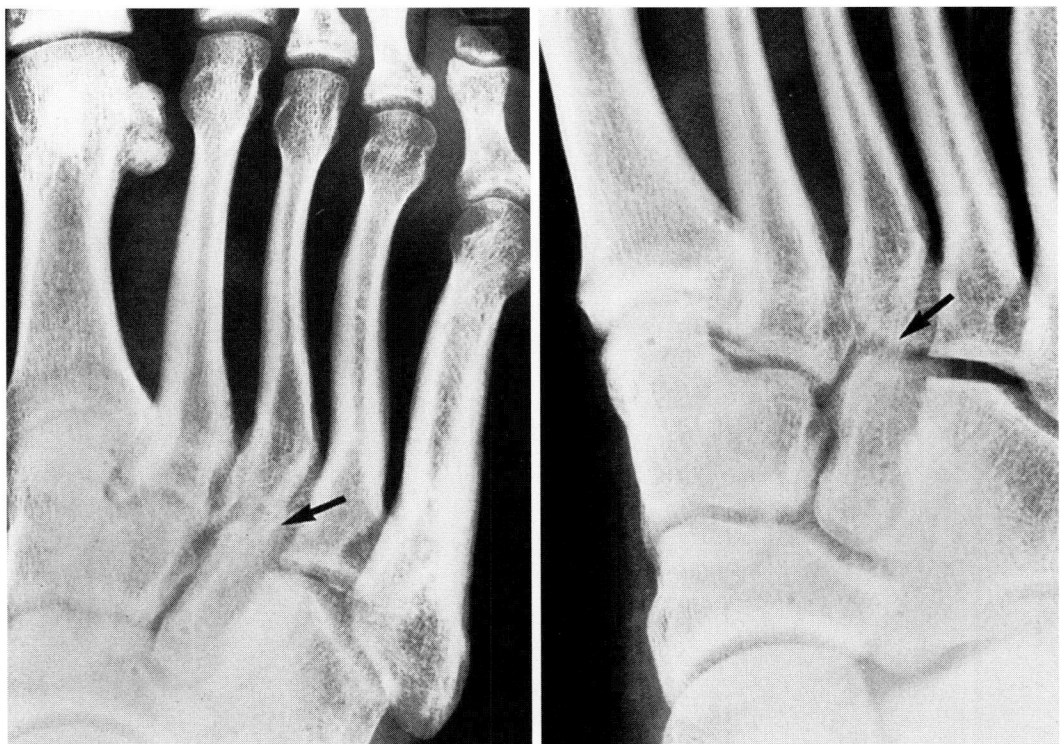

Figure 7–572. *Left,* Simulated fusion between the base of the third metatarsal and the lateral cuneiform. *Right,* Situation clarified by filming in greater obliquity.

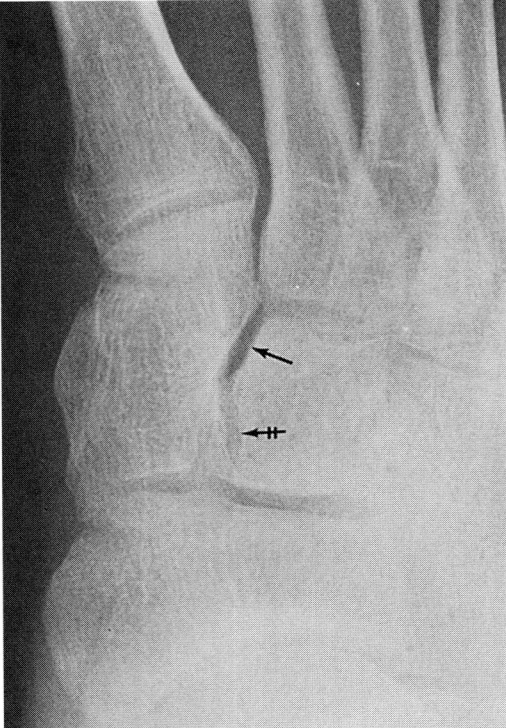

Figure 7–573. Normal spacing between the first and second cuneiforms (←), not to be confused with traumatic alteration. The groove on the medial surface is also normal (←⧺).

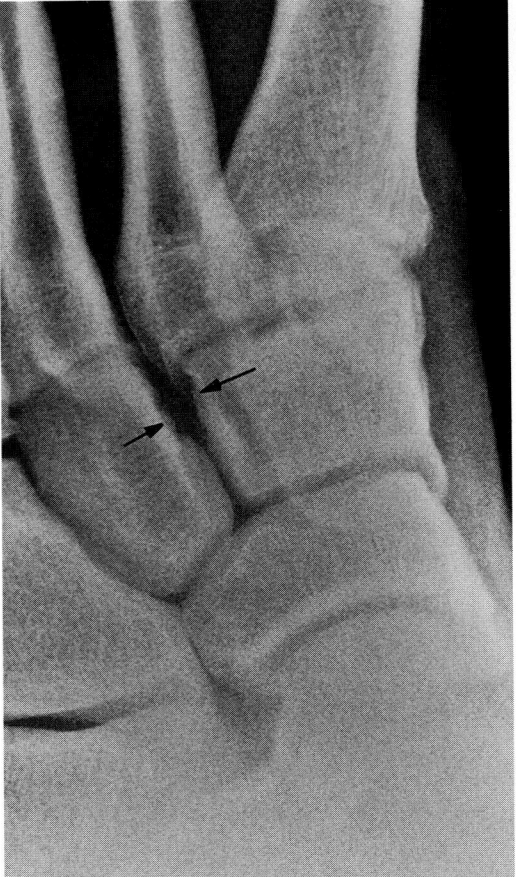

Figure 7–574. Normal fossa between the second and third cuneiforms.

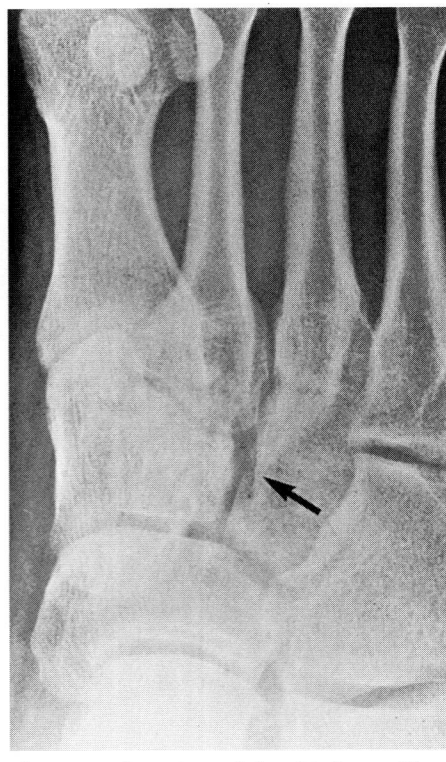

Figure 7–575. Contour alteration of the third cuneiform, mistaken for a fracture.

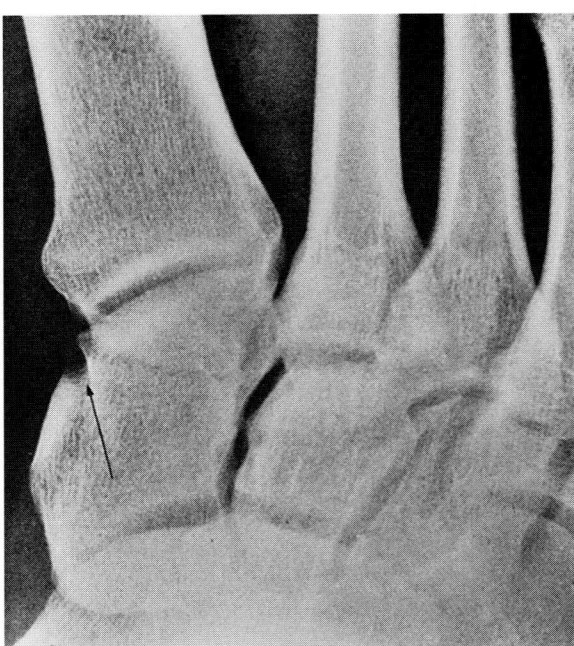

Figure 7–576. Groove for the tibialis anterior tendon, not an erosion.

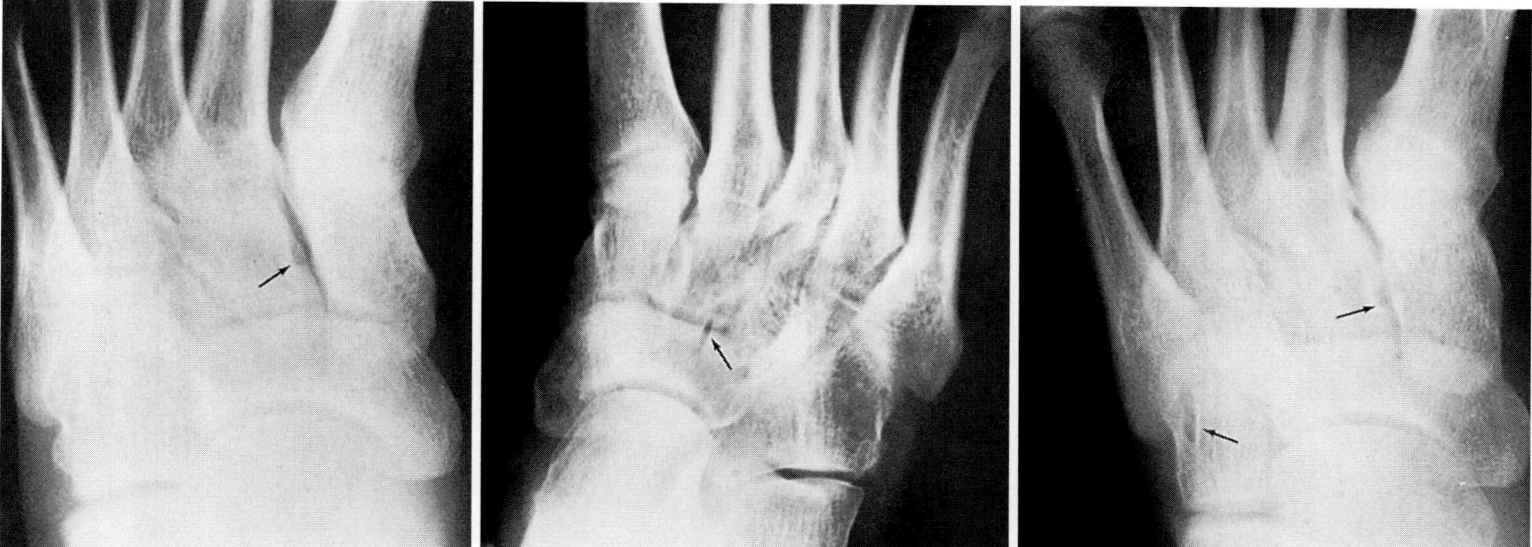

Figure 7–577. Normal radiolucencies seen in and between the cuneiforms.

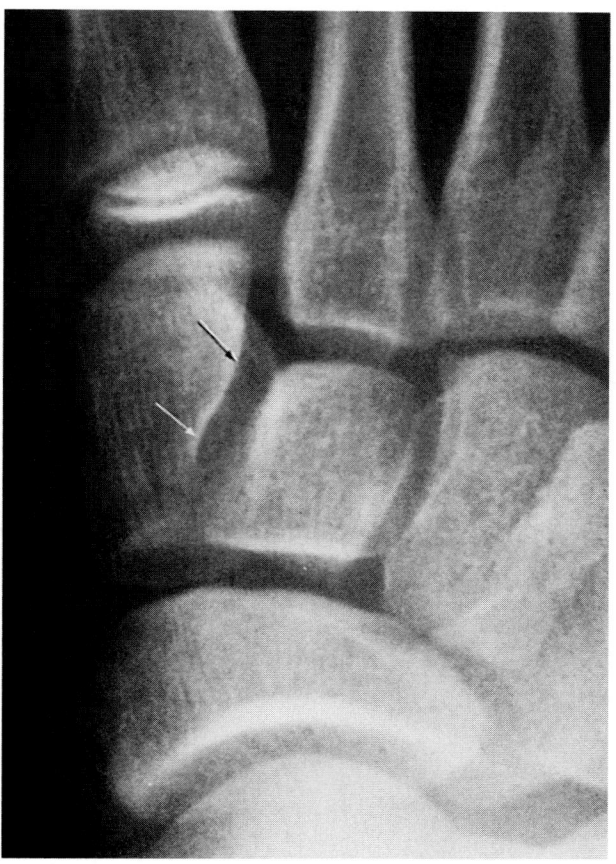

Figure 7–578. Prominent fossa on lateral aspect of first cuneiform.

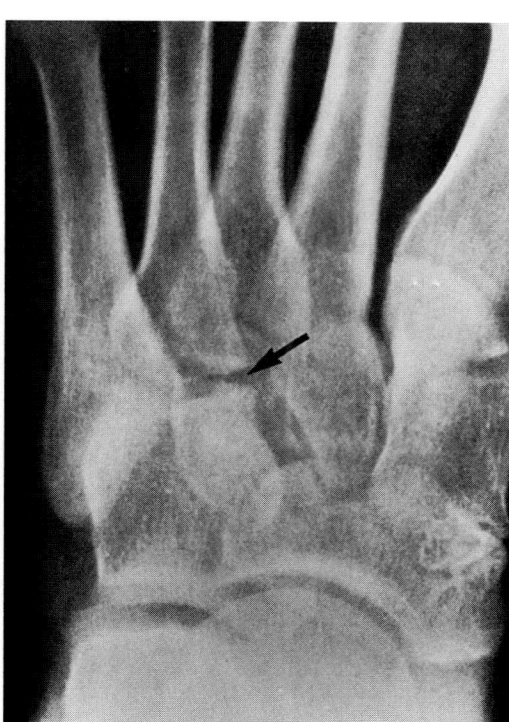

Figure 7–579. Simulated fracture produced by a well-demonstrated joint between the fourth metatarsal and the third cuneiform.

The Tarsals

THE CUBOID

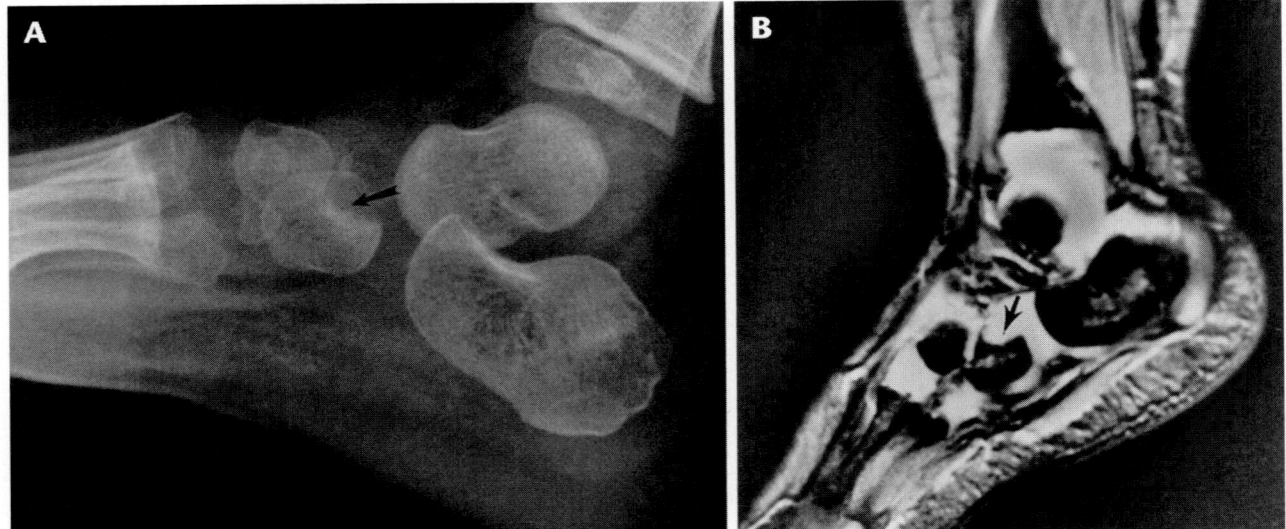

Figure 7–580. Normal irregularity of the posterior aspect of: **A,** The cuboid in a 2-year-old child with a fracture of the calcaneus. **B,** Gradient echo T2*-weighted MR image shows the fossa to be cartilaginous.

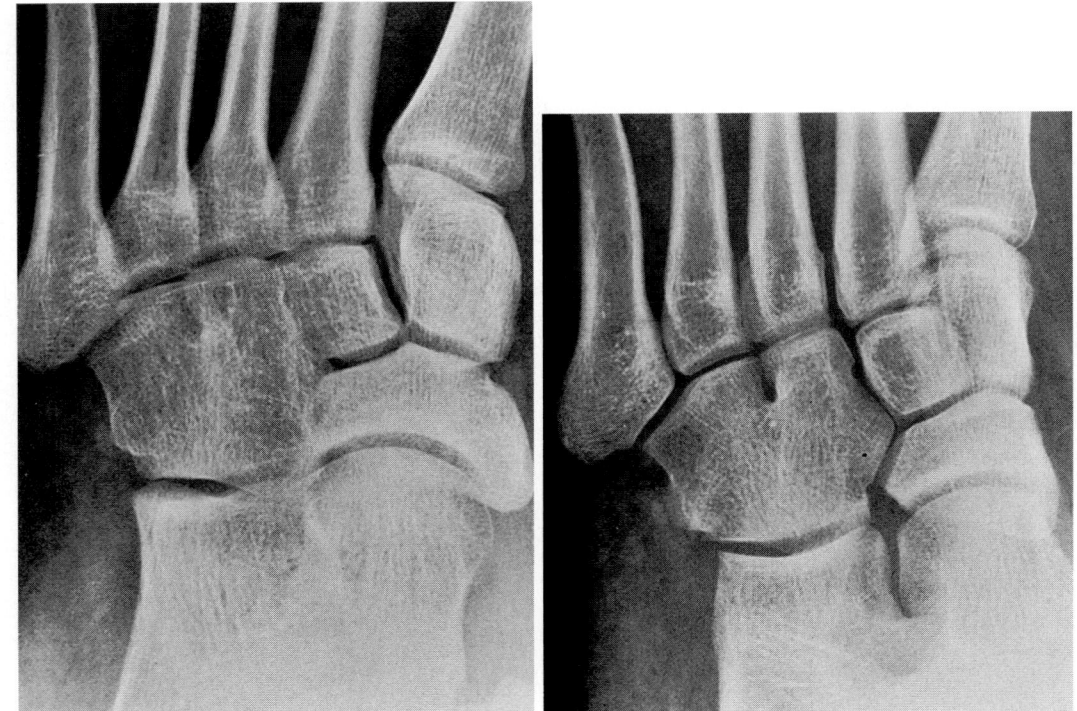

Figure 7–581. Congenital fusion of the cuboid and the third cuneiform. Several cases of naviculocuneiform coalition have been reported. (Ref: Miki J et al: Naviculocuneiform coalition. *Clin Orthop* 196:256, 1985.)

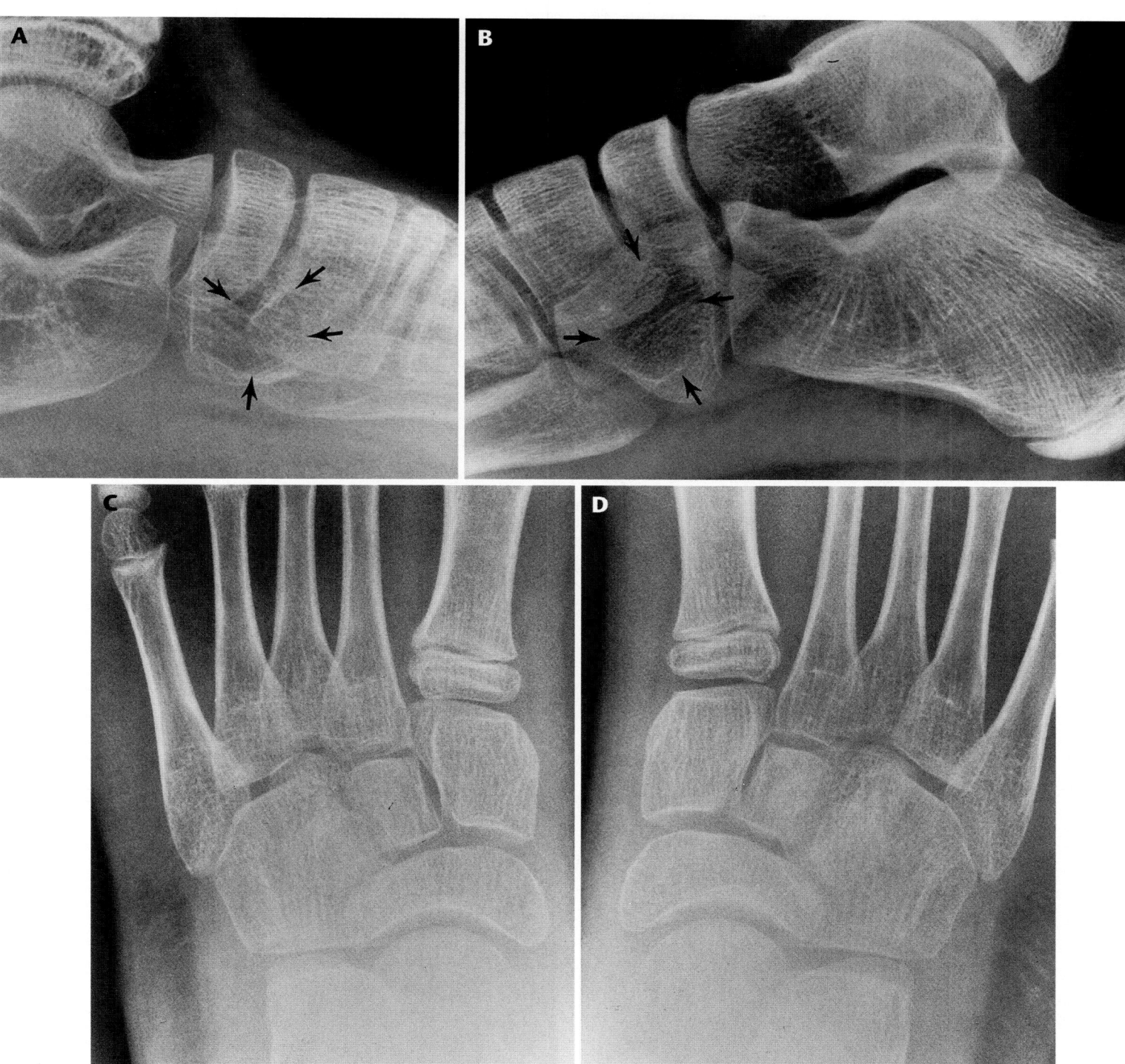

Figure 7–582. Simulated cysts in the cuboids of a 12-year-old boy in lateral projection (**A** and **B**). Anteroposterior projections (**C** and **D**) show no abnormality.

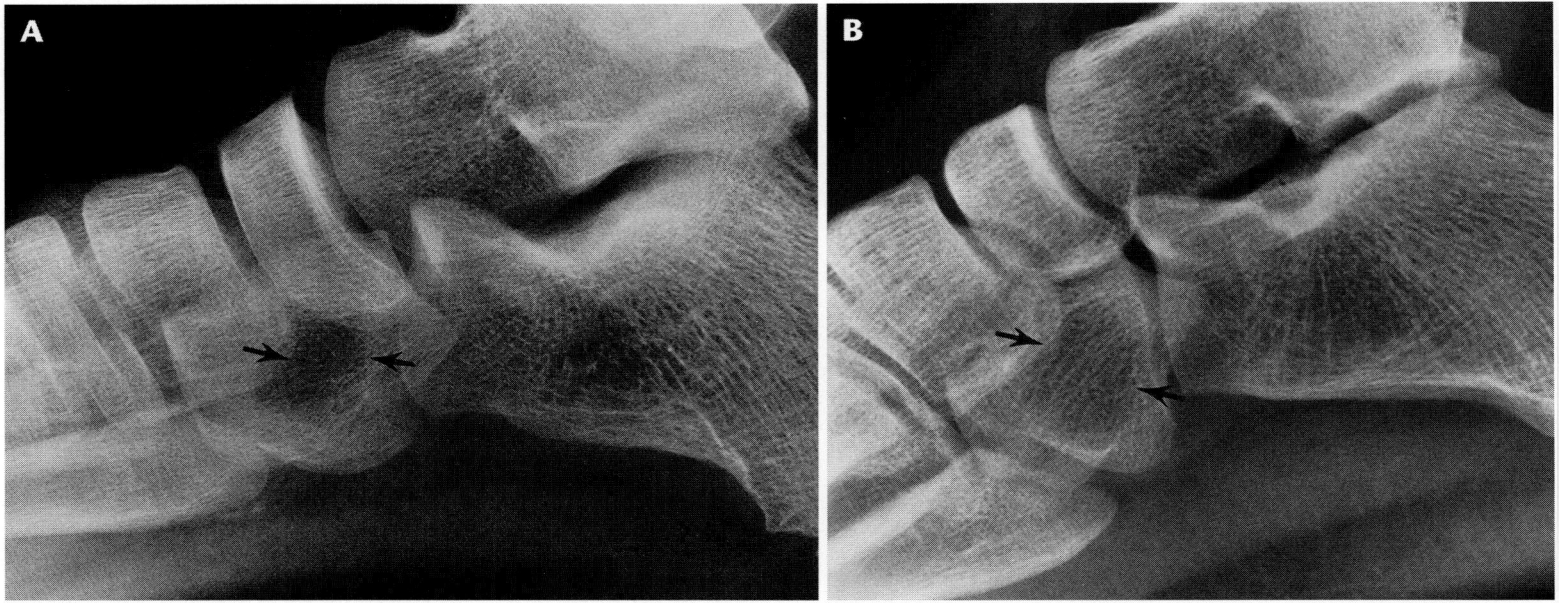

Figure 7–583. The same entity as the preceding figure in a 10-year-old (**A**) and an 11-year-old (**B**).

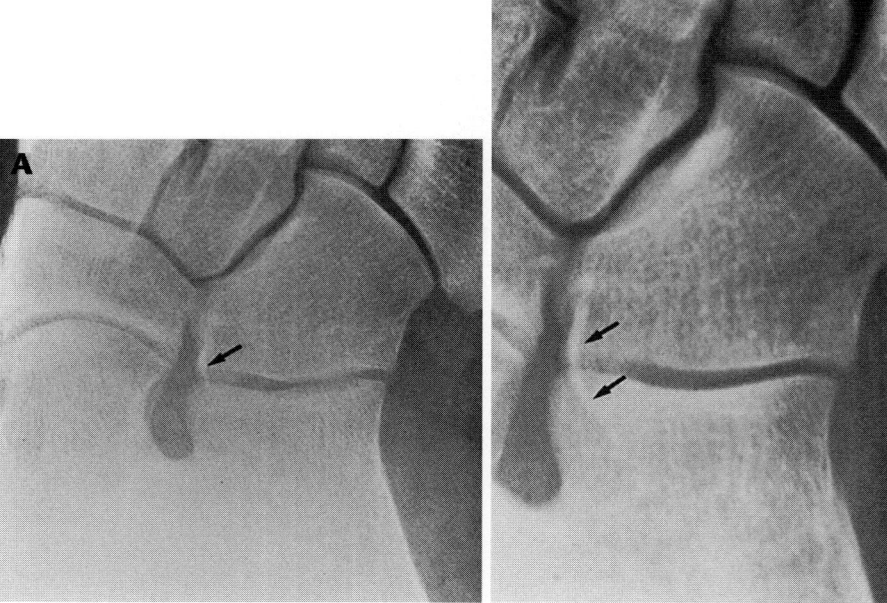

Figure 7–584. A, Simulated fracture of the cuboid. **B,** Magnification view shows that the simulated fracture is due to the dense cortex of the upper margin of the bone.

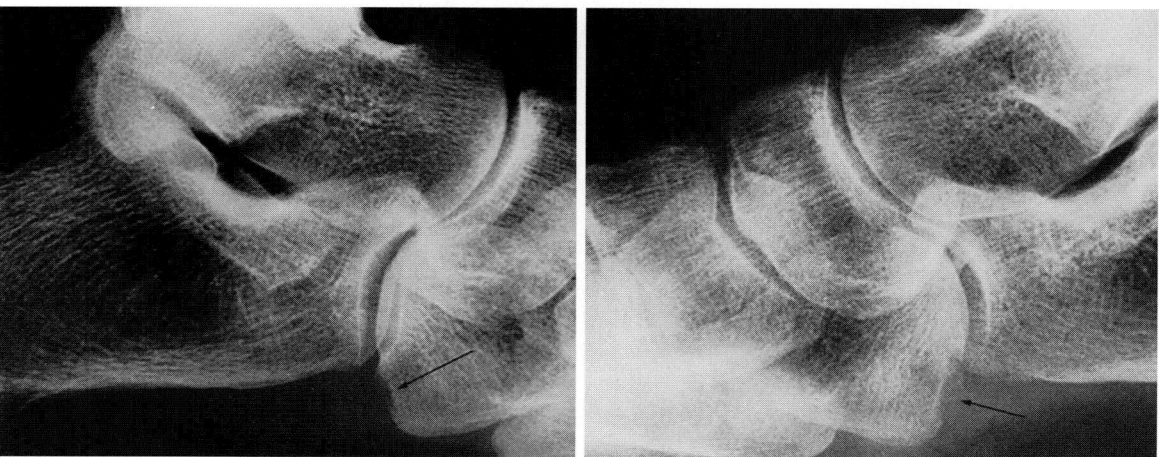

Figure 7–585. Fossae in the posterior aspect of the cuboid, which should not be mistaken for erosions.

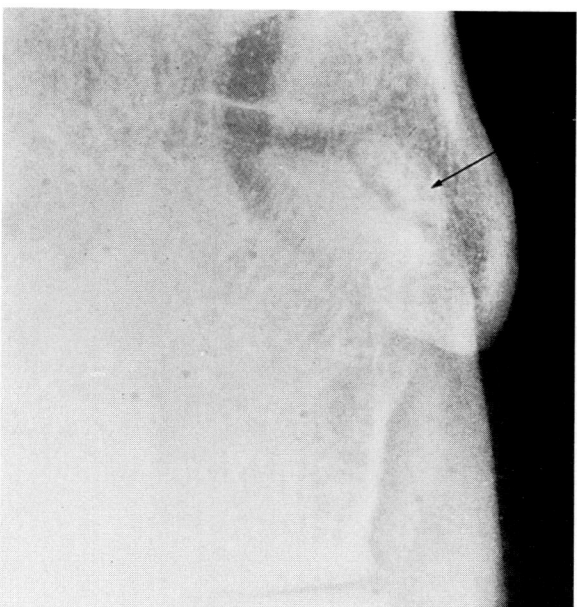

Figure 7–586. Accessory bone of the lateral aspect of the distal end of the cuboid.

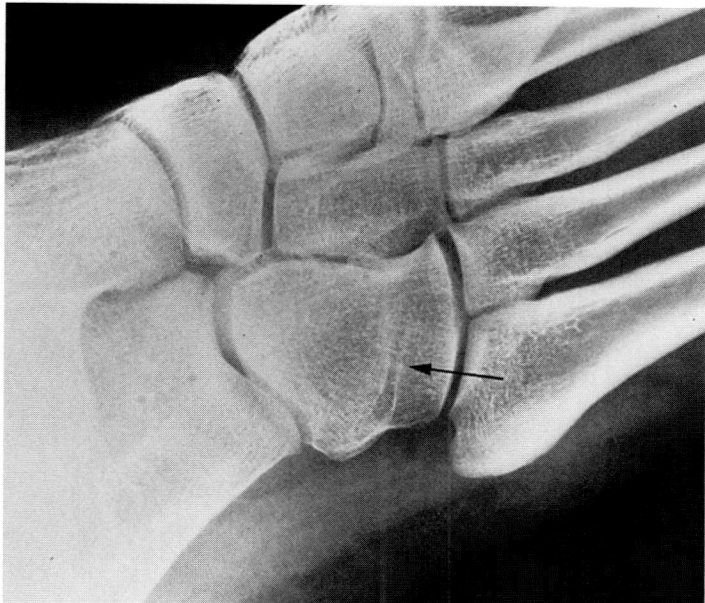

Figure 7–587. Groove for the peroneus longus tendon.

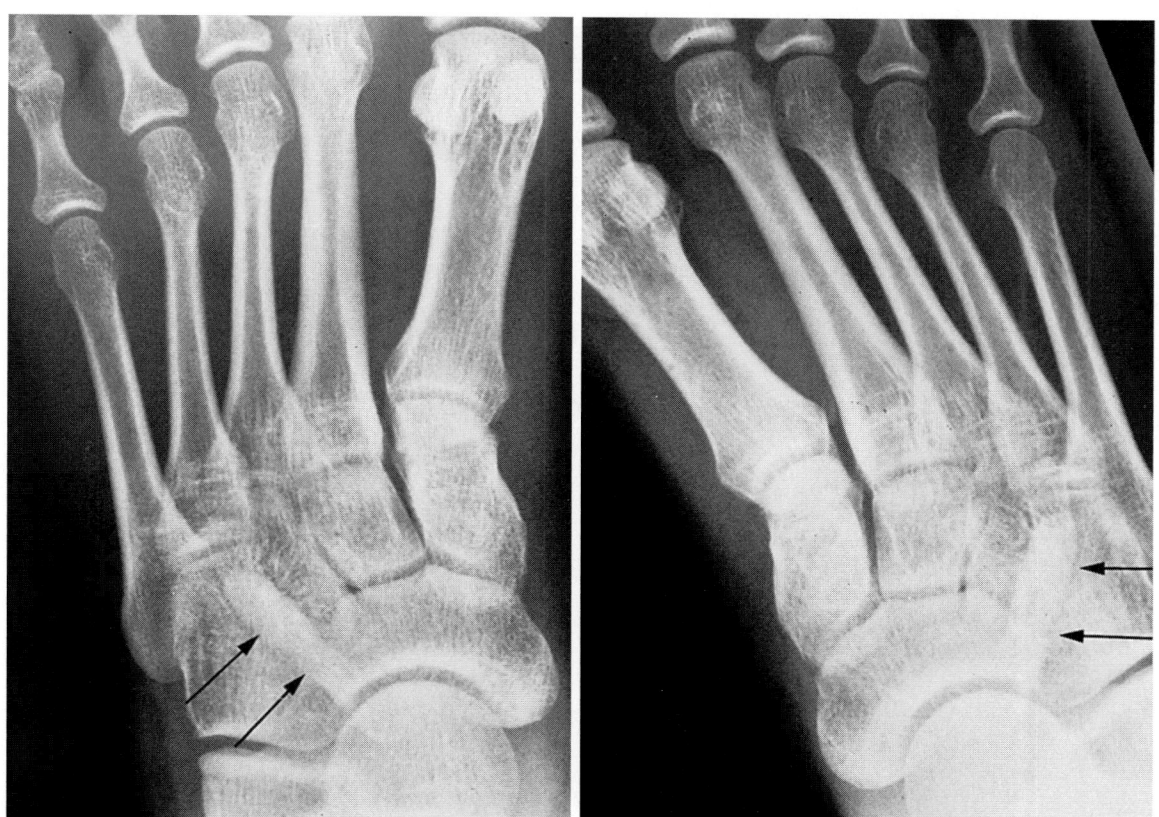

Figure 7–588. Overlapping shadows of cuboid and cuneiforms, producing an unusual shadow bilaterally.

The Metatarsals

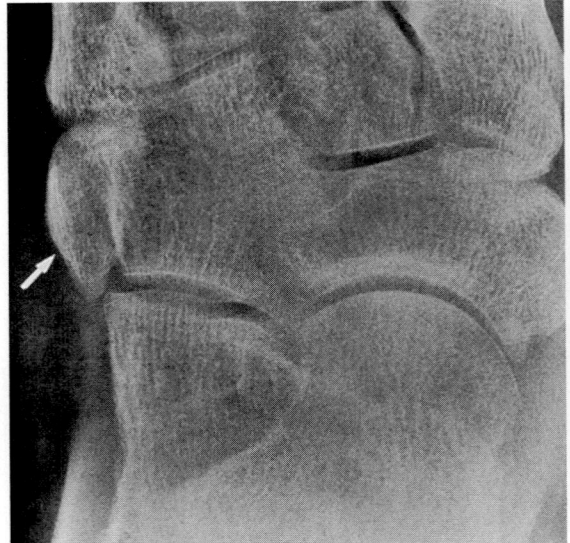
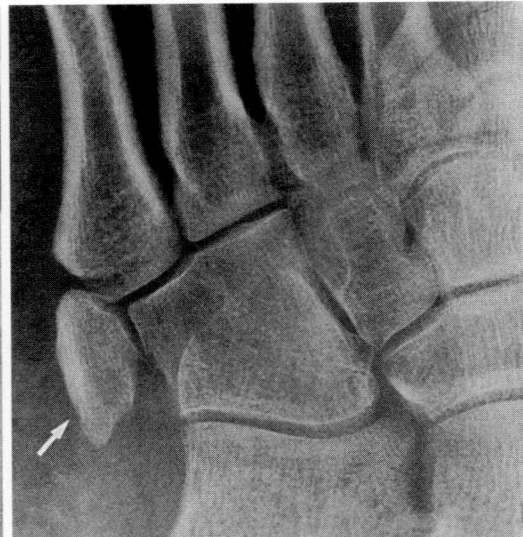
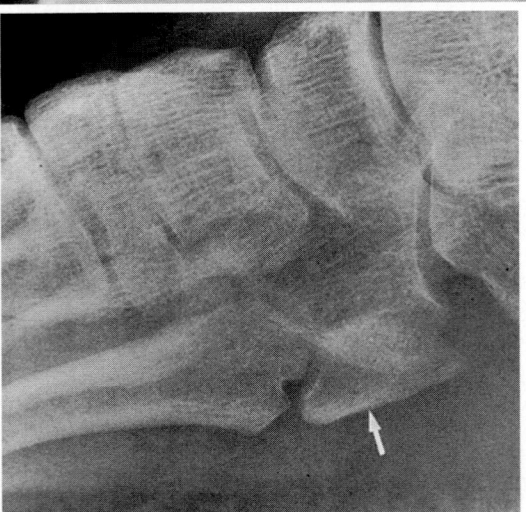

Figure 7–589. Os vesalianum, which lies in the peroneus brevis tendon. (Ref: Smith CD et al: The os vesalianum: An unusual cause of lateral foot pain. *Orthopedics* 7:86, 1984.)

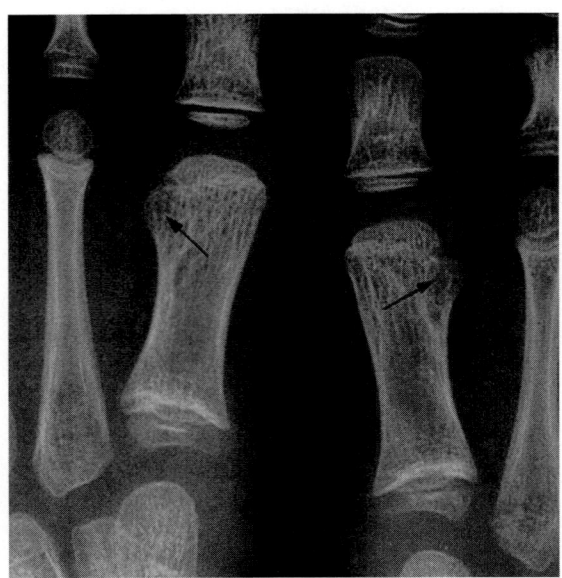

Figure 7–590. Knoblike expansions of the lateral aspects of the first metatarsals in a 3-year-old child. See Figure 6–317 for a similar appearance in the first metacarpal.

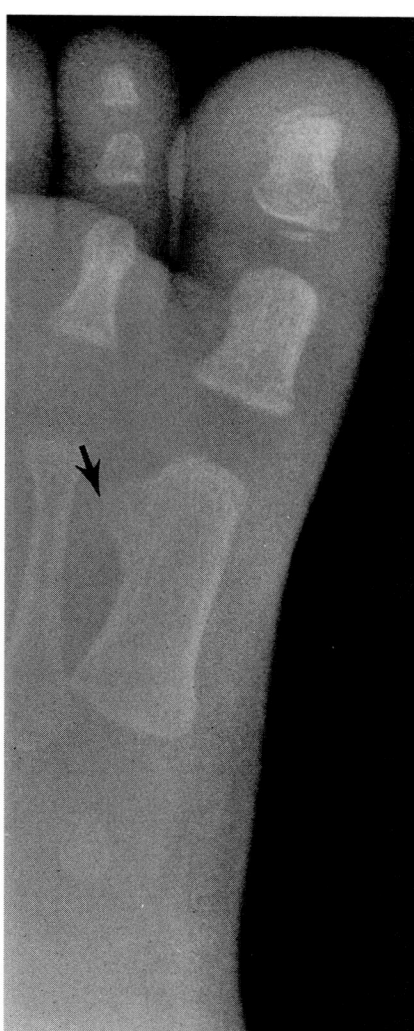

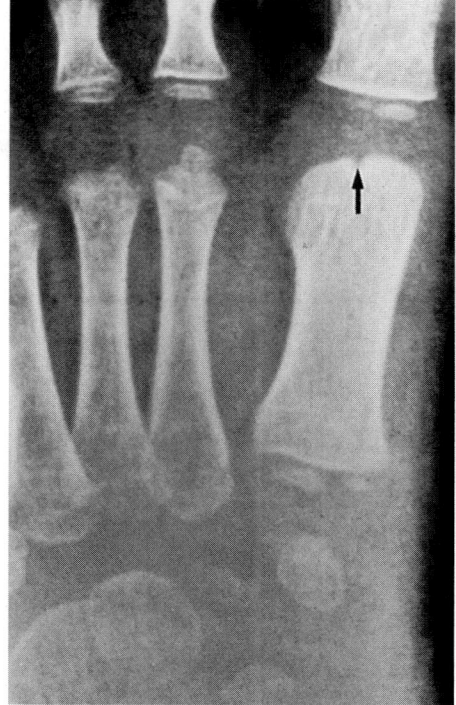

Figure 7–592. Developmental notch in the distal end of the first metatarsal in a young child.

Figure 7–591. The same entity as described in Figure 7–590 in an 18-month-old child.

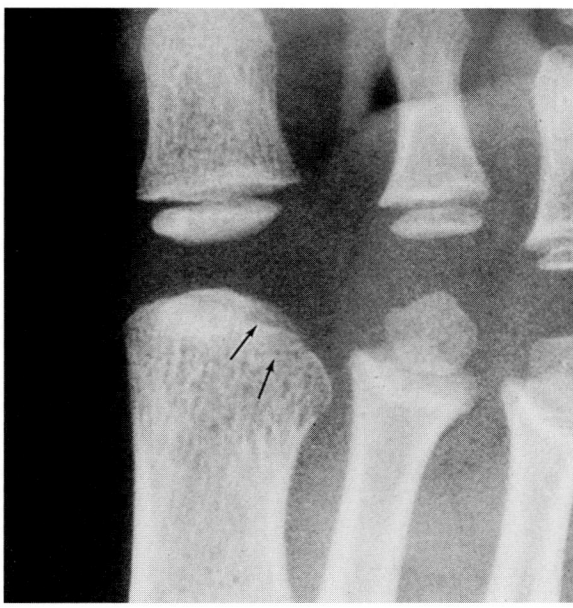

Figure 7–593. Oblique fissures in the metaphysis of the distal end of the first metatarsal, not to be mistaken for fractures.

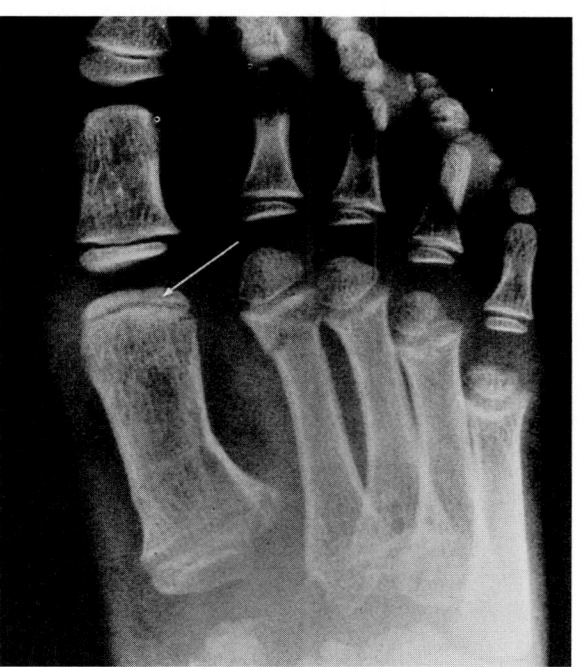

Figure 7–594. Accessory ossification center at the distal end of the first metatarsal.

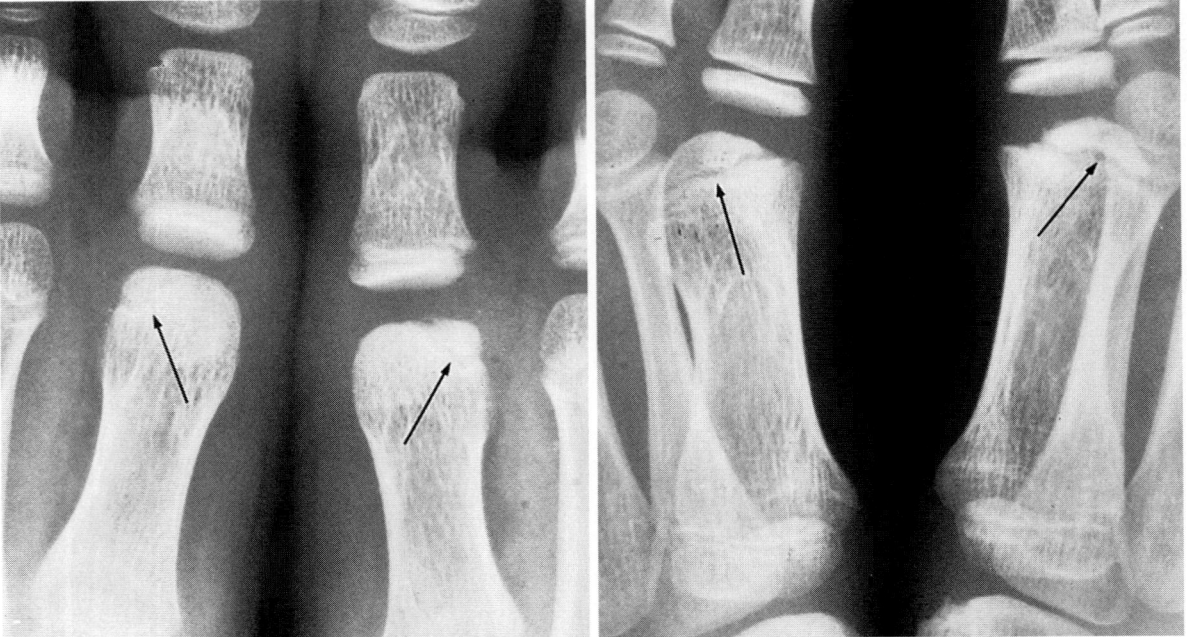

Figure 7–595. Accessory ossification centers in the distal ends of the first metatarsals in an 8-year-old boy.

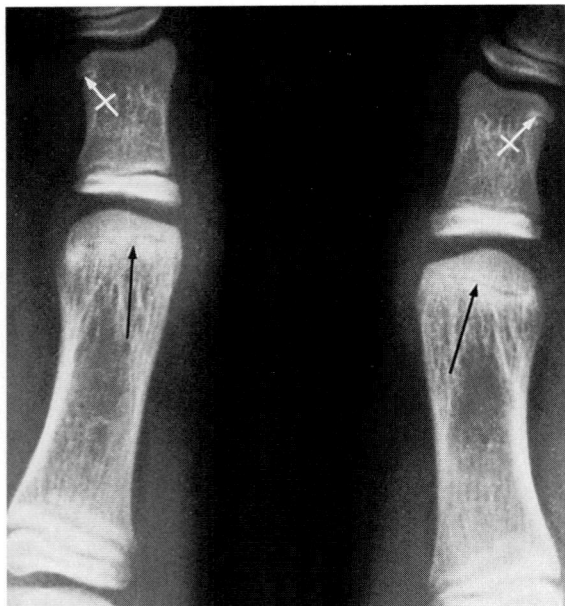

Figure 7–596. Bilateral symmetrical accessory ossification centers at the distal ends of the first metatarsals in an 11-year-old boy (←). Note clefts in the distal ends of the proximal phalanges as well (↤).

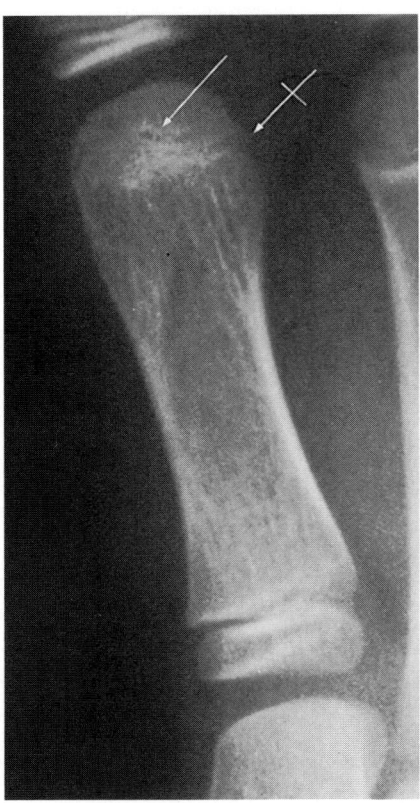

Figure 7–597. Accessory ossification center of the distal end of the first metatarsal (→) in an 8-year-old boy with an epiphyseal spur (↦).

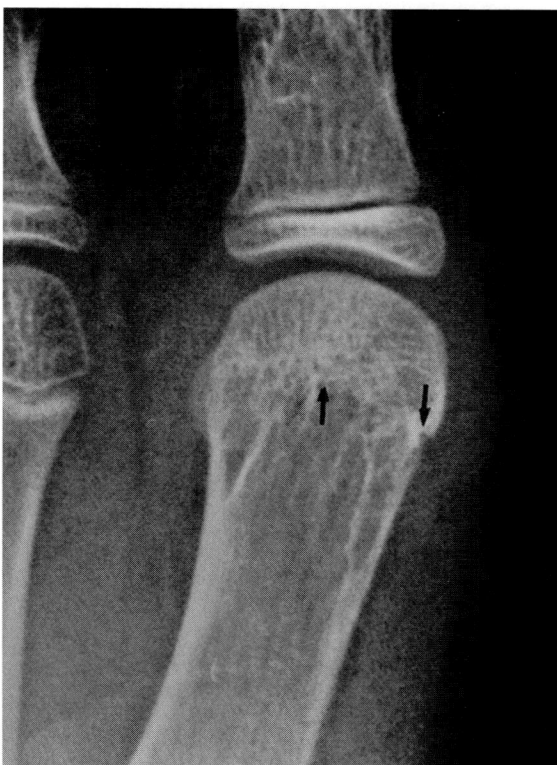

Figure 7–598. Partial closure of the pseudoepiphysis at the head of the first metatarsal in a 6-year-old girl, which may simulate a fracture.

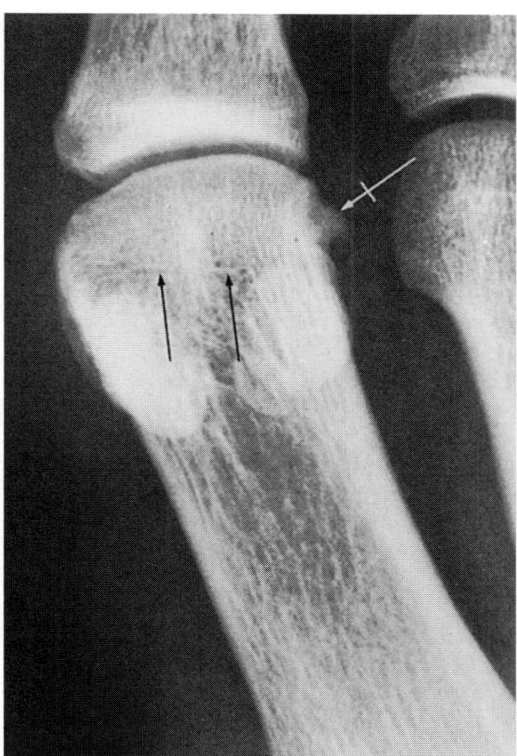

Figure 7–599. Closed accessory ossification center of distal end of the first metatarsal (←) with an epiphyseal spur (↔).

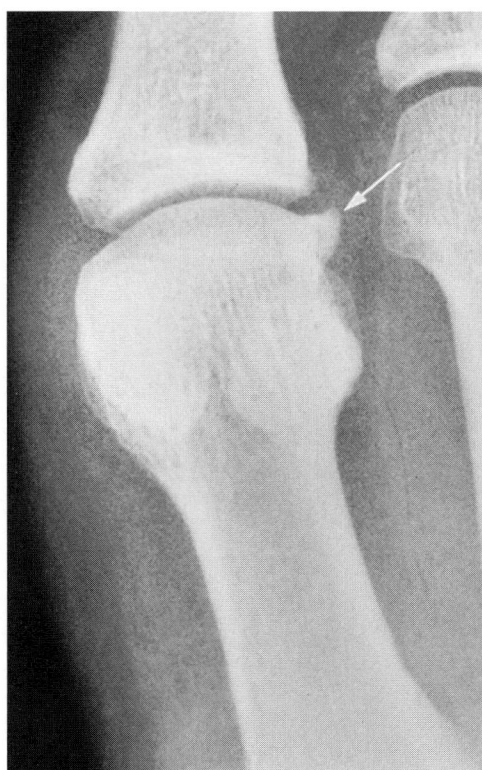

Figure 7–600. The dorsofibular process of the head of the first metatarsal, a normal variant. (Ref: Fischer E: Der dorsofibulare Fortsatz am Kopf des l. Metatarsale, eine ossare variante. *Radiologe* 28:45, 1988.)

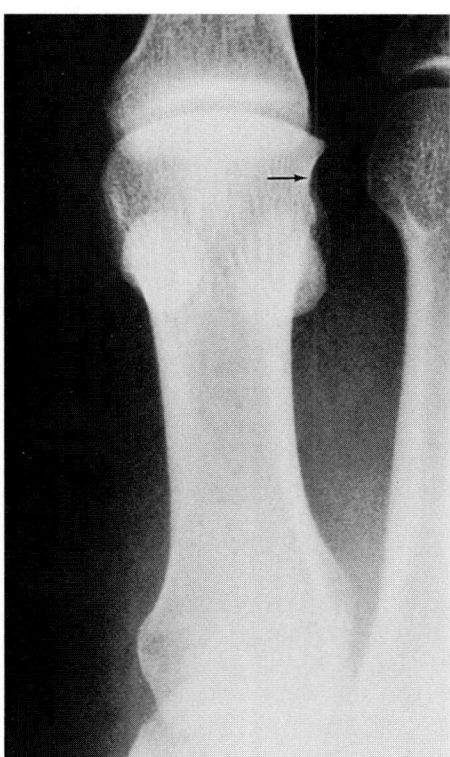

Figure 7–601. Exaggeration of normal fossa in the head of the first metatarsal.

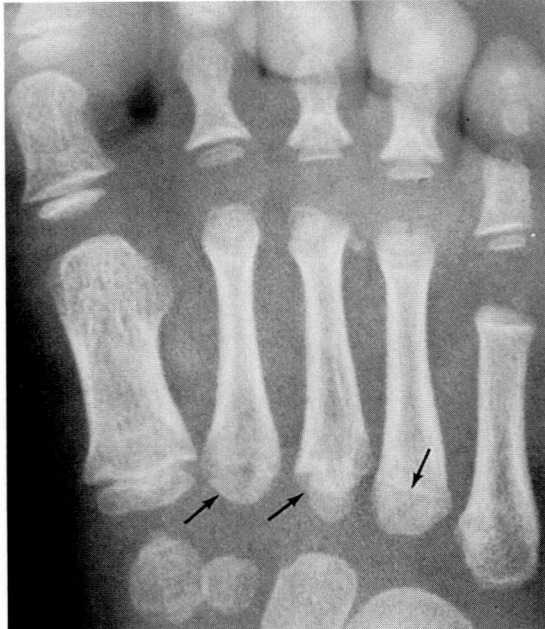

Figure 7–602. Accessory ossification centers at the bases of the second, third, and fourth metatarsals. These are of no clinical significance.

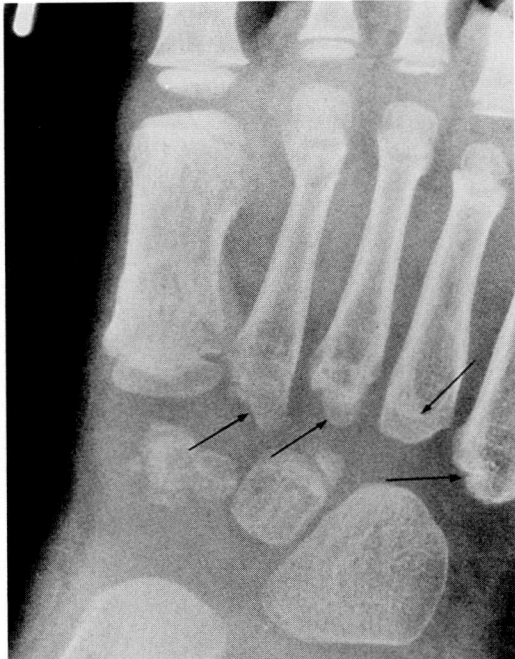

Figure 7–603. Accessory ossification centers at the bases of the second to fifth metatarsals, with partial fusion, in a 4-year-old boy.

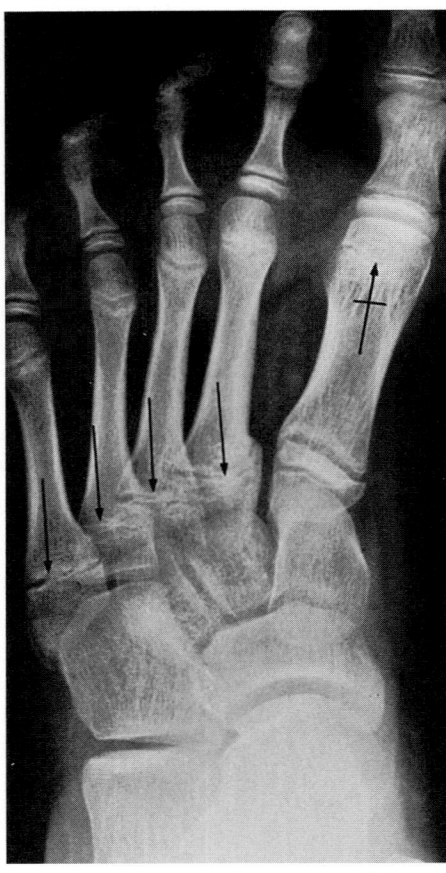

Figure 7–604. Accessory ossification centers at the bases of metatarsals two through five (←) and an accessory center at the distal end of the first metatarsal (↤) in a 12-year-old boy.

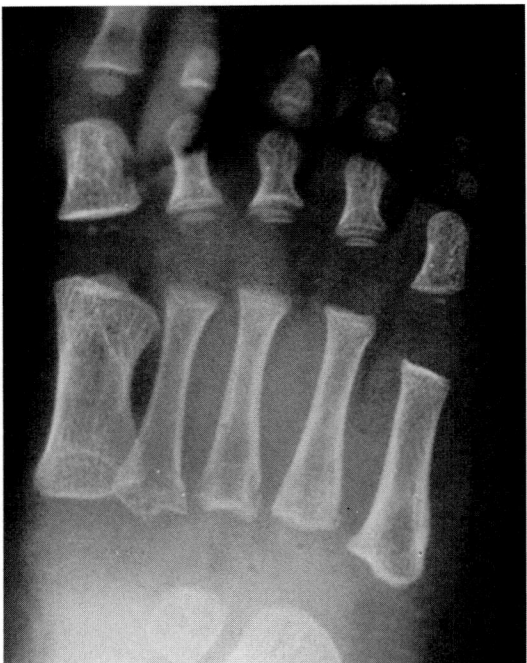

Figure 7–605. Normal irregularities of the bases of the metatarsals in a 3-year-old boy.

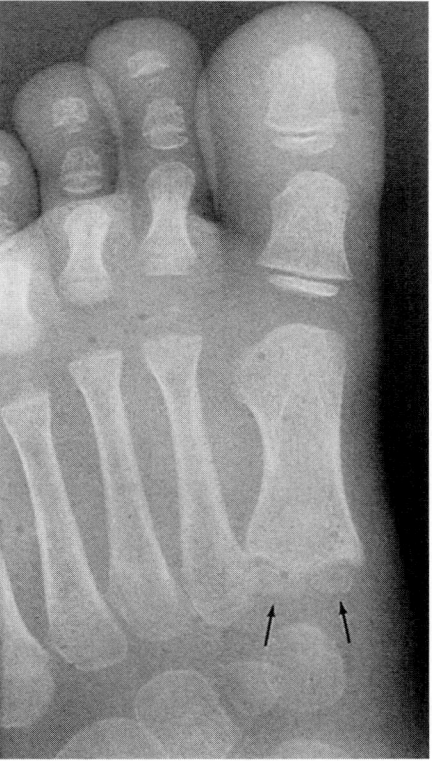

Figure 7–606. Duplication of the ossification center of the base of the first metatarsal.

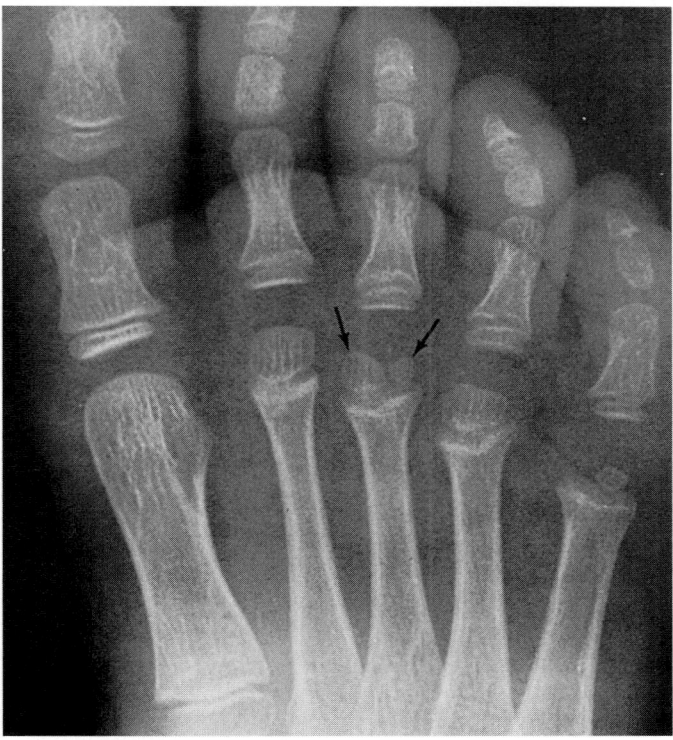

Figure 7–607. Duplication of the ossification center of the head of the third metatarsal, not a fracture.

Figure 7–608. Duplication of the ossification centers of the heads of the third, fourth, and fifth metatarsals.

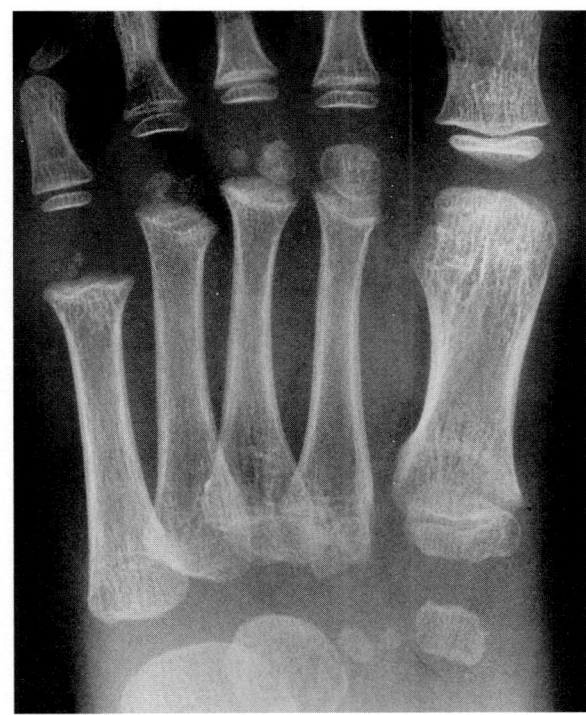

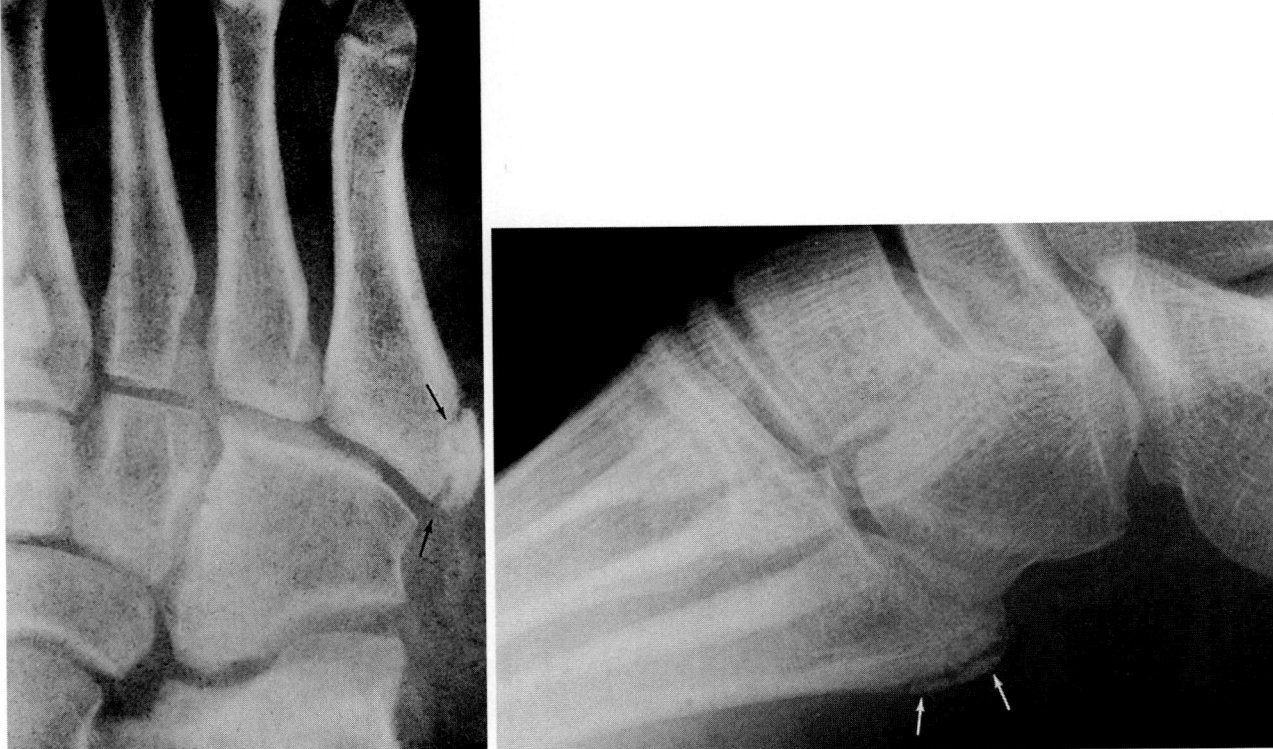

Figure 7–609. The normal apophysis of the tuberosity of the base of the fifth metatarsal, which resembles a fracture. Most fractures of this area are transverse rather than longitudinal.

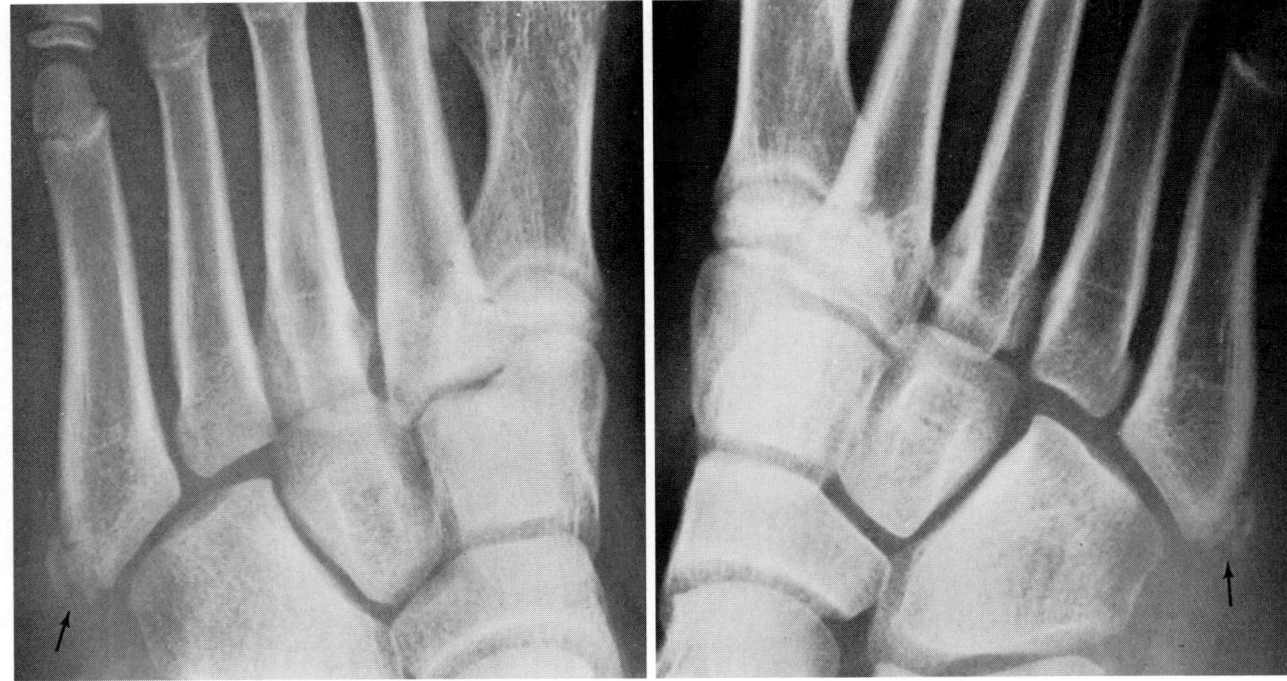

Figure 7–610. Multicentric ossification centers of the tuberosities of the fifth metatarsals in a 12-year-old girl, simulating fractures.

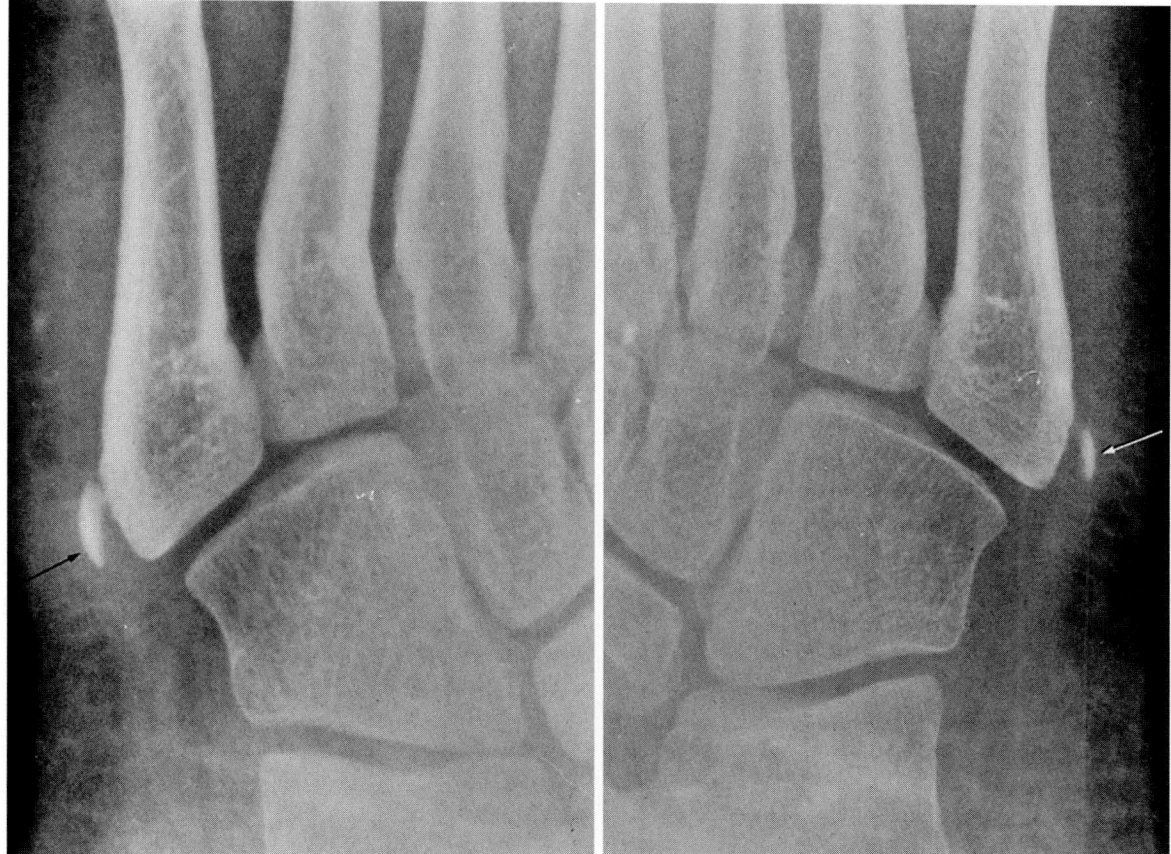

Figure 7–611. The lateral position of the apophysis of the base of the fifth metatarsal in the oblique projection should not be misconstrued as an avulsion injury.

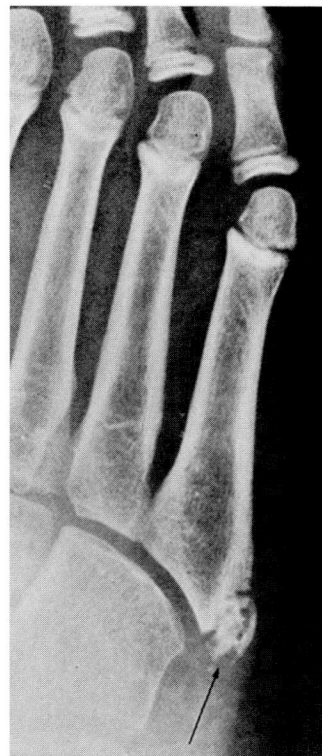

Figure 7–612. Irregular mineralization of the apophysis of the base of the fifth metatarsal.

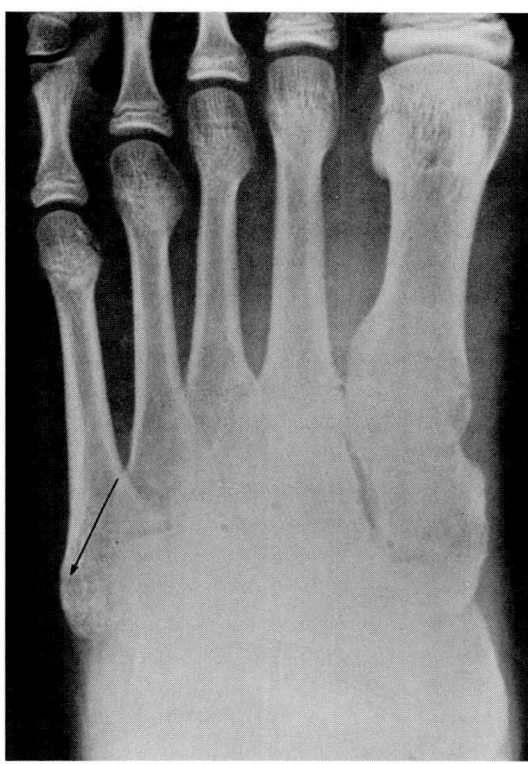

Figure 7–613. The fusing apophysis at the base of the fifth metatarsal may simulate a fracture in the frontal projection.

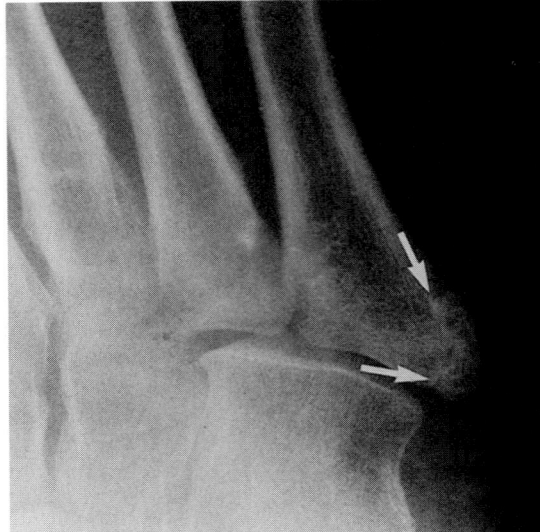

Figure 7–614. Closing apophysis that might be mistaken for a fracture at the base of the fifth metatarsal in an 11-year-old boy.

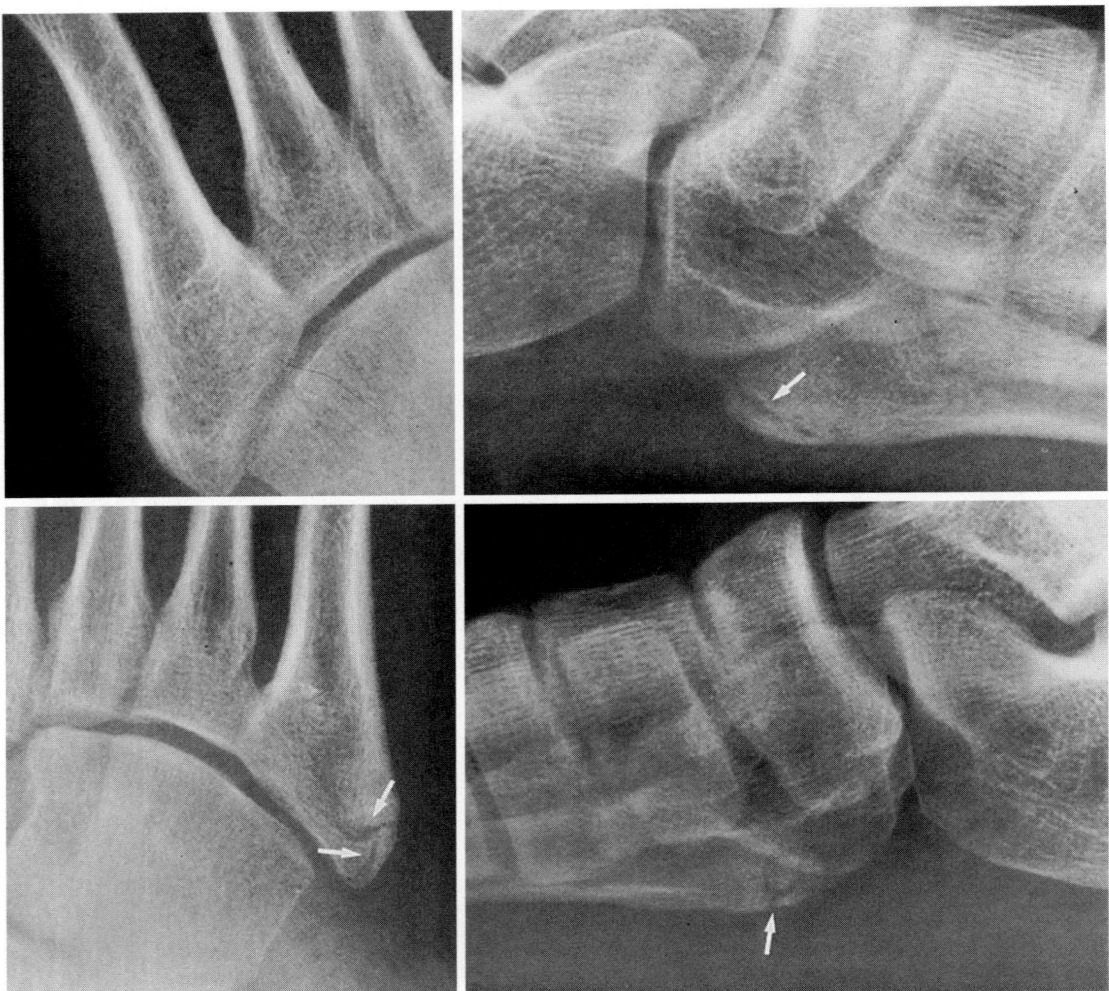

Figure 7–615. Asymmetric closure of the apophysis of the base of the fifth metatarsal in an 11-year-old boy. *Top,* Left foot. *Bottom,* Right foot.

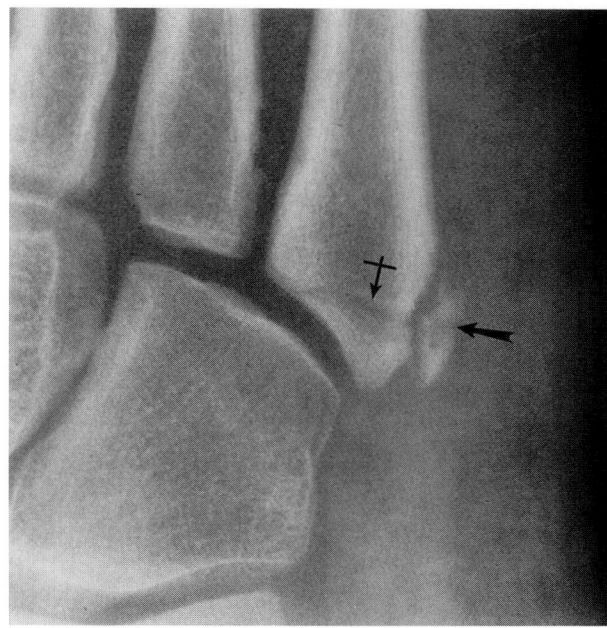
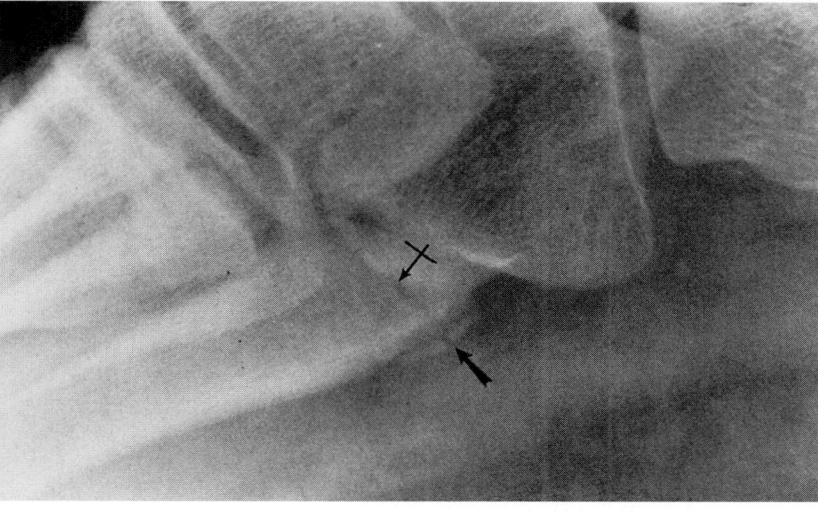

Figure 7–616. The apophysis at the base of the fifth metatarsal (←) plus a fracture (↔) in a 13-year-old girl.

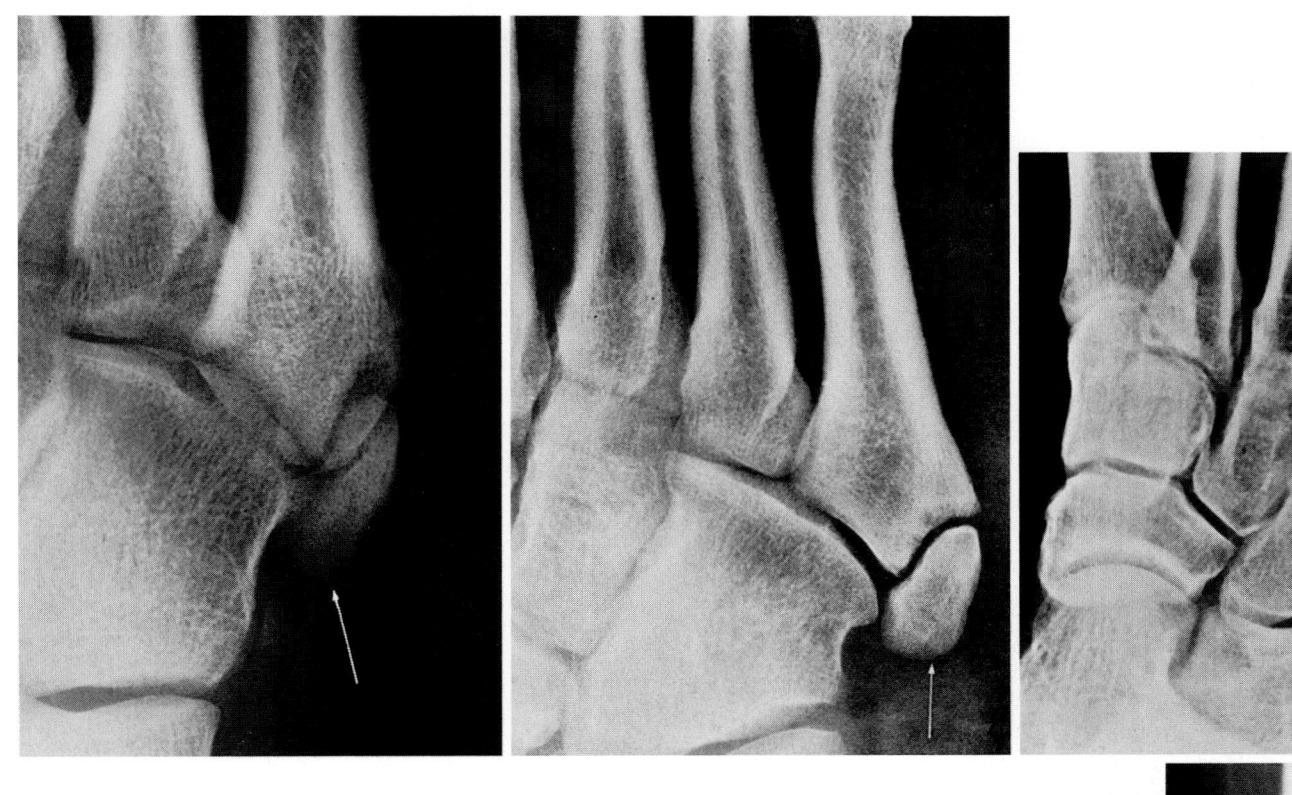
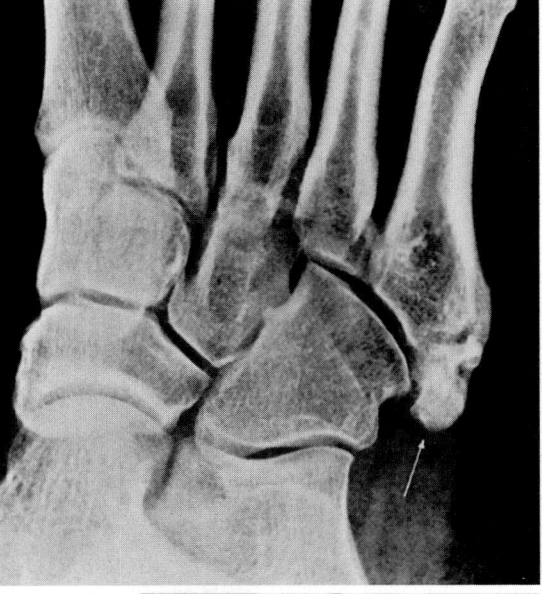
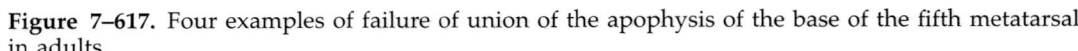
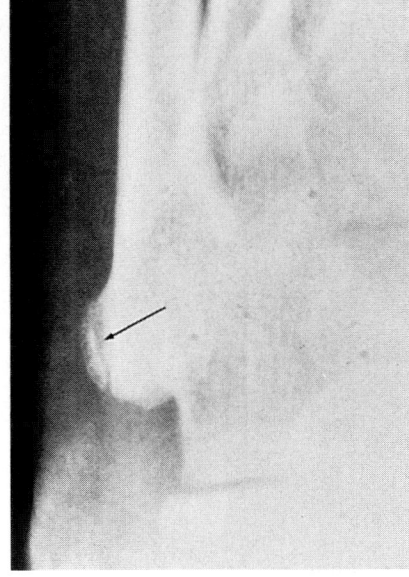

Figure 7–617. Four examples of failure of union of the apophysis of the base of the fifth metatarsal in adults.

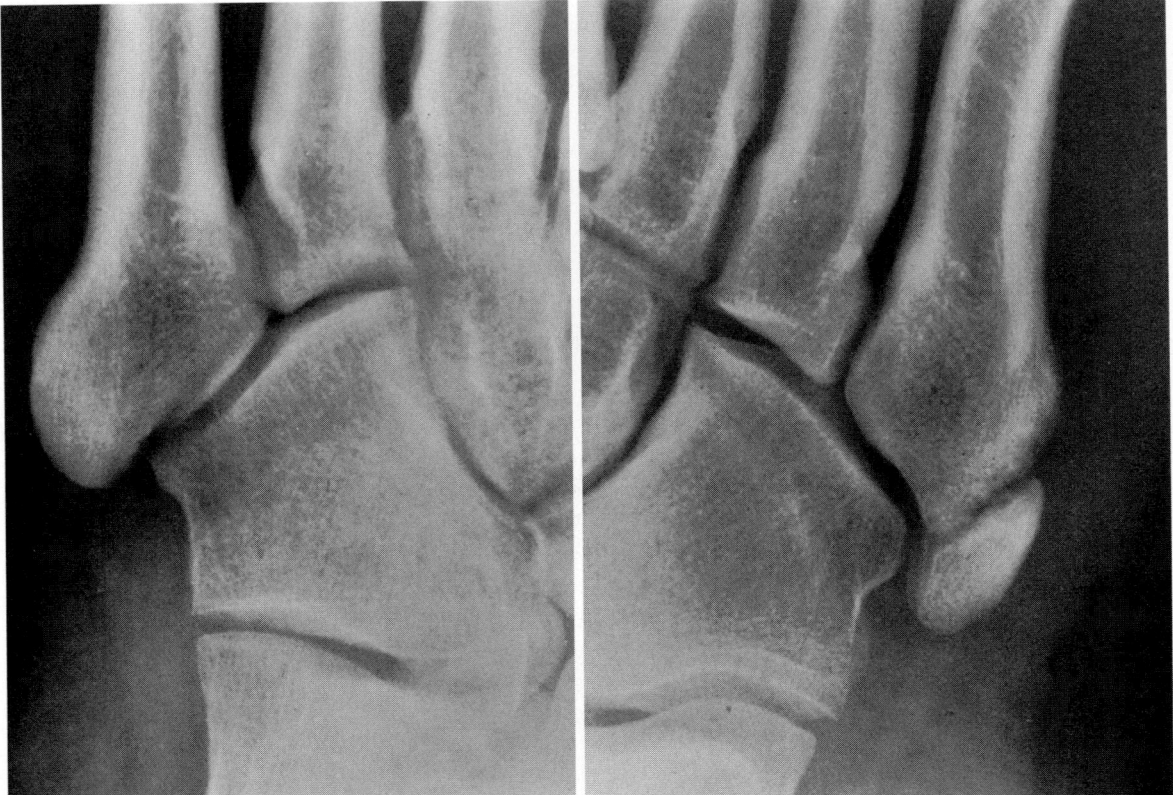

Figure 7–618. Asymmetric closure of the apophyses at the bases of the fifth metatarsals in a 20-year-old man.

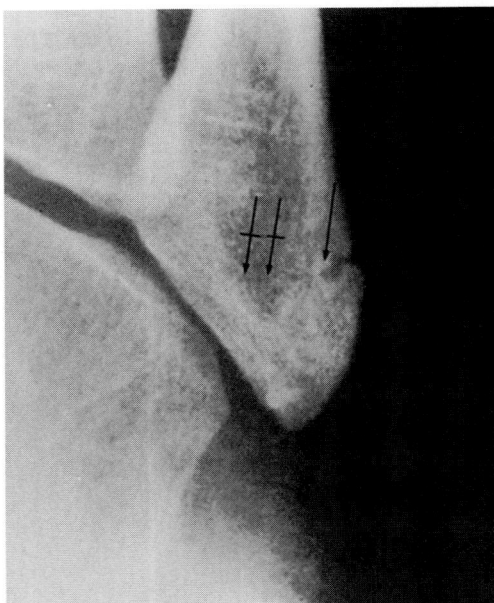

Figure 7–619. Closing apophysis at the base of the fifth metatarsal (←). Note how the trabeculations of the bone appear to line up in continuity with the apophyseal plate and simulate a fracture of the base (↔).

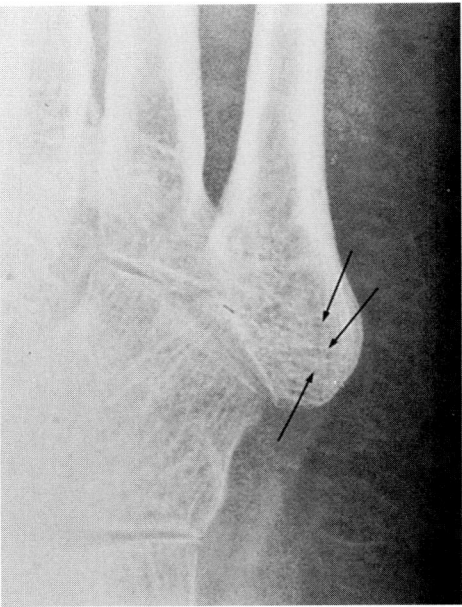

Figure 7–620. Note the horizontal trabeculations in the base of the fifth metatarsal. It is these lines that create the illusion of a transverse fracture, as shown in Figure 7–619.

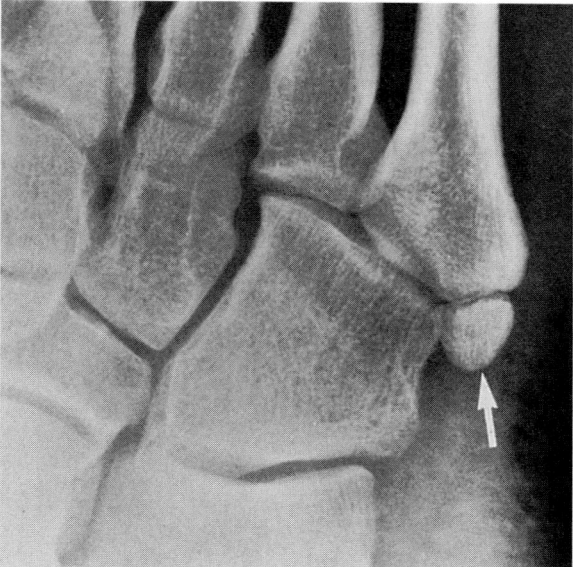

Figure 7–621. Apophysis at the tip rather than at the side of the base of the fifth metatarsal in a 14-year-old boy. (Ref: Dameron JB: Fractures and anatomical variation of the proximal portion of the fifth metatarsal. *J Bone Joint Surg* 57A:788, 1975.)

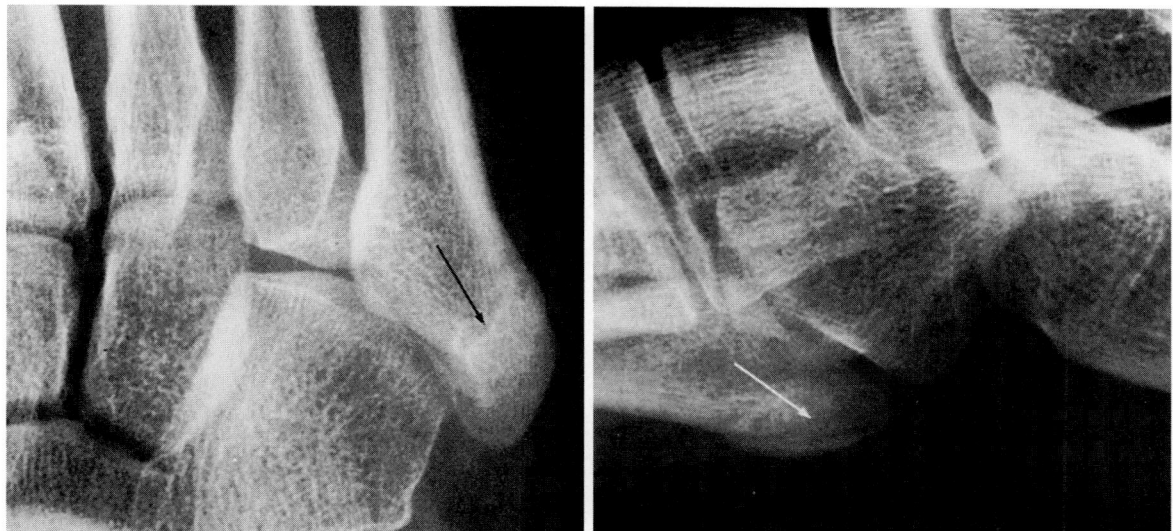

Figure 7–622. Very large apophyses at the bases of the fifth metatarsals in an 11-year-old boy.

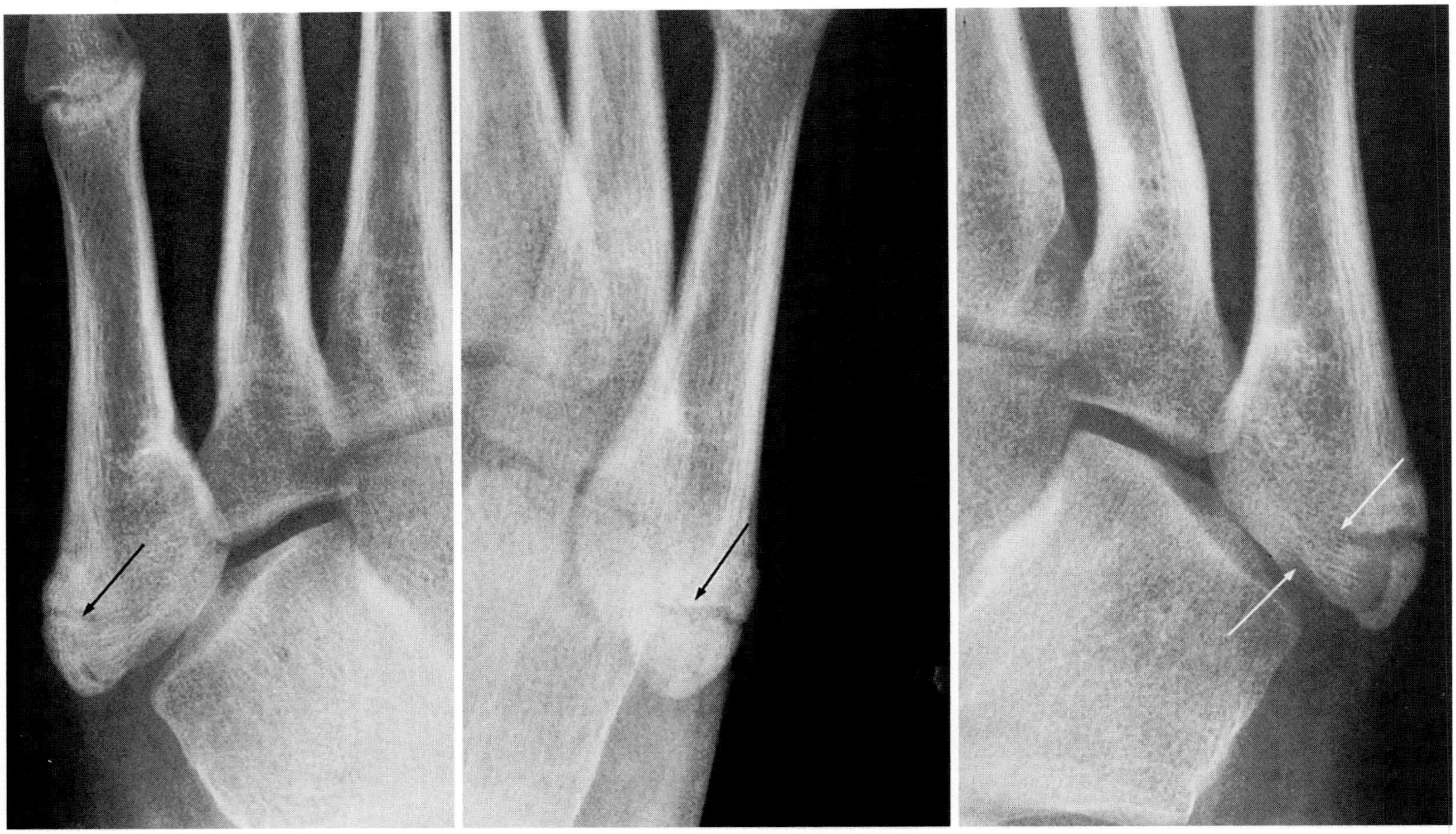

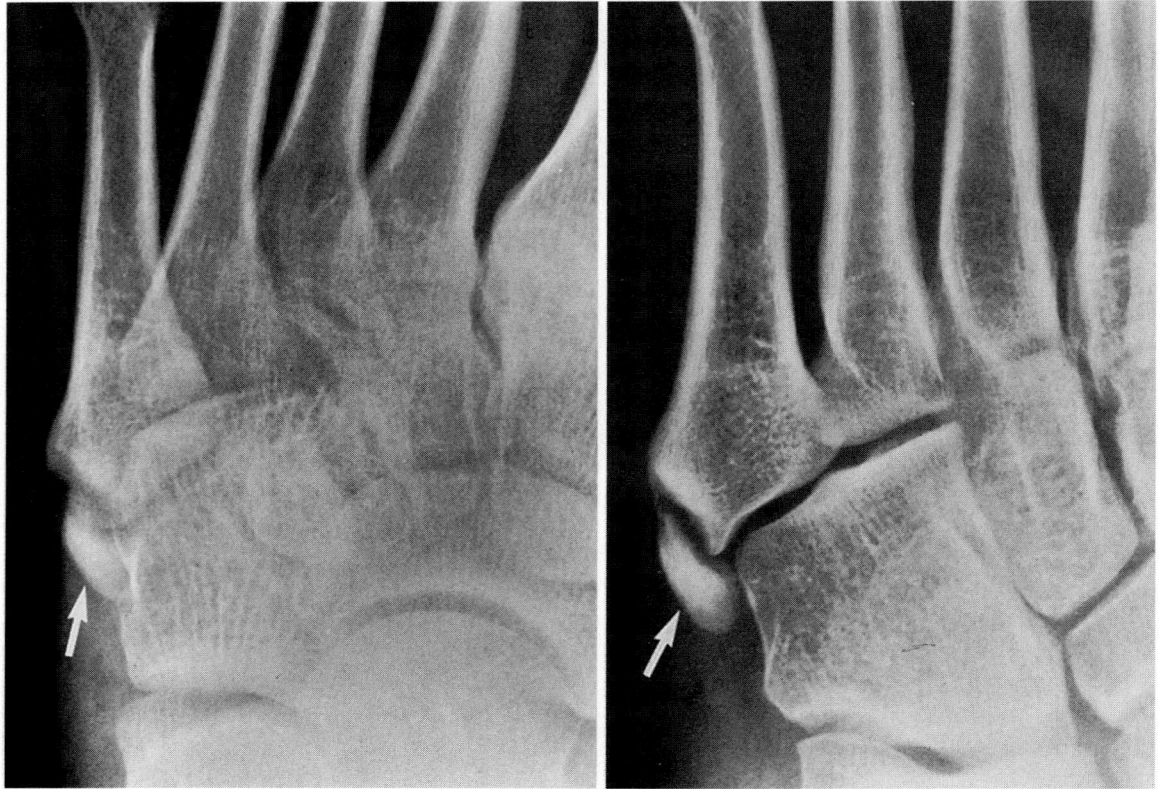

Figure 7–623. Bilateral closing apophyses of the type shown in Figure 7–622 in a 12-year-old boy, which could be mistaken for fractures. *Left and center,* Left foot. *Right,* Right foot.

Figure 7–624. Unfused apophysis at the base of the fifth metatarsal in a 19-year-old man. Note that the apophysis is located at the end of the metatarsal rather than in its usual lateral position. This is an unusual but not rare variation in the position of the apophysis.

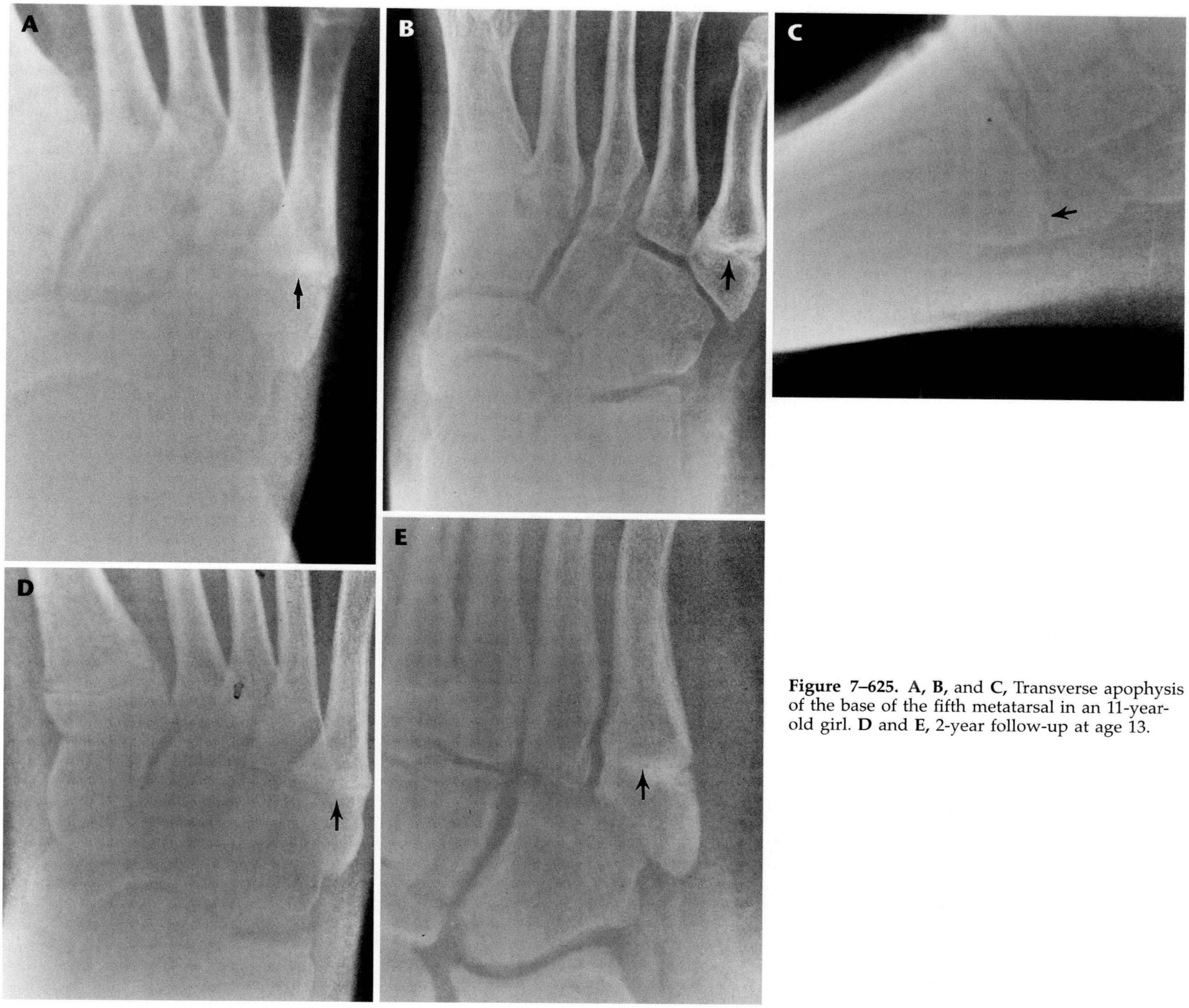

Figure 7–625. **A, B,** and **C,** Transverse apophysis of the base of the fifth metatarsal in an 11-year-old girl. **D** and **E,** 2-year follow-up at age 13.

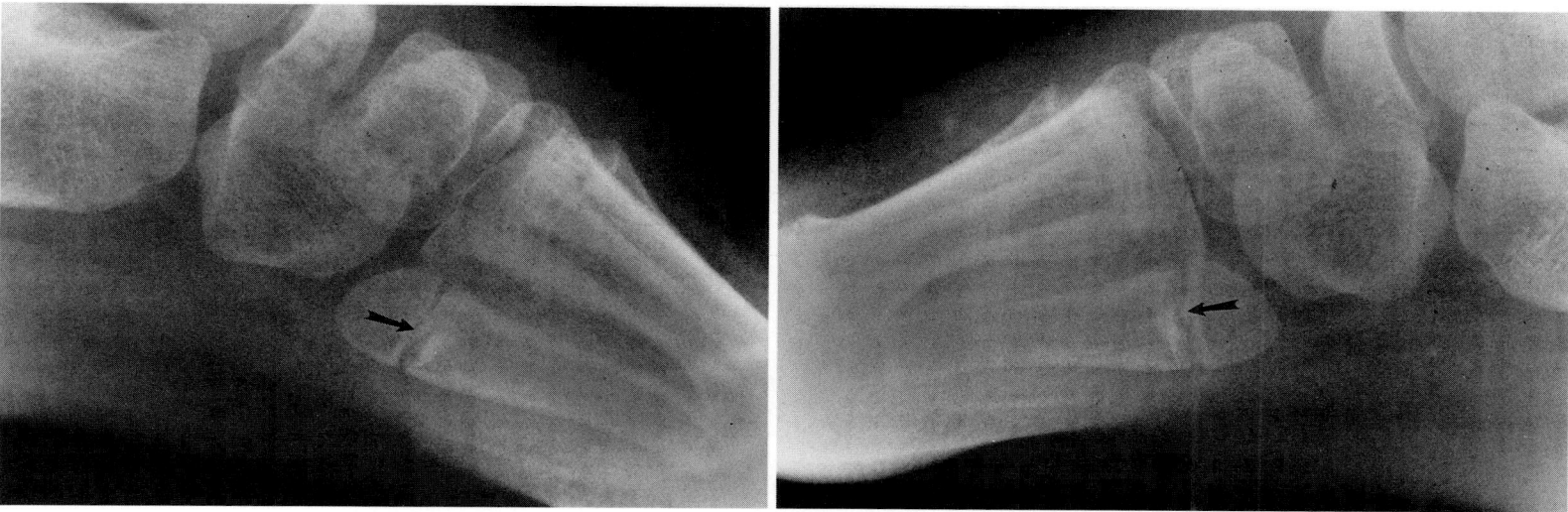

Figure 7–626. Bilateral transverse apophyses at the bases of the fifth metatarsals in an 8-year-old girl.

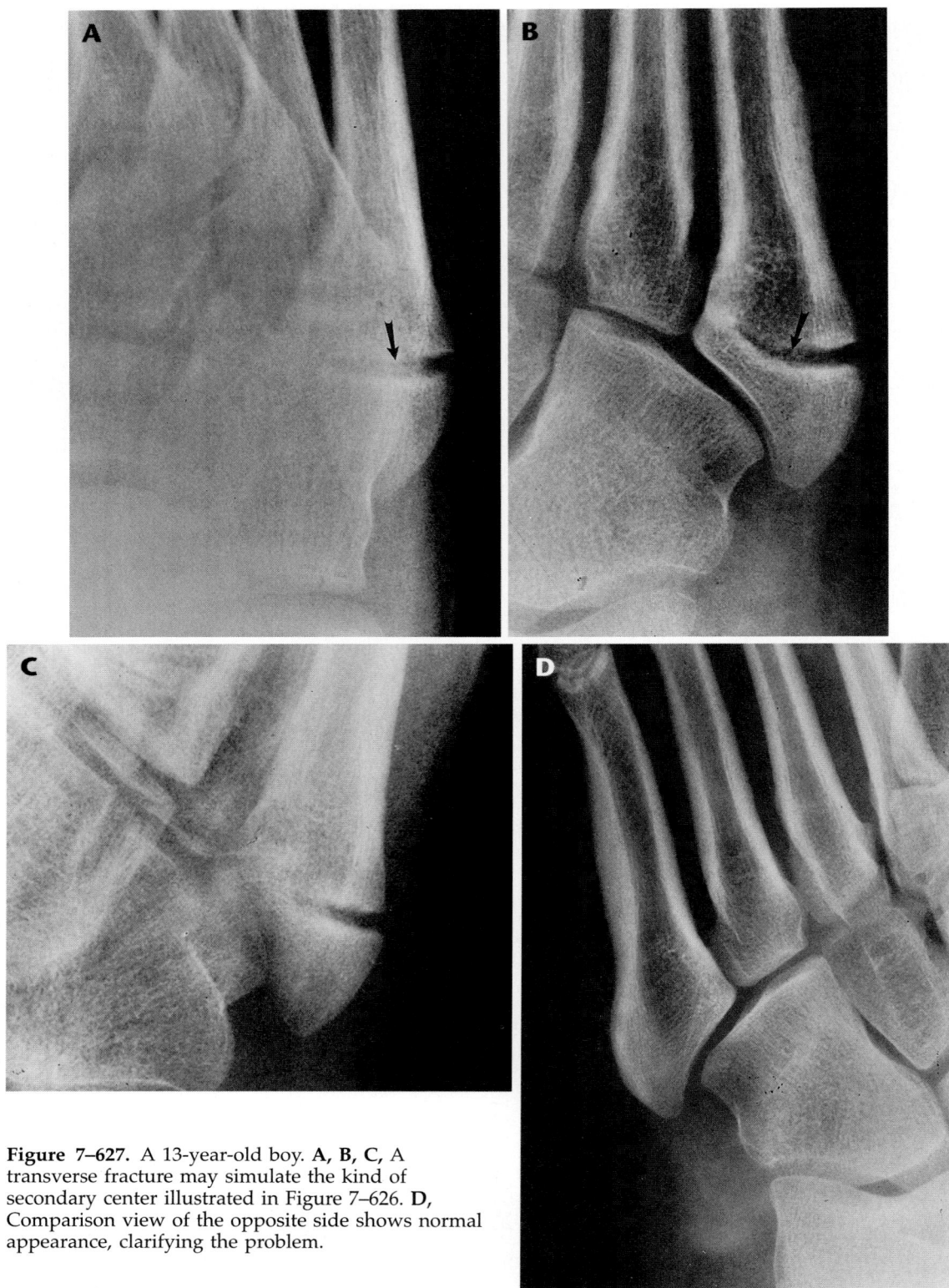

Figure 7–627. A 13-year-old boy. **A, B, C,** A transverse fracture may simulate the kind of secondary center illustrated in Figure 7–626. **D,** Comparison view of the opposite side shows normal appearance, clarifying the problem.

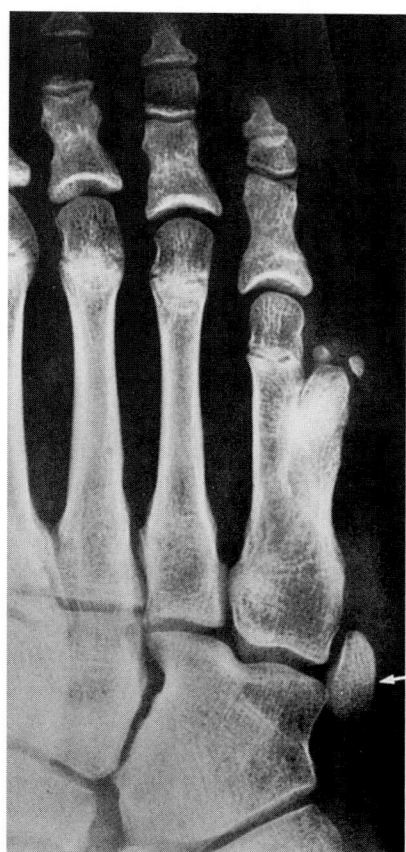

Figure 7–628. Duplication anomaly of the fifth metatarsal with nonunion of the basal apophysis (*arrow*).

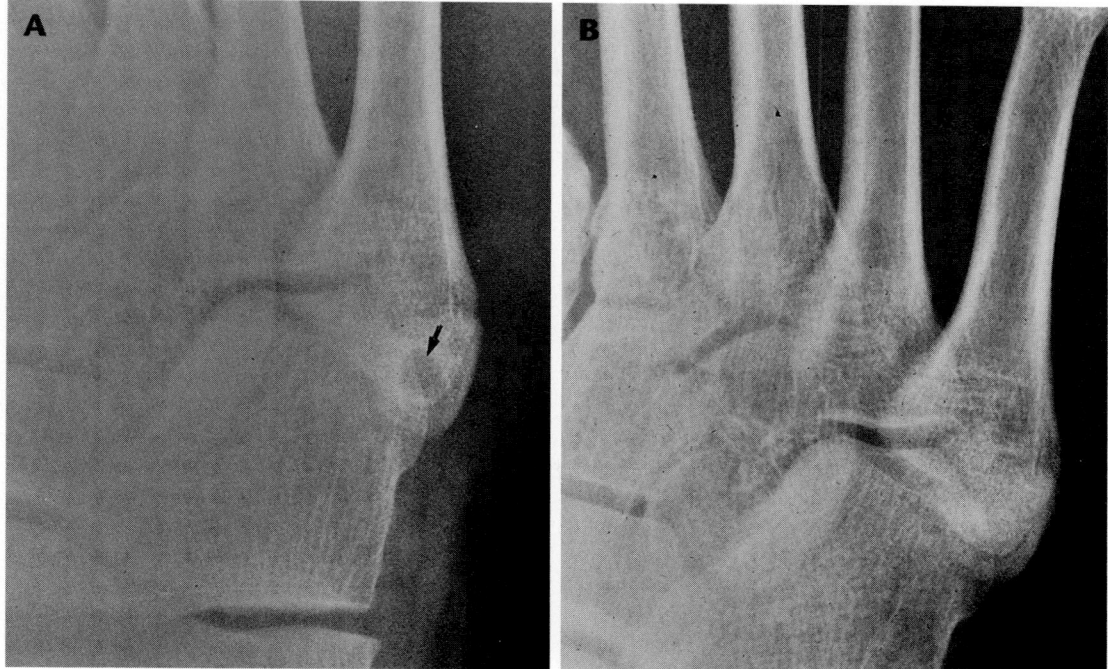

Figure 7–629. A, Cystlike radiolucency in the base of the fifth metatarsal in a 14-year-old girl. **B,** Follow-up in 5 months shows normal appearance. For a similar sequence, see Figure 7–370.

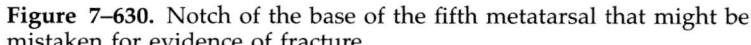

Figure 7–630. Notch of the base of the fifth metatarsal that might be mistaken for evidence of fracture.

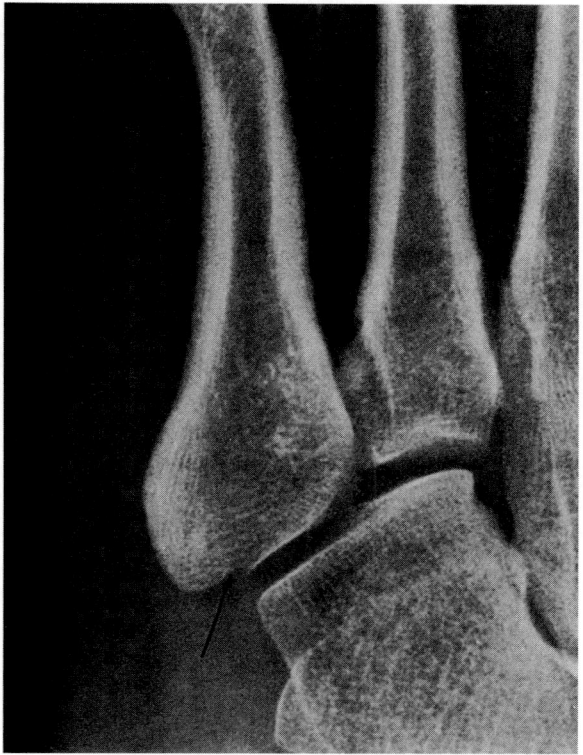

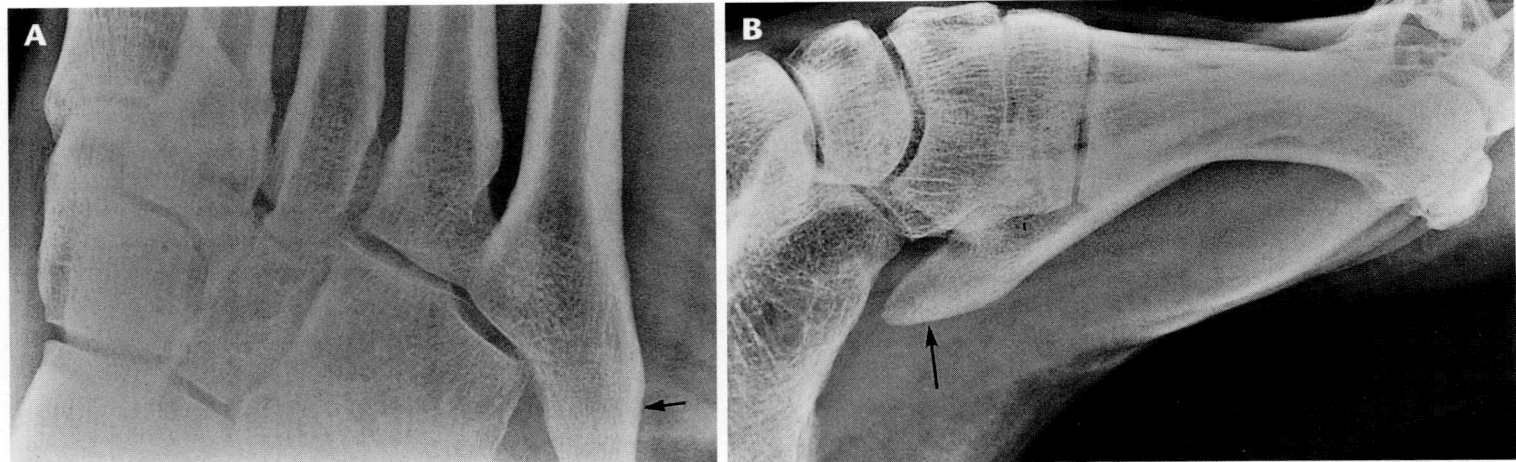

Figure 7–631. A, B, Os vesalianum fused to base of fifth metatarsal.

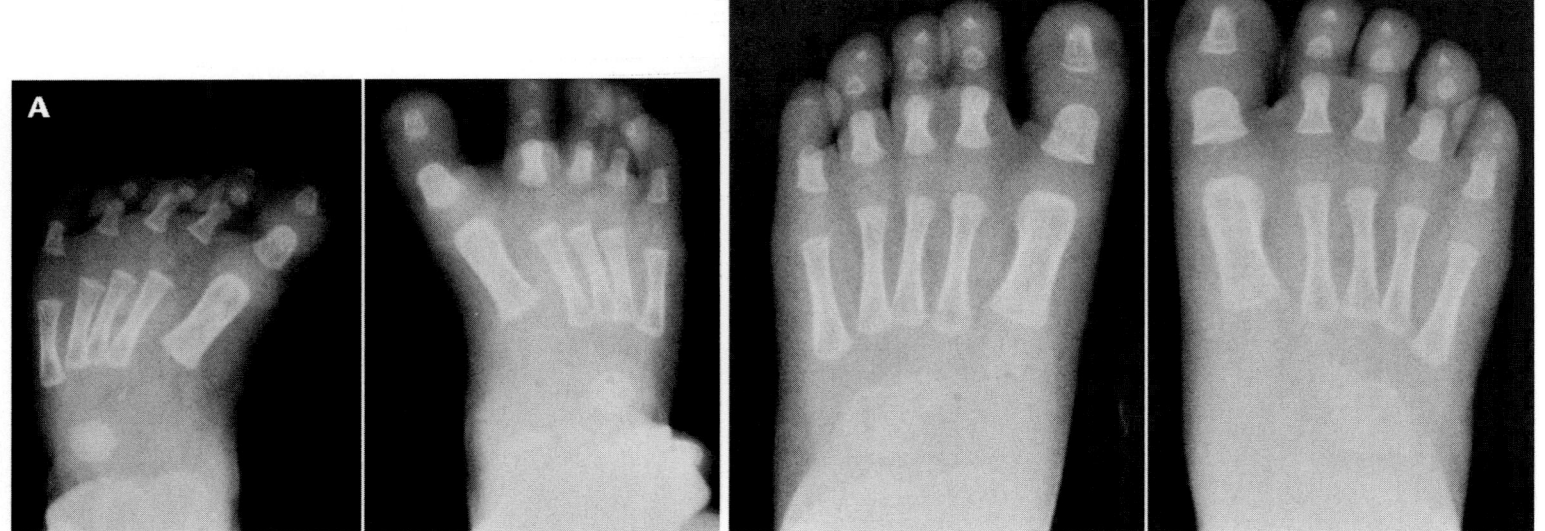

Figure 7–632. Metatarsus adductus is physiologic in many infants and will correct spontaneously with weight-bearing. **A,** 4 months of age. **B,** 16 months of age. (Ref: Berg EE: A reappraisal of metatarsus adductus and skewfoot. *J Bone Joint Surg* 68A:1185, 1986.)

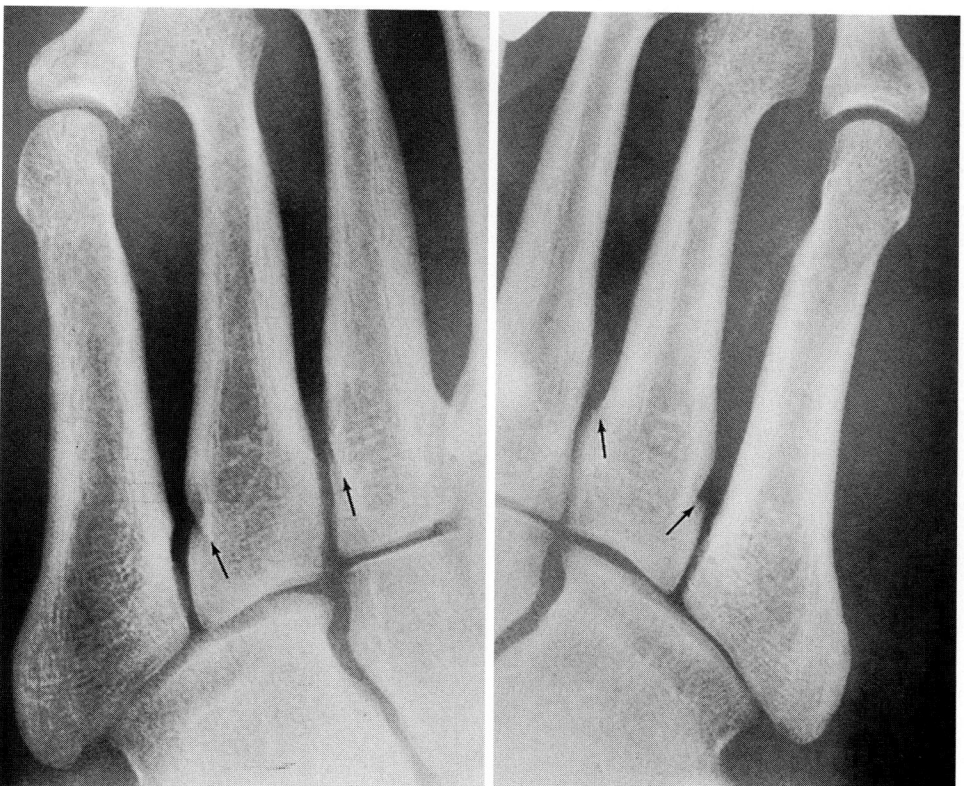

Figure 7–633. Normal clefts seen at the bases of the metatarsals.

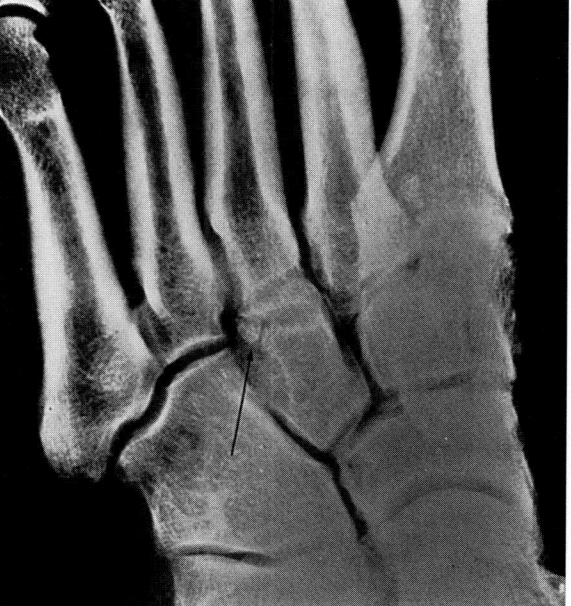

Figure 7–634. Accessory ossicle at the base of the third metatarsal.

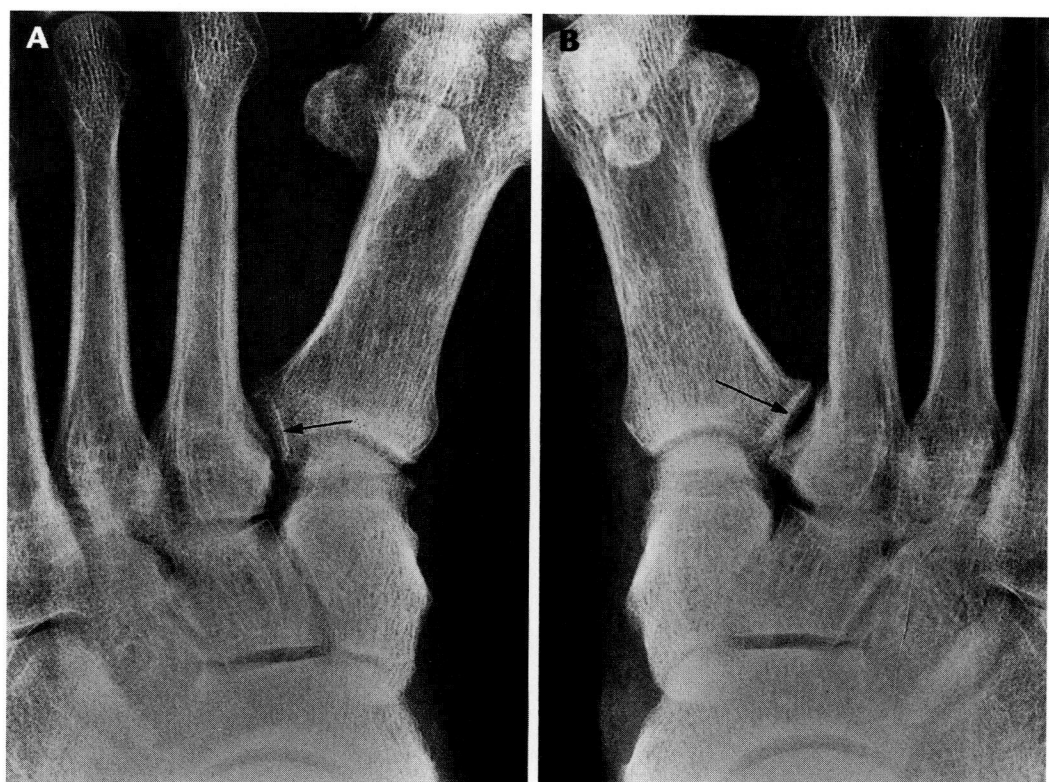

Figure 7–635. A, B, Unusual bilateral articulations between the bases of first and second metatarsals.

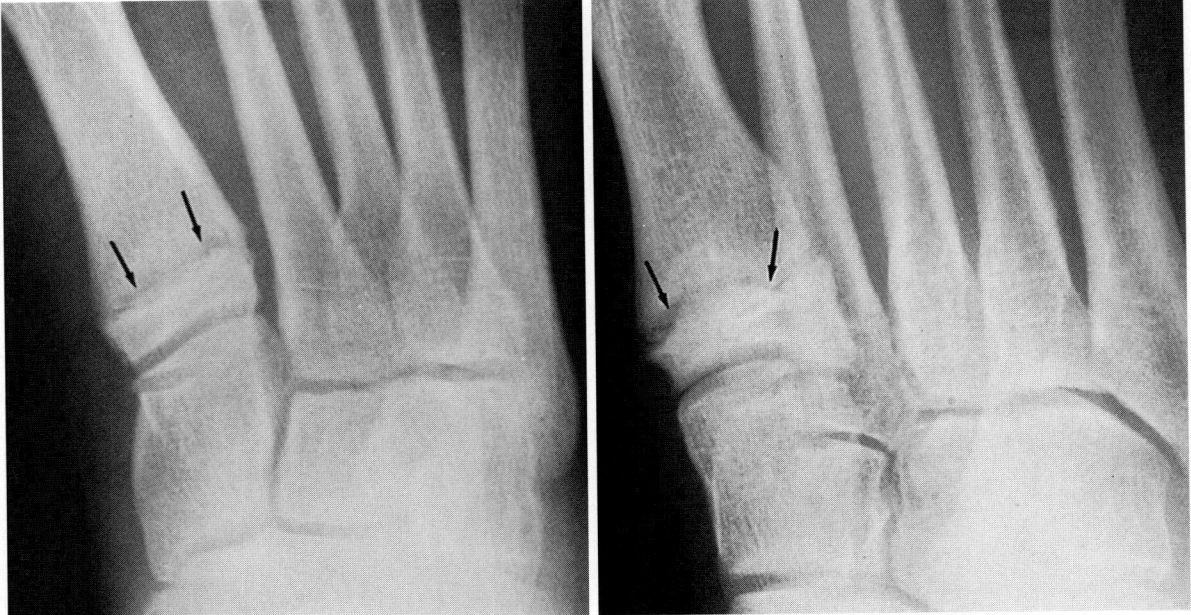

Figure 7–636. Normal irregularity of the epiphyseal line at the base of the first metatarsal in an adolescent boy, which should not be mistaken for evidence of a fracture.

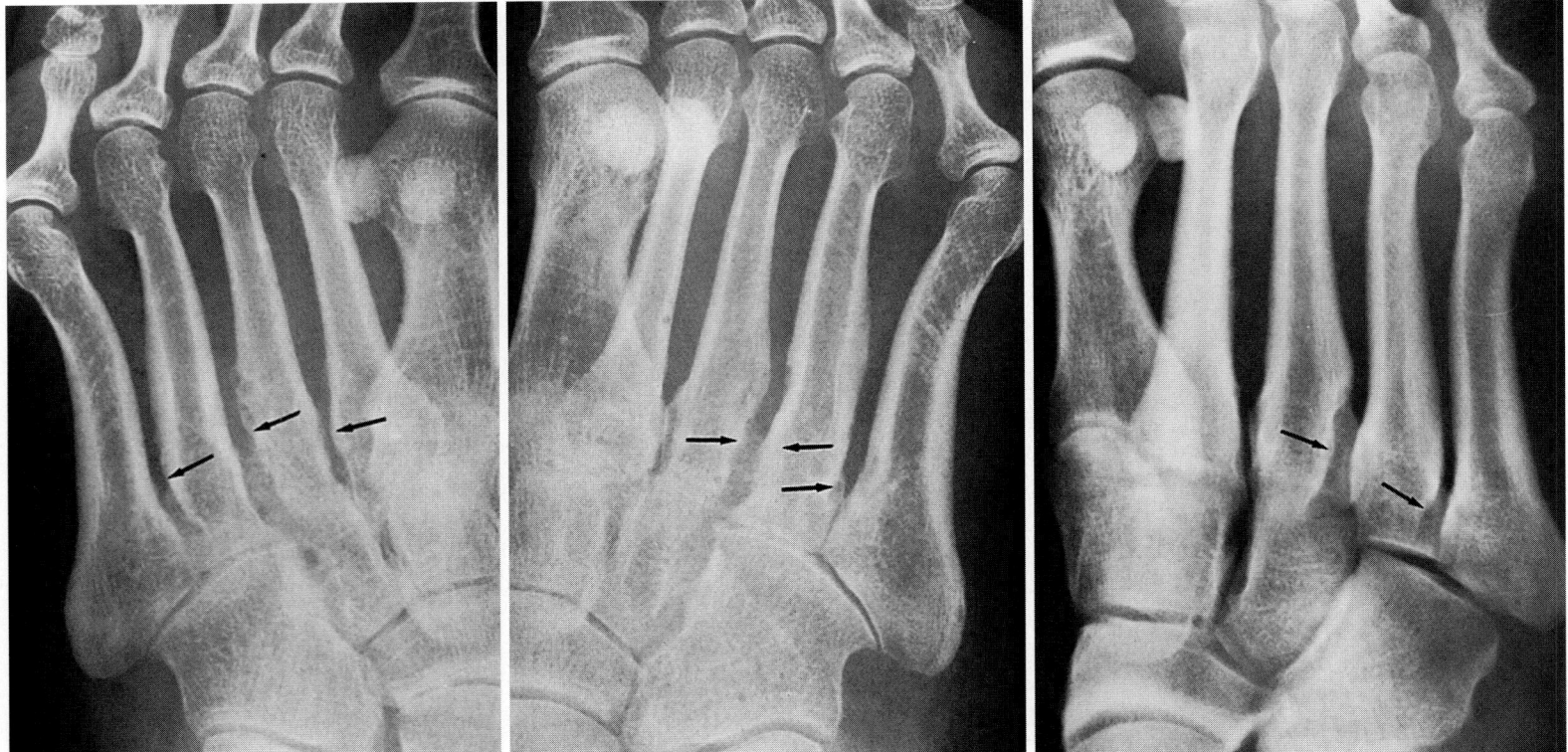

Figure 7–637. Three examples of normal irregularities of the bases of the second, third, and fourth metatarsals, evident in oblique projection.

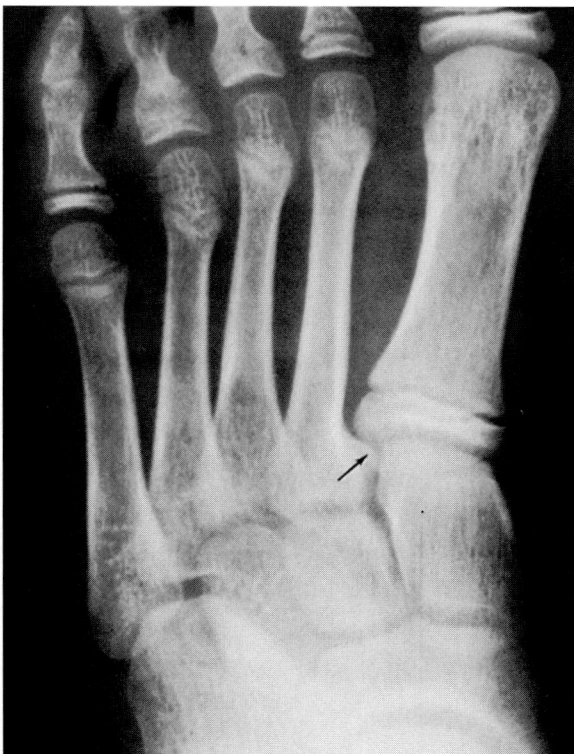

Figure 7–638. Simulated torus fracture produced by the tuberosity at the base of the second metatarsal in a 13-year-old girl.

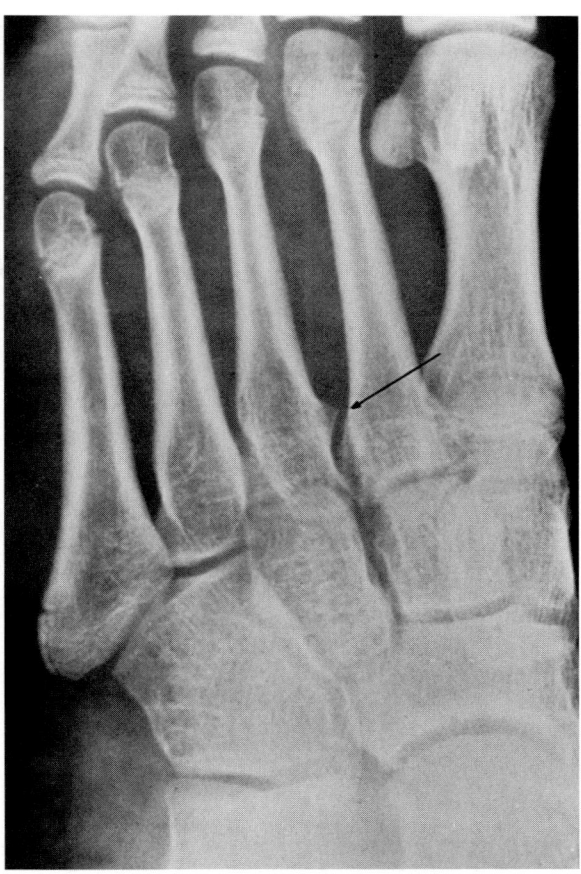

Figure 7–639. Developmental spur at the base of the third metatarsal.

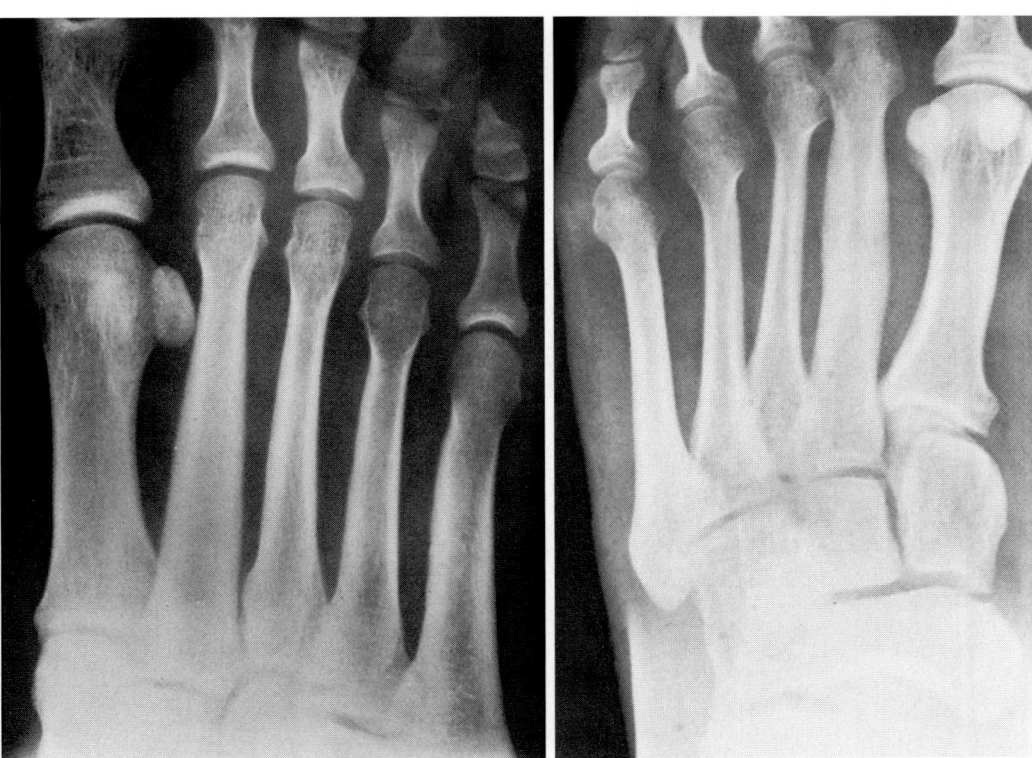

Figure 7–640. Two examples of increase in size and cortical thickness of the shaft of the second metatarsal, seen in patients with short first metatarsals. This is apparently a compensatory weight-bearing mechanism.

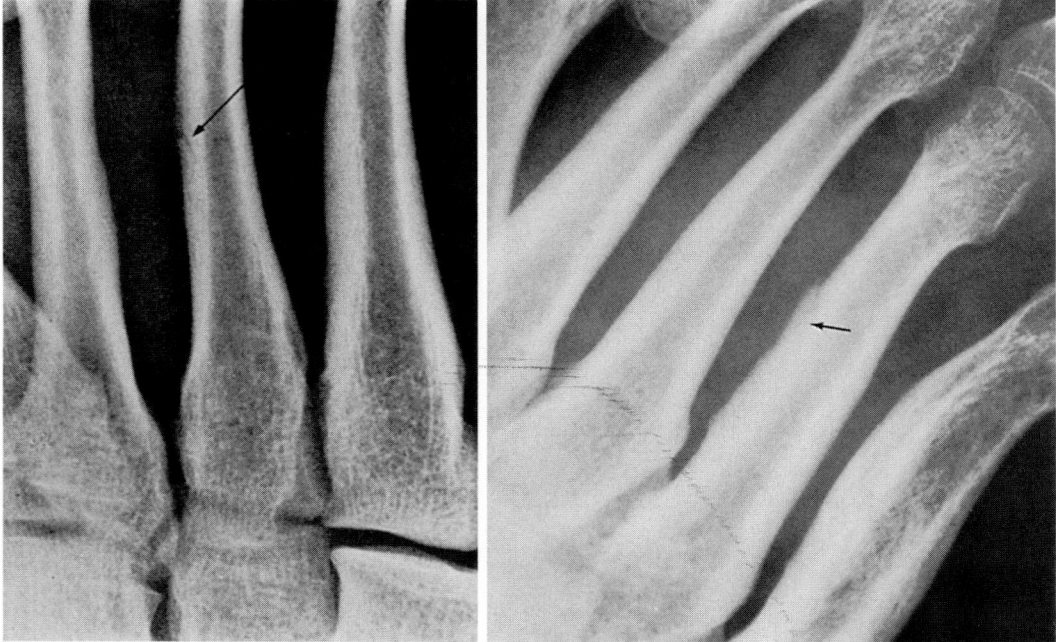

Figure 7–641. Two examples of the nutrient channels for the metatarsals.

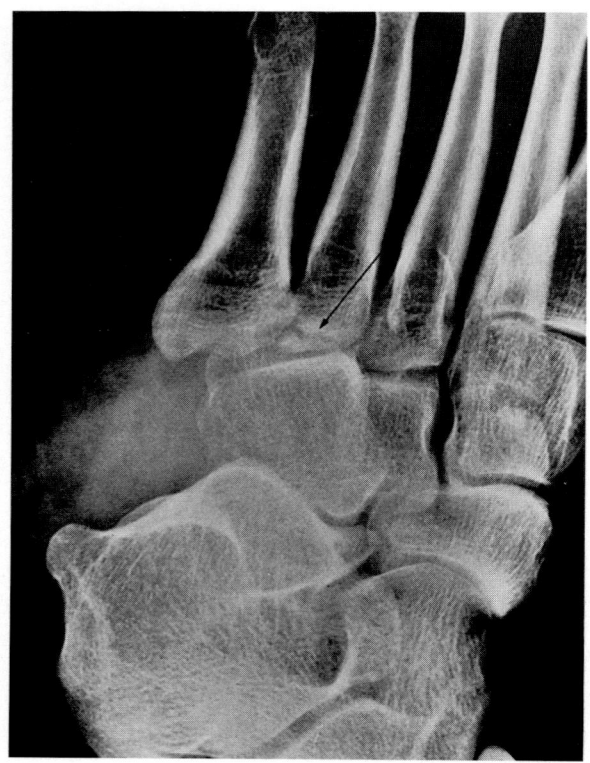

Figure 7–642. Simulated fracture of the base of the fourth metatarsal, resulting from overlapping of the cuboid.

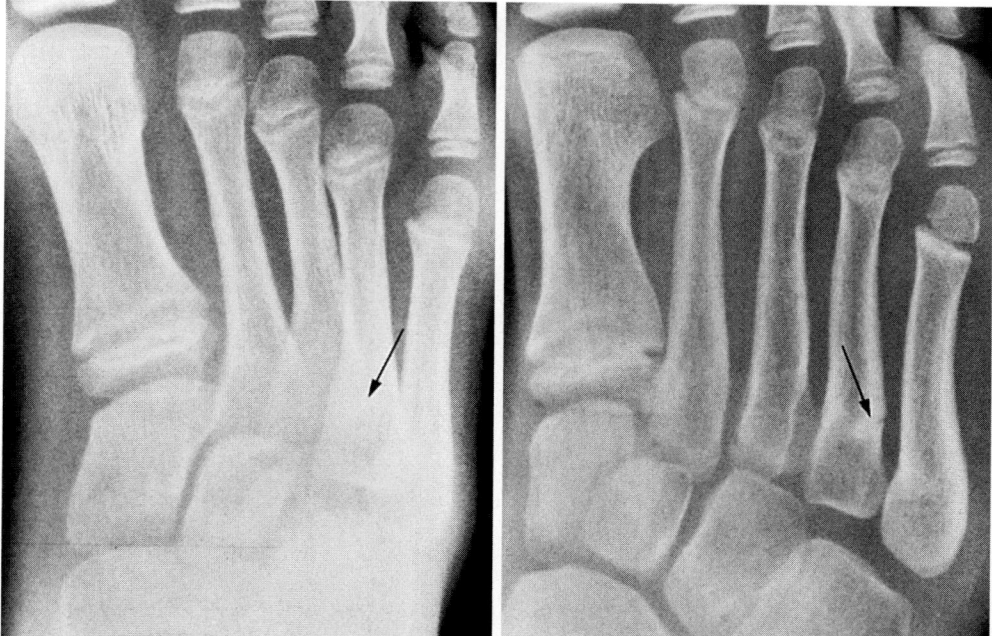

Figure 7–643. Developmental cleft at the base of the fourth metatarsal in a young child.

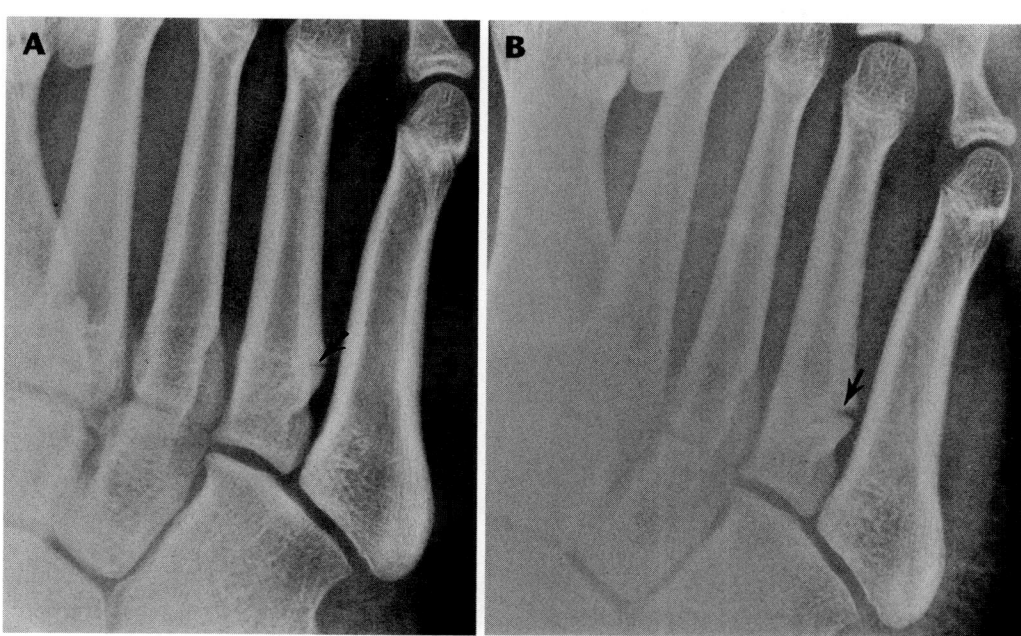

Figure 7–644. A, Similar entity as illustrated in Figure 7–643. This adolescent girl was examined for minor trauma. A cleft is seen in the proximal shaft of the fourth metatarsal. **B,** Follow-up examination in one month shows no change. The patient is asymptomatic.

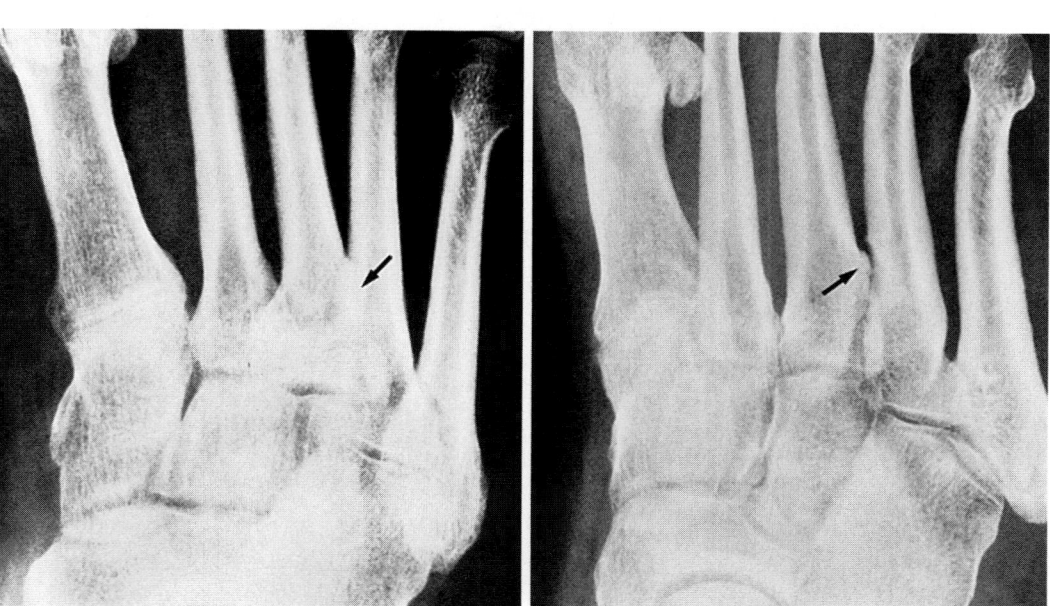

Figure 7–645. Anomalous articulation between the third and fourth metatarsals.

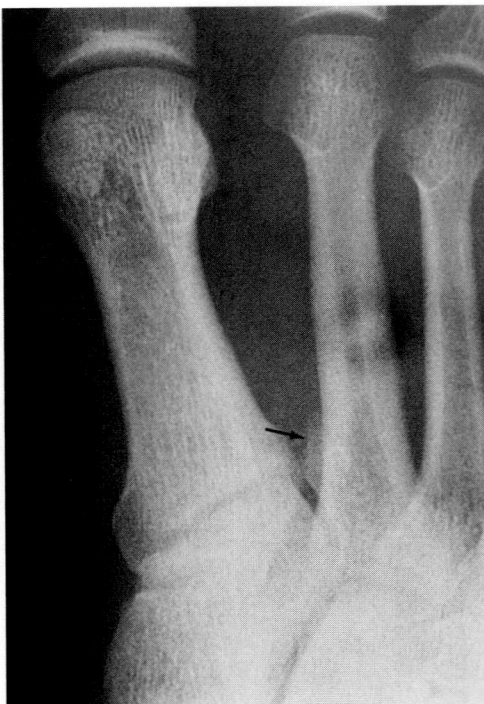

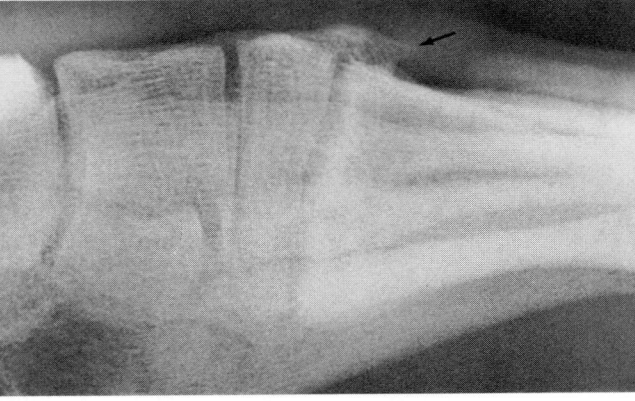

Figure 7–646. Os intermetatarseum. This accessory bone appears on the dorsal aspect of the foot and is variable in size and shape. It may be separate or attached to the base of the first or second metatarsal. (Ref: Kohler A, Zimmer EA: *Borderlands of normal and early pathologic findings in skeletal radiography,* 4th ed. New York, Thieme, 1993, p. 840.)

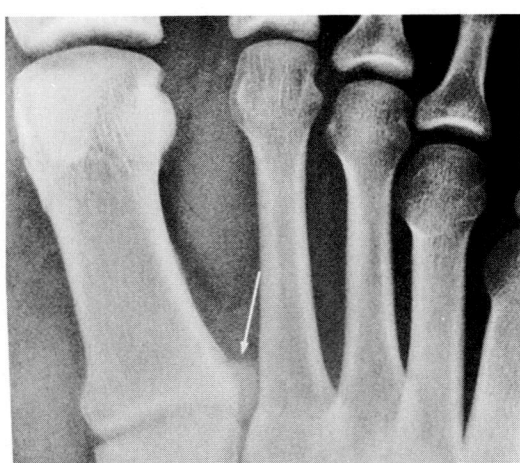

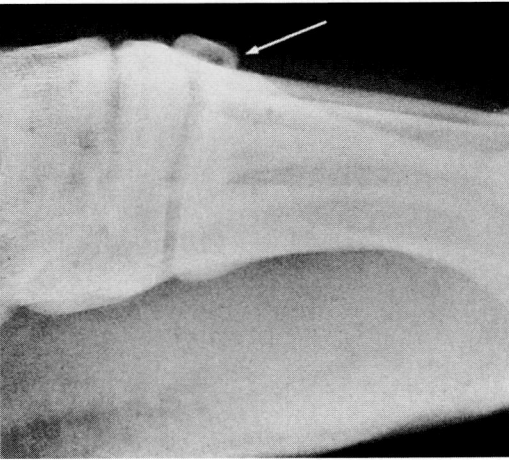

Figure 7–647. Os intermetatarseum arising from the base of the first metatarsal, unlike the example in Figure 7–646, which arose from the base of the second metatarsal.

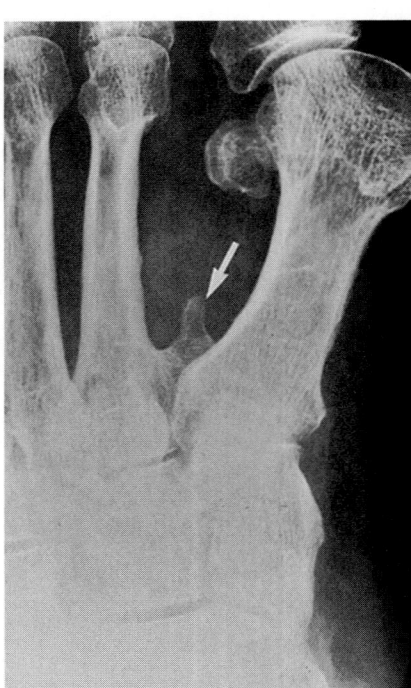

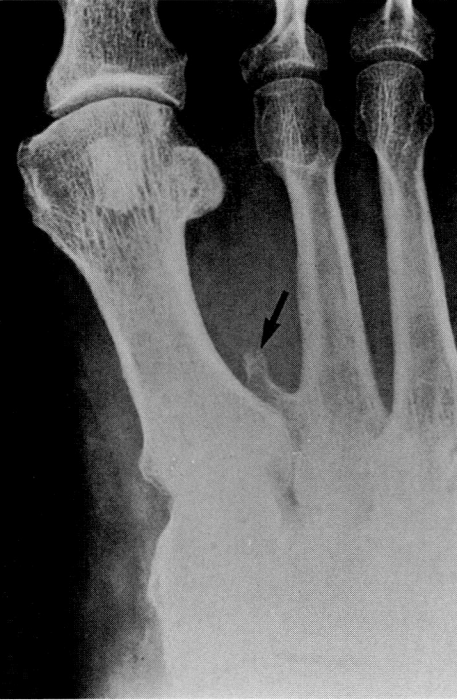

Figure 7–648. Bilateral os intermetatarseum.

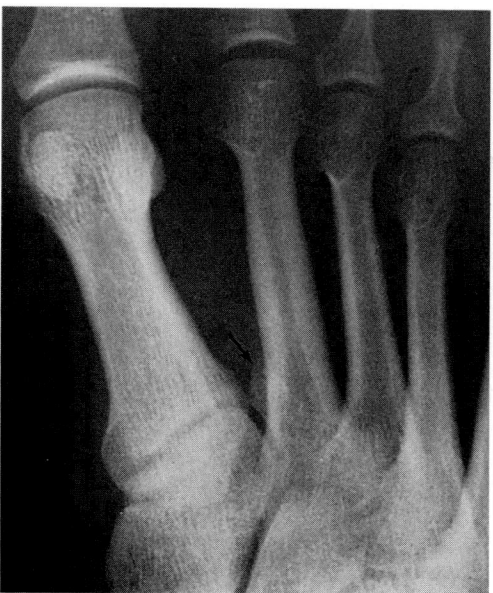

Figure 7–649. Variation in configuration of the os intermetatarseum.

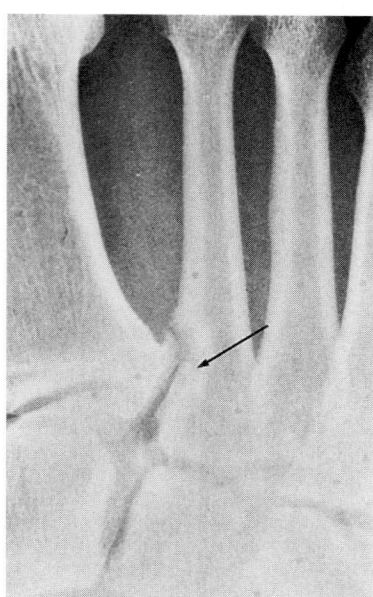

Figure 7–650. Fossa in the base of the second metatarsal secondary to the presence of a small os intermetatarseum.

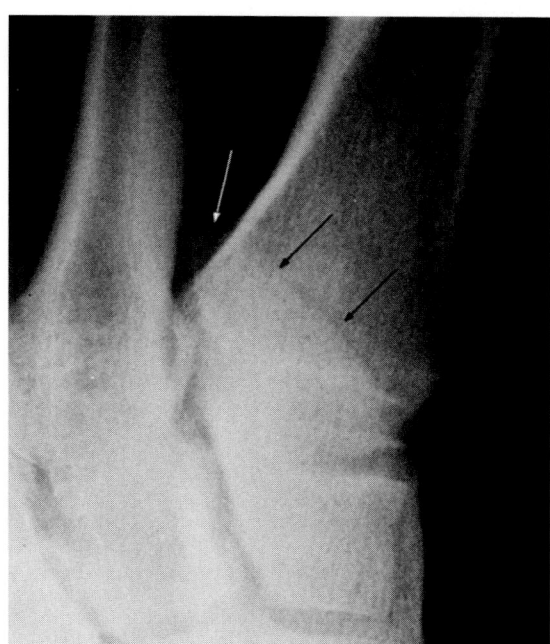

Figure 7–651. Simulated fracture of the first metatarsal, produced by the os intermetatarseum.

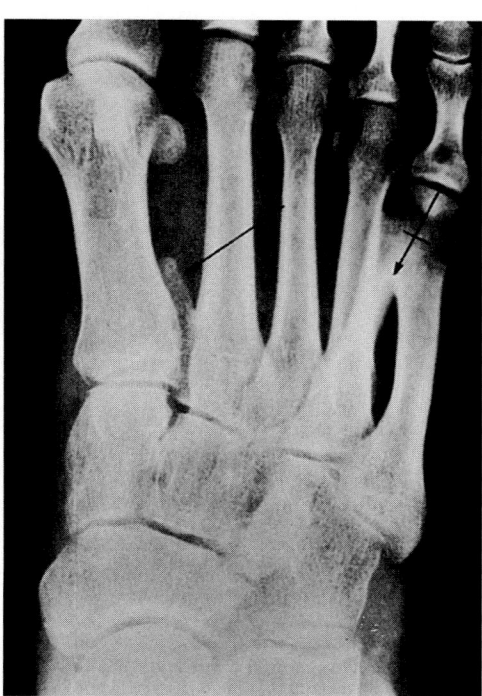

Figure 7–652. Os intermetatarseum (→) and developmental fusion between the fourth and fifth metatarsals (↦).

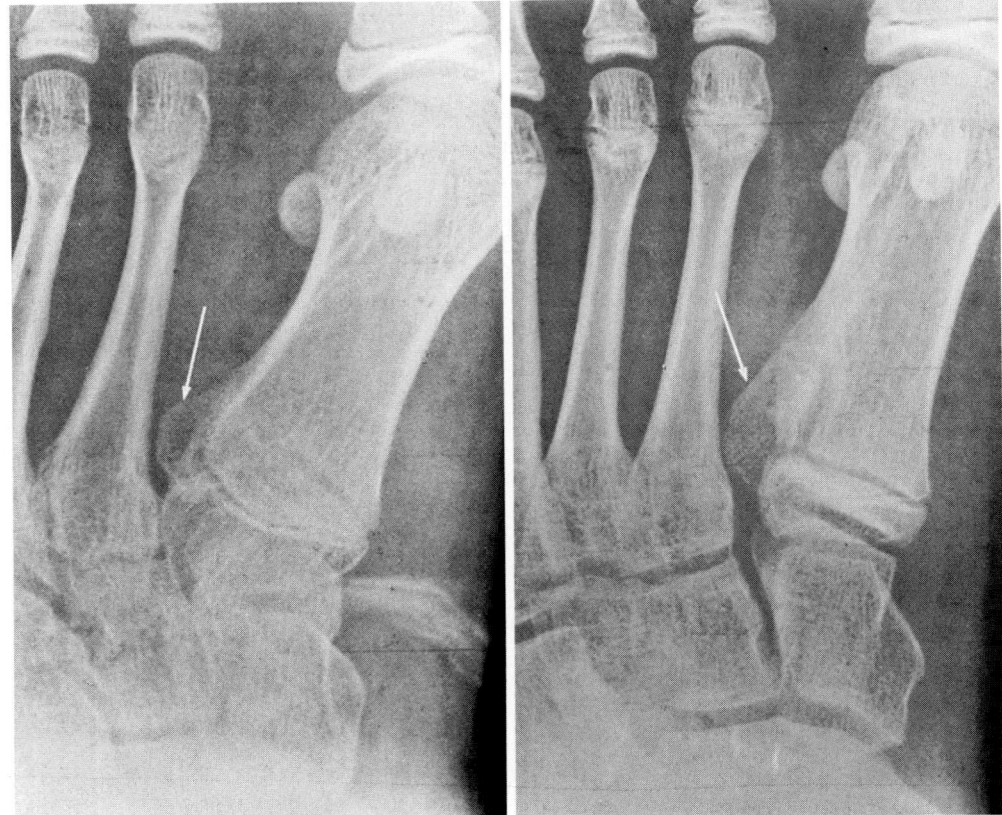

Figure 7–653. Unusual os intermetatarseum.

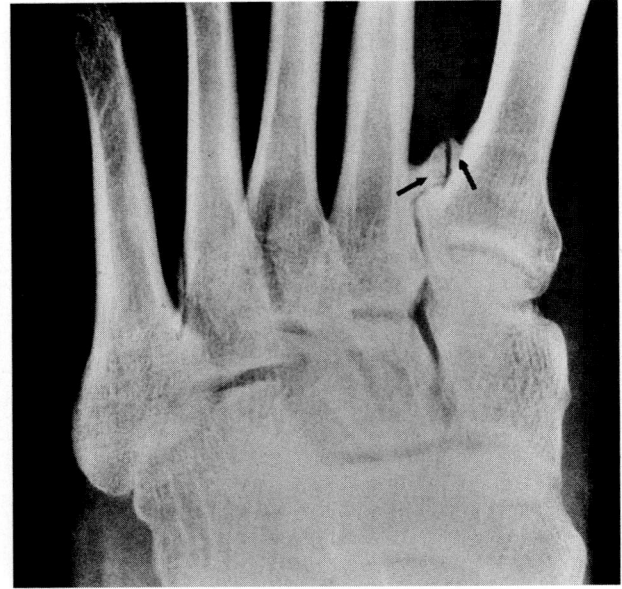

Figure 7–654. Bipartate os intermetatarseum.

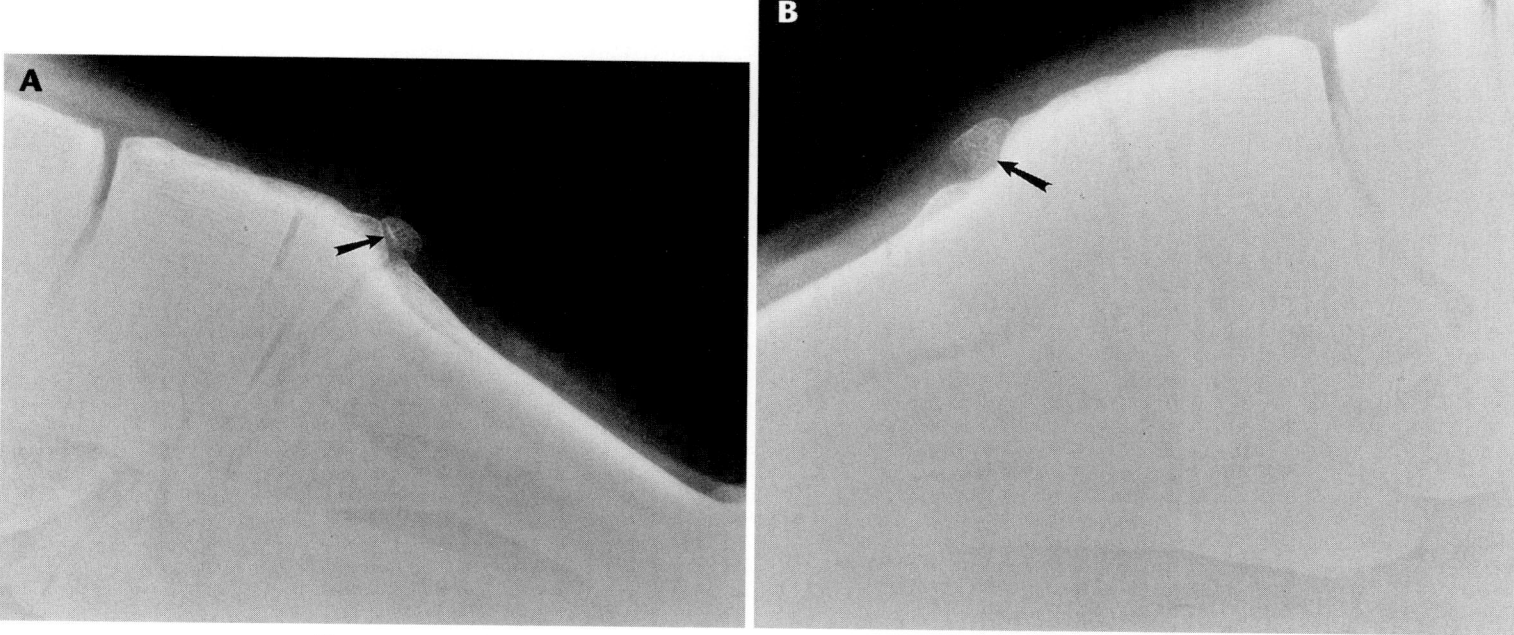

Figure 7–655. A, B, Bilateral os intermetatarseums seen in lateral projection of the feet.

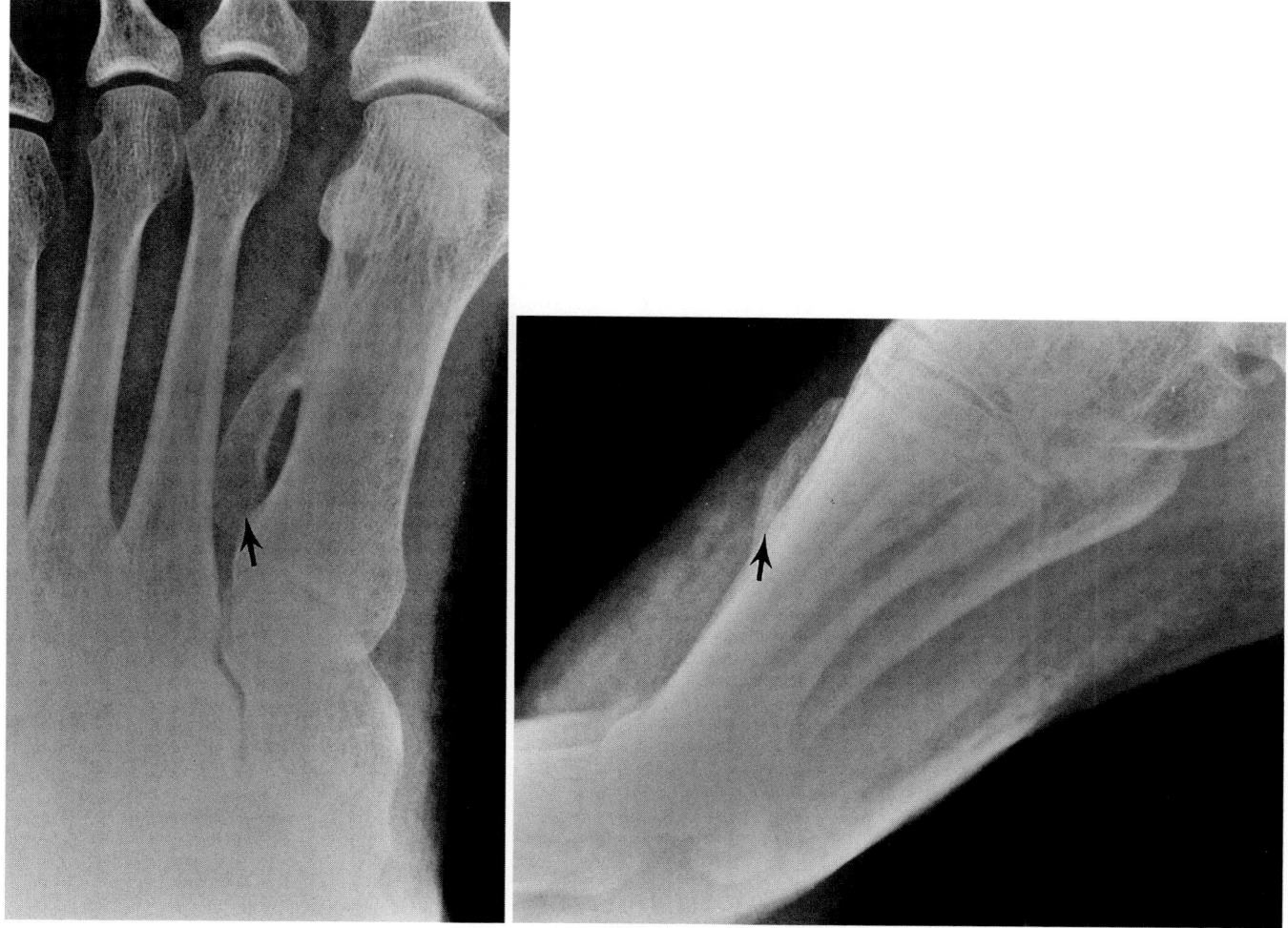

Figure 7–656. An unusual os intermetatarseum.

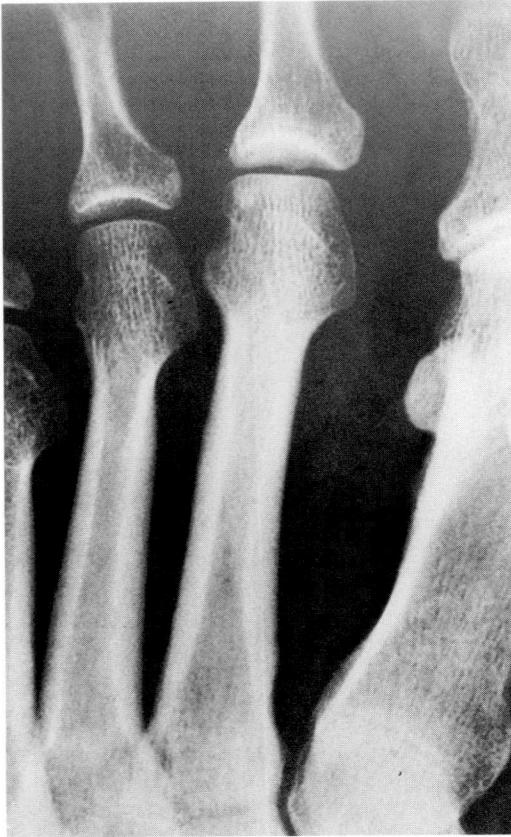

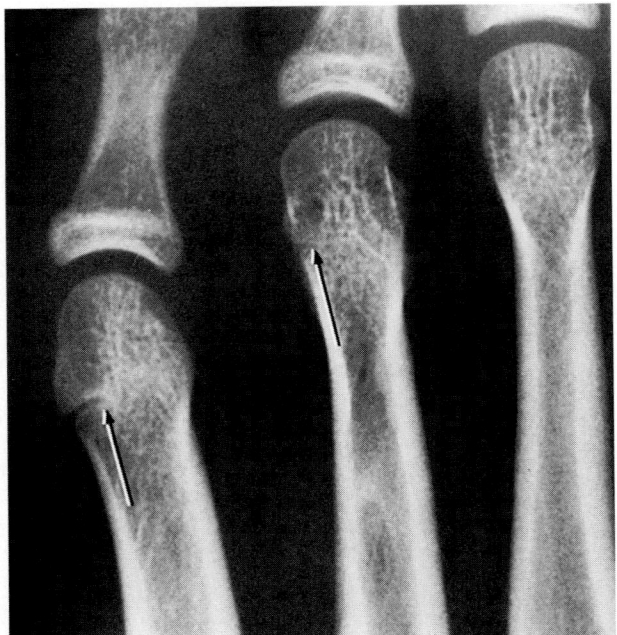

Figure 7–658. Partial closure of the physes of the fourth and fifth metatarsals in a 14-year-old girl.

Figure 7–657. Flat configuration of the head of the second metatarsal and resultant widening of the joint space should not be misconstrued as evidence of aseptic necrosis (Freiberg's disease). (Ref: Jenson EL, de Carvalho A: A normal variant simulating Freiberg's disease. *Acta Radiol* 28:85, 1987.)

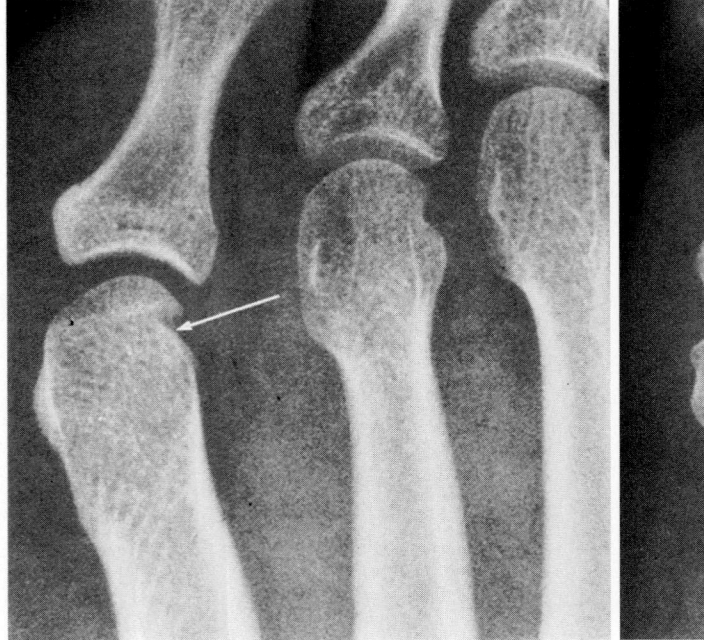

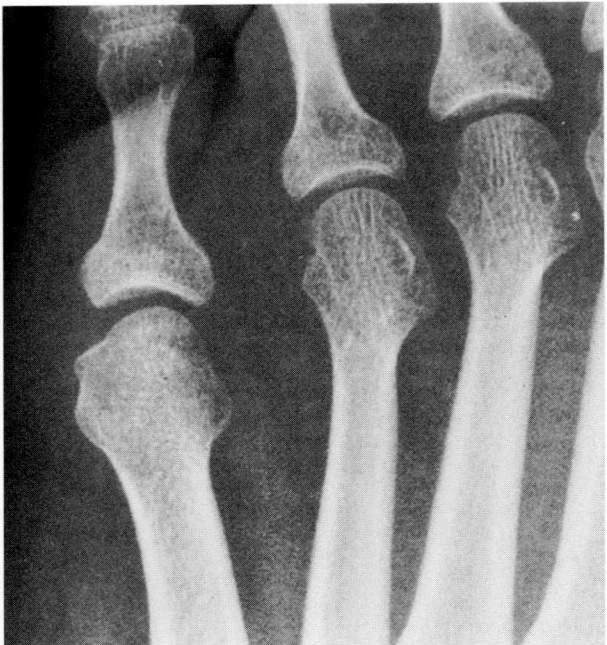

Figure 7–659. *Left,* Deep cleft in the head of the fifth metatarsal in a 23-year-old woman in oblique projection (*arrow*). *Right,* Frontal projection shows unusual configuration of the head of the metatarsal.

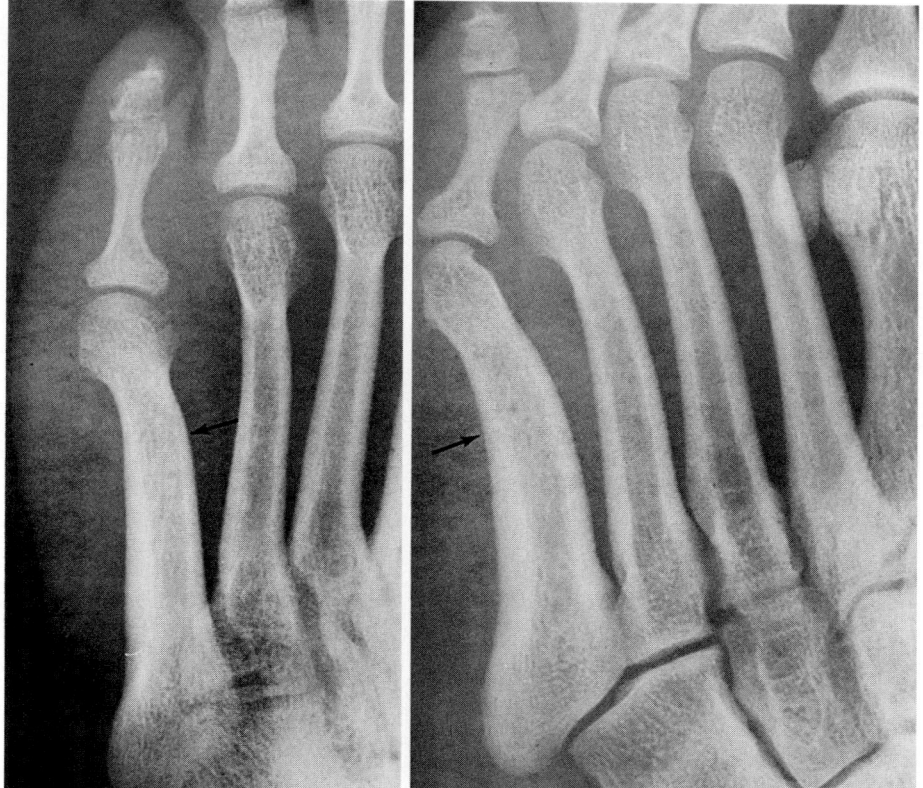

Figure 7–660. Exaggeration of the normal curvature of the fifth metatarsal.

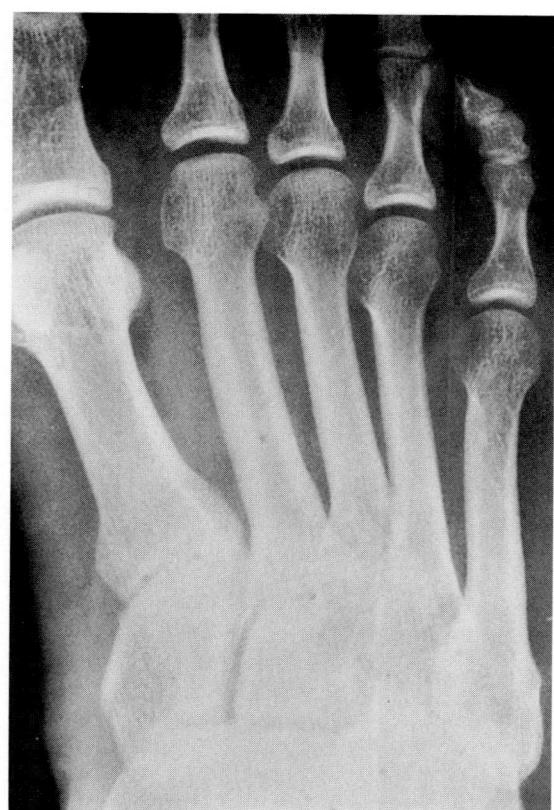

Figure 7–661. Developmentally short fifth metatarsal.

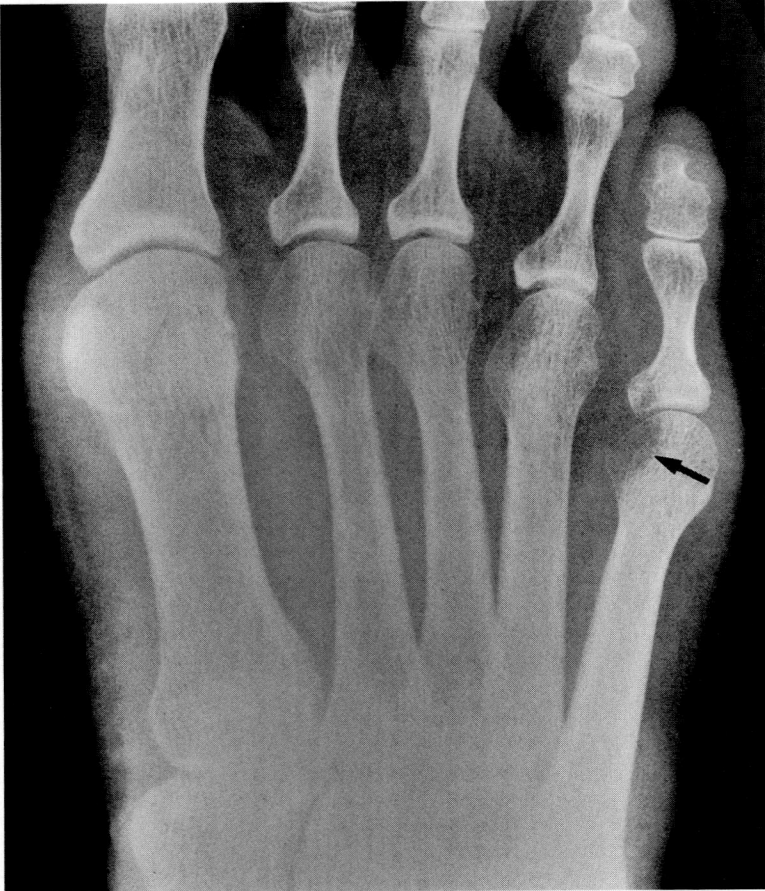

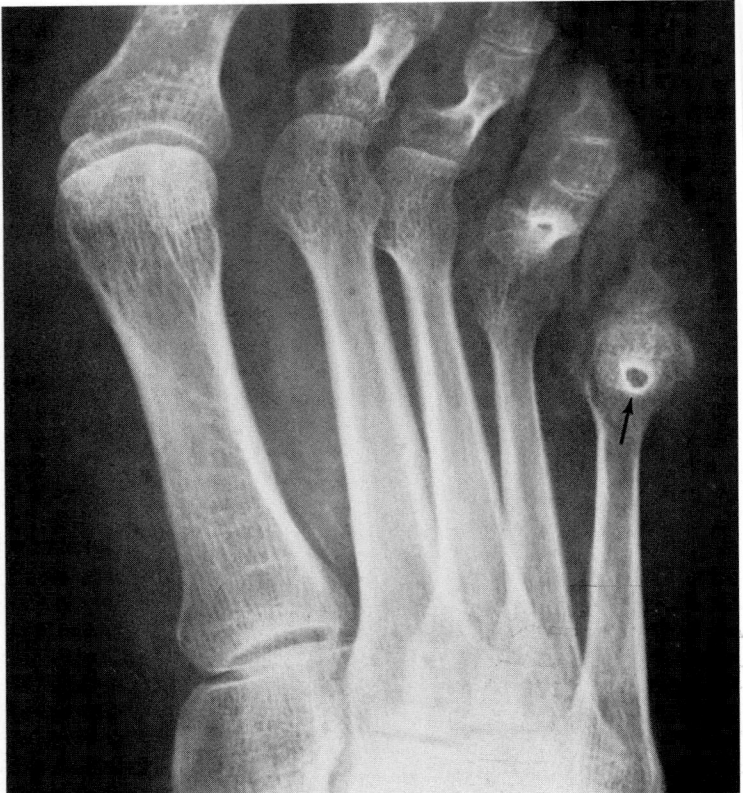

Figure 7–663. Axial projection of the shafts of the proximal phalanges, simulating a cyst in the head of the fifth metatarsal.

Figure 7–662. Normal lucency in the medial aspect of the head of the fifth metatarsal that should not be mistaken for an erosion.

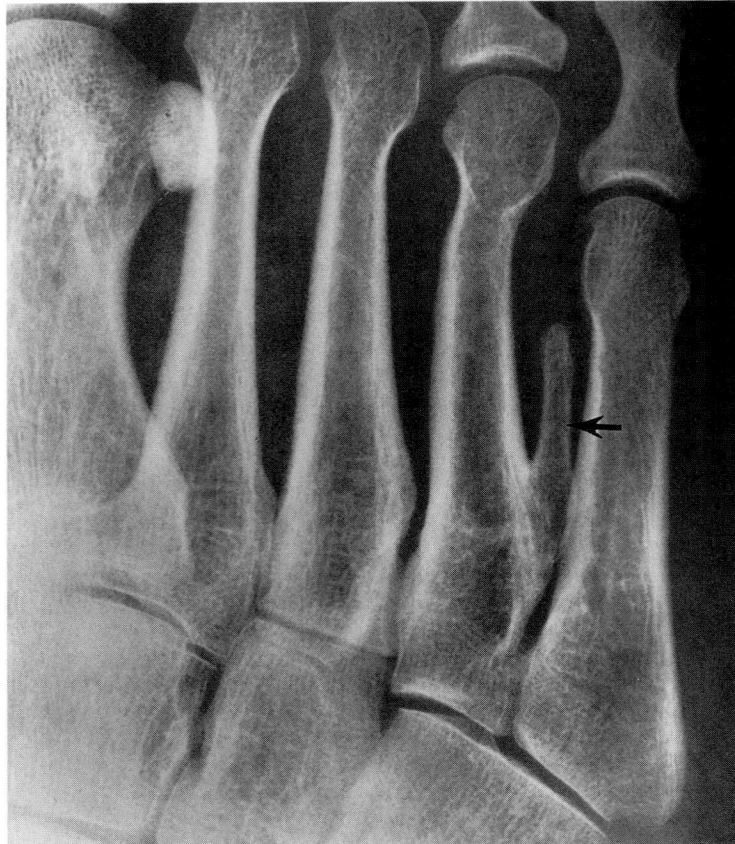

Figure 7–664. Duplication of the fourth metatarsal.

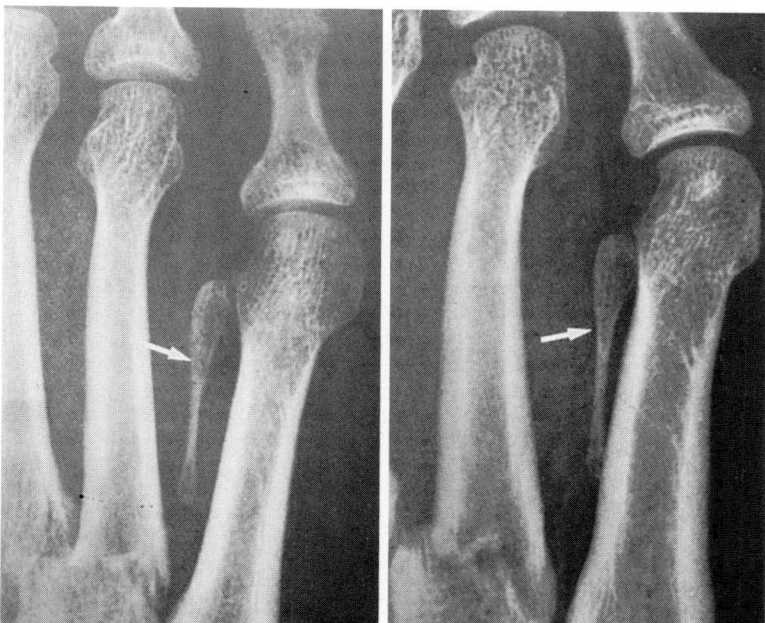

Figure 7–665. Supernumerary metatarsal between the fourth and fifth metatarsals.

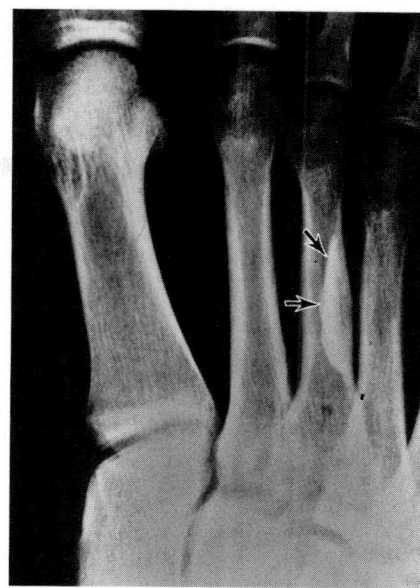

Figure 7–666. Healed benign cortical deficit of the third metatarsal.

Figure 7–667. A, B, An additional example of a healed benign cortical defect of the metatarsal.

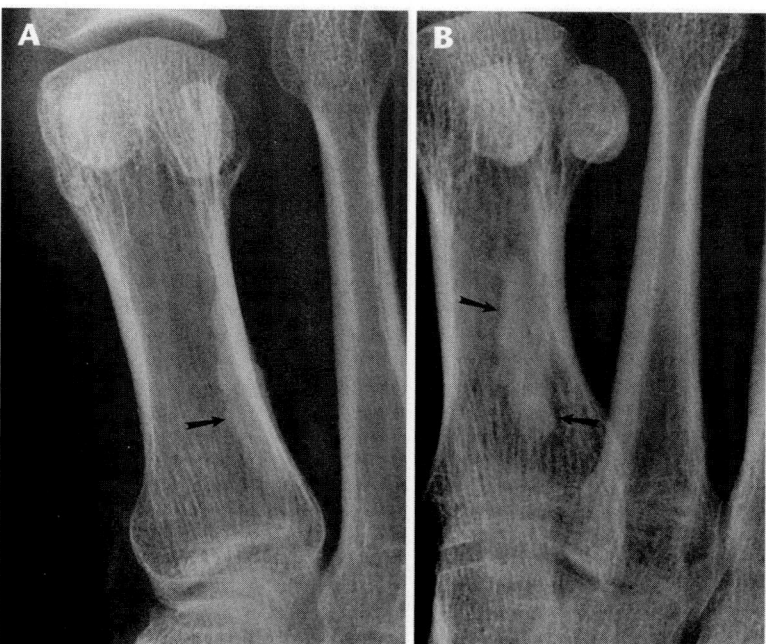

The Sesamoid Bones

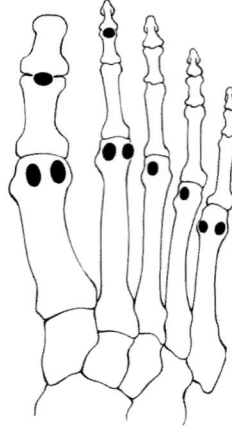

Figure 7–668. The sesamoid bones of the foot. (Refs: Kohler A, Zimmer EA: *Borderlands of the normal and early pathologic findings in skeletal roentgenology,* 3rd ed. New York, Grune & Stratton, 1968; Potter G et al: The hallux sesamoids revisited. *Skeletal Radiol* 21:437, 1992.)

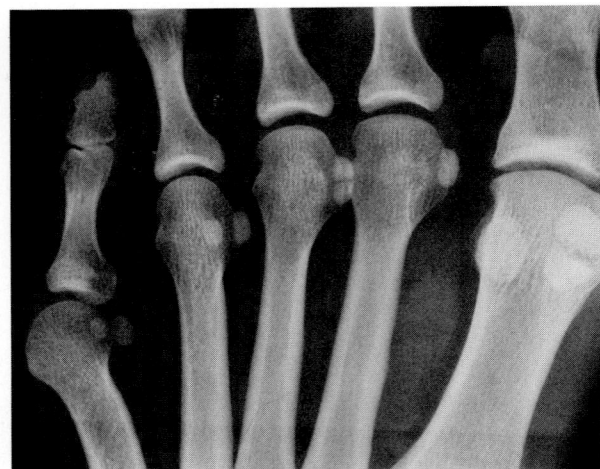
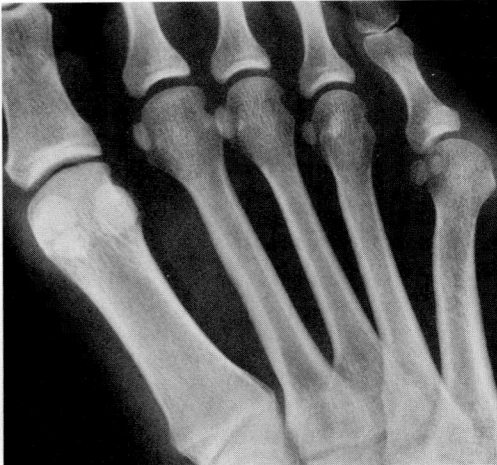

Figure 7–669. Multiple sesamoids of both feet.

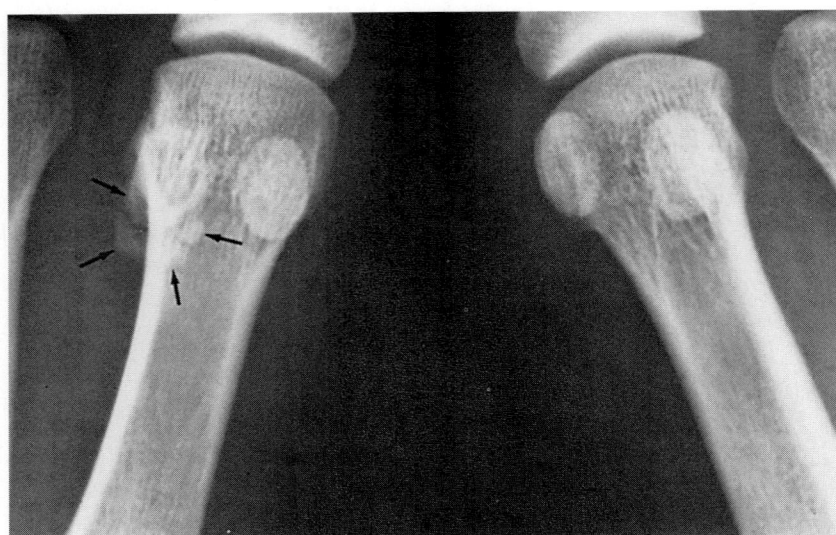

Figure 7–670. Multipartite sesamoid bone, simulating a comminuted fracture.

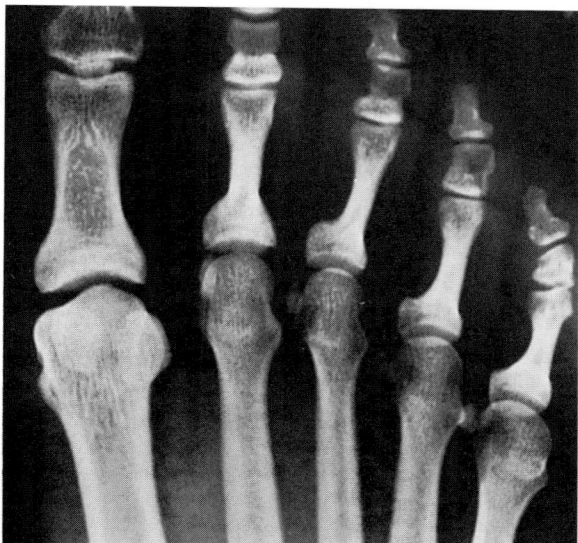

Figure 7–671. Multiple sesamoids of the metatarsal heads.

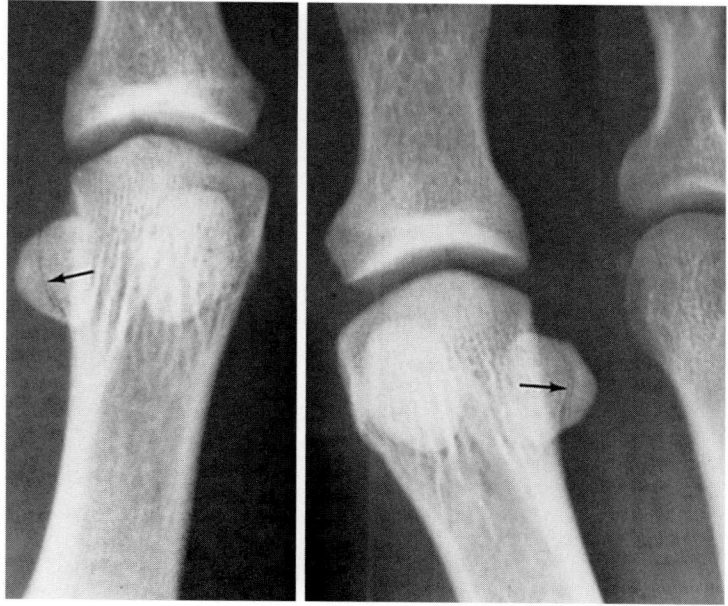

Figure 7–672. Fissure-like lucencies in the sesamoids of the first toes, simulating fractures.

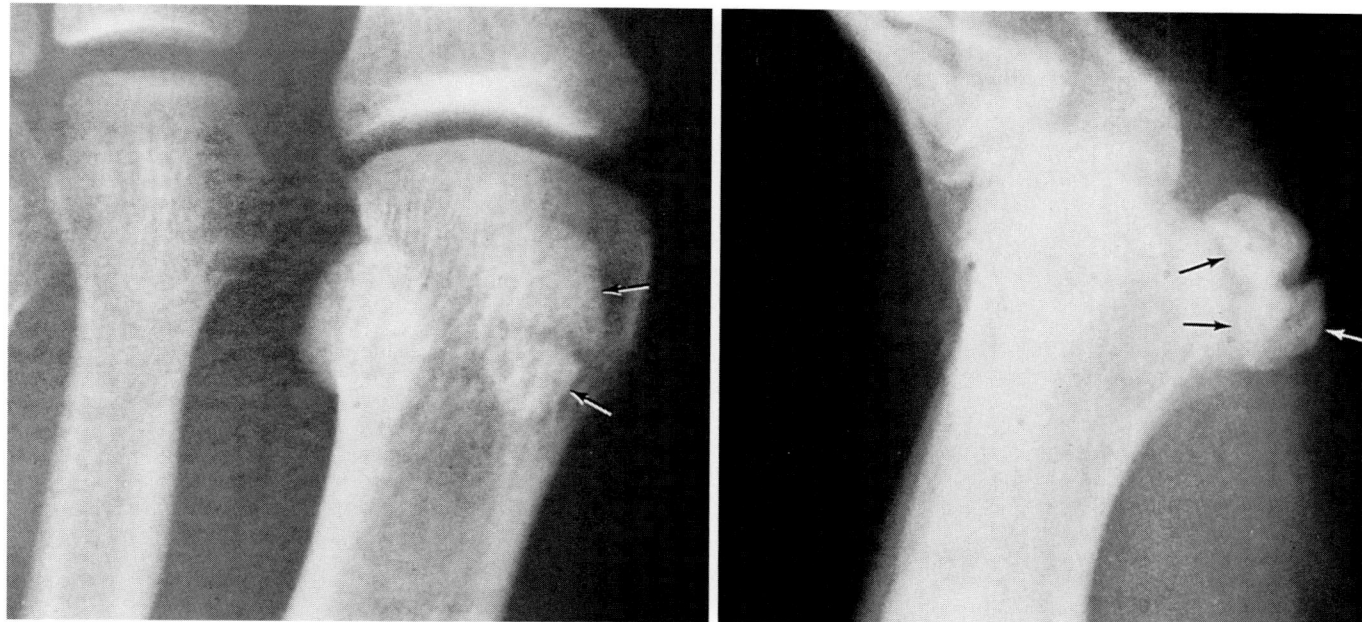

Figure 7–673. Frontal and lateral projections of a bipartite sesamoid bone of the first toe, with equal size of the members. (Ref: Feldman F et al: The case of the wandering sesamoid and other sesamoid afflictions. *Radiology* 96:275, 1970.)

Figure 7–674. Developing sesamoids in a 12-year-old boy, seen in lateral projection.

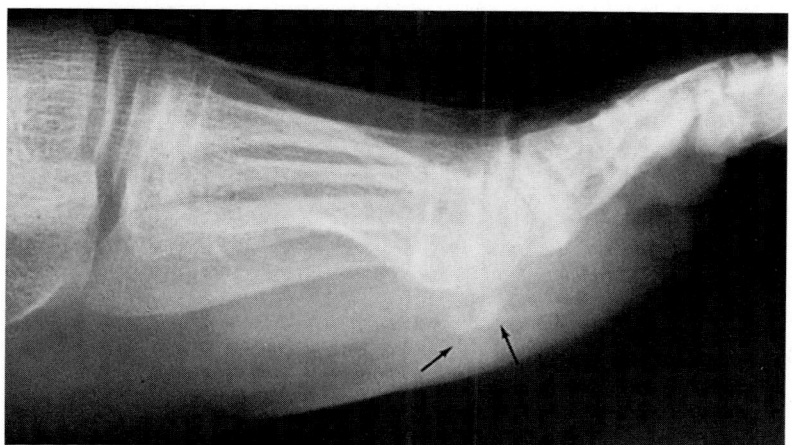

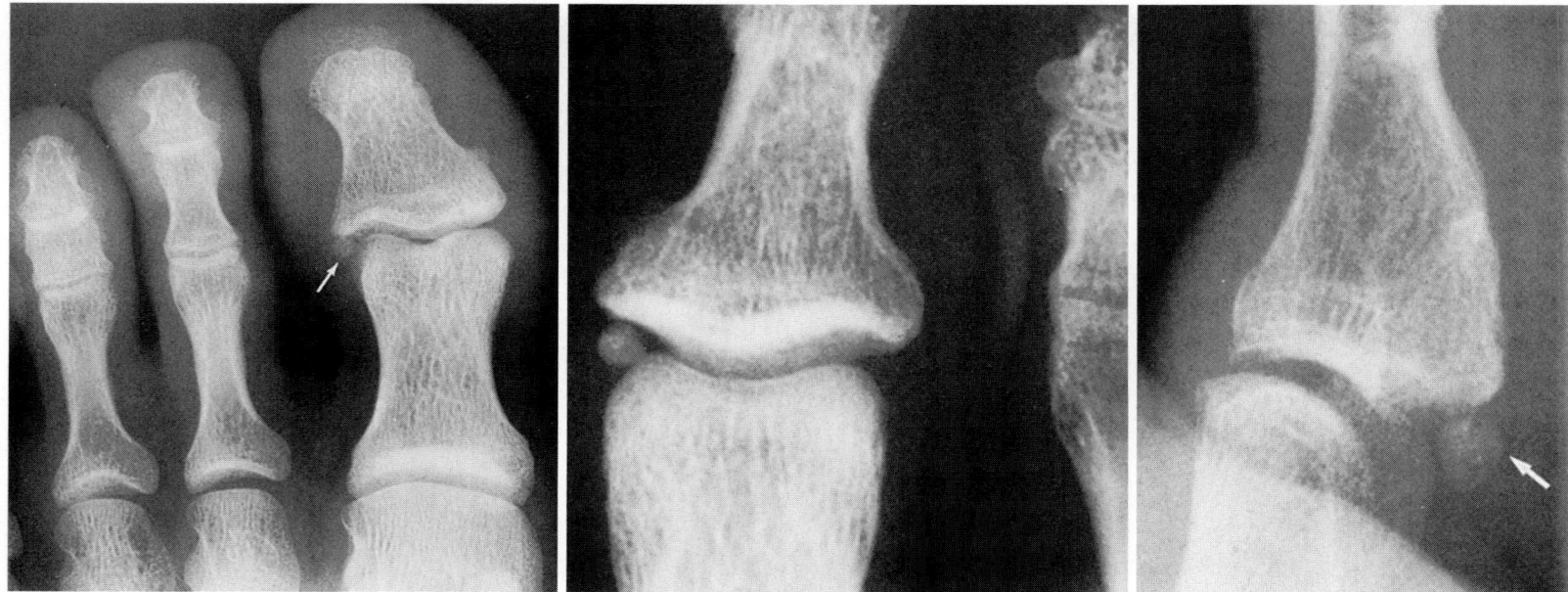

Figure 7–675. Three examples of sesamoids at the distal interphalangeal joint of the first toe.

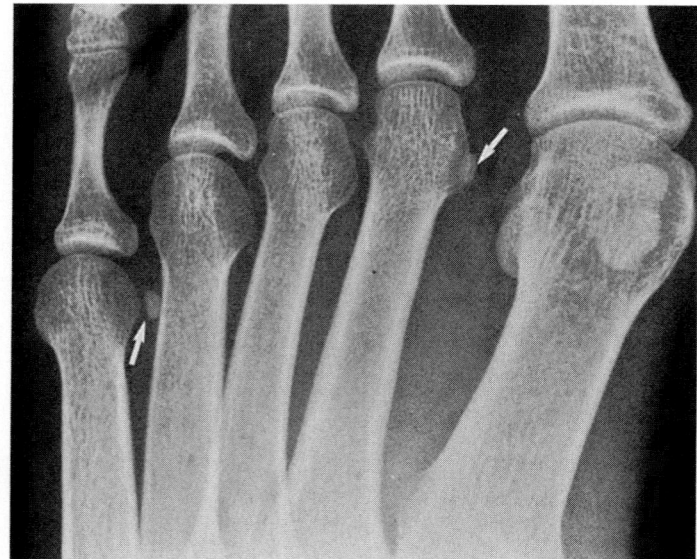

Figure 7–676. Sesamoids at the second and fifth metatarsal heads.

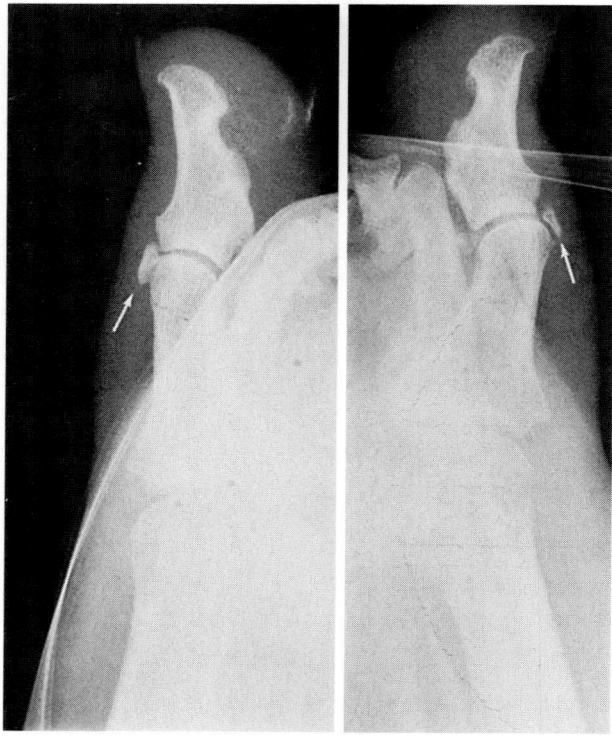

Figure 7–677. Bony ossicles, resembling sesamoids, on the dorsal aspect of both interphalangeal joints of the great toes in a 36-year-old woman.

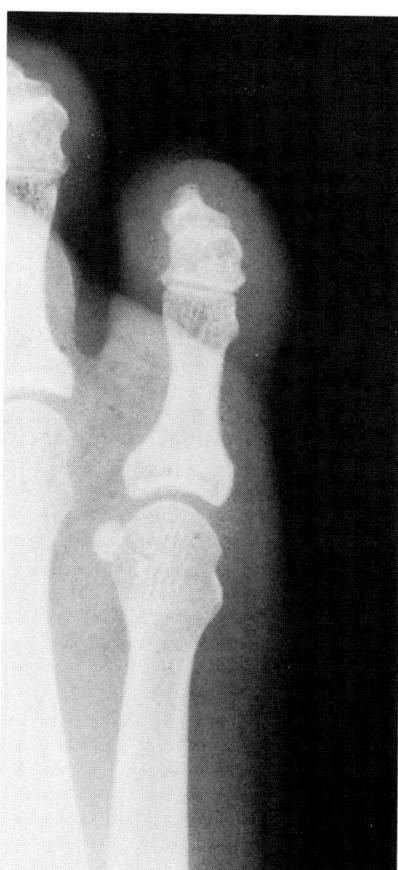

Figure 7–678. Sesamoid at the fifth metatarsophalangeal joint.

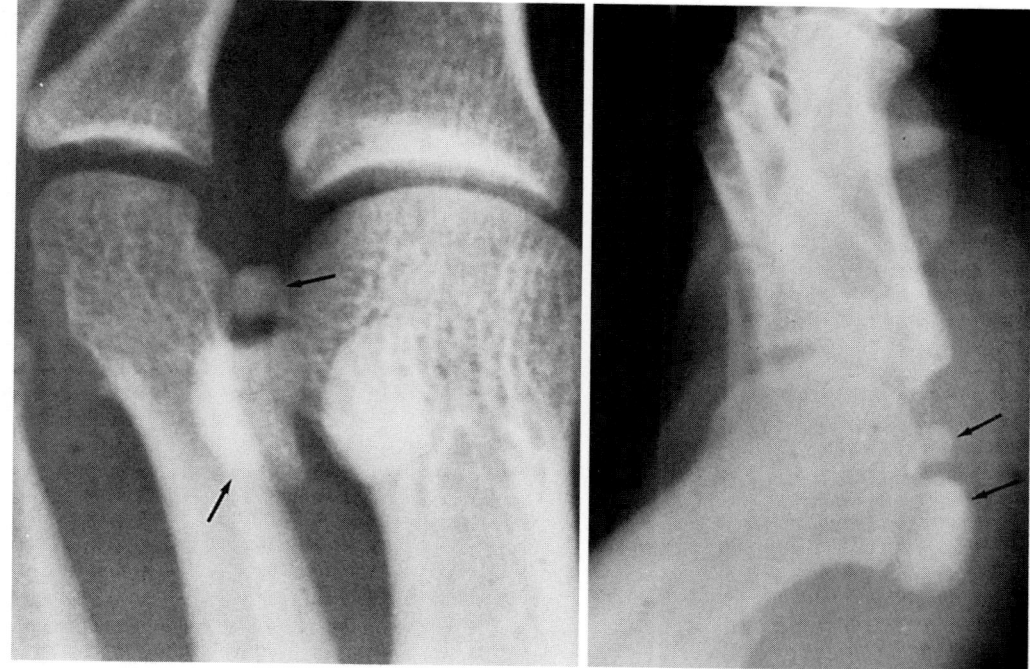

Figure 7–679. Bipartite sesamoid of the first toe, with unequal size of the members.

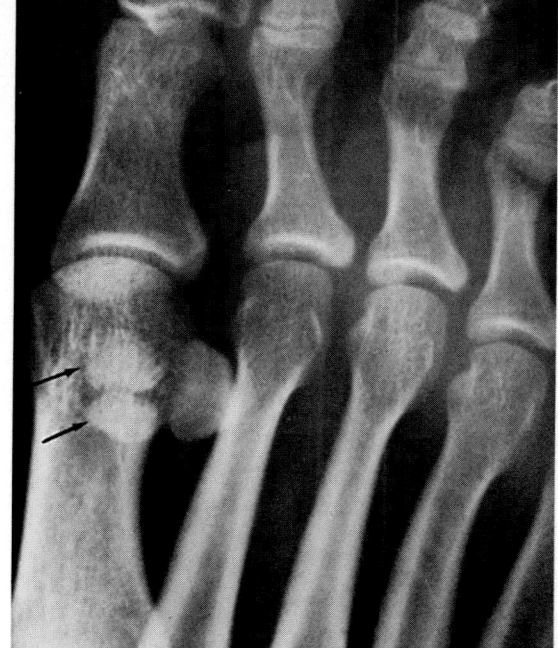

Figure 7–680. Symmetric oval bipartite sesamoids of the first toe.

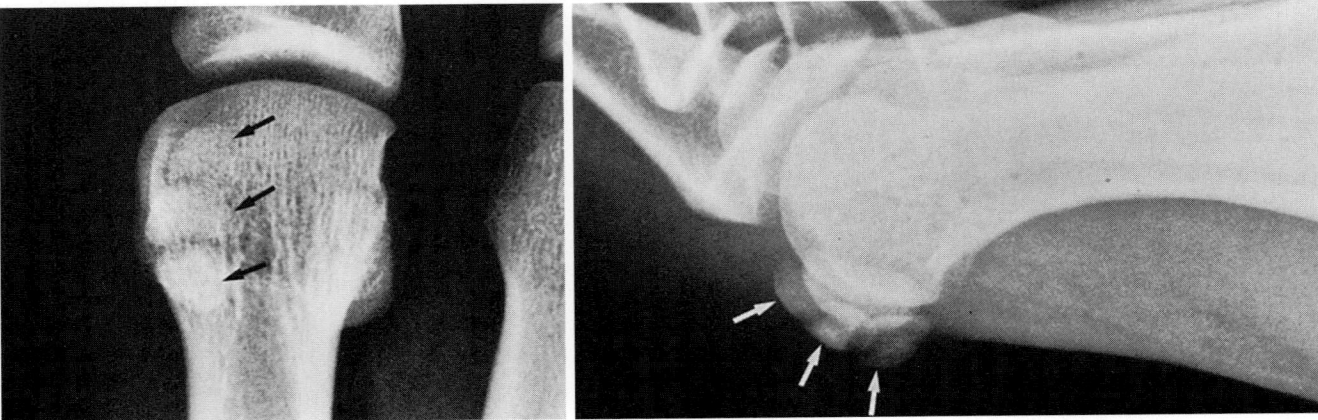

Figure 7–681. Tripartite sesamoid of the first toe.

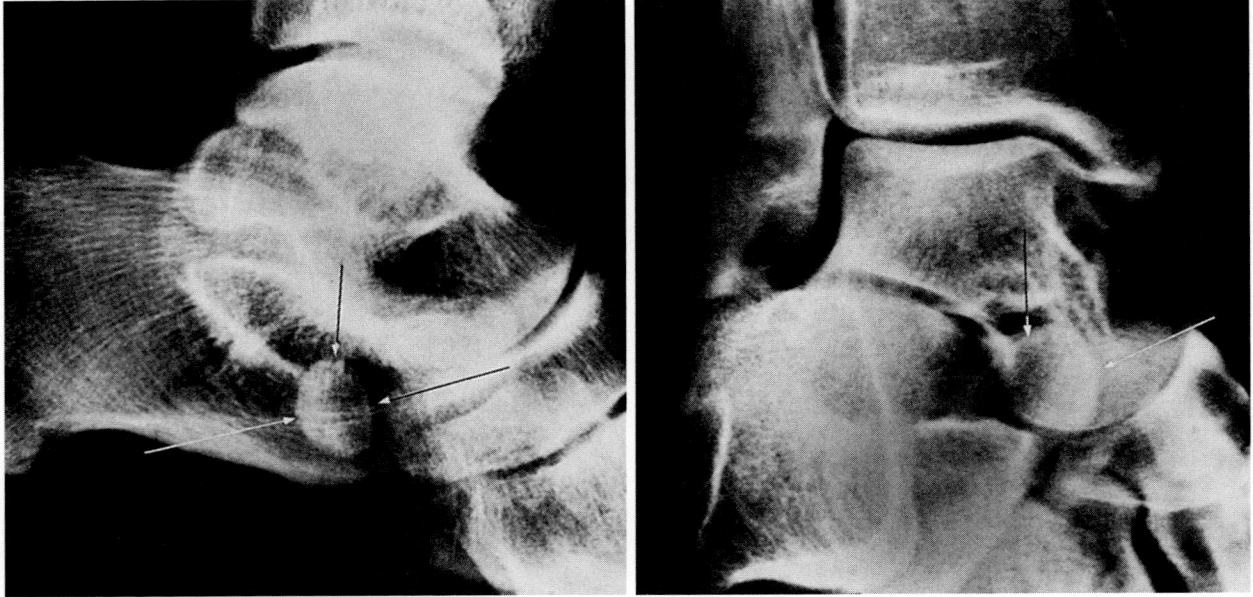

Figure 7–682. Large sesamoid bone in the tibialis posterior tendon or an os sustentaculum tali.

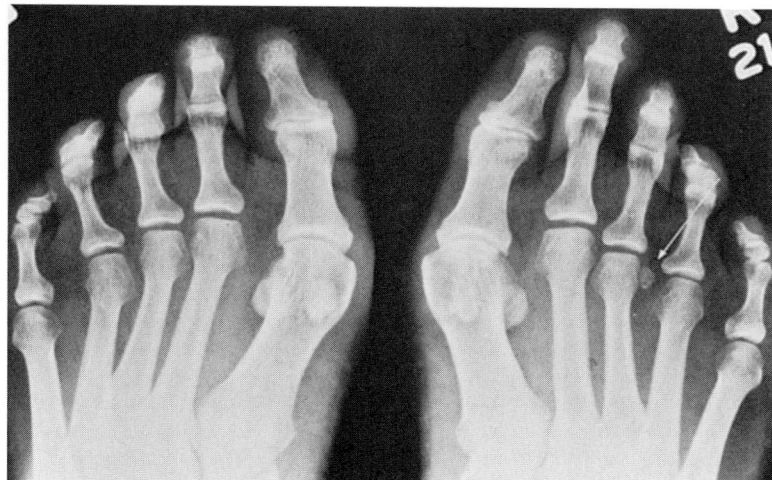

Figure 7–683. Isolated sesamoid at the head of the third metatarsal.

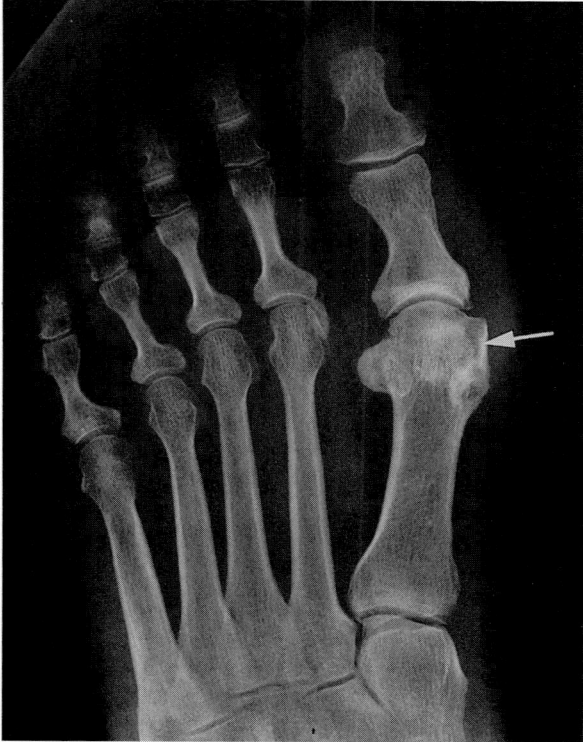

Figure 7–684. Prominent facet for the medial sesamoid at the first metatarsal (*arrow*).

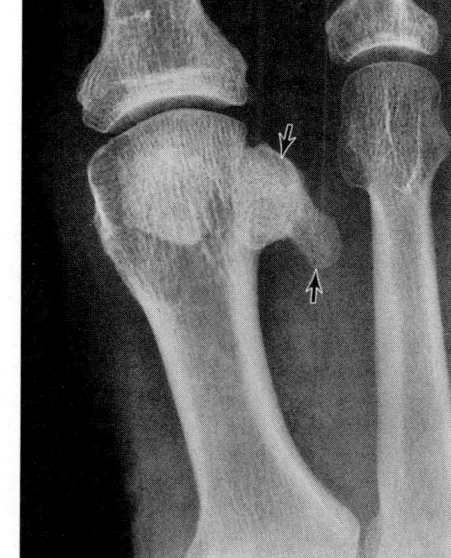

Figure 7–685. Unusual sesamoid at the head of the first metatarsal.

The Toes

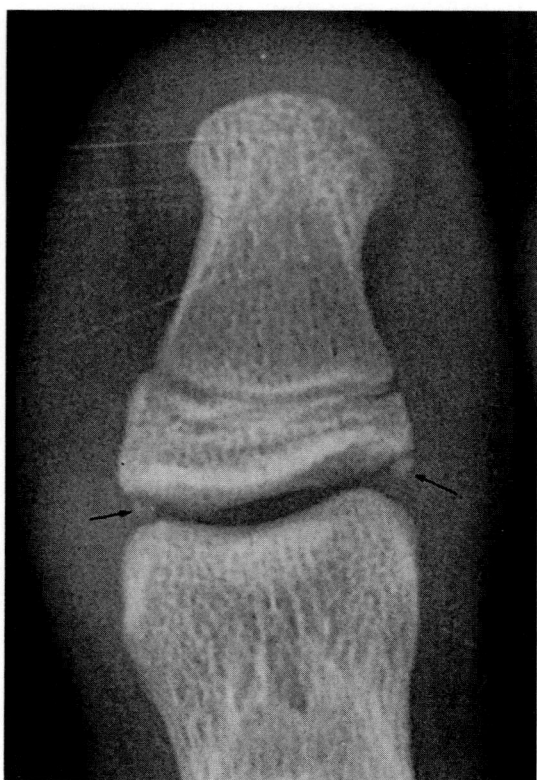

Figure 7–686. Accessory ossification centers at the base of the distal phalanx of the first toe in a 10-year-old boy.

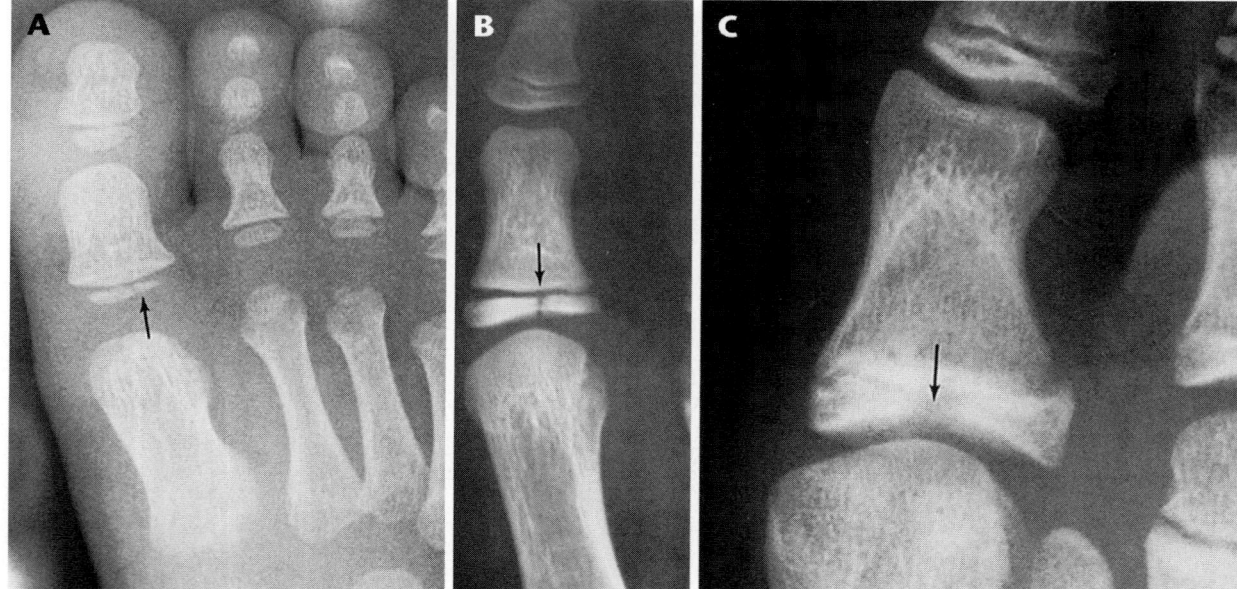

Figure 7–687. Divided epiphysis at the base of the proximal phalanx of the first toe (not a fracture). **A,** 3-year-old boy. **B,** 11-year-old boy. **C,** 13-year-old boy. (Ref: Lyritis C: Developmental disorders of the proximal epiphysis of the hallux. *Skeletal Radiol* 10:250, 1983.)

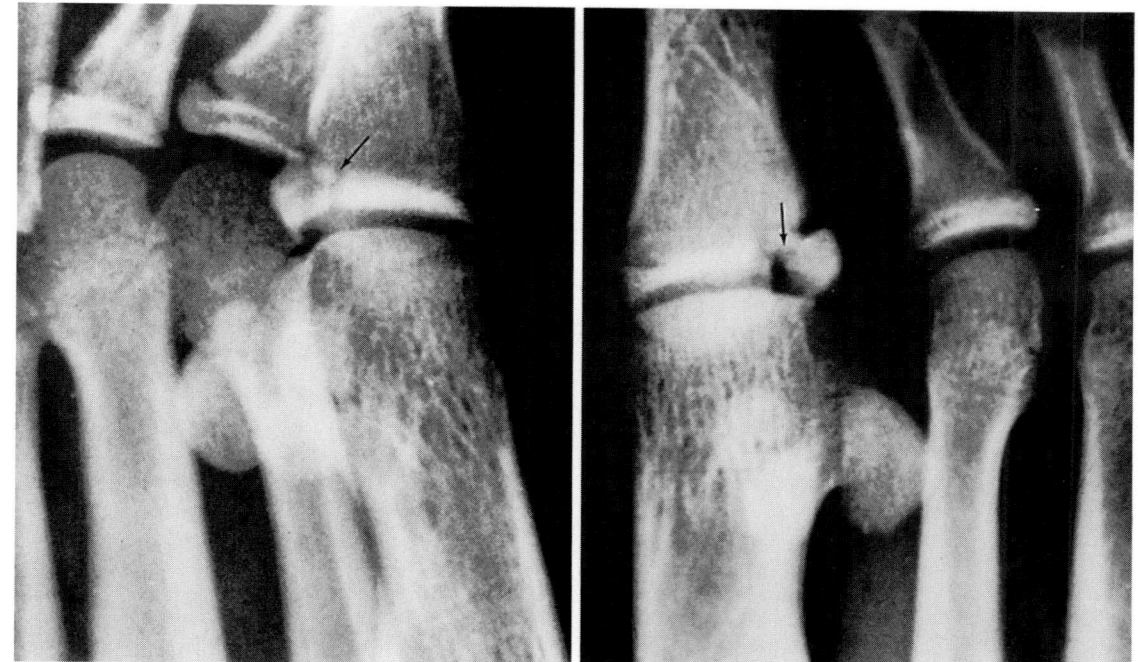

Figure 7–688. Sixteen-year-old boy with cleft in the ossification center at the base of the proximal phalanx of the first toe, in the plane opposite to that of Figure 7–687.

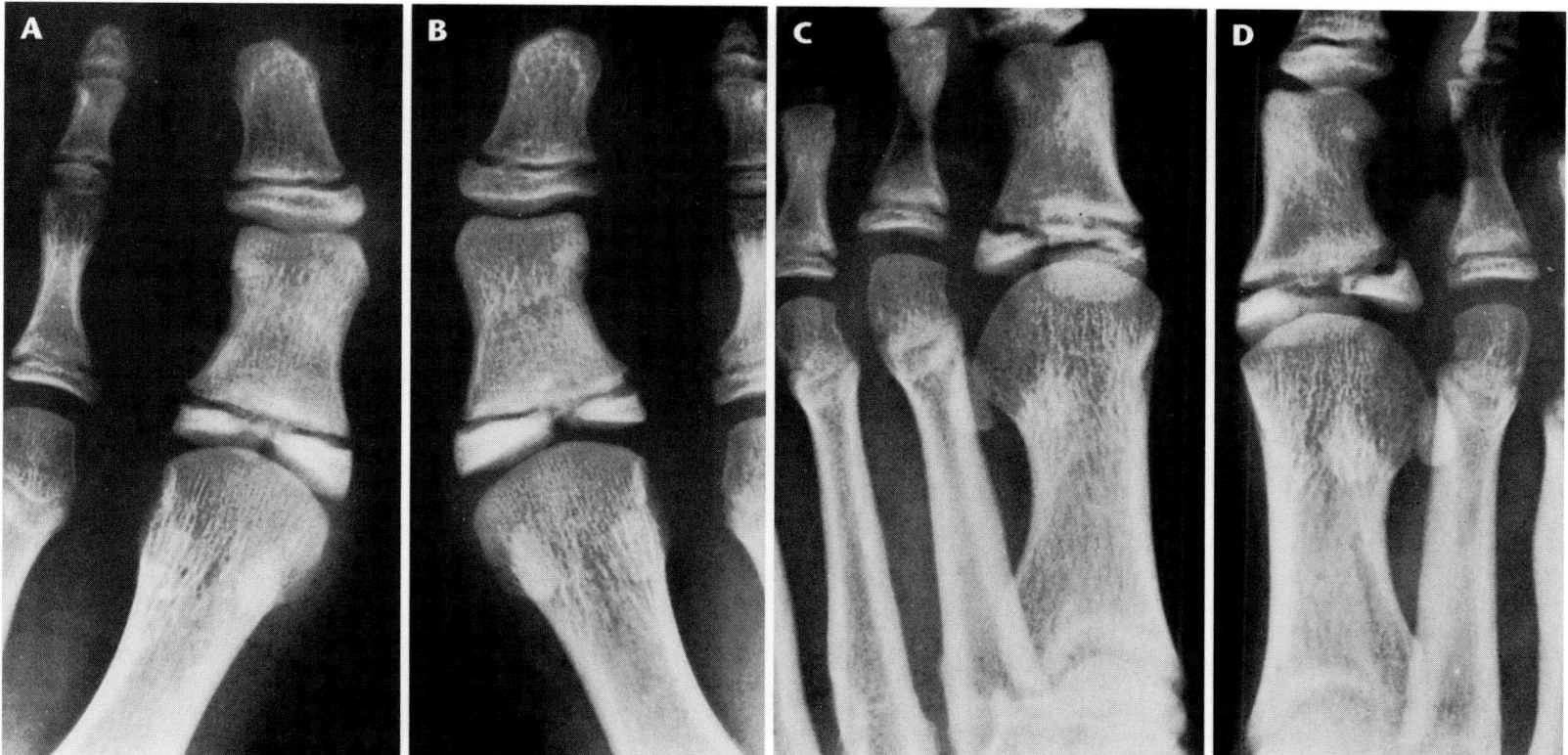

Figure 7–689. A and **B,** Bilateral cleft epiphyses of the proximal phalanges of the first toes. **C** and **D,** The appearance in the oblique projection could be mistaken for a comminuted fracture.

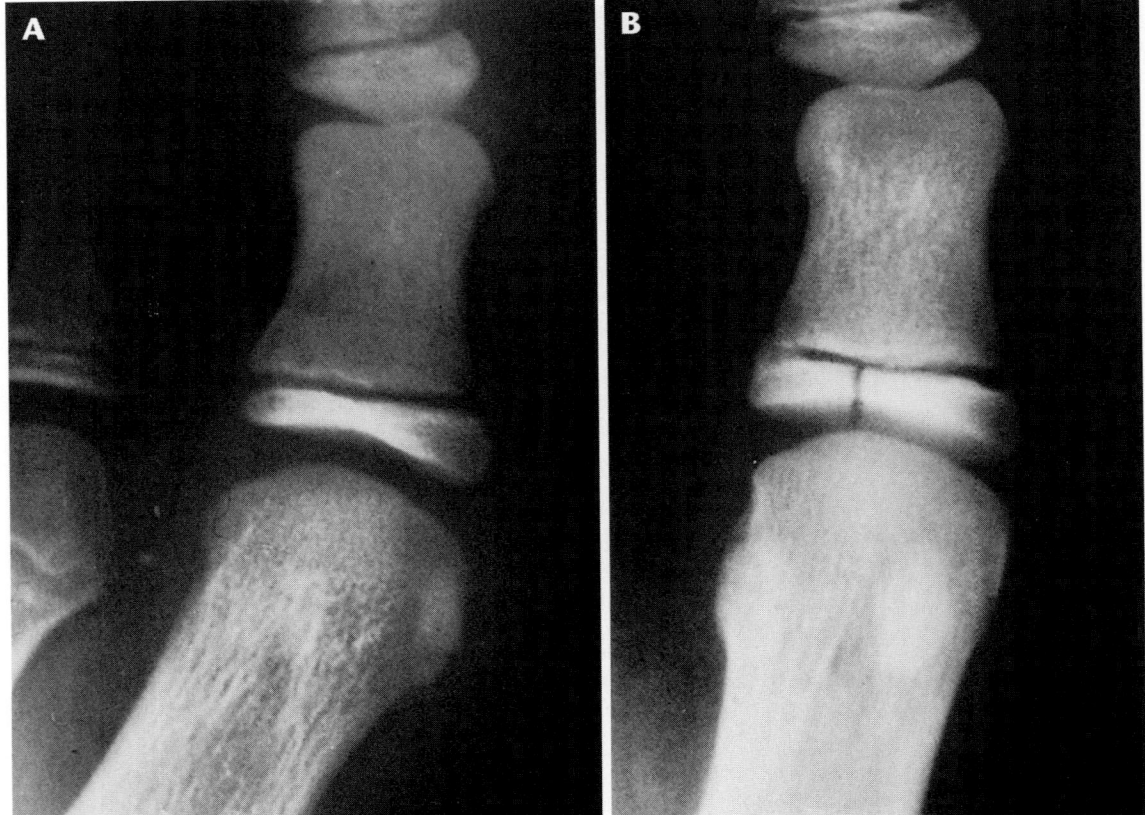

Figure 7–690. A, Single ossification centers at the base of the first toe in an 11-year-old boy. **B,** One year later, the epiphysis has developed a cleft. This is a normal phenomenon that may be seen in any epiphysis. (Ref: Harrison RB, Keats TE: The cleft epiphysis. *Skeletal Radiol* 5:23, 1980.)

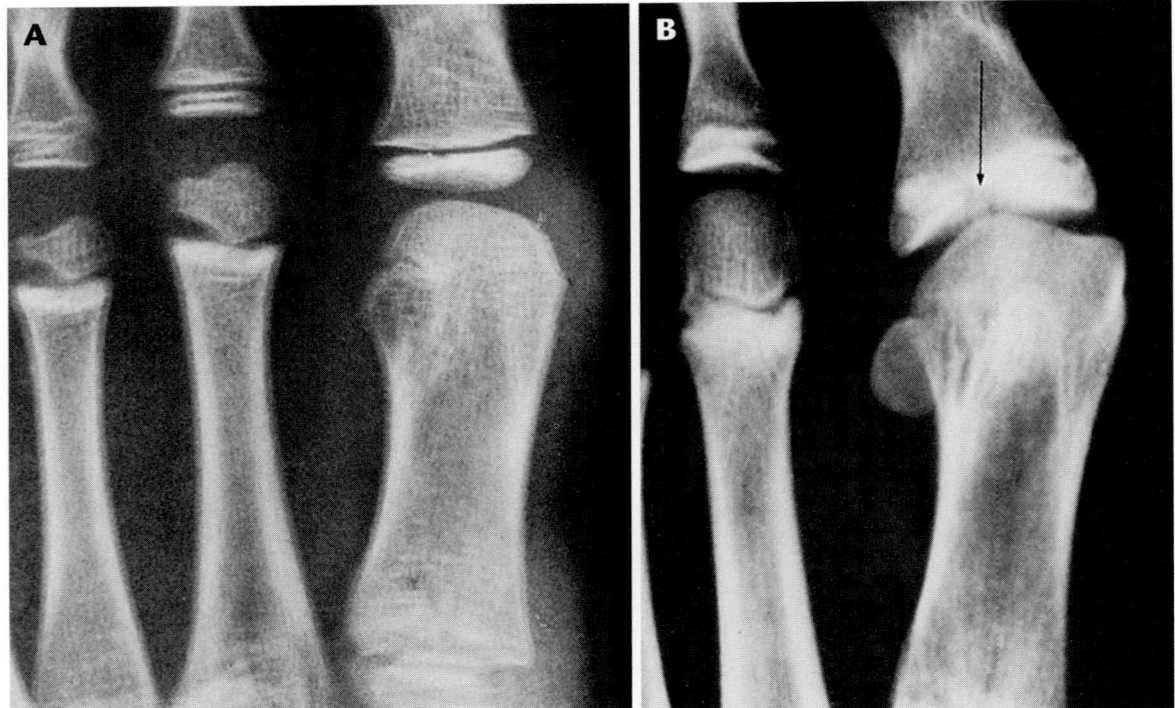

Figure 7–691. Development of cleft epiphysis. **A,** Age 3. **B,** Age 13.

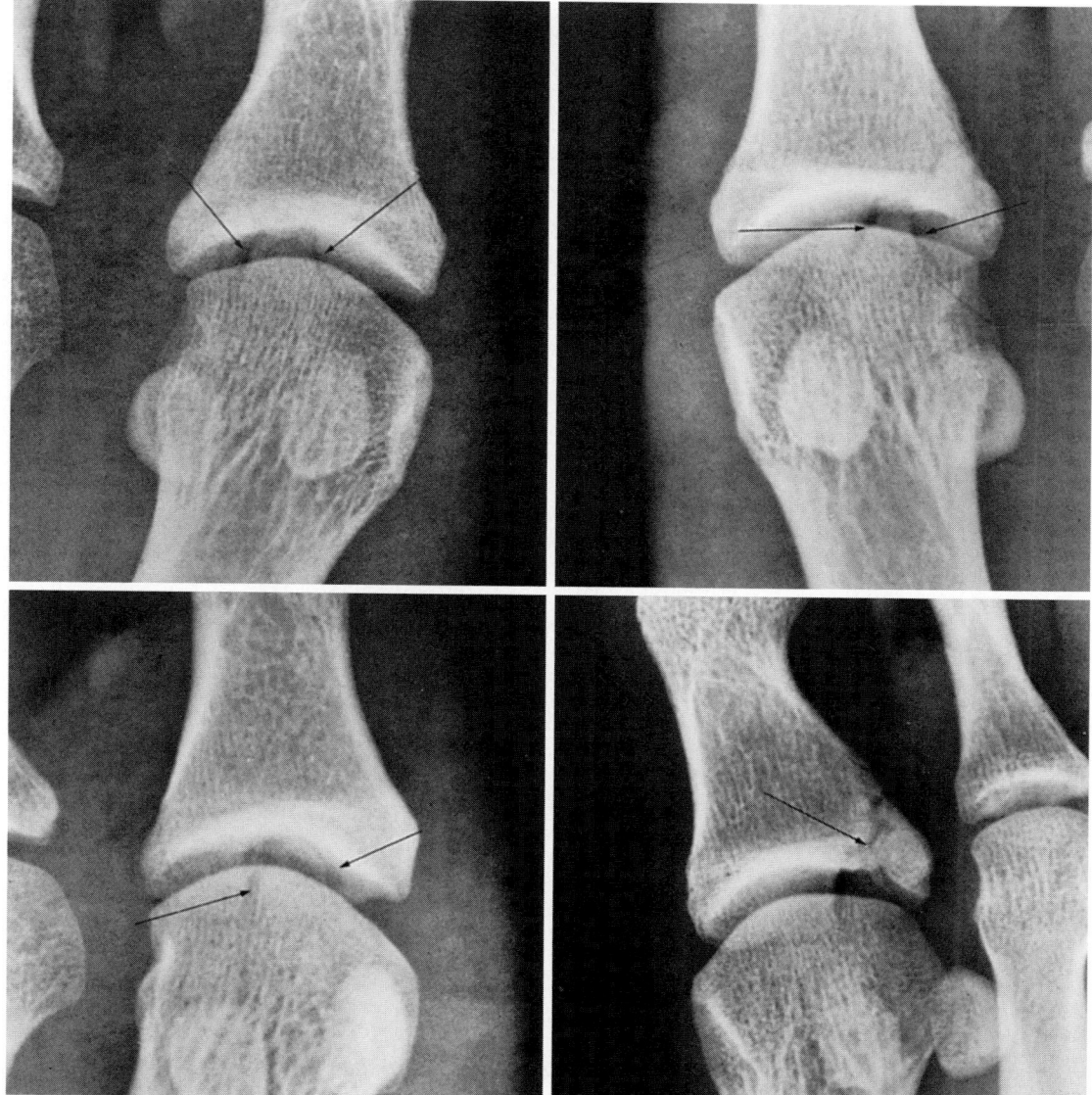

Figure 7–692. Bilateral persistence of the type of cleft epiphysis illustrated in Figure 7–691.

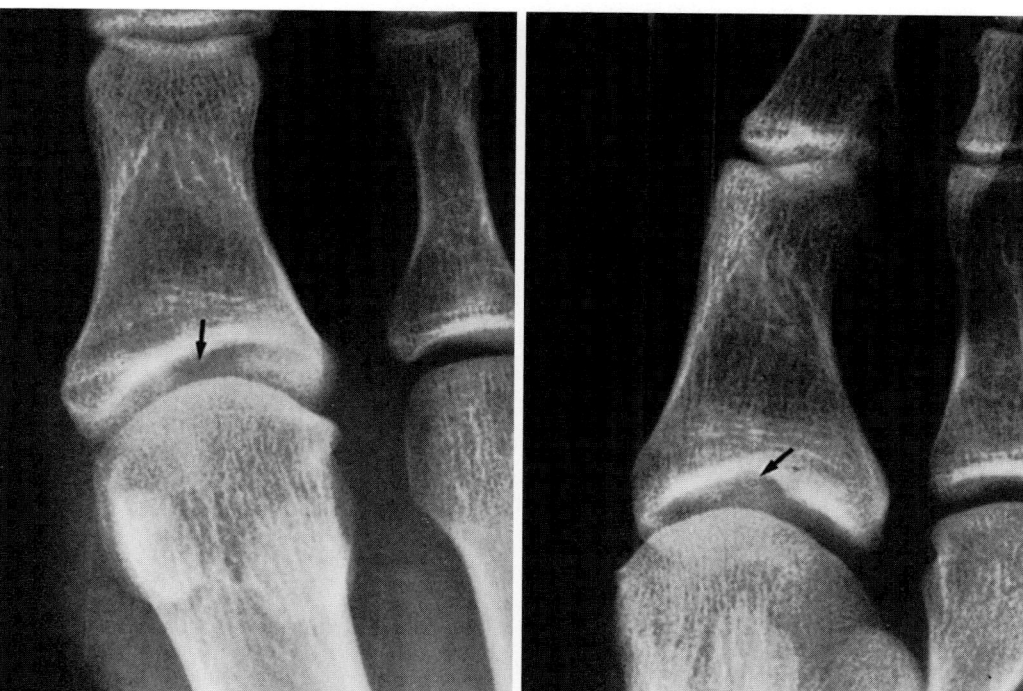

Figure 7–693. Fossa in the base of the proximal phalanx of the first toe, possibly related to residual of cleft epiphysis.

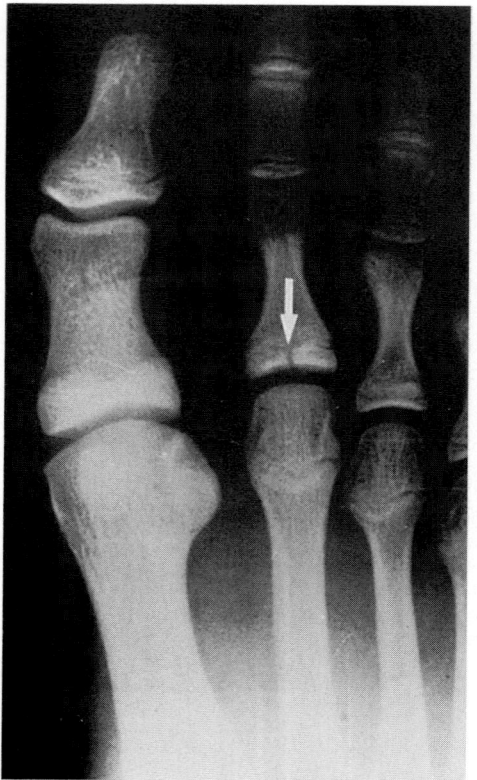

Figure 7–694. Cleft epiphysis of the base of the proximal phalanx of the second toe.

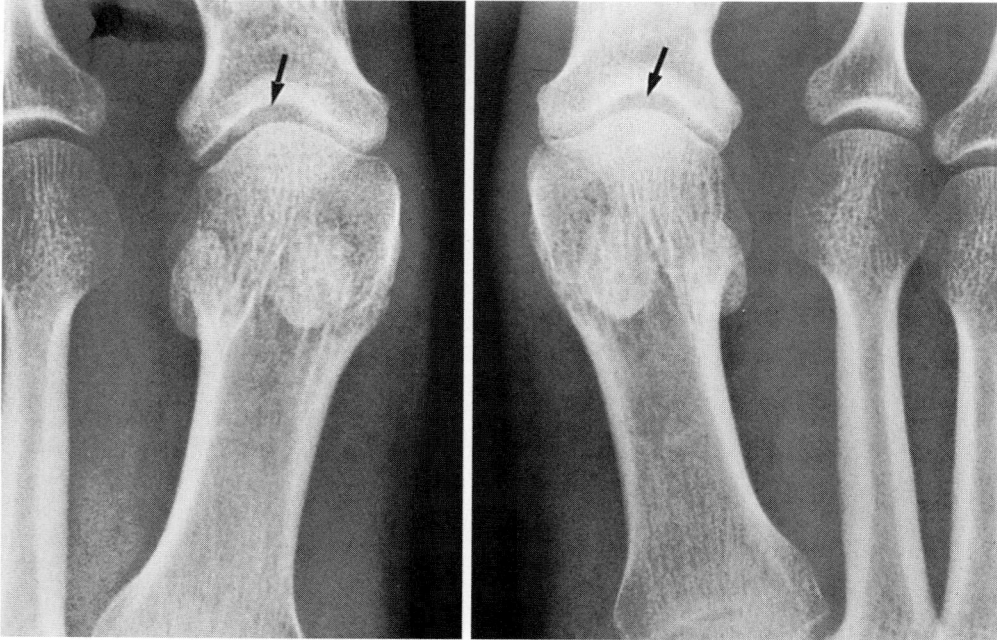

Figure 7–695. Unusually deep fossae bilaterally at the bases of the proximal phalanges of the first toes.

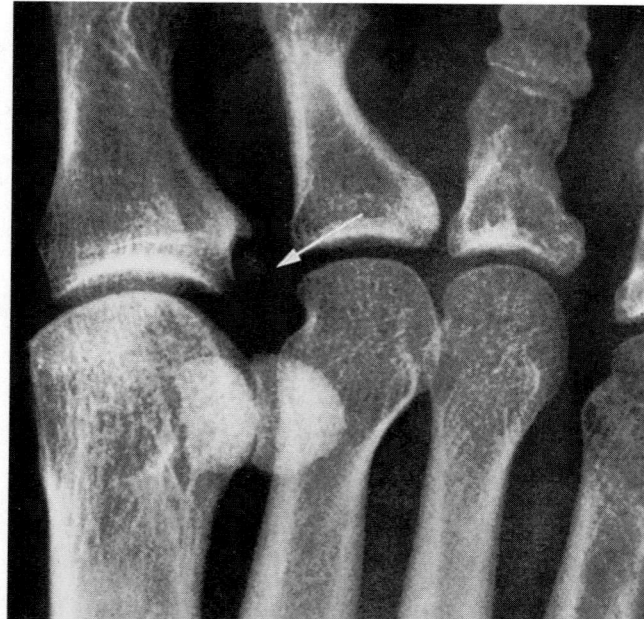

Figure 7–696. Fossa at the lateral aspect of the base of the proximal phalanx of the first toe, with small ossicle within (*arrow*). Note the similarity to Figure 7–688.

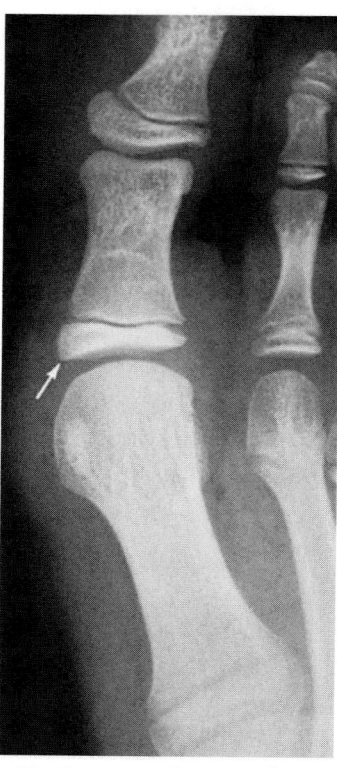

Figure 7–697. Normally dense epiphysis at the base of the proximal phalanx of the first toe in a 12-year-old boy. This should not be mistaken for evidence of osteochondritis.

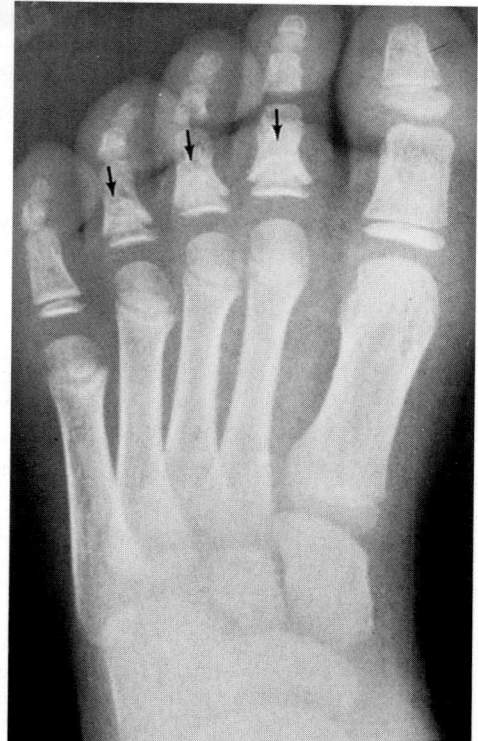

Figure 7–698. Cone epiphyses are very common in the proximal phalanges of children and are not necessarily associated with abnormality.

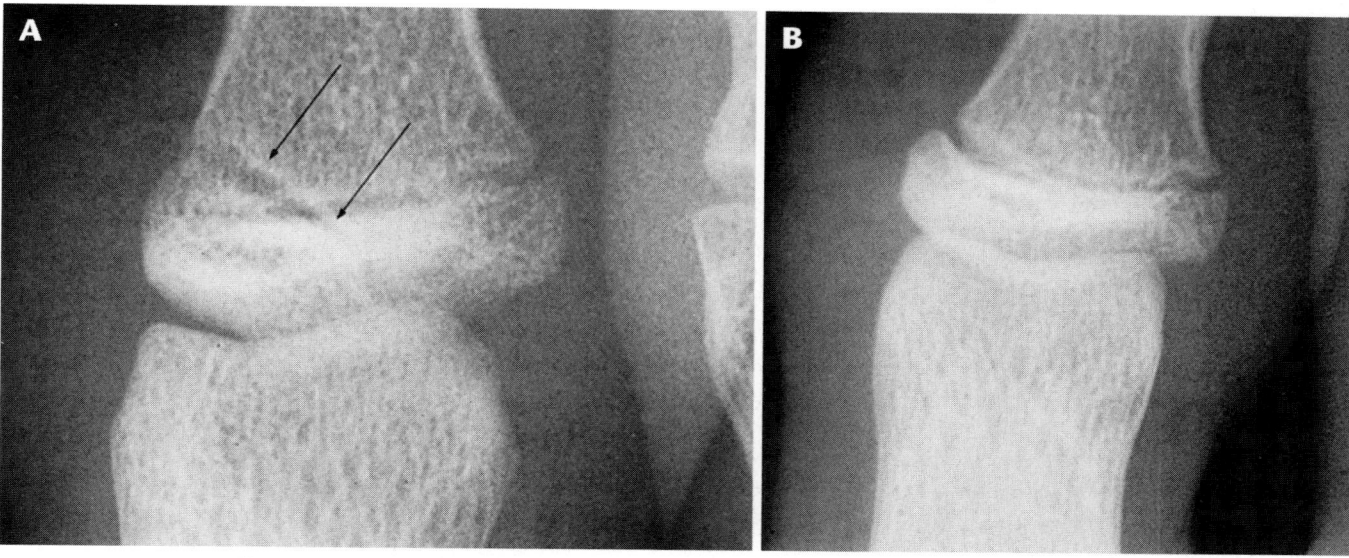

Figure 7–699. A, Simulated fracture of the epiphysis of the first toe, by oblique projection. **B,** No fracture seen in the frontal plane.

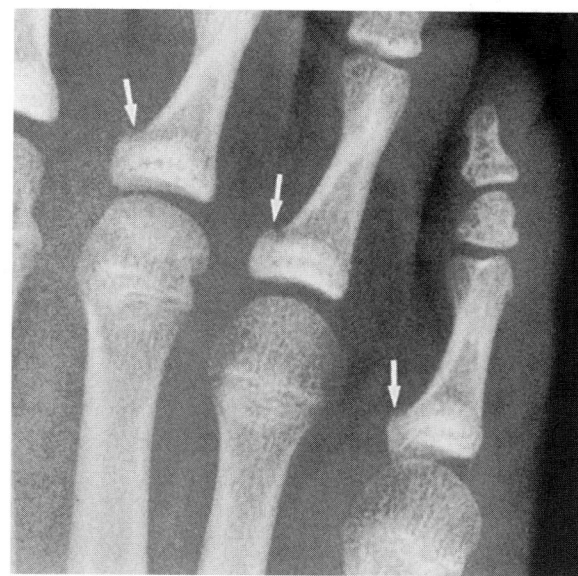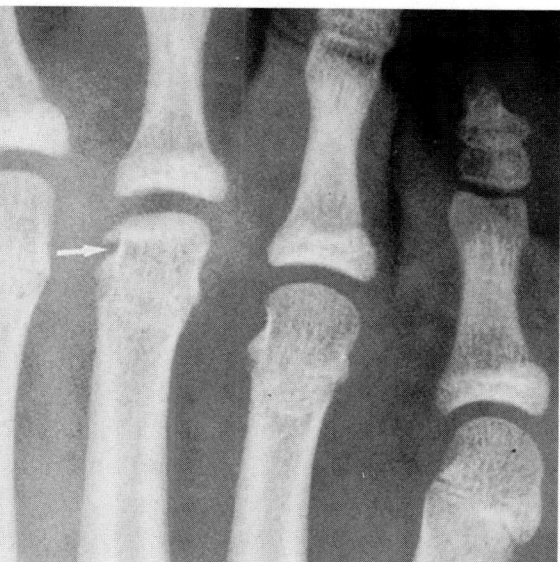

Figure 7–700. *Left,* Simulated fractures of the bases of the proximal phalanges, in the oblique projection in an 11-year-old girl (*arrows*). *Right,* Frontal projection shows no fractures. Note deep fossa in the head of the third metatarsal (*arrow*).

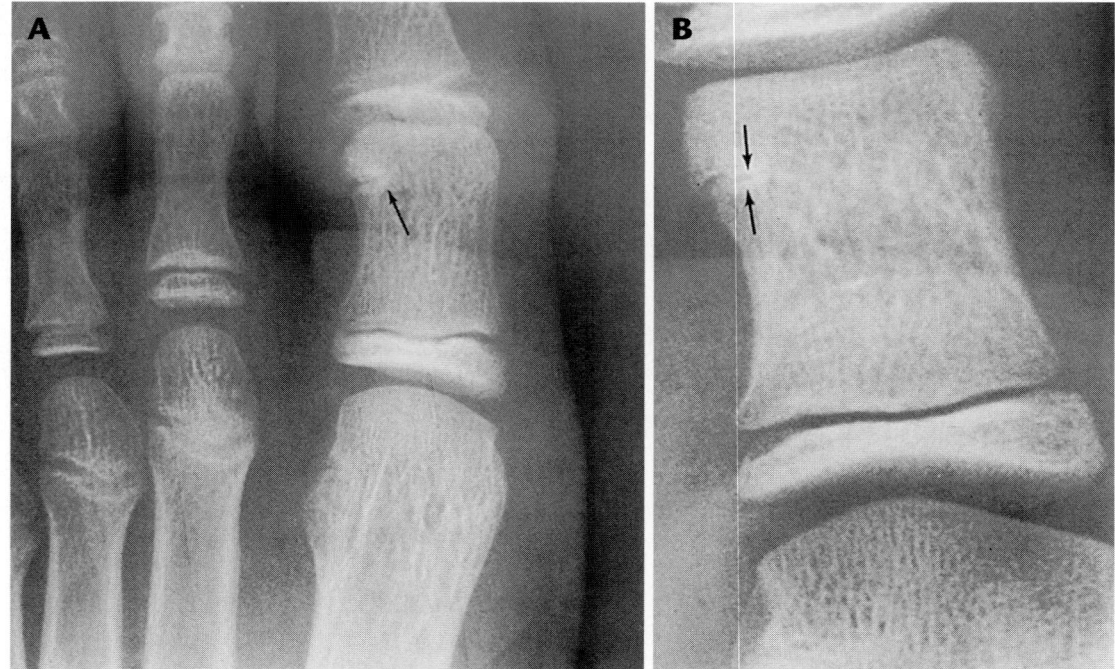

Figure 7–701. Incomplete developmental fissures through the proximal phalanx of the first toe. **A,** 10-year-old boy. **B,** 12-year-old boy.

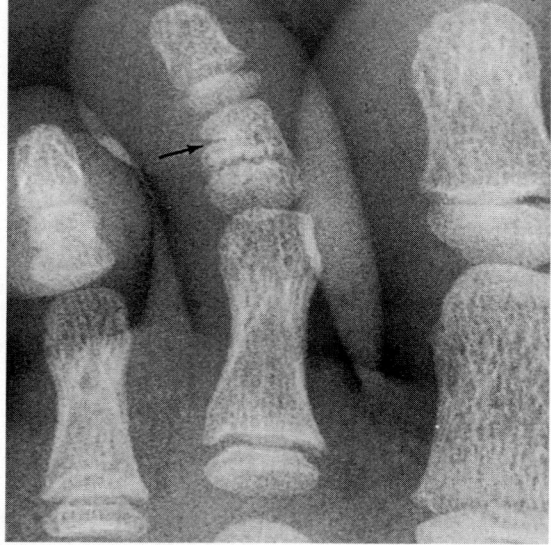

Figure 7–702. Incomplete developmental fissure in the middle phalanx of the second toe in an 8-year-old boy.

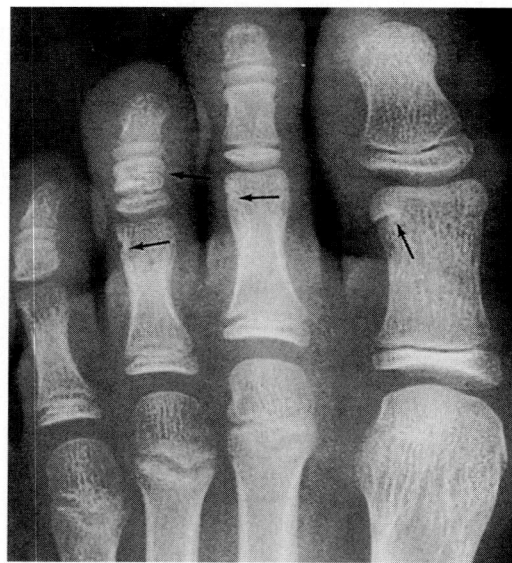

Figure 7–703. Fissures in the first, second, and third toes of a 10-year-old boy.

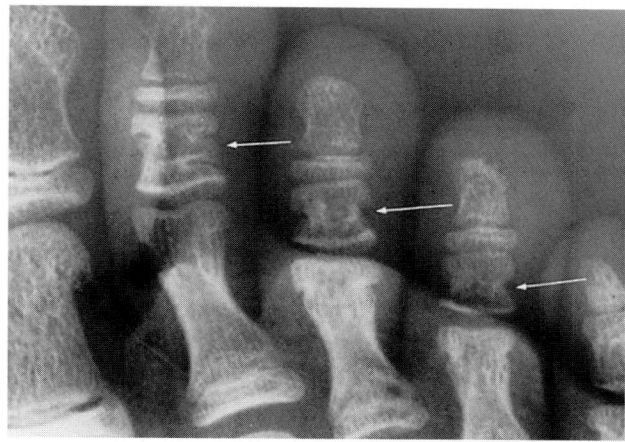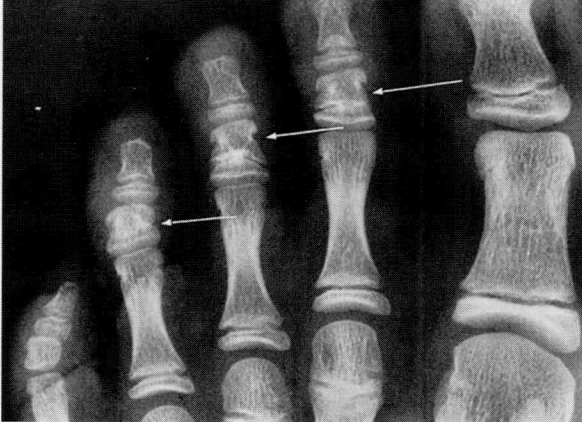

Figure 7–704. Two examples of marked irregularity in development of the phalanges in 12-year-old girls. This is a normal and transient phenomenon.

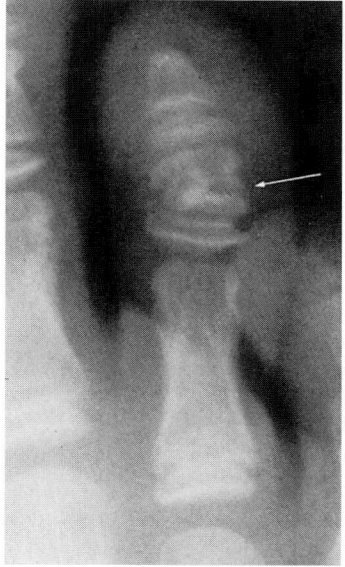

Figure 7–705. Developmental irregularity of the middle phalanx of the fourth toe in an 11-year-old girl, interpreted as a fracture.

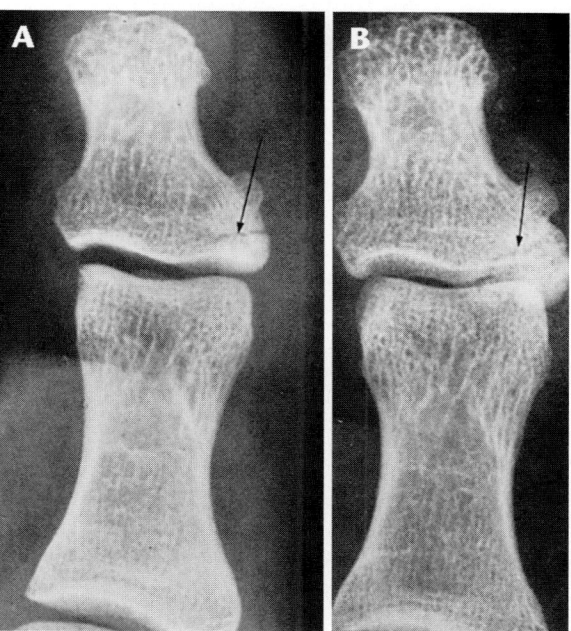

Figure 7–706. **A,** Failure of fusion of a portion of the epiphysis at the base of the distal phalanx of the first toe, originally interpreted as a fracture despite absence of pertinent history or physical findings. **B,** 3-year follow-up shows no change.

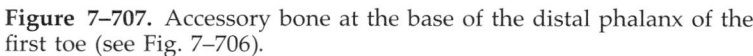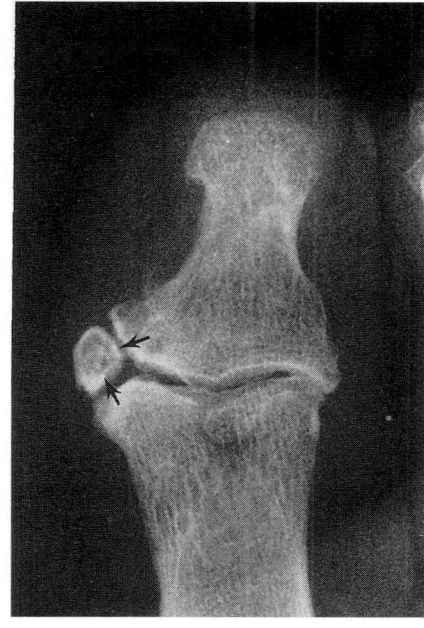

Figure 7–707. Accessory bone at the base of the distal phalanx of the first toe (see Fig. 7–706).

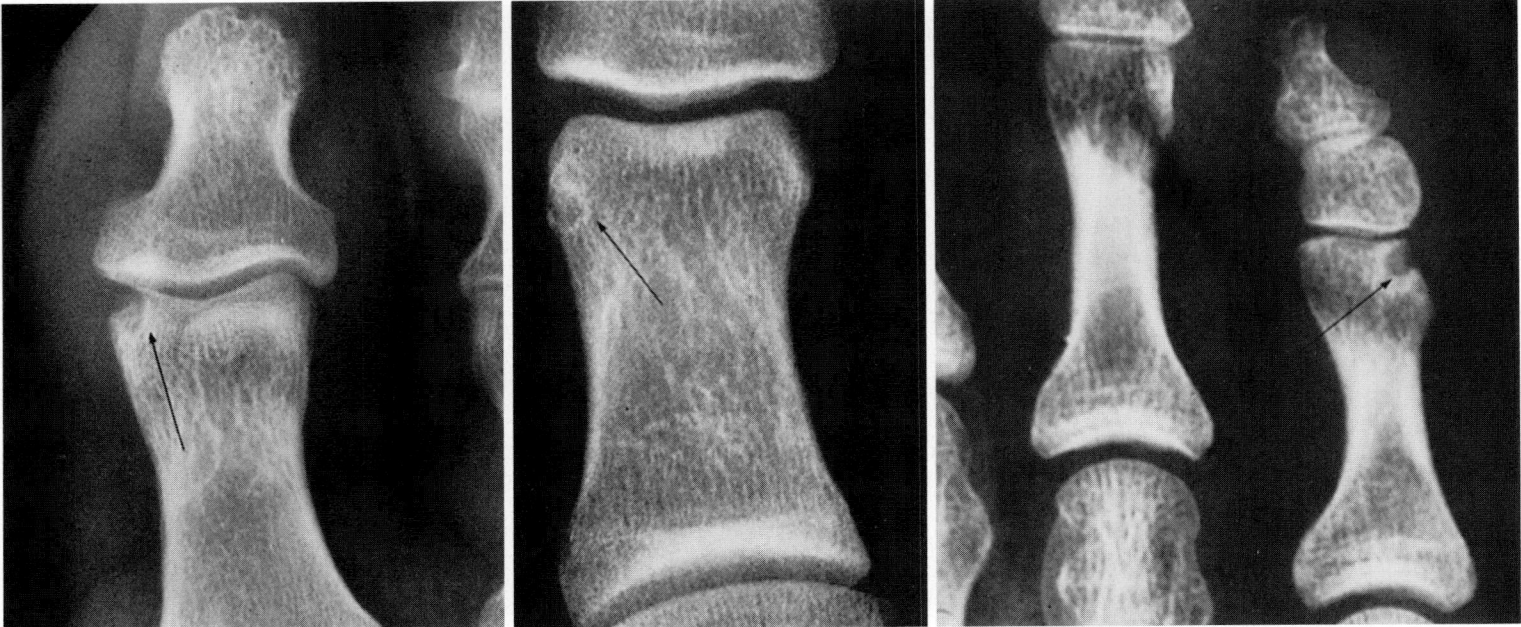

Figure 7–708. Three examples of ringlike defects seen near the joints of the toes. These represent small areas of fat necrosis, but are apparently of no importance clinically. (Ref: Keats TE et al: Idiopathic punctate necrosis of the phalanges of the feet. *Skeletal Radiol* 18:25, 1989.)

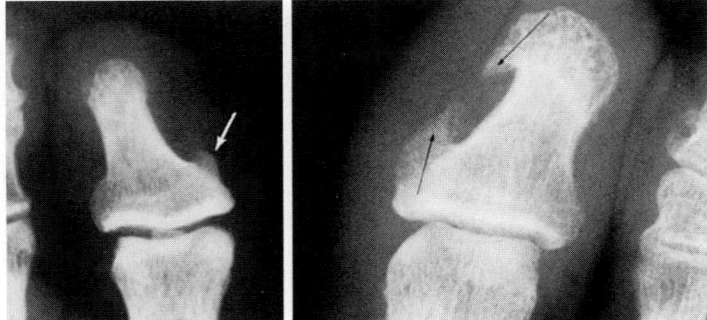

Figure 7–709. Two examples of spurlike enlargements of the distal phalanx of the great toe. They are of no clinical significance. *Right,* Note the ossifications between the spurs that are located in the lateral supporting ligament. (Ref: Lee M et al: Bone excrescence at the medial base of the distal phalanx of the first toe: Normal variant, reactive change, or neoplasia? *Skeletal Radiol* 21:161, 1992.)

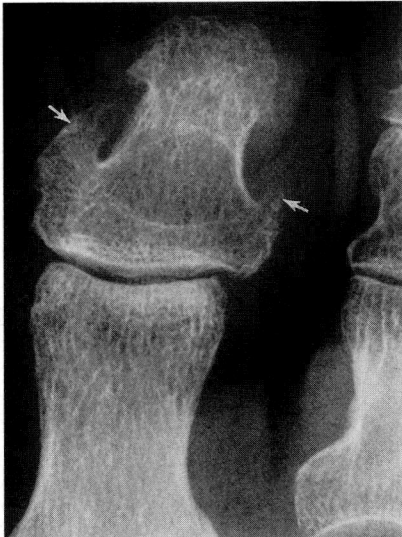

Figure 7–710. The same entity as the preceding figure, with osseous excrescences on both sides of the distal phalanx.

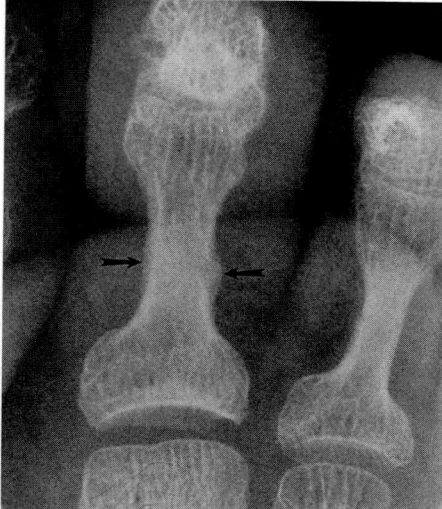
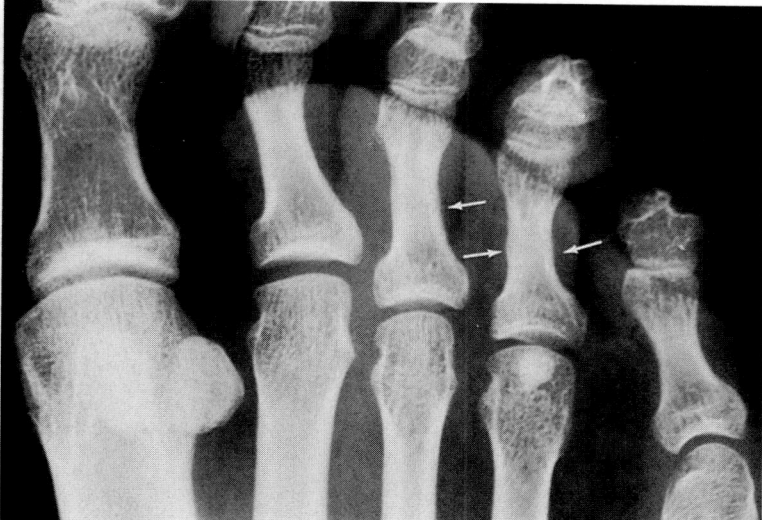

Figure 7–711. Normal irregularities seen along the shafts of the proximal phalanges, not to be confused with periostitis.

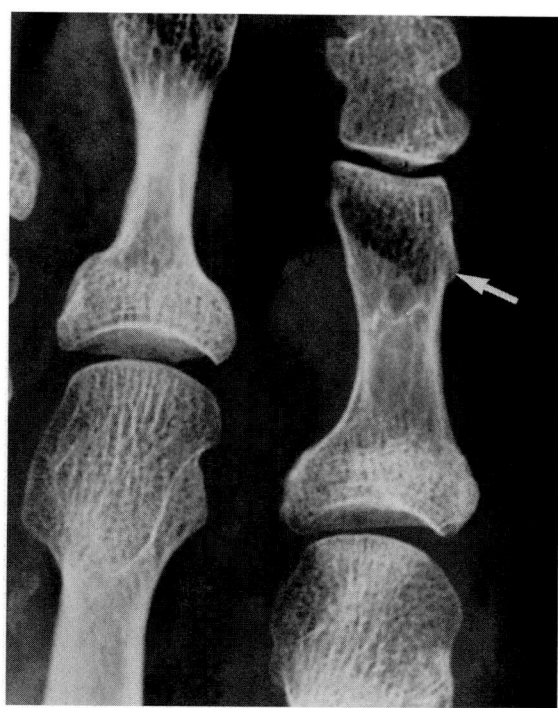

Figure 7–712. Normal irregularity on the lateral aspect of the shaft of the proximal phalanx of the fifth toe. This change was present on the opposite side as well.

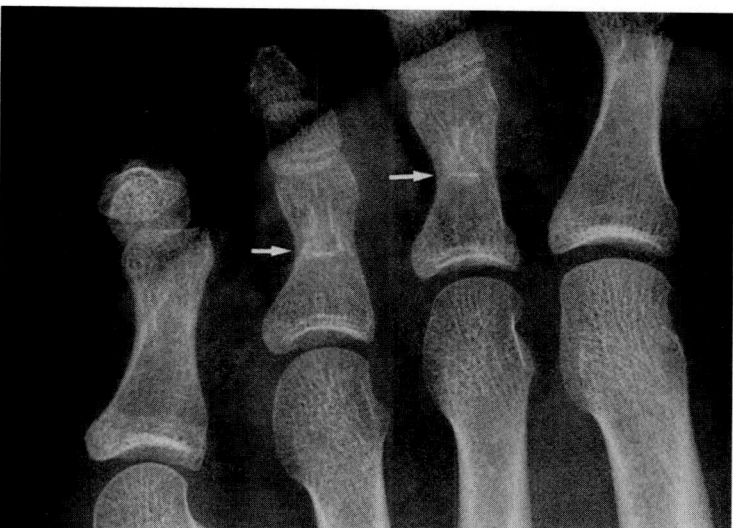

Figure 7–713. Simulated fractures of the proximal phalanges of the third and fourth toes.

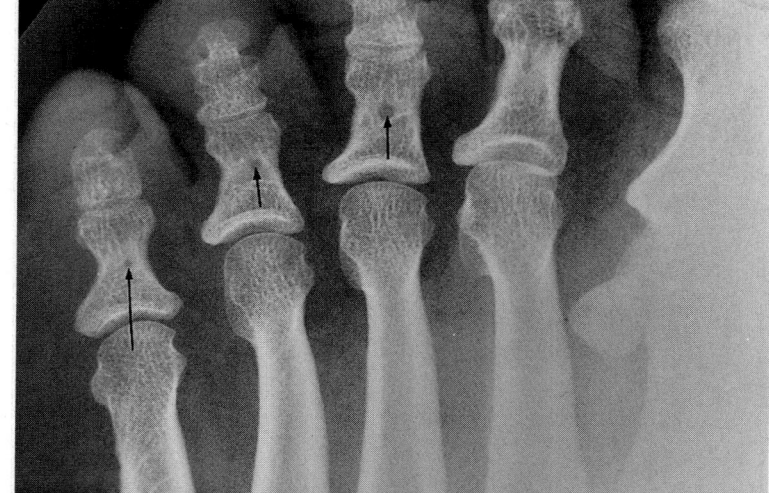

Figure 7–714. Nutrient foramina of the proximal phalanges.

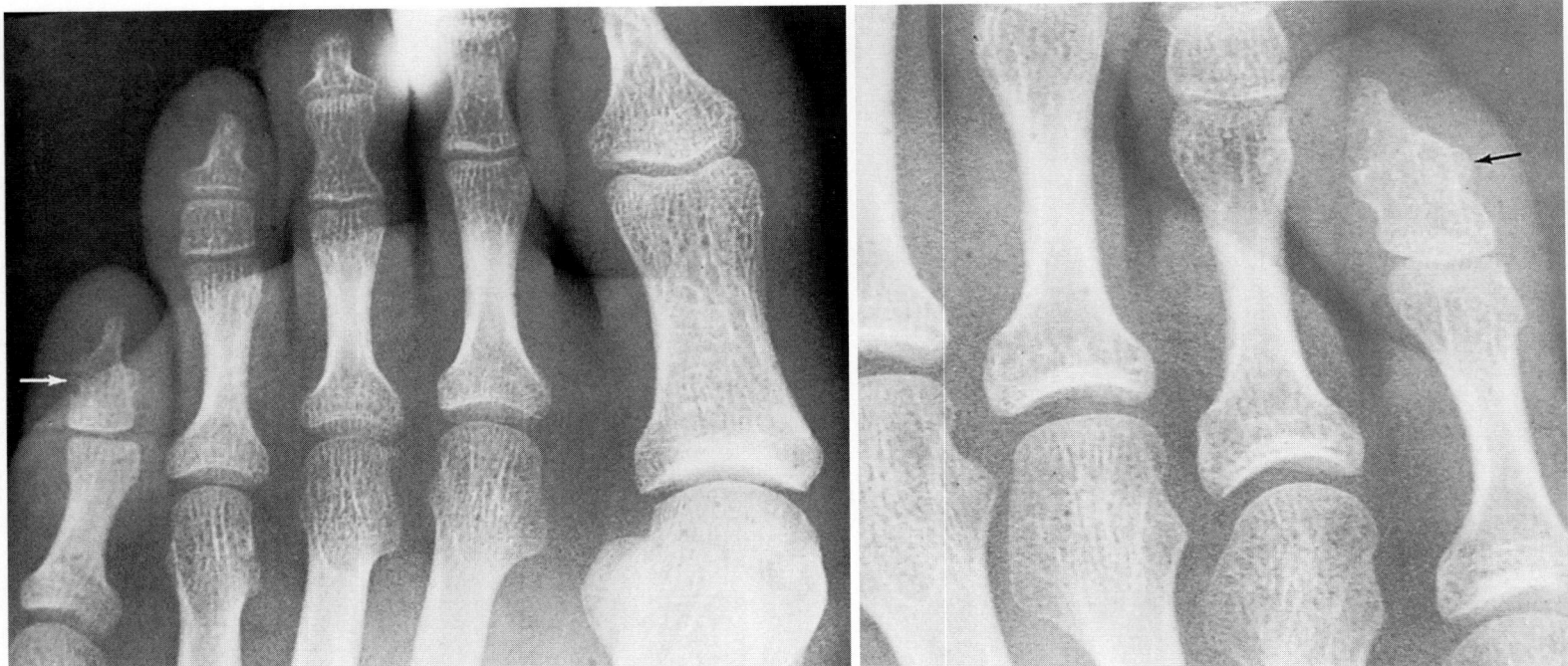

Figure 7–715. Two examples of fifth toes with only two phalanges. This is a common anatomic variant and not the product of disease. (Ref: Ellis R et al: The two-phalanged fifth toe. *JAMA* 206:2526, 1968.)

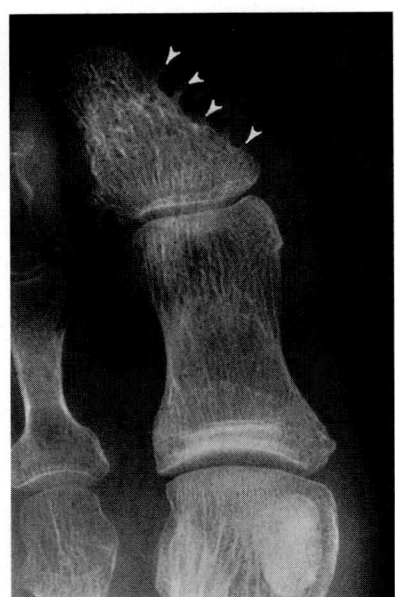

Figure 7–716. Marked excrescences of the distal phalanx of the first toe.

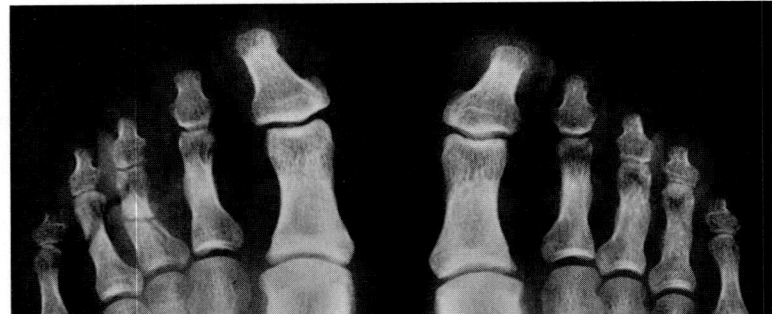

Figure 7–717. Two-phalanged toes, an anatomic variation.

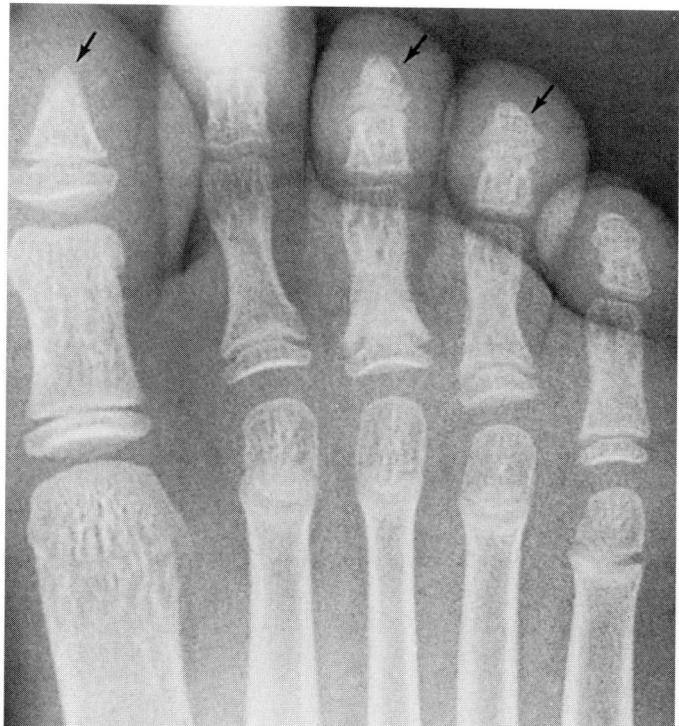

Figure 7–718. Pointed distal phalanges in a healthy 6-year-old girl.

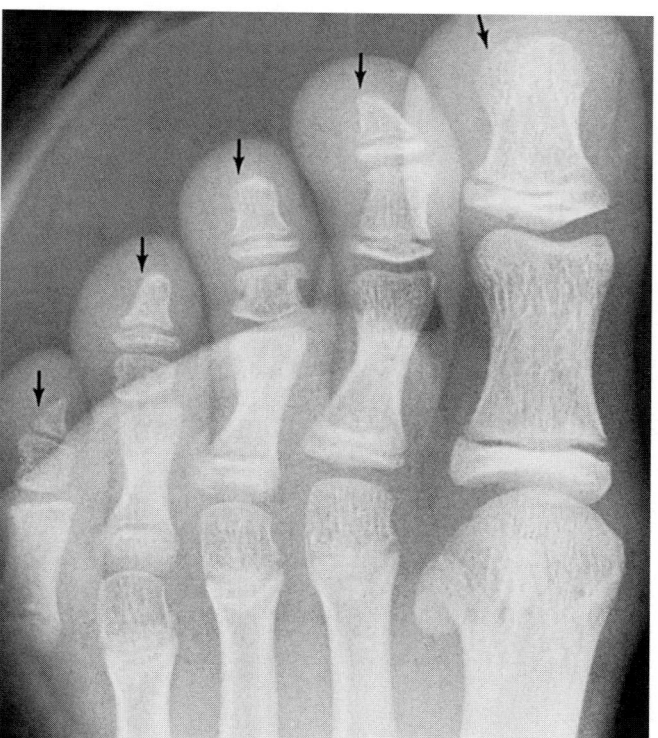

Figure 7–719. Pointed distal phalanges in a healthy 11-year-old boy. Absence of the distal tufts may be normal, unassociated with disease.

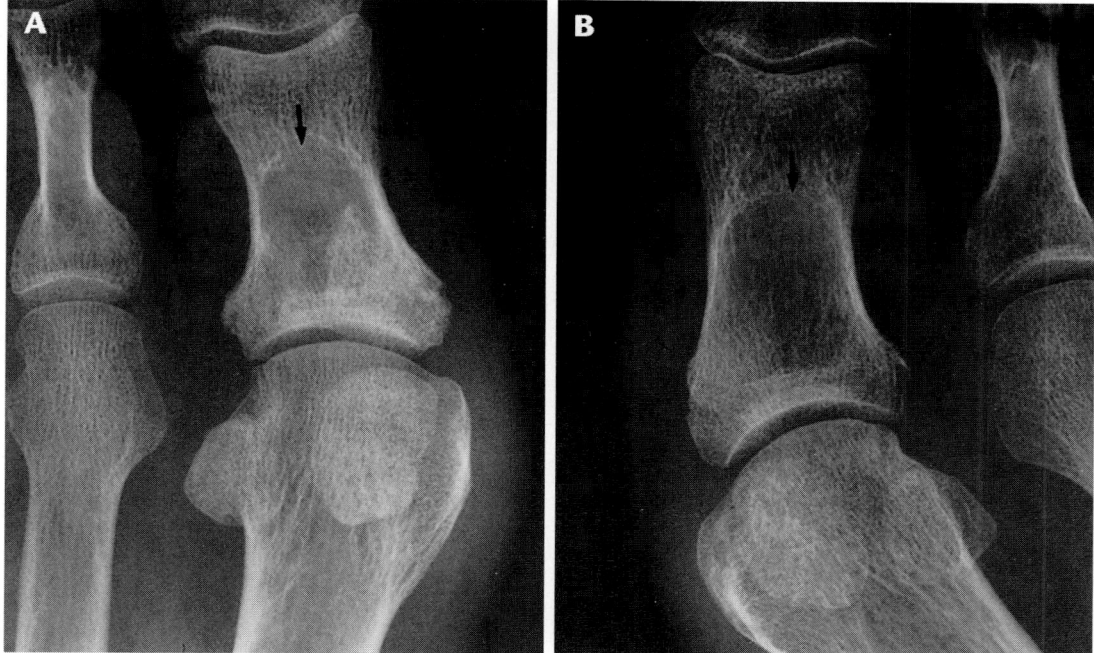

Figure 7–720. A, B, Pseudocysts of the proximal phalanges of the first toes in an osteoporotic woman.

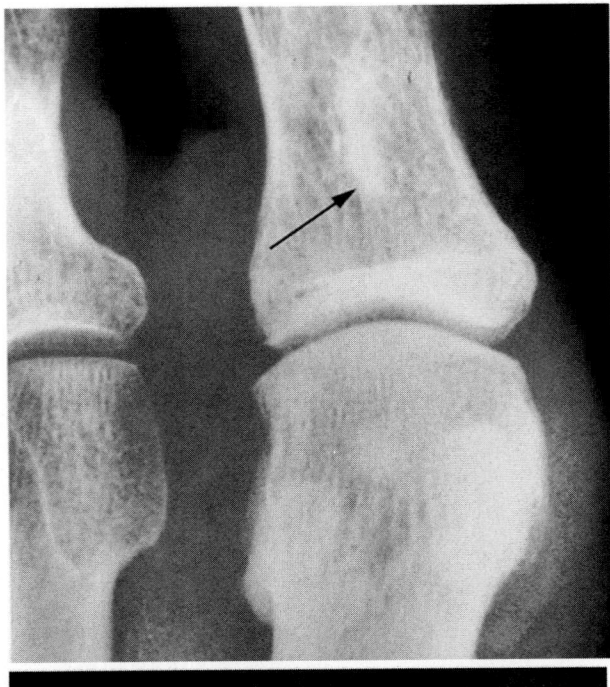
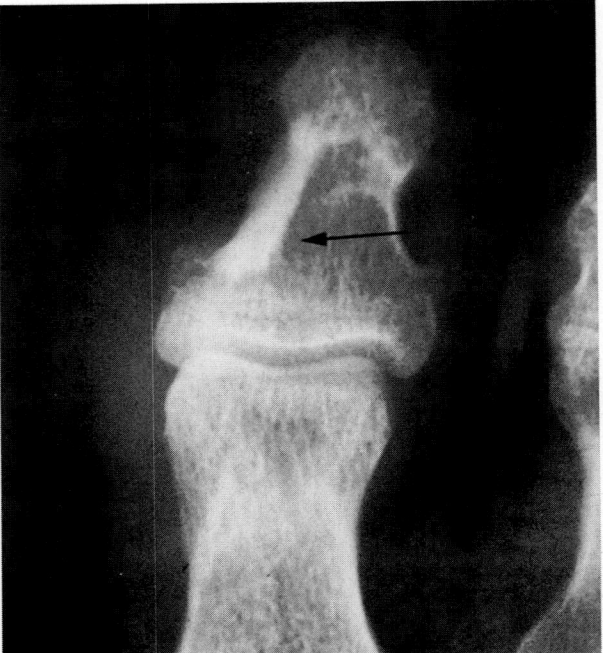
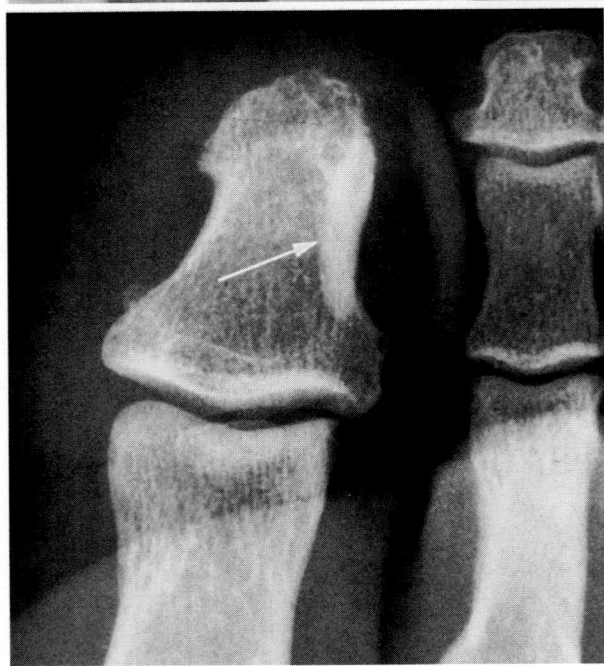

Figure 7–721. Three examples of phalangeal sclerosis, a finding of no clinical significance. *Top left,* Proximal phalanx. *Top right* and *bottom,* Distal phalanges. (Ref: Carter BC et al: Skeletal manifestations of idiopathic bone sclerosis. *Australas Radiol* 32:242, 1988.)

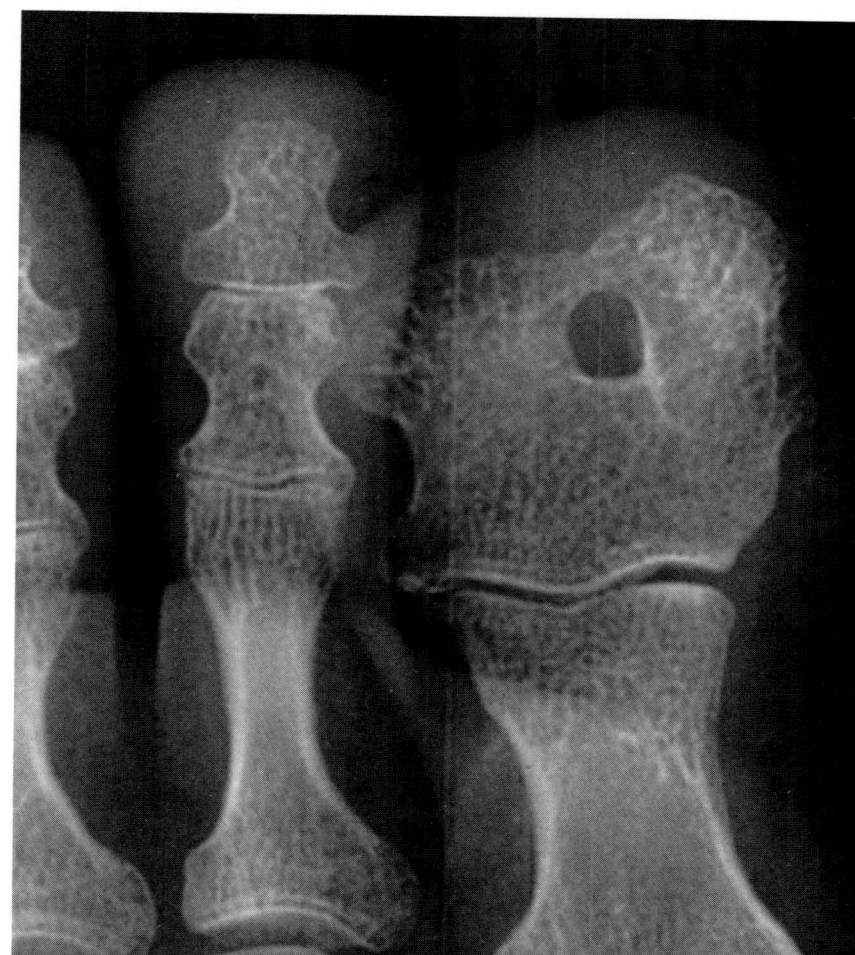

Figure 7–722. Duplication anomaly of the first toe with an articulation with the second toe.

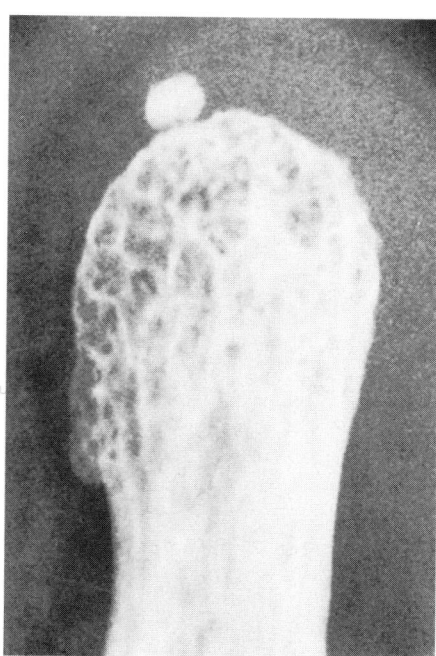

Figure 7–723. Subungual calcification in the normal nail bed of the toes. This phenomenon is seen in adults in middle age and late life and is of no clinical significance. (From Fischer E: Subunguale Verkalkungen im normalen Nagelbett der Zehen. *Radiologie* 24:31, 1984.)

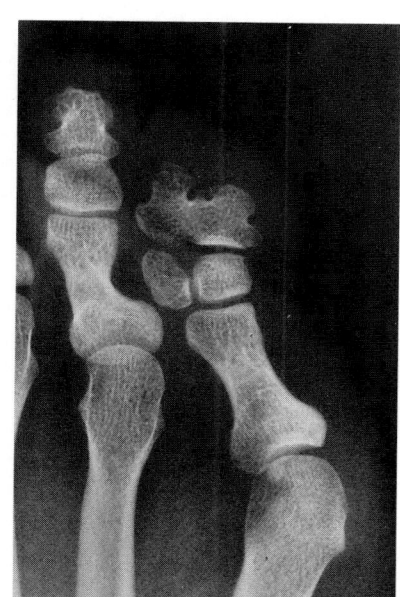

Figure 7–724. Duplication of the fifth toe.

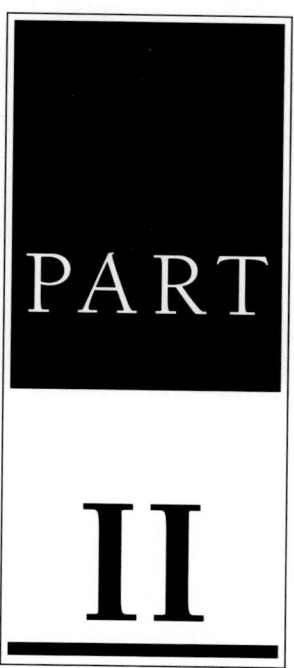

PART

II

The Soft Tissues

CHAPTER

8

The Soft Tissues of the Neck

Pages
906 to 930

Figures
8–1 to 8–74

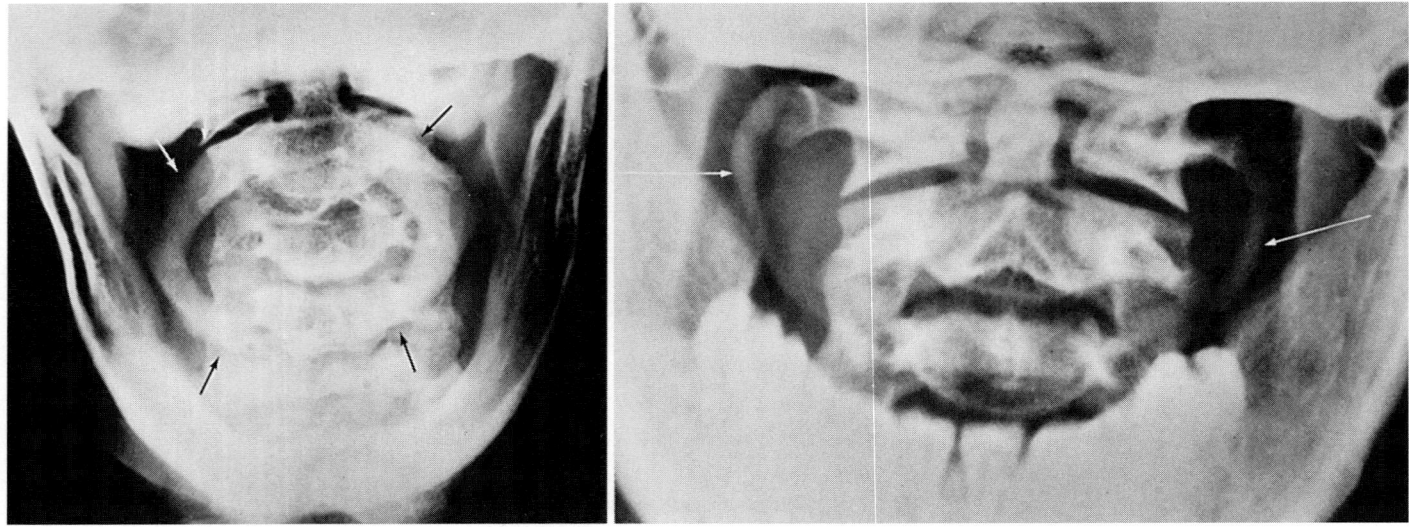

Figure 8–1. Shadows of the lips seen in frontal projection of the mandible. (Ref: Bohrer SP, Brody JA: More than just lip service. *Skeletal Radiol* 21:305, 1992.)

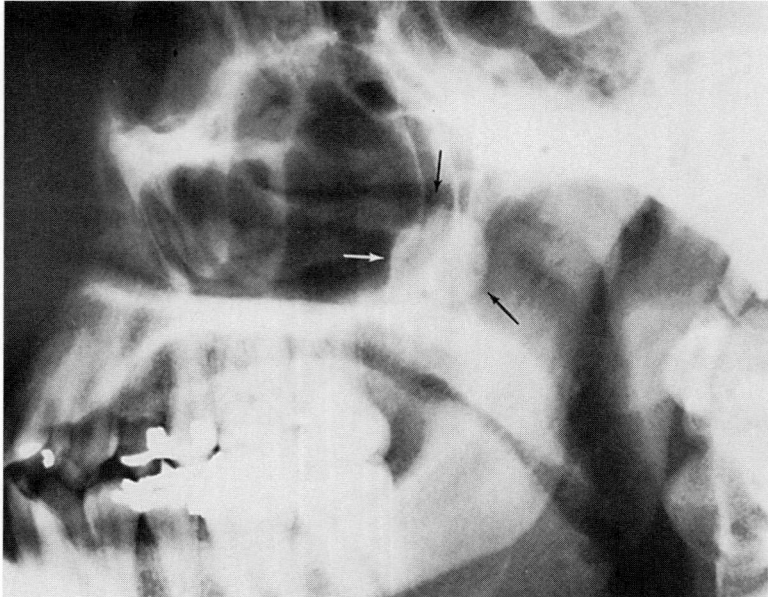

Figure 8–2. Pseudotumor of the nasal passage, produced by superimposition of the coronoid process of the mandible on the inferior turbinate. (Ref: Sistrom CL, Keats TE, Johnson CM: The anatomic basis of the pseudotumor of the nasal cavity. *Am J Roentgenol* 147:782, 1986.)

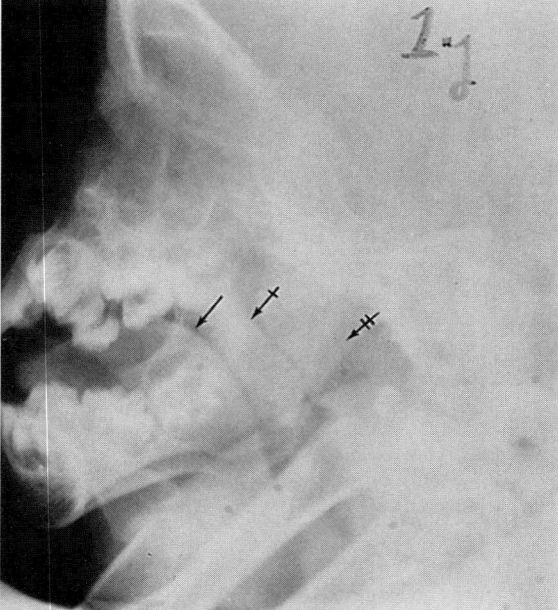

Figure 8–3. Normal configuration of the soft tissues of the mouth and oropharynx in a 1-year-old infant during swallowing, showing tongue (→), soft palate (↦), and adenoids (⇸).

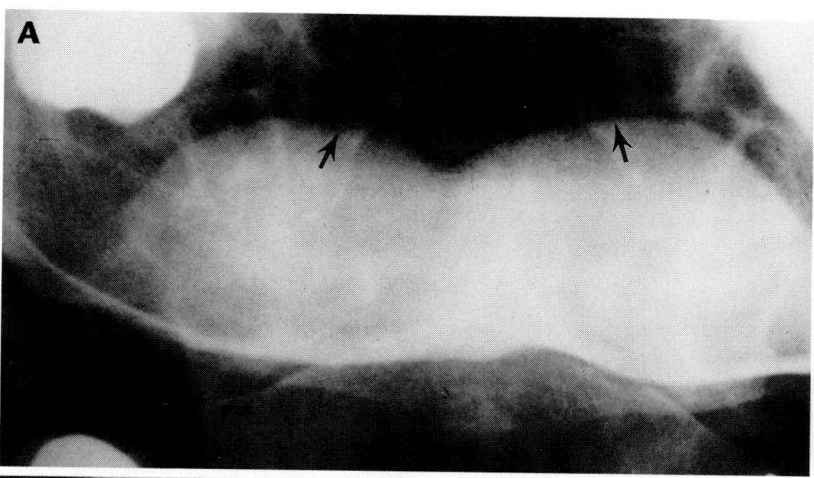

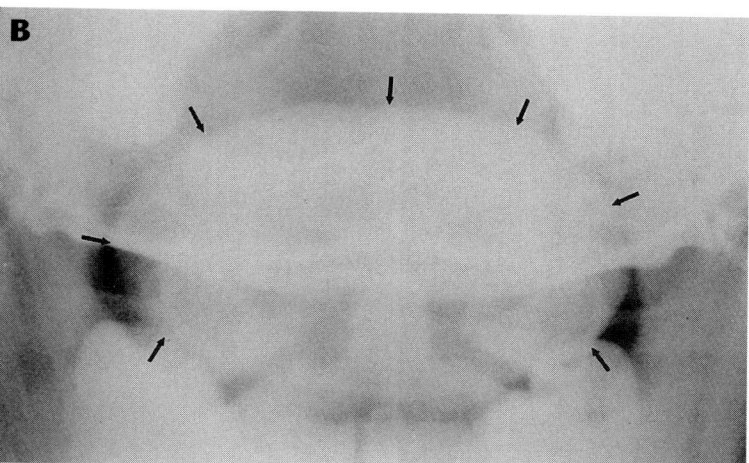

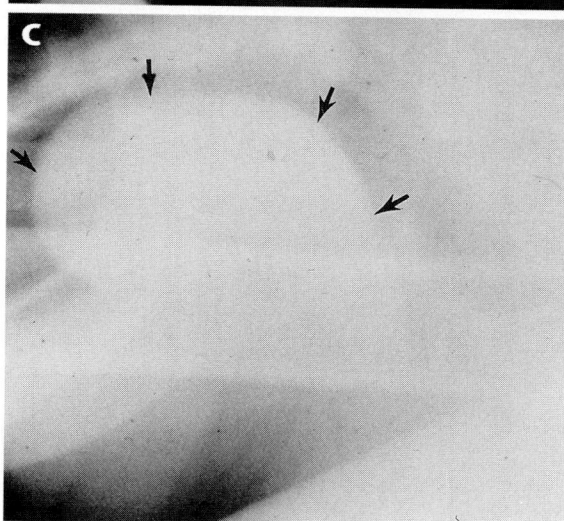

Figure 8–4. A, Summation shadow of the occiput and upper lip. **B,** Tongue in frontal projection. **C,** Tongue in lateral projection. (Courtesy of Dr. Stan Bohrer).

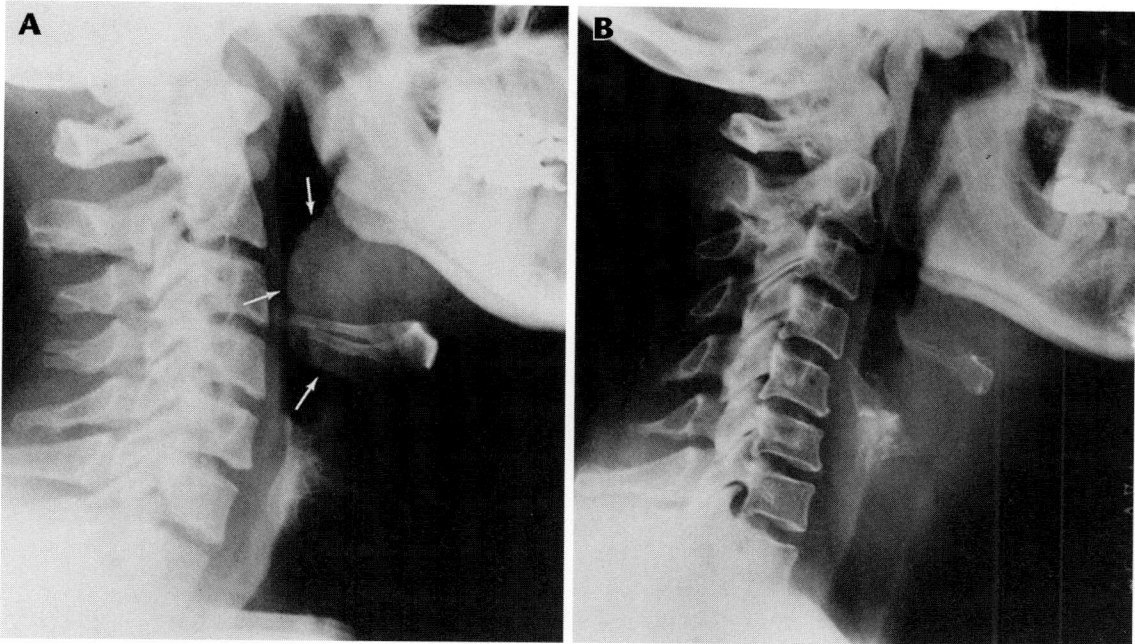

Figure 8–5. A, Pseudomass of the pharynx, produced by the base of the tongue, filmed during the act of swallowing. **B,** Normal configuration of soft tissues at rest in another patient for contrast with **A.**

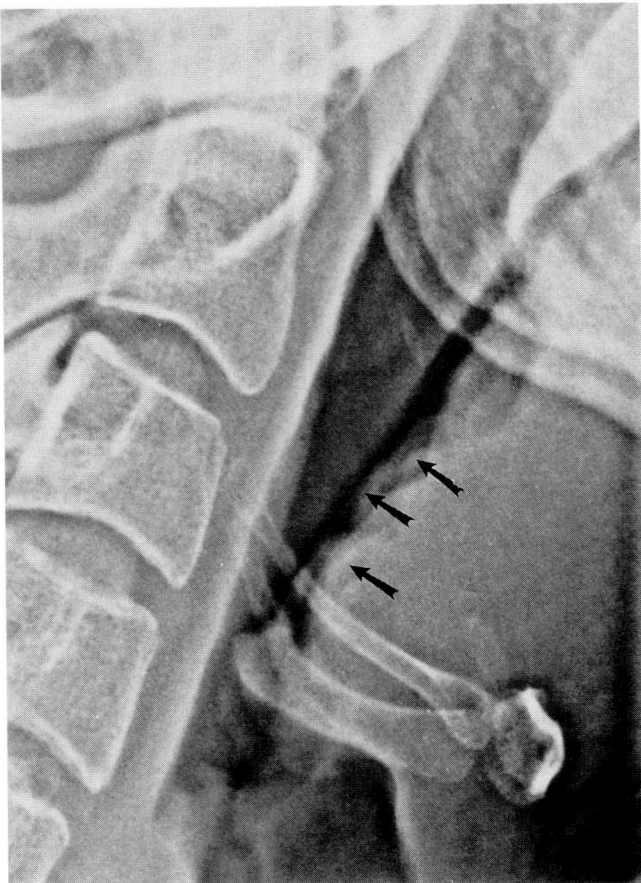

Figure 8–6. Normal irregularity of the surface of the base of the tongue caused by lymphoid tissue.

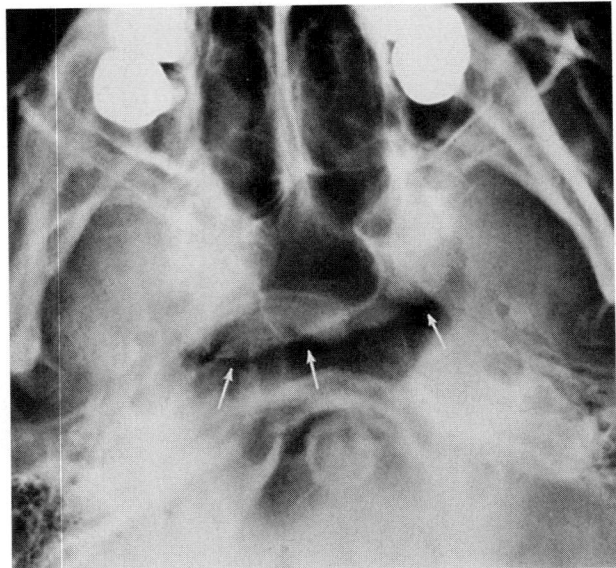

Figure 8–7. Base of the tongue seen in the basal view of the skull.

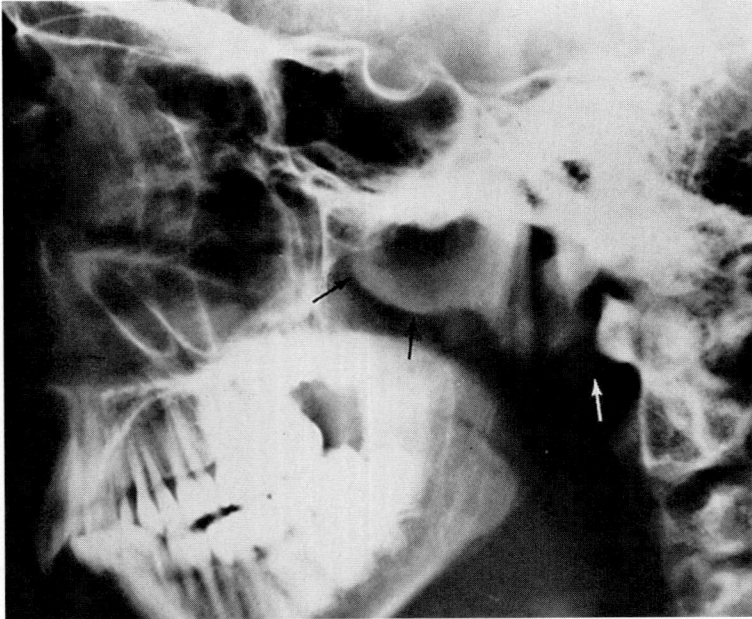

Figure 8–8. Large but normal adenoids in a young adult. The lucency within is due to superimposition of the nasopharyngeal air shadow.

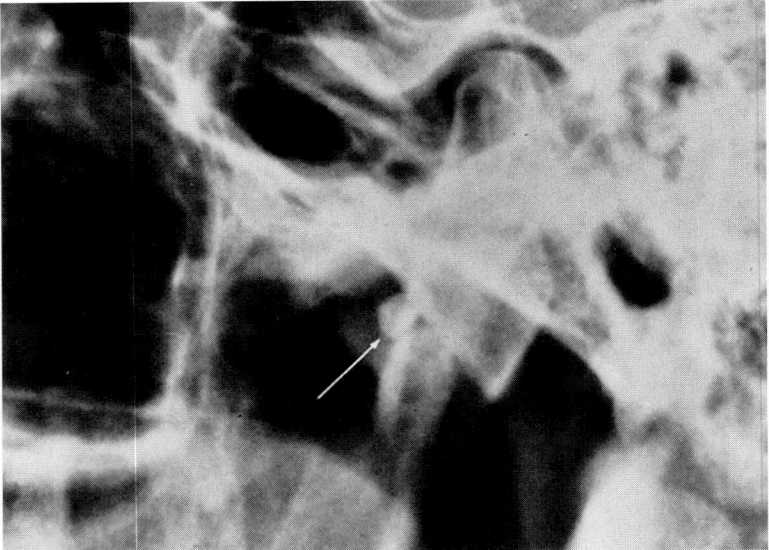

Figure 8–9. Calcification in the adenoids.

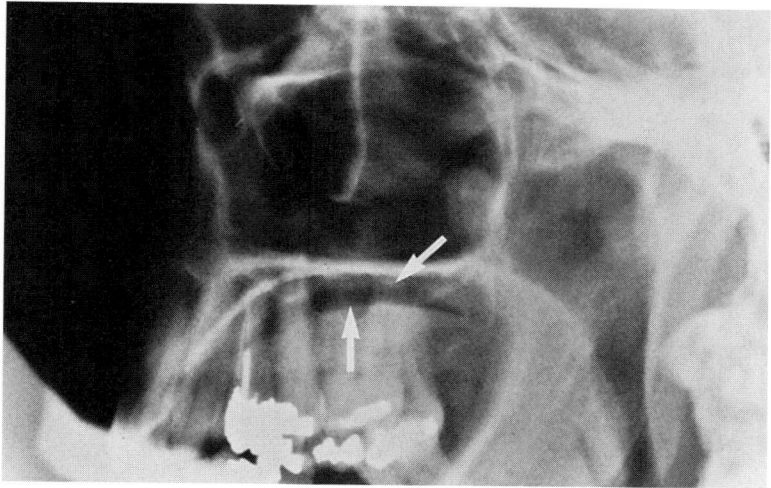

Figure 8–10. Air between the hard palate and the tongue.

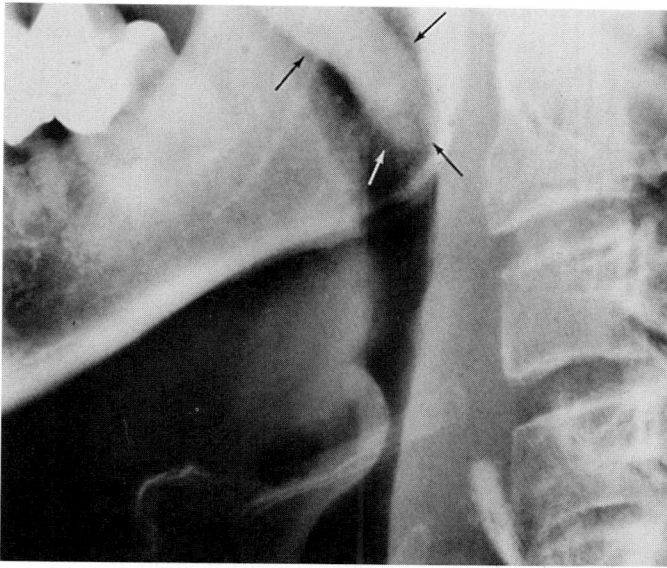

Figure 8–11. Prominent soft palate and uvula.

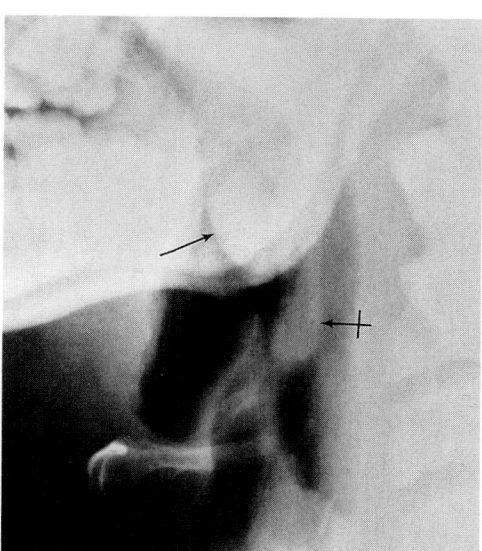

Figure 8–12. Large soft palate (←) and uvula (↔).

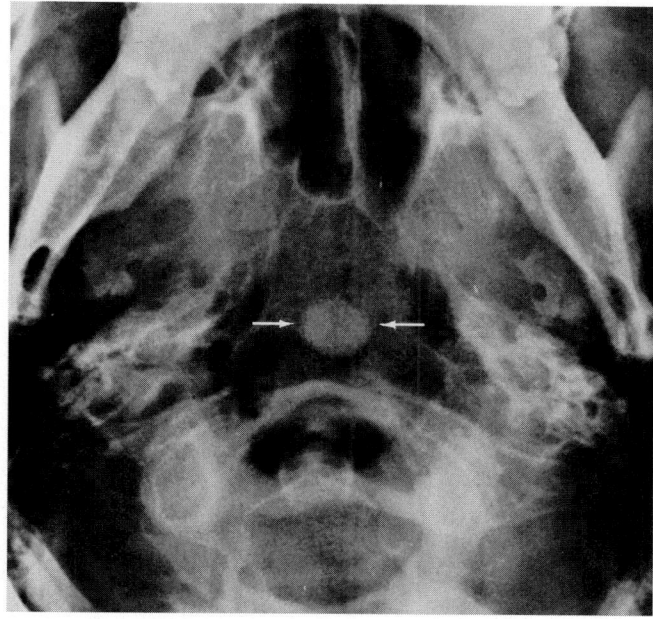

Figure 8–13. Shadow of the uvula seen in the basal view of the skull.

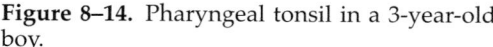

Figure 8–14. Pharyngeal tonsil in a 3-year-old boy.

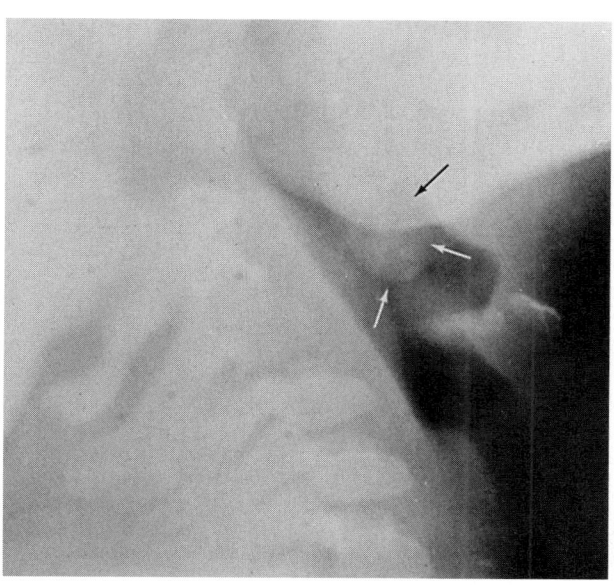

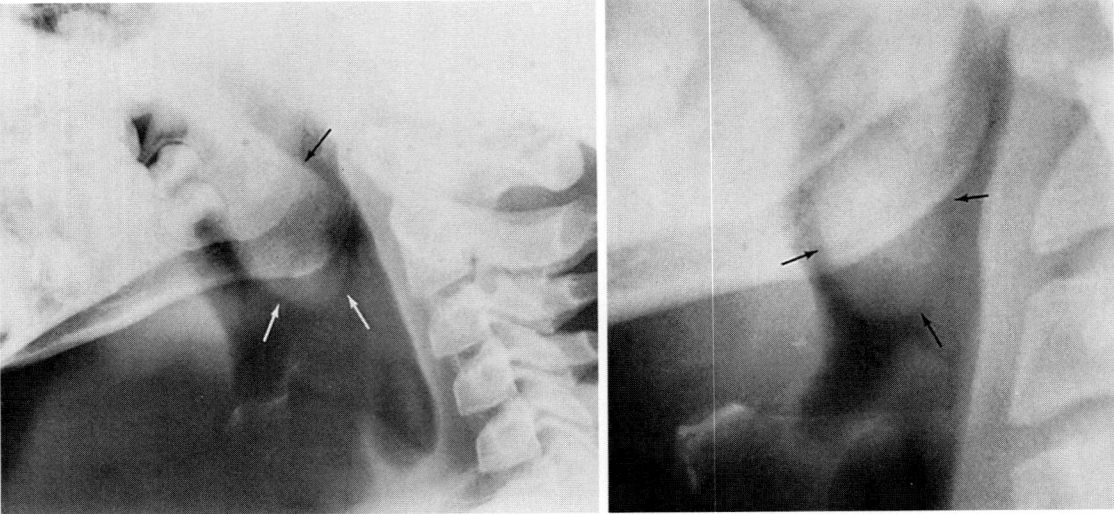

Figure 8–15. Two examples of large pharyngeal tonsils, which may simulate a tumor of the pharynx.

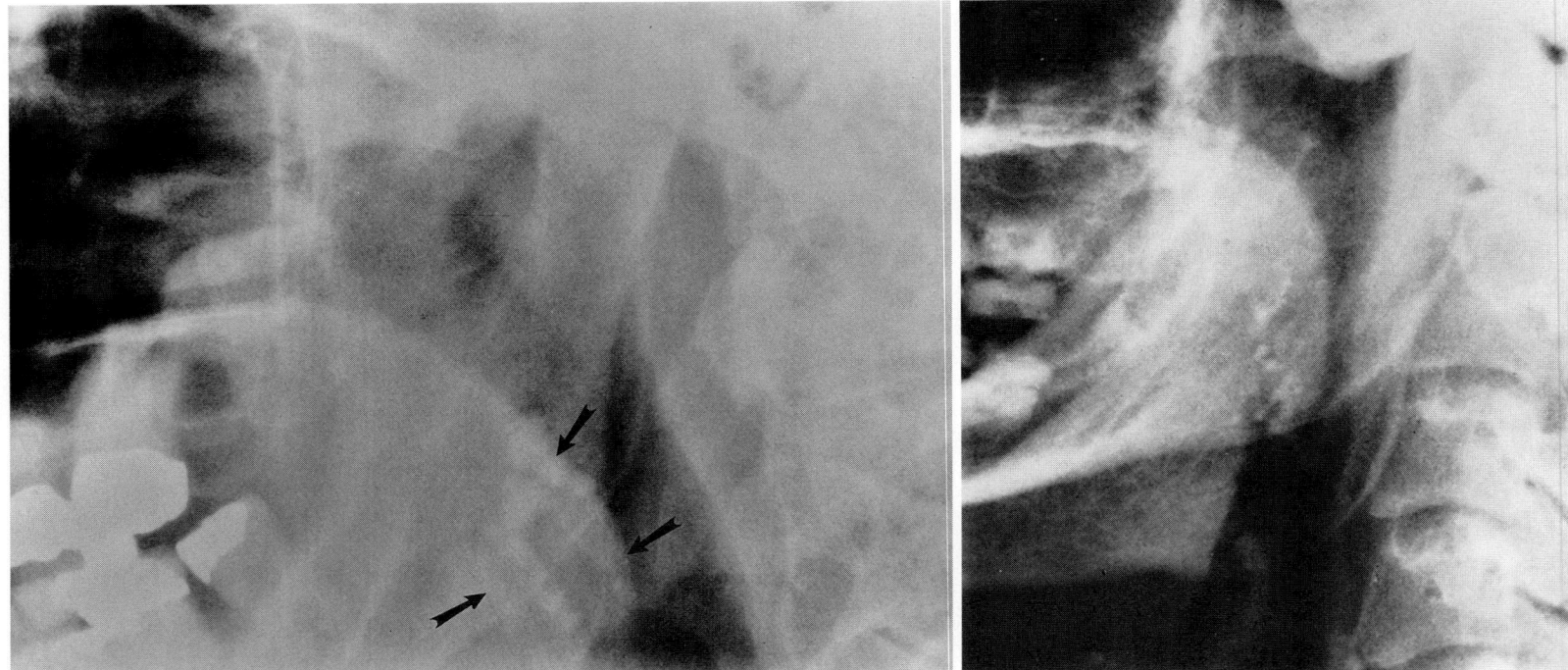

Figure 8–16. Two examples of calcification in the tonsilar crypts. (Ref: Aspestrand F, Kolbenstredt A: Calcifications of the palatine tonsillary region: CT demonstration. *Radiology* 165:479, 1987.)

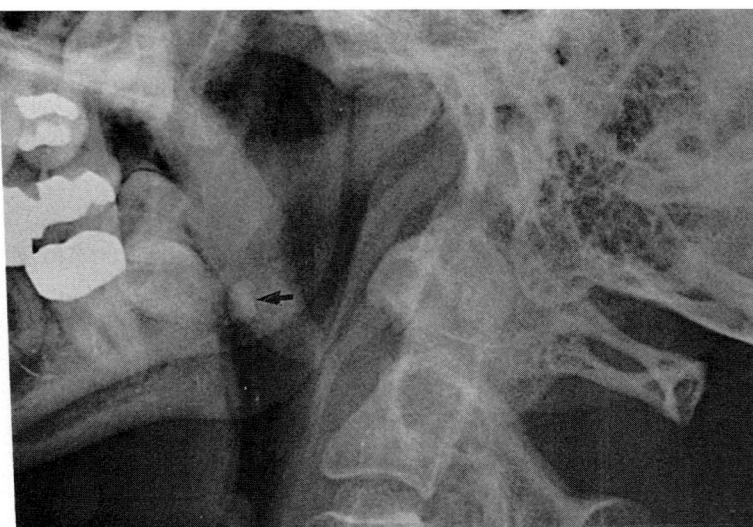

Figure 8–17. Parotid or tonsilar stone.

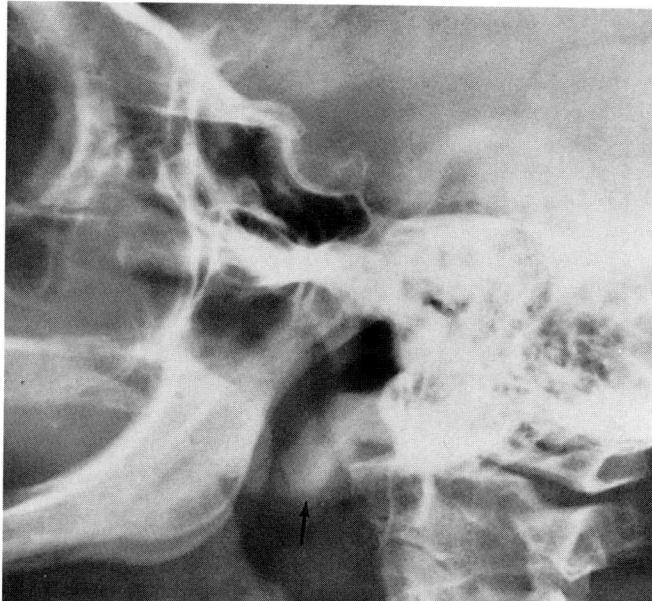

Figure 8–18. Shadow of the ear lobe, simulating a mass in the nasopharynx.

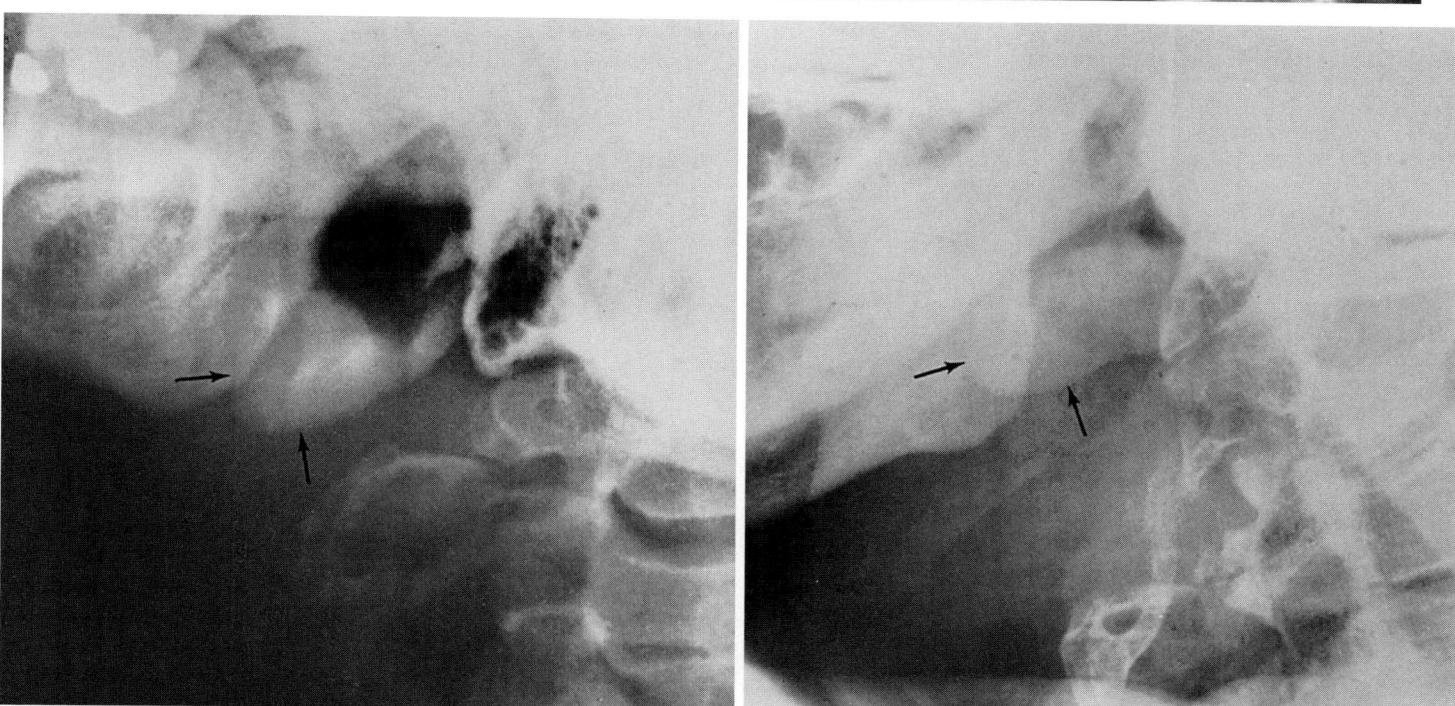

Figure 8–19. Ear lobe, simulating mass lesions, seen in preliminary films for submaxillary sialography.

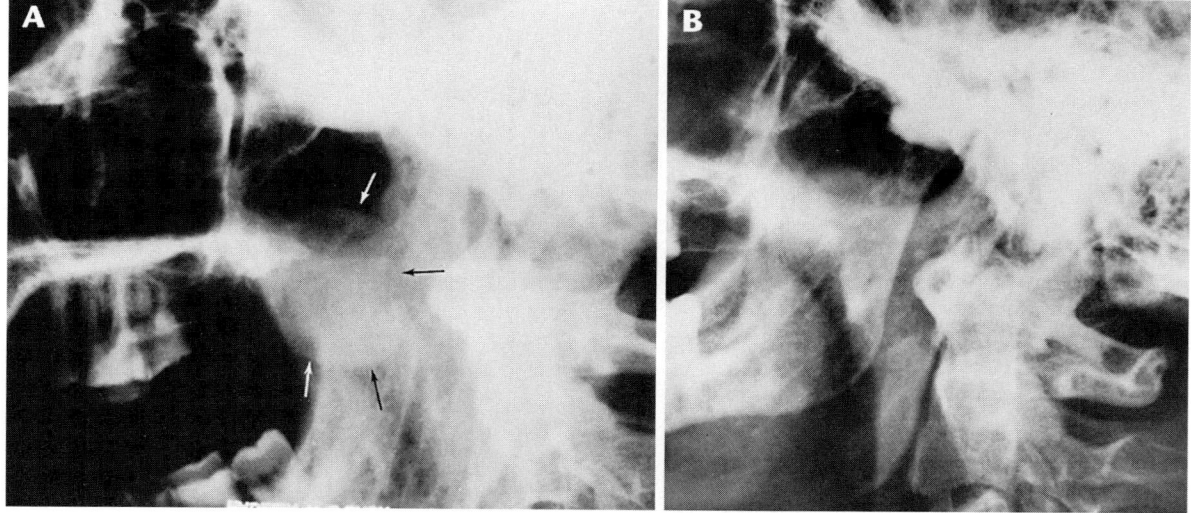

Figure 8–20. A, Simulated soft tissue mass produced by the soft palate during phonation. **B,** Same patient at rest. No mass present.

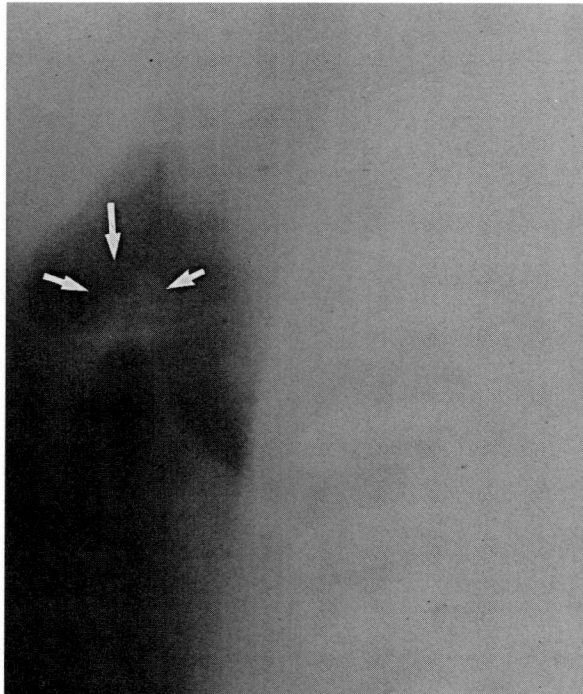

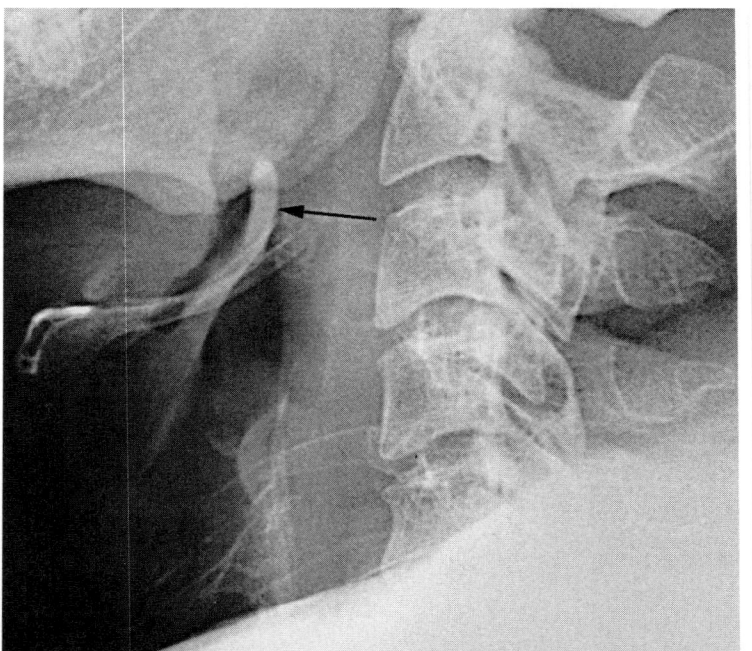

Figure 8–22. Elongated epiglottis.

Figure 8–21. Bulbous distal end of epiglottis is a normal variation, not to be mistaken for the swelling of epiglottis. Note normal aryepiglottic folds. The patient had croup.

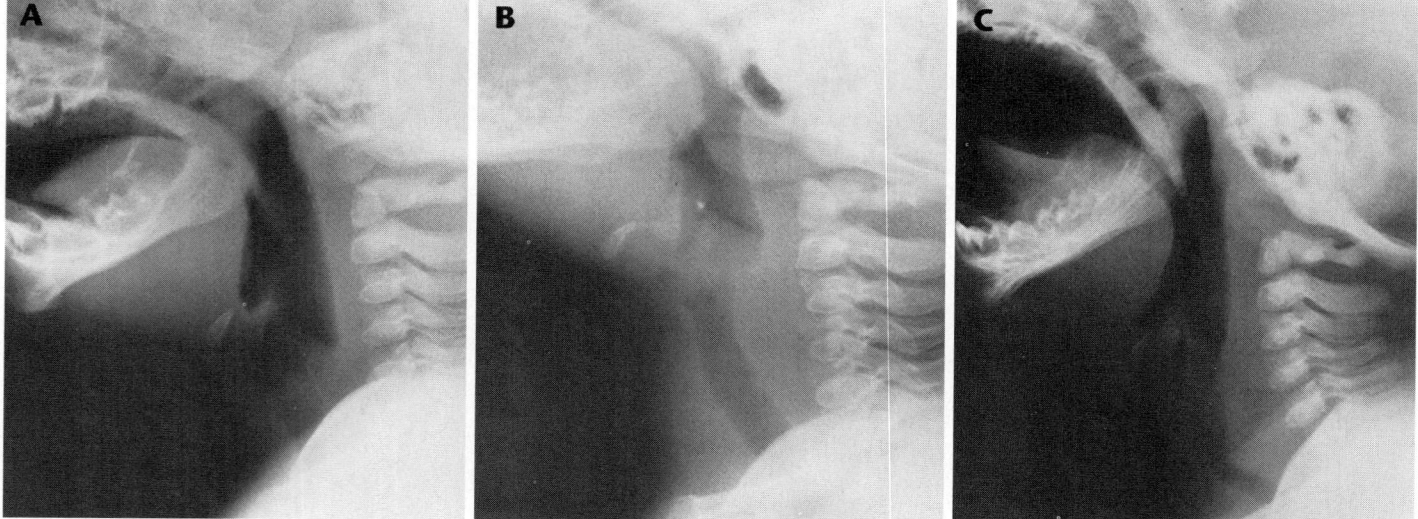

Figure 8–23. Normal alterations of the retropharyngeal soft tissues with respiration in infancy. **A,** Quiet breathing. **B,** Expiration. **C,** Inspiration. The expiratory film resembles the changes of retropharyngeal abscess and is a potential source of misinterpretation.

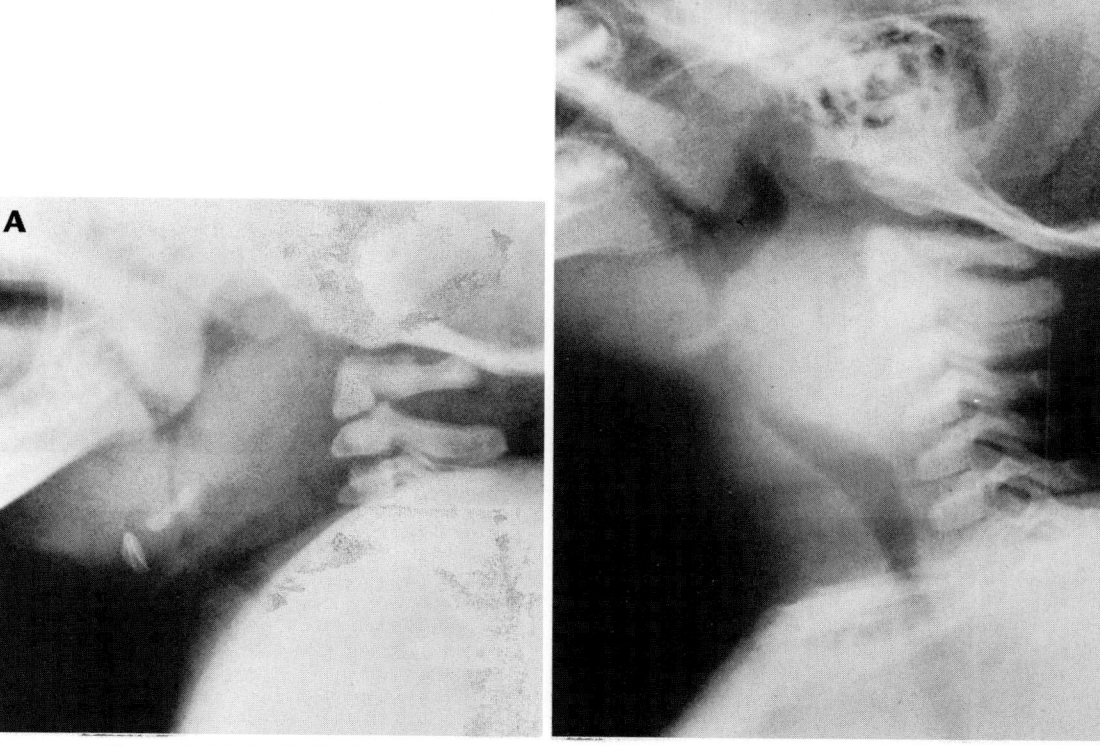

Figure 8–24. **A, B,** Expiratory prominence of the retropharyngeal soft tissues in infants. Note the small air collection in the soft tissues of the patient illustrated in **B.** Both the prominence of the soft tissues and the air disappear on inspiration. (Ref: Currarino G, Williams B: Air collections in the retropharyngeal soft tissues observed in lateral expiratory films of the neck in 9 infants. *Pediatr Radiol* 23:186, 1993.)

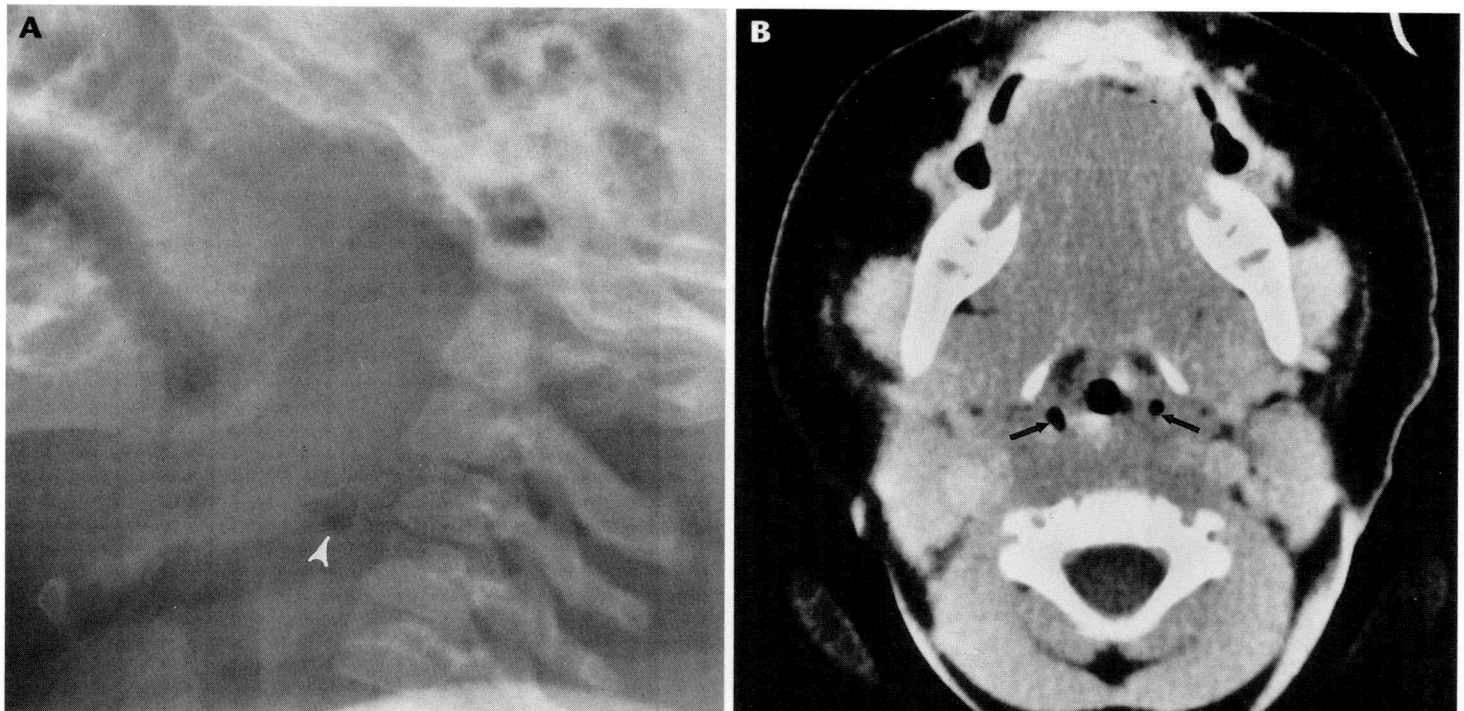

Figure 8–25. Air in the pyriform sinuses in a 1-year-old infant, which explains the appearance seen in the preceding figure, *B.* **A,** Lateral projection. **B,** Axial CT.

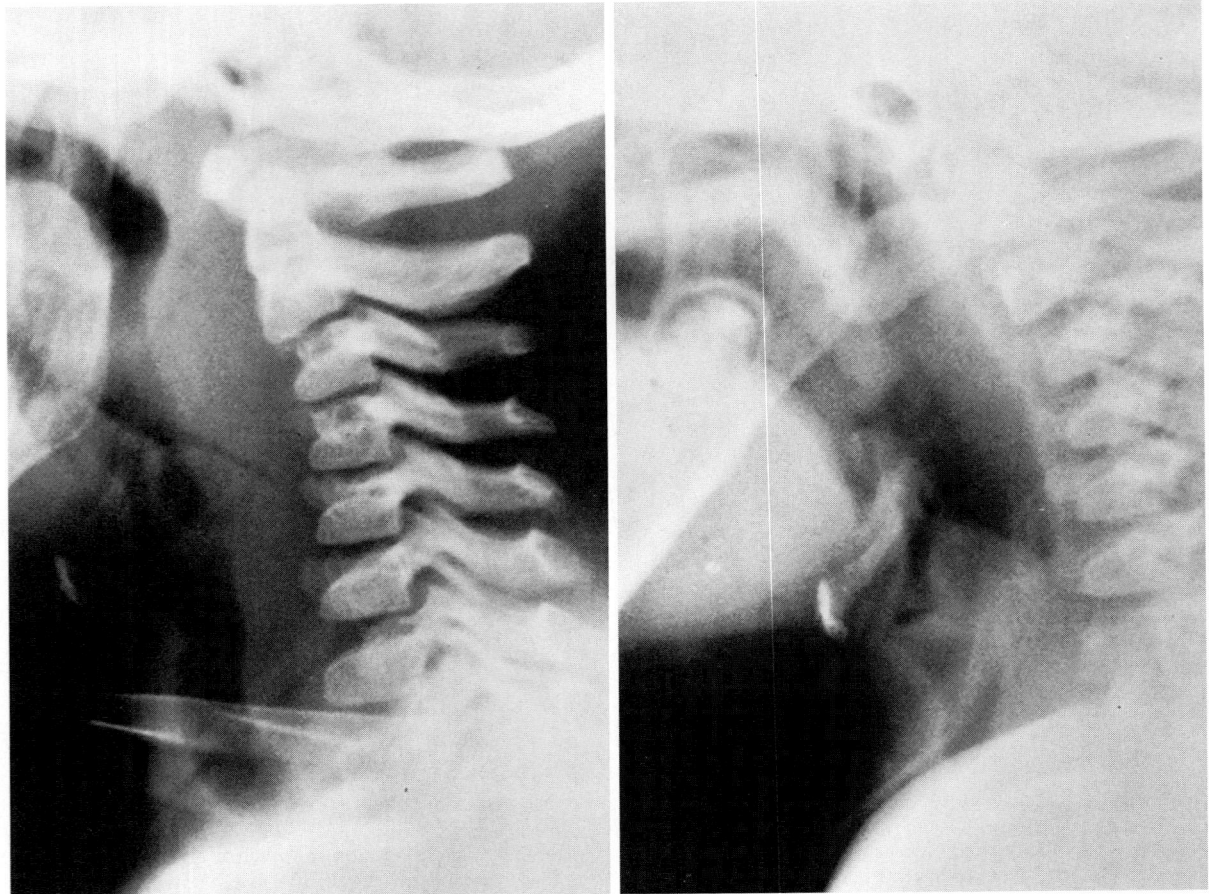

Figure 8–26. Retropharyngeal soft tissue changes with respiration in a 1-year-old. *Left,* Expiration. *Right,* Inspiration.

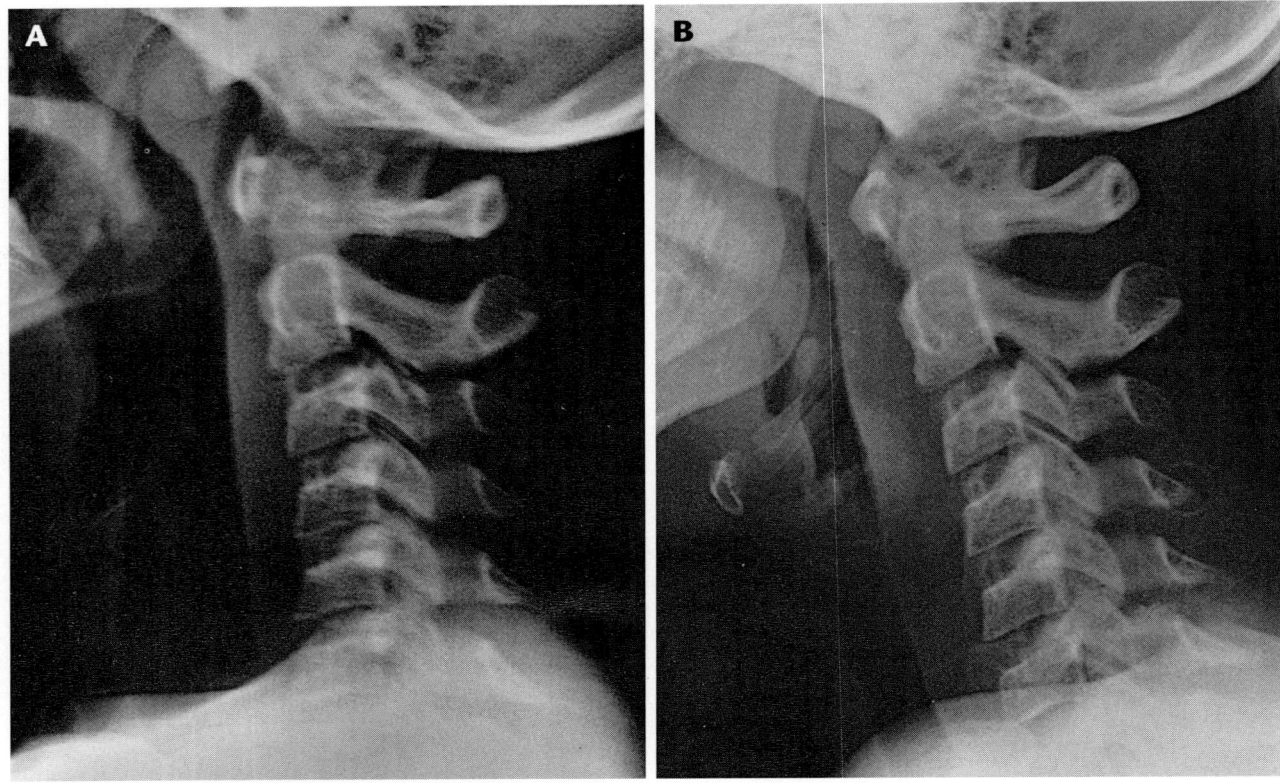

Figure 8–27. Residual normal prominence of retropharyngeal soft tissues in a 10-year-old. **A,** Inspiration. **B,** Expiration. Note similarity to the changes of retropharyngeal abscess.

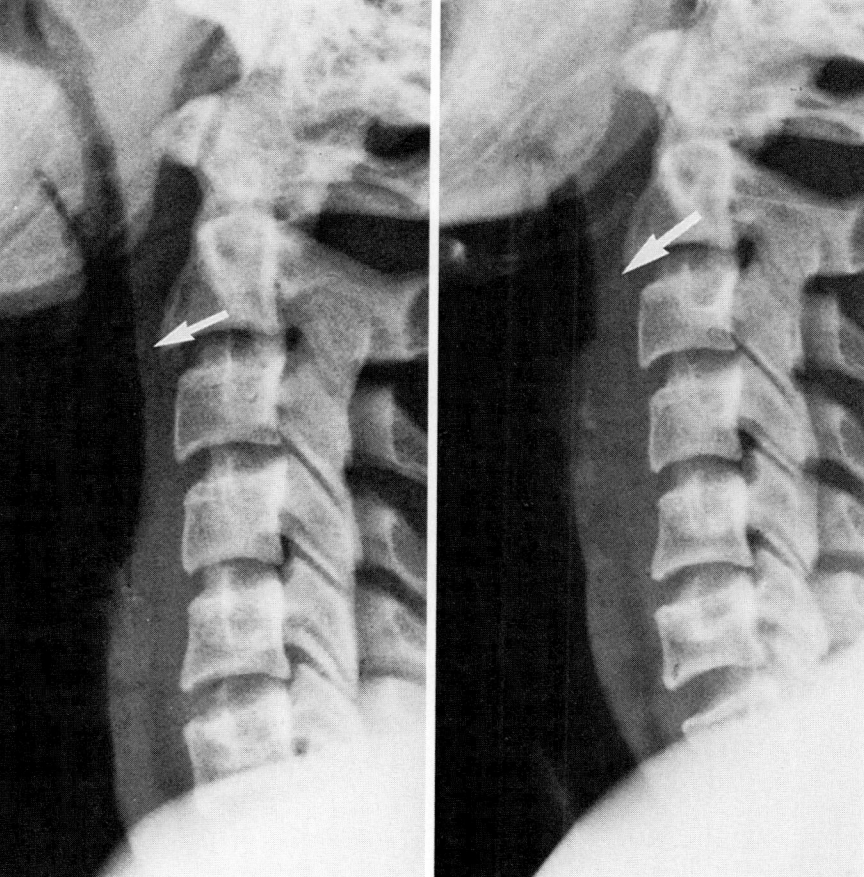

Figure 8–28. Thickening of the retropharyngeal tissues may be seen to a lesser degree in adults. *Left,* Inspiration. *Right, Expiration.* Transposition of the carotids anterior from their normal lateral positions into the retropharyngeal soft tissues has been described in elderly patients resulting in striking thickening of the retropharyngeal soft tissues at C2 and C3. (Ref: Fix TJ et al: Carotid transpositions. *Am J Roentgenol* 167:1305, 1996.)

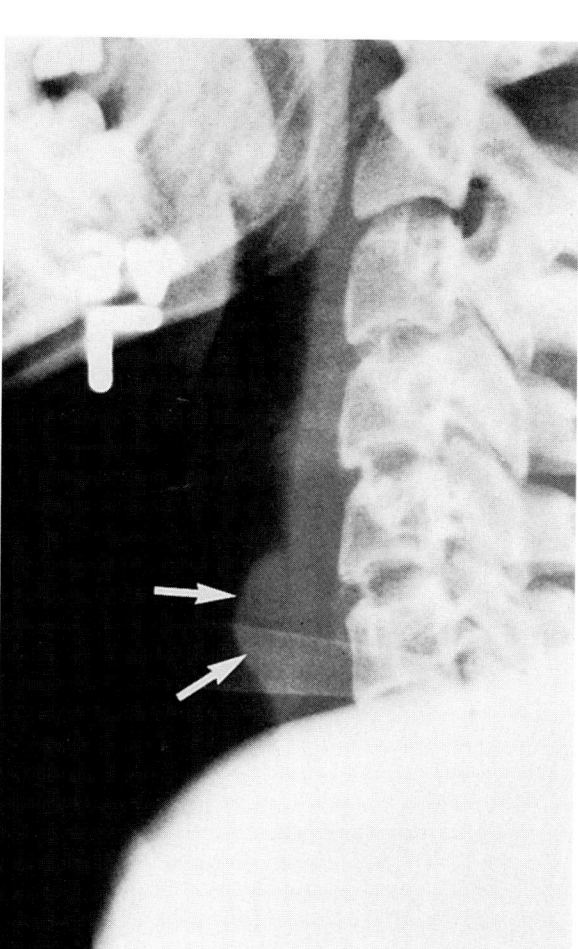

Figure 8–29. Localized anterior bulging of soft tissues and impression on the posterior aspect of the trachea in an adult in expiration.

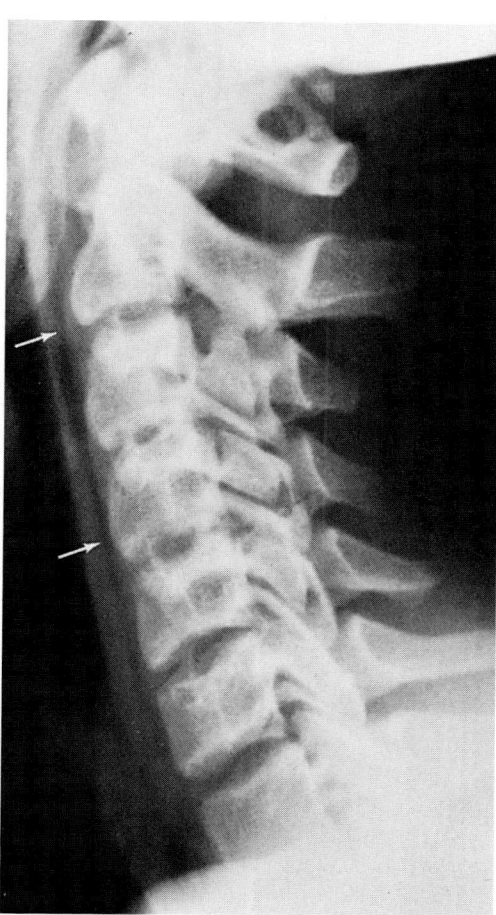

Figure 8–30. Prominent prevertebral fat stripe, not to be mistaken for gas in the soft tissues. (Ref: Whalen JP, Woodruff CL: The cervical prevertebral fat stripe: A new aid in evaluating the cervical prevertebral soft tissue space. *Am J Roentgenol* 109:445, 1970.)

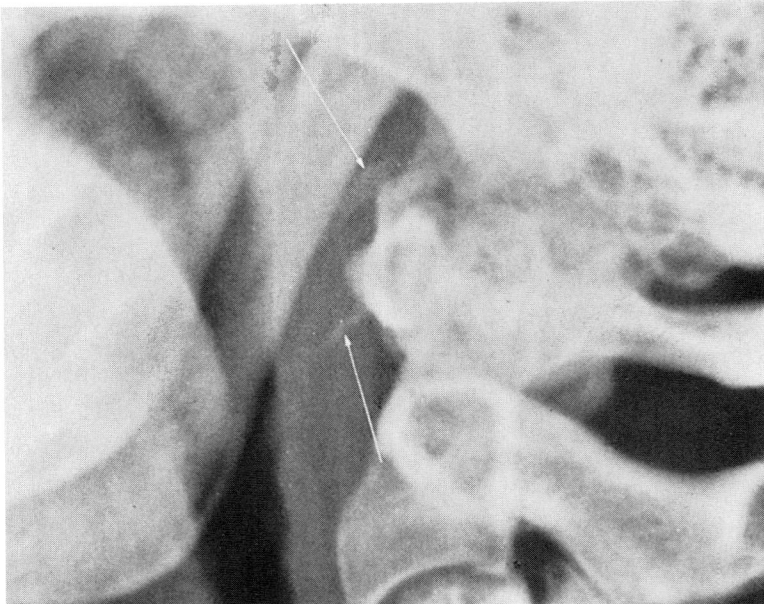

Figure 8–31. Styloid processes, which should not be mistaken for foreign bodies.

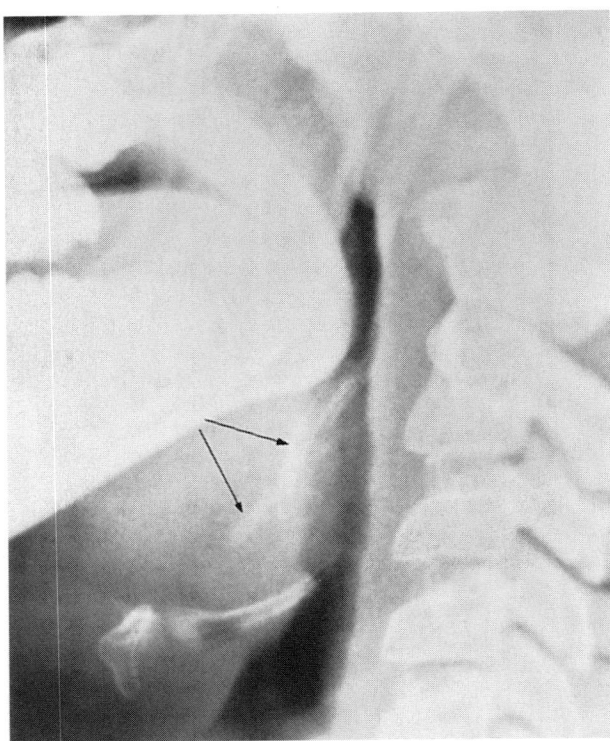

Figure 8–32. Stylohyoid ligament calcification in an 11-year-old girl.

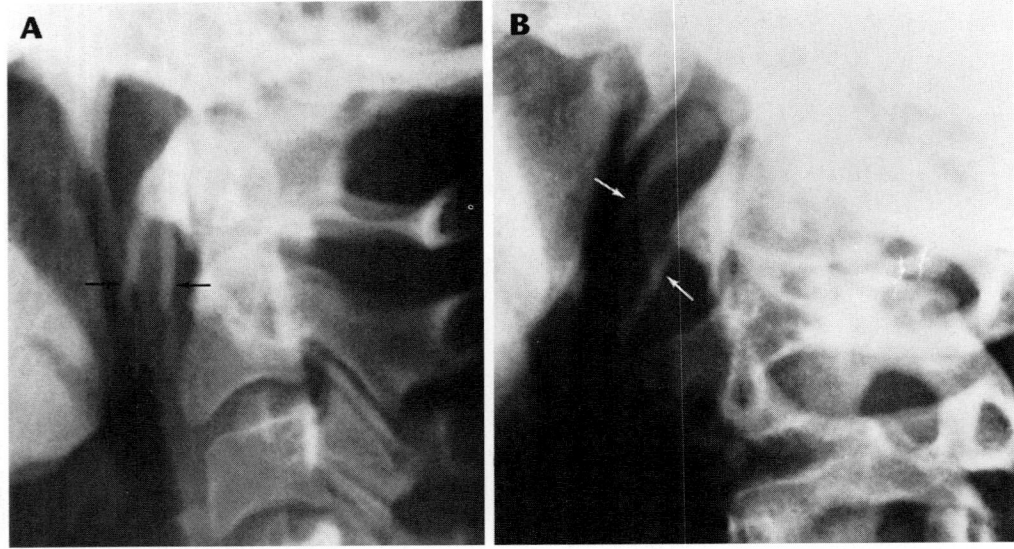

Figure 8–33. Calcified stylohyoid ligaments in lateral (**A**) and oblique (**B**) projections.

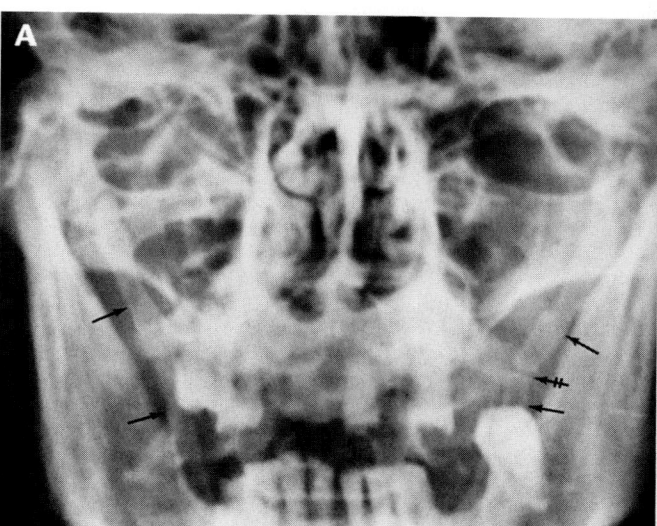
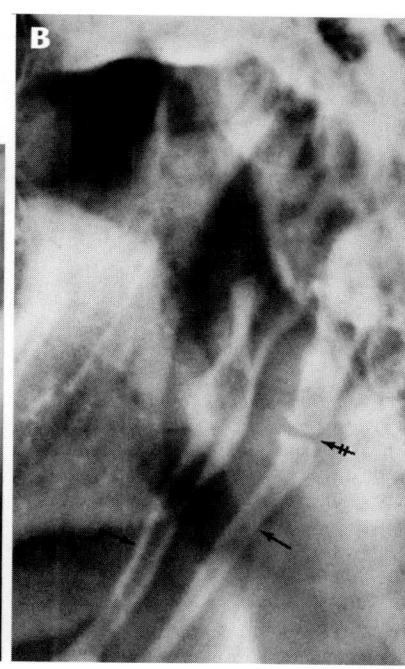

Figure 8–34. Extensively calcified stylohyoid ligaments in frontal (**A**) and lateral (**B**) projections (←). Note the articulation at the junction of the ligament and the styloid process (⟻). (Ref: Genez BM et al: Case report 584: Ossified stylohyoid complex with pseudarthroses. *Skeletal Radiol* 18:623, 1989.)

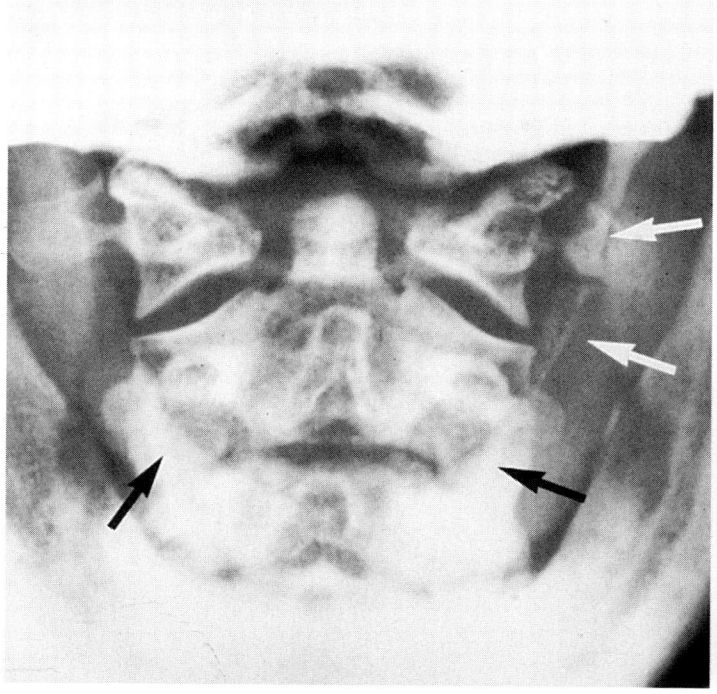
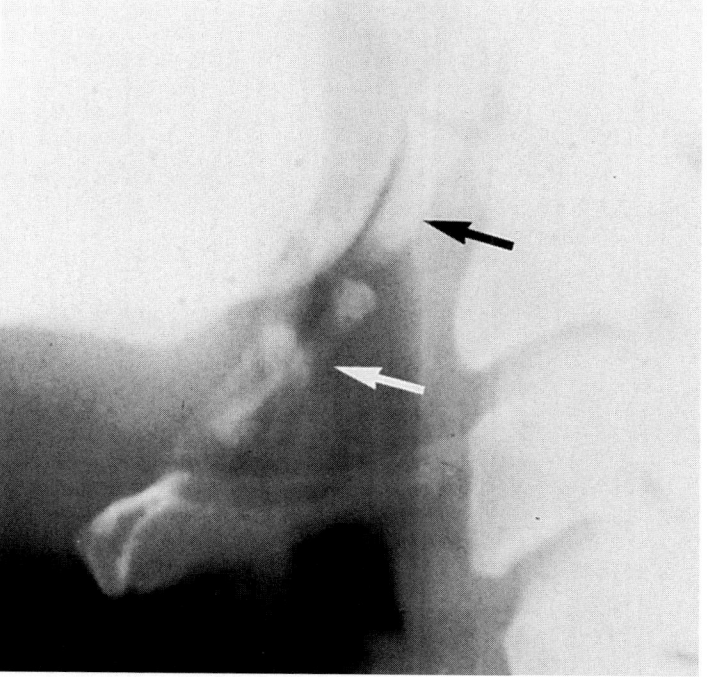

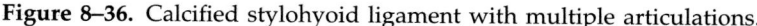
Figure 8–35. Calcified stylohyoid ligaments with multiple segments.

Figure 8–36. Calcified stylohyoid ligament with multiple articulations.

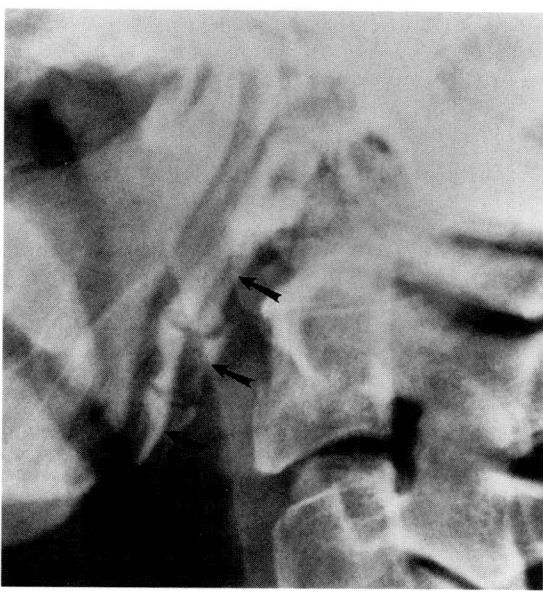

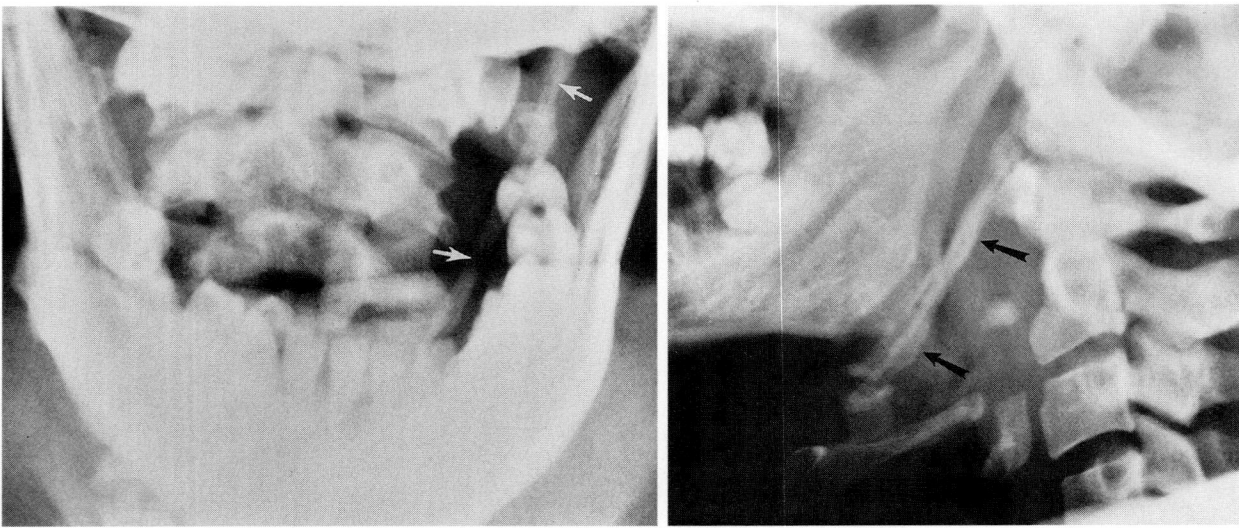

Figure 8–37. Large calcified stylohyoid ligaments.

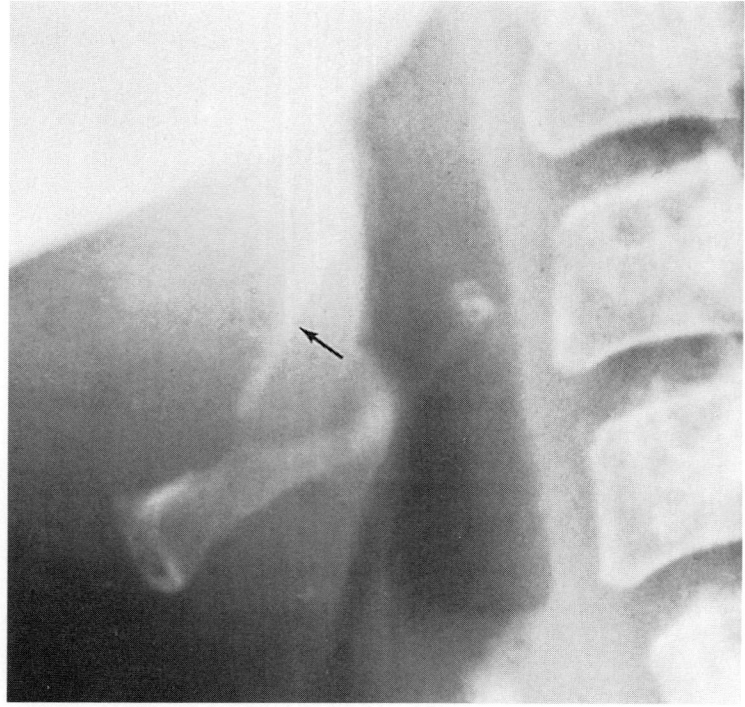

Figure 8–38. Partial calcification of the stylohyoid ligaments, simulating a foreign body.

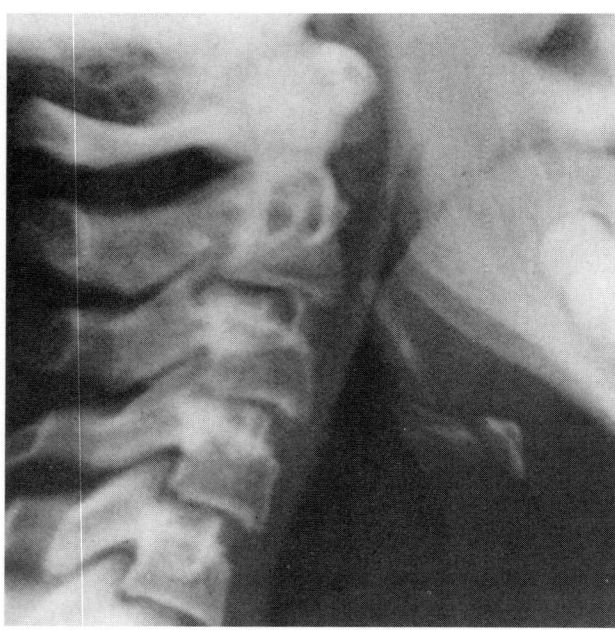

Figure 8–39. Unilateral calcified stylohyoid ligament in an 11-year-old girl, mistaken for a foreign body.

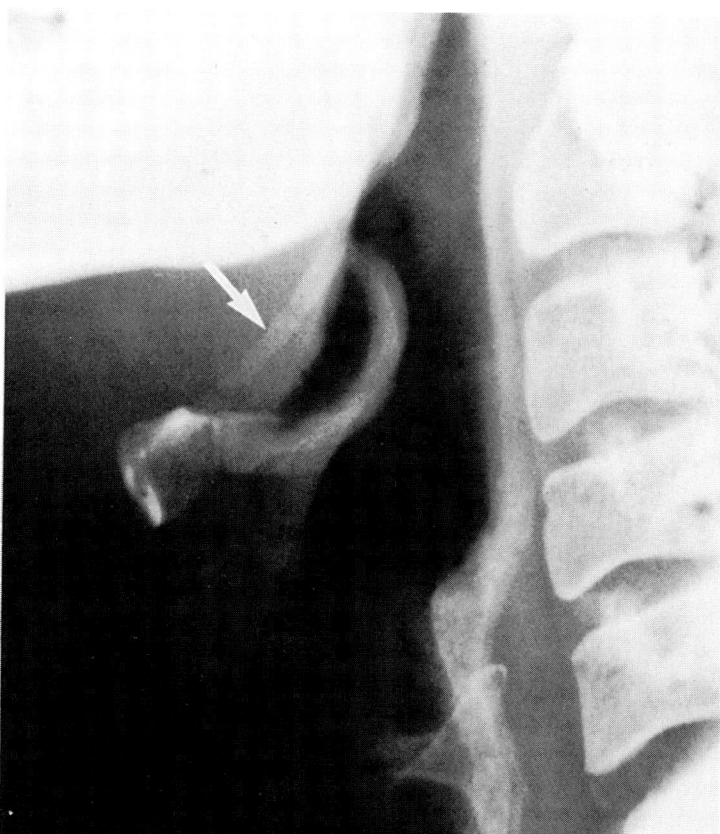

Figure 8–40. Stylohyoid ligament calcification mistaken for an impacted chicken bone.

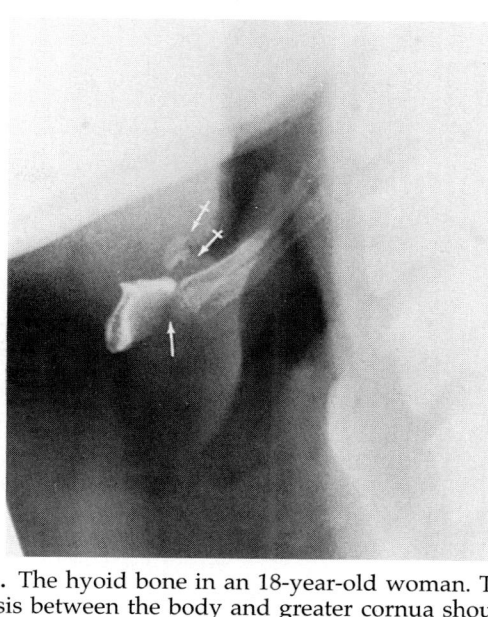

Figure 8–41. The hyoid bone in an 18-year-old woman. The synchondrosis between the body and greater cornua should not be mistaken for a fracture (→). Note also the lesser cornua (↔).

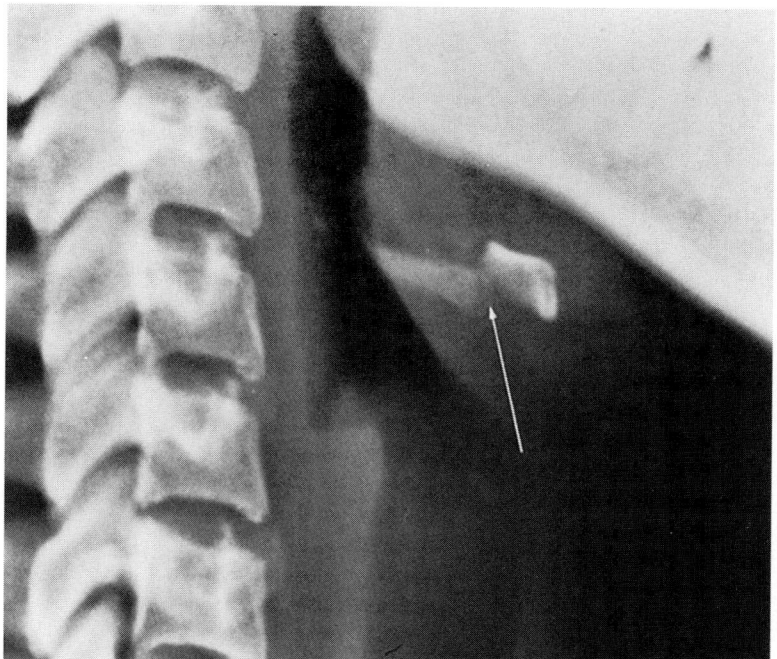

Figure 8–42. Simulated fracture of the hyoid in a 12-year-old girl.

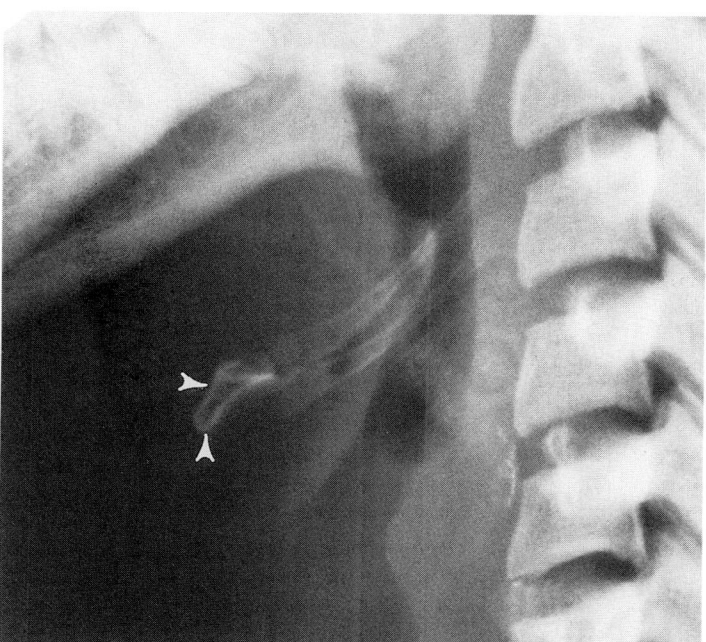

Figure 8–43. Variation in anatomy of the hyoid bone. Note inclination of the body of the hyoid compared with the preceding figure.

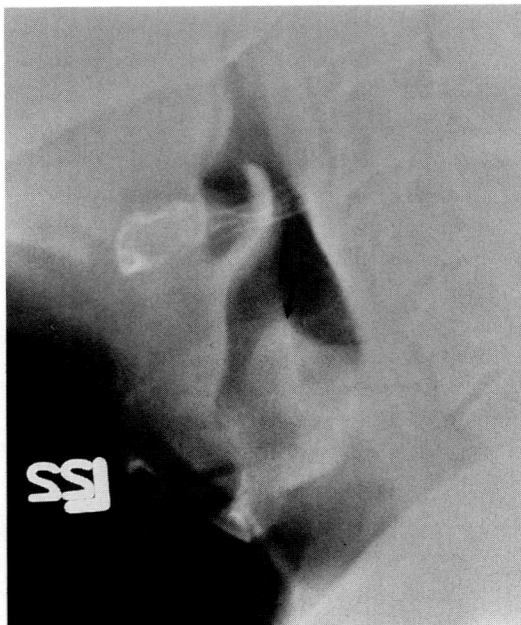

Figure 8–44. Arytenoid "bump."

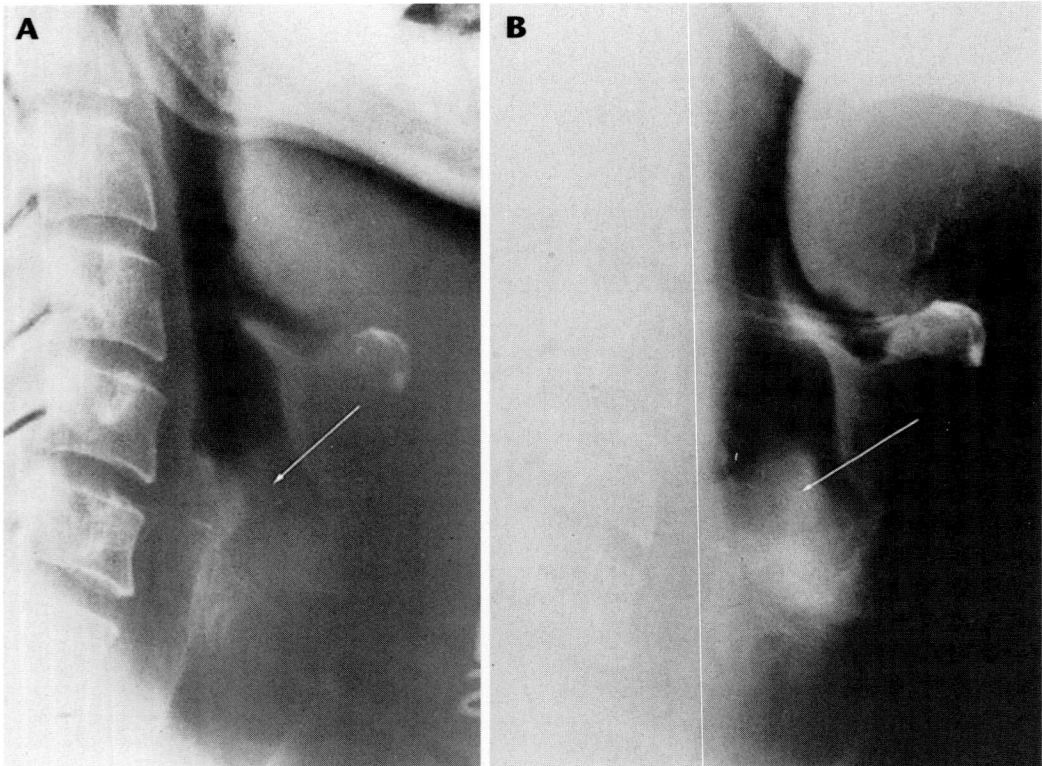

Figure 8–45. Variations in the arytenoid with phonation. **A,** Quiet breathing. **B,** Phonation.

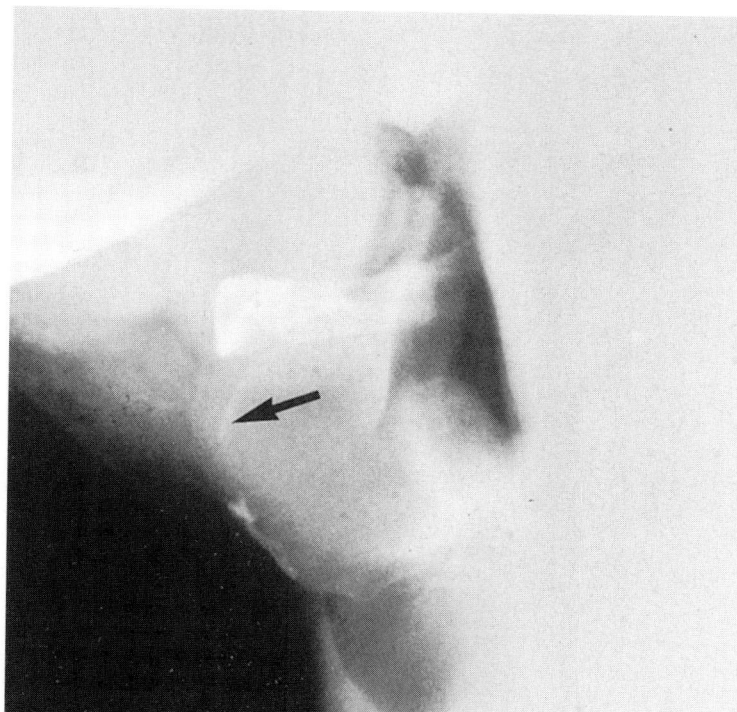

Figure 8–46. Calcification in the thyrohyoid ligament.

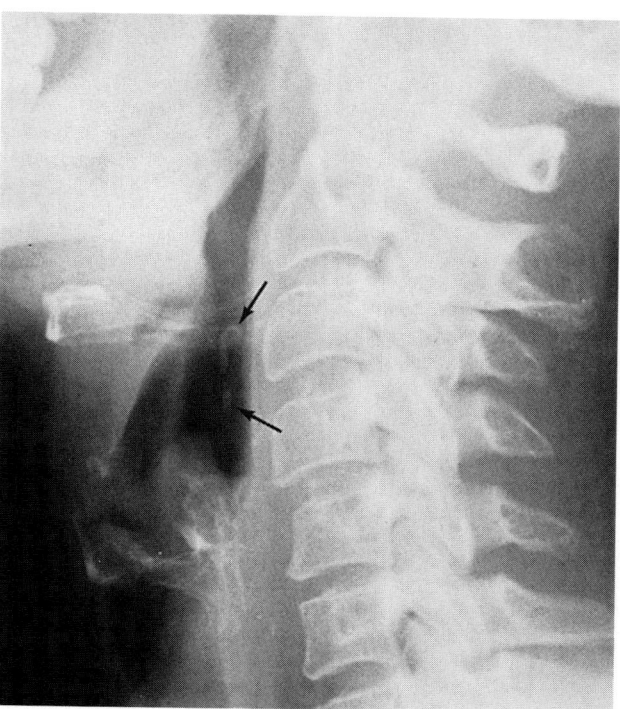

Figure 8–47. Calcification in the arytenoid cartilage. (Ref: Jurik AG: Ossification and calcification of the laryngeal skeleton. *Acta Radiol Diagn* 25:17, 1984.)

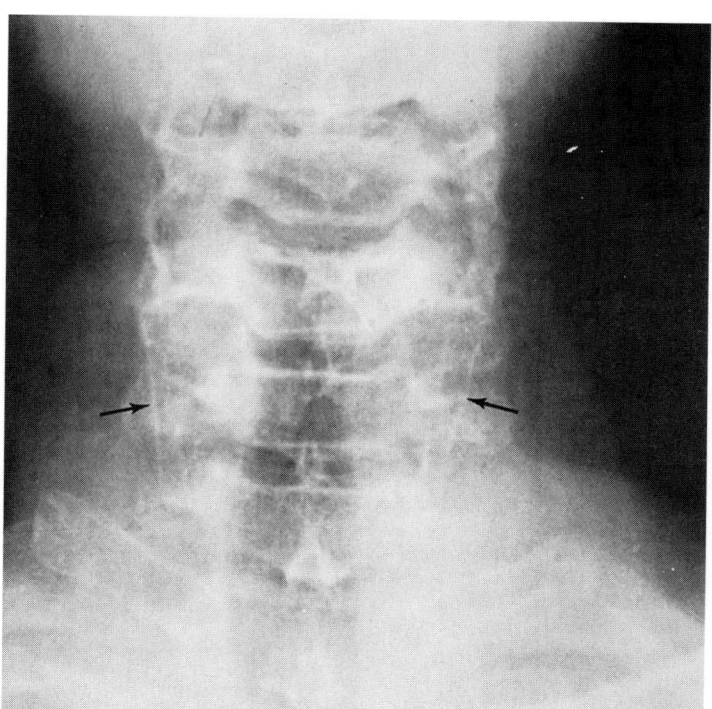

Figure 8–48. Calcification of the thyroid cartilages, simulating carotid artery calcification.

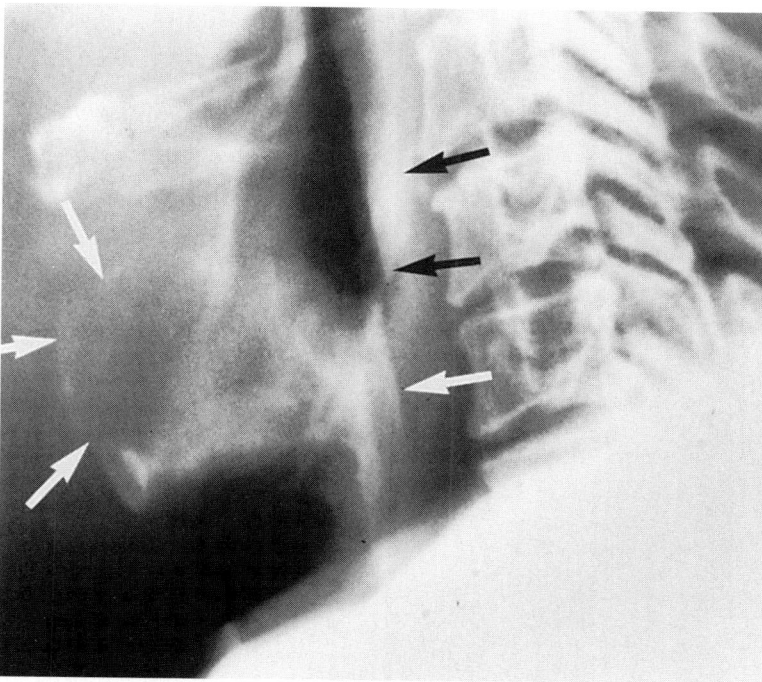

Figure 8–49. Calcification of the entire thyroid cartilage.

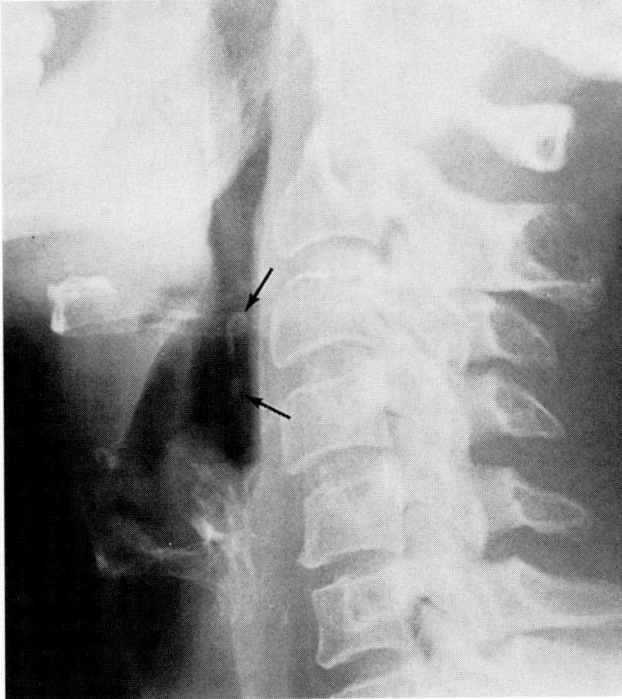

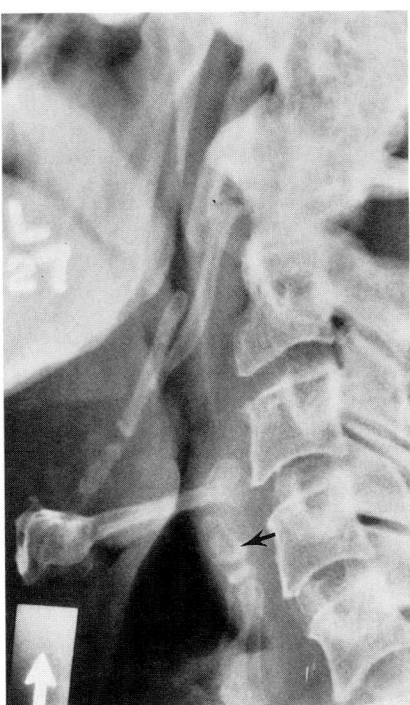

Figure 8–50. Calcification of the superior cornua of the thyroid cartilage, which might be mistaken for a foreign body.

Figure 8–51. Superior cornua of the thyroid cartilage as a separate ossicle. Note also the calcification of the stylohyoid ligaments.

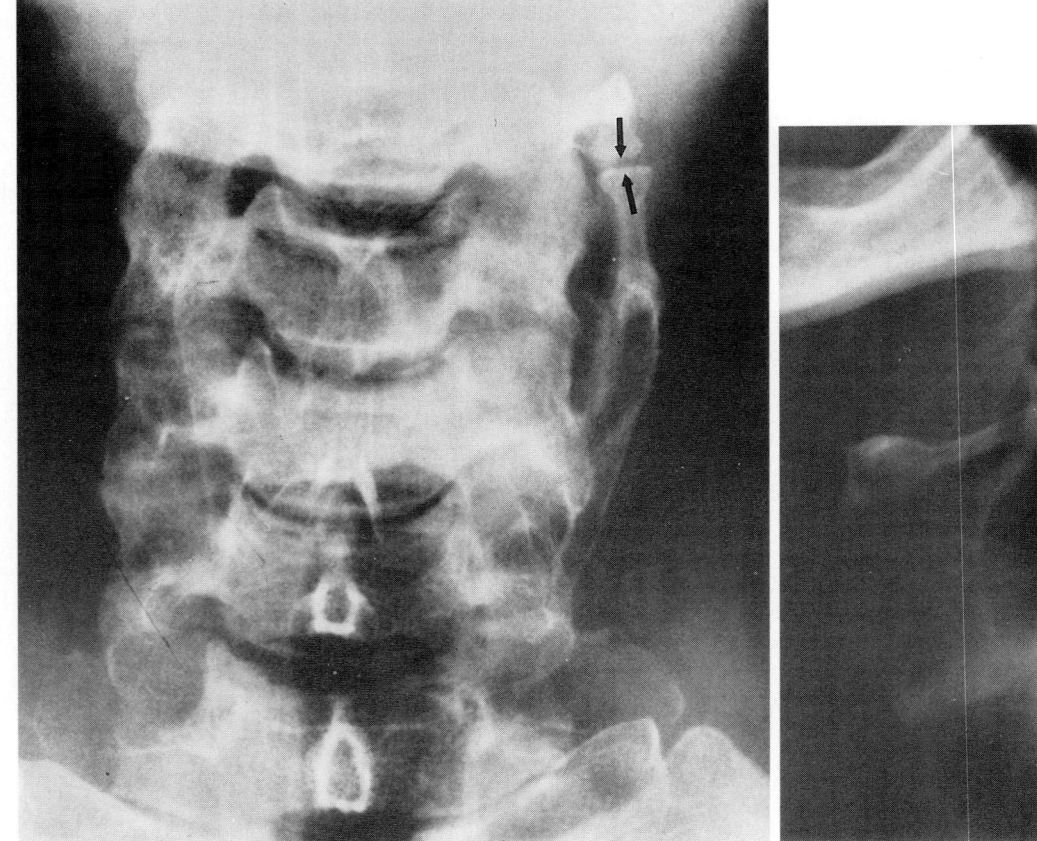

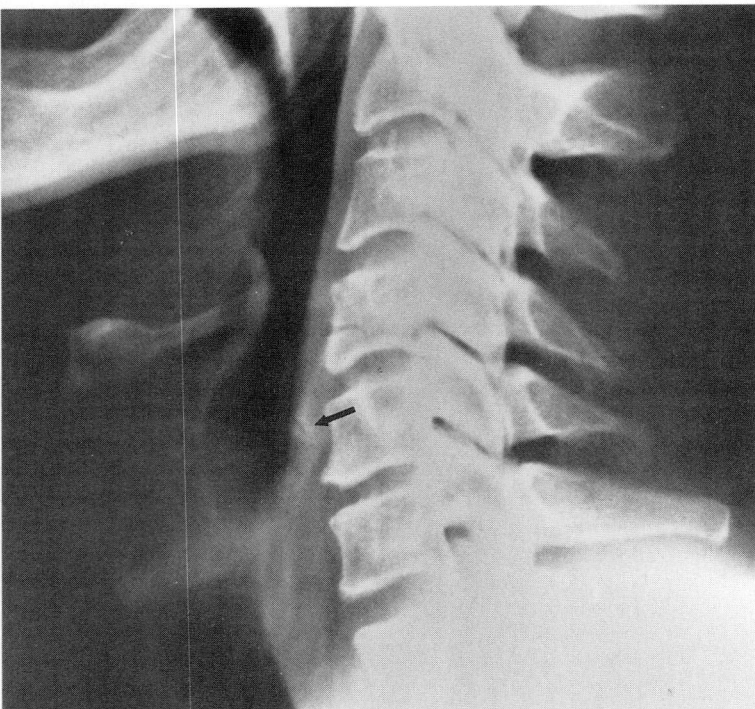

Figure 8–52. Superior cornua of the thyroid cartilage as a separate ossicle with an articulation.

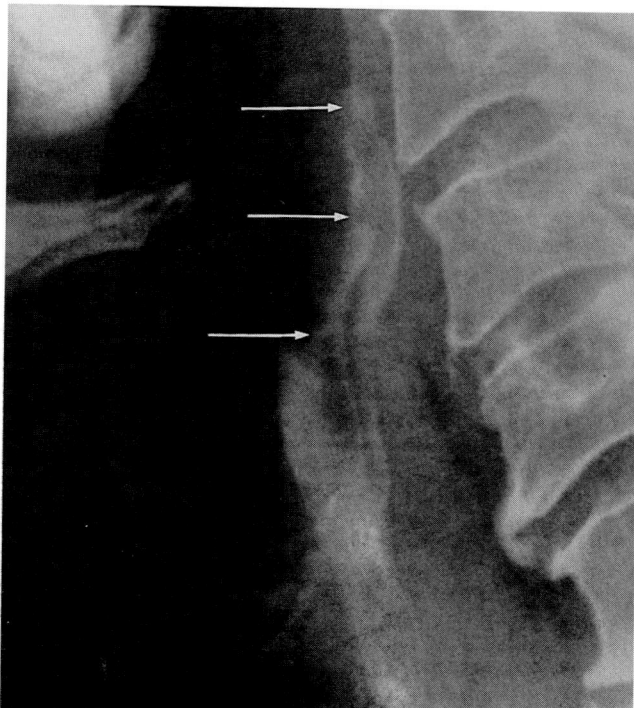

Figure 8–53. Huge superior cornua of the thyroid cartilage.

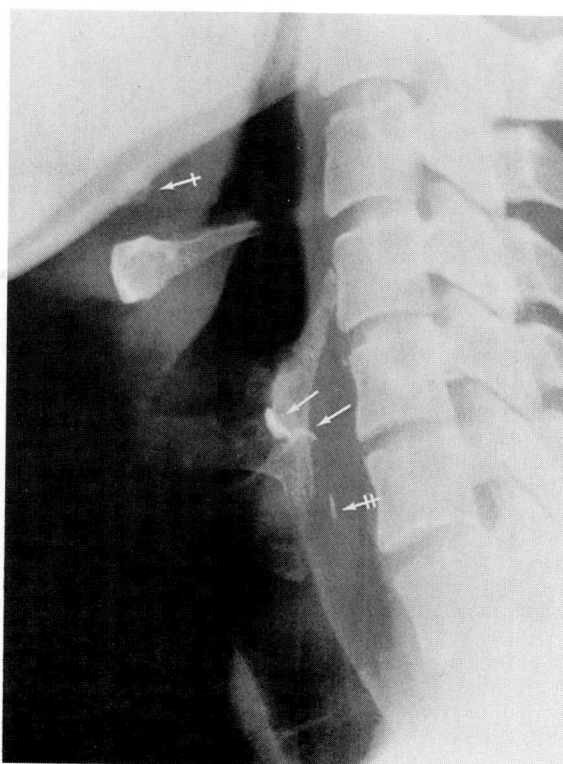

Figure 8–54. Calcification in the arytenoid cartilages (→). Note also a submaxillary gland calculus (↦). The *lowest arrow* (⇥) indicates calcification in the posterior lamina of the cricoid cartilage.

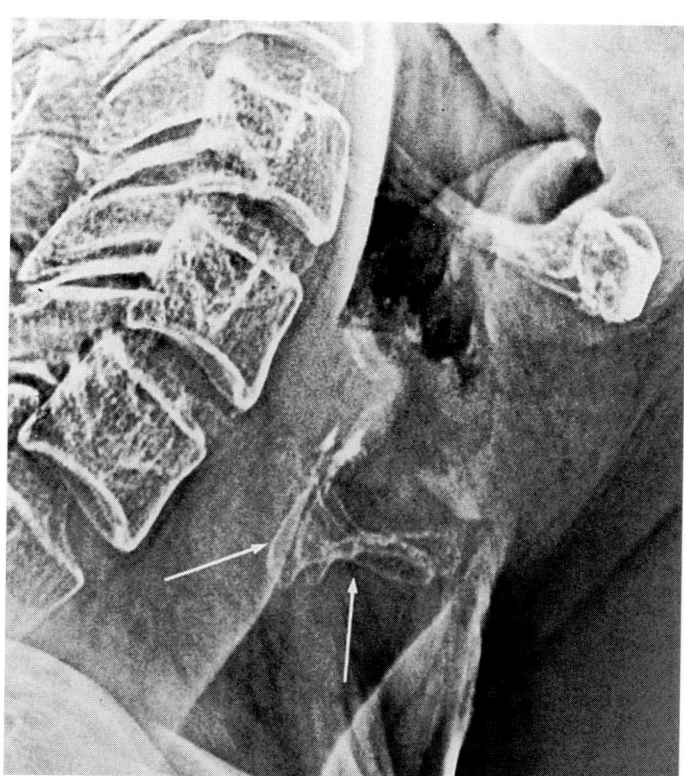

Figure 8–55. Calcification of the cricoid cartilages.

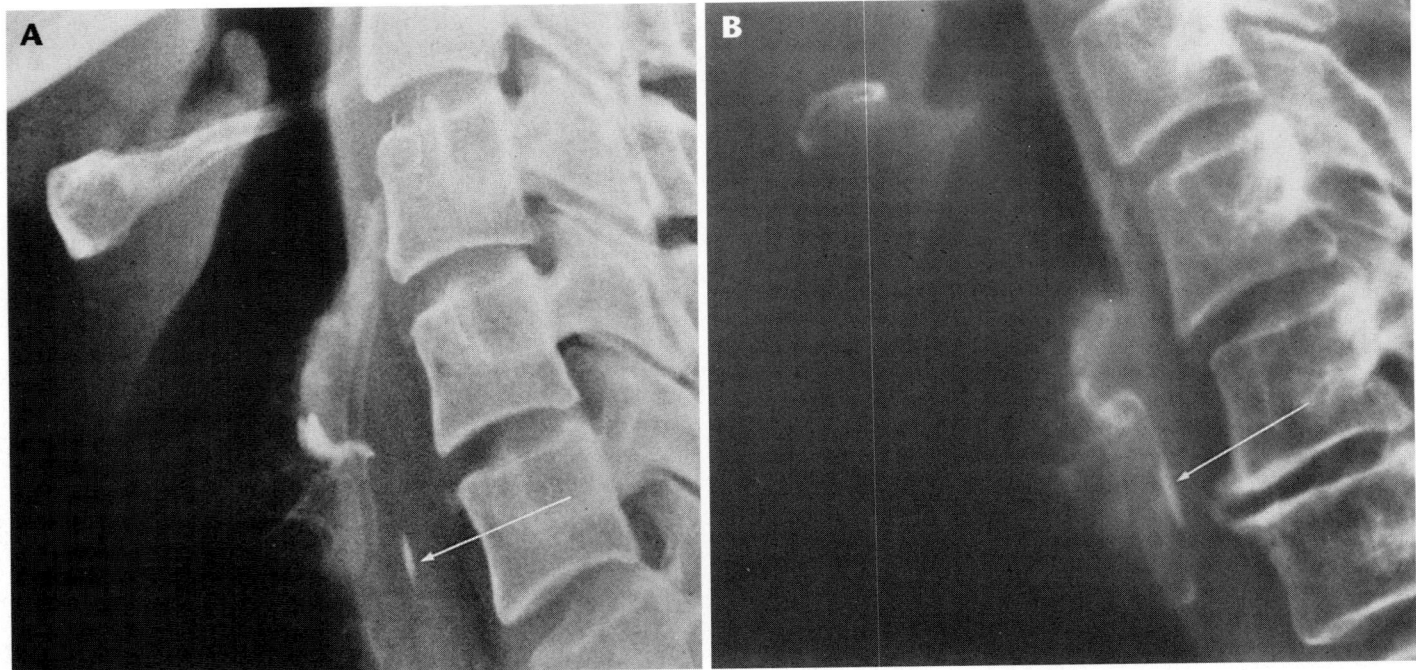

Figure 8–56. A, Calcification of the posterior cricoid lamina when seen in isolation may be easily confused with a foreign body. **B,** In a patient with more extensive calcification of the larynx, the relationship to the density seen in **A** is more easily identified.

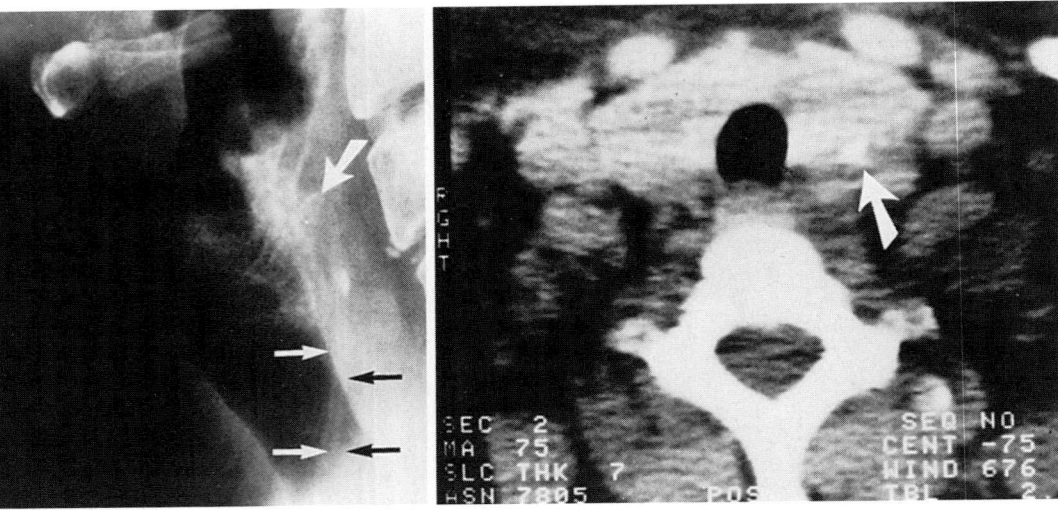

Figure 8–57. *Left,* Unusually long tubular calcification arising from the cricoid cartilage and descending anteriorly and inferiorly. *Right,* CT shows the same structure. The nature of this variant is unknown. (From Nidecker A et al: The cricoid cartilage: Observations on some roentgen variants. *ORL J Otorhinolaryngol Relat Spec* 44:170, 1982.)

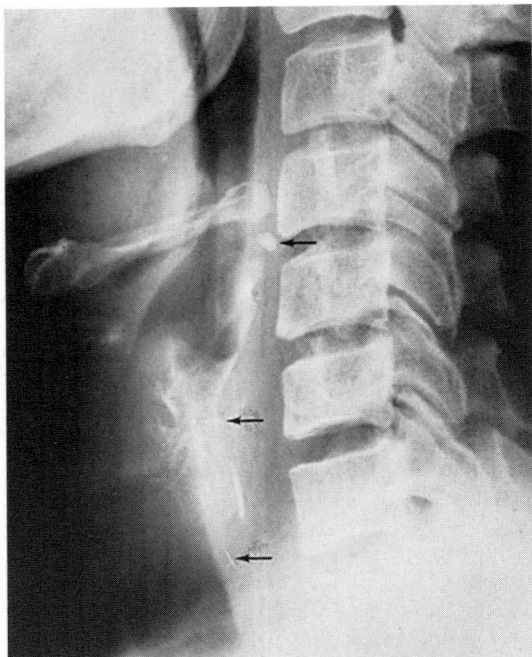

Figure 8–58. Physiologic calcification of the soft tissues of the neck. The *upper arrow* indicates calcification in the thyrohyoid ligament (cartilago triticea). The *middle arrow* shows calcification in the arytenoid cartilage. The *lower arrow* indicates calcification in the tracheal cartilage.

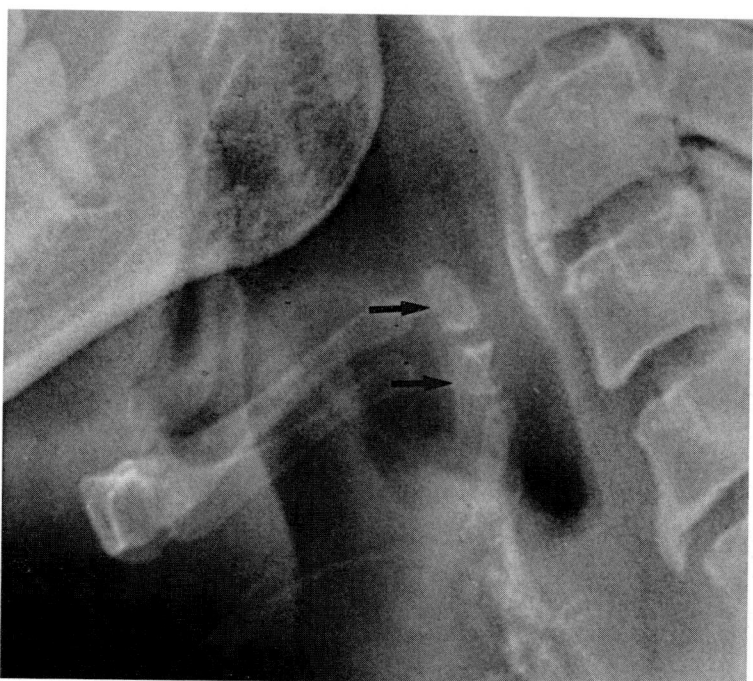

Figure 8–59. Large cartilago triticea.

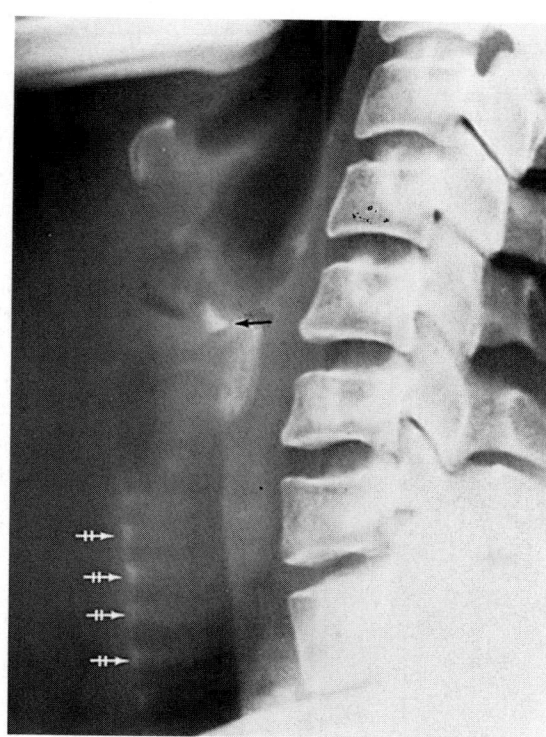

Figure 8–60. Calcified arytenoid (←) and calcification of tracheal cartilages (↔) in a 37-year-old woman.

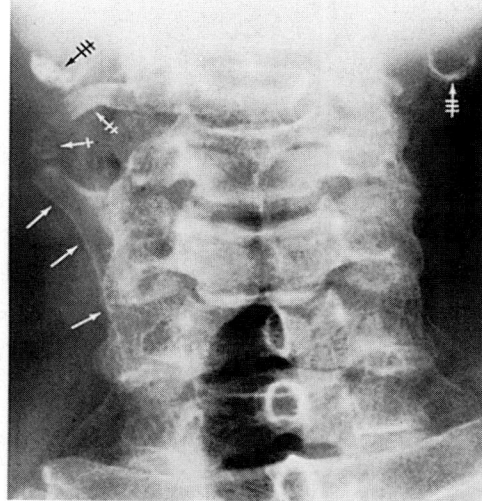

Figure 8–61. Physiologic calcifications in the frontal projection: Thyroid cartilage (→), cartilago triticea (↦), hyoid bone (↦), and carotid artery calcification (↦).

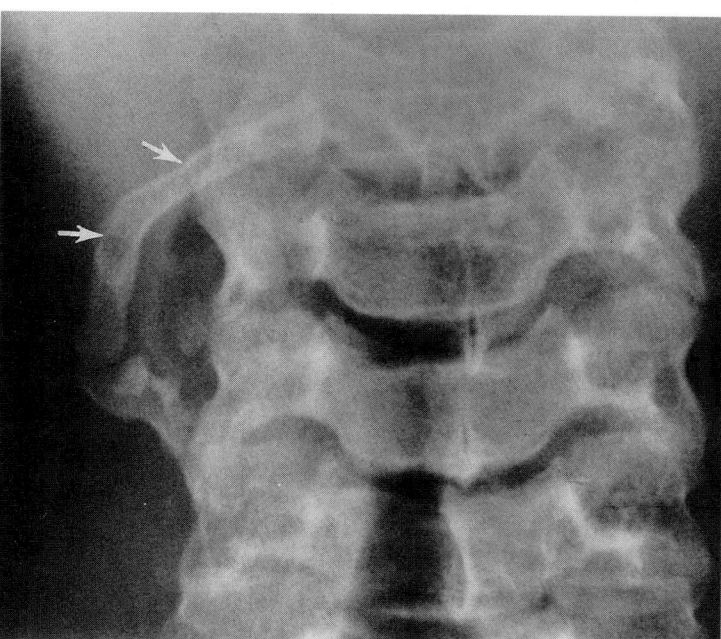

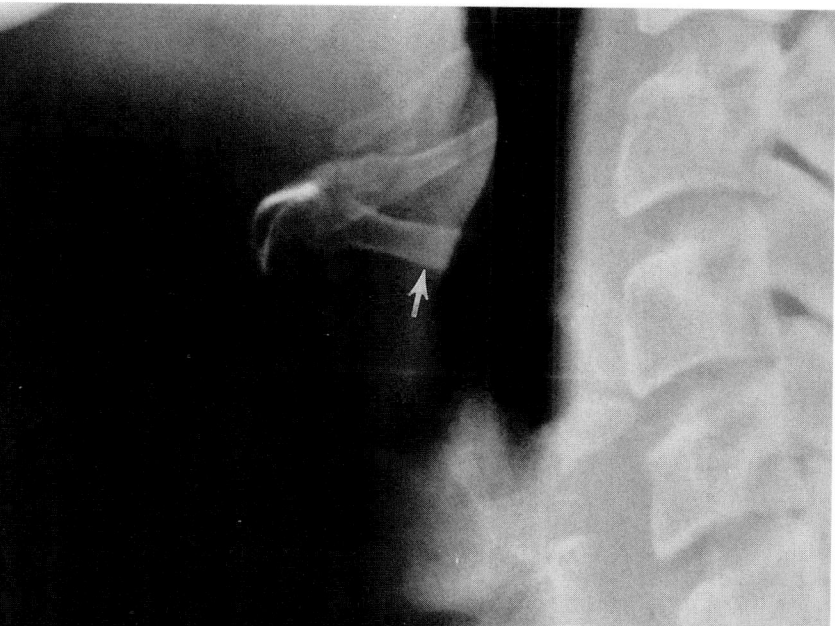

Figure 8–62. Marked calcification in the thyrohyoid ligament in a 28-year-old woman.

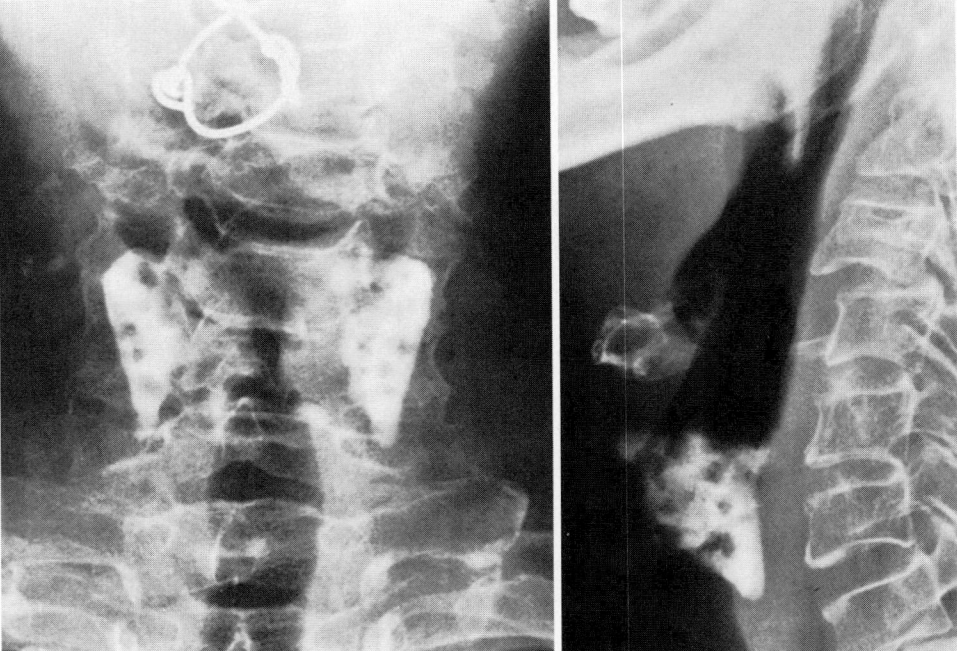

Figure 8–63. Very dense calcification of the thyroid cartilages.

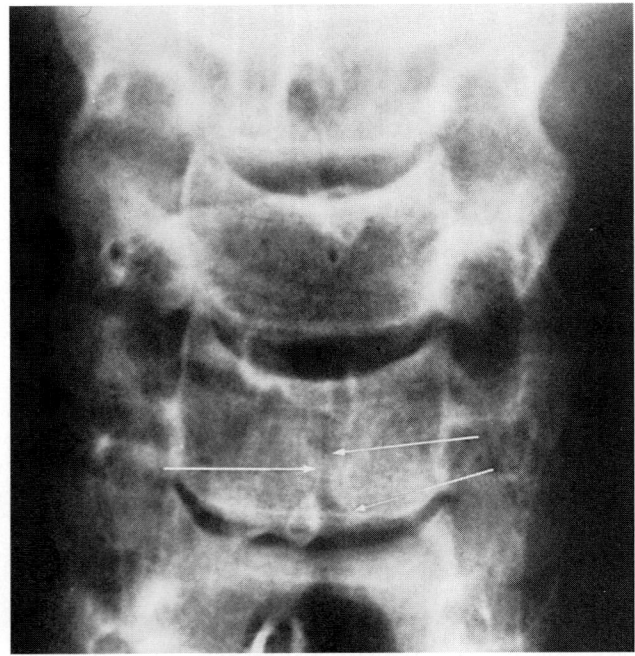

Figure 8–64. Shadow of the glottis was originally misinterpreted as a fracture of the vertebral body.

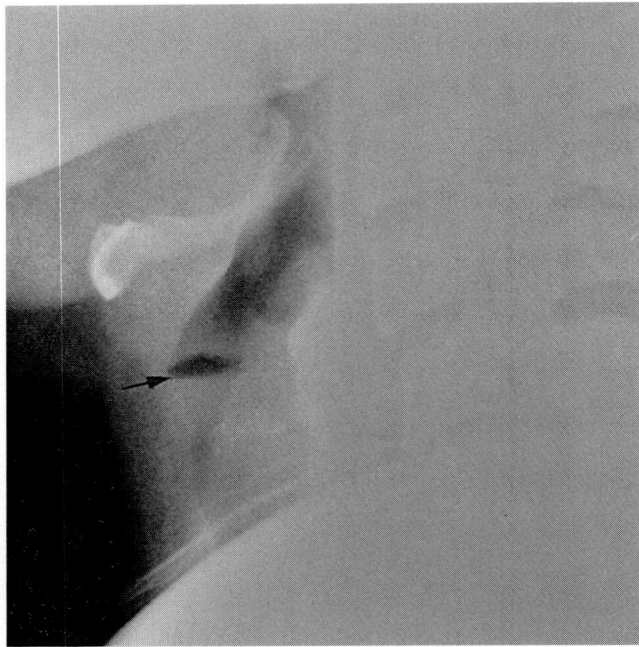

Figure 8–65. Air in laryngeal ventricle mistaken for an abscess.

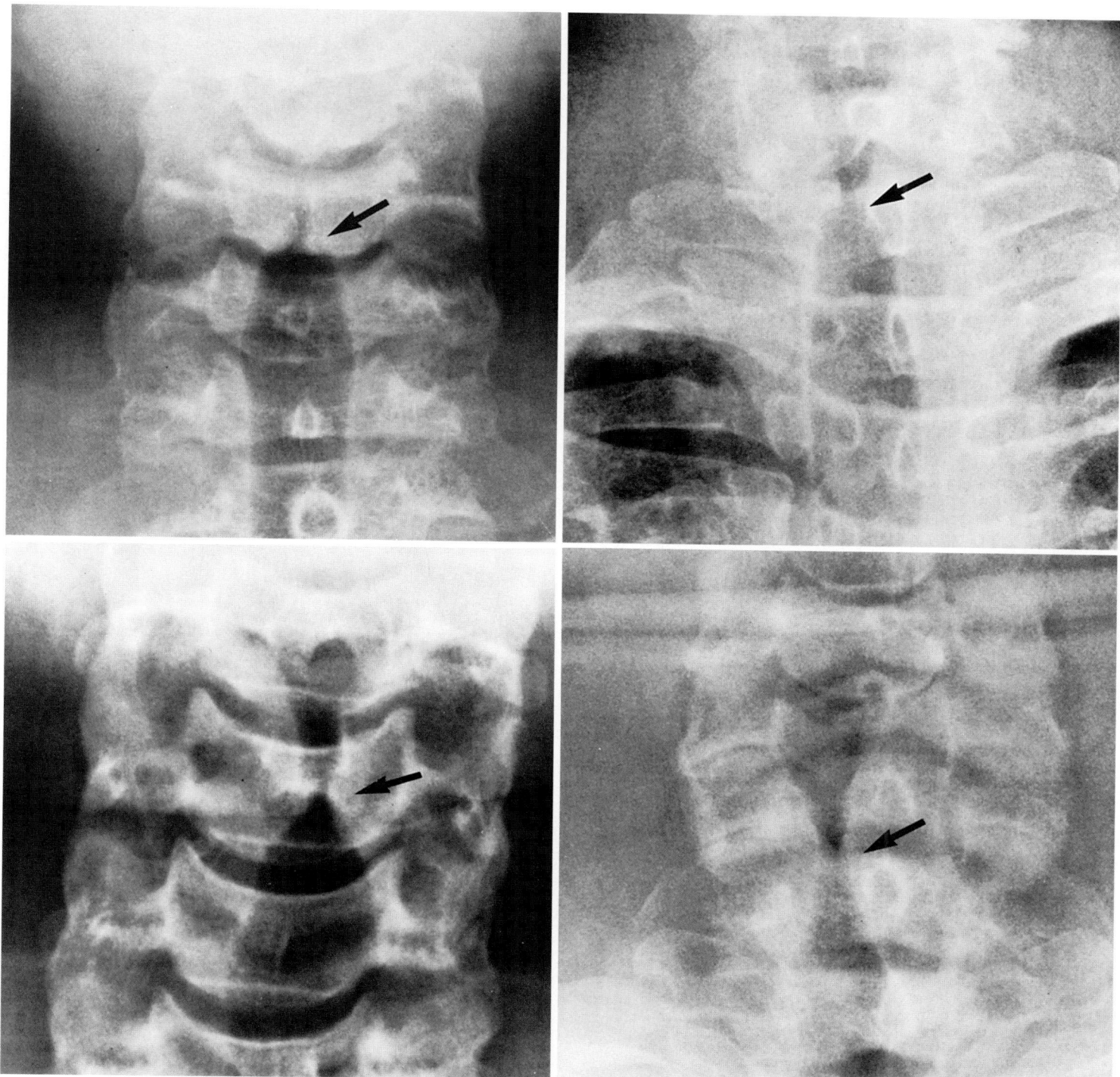

Figure 8–66. Variations in appearance of the normal closed glottis in frontal projection. (Ref: Wittrum C, Kenny JB: The radiographic appearances of the larynx on the chest radiograph. *Br J Radiol* 67:755, 1994.)

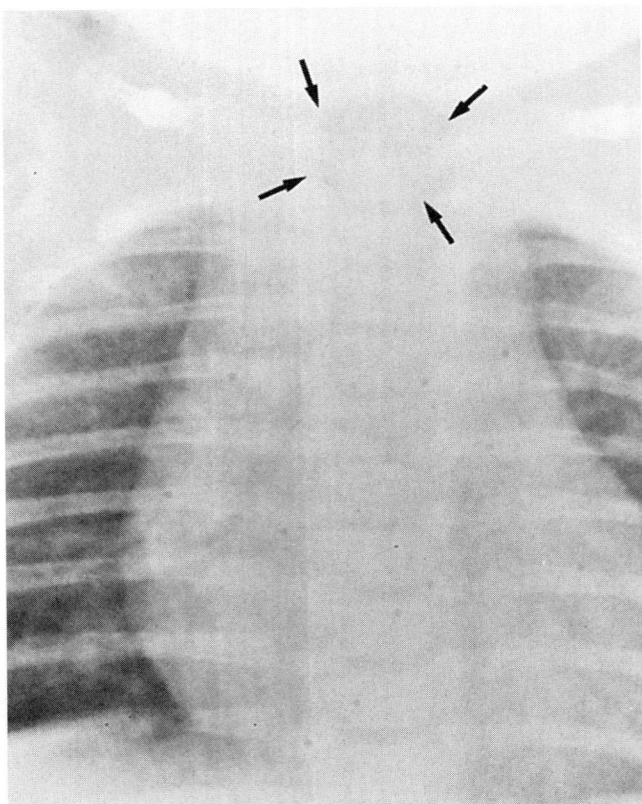

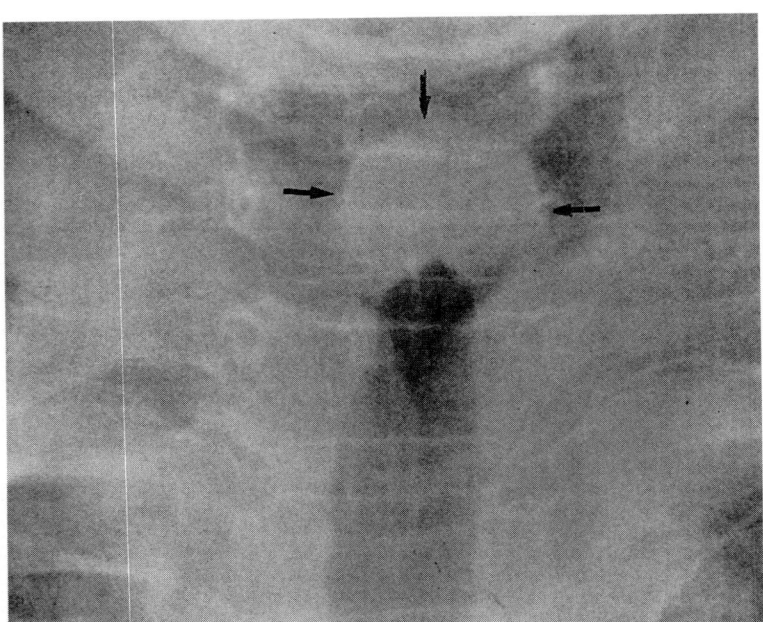

Figure 8–68. Pseudomass produced by deep pyriform sinuses.

Figure 8–67. The suprasternal fossa in a newborn infant may simulate the distended proximal pouch of an esophageal atresia. (Ref: Hernandez R et al: The suprasternal fossa on chest radiographs in newborns. *Am J Roentgenol* 130:745, 1978.)

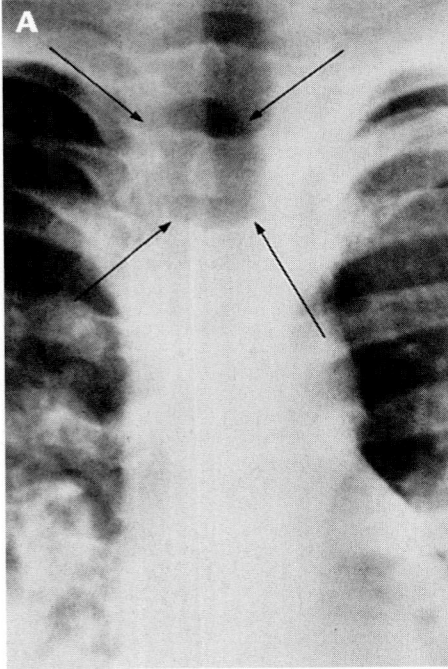

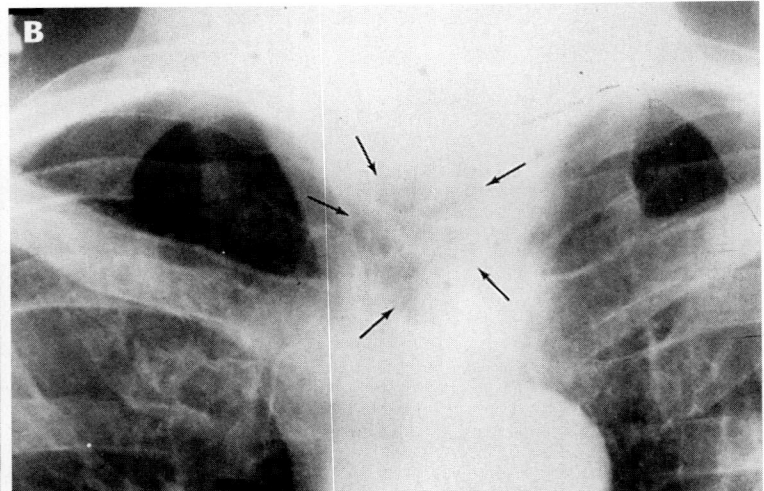

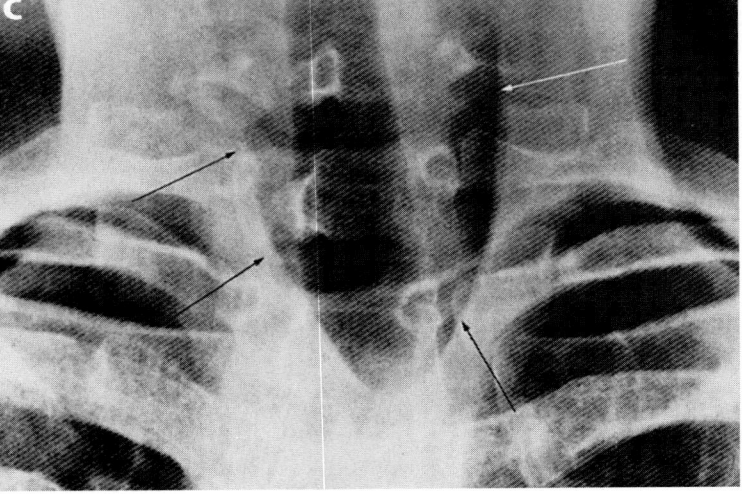

Figure 8–69. Suprasternal fossa in older children (**A**) or thin adults (**B** and **C**) may be quite deep and may cast a radiolucency that may be mistaken for an air-filled esophageal diverticulum. (Ref: Ominsky S, Berinson HS: The suprasternal fossa. *Radiology* 122:311, 1976.)

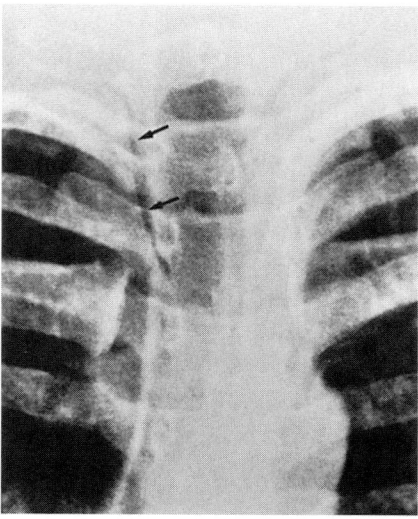

Figure 8–70. Simulated gas in soft tissues, produced by suprasternal fossa.

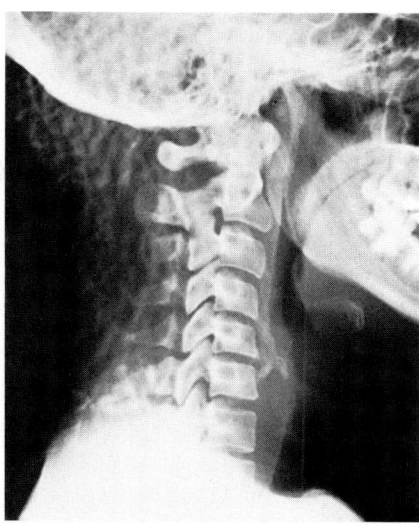

Figure 8–71. Simulated interstitial air in the posterior neck, caused by hair braids.

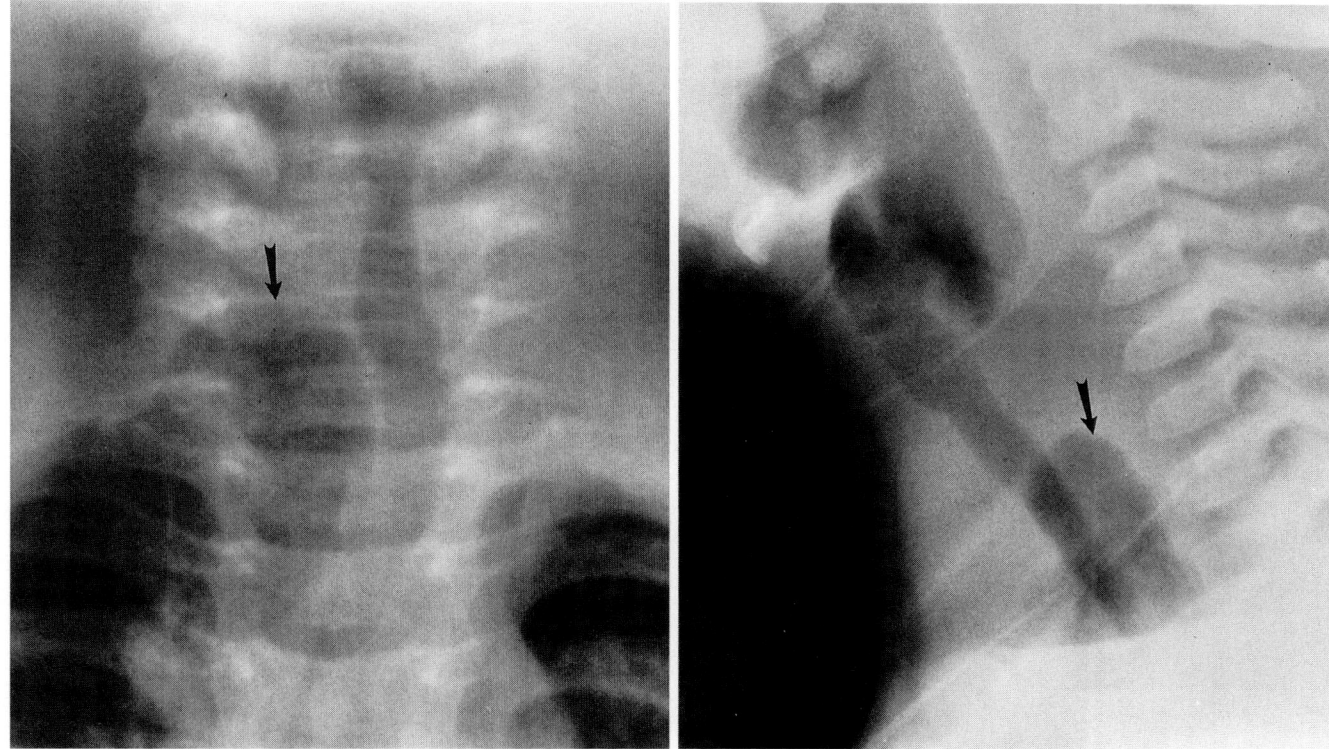

Figure 8–72. Herniation of the apex of the right lung in a 1-year-old infant.

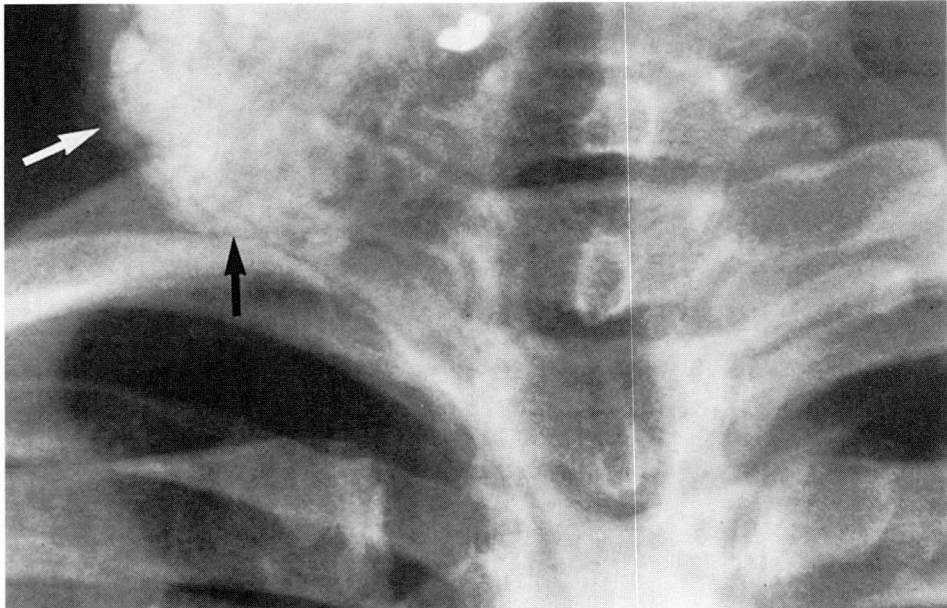

Figure 8–73. Hair braids simulating calcific thyroid mass.

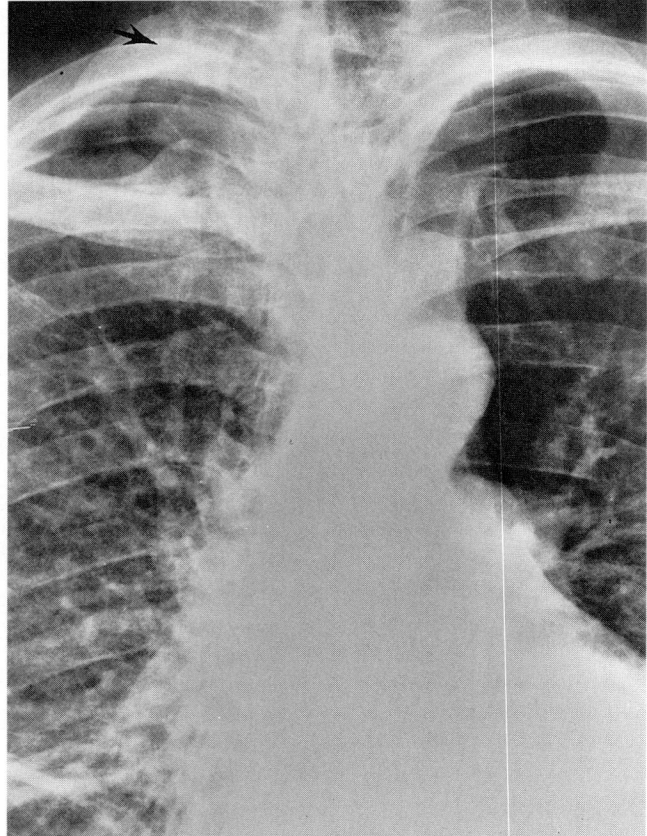

Figure 8–74. Hair braids simulating interstitial emphysema of the soft tissues of the neck.

CHAPTER

9

The Soft Tissues of the Thorax

The Chest Wall

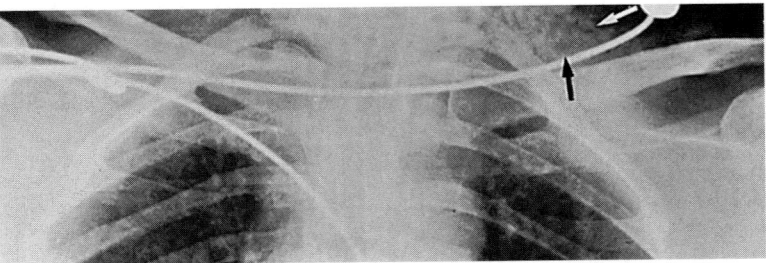

Figure 9–1. Hair braids simulating gas in the soft tissues of the neck.

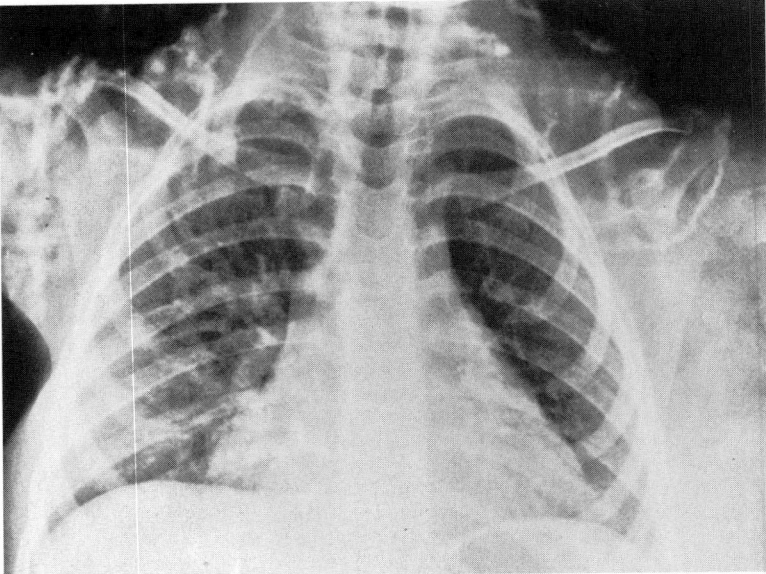

Figure 9–2. Plastic hair braid beads producing unusual appearance of the soft tissues of the neck and shoulders.

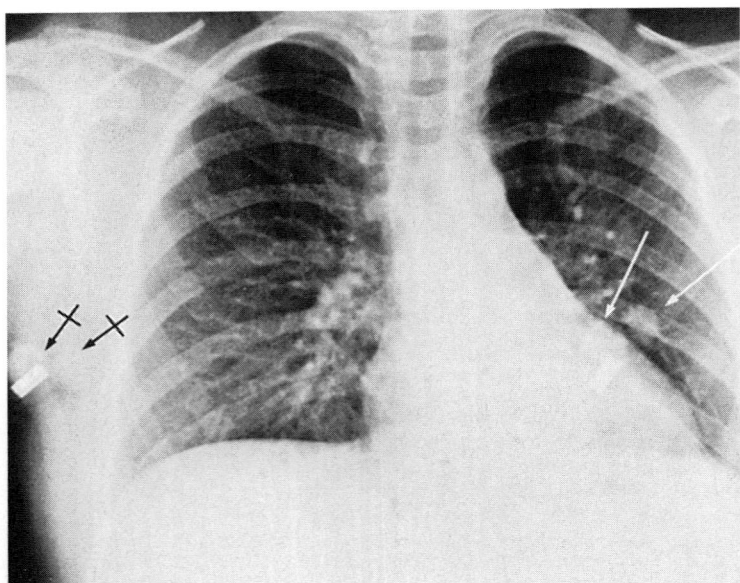

Figure 9–3. Simulated parenchymal lesions caused by hair braids (←). Note similar shadow laterally on right (↤).

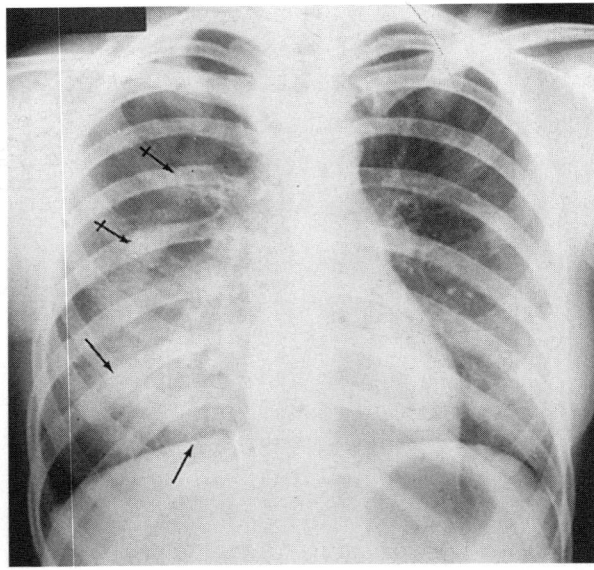

Figure 9–4. The dense juvenile breast may cast shadows simulating parenchymal density (→). Note also shadows cast by hair braids (↦).

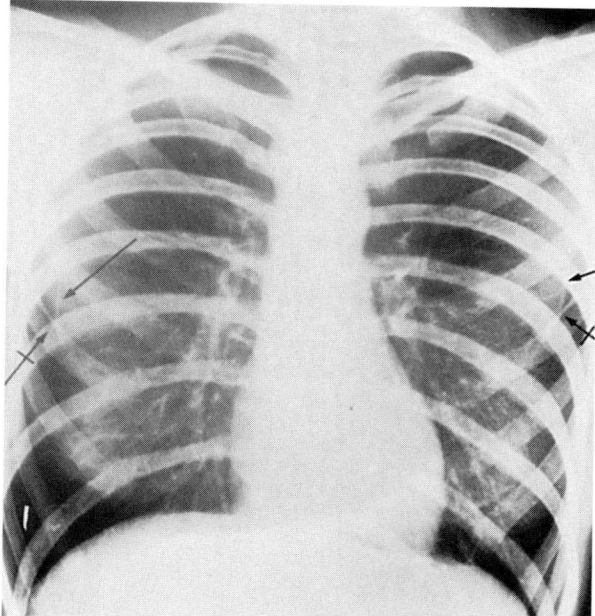

Figure 9–5. Intersecting shadows of the breast (←) and pectoral folds (↤).

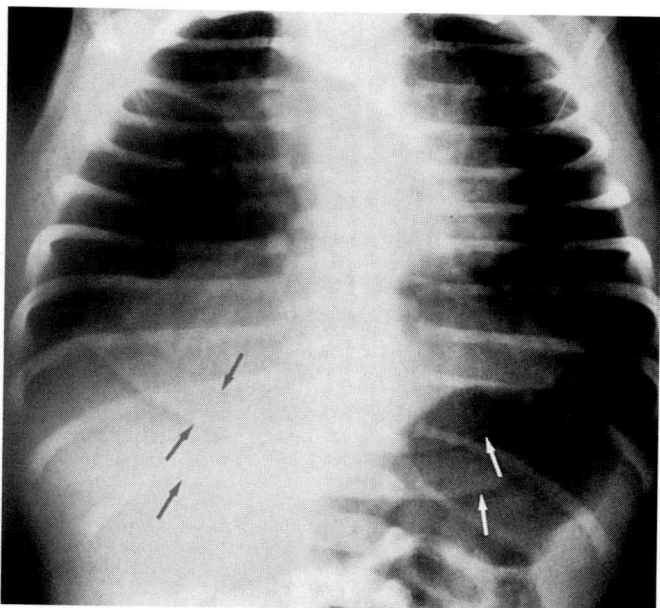

Figure 9–6. Skin folds producing curvilinear densities in the lower thorax and upper abdomen in a 3-week-old infant.

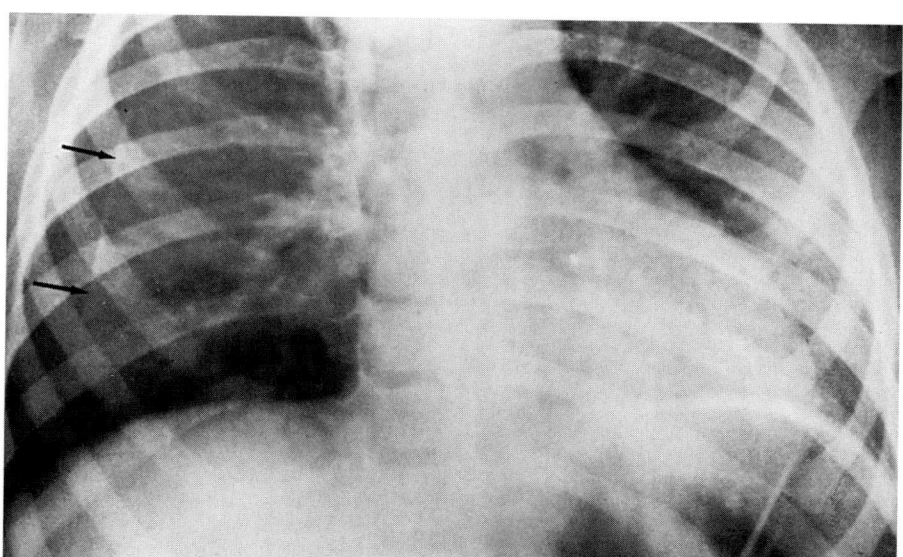

Figure 9–7. Simulated pneumothorax in a 3½-year-old child, caused by a skin fold.

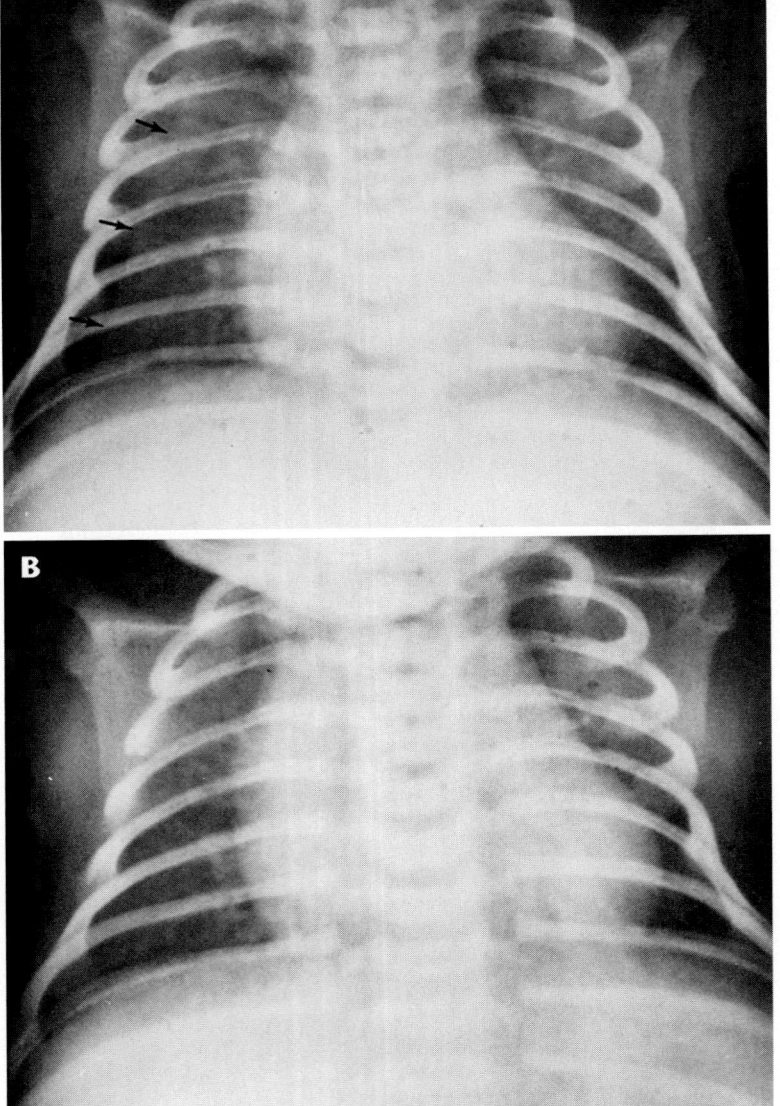

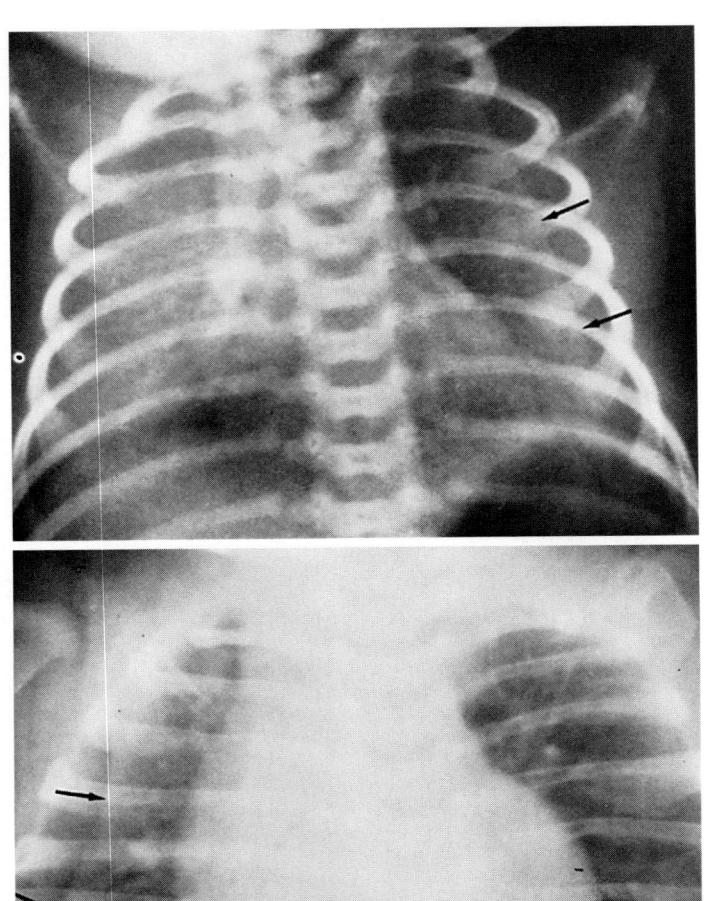

Figure 9–9. Two examples of simulated pneumothoraces in neonates, produced by skin folds.

Figure 9–8. Simulated pneumothorax in a neonate, produced by a skin fold. **A,** Simulated pneumothorax. **B,** Normal appearance 5 hours later.

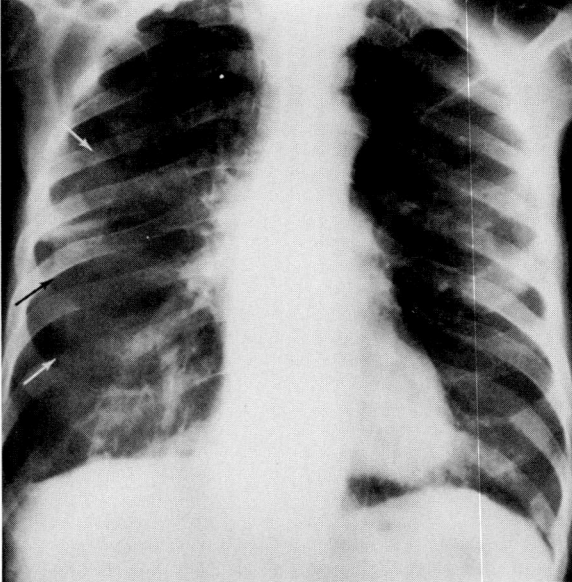

Figure 9–10. Folds of lax skin in the elderly may also simulate a pneumothorax.

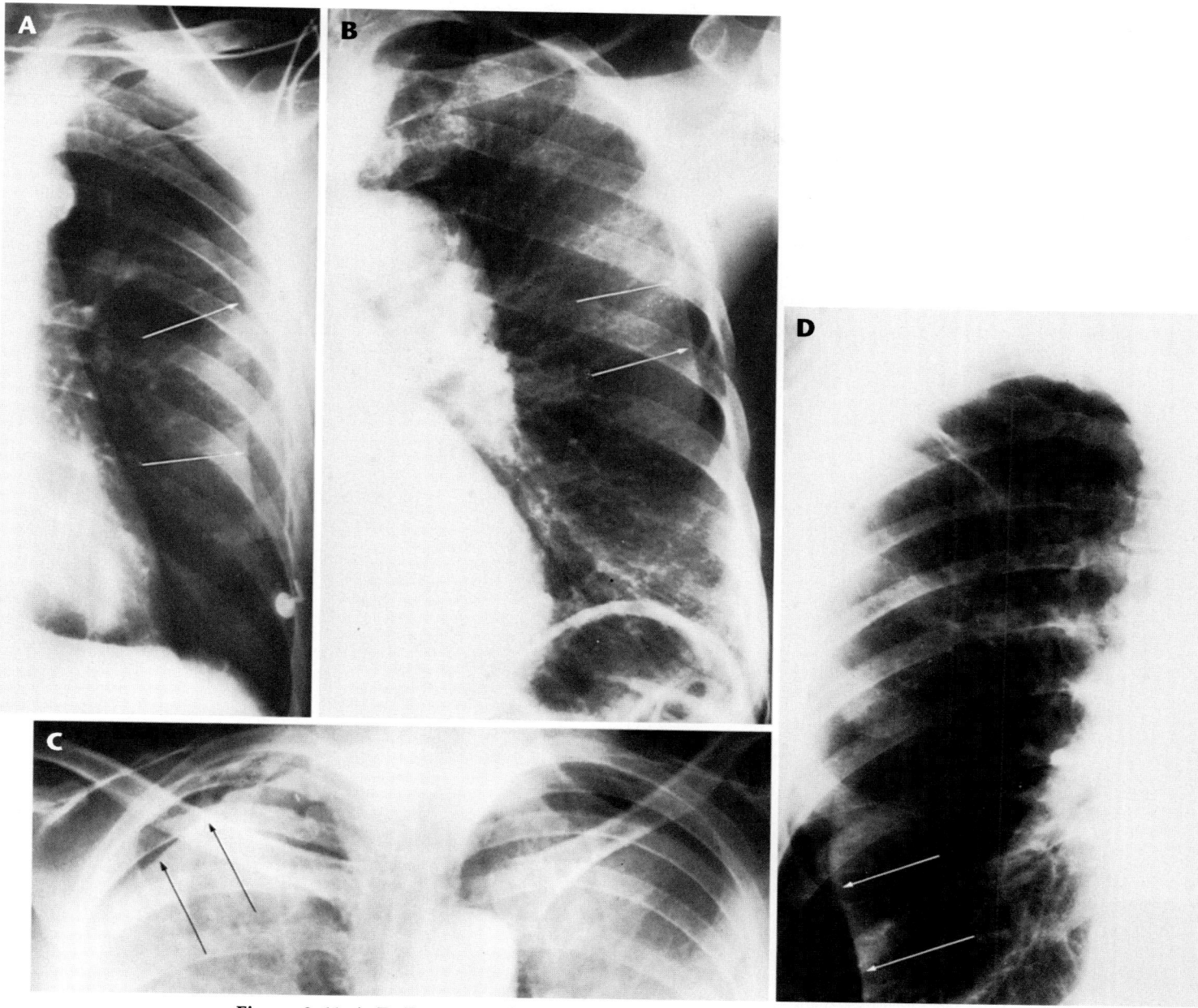

Figure 9–11. A–D, Four examples of skin folds simulating pneumothoraces. The patient illustrated in **D** was intubated. Note the fading margin of the skin fold in contrast to the sharp pleural line seen with a true pneumothorax. (Ref: Fisher JK: Skin fold versus pneumothorax. *Am J Roentgenol* 130:791, 1978.)

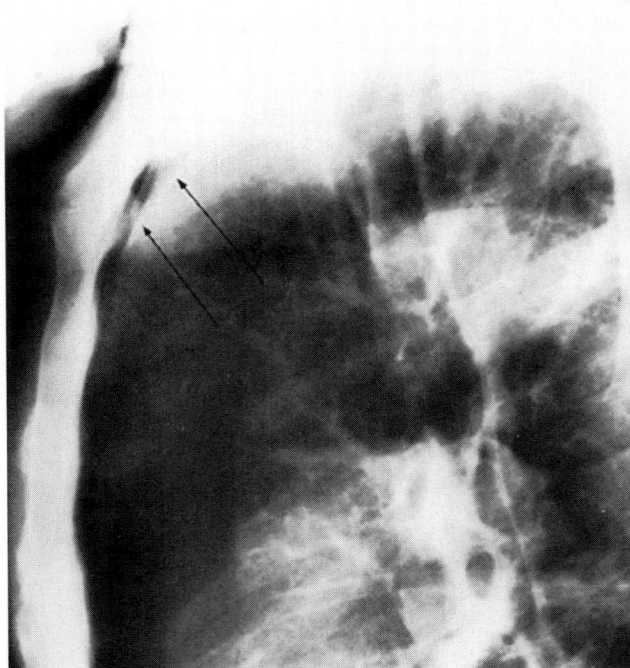

Figure 9–12. Examples of axillary folds simulating pneumothorax in lateral projection.

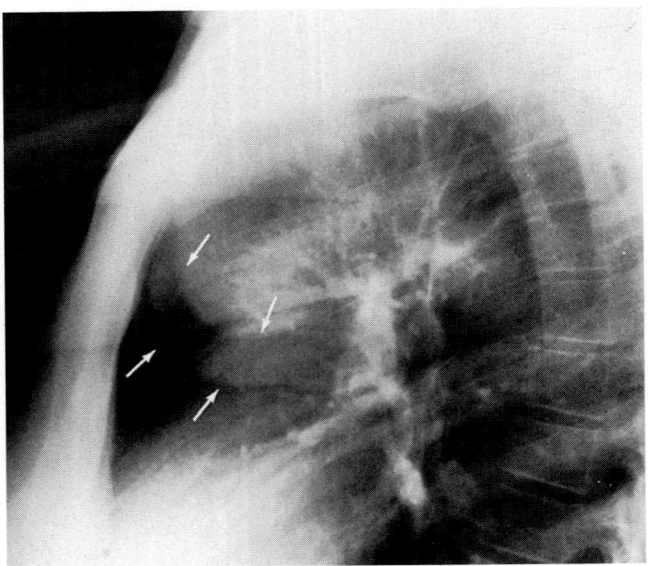

Figure 9–13. Redundant soft tissues of the axilla, producing rounded densities in the mediastinum.

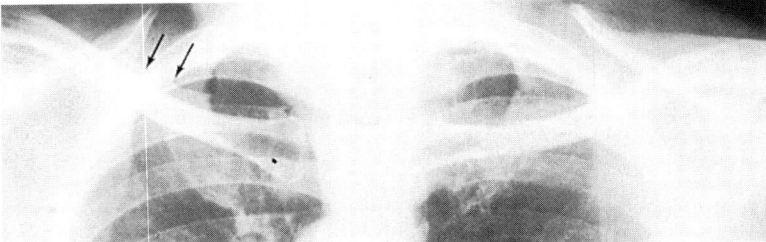

Figure 9–14. Nonsignificant asymmetry of the companion shadows of the clavicles, resulting from faulty positioning. No shadow is seen on the left side.

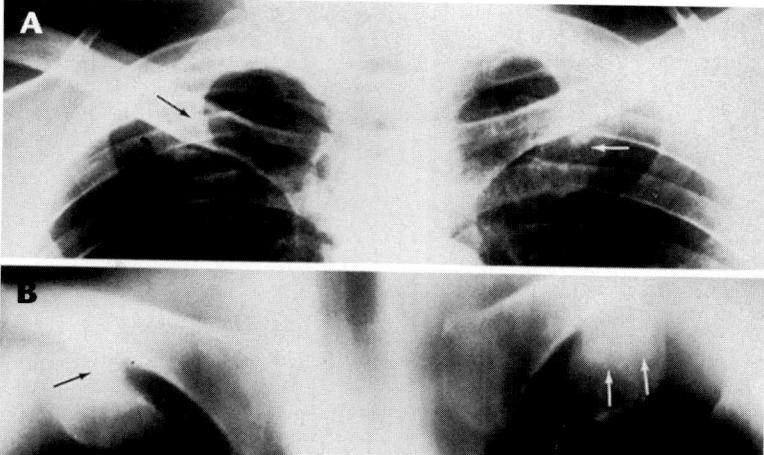

Figure 9–15. Calcification in the costoclavicular fascia, not to be mistaken for parenchymal lesions. **A,** Plain film. **B,** Tomography.

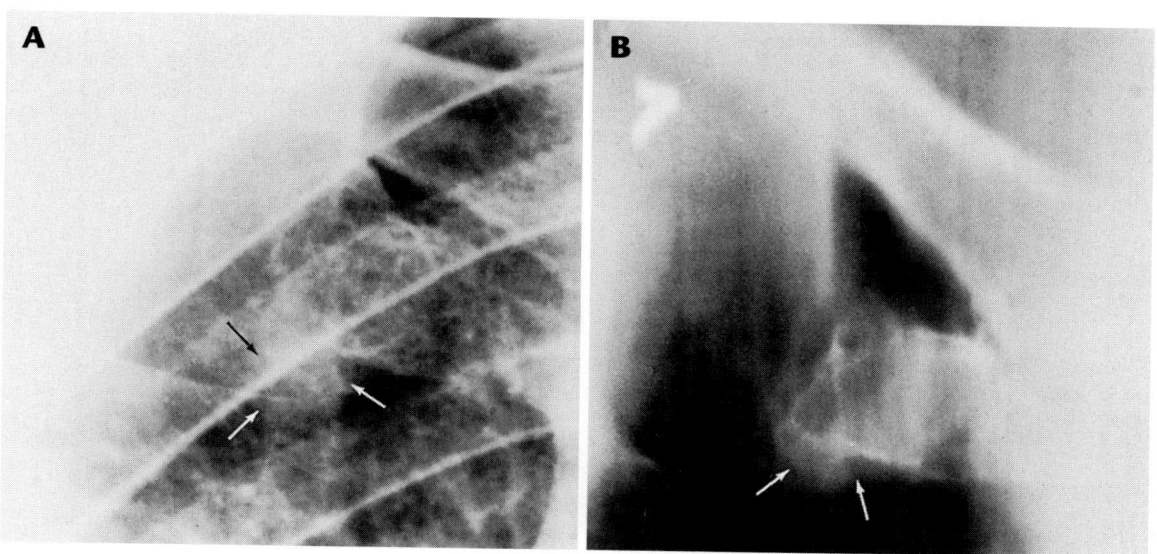

Figure 9–16. Calcified costal cartilage may simulate a parenchymal lesion. **A,** Plain film. **B,** Tomography.

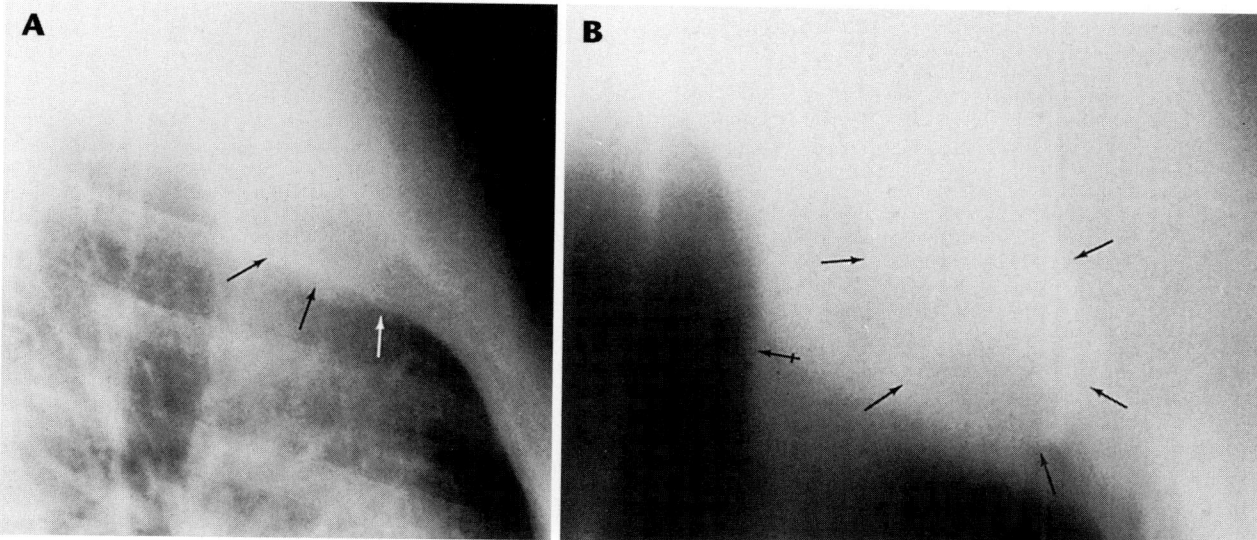

Figure 9–17. Exuberant calcified costal cartilage at the end of the first rib may produce a mass effect behind the sternum in the anterior mediastinum. **A,** Plain film. **B,** Tomography in the lateral projection shows that the mass consists of the calcified cartilage (→). Note the position of trachea for orientation (↔).

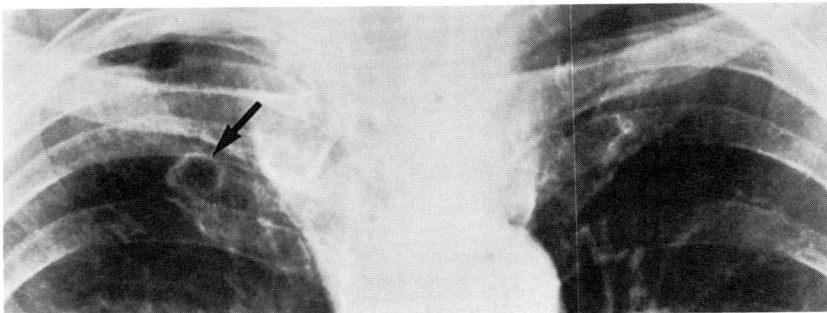

Figure 9–18. Ring shadow of calcified costal cartilage of first rib, simulating a cavity in lung.

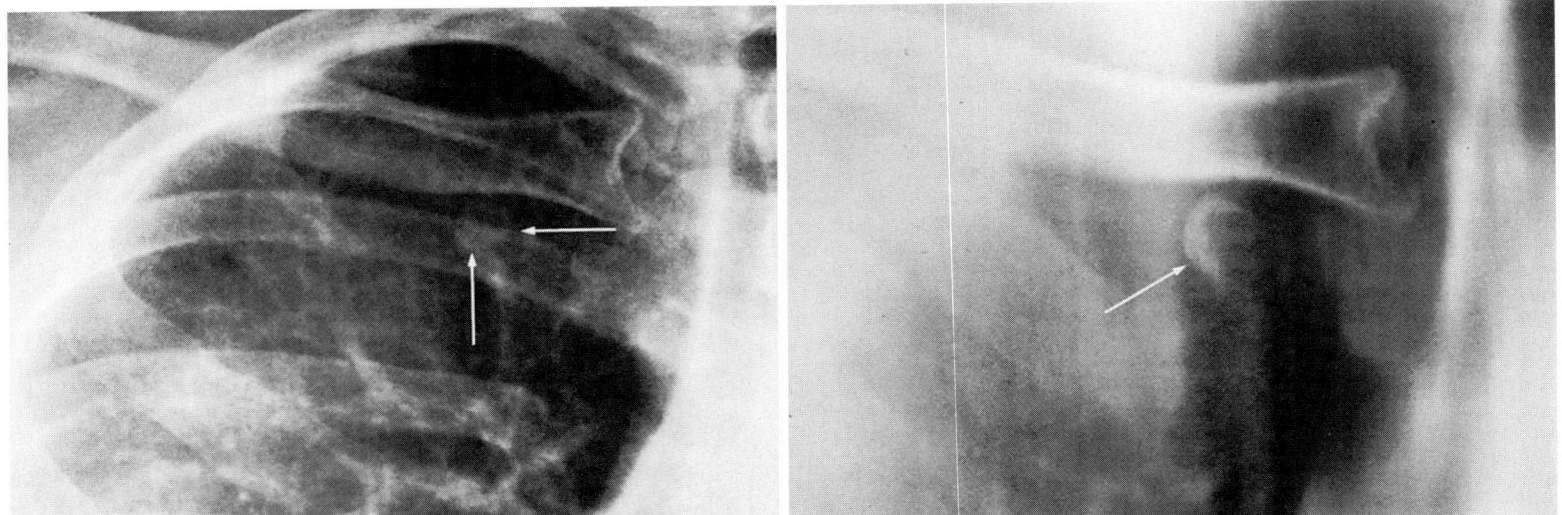

Figure 9–19. Simulated nodule produced by underdevelopment of the anterior end of the first rib, with isolated development of the costal cartilage. *Left*, Plain film. *Right*, Tomogram.

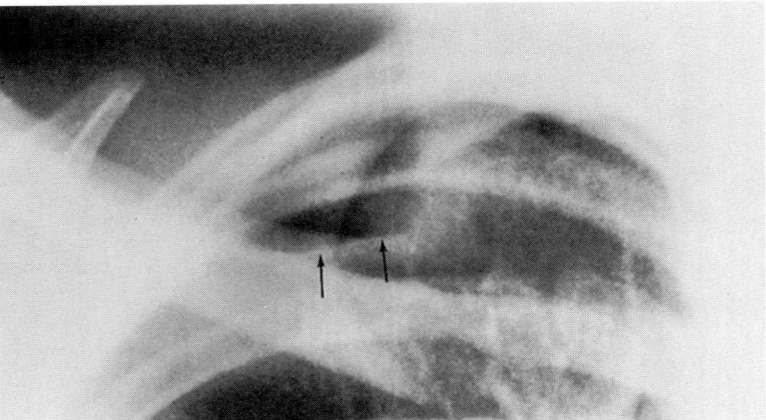

Figure 9–20. The floor of the supraclavicular fossa may be very well defined and simulate an air-fluid level in the lung. (Ref: Christensen EE, Dietz GW: The supraclavicular fossa. *Radiology* 118:37, 1976.)

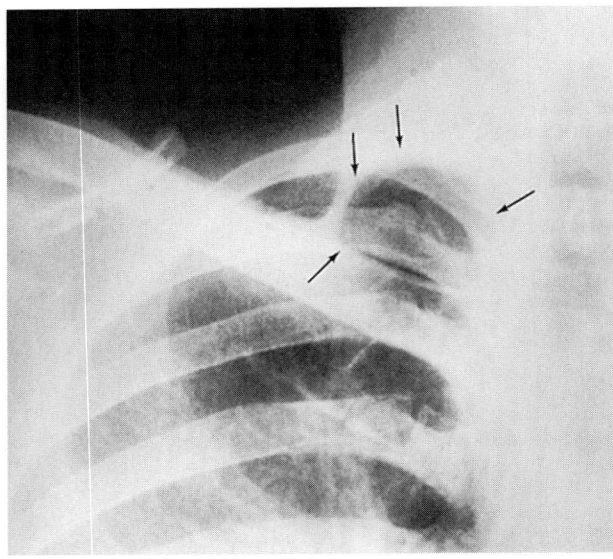

Figure 9–21. The confluence of the shadows of the sternocleidomastoid muscle, the first rib, and the clavicle may simulate a bulla or cavity in the apex of the lung.

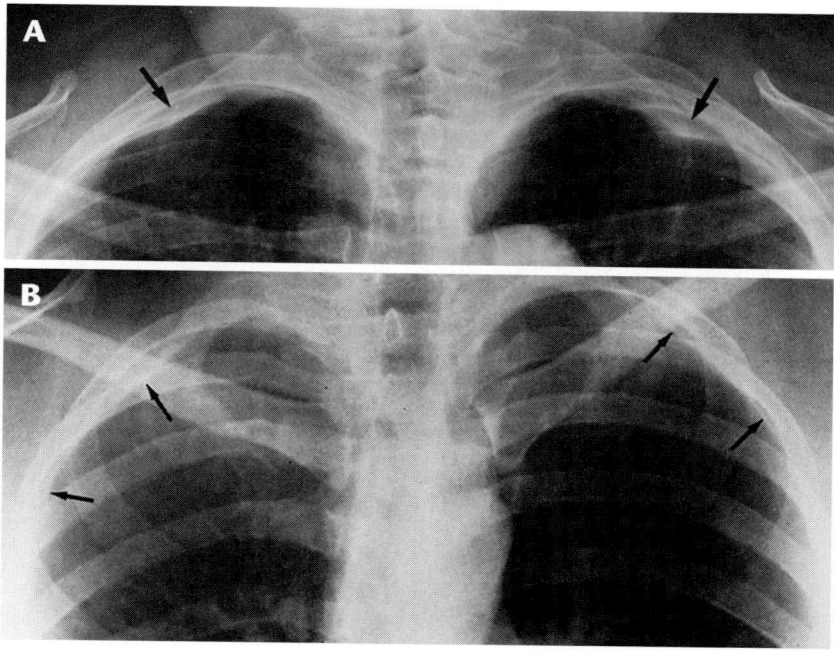

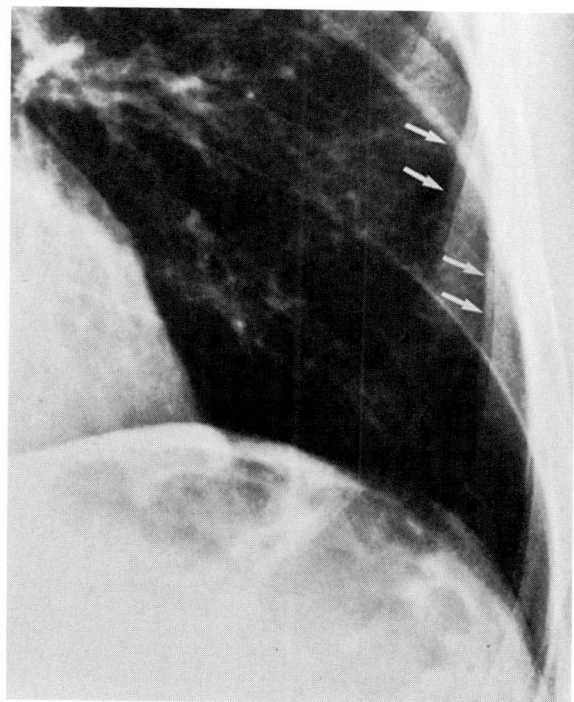

Figure 9–22. Two examples of the shadows of the subcostal muscles that produce an appearance simulating pleural thickening or small pneumothorax.

Figure 9–23. Companion shadows of the ribs.

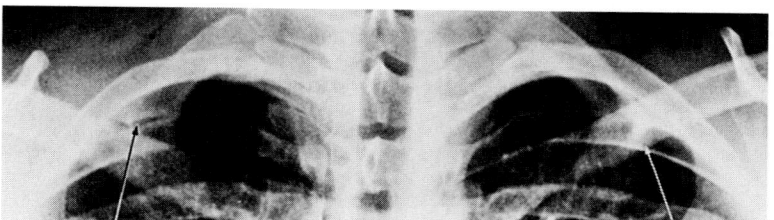

Figure 9–24. Triangular companion shadow of the first rib.

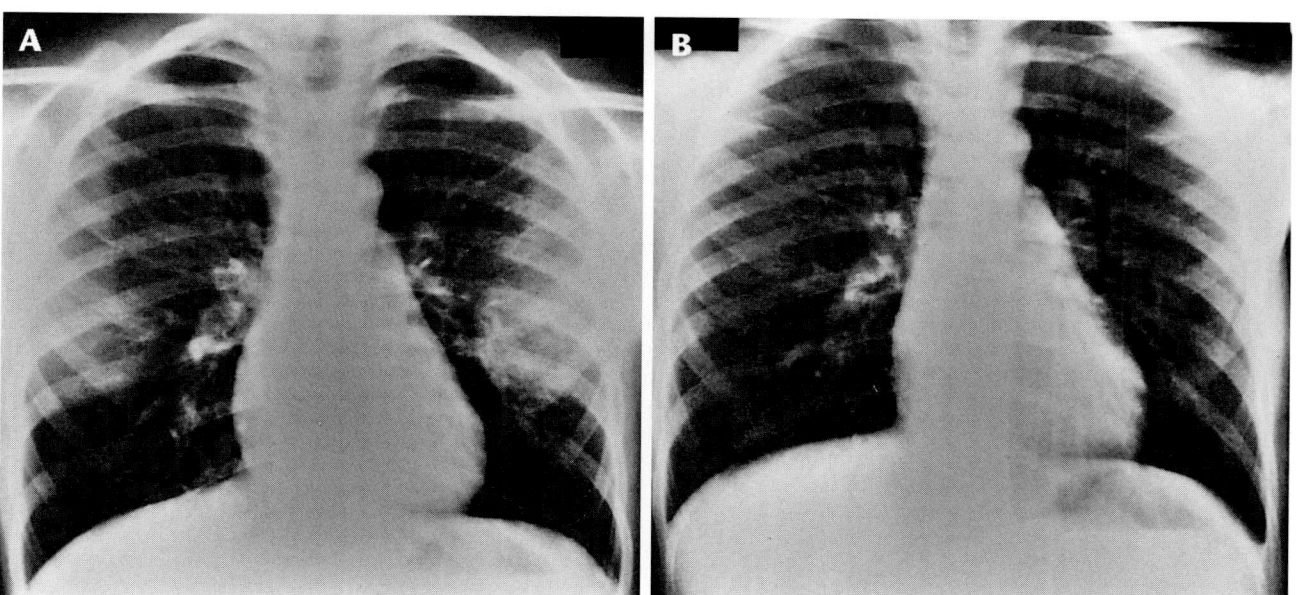

Figure 9–25. A, Posteroanterior film shows bilateral soft tissue shadows resulting from large pectoral muscles. **B,** Anteroposterior film no longer shows pectoral shadows.

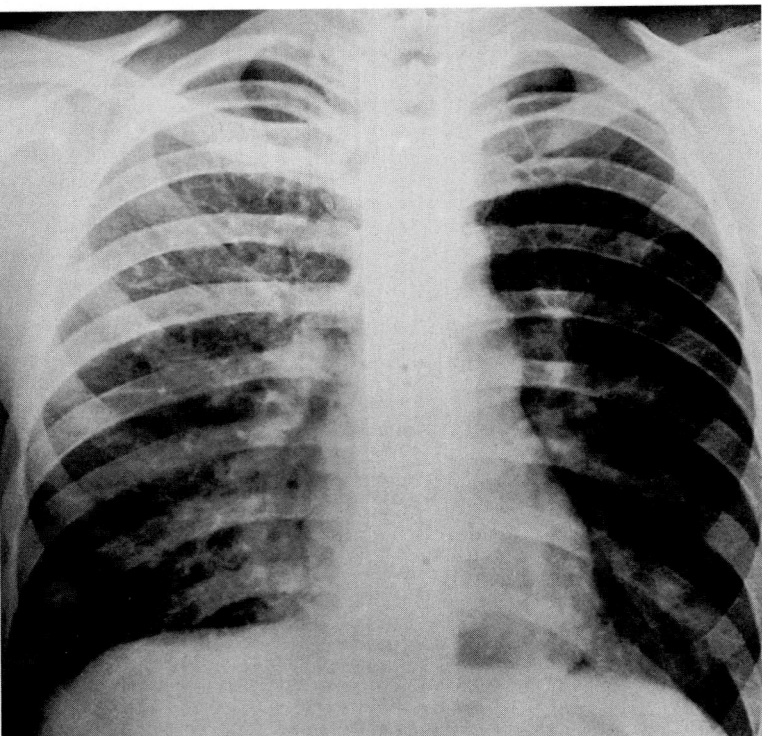

Figure 9–26. Congenital absence of the left pectoralis major muscle, producing increased radiolucency of the left hemithorax.

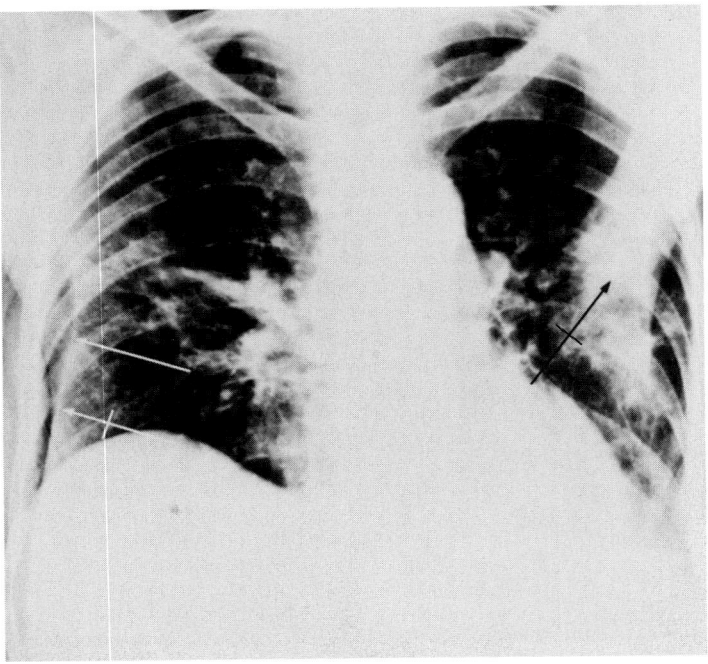

Figure 9–27. Shadow of the pectoralis major muscle, simulating a lung lesion (←). Note also the pseudopneumothorax on the patient's right side, produced by a skin fold (↔).

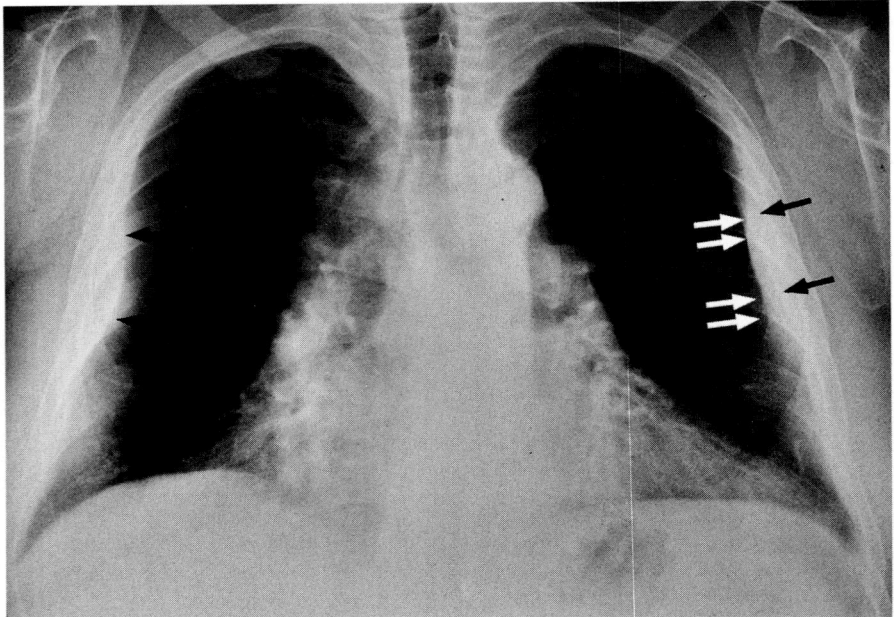

Figure 9–28. Extrapleural fat in a very obese man, simulating pleural thickening. The absence of blunting of the costophrenic angles in this entity is a useful differential clue. (Refs: Vix VA: Extrapleural costal fat. *Radiology* 112:563, 1974; Sargent EN et al: Subpleural fat pads in patients exposed to asbestos: Distinction from non-calcified pleural plaques. *Radiology* 152:273, 1984.)

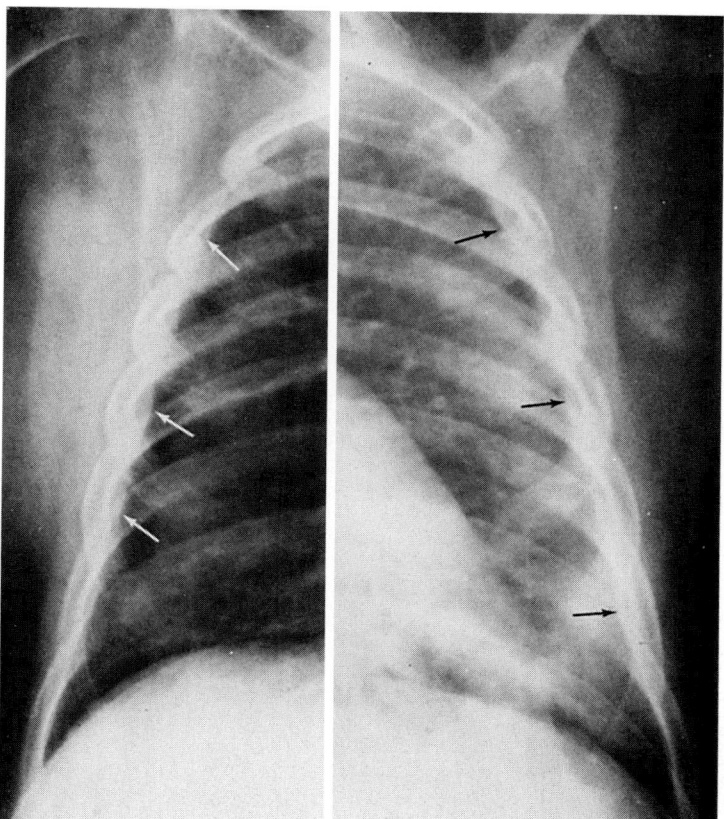

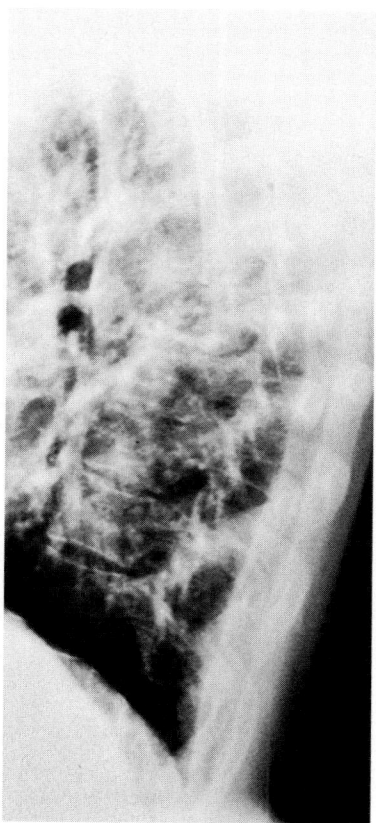

Figure 9–29. Additional example of extrapleural fat deposits in a very obese patient, simulating pleural thickening. The shadow of the extrapleural fat does not reach the costophrenic angles. Occasionally these extrapleural fat deposits may be slightly asymmetric. (Ref: Friedman AC et al: Asbestos-related pleural disease and asbestosis: A comparison of CT and chest radiography. *Am J Roentgenol* 150:269, 1988.)

Figure 9–30. Extrapleural fat seen in an off-lateral projection. Note that it loses its prominence at the bases.

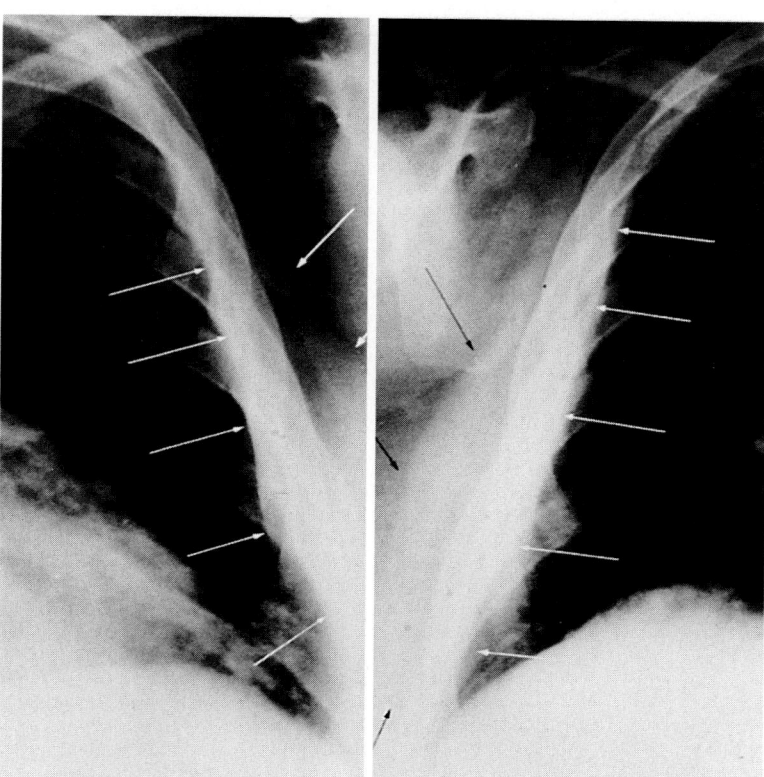

Figure 9–31. The serratus anterior muscle produces a shadow that may be confused with pleural thickening or extrapleural fat. In frontal views, it produces a "bowling pin" configuration. (Ref: Gilmartin D: The serratus anterior muscle on chest radiographs. *Radiology* 131:629, 1979.)

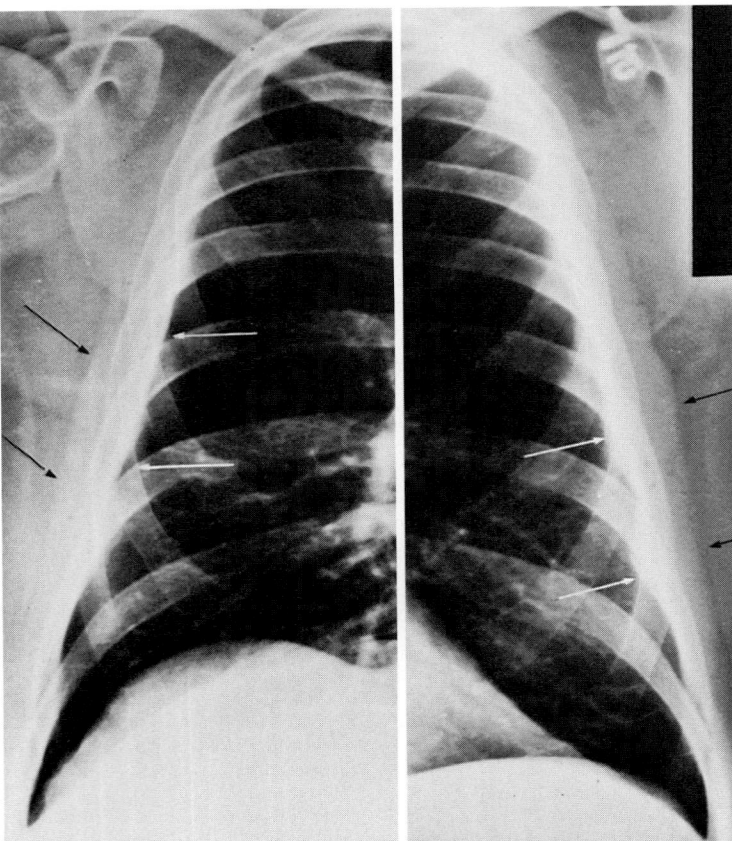

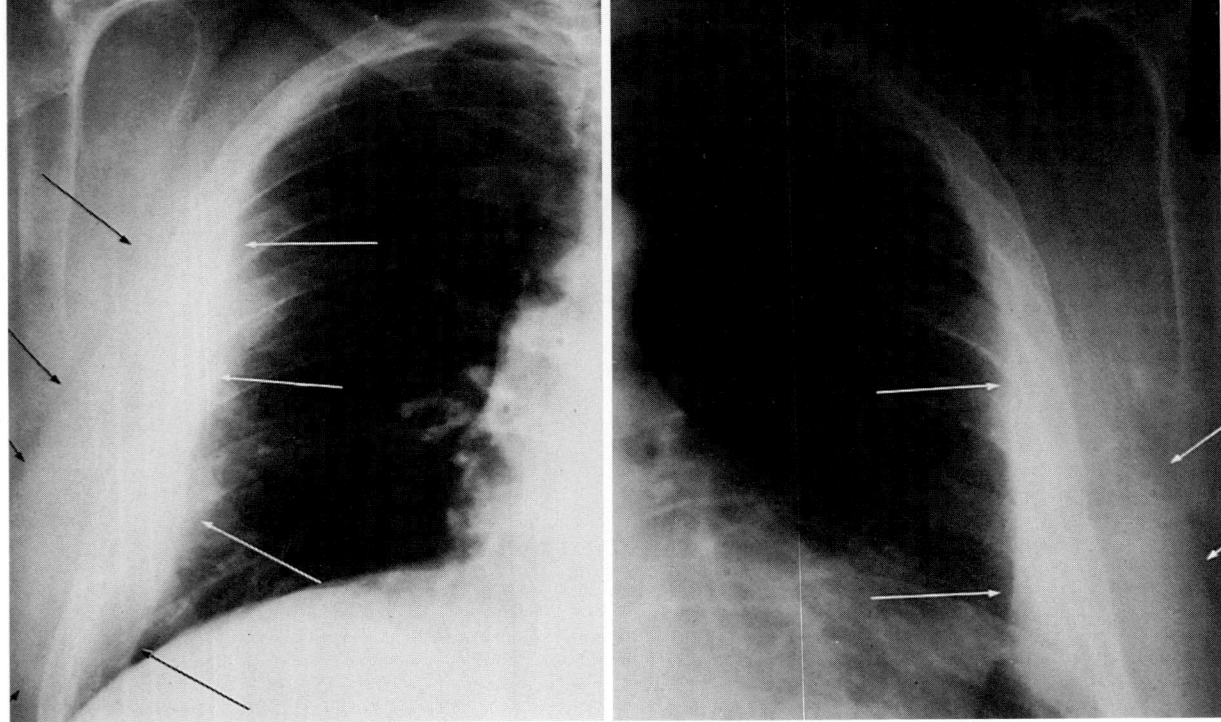

Figure 9–32. Two additional cases showing the varying appearance of the serratus anterior muscle shadows.

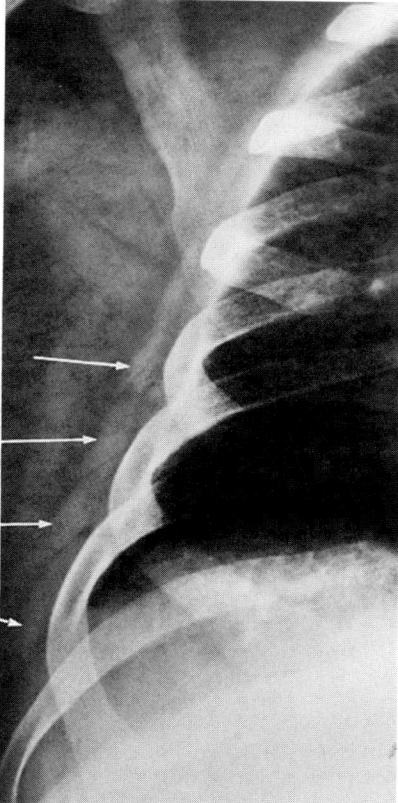

Figure 9–33. A demonstration of the muscle slips of the serratus anterior muscle that constitute the "bowling pin" sign in Figures 9–31 and 9–32.

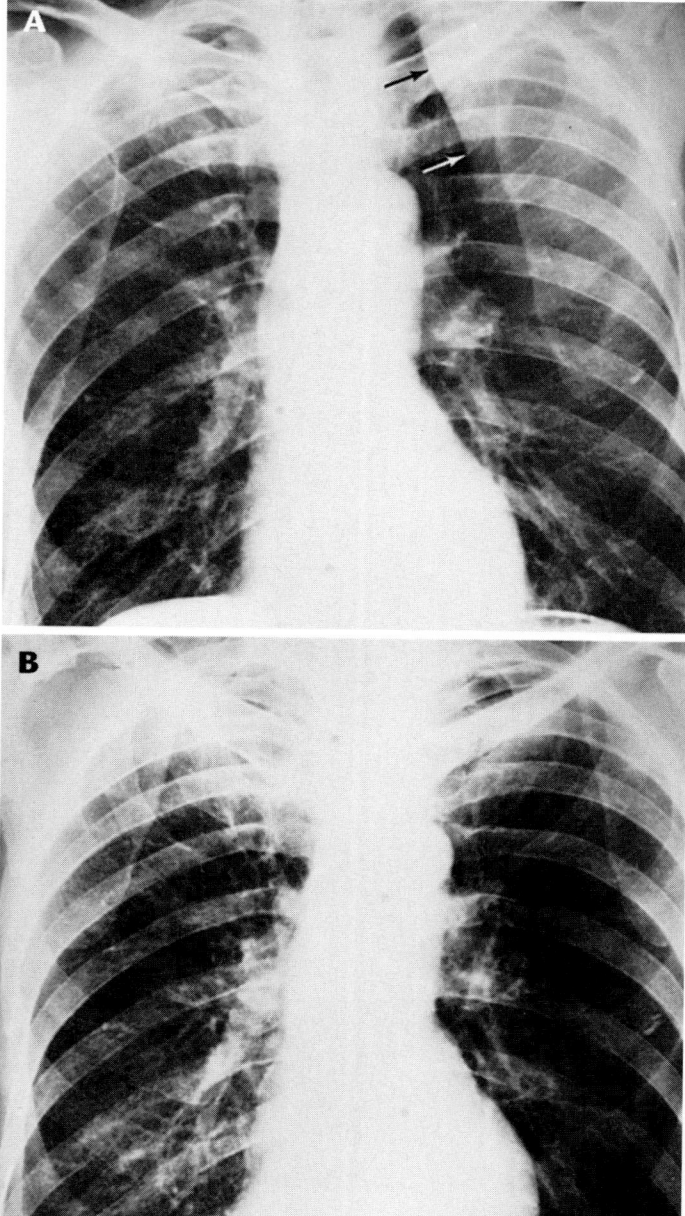

Figure 9–34. A, Simulated parenchymal density produced by soft tissues over the scapula, caused by improper positioning of the arms. **B,** Shadow not seen with proper positioning. (Ref: Lams PM, Jolles H: The scapula companion shadow. *Radiology* 138:19, 1981.)

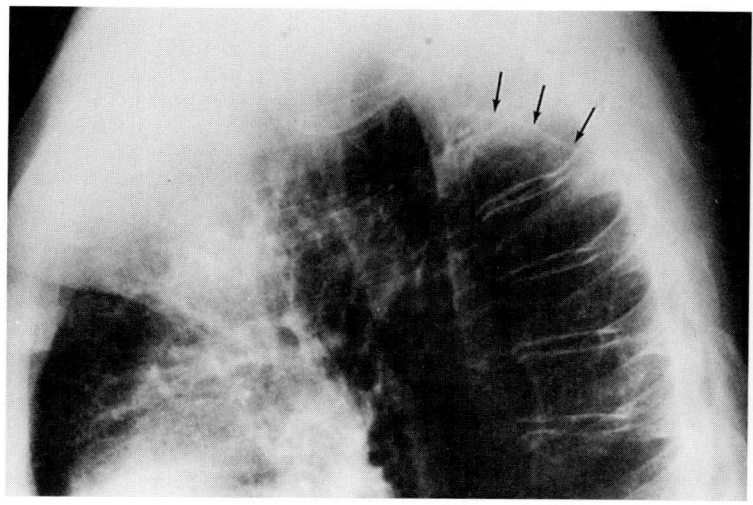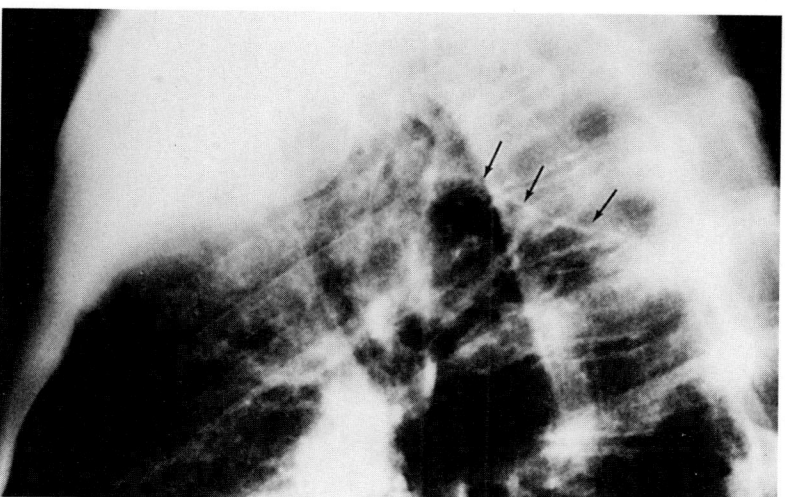

Figure 9–35. In an improperly positioned chest film, the spine of the scapula may overlap the lungs and produce a shadow that may be mistaken for a pneumothorax. (Ref: Harbin WP, Cimmino CV: The radiographic innominate lines of the scapular spine. *Va Med* 101:1050, 1974.)

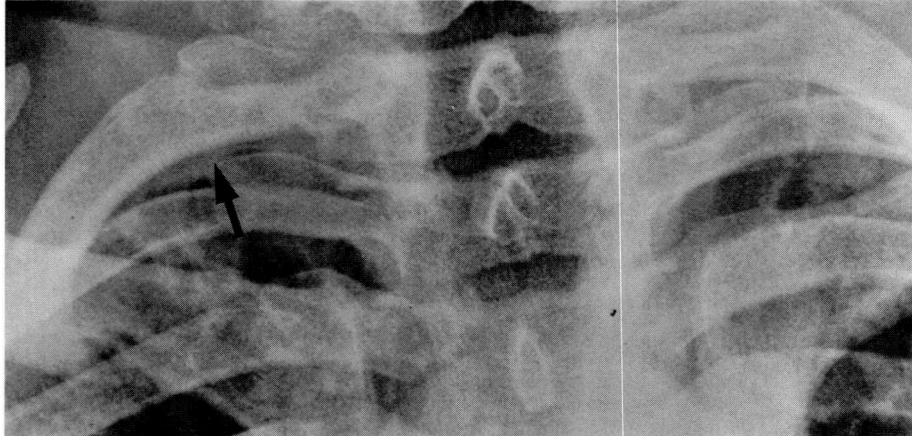

Figure 9–36. Simulated pneumothorax produced by the transverse process of T2.

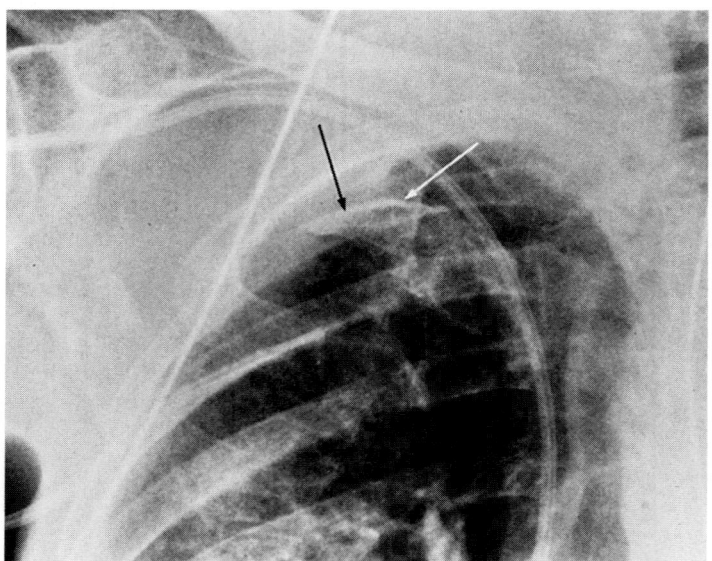

Figure 9–37. Confluence of the first and second ribs, simulating a pneumothorax.

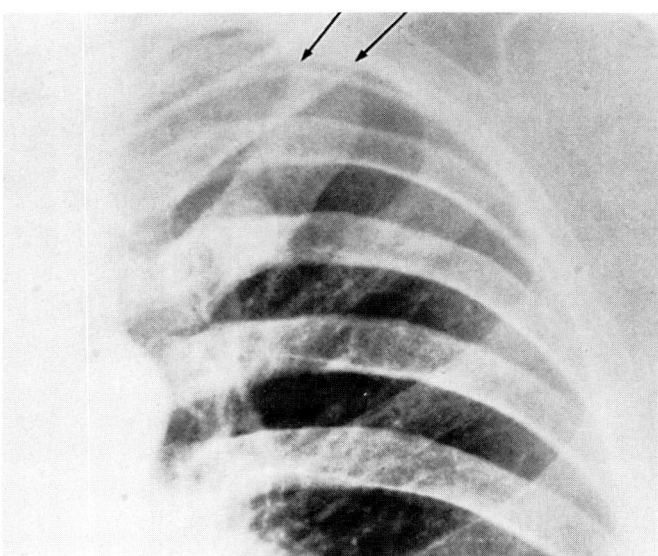

Figure 9–38. Lucency of medullary cavity of the second rib, simulating a pneumothorax.

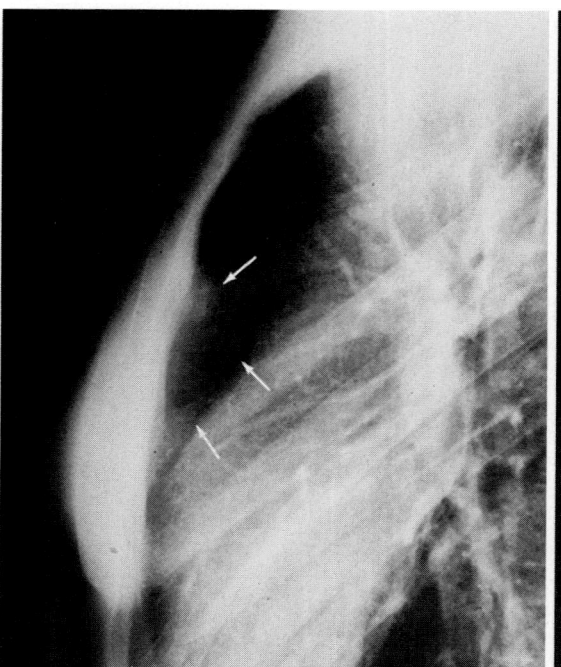

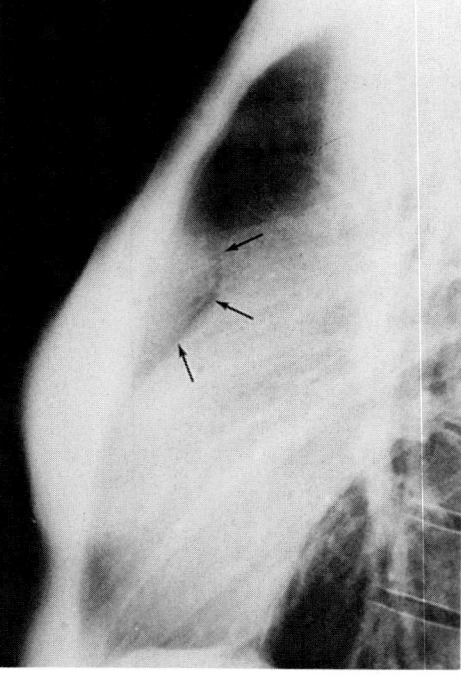

Figure 9–39. Two examples of the mammary anterior mediastinal pseudotumor. The lateral aspects of the dense, small breasts in young women may project into the anterior mediastinum in the lateral projection and simulate a mediastinal mass. (Ref: Keats TE: Mammary anterior mediastinal pseudotumor. *J Can Assoc Radiol* 27:262, 1976.)

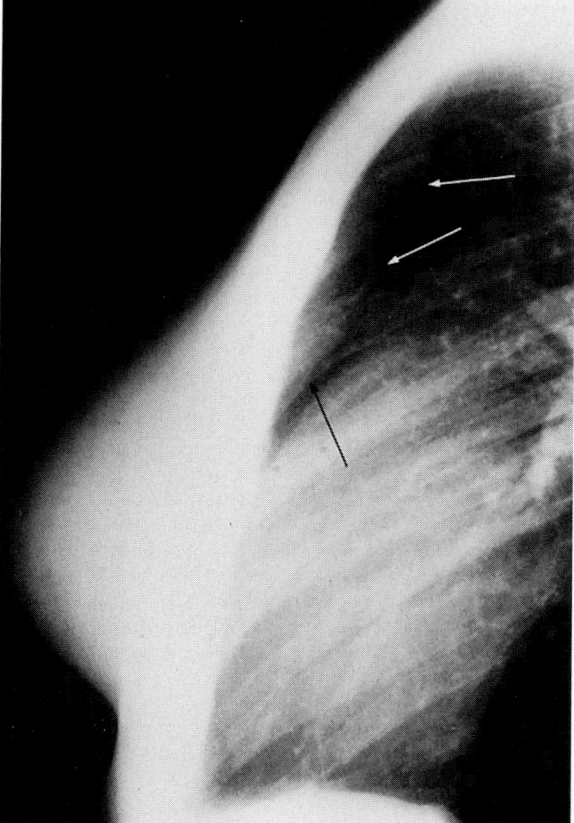

Figure 9–40. The axillary tail of the breast may simulate an anterior mediastinal mass.

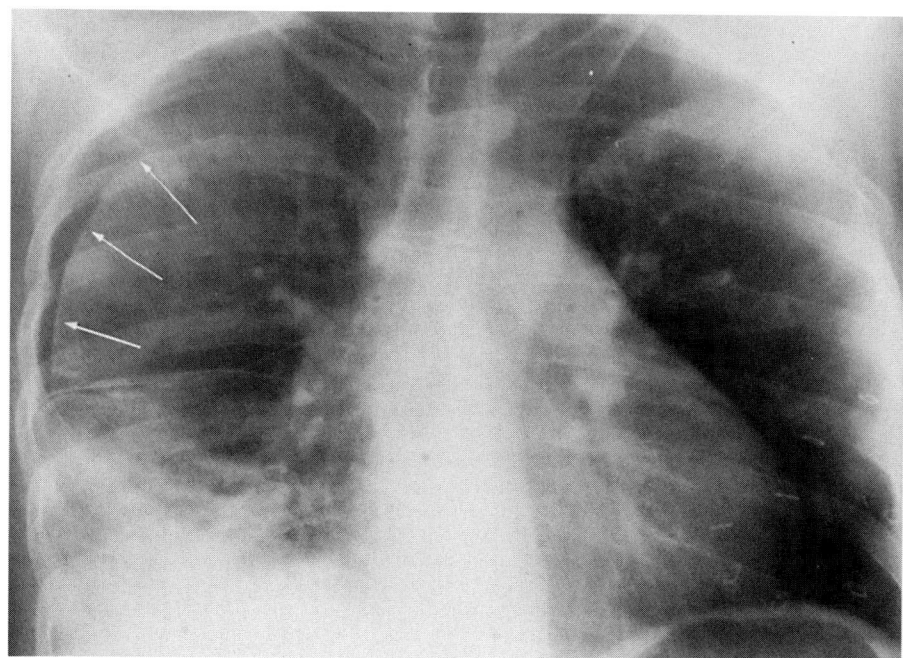

Figure 9–41. The compressed breast in the prone position may simulate a pneumothorax.

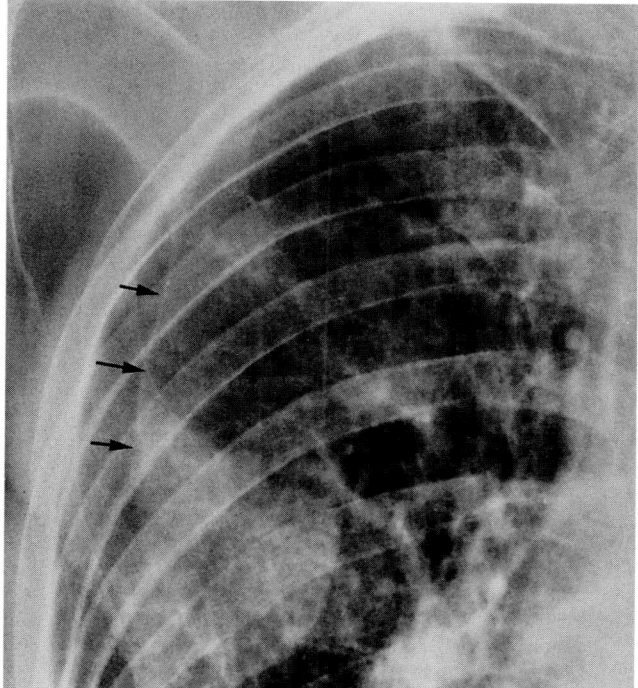

Figure 9–42. The axillary fold simulating a pneumothorax.

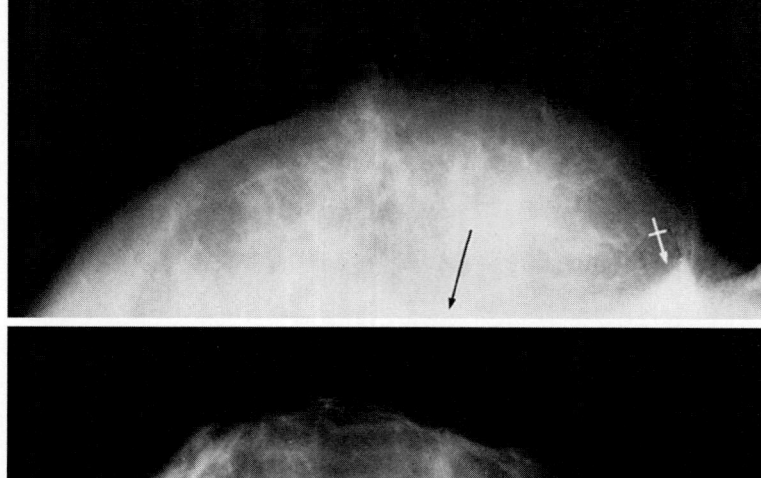

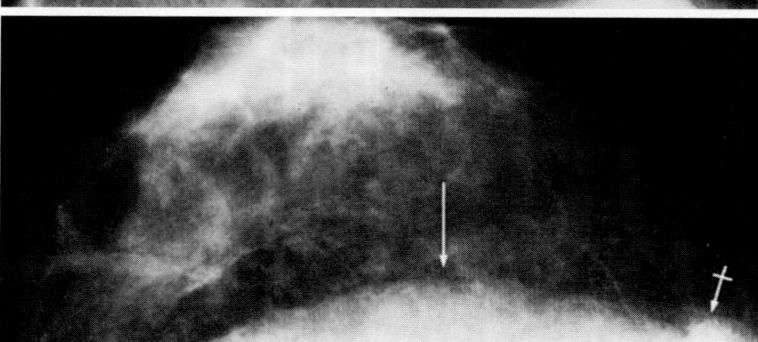

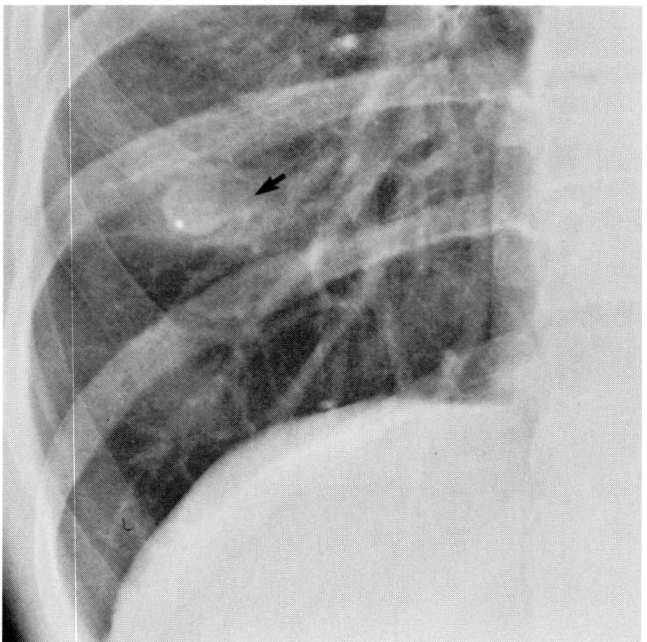

Figure 9–44. Nipple shadow. These characteristically have a fading medial margin. (Ref: Ferris RA, White AF: The round nipple shadow. *Radiology* 121:293, 1976.)

Figure 9–43. Three examples of the sternal insertion of the pectoralis major muscle that might be mistaken for carcinoma on mammography. *Top,* Triangular area of increased density is seen in the medial aspect of the breast on craniocaudal view (↔), continuous with underlying pectoral muscle (←). *Center,* rounded area of increased density is seen in the medial aspect of the breast on craniocaudal view (←). *Bottom,* Craniocaudal view of left breast in a female weightlifter reveals continuity between pectoral muscle (→) and density (↔). (From Britton CA et al: Carcinoma mimicked by sternal insertion of the pectoral muscle. *Am J Roentgenol* 153:955, 1989.)

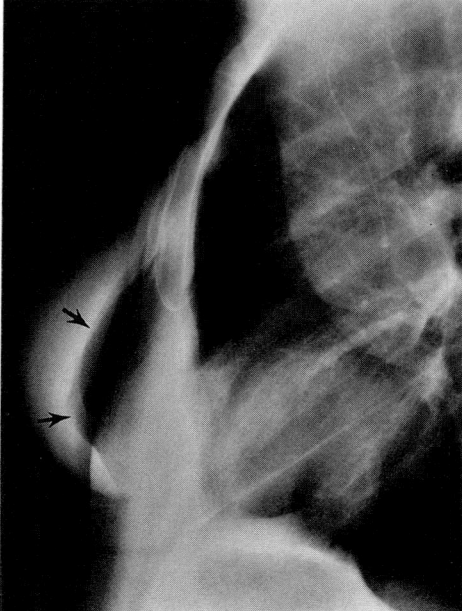

Figure 9–45. Simulated herniation of the lung, produced by an inflatable brassiere.

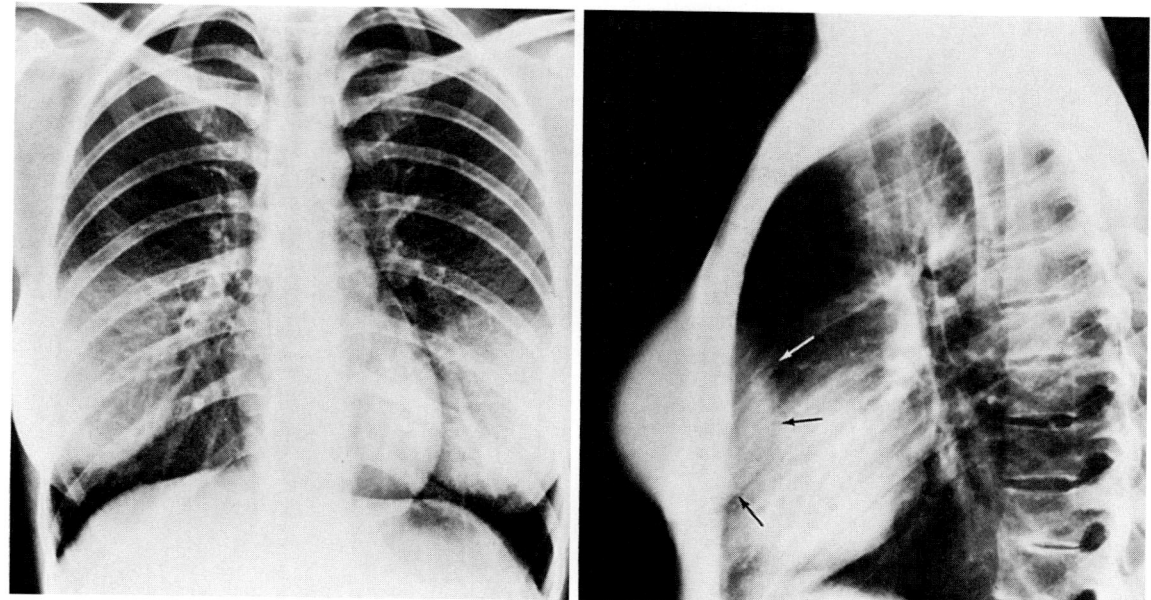

Figure 9–46. Prosthetic mammary implants. Note the similarity in this patient's lateral projection to the pseudotumor in Figure 9–39.

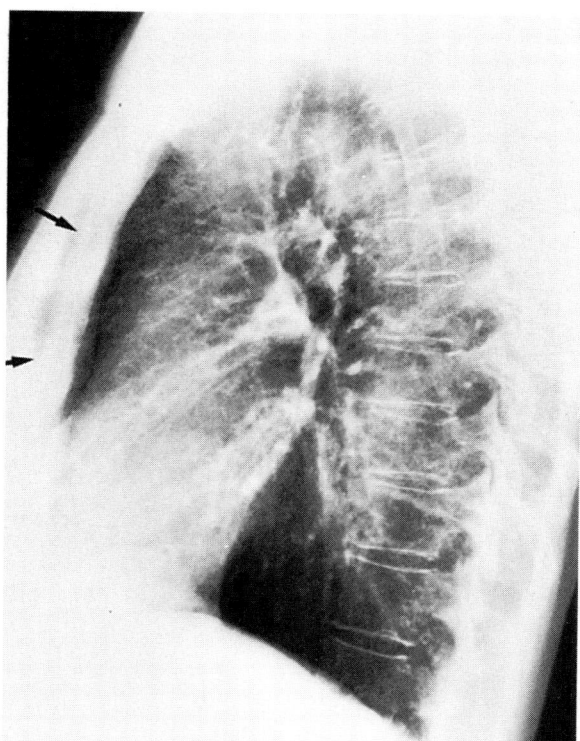

Figure 9–47. Simulated air in soft tissues, produced by rotation.

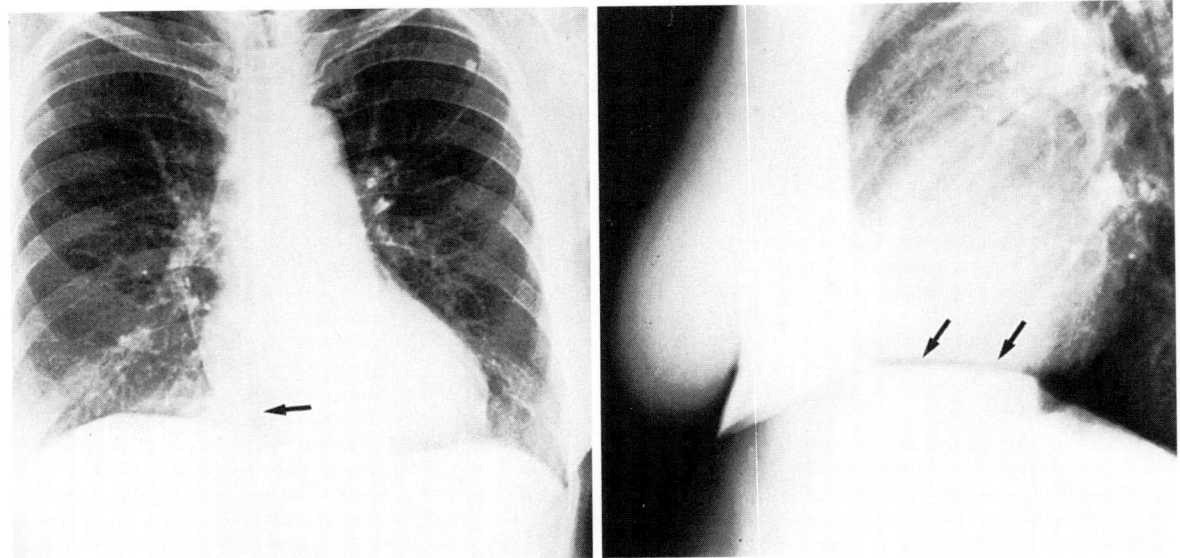

Figure 9–48. Air under the breast, producing a striking radiolucency beneath the heart shadow in the lateral projection.

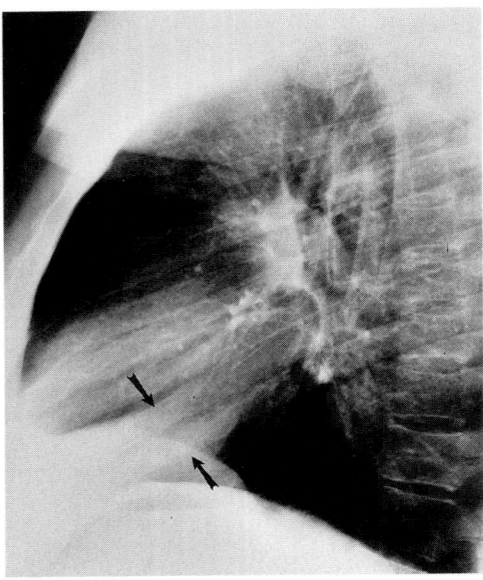

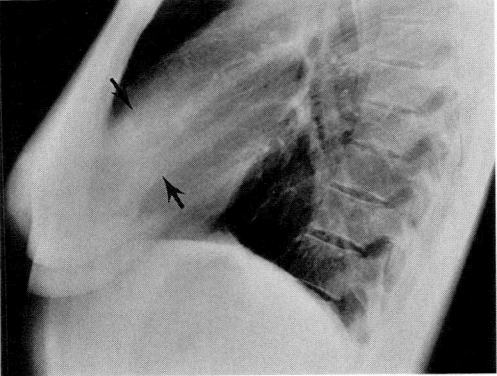

Figure 9–50. Simulated consolidation of the lung, produced by superimposed breast shadows.

Figure 9–49. Breast shadow simulating pulmonary infiltrate.

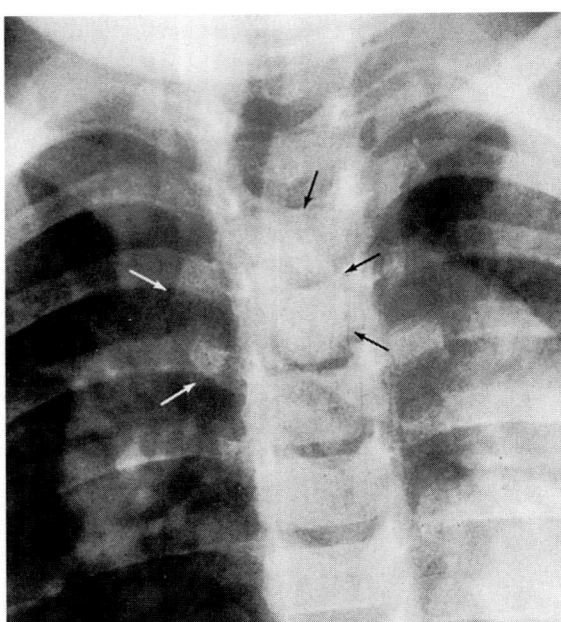

Figure 9–51. Manubrium of a 2½-year-old boy, simulating a soft tissue mass.

The Pleura

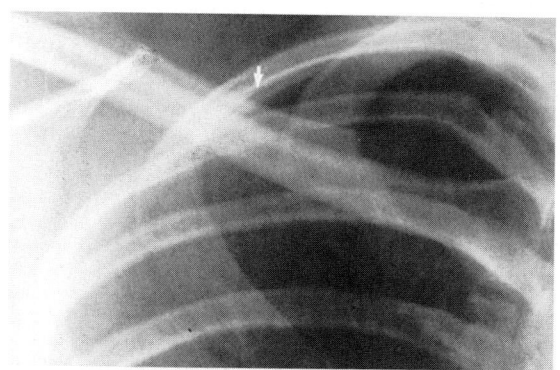

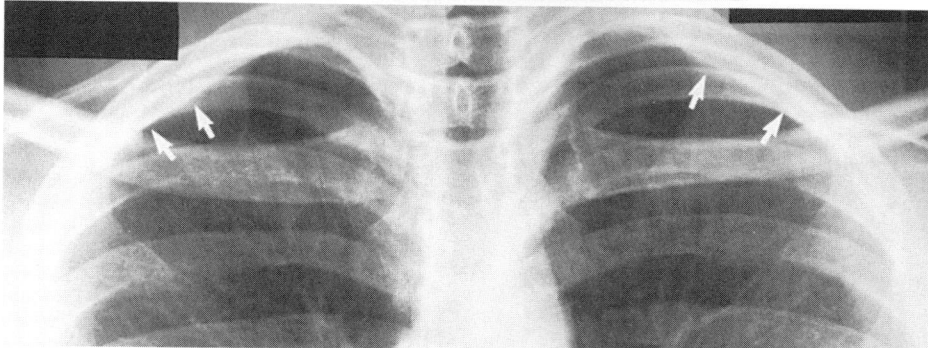

Figure 9–52. Subcostal muscle simulating pleural thickening (*bottom*) or pneumothorax (*top*).

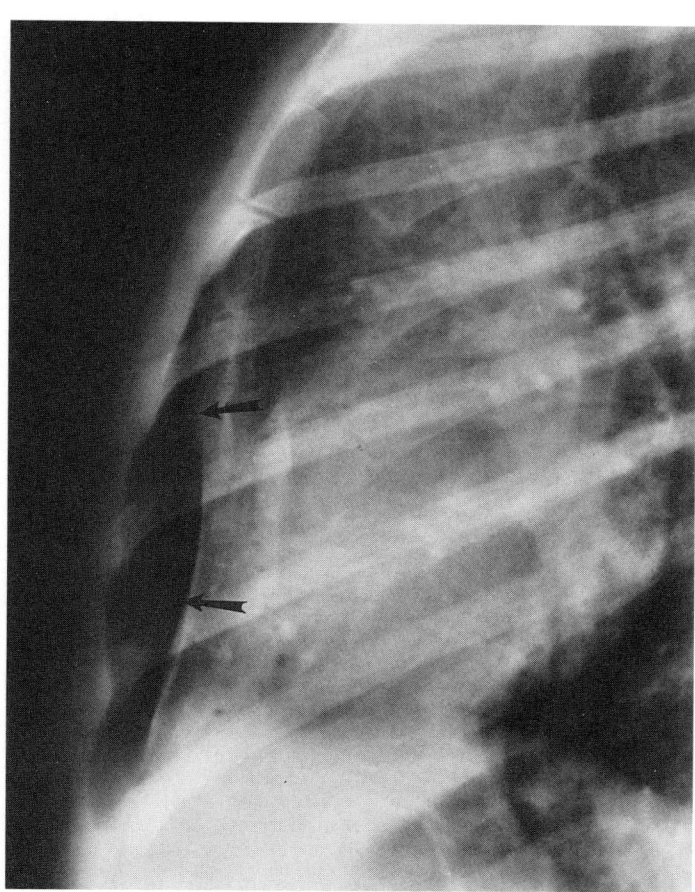

Figure 9–53. Simulated pneumothorax produced by poor positioning in lateral projection.

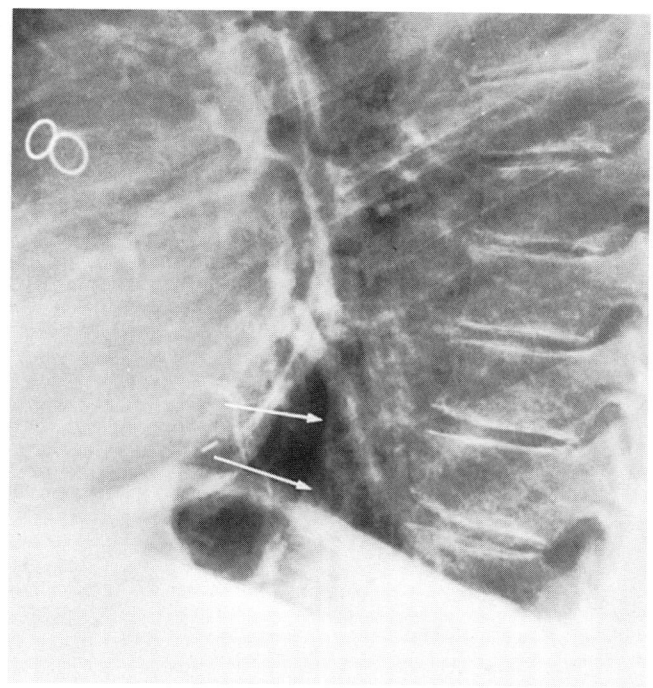

Figure 9–54. Shadow of the descending aorta, simulating localized pneumothorax.

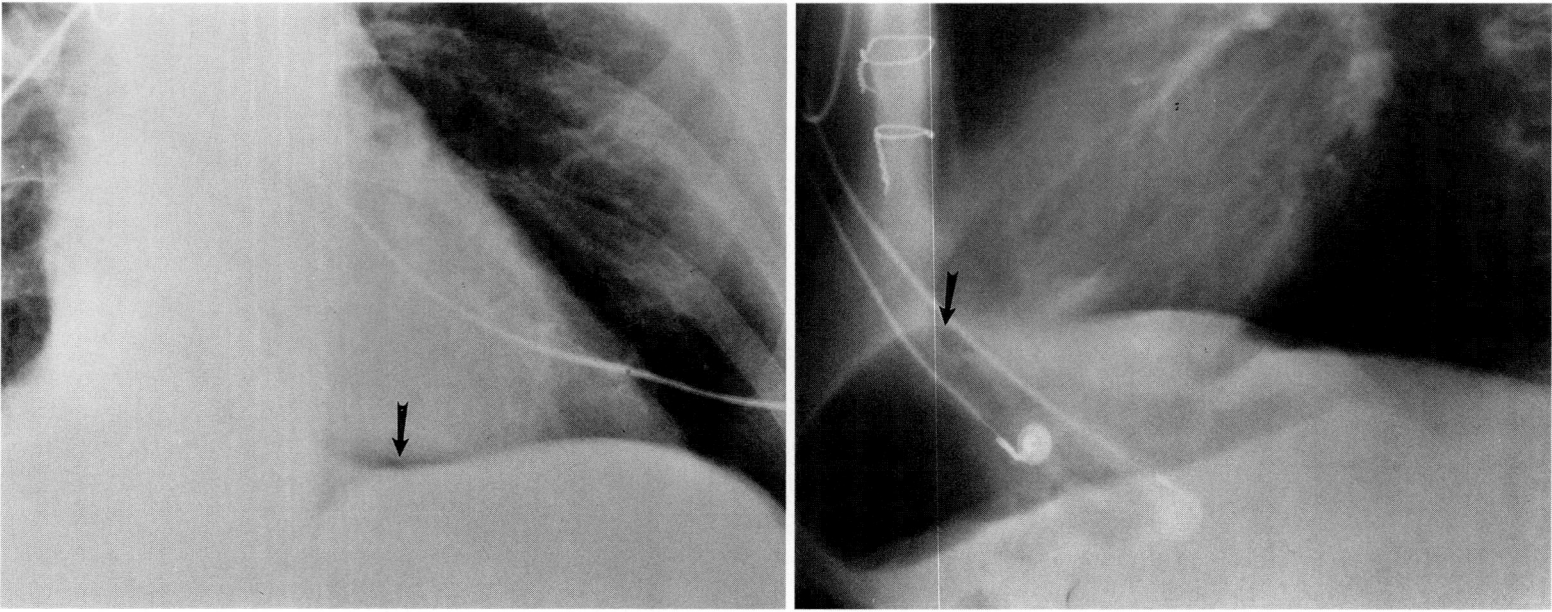

Figure 9–55. Simulated basal pneumothorax produced by high position of the stomach anteriorly.

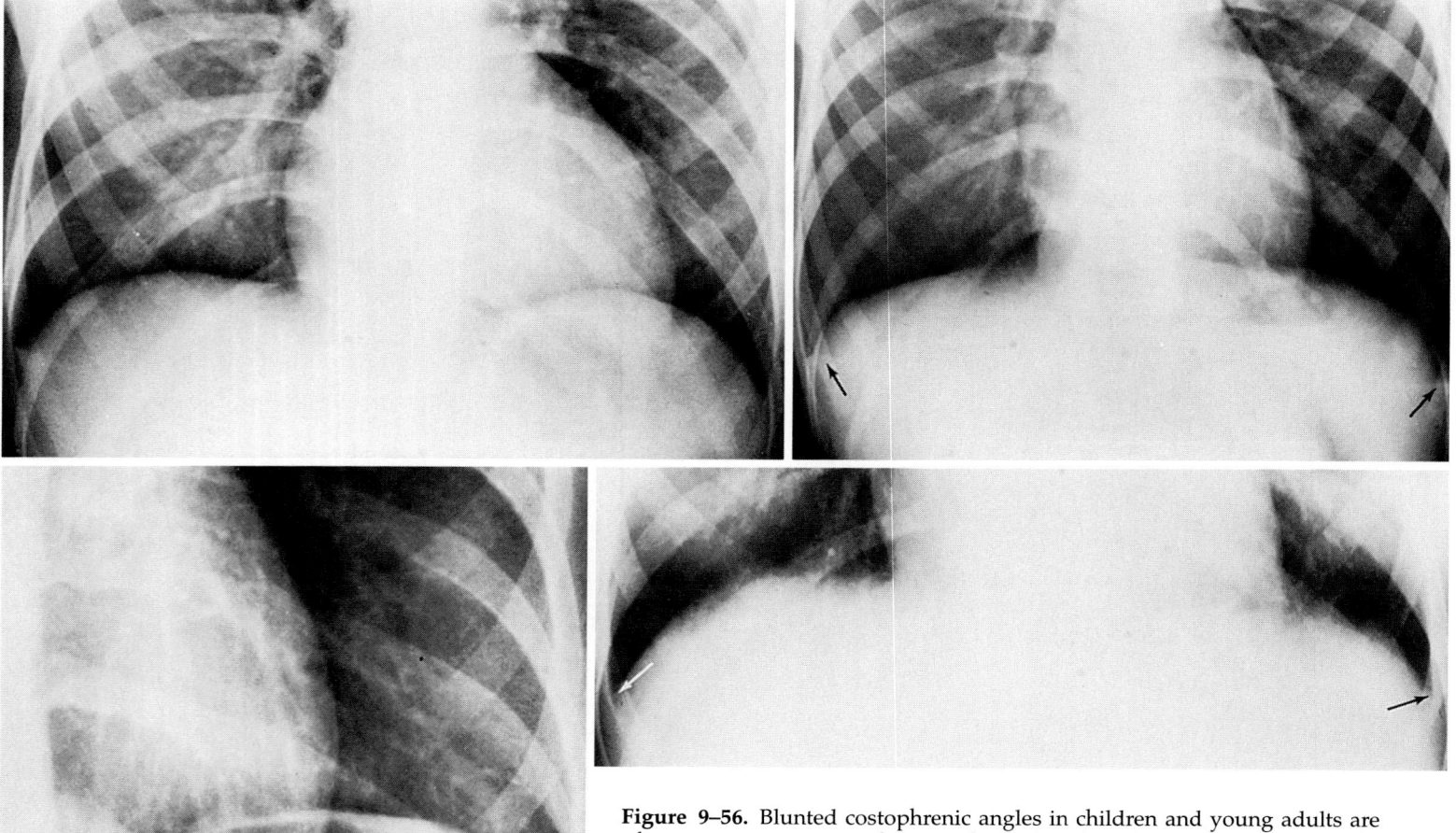

Figure 9–56. Blunted costophrenic angles in children and young adults are often seen as an apparently normal, incidental, and inconsistent finding that many times cannot be reproduced on the same day. It is frequently misinterpreted as evidence of pathologic pleural effusion or pleuritis. It may be due to redundancy of the pleura or may represent the pleural fluid normally present in the pleural space in healthy children and possibly in young adults. (Ref: Ecklof O, Torngren A: Pleural fluid in healthy children. *Acta Radiol [Diagn]* 11:346, 1971.)

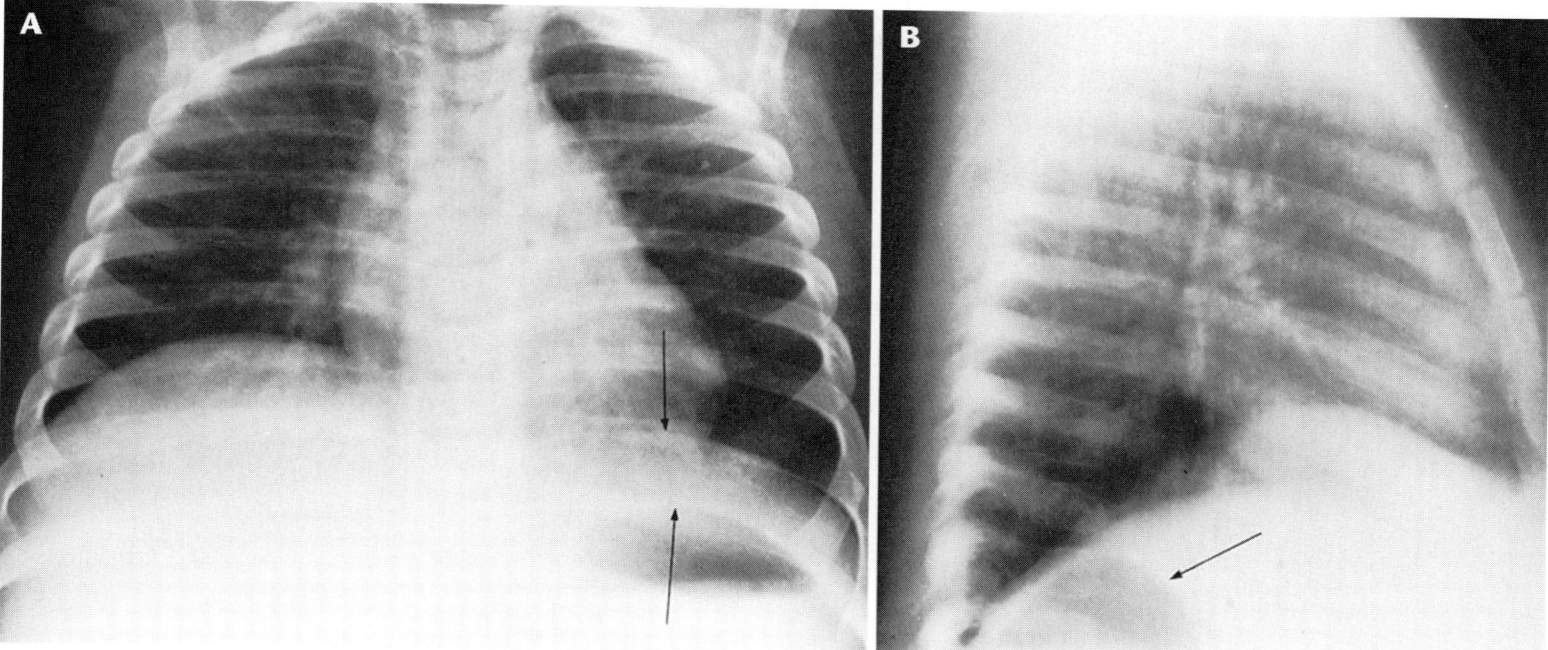

Figure 9–57. A, Simulated subpulmonic effusion as evidenced by increased distance between the stomach air bubble and the dome of the diaphragm. **B,** The apparent separation is due to the marked posterior position of the fundus of the stomach with projection of the diaphragm above.

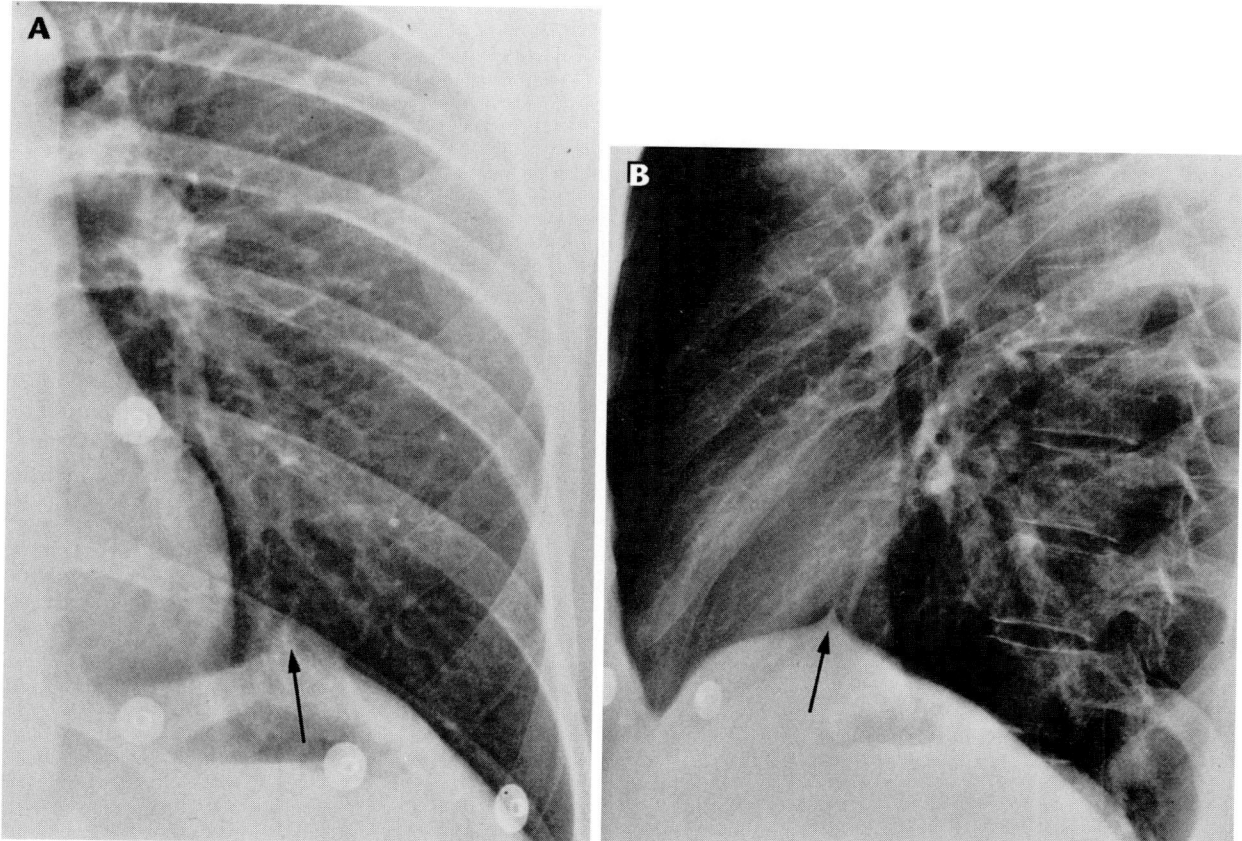

Figure 9–58. A, B, Triangular area of relative obliteration of the diaphragm, said to be due to extension of the areolar tissue into the base of the inferior pulmonary ligament. (Ref: Proto AV, Speckman JM: The left lateral radiograph of the chest. *Med Radiogr Photogr* 55:69, 1979.)

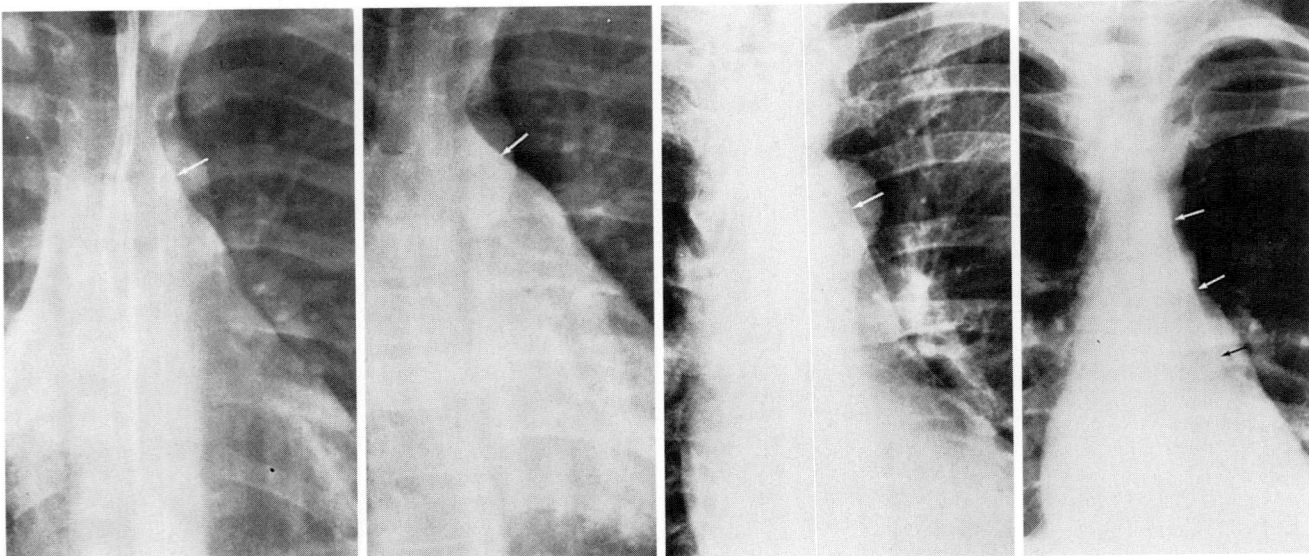

Figure 9–59. Four examples of the aortic pulmonary stripe, a reflection of the mediastinal pleura from the aorta to the pulmonary artery. This should not be confused with displacement of the mediastinal pleura caused by adenopathy. (From Keats TE: The aortic-pulmonary mediastinal stripe. *Am J Roentgenol* 116:107, 1972.)

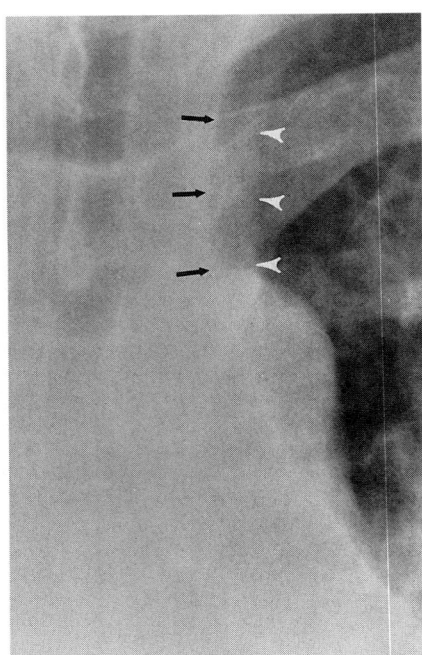

Figure 9–60. The left paratracheal reflection. This shadow (*black arrows*) is seen medial to the left subclavian reflection (*white arrowheads*). This finding is produced by contact of the lung with the mediastinum anterior to the left subclavian artery. (Ref: Proto AV et al: The left paratracheal reflection. *Radiology* 171:625, 1989.)

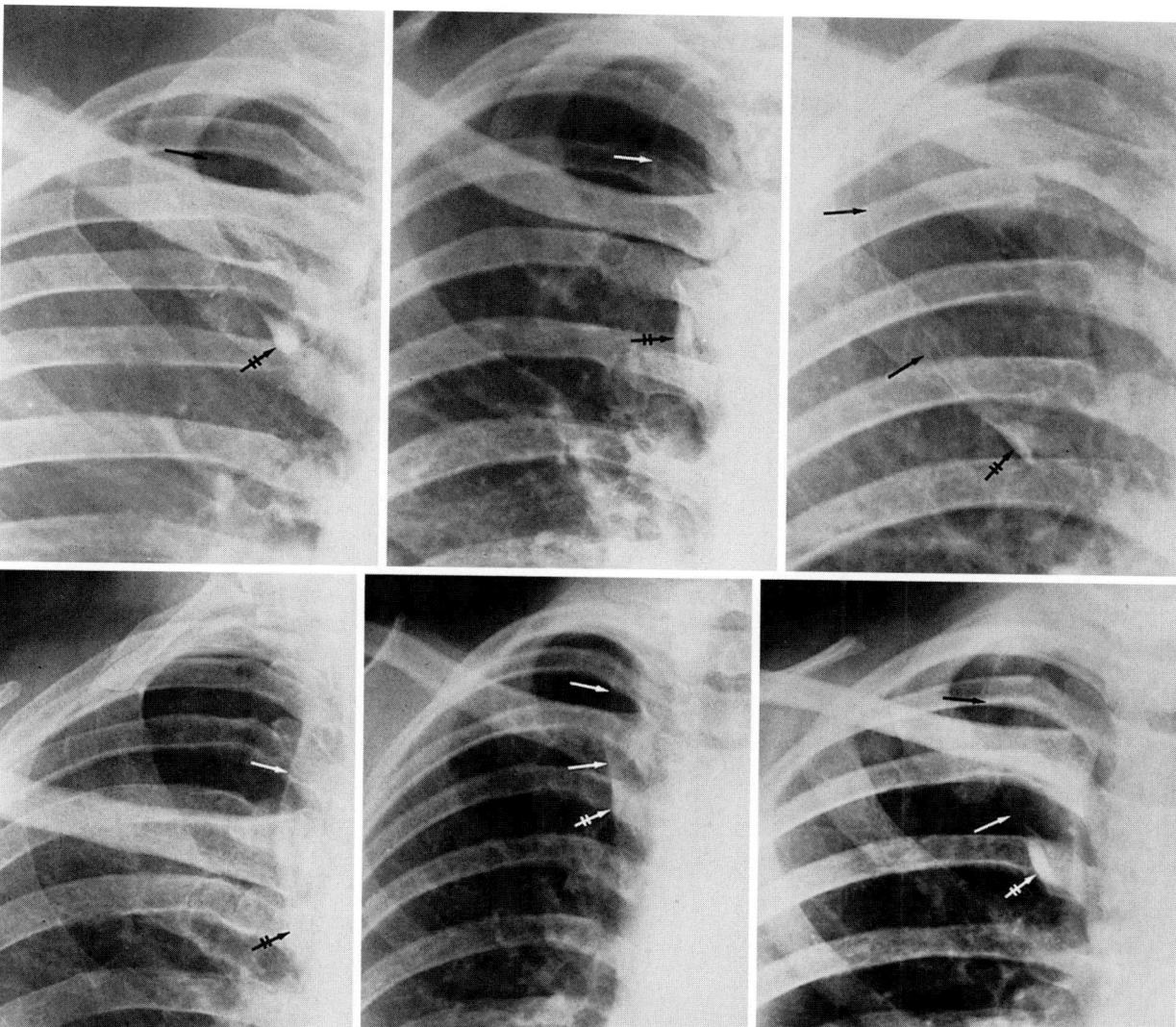

Figure 9–61. A–D. Six examples of azygos lobes to demonstrate the variation in configuration of the pleural line (←) and the position and size of the azygos vein (⬌). Note the opacity of azygos lobes in illustrations **D** and **E,** which may be mistaken for disease. (Ref: Caceras J et al: Increased density of the azygos lobe on frontal chest radiographs simulating disease. *Am J Roentgenol* 160:245, 1993.)

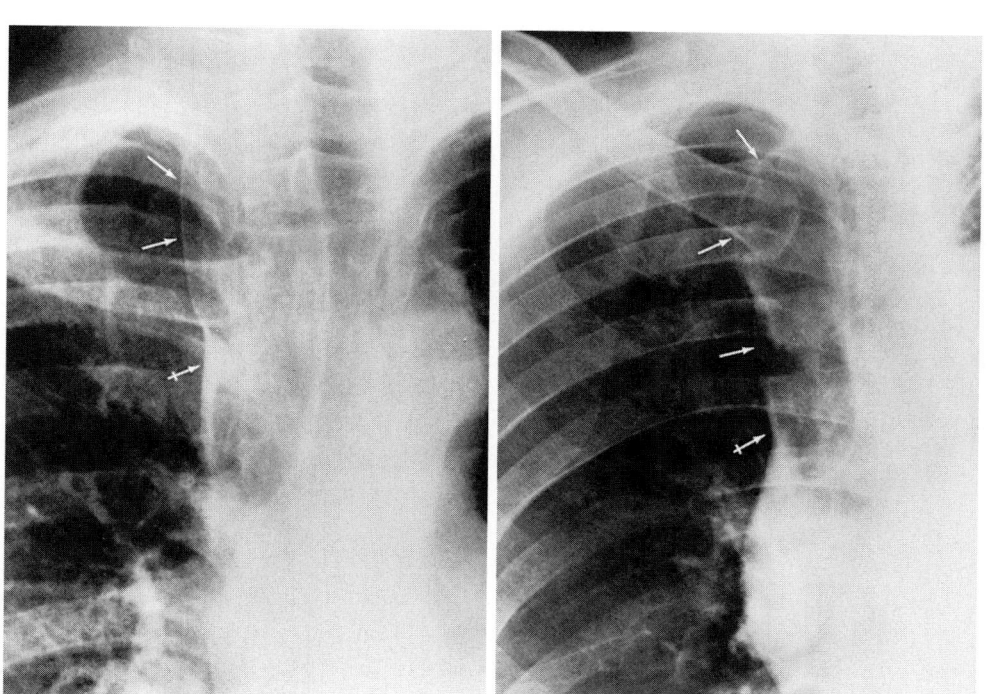

Figure 9–62. Additional examples of azygos lobes to demonstrate the variation in configuration of the pleural line (←) and the position and size of the azygos vein (⬌).

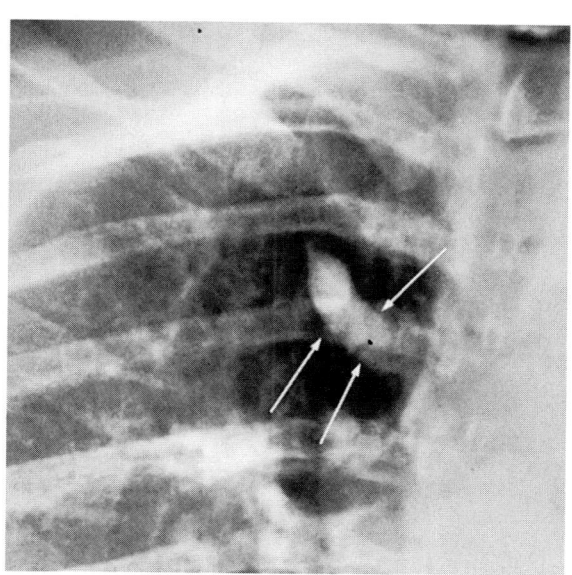

Figure 9–63. The azygos lobe and arch and its continuity with the azygos vein (*arrows*).

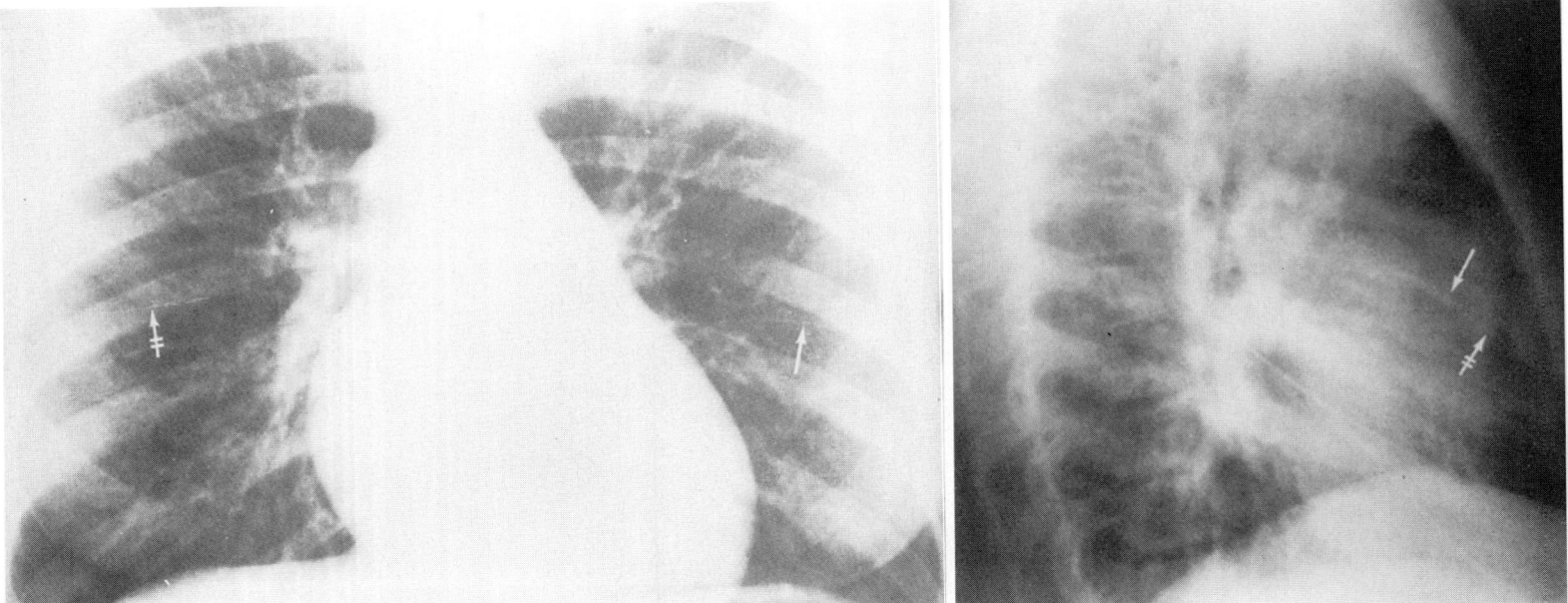

Figure 9–64. The lingular fissure. This fissure separates the lingula from the remainder of the left upper lobe (←). It duplicates the minor fissure on the right (⬅╫). (Ref: Boyden EA: Cleft left upper lobes and the split anterior bronchus. *Surgery* 26:167, 1949.)

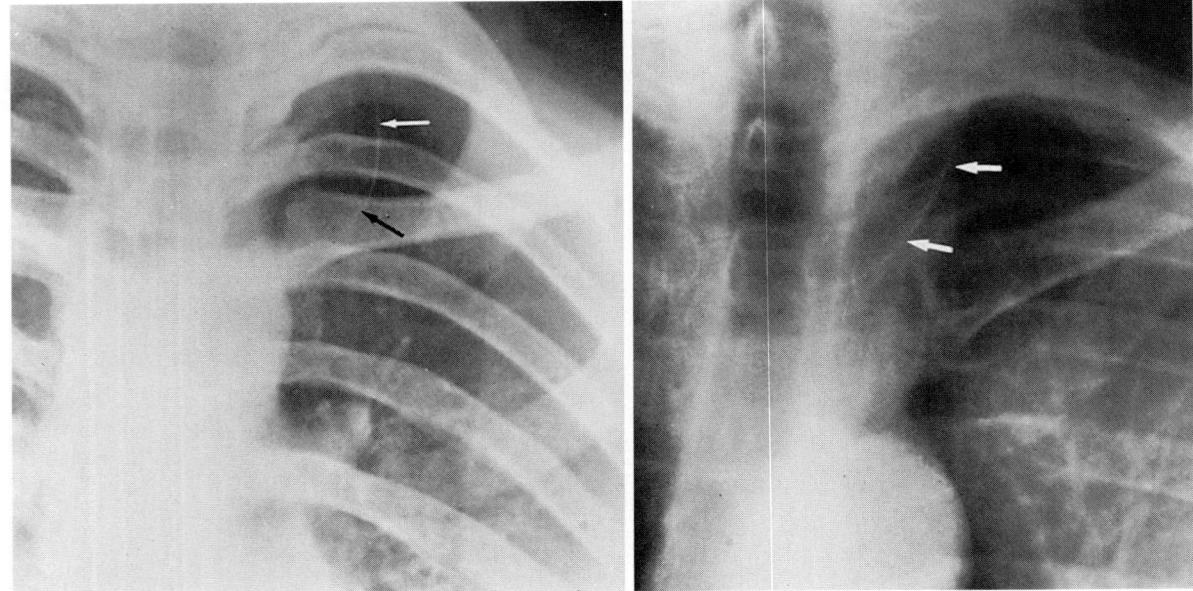

Figure 9–65. Two examples of an accessory fissure of the left upper lobe, the left azygos lobe. (Ref: Takasugi JE, Goodwin JD: Left azygos lobe. *Radiology* 171:133, 1989.)

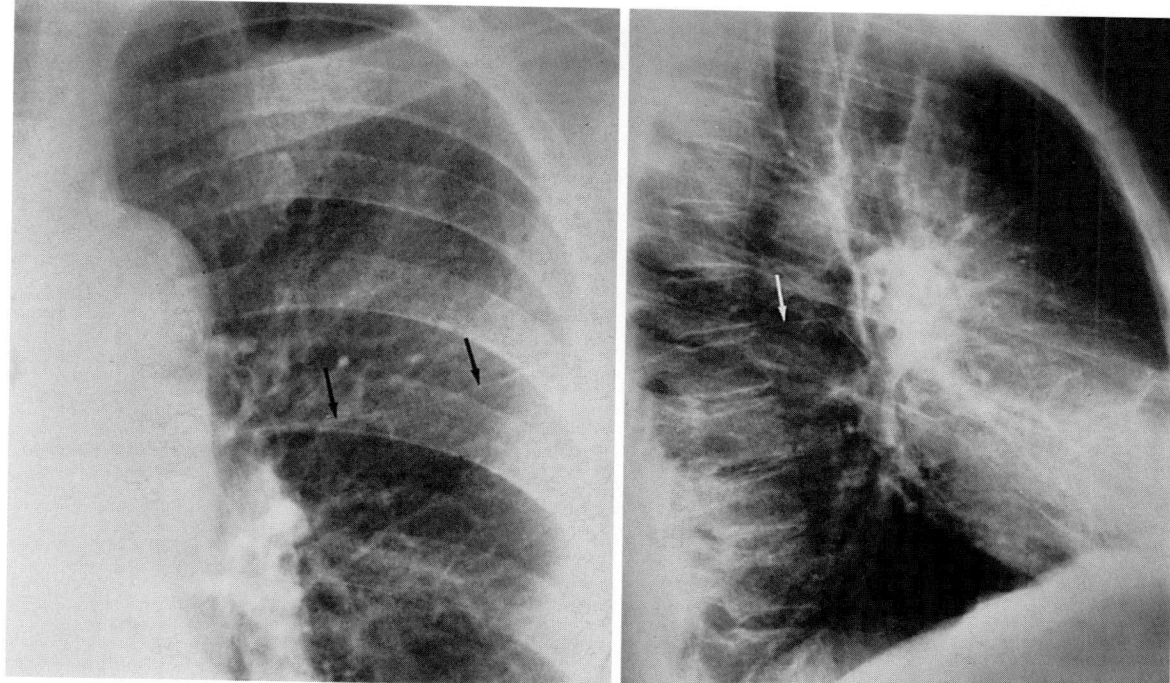

Figure 9–66. The superior accessory fissure of the left lower lobe. This fissure separates the superior and basal segments of the left lower lobe. A similar fissure occurs in the right lower lobe. (Ref: Felson B: The lobes and interlobar pleura: Fundamental roentgen considerations. *Am J Med Sci* 230:572, 1955.)

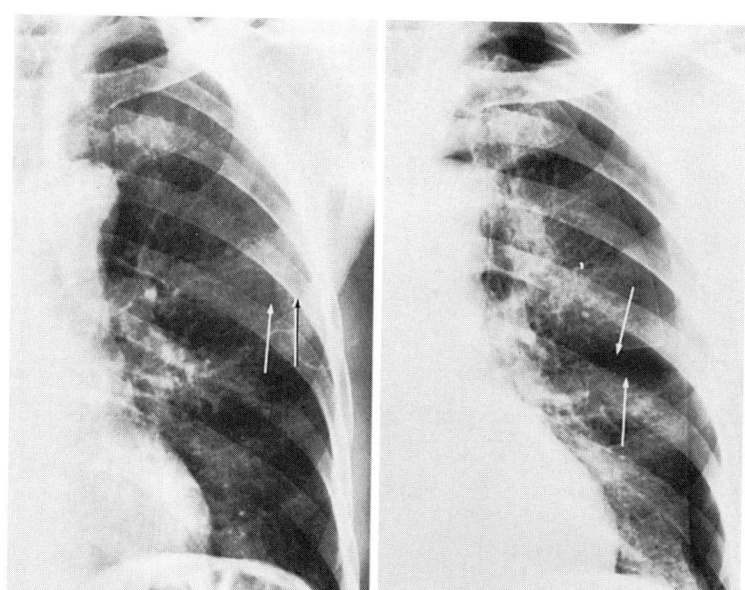

Figure 9–67. Superior accessory fissure by plain film (*left*) and with pneumothorax (*right*).

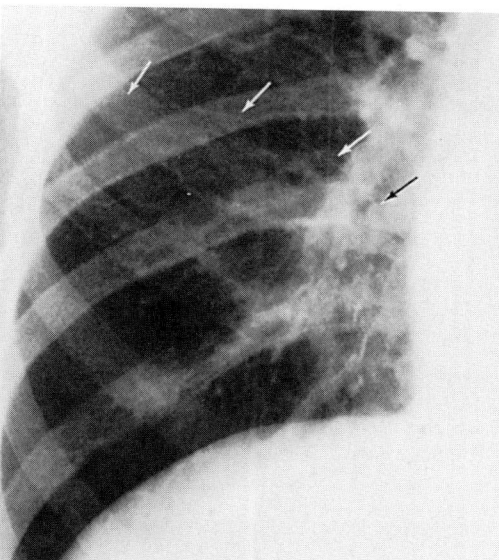

Figure 9–68. Cephalic curvature of the minor interlobar fissure may be seen as a normal variation.

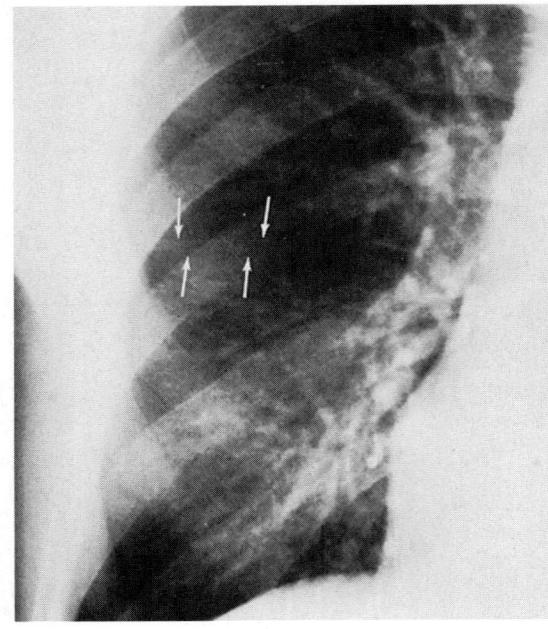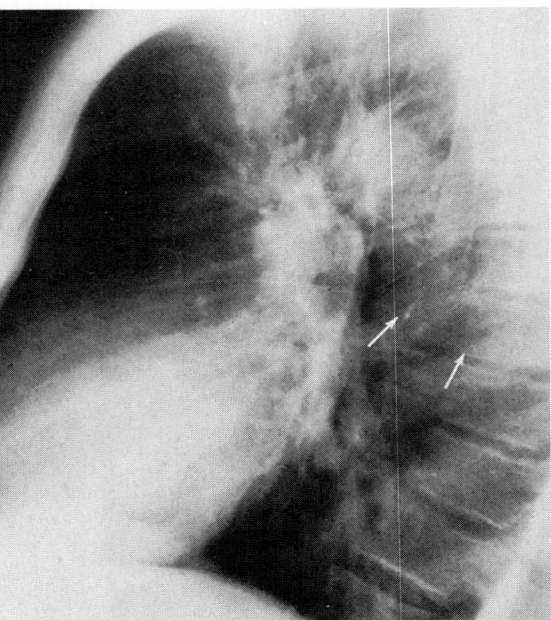

Figure 9–69. Accessory fissure for the superior segment of the right lower lobe. Note the presence of two pleural lines in the frontal projection. (Ref: Godwin JD, Tarver RD: Accessory fissures of the lung. *Am J Roentgenol* 144:39, 1985.)

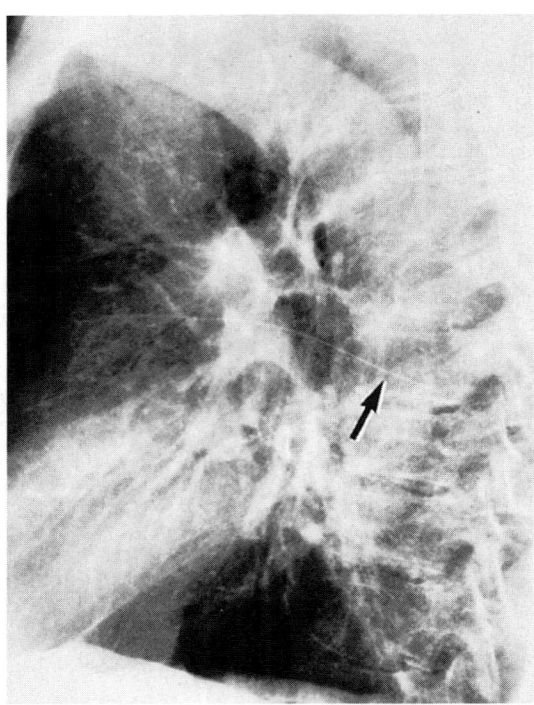

Figure 9–70. Minor fissure may normally be seen posteriorly in films made with slight rotation, and may be mistaken for the accessory fissure seen in the preceding figure.

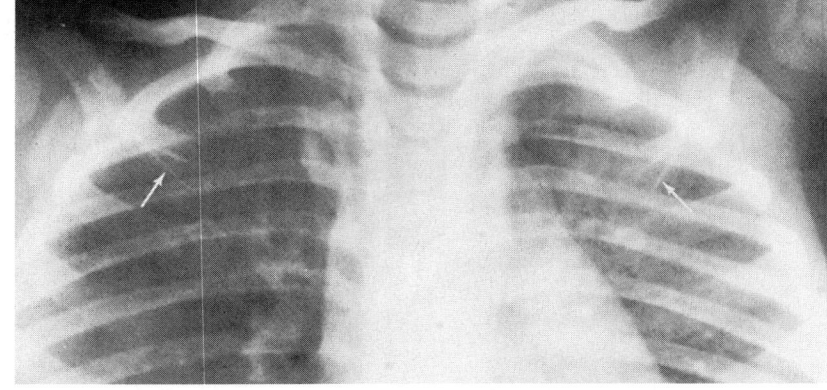

Figure 9–71. Superimposed scapular spines may simulate interlobar pleural surfaces.

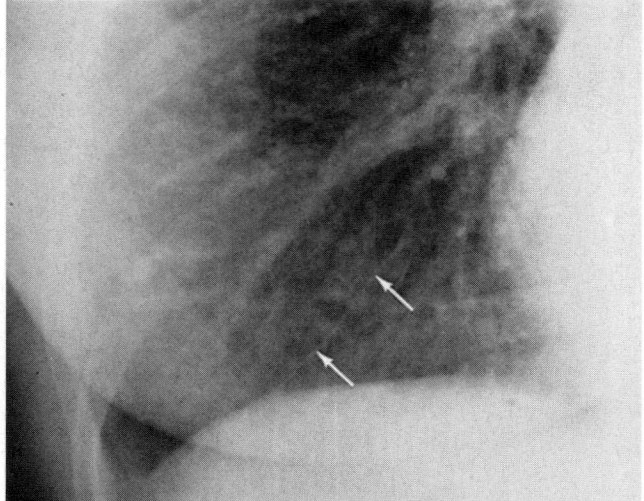

Figure 9–72. Inferior accessory fissure. When complete, it isolates the medial basal segment of the lower lobe. (Ref: Felson B: The lobes and interlobar pleura: Fundamental roentgen considerations. *Am J Med Sci* 230:572, 1955.)

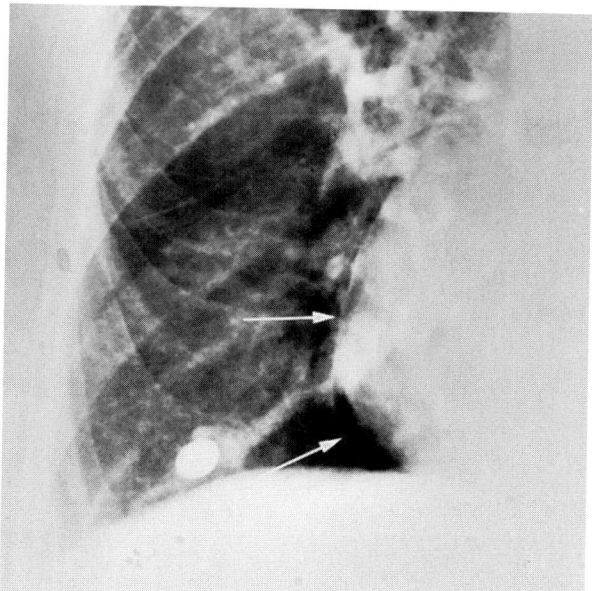

Figure 9–73. Sagittal orientation of the major fissure. Note how it may simulate pneumopericardium. (Ref: Gross BH et al: Sagittal orientation of the anterior minor fissure: Radiography and CT. *Radiology* 166:717, 1988.)

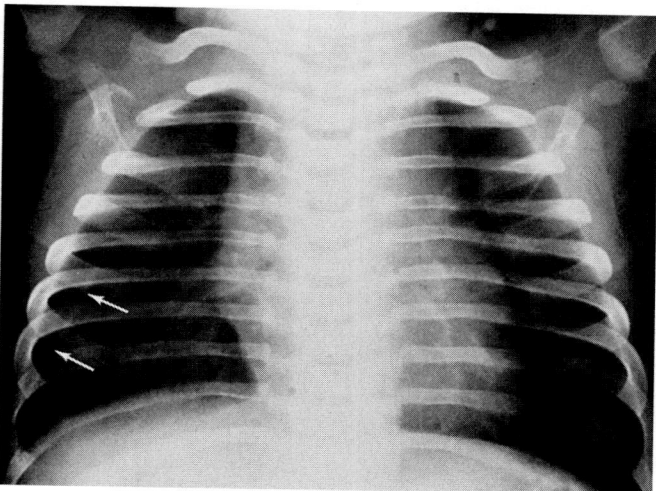

Figure 9–74. Vertical fissure line. This line represents the caudal end of the major interlobar fissure. It may be seen in films of healthy children when it is ectopic and lies forward so part of it is in axial projection. It should not be mistaken for a pneumothorax. (Ref: Davis LA: The vertical fissure line. *Am J Roentgenol* 84:451, 1960.)

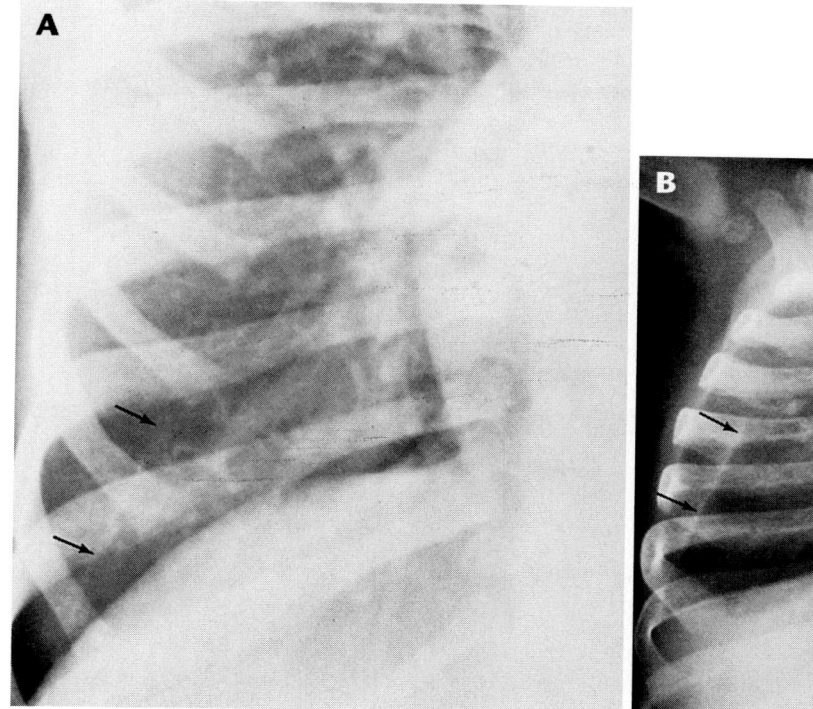

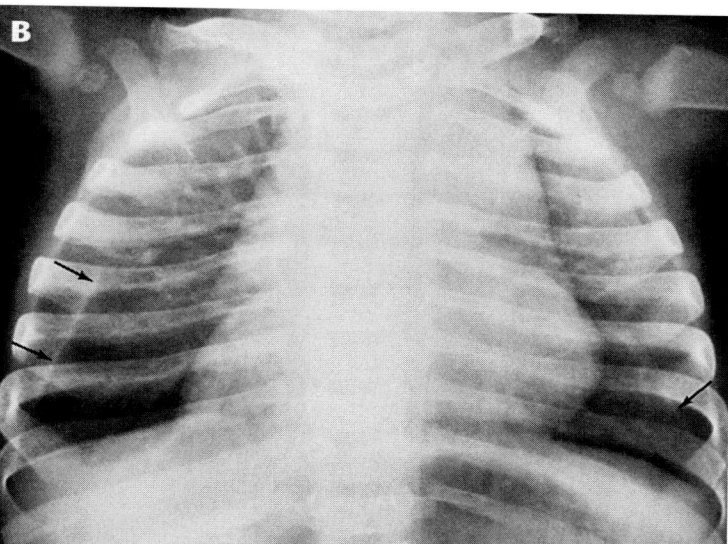

Figure 9–75. Vertical fissure line. **A,** Unilateral. **B,** Bilateral. (Ref: Webber MM, O'Loughlin BJ: Variations of the pleural vertical fissure line. *Radiology* 82:461, 1964.)

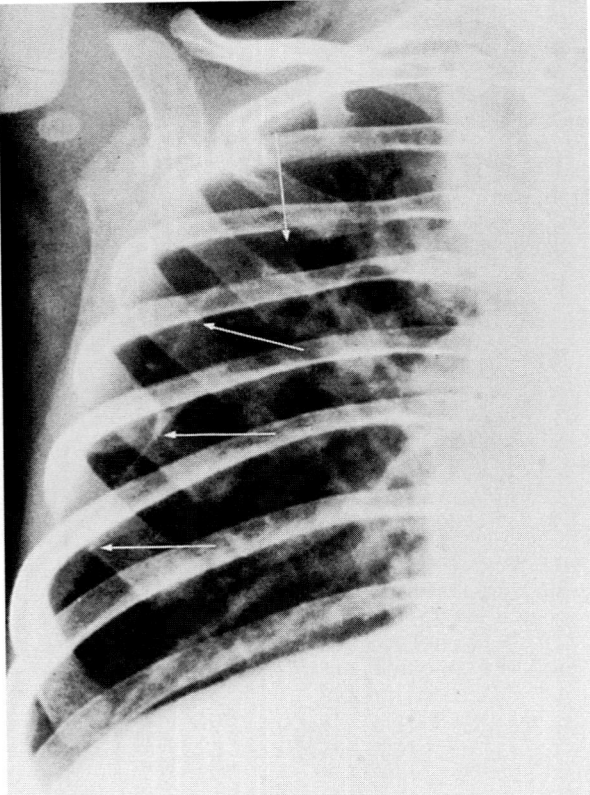

Figure 9–76. Vertical fissure line with extension over the apex of the right lower lobe.

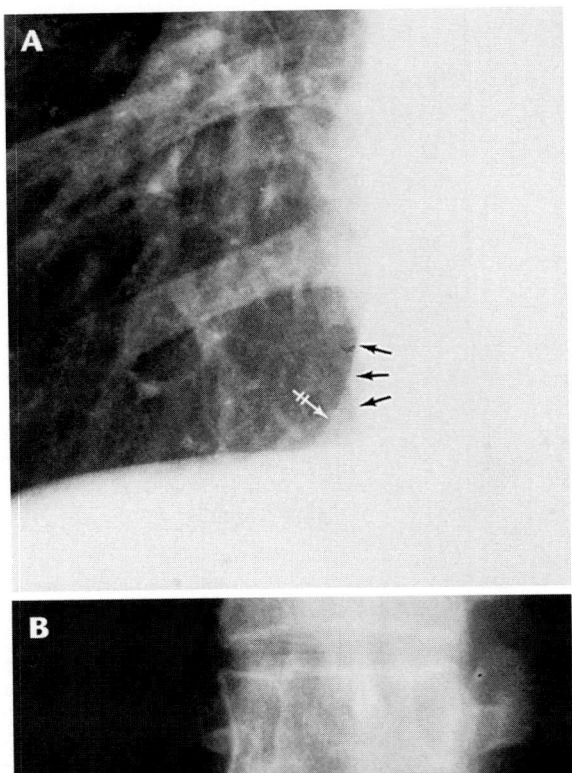

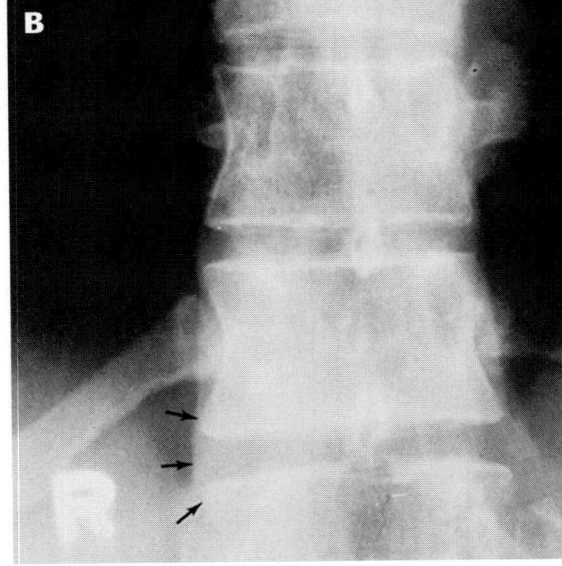

Figure 9–77. Pleural reflection over the inferior vena cava. **A,** Apparent paraspinous mass (←) produced by pleural reflection over the inferior vena cava (◄╫). **B,** Detailed view with greater penetration shows no paraspinous mass.

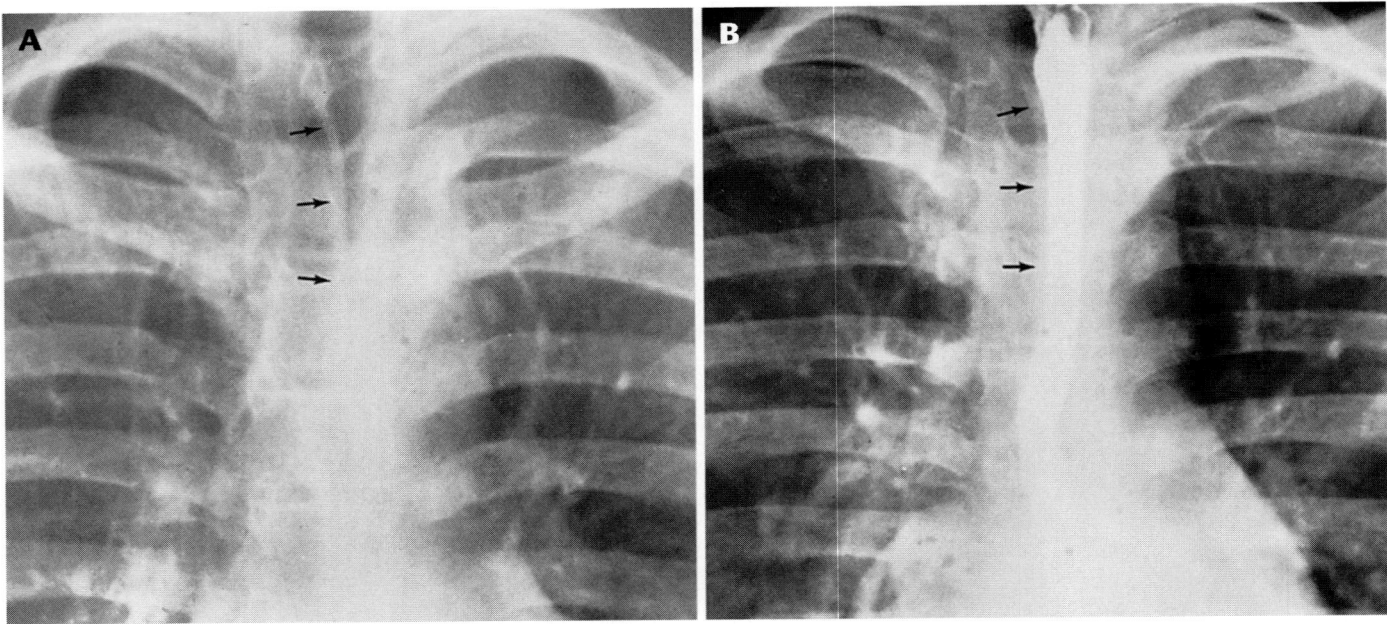

Figure 9–78. Esophageal pleural stripe that represents the right esophageal wall and its adjacent pleural covering. **A,** Plain film. **B,** Esophagram. (Ref: Cimmino CV: The esophageal-pleural stripe on chest teleroentgenograms. *Radiology* 67:754, 1956.)

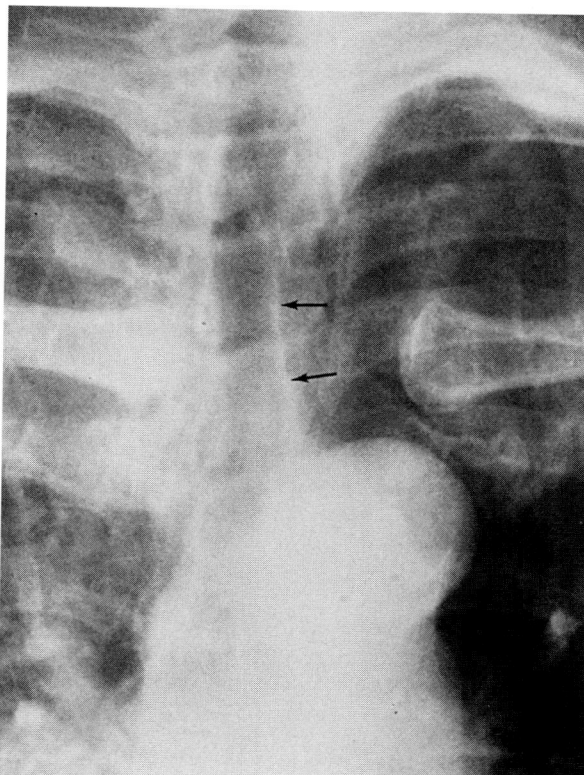

Figure 9–79. Posterior mediastinal stripe, the interface of the right and left lungs, seen in frontal projection. (Ref: Cimmino CV, Snead LO Jr: The posterior mediastinal line on chest roentgenograms. *Radiology,* 84:516, 1965.)

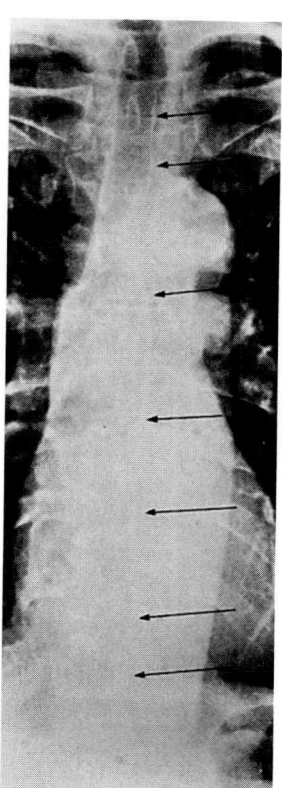

Figure 9–80. Posterior medastinal line seen in its entirety.

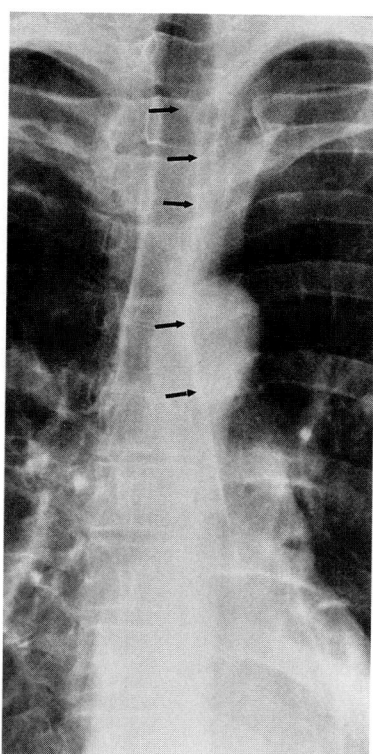

Figure 9–81. Anterior mediastinal stripe, representing the interface between the right and left lungs, seen in frontal projection (←). (Ref: Cimmino CV: The anterior mediastinal line on chest roentgenograms. *Radiology* 82:459, 1964.)

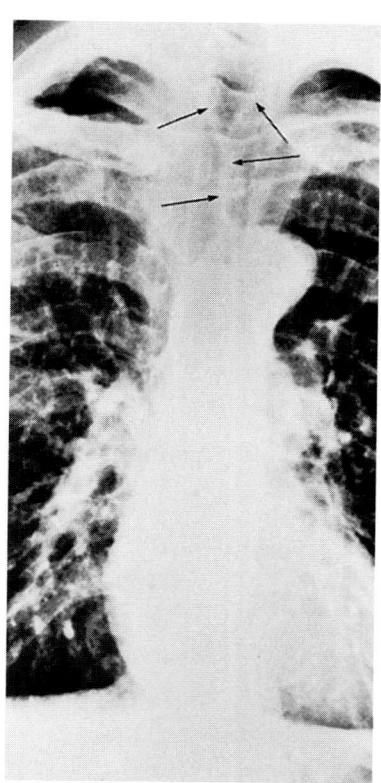

Figure 9–82. Anterior mediastinal stripe and its lateral extensions.

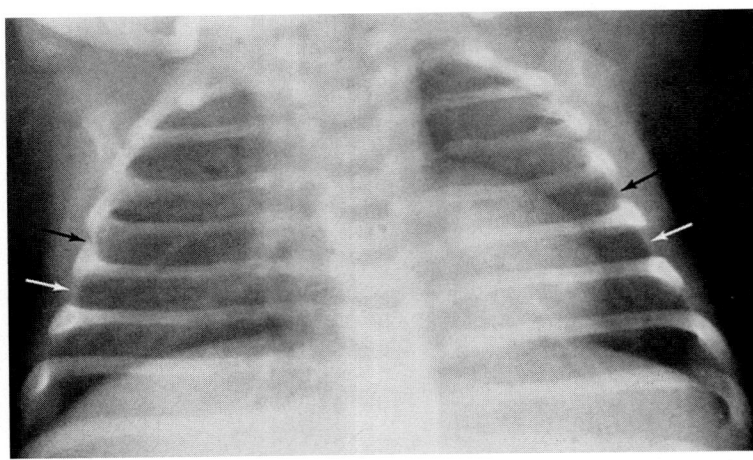

Figure 9–83. Bulging of the interspaces in a normal child. Although intercostal bulging of the lung is said to be an early sign of obstructive emphysema, it may also be seen in normal, thin children who inspire fully. (Ref: Kattan KR et al: Intercostal bulging of the lung without emphysema. *Am J Roentgenol* 112:542, 1971.)

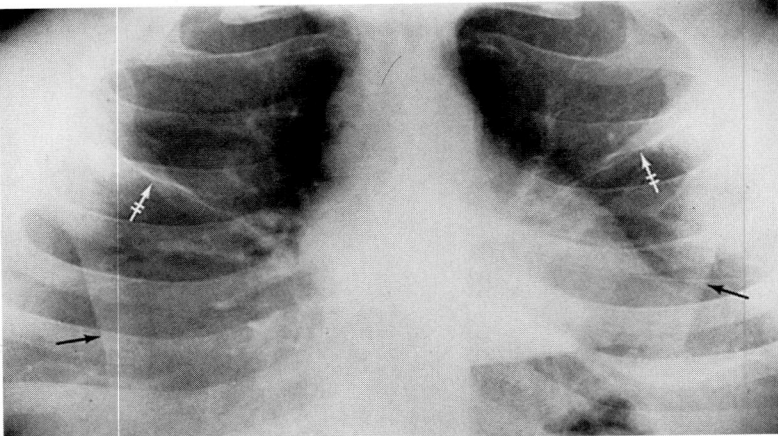

Figure 9–84. Scapulae seen in lordotic projection may simulate pulmonary pathology (←), particularly the shadow of the spine of the scapula (⇤).

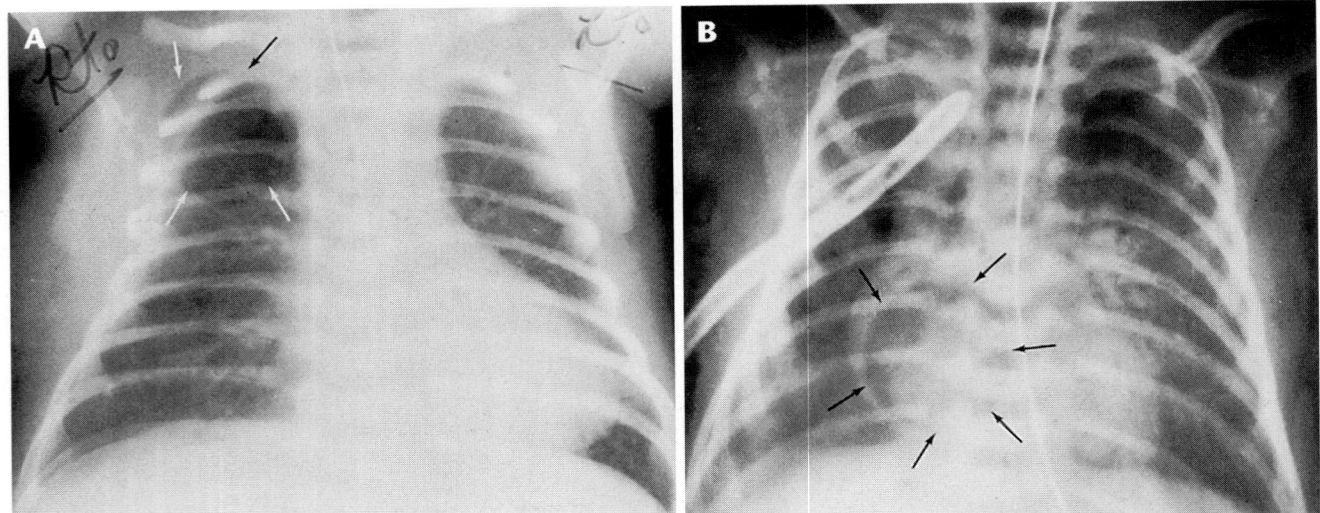

Figure 9–85. Films made of infants in isolettes may show radiolucencies produced by the opening in the isolette covers. These may simulate abnormalities such as air cysts, as in **A,** or pneumopericardium, as in **B.**

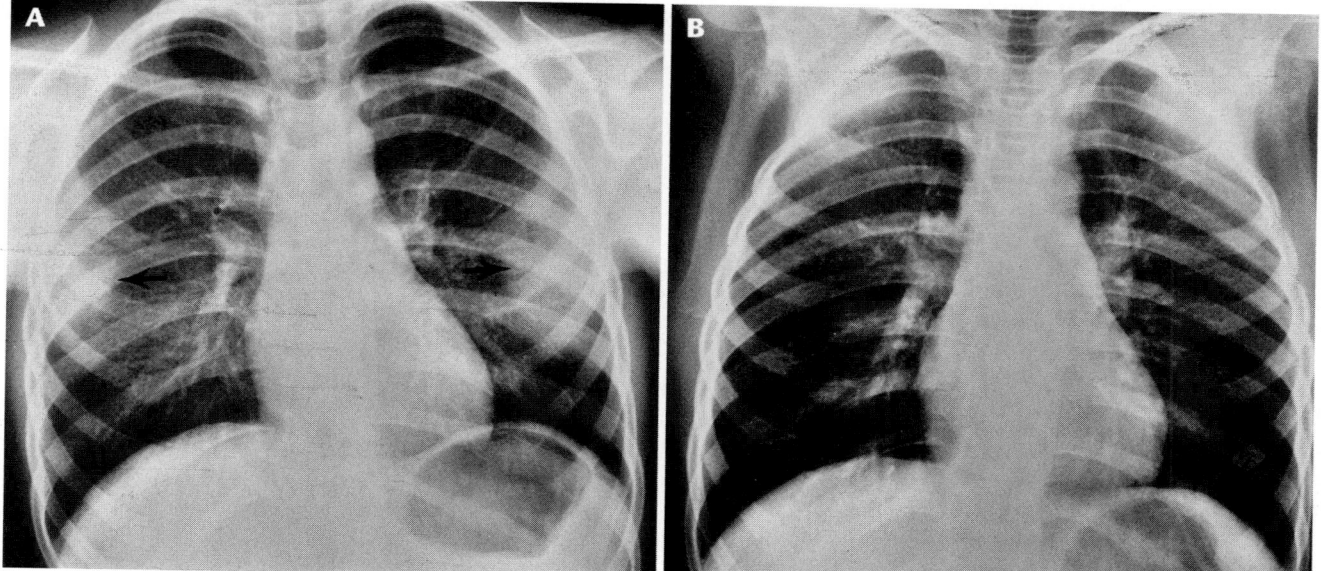

Figure 9–86. A, Simulated pneumonia produced by pectoral muscle shadows with arms down. **B,** Film made 5 minutes later with arms elevated shows disappearance of pectoral shadows.

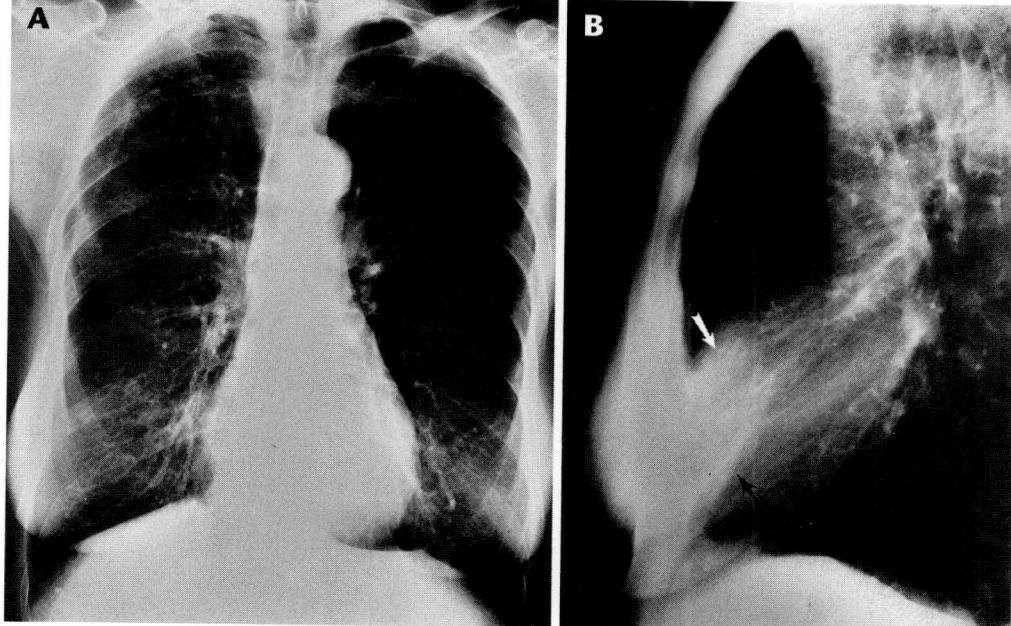

Figure 9–87. A, B, Breast shadows simulating pulmonary consolidation in the lateral projection (**B**).

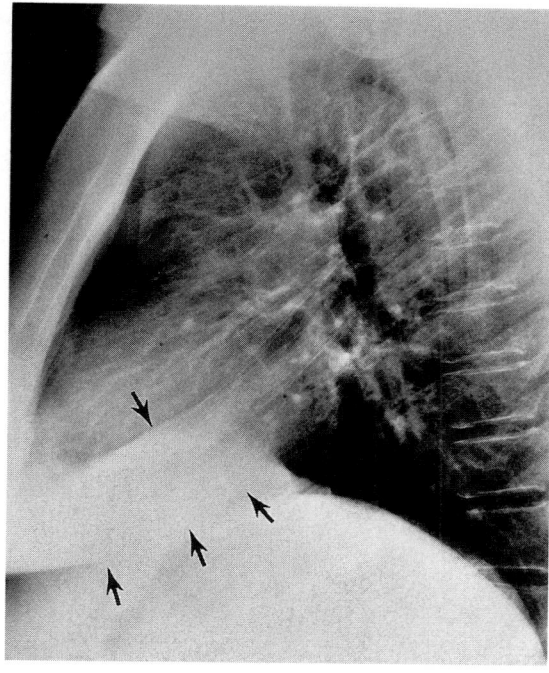

Figure 9–88. Simulated consolidation of the lung, produced by superimposed breast shadows.

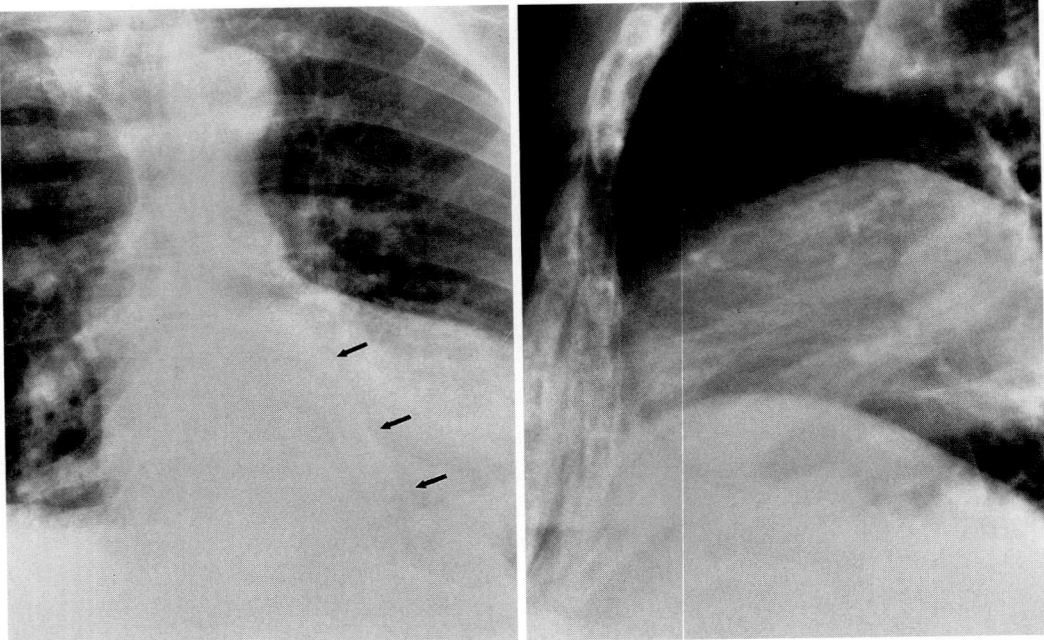

Figure 9–89. Dense calcification of the costal cartilages mistaken for a left lower lobe consolidation or atelectasis in the frontal film.

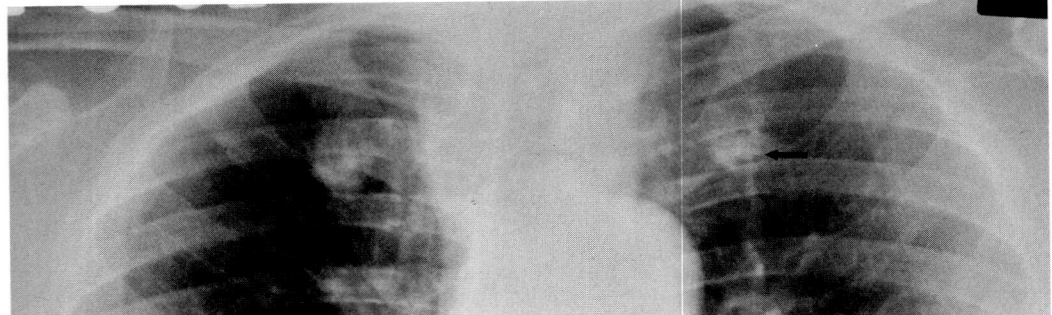

Figure 9–90. Costal cartilage calcification of the first rib, not to be mistaken for parenchymal lesions.

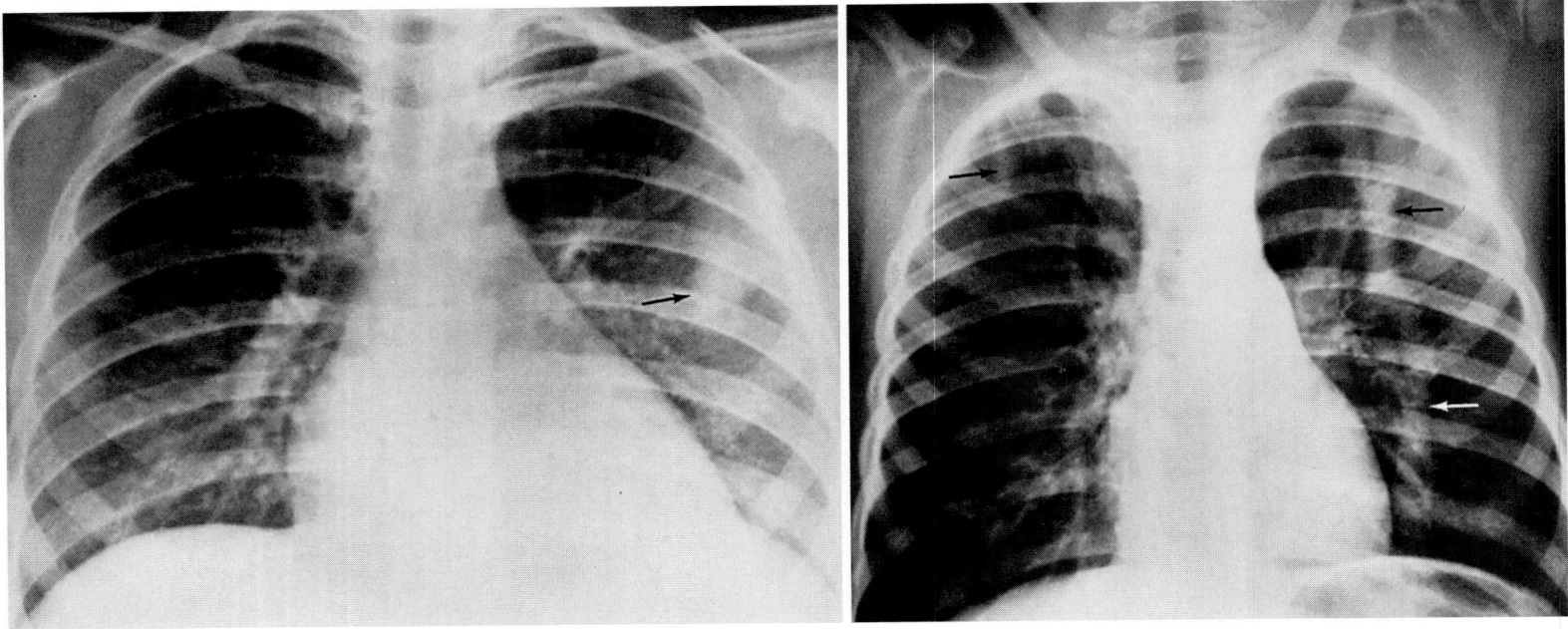

Figure 9–91. Two examples of hair braids simulating parenchymal abnormality.

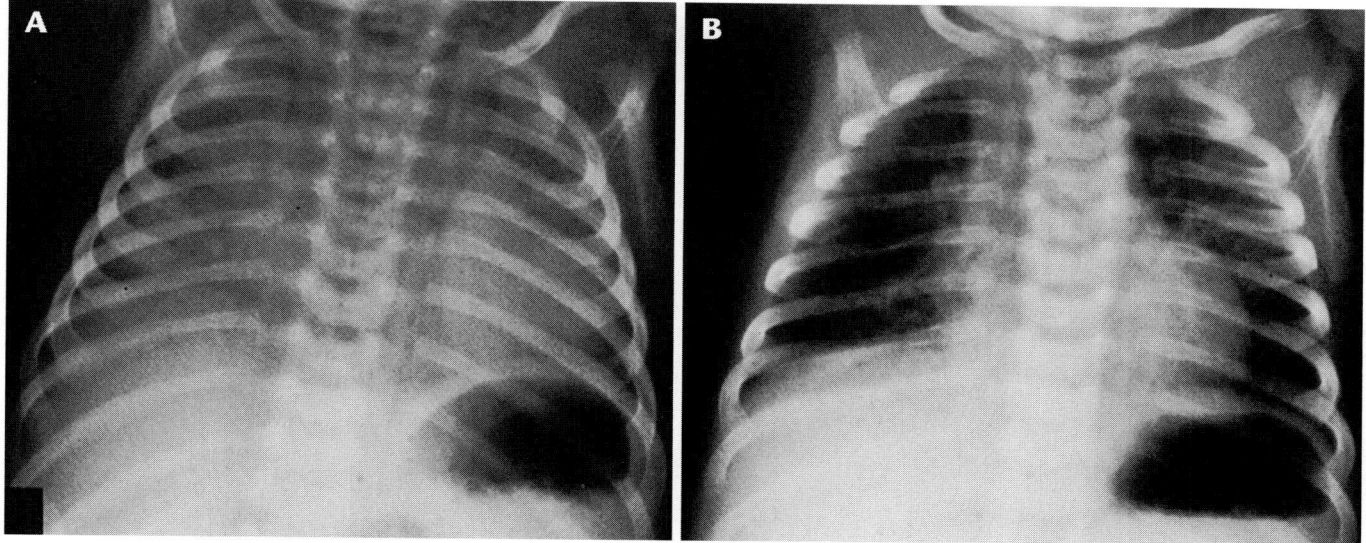

Figure 9–92. Filming infant chests in even minor degrees of expiration may result in misinterpretation caused by the marked opacity of the parenchyma, as illustrated in this normal infant. **A,** Expiration. **B,** Inspiration.

Figure 9–93. Expiratory film with superimposition of the right hemidiaphragm on the heart, producing an image simulating atelectasis of the right middle lobe.

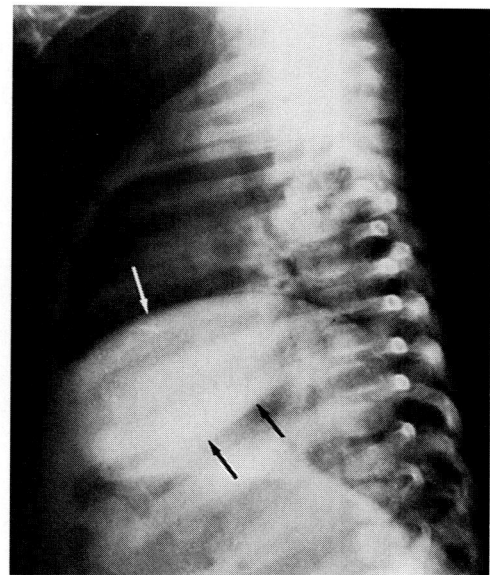

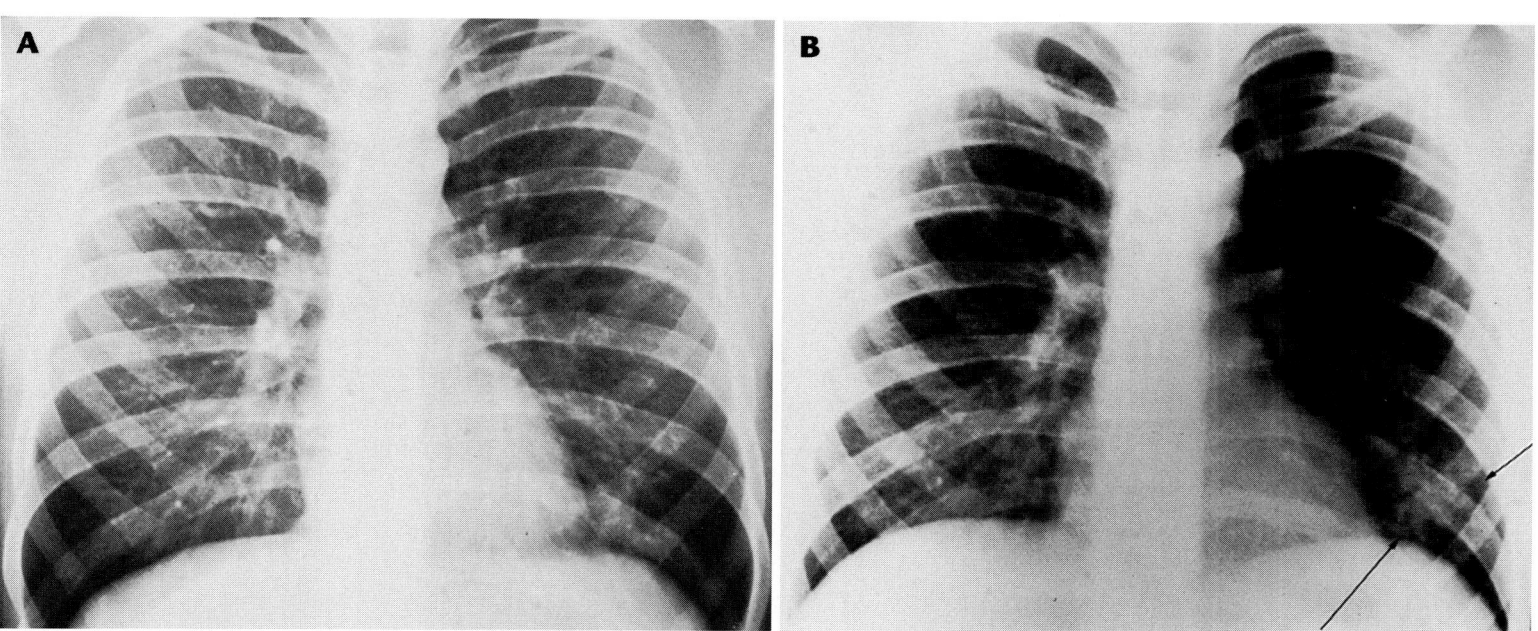

Figure 9–94. Filming in expiration may simulate basal pneumonitis in the adult. **A,** Inspiration. **B,** Expiration.

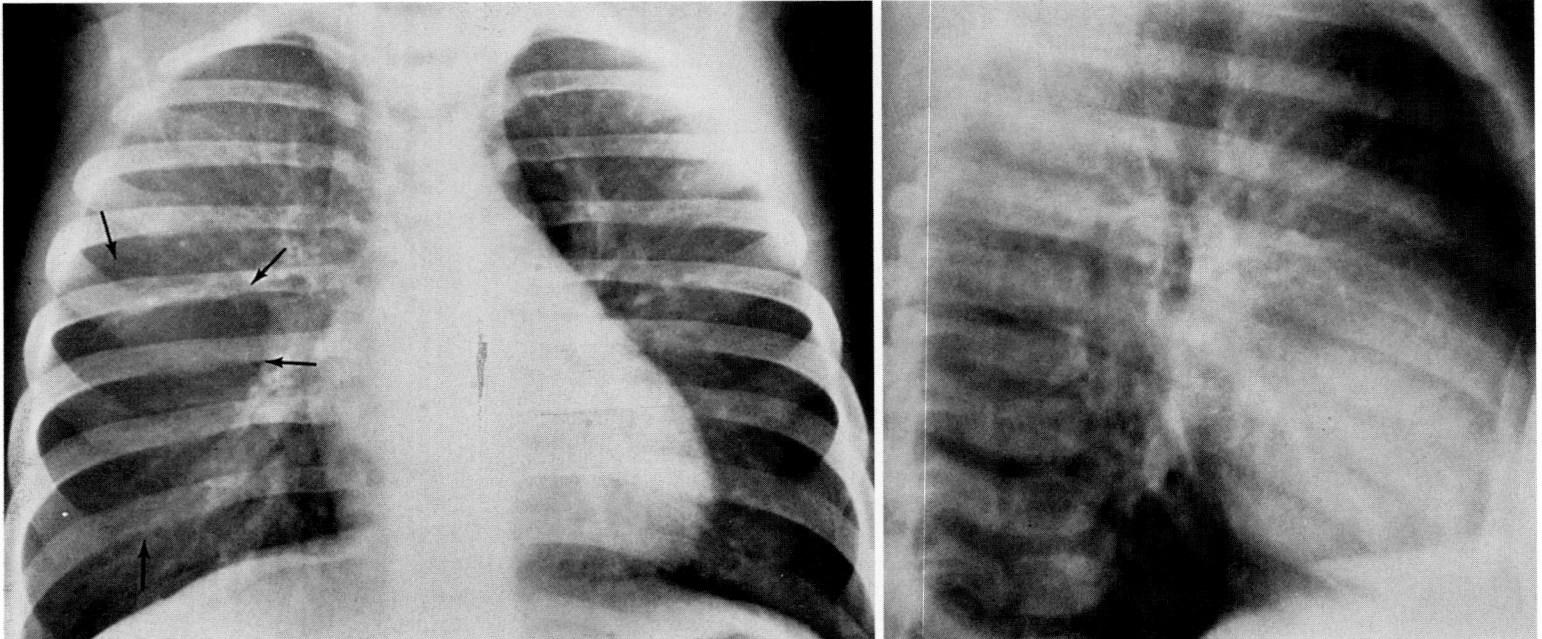

Figure 9–95. Simulated air trapping in the right middle lobe. This misleading appearance is not infrequent and results from the pattern of division of the major vascular trunks. There is no evidence of air trapping in the lateral projection. (Refs: Milne ENC, Bass H: The right midlung window. *J Can Assoc Radiol* 20:3, 1969; Goodman LR et al: The right midlung window. *Radiology* 143:135, 1982.)

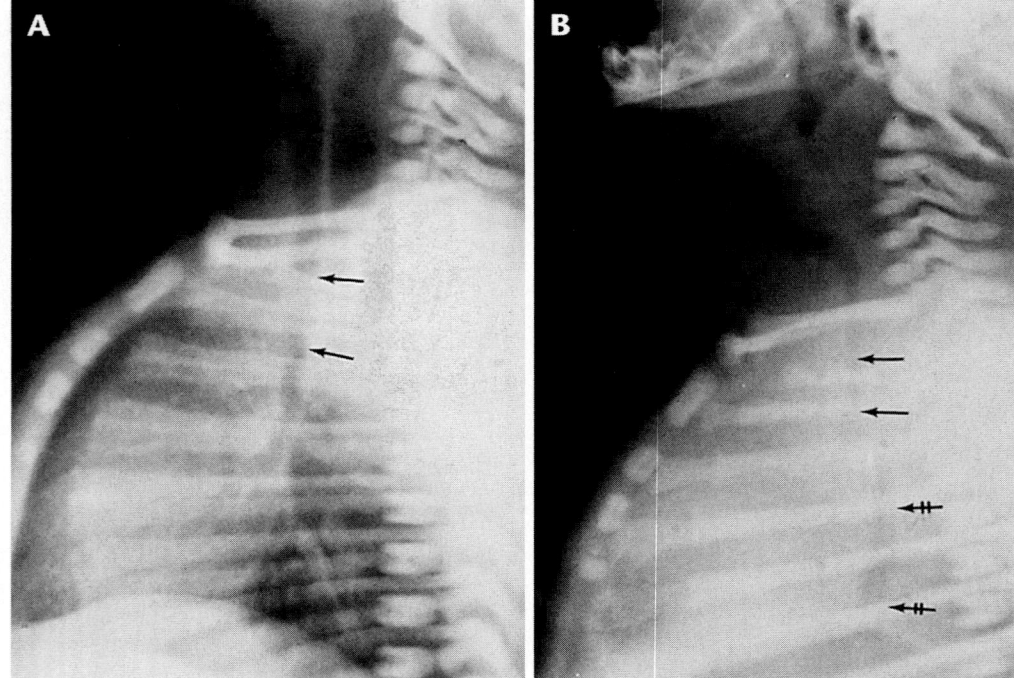

Figure 9–96. Effects of respiration on the trachea in infancy. The trachea (←) widens on inspiration (**A**) and narrows on expiration (**B**). The hatched arrows (◄╫) in **B** indicate swallowed air in the esophagus. Note also the normal anterior buckling of the airway in the neck on expiration. (Ref: Wittenberg MH et al: Tracheal dynamics in infants with respiratory distress, stridor, and collapsing trachea. *Radiology* 88:613, 1967.)

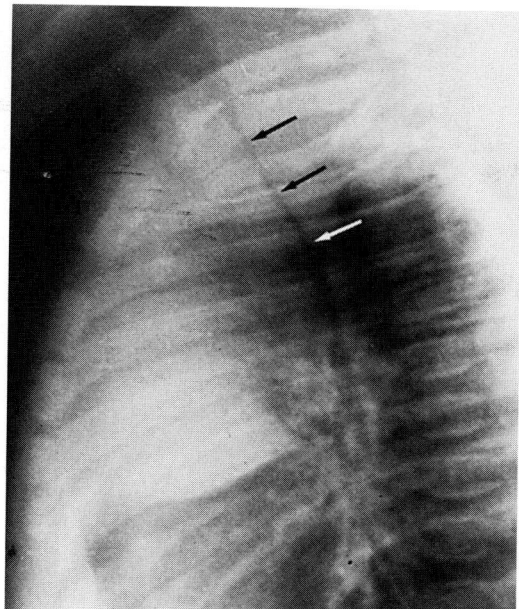

Figure 9–97. Tracheal narrowing on expiration in a 3-week-old infant, illustrating how marked this physiologic event may normally be.

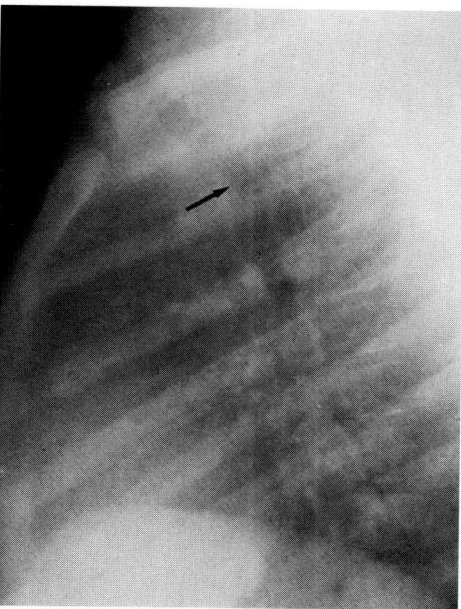

Figure 9–98. Normal anterior tracheal indentation in a 2-year-old child. This is a common finding just below the thoracic inlet. It changes with respiration and is usually of no clinical significance. There is evidence that it is the product of intermittent cephalic movement of the thymus from the anterior mediastinum into the neck with respiration. It is seen commonly in children under the age of 2 years. (Refs: Swischuk LE: Anterior tracheal indentations in infancy and early childhood. Normal or abnormal? *Am J Roentgenol* 112:12, 1971; Mandell CA et al: Cervical trachea: Dynamics in response to herniation of the normal thymus. *Radiology* 186:383, 1993.)

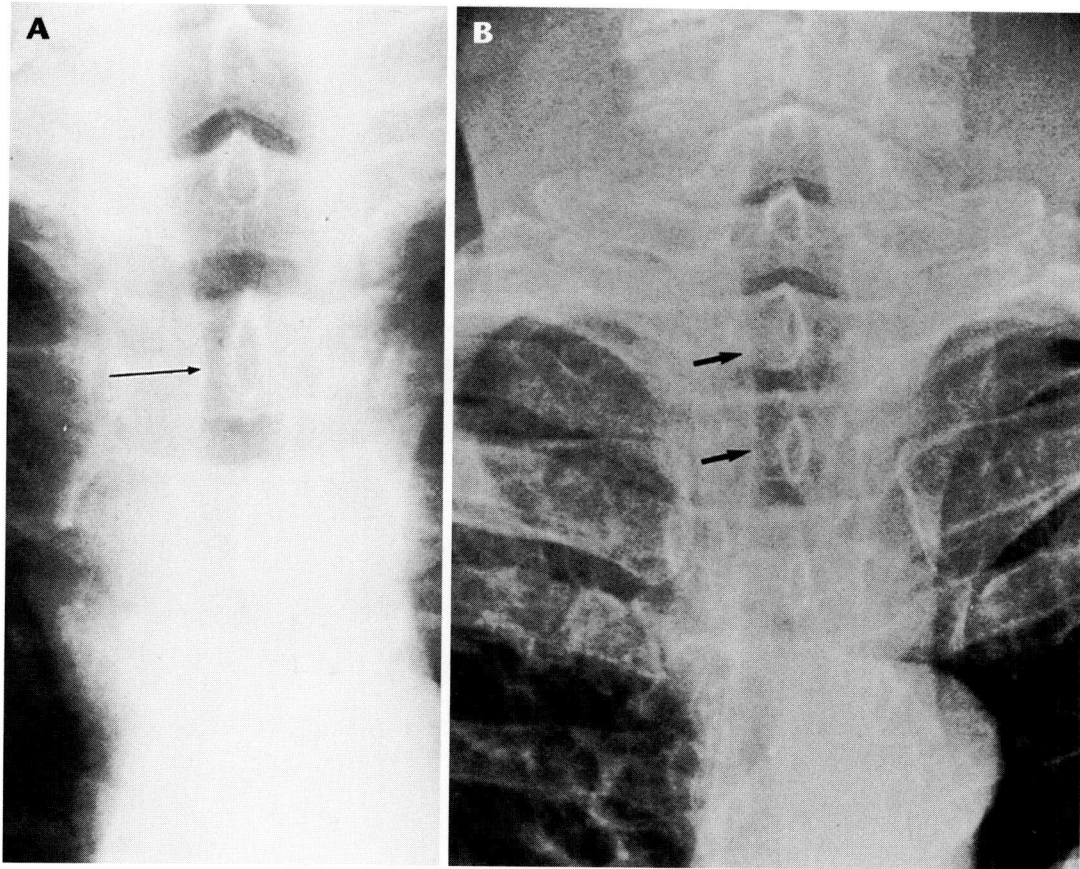

Figure 9–99. A shallow impression on the right side of the trachea at the thoracic inlet is seen in many normal children (**A**) and adults (**B**).

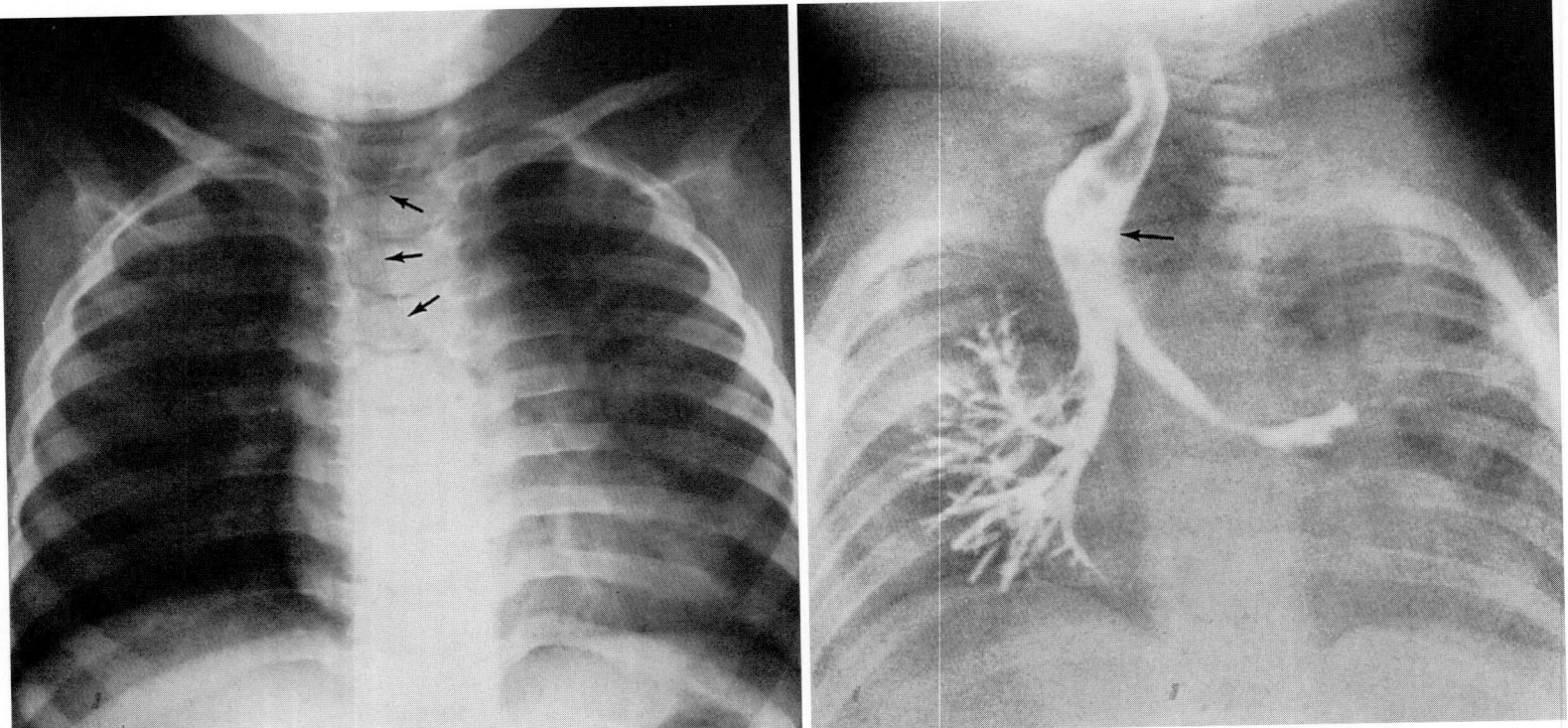

Figure 9–100. Lateral buckling of the trachea at the thoracic inlet occurs normally in infants and children up to 5 years of age. The displacement is to the side opposite the aortic arch and is best seen in expiration. (Ref: Chang LWM et al: Normal lateral deviation of the trachea in infants and children. *Am J Roentgenol* 109:247, 1970.)

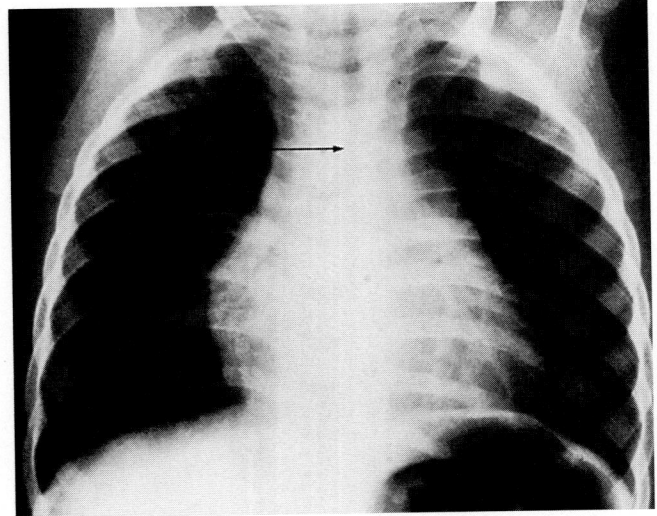

Figure 9–101. Deviation of the trachea to the left in the presence of a right aortic arch.

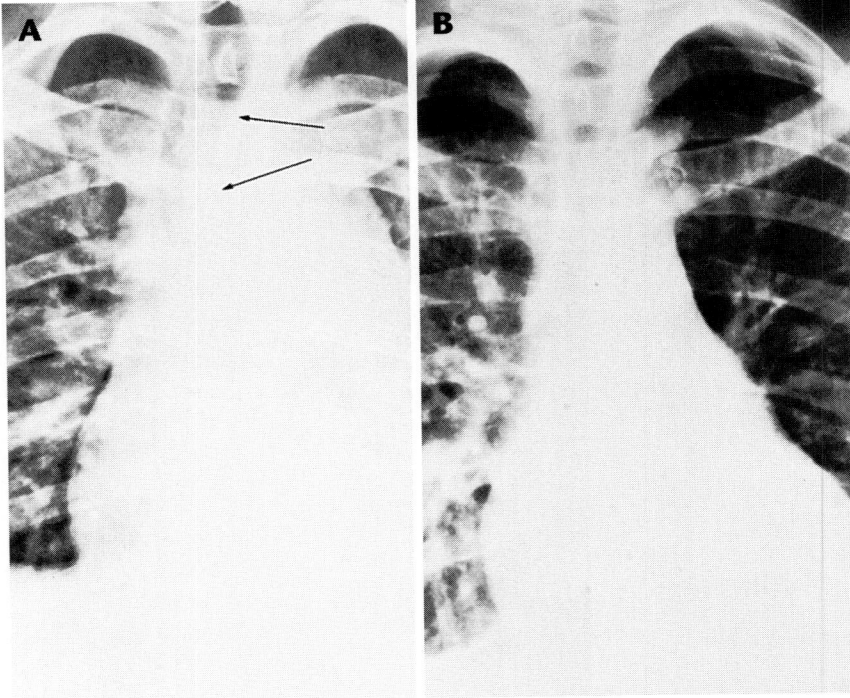

Figure 9–102. A, Tracheal buckling on expiration in an adult. **B,** Inspiration does not show buckling.

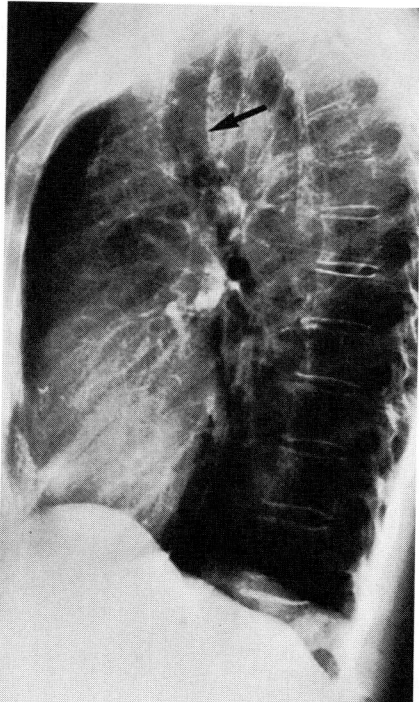

Figure 9–103. Normal anterior bowing of the trachea in the adult, associated with ectasia of the aorta.

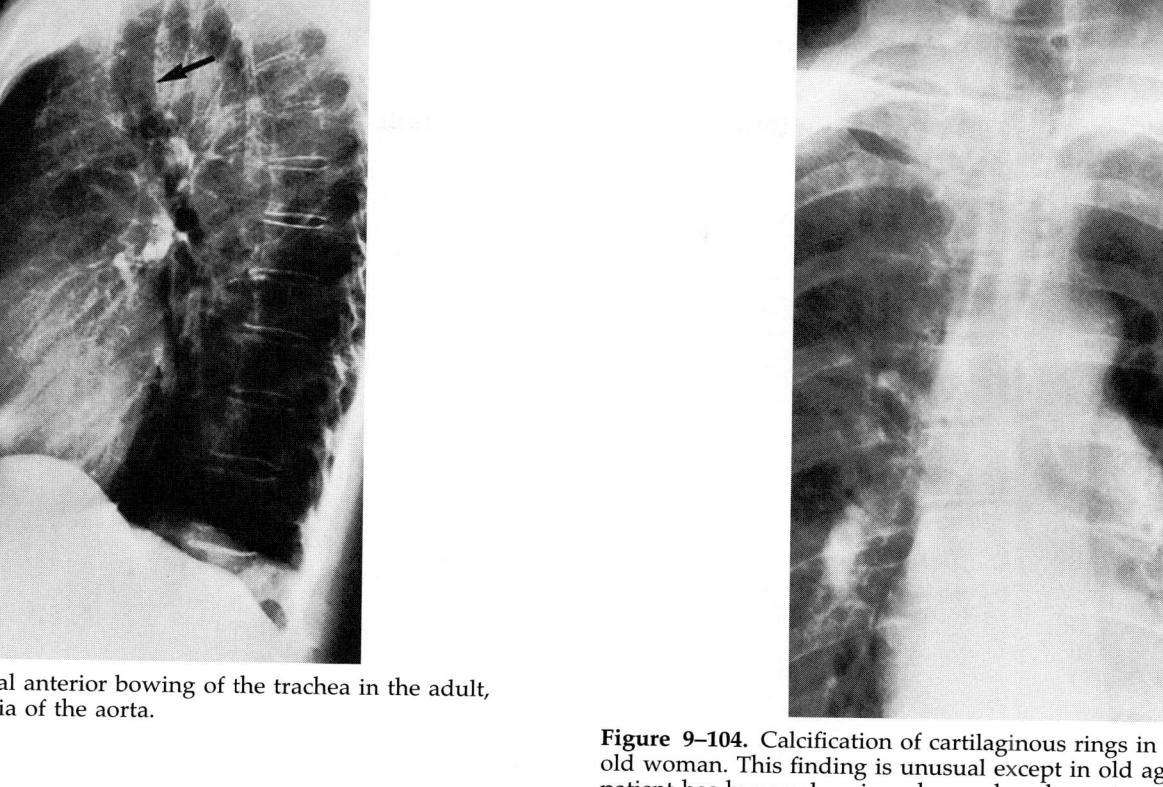

Figure 9–104. Calcification of cartilaginous rings in a healthy 47-year-old woman. This finding is unusual except in old age, unless the patient has hypercalcemia or hyperphosphatemia.

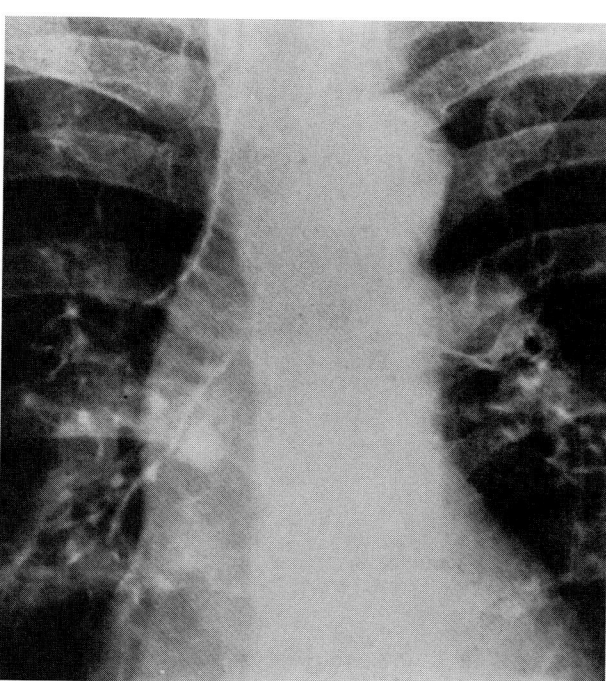

Figure 9–105. "Physiologic" calcification of the tracheobronchial cartilages in a 56-year-old woman. Tracheal calcification is a feature particularly seen in elderly women. (Ref: Kurihara Y et al: Radiologic evidence of sex differences. (*Am J Roentgenol* 167:1037, 1996.)

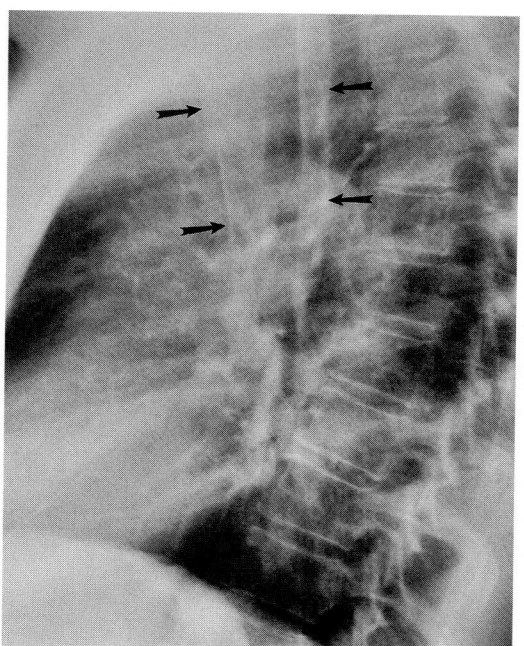

Figure 9–106. Superimposition of the scapulae simulating thickening of the paratracheal soft tissues.

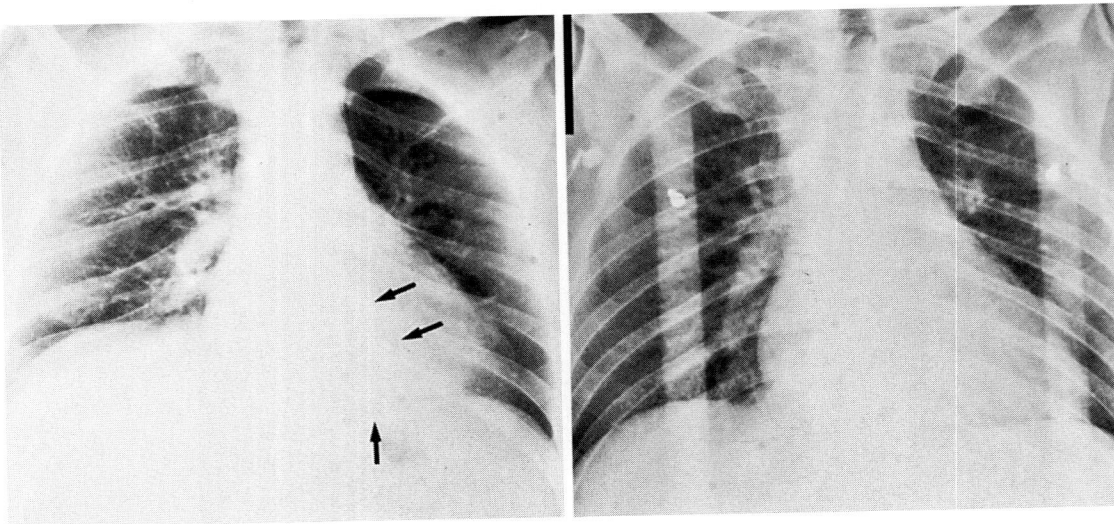

Figure 9–107. *Left,* Portable chest films that are made with lordotic projection will produce an illusory consolidation of the left lower lobe, with loss of the medial portion of the left hemidiaphragm. *Right,* Film made with proper projection does not show the pseudoconsolidation. (Ref: Zylak CJ et al: Illusory consolidation of the left lower lobe: A pitfall in portable radiology. *Radiology* 167:653, 1988.)

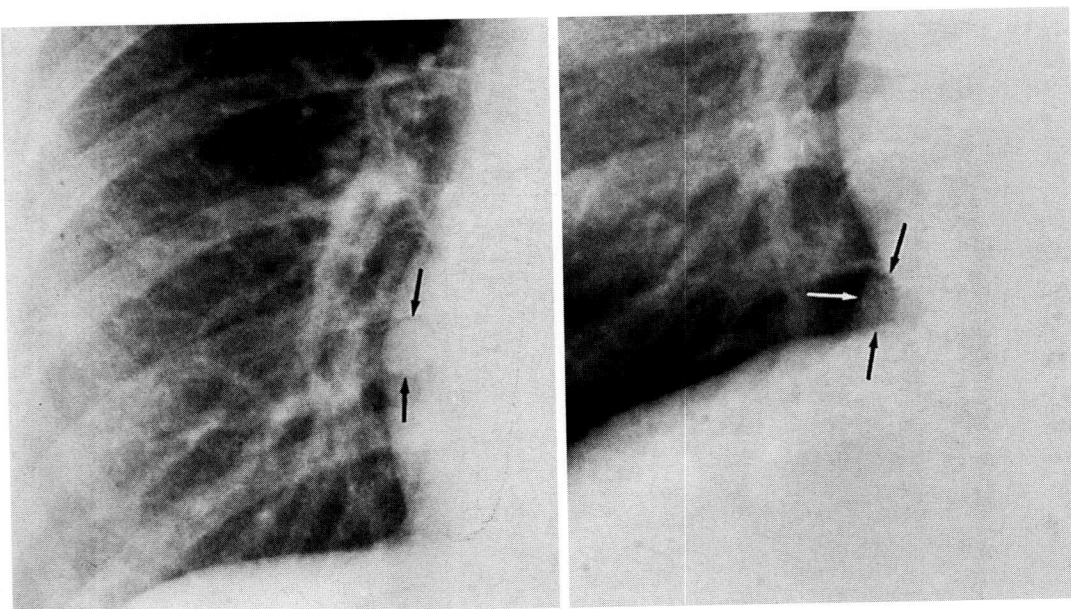

Figure 9–108. Two examples of large transverse processes that simulate nodular pulmonary lesions.

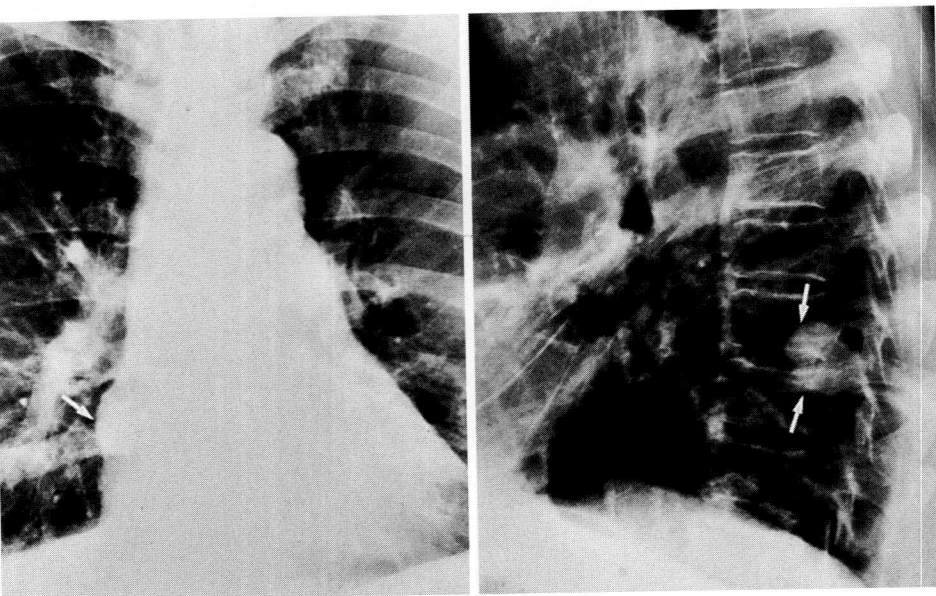

Figure 9–109. Large hypertrophic spur simulating a parenchymal lesion in both frontal and lateral projections.

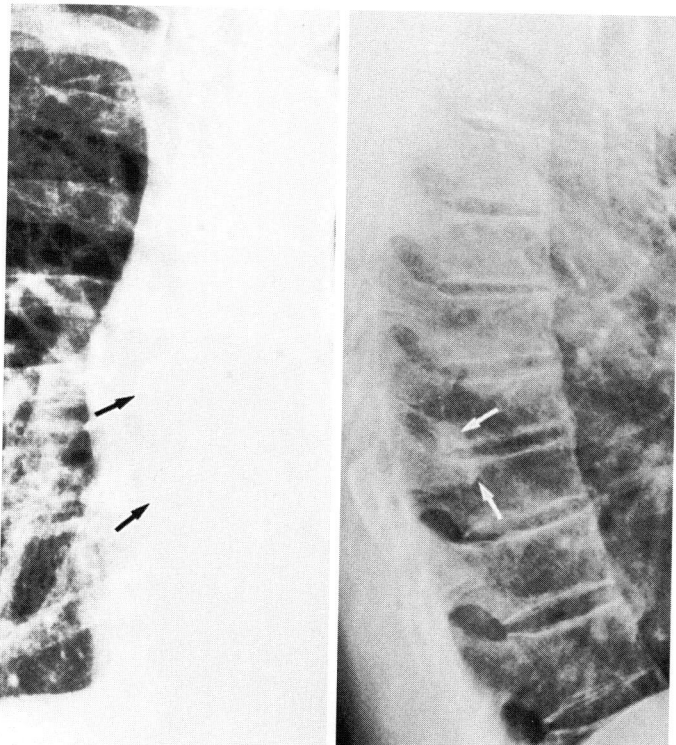

Figure 9–110. Hypertrophic spurs simulating lung nodules.

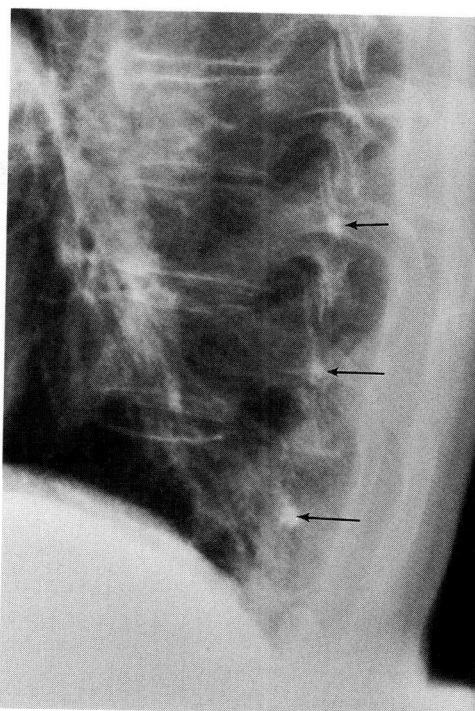

Figure 9–111. Transverse processes producing nodular shadows.

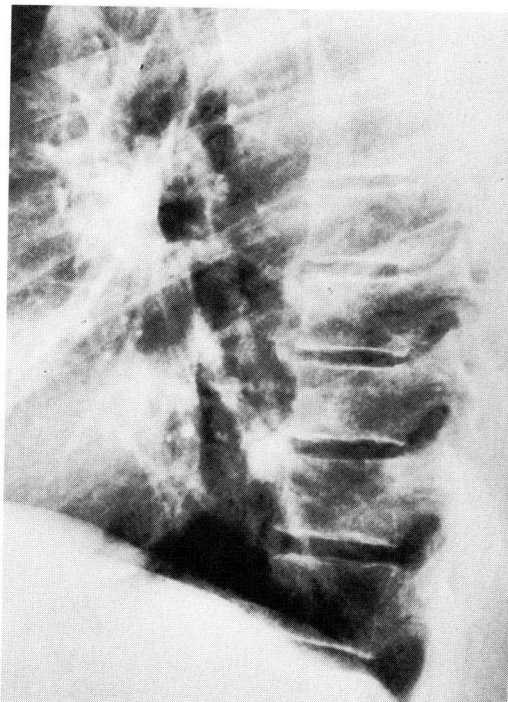

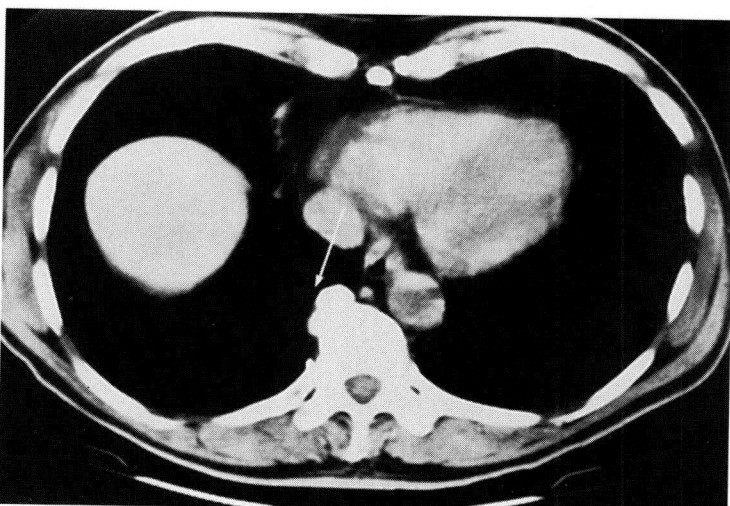

Figure 9–112. Hypertrophic spur simulating a lung nodule. *Left,* Lateral projection. *Above,* CT.

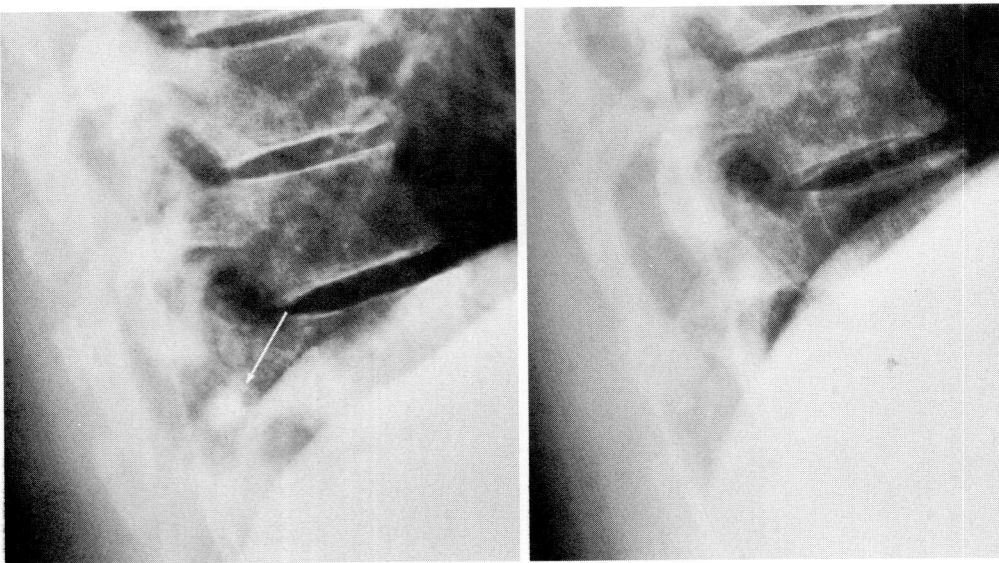

Figure 9–113. *Left,* Large transverse process simulating lung nodule. *Right,* Film, made with slight rotation does not reproduce the pseudonodule.

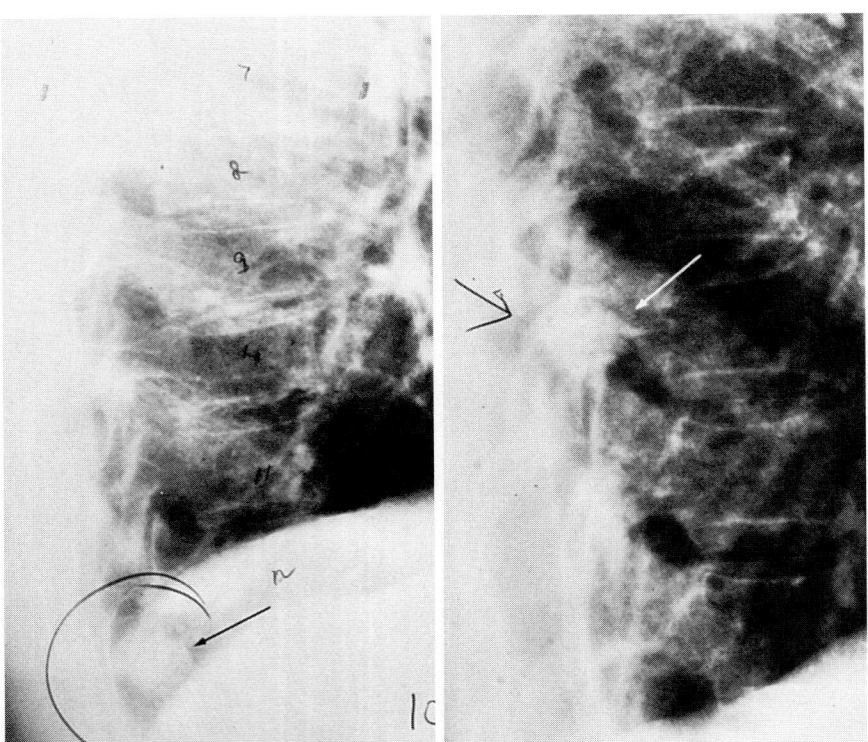

Figure 9–114. Two examples of hypertrophy of interarticulating facets, producing pseudonodules.

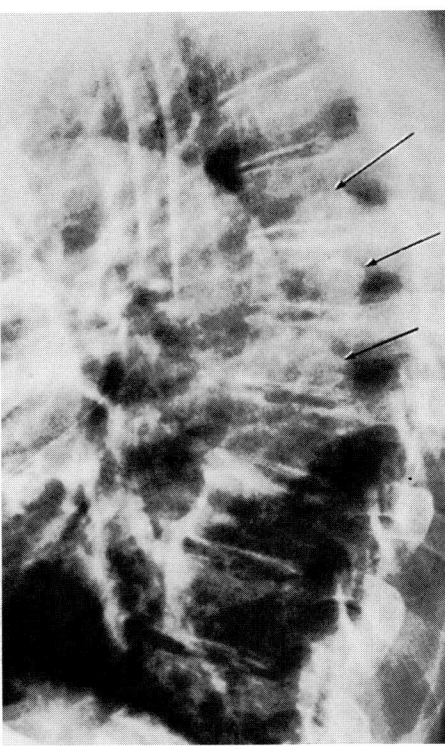

Figure 9–115. Vertebral hypertrophic spurs may simulate pulmonary lesions.

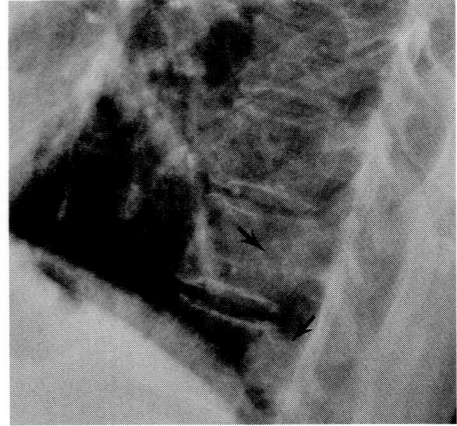

Figure 9–116. Neural arches simulating lung nodules.

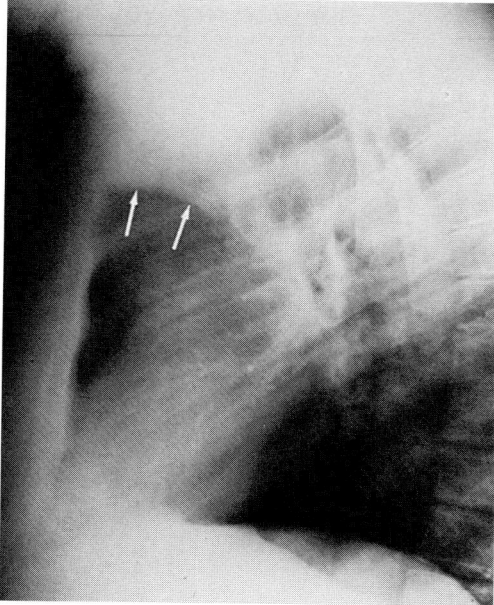

Figure 9–117. Soft tissues of the arm seen in lateral projection, simulating atelectasis of the upper lobe.

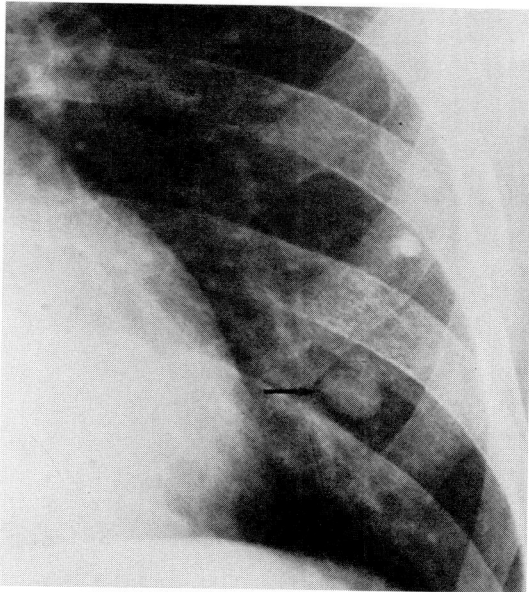

Figure 9–118. Prominent nipple shadow in a male, simulating a nodular pulmonary lesion.

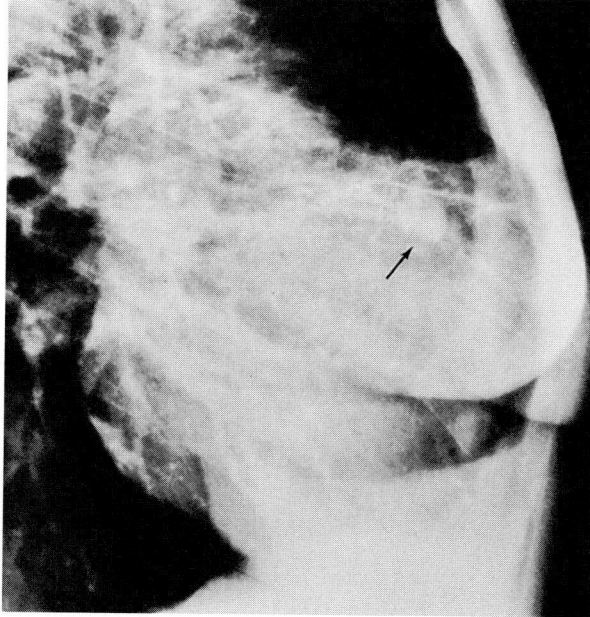

Figure 9–119. Nipple shadows can cause confusing images in the lateral projection when patients are poorly positioned.

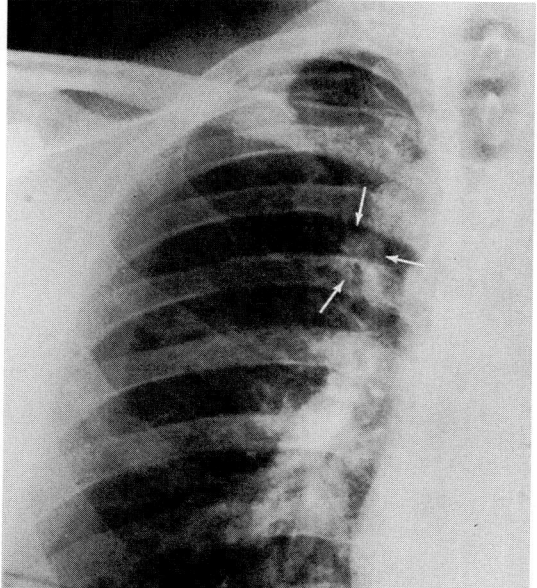

Figure 9–120. Skin lesions may produce nodular shadows that simulate parenchymal nodules, in this case a large nevus.

Figure 9–121. Two examples of simulated cavitary lesions produced by superimposition of vascular shadows. This phenomenon is common in the perihilar areas.

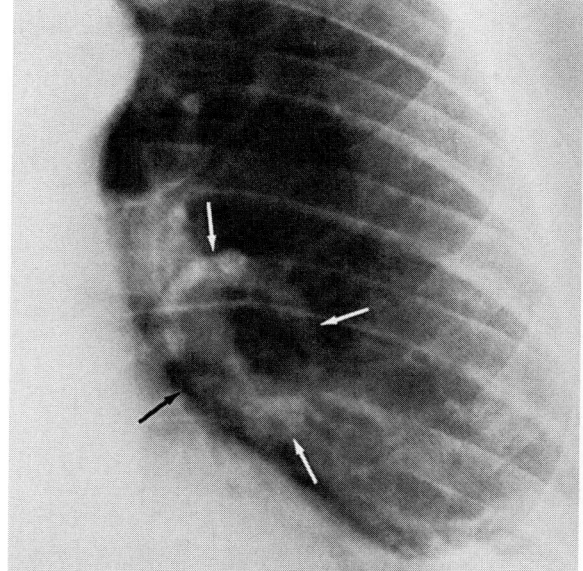
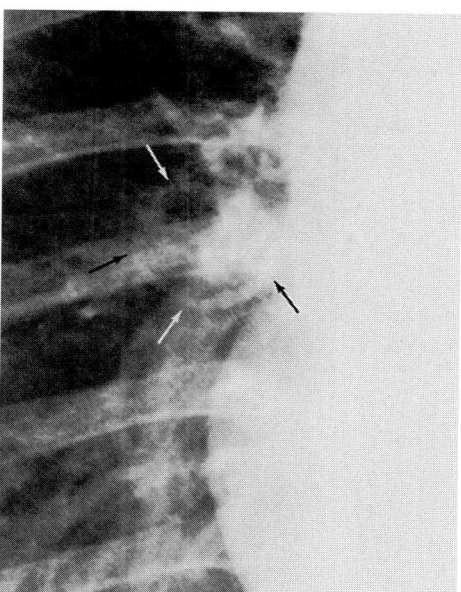

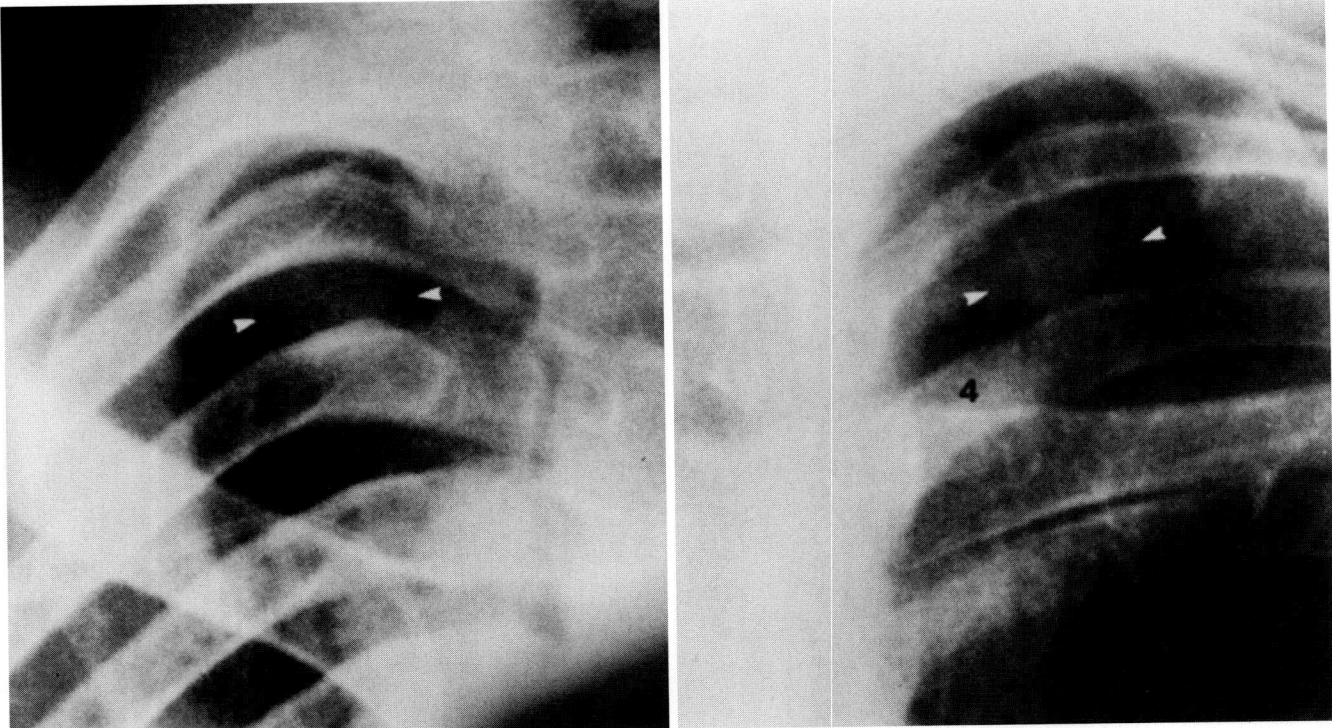

Figure 9–122. Apical opacities produced by the subclavian arteries, which may be mistaken for a a parenchymal abnormality. (From Proto AV: Conventional chest radiographs: Anatomic understanding of newer observations. *Radiology* 183:593, 1992.)

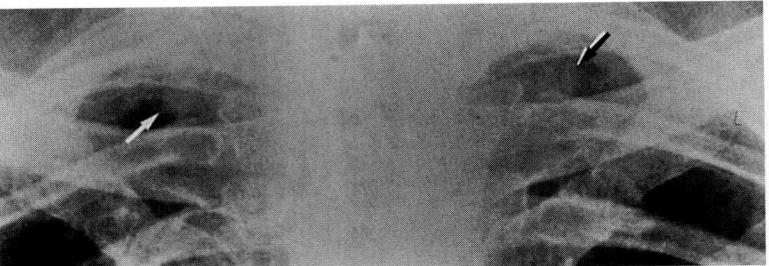

Figure 9–123. Same entity as illustrated in the preceding figure.

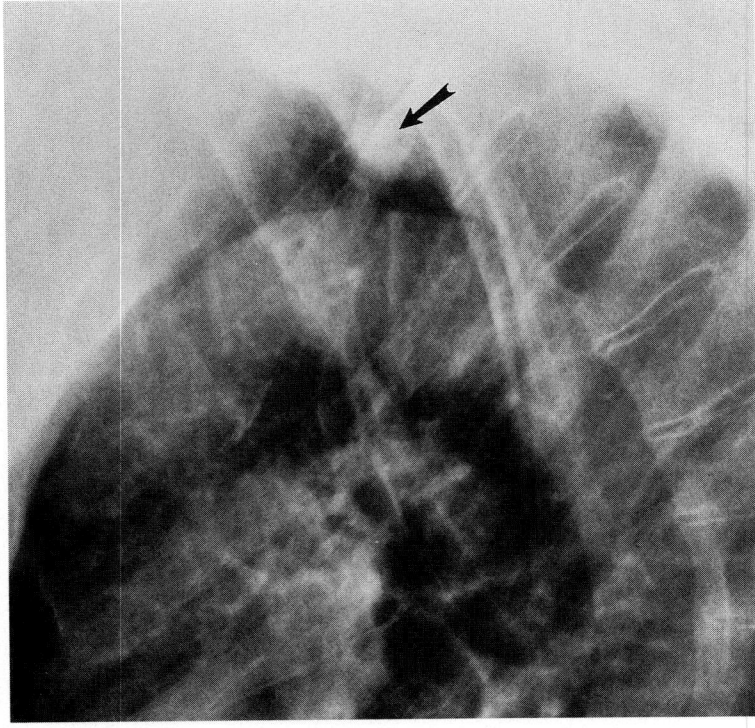

Figure 9–124. Simulated nodule produced by branches of the aortic arch. (Ref: Caceras J et al: Pulmonary nodules simulated on the lateral chest radiograph by branches of the aortic arch. *Am J Roentgenol* 151:465, 1988.)

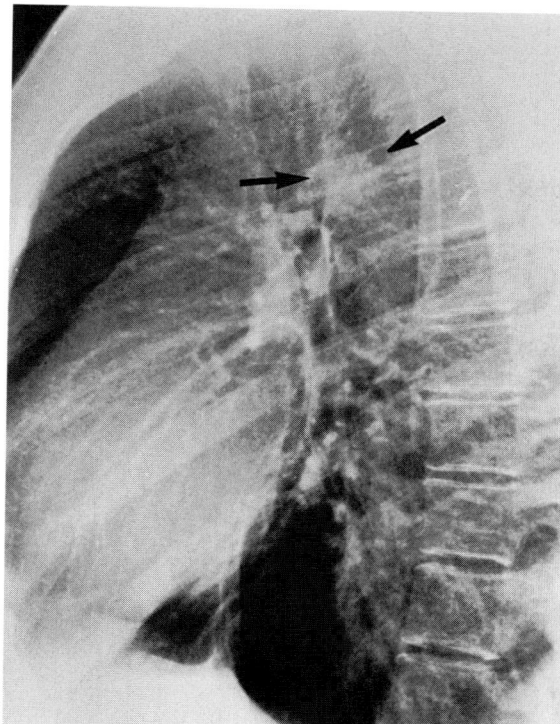

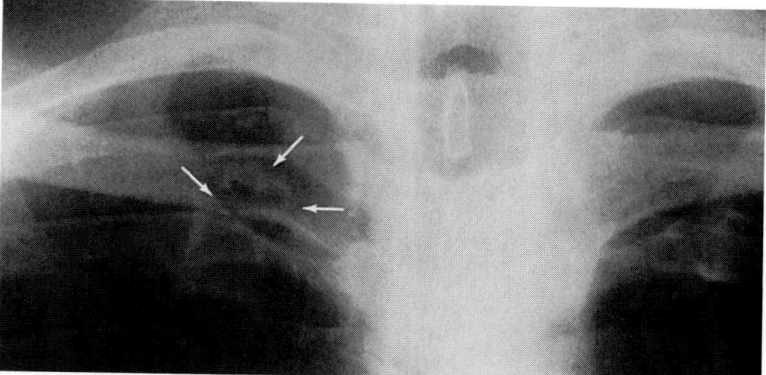

Figure 9–126. Rhomboid fossa of the clavicle, simulating a cavitary lesion of the right upper lobe.

Figure 9–125. Pseudolesion of the lung, produced by superimposition of normal upper lobe vascular structures on the arch of the aorta (see Fig. 9–144). (Ref: Stark P et al: Pseudolesion of the chest: A conglomerate shadow on the lateral radiograph, *Chest* 87:541, 1985.) (see also Fig. 9–144 and Fig. 9–124.)

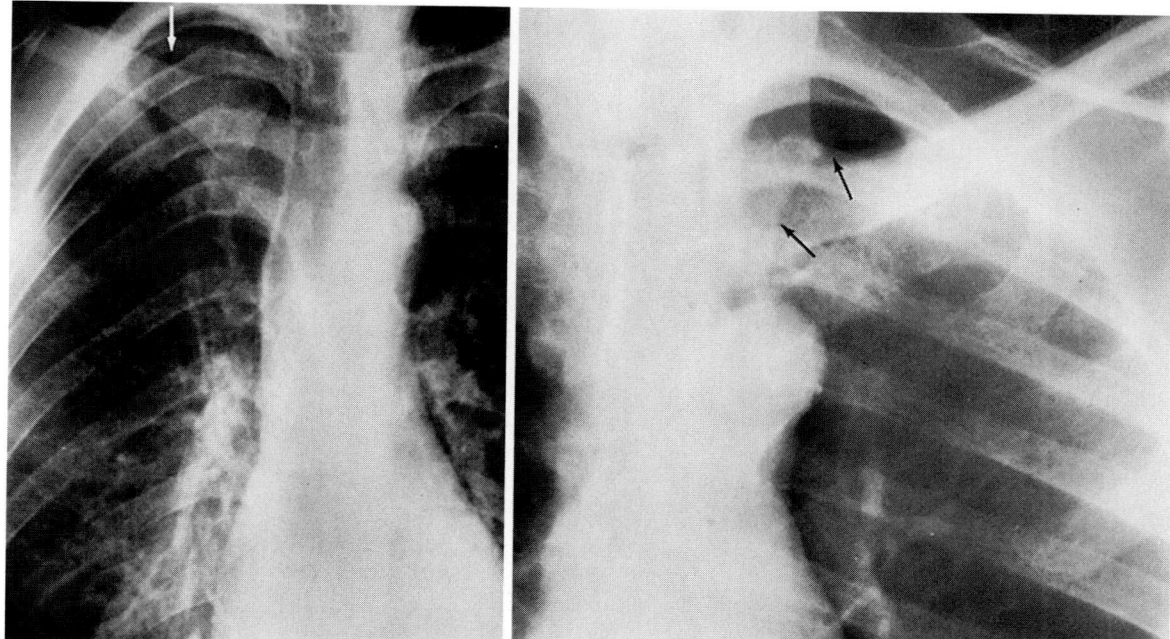

Figure 9–127. Shadows of the subclavian arteries may simulate a pleural or parenchymal density.

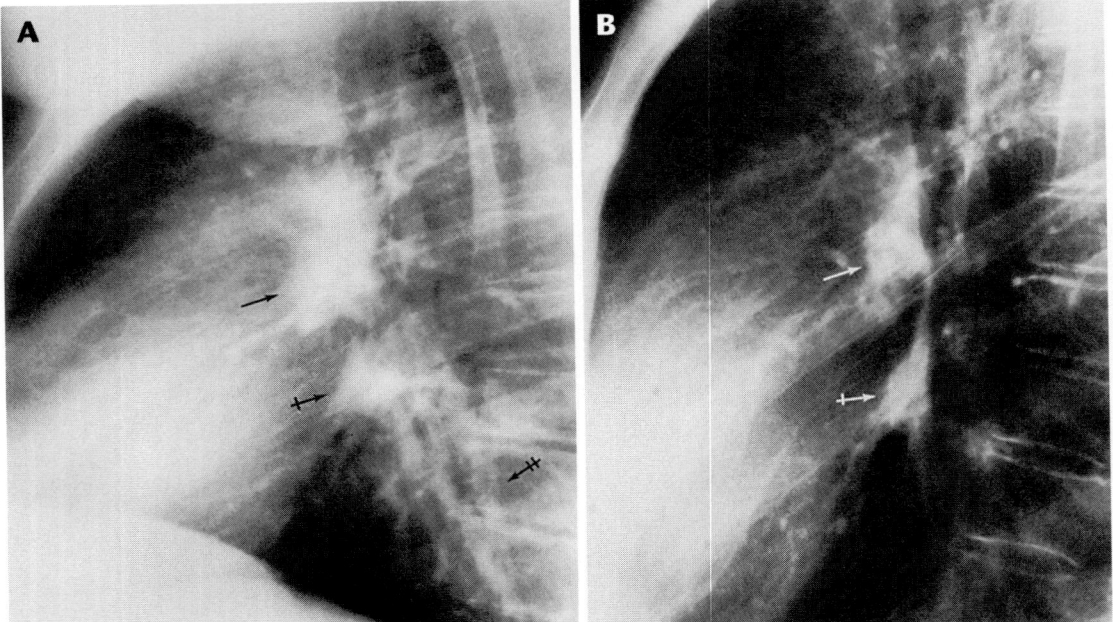

Figure 9–128. Films made in expiratory phases of respiration show greater prominence of the pulmonary arteries (→) and the confluence of the pulmonary veins (↦). Note also the vascular prominence in the posterior base in **A** (↦). The shadow of these vessels is often misinterpreted as evidence of pneumonitis. The problem does not present itself in films made with good inspiration, as in **B**.

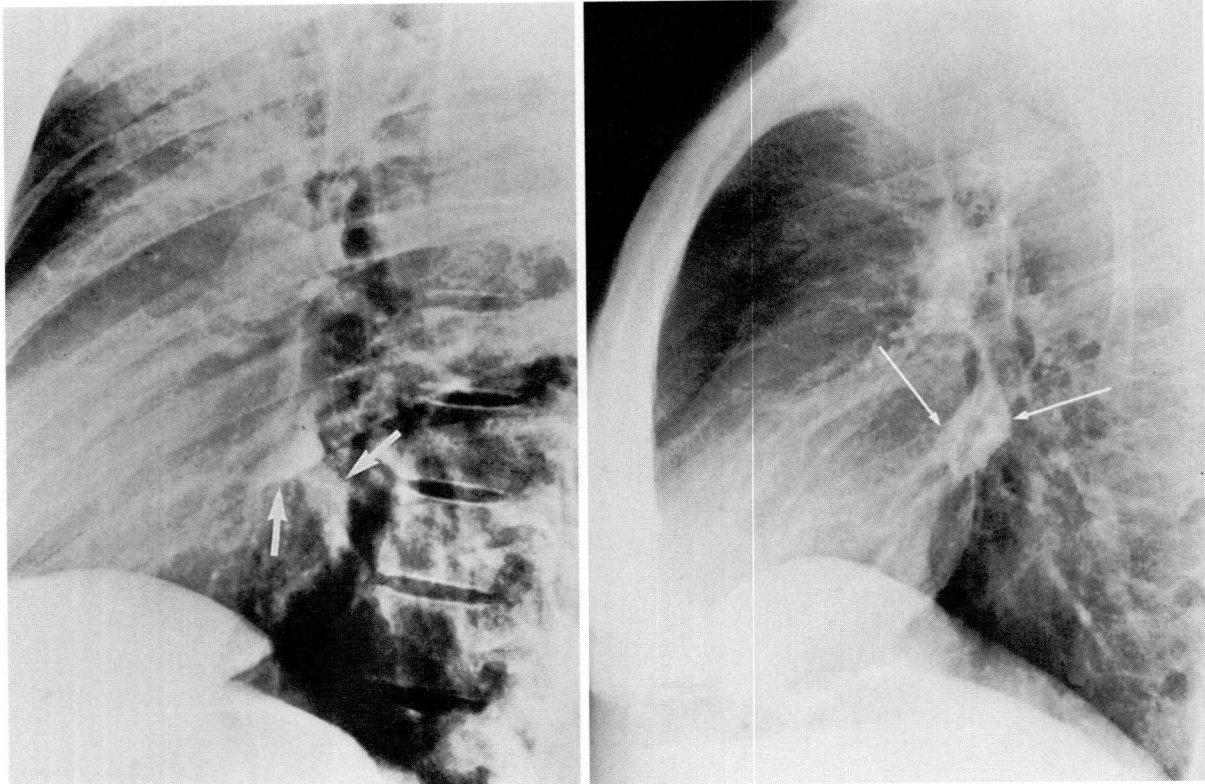

Figure 9–129. Pulmonary veins in lateral projection may assume a somewhat nodular configuration.

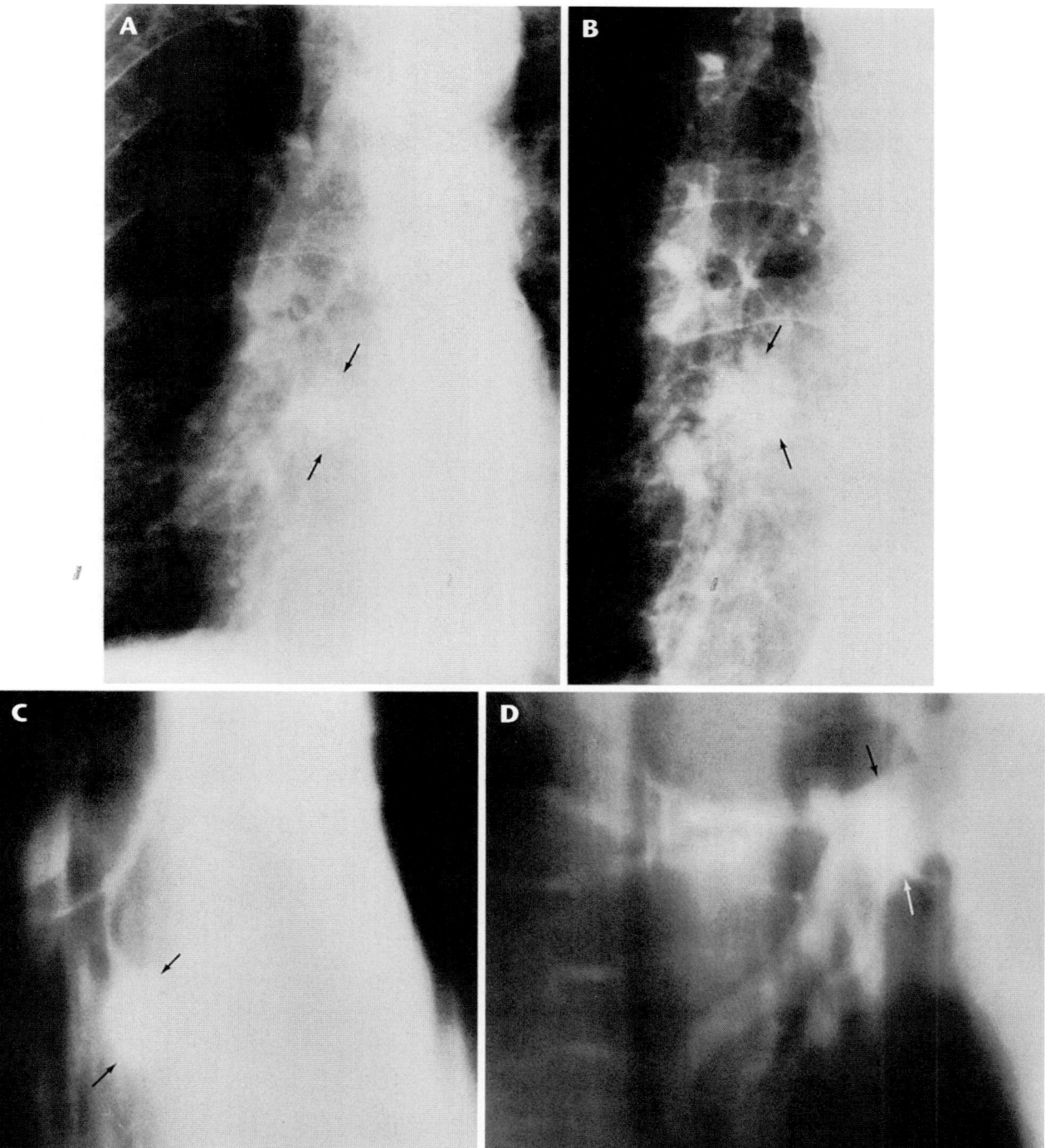

Figure 9–130. Confluence of the pulmonary veins at the left atrium may present as a nodular density, which should not be confused with a mass lesion. **A,** Plain frontal film. **B,** Oblique projection. **C,** Frontal tomogram. **D,** Lateral tomogram.

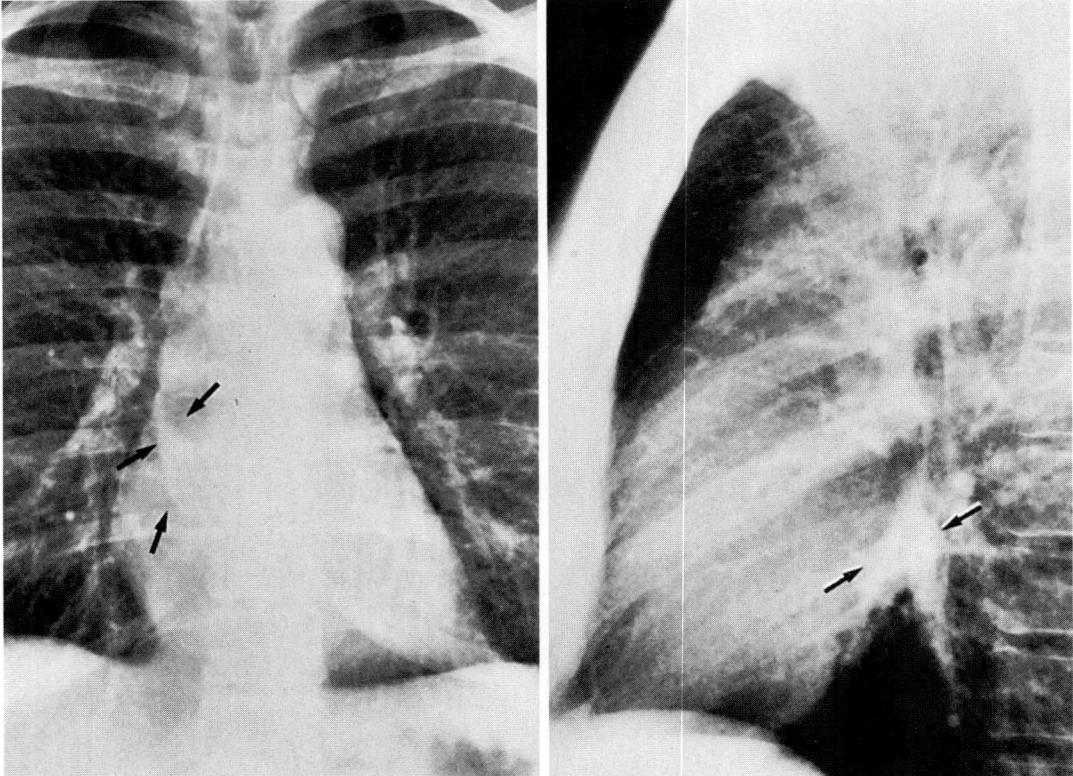

Figure 9–131. Confluence of the pulmonary veins.

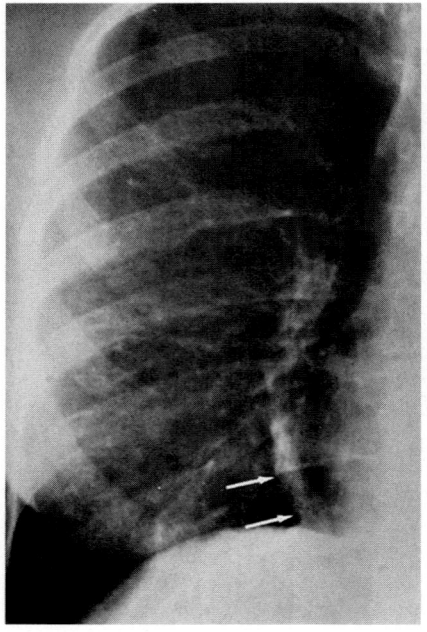

Figure 9–132. Scimitar vein, an anomalous vessel that drains into the inferior vena cava below the diaphragm. This vein may be an isolated finding, as in this case, or associated with hypoplasia of the right lung. (Ref: Roehm JO Jr et al: Radiographic features of the scimitar syndrome. *Radiology* 86:856, 1966.)

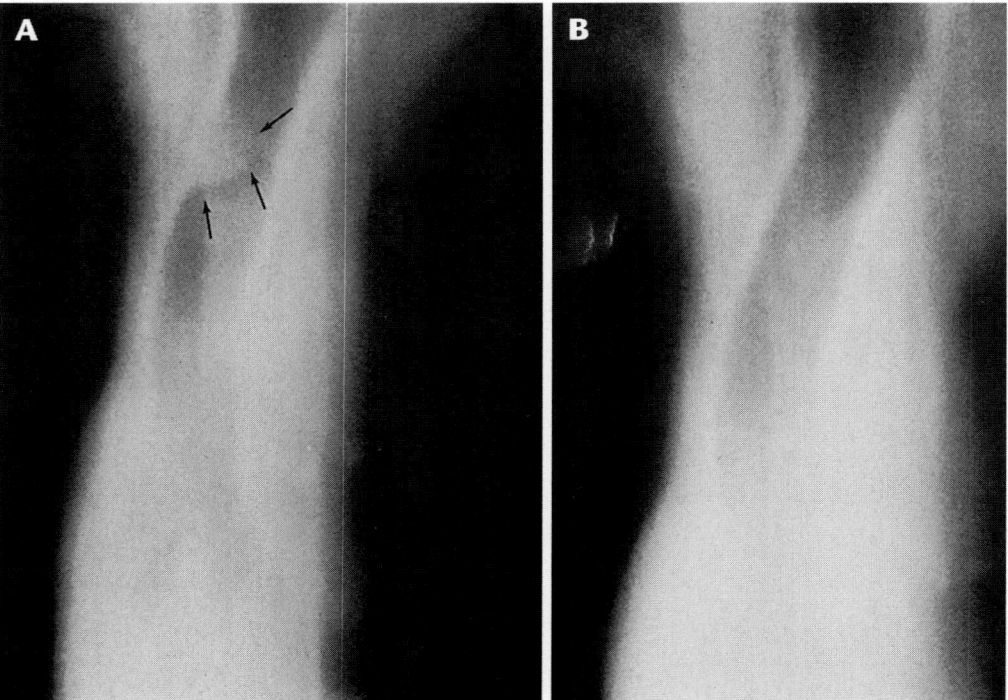

Figure 9–133. Mucus plugs in the trachea may simulate significant lesions, such as neoplasms. **A,** Tomogram of the trachea, showing filling defect. **B,** Tomogram after coughing up mucus plug. (Ref: Karasick D et al: Mucoid pseudotumors of the tracheobronchial tree in two cases. *Am J Roentgenol* 132:459, 1979.)

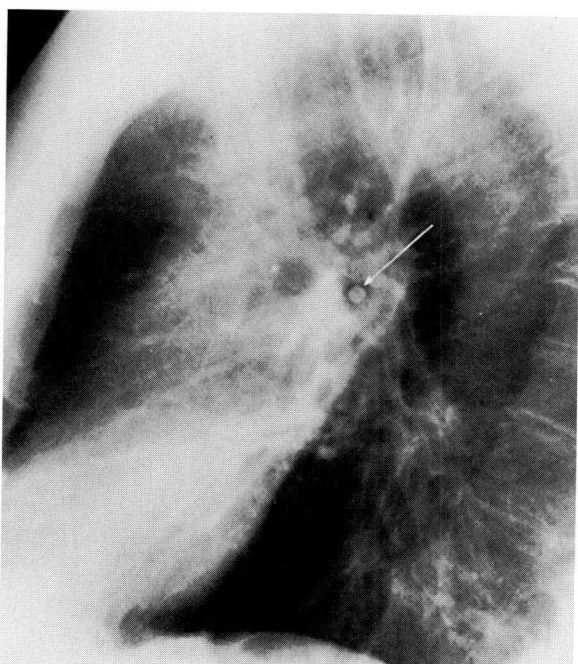

Figure 9–134. Arterial shadow superimposed on the bronchus, simulating a broncholith.

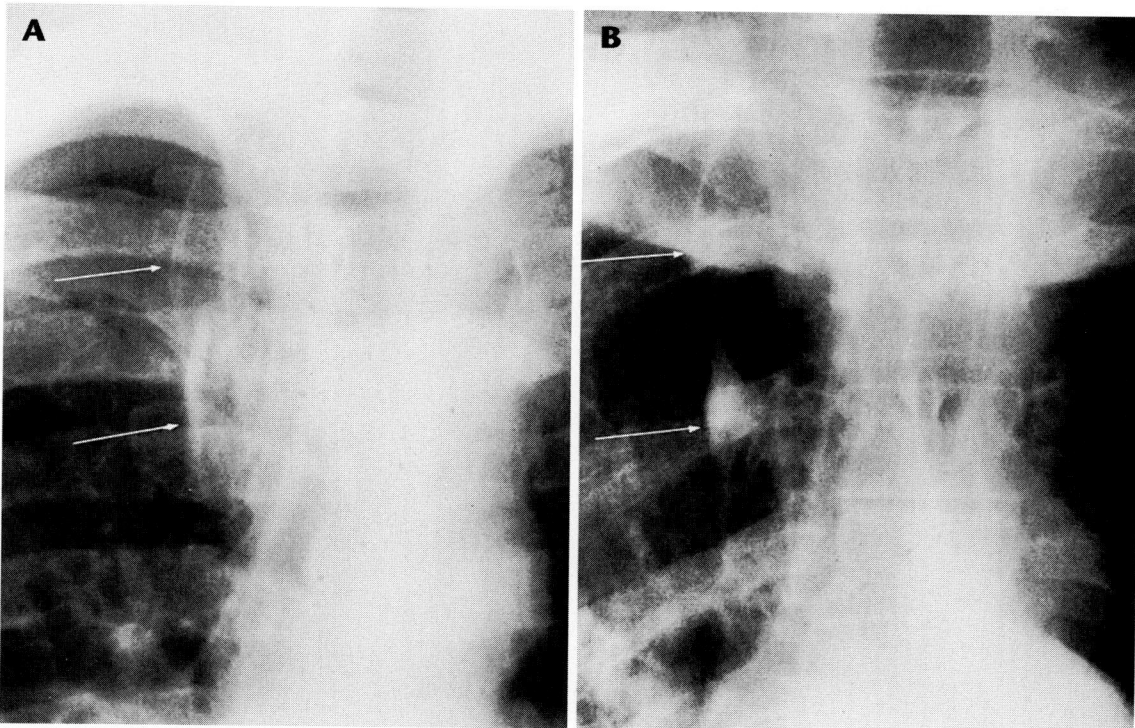

Figure 9–135. A, The azygos lobe may simulate an infiltrate in a standard frontal film. **B,** Same area seen in lordotic projection, showing the usual appearance of the azygos lobe.

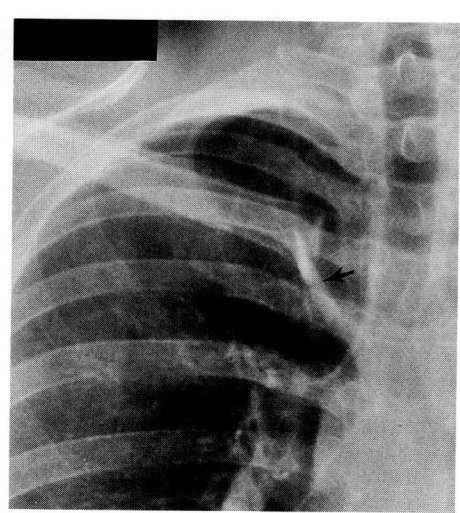

Figure 9–136. Unusual configuration of the azygos lobe, which may simulate a parenchymal lesion.

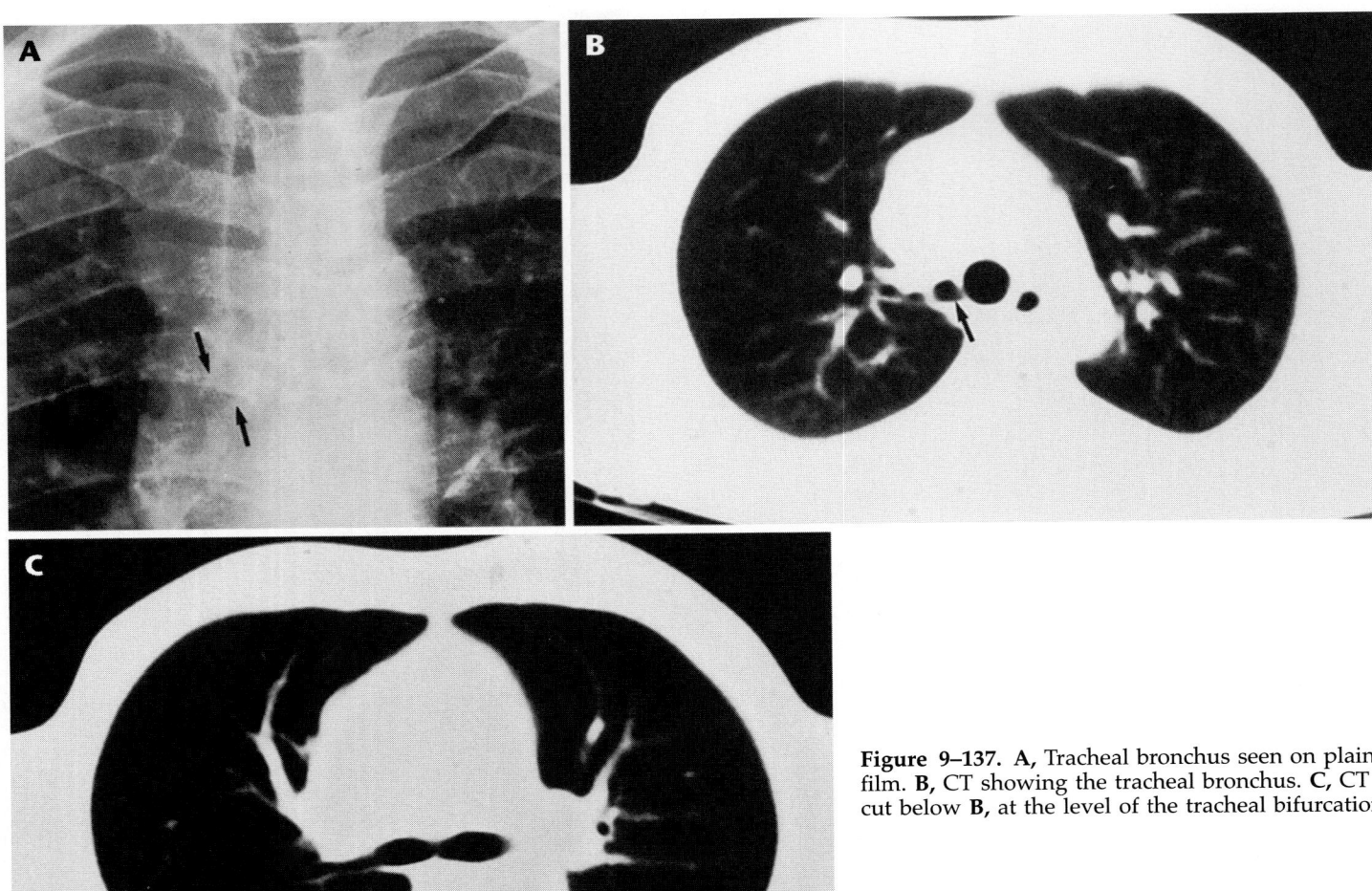

Figure 9–137. A, Tracheal bronchus seen on plain film. **B,** CT showing the tracheal bronchus. **C,** CT cut below **B,** at the level of the tracheal bifurcation.

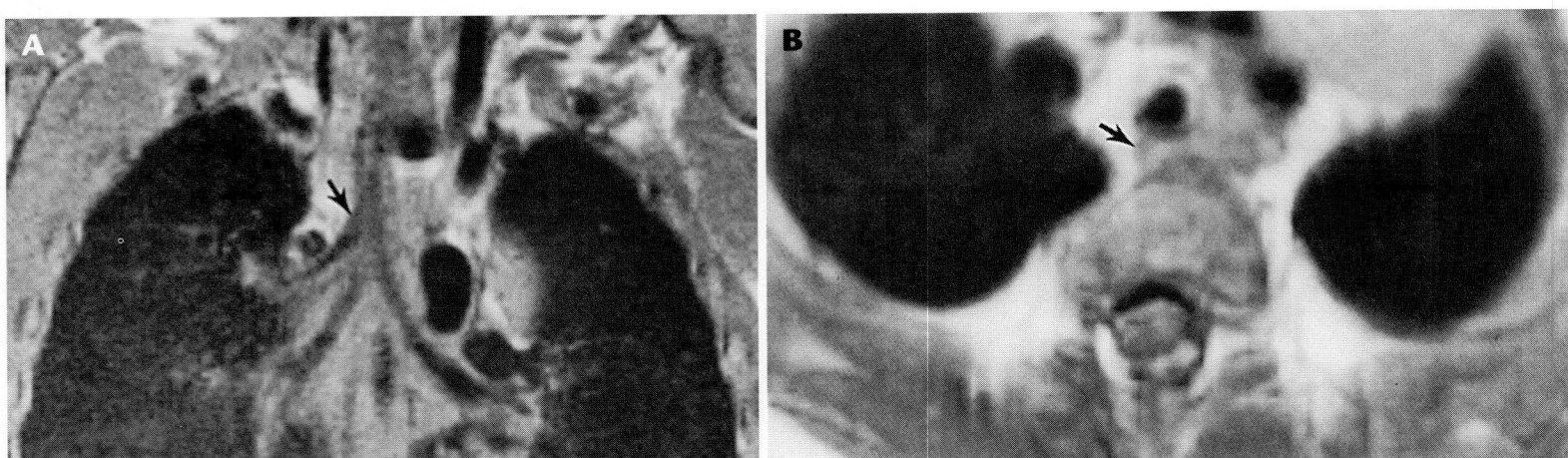

Figure 9–138. Tracheal bronchus shown by MRI. **A,** Coronal section. **B,** Axial section.

The Mediastinum

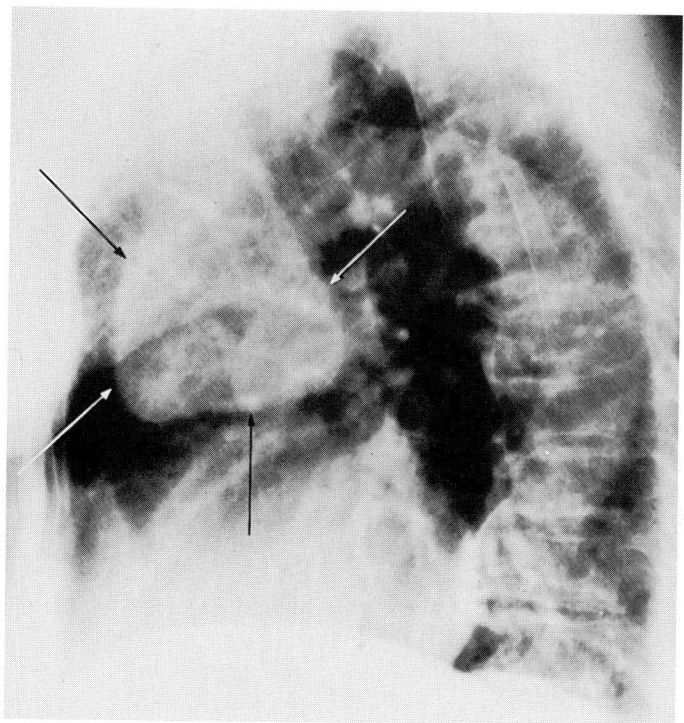

Figure 9–139. Arm fold superimposed on anterior mediastinum, producing a mass effect. (Ref: Vaezy A, Delaney DJ: Chest wall mass mimicking pulmonary tumor. *South Med J* 72:499, 1979.)

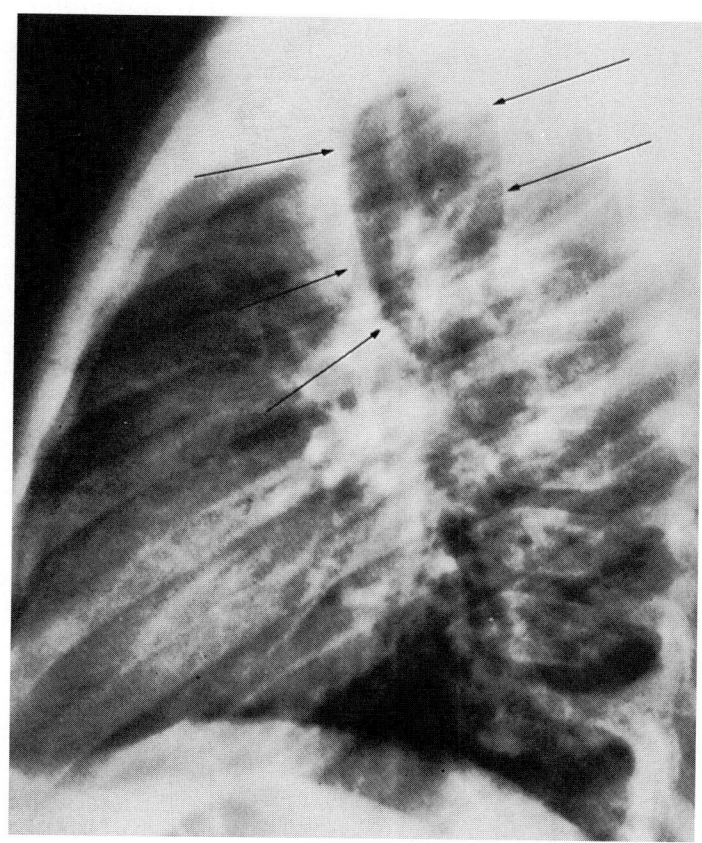

Figure 9–140. Scapula and arm fold producing a simulated lucent mass.

Figure 9–141. A, Spurious widening of the mediastinum, produced by lordotic projection. **B,** Conventional posteroanterior projection shows a normal appearance. (Ref: Itollman AJ, Adams FG: Lordotic projectional widening of the mediastinum. *Clin Radiol* 40:360, 1989.)

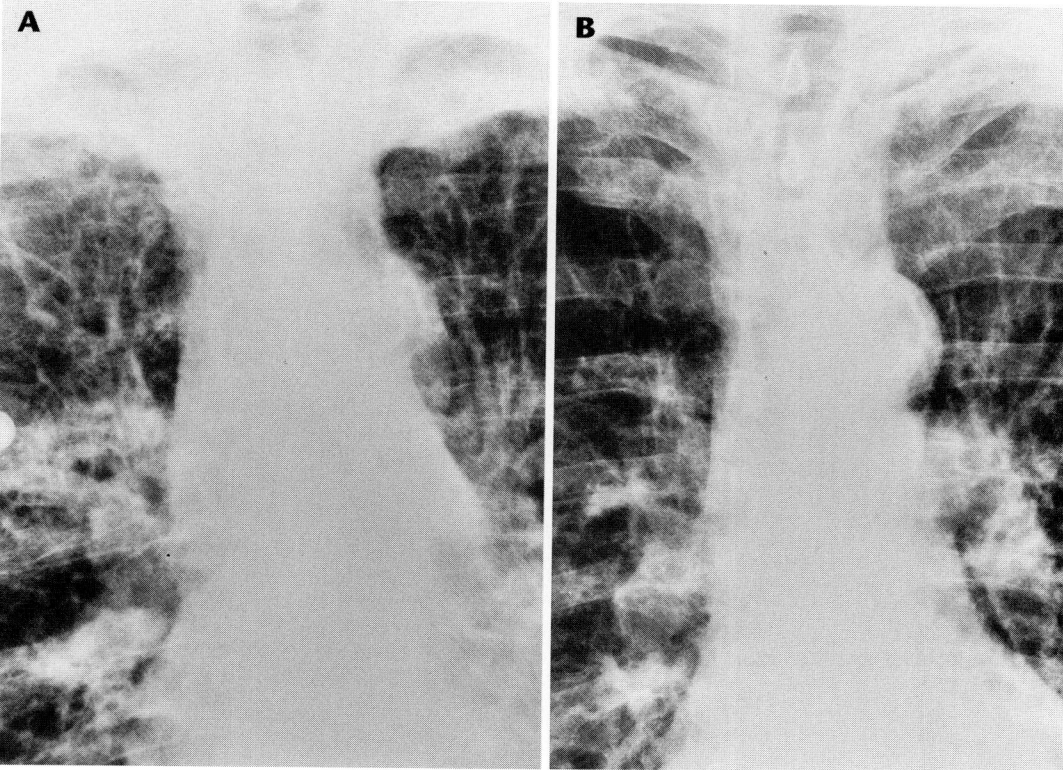

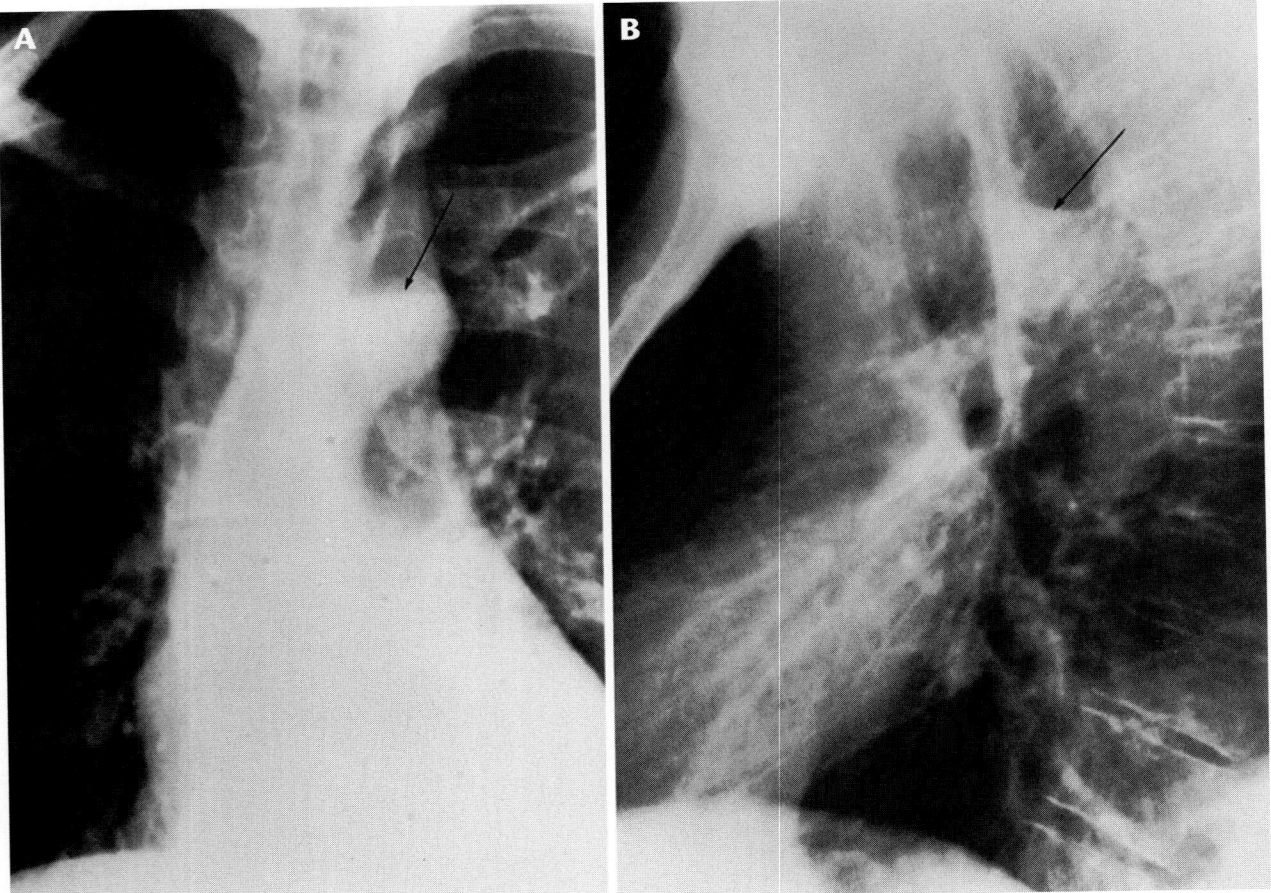

Figure 9–142. A, Superimposition of a rib shadow on the aortic arch simulates an air-fluid level. **B,** The top of the arch of the aorta may simulate an air-fluid level in the esophagus.

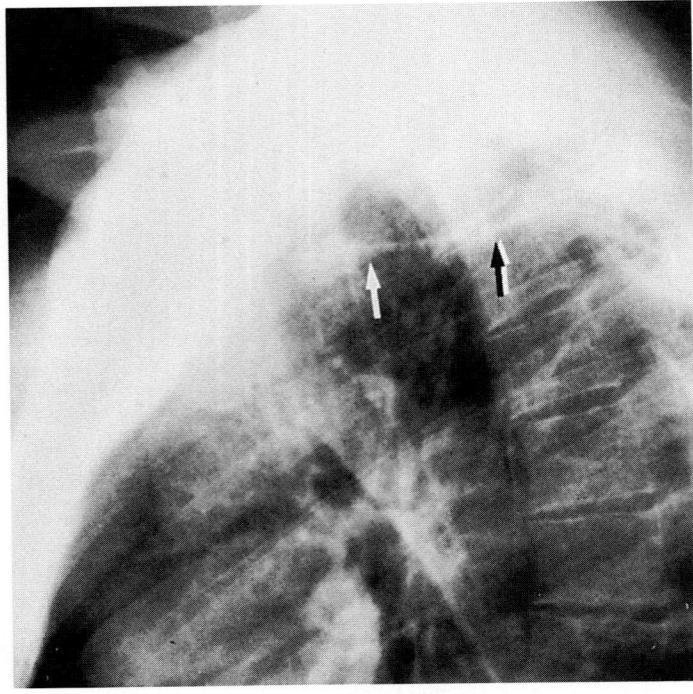

Figure 9–143. Spine of the scapula, simulating a cavitary lesion with air-fluid level.

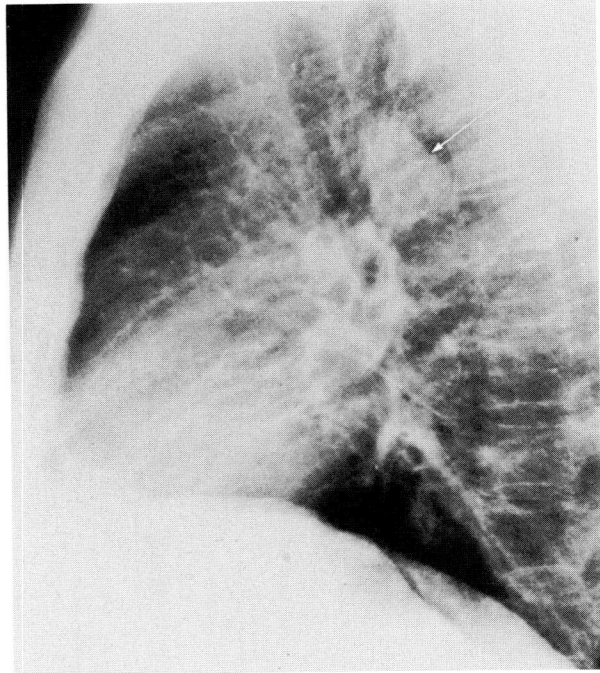

Figure 9–144. Superimposition of the shadows of the aorta and scapula produces a triangular shadow of increased density (see Fig. 9–125).

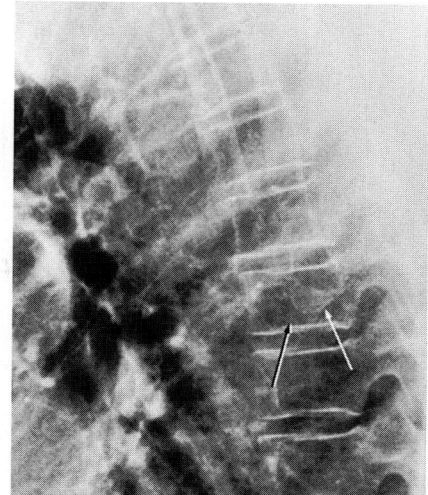

Figure 9–145. Angle of the scapula simulating a lung nodule.

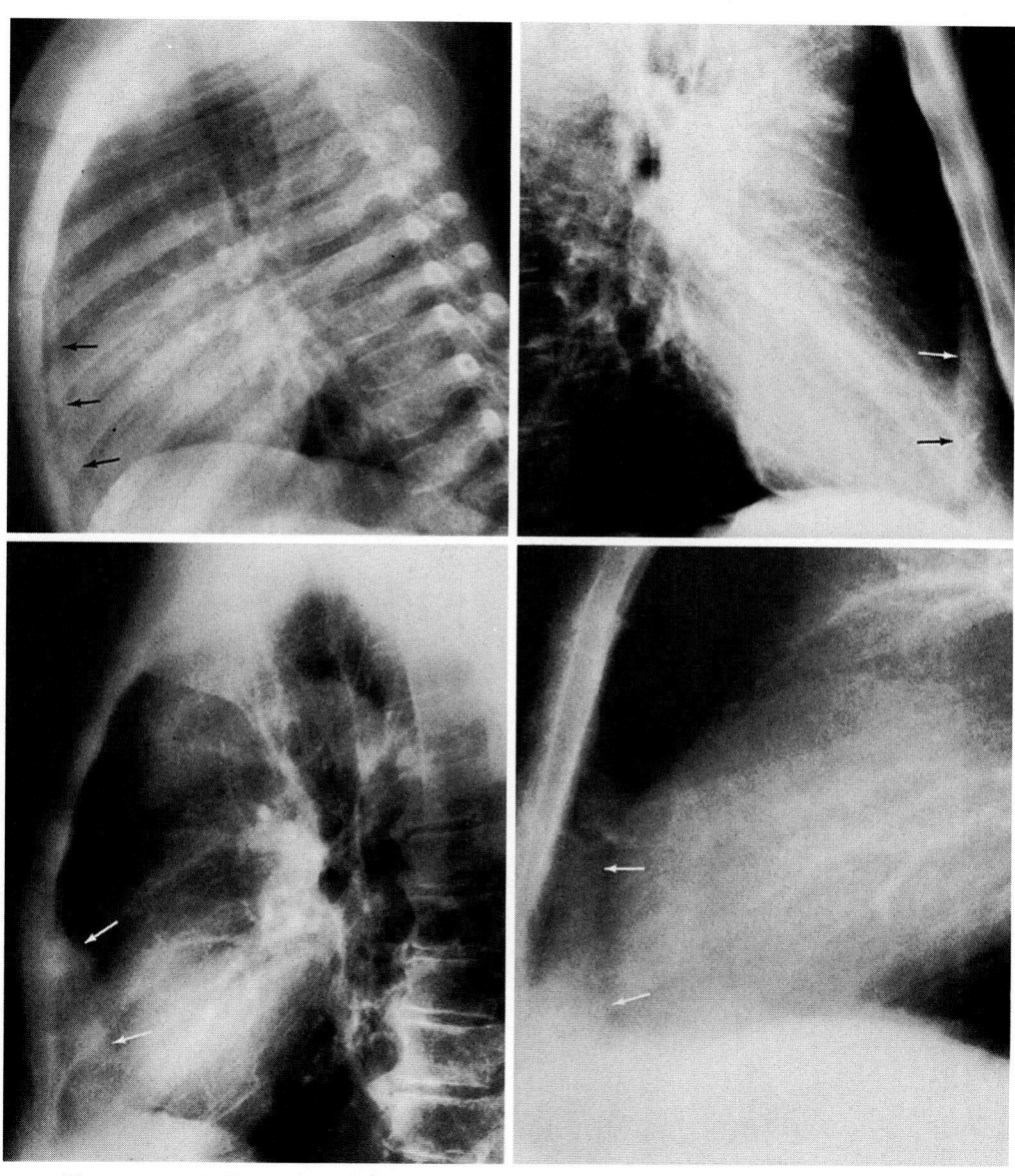

Figure 9–146. Examples of the retrosternal line produced by the interface between the two lungs and the mediastinal fat. (Ref: Whalen JP et al: The retrosternal line: A new sign of an anterior mediastinal mass. *Am J Roentgenol* 117:861, 1973.)

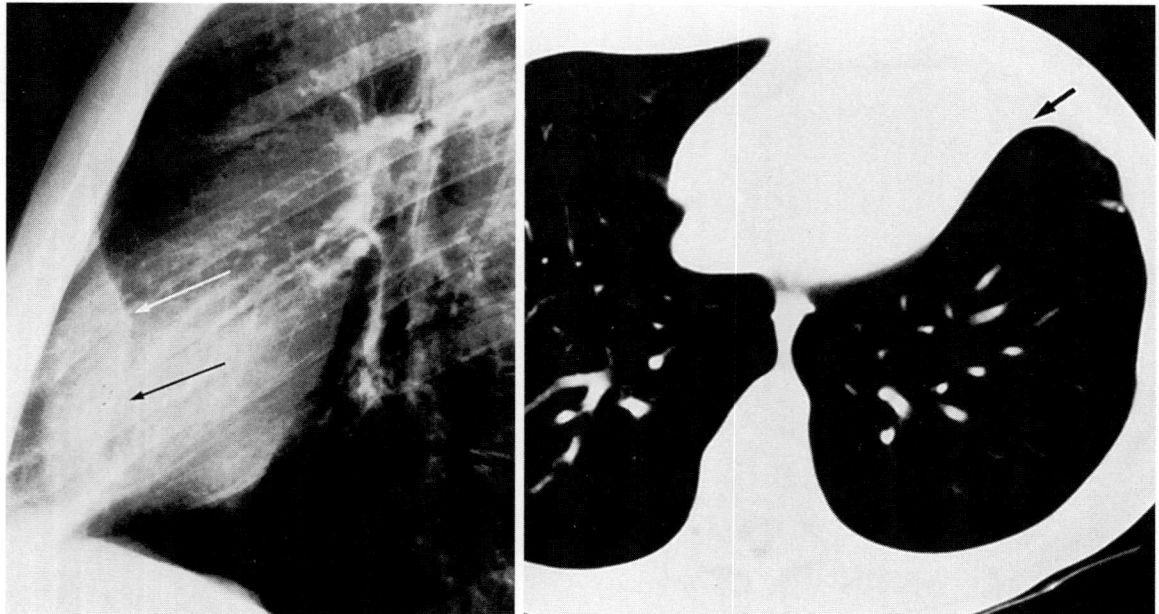

Figure 9–147. *Left,* Prominent retrosternal line. *Right,* CT shows the mechanism of production of the line. The right lung extends to the anterior chest wall. The left lung is excluded by the heart and mediastinal fat (*arrow*). The difference in anterior extension of the two lungs creates the retrosternal line.

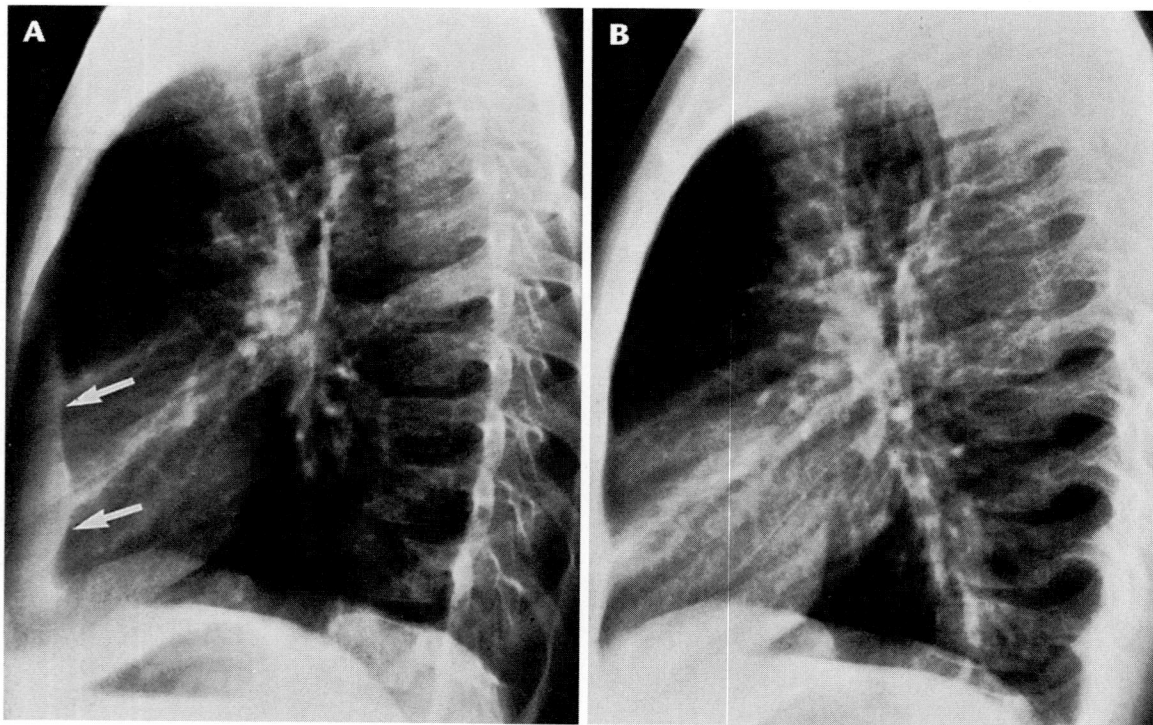

Figure 9–148. A, Unusually prominent retrosternal line produced by rotation at the time of filming. **B,** True lateral shows usual appearance.

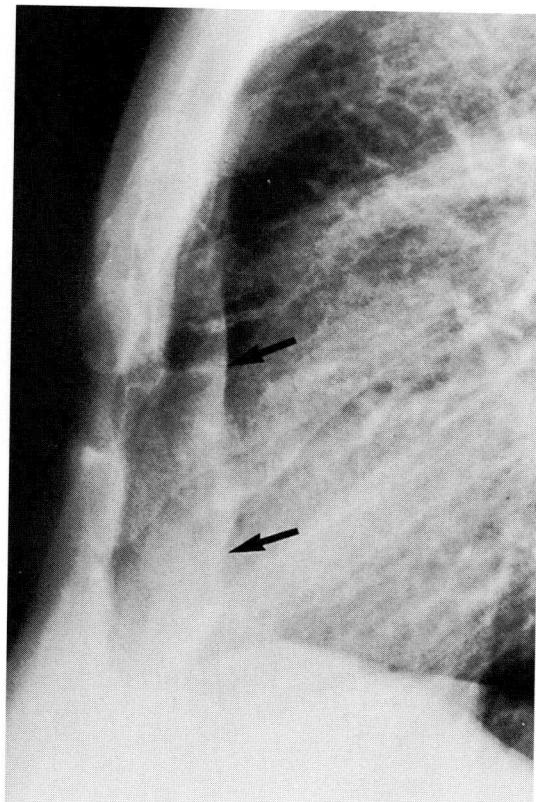

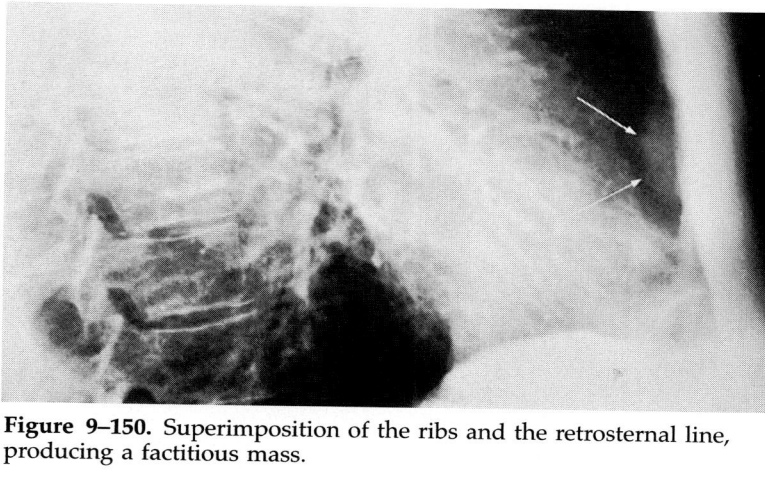

Figure 9–150. Superimposition of the ribs and the retrosternal line, producing a factitious mass.

Figure 9–149. Very prominent retrosternal line.

Figure 9–151. In some individuals with well-defined retrosternal lines, an additional line (the right parasternal stripe) may be seen through the right side of the heart. This line indicates the medial edge of the right lung. (Ref: Keats TE: The right parasternal stripe: A new mediastinal shadow and a contribution to the nature of the retrosternal line. *Am J Roentgenol* 120:898, 1974.)

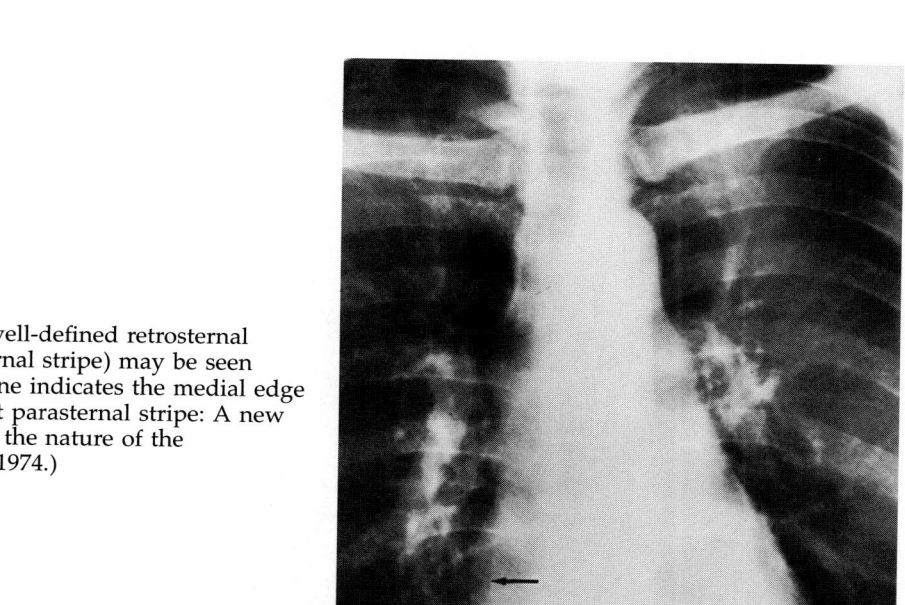

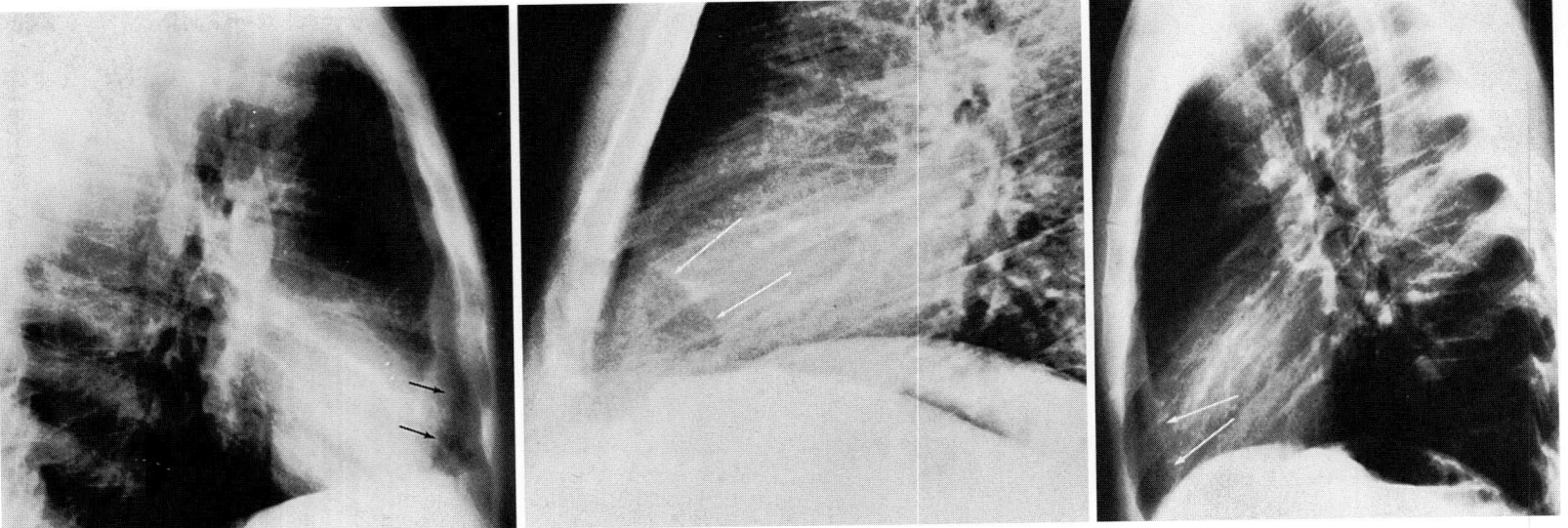

Figure 9–152. Three examples of clinically unimportant triangular radiolucencies in the anterior mediastinum in adults. The mechanism of production of these shadows is not proved, but they are probably the result of the same anatomy that produces the retrosternal line, illustrated in Figure 9–146.

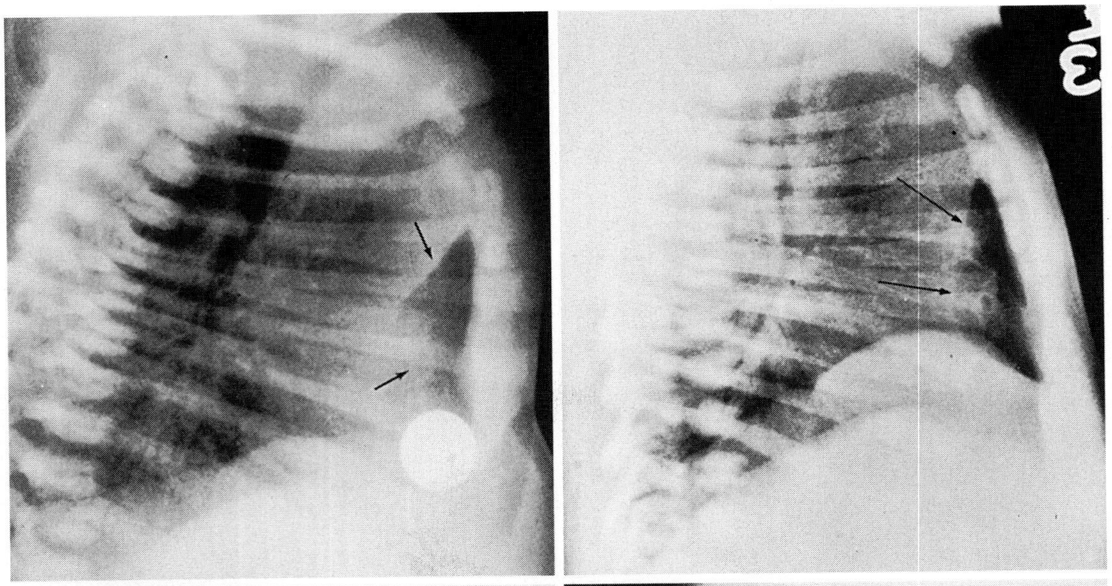

Figure 9–153. Five examples of triangular anterior mediastinal radiolucencies seen in young children with large thymuses. They may represent the same entity illustrated in Figure 9–152 or are possibly related to the presence of the thymus. (Ref: Quattromani FL et al: Fascial relationship of the thymus. *Am J Roentgenol* 137: 1209, 1981.)

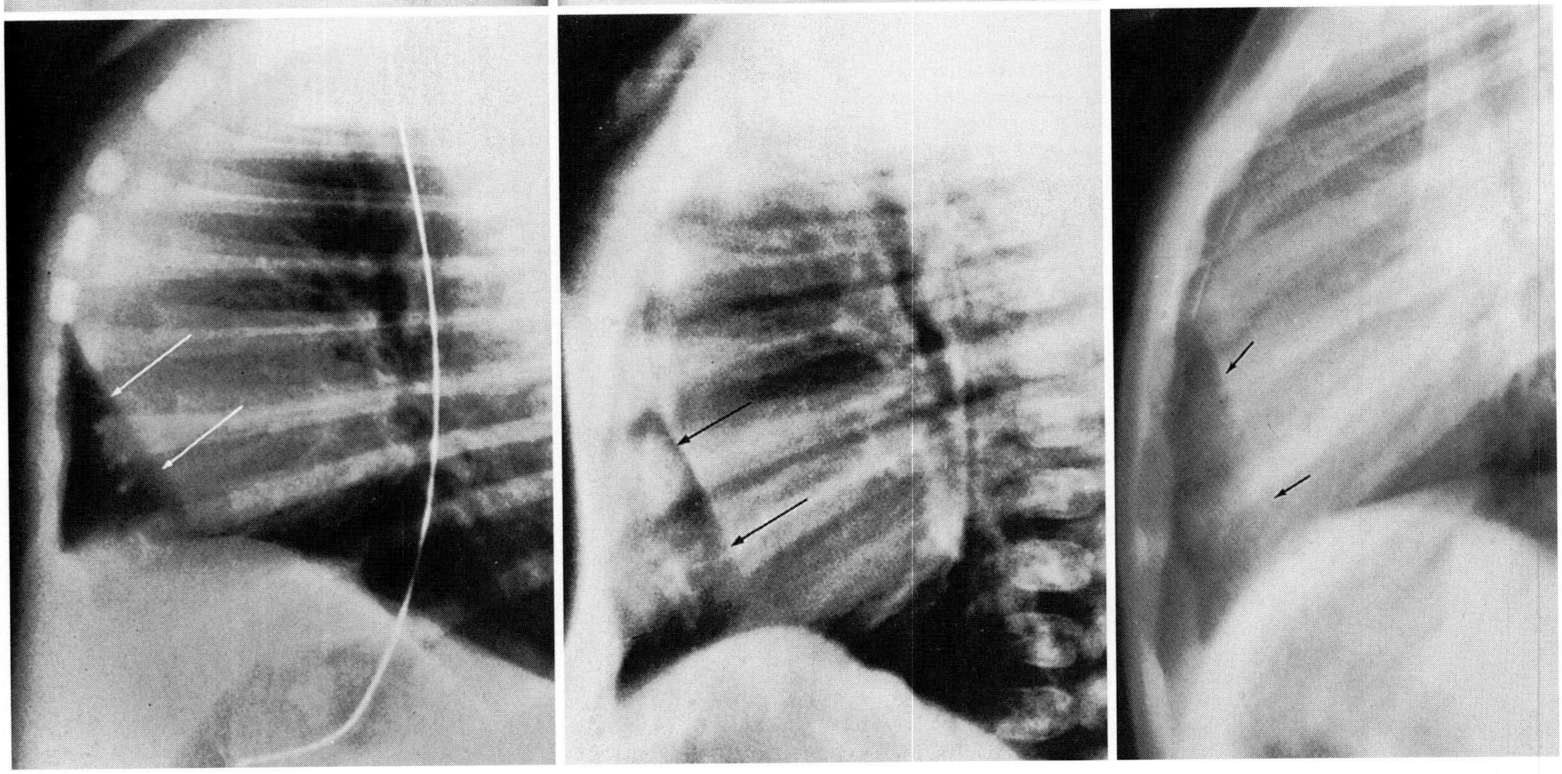

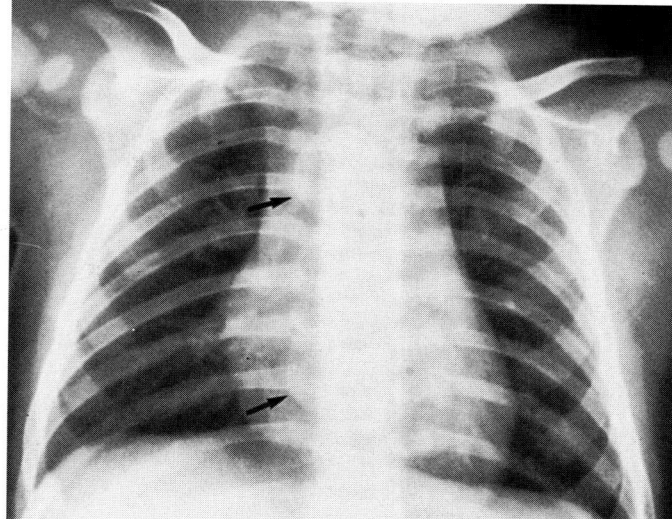

Figure 9–154. Sternal ossification centers in an infant, which may be confused with mediastinal masses.

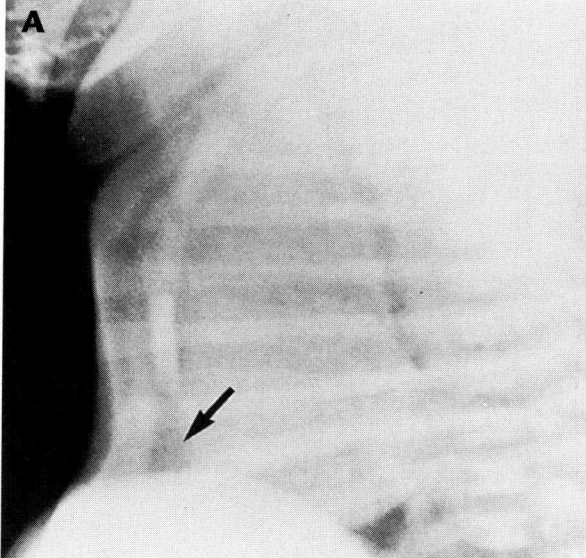
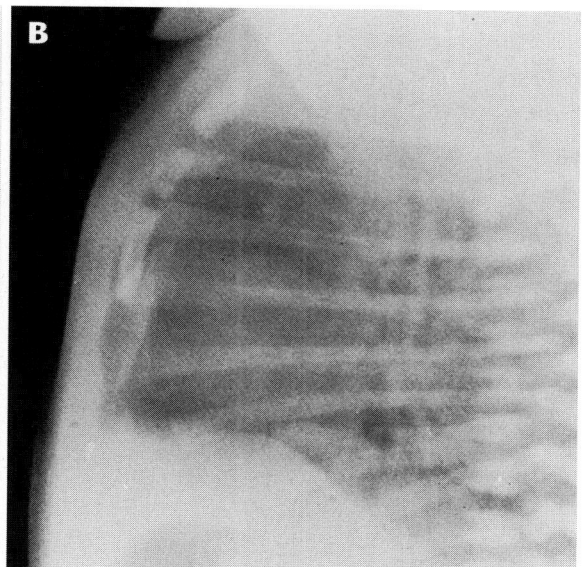

Figure 9–155. A, Simulated pneumomediastinum produced by sternal retraction. **B,** Follow-up examination shows normal appearance.

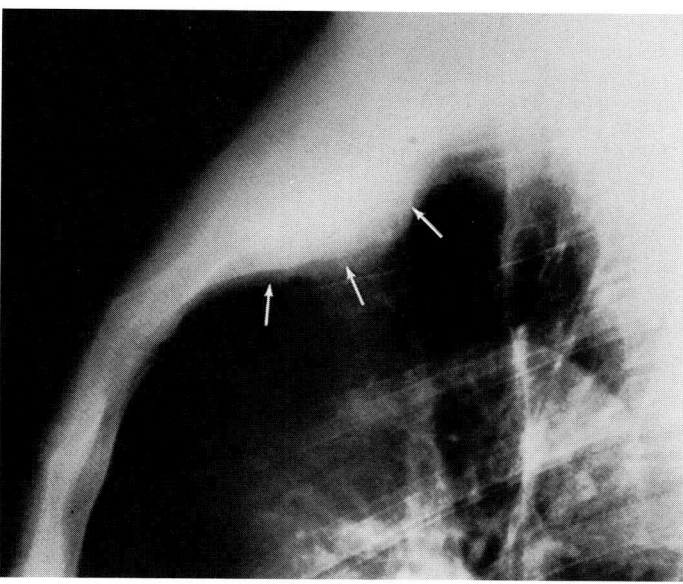

Figure 9–156. The anterior extra pleural line represents a deviation of the pleura produced by the innominate artery and vein and the costal cartilages of the first ribs. It should not be mistaken for a lesion of the sternum or a mediastinal mass. (Ref: Whalen JP et al: Anterior extrapleural line: Superior extension. *Radiology* 115:525, 1975.)

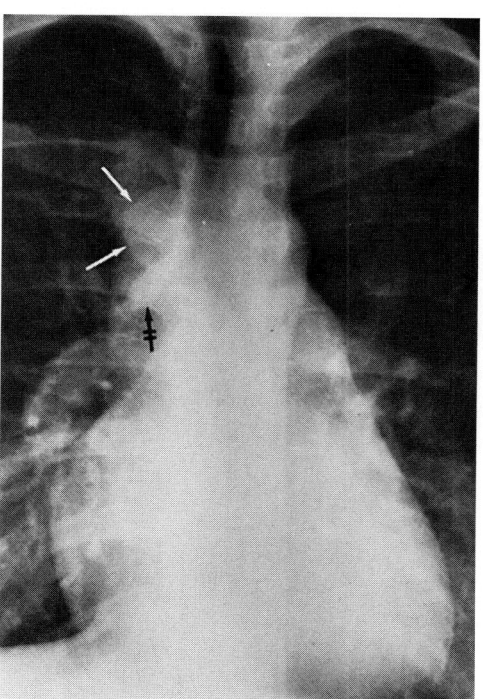

Figure 9–157. The manubrium, simulating a mediastinal mass (←) produced by slight scoliosis. The azygos arch is seen below (⊣⊢).

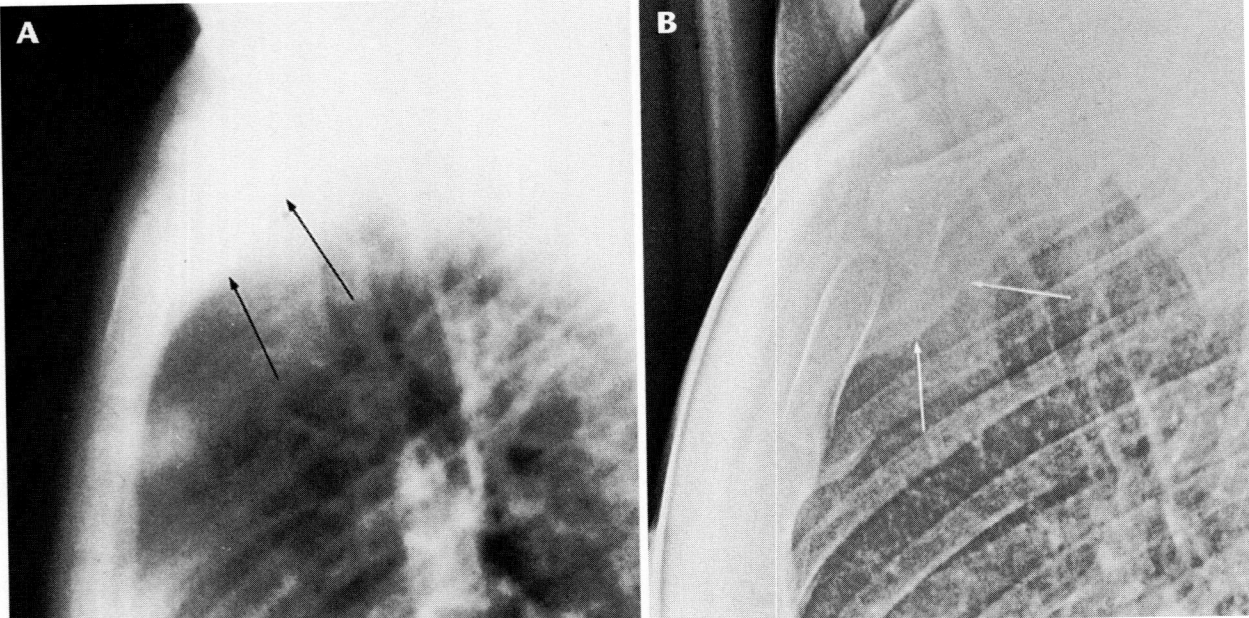

Figure 9–158. The anterior extrapleural line in a child, misinterpreted as a mass lesion. **A,** Conventional film. **B,** Xerogram.

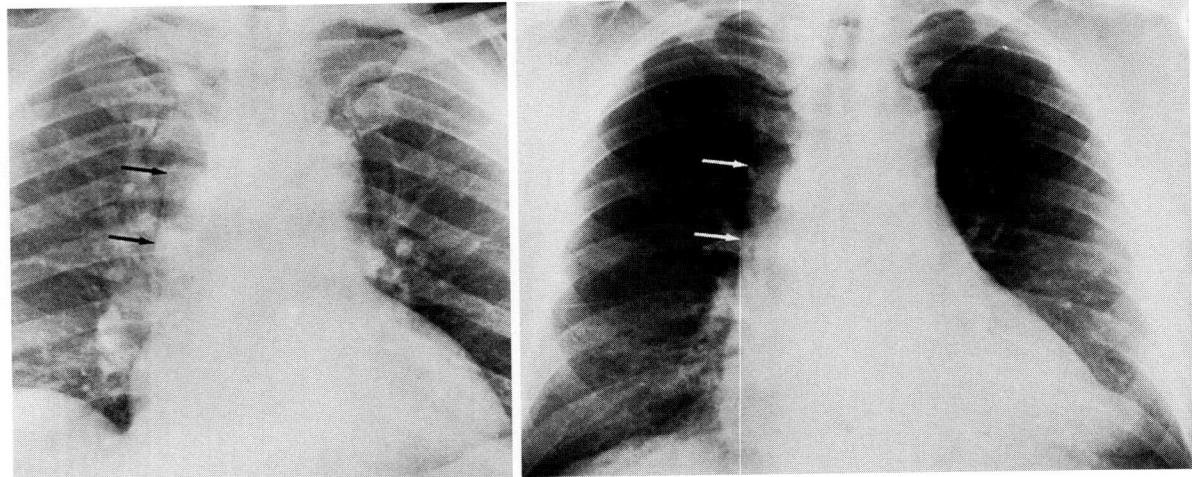

Figure 9–159. Two examples of mediastinal fat, producing widening of the mediastinum. This may be seen in obesity, in Cushing's disease, and in patients receiving steroids. (Ref: Price JE Jr, Rigler LG: Widening of the mediastinum resulting from fat accumulation. *Radiology* 96:497, 1970.) Seen in lateral projection, such fat may simulate the thymus. (Ref: Steckel RJ: Mediastinal pseudotumors associated with exogenous obesity. *Radiology* 119:74, 1976.)

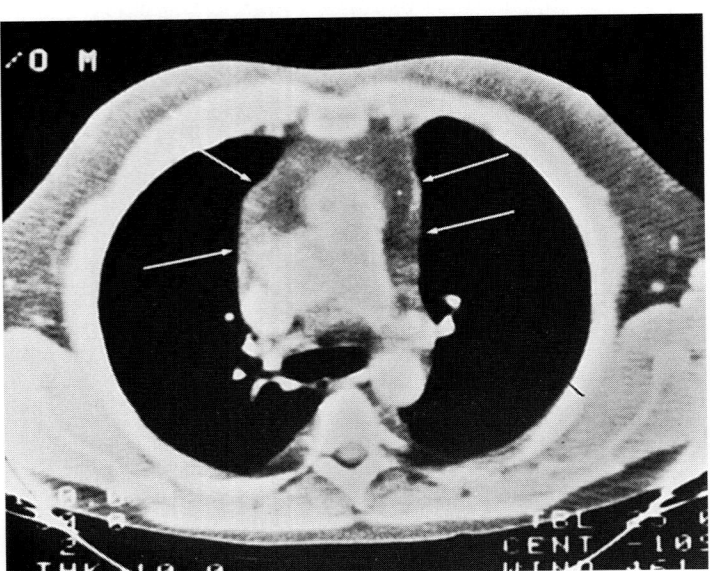

Figure 9–160. CT showing extensive mediastinal lipomatosis.

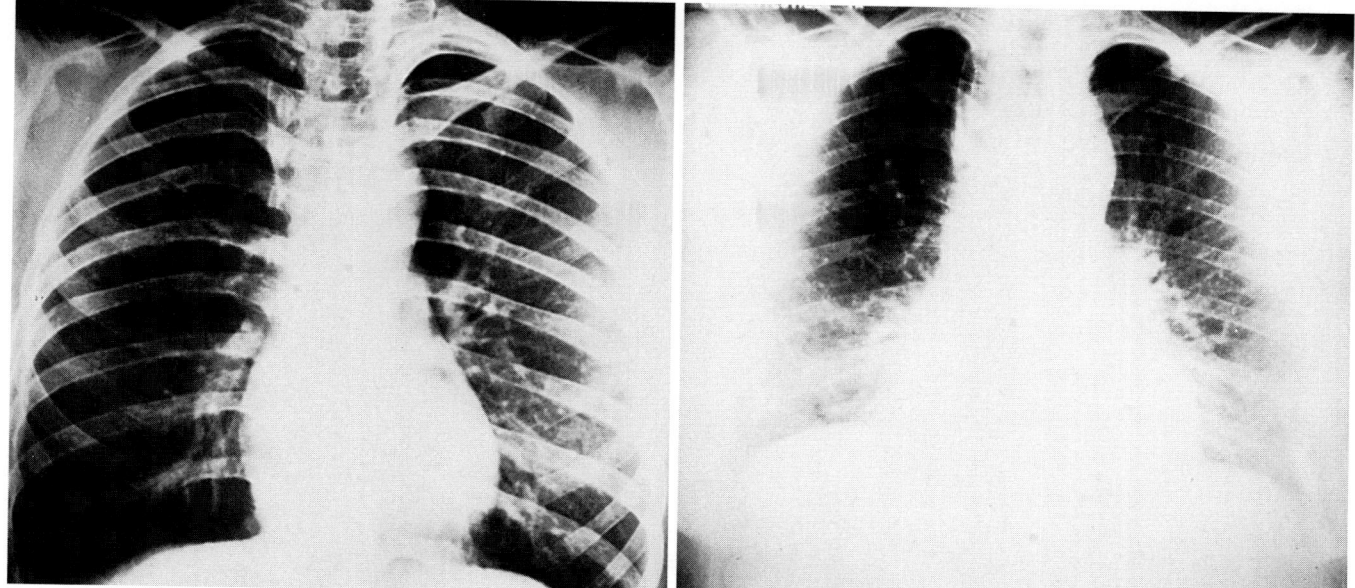

Figure 9–161. Alterations in configuration of the mediastinum over a period of 25 years, as a result of mediastinal deposition of fat. An azygos lobe is present.

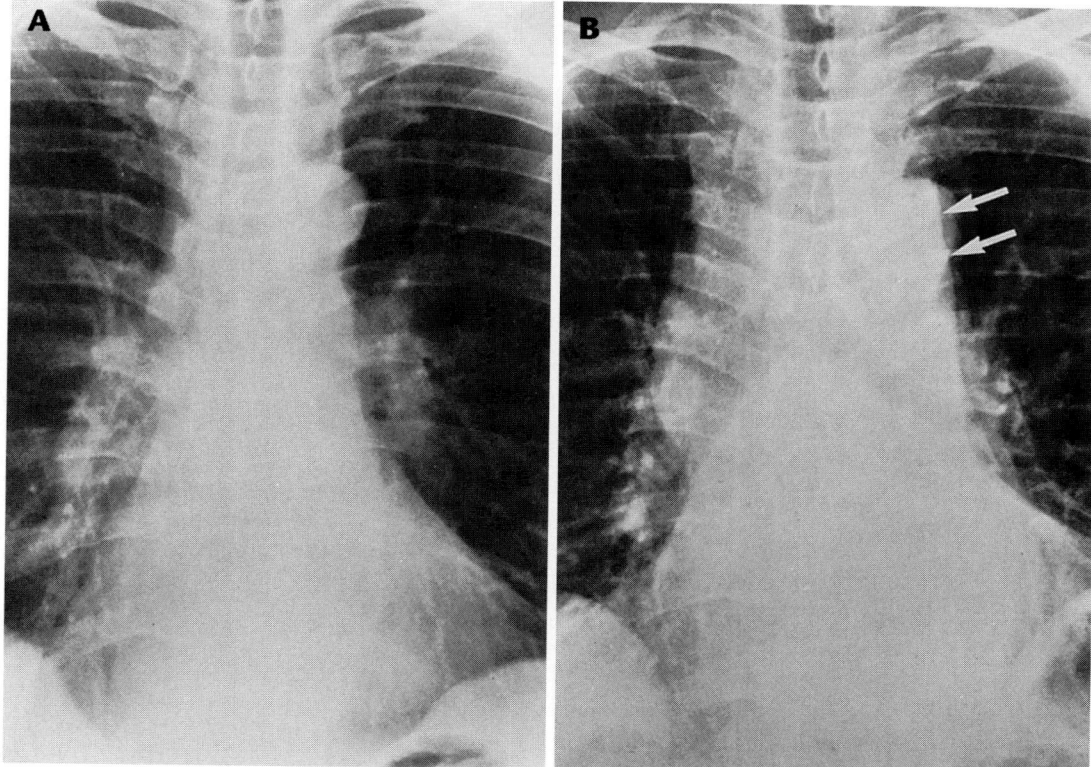

Figure 9–162. A, B, Progressive mediastinal lipomatosis over a 10-year period, secondary to steroids. Note displacement of the aortic pulmonary stripe in (**B**) (←).

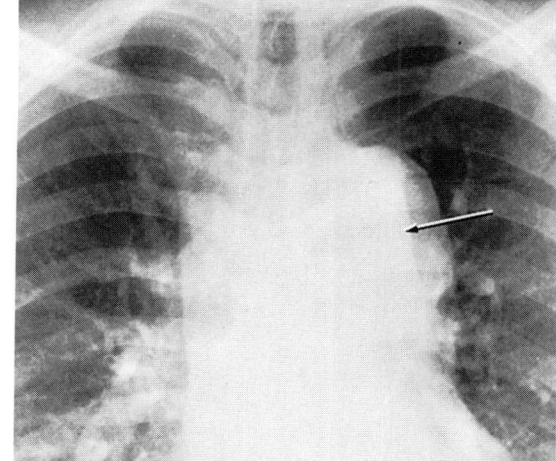

Figure 9–163. Mediastinal lipomatosis with marked displacement of the aortic pulmonary stripe.

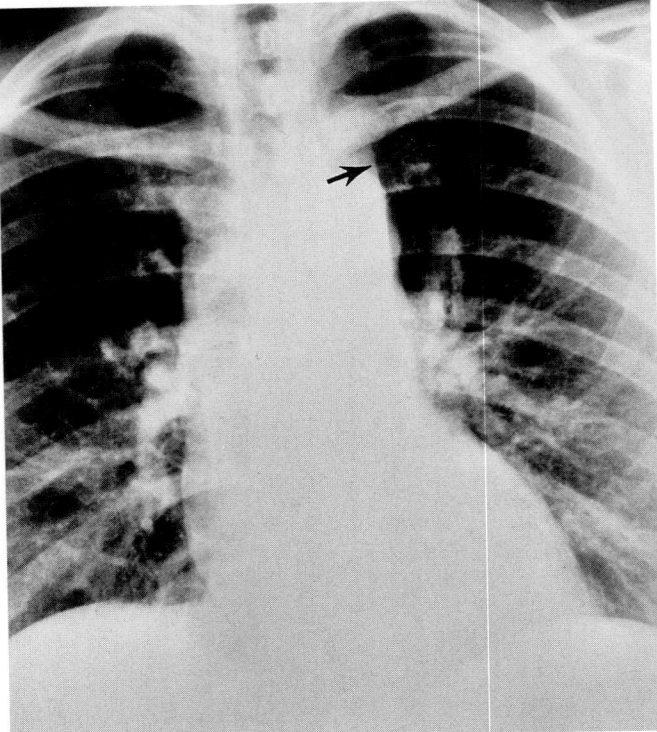

Figure 9–164. Mediastinal lipomatosis displacing the aortic pulmonary stripe above the level of the aortic arch.

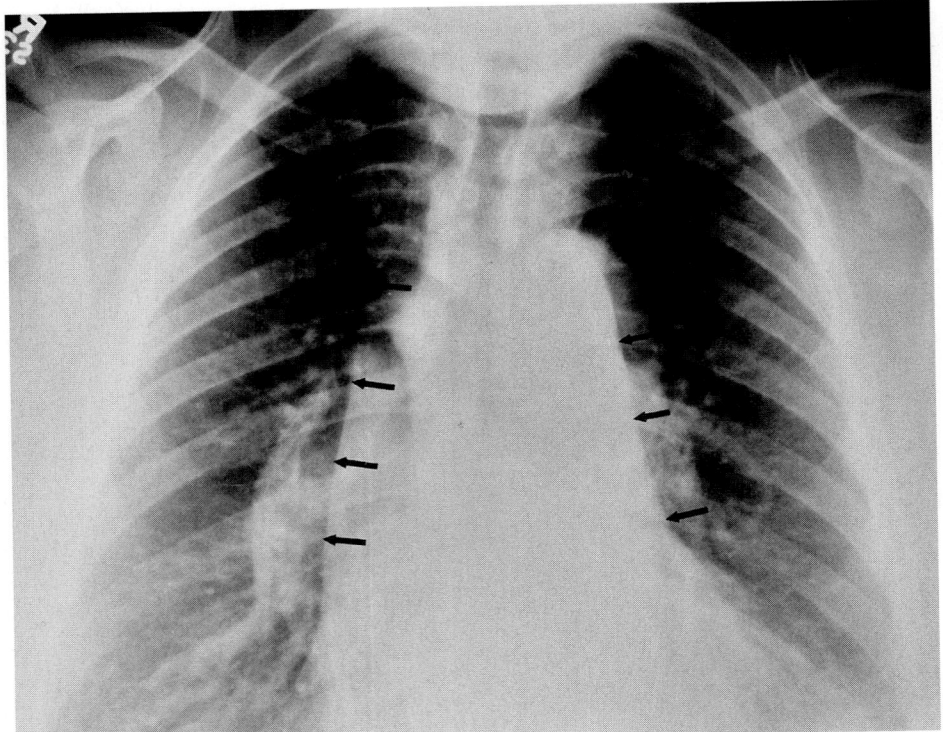

Figure 9–165. Mediastinal lipomatosis producing mediastinal linear densities.

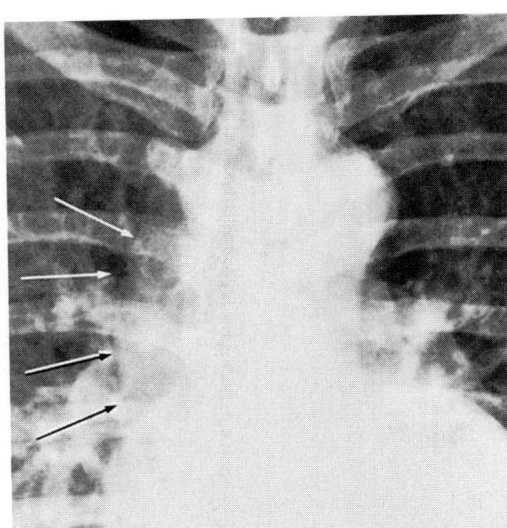

Figure 9–166. Mediastinal fat simulating a dilated ascending aorta *(arrows)*.

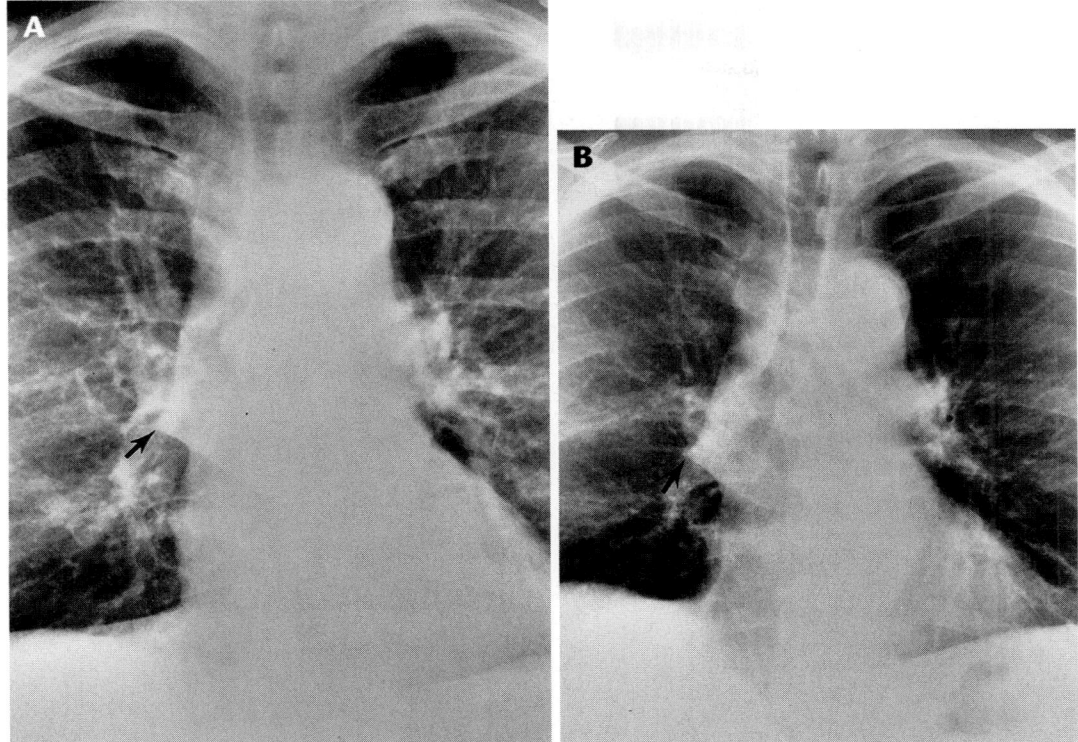

Figure 9–167. A, Extension of mediastinal fat into the medial aspect of the minor interlobar fissure. **B,** Four-year follow-up.

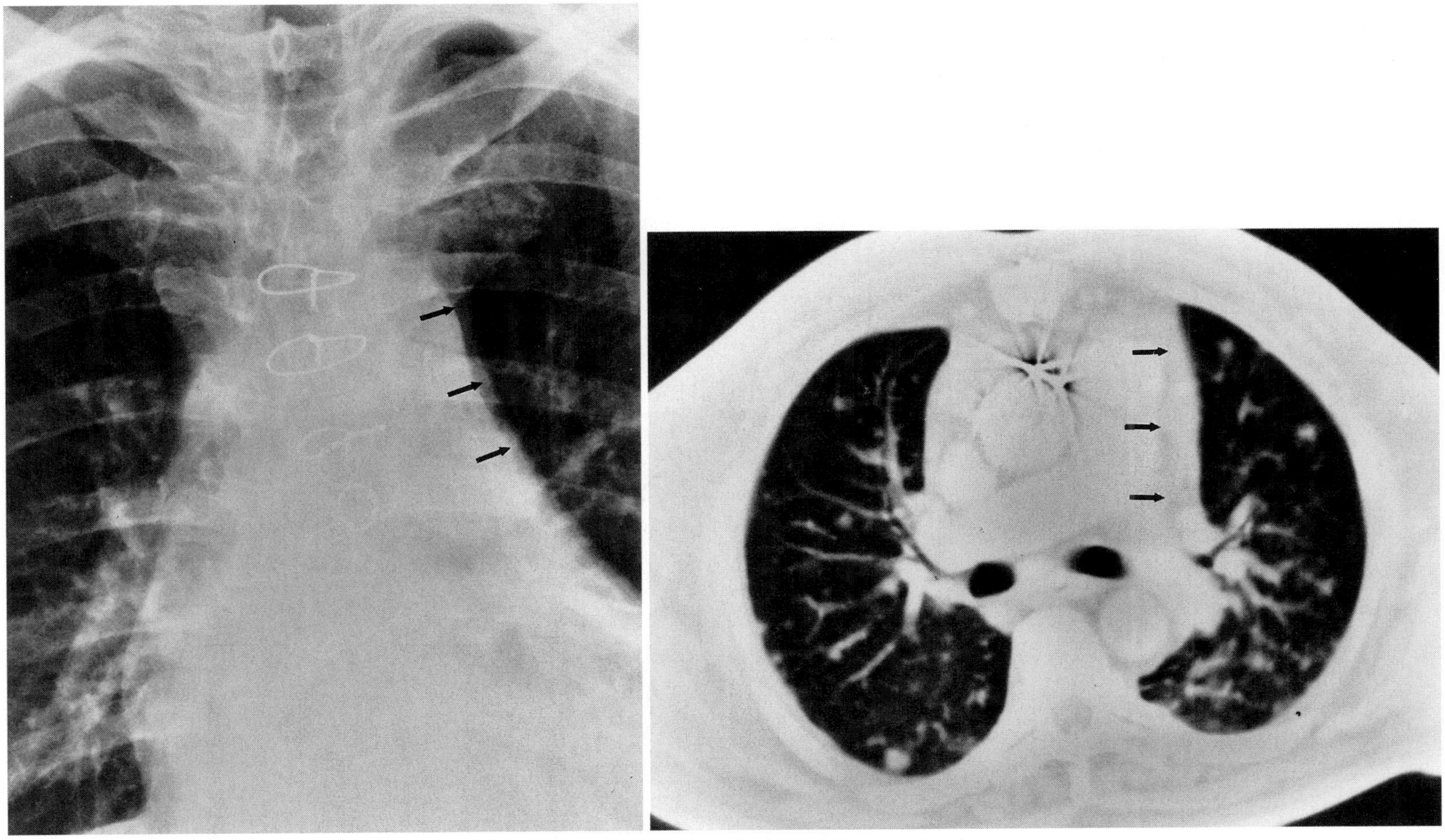

Figure 9–168. Mediastinal fat paralleling the left mediastinal border.

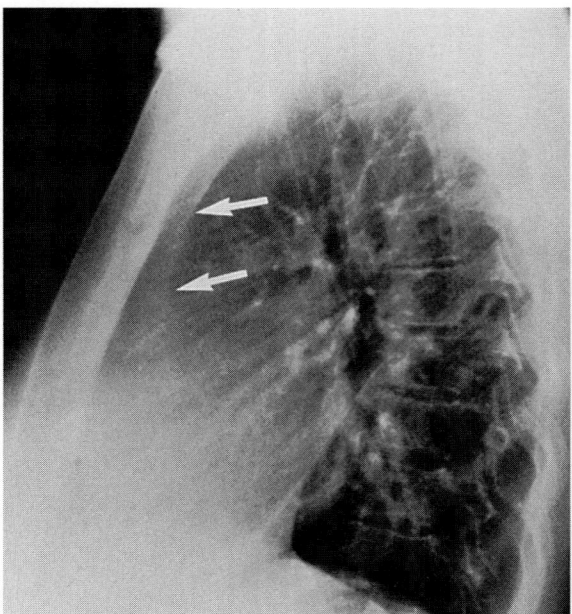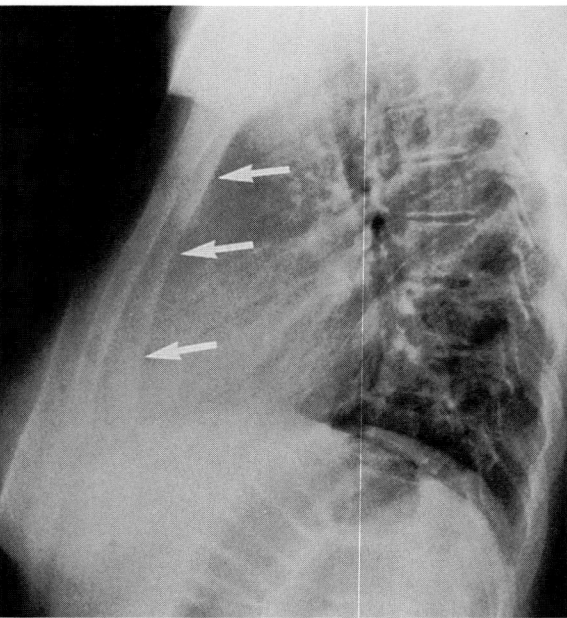

Figure 9–169. Fat seen in the anterior mediastinum, which increased over a 2-year period of progressive obesity.

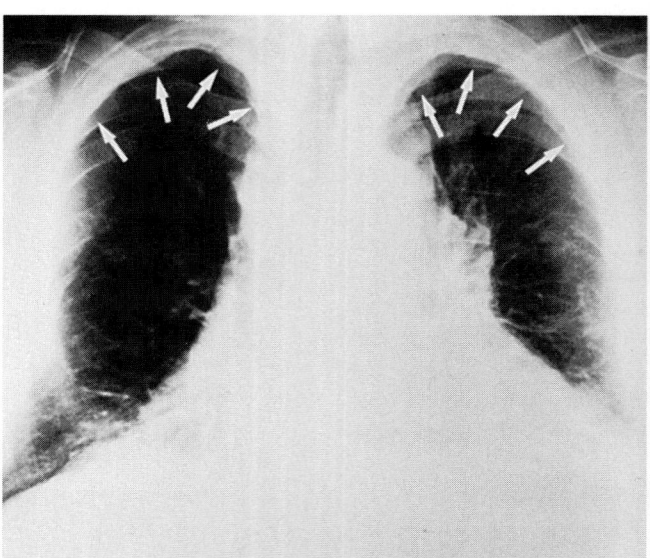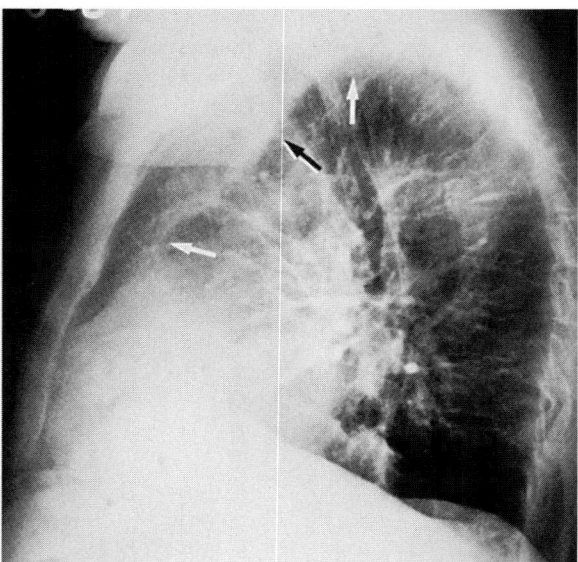

Figure 9–170. Mediastinal lipomatosis. Note also the extension of the fat over the apex of the lungs and into the extrapleural spaces (*arrows*).

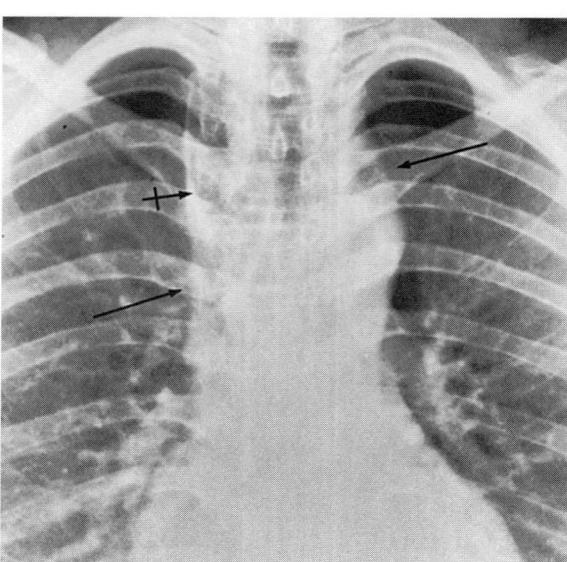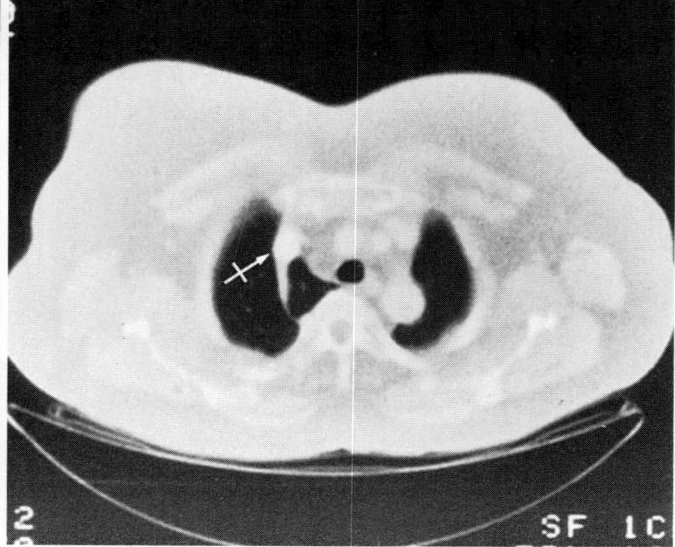

Figure 9–171. *Left,* Confusing appearance produced by mediastinal lipomatosis (←) and an azygos lobe (↔). *Right,* CT shows the course of the azygos vein.

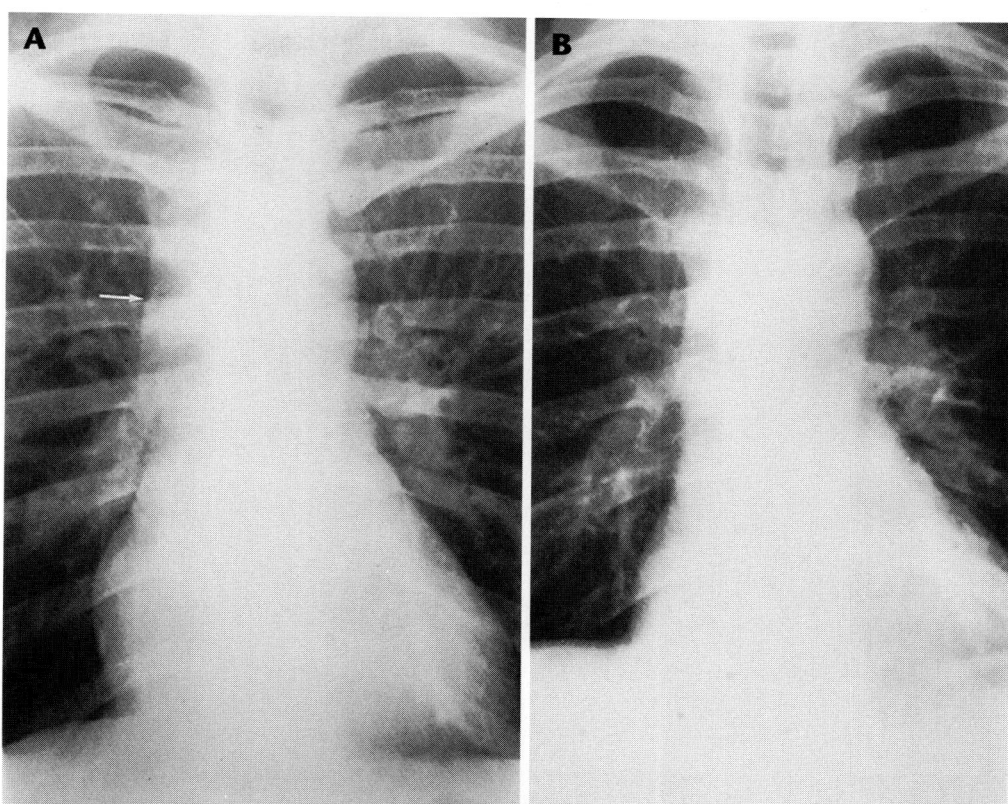

Figure 9–172. A, Widening of the right side of the mediastinum produced by distention of the superior vena cava after forceful Valsalva maneuver. **B,** Same patient in suspended respiration without Valsalva maneuver.

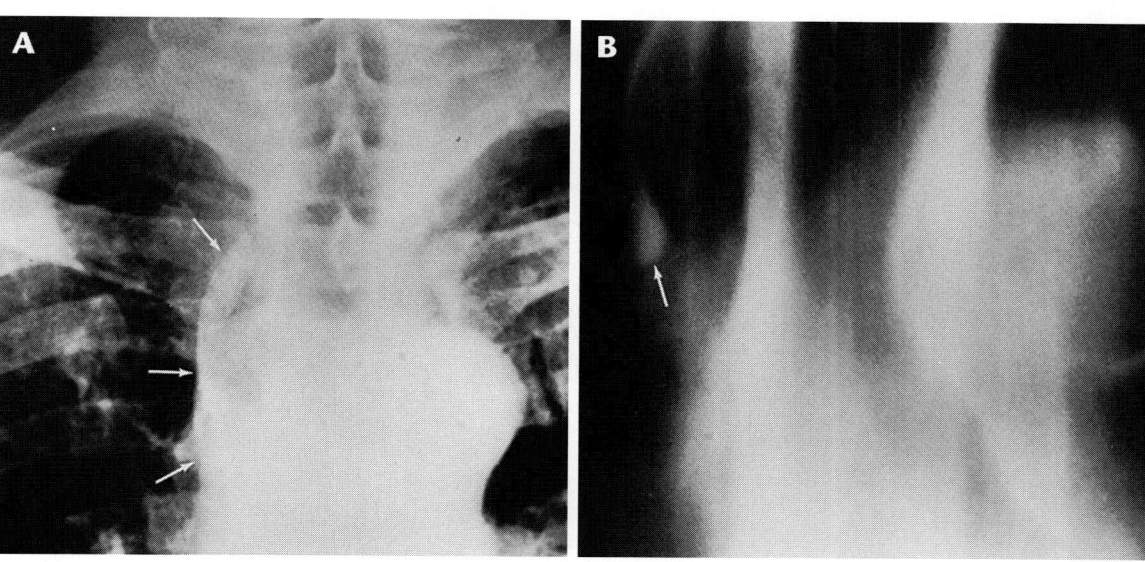

Figure 9–173. Azygos lobe simulating a distended air-filled esophagus. **A,** Plain film. **B,** Tomography.

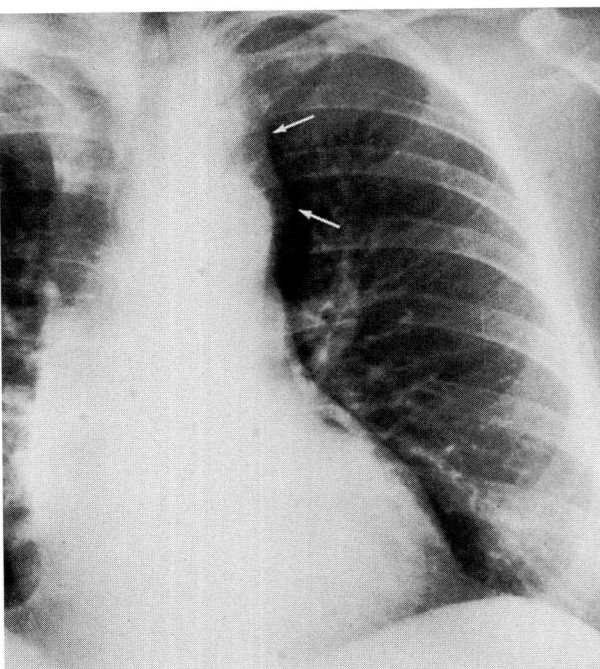

Figure 9–174. Widening of the superior mediastinum produced by anomalous venous drainage of the left upper lobe. The anomalous vertical vein is evident. (Ref: Adler SC, Silverman JF: Anomalous venous drainage of the left upper lobe. *Radiology* 108:563, 1973.)

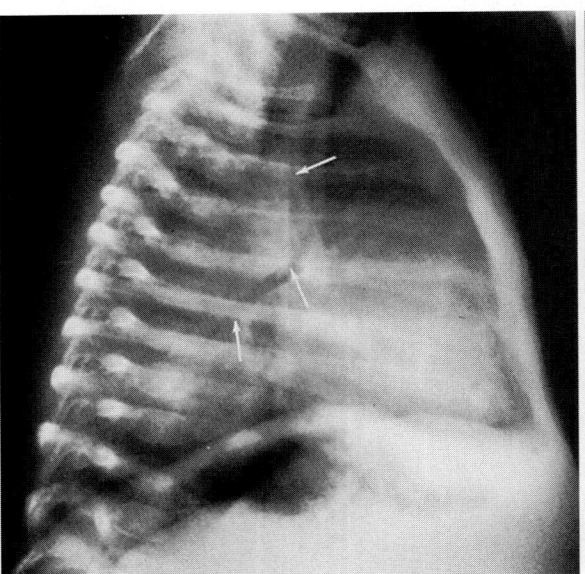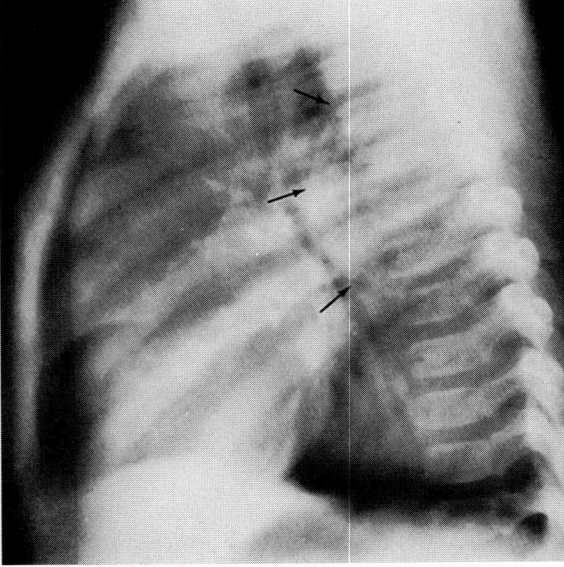

Figure 9–175. The spurious posterior mediastinal mass, seen in infants as the result of superimposition of the scapulae and the axillary soft tissues, combined with the anterior curve of the trachea and the lower lobe continuation of the left main bronchus. (Refs: Alazraki NP, Friedman PJ: Posterior mediastinal "pseudo-mass" of the newborn. *Am J Roentgenol* 116:571, 1972; Balsand D et al: The scapula as a cause of spurious posterior mediastinal mass on lateral chest films of infants. *J Pediatr Surg* 9:501, 1972.)

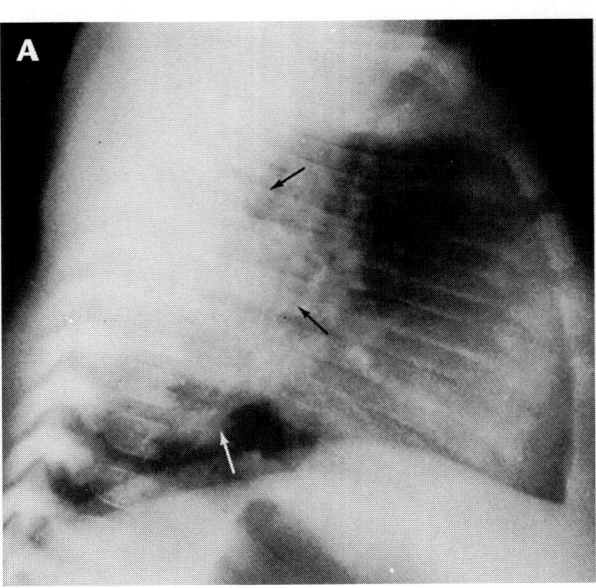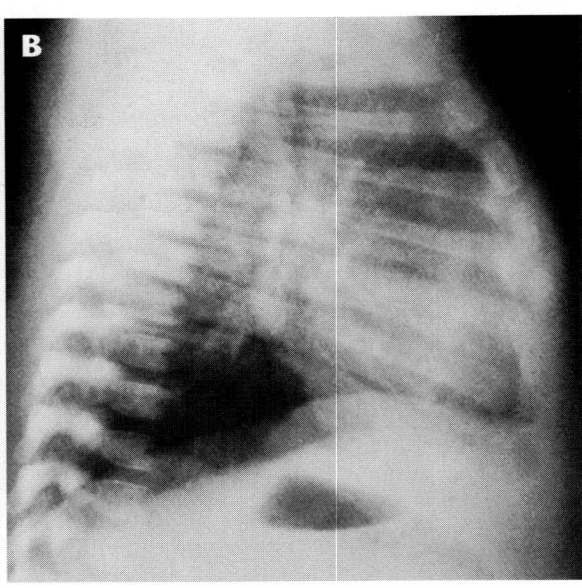

Figure 9–176. The pseudomass of the mediastinum in infants, illustrated in Figure 9–175, will be accentuated by filming in the expiratory phase of respiration. **A,** Expiration. **B,** Full inspiration. No mass effect seen.

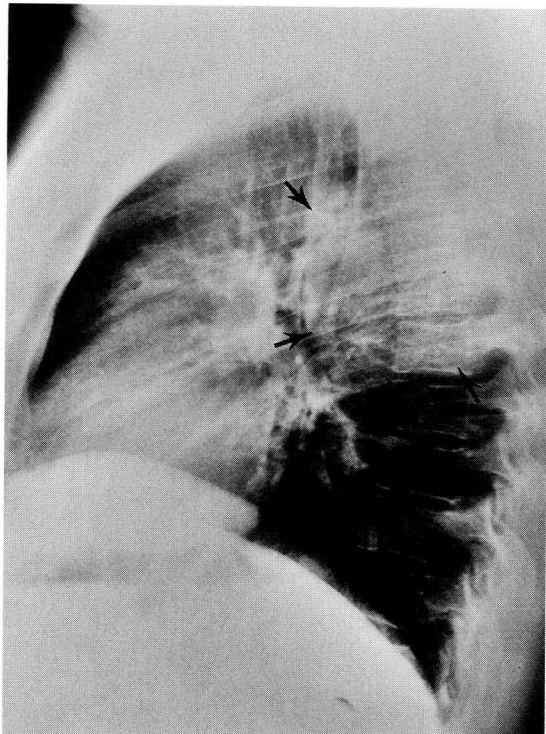

Figure 9–177. Posterior mediastinal pseudomass in an adult.

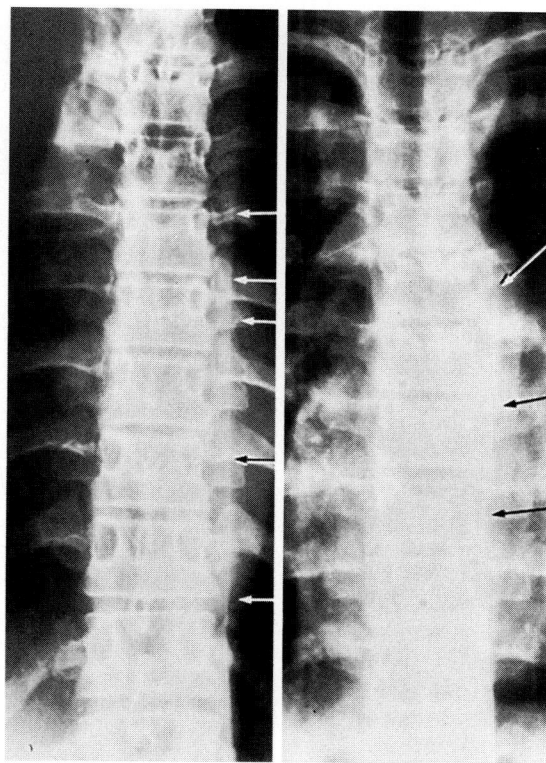

Figure 9–178. Normal paravertebral stripe. Note that it is not normally seen in the upper thoracic region, being lost at T4–T5. This is best seen in the patient on the right.

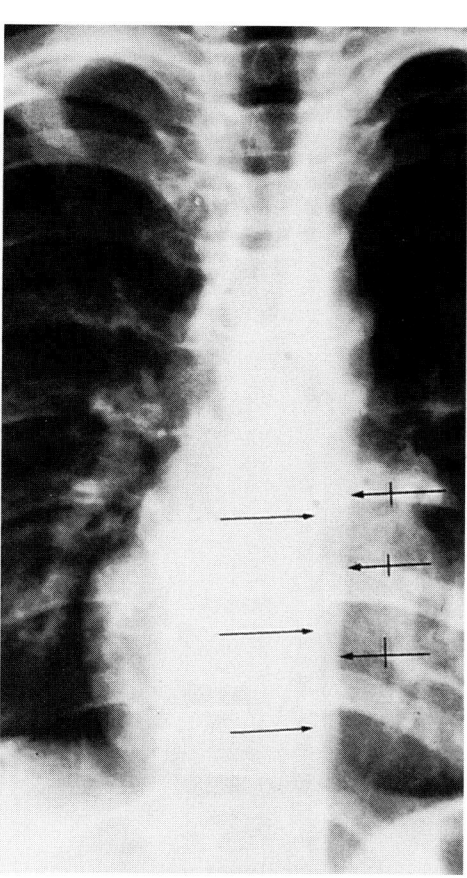

Figure 9–179. Normal left paravertebral soft tissues. *Arrow* indicates the paravertebral stripe; *crossed arrow* indicates the descending aorta. (Ref: Lien HH, Kolbenstvedt A: The thoracic paraspinal shadow: Normal appearances. *Clin Radiol* 33:31, 1982.) Occasionally one may see a localized loss of the infrabronchial descending aortic interface as a normal variant. (Ref: Van Gelderen WFC: Localized loss of the infrabronchial descending interface as a normal variant. *Br J Radiology* 65:865, 1992.)

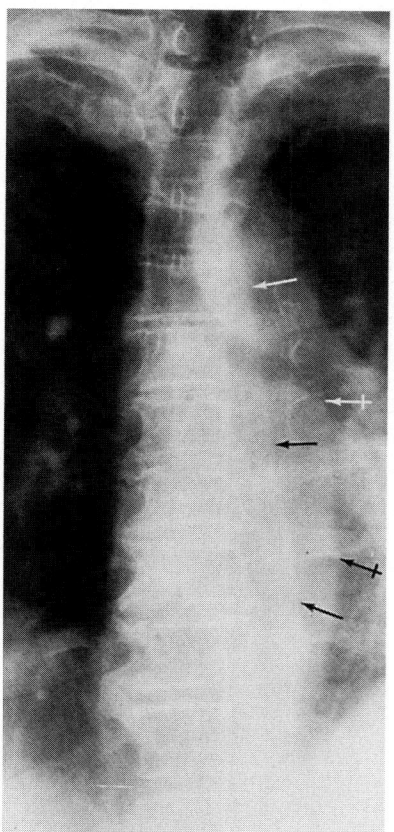

Figure 9–180. The left paramediastinal stripe (→), representing the reflection of the pleura against the spine, may be deviated laterally by ectasia of the thoracic aorta (↦) and is therefore not necessarily an indication of vertebral or mediastinal abnormality. (Ref: Genereux GP: The posterior pleural reflections. *Am J Roentgenol* 141:141, 1983.)

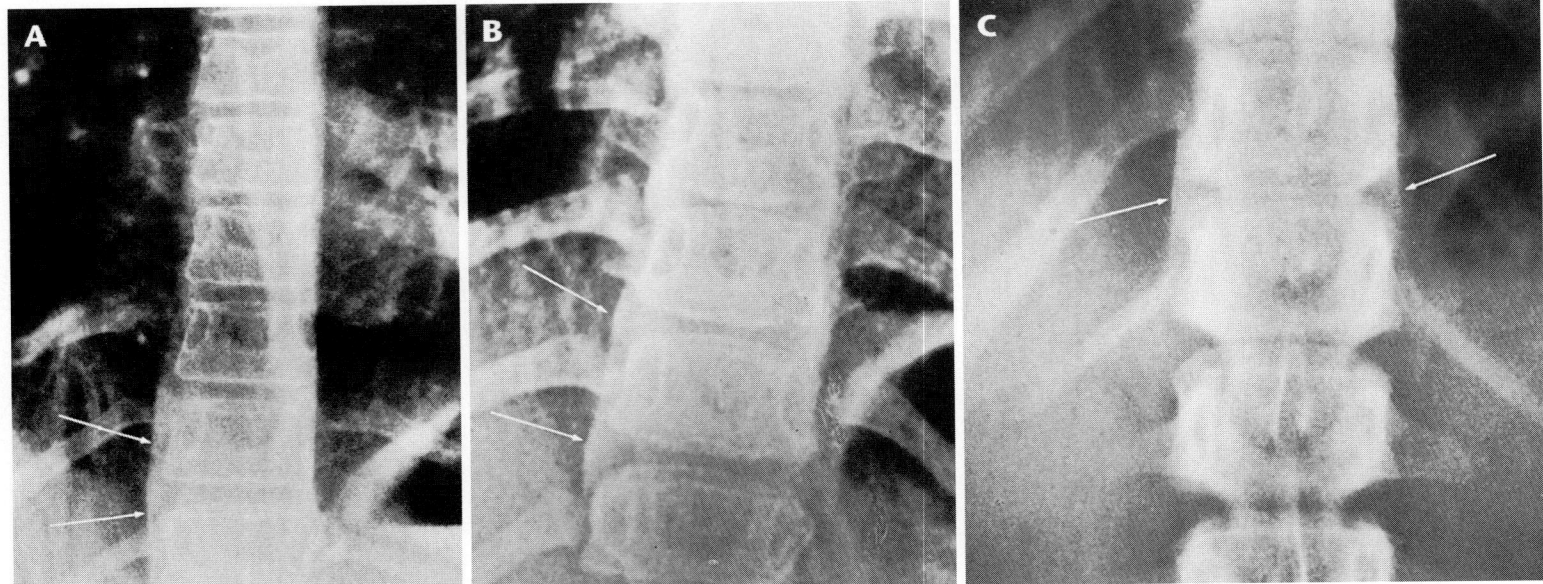

Figure 9–181. Paravertebral stripe may be seen on the right, particularly in young individuals (**A** and **B**), or bilaterally (**C**), and should not be confused with a paraspinous mass. A similar shadow on the right may also be due to a wide inferior vena cava. (Ref: Eklof O et al: Malignant versus benign paravertebral widening in children. *Pediatr Radiol* 11:193, 1981.)

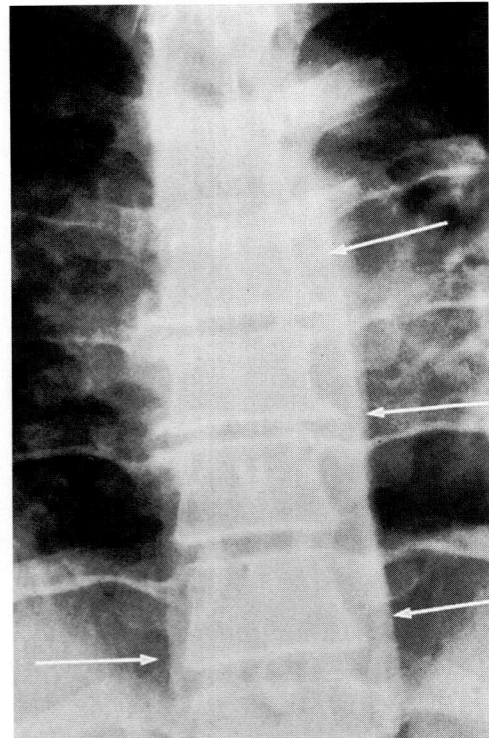

Figure 9–182. Right and left paravertebral stripes in a 49-year-old woman.

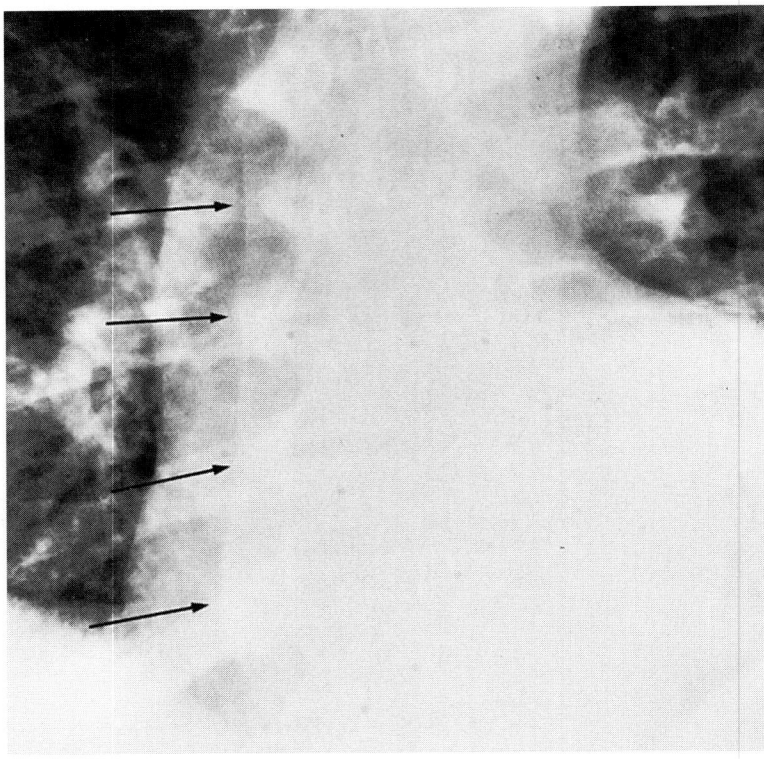

Figure 9–183. Displacement of the right paravertebral stripe by hypertrophic lipping of the spine.

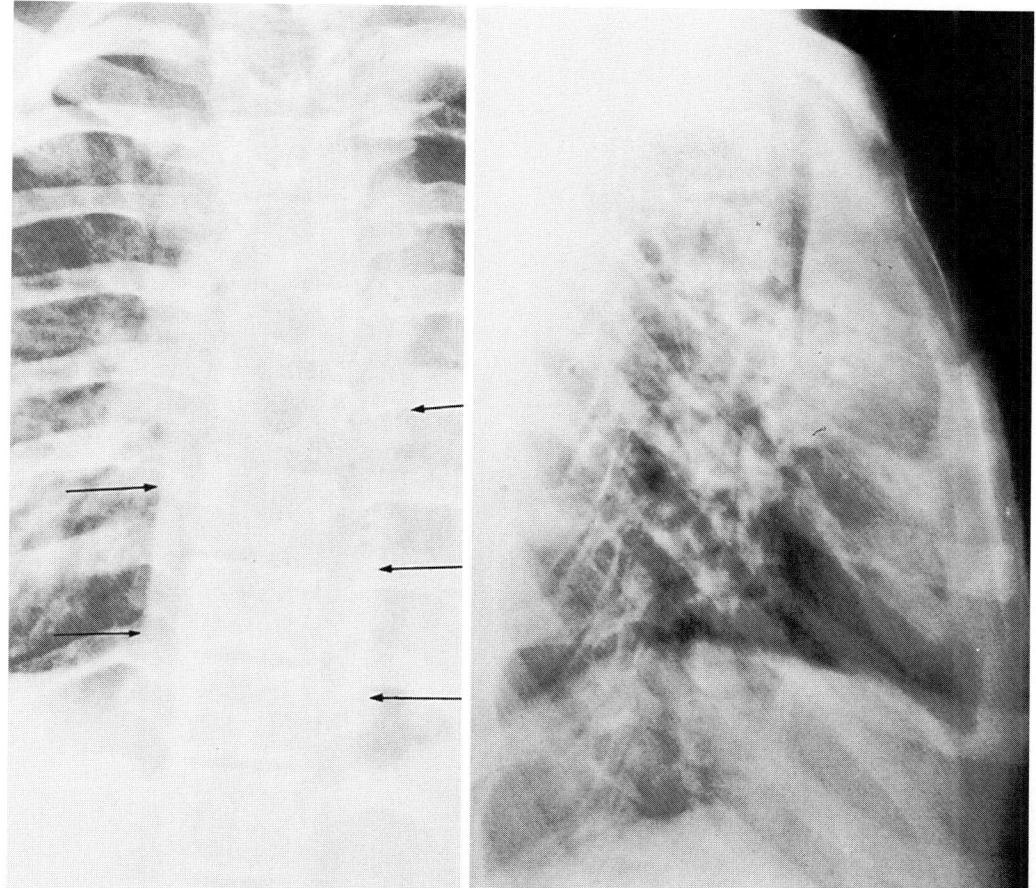

Figure 9–184. A very narrow chest will result in striking visualization of both paravertebral stripes.

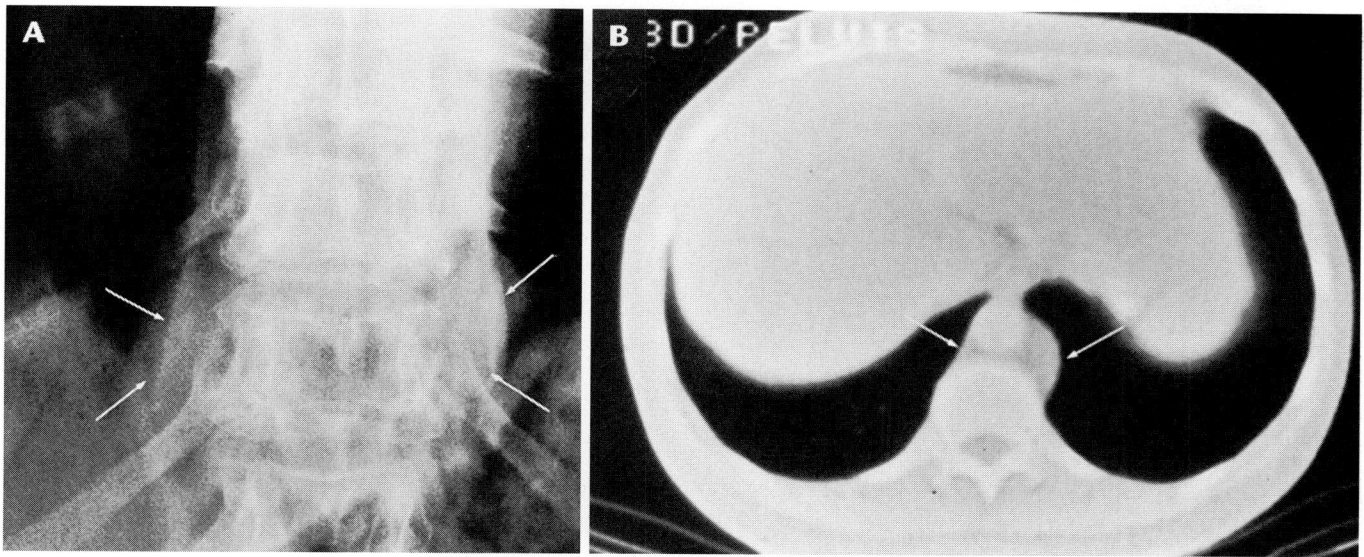

Figure 9–185. Paraspinous fat deposition will displace the paravertebral stripes. **A,** Plain film. **B,** CT. (Refs: Streiter ML et al: Steroid-induced thoracic lipomatosis: Paraspinal involvement. *Am J Roentgenol* 139:679, 1982; Glickstein MC et al: Paraspinal lipomatosis. *Radiology* 163:79, 1987.)

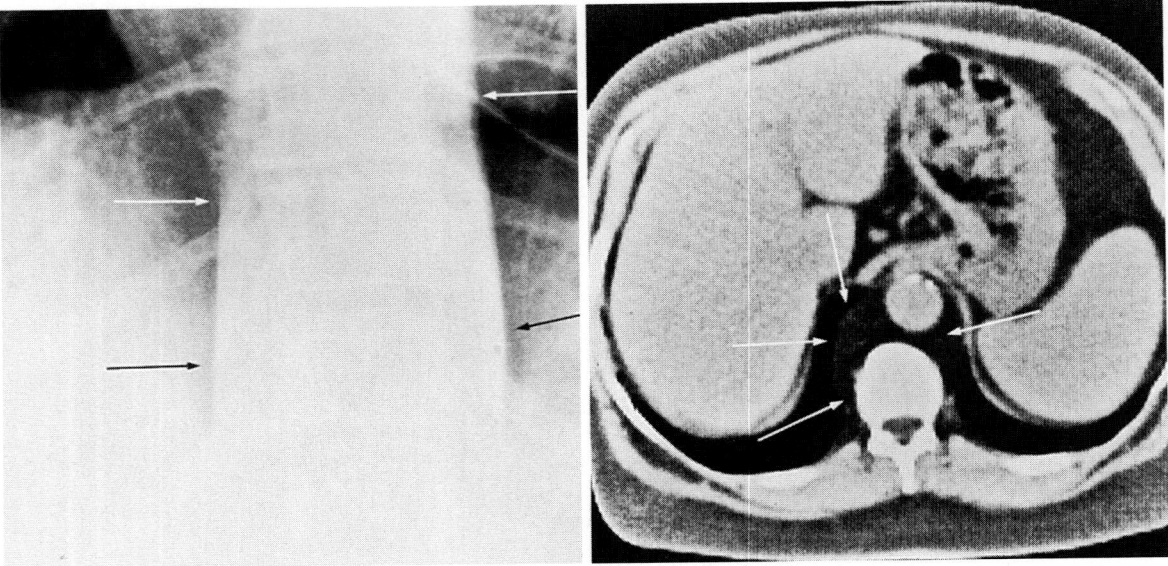

Figure 9–186. *Left*, Striking paraspinal lipomatosis that is bilaterally symmetric. *Right*, CT.

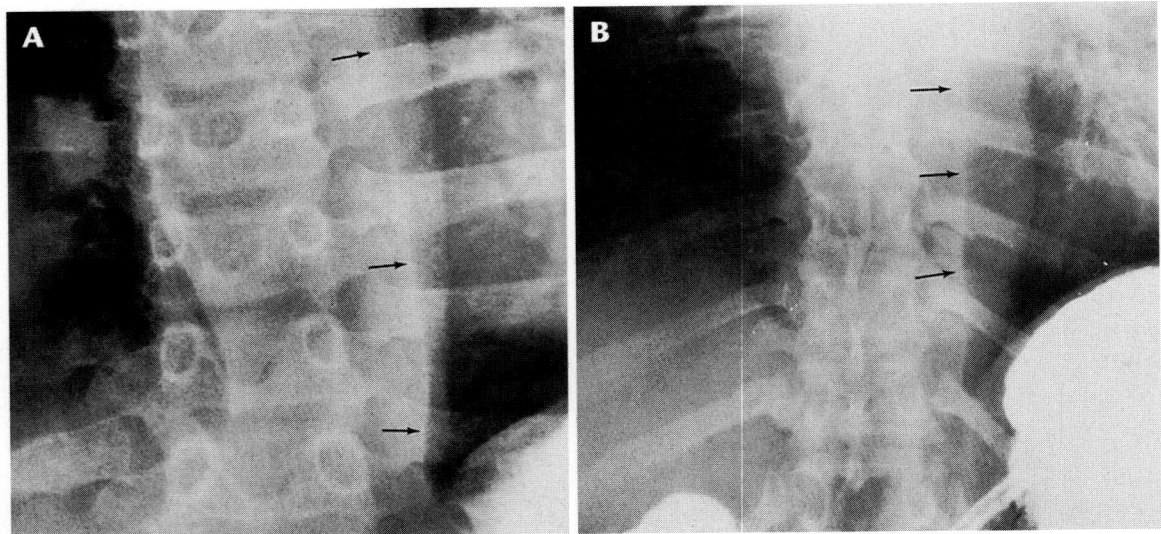

Figure 9–187. Marked obesity resulting in displacement of the paravertebral stripe, caused by fat deposition. **A**, 300-lb, 14-year-old boy. **B**, 250-lb, 46-year-old man.

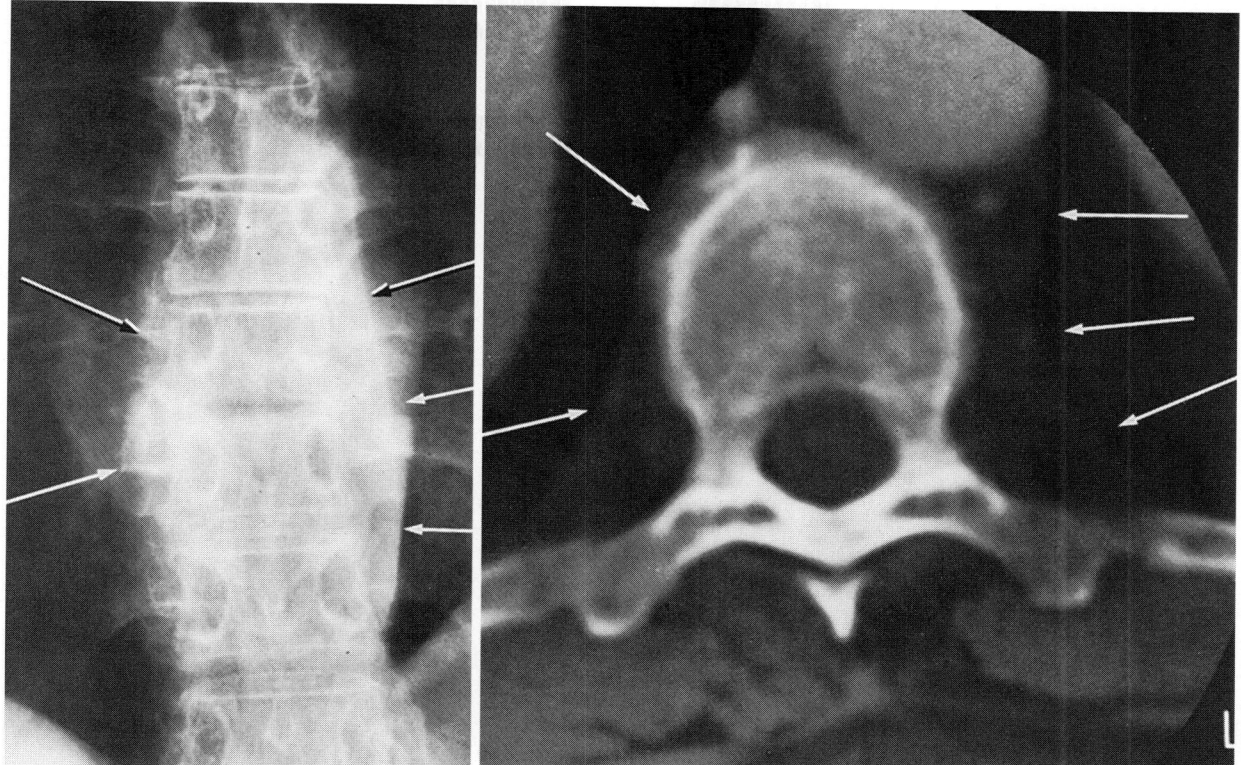

Figure 9–188. Paraspinous fat deposits may not be evenly distributed or symmetric, as illustrated in this case. *Left*, Plain film. *Right*, CT.

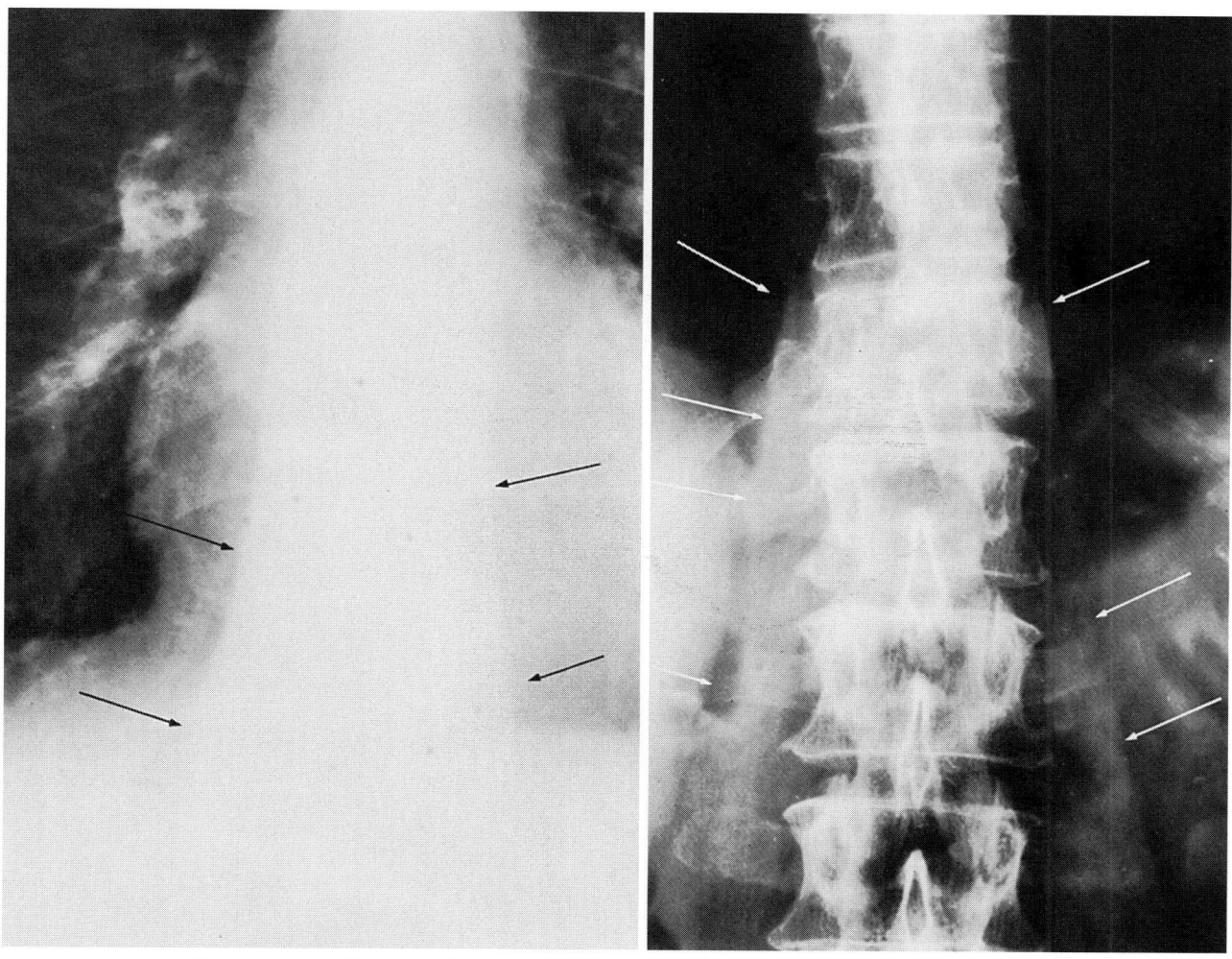

Figure 9–189. Origin of the psoas muscles from the lower thoracic spine, producing paraspinous soft tissue shadows.

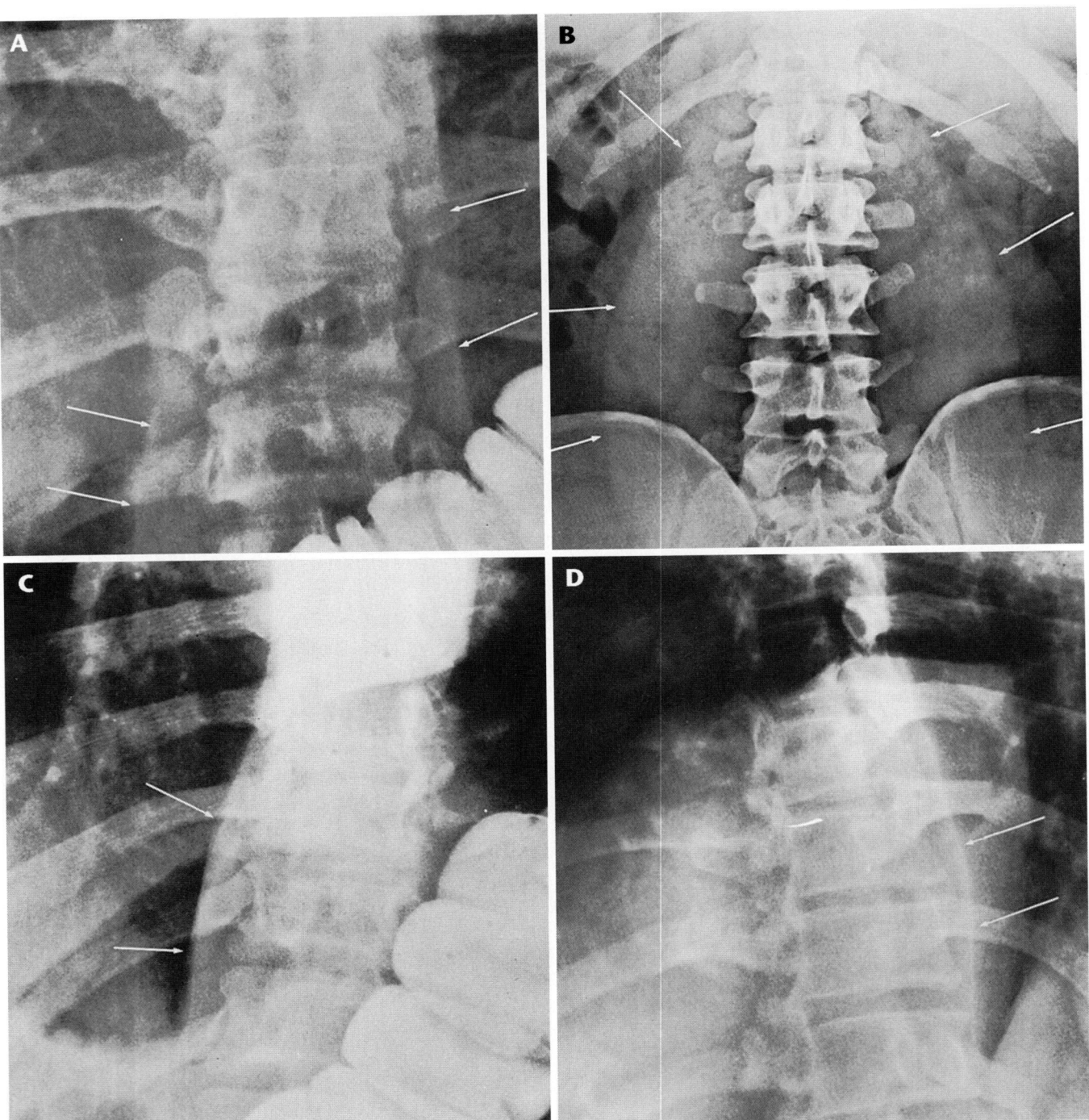

Figure 9–190. Thoracic origin of very large psoas muscles, producing paravertebral soft tissue bulges. **A** and **B,** Frontal projections. **C** and **D,** Oblique projections.

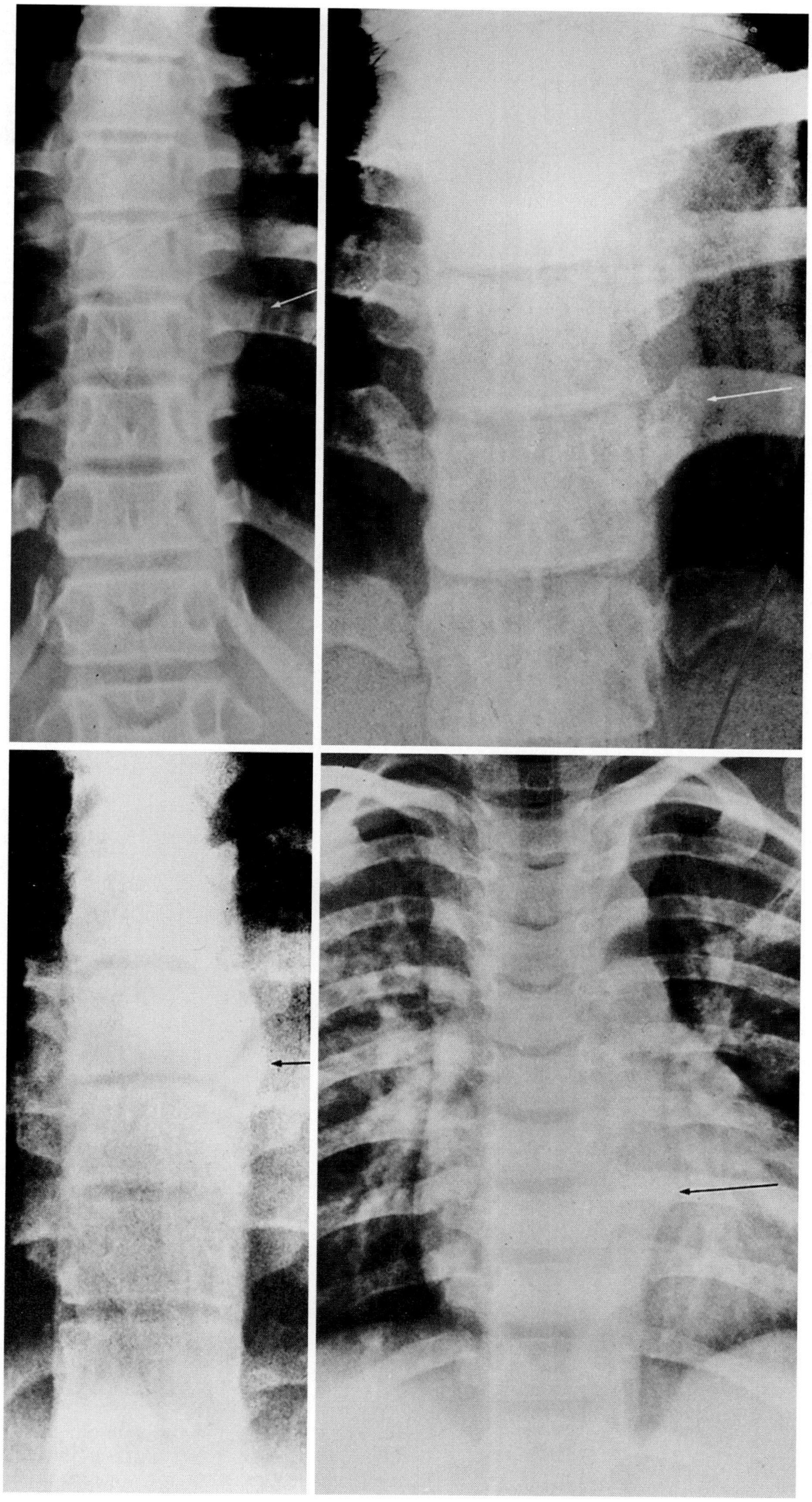

Figure 9–191. Four examples of discrete left paravertebral soft tissue bulges that have not been demonstrable by CT or aortography. In some pathologic states similar shadows may be seen related to the hemiazygous system. These shadows may be the product of intermittent filling of veins. (Ref: Castellino RA et al: Dilated azygous and hemiazygous veins presenting as paravertebral intrathoracic masses. *N Engl J Med* 278:1087, 1968.) A similar shadow may be produced by a mediastinal lymph node (see Fig. 9–192).

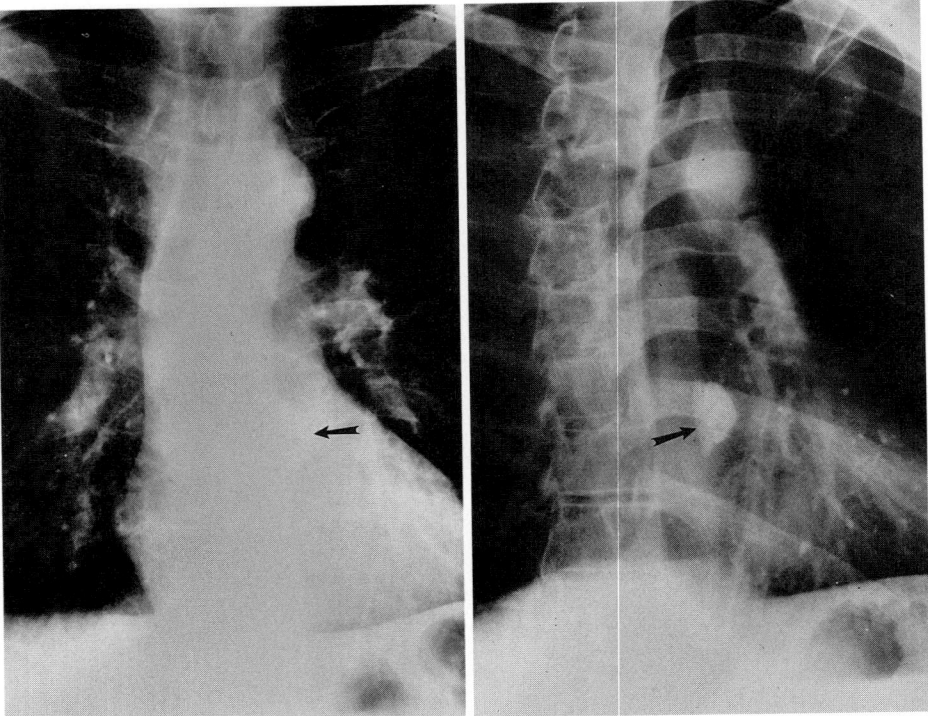

Figure 9–192. PA and right anterior oblique views of the chest showing a calcified mediastinal lymph node producing a shadow similar to those illustrated in Figure 9–191.

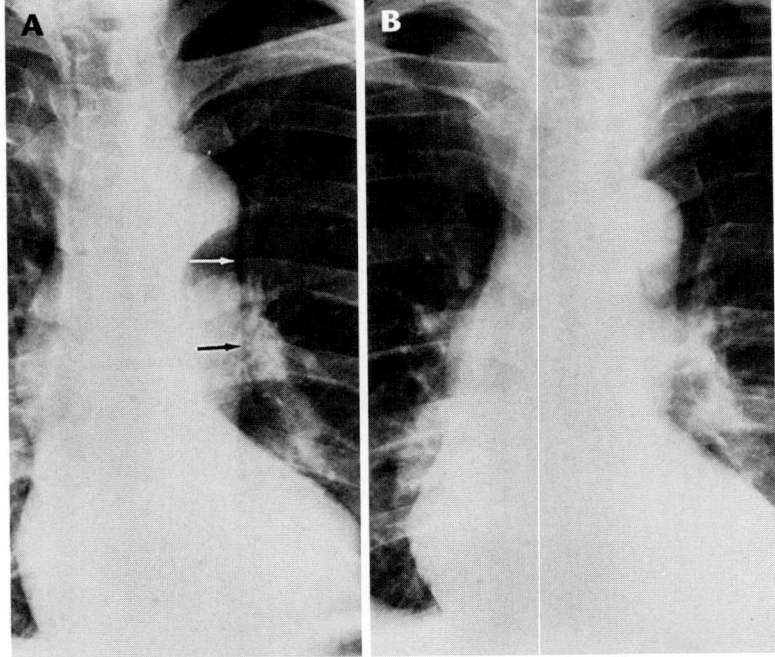

Figure 9–193. A, Simulated pneumomediastinum is evidenced by radiolucency adjacent to the aorta, produced by lucent lung in the interval between the aorta and adjacent pulmonary vessels. **B,** With slight rotation to the left the nature of this factitious lesion is evident.

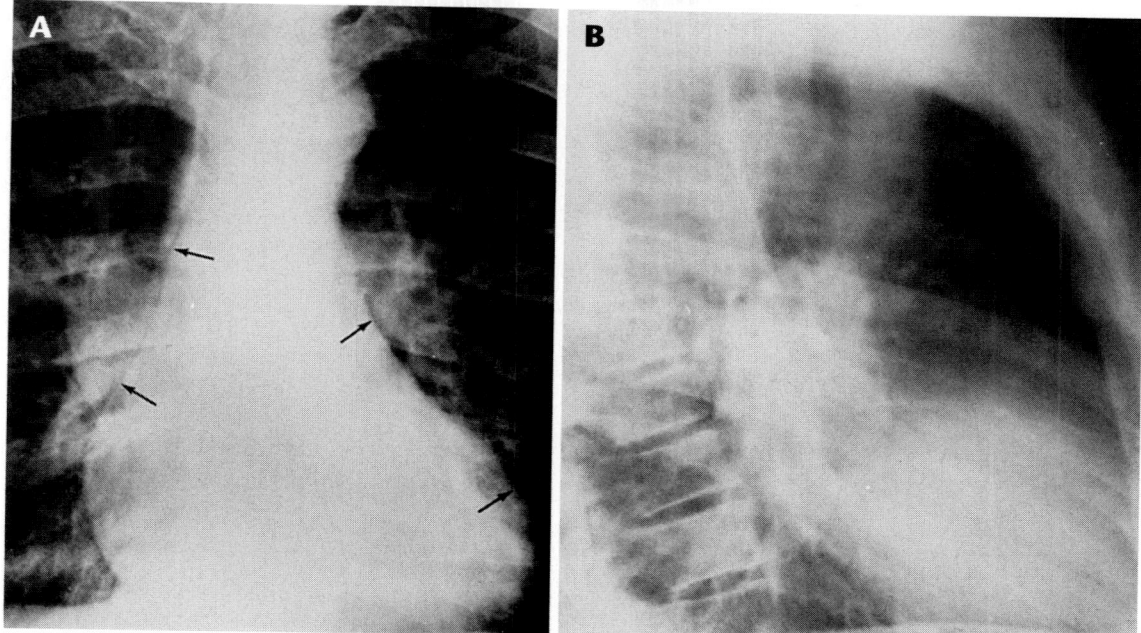

Figure 9–194. **A,** Simulated pneumomediastinum evidenced by a lucent halo around the heart produced by the Mach effect. **B,** No evidence of pneumomediastinum is seen in lateral projection. (Ref: Friedman AC et al: Mach bands and pneumomediastinum. *J Can Assoc Radiol* 32:232, 1981.)

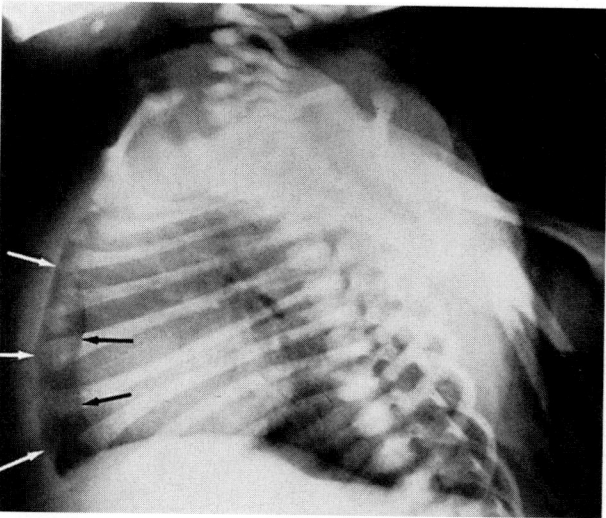

Figure 9–195. Simulated pneumomediastinum in an infant, produced by slight rotation of the chest at the time of filming, projecting lucent lung in front of the cardiac shadow.

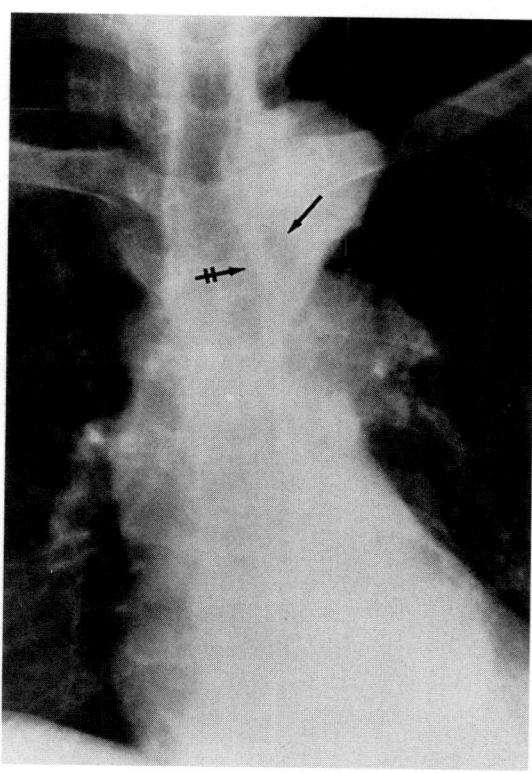

Figure 9–196. Air in the esophagus producing a lucency beneath the aortic arch (←). This is seen when the esophagus is displaced to the left by adhesions to a tortuous aorta. Barium may be retained in this pocket as well. Note position of pleural esophageal reflection (⊪→). (Ref: Cimmino CV: A roentgenologic study in mediastinal anatomy affected by air in the midesophagus. *Am J Roentgenol* 94:333, 1965.)

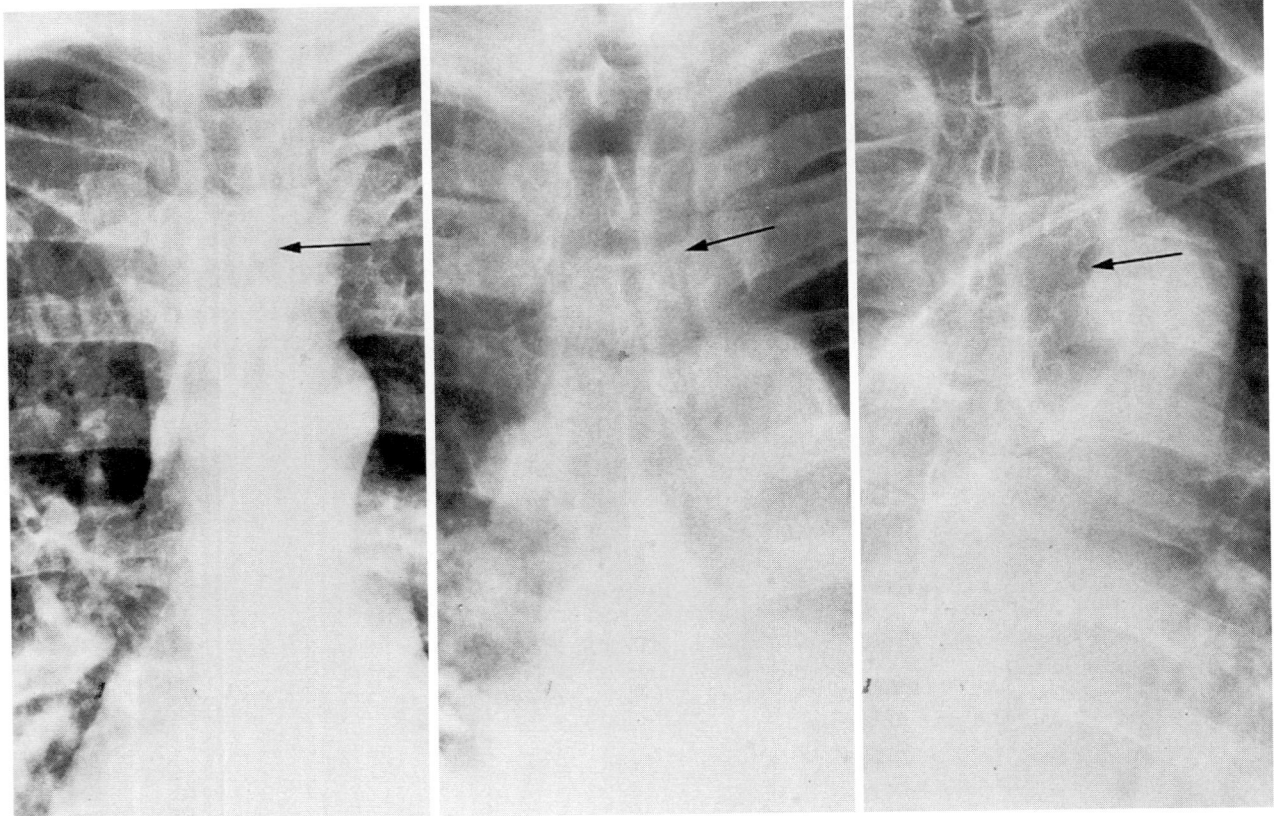

Figure 9–197. Three examples of patients with transient reflux of gas in the esophagus that should not be confused with mediastinal gas. (Ref: Proto A, Lane KJ: Air in the esophagus: A frequent radiographic finding. *Am J Roentgenol* 129:433, 1977.)

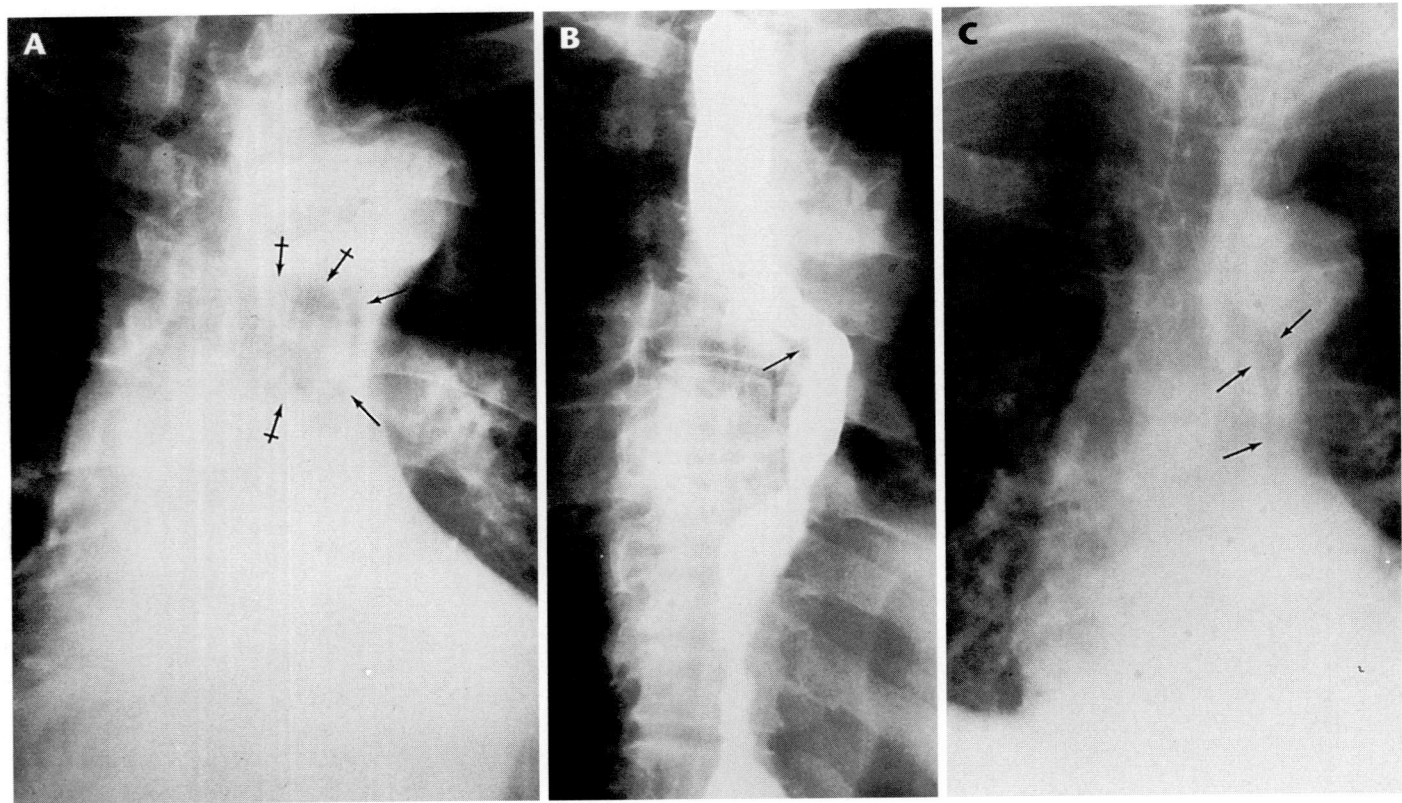

Figure 9–198. **A** and **C,** Examples of air trapped in the midesophagus (→) as in Figure 9–196. Note in **A** that the shift of the esophagus to the left has permitted a portion of the right lung to cross the left side, producing an additional area of radiolucency (↔). **B,** Barium esophagram of the patient shown in **A**. Note that the knuckle in the aorta corresponds to the air shadow in the plain film. (Ref: Proto AV: Air in the esophagus: A frequent radiologic finding. *Am J Roentgenol* 129:433, 1977.)

The Heart and Great Vessels

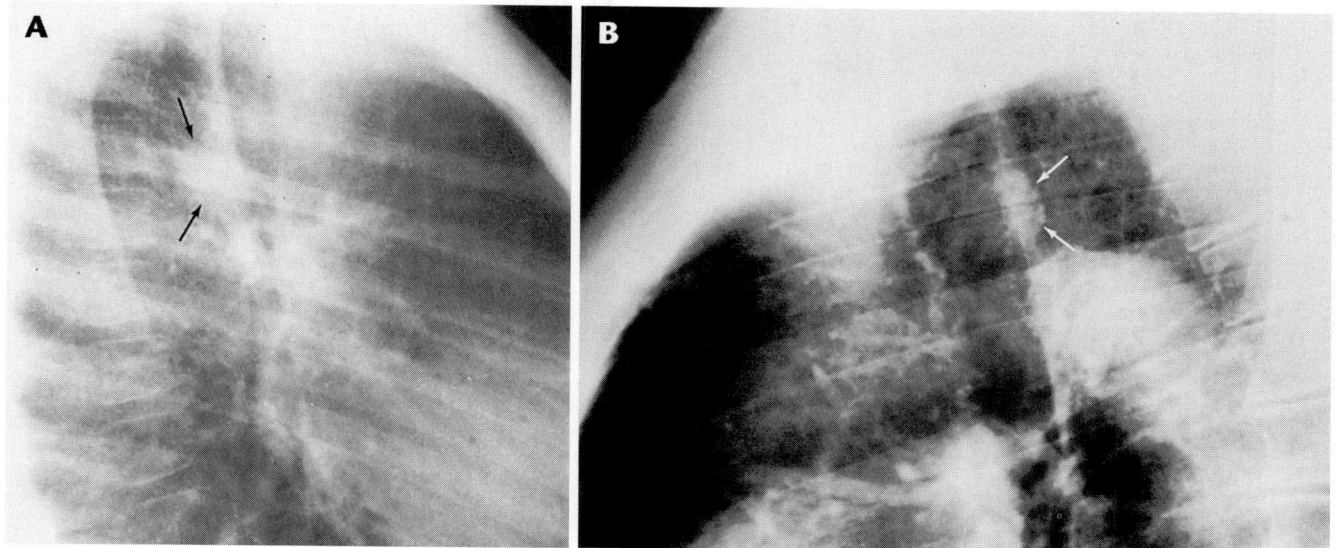

Figure 9–199. Azygos arch may be seen in the lateral projection as a nodular density, immediately behind the trachea. **A,** Child. **B,** Adult.

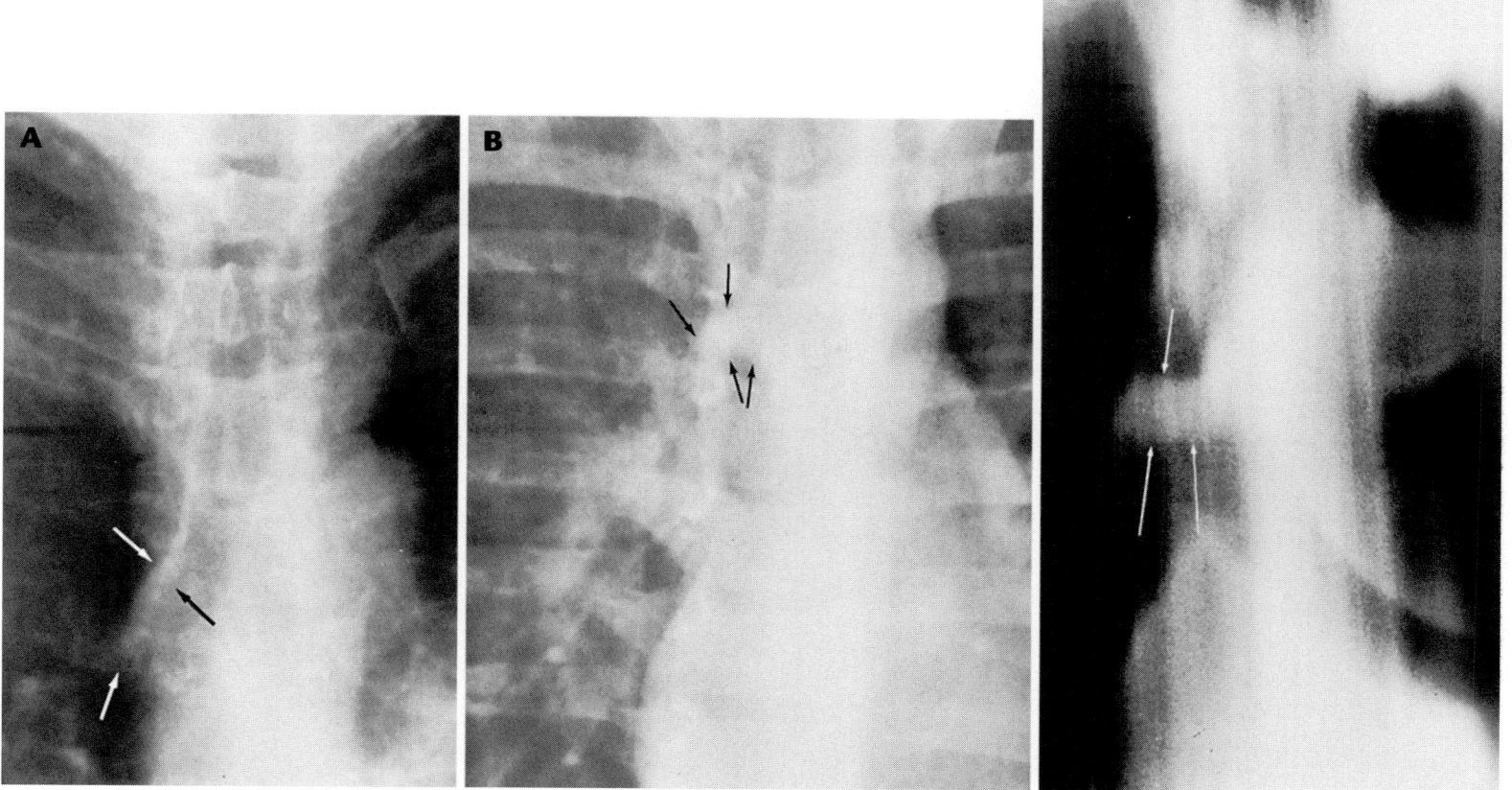

Figure 9–200. Shadows of the normal azygos vein. **A,** Arch of the azygos vein. **B,** Posterior portion of the azygos arch, the "azygos knob." **C,** Posterior portion of the azygos arch shown by tomography. (Ref: Heitzman ER et al: The azygos vein and its pleural reflections. *Radiology* 101:259, 1971.)

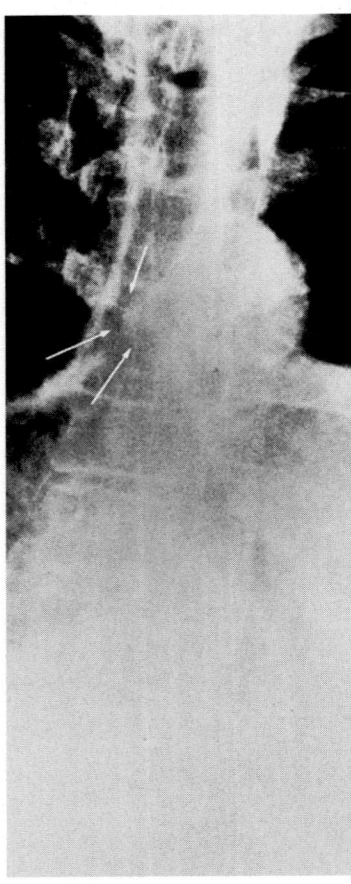

Figure 9–201. Azygos knob may be seen without tomography.

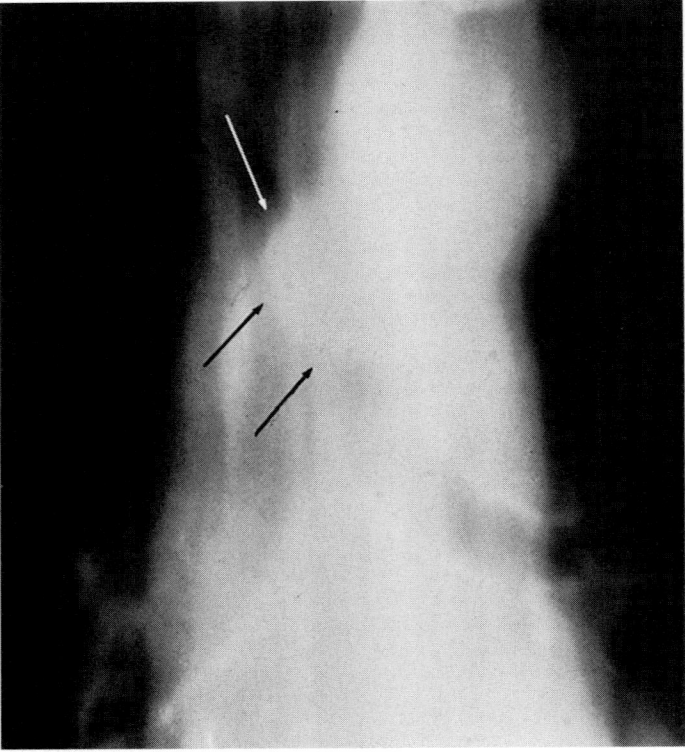

Figure 9–202. On tomography the azygos knob may simulate an intratracheal mass. (Ref: Austin JHM, Thorson MK: Normal azygous arch: Retrotracheal visualization on frontal chest tomograms. *Am J Roentgenol* 137:1205, 1981.)

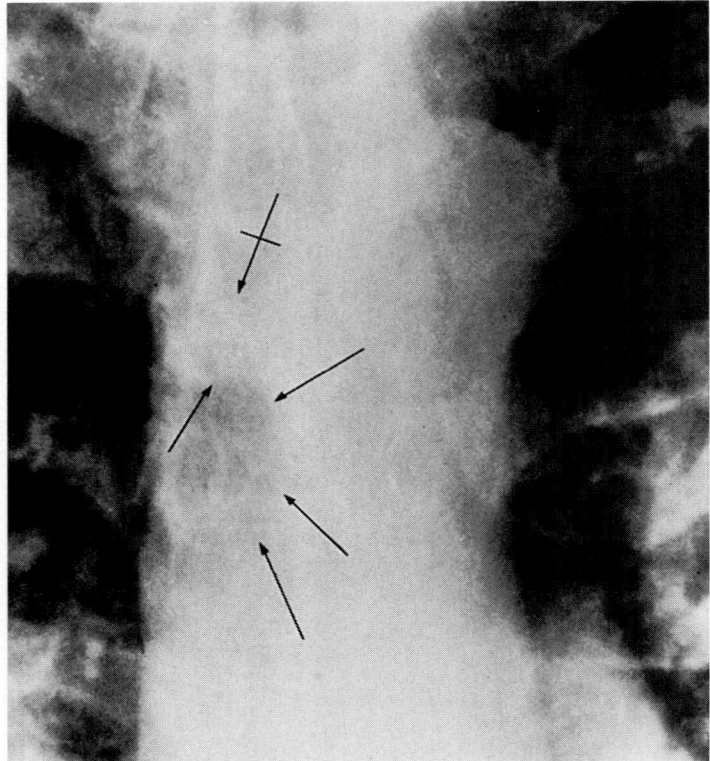

Figure 9–203. Azygopulmonary recess (→). *Hatched arrow* (↔) indicates the posterior portion of the azygos arch.

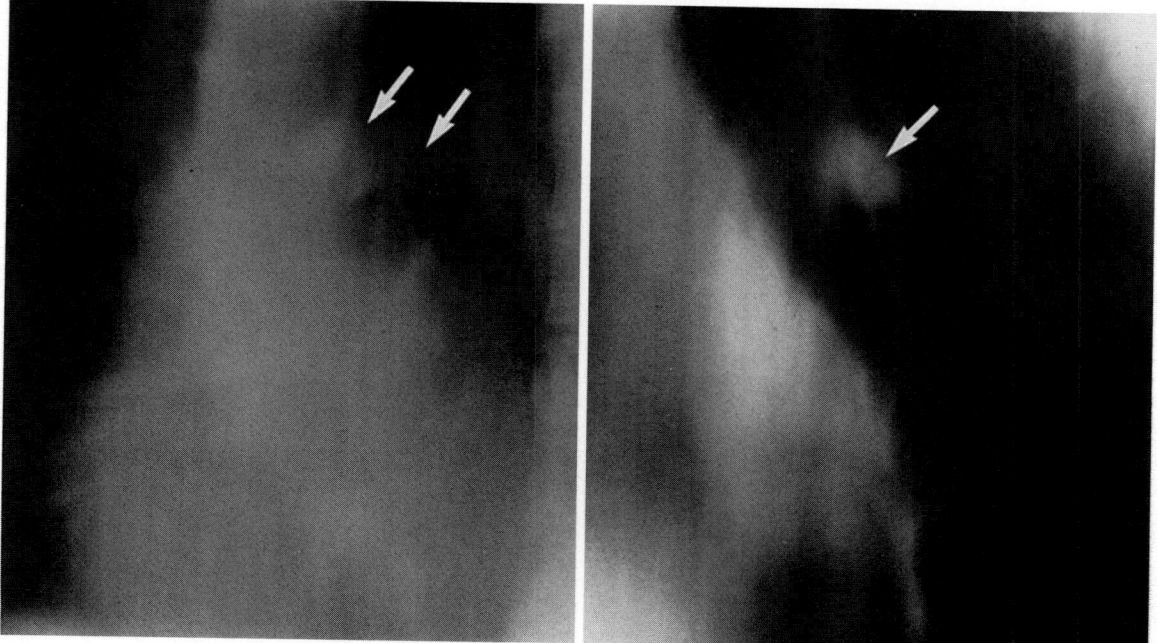

Figure 9–204. Azygos arch seen in lateral projection by tomography.

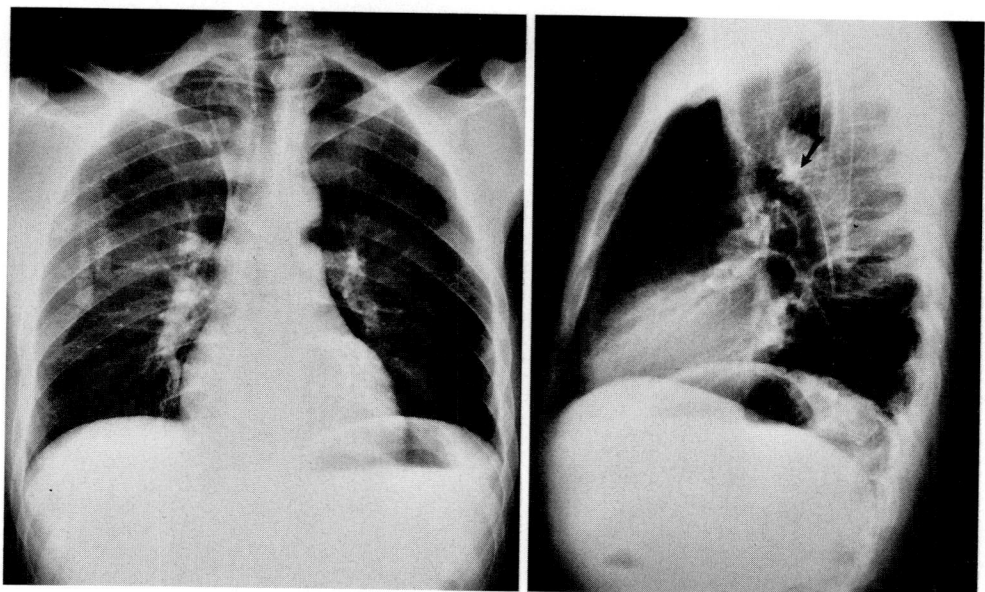

Figure 9–205. Catheter placed in the azygos vein. Note the coincidence of the catheter position with the shadows seen in the lateral projection in Figures 9–199 and 9–204.

Figure 9–206. In congenital absence of the inferior vena cava with azygos continuation, the arch of the azygos is large and may be mistaken for a mediastinal mass. (Refs: Heller RM et al: A useful sign in the recognition of azygos continuation of the inferior vena cava. *Radiology* 101:519, 1971; Pallin J et al: Azygos continuation of the inferior vena cava masquerading as neoplasm. *South Med J* 82:259, 1989.)

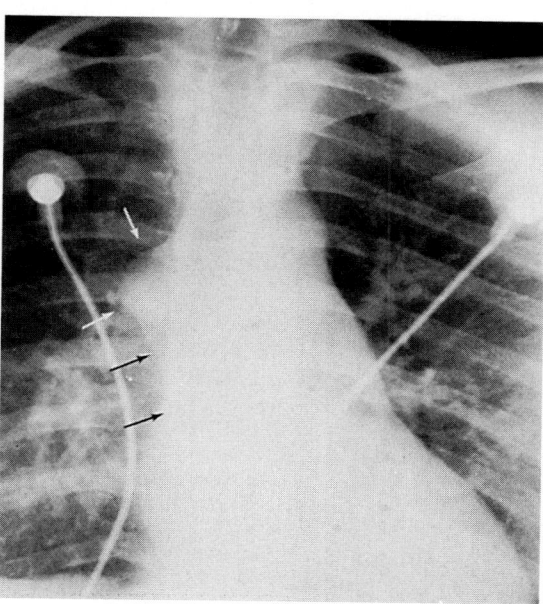

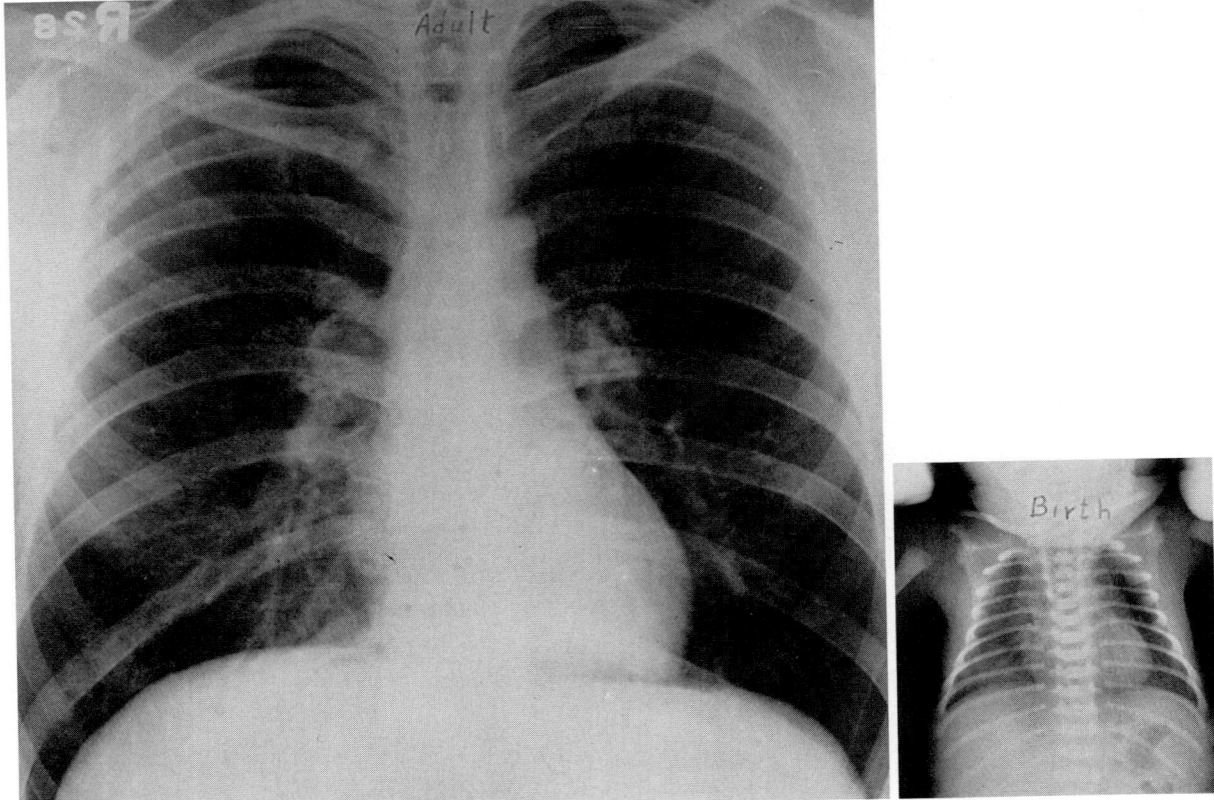

Figure 9–207. Proportional difference between the sizes of the heart and thorax in a newborn and an adult. The heart in infancy occupies a proportionately larger area of the thorax than it does in the adult, and adult criteria for heart size cannot be applied to infants and children. (From Keats TE: Pediatric radiology: Some potentially misleading variations from the adult. *Va Med* 93:630, 1966.)

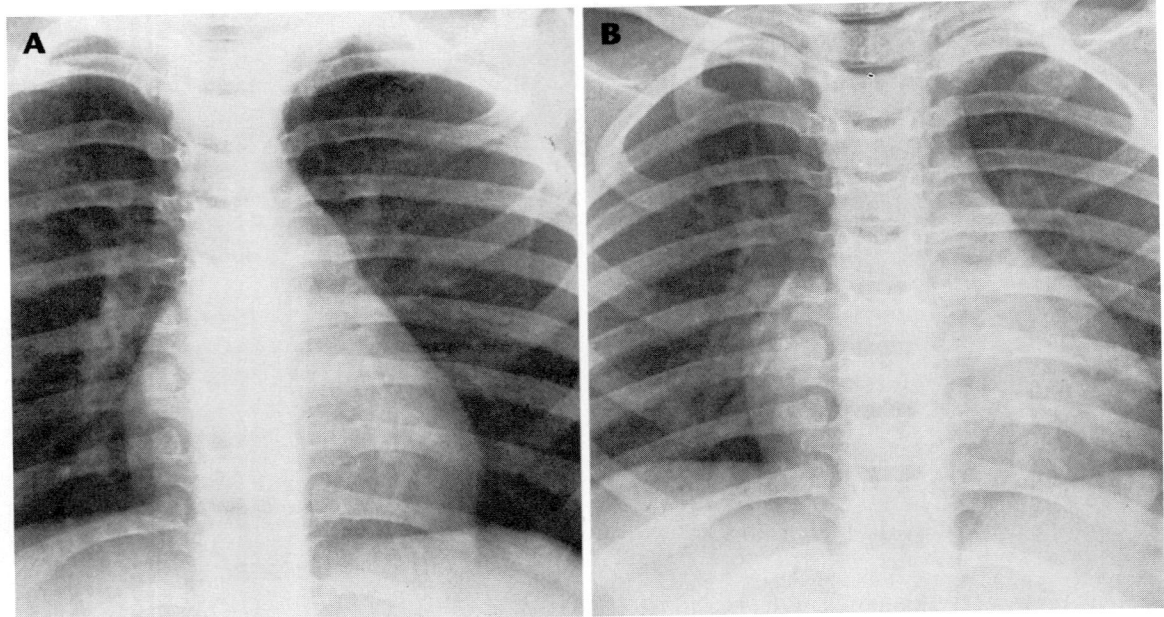

Figure 9–208. Normal variability in heart size with changes in the cardiac cycle in a child. **A,** Systole. **B,** Diastole.

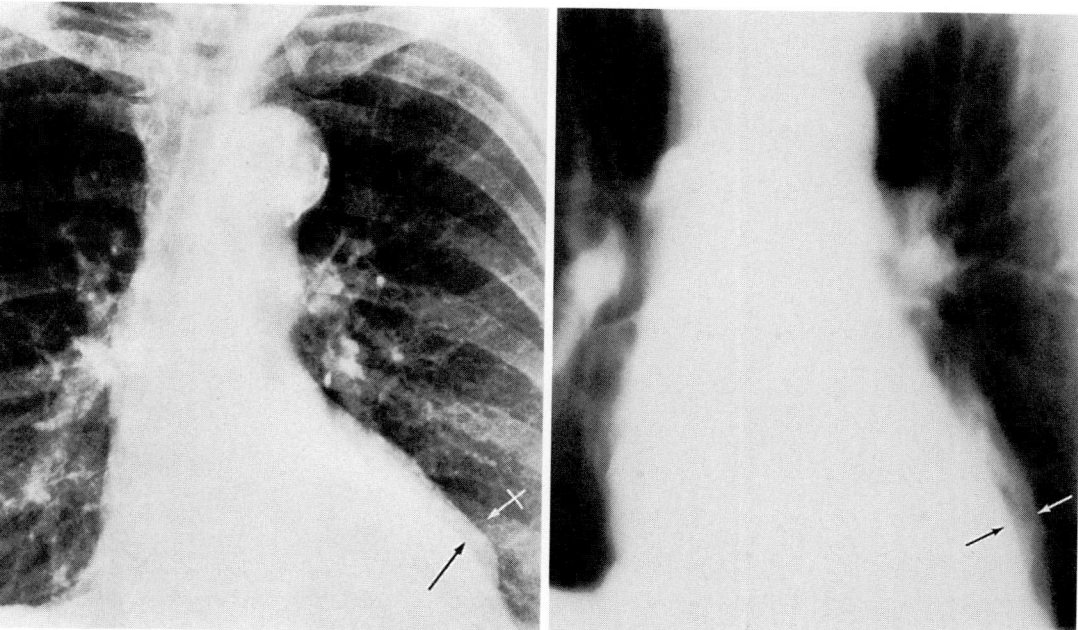

Figure 9–209. Normal variability in heart size with changes in the cardiac cycle in the adult. **A,** Systole. **B,** Diastole.

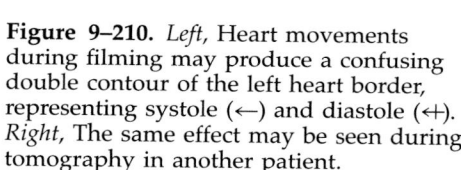

Figure 9–210. *Left,* Heart movements during filming may produce a confusing double contour of the left heart border, representing systole (←) and diastole (↔). *Right,* The same effect may be seen during tomography in another patient.

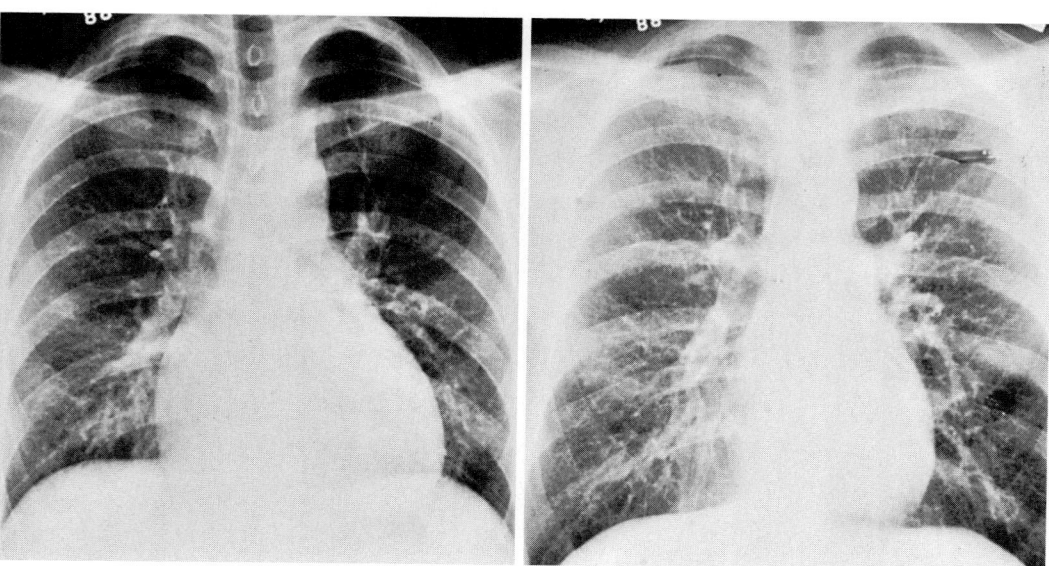

Figure 9–211. Decrease in heart size resulting from the Valsalva effect. *Left,* Baseline. *Right,* After the Valsalva maneuver.

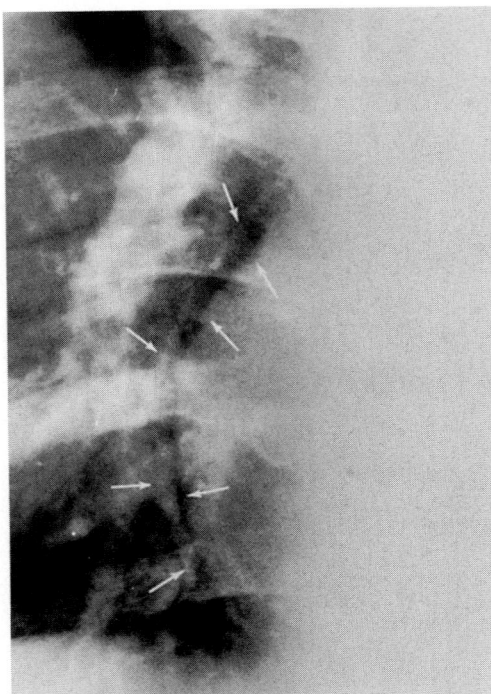

Figure 9–212. Shadows of the bronchus and pulmonary vessel adjacent to the right heart border simulate pneumopericardium.

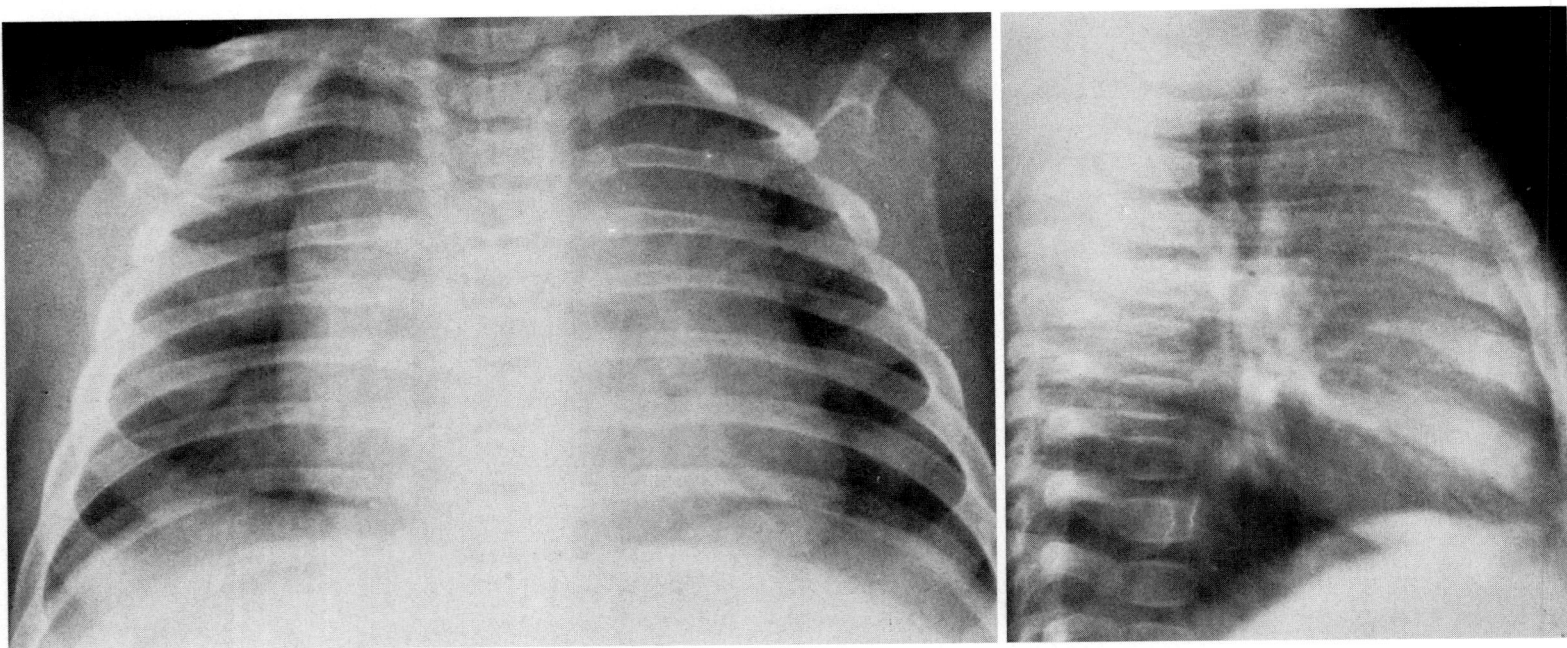

Figure 9–213. Large thymus simulating cardiomegaly. Note the normal heart size in the lateral projection.

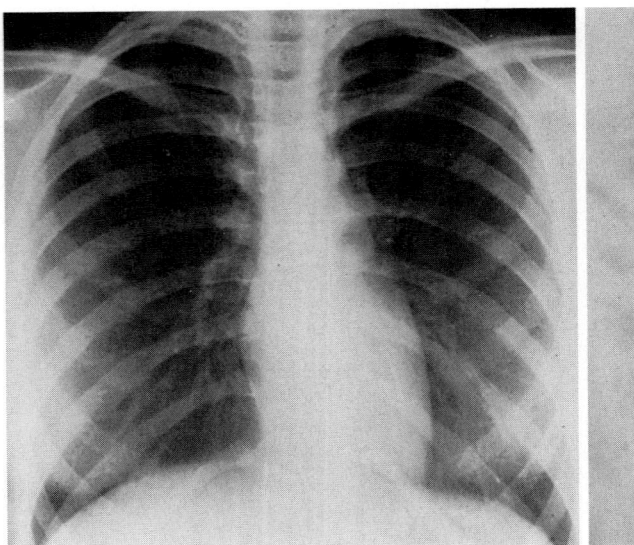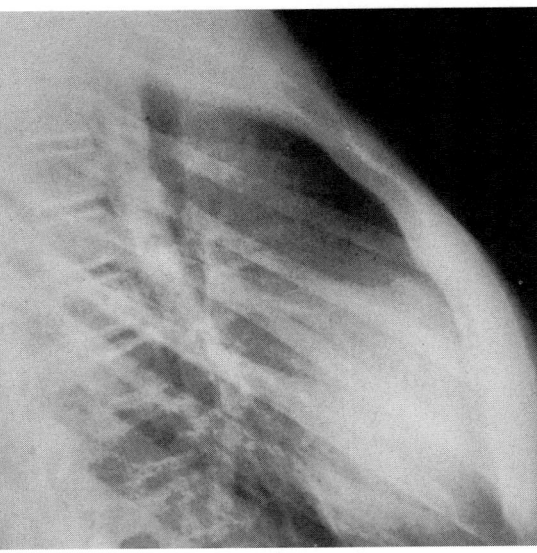

Figure 9–214. Very small hearts are not necessarily of significance and are often seen in young, asthenic women. (Ref: Swischuk LE: Microcardia: An uncommon diagnostic problem. *Am J Roentgenol* 103:115, 1968.)

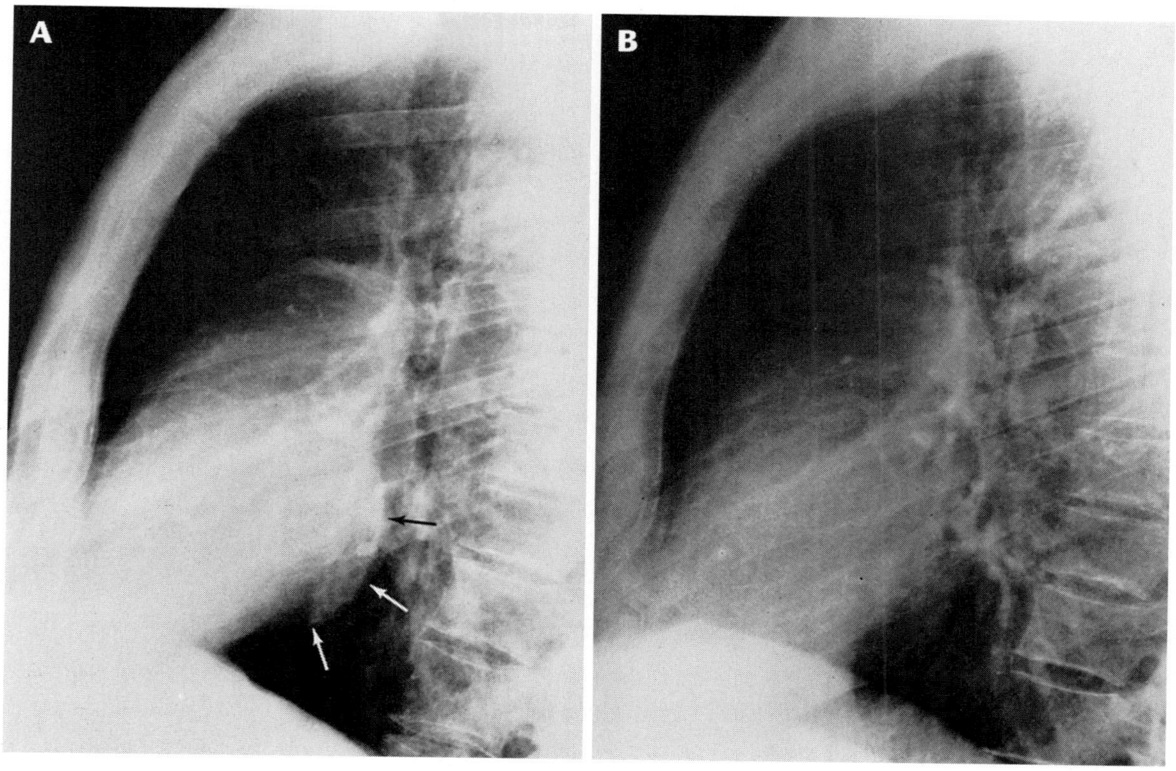

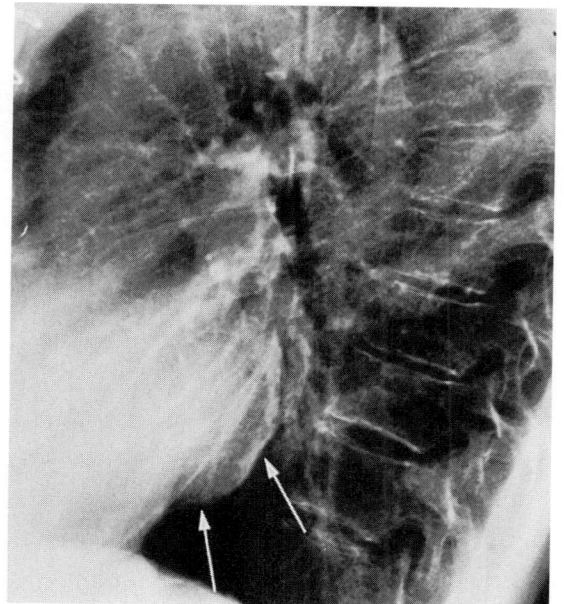

Figure 9–215. Pseudomyocardial aneurysm of the posterior wall of the left ventricle. **A,** A discrete bulge is seen on the posterior wall of the left ventricle that is not seen in an exposure made later in the same session (**B**). This bulge is seen fluoroscopically and shows apparent paradoxic movement. It represents a transient phase of contraction of the left ventricle late in systole and is a normal phenomenon. (From Keats TE, Martt JM: False paradoxic movement of the posterior wall of the left ventricle simulating myocardial aneurysm. *Radiology* 78:381, 1962.)

Figure 9–216. Additional example of the pseudoaneurysm of the posterior wall of the left ventricle.

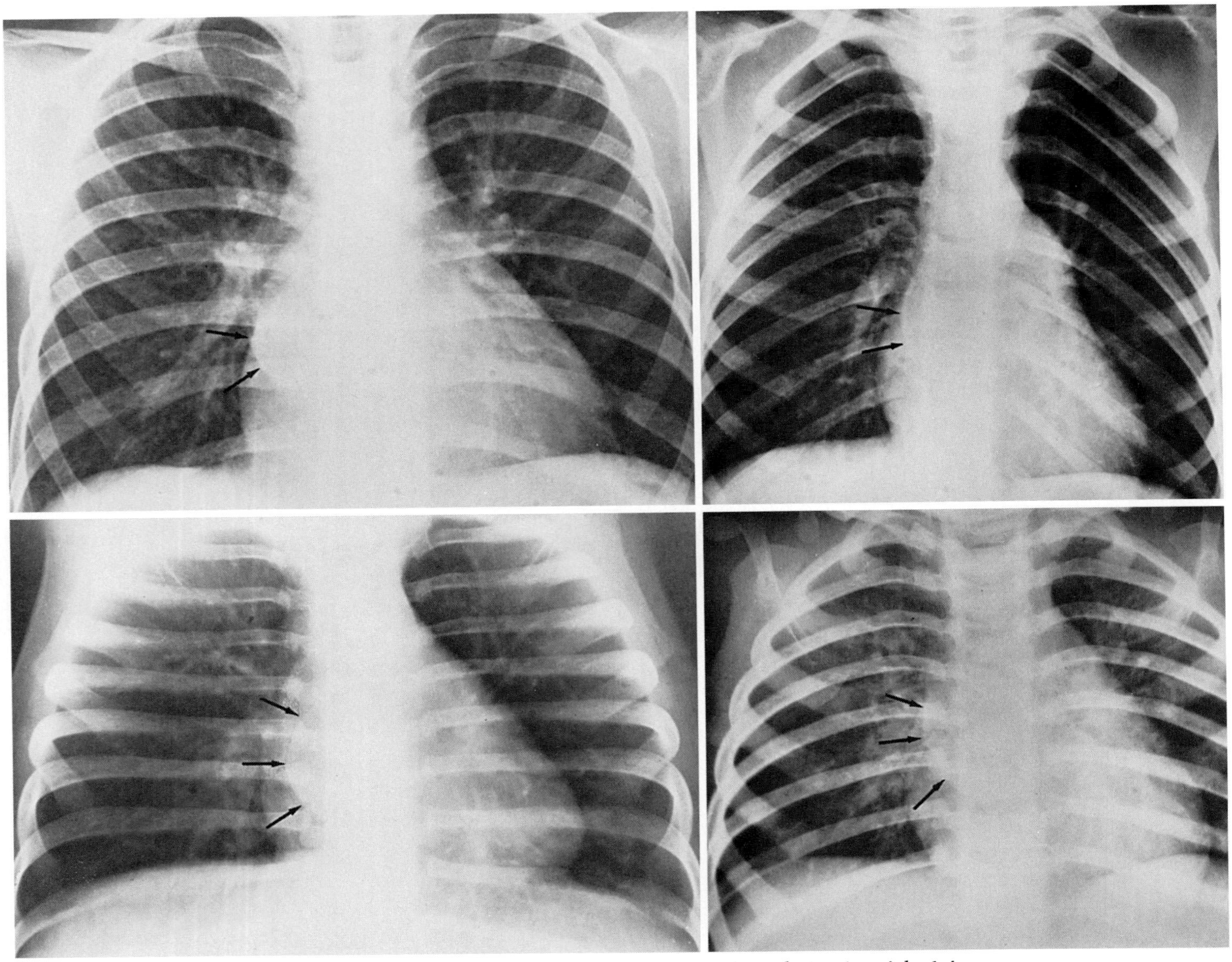

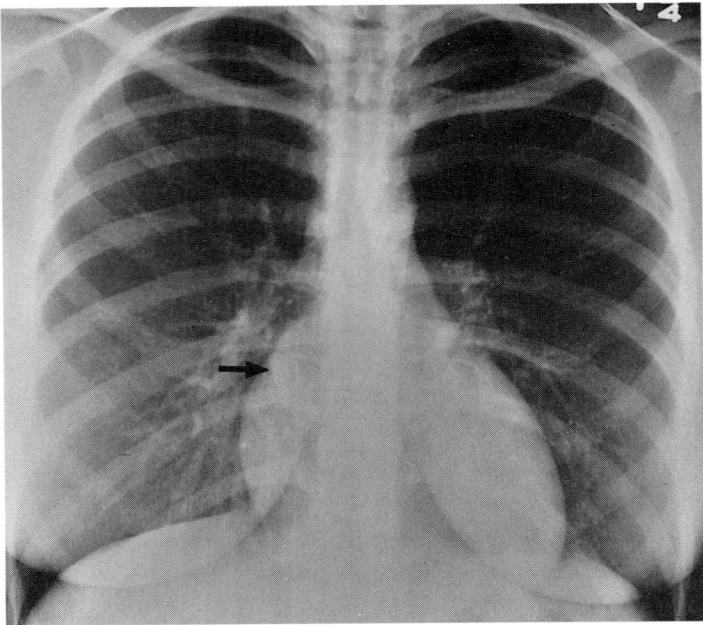

Figure 9–217. Four examples of the visualization of the right border of the left atrium in normal children. This may be seen also in adults and should not be taken as evidence of left atrial enlargement in itself unless correlative evidence is present in the other projections. (Ref: Rosario-Medina W et al: Normal left atrium: Appearance in children on frontal chest radiographs. *Radiology* 161:345, 1986.)

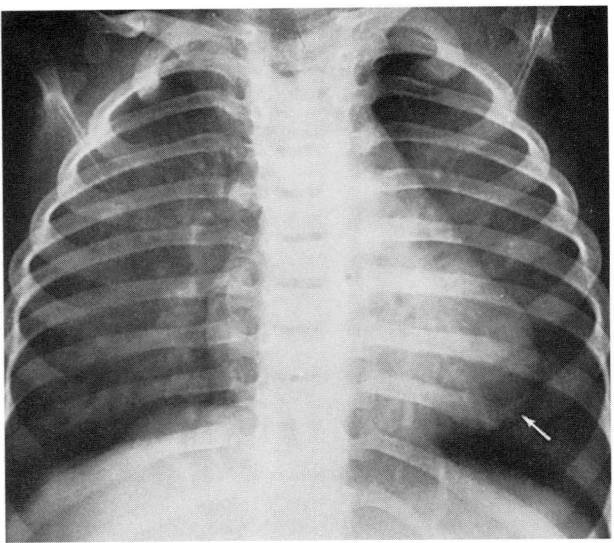

Figure 9–218. The normal left atrium in a 19-year-old woman.

Figure 9–219. Elevation of the cardiac apex in a normal 2-year-old child, produced by very deep inspiration. This configuration should not be confused with the alteration caused by ventricular hypertrophy.

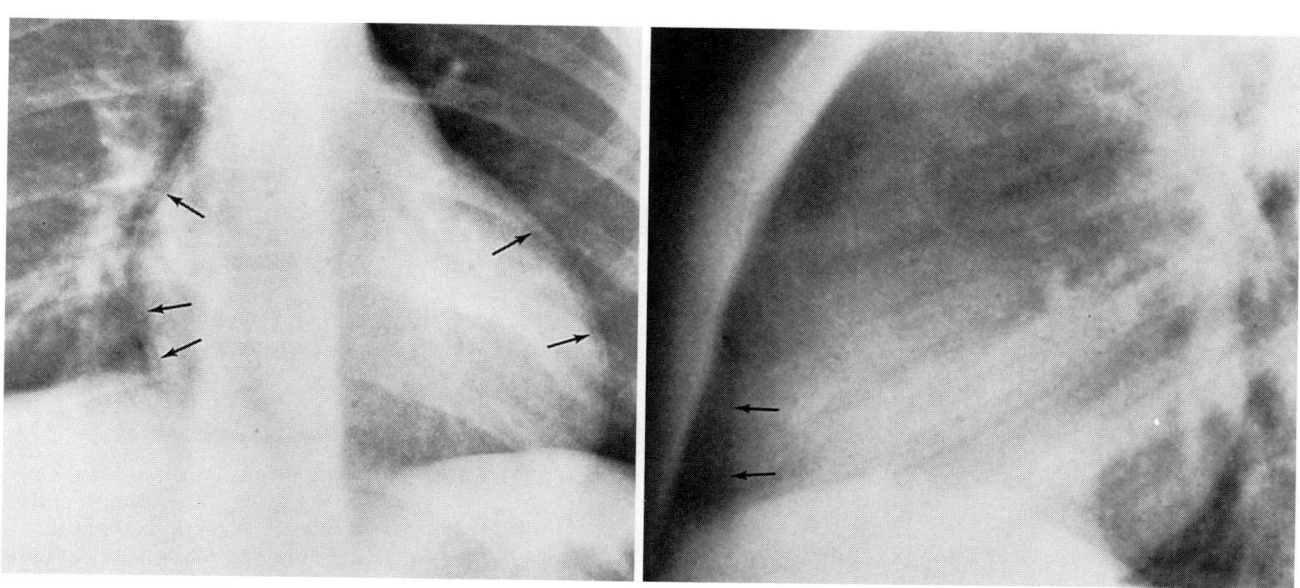

Figure 9–220. Two examples of the subepicardial fat line seen as a lucent crescent beyond the heart shadow (←). The pericardium (↔) is sandwiched between the subepicardial fat and the epicardial fat. (Ref: Lane EJ Jr, Carsky EW: Epicardial fat: Lateral plain film analysis in normals and in pericardial effusion. *Radiology* 91:1, 1968.)

Figure 9–221. Subepicardial fat, which could be mistaken for pneumopericardium, seen in frontal and lateral projections in a 7-year-old boy. (Ref: Kremens V: Demonstration of pericardial shadow on routine chest roentgenogram: A new roentgen finding. *Radiology* 64:72, 1955.)

Figure 9–222. Congenital absence of the left pericardium. This appearance is quite characteristic. The heart is shifted to the left in the absence of pectus excavatum of the sternum, and there is a large bulge in the left contour of the heart in the area normally occupied by the main pulmonary artery (*arrow*). (Ref: Tabakin BJ et al: Congenital absence of the left pericardium. *Am J Roentgenol* 94:122, 1965.)

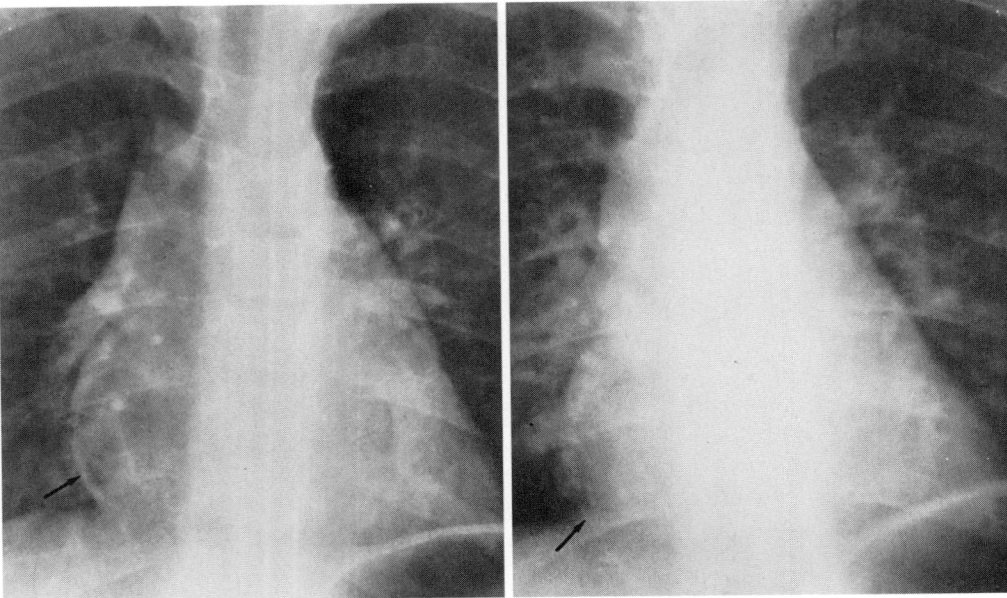

Figure 9–223. Visualization of the pericardium at the right side of the heart border in a 4-year-old boy on two different occasions. Its visualization is due to the presence of subepicardial fat. The pericardial shadow should not be misinterpreted as calcification in the pericardium. (Ref: Keats TE: Four normal anatomic variations of importance to radiologists. *Am J Roentgenol* 78:89, 1957.)

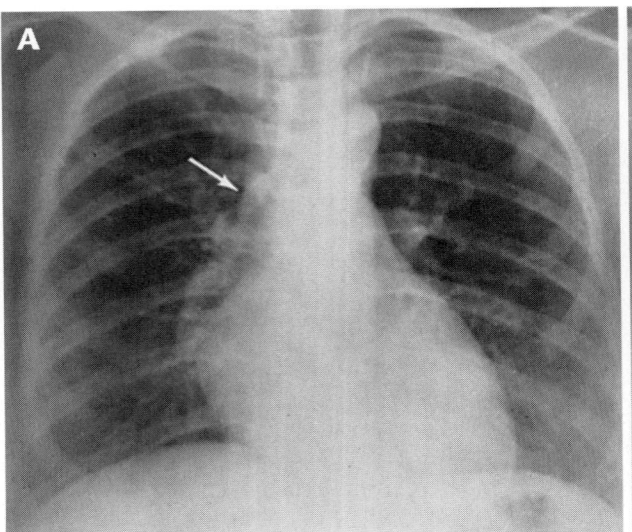
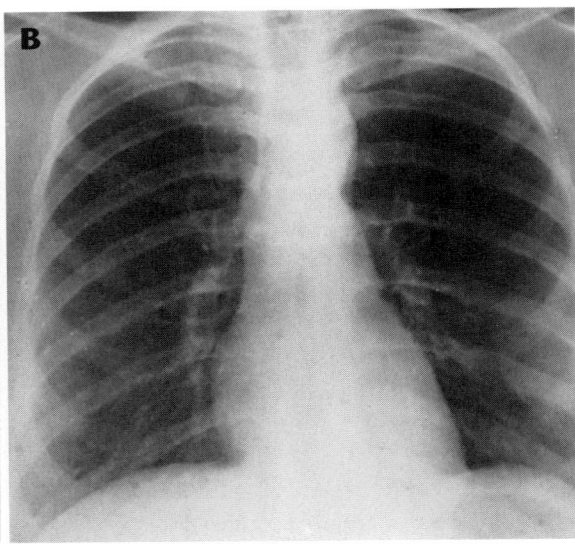

Figure 9–224. Normal cardiac changes in pregnancy. **A,** In addition to cardiac enlargement, there is a rather selective dilation of the right atrium in some normal women during pregnancy. In addition, the arch of the azygos vein enlarges (←). **B,** Regression of these changes shortly after parturition (Refs: Keats TE, Martt JM: Selective dilatation of the right atrium in pregnancy. *Am J Roentgenol* 91:307, 1964; Keats TE et al: Mensuration of the azygos vein and its application to the study of cardiopulmonary disease. *Radiology* 90:990, 1968.)

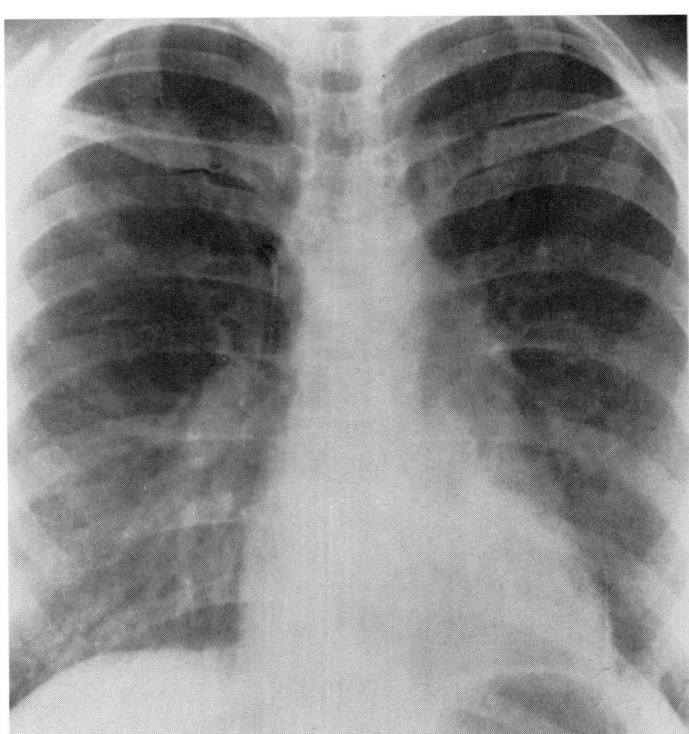
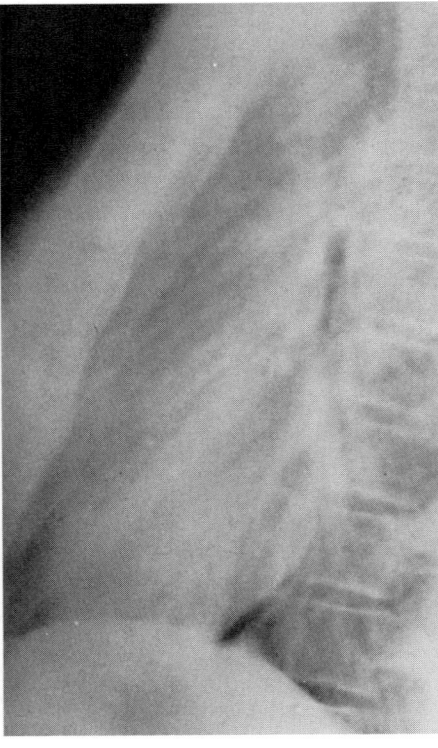

Figure 9–225. Straight back syndrome, producing flattening of the heart and prominence of the pulmonary artery. Individuals with congenital absence of the normal dorsal kyphosis and narrow sagittal diameter of the chest present striking alterations in cardiac contour compounded by the coexistence of physical findings that may mimic organic heart disease. (Ref: de Leon A et al: The straight back syndrome. *Circulation* 17:197, 1965.) Note also the partial obliteration of the descending aorta, which is an associated finding in patients with narrow chests. (Ref: Okawada T et al: Partial obliteration of the descending aortic contours: A pitfall on plain chest radiographs. *Clin Radiol* 48:192, 1993.)

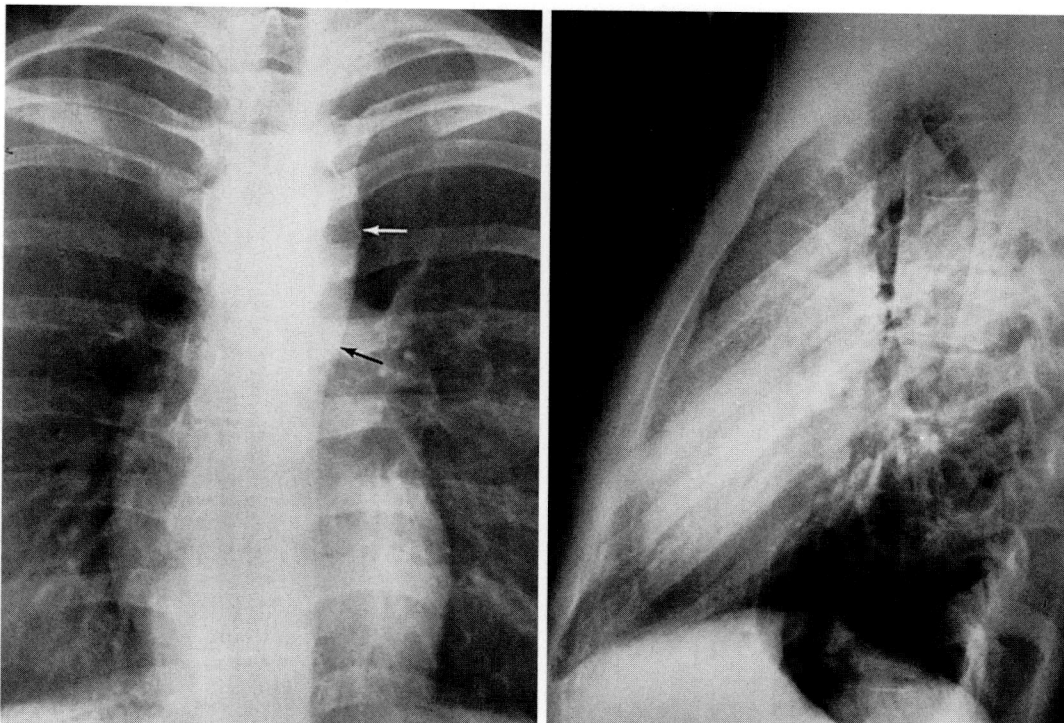

Figure 9–226. Straight back syndrome showing distortion of the aortic arch and descending aorta.

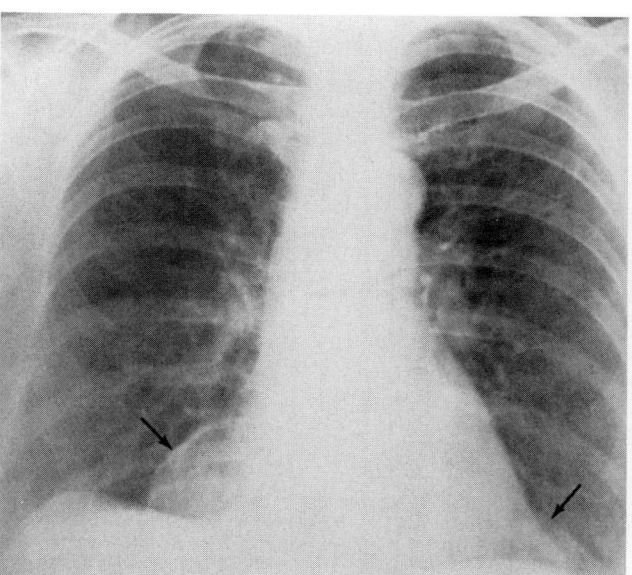
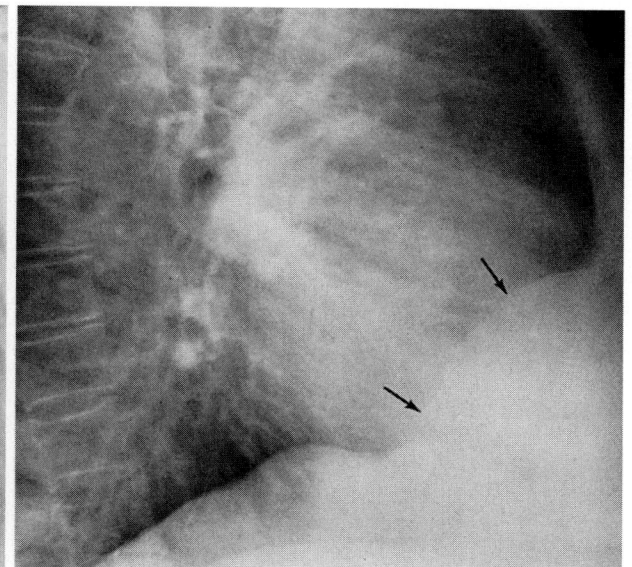

Figure 9–227. Normal epipericardial fat pads. These fat collections may be confused with cysts and neoplasms. They vary in size with the weight of the patient. (Ref: Holt JF: Epipericardial fat shadows in differential diagnosis. *Radiology* 48:472, 1947.)

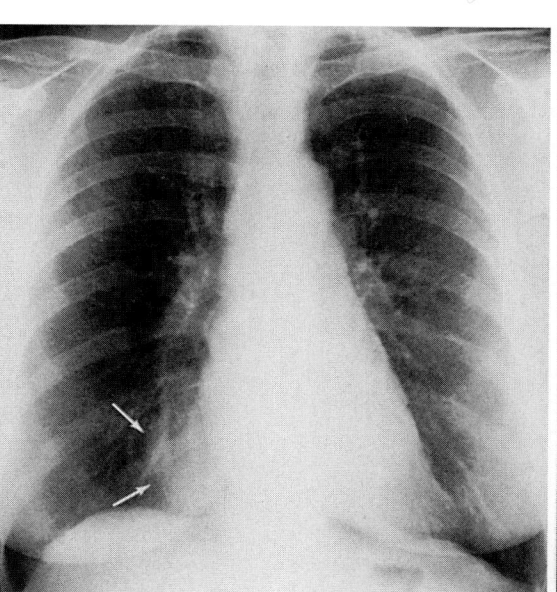
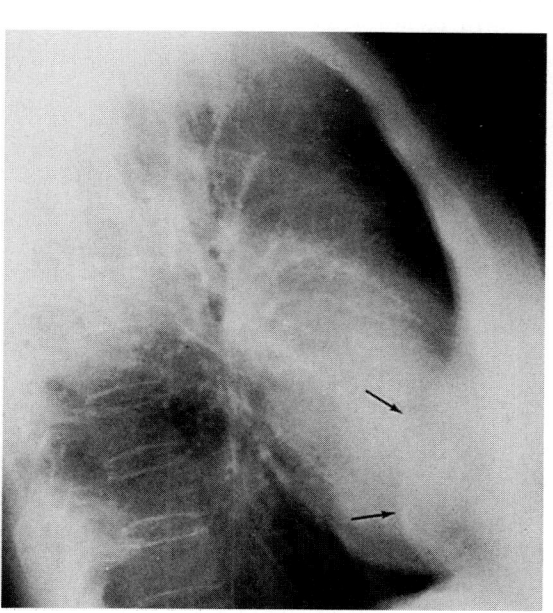

Figure 9–228. Unusual configuration of the epipericardial fat pad.

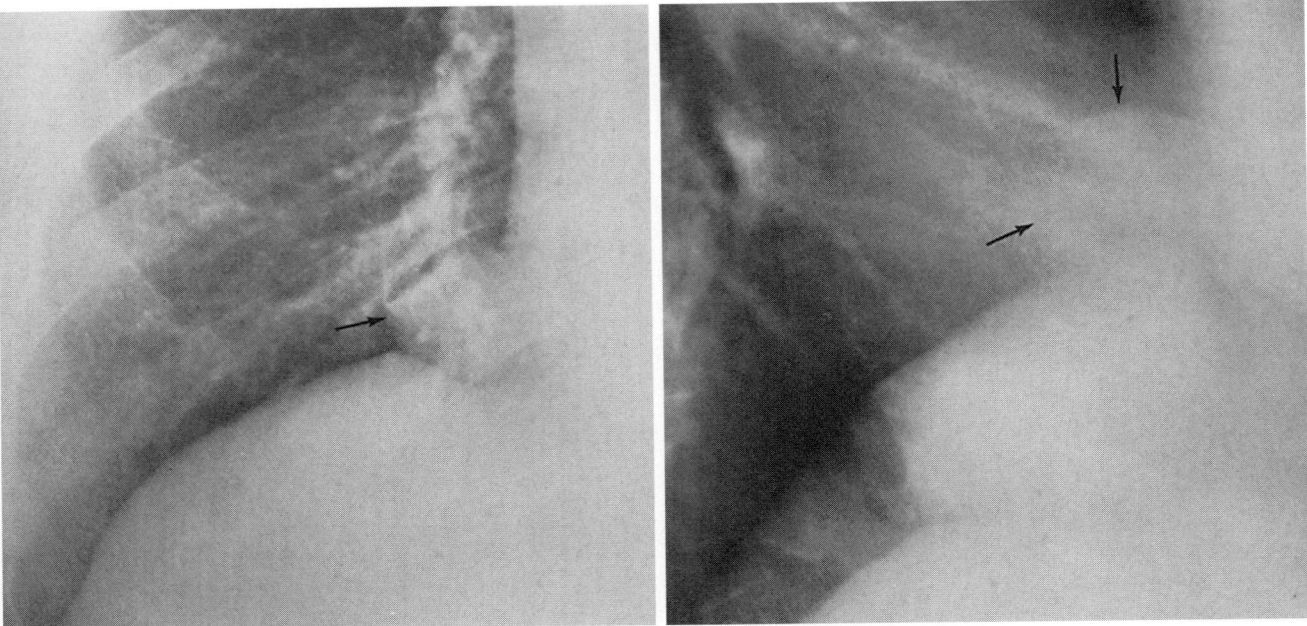

Figure 9–229. Small, discrete, round epipericardial fat pad in the right cardiophrenic angle.

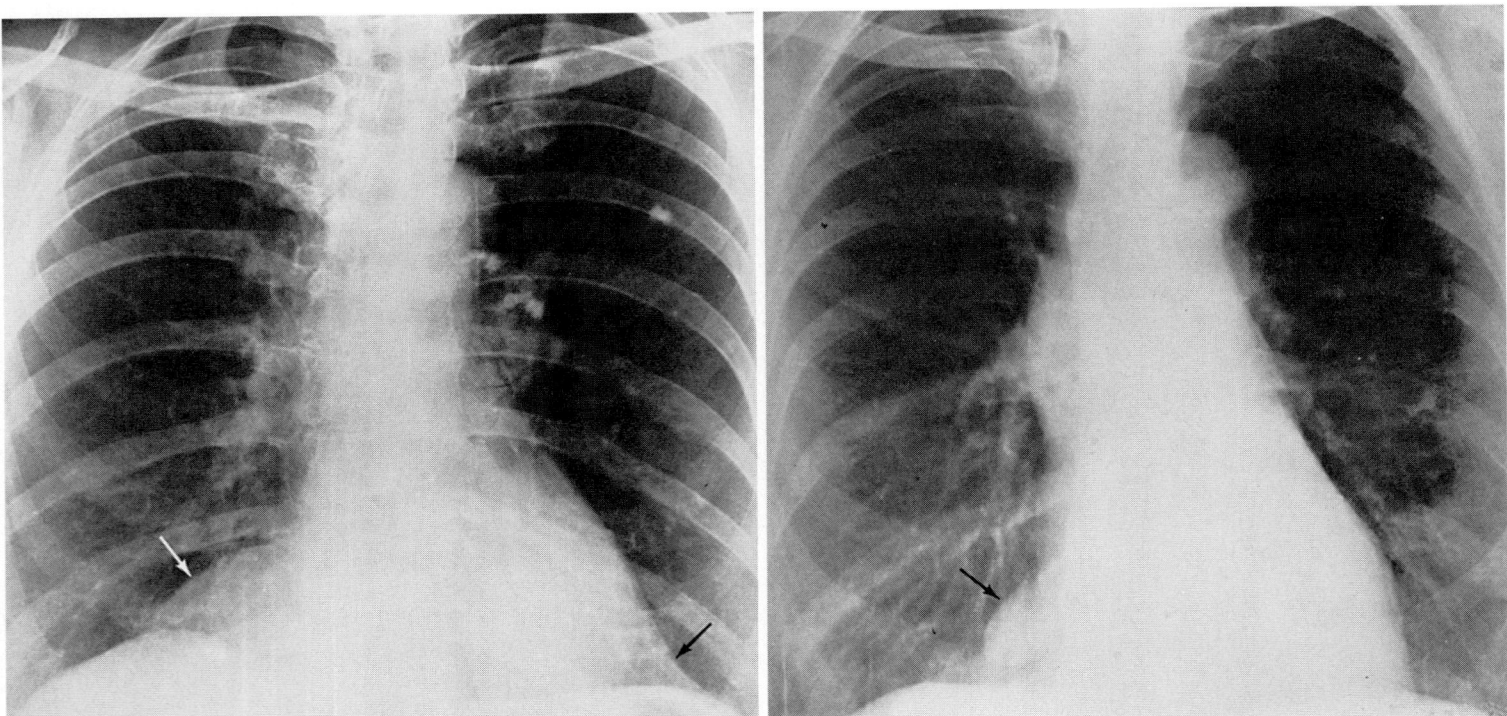

Figure 9–230. Additional examples of epipericardial fat pads. (Ref: Nahon JR: Roentgen characteristics of the epipericardial fat pad with a case report. *Radiology* 65:745, 1955.)

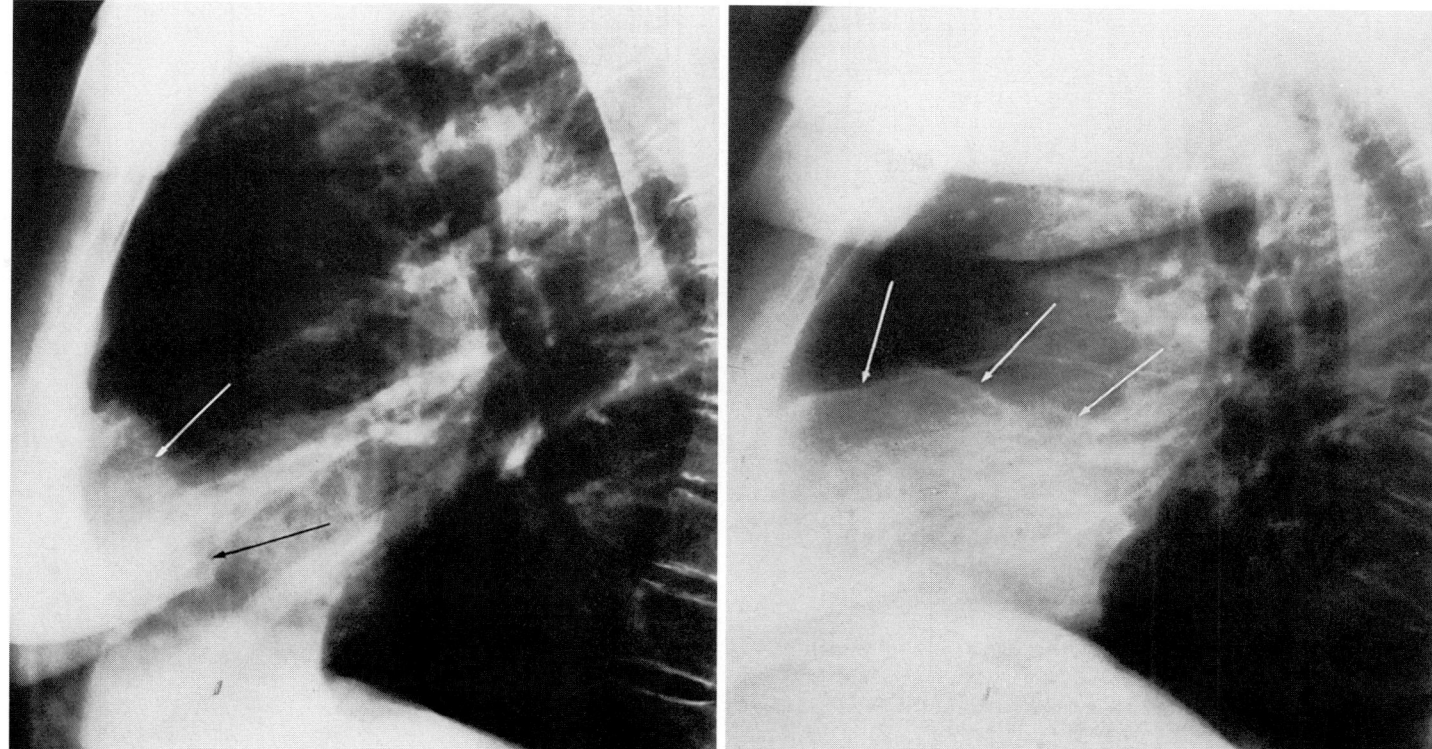

Figure 9–231. Increasing size of epipericardial fat pad over a 6-year period of progressive obesity.

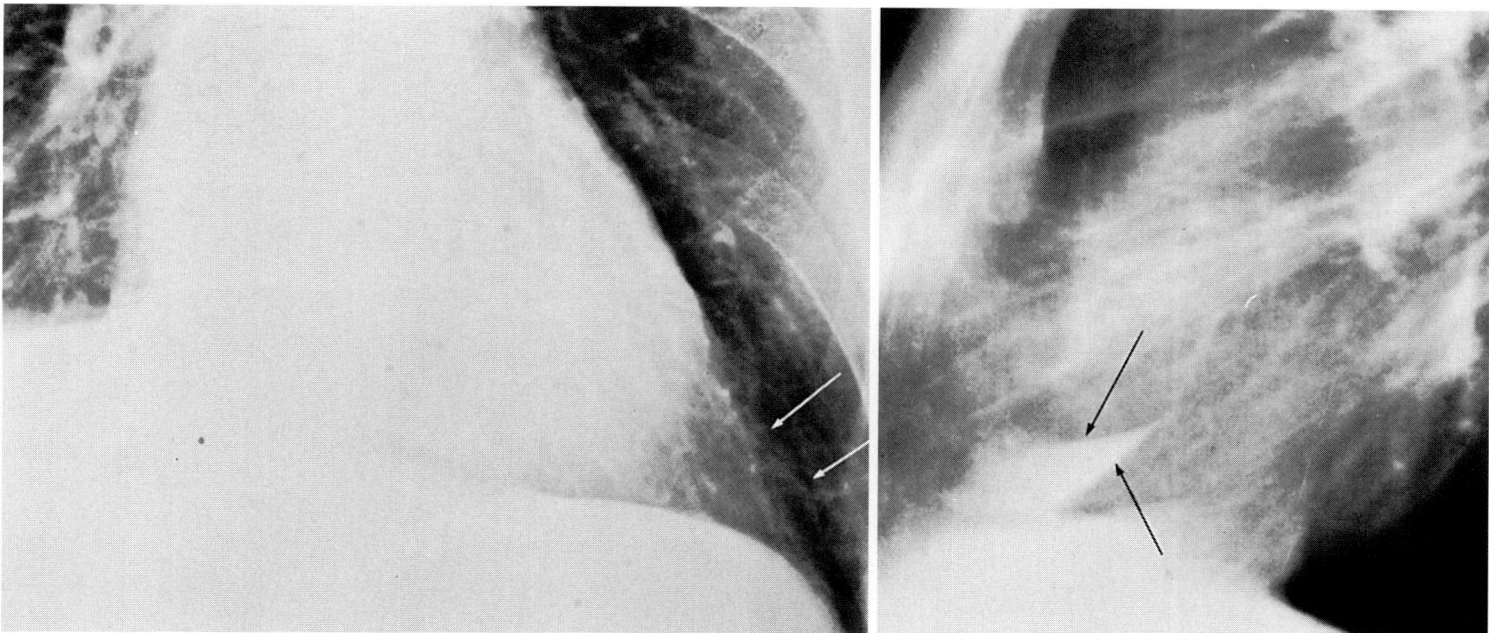

Figure 9–232. Extension of the epipericardial fat pad into the major interlobar fissure. (Ref: Gale ME, Greif WL: Intrafissural fat: CT correlation with chest radiography. *Radiology* 160:333, 1986.)

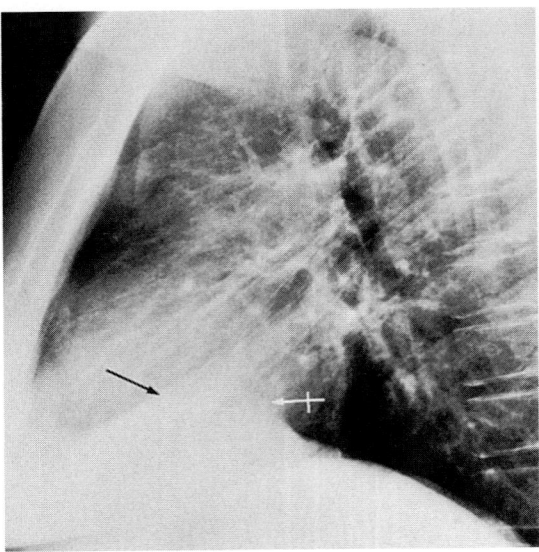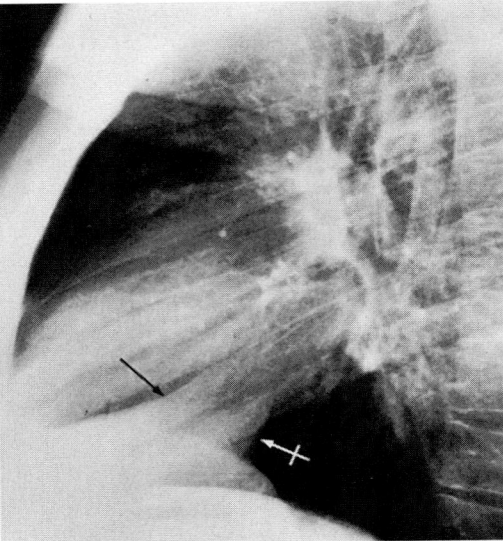

Figure 9–233. Two examples of triangular shadows at the lung base produced by extension of the epipericardial fat pad into the left major fissure anteriorly (←) and the shadow of the inferior vena cava posteriorly (↔). (Ref: Fisher ER, Godwin JD: Extrapleural fat collections: Pseudotumors and other confusing manifestations. *Am J Roentgenol* 161:47, 1993.)

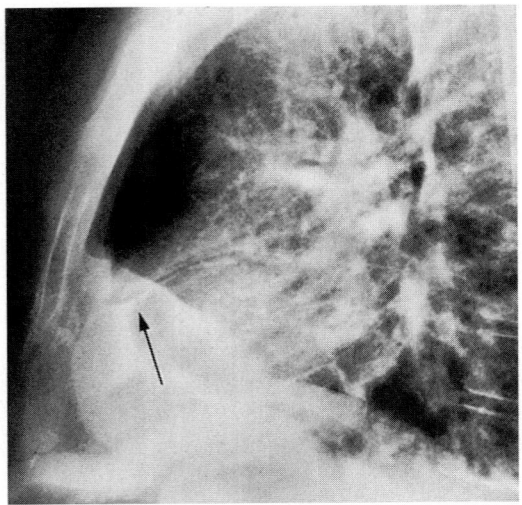

Figure 9–234. Extension of an epipericardial fat pad into the minor interlobar fissure.

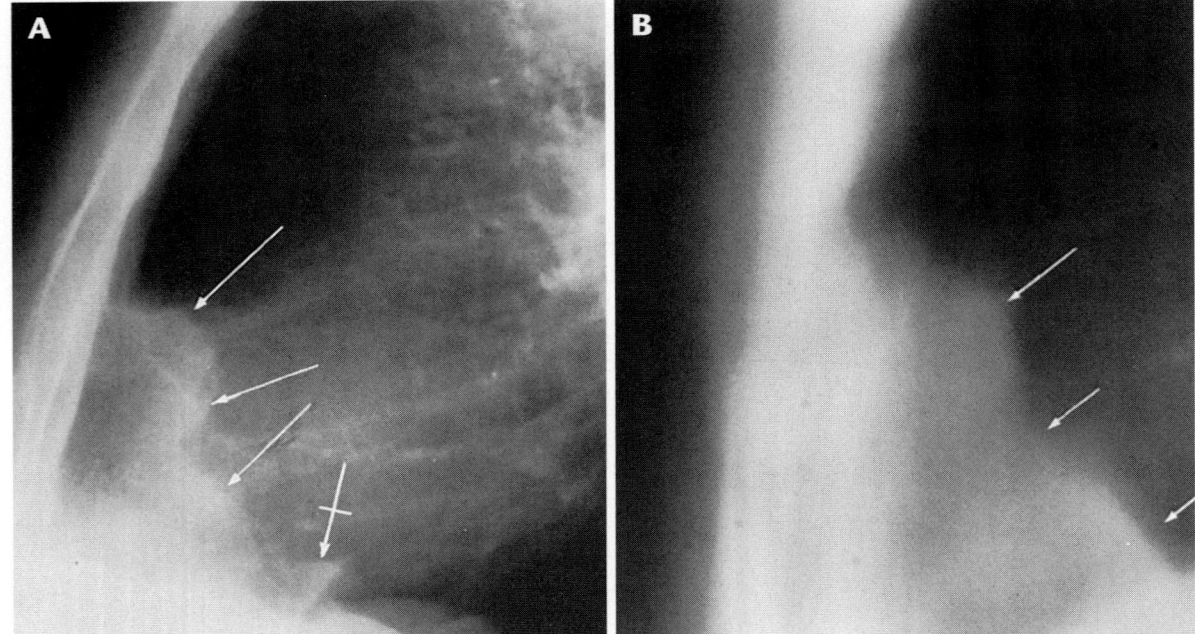

Figure 9–235. Irregular epipericardial fat pad misinterpreted as a neoplasm and removed by thoracotomy (→). **A,** Plain film, lateral view. Note extension into the major interlobar fissure (↔). **B,** Tomogram.

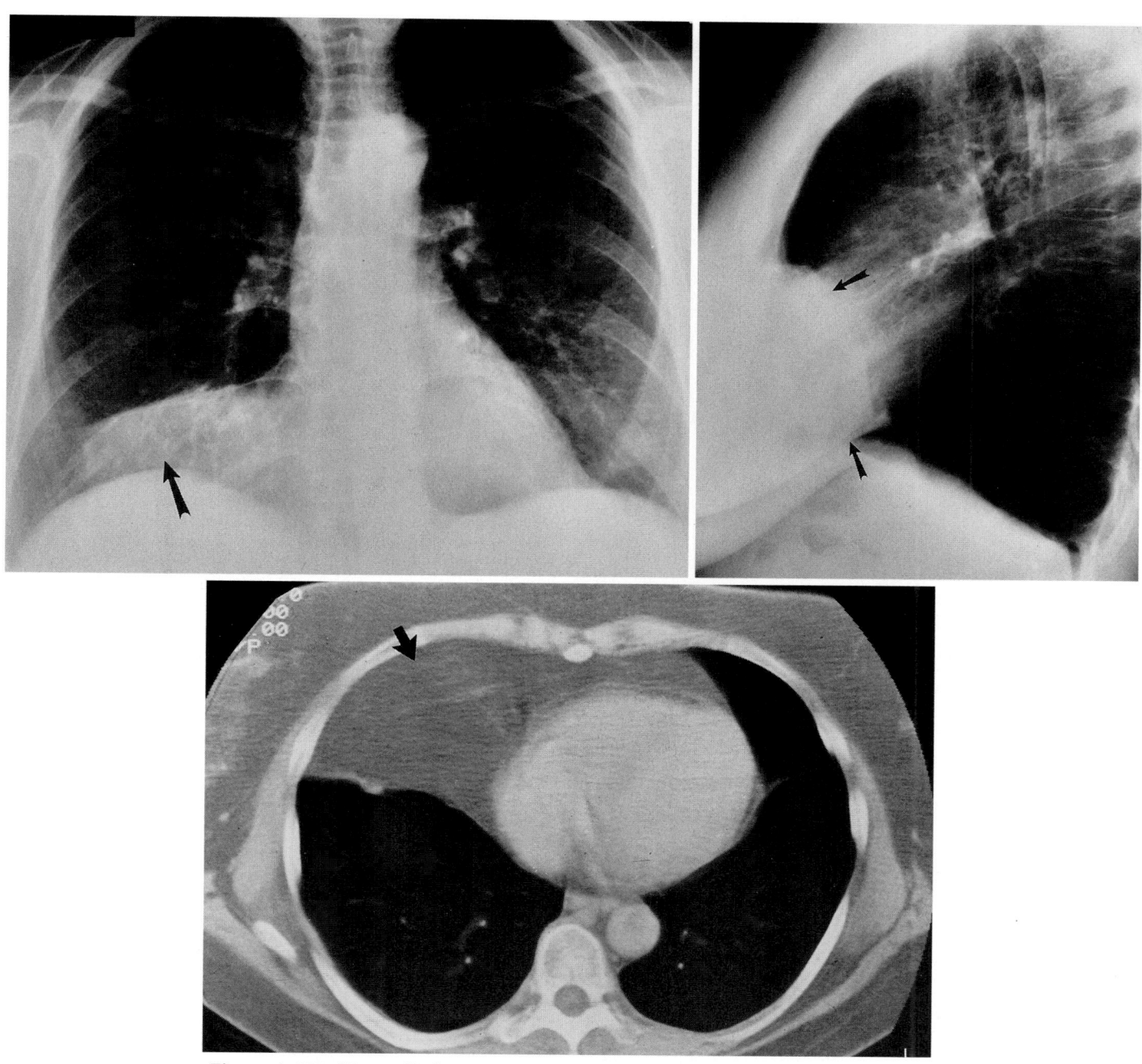

Figure 9–236. *Left,* Baseline film. *Right,* 10 years later right middle lobe atelectasis was misdiagnosed because of superimposition of epipericardial fat pad with extension into the major interlobar fissure (*arrow*).

Figure 9–237. Unusually large epipericardial fat pad on the right with CT demonstration.

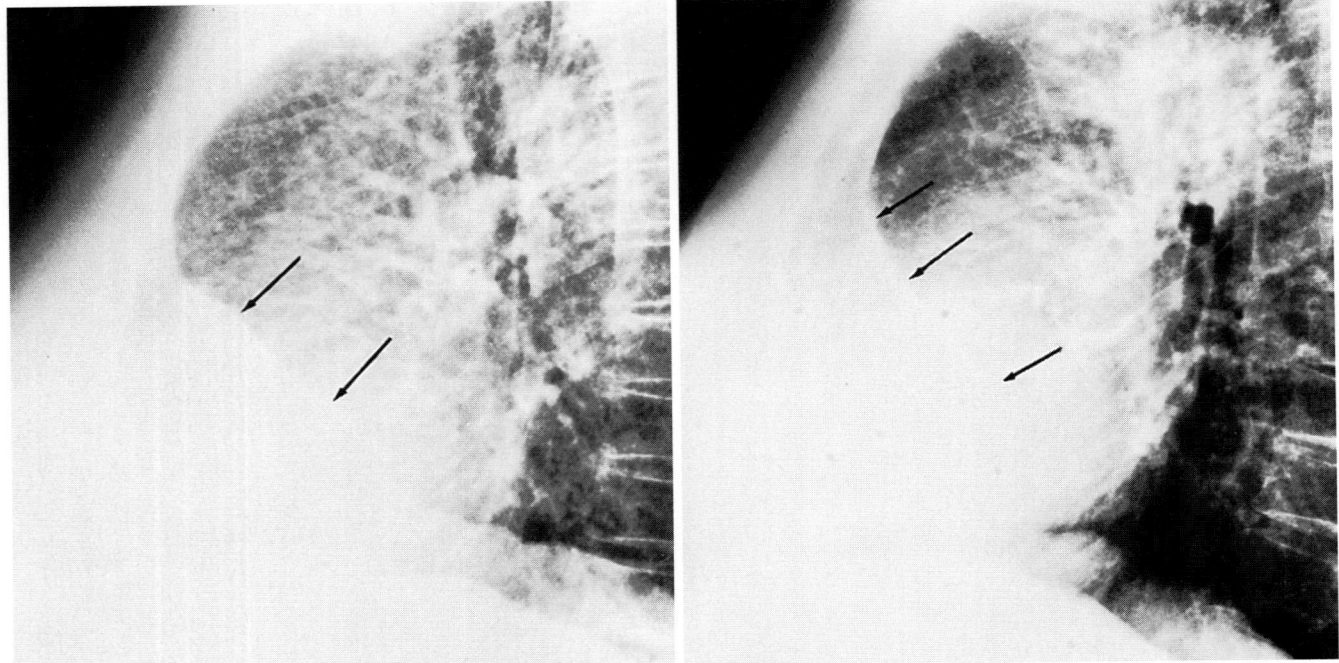

Figure 9–238. Unusual configuration of the epipericardial fat pad, showing increasing size over a 1-year period of increasing obesity.

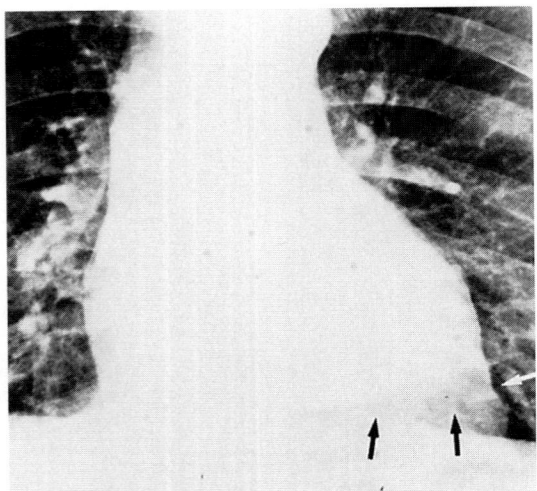

Figure 9–239. Lucency under the heart produced by the pressure of epipericardial fat.

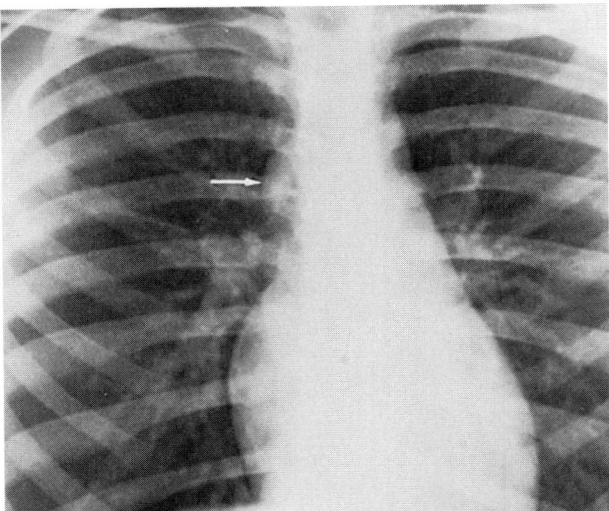

Figure 9–240. Normal but prominent azygos arch in a young adult. This structure can be distinguished from an enlarged azygos node by noting its change in size between the supine and upright positions. (Ref: Keats TE et al: Mensuration of the arch of the azygos vein and its application to the study of cardiovascular disease. *Radiology* 90:990, 1968.)

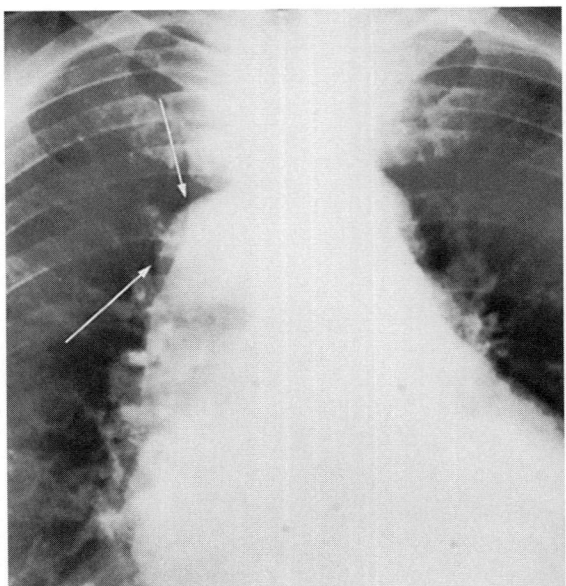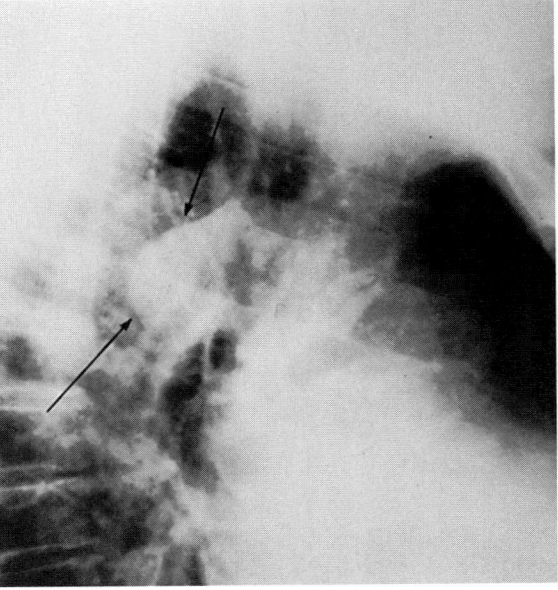

Figure 9–241. Marked dilatation of the arch of the azygos vein in congenital interruption of the inferior vena cava. Absence of a shadow of the inferior vena cava in the lateral projection has been described. However, this sign is not always useful in diagnosis, since it may not be seen in some normal individuals. (Ref: Heller R et al: A useful sign in recognition of azygos continuation of the inferior vena cava. *Radiology* 101:519, 1971.)

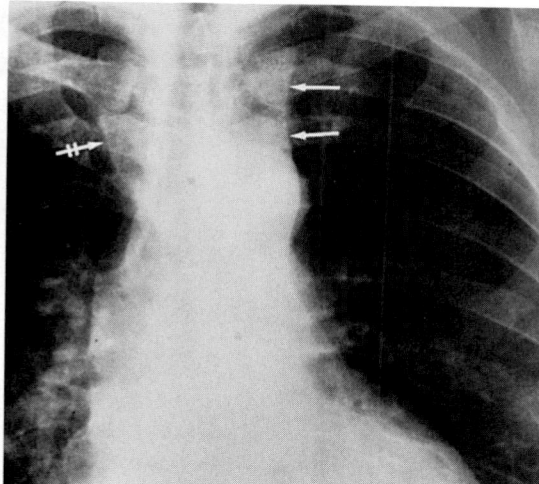

Figure 9–242. Shadow of the left subclavian artery in a 75-year-old man (←). The edge of the manubrium is seen on the opposite side (⊬).

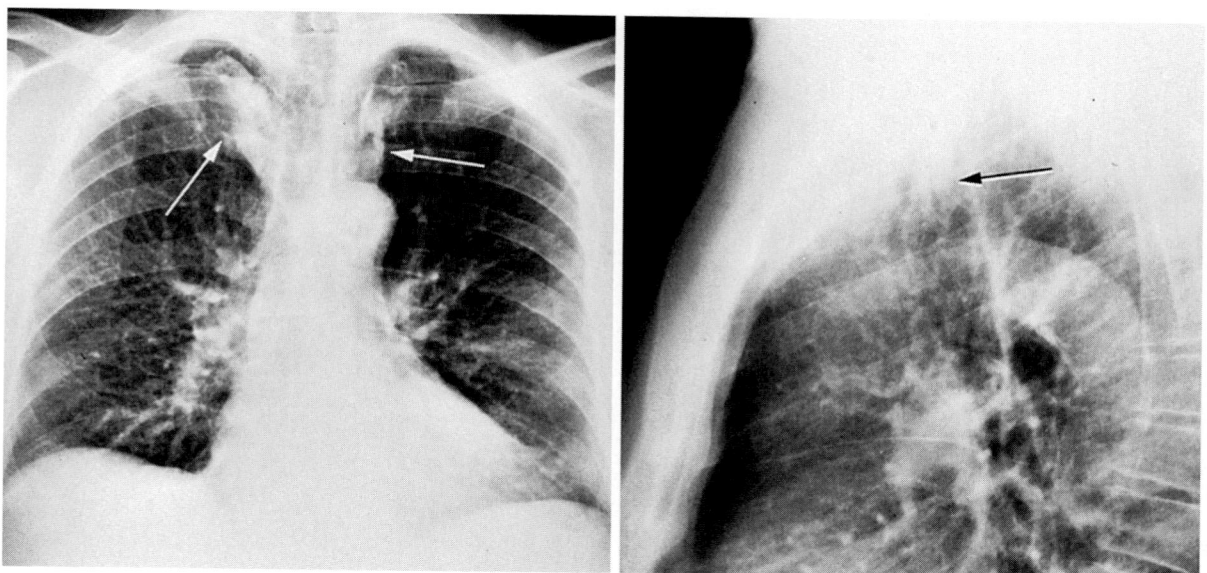

Figure 9–243. Marked calcification in the great vessels.

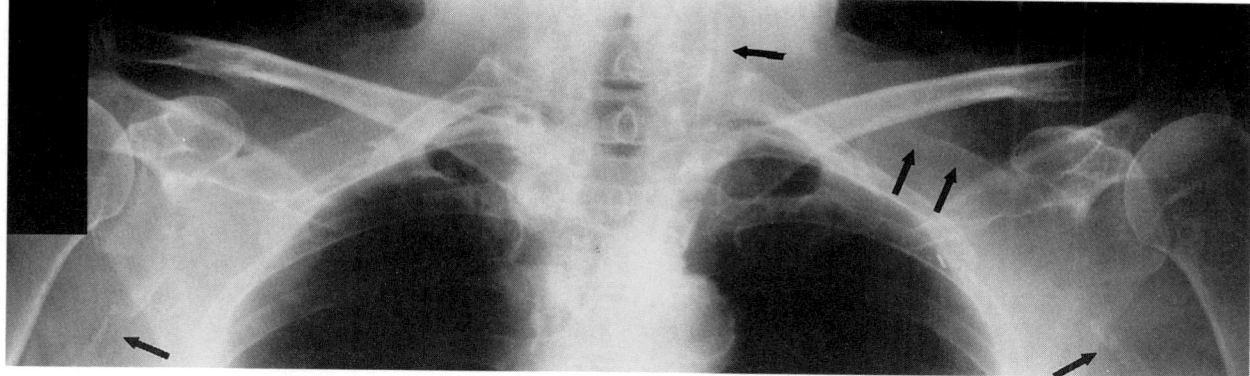

Figure 9–244. Marked calcification of the carotid and subclavian arteries.

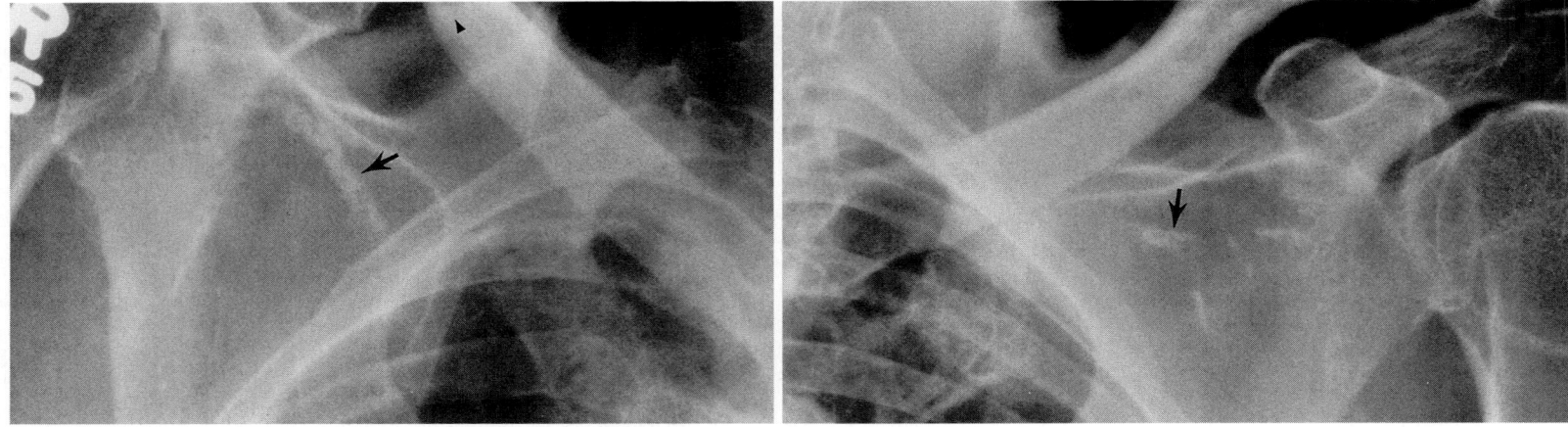

Figure 9–245. Marked calcification of the subclavian arteries.

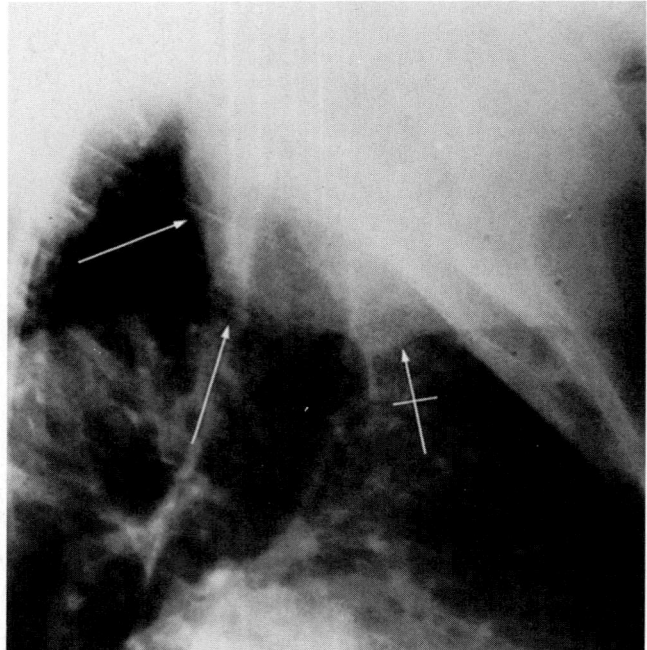

Figure 9–246. Mass effect produced by dilated brachiocephalic vessels (↔) and arm shadow (→).

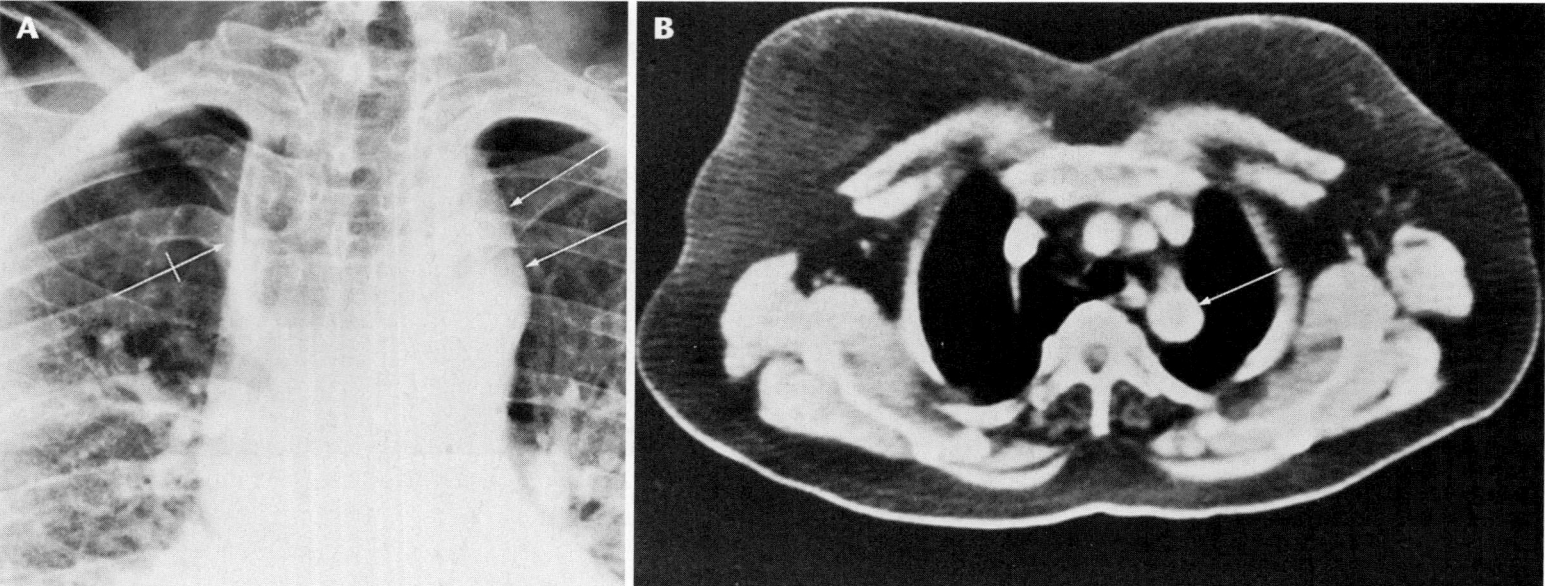

Figure 9–247. A, Broadened mediastinal outline on the left is due to a very large left subclavian artery (→). An azygos lobe is present (↔). **B,** CT shows the large artery.

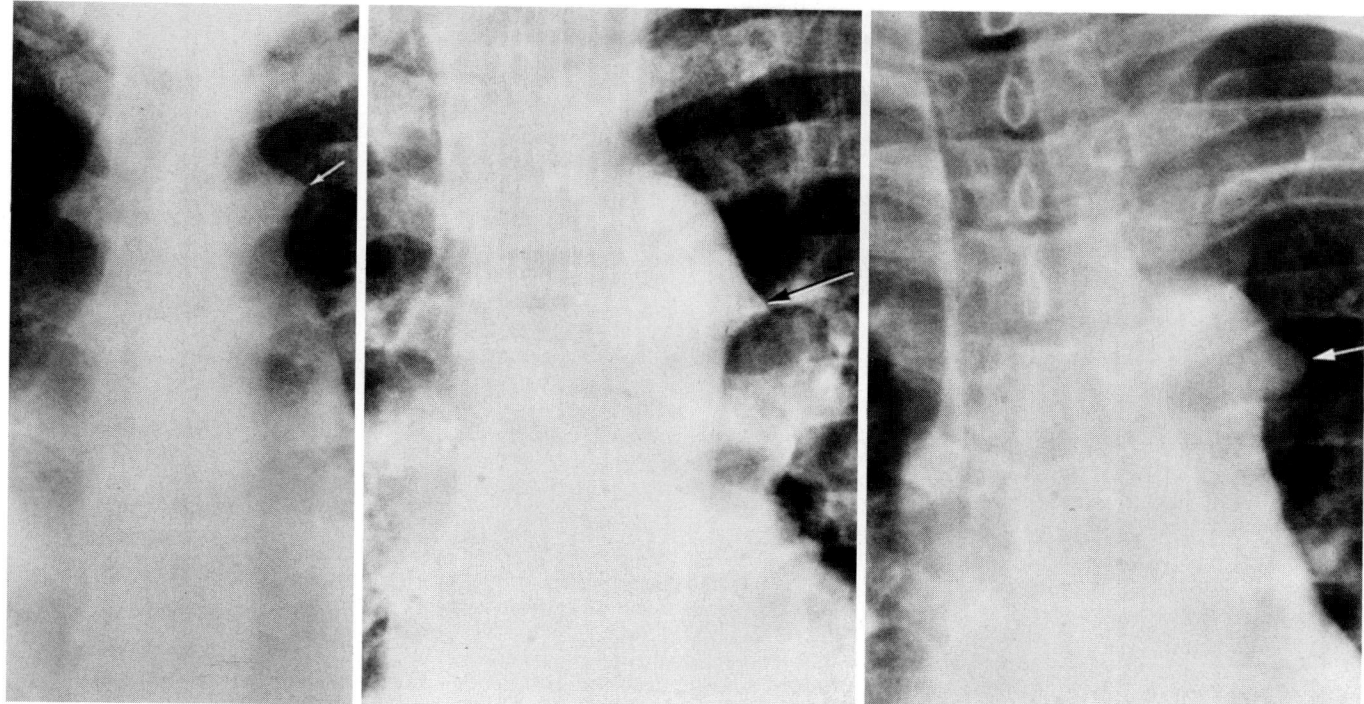

Figure 9–248. Three examples of the aortic nipple. This normal shadow is due to the highest intercostal vein and is seen in children and adults. (Ref: Ball JB Jr, Proto AV: The variable appearance of the left superior intercostal vein. *Radiology* 144:445, 1982.) The nipple should not exceed 4.5 mm in diameter. (Ref: Friedman AC et al: The normal and abnormal left superior intercostal vein. *Am J Roentgenol* 131:599, 1978.)

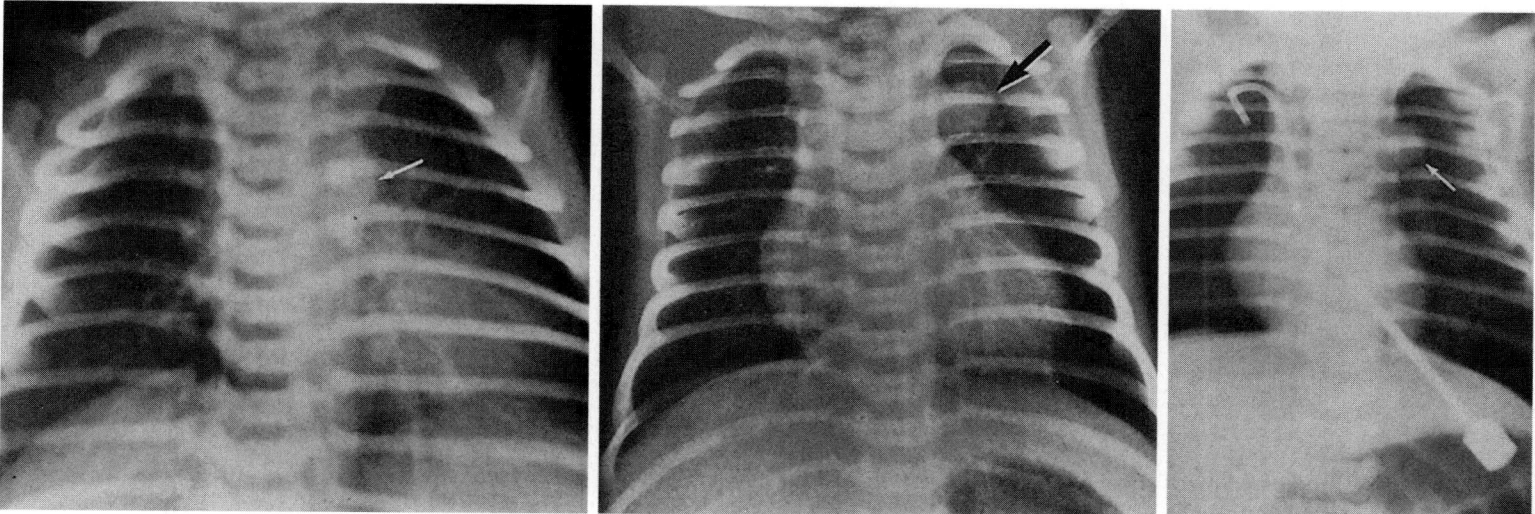

Figure 9–249. Three examples of the ductus bump in neonates. This density is seen in normal infants in the first day of life and usually disappears by the third day. It represents a reflection of neonatal adjustment to extrauterine life and is the shadow of the ductus functioning briefly before closure. (Ref: Berdon WE et al: The ductus bump: A transient physiologic mass in chest roentgenograms in newborn infants. *Am J Roentgenol* 95:91, 1965.)

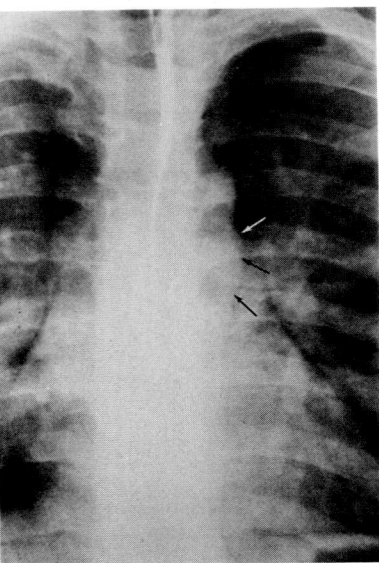

Figure 9–250. Infundibulum of the ductus, the point of insertion of the ductus in early life. Its presence does not indicate patency of the ductus. (Ref: Keats TE, Steinbach HL: Patent ductus arteriosus: A critical evaluation of its roentgen signs. *Radiology* 64:528, 1955.) The infundibulum may produce a figure-of-3 configuration, as illustrated in this case, that should not be misinterpreted as evidence of coarctation of the aorta or of aortic rupture. (Refs: Yousefzadeh DK et al: The aortic isthmus. *Radiology* 140:710, 1981; Morse SS et al: Atypical ductus diverticulum mistaken for aortic rupture. *Am J Roentgenol* 150:753, 1988.)

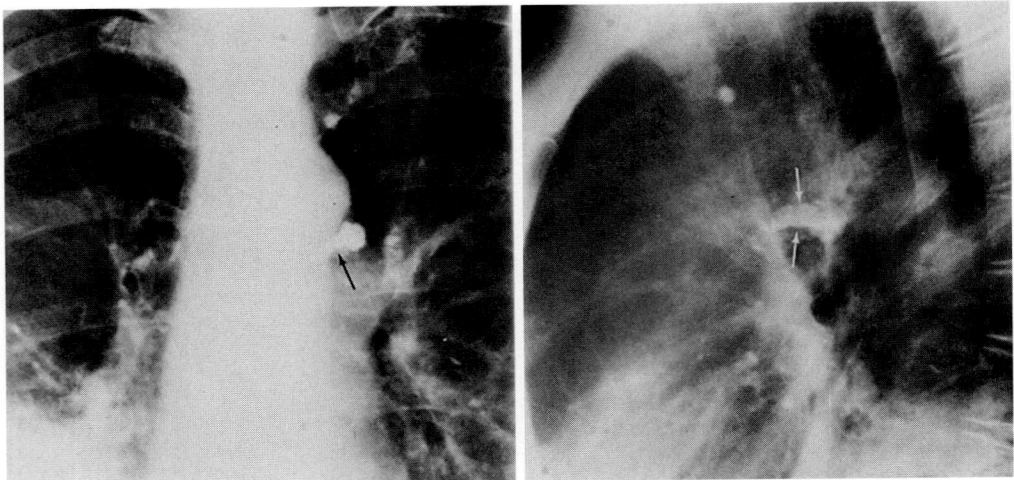

Figure 9–251. Calcification in the ligamentum arteriosum.

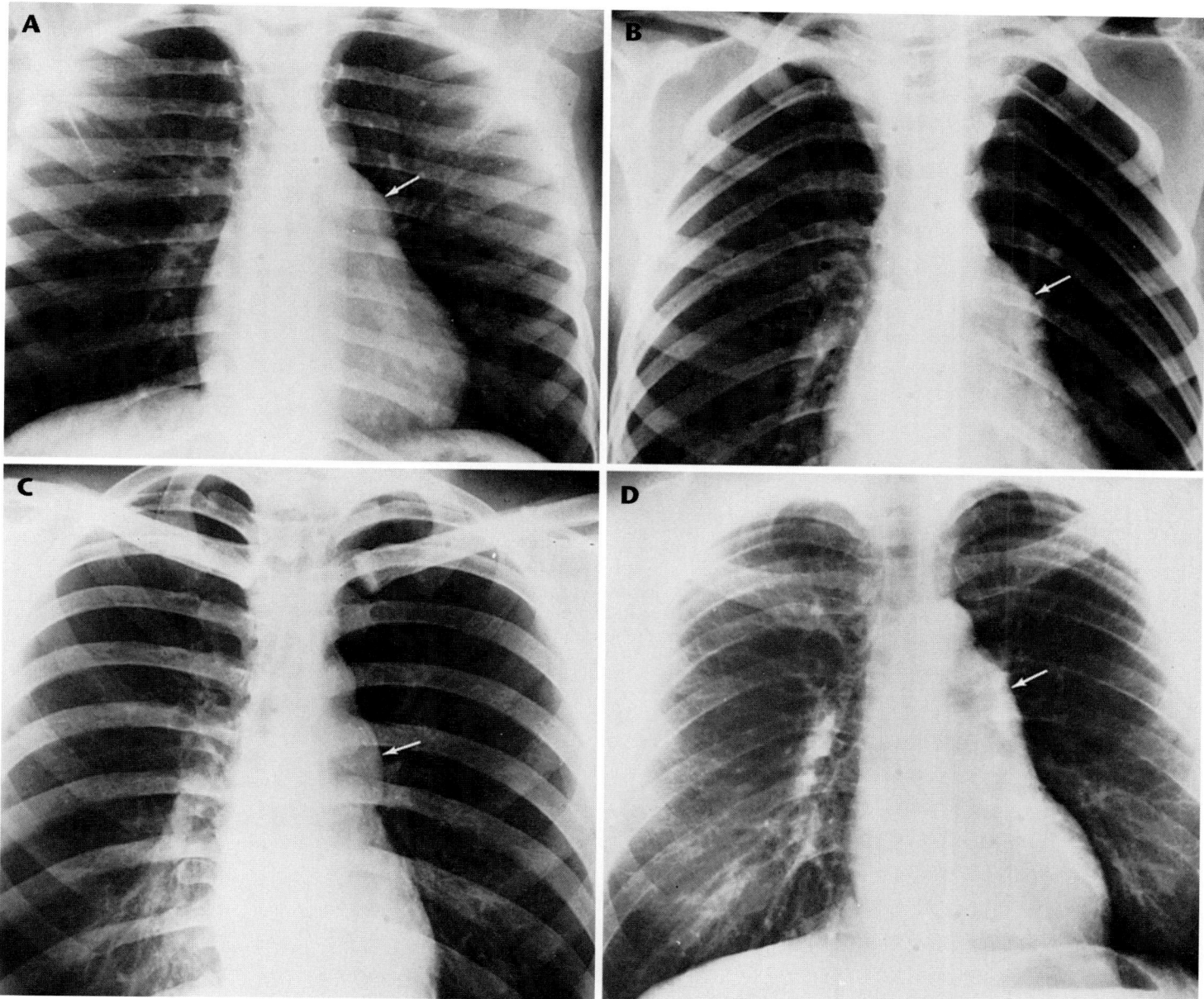

Figure 9–252. Four examples of normal variation in size of the pulmonary artery in children and young adults. The pulmonary artery is extremely variable in size, and its prominence in the young is a common finding. It should not be a source of concern in itself. **A,** 5-year-old boy. **B,** 8-year-old boy. **C,** 9-year-old girl. **D,** 18-year-old boy.

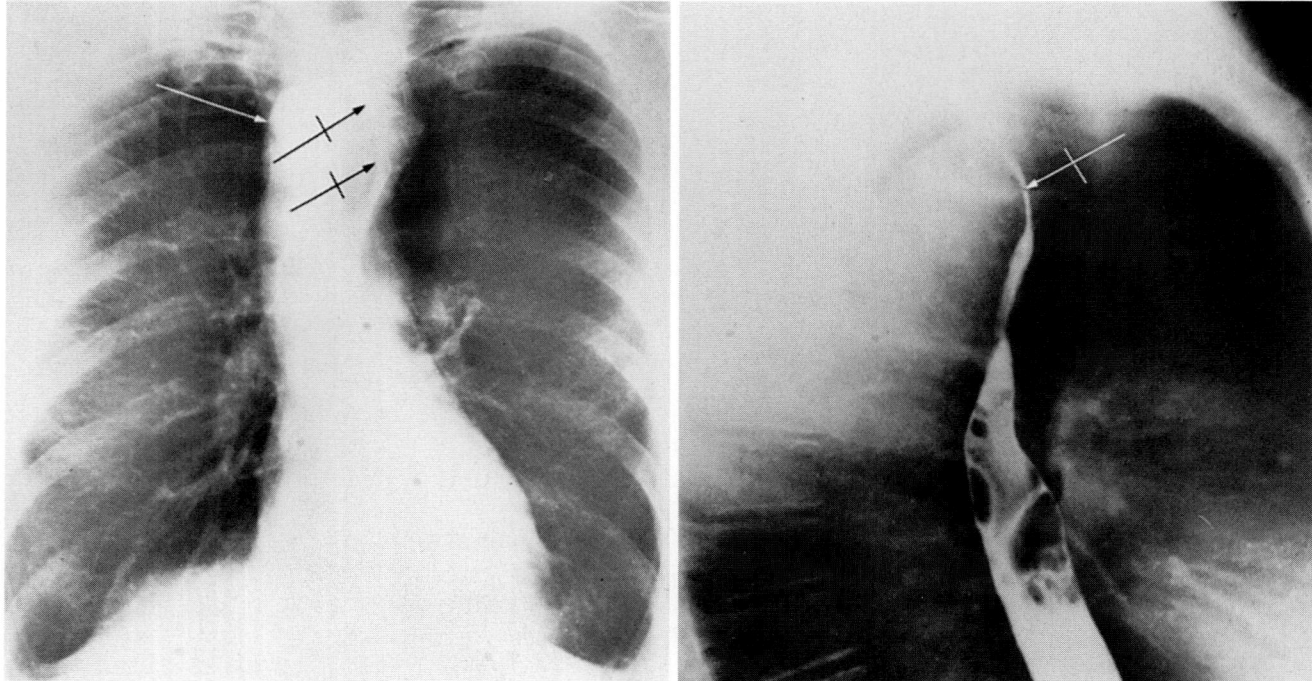

Figure 9–253. Right aortic arch (→) with retroesophageal course is not necessarily associated with congenital heart disease and may be mistaken for a mediastinal mass. It displaces the esophagus to the left and anteriorly (↦).

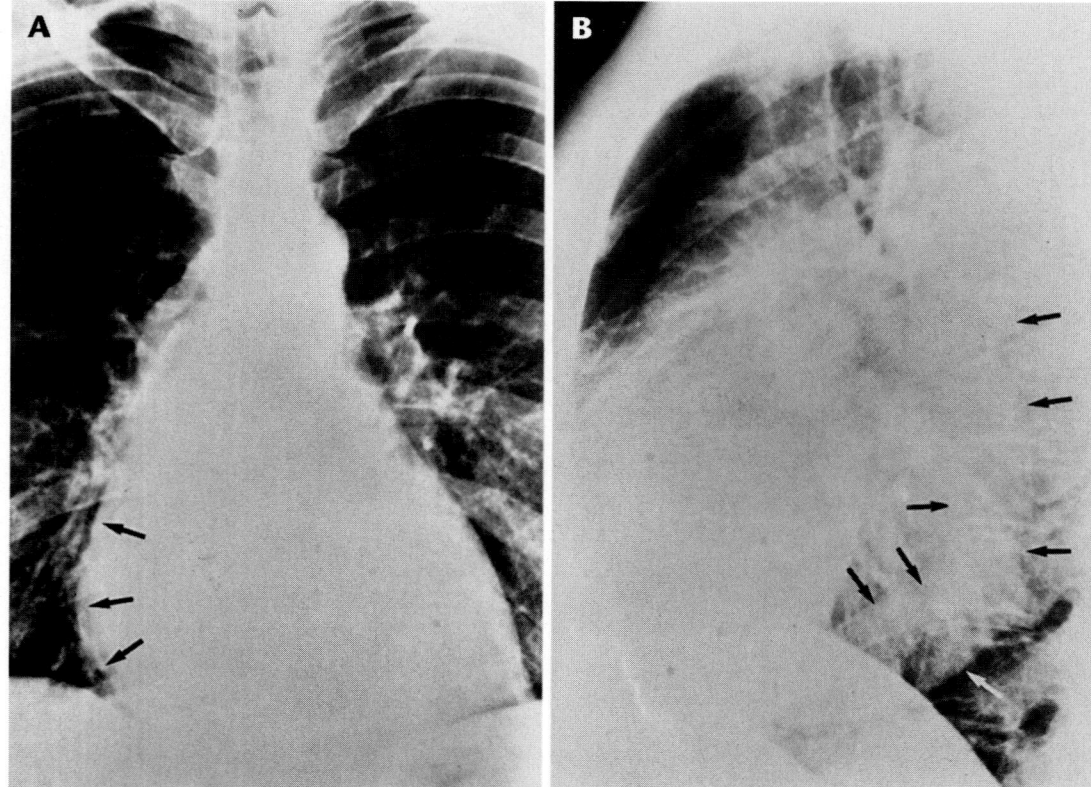

Figure 9–254. A, Tortuous aorta presenting on the right heart border (*arrows*). **B,** Lateral projection shows tortuosity.

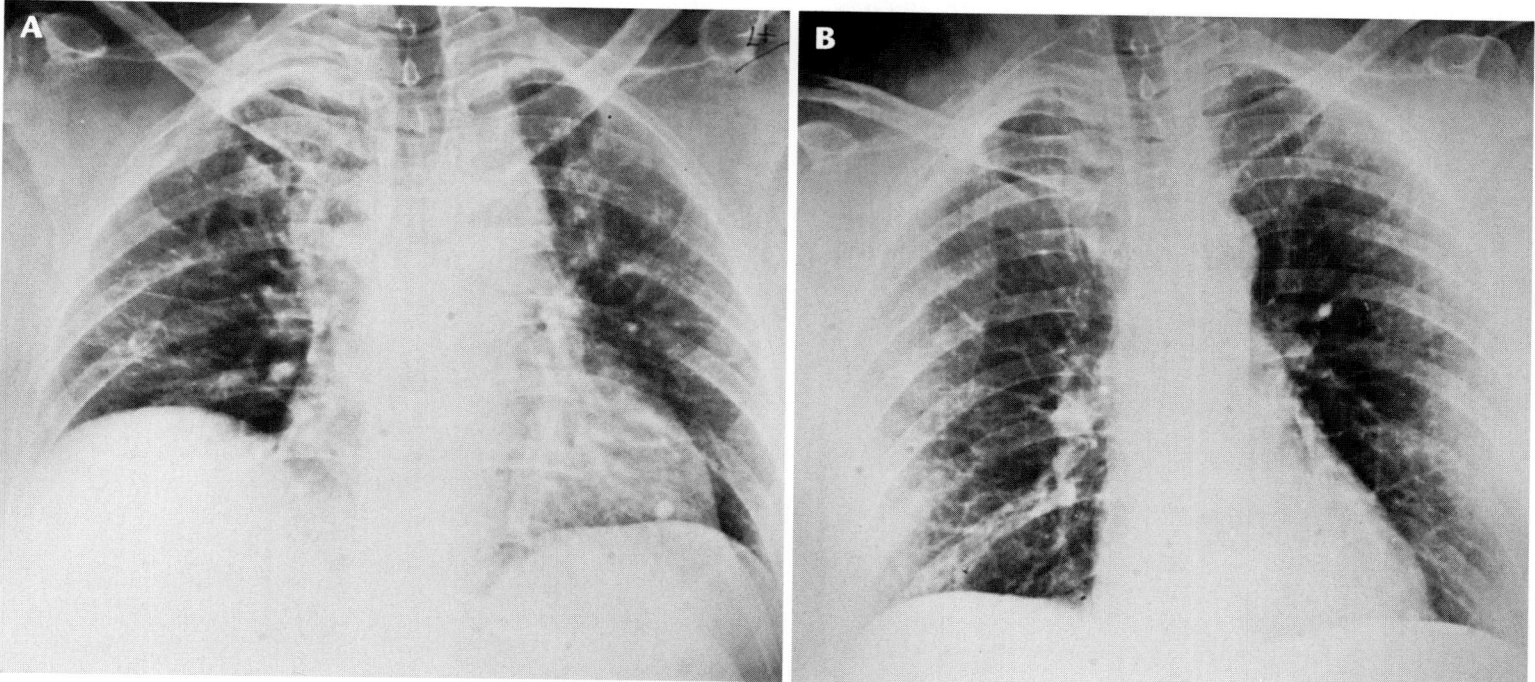

Figure 9–255. A, Widened mediastinum in this acutely injured patient is due to filming in expiration and was misinterpreted as evidence of aortic rupture. **B,** Inspiratory film made within an hour of **A** shows normal appearance.

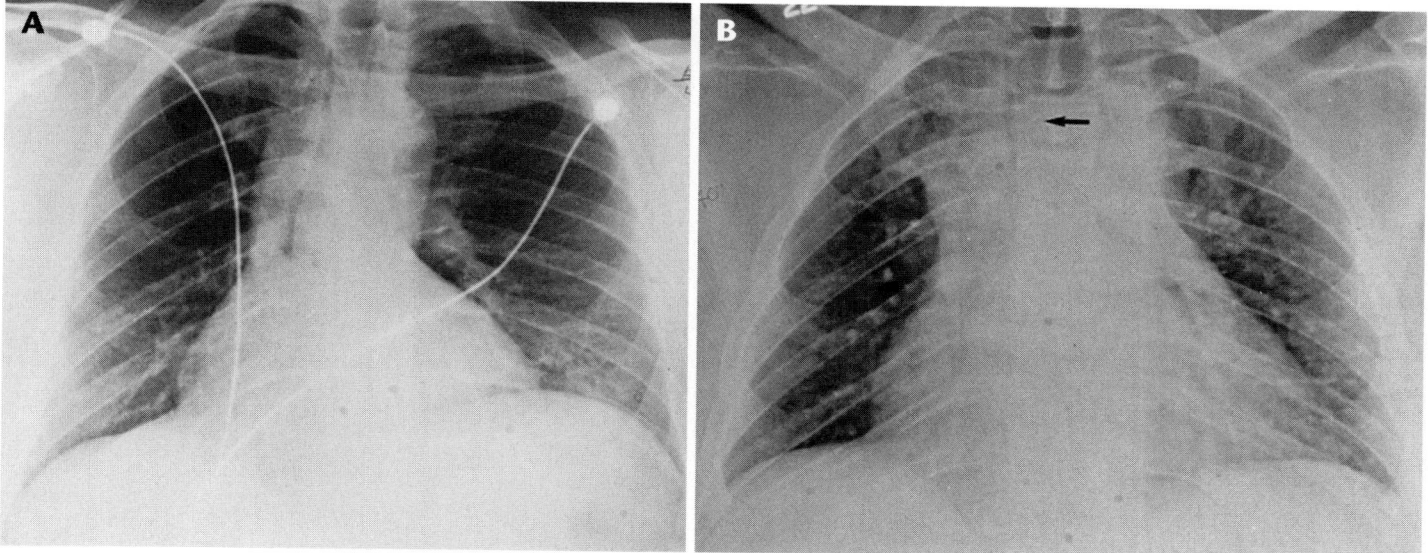

Figure 9–256. Normal widening of the mediastinal silhouette in the supine position. This finding coupled with buckling of the trachea to the right in expiration (←) may lead to an erroneous diagnosis of traumatic rupture of the aorta (see Fig. 9–102). **A,** Upright. **B,** Supine.

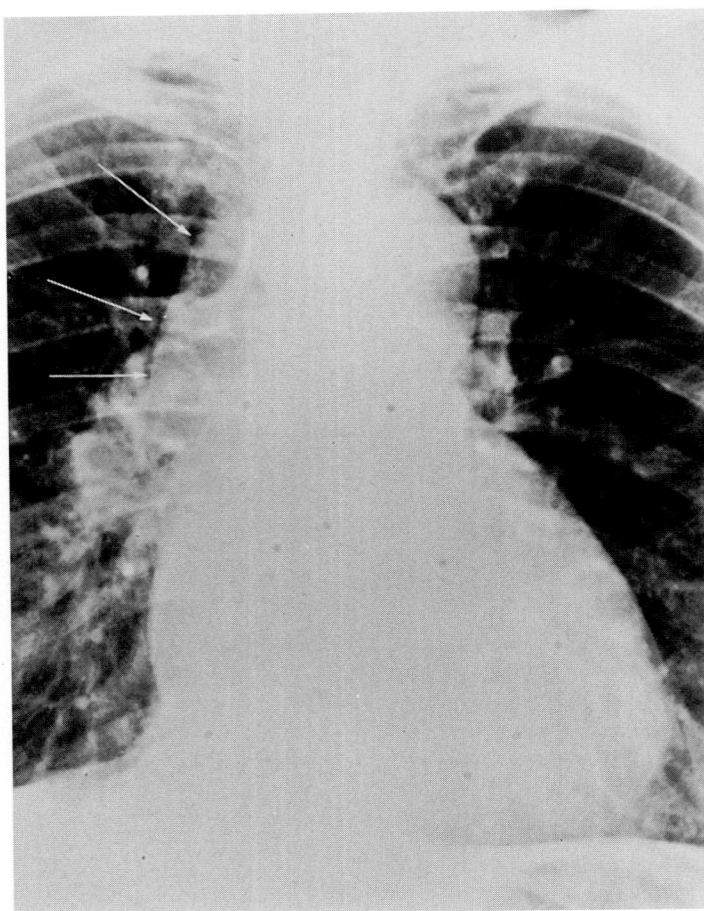

Figure 9–257. Lateral displacement of the superior vena cava by an ectatic aortic arch. (Ref: Drasin E et al: Nondilated superior vena cava presenting as a superior mediastinal mass. *J Can Assoc Radiol* 23:273, 1972.)

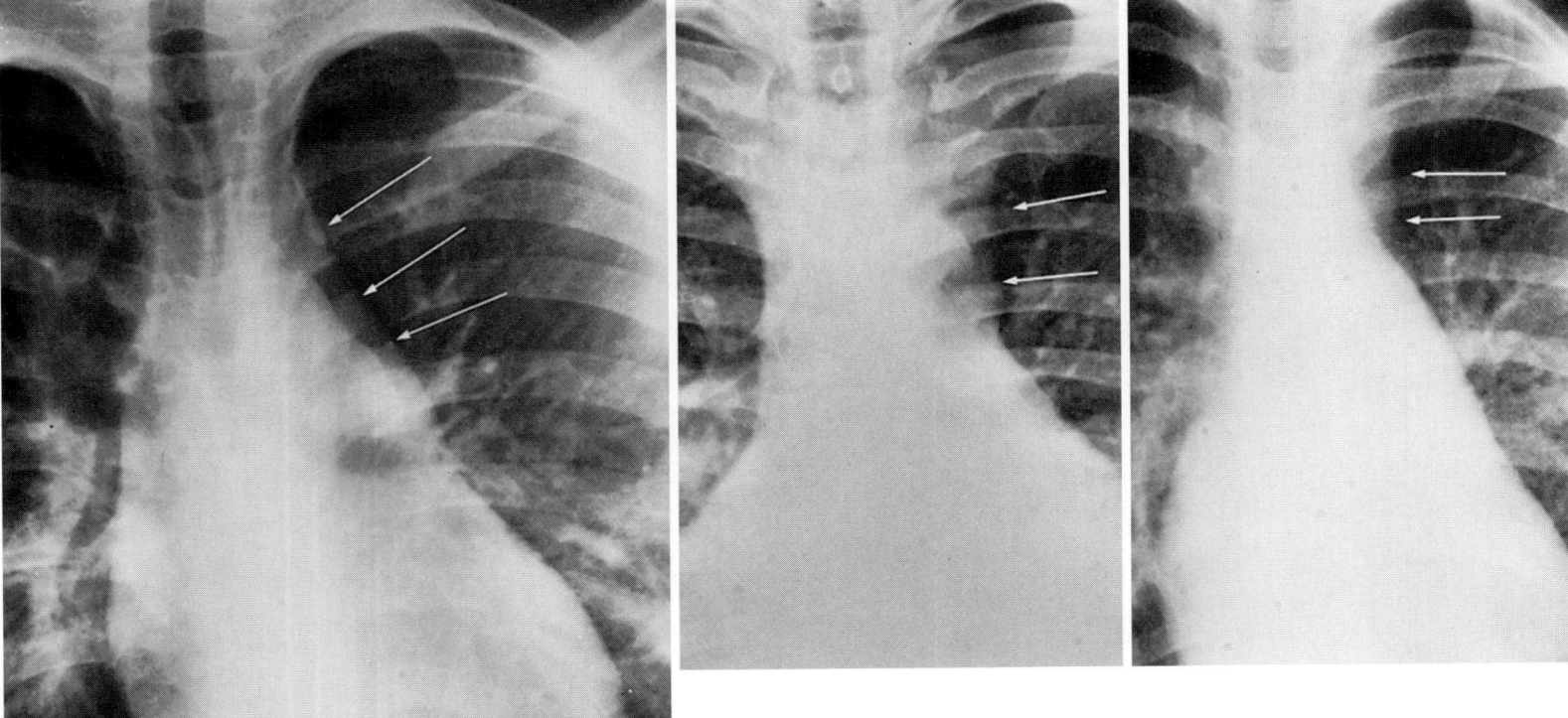

Figure 9–258. Three examples of left superior vena cava.

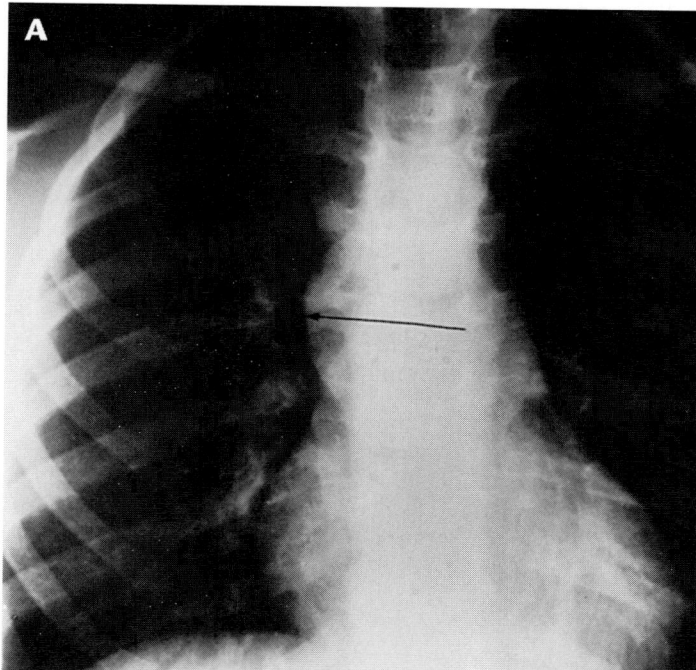

Figure 9–259. Idiopathic dilatation of the superior vena cava is a developmental variant of no significance. **A,** Plain film. **B,** Tomogram. **C,** Angiocardiogram. (Ref: Polansky S et al: Idiopathic dilatation of the superior vena cava in children. *Pediatr Radiol* 2:167, 1974.)

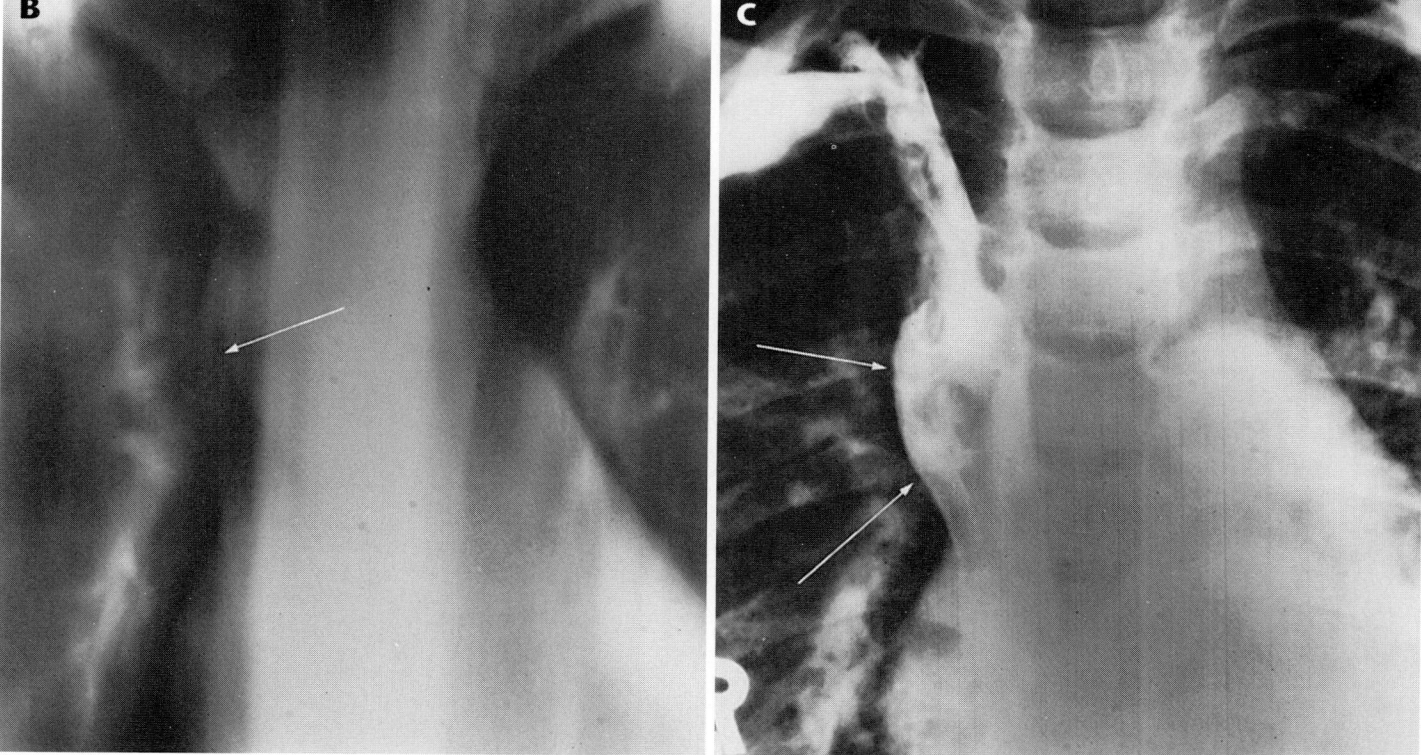

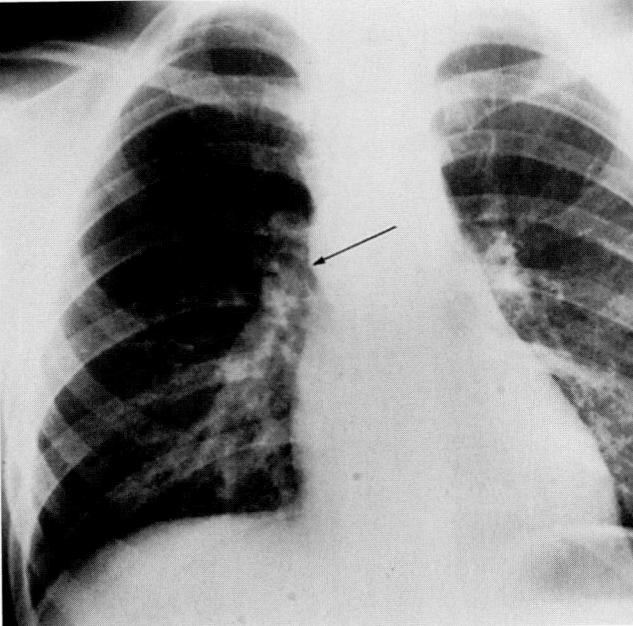

Figure 9–260. Another example of idiopathic dilatation of the superior vena cava. Note similarity to preceding case.

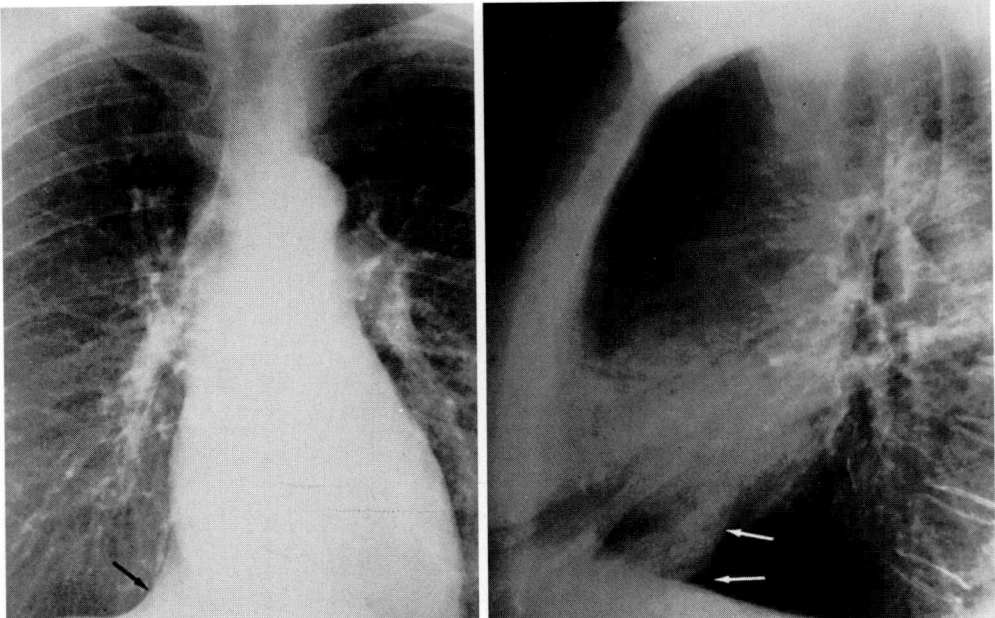

Figure 9–261. Prominent but normal shadow of the inferior vena cava.

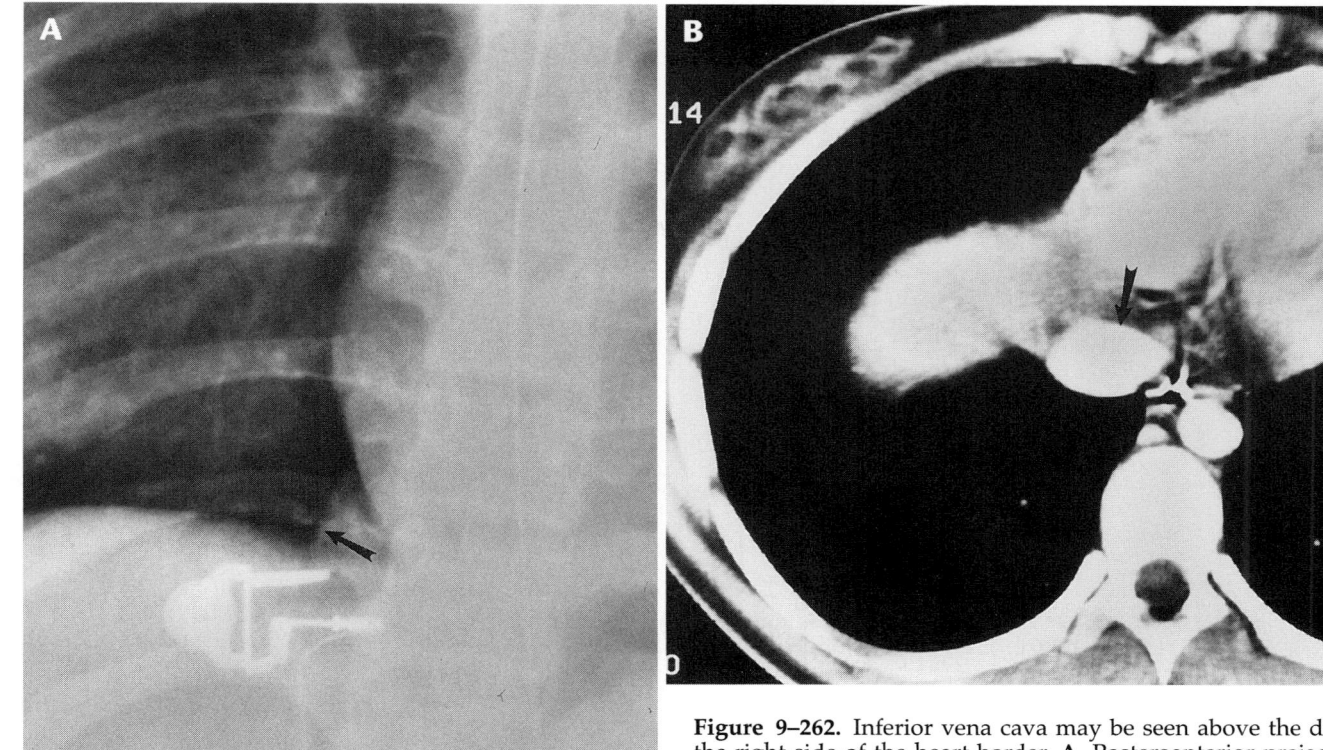

Figure 9–262. Inferior vena cava may be seen above the diaphragm adjacent to the right side of the heart border. **A,** Posteroanterior projection. **B,** CT.

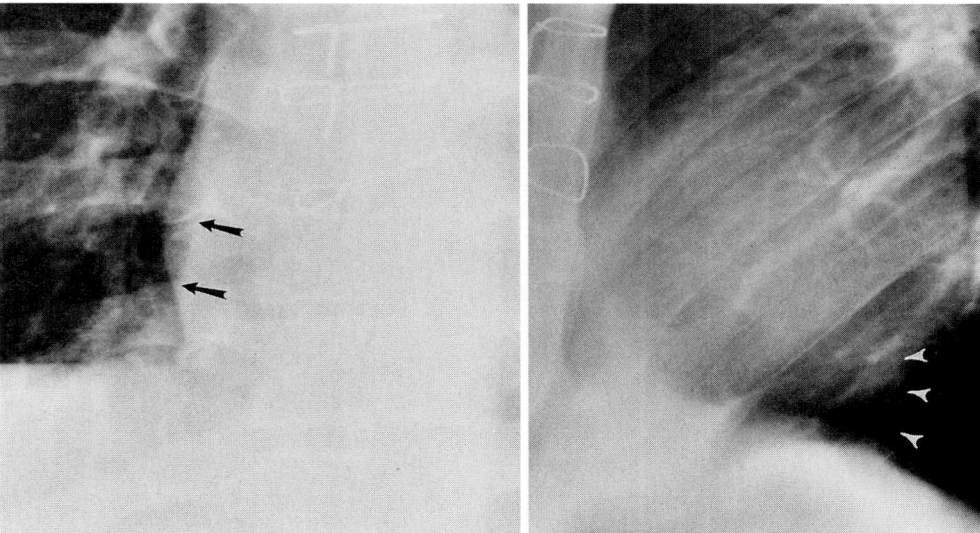

Figure 9–263. Inferior vena cava may be seen through the shadow of the right atrium.

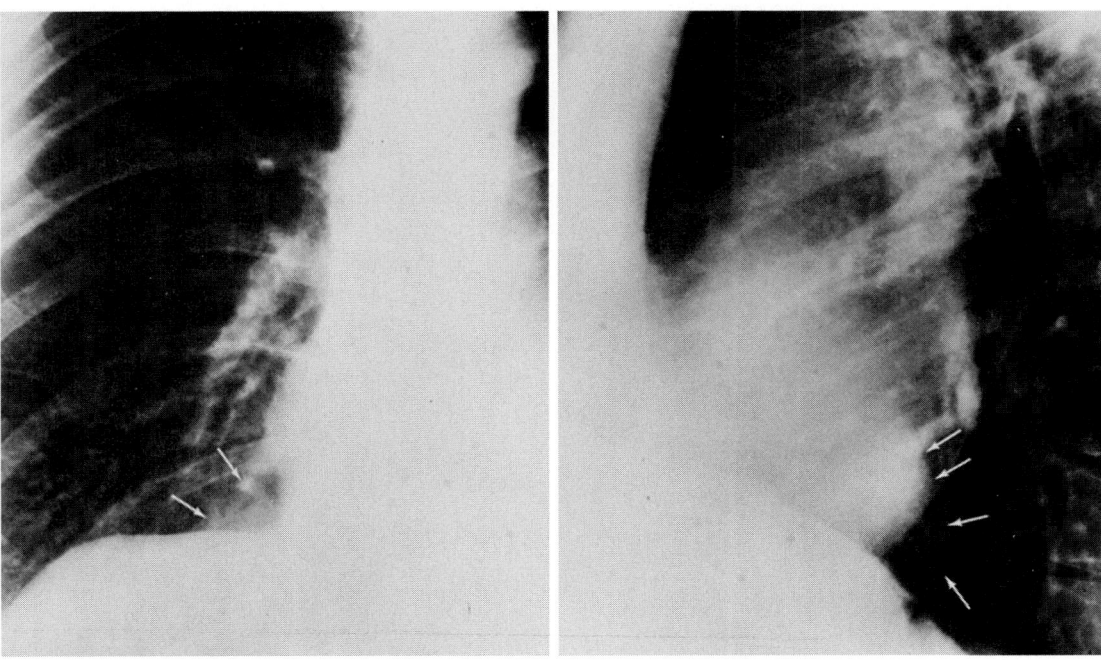

Figure 9–264. Idiopathic dilatation of the inferior vena cava, so-called varix of the inferior vena cava, a finding of no clinical significance in itself. (Ref: Oh KS et al: Inferior vena cava varix. *Radiology* 109:161, 1973.)

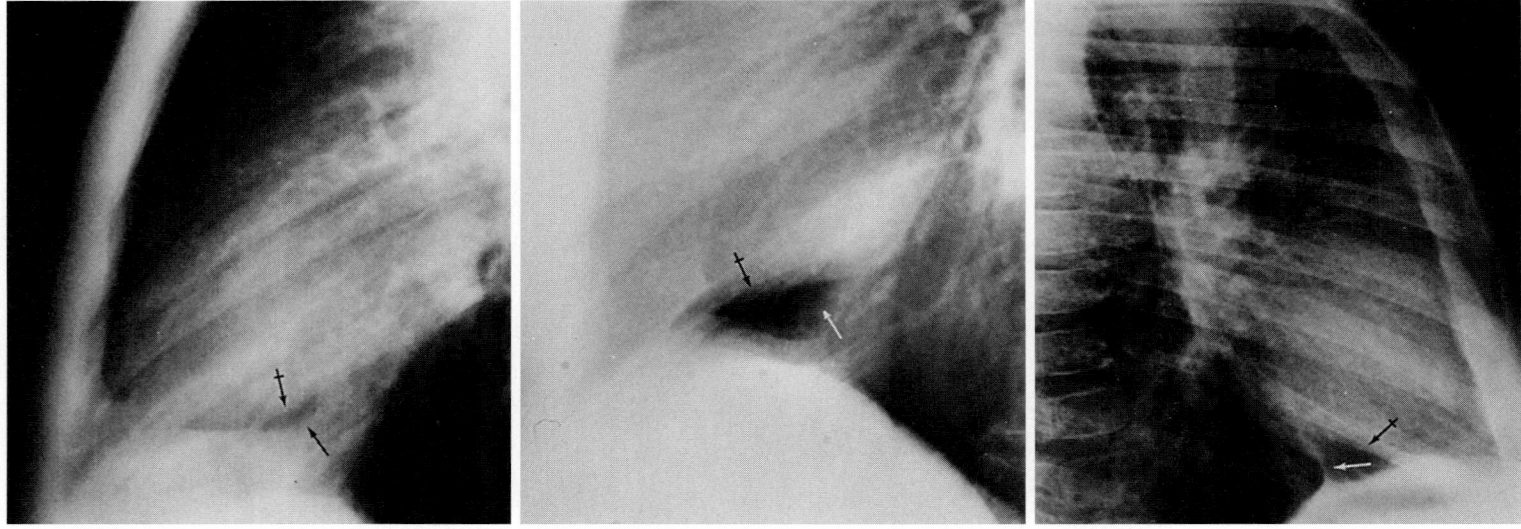

Figure 9–265. Three examples of confusing radiolucencies produced by the inferior vena cava. With maximum inspiration it is possible to clear a portion of the diaphragmatic surface of the heart and expose the anterior wall of the inferior vena cava (→). This results in a triangular area of radiolucency (↦), which may be confusing if its origin is not appreciated. (Ref: Tonkin IL et al: Radiographic isolation of the inferior vena cava. *Am J Roentgenol* 129:657, 1977.)

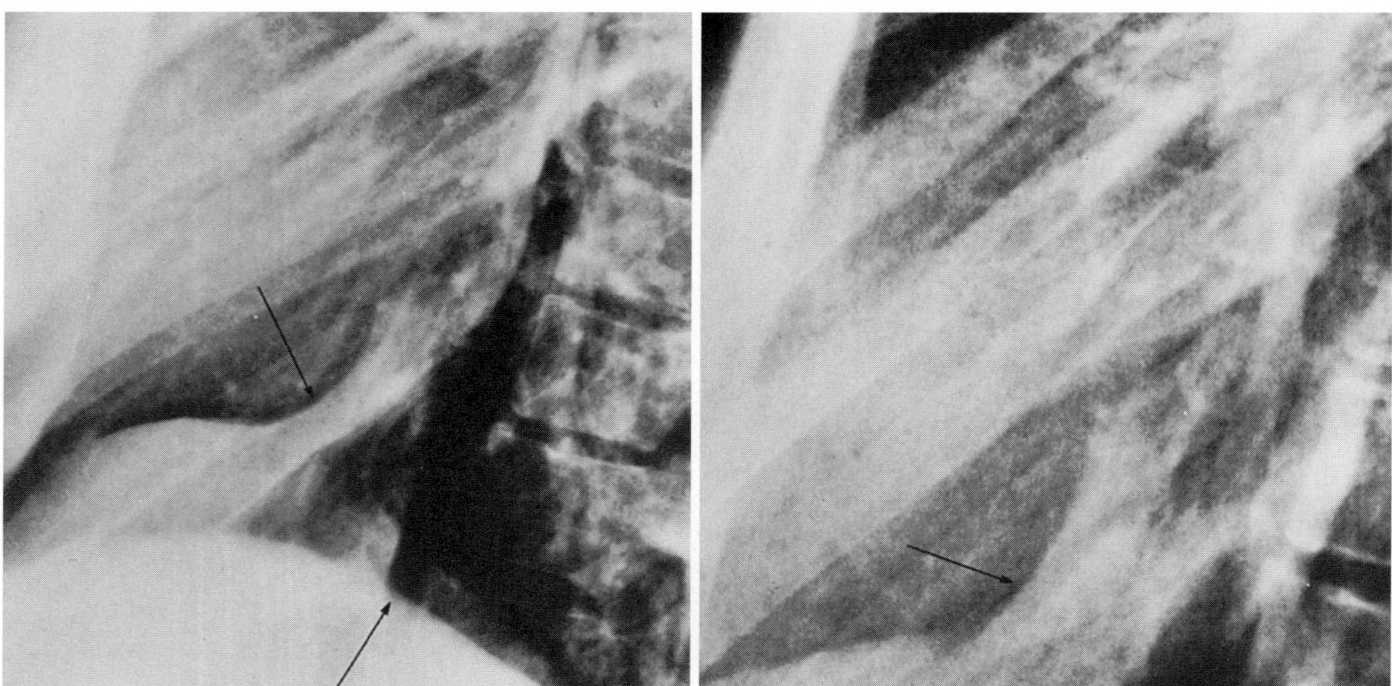

Figure 9–266. Shadow of the inferior vena cava, producing an appearance simulating atelectasis. The upper margin is probably produced by superimposition of the heart shadow.

The Thymus

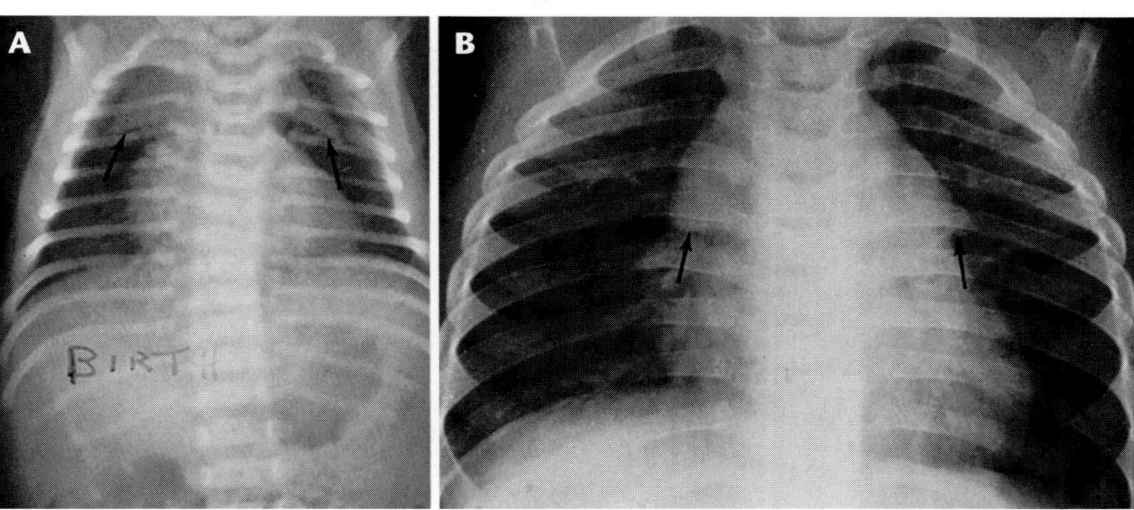

Figure 9–267. Variations in the configuration of the thymus. **A,** At birth, an appearance of the thymus simulating pneumomediastinum. **B,** Same individual at 16 months. The thymus is still prominent but more closely applied to the mediastinum.

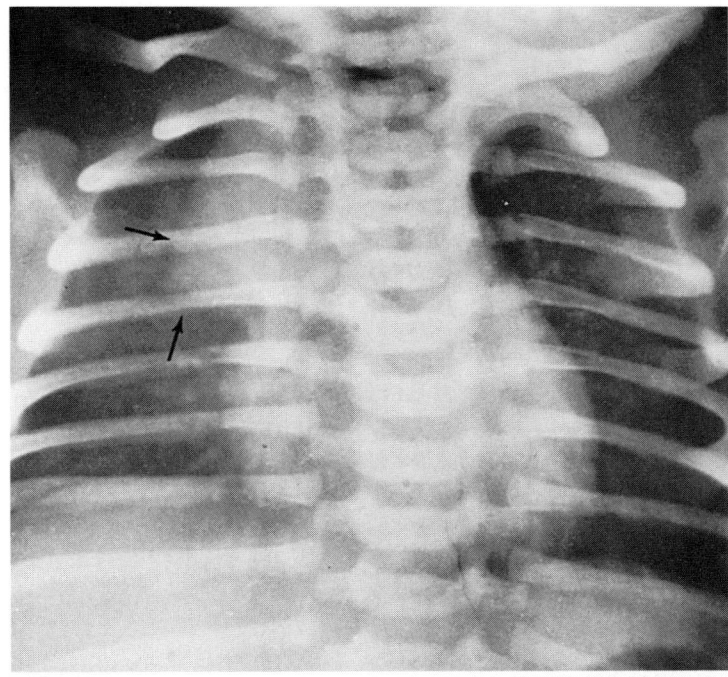

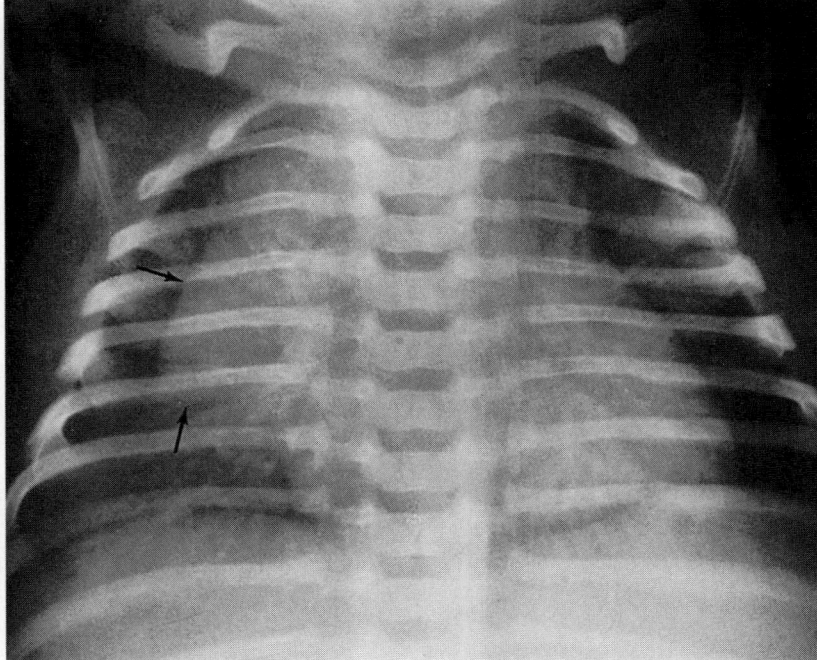

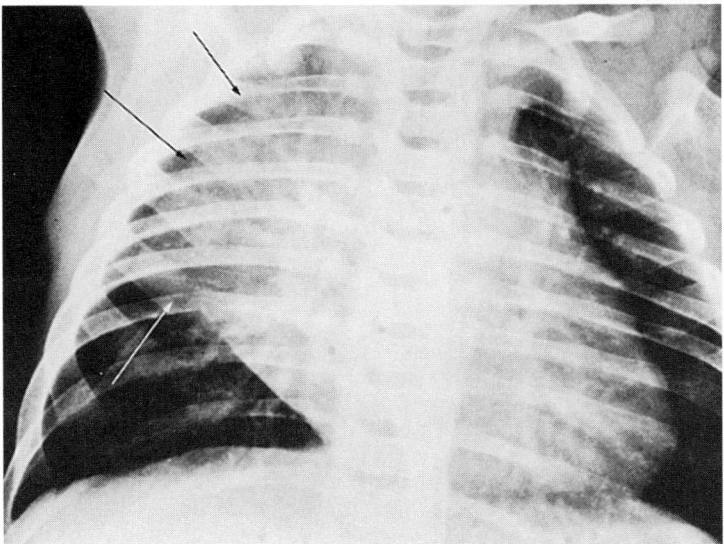

Figure 9–268. Three examples of unilateral presentation of the thymus to the right side.

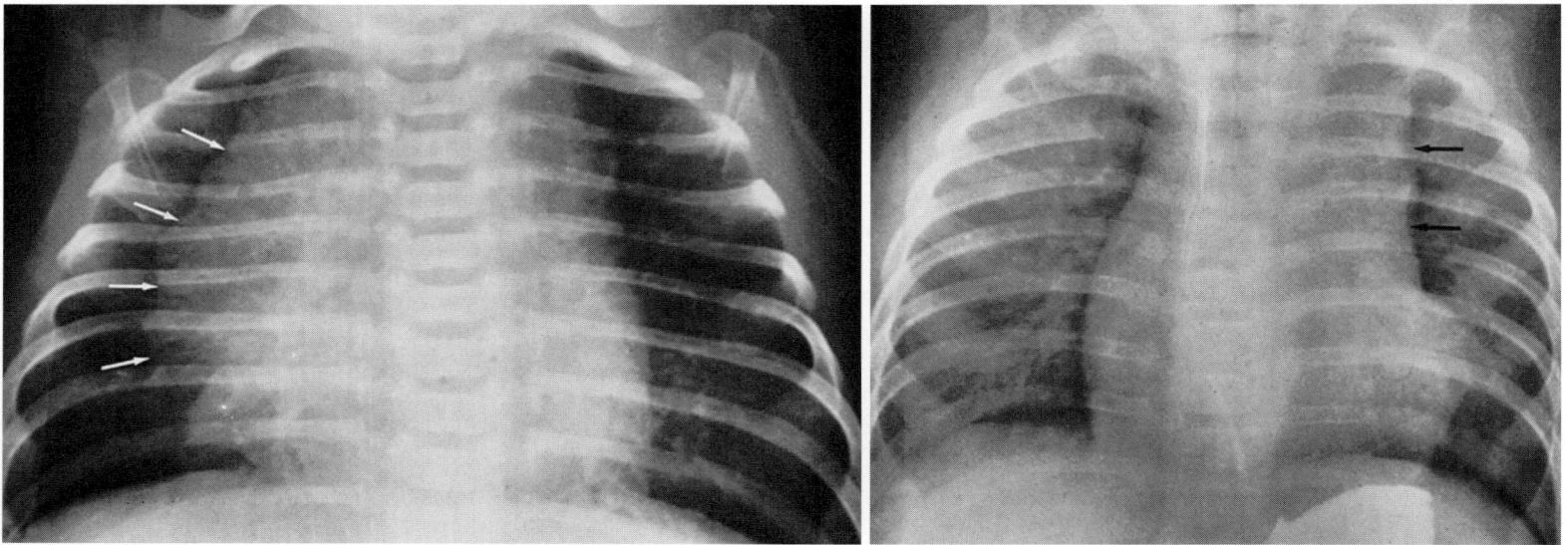

Figure 9–269. Two examples of the thymic wave sign. The undulating configuration of the edge of the thymus is due to impression of the anterior portion of the ribs. (Ref: Mulvey RB: The thymic "wave" sign. *Radiology* 81:834, 1963.)

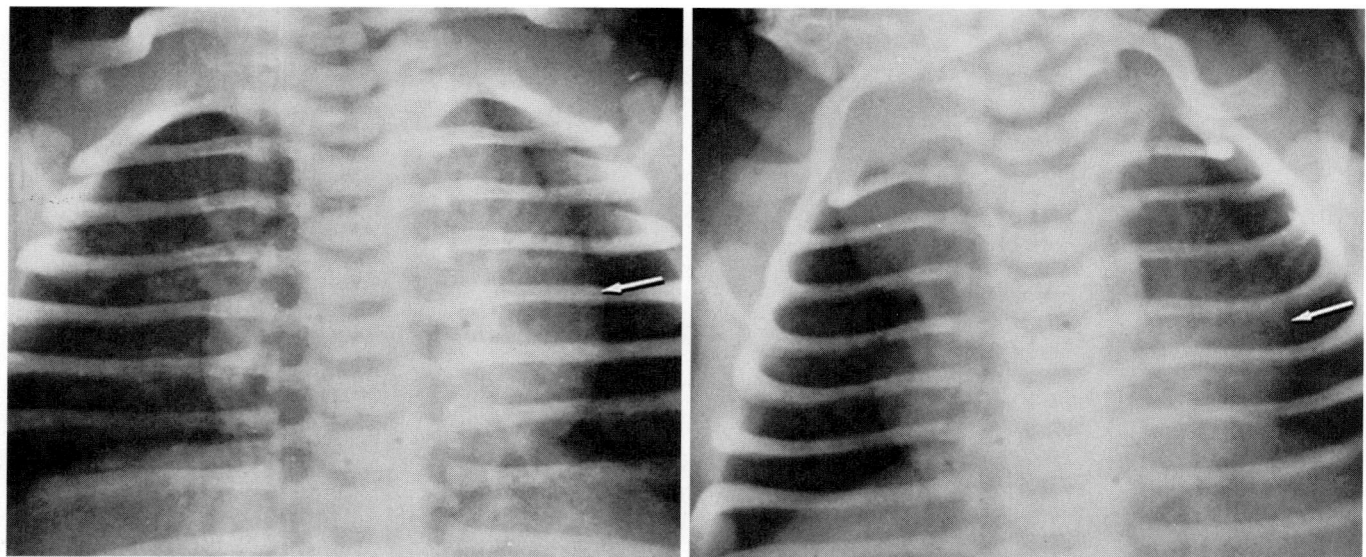

Figure 9–270. Two examples of large left lobes of the thymus, producing an appearance suggesting dextrocardia.

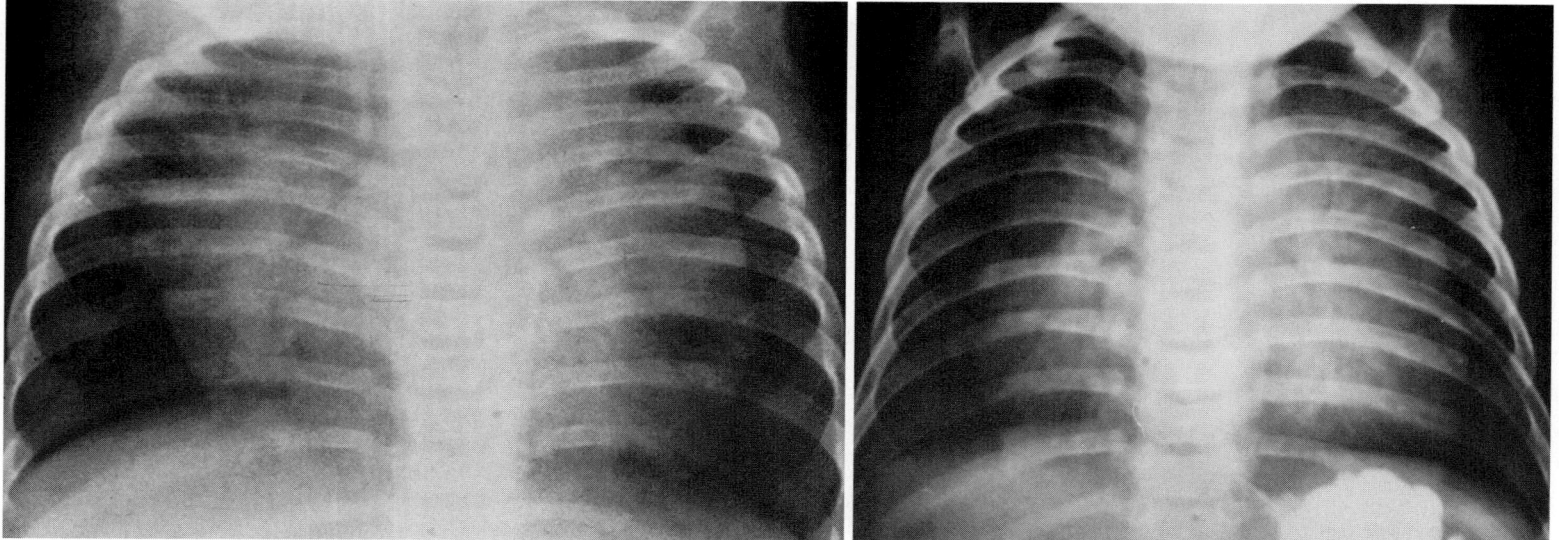

Figure 9–271. Two examples of very large thymuses simulating cardiomegaly.

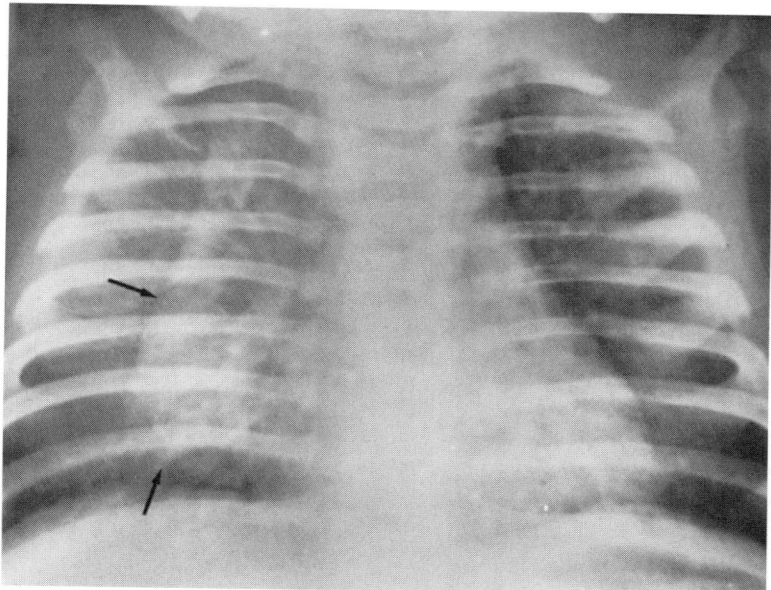

Figure 9–272. Unilateral presentation of the thymus to the right and extending almost to the diaphragm.

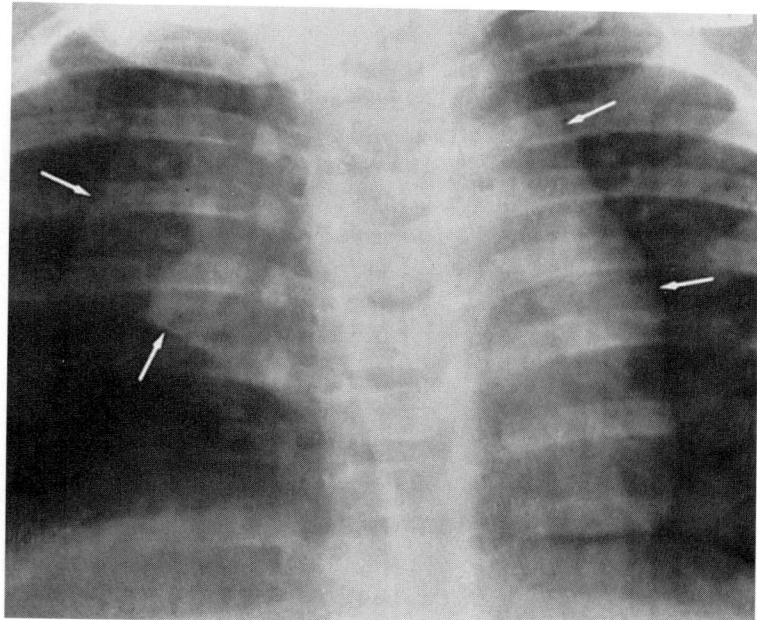

Figure 9–273. Huge thymus in a 9-month-old baby.

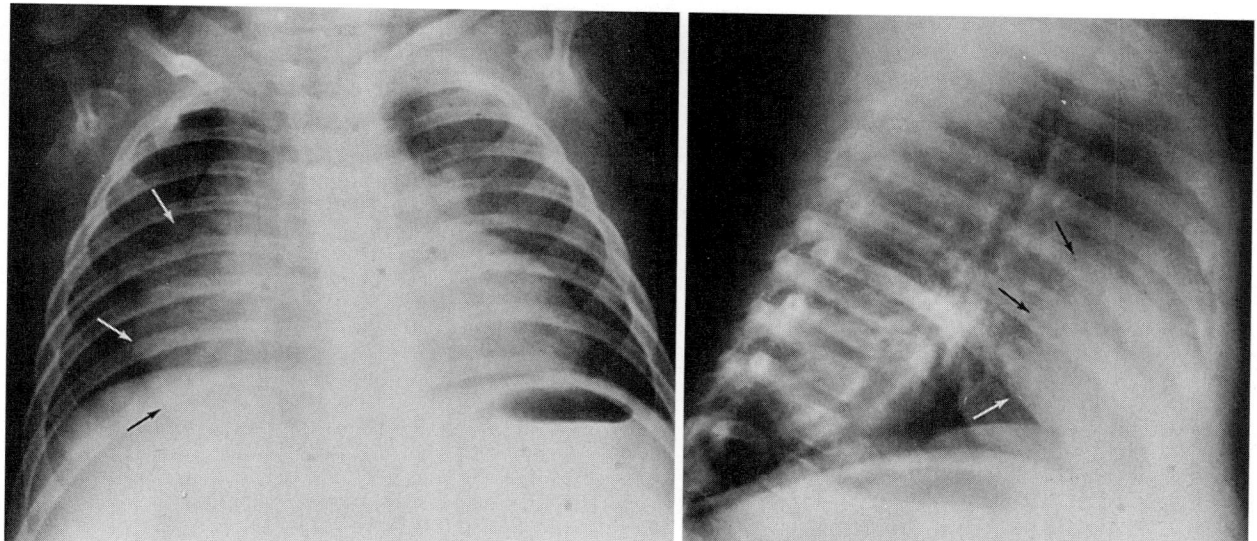

Figure 9–274. Huge thymus simulating cardiomegaly in the frontal plane. Note the radiolucency on the right in contrast to the heart on the left.

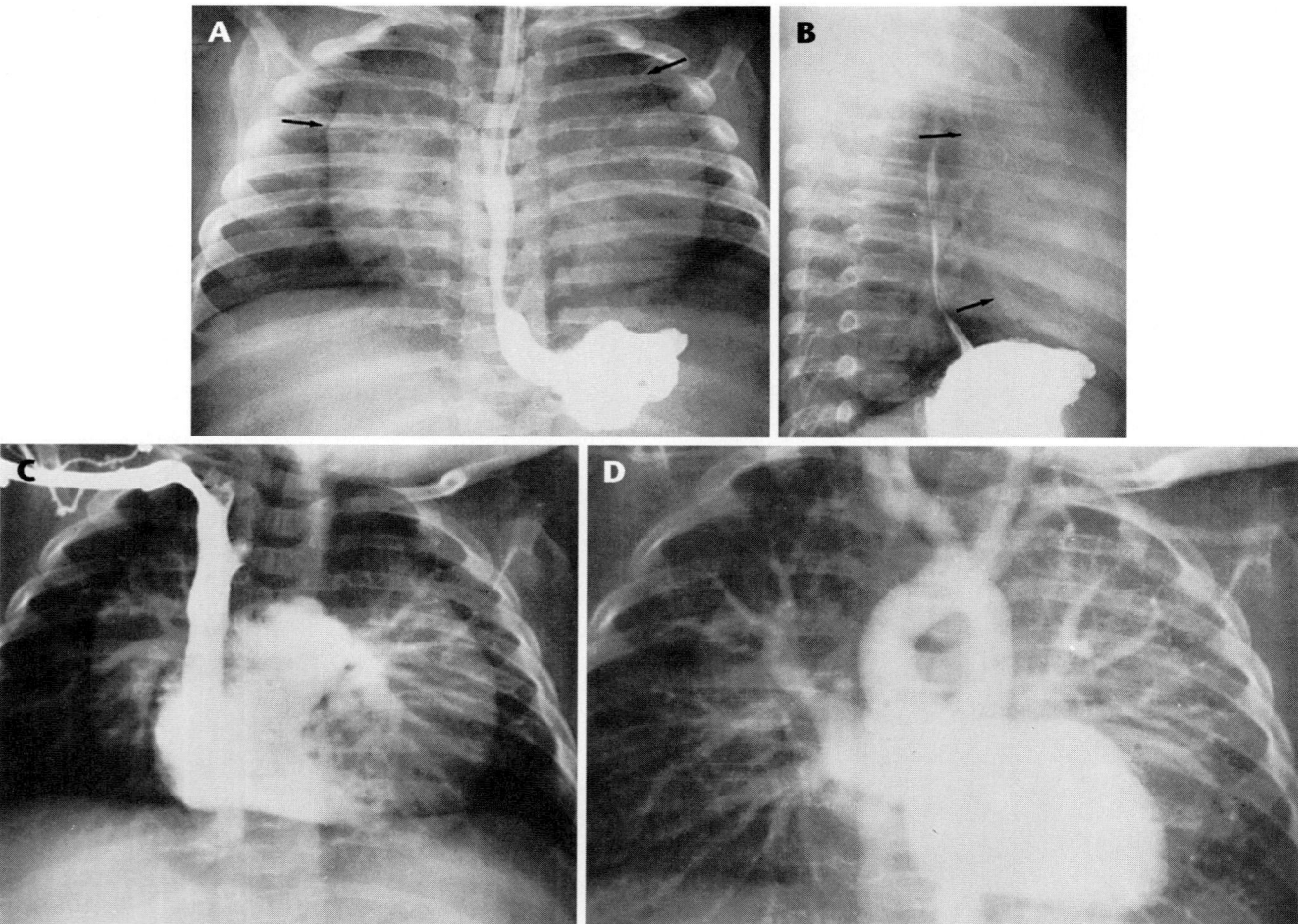

Figure 9–275. A, Large thymus simulating cardiomegaly. **B,** Lateral projection fails to show corresponding cardiomegaly and indicates the large thymic outline anteriorly. **C** and **D,** Dextro- and levoangiocardiograms show normal cardiac size within the huge thymus.

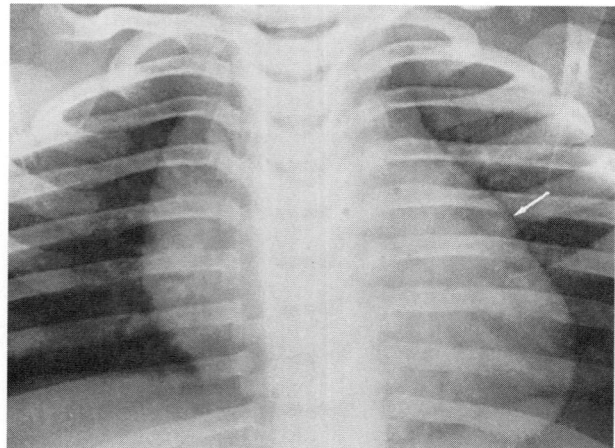

Figure 9–276. Left lobe of the thymus simulating enlargement of the left atrial appendage.

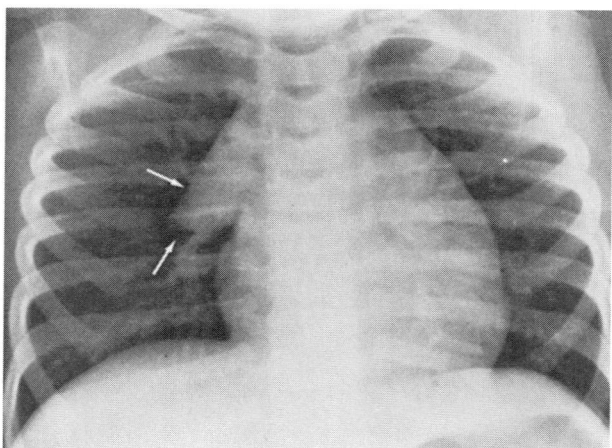

Figure 9–277. Unilateral "sail" configuration of the right lobe of the thymus.

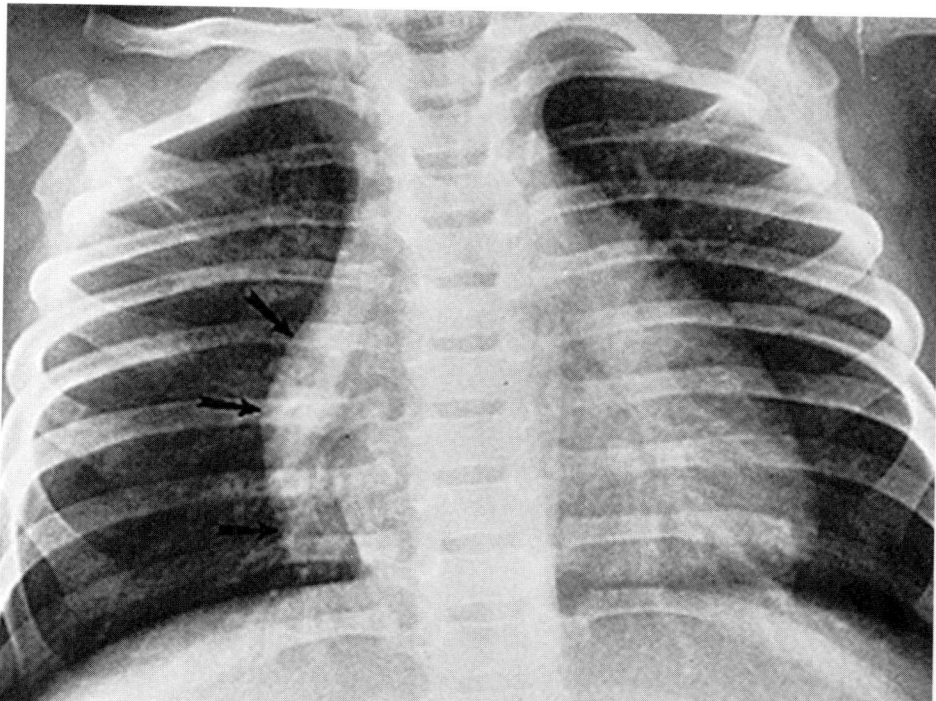
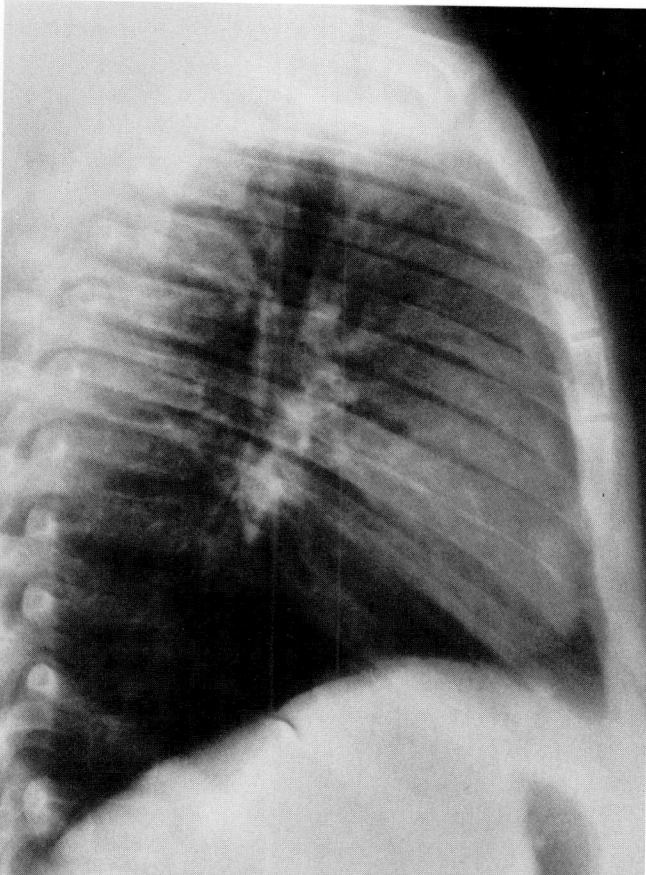

Figure 9–278. Extension of the thymus to the apex of the right atrium.

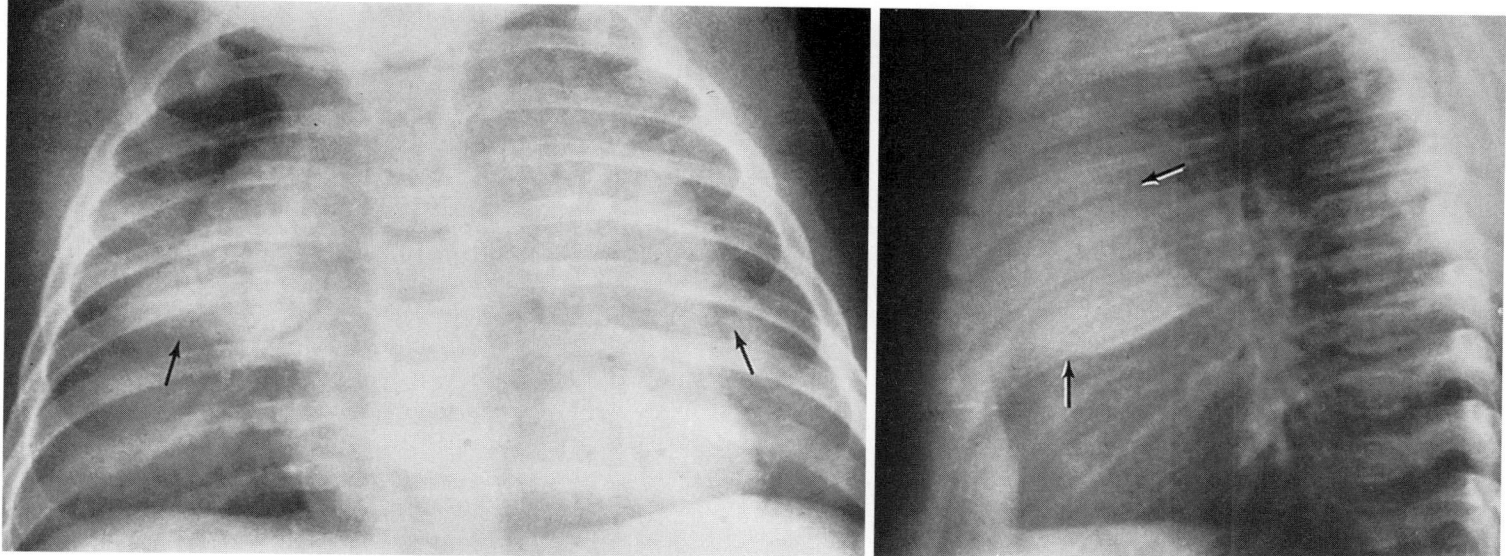

Figure 9–279. Unusual configuration of the thymus. Note the large shadow of the thymus in the lateral projection.

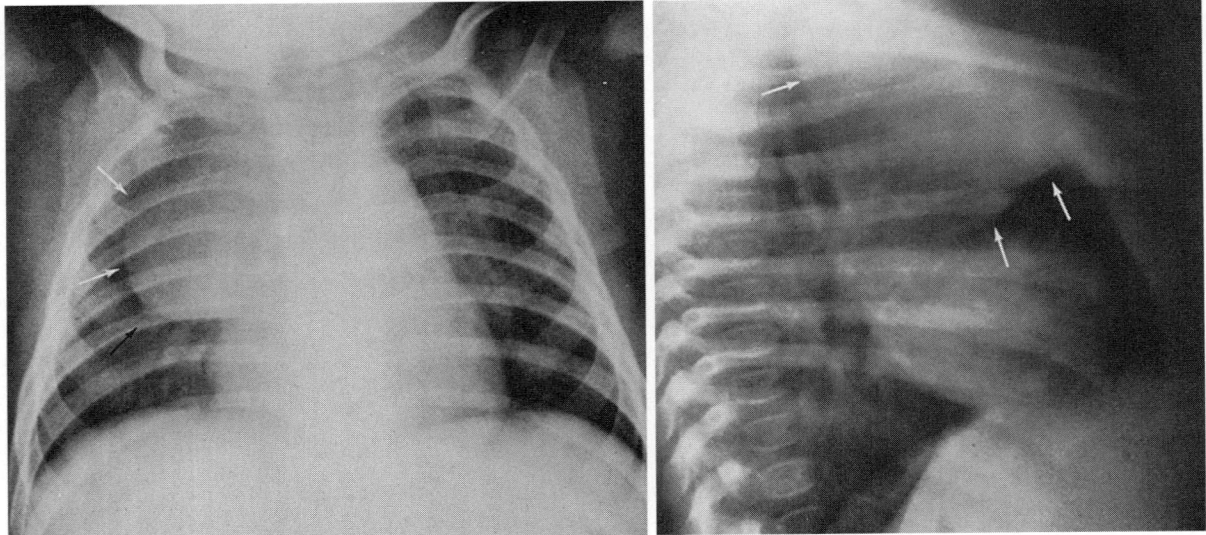

Figure 9–280. Unusually rounded configuration of the thymus.

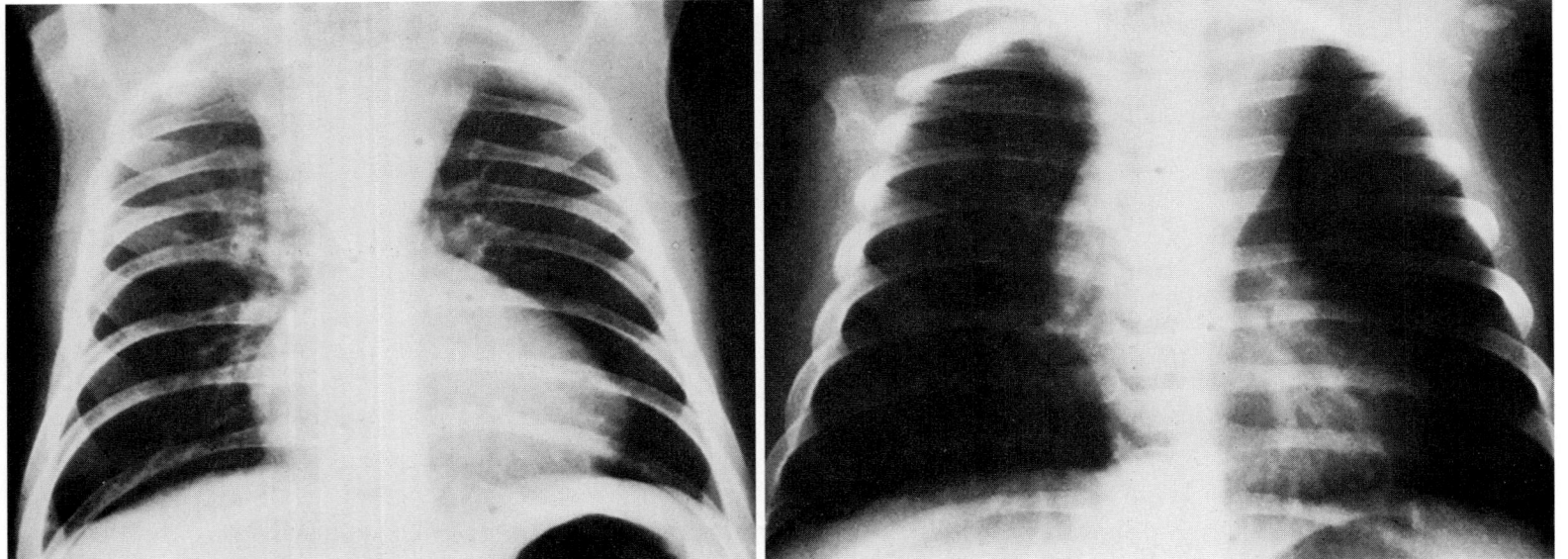

Figure 9–281. Two examples of the thymus producing an appearance resembling the "snowman heart" of total anomalous pulmonary venous return.

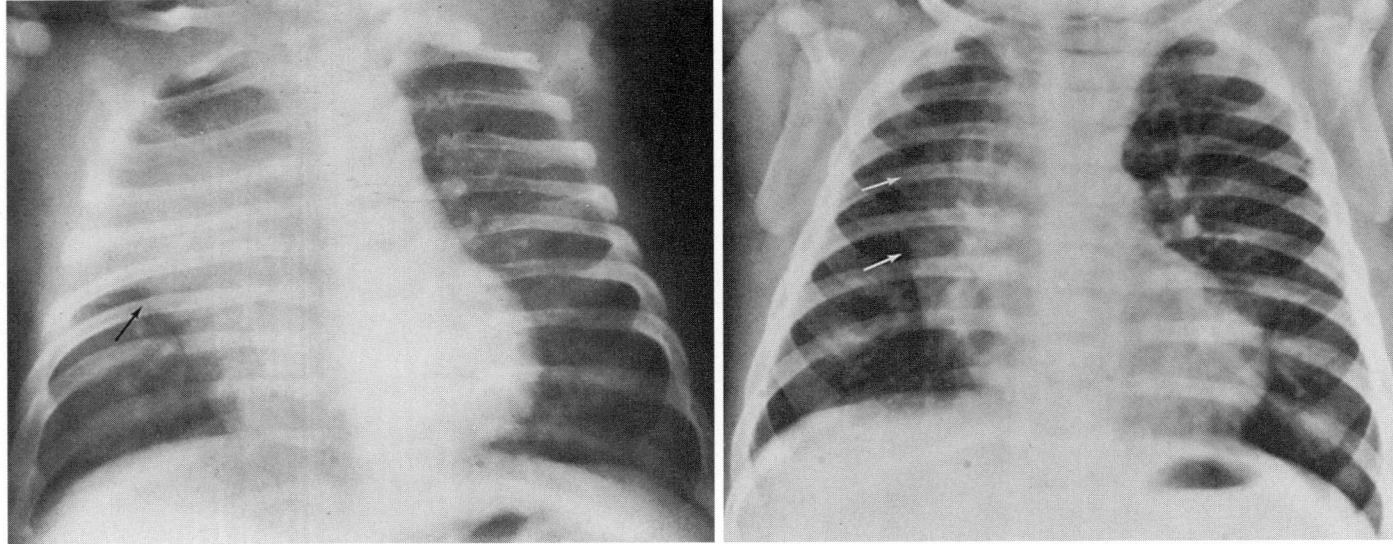

Figure 9–282. Examples of the thymus presenting entirely to the right side.

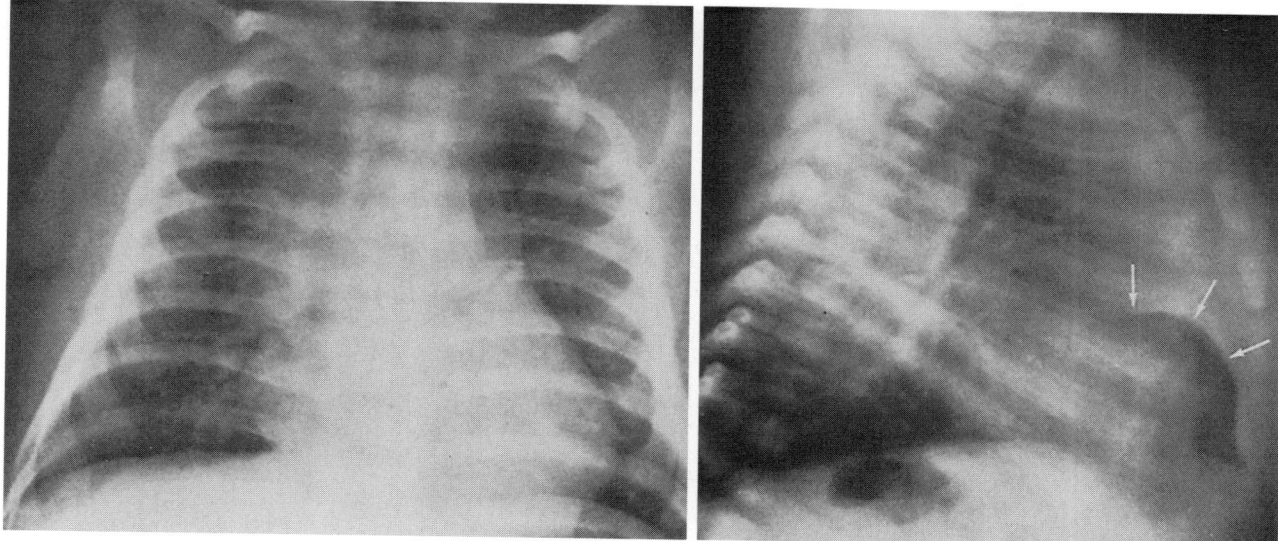

Figure 9–283. Thymus in a neonate, producing a relative radiolucency anteriorly in the lateral projection, which was originally mistaken for a hernia through Morgagni's foramen.

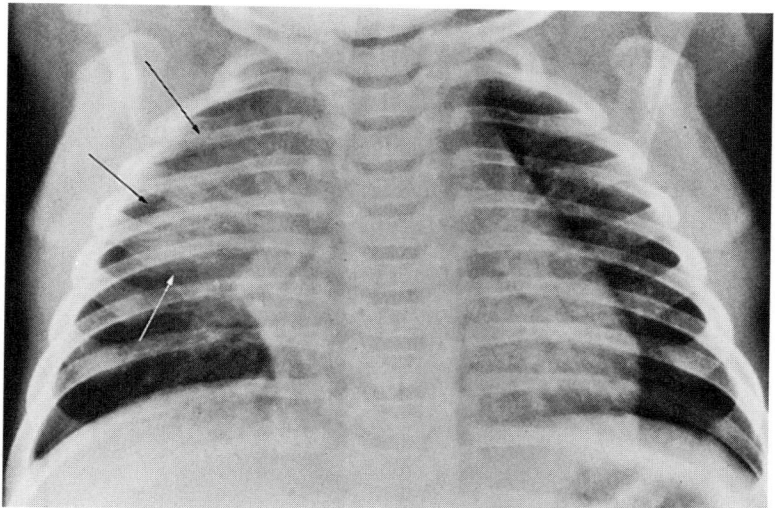

Figure 9–284. Right lobe of the thymus simulating right upper lobe pneumonitis. The thymus may simulate upper lobe atelectasis as well. (Ref: Lanning P, Heikkinen E: Thymus simulating left upper lobe atelectasis. *Pediatr Radiol* 9:177, 1980.)

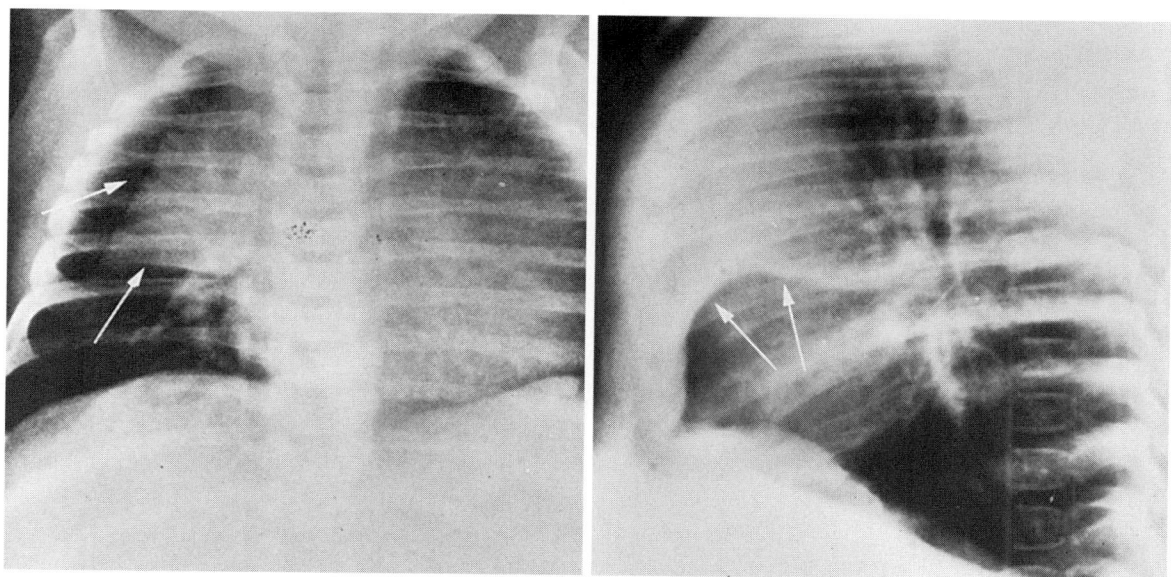

Figure 9–285. Large thymus misdiagnosed as right upper lobe pneumonia because of its appearance in the lateral projection.

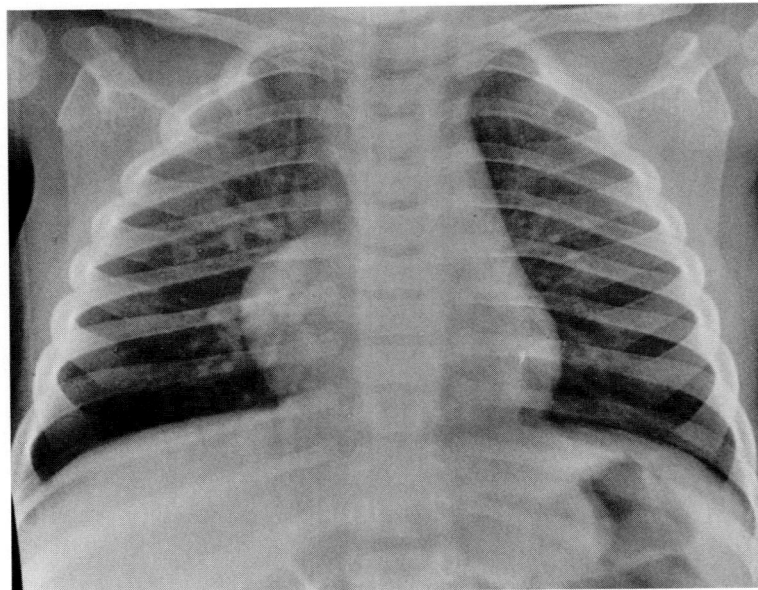

Figure 9–286. Absence of visible thymus on the right simulates dextrocardia.

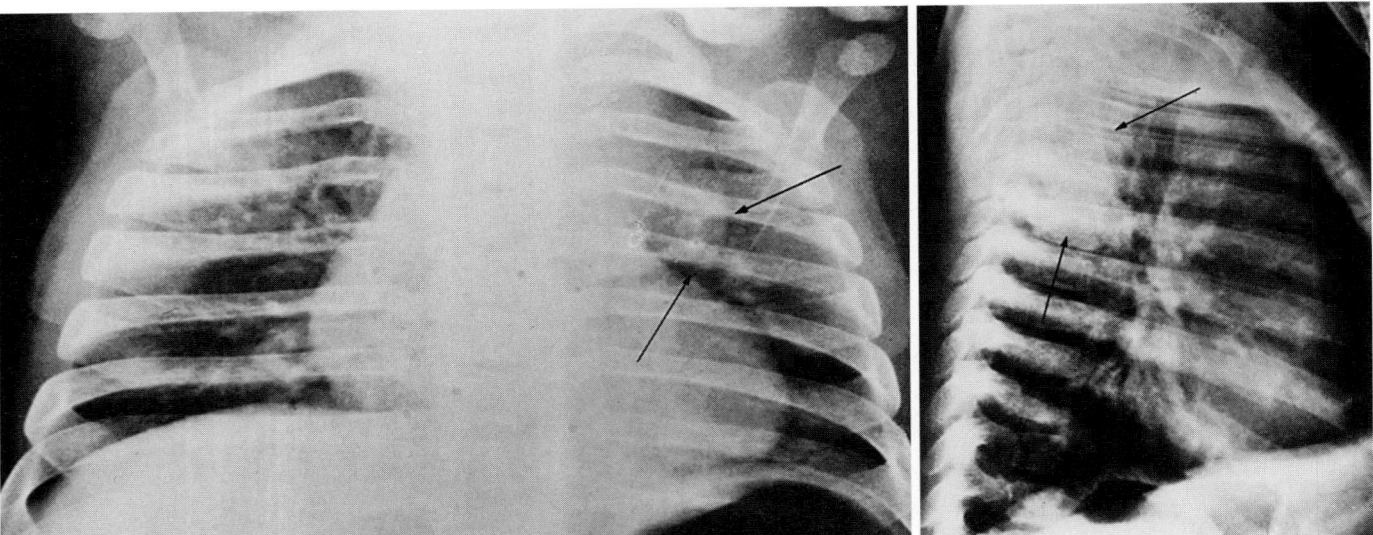

Figure 9–287. Posterior mediastinal thymus, a rare variant. At surgery the thymus was connected to the anterior mediastinum by a thin pedicle. (Refs: Cohen MD et al: The diagnostic dilemma of the posterior mediastinal thymus: CT manifestations. *Radiology* 146:691, 1983; Bar-Ziv J et al: Posterior mediastinal accessory thymus. *Pediatr Radiol*, 14:165, 1984; Siegel MJ et al: Normal and abnormal thymus in childhood: MR imaging. *Radiology* 172:367, 1989.)

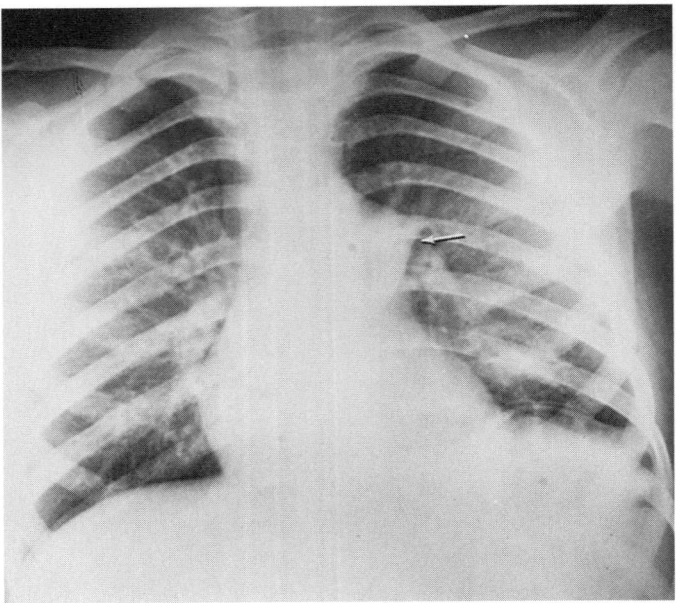

Figure 9–288. The thymus does not always regress in early childhood and may persist into early adolescence. Its presence in late childhood, therefore, should not be construed as evidence of abnormality. Note residual thymus in a 14-year-old boy. (Ref: Oh KS et al: Normal mediastinal mass in late childhood. *Radiology* 101:625, 1971.)

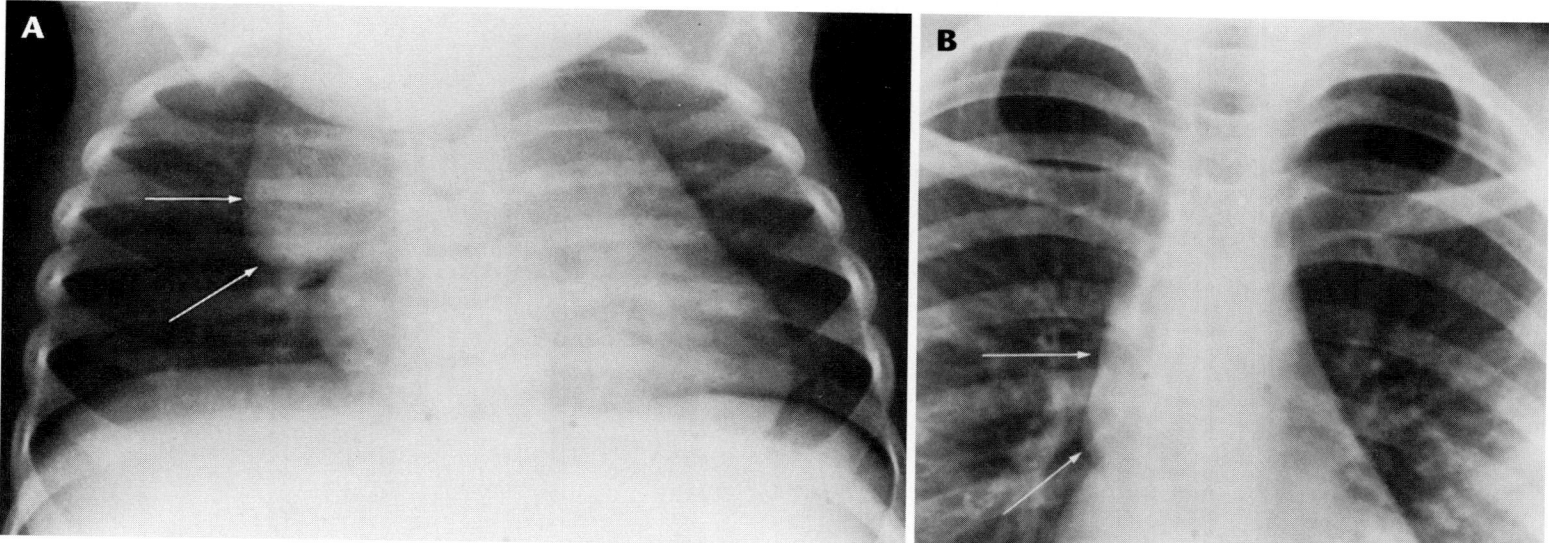

Figure 9–289. Late persistence of the thymus. A, 1-year-old. B, 9-year-old.

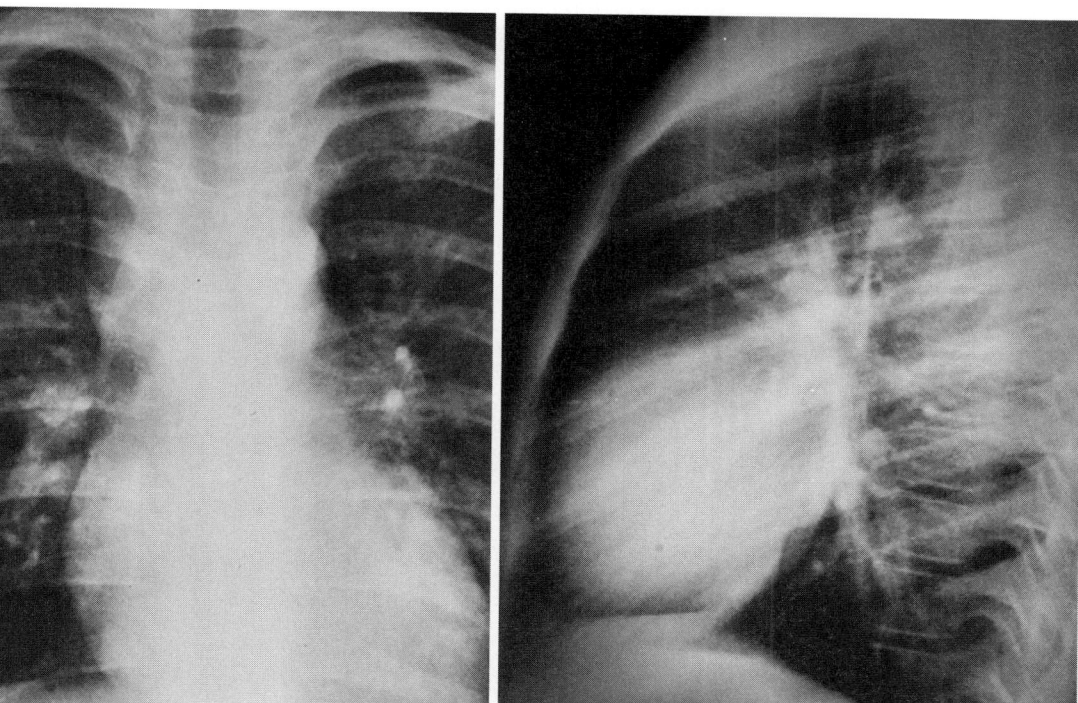

Figure 9–290. Residual thymus in a 6-year-old girl.

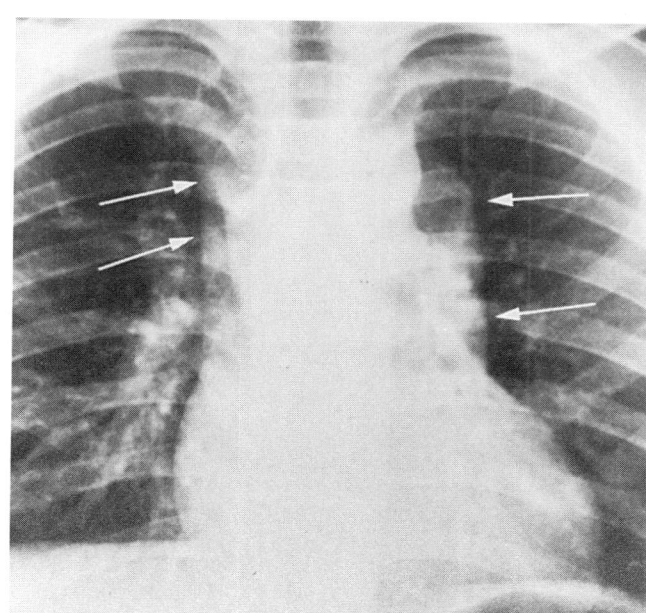

Figure 9–291. Residual thymus in a 6-year-old boy.

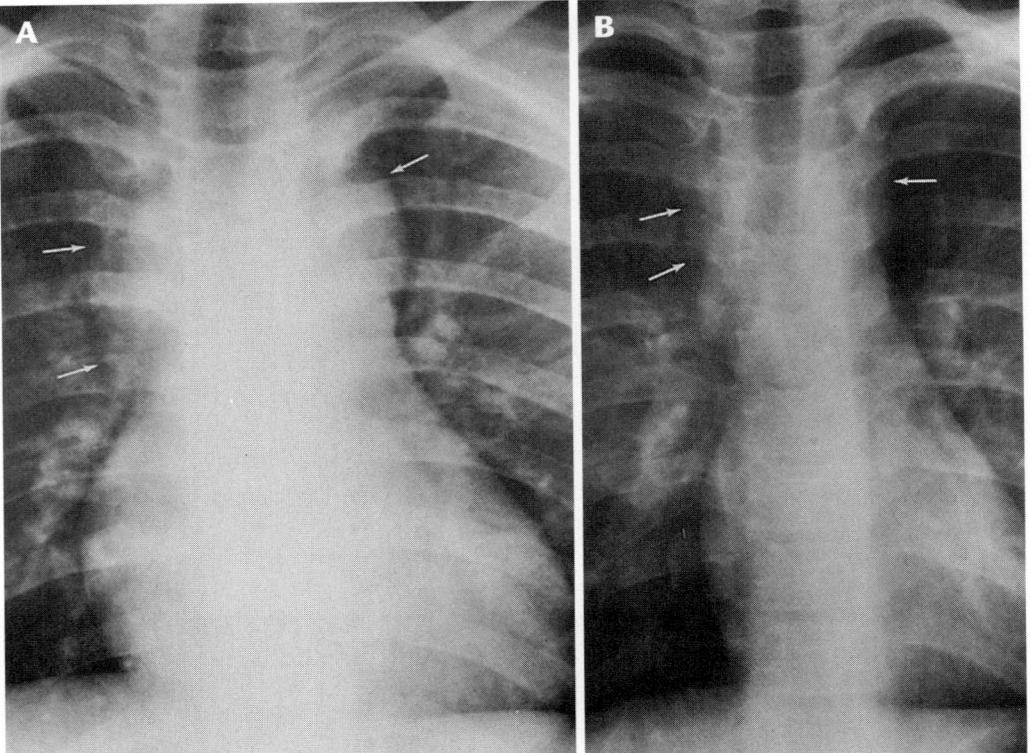

Figure 9–292. A, Residual thymus in an 8-year-old girl. **B,** 2-year follow-up.

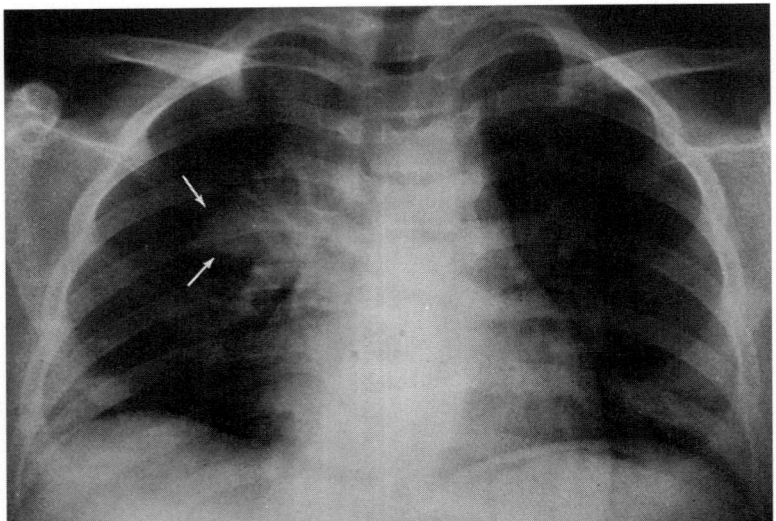

Figure 9–293. Residual thymus in a 9-year-old boy.

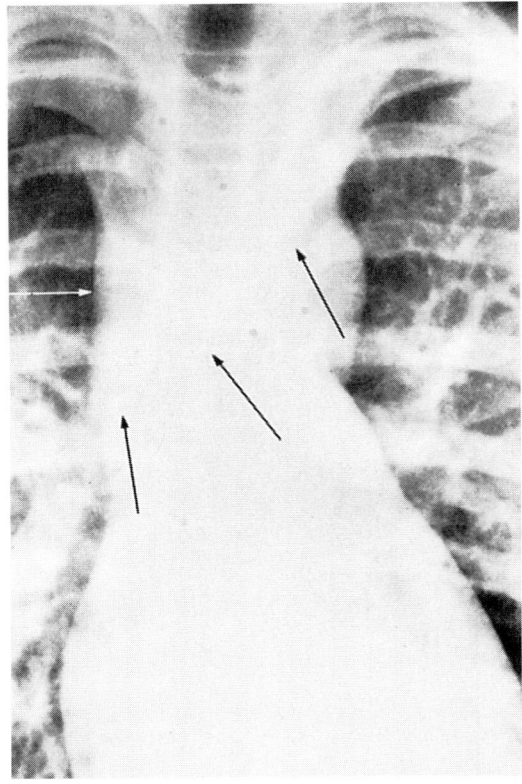

Figure 9–294. Residual thymus in a 9-year-old boy, which can be traced across the mediastinum.

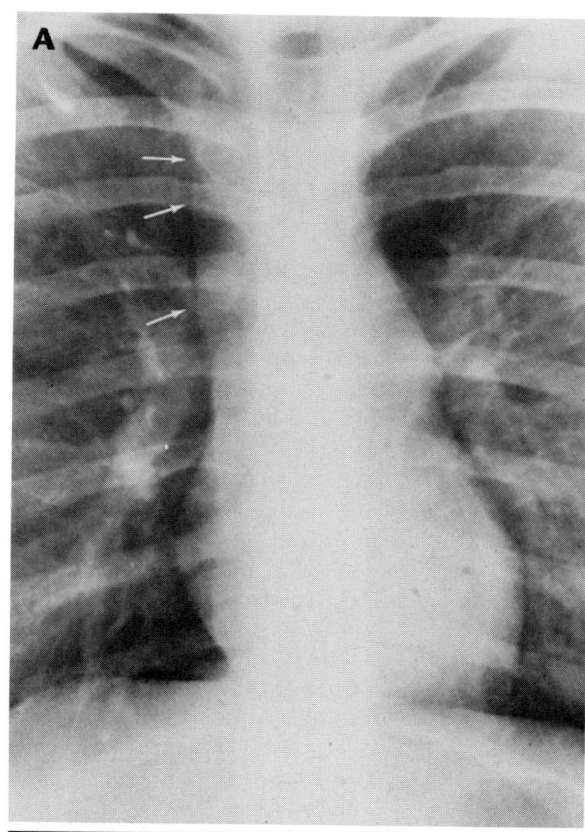

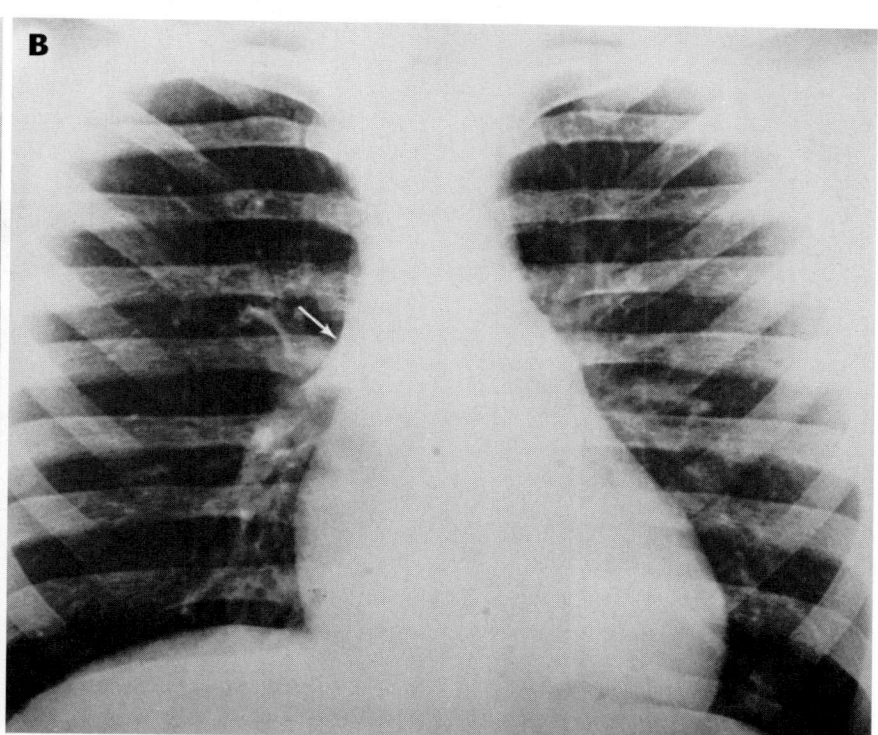

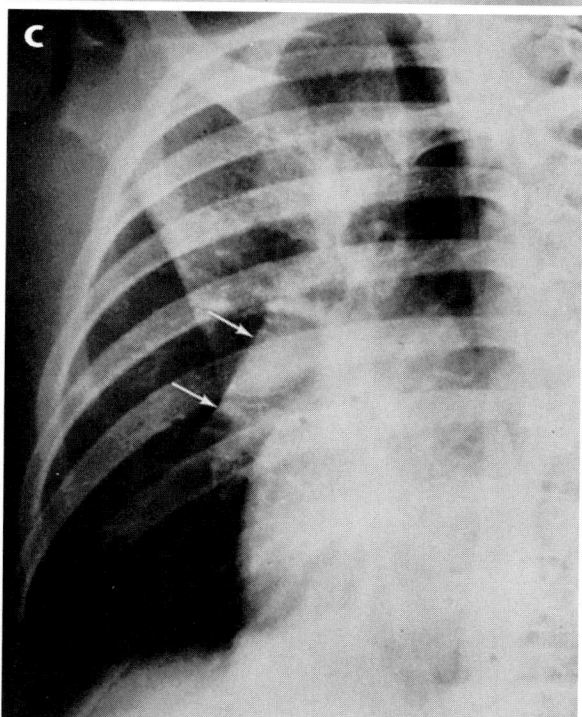

Figure 9–295. A, Residual thymus in an 11-year-old boy. B and C, Frontal and left anterior oblique projections in a 14-year-old boy showing residual thymus.

Figure 9–296. Residual thymus in a 13-year-old girl.

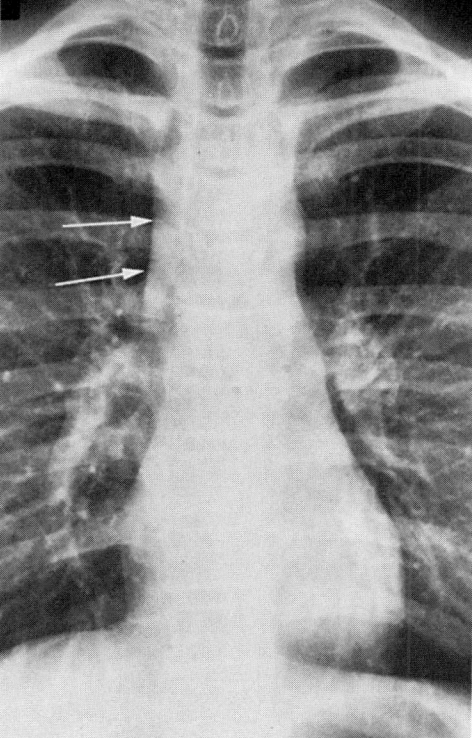

1041

CHAPTER

10

The Diaphragm

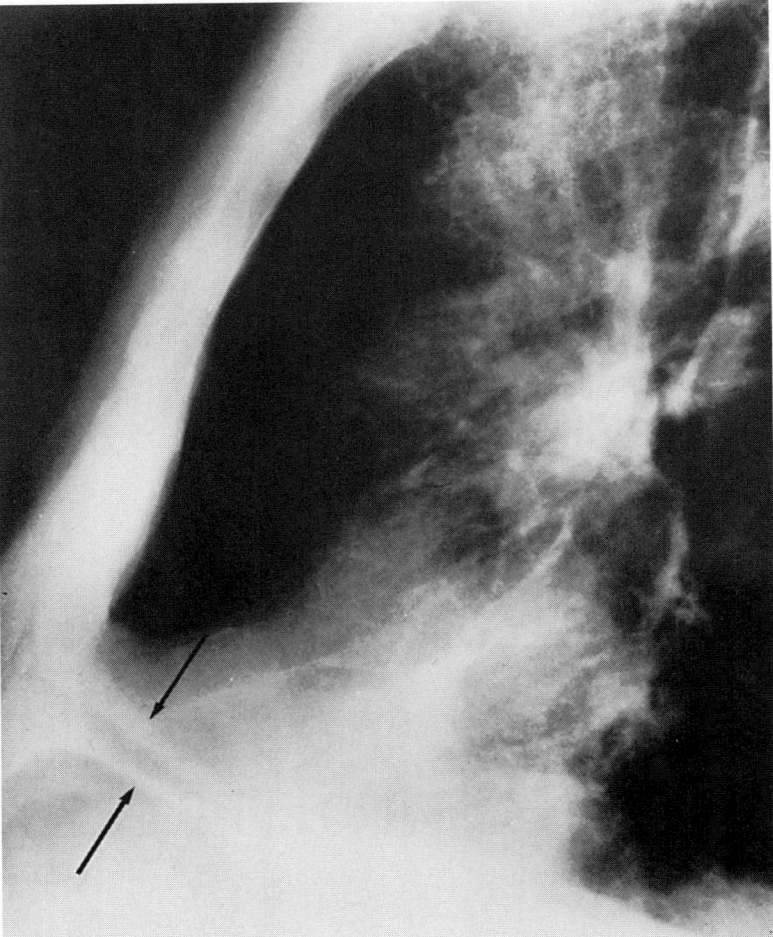

Figure 10–1. Sternal insertions of the diaphragm, which consist of a pair of short, narrow slips that arise from the back of the xiphoid and pass backward to be inserted into the central tendon of the diaphragm. (Ref: Kleinman PK, Raptopoulos V: The anterior diaphragmatic attachments. *Radiology* 155:289, 1985.)

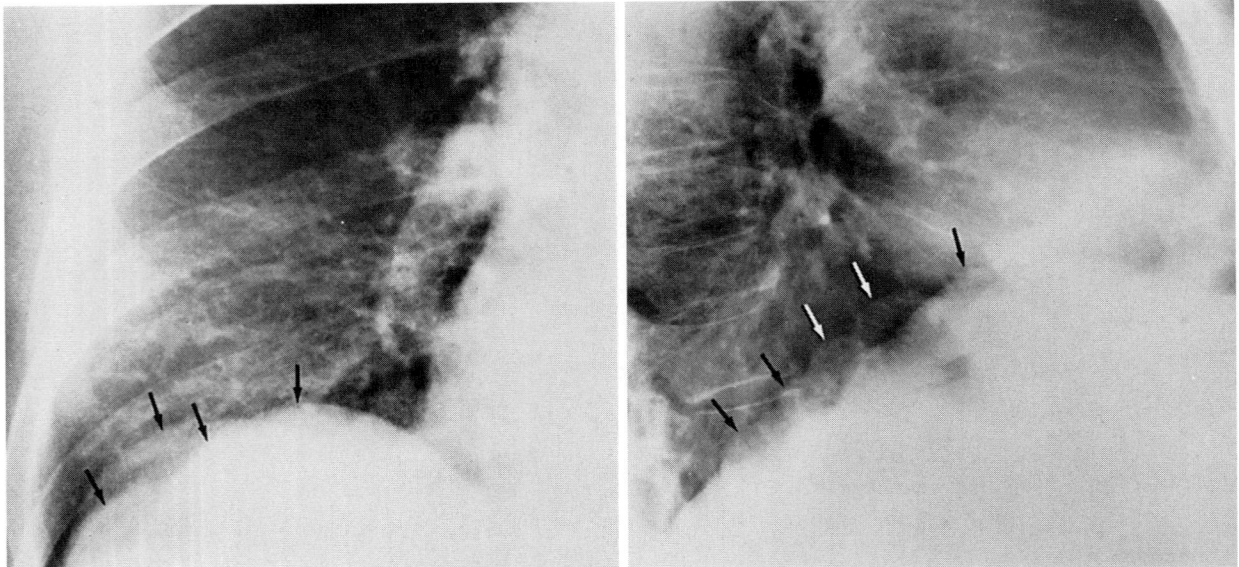

Figure 10–2. "Scalloping" of the diaphragm is caused by hypertrophy and contraction of individual muscle bundles in the diaphragm. This case shows multiple small convexities.

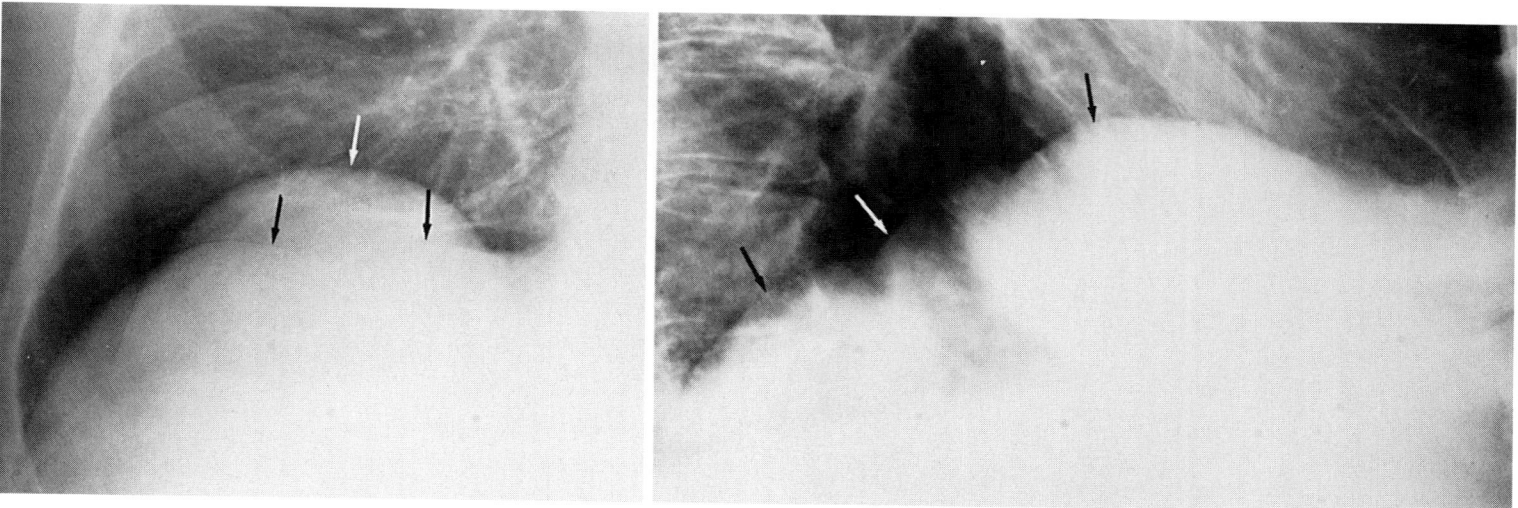

Figure 10–3. "Scalloping" of the diaphragm, with several large convexities.

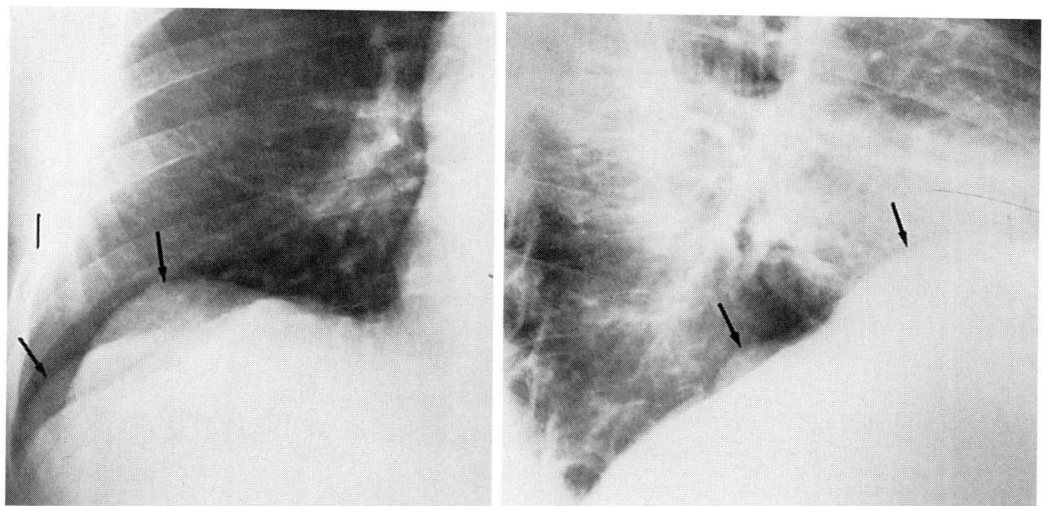

Figure 10–4. "Scalloping" of the diaphragm.

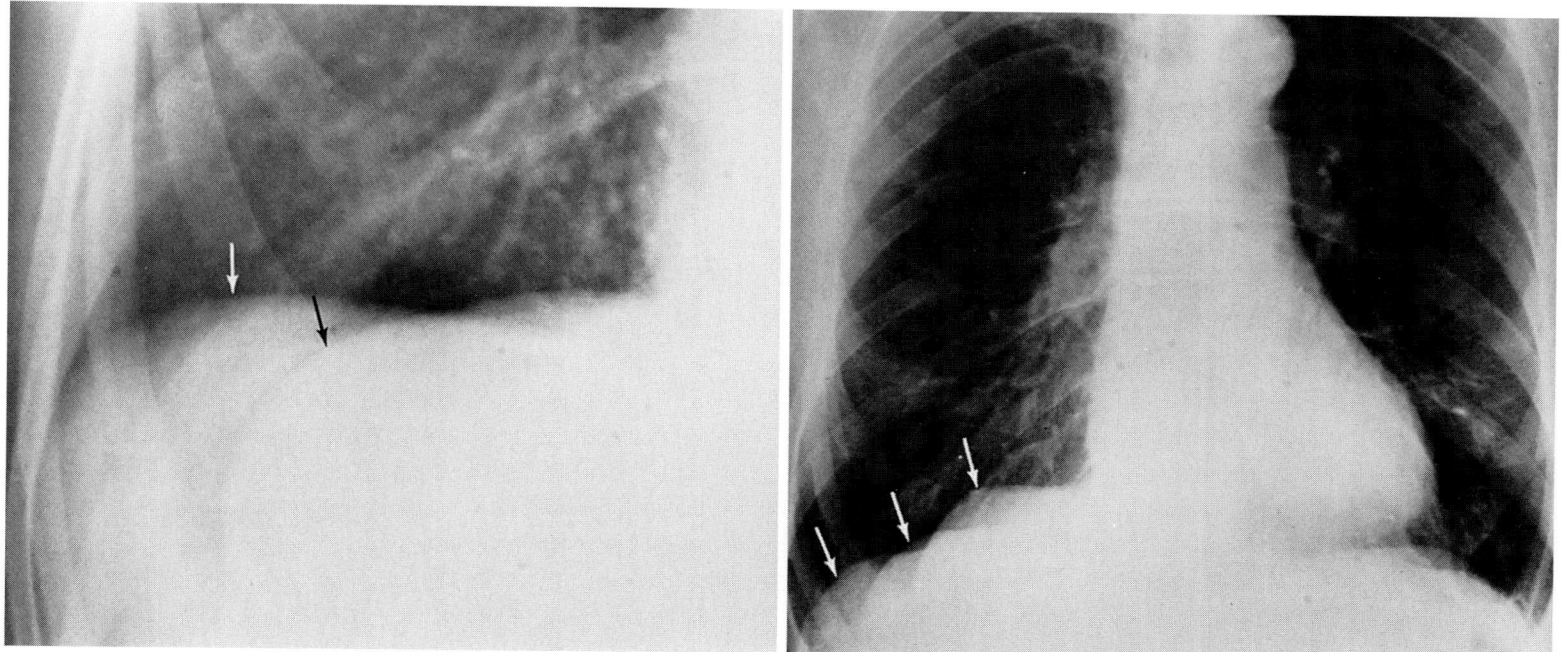

Figure 10–5. Additional variations of "scalloped" diaphragms.

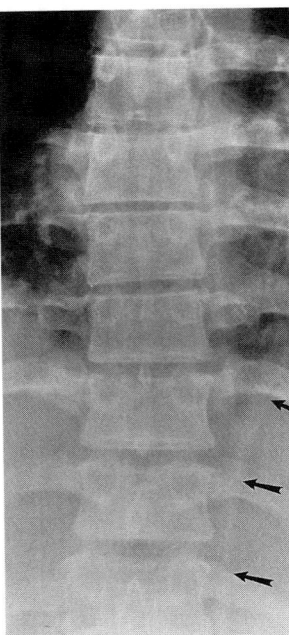

Figure 10–6. Crus of the left hemidiaphragm.

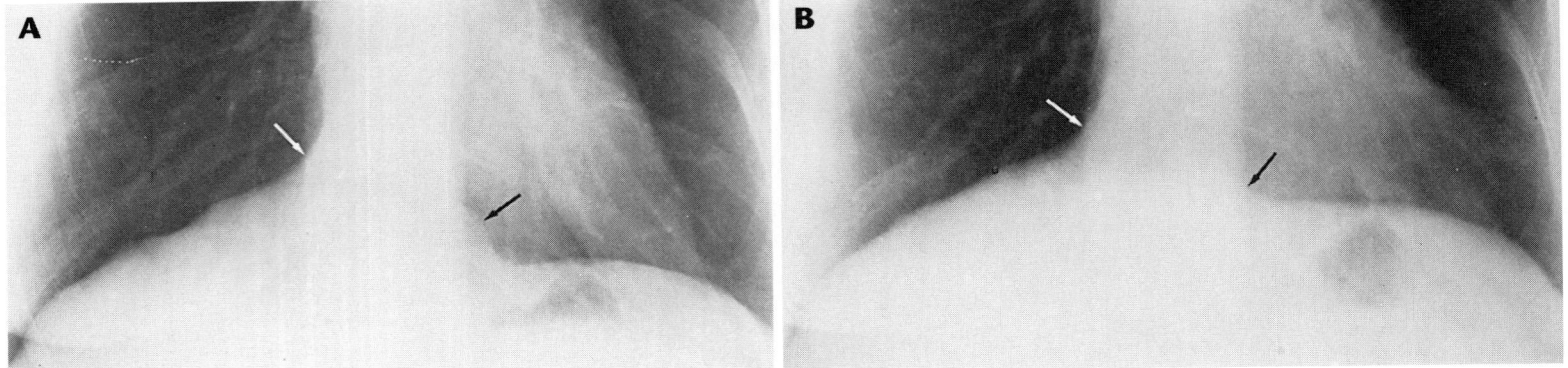

Figure 10–7. High insertions of the medial attachments of the diaphragm, simulating mass lesions. **A,** Inspiration. **B,** Partial expiration, in which the attachments are not seen as clearly.

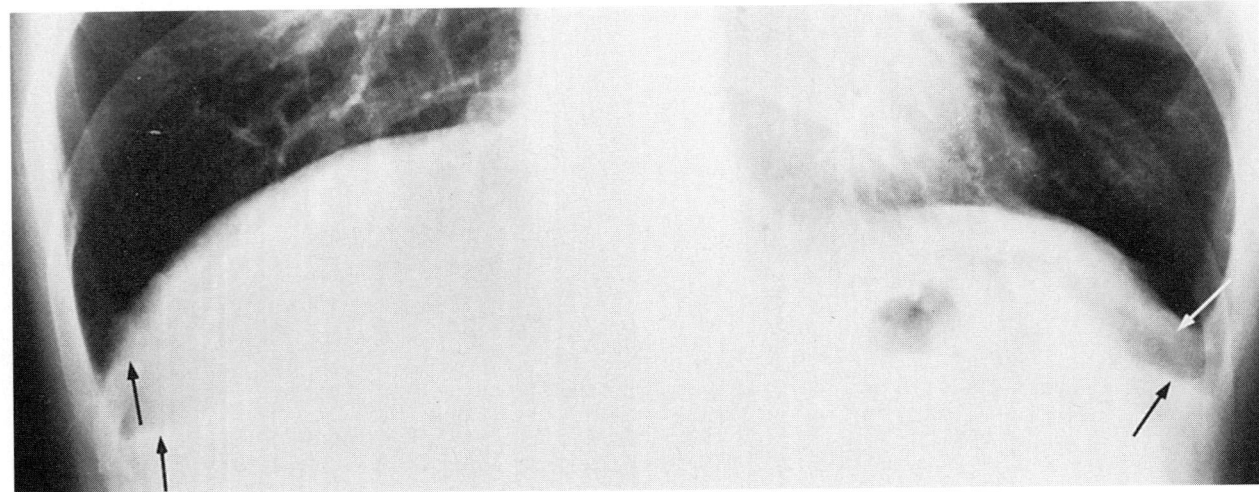

Figure 10–8. Muscular slips of the diaphragm seen in maximal inspiration.

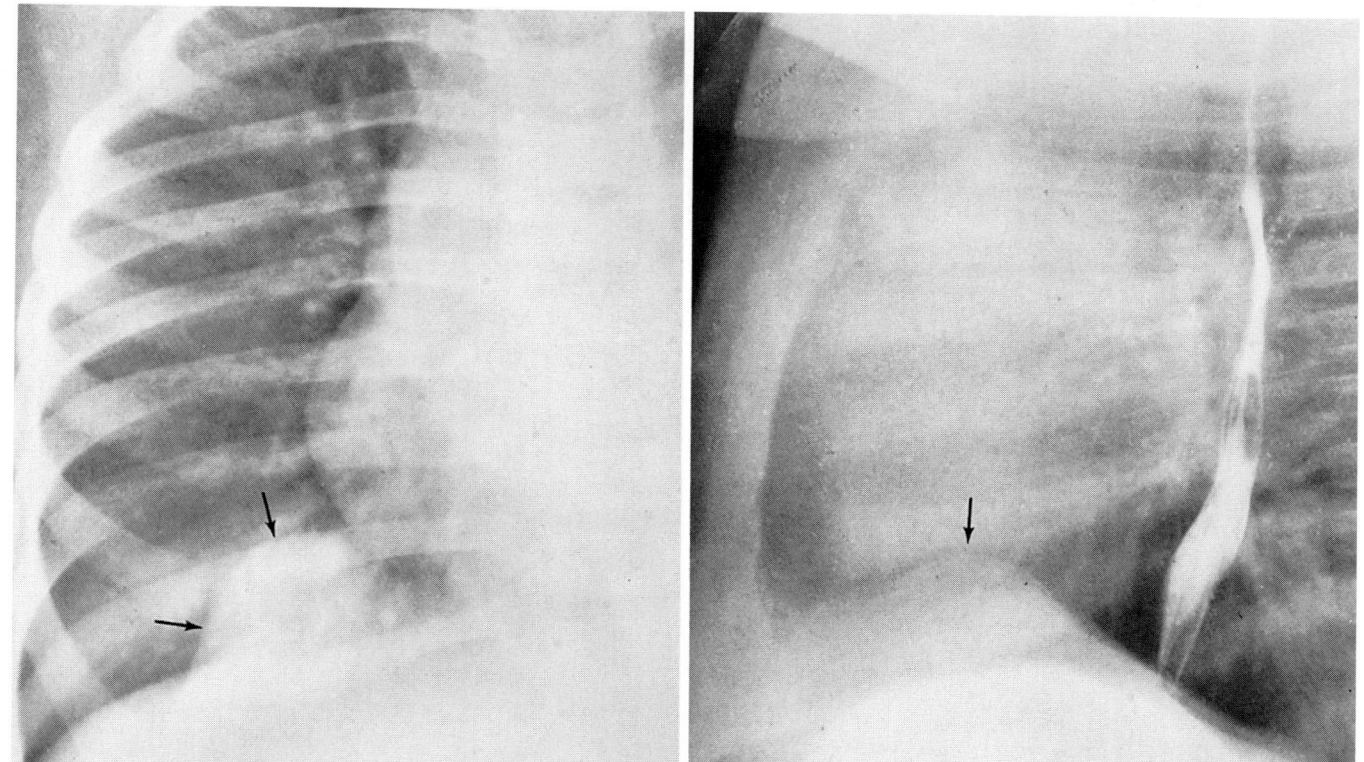

Figure 10–9. Localized eventration of the diaphragm in a child. Without benefit of the lateral projection, this variation could be mistaken for a mass lesion.

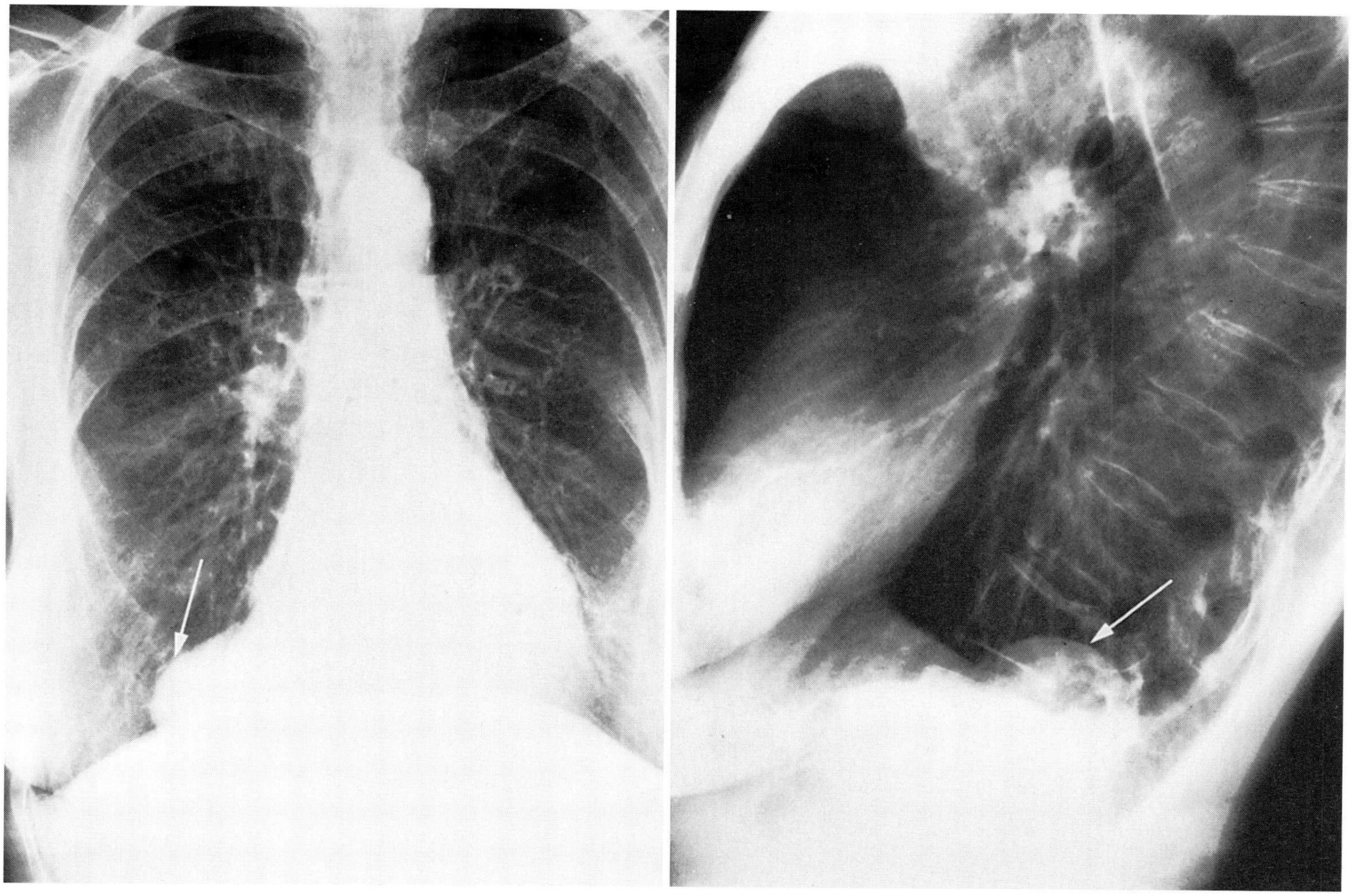

Figure 10–10. Intrathoracic migration of the right kidney through the right foramen of Bochdalek in a 70-year-old woman that was not present on an examination made 20 years earlier. Diaphragmatic defects and pseudolesions such as fat or visceral herniations through diaphragmatic defects increase in number and severity in the seventh and eighth decades of life. (Ref: Laskey Cl et al: Aging of the diaphragm: A CT study. *Radiology* 171:385, 1989.)

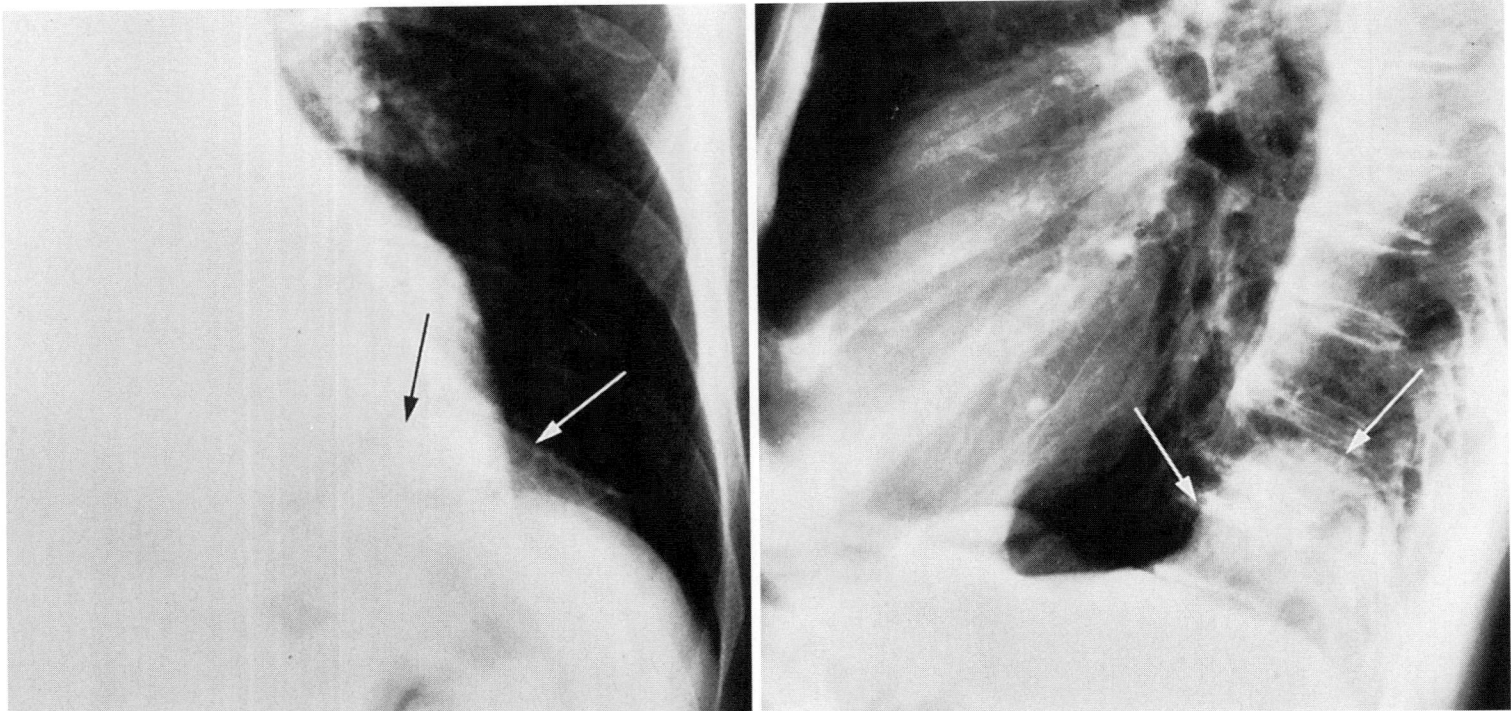

Figure 10–11. Another example of the entity illustrated in Figure 10–10 on the left side.

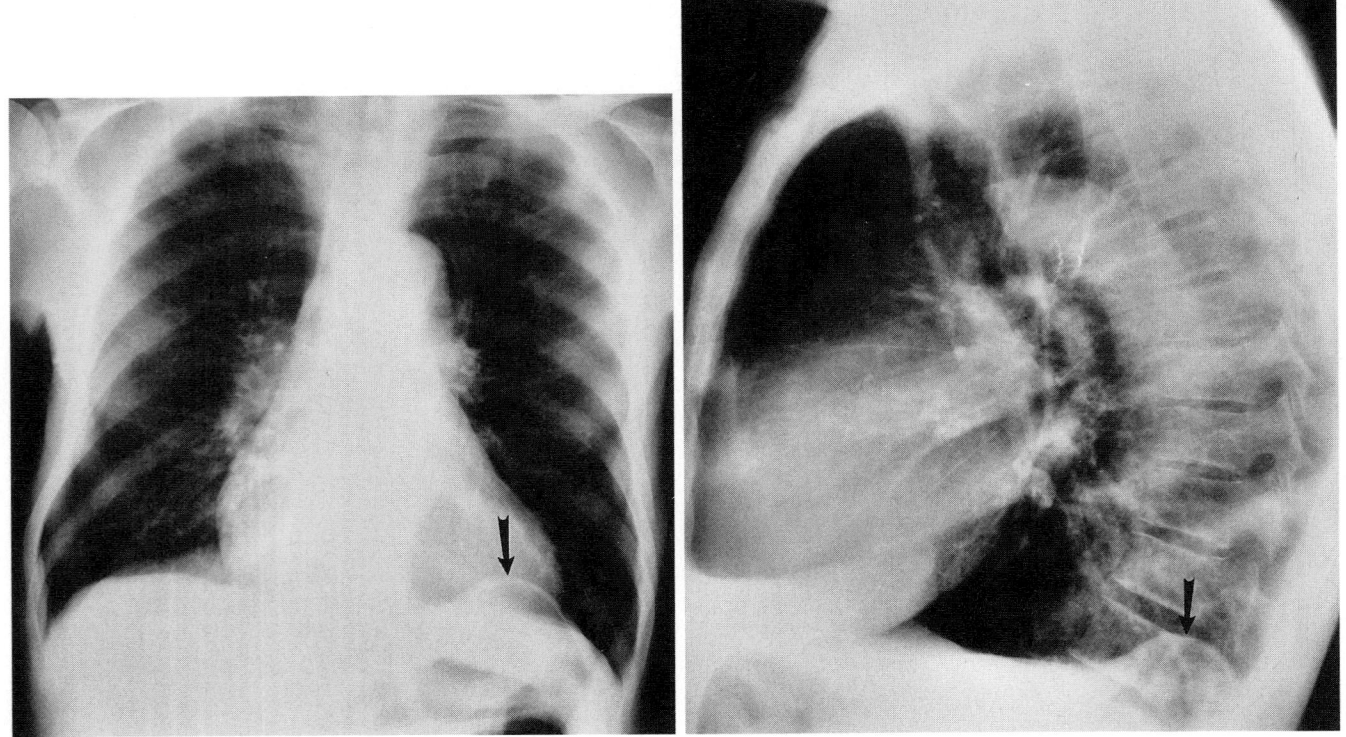

Figure 10–12. Intrathoracic migration of the colon through the foramen of Bochdalek in an 83-year-old woman.

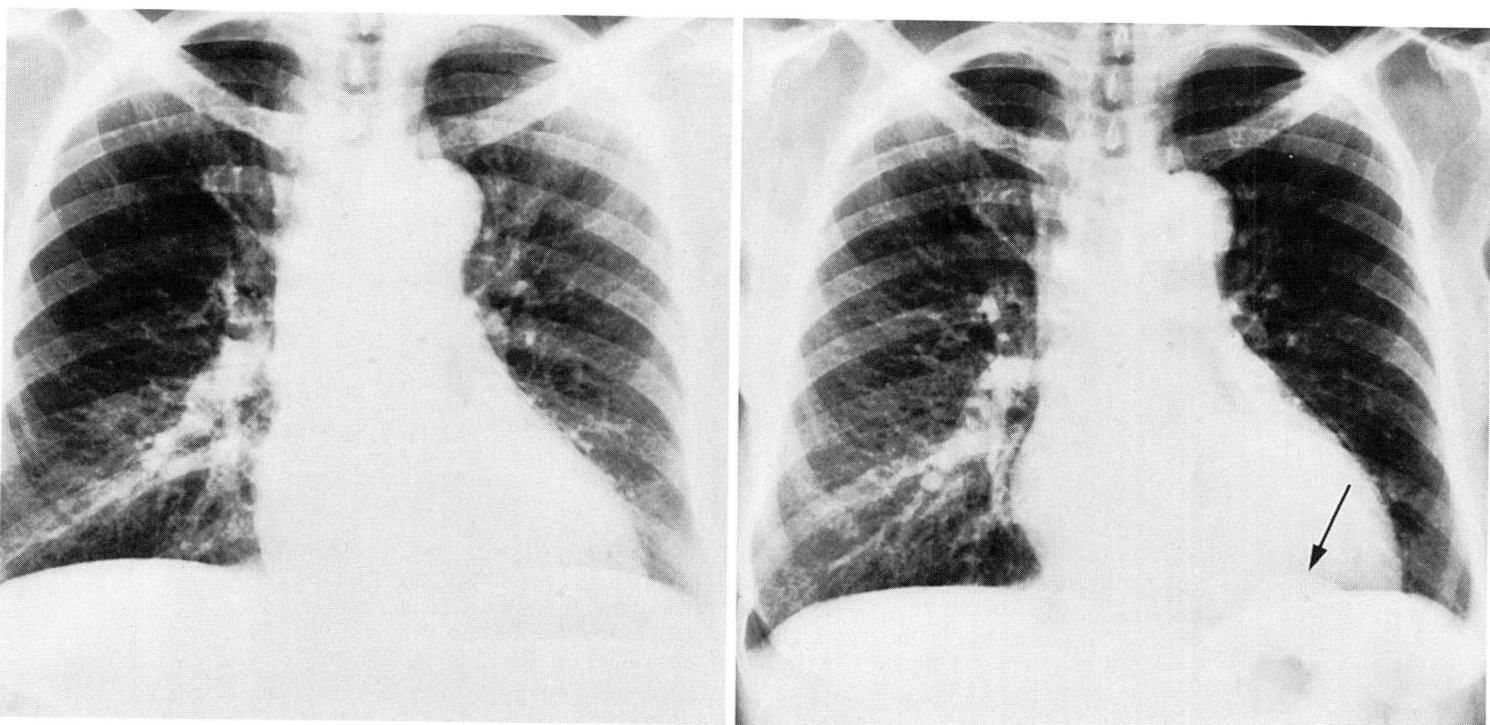

Figure 10–13. Intrathoracic migration of the kidney through the foramen of Bochdalek is not seen on shallow inspiration (*left*), but is visualized with maximal inspiration (*right*).

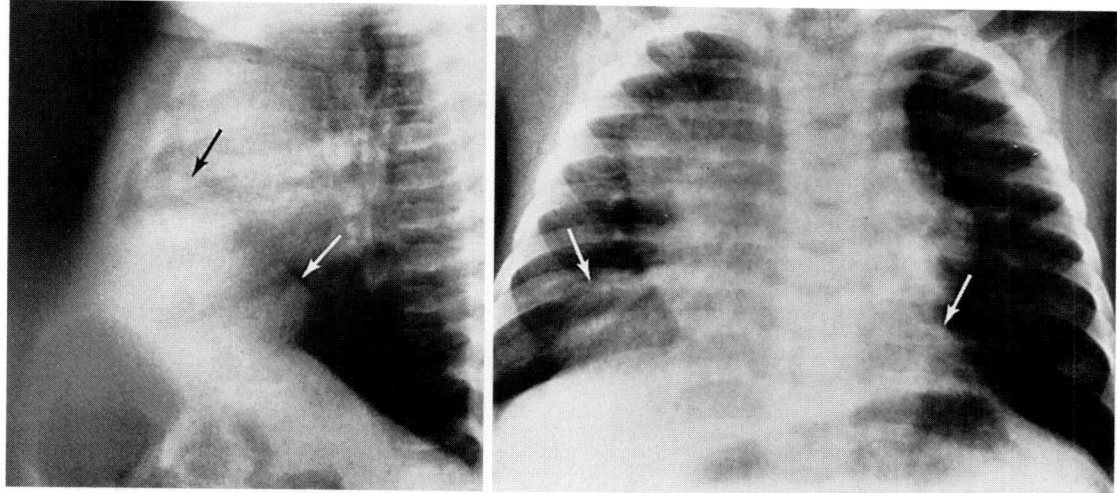

Figure 10–14. Bilateral anterior diaphragmatic eventration in a newborn. This condition may be asymptomatic. Note upward displacement of the heart. (Ref: Avnet NE: Roentgenologic features of congenital bilateral interior diaphragmatic eventration. *Am J Roentgenol* 88:743, 1962.)

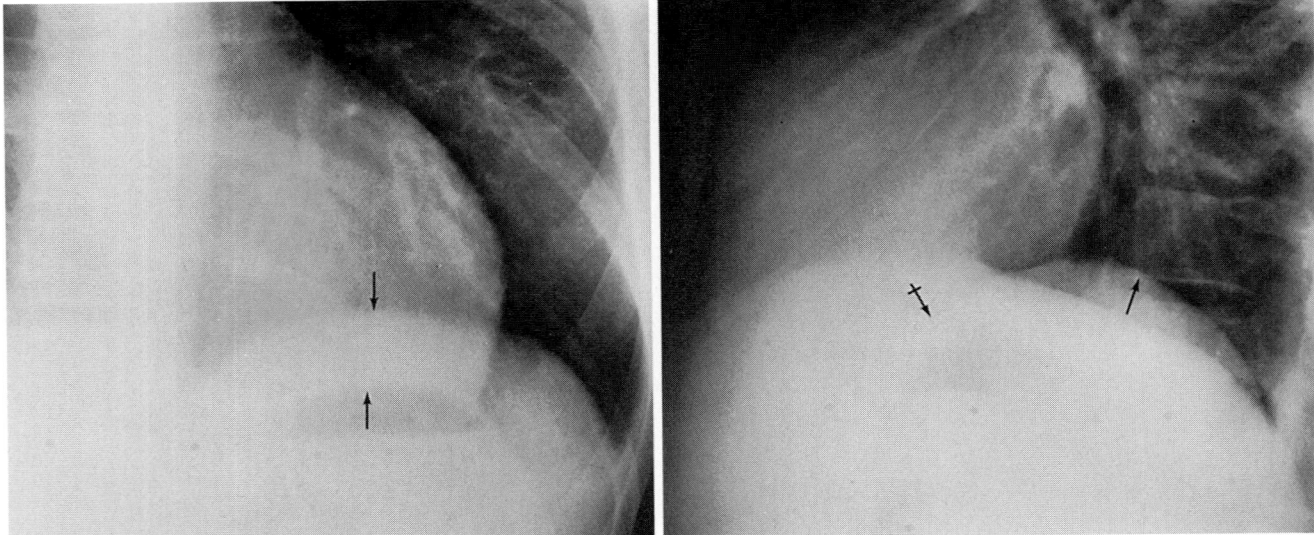

Figure 10–15. Increased distance between the stomach gas bubble and the diaphragm suggests a subpulmonic effusion. The lateral projection indicates that this appearance is due to the fact that the posterior portion of the left hemidiaphragm (→) is higher than the anterior portion (↔), which is adjacent to the gas bubble.

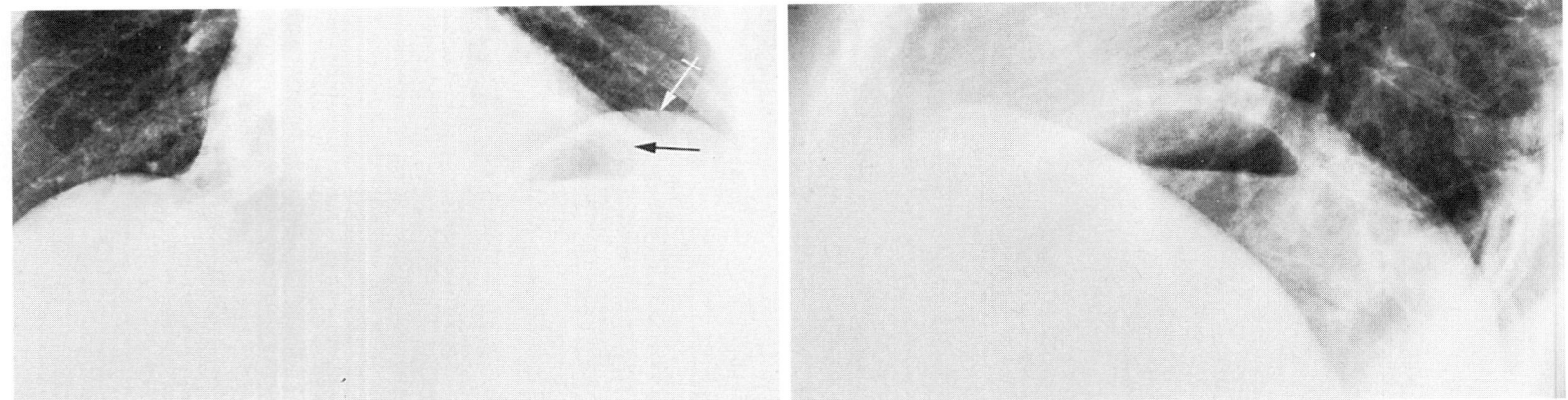

Figure 10–16. Increased distance between the stomach gas bubble and the diaphragm in lateral projection caused by the medial position of the gas bubble (←) in relation to the highest point of the dome of the diaphragm (↔).

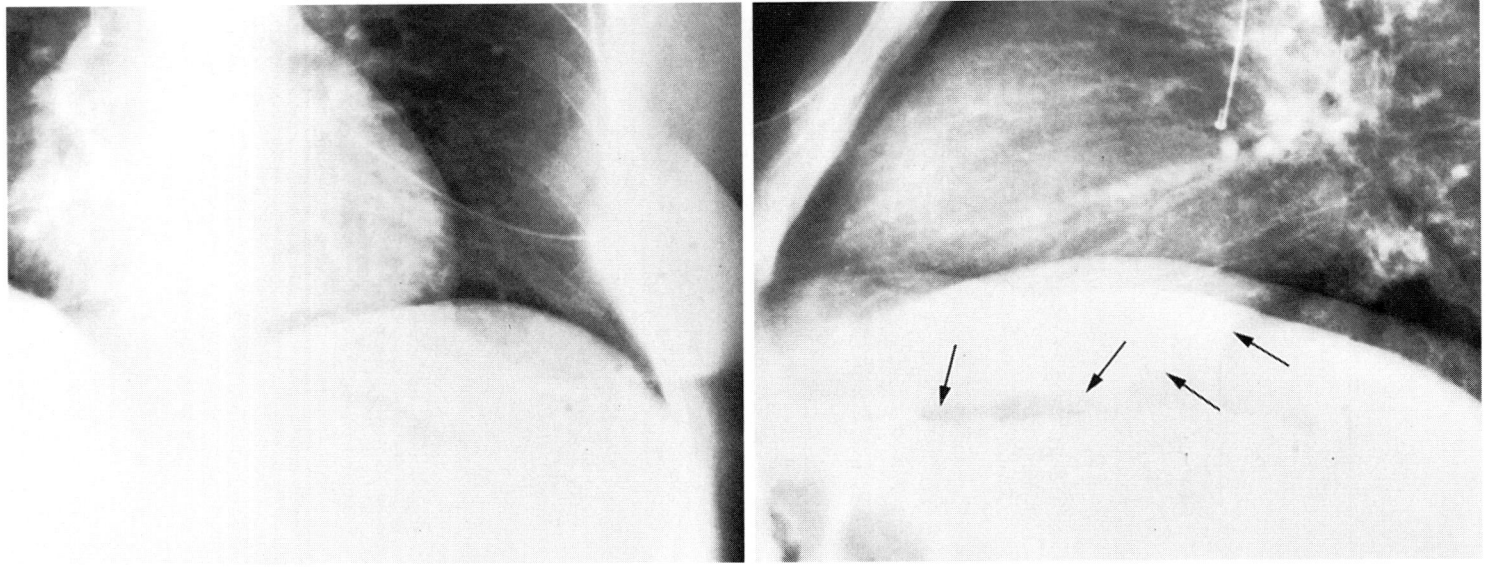

Figure 10–17. Increased distance between the stomach gas bubble and the diaphragm in lateral projection caused by the impression of the heart on the gas bubble (*arrows*).

CHAPTER

11

The Soft Tissues of the Abdomen

The Abdomen in General

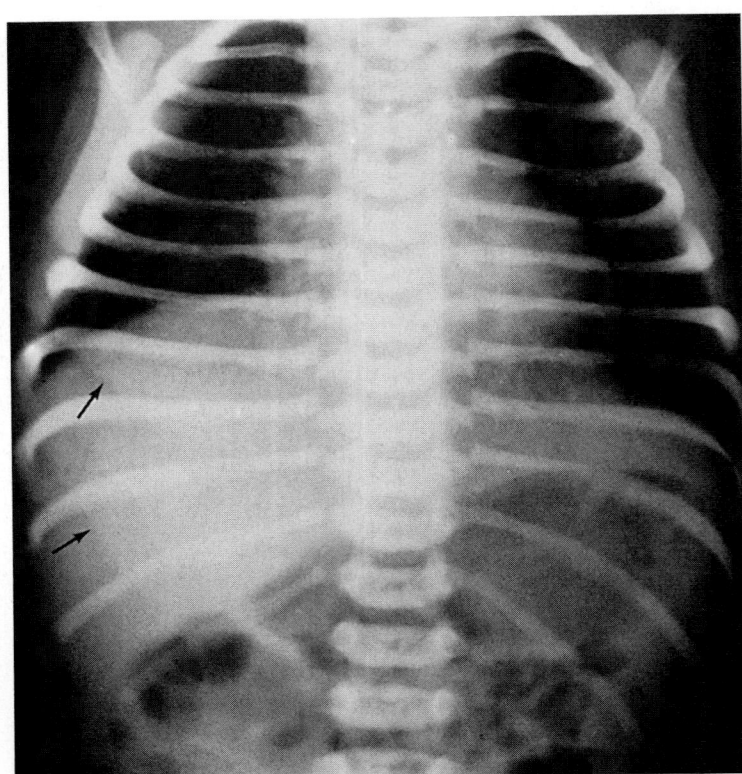

Figure 11–1. Skin folds in an infant, producing an unusual appearance of the hepatic shadow.

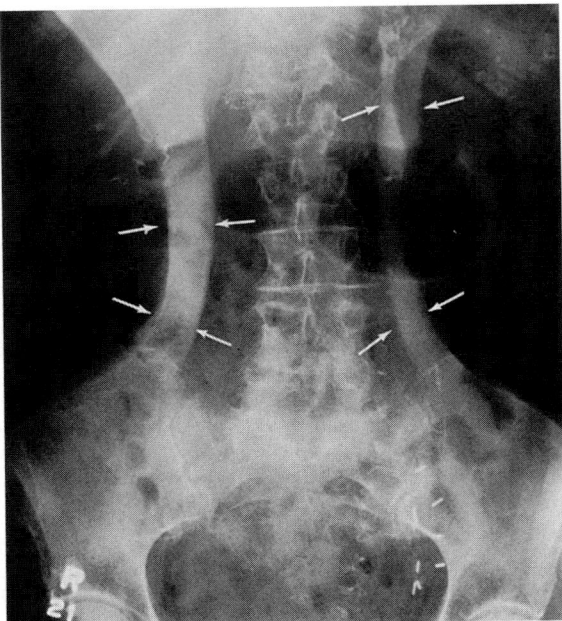

Figure 11–2. Posterior skin folds in an elderly patient, lending a striking appearance to the abdomen.

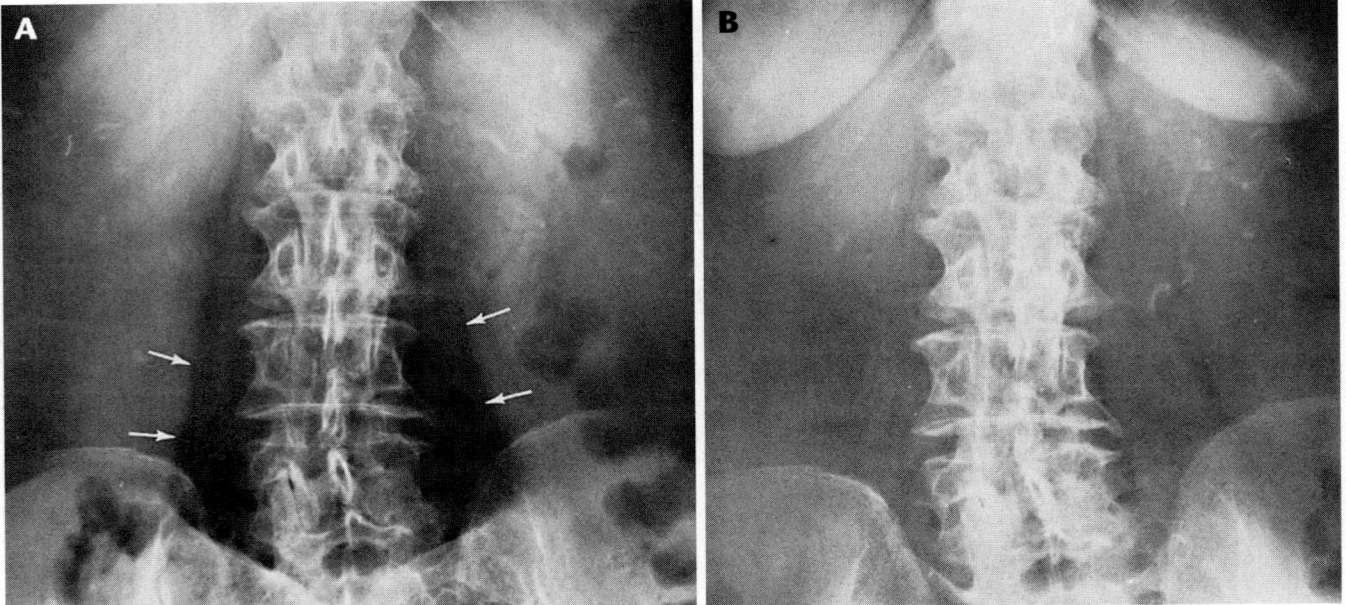

Figure 11–3. A, Simulated lucency of the psoas muscles produced by folding of the soft tissues of the back. **B,** This appearance is not seen in the subsequent film after alteration of the patient's position.

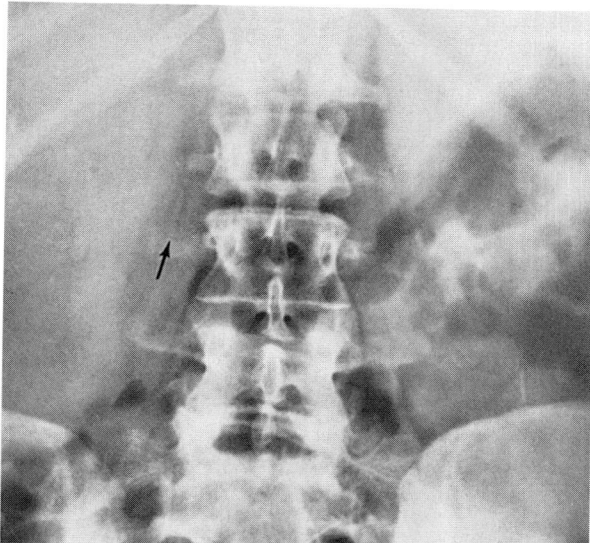

Figure 11–4. Lucent stripes in the shadow of the psoas muscle caused by fat between the muscle bundles.

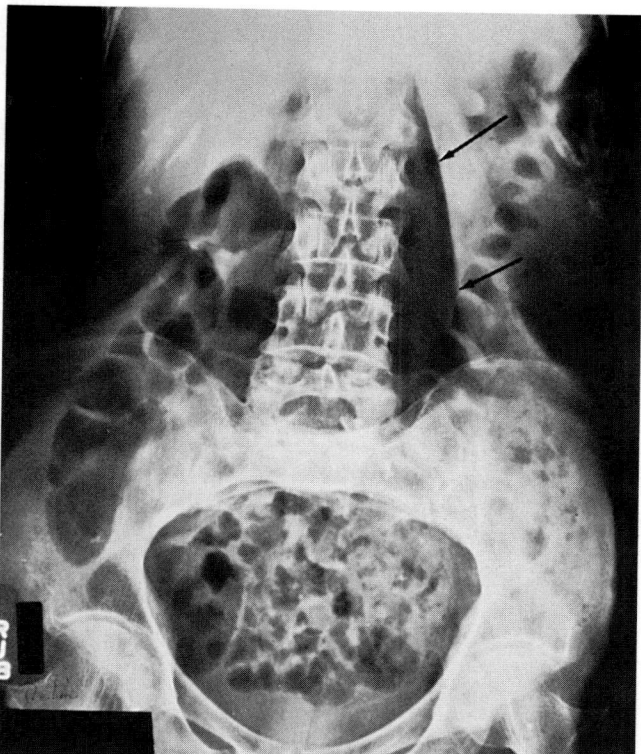

Figure 11–5. Skin fold simulating a lucent psoas shadow.

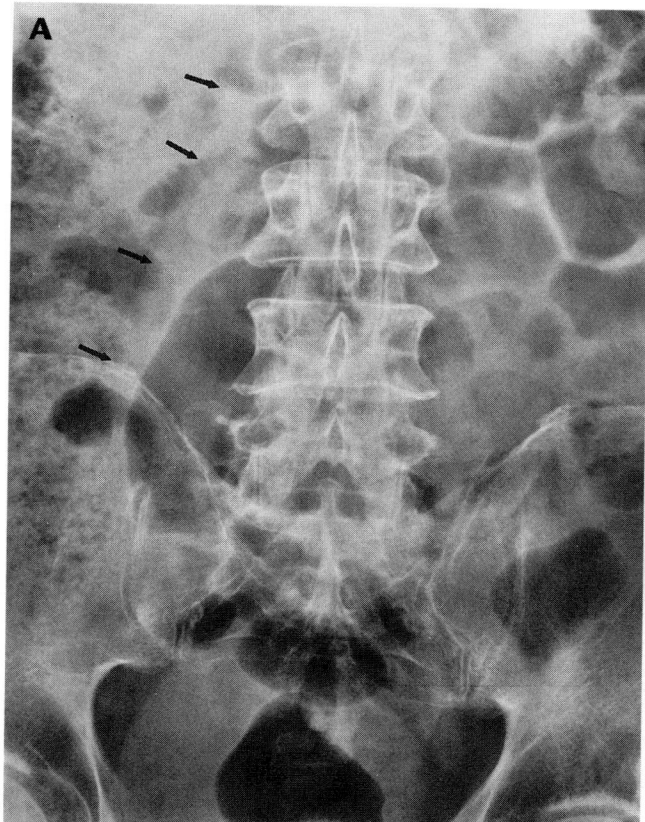

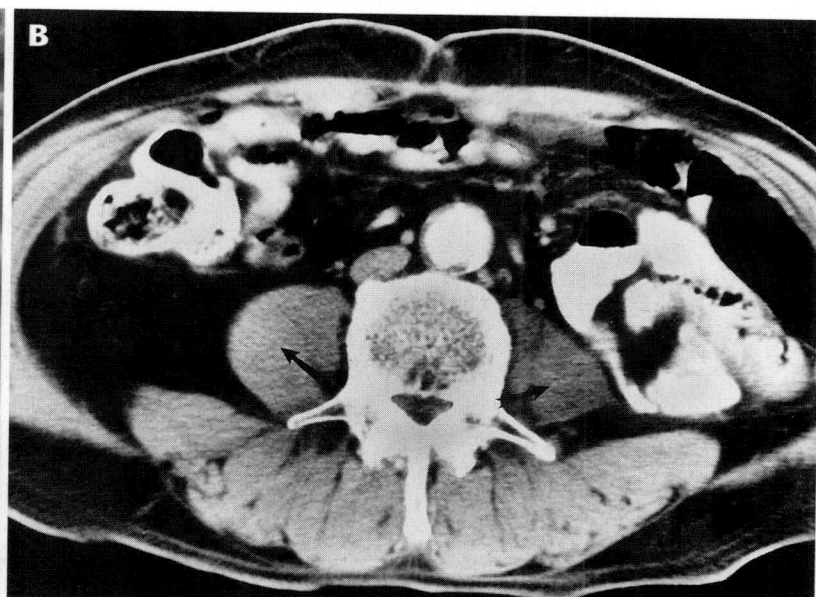

Figure 11–6. A, Good visualization of the right psoas muscle shadow but not the left. **B,** CT shows a large right psoas muscle and a smaller left muscle. Such nonvisualization may also be due to the obliquity of the muscle itself. (Ref: Williams SM et al: Psoas sign: Reevaluation. *Radiographics* 5:525, 1985.)

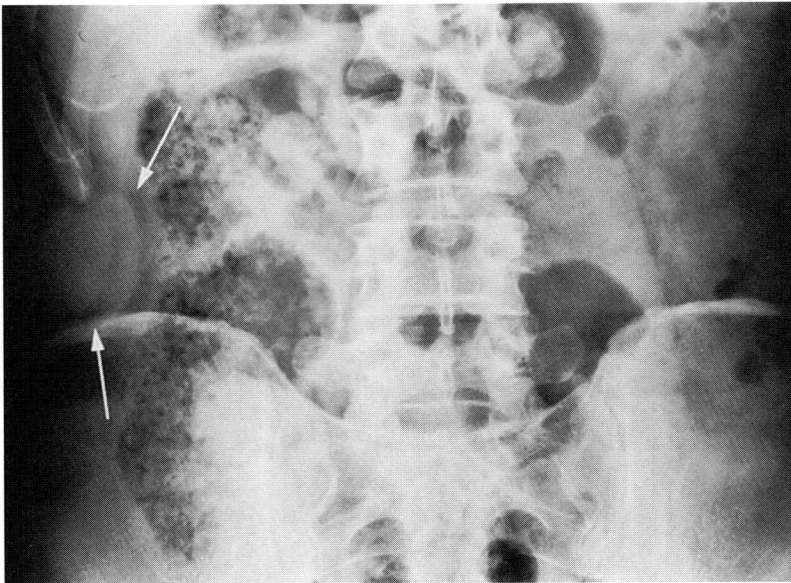

Figure 11–7. Simulated mass in the right flank, produced by muscle splinting on that side.

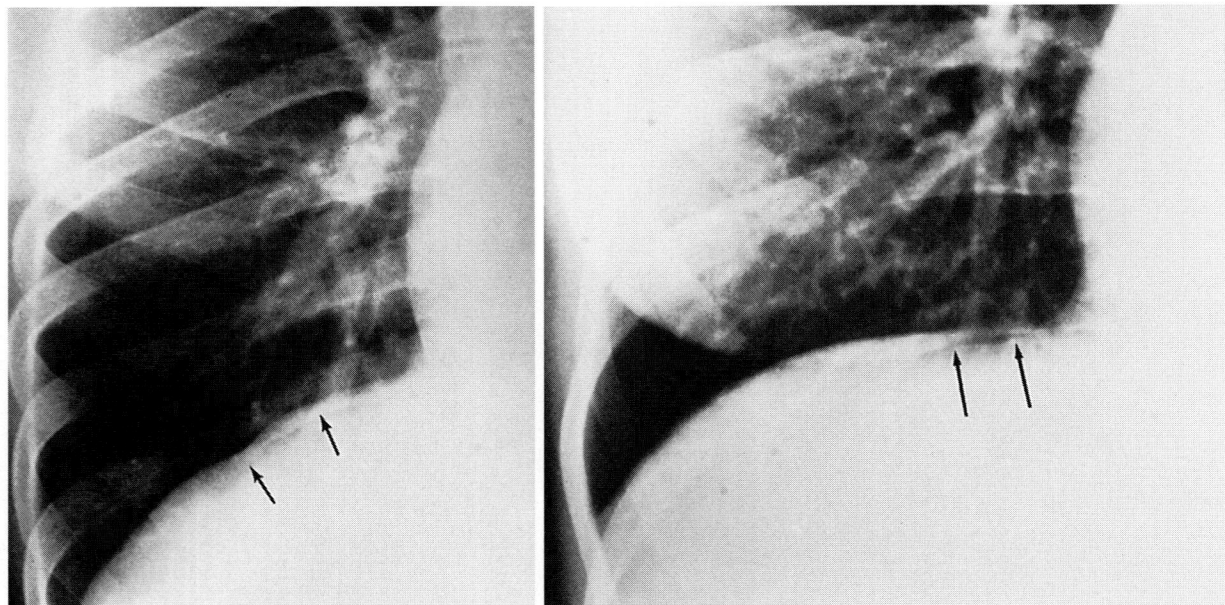

Figure 11–8. Two examples of simulated pneumoperitoneum caused by the Mach effect of the rib superimposed on the diaphragm.

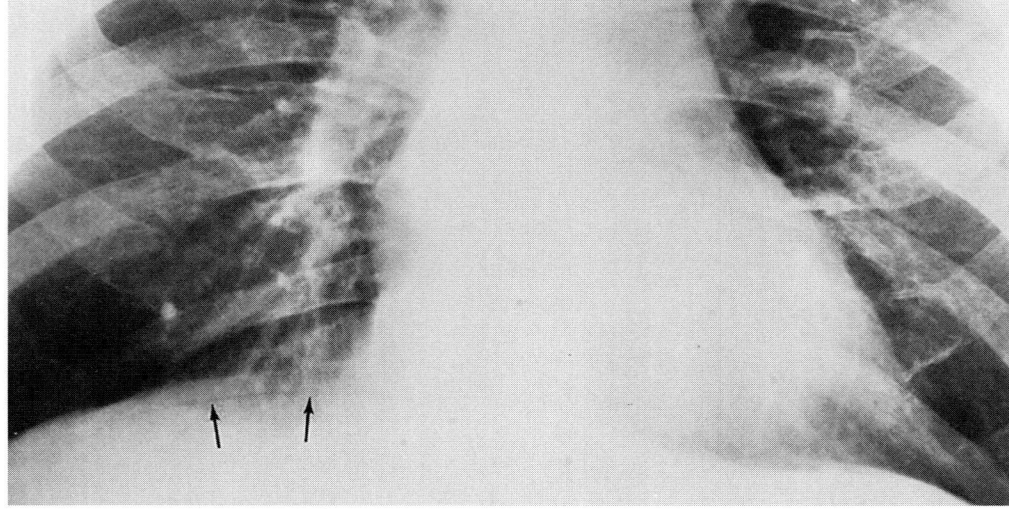

Figure 11–9. Simulated pneumoperitoneum caused by subdiaphragmatic fat. (Ref: Rao KG, Woodlief RM: Excessive right subdiaphragmatic fat: A potential diagnostic pitfall. *Radiology* 138: 15, 1981.)

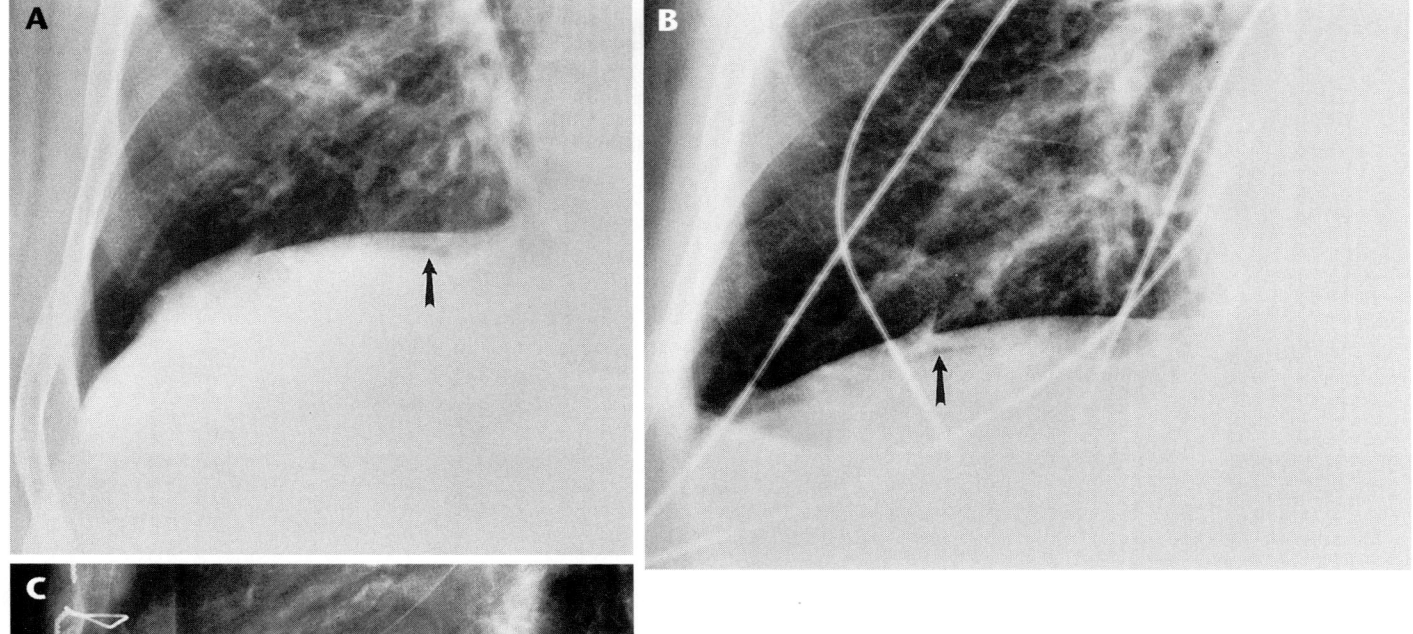

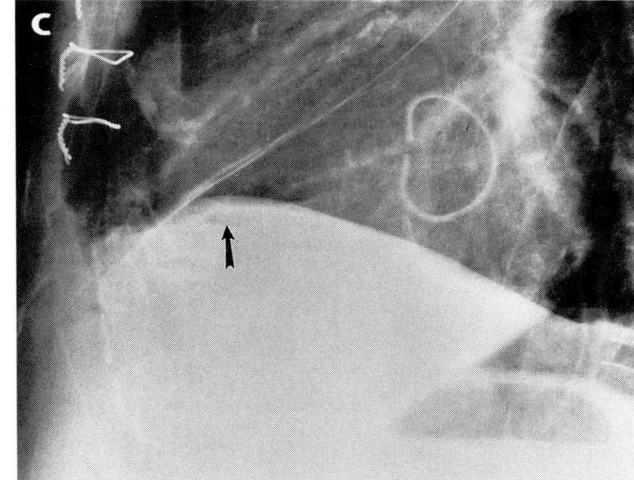

Figure 11–10. Simulated pneumoperitoneum produced by subdiaphragmatic fat. **A** and **B**, Frontal films on two different days. **C**, Lateral projection.

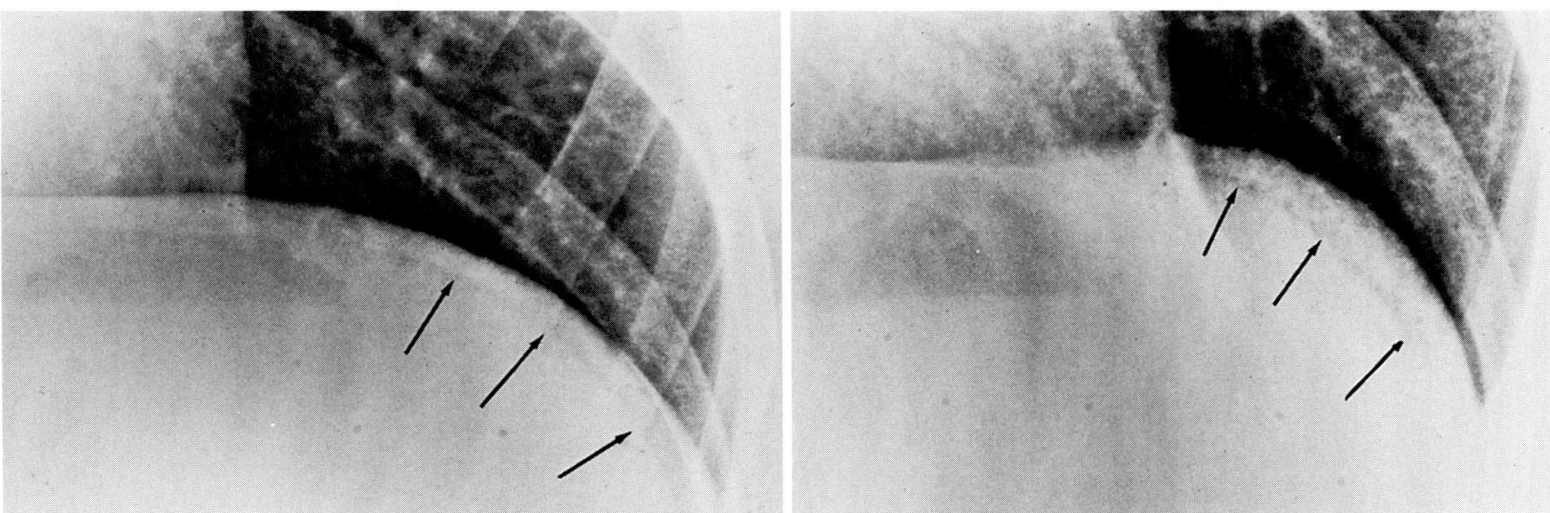

Figure 11–11. Fat may also be seen beneath the left hemidiaphragm, as illustrated in these two cases.

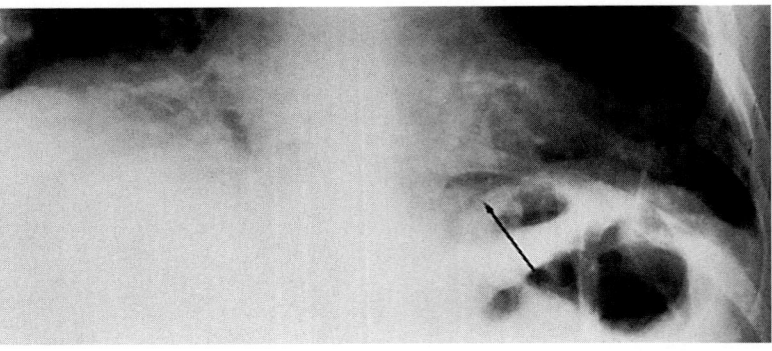
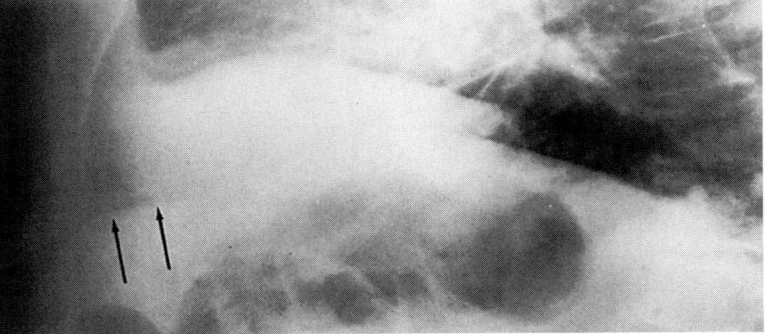

Figure 11–12. *Left,* Fat between the fundus of the stomach and the diaphragm. *Right,* Lateral projection shows fat anteriorly beneath the diaphragm.

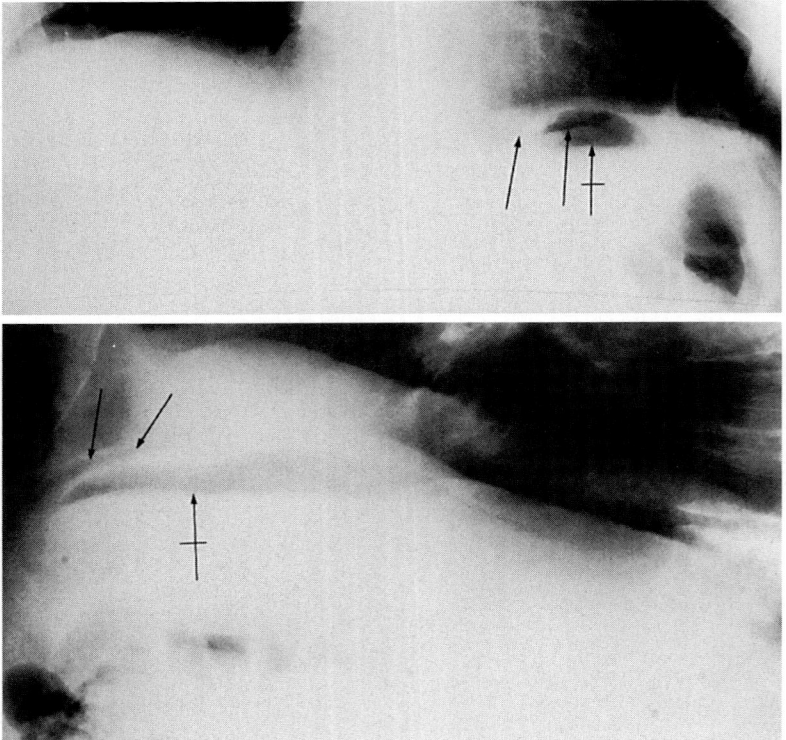

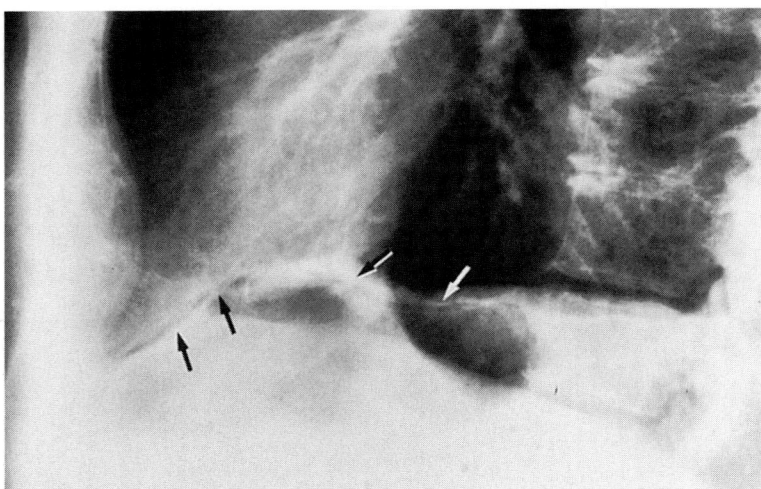

Figure 11–14. Simulated pneumoperitoneum produced by fat between the junction of the stomach and the diaphragm.

Figure 11–13. Simulated pneumoperitoneum produced by fat between the fundus of the stomach and the diaphragm. *Top,* Two air-fluid levels are seen in the upright frontal film. *Arrow* (←) indicates fat; *hatched arrow* (↔) indicates stomach. *Bottom,* Lateral projection shows the anterior position of the stomach with a large air-fluid level (↔) and fat interposed between the stomach and the diaphragm (←). Note how far anteriorly the normal stomach may extend.

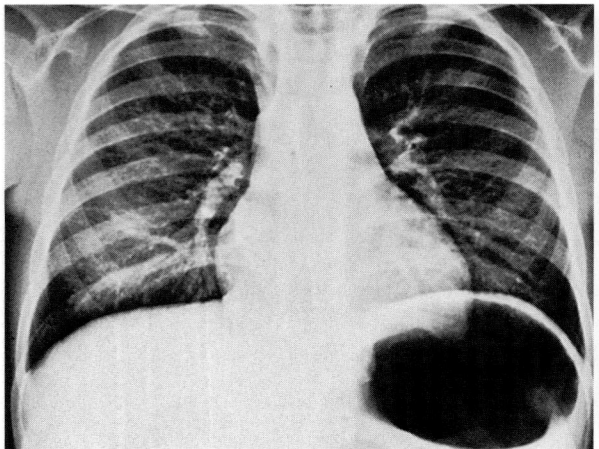
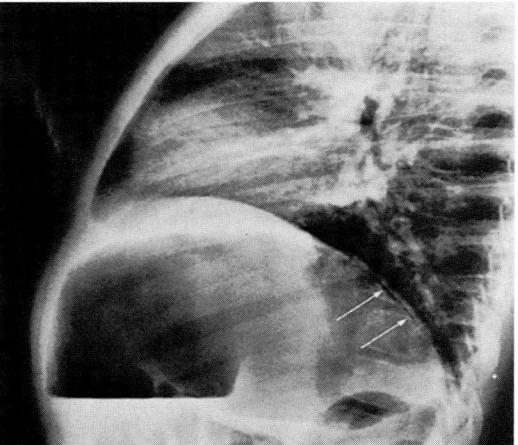

Figure 11–15. Simulated pneumoperitoneum produced by lucent interval between the two diaphragmatic shadows and an air-filled stomach.

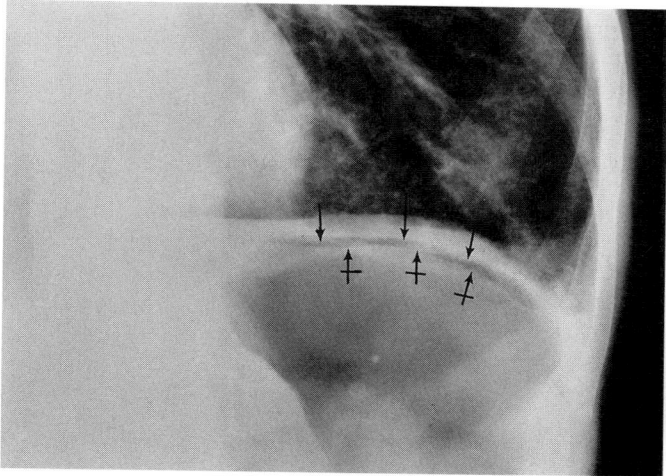

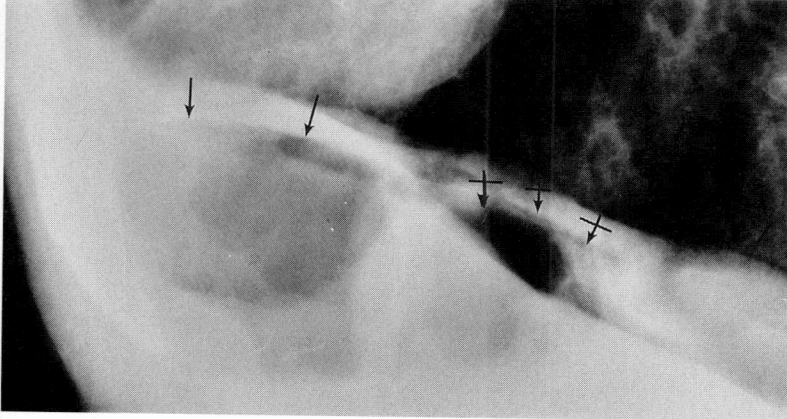

Figure 11–16. Simulated pneumoperitoneum on the left produced by superimposition of the colon (←) on the stomach (↔).

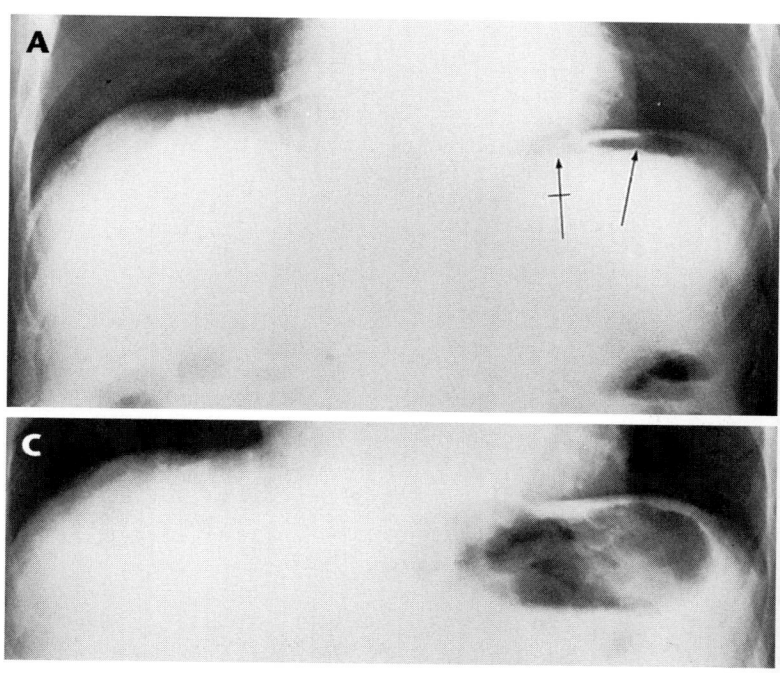

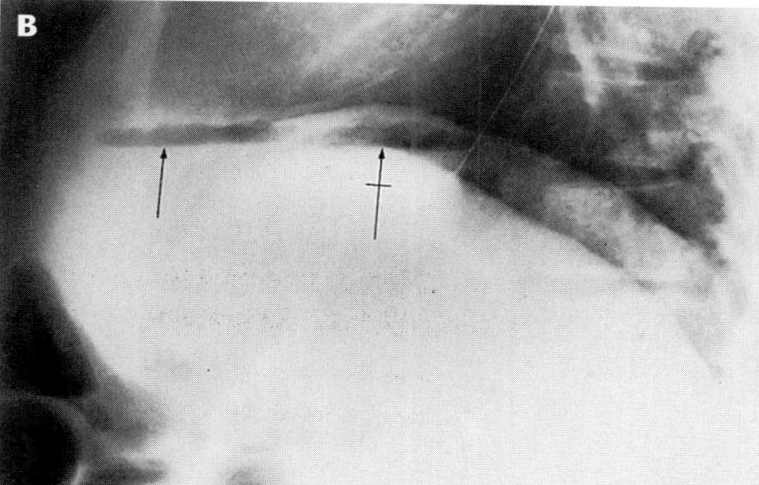

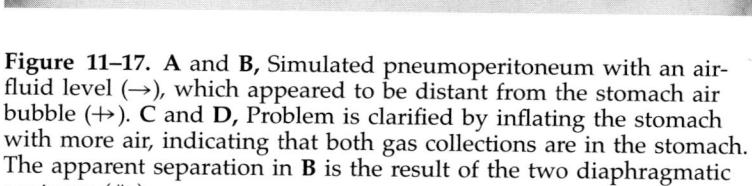

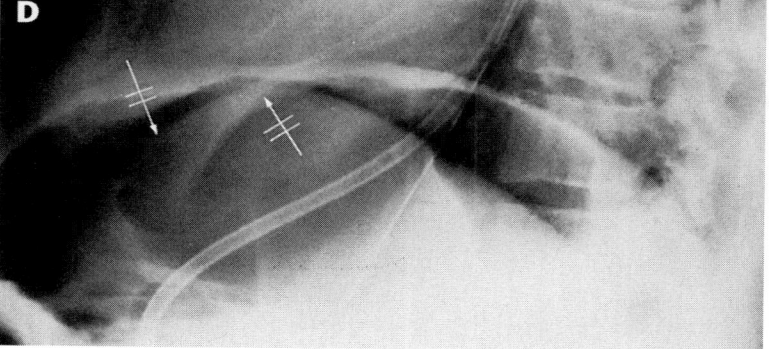

Figure 11–17. A and **B,** Simulated pneumoperitoneum with an air-fluid level (→), which appeared to be distant from the stomach air bubble (↔). **C** and **D,** Problem is clarified by inflating the stomach with more air, indicating that both gas collections are in the stomach. The apparent separation in **B** is the result of the two diaphragmatic contours (⊪).

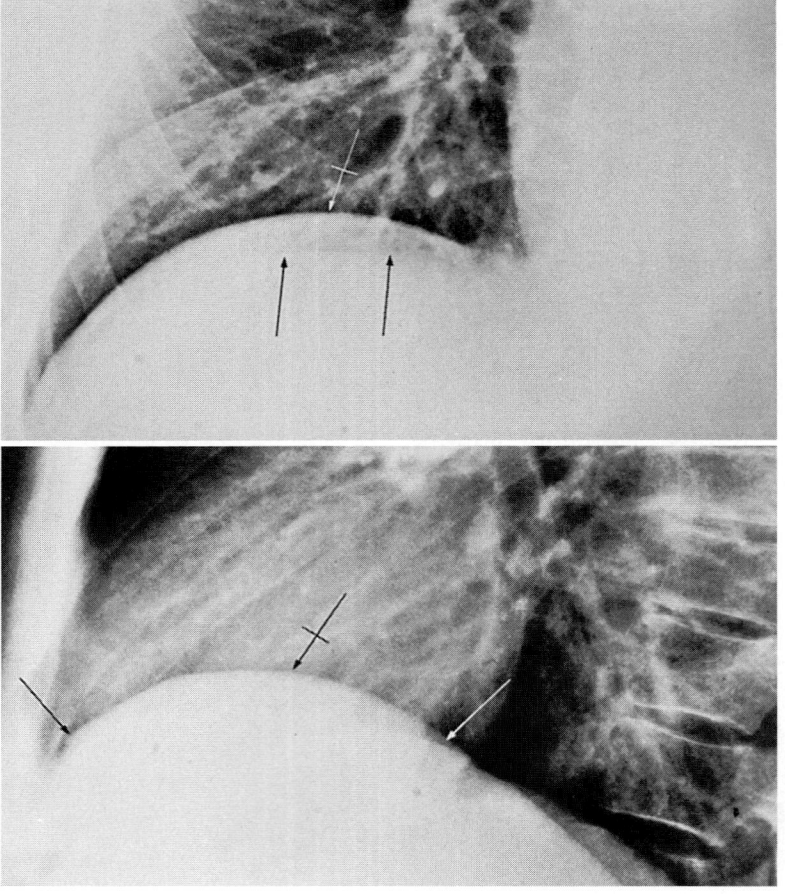

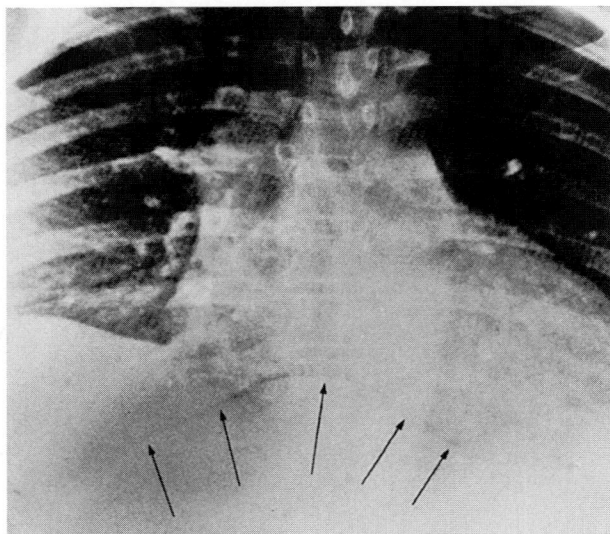

Figure 11–19. Air beneath the breasts, simulating pneumoperitoneum.

Figure 11–18. Simulated air-fluid level beneath the right hemidiaphragm, resulting from through projection of the different heights of the base of the diaphragm (→) and its dome (↦).

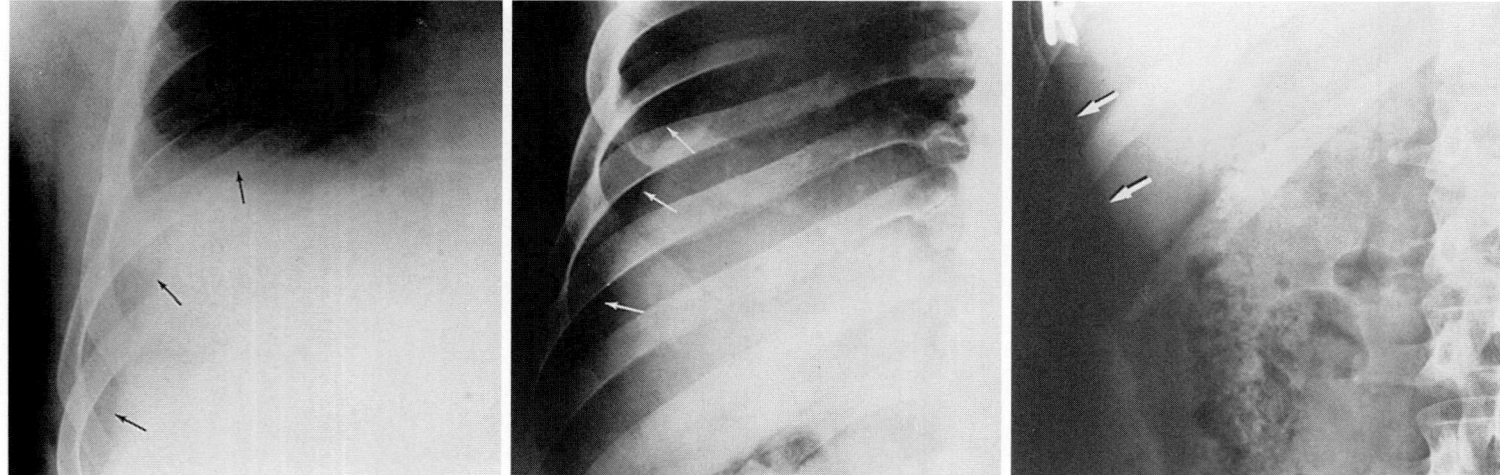

Figure 11–20. Simulated pneumoperitoneum produced by fat around the lateral and superior aspect of the liver. The right side of the liver may also be visualized by ascites. (Ref: Proto AV, Lane EJ: Visualization of differences in soft-tissue densities. *Radiology* 121:19, 1976.)

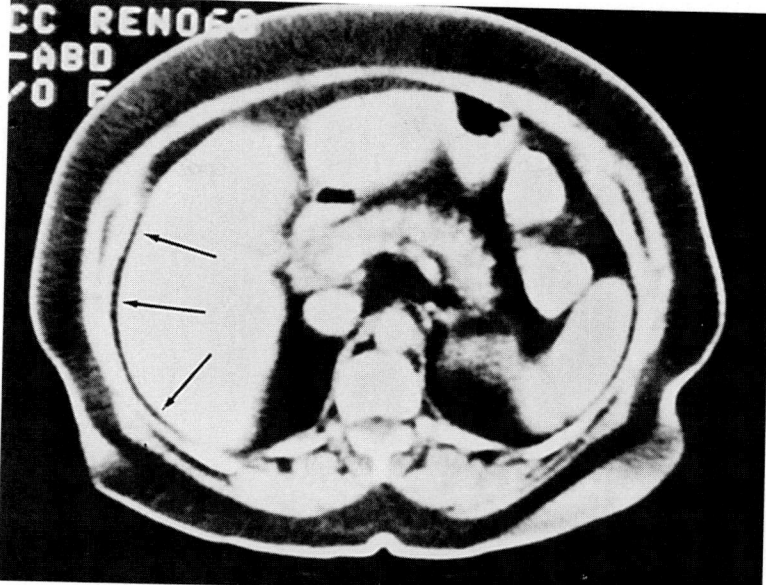

Figure 11–21. CT showing the fat around the liver that produces the radiolucency seen in Figure 11–20.

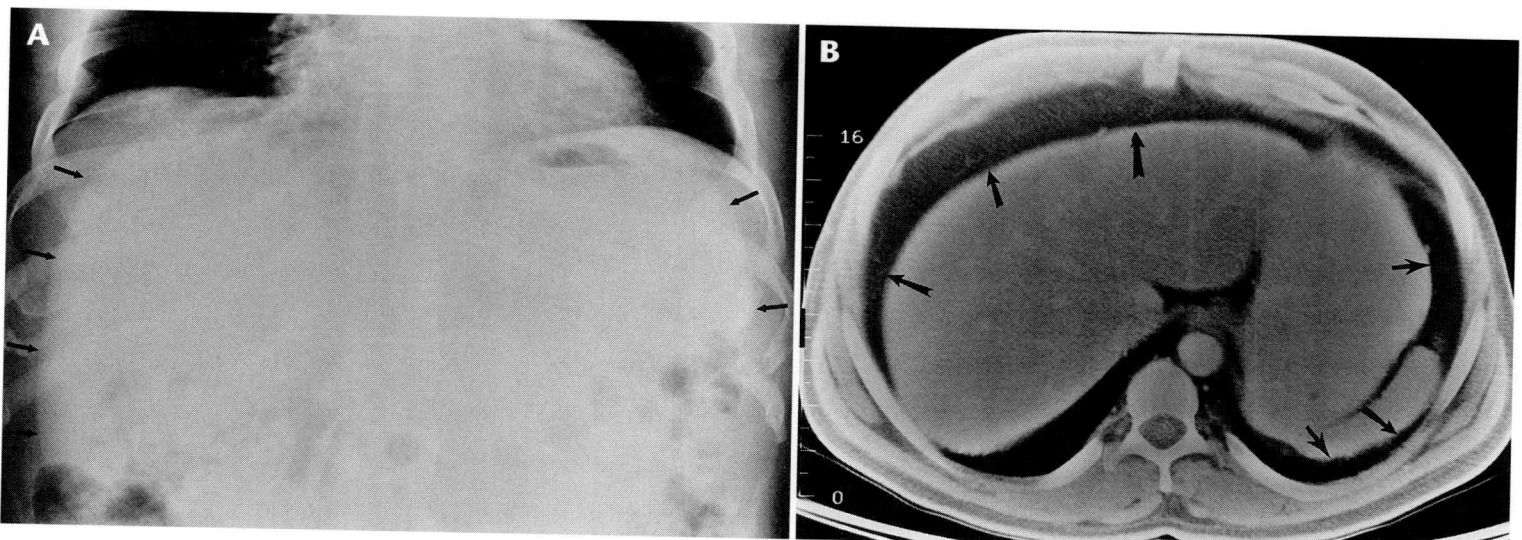

Figure 11–22. The liver and spleen are demonstrated with unusual clarity (**A**), owing to surrounding fat, as confirmed by CT (**B**).

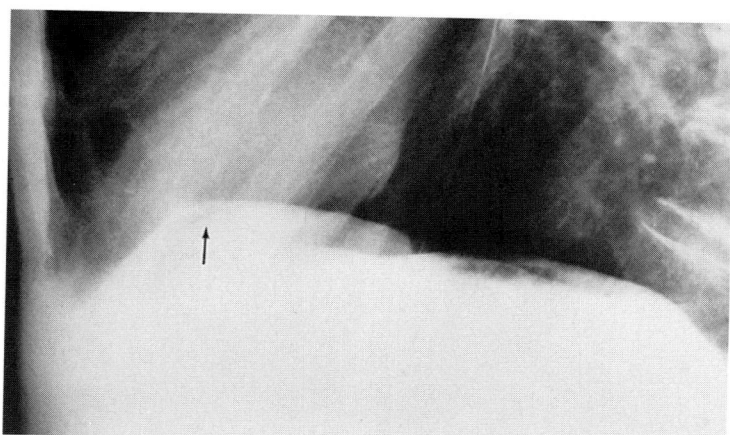

Figure 11–23. Colonic interposition on the right simulating pneumoperitoneum.

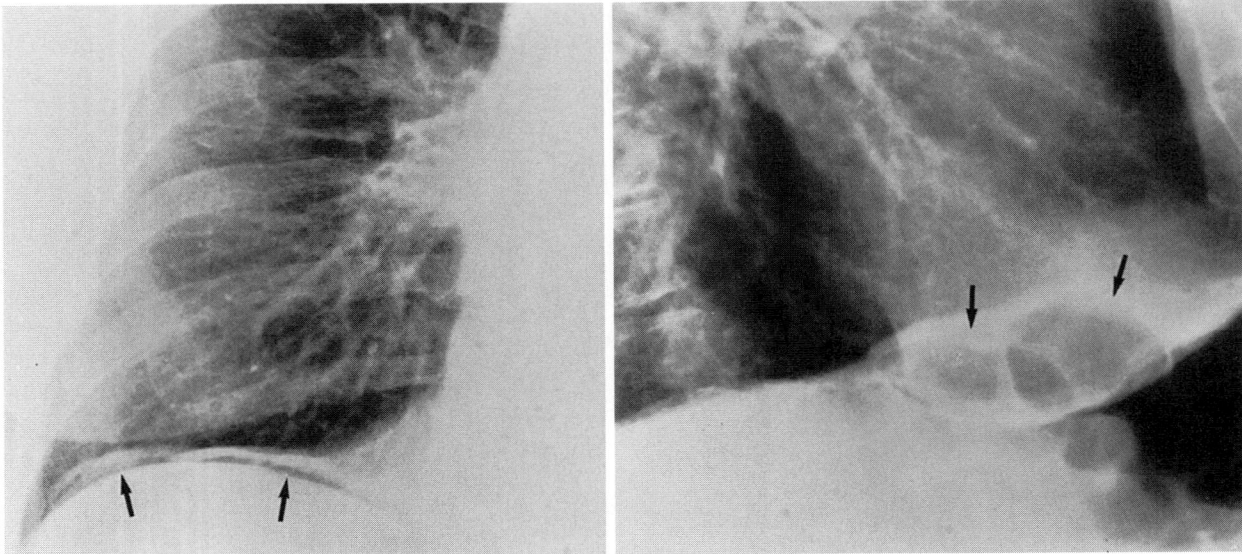

Figure 11–24. Colonic interposition simulating pneumoperitoneum in the frontal film.

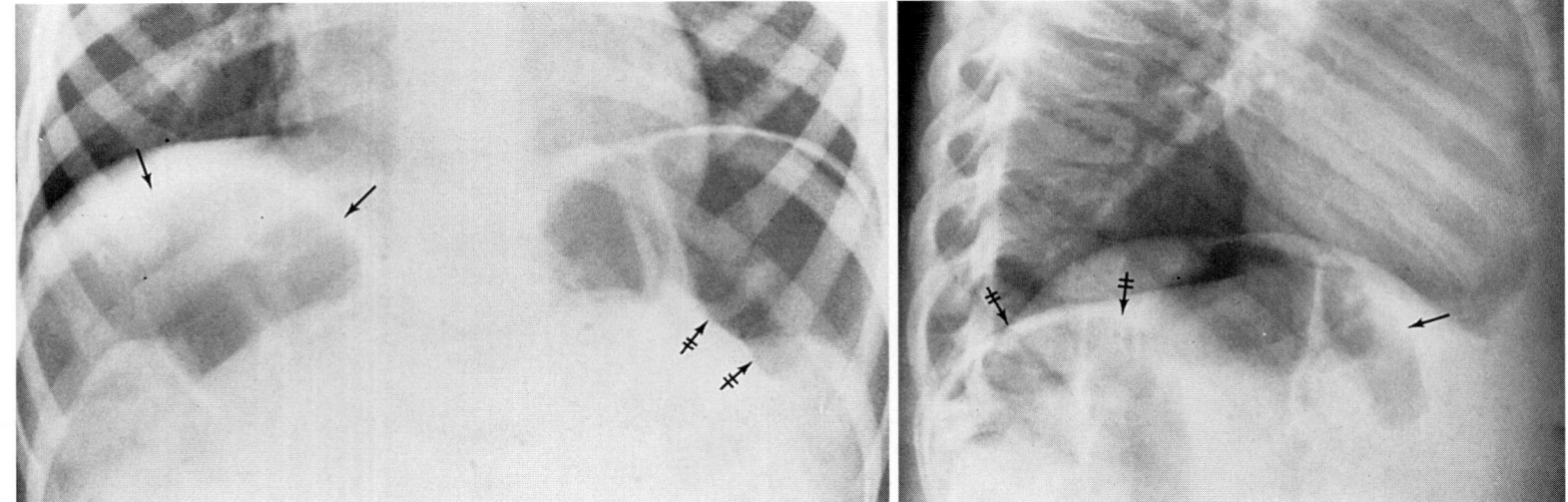

Figure 11–25. Colonic interposition between the liver and the diaphragm (←) and between the spleen and the diaphragm (⇇#) in a 3-year-old child. This is a common finding in children and is not usually productive of symptoms. It should not be confused with pneumoperitoneum. (Ref: Behlke FM: Hepatodiaphragmatic interposition in children. *Am J Roentgenol* 91:669, 1964.)

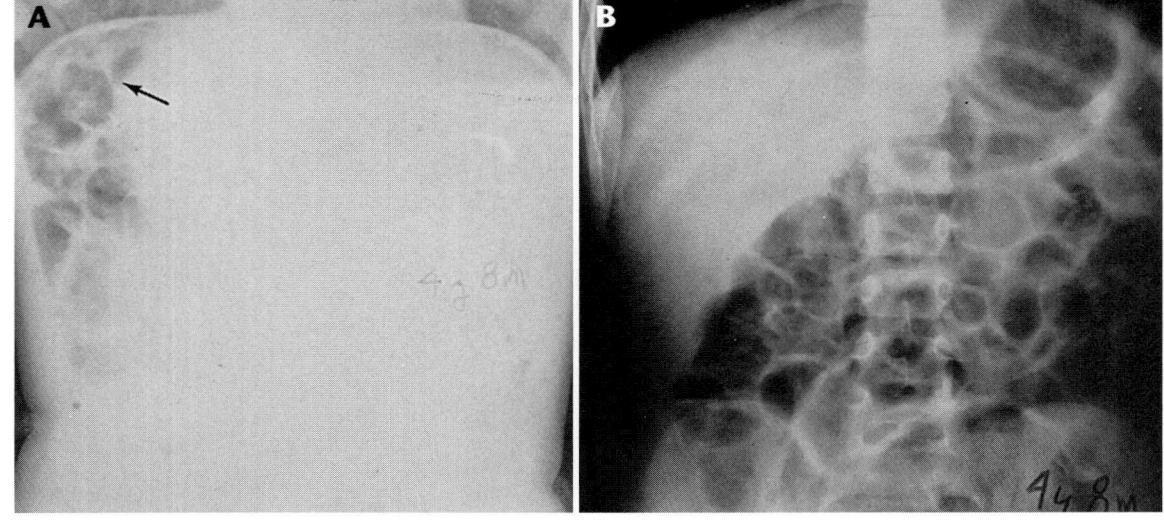

Figure 11–26. Colonic interposition between the liver and diaphragm in a 4-year-old boy (**A**) and its spontaneous reduction on the same day (**B**).

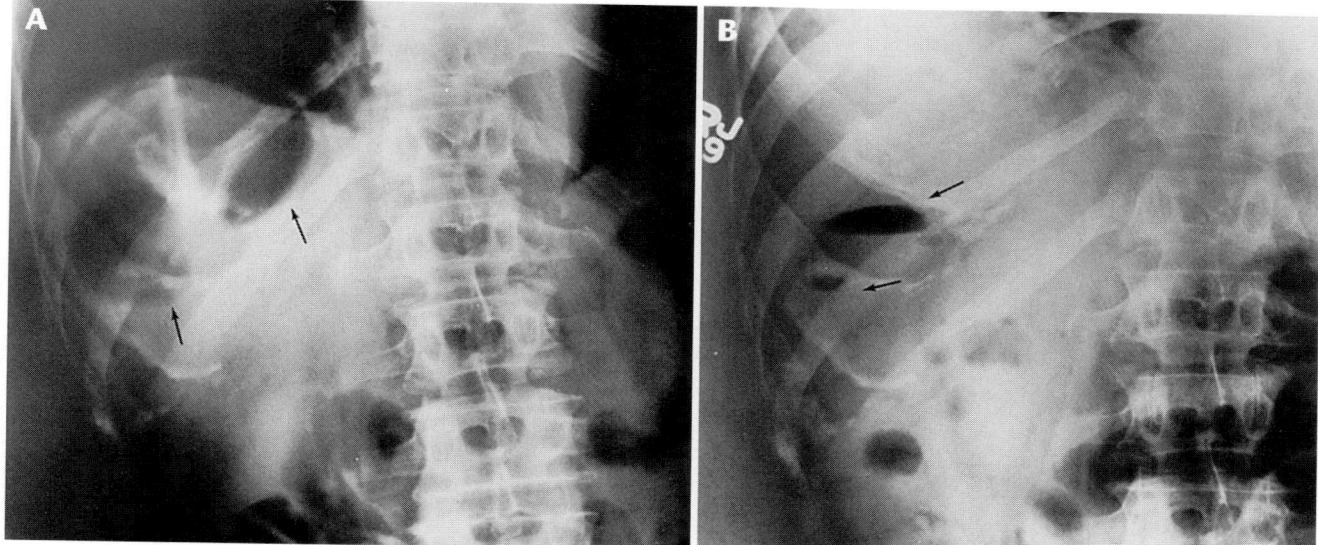

Figure 11–27. Colonic interposition simulating a subphrenic abscess. **A,** Supine film. **B,** Upright film.

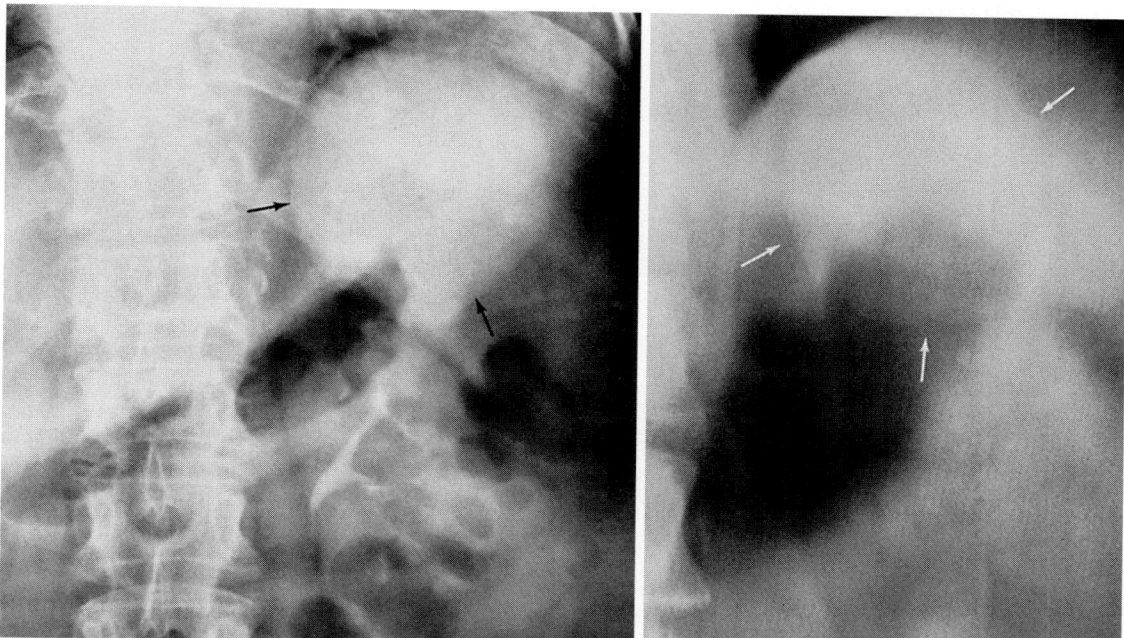

Figure 11–28. In the supine position, the fluid-filled fundus of the stomach simulates a mass lesion. *Left,* Plain film. *Right,* Tomogram. This pseudotumor may opacify on angiography and thus further obscure its proper identification. (Ref: Bjorn-Hansen RW, O'Brien DS: Aortographic opacification of the gastric fundus simulating neoplasm. *Am J Roentgenol* 100:408, 1967.)

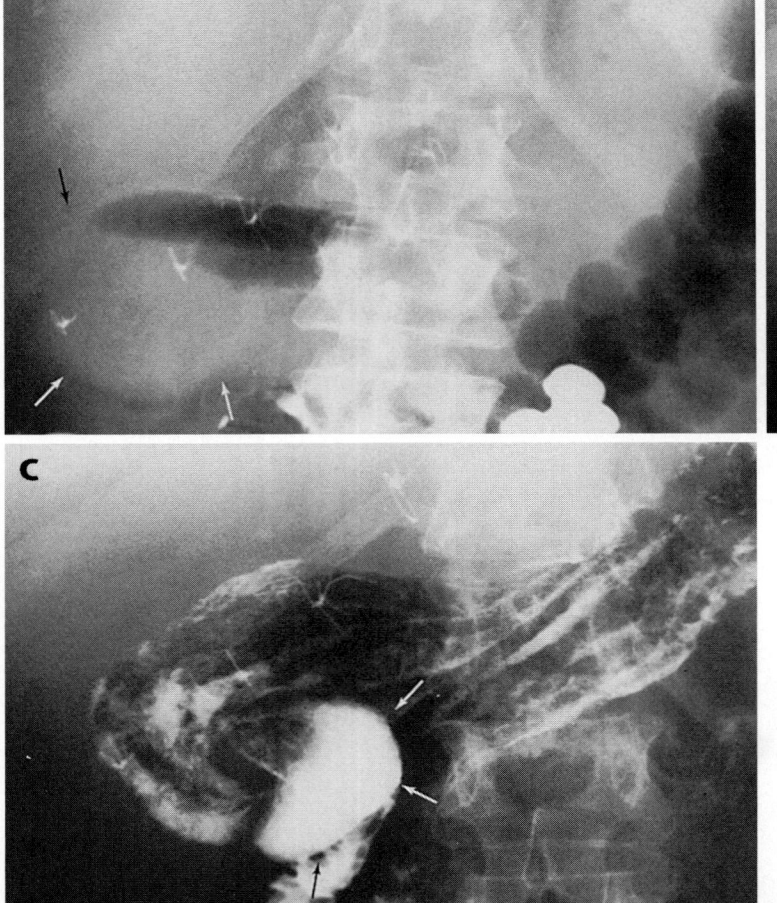
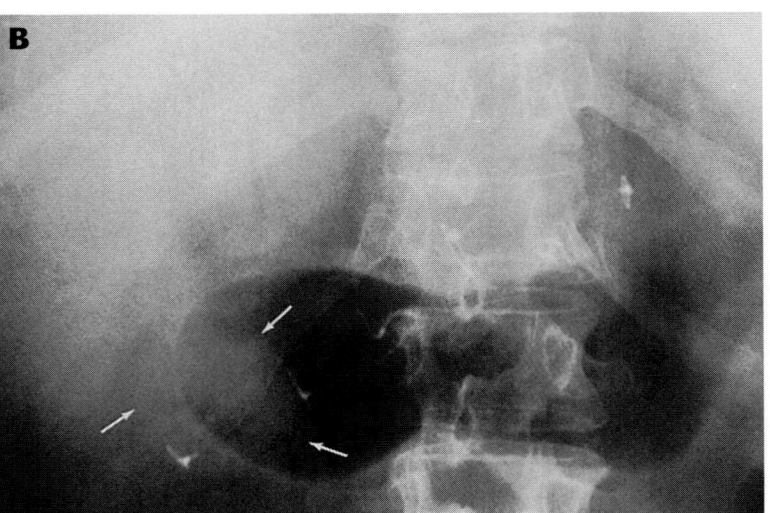
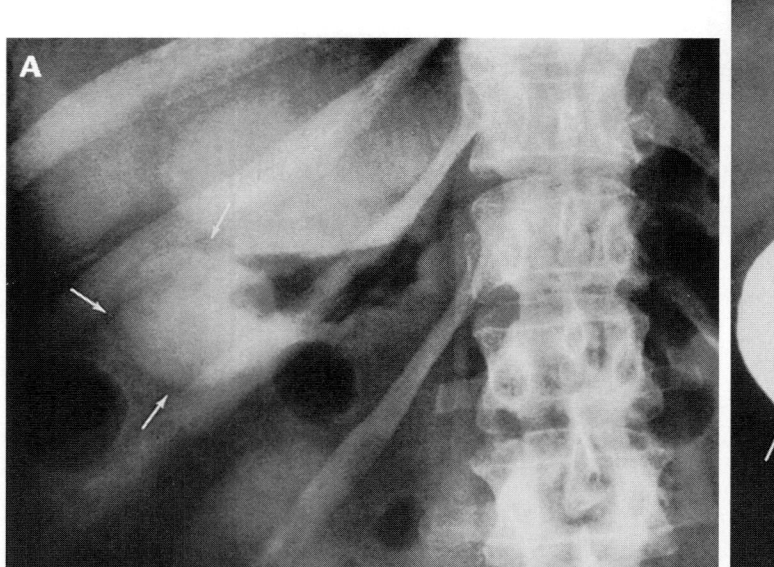
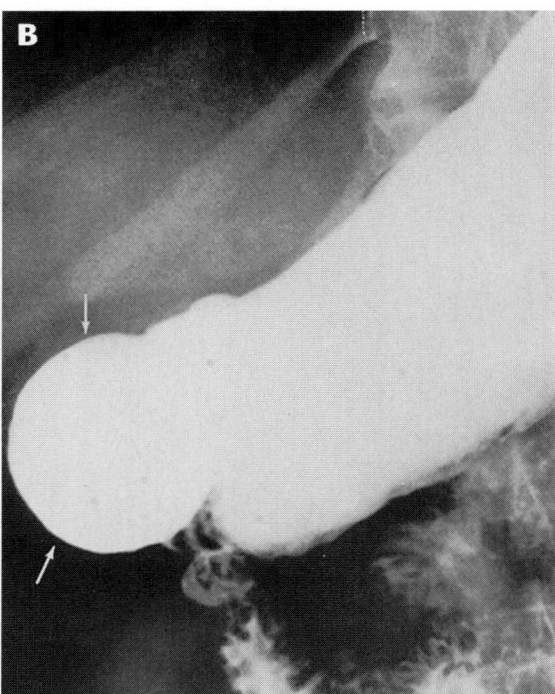

Figure 11–29. **A,** Fluid-filled duodenal bulb may present as a right upper quadrant mass in the prone position. **B,** Supine position shows the mass less distinctly. **C,** Barium examination shows the mass effect to be due to the duodenal bulb.

Figure 11–30. **A,** In the prone position, the fluid-filled gastric antrum may also simulate a right upper quadrant mass. **B,** Antrum filled with barium in same position as **A.** (Ref: Balthazar E: Right upper quadrant pseudotumor, a fluid-filled viscus. *Radiology* 112:11, 1974.)

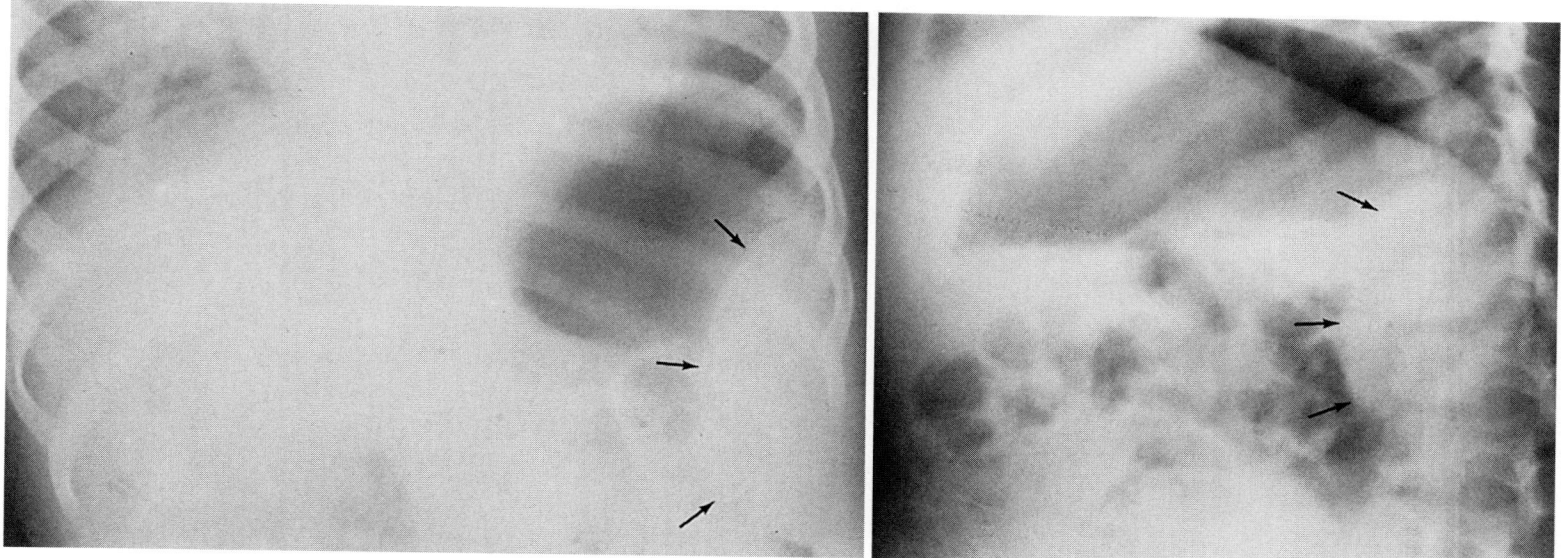

Figure 11–31. Gas-filled gastric fundus displacing the shadow of the spleen (*arrows*) from the diaphragm, simulating a mass.

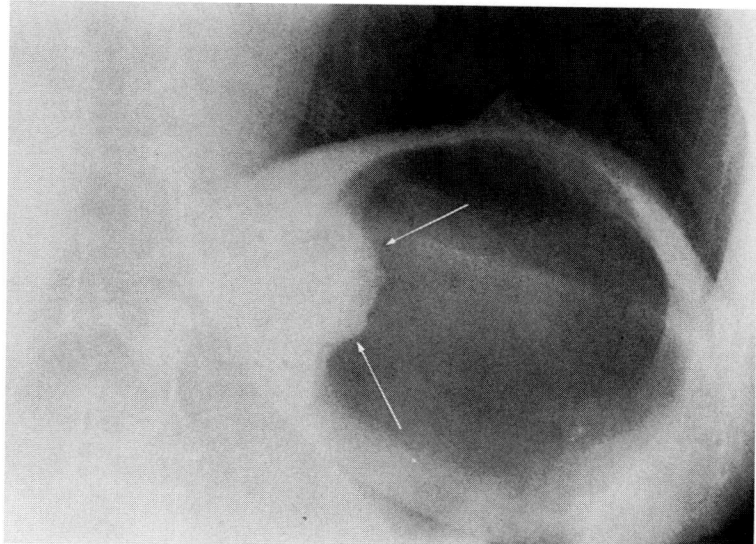

Figure 11–32. Left lobe of the liver presenting into the stomach gas bubble, simulating a neoplasm (see Fig. 11–83).

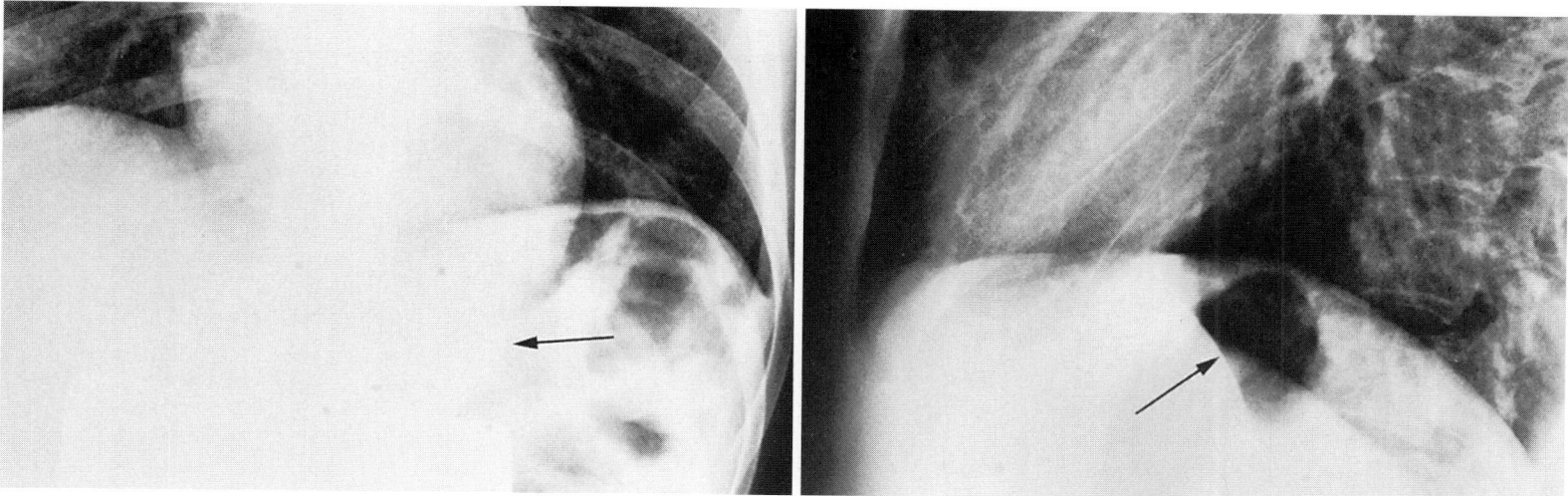

Figure 11–33. Liver shadow encroaching on the stomach gas bubble in both projections.

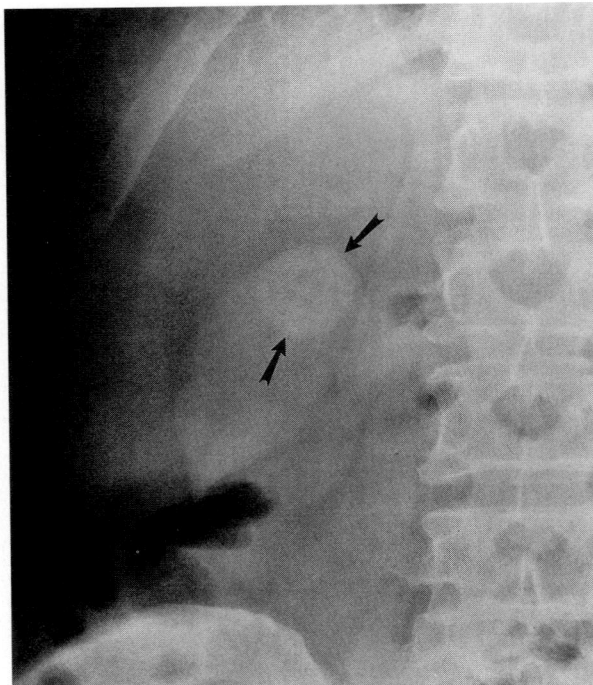

Figure 11–34. Fluid-filled antrum of the stomach with the lucent folds of the pylorus, simulating a gallstone with fissures within (see Fig. 11–197).

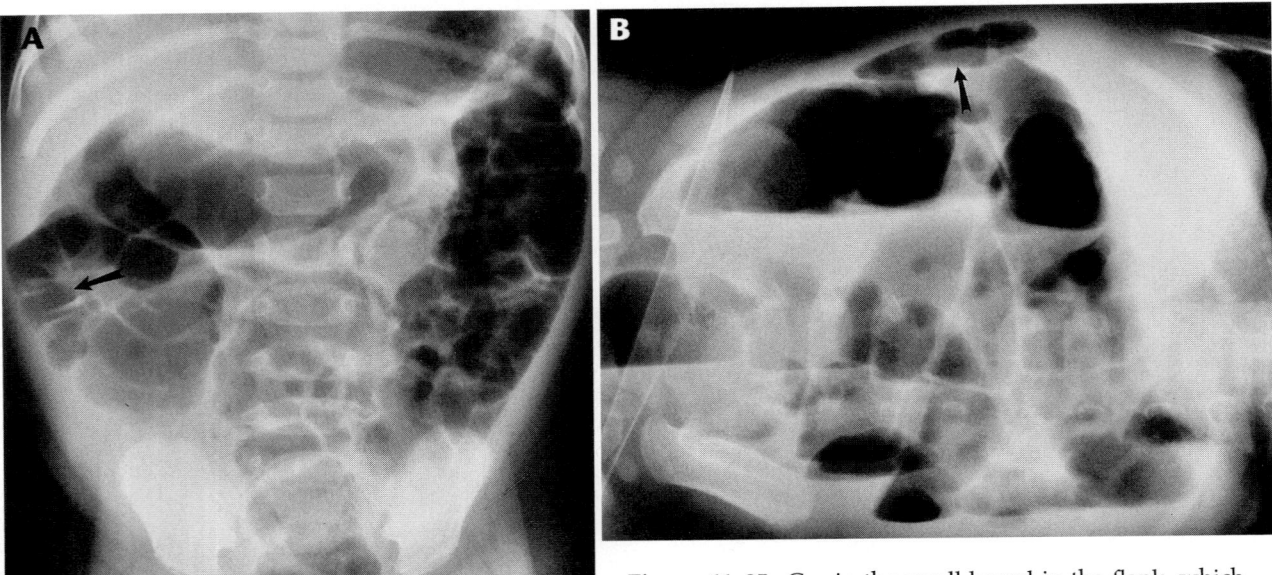

Figure 11–35. Gas in the small bowel in the flank, which can simulate colon or free air in the peritoneal cavity. **A,** Supine film. **B,** Left lateral decubitus.

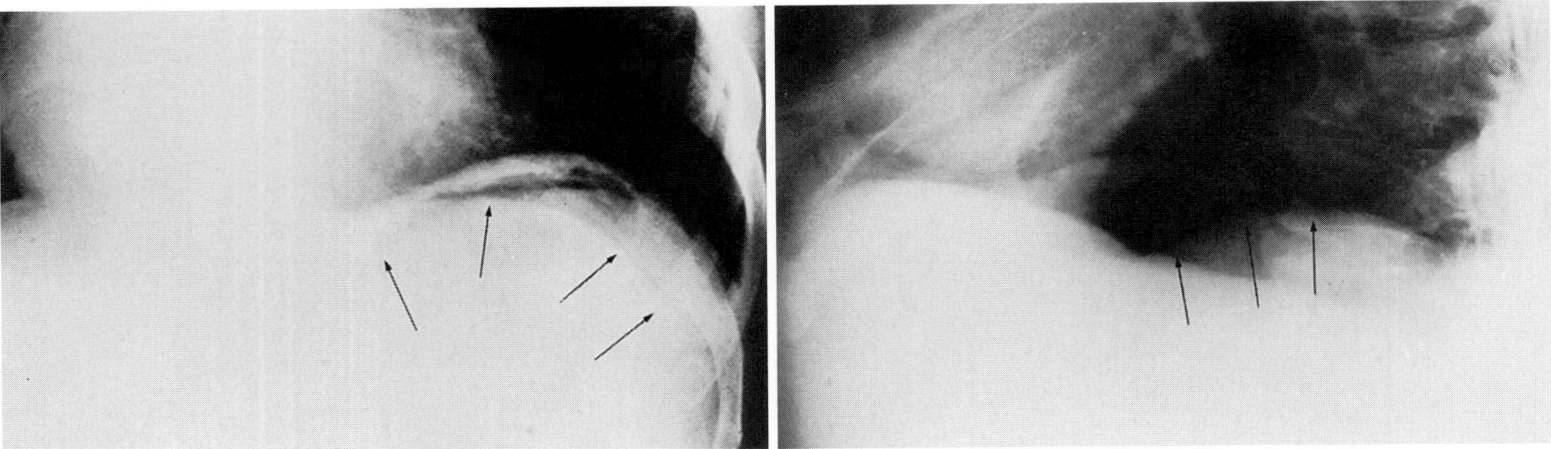

Figure 11–36. Fluid-filled splenic flexure of the colon, simulating a mass encroaching on the stomach.

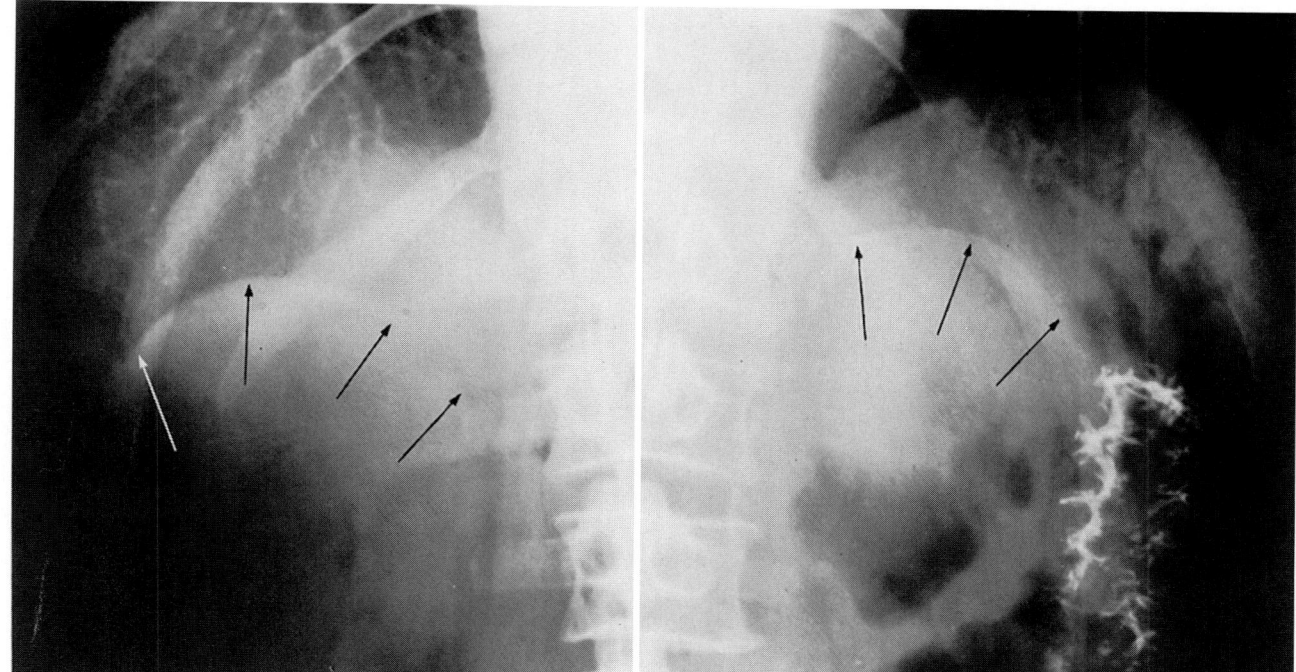

Figure 11–37. Posterior lung margins simulating an abdominal mass.

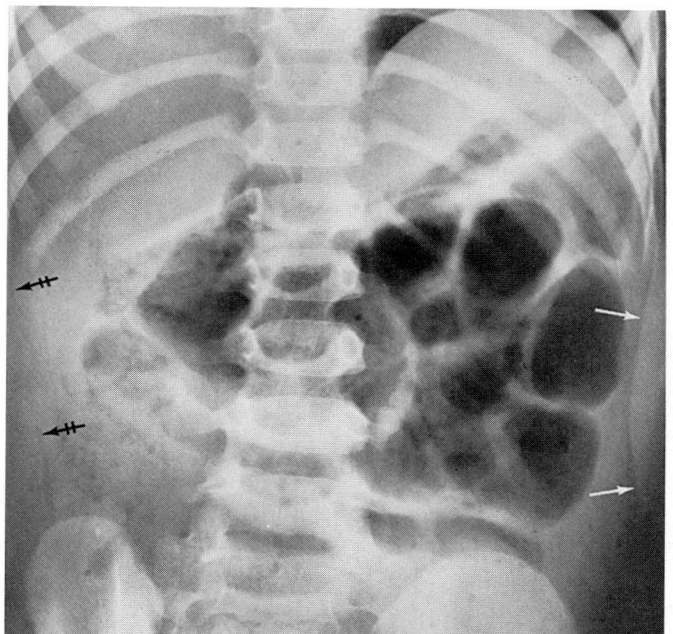

Figure 11–38. Simulated properitoneal fat line produced by the contact of the patient's arm with the abdomen (←). A true properitoneal fat line is seen on the opposite side (↢).

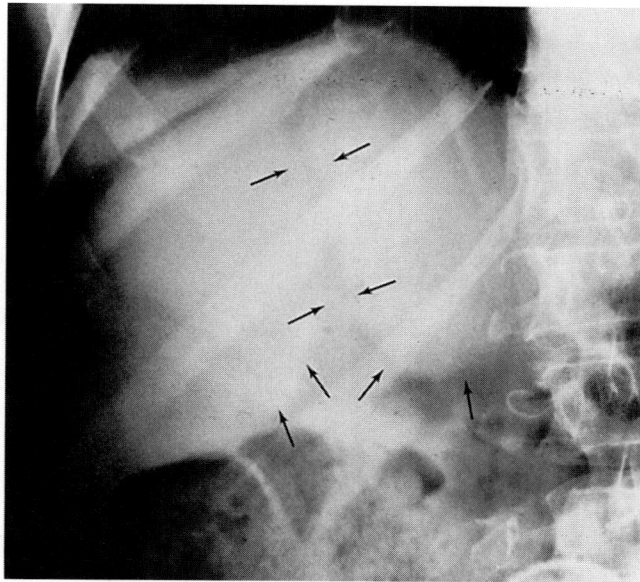

Figure 11–39. Fat around the ligamentum teres of the liver, producing a bilobed appearance of the liver or a simulated mass. (Ref: Haswell DM et al: Plain film recognition of the ligamentum teres hepatis. *Radiology* 114:263, 1975.)

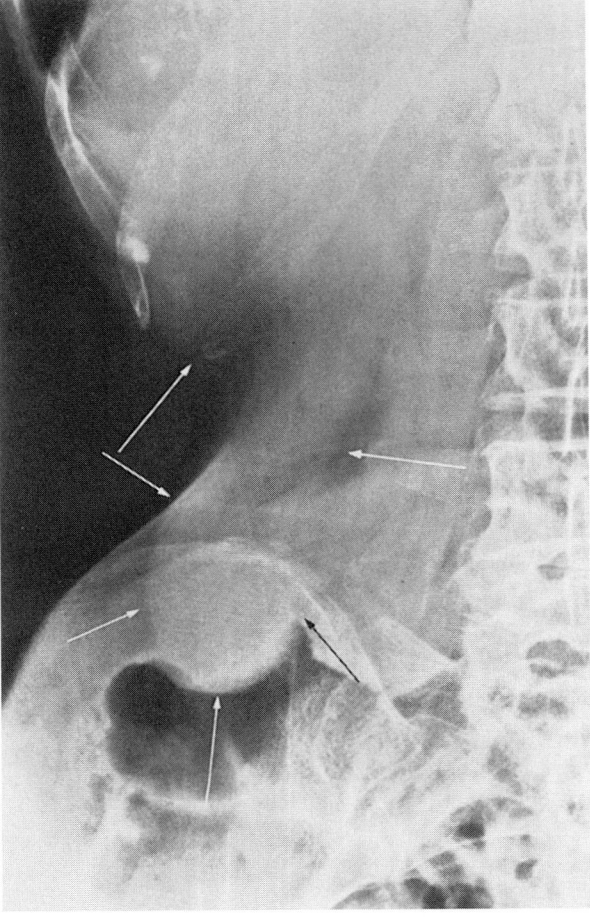

Figure 11–40. Riedel's lobe of the liver, which may be mistaken for a right lower quadrant mass (see Fig. 11–194).

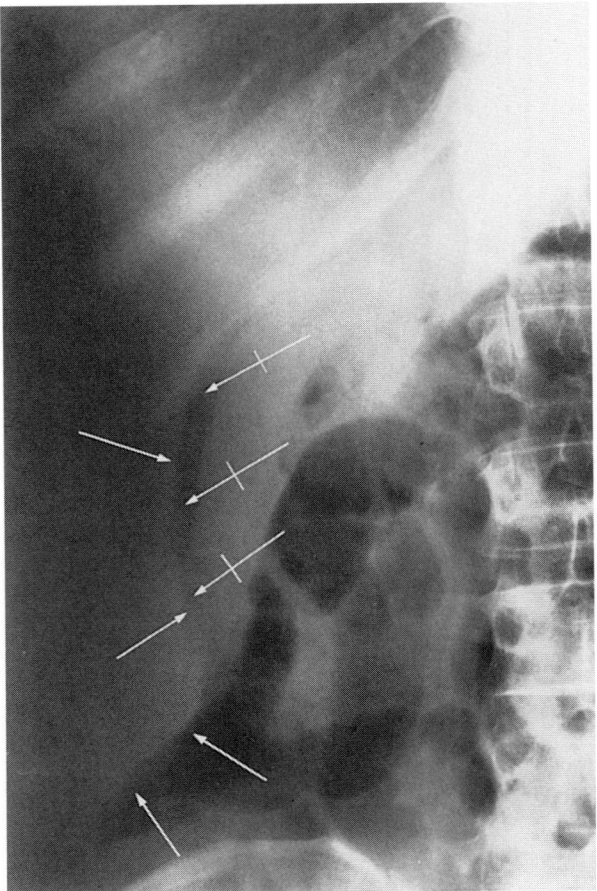

Figure 11–41. Riedel's lobe of the liver (→) and perinephric fat (↦) produce an appearance suggesting gas in the perirenal space.

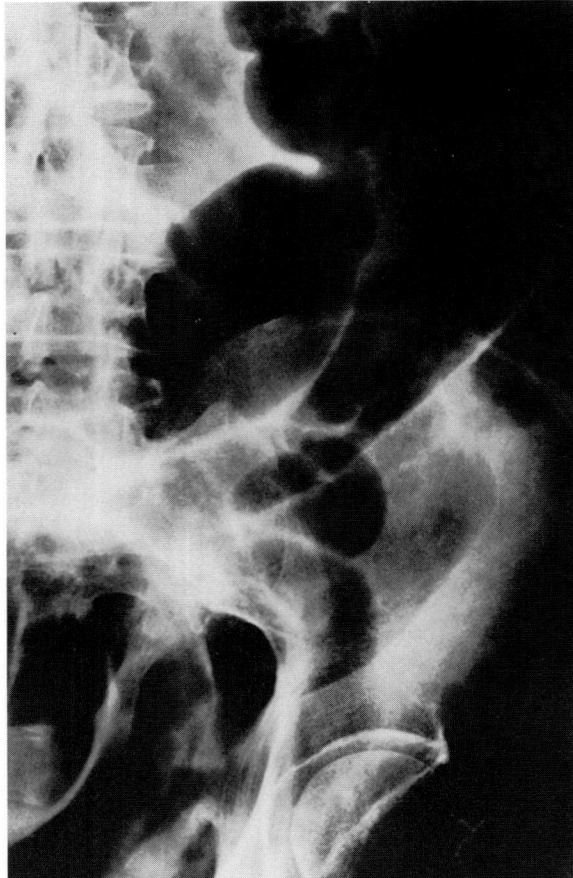

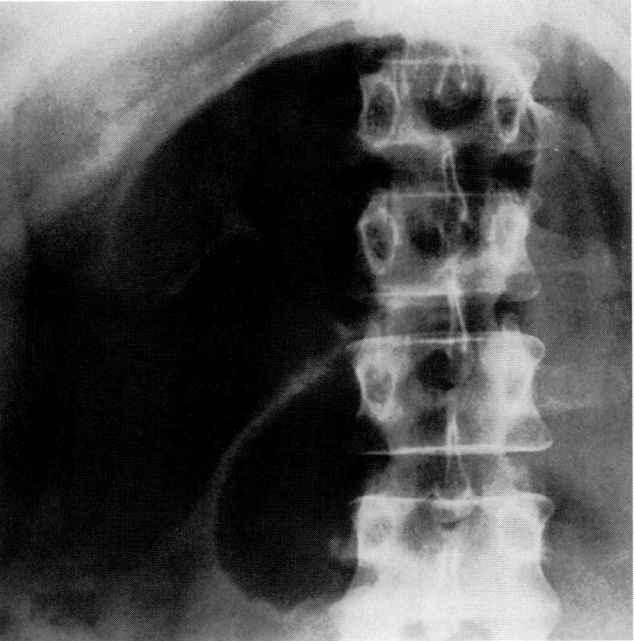

Figure 11–42. Two examples of the double wall sign. The ability to see both sides of the bowel wall is not reliable evidence of pneumoperitoneum. In these cases it is due to two loops of distended intestine in contact with each other. (Ref: deLacy G et al: Pneumoperitoneum, the misleading double wall sign. *Clin Radiol* 28:445, 1977.)

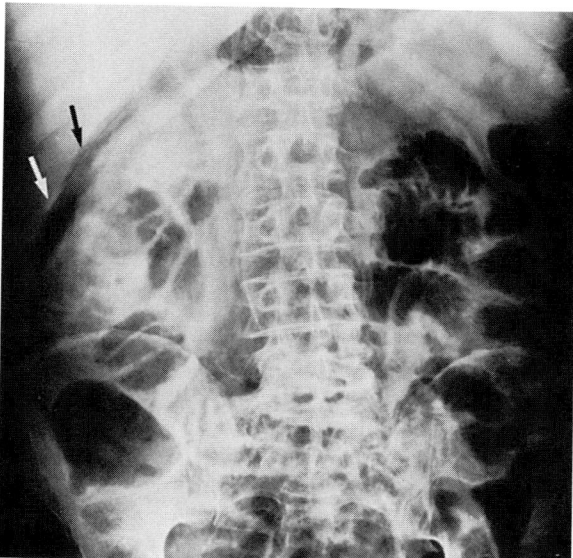

Figure 11–43. Extensive mesenteric fat simulating pneumoperitoneum.

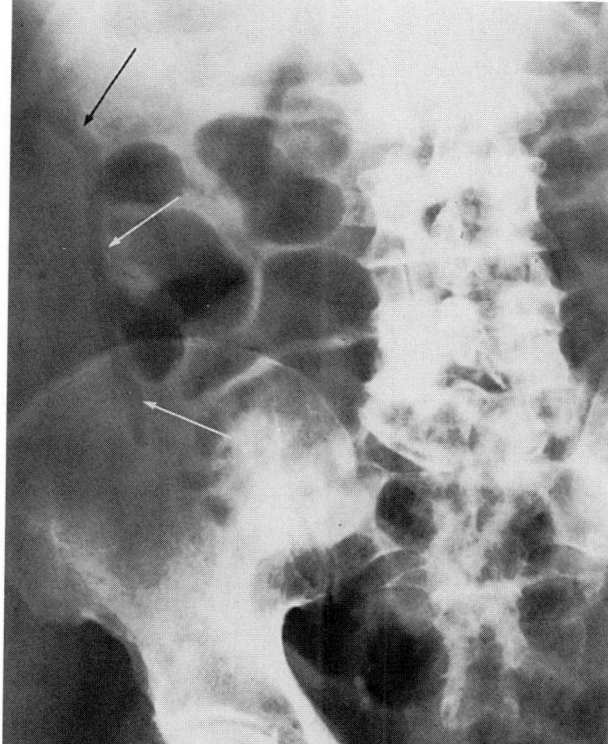

Figure 11–44. Air in the appendix is a normal phenomenon and should not be considered as evidence of acute appendicitis. (Ref: Shaffer HA, Harrison GB: Gas in the appendix. *Arch Surg* 114:587, 1979.) Gas may also be seen in the appendix with a subhepatic cecum. (Ref: Hussain SM, Ginal AZ: Case of the month: All's well that ends well. *Brit J Radiol* 68:435, 1995.)

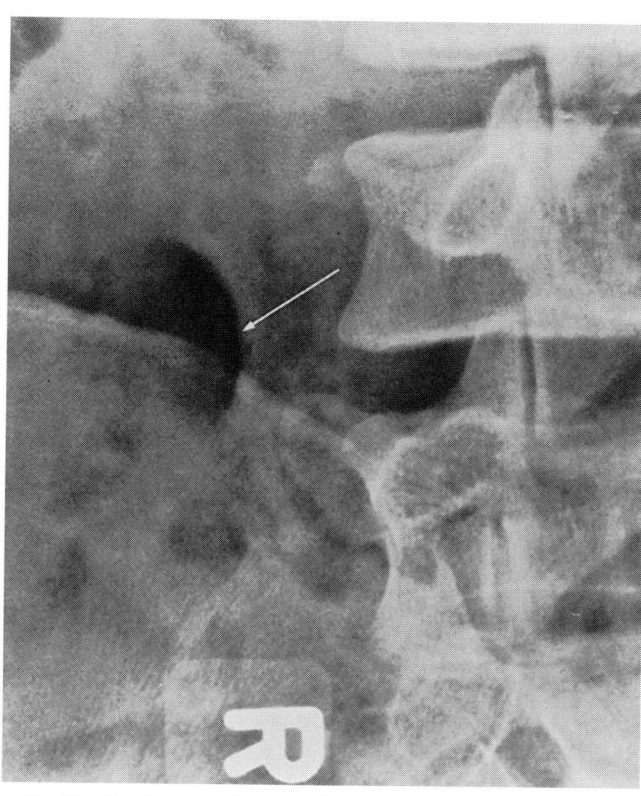

Figure 11–45. Shadow of the umbilicus seen in the oblique projection of the abdomen.

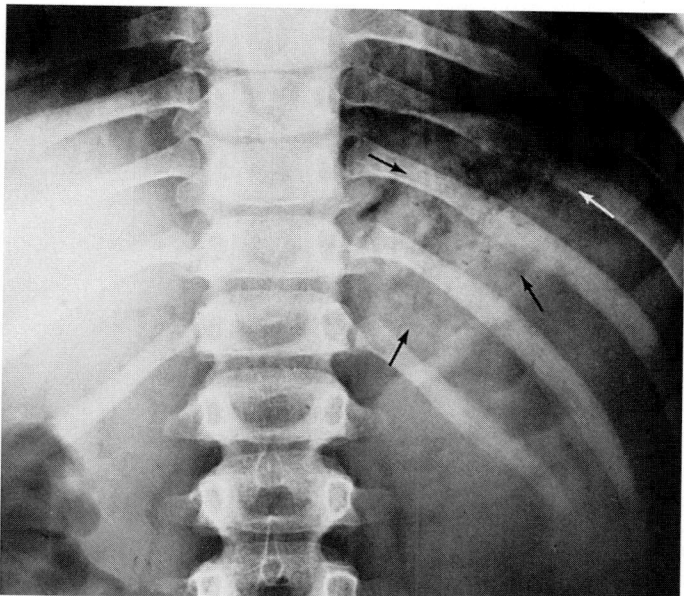

Figure 11–46. Gastric contents simulating the changes of bronchiectasis at the base of the left lung.

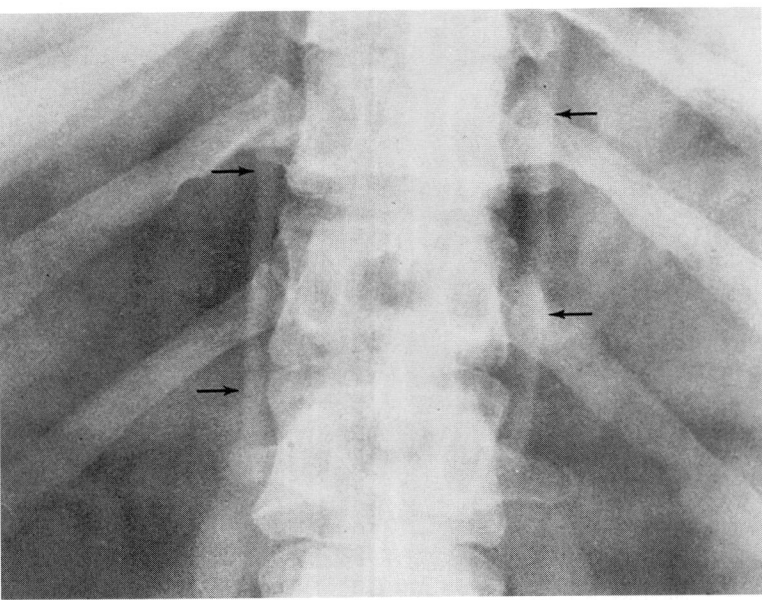

Figure 11–47. Visualization of the diaphragmatic attachments.

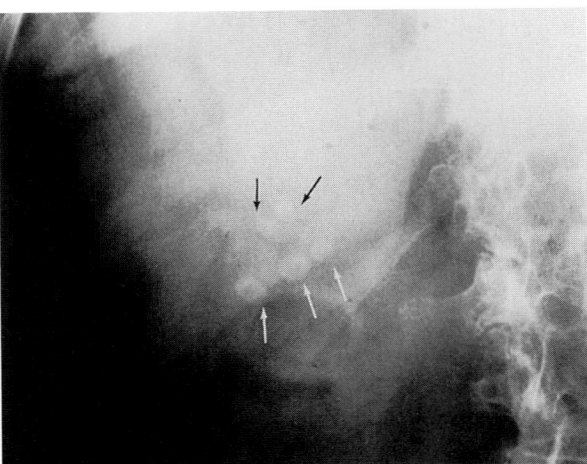

Figure 11–48. Ring-shaped calcified costal cartilage simulating gallstones.

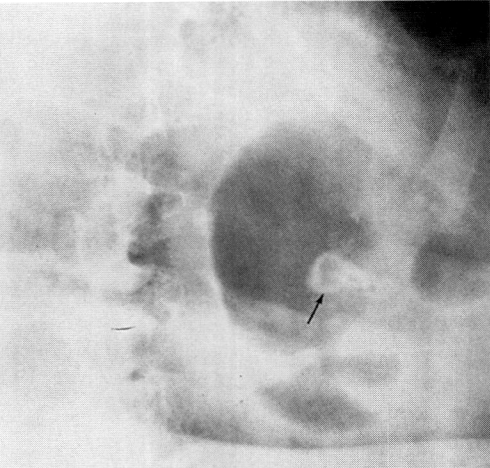

Figure 11–49. Calcified costal cartilage in the left upper quadrant, simulating a renal calculus.

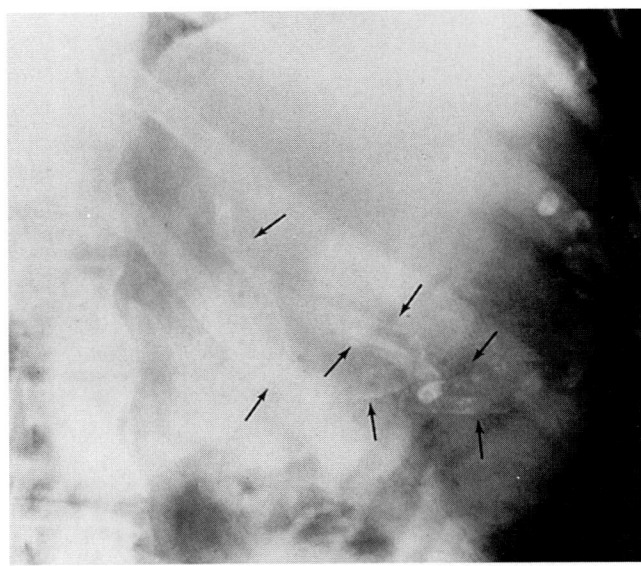

Figure 11–50. Calcification in a tortuous splenic artery.

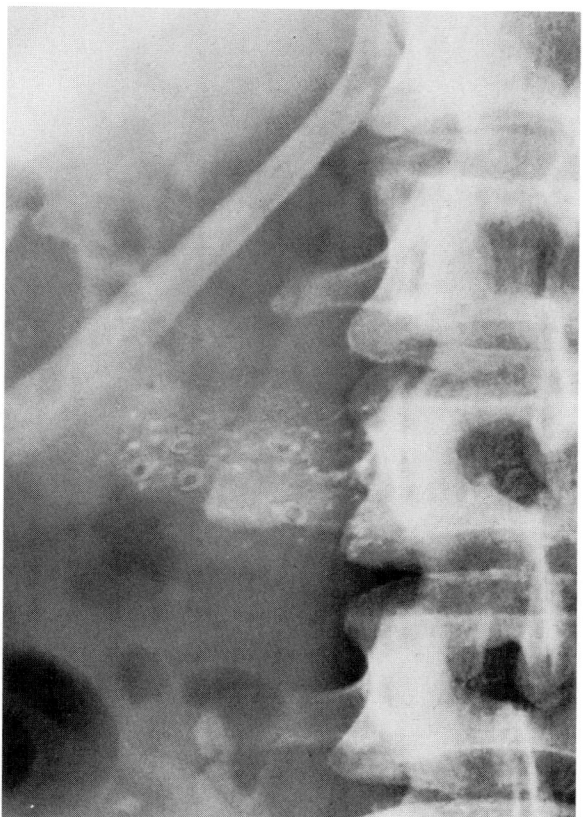

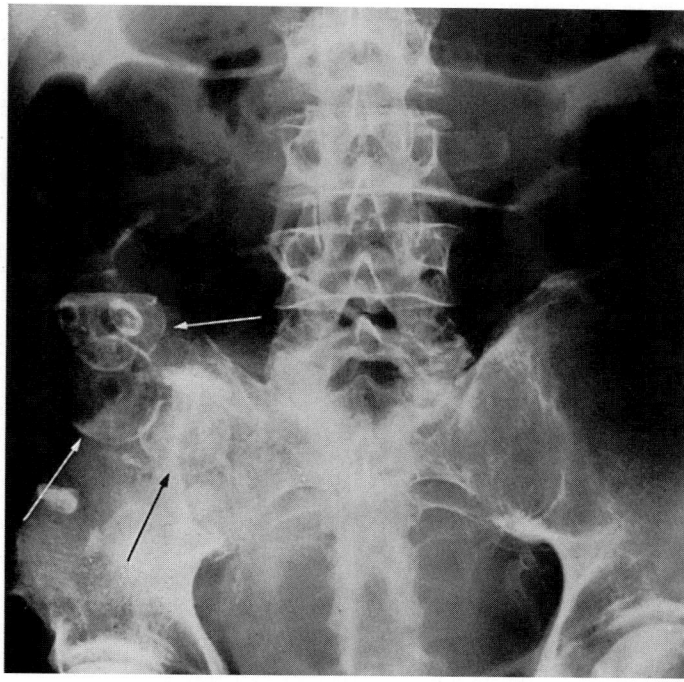

Figure 11–52. Enteroliths in the cecum, formed around ingested prune pits.

Figure 11–51. Ingested seeds in the transverse colon, simulating pancreatic calcification.

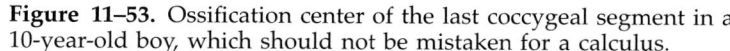

Figure 11–53. Ossification center of the last coccygeal segment in a 10-year-old boy, which should not be mistaken for a calculus.

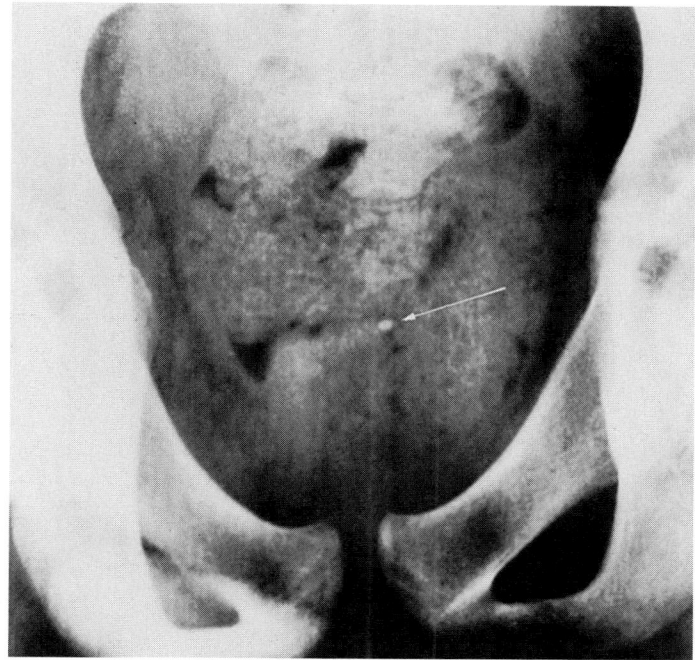

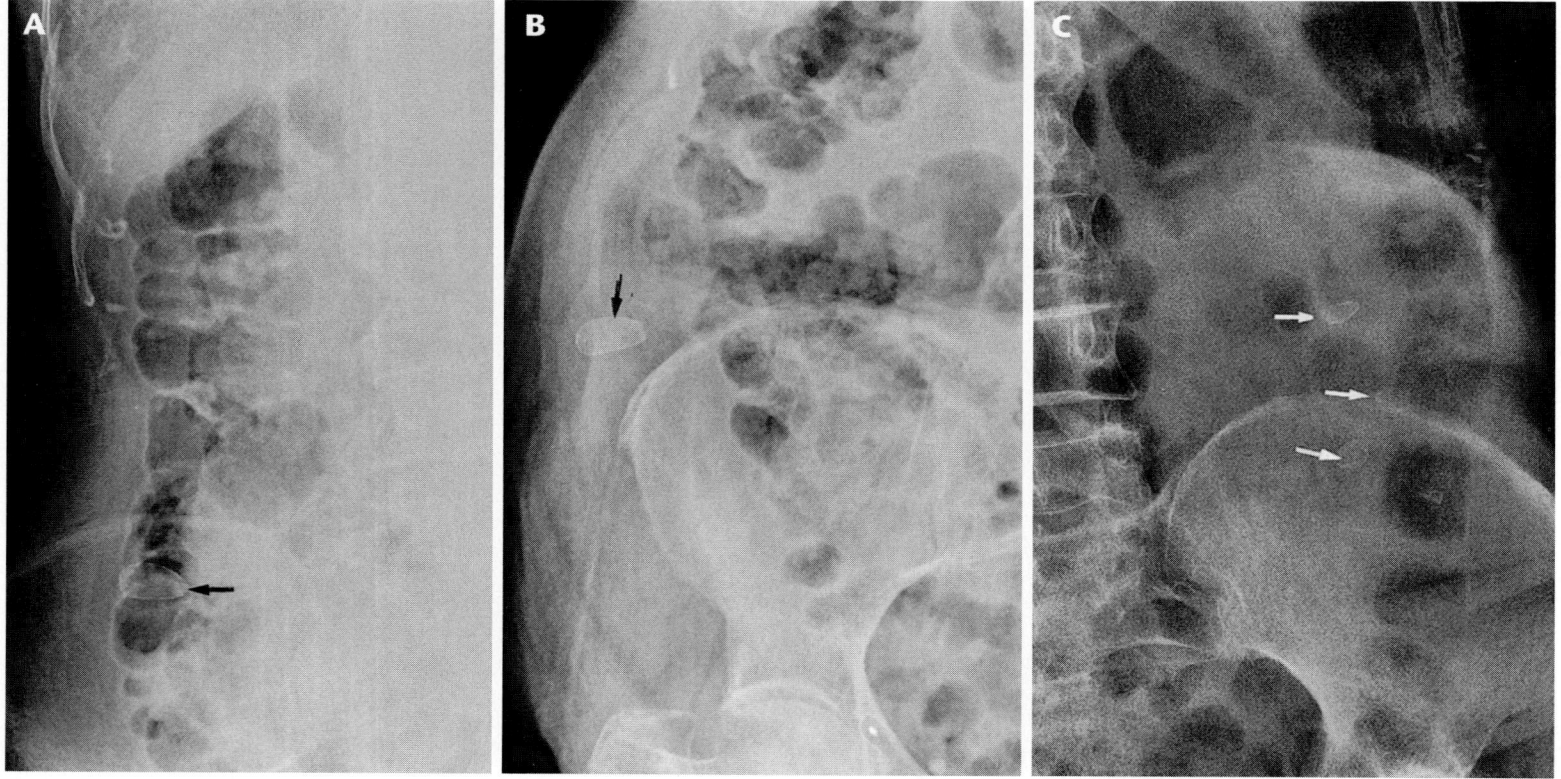

Figure 11–54. Calcified epiploic appendage still attached to colon. **A,** Frontal film. **B,** Oblique projection. **C,** Same entity in another patient.

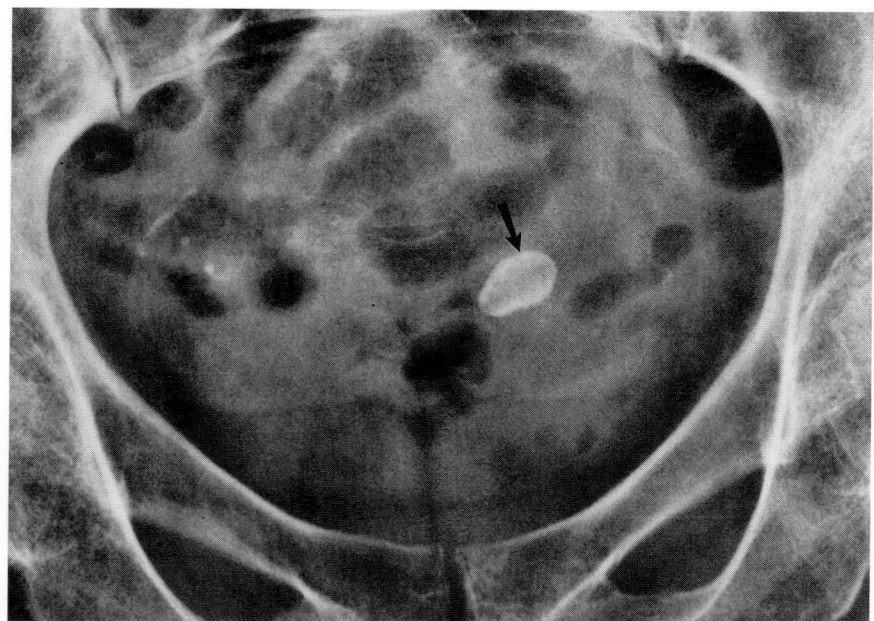

Figure 11–55. Calcified epiploic appendage. These have a characteristic oval shape with a more lucent center.

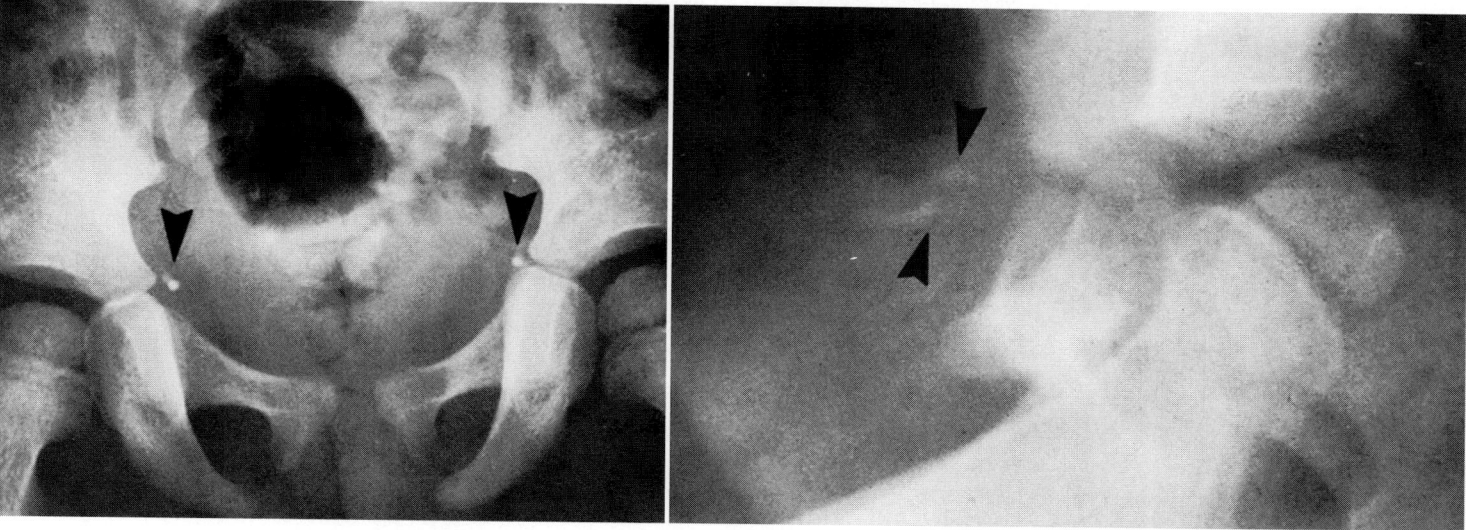

Figure 11–56. Dystrophic calcification in obliterated umbilical arteries in a 2-year-old child, an unusual normal finding in infants. (From Currarino G, Weinberg A: Dystrophic calcification in obliterated umbilical artery. *Pediatr Radiol* 15: 346, 1985.)

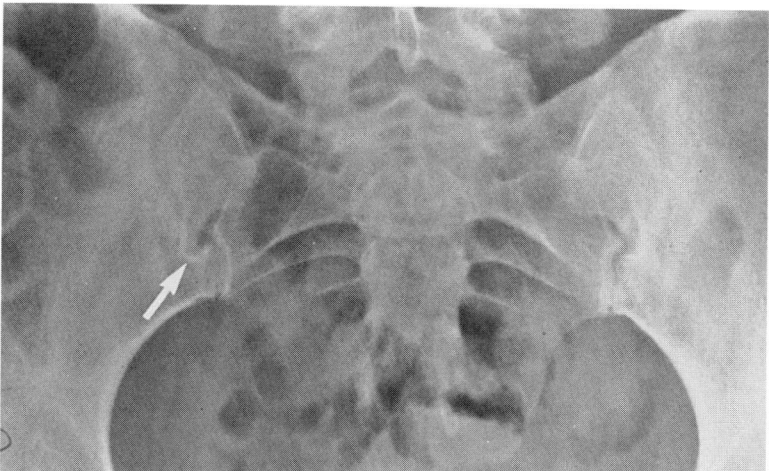

Figure 11–57. Edge of the sacroiliac joint simulating calcification in the appendix. The appearance is less marked on the opposite side.

The Gastrointestinal Tract

The Esophagus

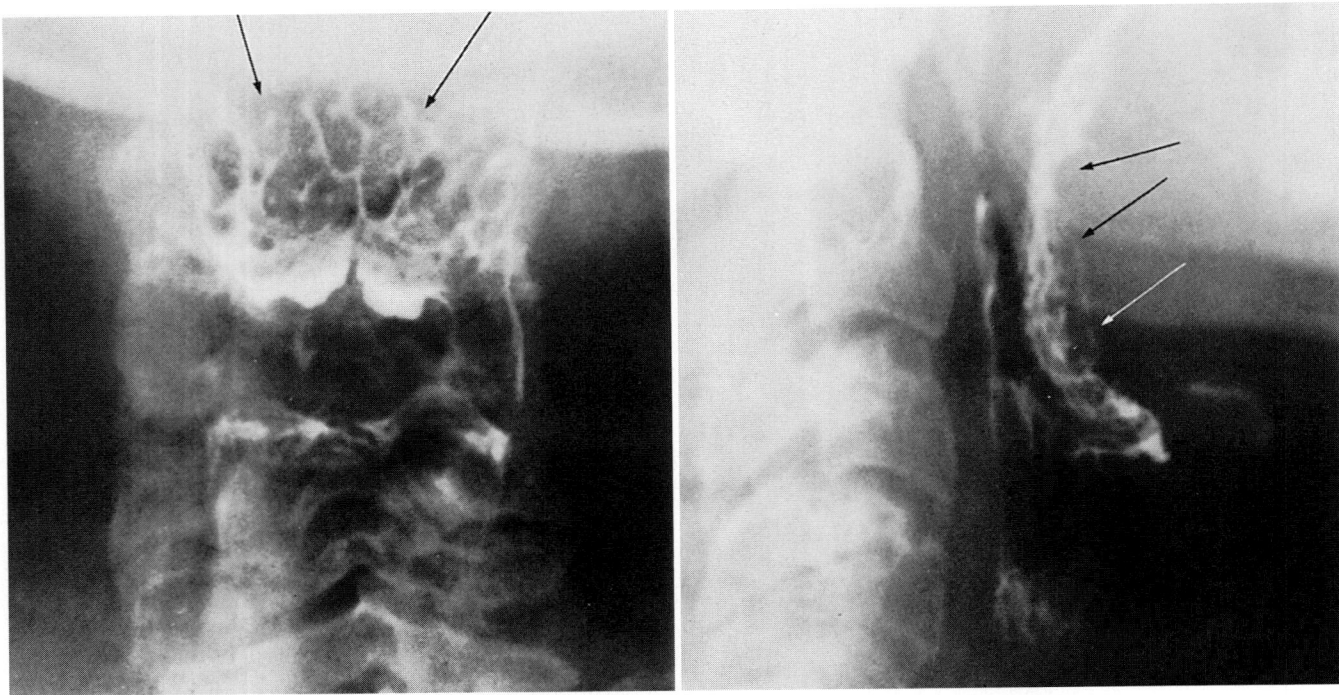

Figure 11–58. Lingual tonsil, which consists of a fine fibrous network containing lymphoid tissue scattered over the pharyngeal part of the tongue. (Ref: Gromet NL: Lymphoid hyperplasia in the base of the tongue. *Radiology* 144:825, 1982.)

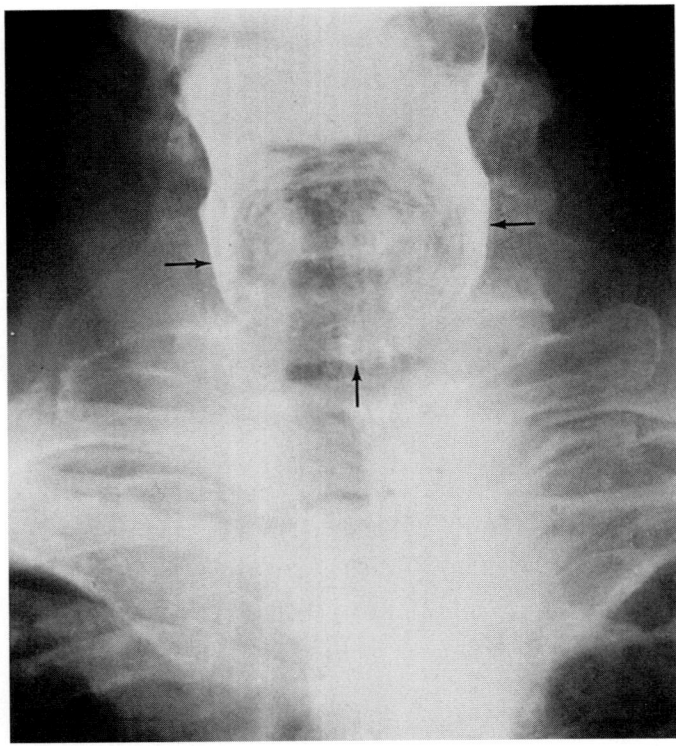

Figure 11–59. Pseudomass of the pharynx produced by the larynx and barium in the pyriform sinuses during the early phase of swallowing. (Ref: Howie JL: Postcricoid pseudotumor. *J Can Assoc Radiol* 31:225, 1980.)

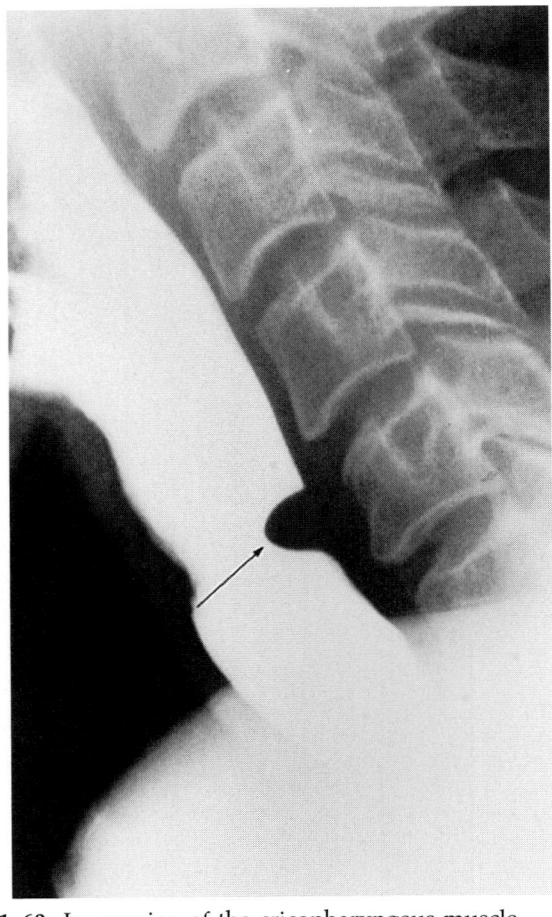

Figure 11–60. Impression of the cricopharyngeus muscle.

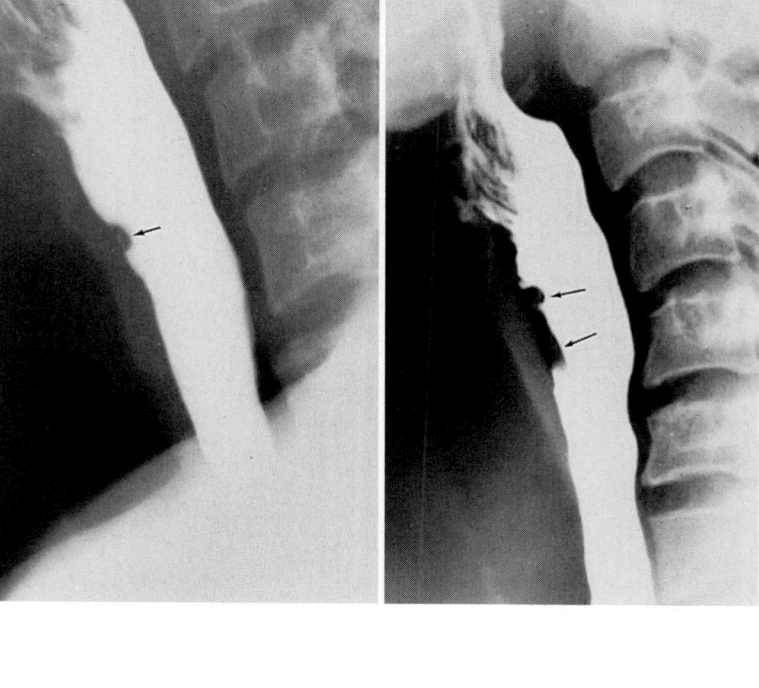

Figure 11–61. Four examples of the variable appearance of the postcricoid impression, which is due to the prolapse of lax mucosal folds over the ventral submucosal venous plexus (*arrows*). It is not seen after the barium bolus is passed. (Ref: Pitman RG, Frazer GM: The postcricoid impression on the esophagus. *Clin Radiol* 16:34, 1965.)

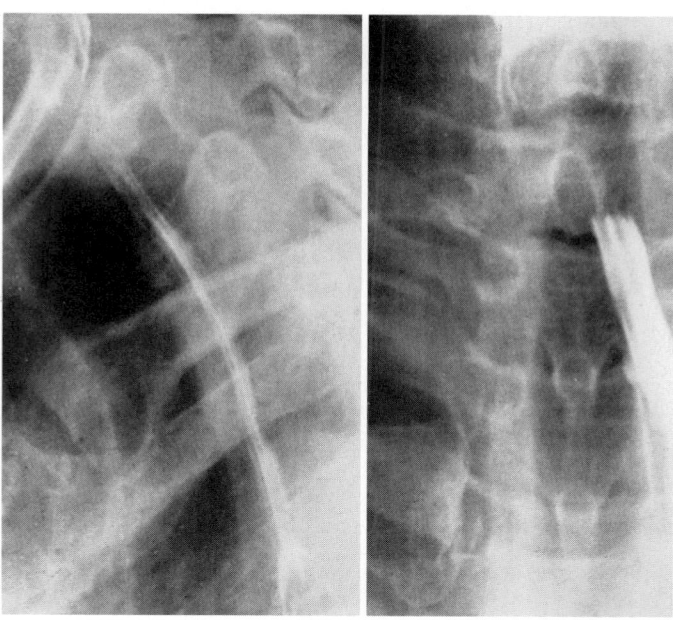

Figure 11–62. Marked shift of the esophagus to the left at the thoracic inlet caused by narrowness of the bony inlet. This variation is often confused with displacement by a mass lesion. (Ref: Kendall BE et al: A physiologic variation in the barium-filled gullet. *Br J Radiol* 35:769, 1962.)

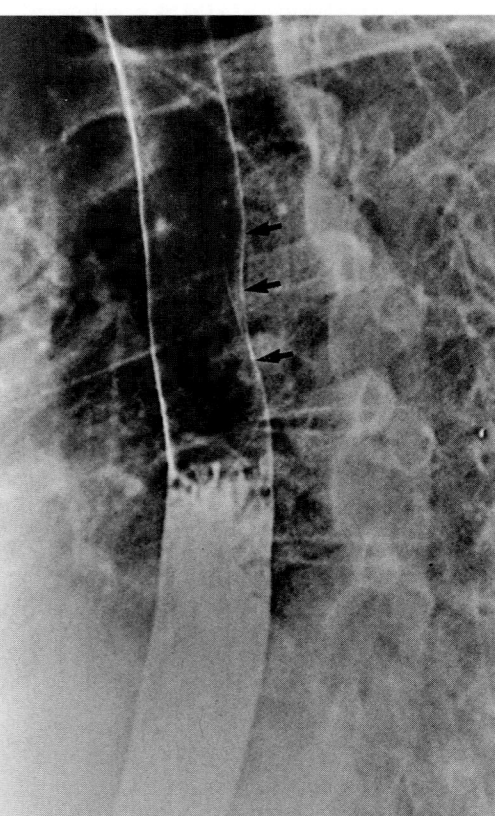

Figure 11–63. Upright double-contrast esophagram shows smooth extrinsic impression on the posterolateral wall of the upper esophagus produced by the prominent right inferior supra azygous recess. (Ref: Sam JW et al: The right inferior supra azygous recess. *Am J Roentgenol* 171:1583, 1998.)

Figure 11–64. Pulmonary venous indentation on the esophagus, caused by pressure of the inferior pulmonary vein, a normal variant. The *asterisk* indicates the venous impression; the *arrow* marks the aortic arch. (From Yeh H-C, Wolf BS: A pulmonary venous indentation on the esophagus—a normal variant. *Radiology* 116:299, 1975.)

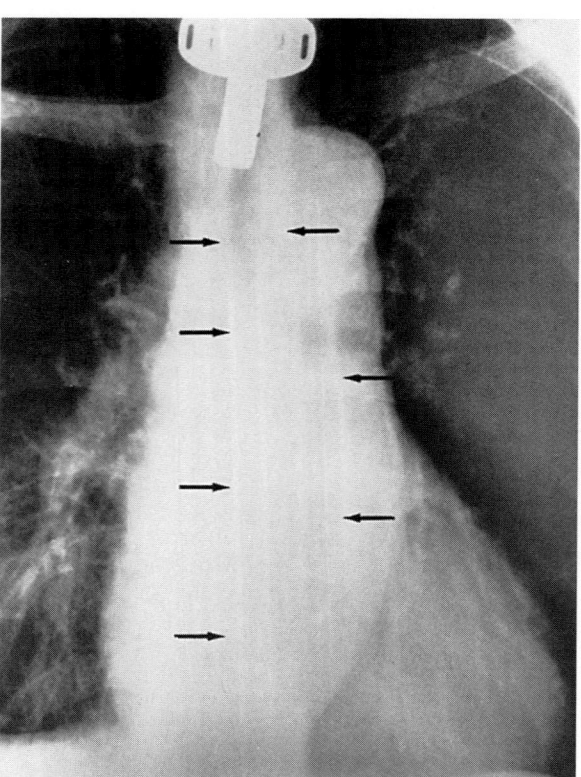

Figure 11–65. Visualization of the esophageal walls in a postlaryngectomy patient with esophageal speech.

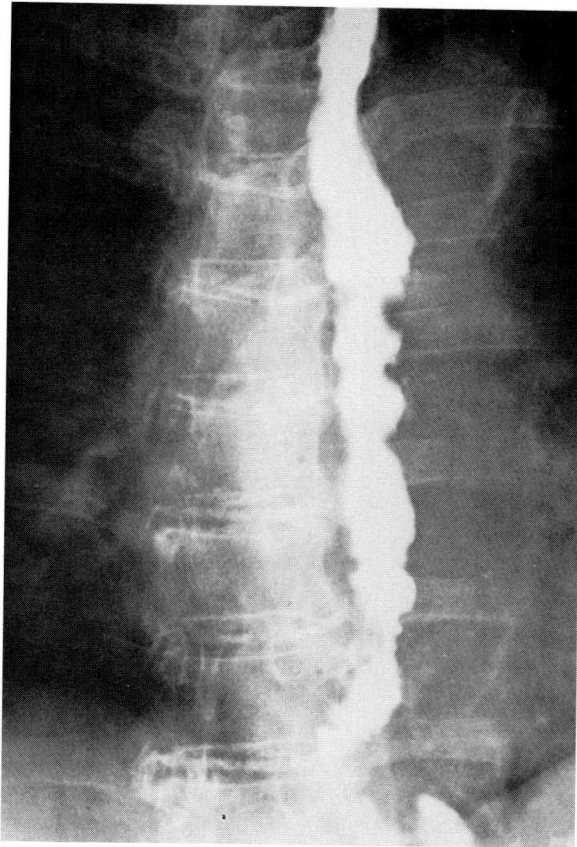

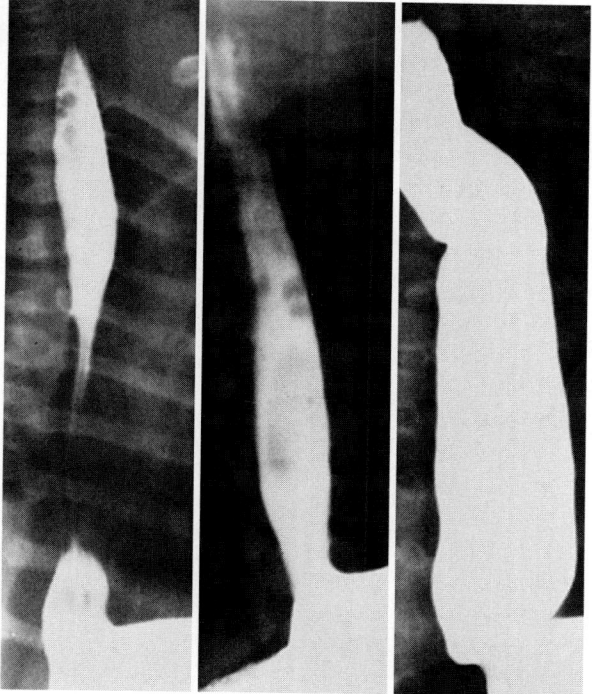

Figure 11–67. Illustration of the great normal distensibility of the infantile esophagus, which might be mistaken for megaesophagus.

Figure 11–66. Presbyesophagus. Tertiary contractions ("curling") of the esophagus are frequently found in the elderly and are not usually of significance. (Ref: Zboralske FF et al: Presbyesophagus: Cineradiographic manifestations. *Radiology* 82:463, 1964.)

Figure 11–68. Transverse striations of the esophagus may be seen as a normal variation as well as in pathologic states, particularly in association with gastroesophageal reflux. (Refs: Gohel VK et al: Transverse folds in the human esophagus. *Radiology* 128:303, 1978; Williams SM et al: Transverse striations of the esophagus: Association with gastroesophageal reflux. *Radiology* 146:25, 1983.)

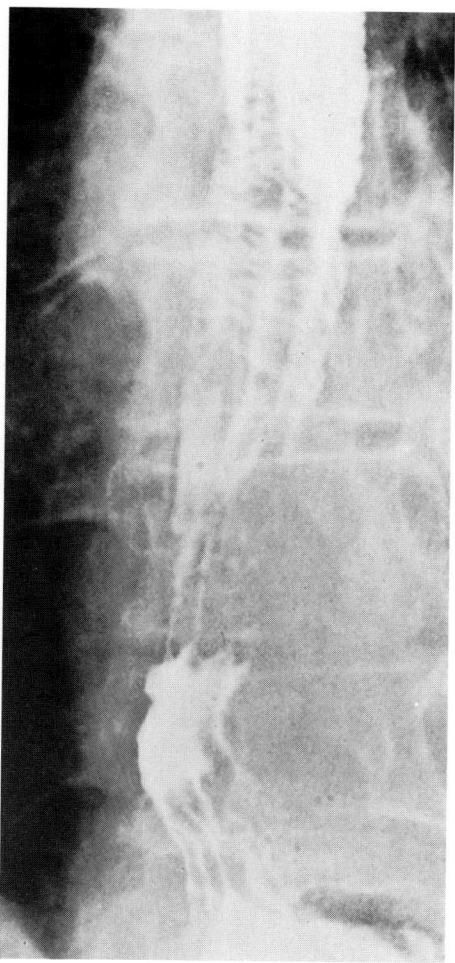

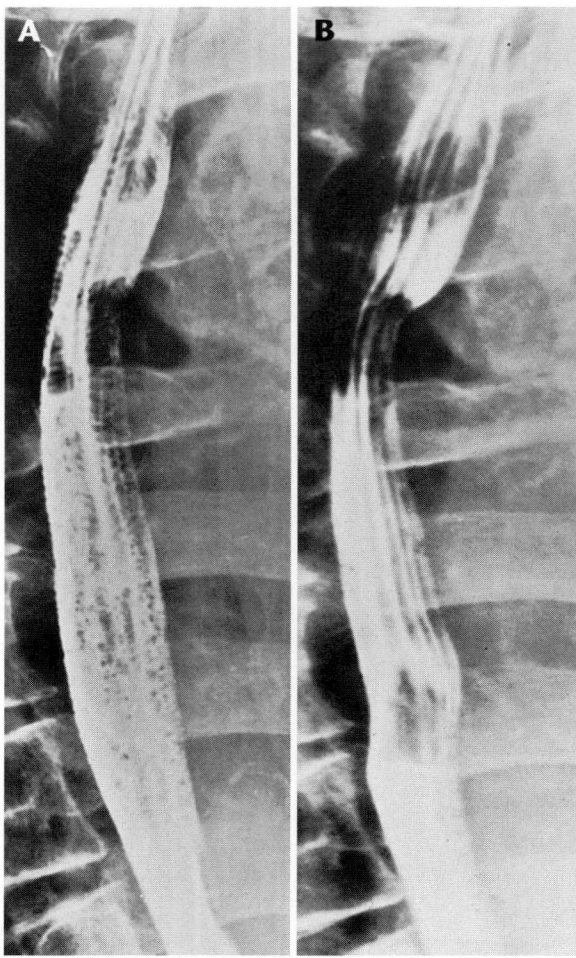

Figure 11–69. Transverse striations seen in **A** are transient, as illustrated in these two films made with the same barium swallow.

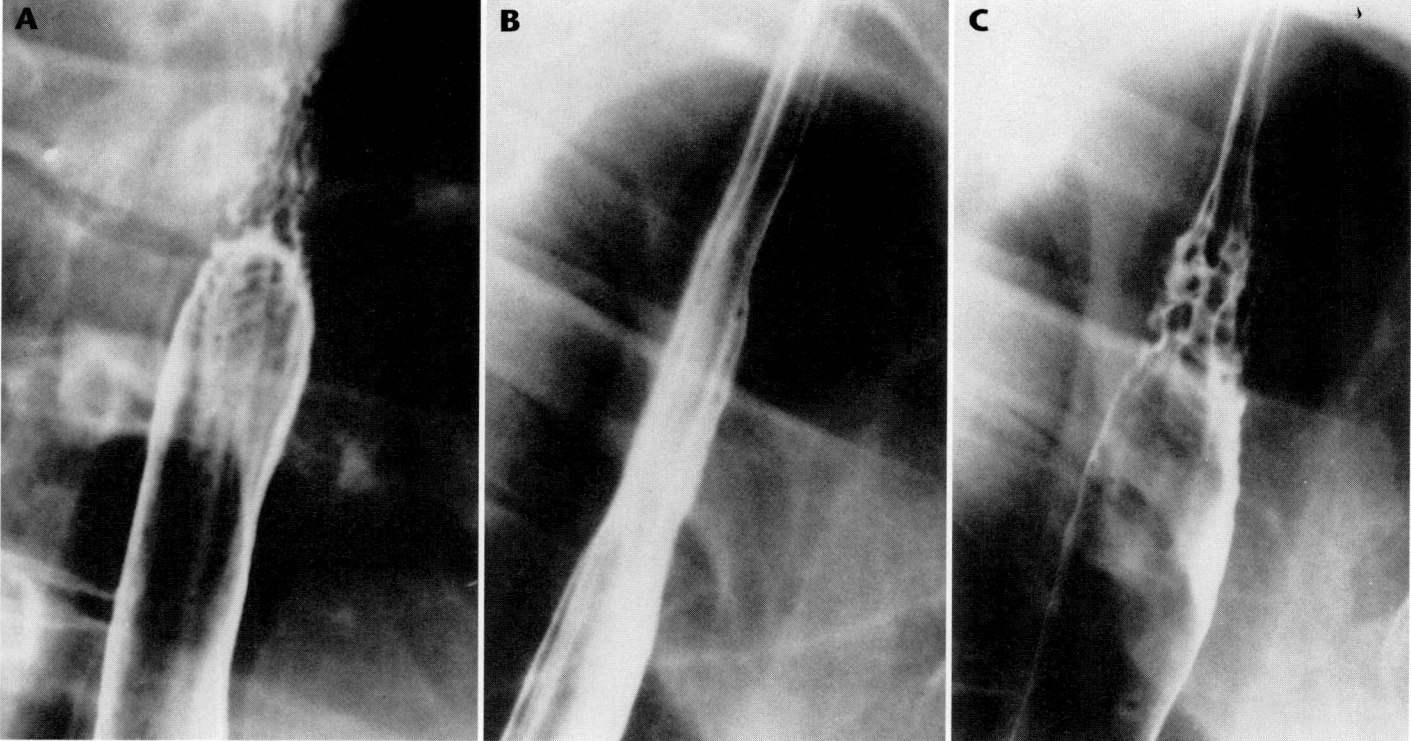

Figure 11–70. Focal spiculation of the upper thoracic esophagus, a normal variant. This entity is seen above the level of the aortic arch and should not be mistaken for a focal area of esophagitis. **A,** Spiculation at edge of peristaltic wave. **B,** Spiculation seen in another patient. **C,** Same patient as in **B,** with a view obtained moments later with greater distention, shows normal appearance. (From Levine MS et al: Focal spiculation of the upper thoracic esophagus: Normal variant at double contract esophagography. *Radiology* 183:807, 1992.)

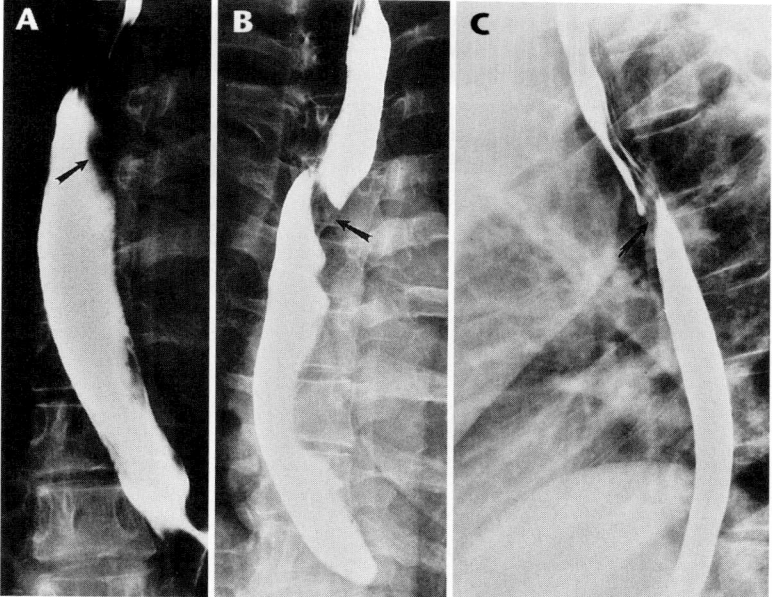

Figure 11–71. Impression of the left main bronchus on the esophagus. **A,** Full column. **B** and **C,** Partial column.

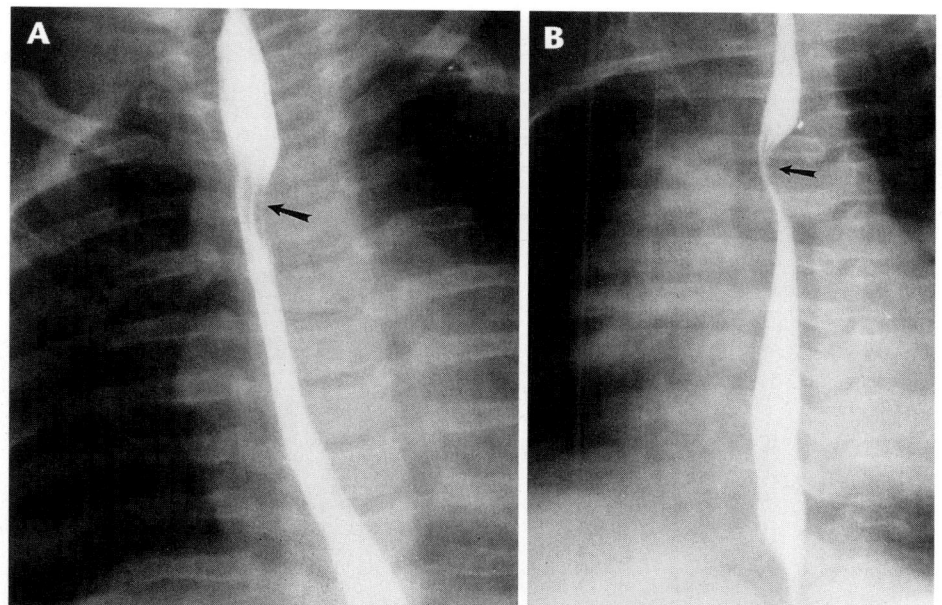

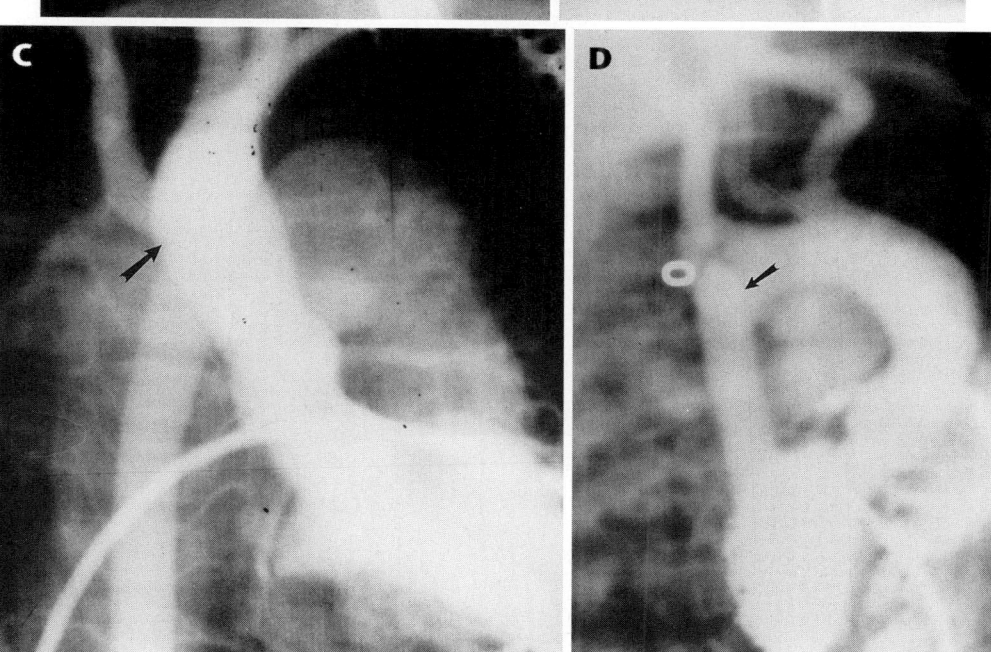

Figure 11–72. A and **B,** Esophageal impression of an aberrant (*right*) subclavian artery. **C** and **D,** Angiocardiogram shows anomalous origin of the right subclavian artery from the proximal descending aorta. (Ref: Freed K, Low WHS: The aberrant subclavian artery. *Am J Roentgenol* 168:481, 1997.)

The Stomach

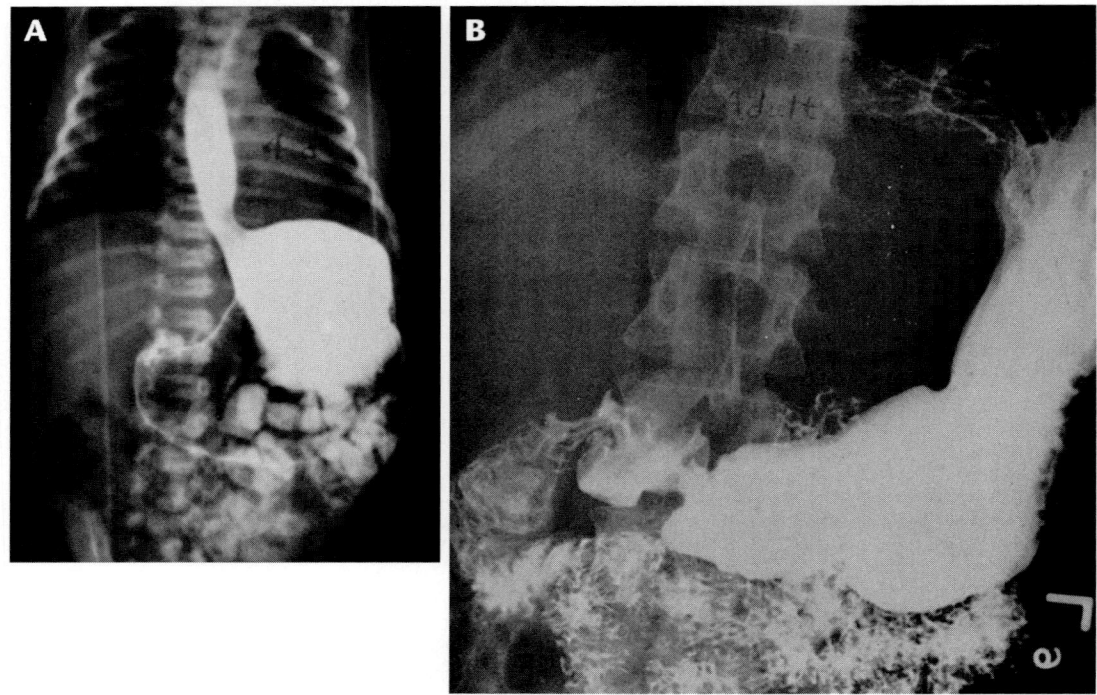

Figure 11–73. Proportional differences in size between the stomach and total abdomen in an infant (**A**) and an adult (**B**). The infant's stomach is proportionately larger, an important concept in avoiding misinterpretation of the size of the air-distended stomach of the infant. (From Keats TE: Pediatric radiology: Some potentially misleading variations from the adult. *VA Med* 93:630, 1966.)

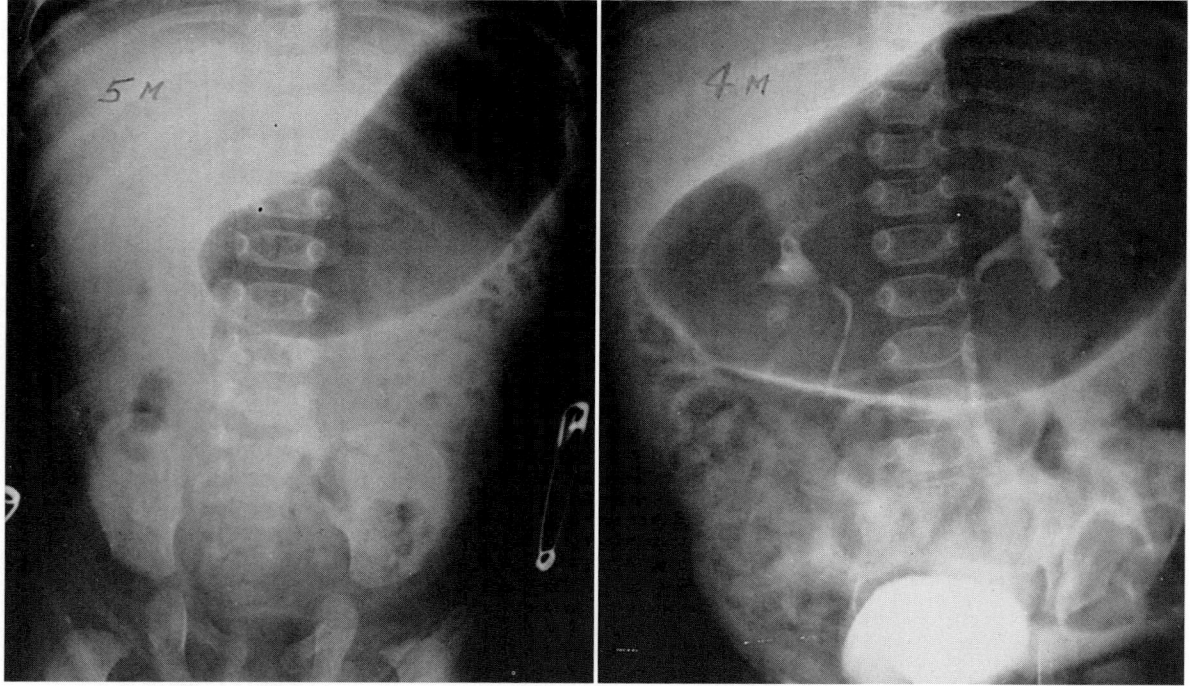

Figure 11–74. Normal but marked gaseous distention of the stomach in crying infants.

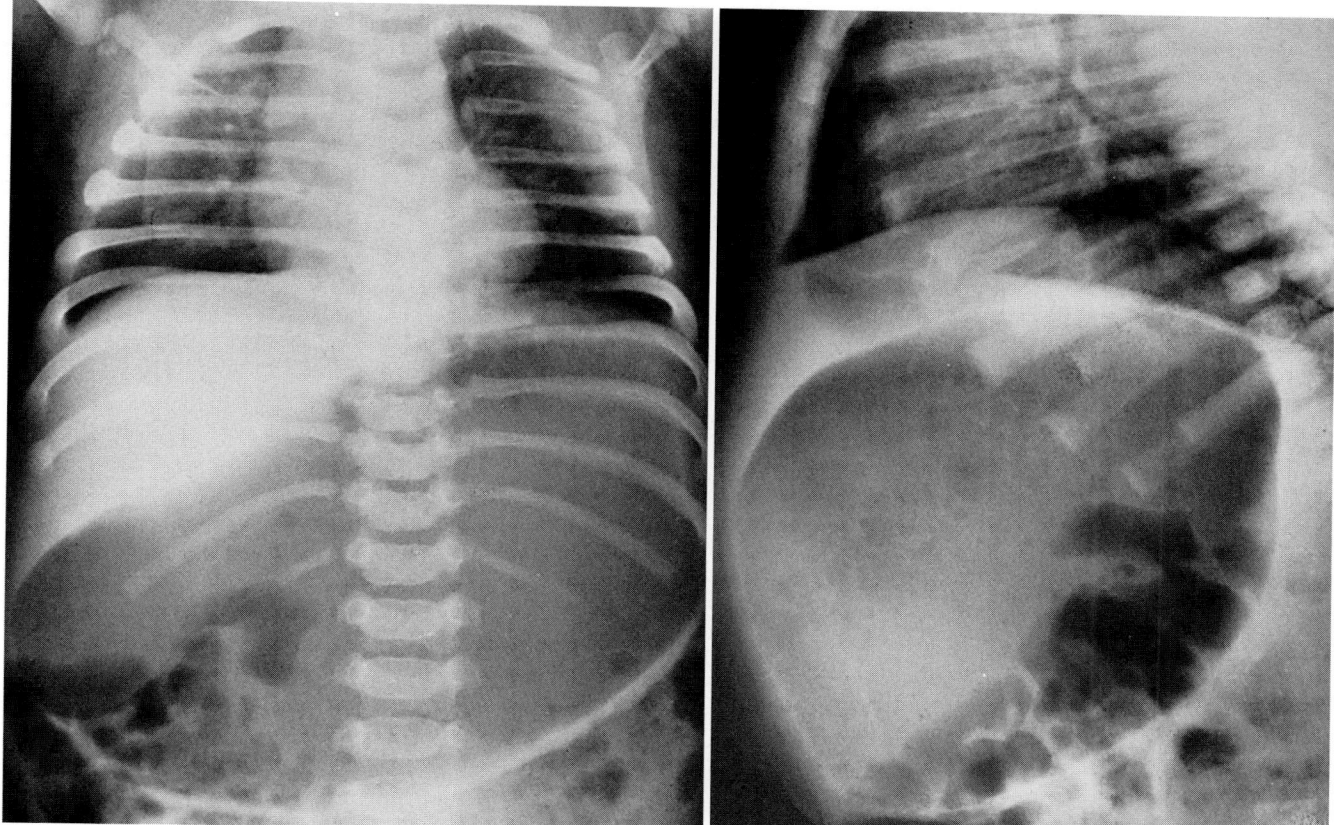

Figure 11–75. Normal but marked gaseous distention of the stomach in a crying infant.

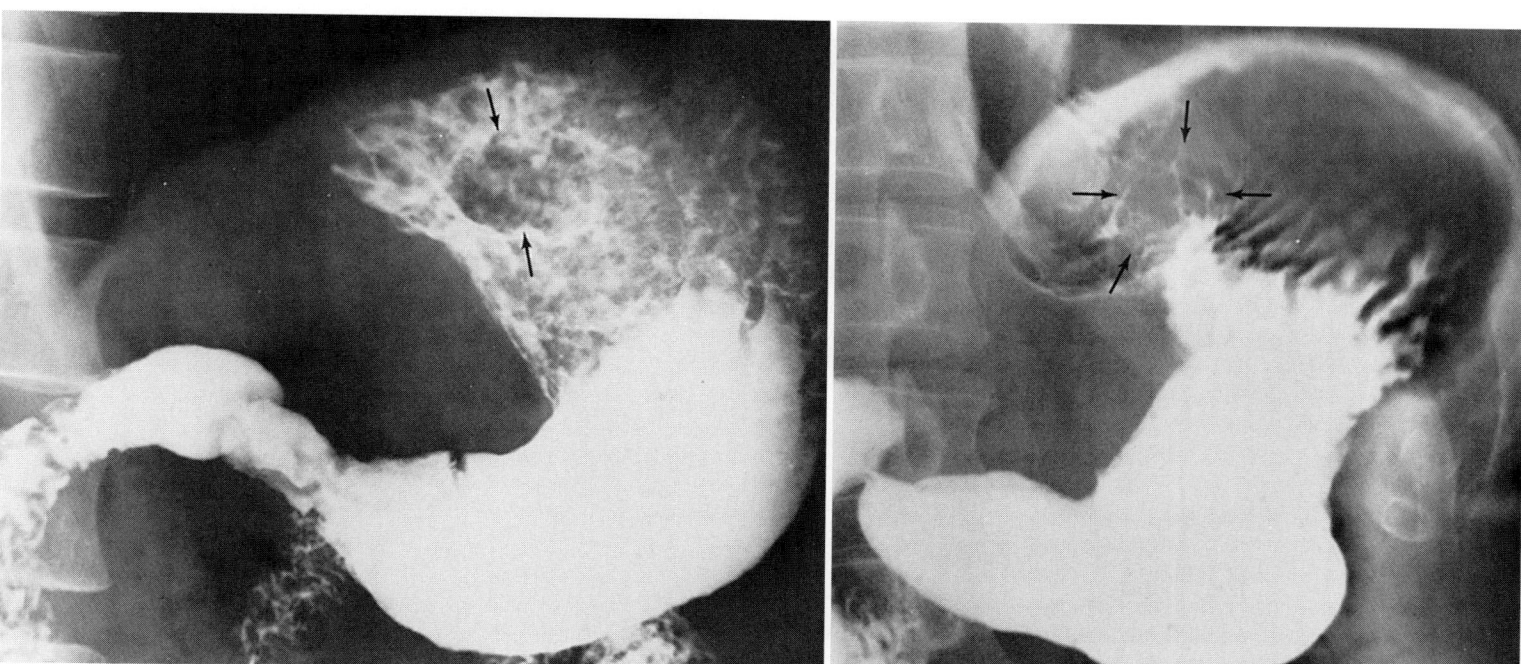

Figure 11–76. Two examples of the cardioesophageal junction seen en face, simulating a polypoid filling defect in the stomach.

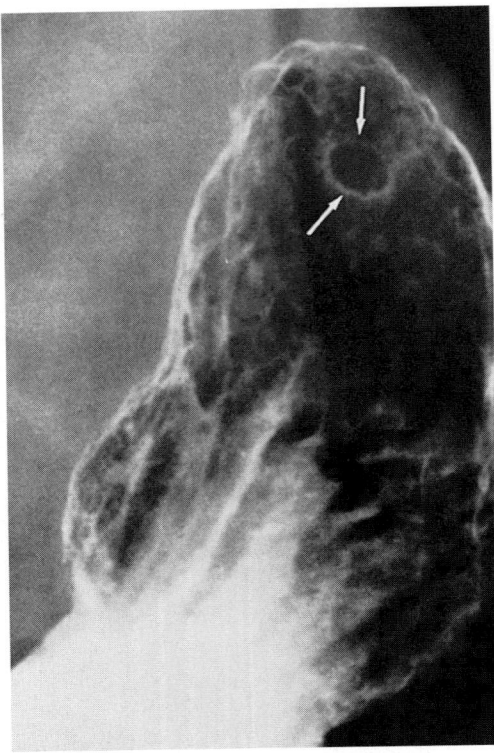

Figure 11–77. Esophagogastric junction presenting as a polypoid filling defect.

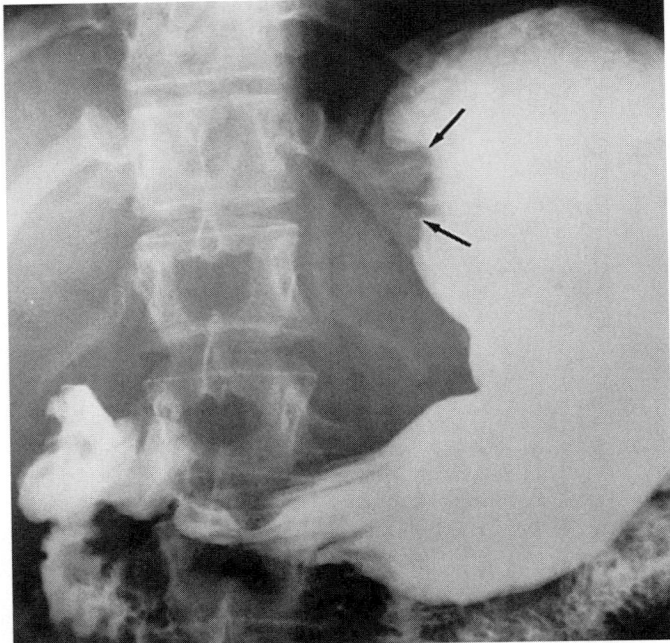

Figure 11–78. Invagination of the esophageal mucosa at the cardia, simulating a mass lesion. (Ref: de Lorimor AA, Warren JP: Prolapse of the mucosa at the esophagogastric junction. *Am J Roentgenol* 84:1061, 1960.)

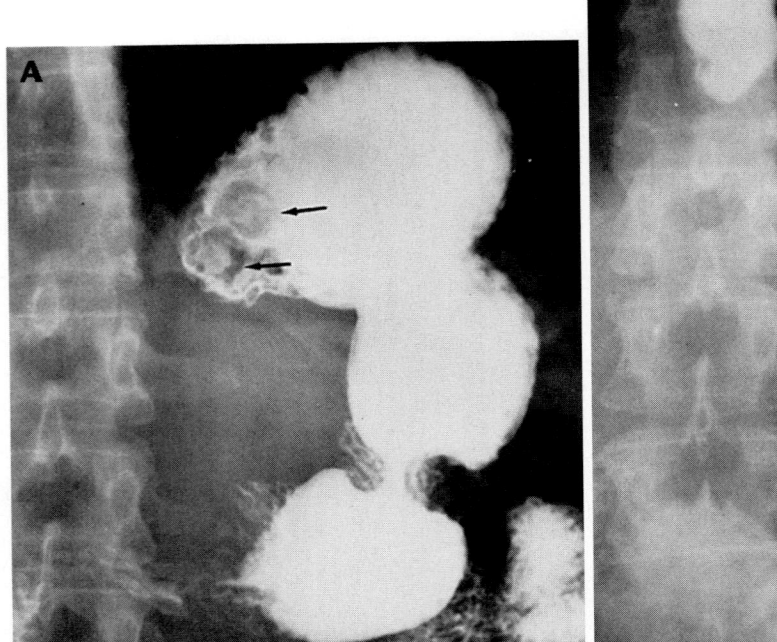

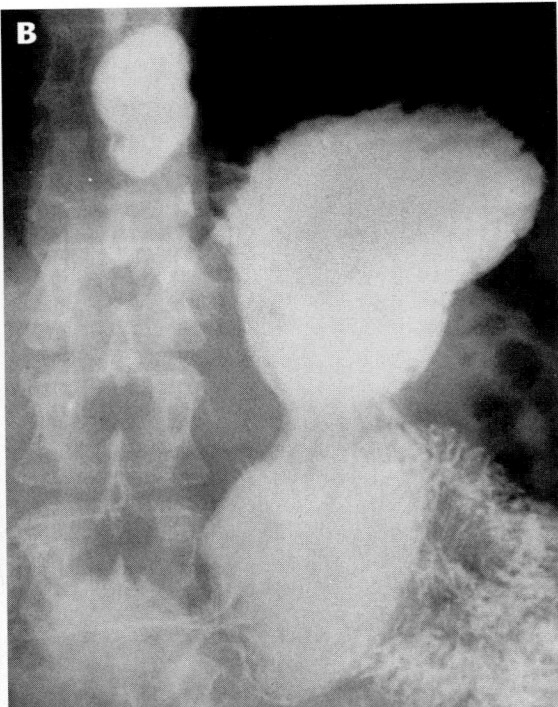

Figure 11–79. Esophageal mucosa simulating a gastric mass in a patient with a hiatal hernia. **A,** Mucosa is prolapsed into the stomach. **B,** Hernia is now present and prolapse is no longer evident. (Ref: Aldridge NH: Transmigration of the lower esophageal mucosa. *Radiology* 79:962, 1962.)

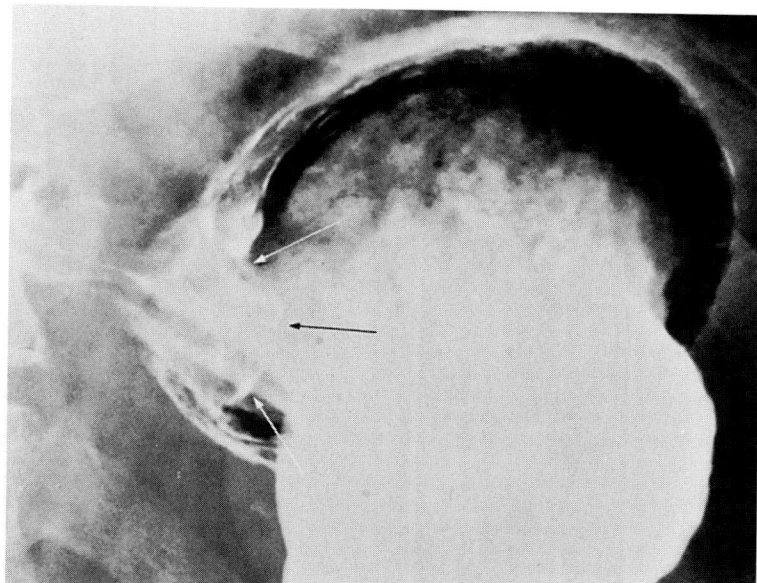

Figure 11–80. Prolapse of the esophageal mucosa into the stomach (proved at surgery).

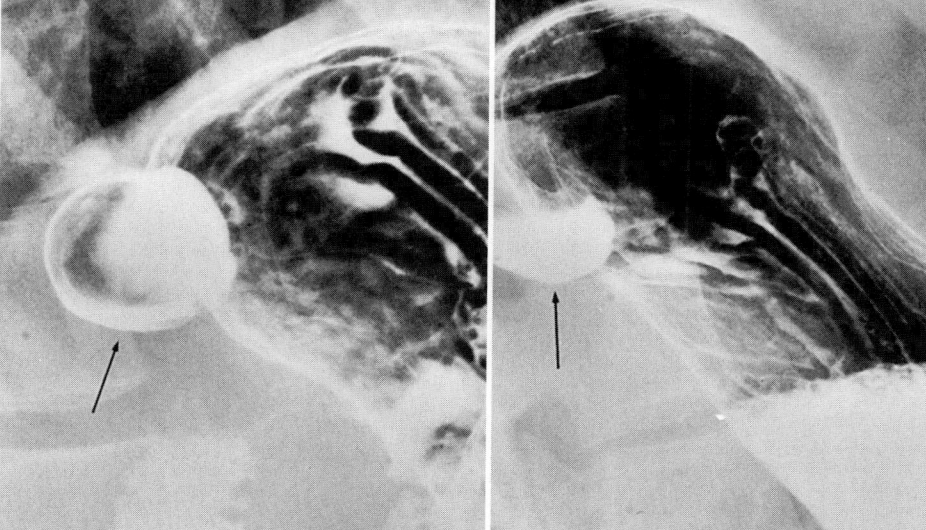

Figure 11–81. Gastric diverticulum in its typical location in the cardia of the stomach.

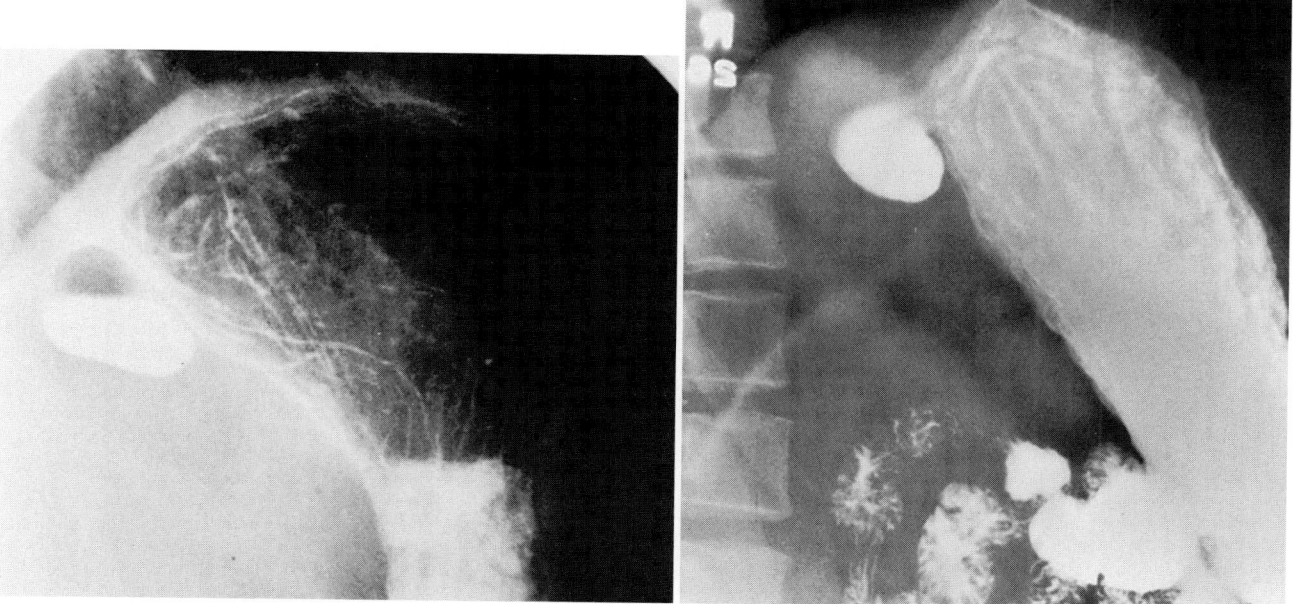

Figure 11–82. Two examples of developmental gastric diverticula in their classic position.

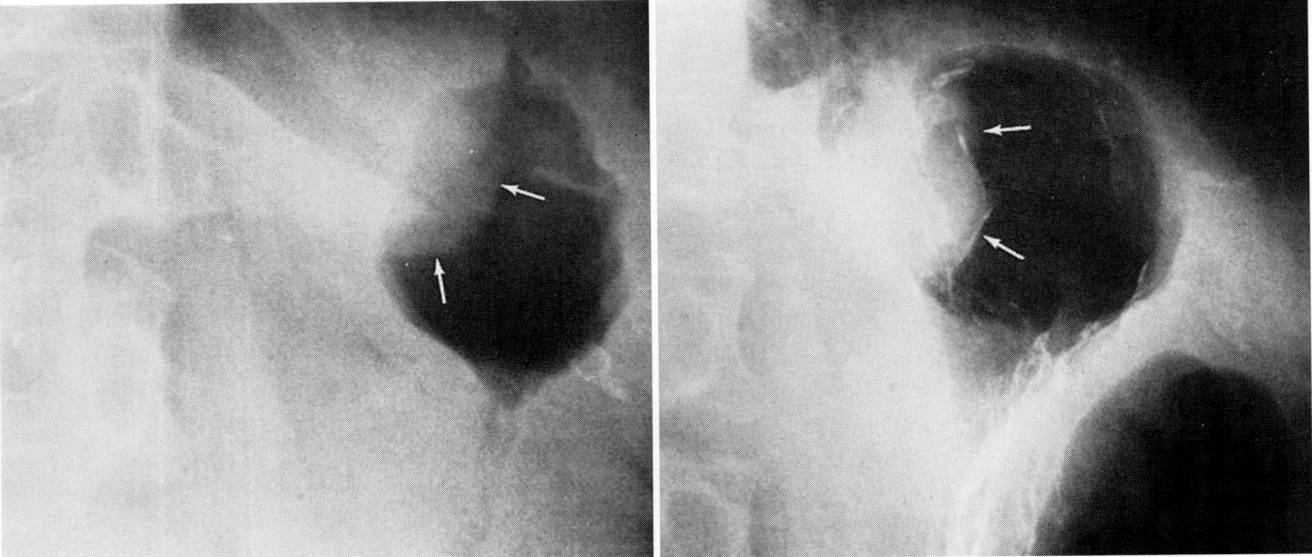

Figure 11–83. Left lobe of the liver presenting into the gastric air bubble (proved at surgery), simulating a neoplasm (see Fig. 11–32).

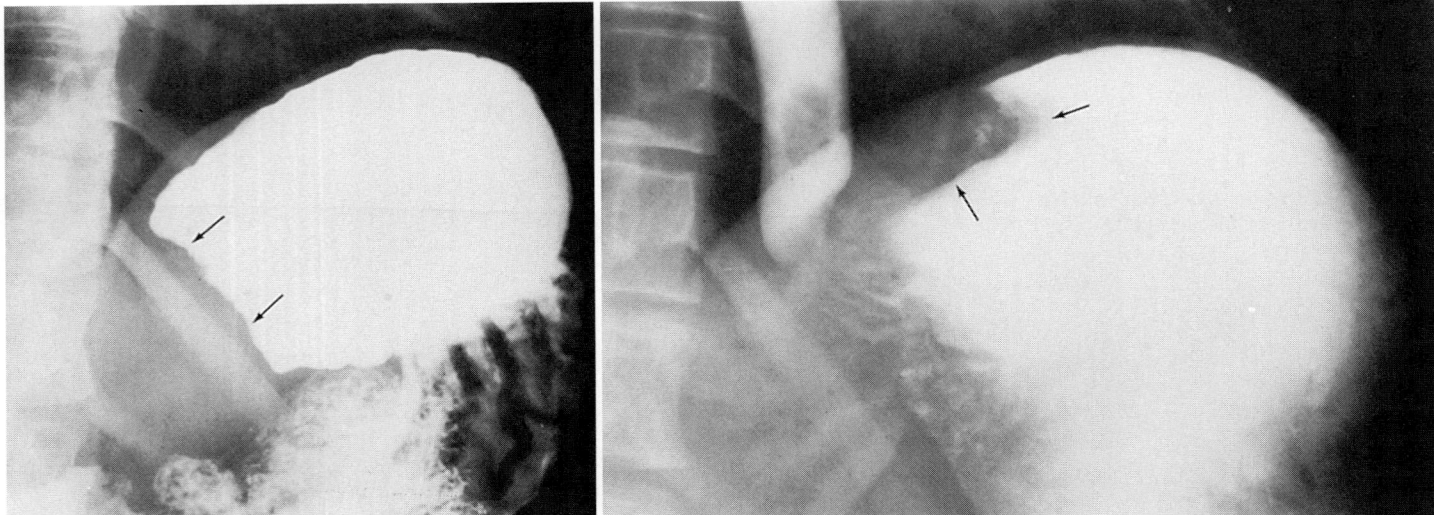

Figure 11–84. Gastric impressions related to the left lobe of the liver.

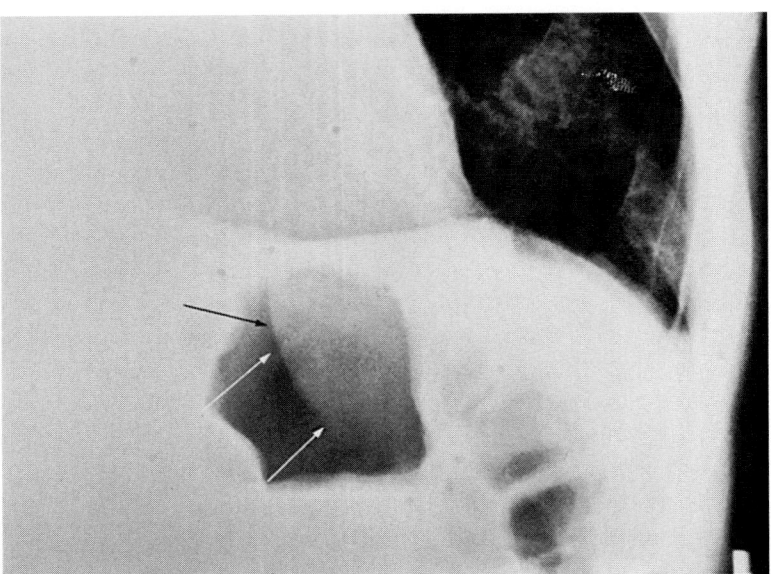

Figure 11–85. Spleen encroaching on the stomach gas bubble.

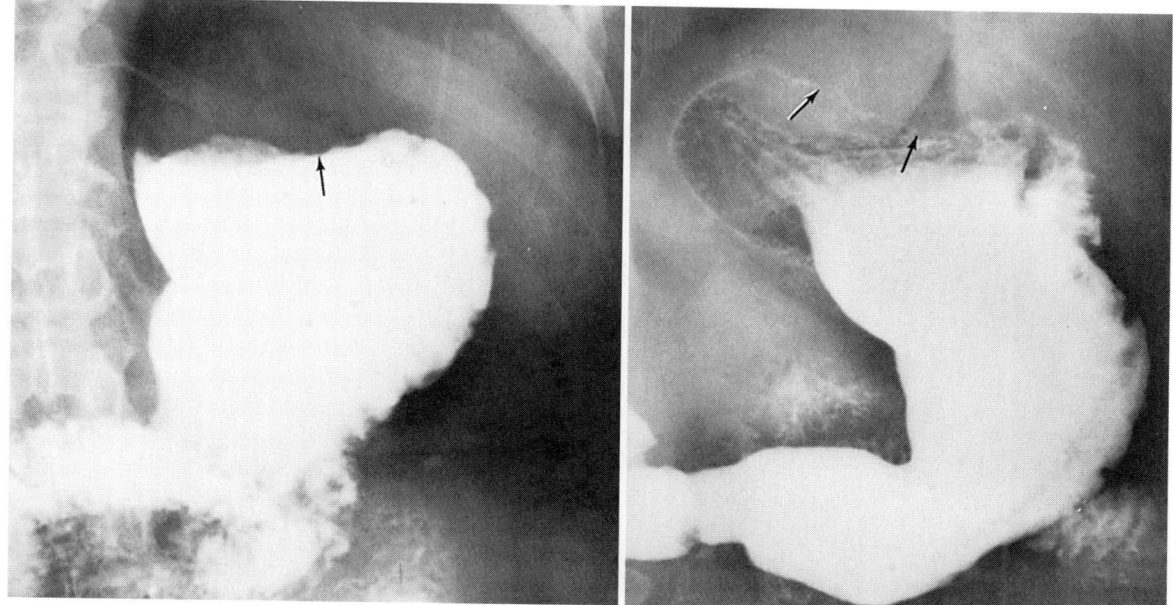

Figure 11–86. Impression of a horizontally oriented spleen simulating a gastric mass.

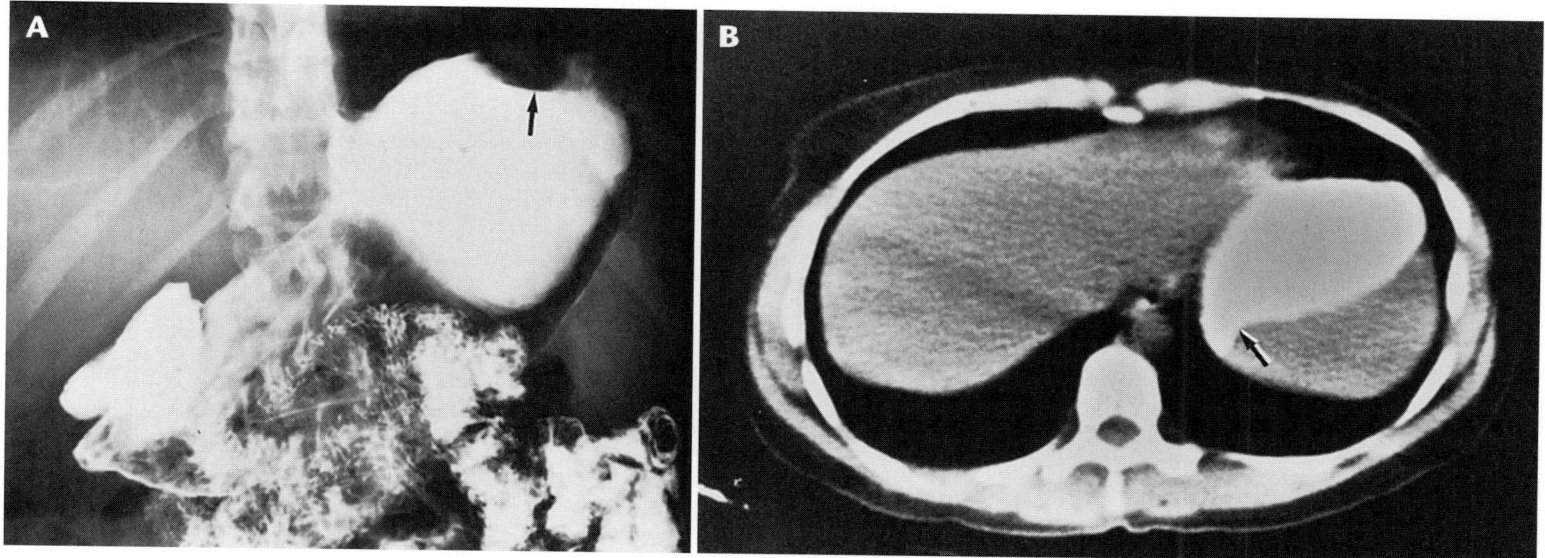

Figure 11–87. Splenic impression on the fundus of the stomach. **A,** GI series. **B,** CT confirmation.

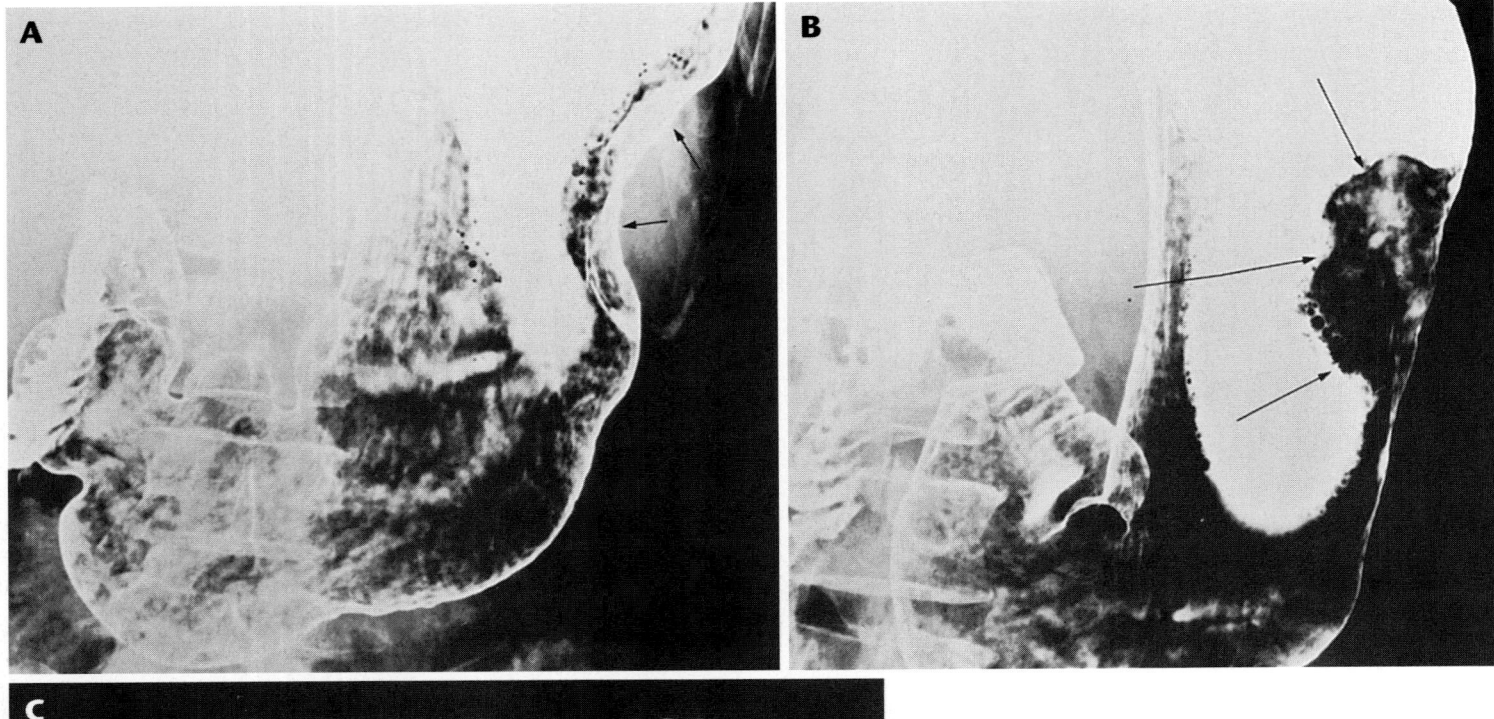

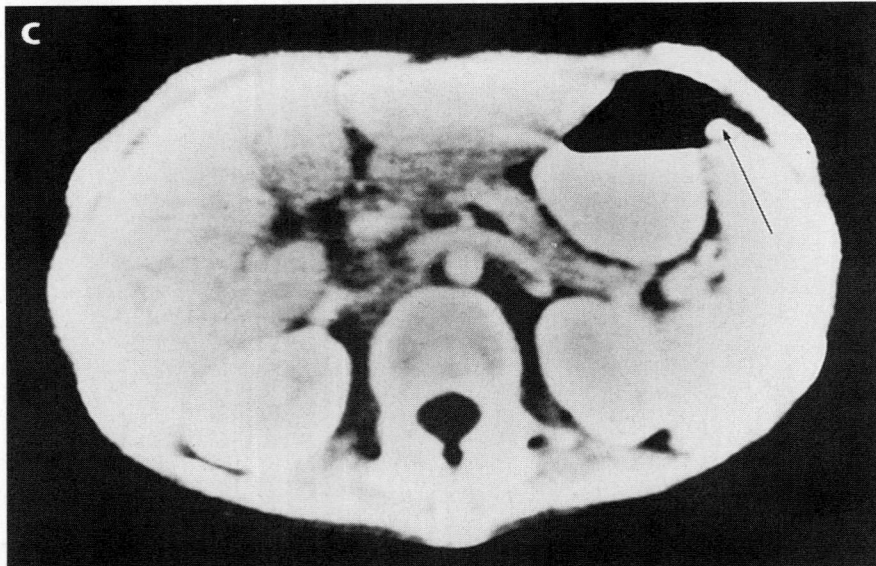

Figure 11–88. Impression of a normal spleen on the stomach. **A,** Anteroposterior projection. **B,** Left posterior oblique projection. **C,** CT shows the anterior tip of the spleen projecting into the stomach gas bubble.

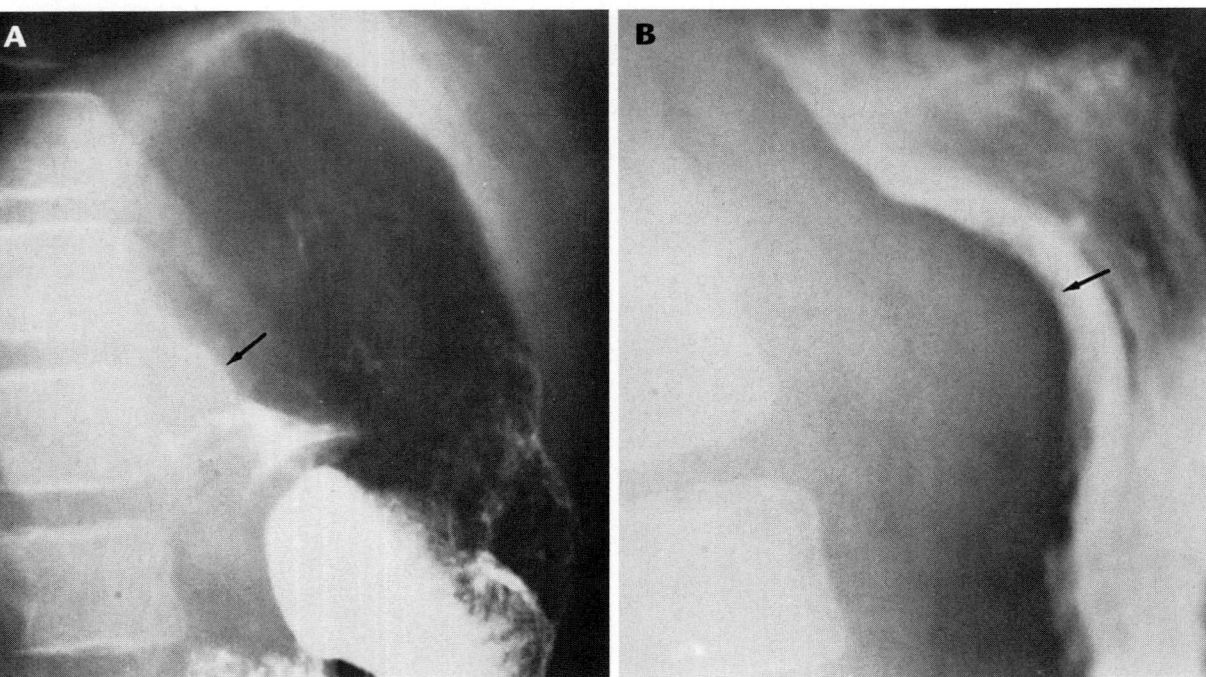

Figure 11–89. Normal impressions of the pancreas on the posterior wall of the stomach in an 8-year-old girl. **A,** Supine lateral projection. **B,** Upright lateral projection.

Figure 11-90. Impression of the costal margin on the stomach, simulating a mass lesion. **A,** Partially filled stomach. **B,** Completely filled stomach (the impression is not as well seen here).

Figure 11-91. Additional examples of the impression of the costal margin, simulating a mass lesion.

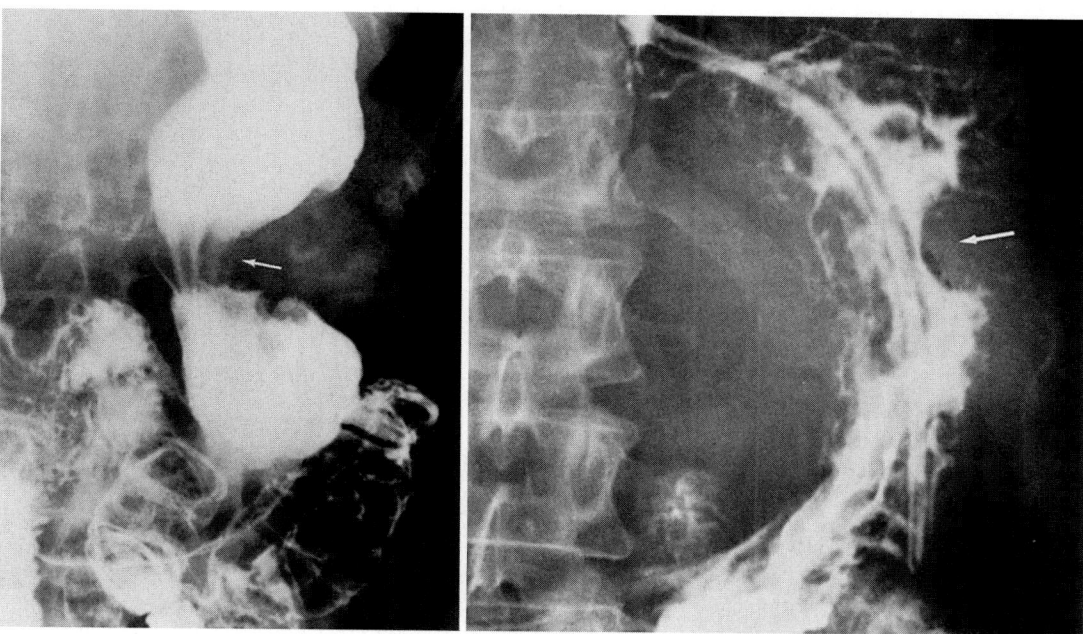

Figure 11-92. Barium in the minute folds of the gastric mucosa (confirmed by gastroscopic examination), simulating small ulcers. This entity may also be seen in the colon (see Fig. 11-177). **A,** Conventional film. **B,** Enlargement. (Ref: Stone DD, Keats TE: Anatomical and physiological characteristics of the État Mammelonné, a normal variant of the gastric mucosa. *Radiology* 107:537, 1973.)

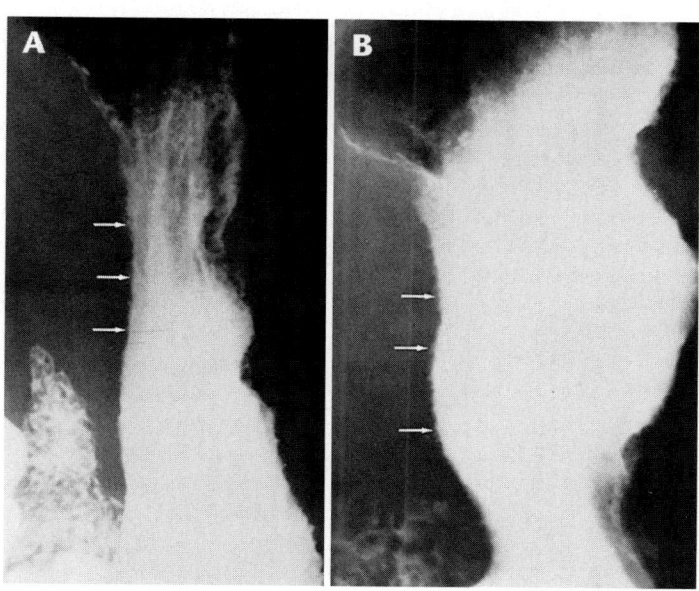

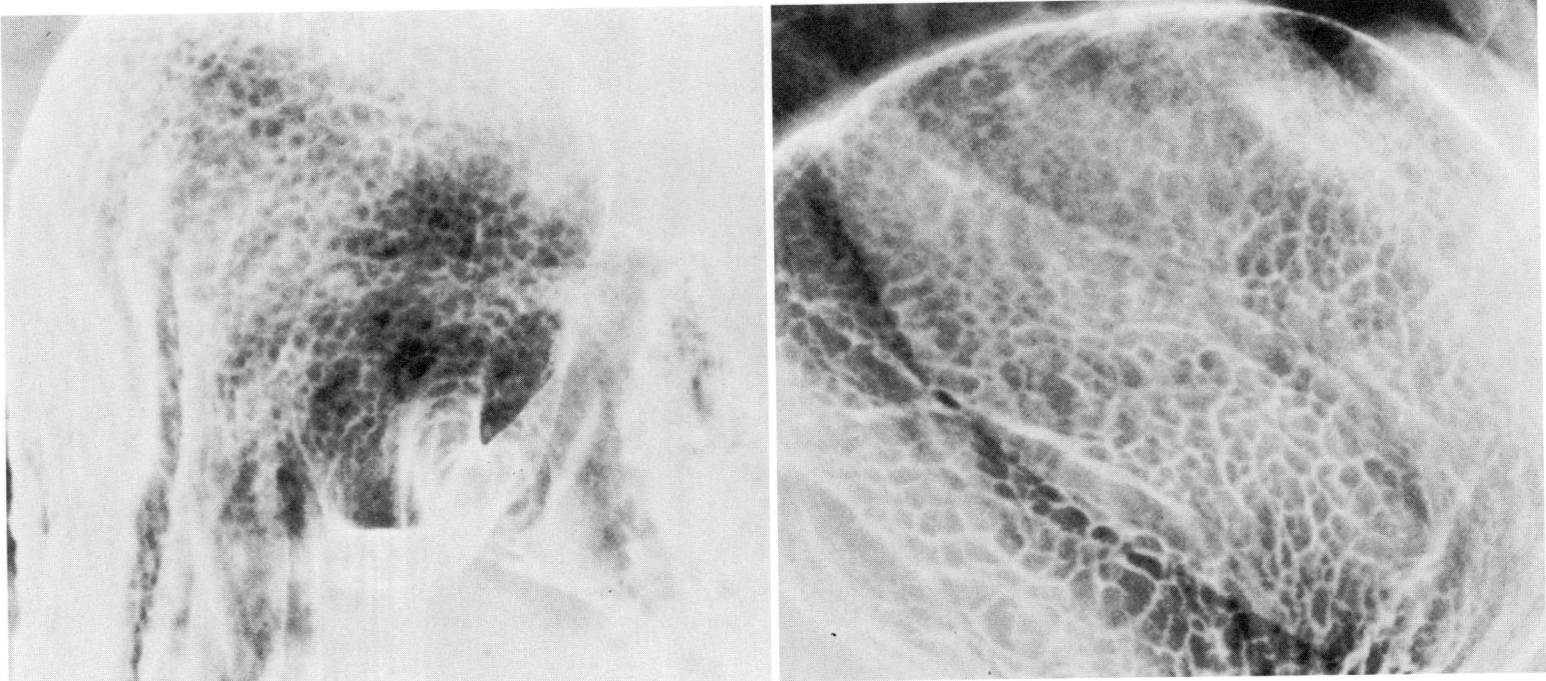

Figure 11–93. Normal appearance of the areae gastricae.

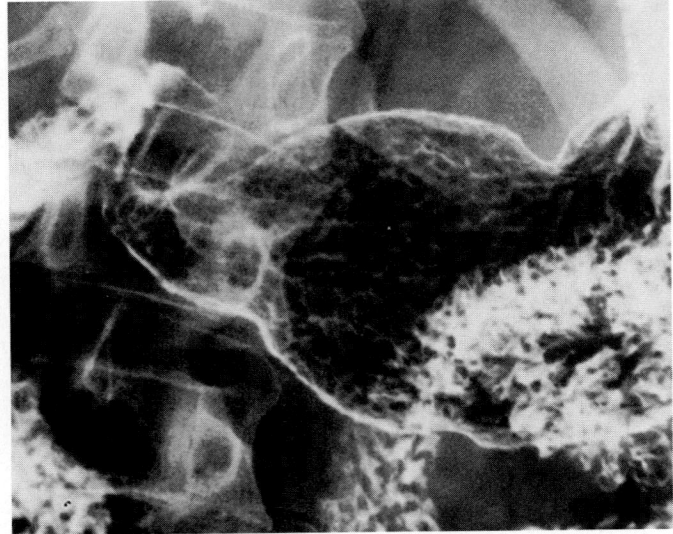

Figure 11–94. Normal gastric mucosal pattern of the stomach by double contrast examination.

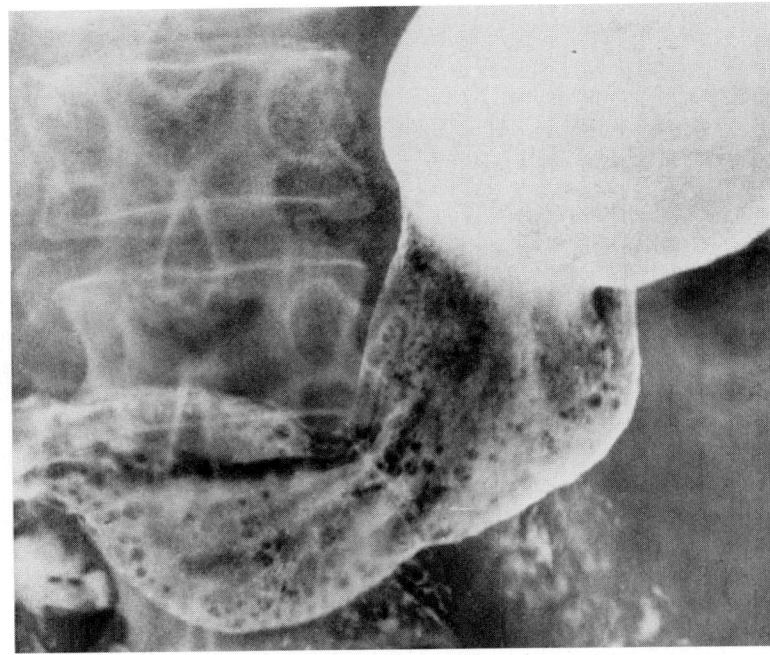

Figure 11–95. Air bubbles in the stomach, simulating polypoid lesions.

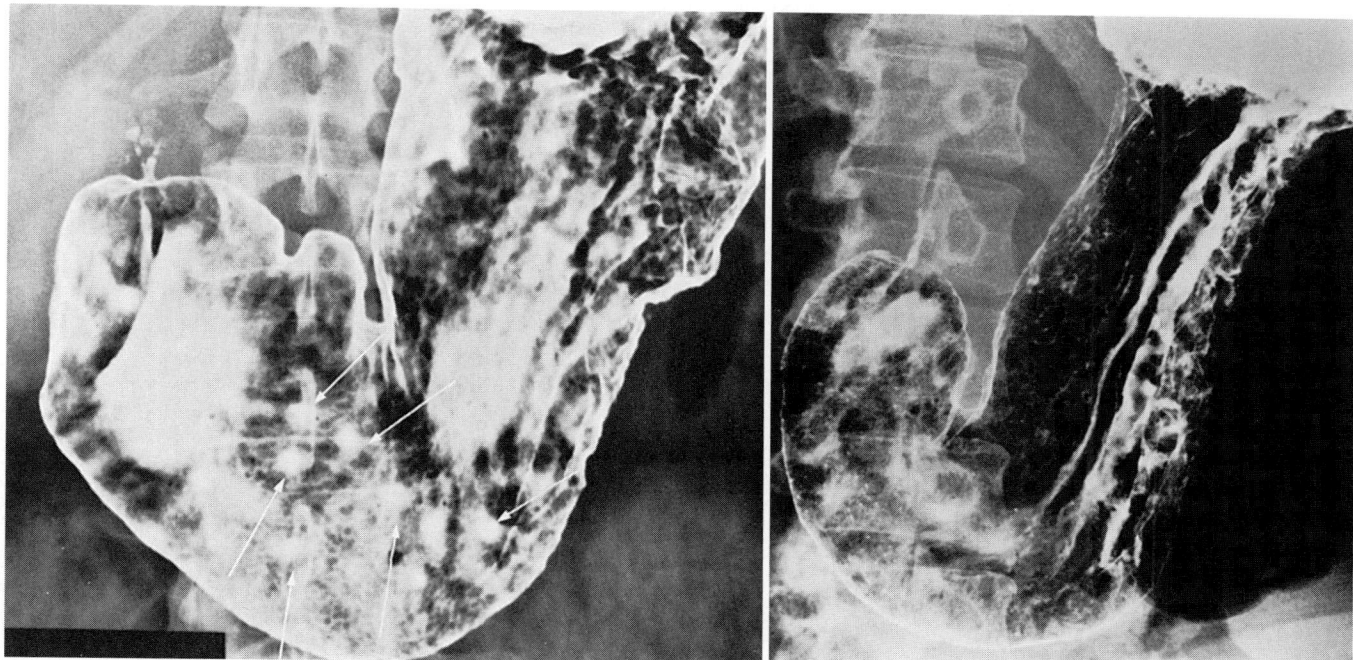

Figure 11–96. Two examples of artifactual gastric erosions produced by particles of barium. Note the absence of surrounding halos. (Refs: Gohel VK et al: Double contrast artifacts. *Gastrointest Radiol* 3:139, 1978; Aronchick J et al: Barium stalactites: Observations on their nature and significance. *Radiology* 149:588, 1983; Samuel E: Radiology of normal and abnormal gastric mucus. *Br J Radiol* 60:987, 1987.)

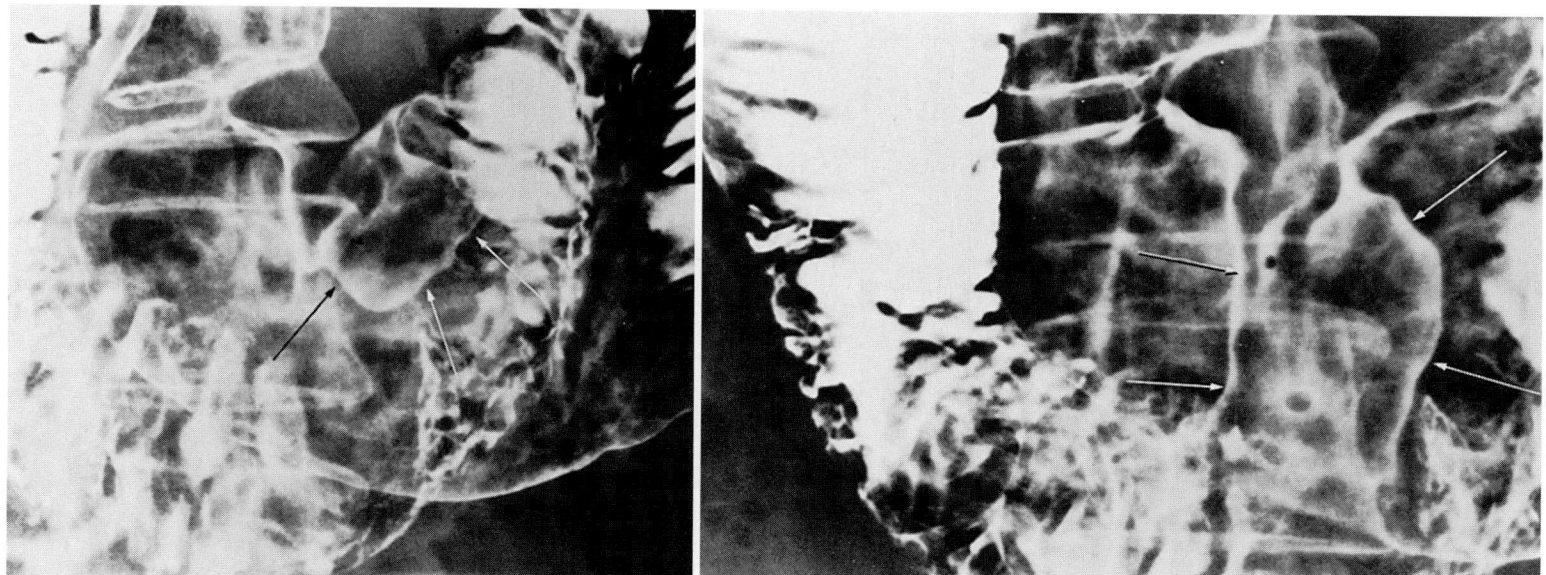

Figure 11–97. Compression films of the stomach, producing "kissing" artifacts simulating mass lesions.

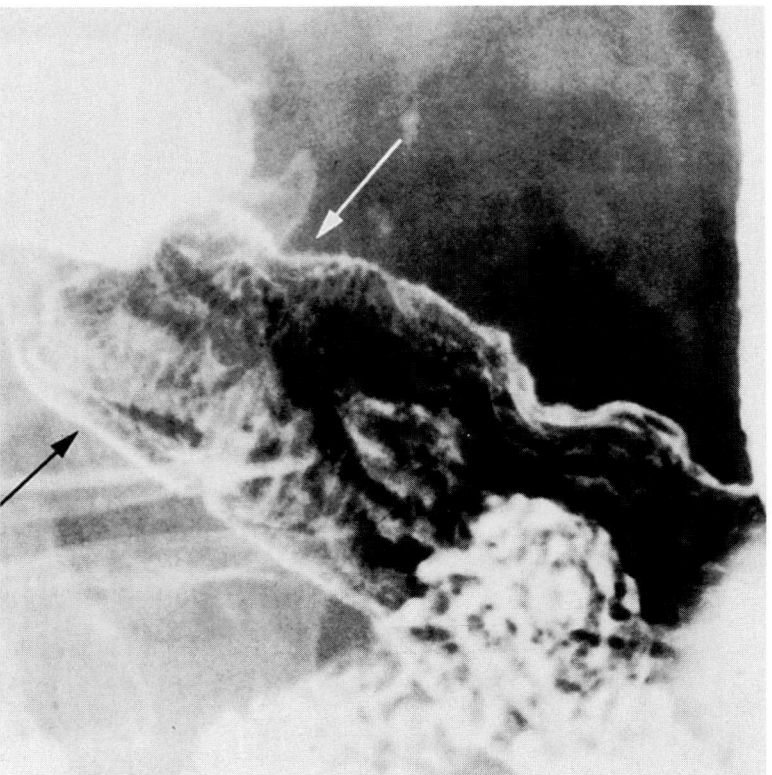

Figure 11–98. Barium dripping simulating a gastric diverticulum. (Ref: Shackelford GD: Barium collections in the stomach mimicking intramural diverticula. *Am J Roentgenol* 139:805, 1982.)

Figure 11–99. Normal transverse mucosal folds of the stomach. (Ref: Cho KC et al: Multiple transverse folds in the gastric antrum. *Radiology* 164:339, 1987.)

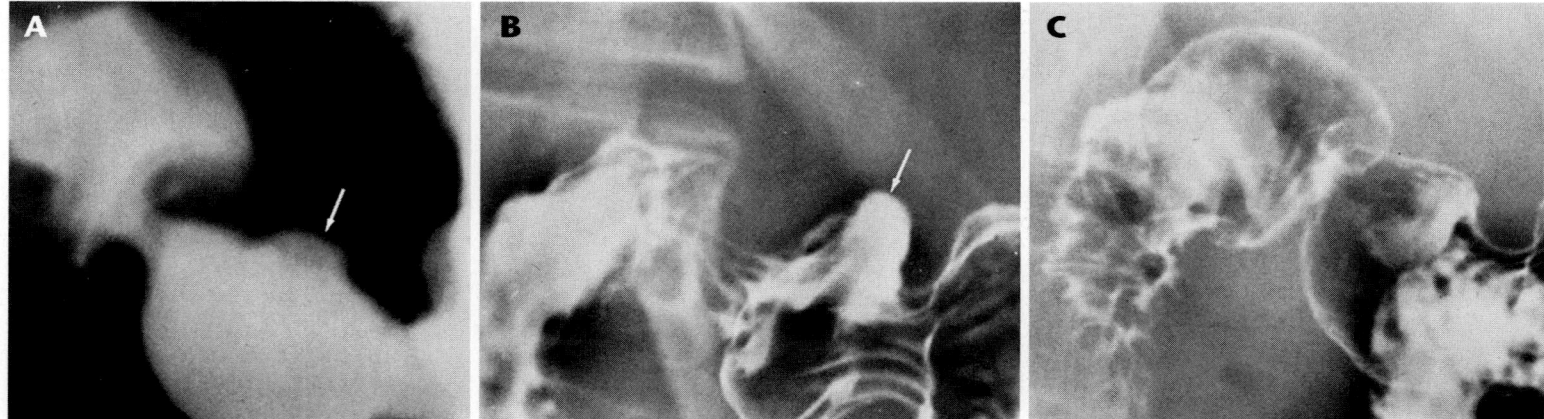

Figure 11–100. Pseudoulceration of the antrum, produced by peristaltic waves seen in **A** and **B**, but not in **C**.

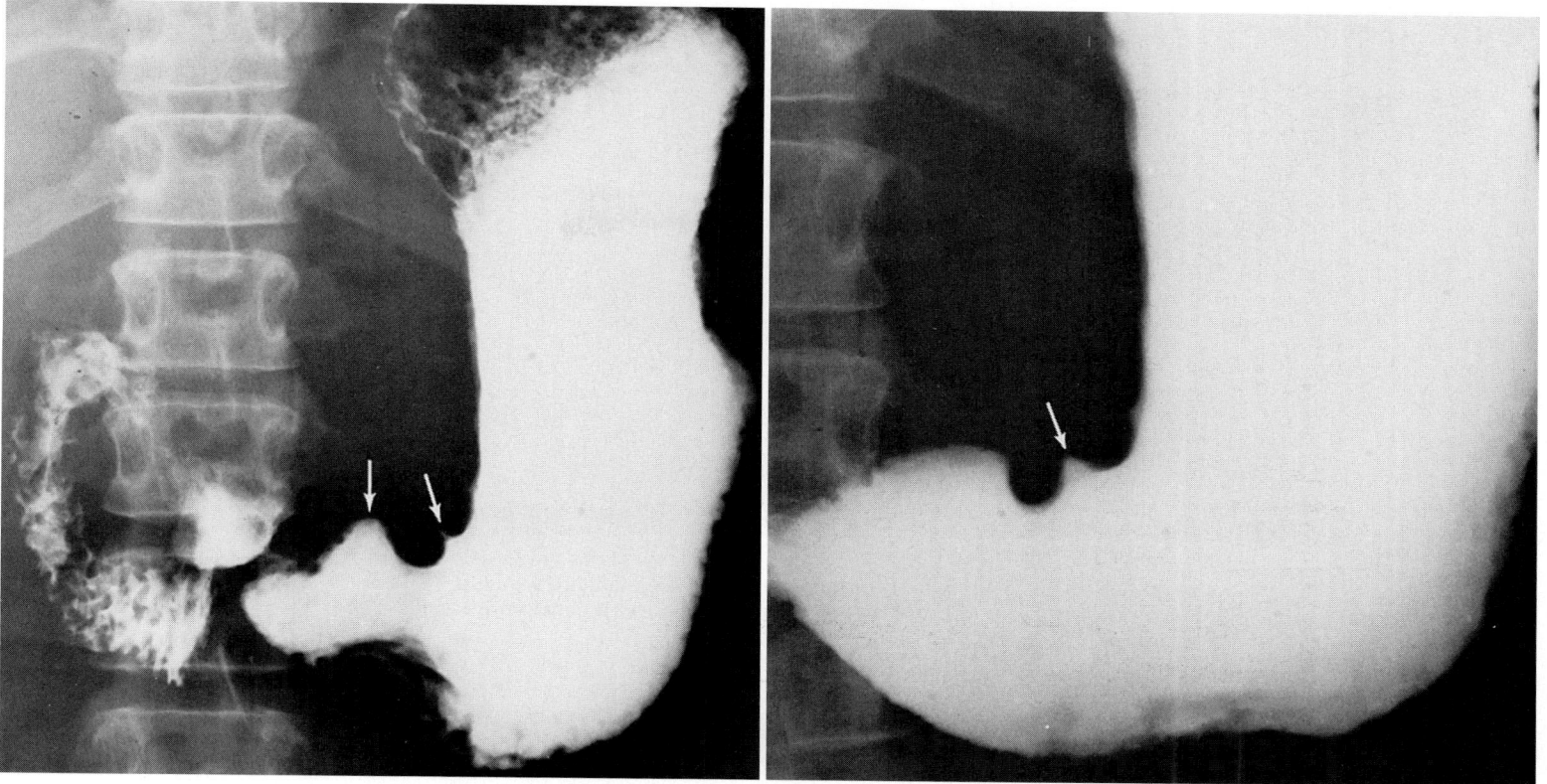

Figure 11–101. Pseudoulceration of the lesser curve of the antrum produced by peristaltic waves. (Ref: Peavy PW et al: Gastric pseudo-ulcers: Membrana angularis and pyloric torus defects. *Radiology* 114:591, 1975.)

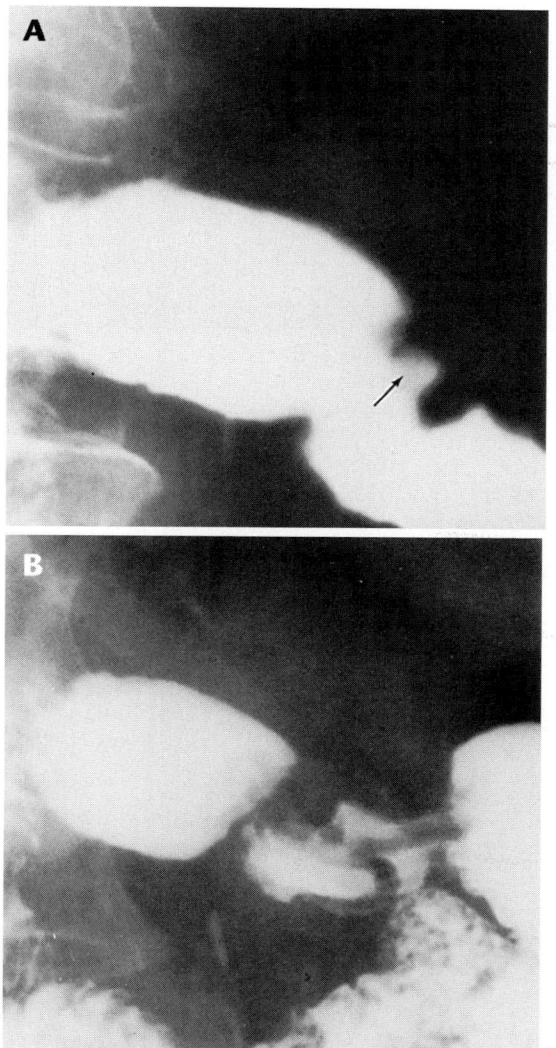

Figure 11–102. Additional examples of pseudoulceration of the antrum seen in **A,** but not in **B.** (Ref: Bremner CG: The lesser curve pyloric niche. *Br J Radiol* 41:291, 1968.)

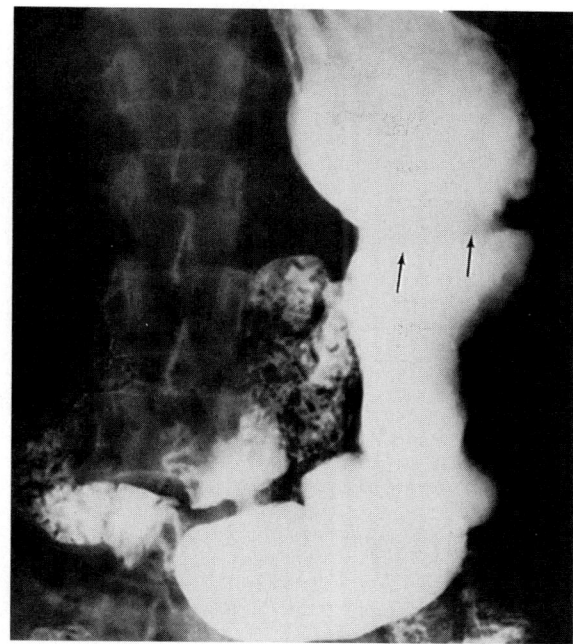

Figure 11–103. Well-defined muscle band in the body of the stomach.

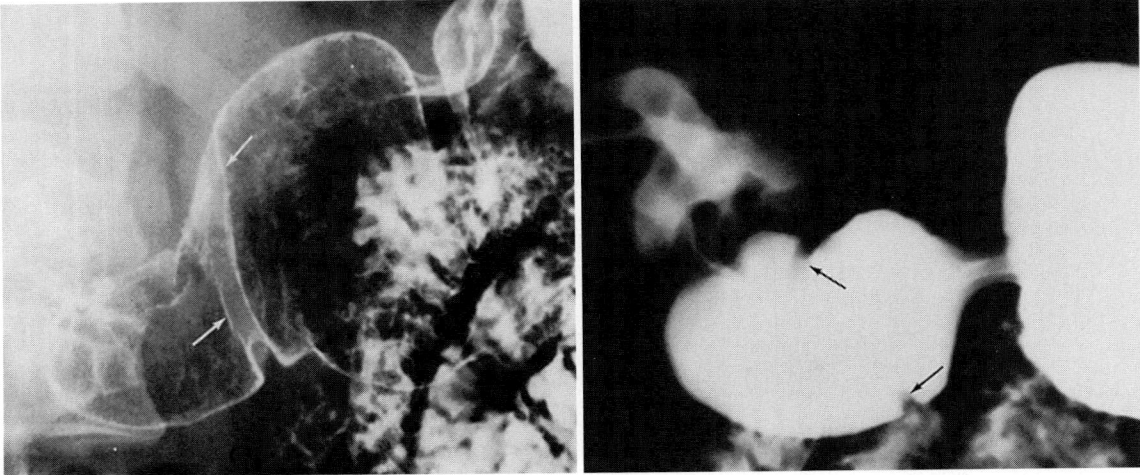

Figure 11–104. Functional and transient peristaltic events of the gastric antrum should not be mistaken for mucosal diaphragms. (Ref: Ghahremani GG: Nonobstructive mucosal diaphragms or rings of the gastric antrum in adults. *Am J Roentgenol* 121:236, 1974.)

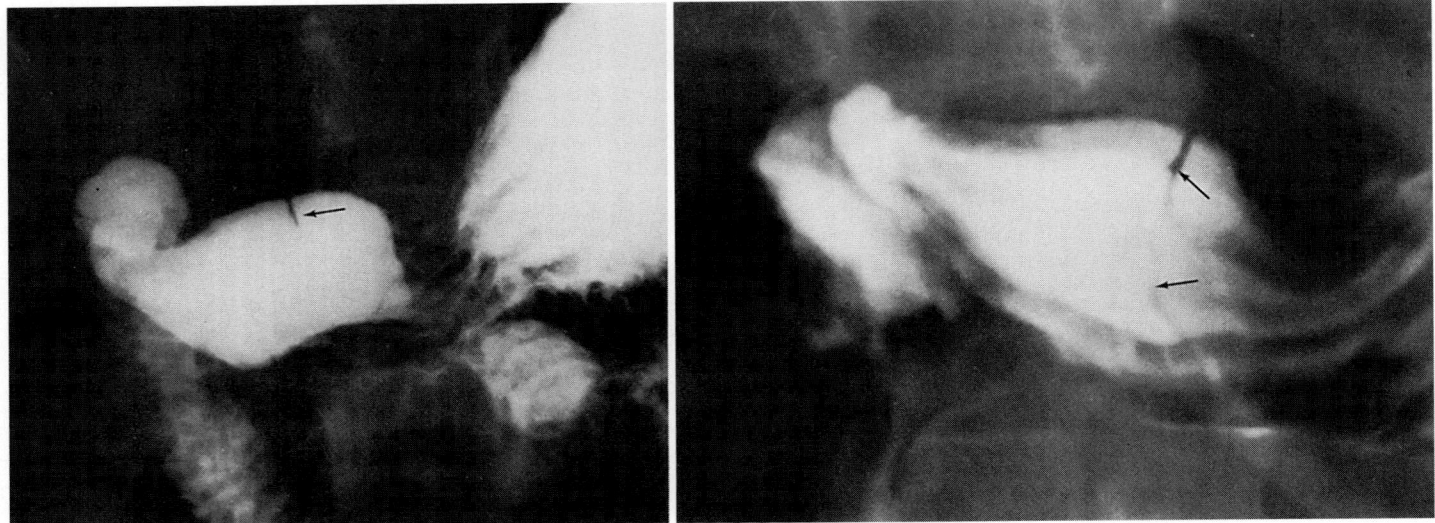

Figure 11–105. Additional examples of simulated antral diaphragms. This entity may be particularly confusing in infants. (Ref: Fujioka M et al: Pseudoweb of the gastric antrum in infants. *Pediatr Radiol* 9:73, 1980.)

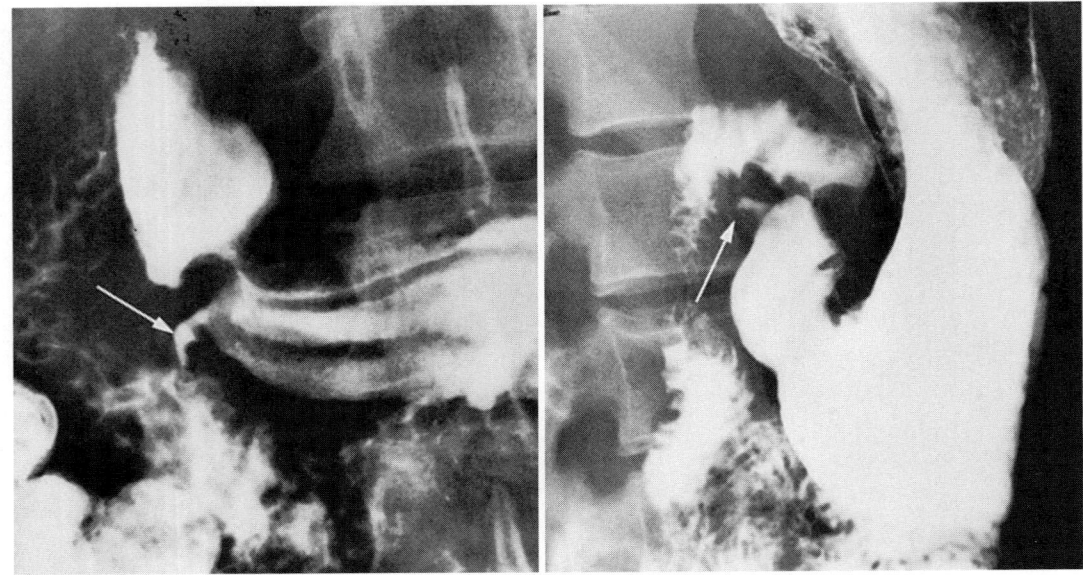

Figure 11–106. Partial gastric diverticulum that could be mistaken for a penetrating ulcer. (Ref: Treichel J et al: Diagnosis of partial gastric diverticula. *Radiology* 119:13, 1976.)

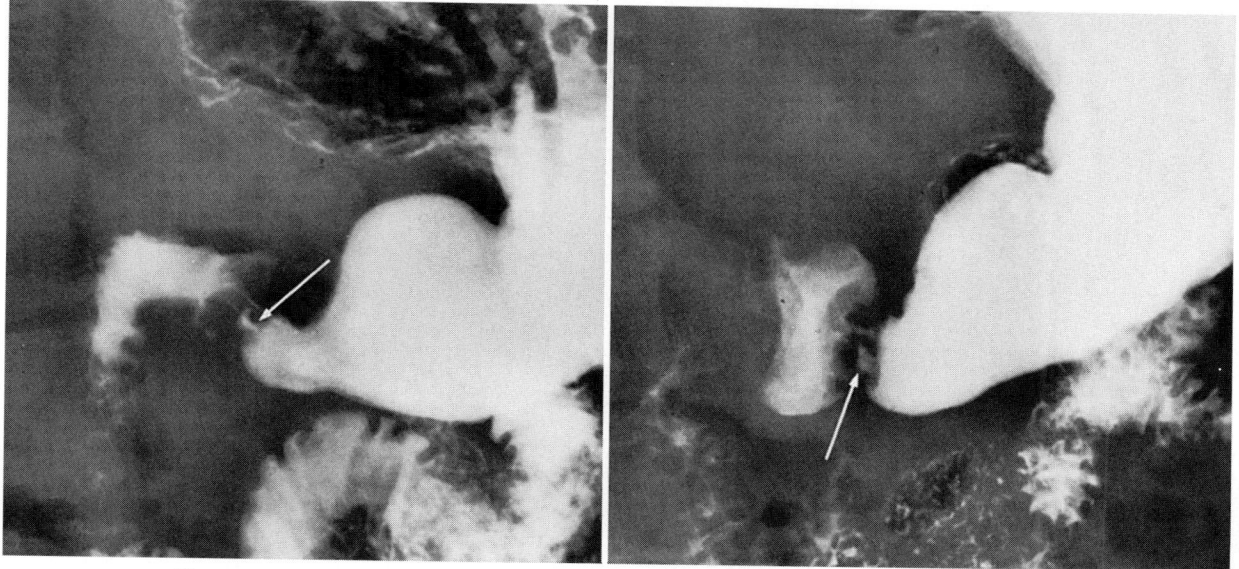

Figure 11–107. Additional example of a partial gastric diverticulum.

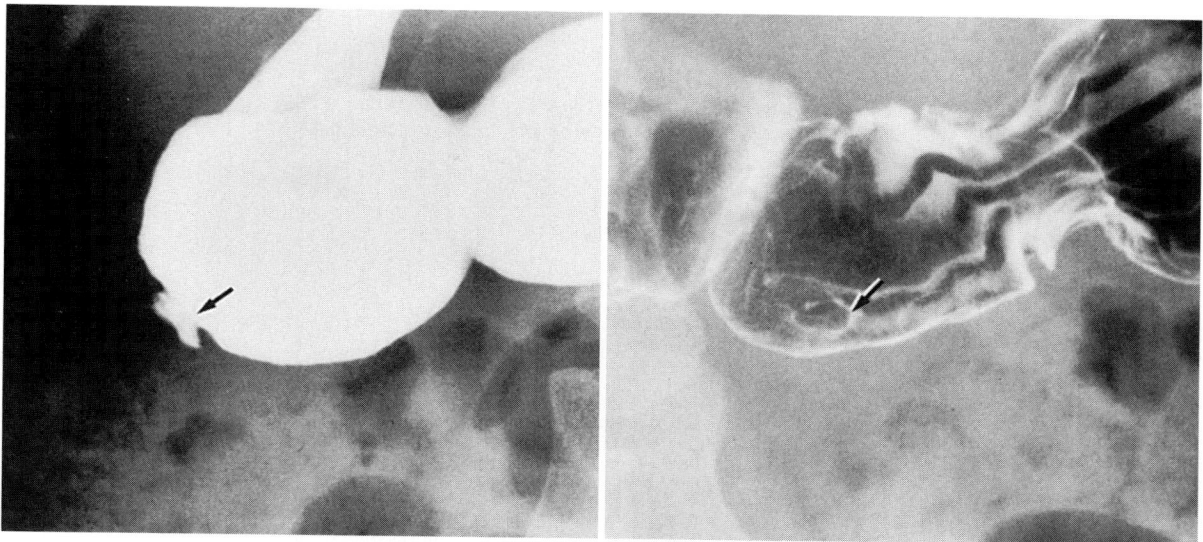

Figure 11–108. Additional example of a partial gastric diverticulum.

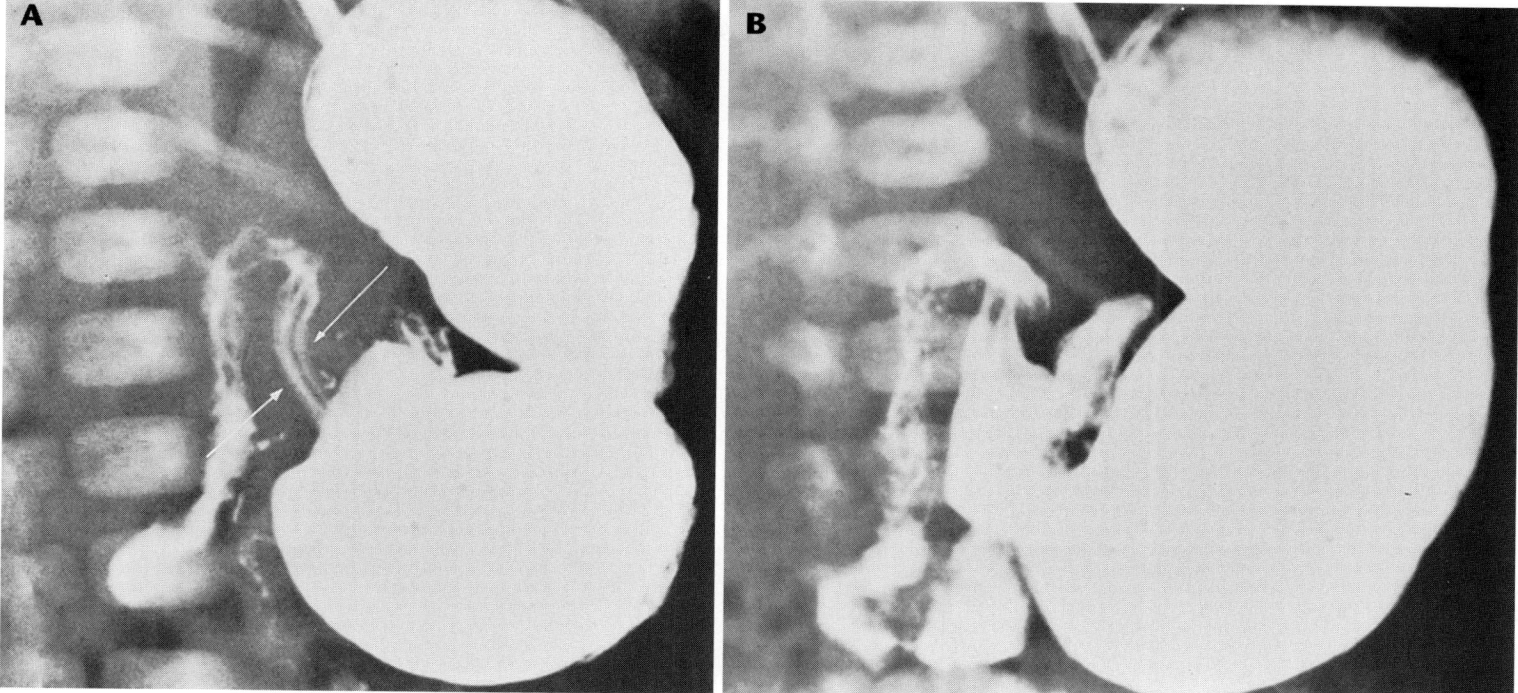

Figure 11–109. A, Transient antral spasm may simulate hypertrophic pyloric stenosis. **B,** Film made later in same session shows an absence of antral narrowing.

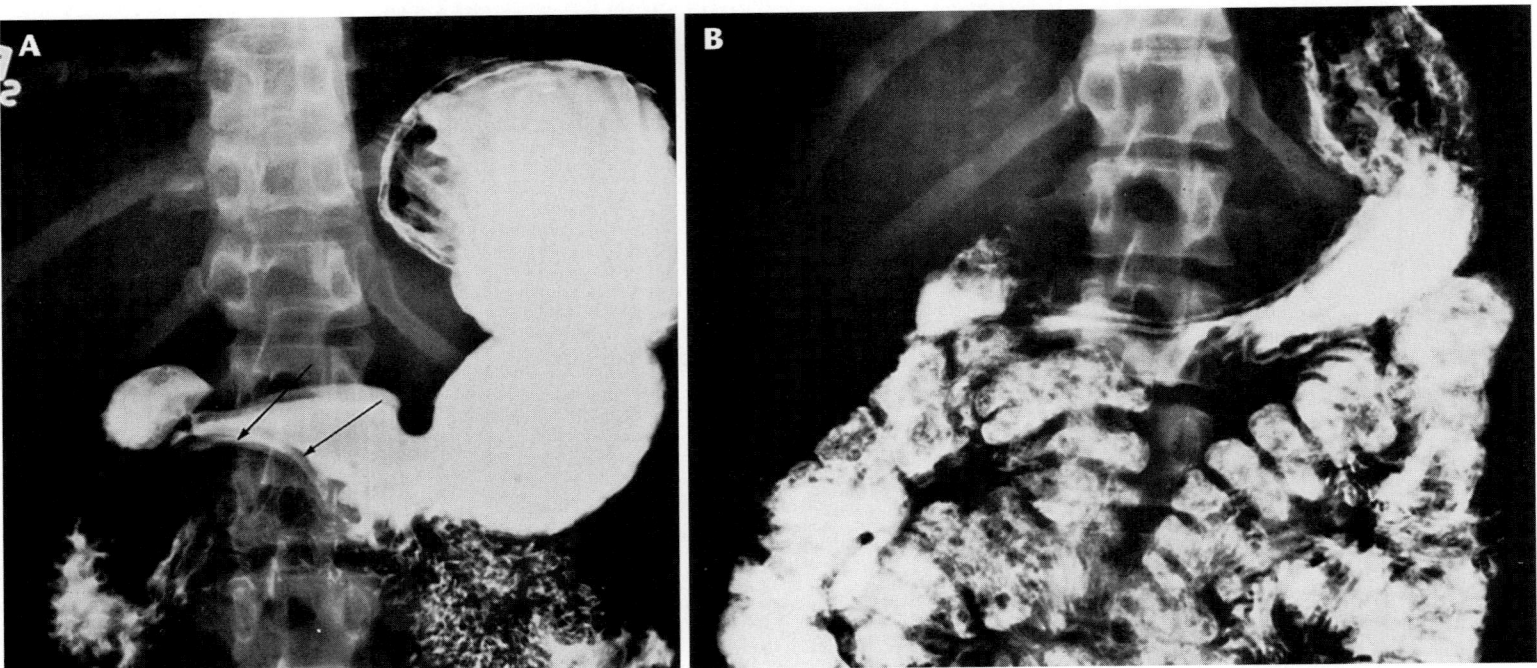

Figure 11–110. A, Impression on greater curvature of the stomach, which simulates pancreatic enlargement. **B,** Impression on the stomach is produced by the filled colon.

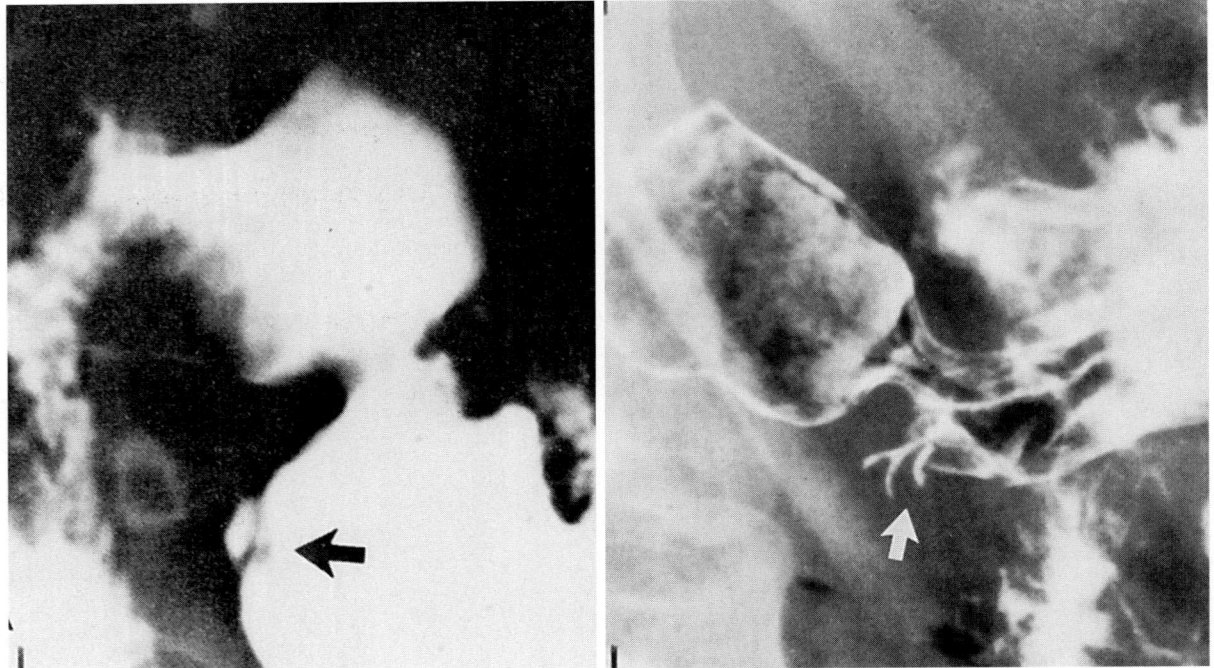

Figure 11–111. *Left,* Aberrant pancreas in the antrum. *Right,* Aberrant pancreas in the same position showing branching ductal pattern. (From Stone DD et al: An unusual case of aberrant pancreas in the stomach. *Am J Roentgenol* 113:125, 1971.)

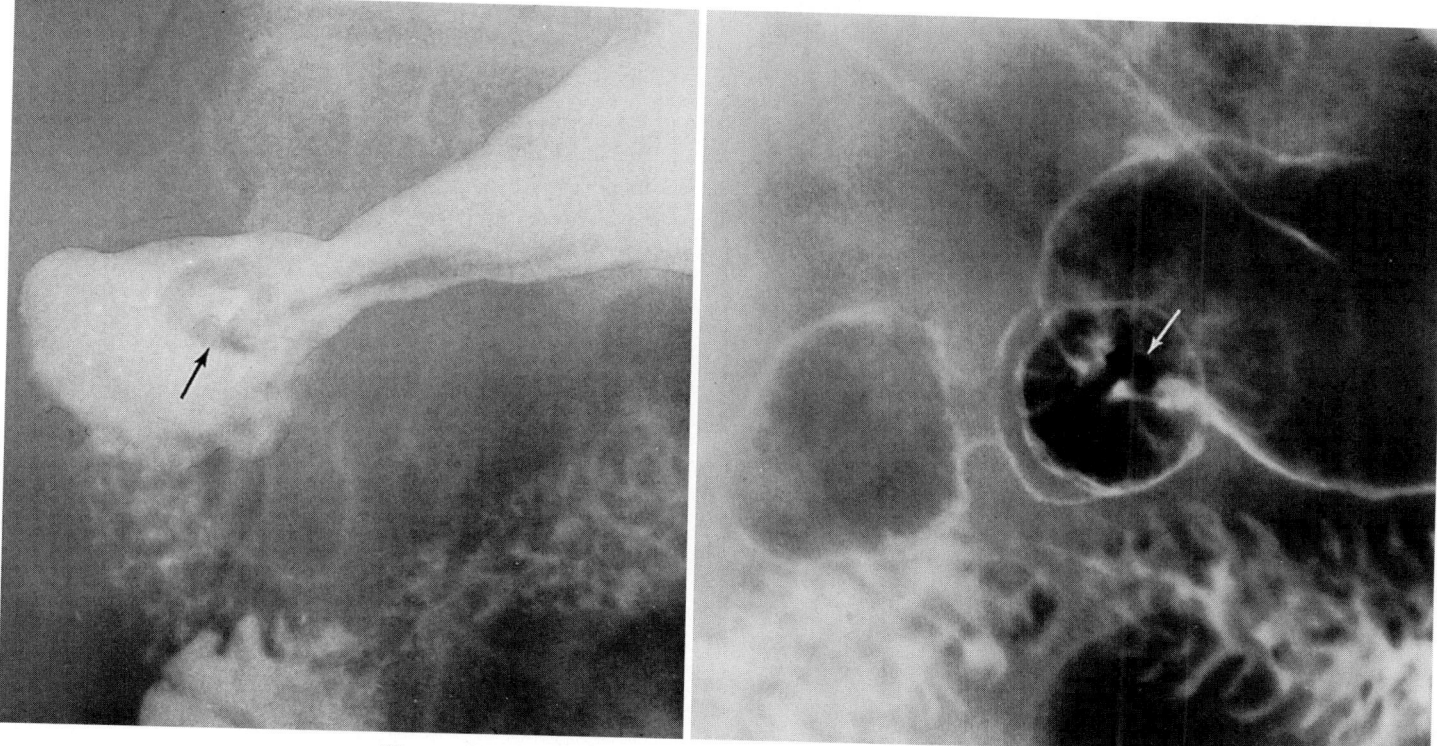

Figure 11–112. Pyloric canal seen en face, simulating an ulcer.

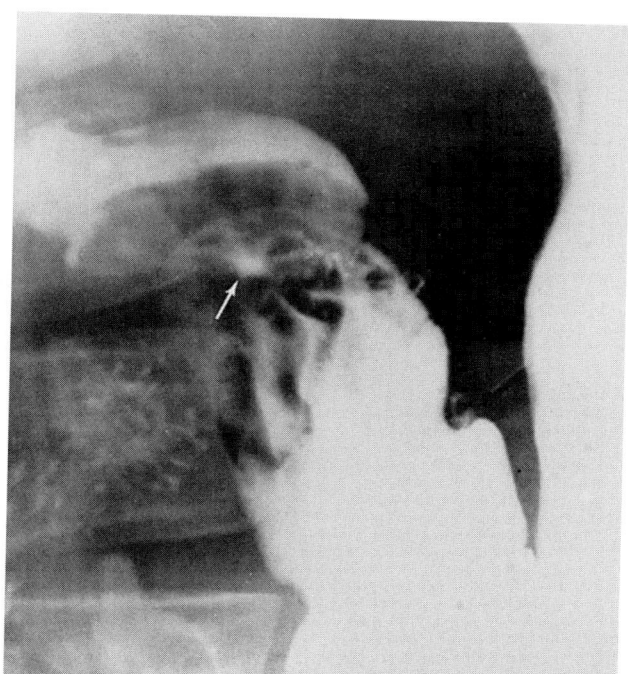

Figure 11–113. Additional example of the pyloric canal ("pyloric star") seen on end, simulating an ulcer.

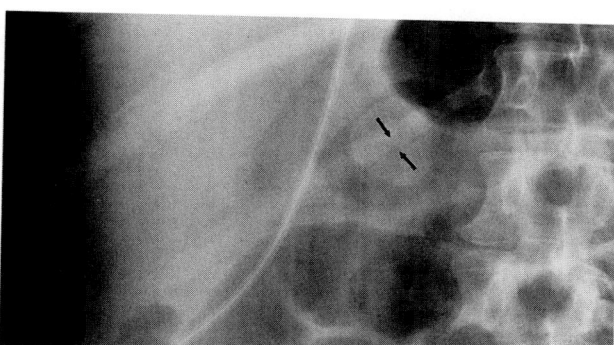

Figure 11–114. Pyloric star seen through the fluid-filled antrum (see Figs. 11–112 and 11–113).

The Duodenum

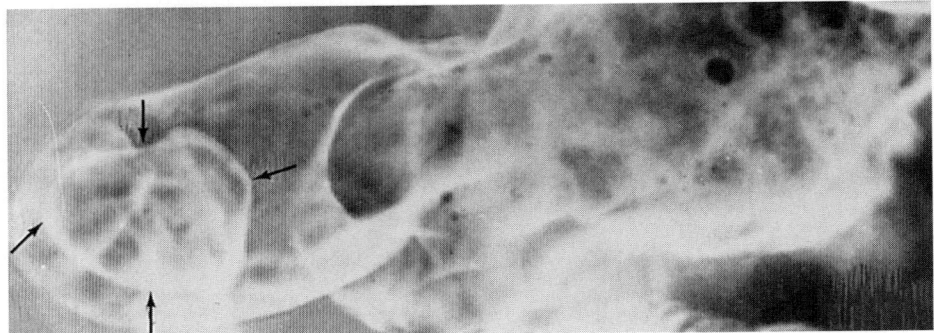

Figure 11–115. Air-filled duodenal bulb projected on the gastric antrum, simulating a polyp. Also note the air bubbles in the stomach, which might be mistaken for polyps.

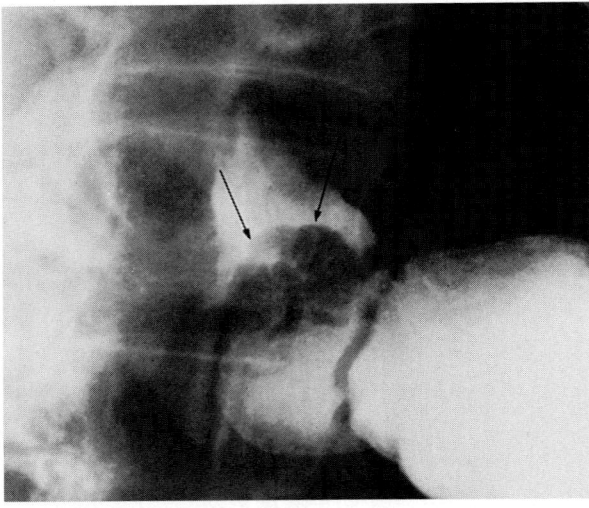

Figure 11–116. Prolapse of the antral mucosa into the base of the duodenal bulb. This entity is not usually of clinical significance.

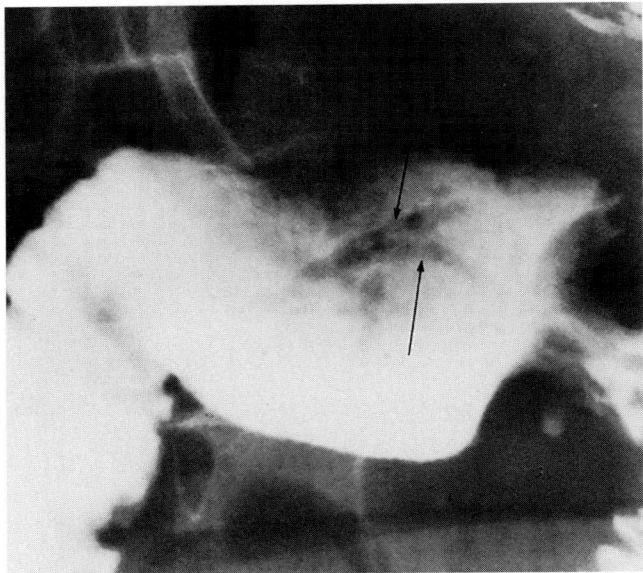

Figure 11–117. Food (spaghetti) in the duodenal bulb, simulating an ascaris.

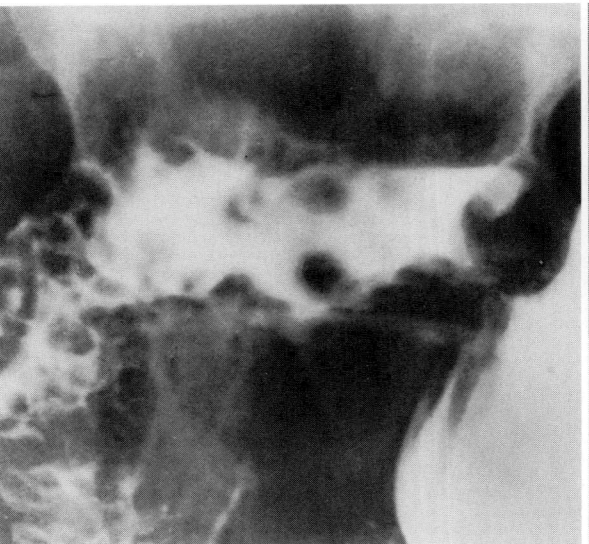
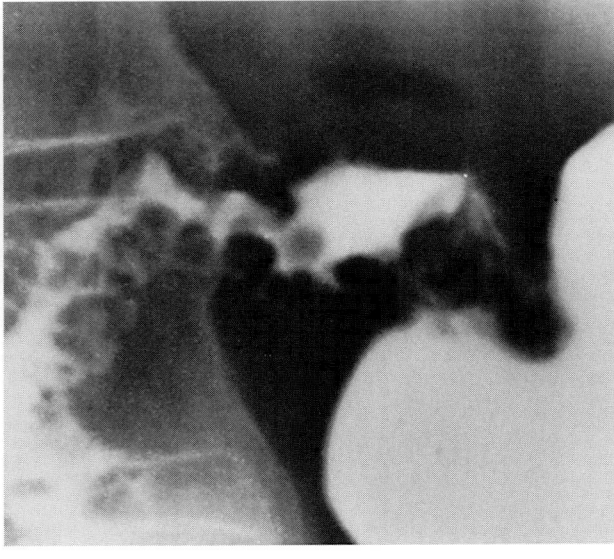

Figure 11–118. Brunner's gland hypertrophy may be seen in dyspeptic patients as well as in asymptomatic individuals and should not be mistaken for polyps. (Ref: Fraser GM et al: Coarse duodenal mucosal folds in patients with dyspepsia and a high gastric acid output. *Clin Radiol* 22:78, 1971.)

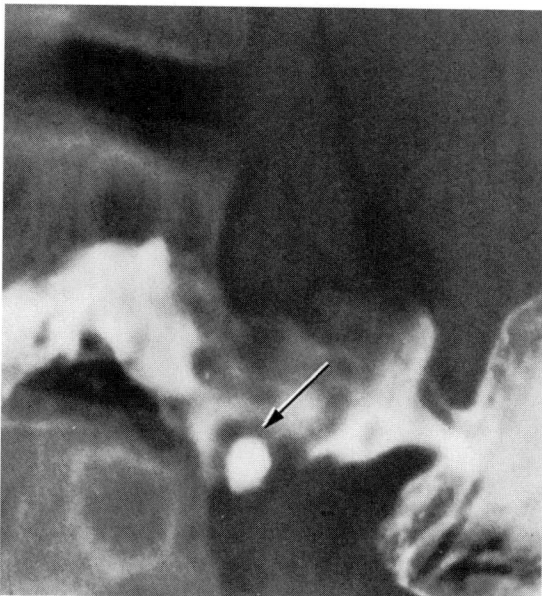

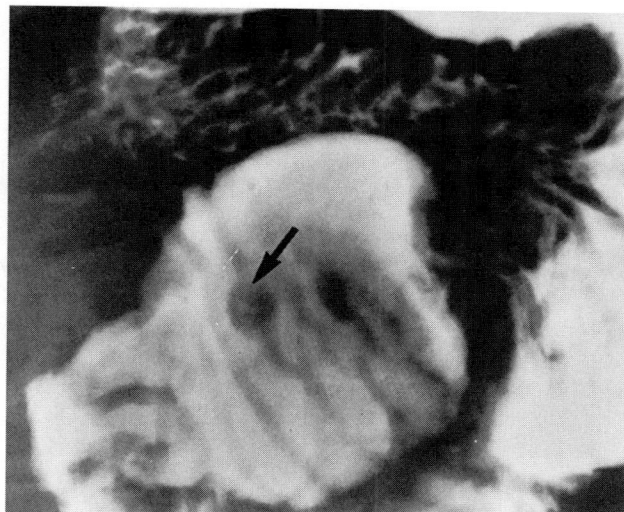

Figure 11–120. Heterotopic pancreatic rest in the duodenal bulb.

Figure 11–119. Aberrant pancreatic rest in the base of the duodenal bulb.

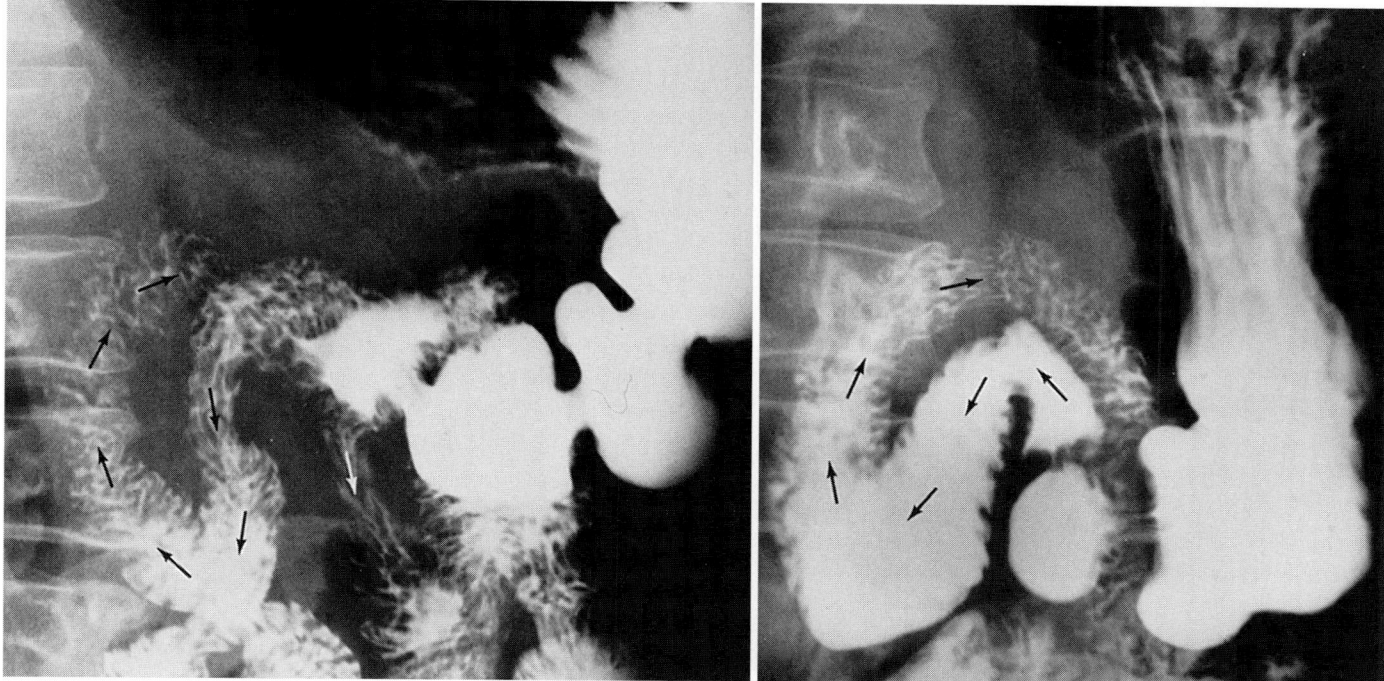

Figure 11–121. Two examples of inversion of the duodenum (duodenum inversum), a clinically unimportant variation in the course of the duodenal loop that does not connote malrotation. (Ref: Faegenburg O, Bosniak M: Duodenal anomalies in the adult. *Am J Roentgenol* 88:642, 1962.)

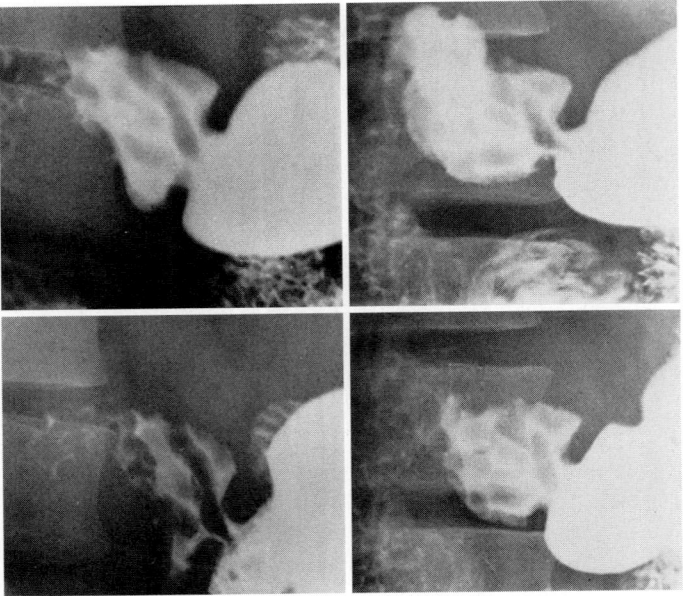

Figure 11–122. Spot films to show normal but prominent mucosal folds of the duodenal bulb. Note the pliability and changing pattern.

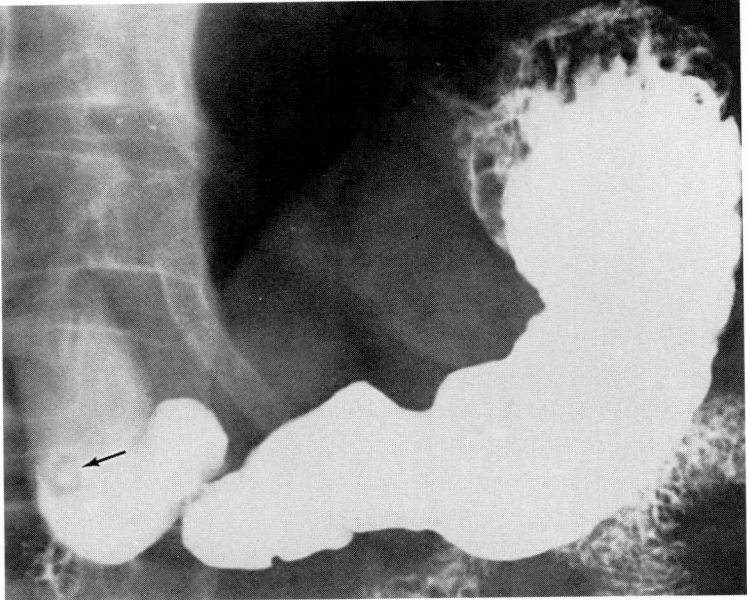

Figure 11–123. Lumen of the second portion of the duodenum seen en face, simulating an intraluminal lesion.

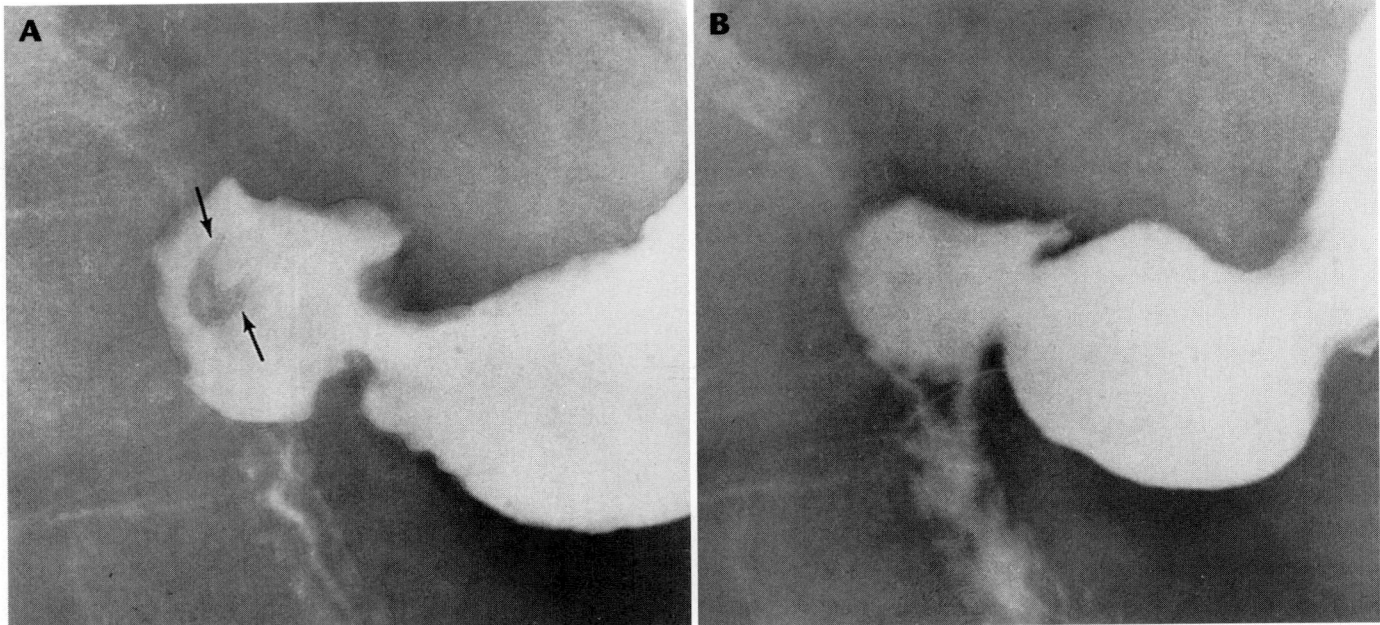

Figure 11–124. A, Lumen of the second portion of the duodenum seen on end, simulating a filling defect. **B,** Pseudolesion is not seen on subsequent film.

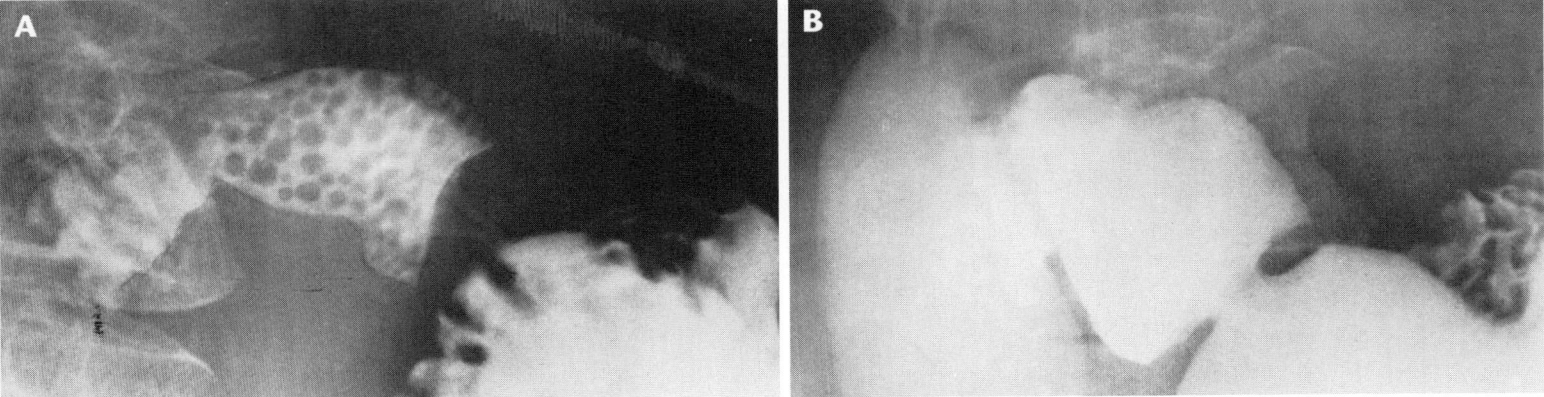

Figure 11–125. A, Air bubbles in the duodenal bulb, simulating polypoid filling defects. **B,** Normal appearance seen on repeat examination.

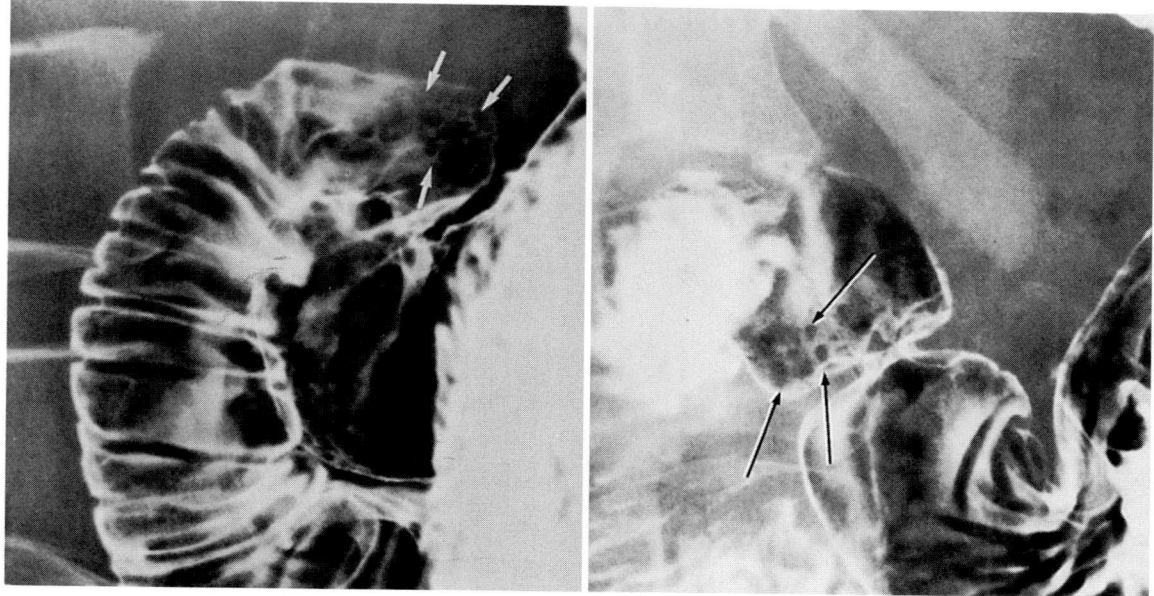

Figure 11–126. Two examples of circular mucosal filling defects said to be due to ectopic gastric mucosa. (Ref: Smithuis RHM, Vos CG: Heterotopic gastric mucosa in the duodenal bulb: Relationship to peptic ulcer. *AJR Am J Roentgenol* 152:59, 1989.) Benign lymphoid hyperplasia may also produce similar filling defects. (Ref: Govoni AF: Benign lymphoid hyperplasia of the duodenal bulb. *Gastrointest Radiol* 1:267, 1976.)

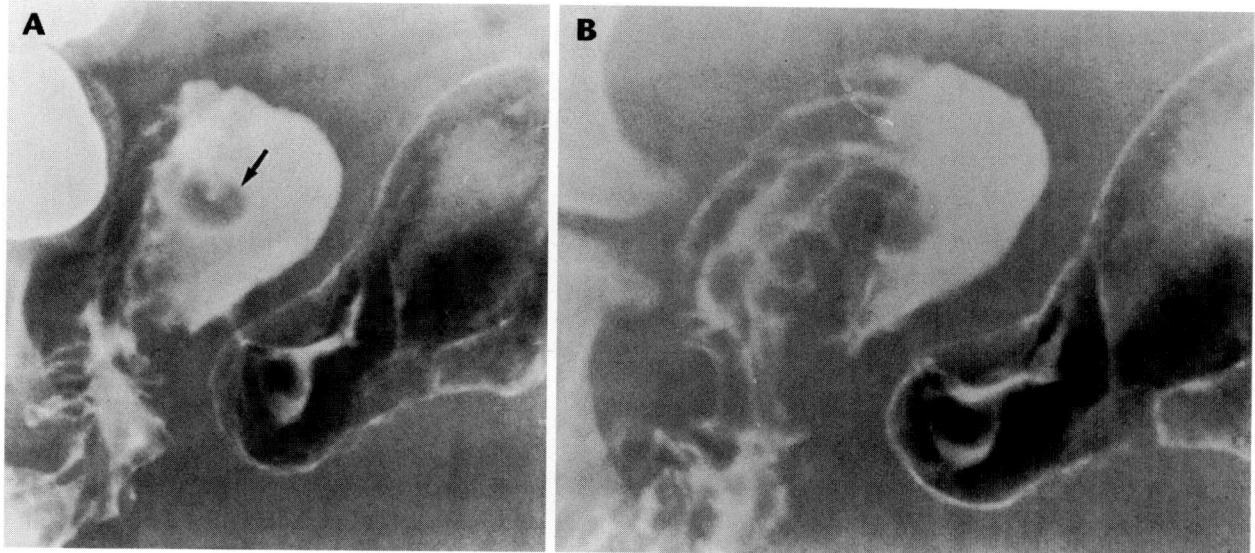

Figure 11–127. A, Simulated "bull's-eye" lesion in the duodenum in a patient with melanoma originally diagnosed as a metastatic deposit. This is produced by the lumen of the second portion of the duodenum, not seen in **B**.

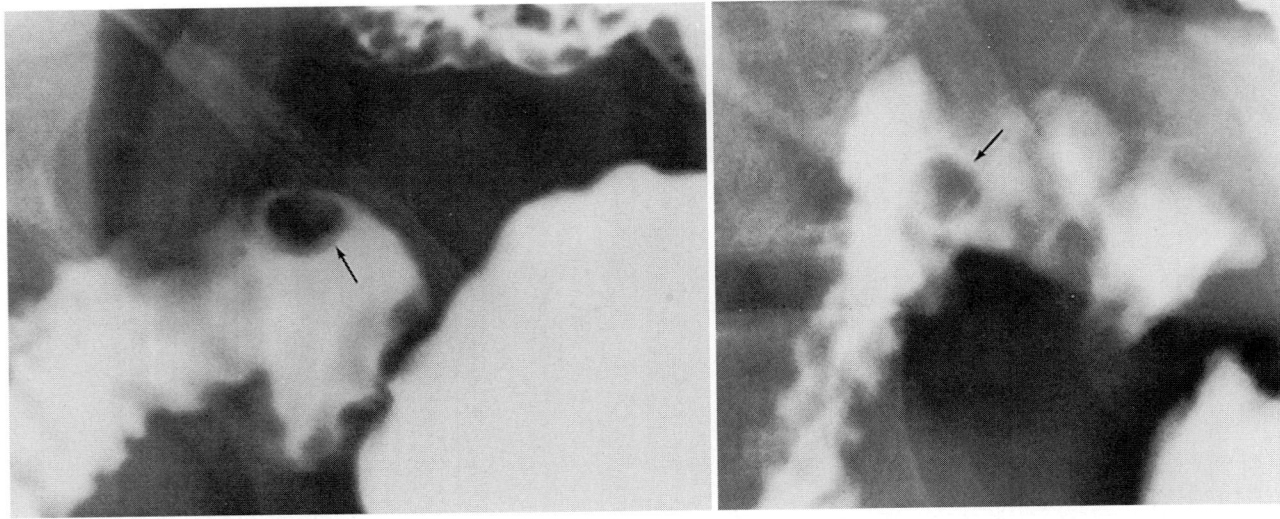

Figure 11–128. Other examples of air bubbles in the duodenal bulb simulating filling defects.

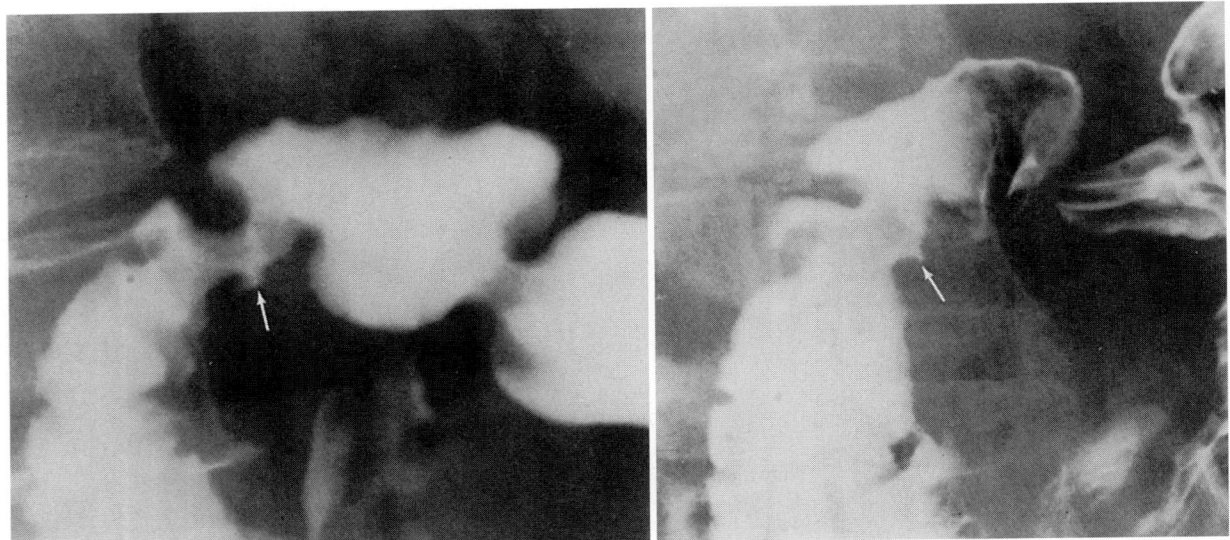

Figure 11–129. Simulated ulcer at the apex of the bulb produced by peristaltic contraction. (Ref: Burrell M, Toffler R: Flexural pseudolesions of the duodenum. *Radiology* 120:313, 1976.)

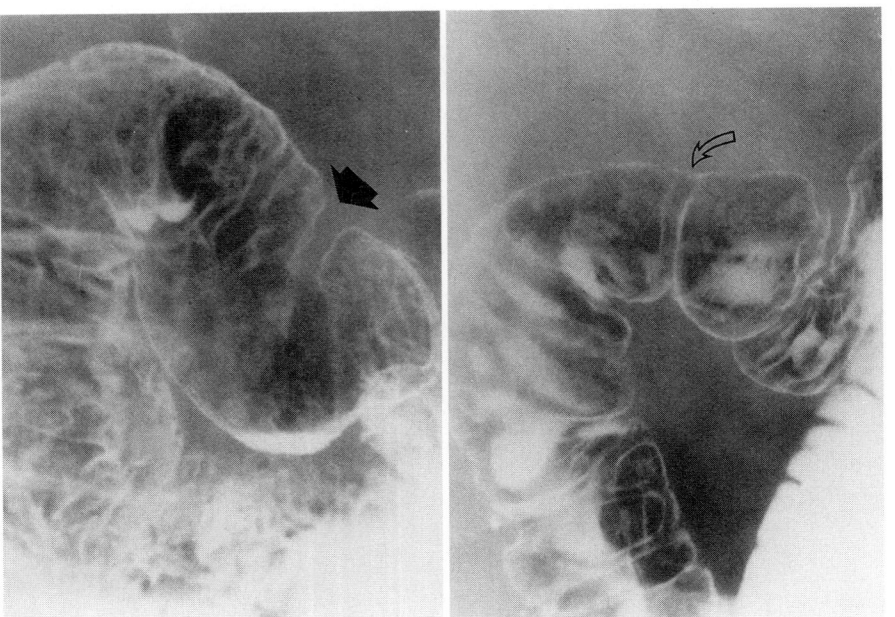

Figure 11–130. Two examples of anomalous peritoneal folds of the duodenum. This fold results in a characteristic smooth, extrinsic indentation upon the anterosuperior surface of the duodenal bulb. (From Low VHS et al: Anomalous peritoneal folds of the duodenum: A normal variant simulating disease. *Australas Radiol* 36:135, 1992.)

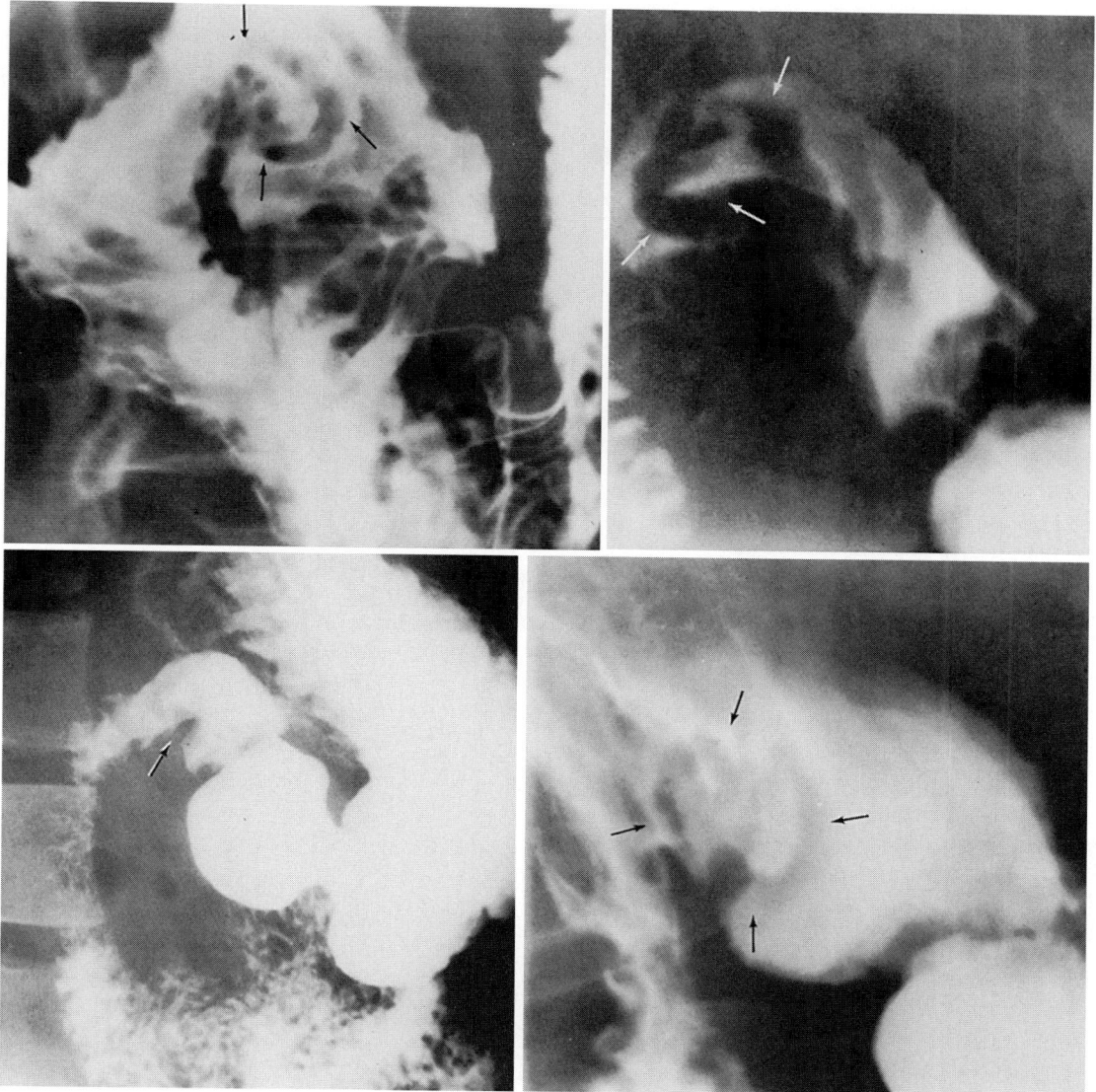

Figure 11–131. Four examples of flexural pseudomasses or ulcers at the apex of the bulb caused by the prominence of the mucosal folds. (Ref: Nelson JA et al: Duodenal pseudopolyp—the flexure fallacy. *Am J Roentgenol* 123:262, 1975.)

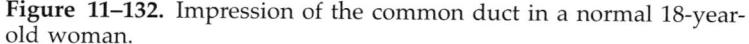

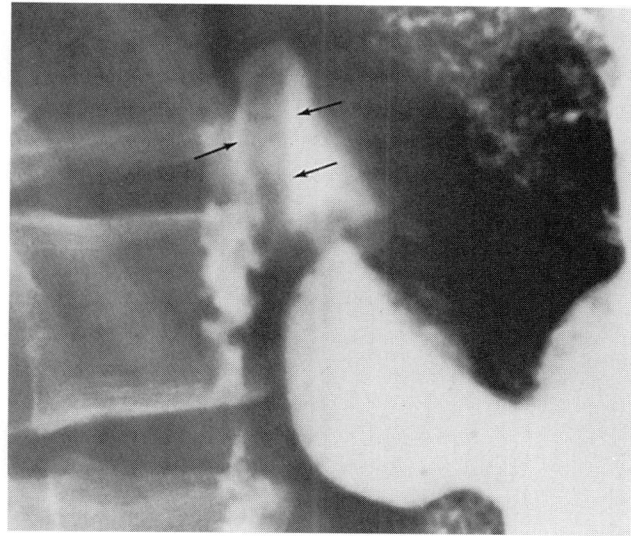

Figure 11–132. Impression of the common duct in a normal 18-year-old woman.

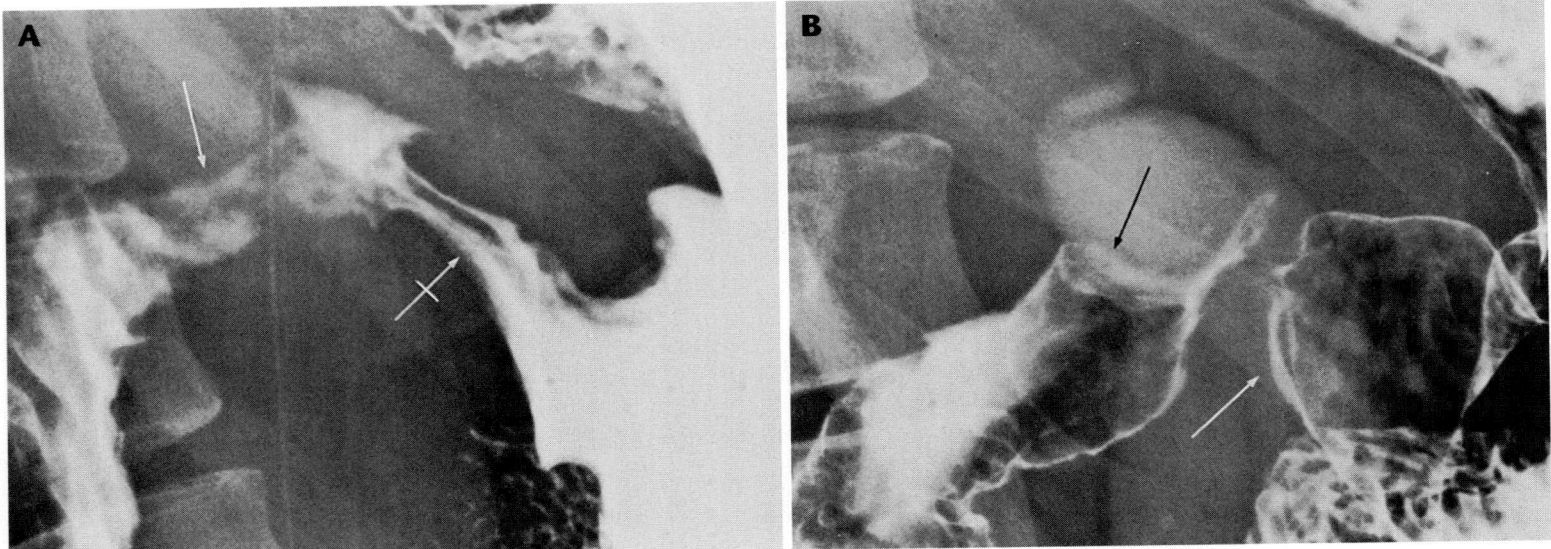

Figure 11–133. A, Impressions of the gallbladder on the superior aspect of the duodenum (←) and the antrum of the stomach (↔). **B,** Cholecystogram shows position of the gallbladder in reference to the impressions in **A.** (Ref: Smeets R, Op Den Orth JO: Gallbladder: Common cause of antral pad sign. *Am J Roentgenol* 132:571, 1979.)

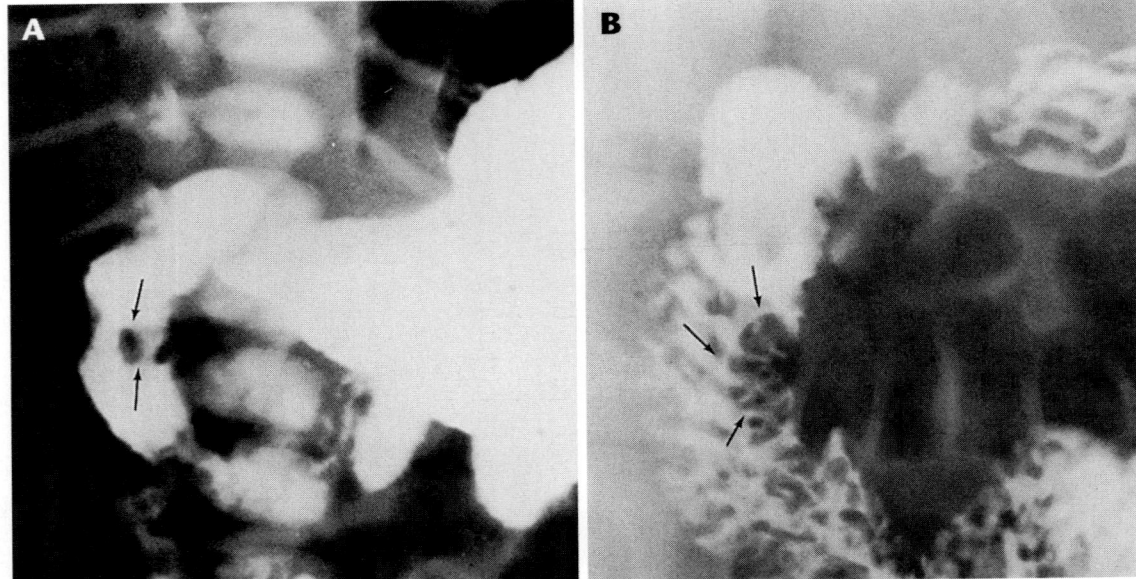

Figure 11–134. Ampula of Vater in normal subjects. **A,** 2-week-old infant. **B,** Adult.

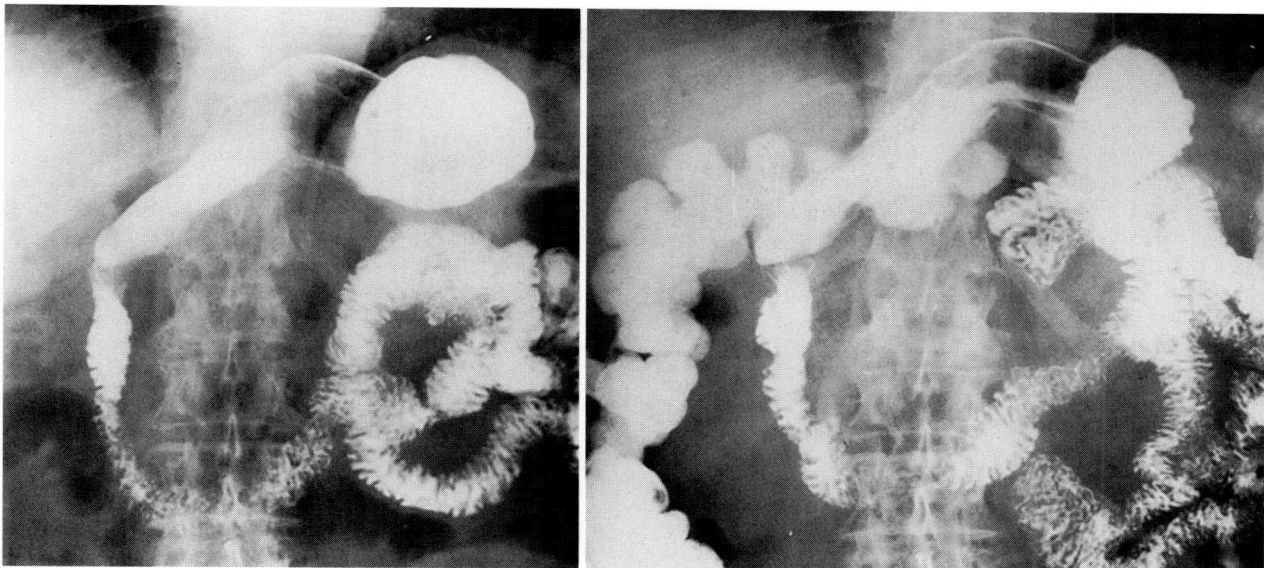

Figure 11–135. Apparent widening of the duodenal loop, produced by high position of the transverse colon, which elevates the stomach and uncovers more of the duodenal loop than is normally seen.

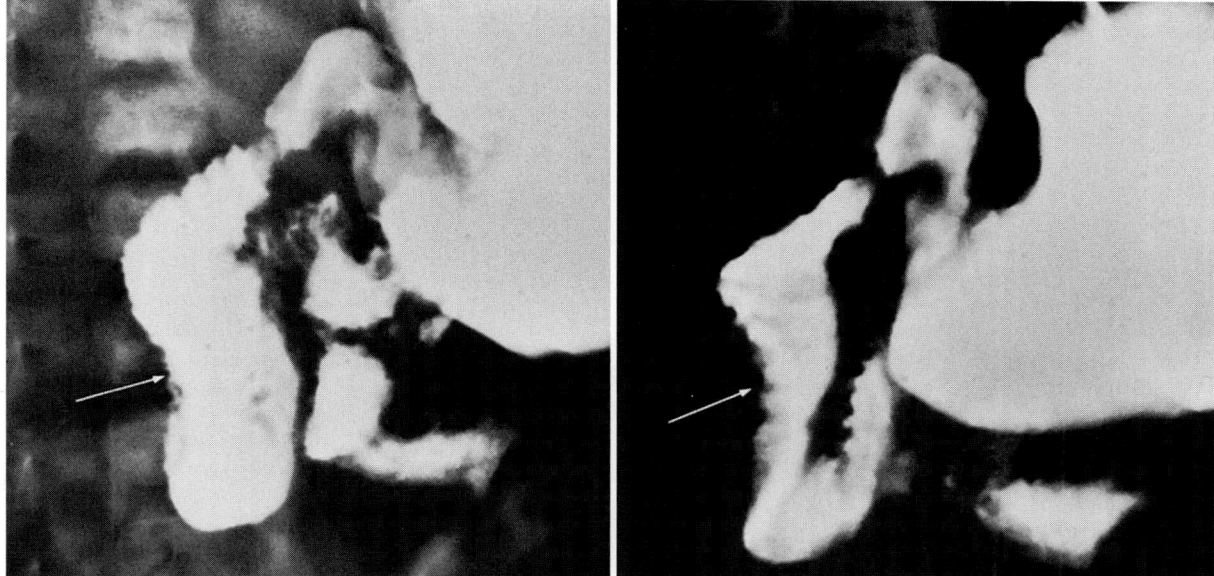

Figure 11–136. Medial displacement of the second portion of the duodenum by the right kidney. (Ref: Yoong P, House R: Deceptive deformity. *Br J Radiol* 53:1012, 1980.)

The Small Intestine

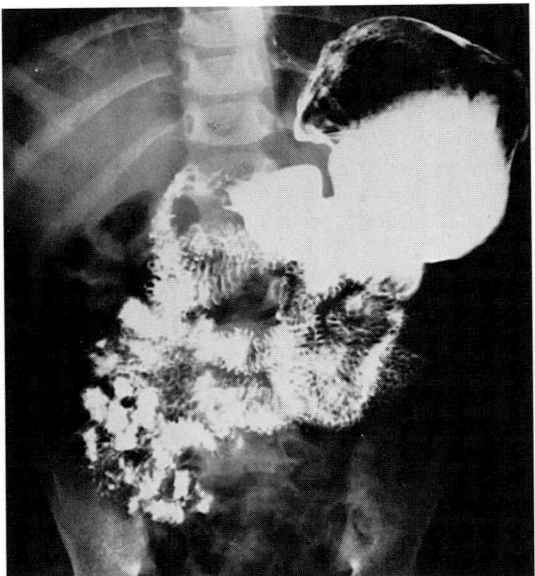

Figure 11–137. Normal prominence of the pattern of the valvulae conniventes of the small bowel in a 2-year-old boy.

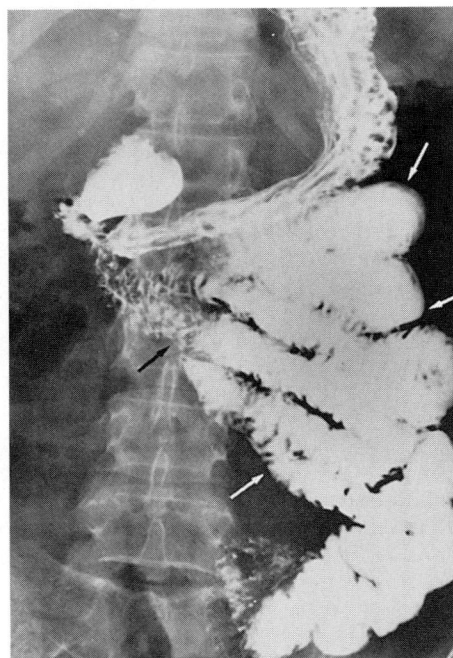

Figure 11–138. Normal grouping of the proximal loops of the jejunum of the left midabdomen, not to be confused with an internal hernia.

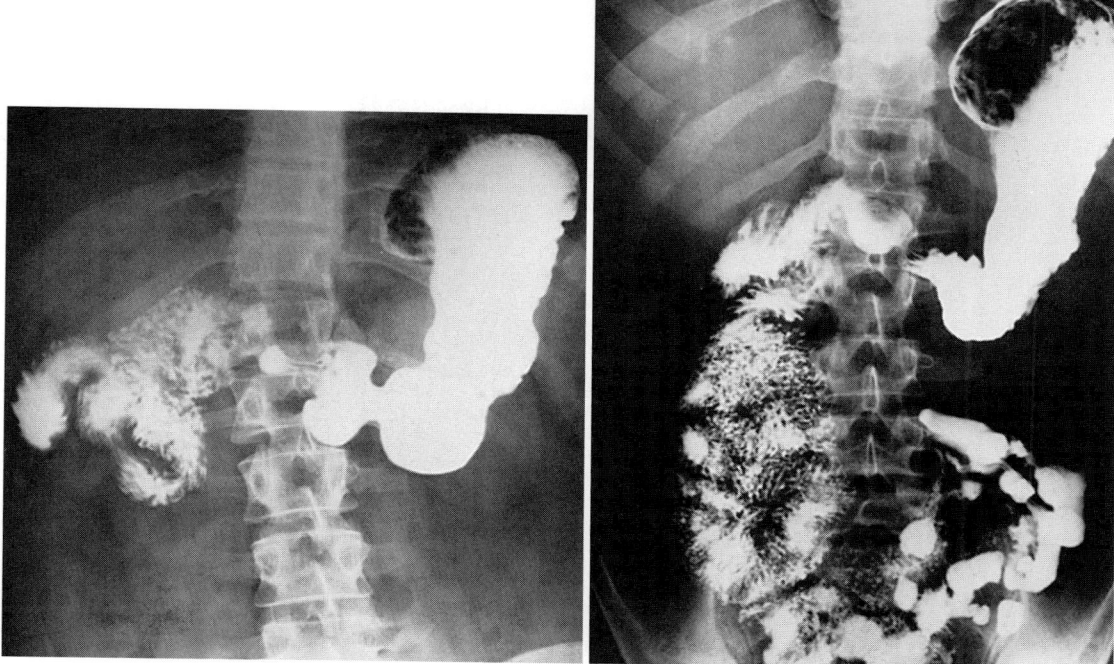

Figure 11–139. Two examples of malrotation of the bowel with ramification of the proximal small bowel on the right rather than on the left (as in Fig. 11–138).

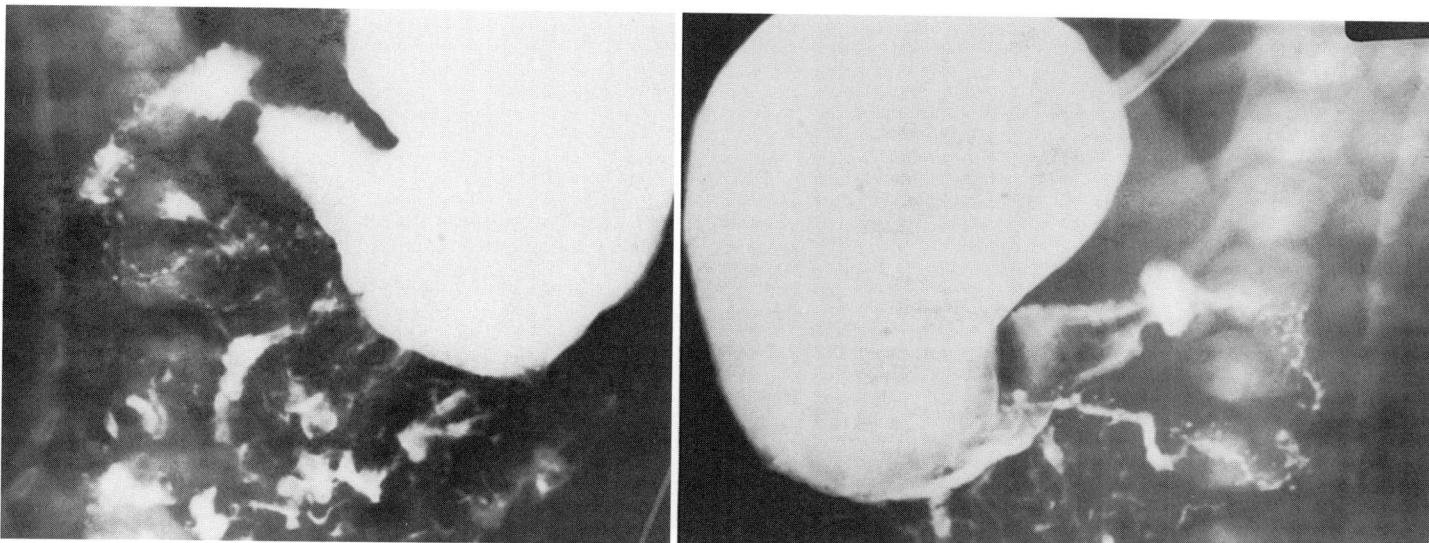

Figure 11–140. Abnormal pattern of the duodenum and proximal small bowel caused by large amount of mucus in the stomach.

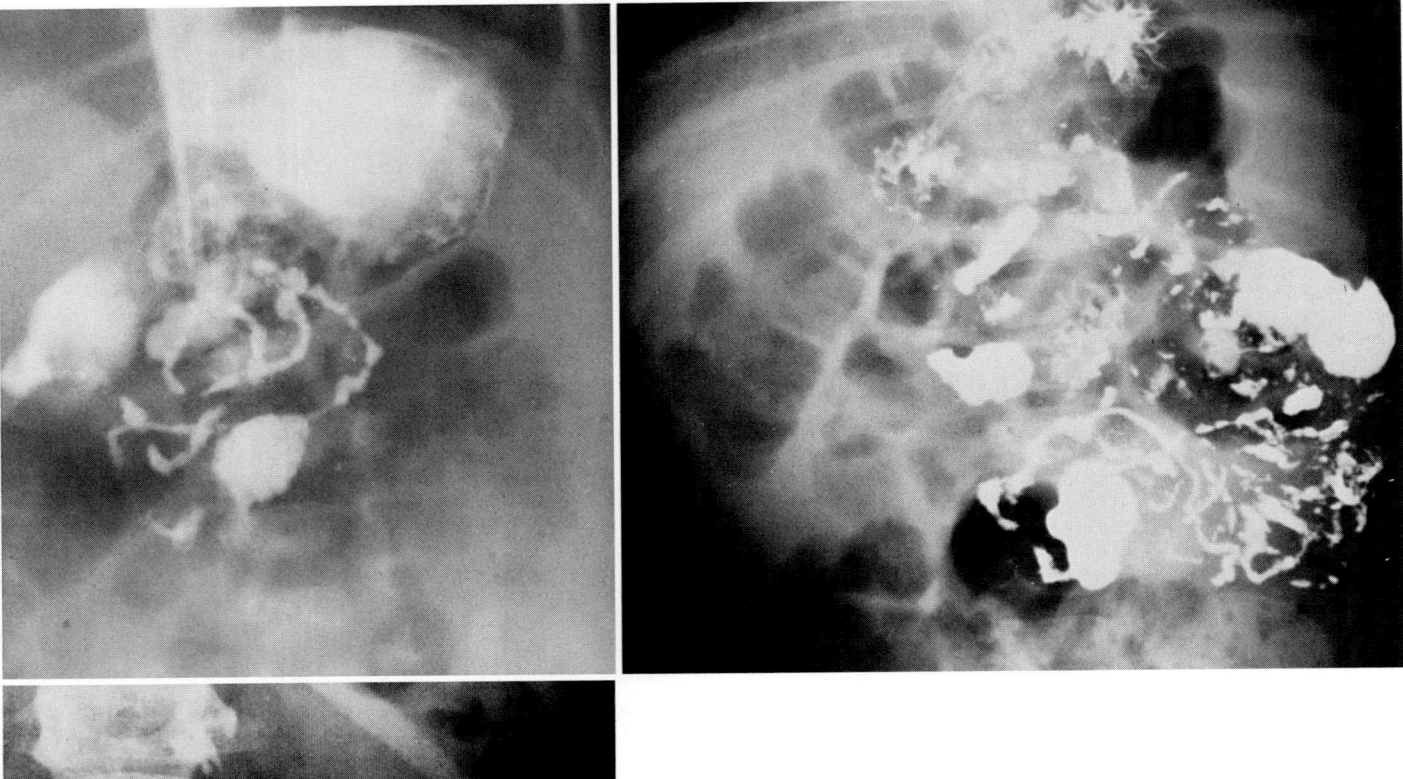

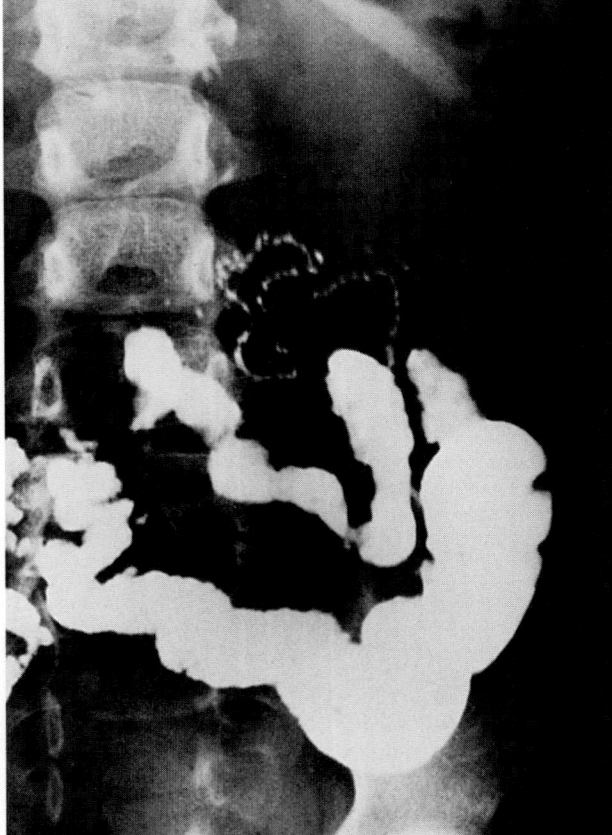

Figure 11–141. Three examples of unusual small bowel patterns in infants, caused by mucus-impregnated barium.

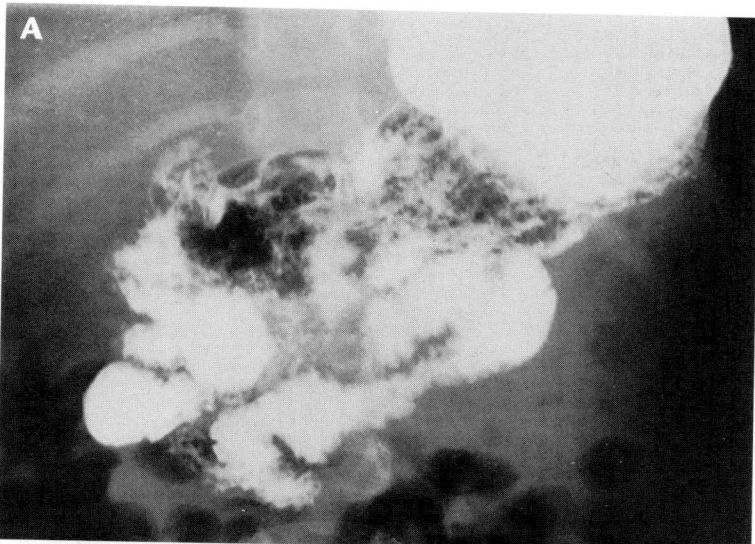

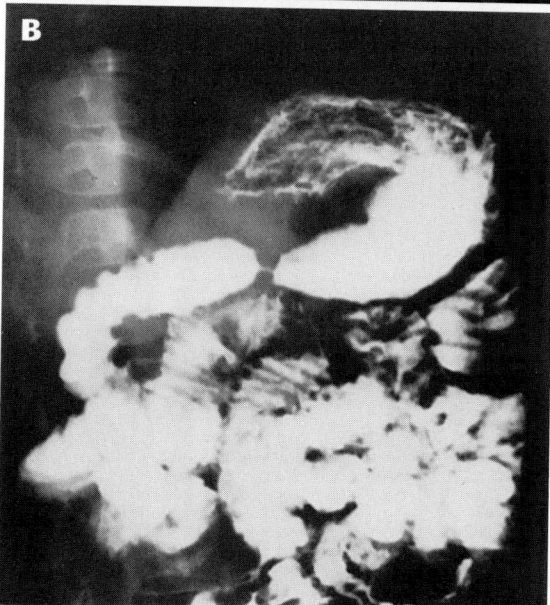

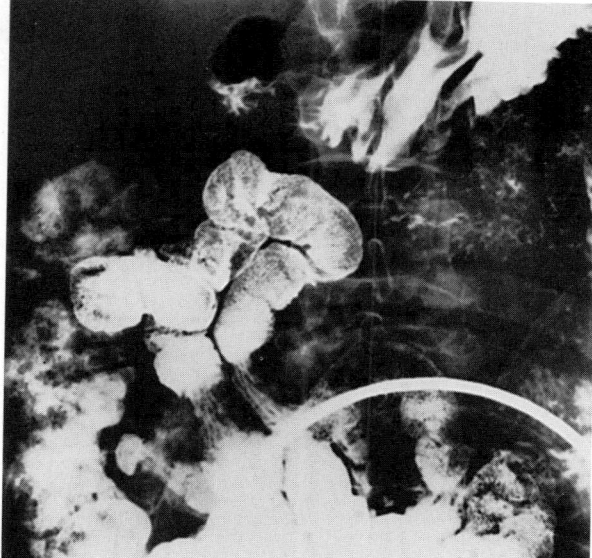

Figure 11–143. Normal mucosal pattern of the adult small bowel shown by double contrast examination.

Figure 11–142. Normal prominent mucosal patterns of the small bowel of young children. **A,** 2-year-old. **B,** 3-year-old.

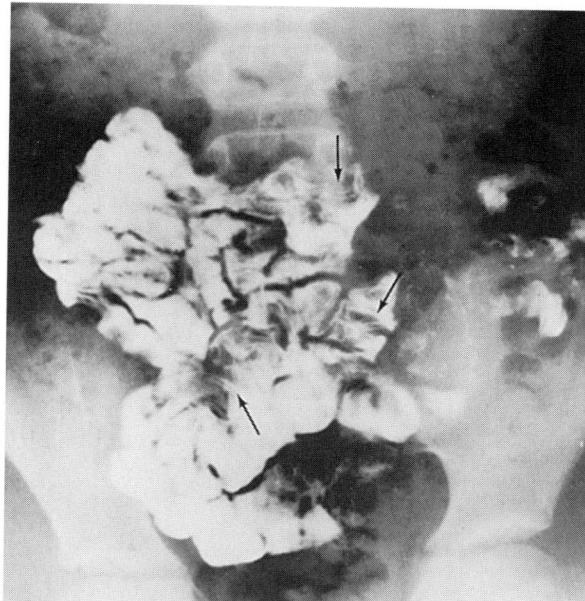

Figure 11–144. Areas of peristaltic contraction may be mistaken for ascariasis in children (see Fig. 11–149).

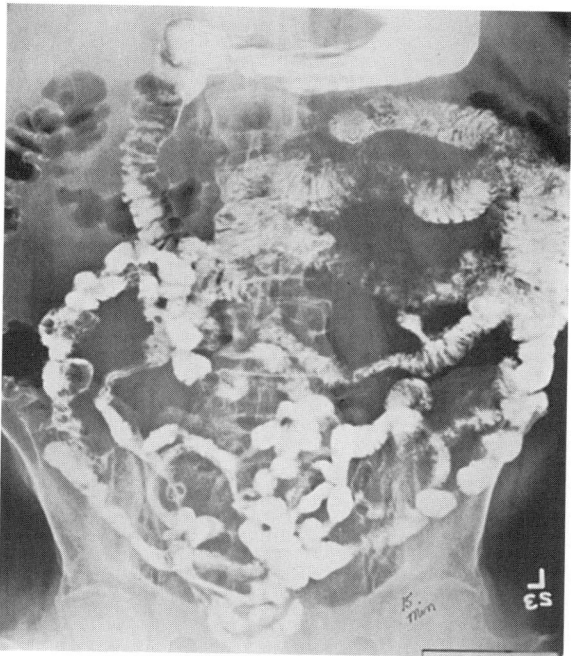

Figure 11–145. Unusual small bowel pattern resulting from a large amount of fat in the mesentery.

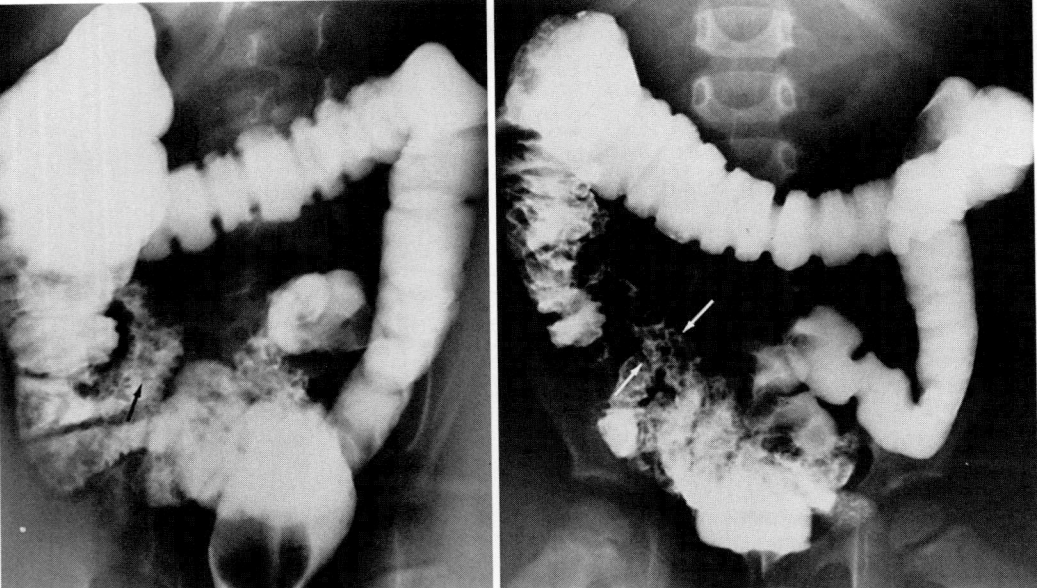

Figure 11–146. The "cobblestone" terminal ileum in a 3-year-old boy. This normal variation is due to the large amounts of lymphoid tissue in this portion of the bowel and should not be mistaken for evidence of inflammatory bowel disease. (Ref: Lassrich MA: Nonspecific changes in the terminal ileum of children. *Fortschr Roentgenstr* 95:757, 1961.)

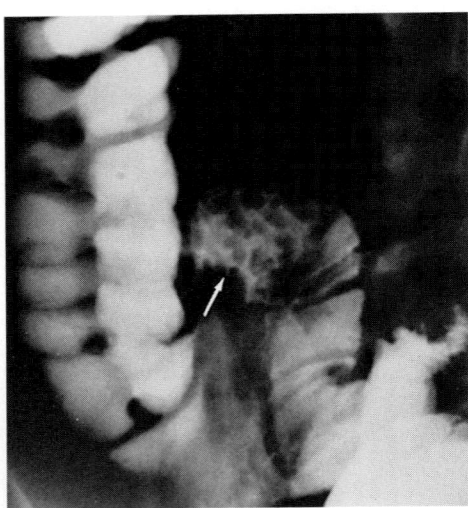

Figure 11–147. Normal lymphoid hyperplasia of the terminal ileum in a 16-year-old boy, a further reflection of the process illustrated in Figure 11–146. These changes are often misinterpreted as evidence of Crohn's disease.

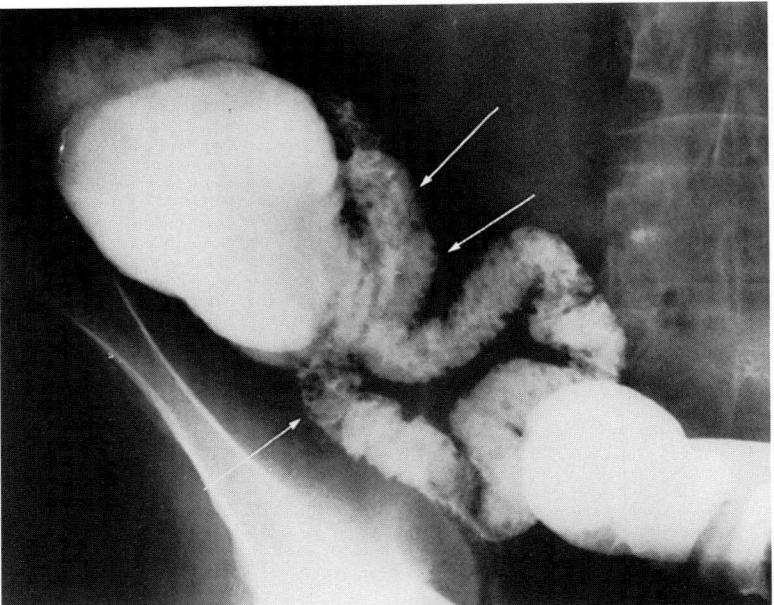

Figure 11–148. Lymphoid hyperplasia in the terminal ileum of a healthy 62-year-old man.

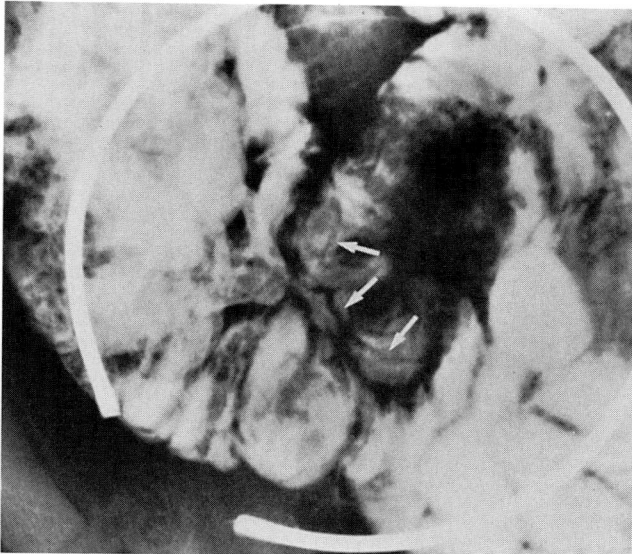

Figure 11–149. Mucosal folds in the terminal ileum, simulating ascariasis.

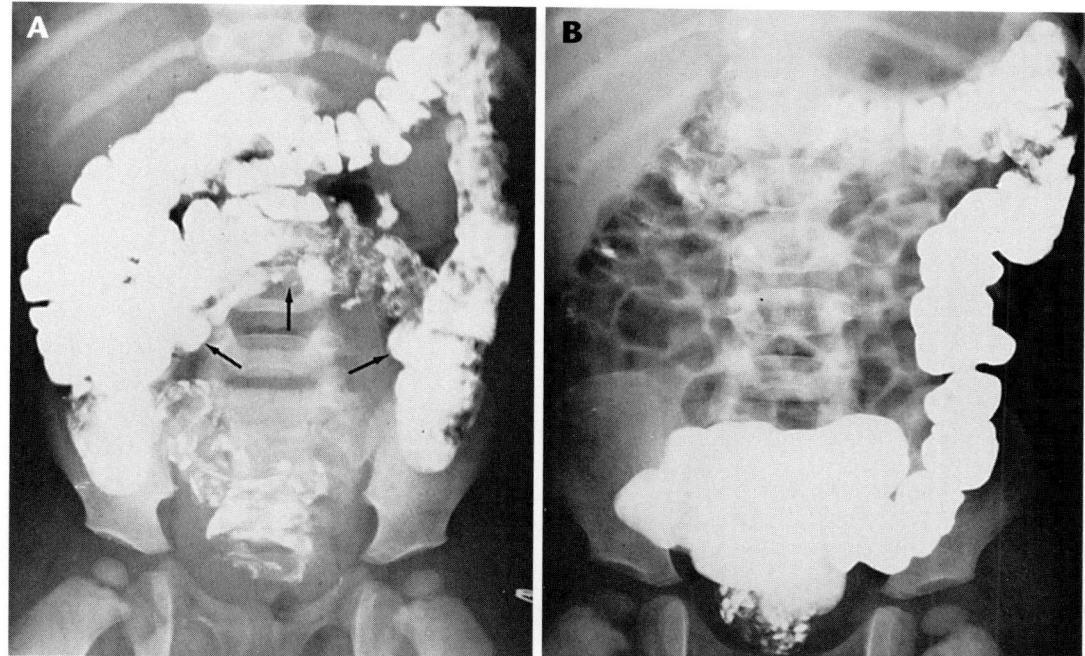

Figure 11–150. A, Distended urinary bladder in a young child, displacing the small bowel and colon. **B,** Disappearance of displacement after catheterization and removal of 300 mL of urine (see Fig. 11–157).

The Colon

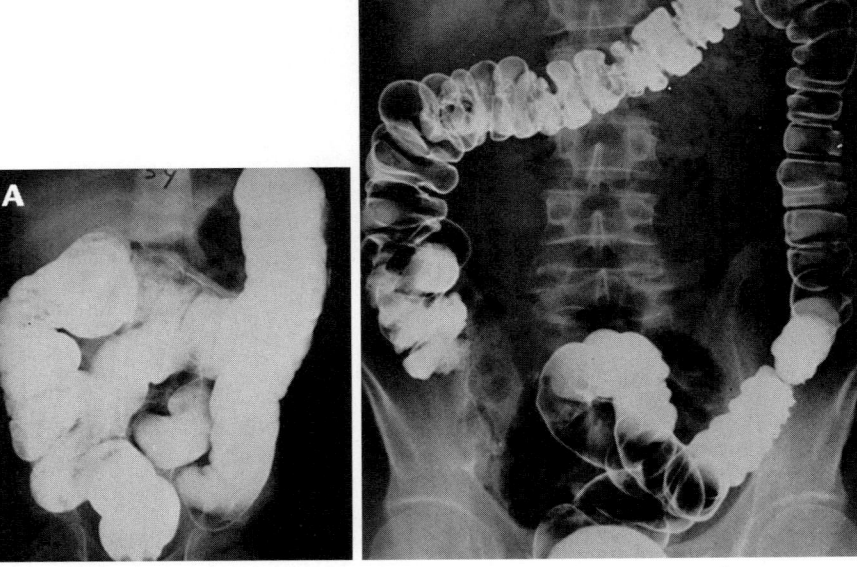

Figure 11–151. Proportional difference in the size of the colon and the abdomen in a 3-year-old child (**A**) and an adult (**B**). The colon of the infant, as well as that of the child, occupies a proportionately larger area of the abdomen, and its size should not be mistaken for megacolon. (From Keats TE: Pediatric radiology: Some potentially misleading variations from the adult. *VA Med* 93:630, 1966.)

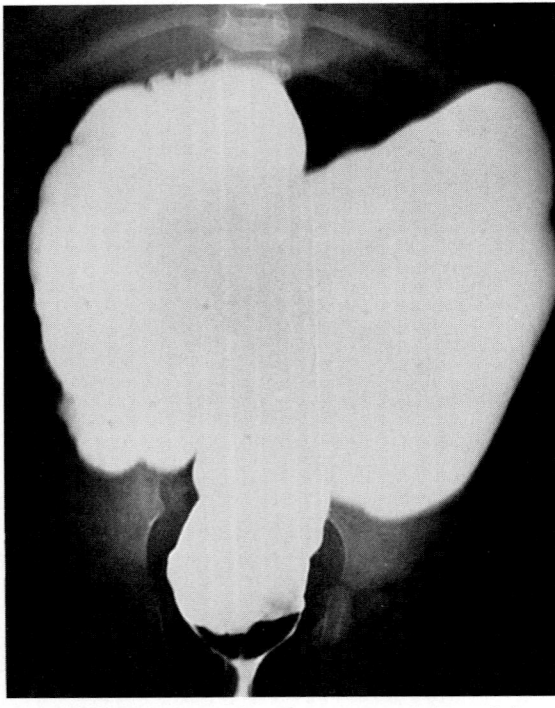

Figure 11–152. Illustration of the great distensibility of the normal juvenile colon, shown here in a 2½-year-old child.

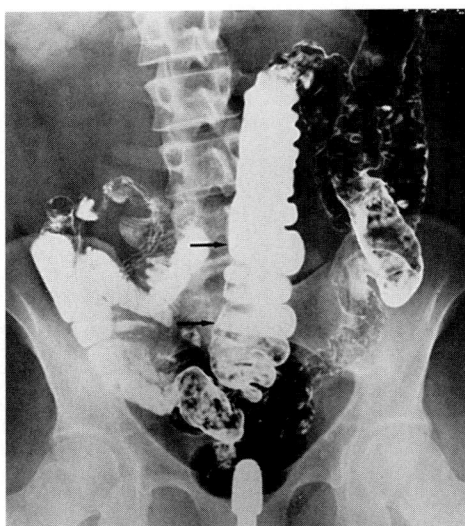

Figure 11–153. Malrotation of the bowel. The colon lies entirely in the left side of the abdomen. The *arrows* indicate the ascending colon.

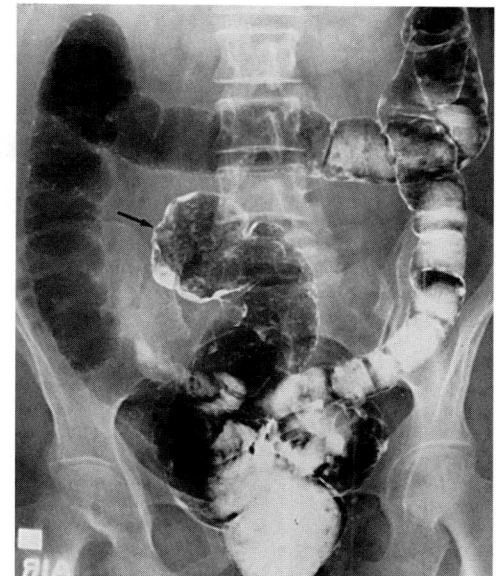

Figure 11–154. "Overrotation" of the colon, with an elongated ascending portion and the cecum presenting in the midabdomen (*arrow*).

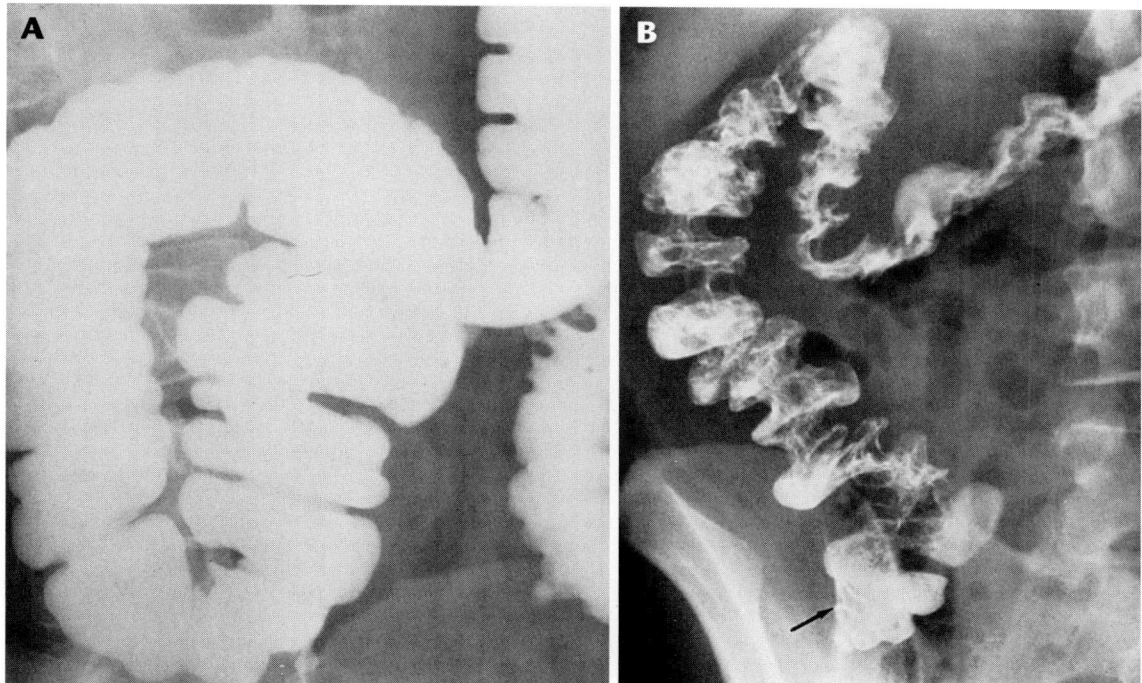

Figure 11–155. A, B, Mobile cecum. Note the change of position following evacuation (**B**). Although not clinically significant in itself, such mobility predisposes to volvulus.

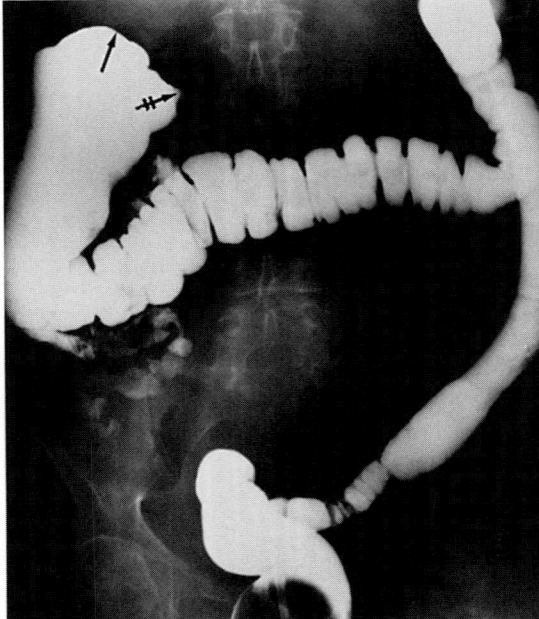

Figure 11–156. Subhepatic cecum (←) and appendix (⊪).

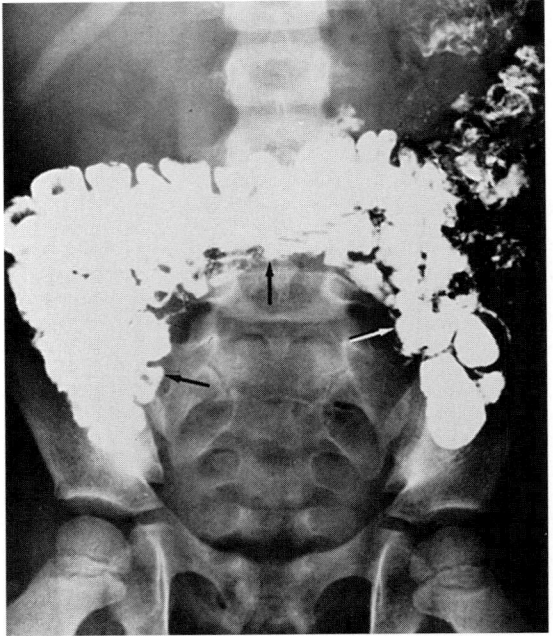

Figure 11–157. Displacement of the colon and small bowel by a distended urinary bladder in a 5-year-old boy.

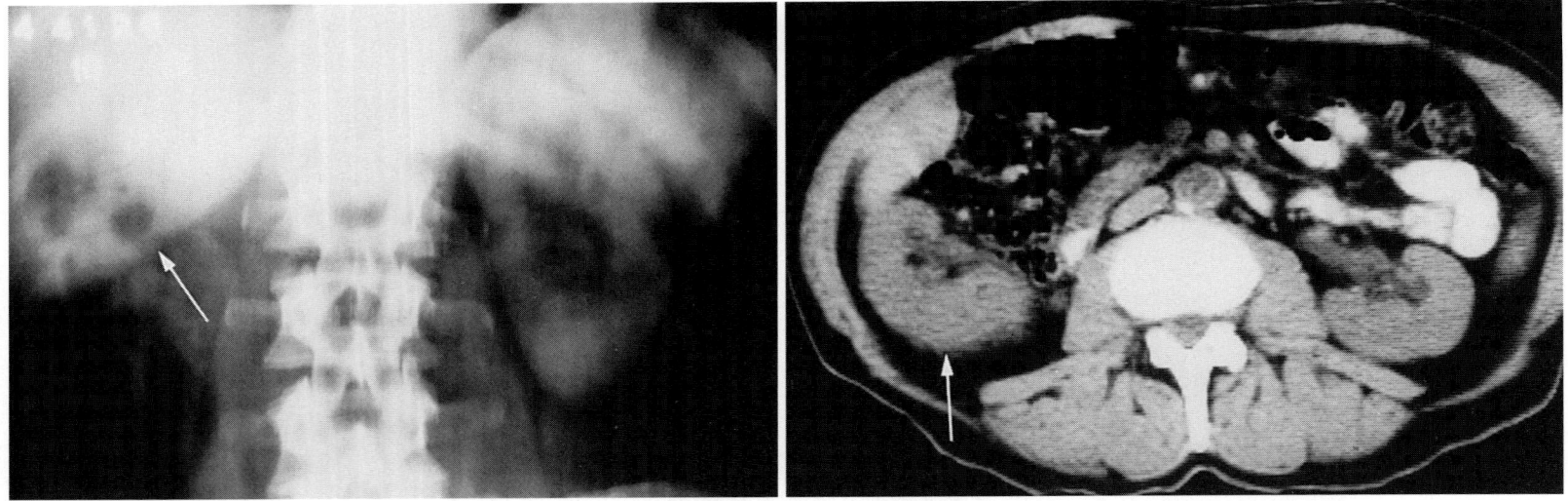

Figure 11–158. Lateral displacement of the right kidney by the colon. *Left,* Plain film tomogram from an intravenous urogram. *Right,* CT scan shows the lateral displacement of the kidney by the ascending colon. (From Silverman PM et al: Lateral displacement of the right kidney by the colon: An anatomic variation demonstrated by CT. *Am J Roentgenol* 140:313, 1983.)

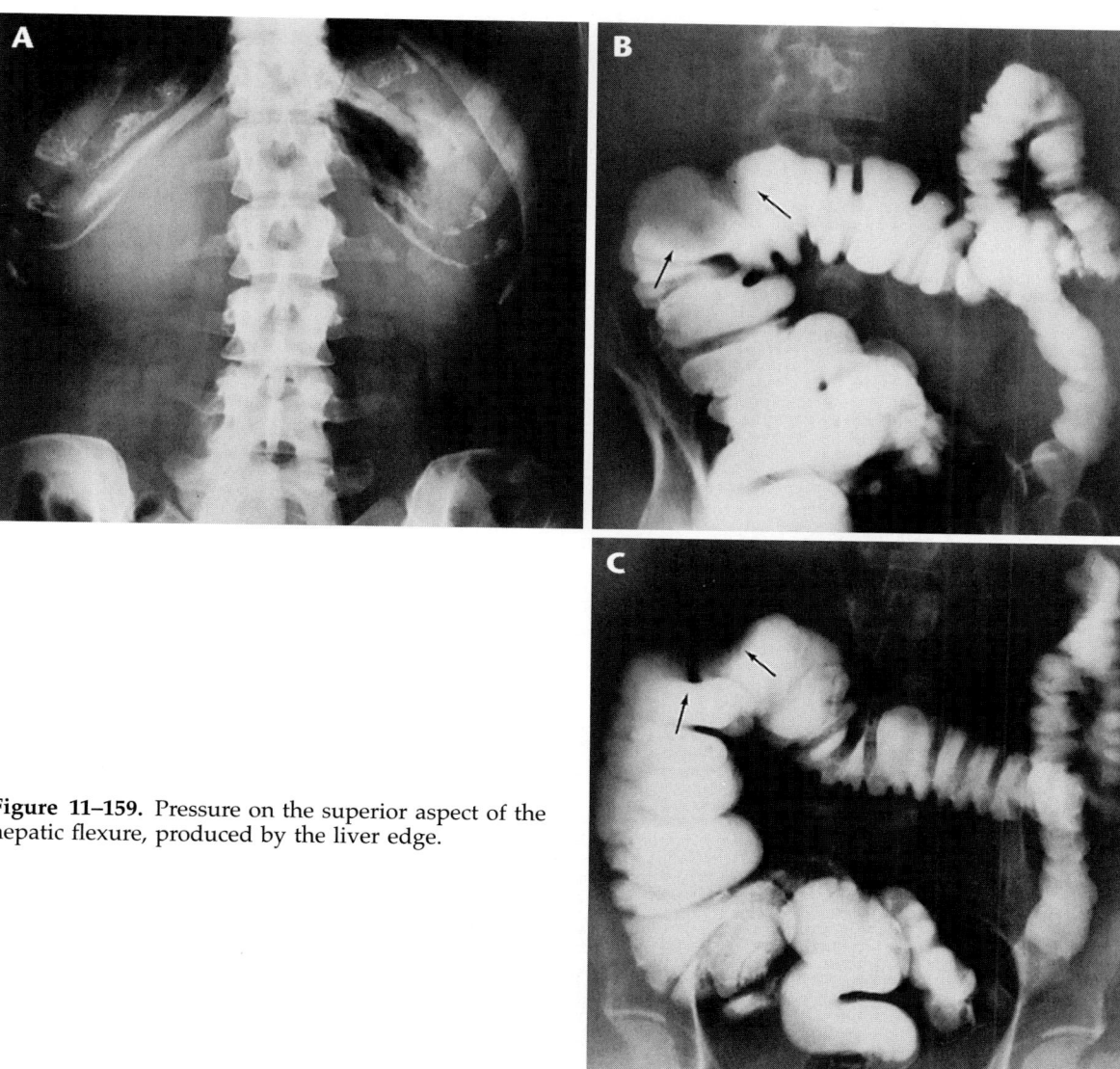

Figure 11–159. Pressure on the superior aspect of the hepatic flexure, produced by the liver edge.

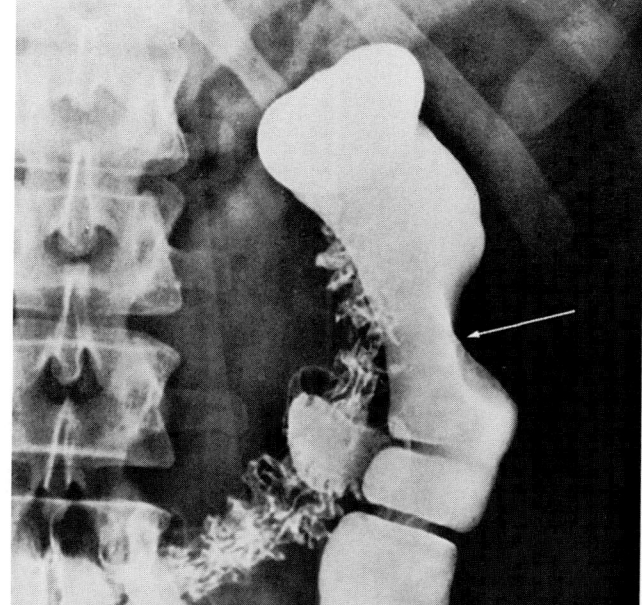

Figure 11–160. Pressure defect on the proximal descending colon, produced by the spleen.

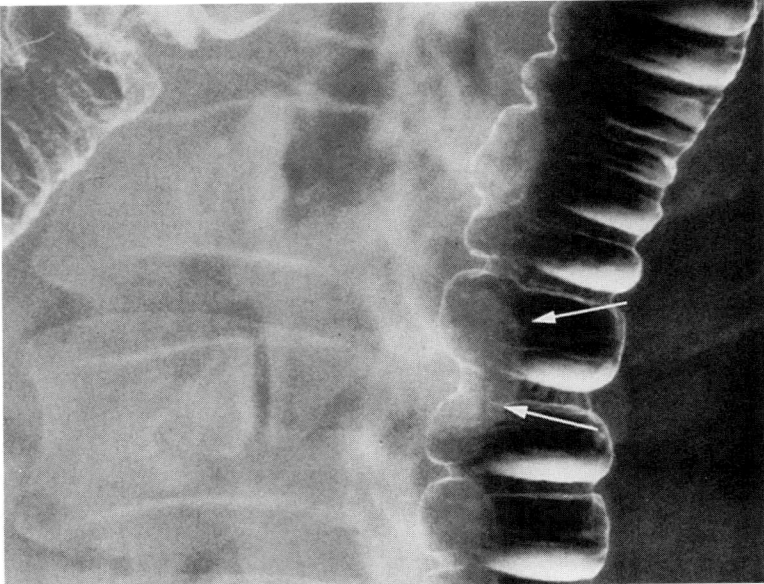

Figure 11–161. Simulated mass in the descending colon, produced by the spinous process of the adjacent lumbar vertebra.

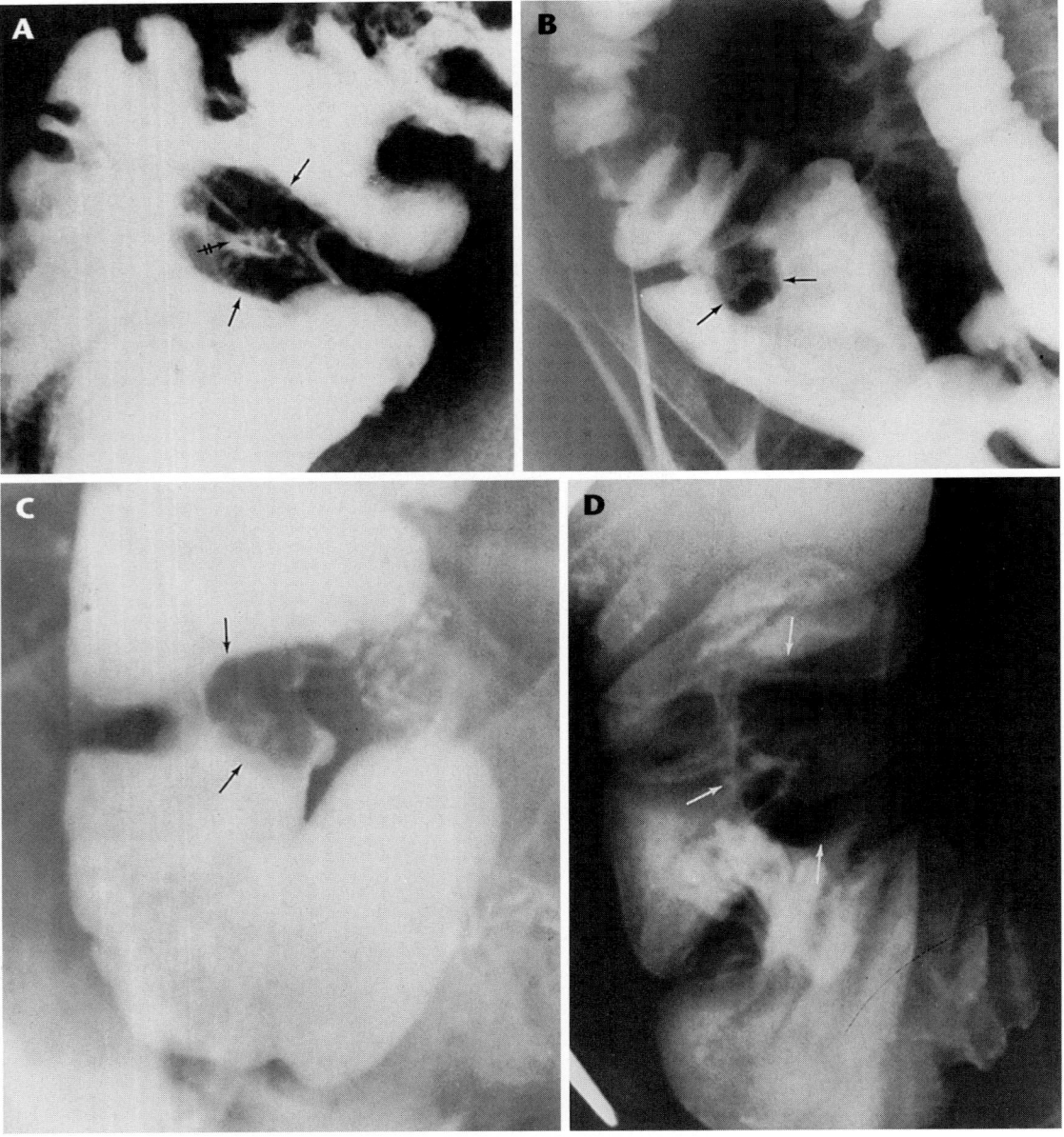

Figure 11–162. Four examples of large ileocecal valves that simulate polypoid masses.

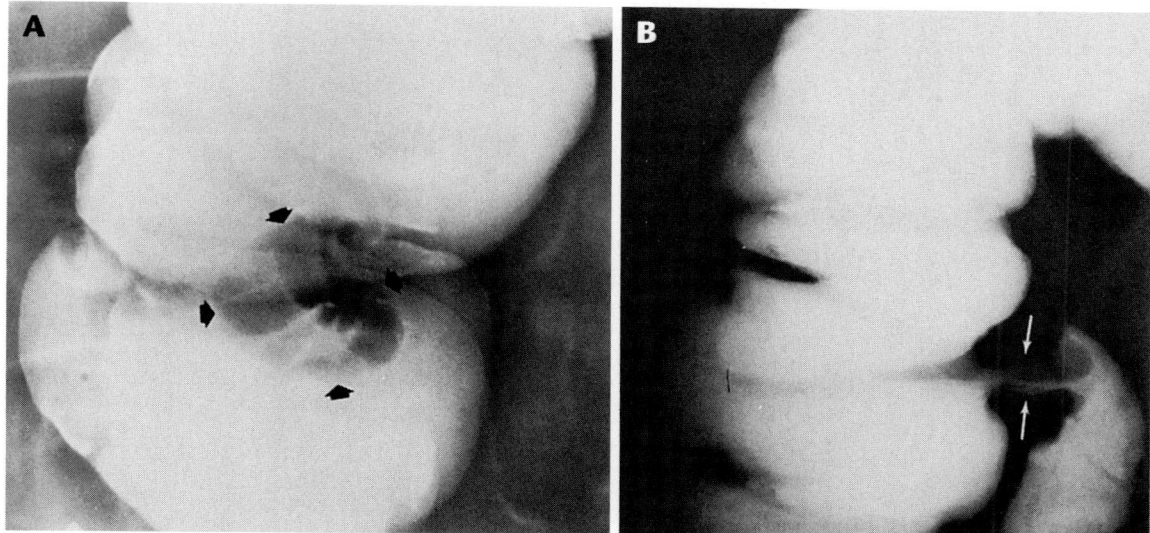

Figure 11–163. Retrograde prolapse of the ileocecal valve, simulating a neoplasm of the terminal ileum. **A,** Before prolapse. **B,** After prolapse. (From Hatten HP Jr et al: Retrograde prolapse of the ileocecal valve. *Am J Roentgenol* 128:755, 1977.)

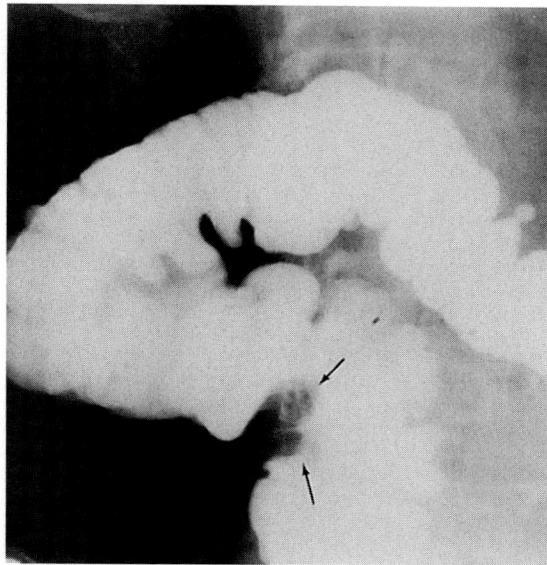

Figure 11–164. Mobile cecum with the ileocecal valve entering from the right side.

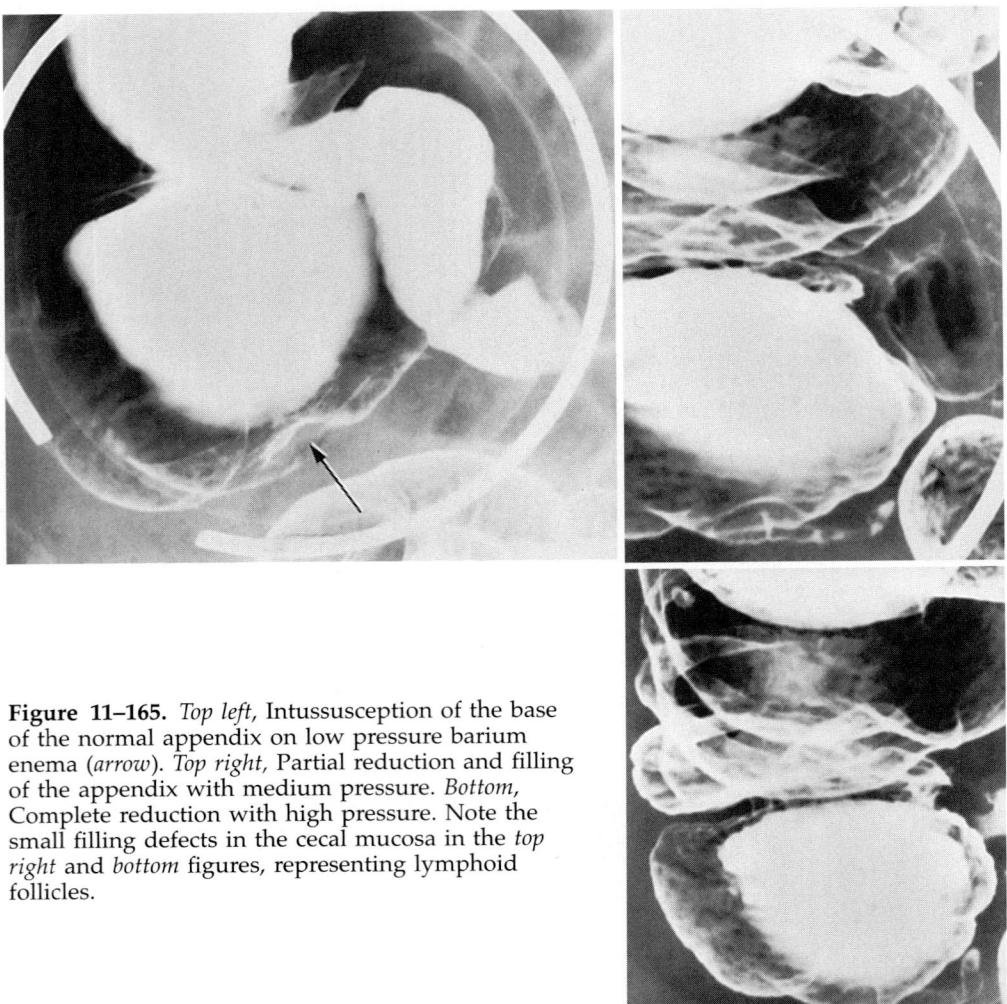

Figure 11–165. *Top left,* Intussusception of the base of the normal appendix on low pressure barium enema (*arrow*). *Top right,* Partial reduction and filling of the appendix with medium pressure. *Bottom,* Complete reduction with high pressure. Note the small filling defects in the cecal mucosa in the *top right* and *bottom* figures, representing lymphoid follicles.

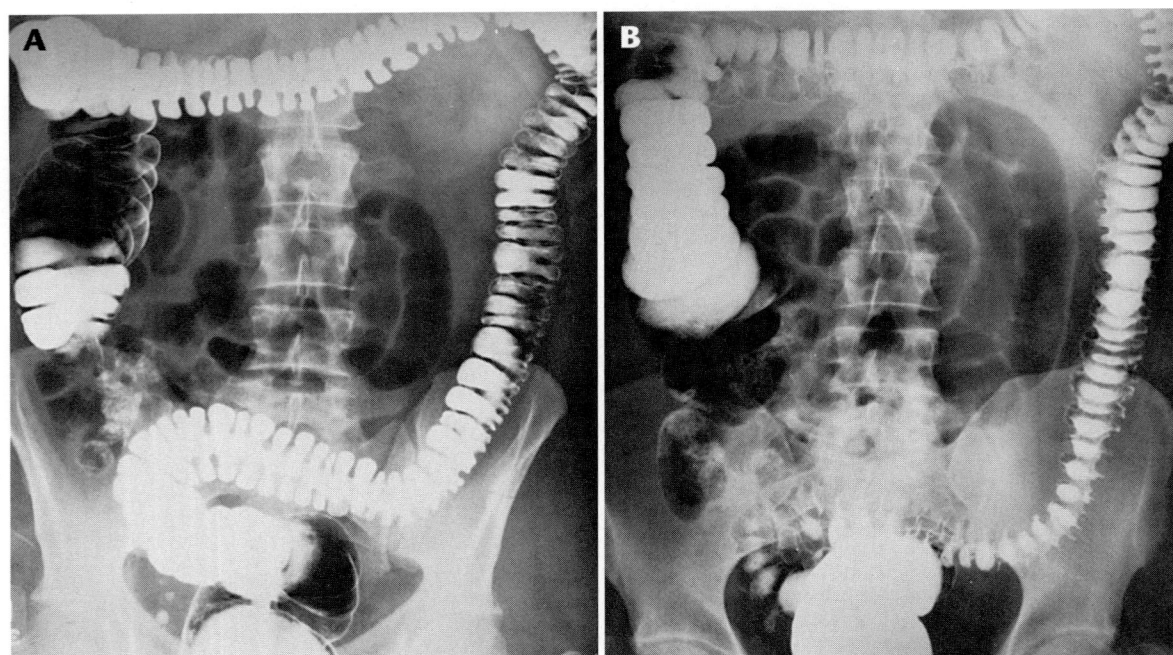

Figure 11–166. Prominent but normal haustral pattern in a healthy 40-year-old man. Note the simulation of diverticula. **A,** Preevacuation. **B,** Postevacuation.

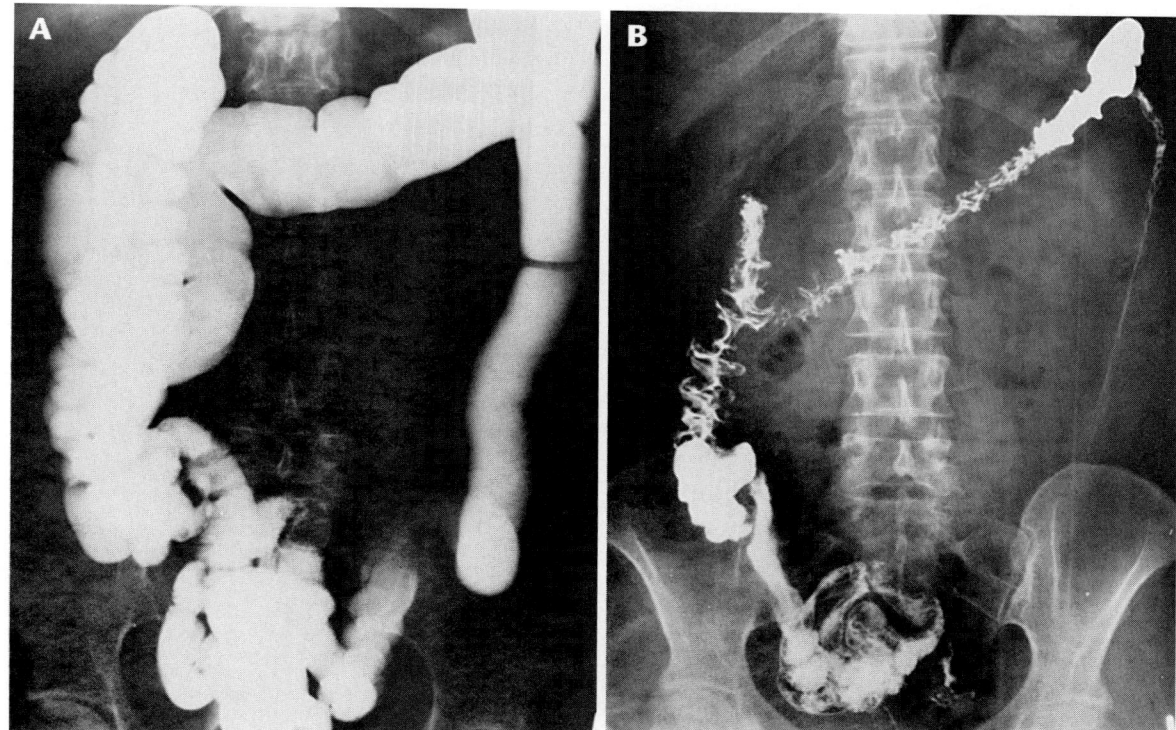

Figure 11–167. Paucity of haustral markings in the left half of the colon is not uncommon in normal individuals and those with prolonged cathartic abuse. This appearance may simulate that of chronic ulcerative colitis. **A,** Preevacuation. **B,** Postevacuation. (Ref: Plum GE et al: Prolonged cathartic abuse resulting in roentgen evidence suggestive of enterocolitis. *Am J Roentgenol* 83:919, 1960.)

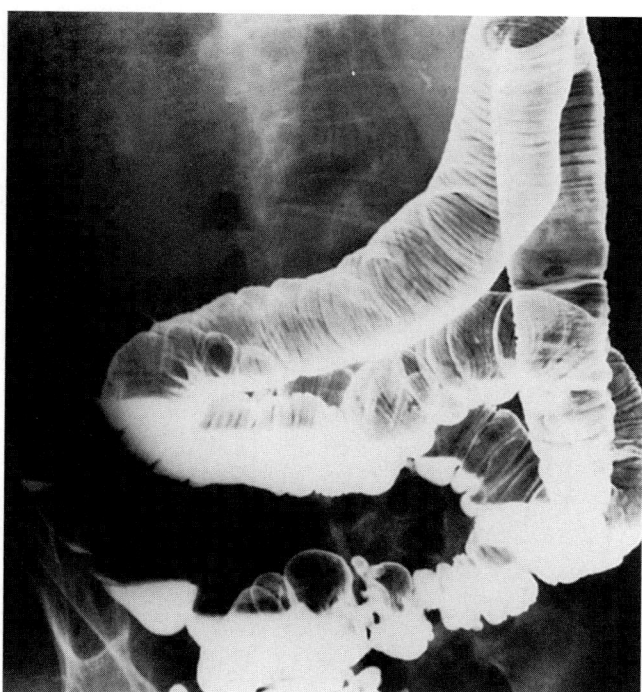

Figure 11–168. Colon shown by double contrast with a pattern that simulates the small bowel, probably the result of barium in the innominate grooves.

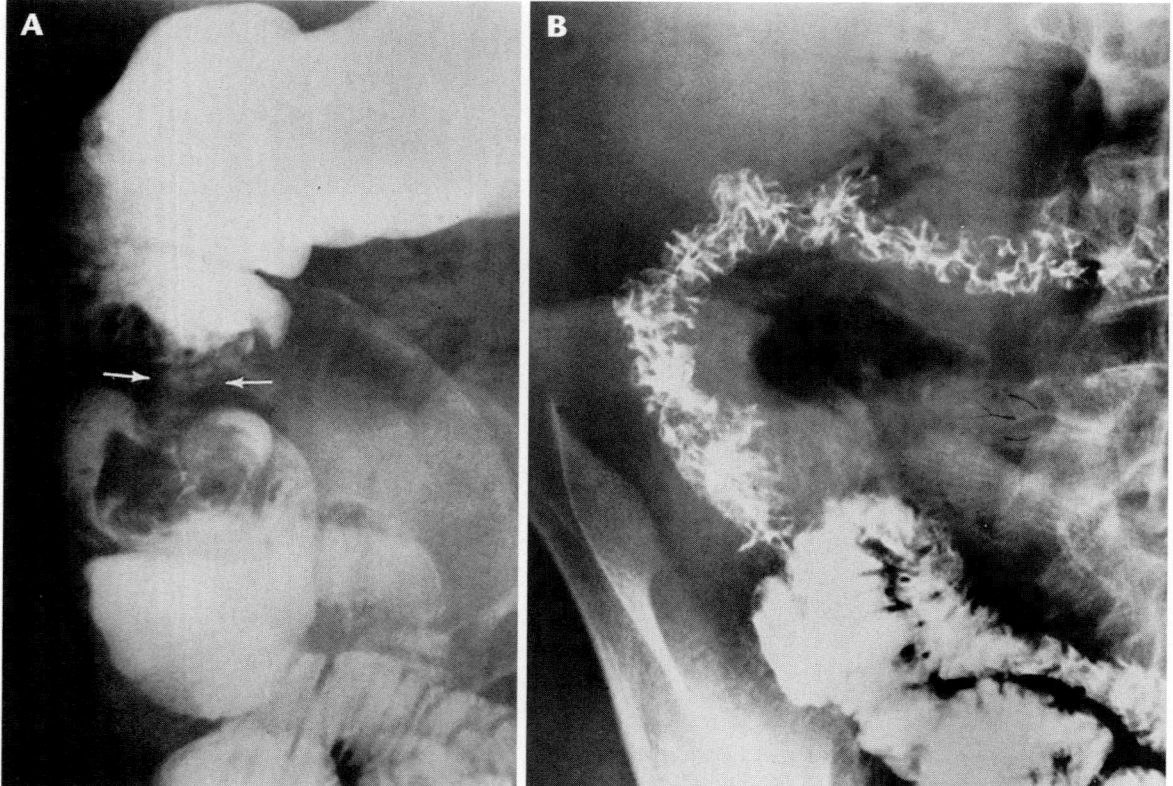

Figure 11–169. A, Physiologic colonic sphincter, simulating colonic neoplasm. **B,** The alteration is not seen in the postevacuation film. (Ref: Templeton A: Colon sphincters simulating organic disease. *Radiology* 75:237, 1960.)

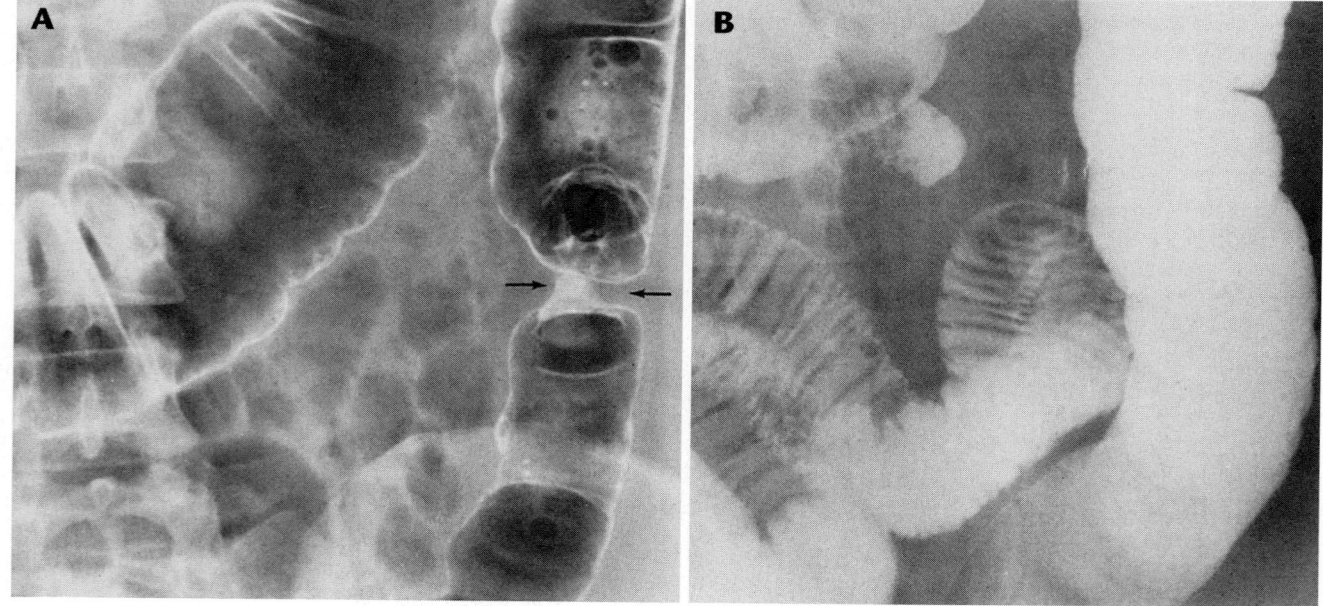

Figure 11–170. A, Additional example of a physiologic sphincter simulating a neoplasm. It is not seen in the follow-up examination (**B**). (Ref: Cimmino CV: Roentgen-diagnostic value of spasm of certain colonic "sphincters." *VA Med* 92:317, 1965.)

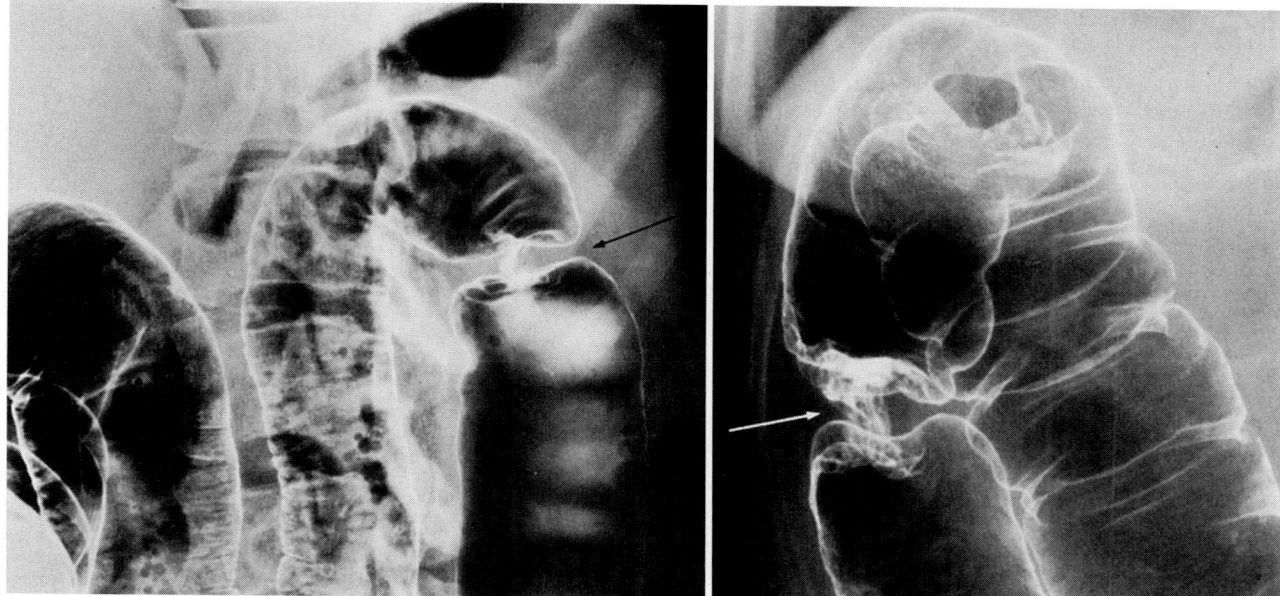

Figure 11–171. Two examples of a physiologic sphincter closely resembling an annular carcinoma.

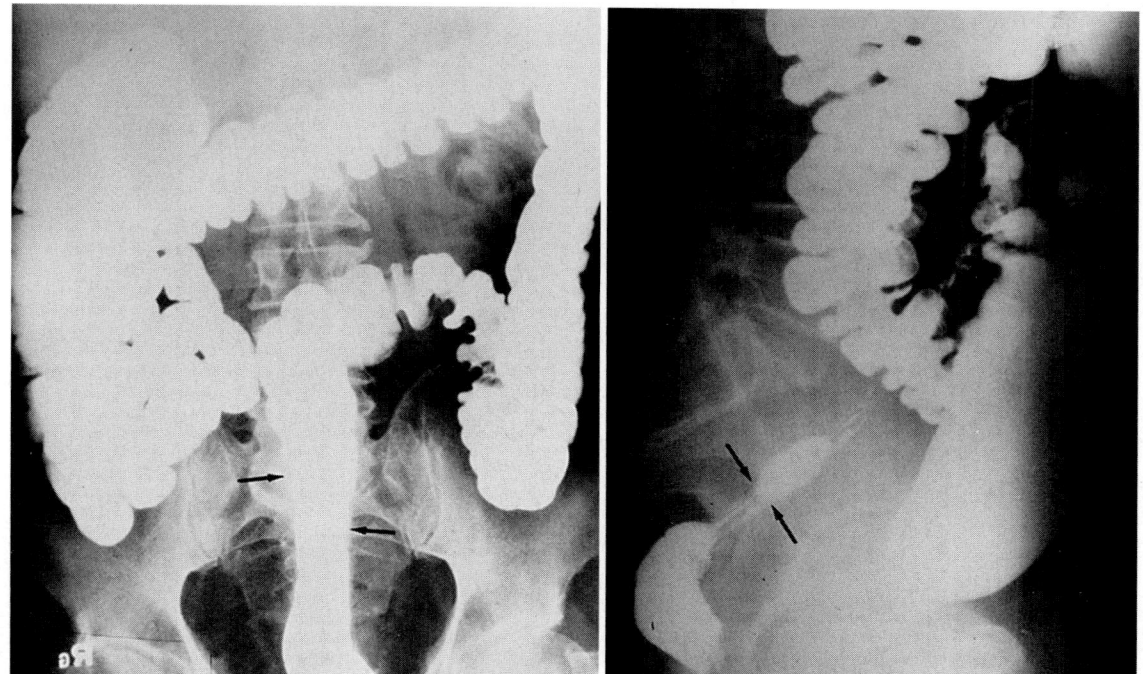

Figure 11–172. Elongation, elevation, and narrowing of the pelvic colon secondary to fat accumulation in the pelvis. This entity should not be confused with the changes caused by pelvic neoplasm. The bladder is similarly altered (see Fig. 13–81). (Ref: Fogg LB, Smyth JW: Pelvic lipomatosis: A condition simulating pelvic neoplasm. *Radiology* 90:558, 1968.)

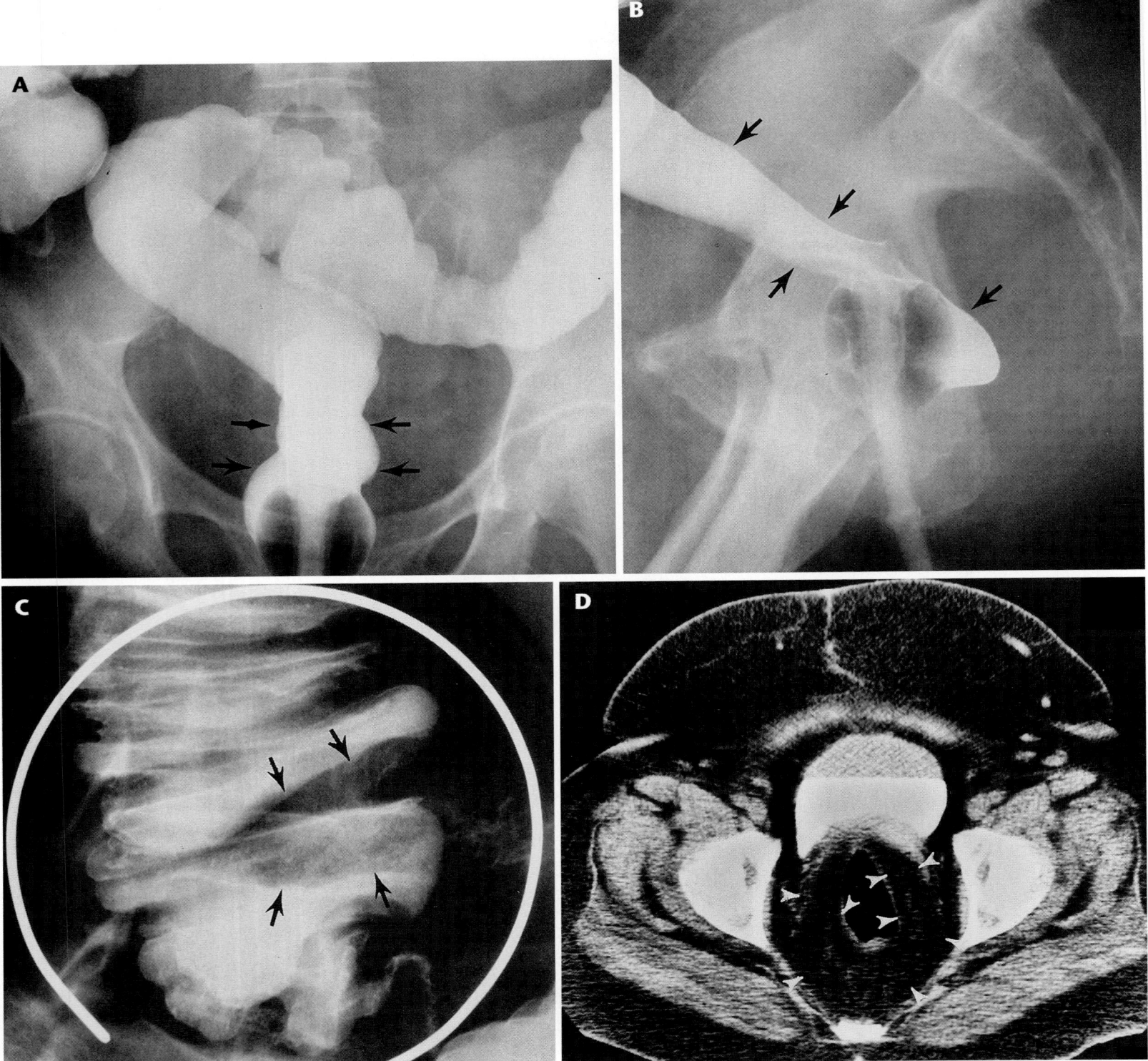

Figure 11–173. Pelvic and ileocecal lipomatosis in the same patient. **A** and **B,** Narrowing and straightening of the rectum and sigmoid by fat. **C,** Fatty infiltration of the ileocecal valve. **D,** CT showing huge amounts of perirectal fat.

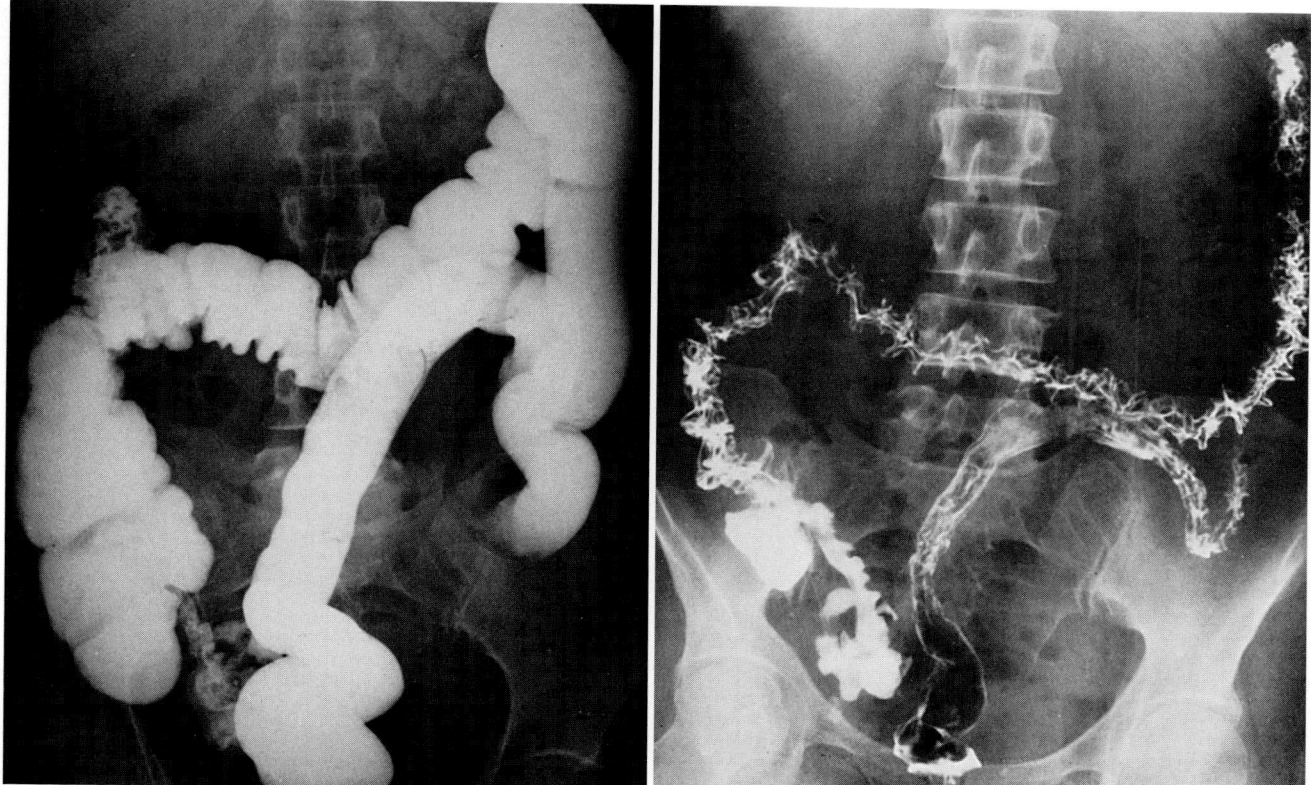

Figure 11–174. Additional example of the colonic changes caused by pelvic lipomatosis.

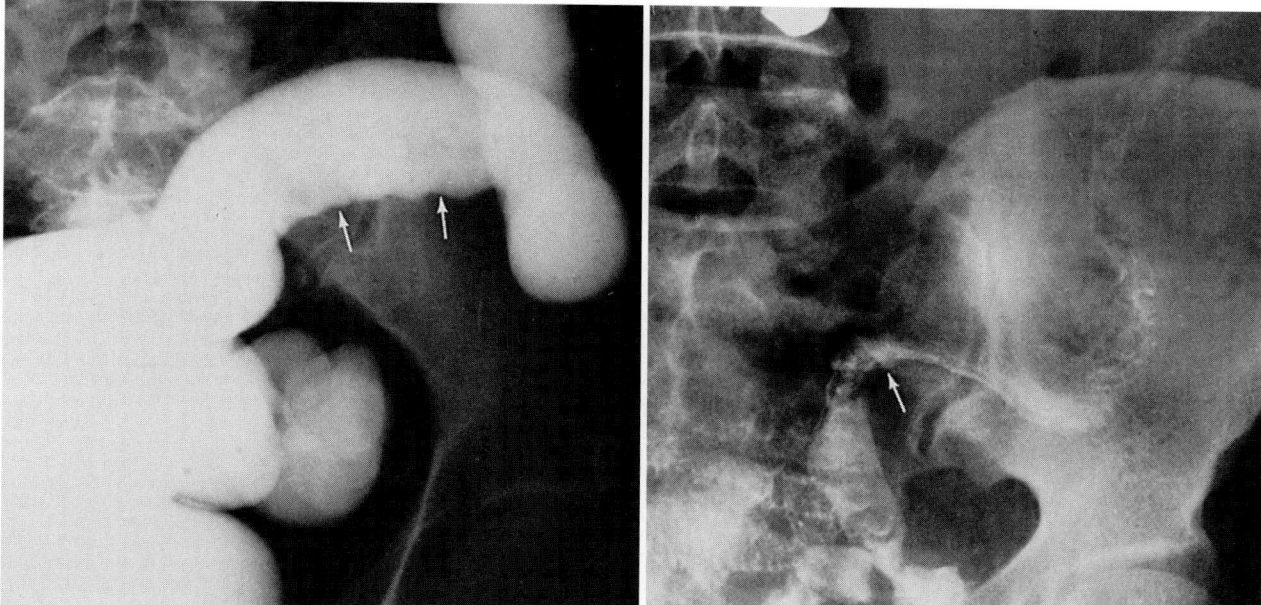

Figure 11–175. Preevacuation and postevacuation films showing displacement of the sigmoid colon by the iliopsoas muscle. A similar defect may be seen in the ascending colon and the terminal ileum in some patients. (Refs: Martel W: Displacement of the intestine by the iliopsoas muscle. *Am J Roentgenol* 94:399, 1965; Duprat G Jr et al: Bowel displacement due to psoas muscle hypertrophy. *Can Assoc Radiol* 34:64, 1983.)

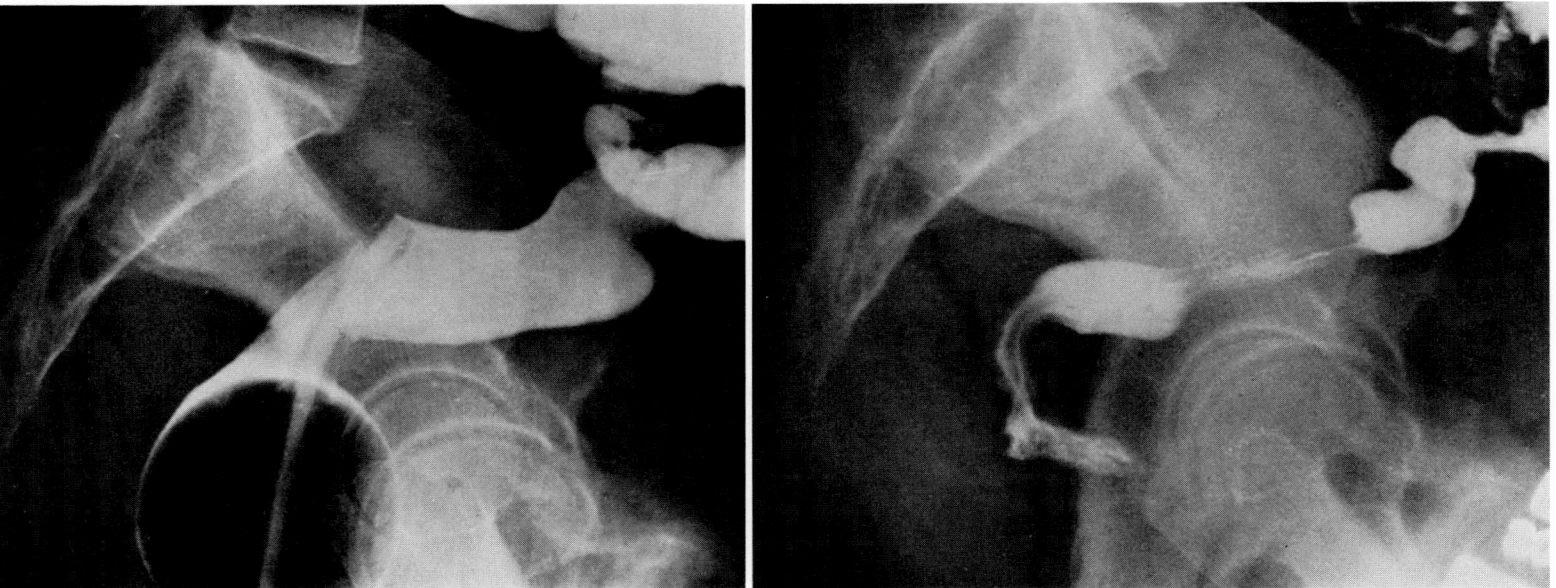

Figure 11–176. Pre- and postevacuation films of the rectum in lateral projection, showing an increase in the retrorectal space that is caused by obesity, not interposed pathology. This may also be seen in Cushing's disease. (Refs: Fennessy JJ et al: Early roentgen manifestations of mild ulcerative colitis and proctitis. *Radiology* 87:848, 1966; Yagan R, Marmslya G: Increased retrorectal space on barium enema in pelvic lipomatosis. *Appl Radiol* 17:36, 1988.)

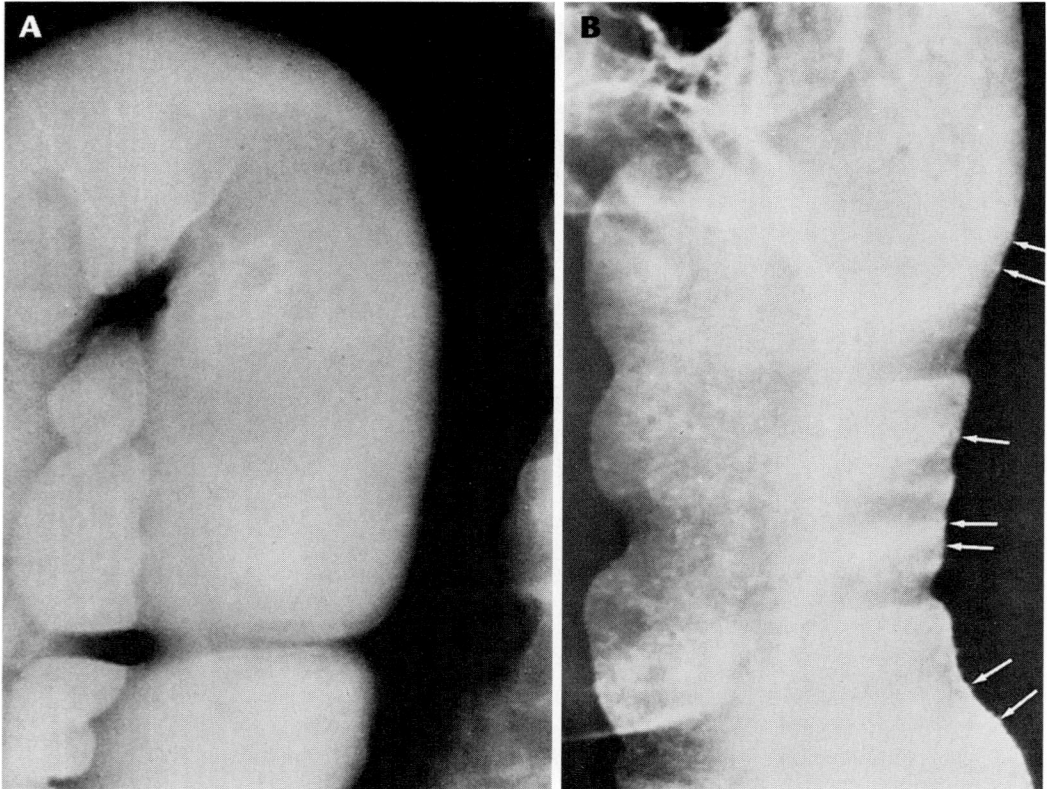

Figure 11–177. Barium in the innominate folds of the hepatic flexure, simulating mucosal ulceration. **A,** Preevacuation film does not demonstrate the folds. **B,** Postevacuation film nicely shows the barium in the folds. (Ref: Williams I: Innominate grooves in the surface of mucosa. *Radiology* 84:877, 1965.)

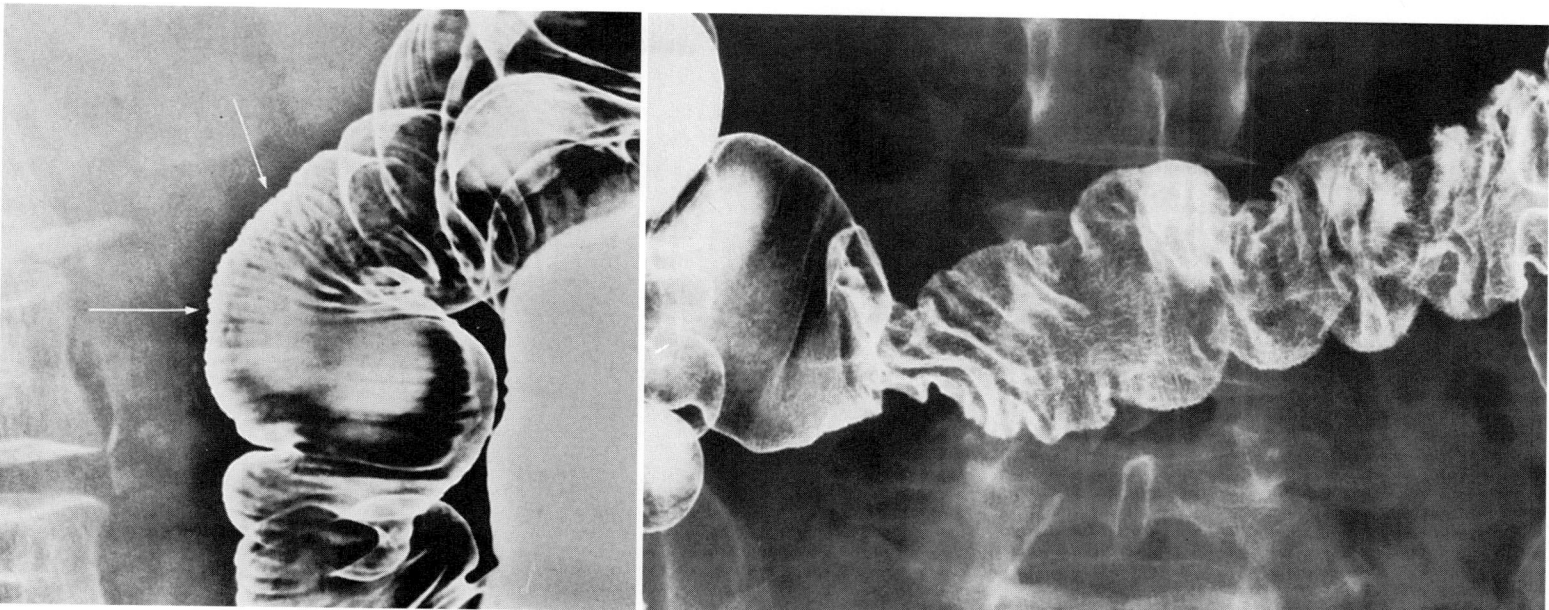

Figure 11–178. Two examples of the innominate grooves of the colon. These can be distinguished from ulcerations by their inconsistency. (Refs: Frank DF et al: Pseudoulcerations of the colon on barium examination. *Gastrointest Radiol* 2:129, 1977; Cole FM: Innominate grooves of the colon: Morphological characteristics and etiologic mechanisms. *Radiology* 128:41, 1978.)

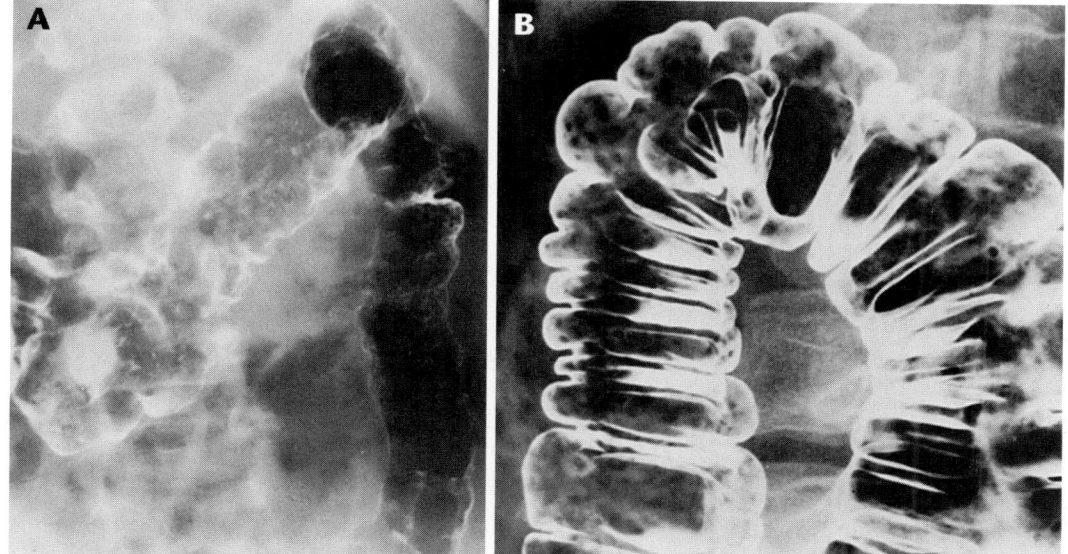

Figure 11–179. Lymphoid follicles in healthy children. **A,** 3-year-old. **B,** 13-year-old. These lesions are not believed to be of significance but may be confused with polyposis coli. (Ref: Laufer I, deSa D: Lymphoid follicular pattern: A normal feature of the pediatric colon. *Am J Roentgenol* 130:51, 1978.)

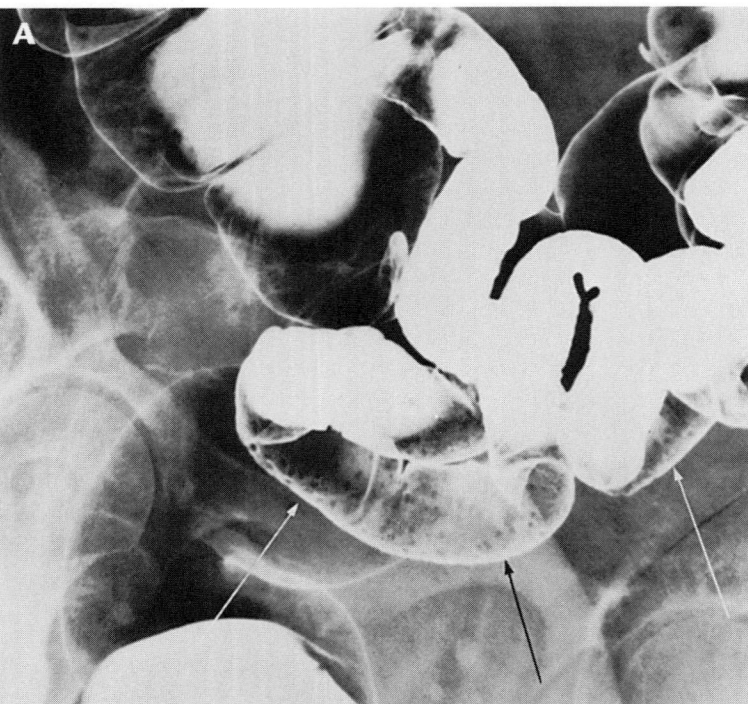

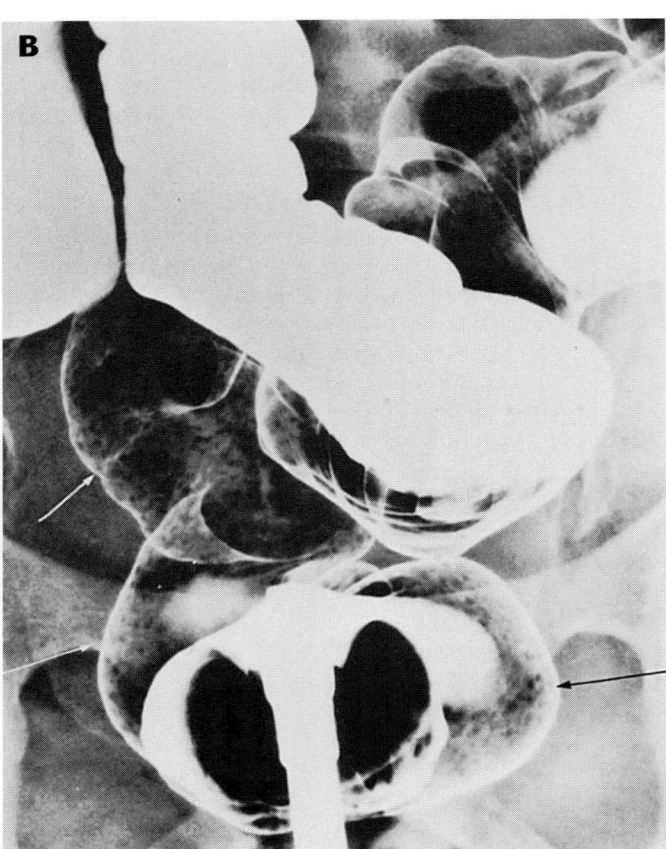

Figure 11–180. Two examples of lymphoid follicles of the colon in adults, a finding of no clinical significance. **A,** 63-year-old man. **B,** 43-year-old man. (Ref: Kelvin FM et al: Lymphoid follicular pattern of the colon in adults. *Am J Roentgenol* 133:821, 1979.)

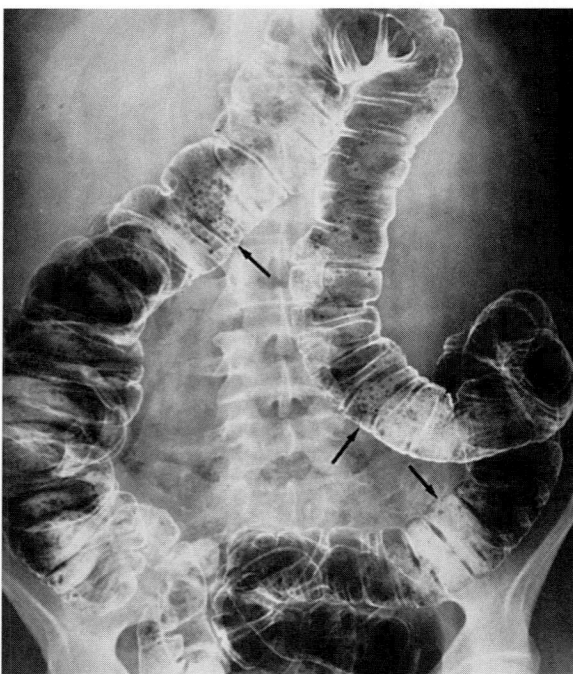

Figure 11–181. Fat droplets in the colon after castor oil ingestion, simulating polypoid lesions.

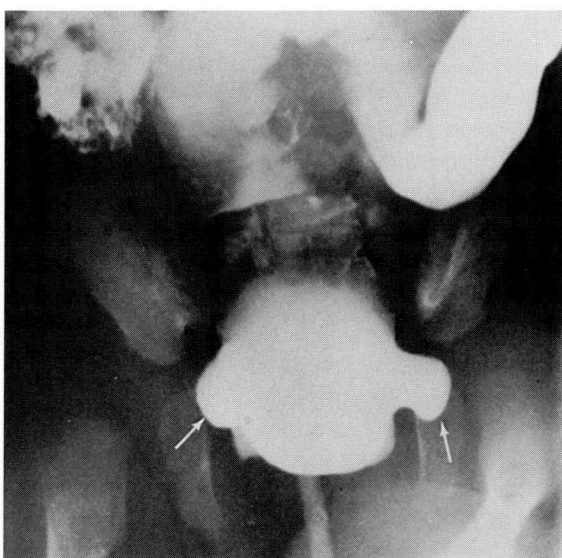

Figure 11–182. "Rectal ears" in a 1-month-old infant. These are transitory protrusions of the rectum into the inguinal rings. (Ref: Kassner EG et al: "Rectal ears." *J Can Assoc Radiol* 26:125, 1975.)

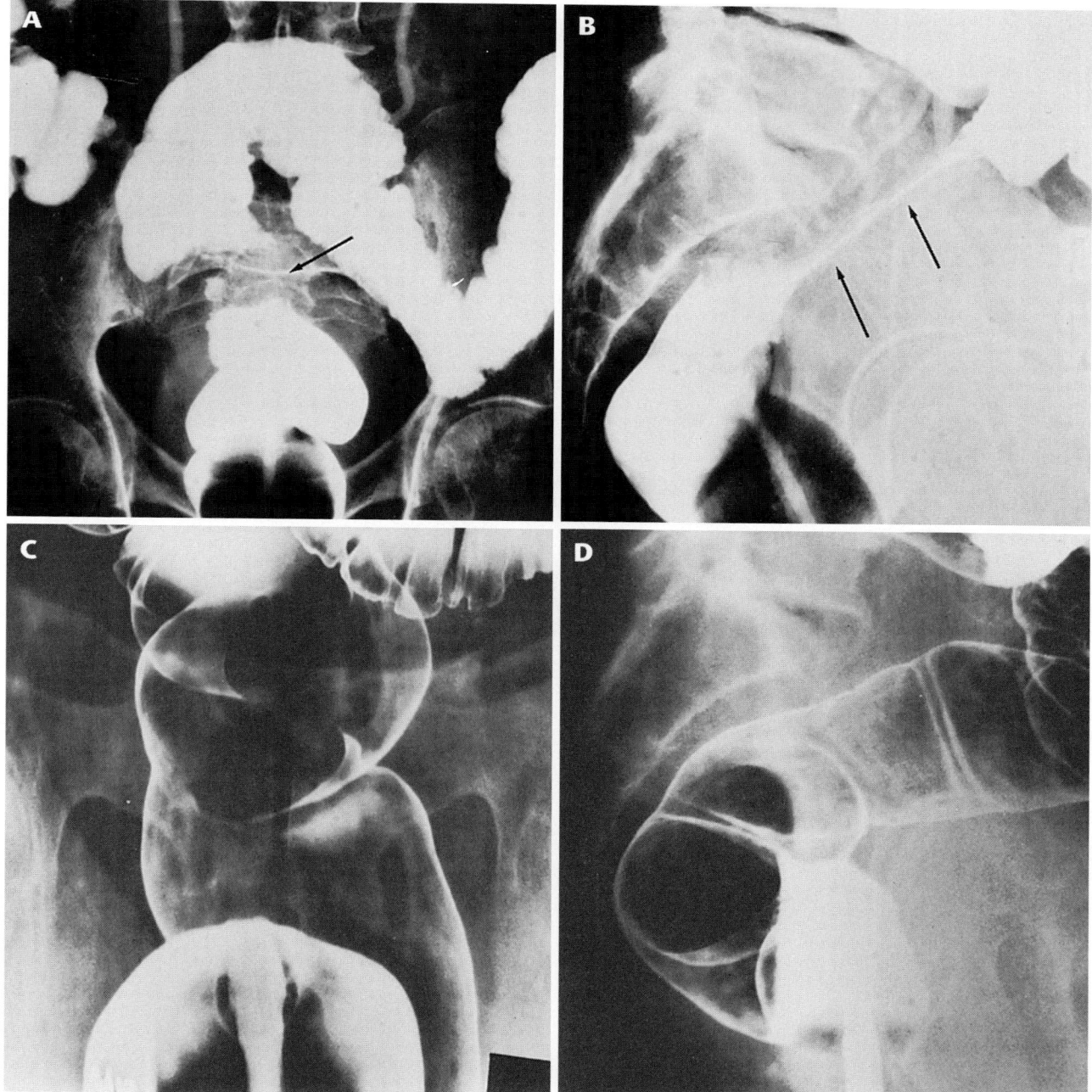

Figure 11–183. Pressure effect of a full bladder on the sigmoid colon. **A** and **B,** Full bladder. **C** and **D,** After bladder is emptied. (Ref: Kleinhaus J, Kaftori J: Rectosigmoid pseudostenosis due to urinary retention. *Radiology* 127:645, 1978.)

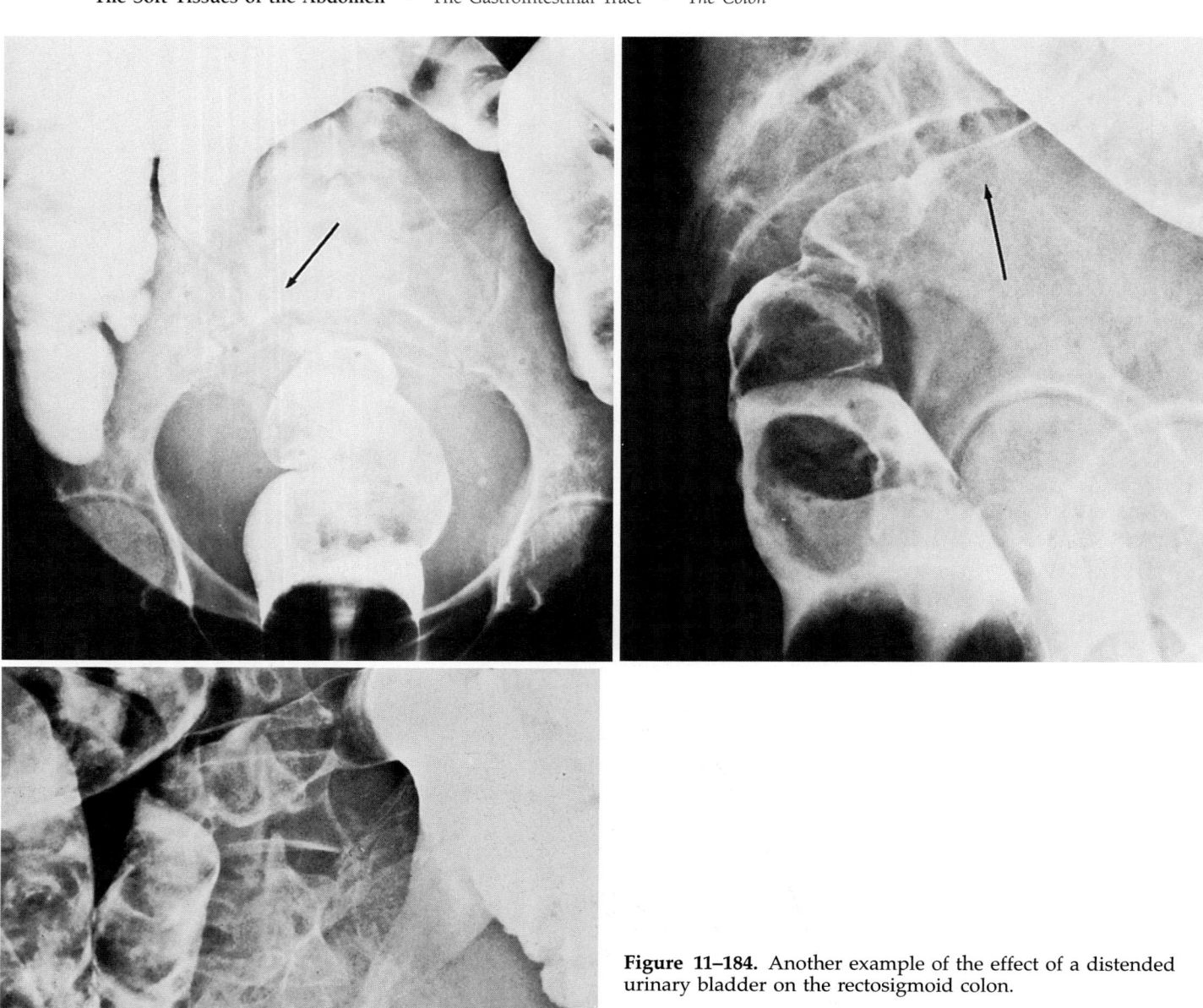

Figure 11–184. Another example of the effect of a distended urinary bladder on the rectosigmoid colon.

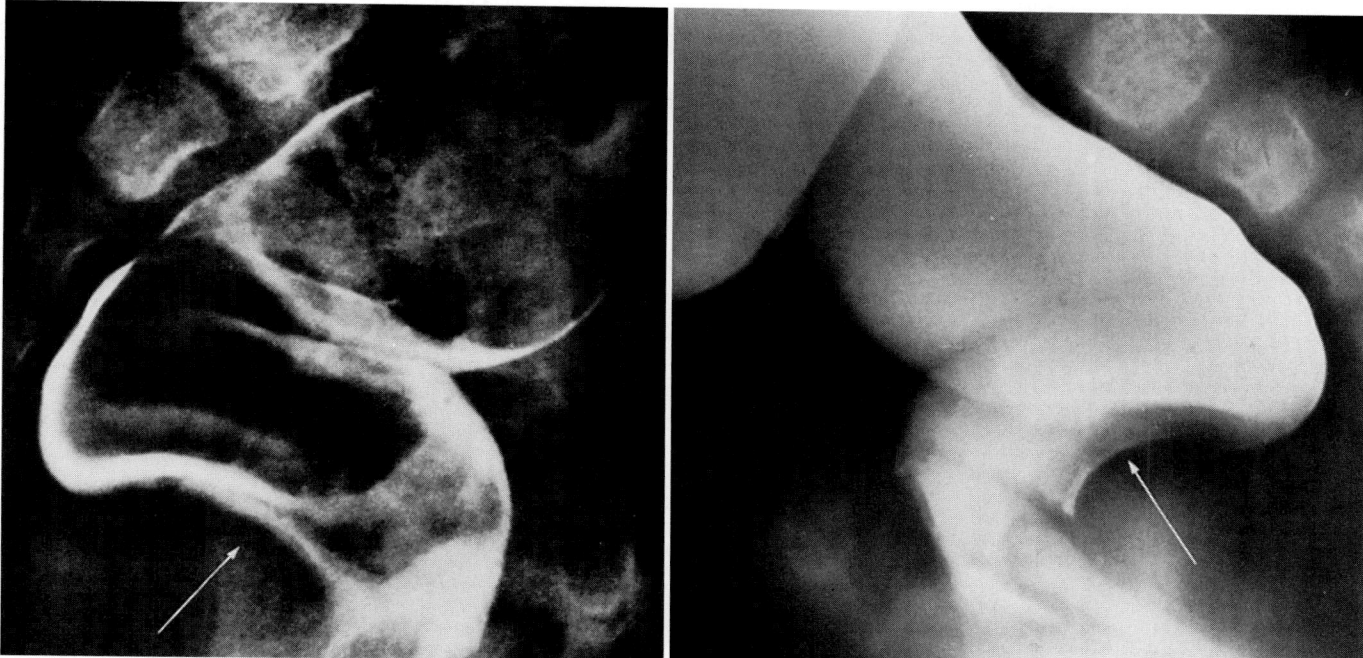

Figure 11–185. Two examples of the impressions of the levator ani muscles on the rectum in children.

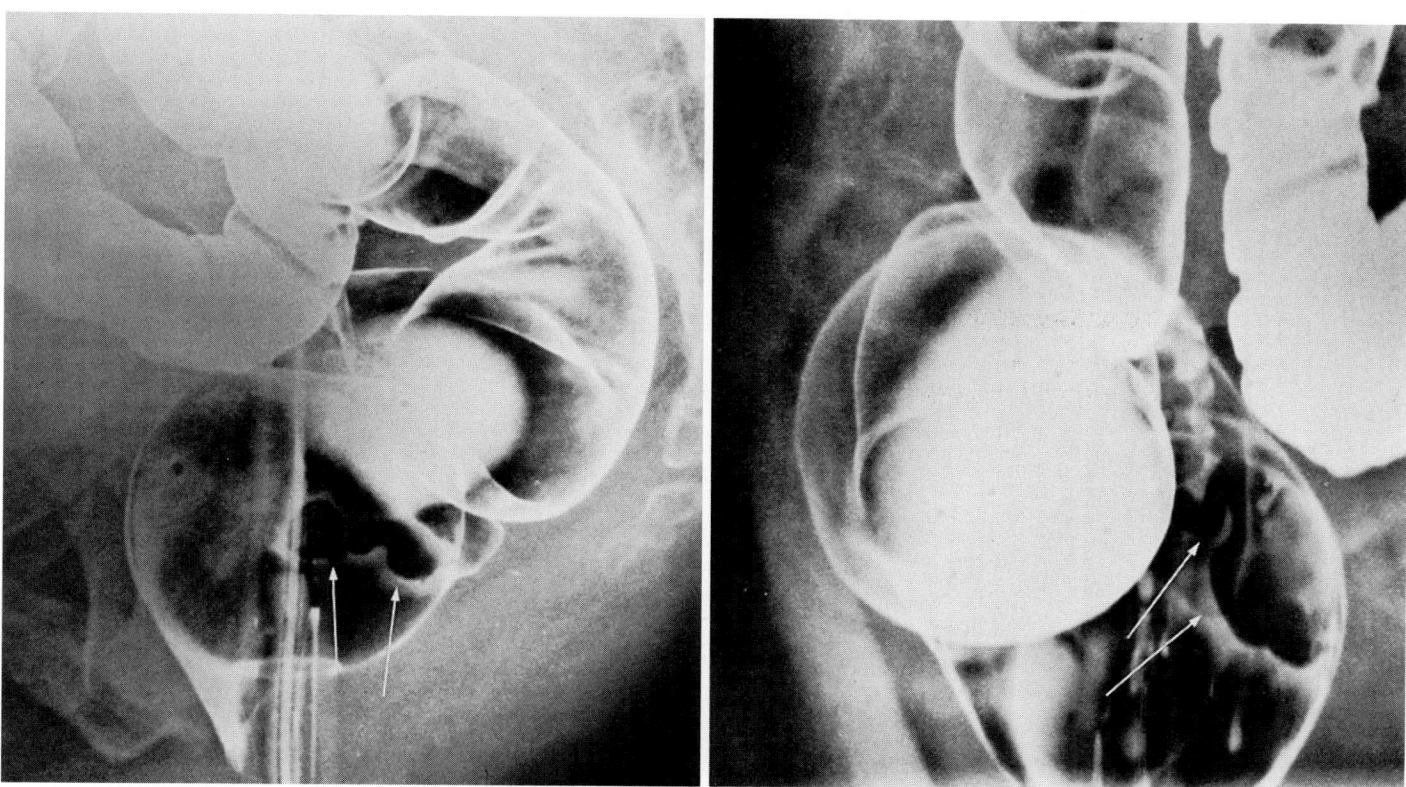

Figure 11–186. Two examples of "kissing" artifacts produced by contact of the rectal balloon and the rectal wall. (Ref: Gohel VK et al: Double contrast artifacts. *Gastrointest Radiol* 3:139, 1978.)

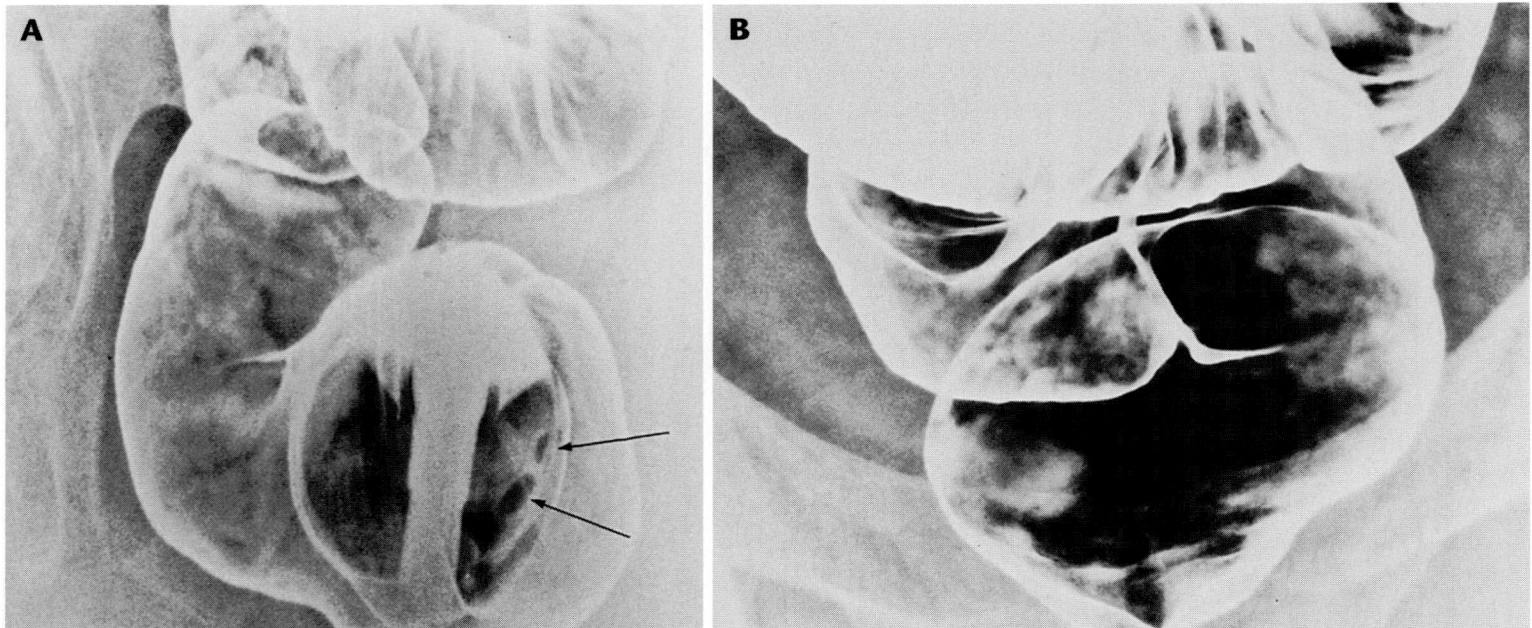

Figure 11–187. A, "Kissing" artifacts of the rectum, produced by balloon contact.
B, After removal of balloon.

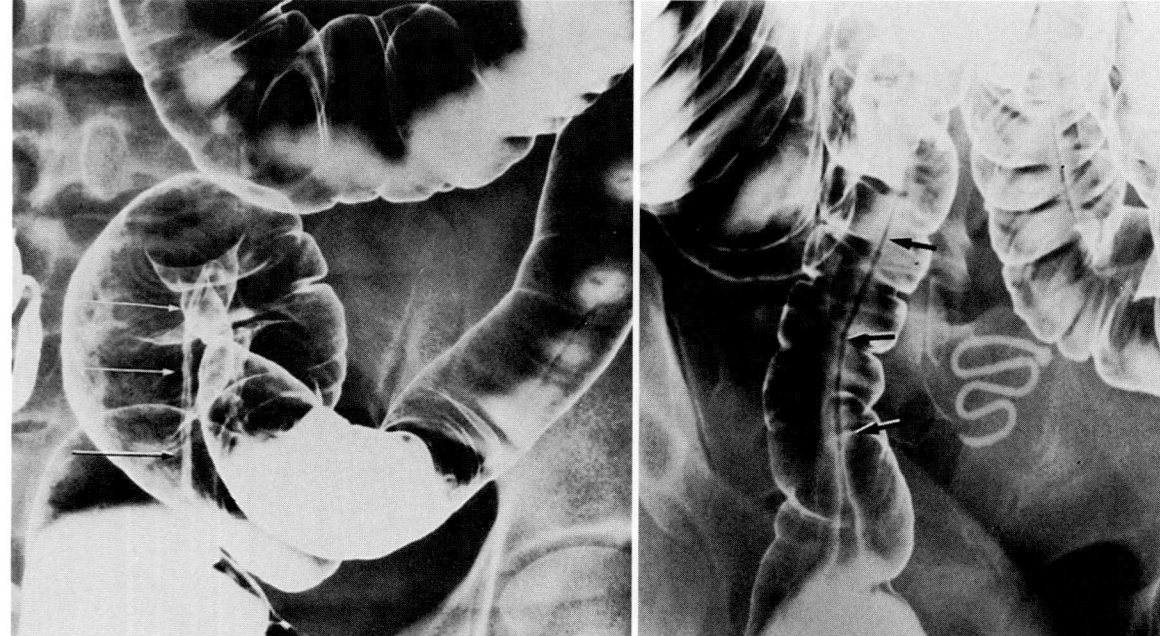

Figure 11–188. Two examples of alterations seen in double contrast examinations, caused by strands of mucus. This should not be confused with linear ulceration.

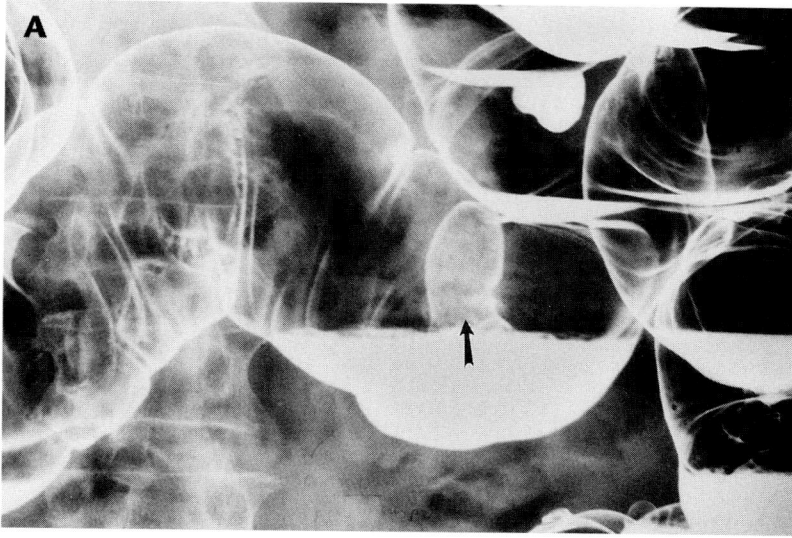

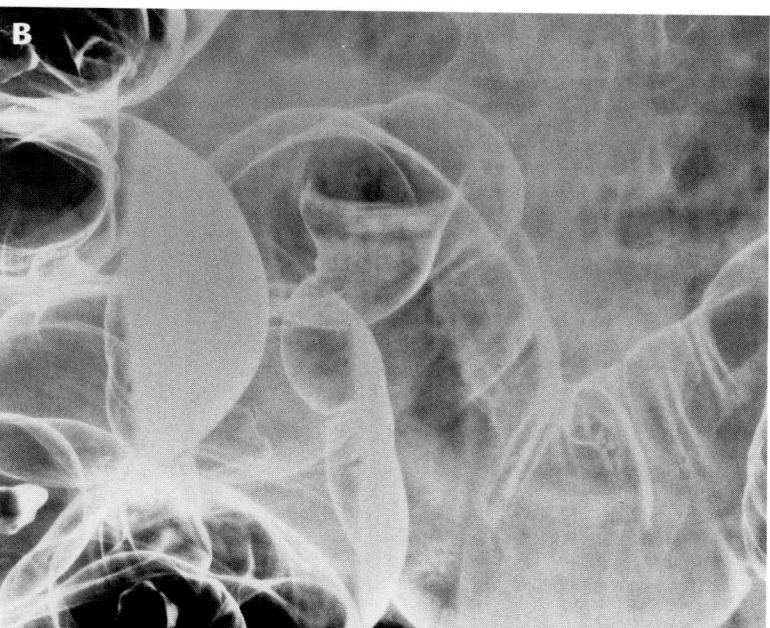

Figure 11–189. A, Kissing artifact, simulating a polyp in the transverse colon, produced by apposition of two folds. **B,** Film made with the patient in the left lateral decubitus position shows no lesion.

Figure 11–190. Two examples of sacral foramina projecting through the colon, simulating filling defects.

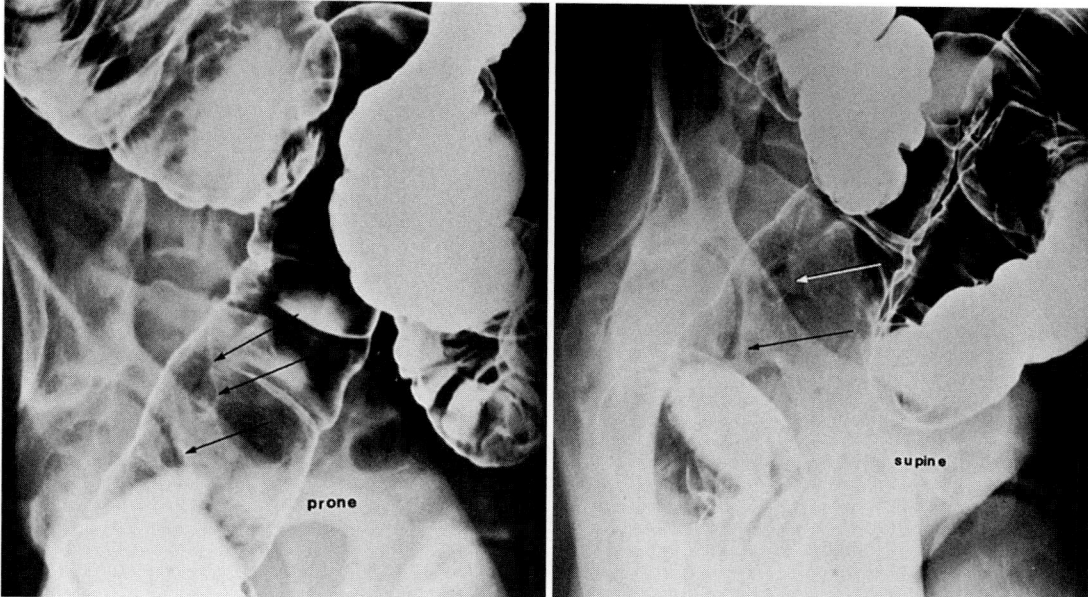

Figure 11–191. Leakage of barium into the vagina during a barium enema simulates extravasation caused by a rupture of the rectum.

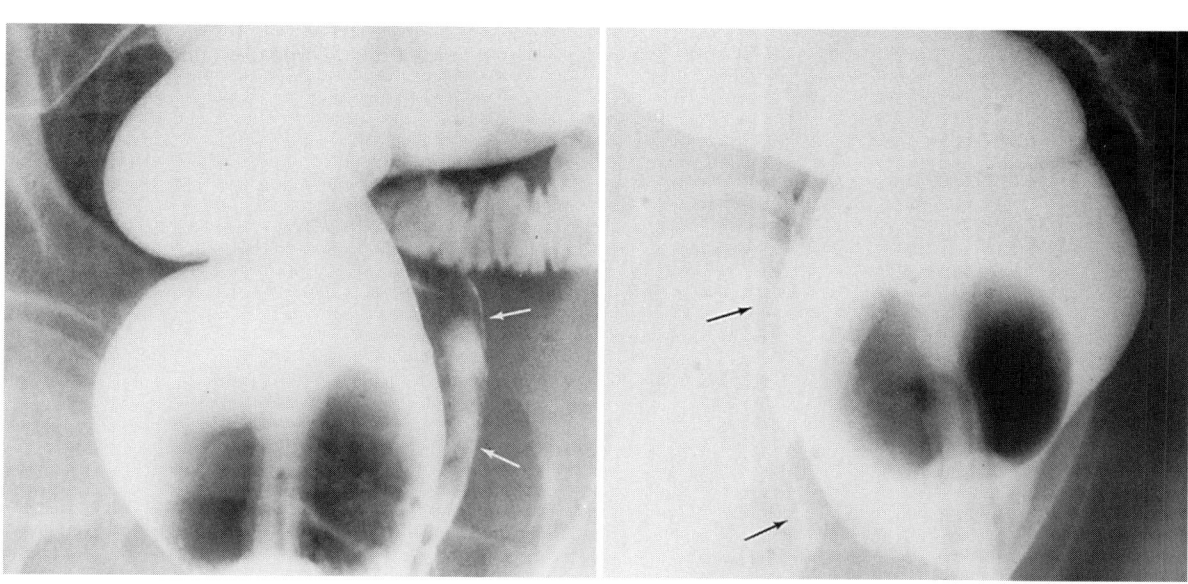

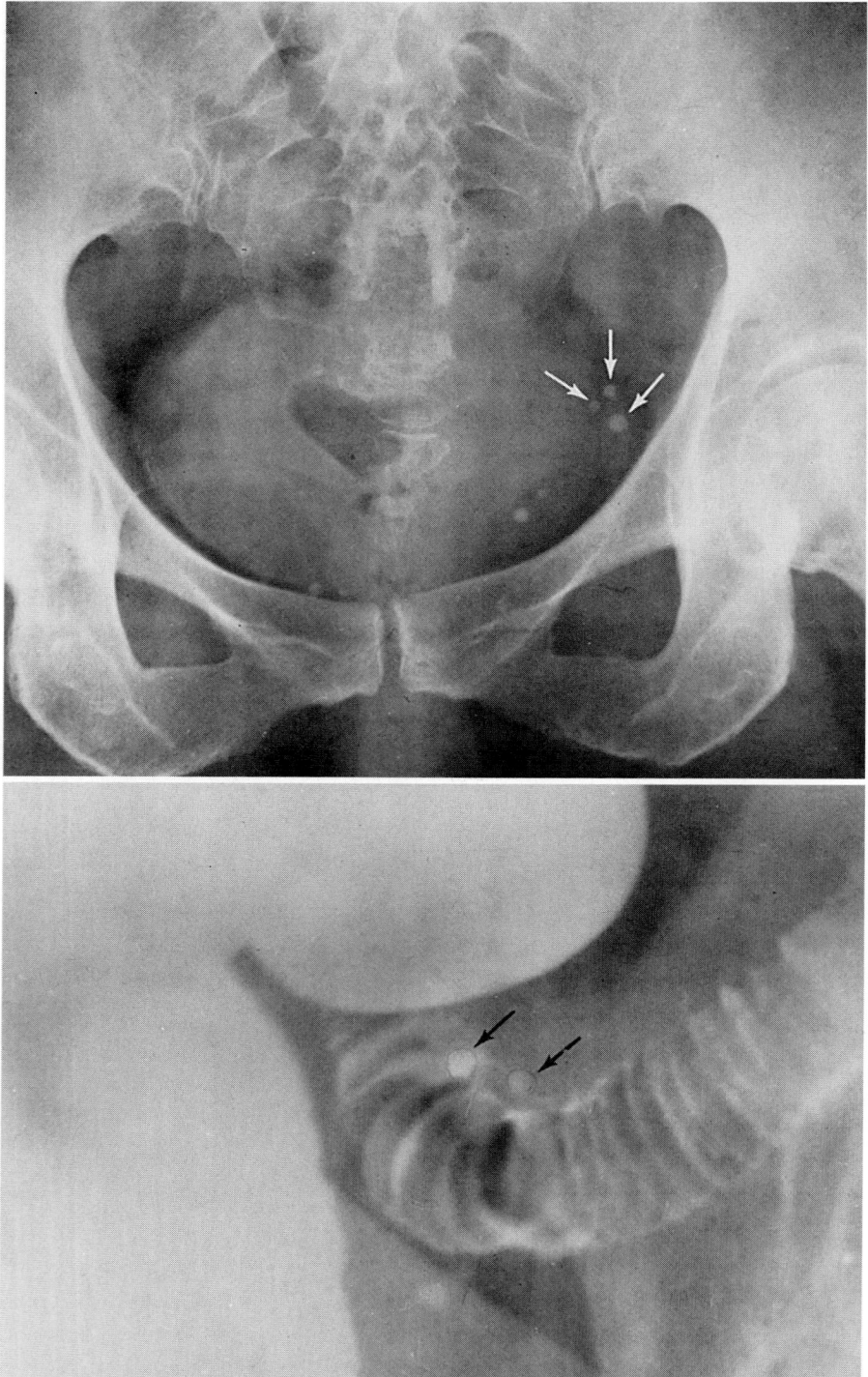

Figure 11–192. Pelvic phleboliths simulating colonic diverticula, on barium enema.

The Liver and Biliary Tract

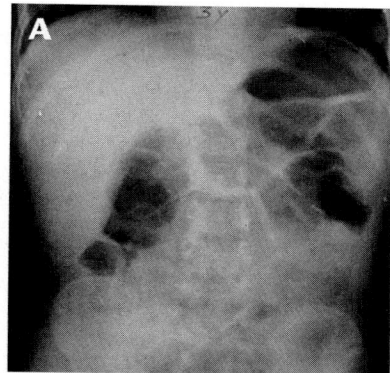

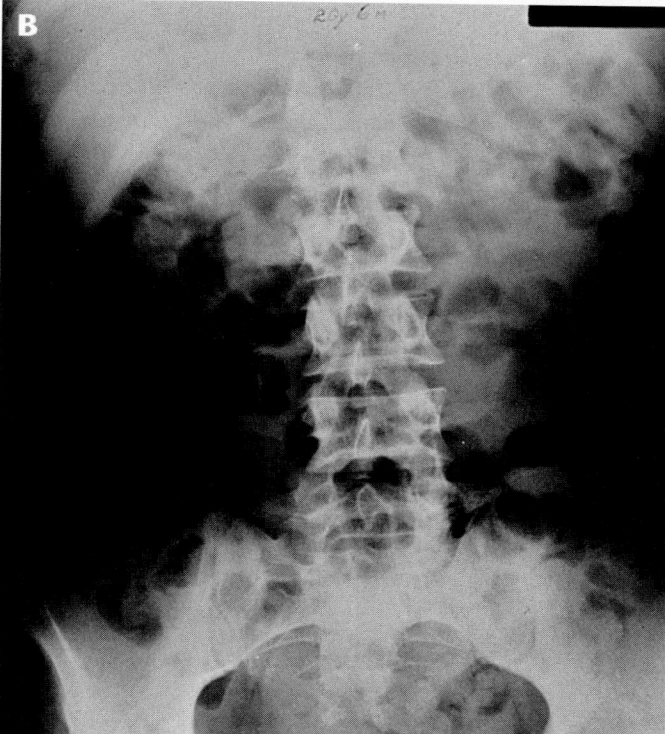

Figure 11–193. Differences in proportion in the size of the liver and the total abdominal area in a child (**A**) and an adult (**B**). The child's liver occupies a proportionately larger portion of the abdomen. (From Keats TE: Pediatric radiology: Some potentially misleading variations from the adult. *VA Med* 93:630, 1966.)

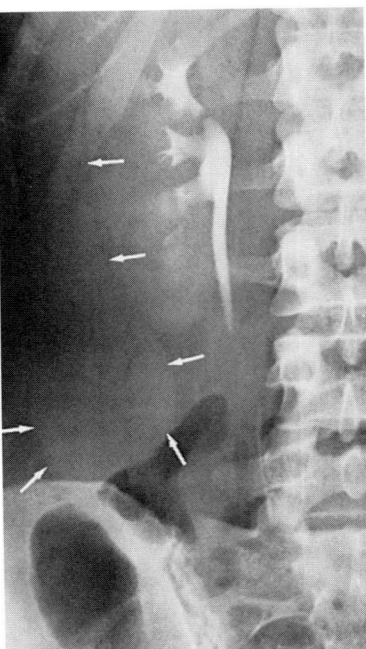

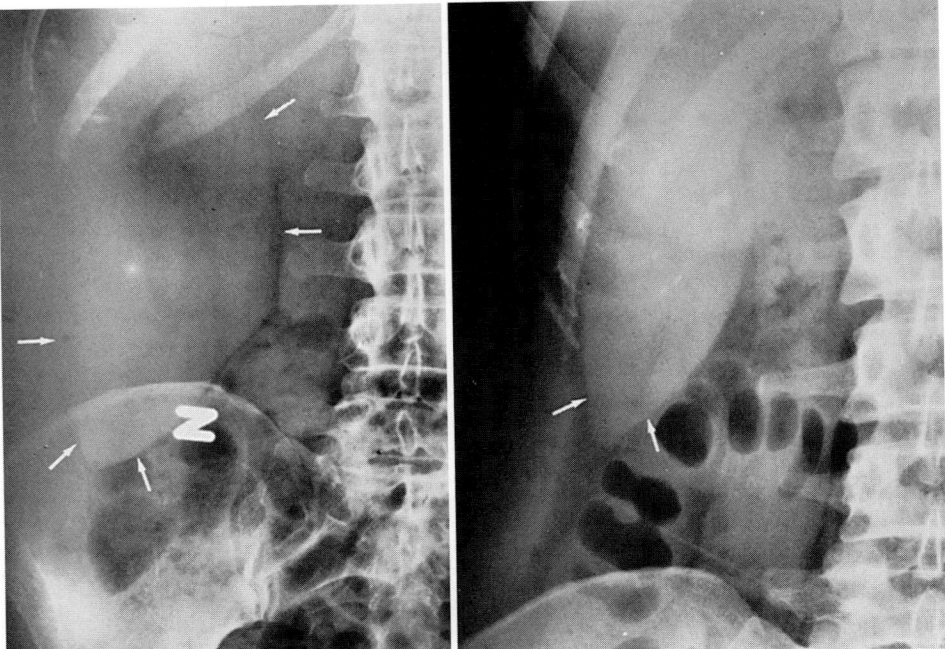

Figure 11–194. Riedel's lobe of the liver simulating an abdominal mass. (Ref: Reitemeier HR et al: Riedel's lobe of the liver. *Gastroenterology* 34:1090, 1958.)

Figure 11–195. Additional examples of Riedel's lobe.

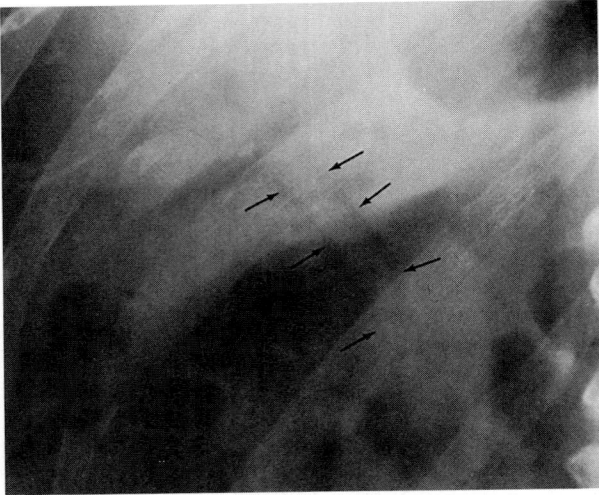

Figure 11–196. Normal common duct visualized tomographically by virtue of its surrounding periductal fat. (Ref: Shaub MS et al: Peribiliary fat. *Am J Roentgenol* 123:330, 1975.) This entity may be confused with pneumobilia. (Ref: Govani AF, Meyers MA: Pseudopneumobilia. *Radiology* 118:526, 1976.)

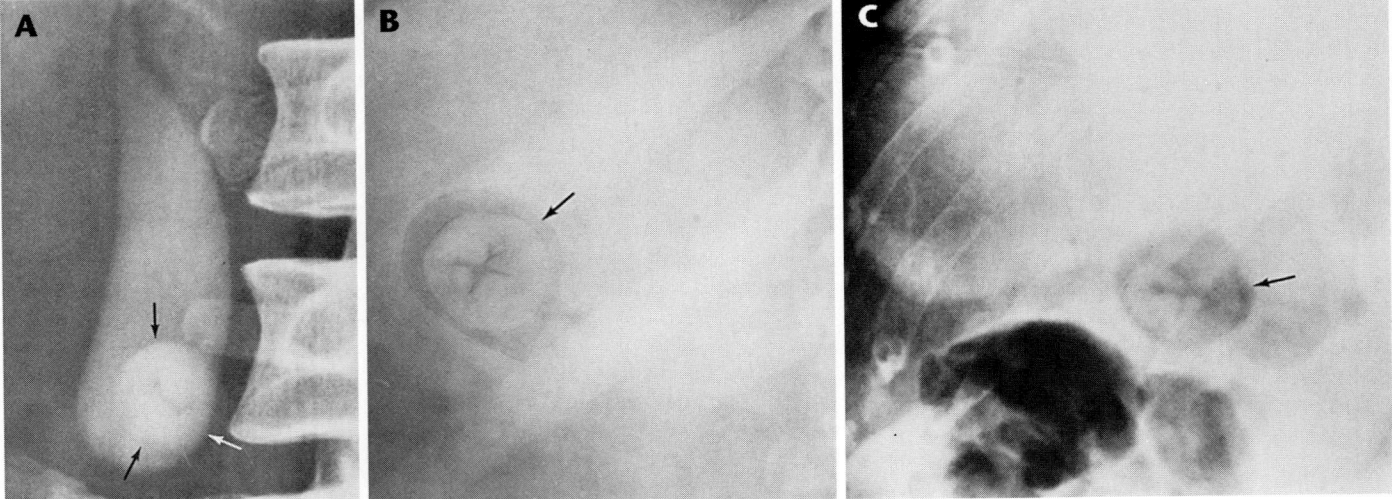

Figure 11–197. A, B, C, Three examples of the pylorus of the stomach, simulating a fissured biliary calculus. In **B** and **C** the air in the duodenal bulb simulates emphysematous cholecystitis with stone.

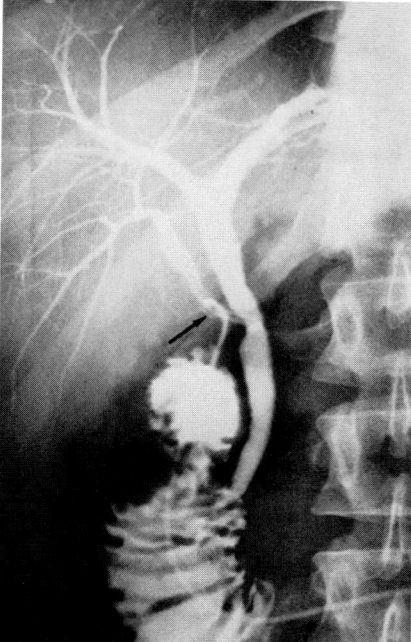

Figure 11–198. Accessory hepatic duct entering low in the common duct.

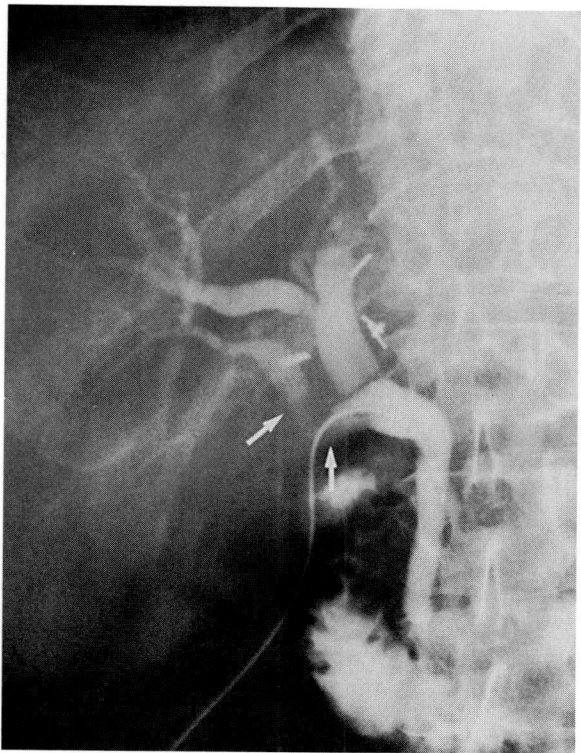

Figure 11–199. Accessory right hepatic duct.

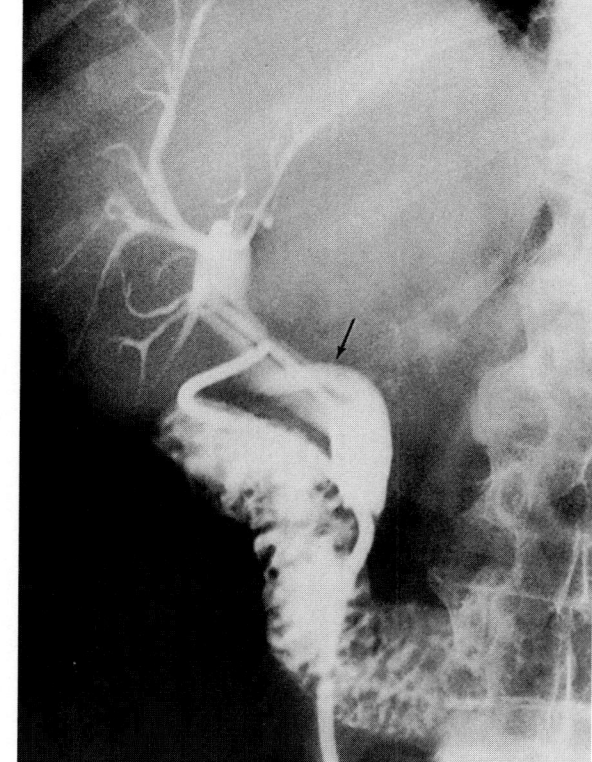

Figure 11–200. Intramural cystic duct remnant. This portion of the cystic duct lies within the wall of the common duct and is not detectable at cholecystectomy.

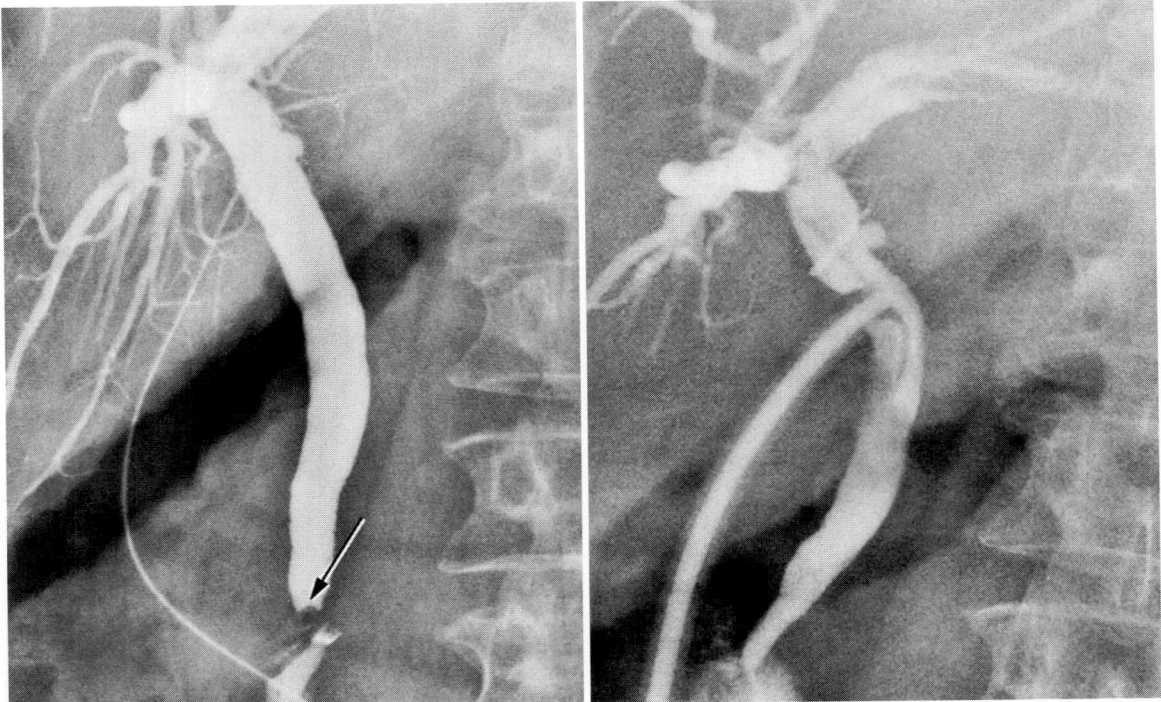

Figure 11–201. *Left,* Pseudocalculus sign seen in cholangiography is produced by muscular contraction of the distal end of the duct and should not be mistaken for a calculus. *Right,* Second film in the same examination does not show the defect. (Ref: Mujahed Z, Evans JA: Pseudocalculus defect in cholangiography. *Am J Roentgenol* 116:337, 1972.) The same defect may be seen on intravenous cholangiography. (Ref: Martinez LO, Cohen G: The pseudocalculus sign in intravenous cholangiography. *South Med J* 65:1066, 1972.)

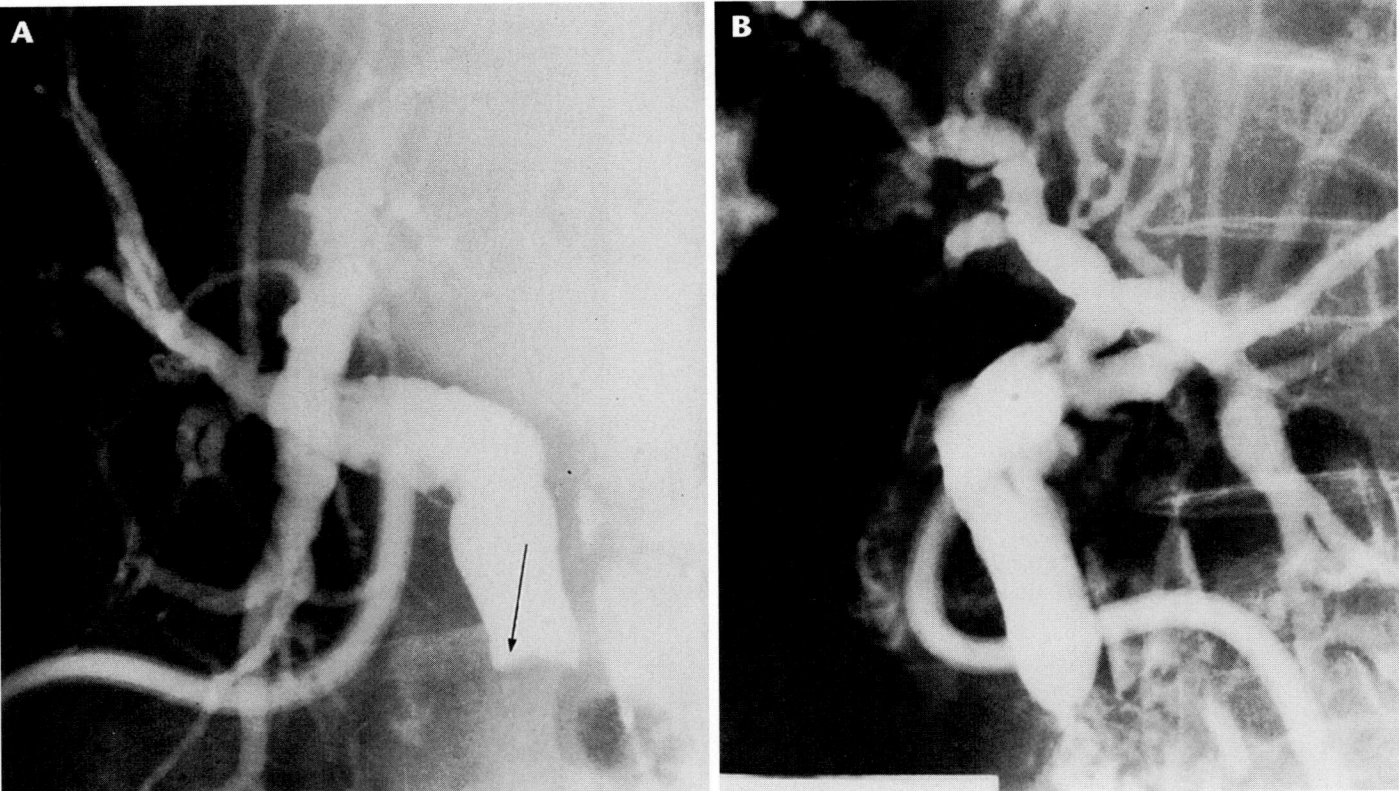

Figure 11–202. A, Pseudocalculus sign in a dilated biliary tree. **B,** Normal appearance after contraction has been relieved.

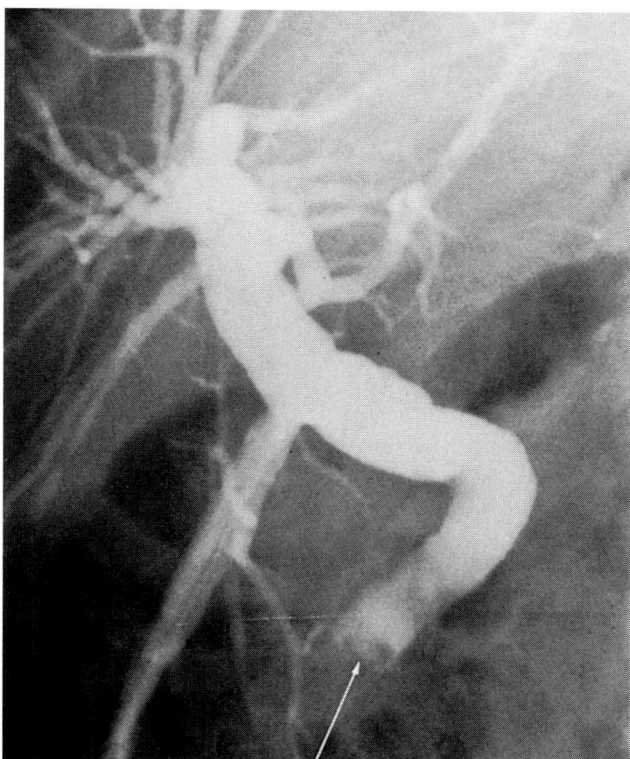

Figure 11–203. Pseudocalculus sign, with a small amount of contrast material in the duct, simulating a stone.

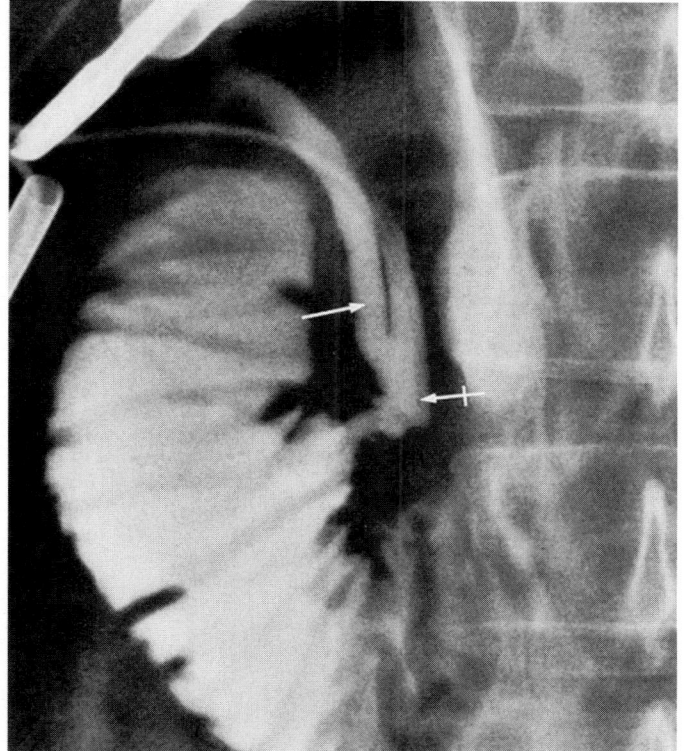

Figure 11–204. Low insertion of the cystic duct (←), resulting in a very short common duct (↔).

Figure 11–205. Duplication of the distal end of the pancreatic duct, shown by endoscopic retrograde cholangiopancreatography.

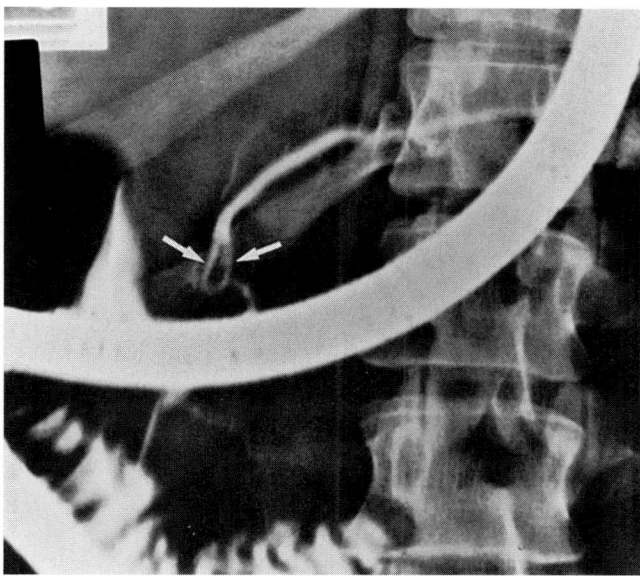

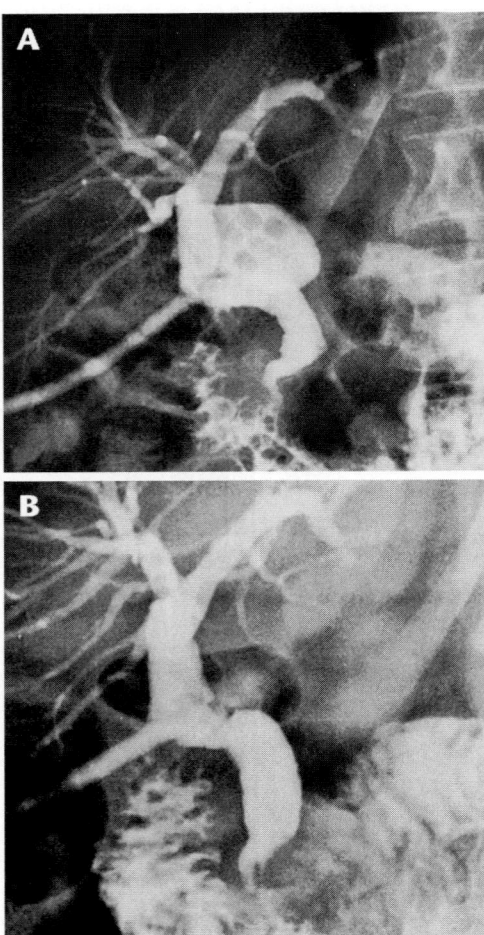

Figure 11–206. A, Contrast and food in the duodenal bulb simulate a gallbladder with stones on cholangiography. **B,** After peristalsis has cleared the duodenum.

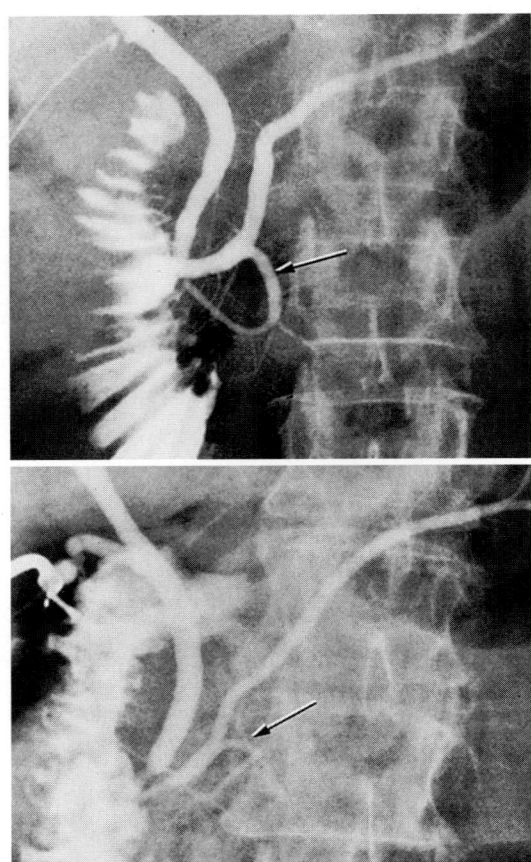

Figure 11–207. Two examples of the accessory duct of Santorini arising from the duct of Wirsung.

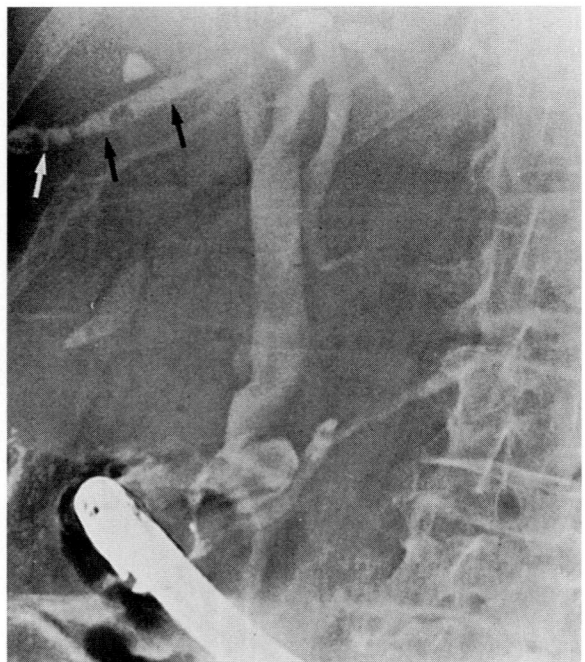

Figure 11–208. Costal cartilage mistaken for stones in the right hepatic duct.

CHAPTER

12

The Soft Tissues of the Pelvis

Pages
1136 to 1144

Figures
12–1 to 12–31

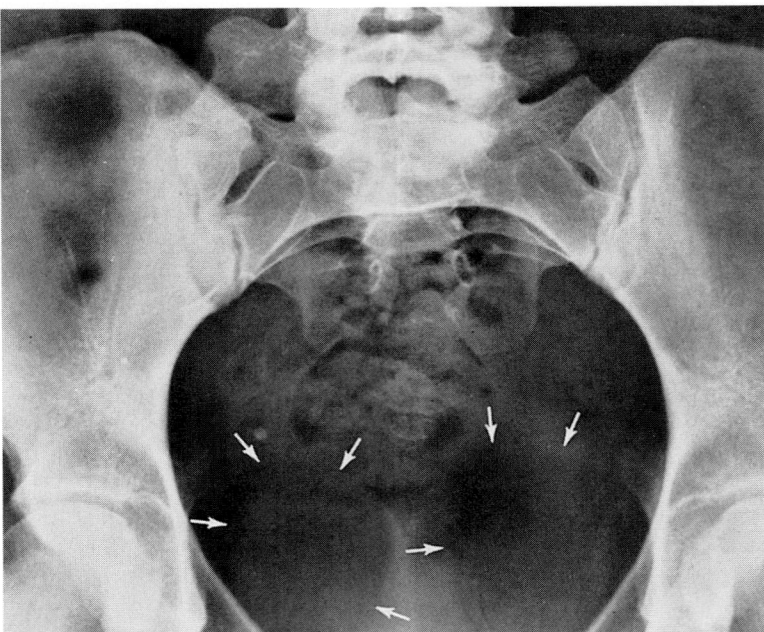

Figure 12–1. Circular areas of radiolucency caused by fat in the buttocks.

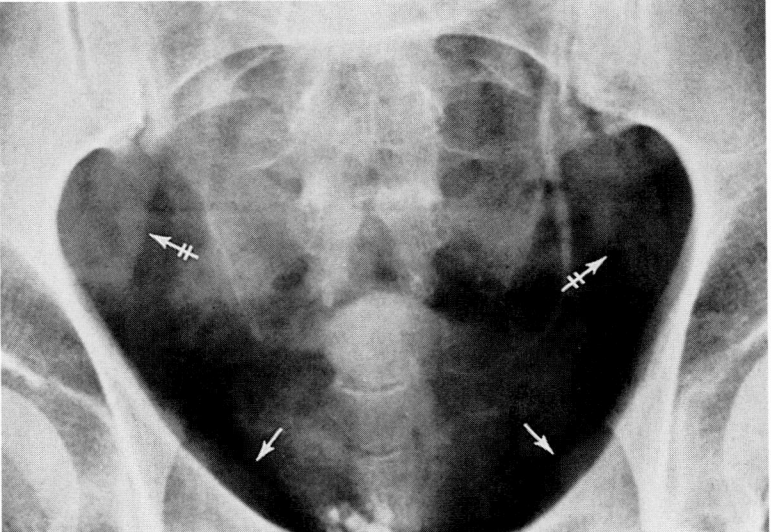

Figure 12–2. Shadows of the levator ani muscles (←). The obturator internus muscles are also seen (↤). (Ref: Levene G, Kaufman JA: The diagnostic significance of roentgenologic soft tissue shadows in the pelvis. *Am J Roentgenol* 79:697, 1958.)

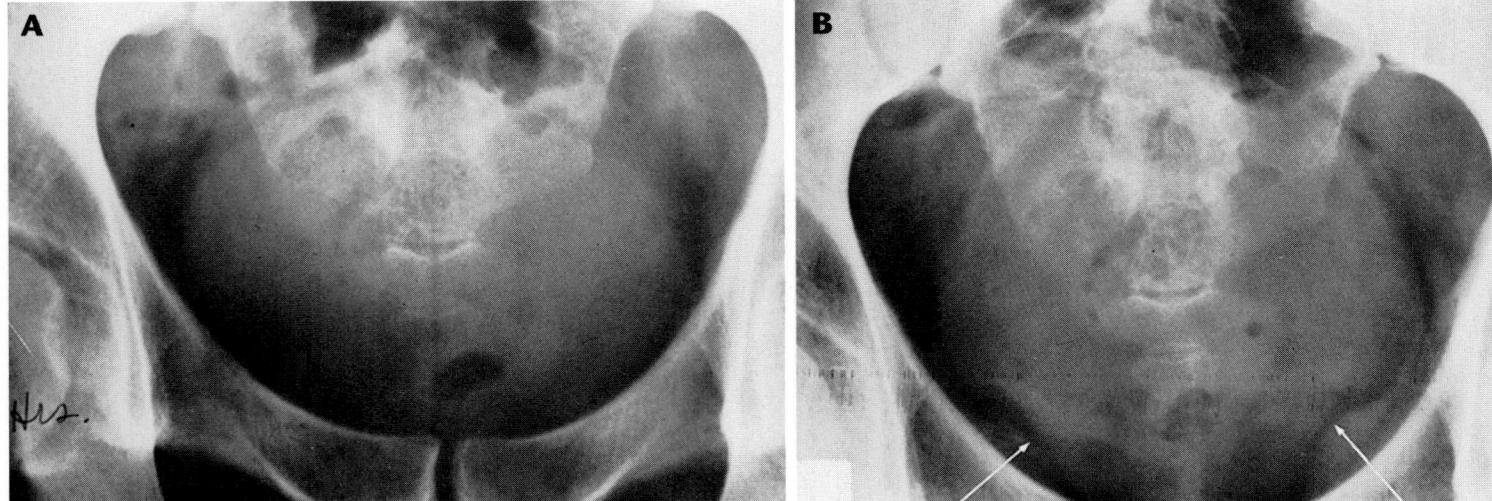

Figure 12–3. Contraction of the levator ani muscles will produce evanescent shadows in the pelvis in a given patient. **A,** Levator ani muscles not seen. **B,** Same patient with muscle contractions, showing intrusion of the bladder outline.

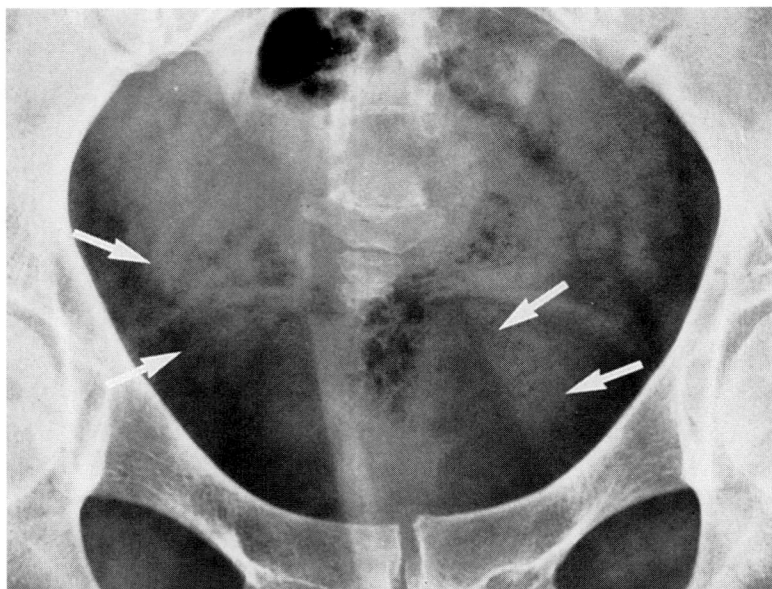

Figure 12–4. Stripes of radiolucency caused by fat accumulations between the muscle bundles of the gluteus maximus.

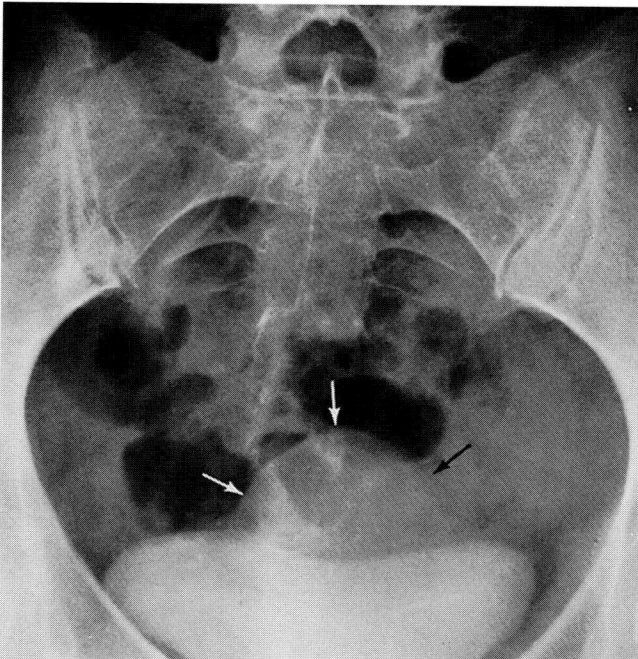

Figure 12–5. Shadow of the uterus seen indenting the superior aspect of the urinary bladder.

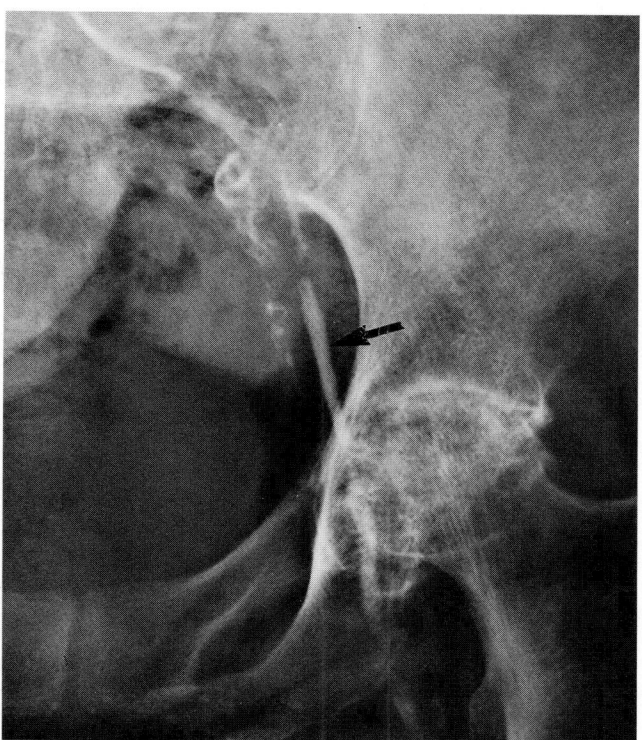

Figure 12–6. Calcified venous thrombus in the iliac vein.

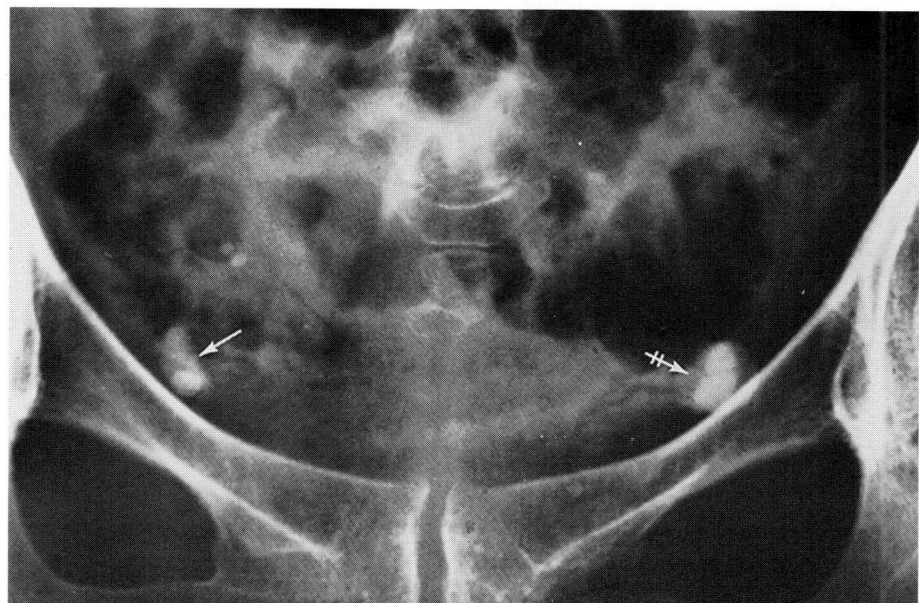

Figure 12–7. Unusual configuration of pelvic phleboliths, elongated on the patient's right (←) and bifid on the left (⊬).

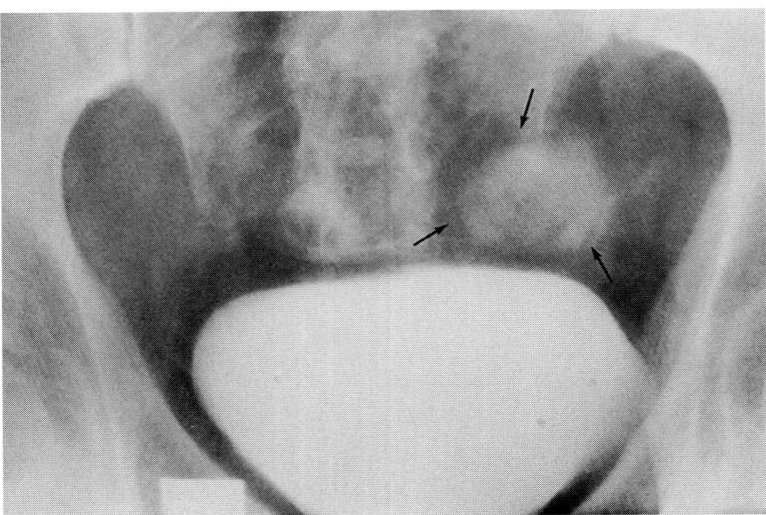

Figure 12–8. Sigmoid colon simulating a pelvic mass.

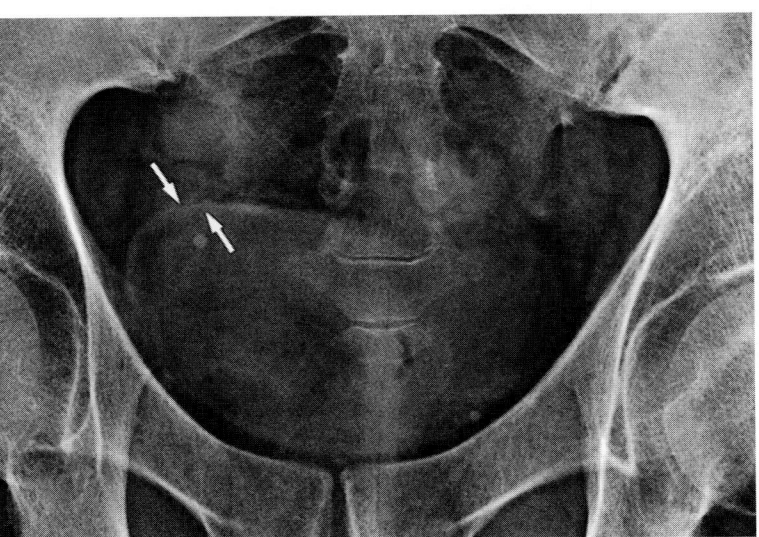

Figure 12–9. Visualization of the bladder wall as a result of the difference in radiographic density between muscle and urine.

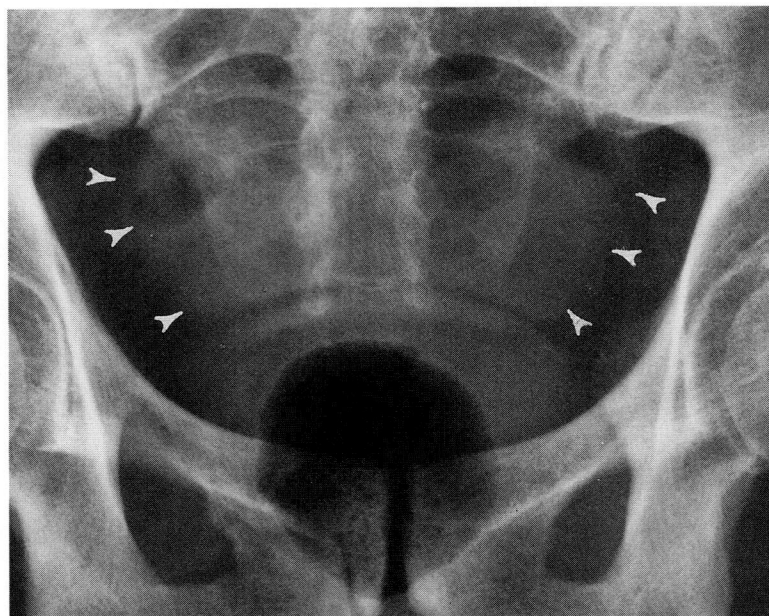

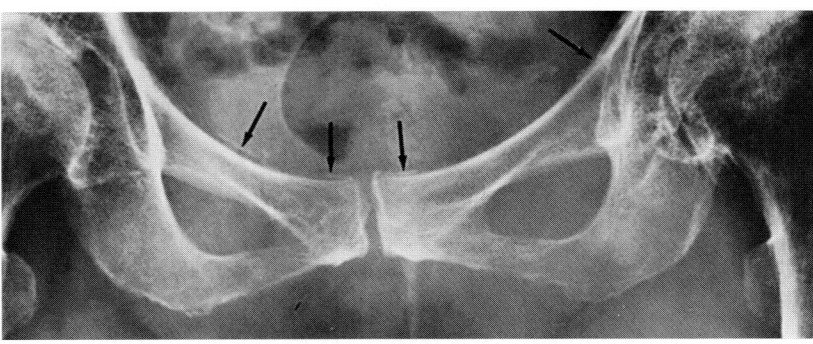
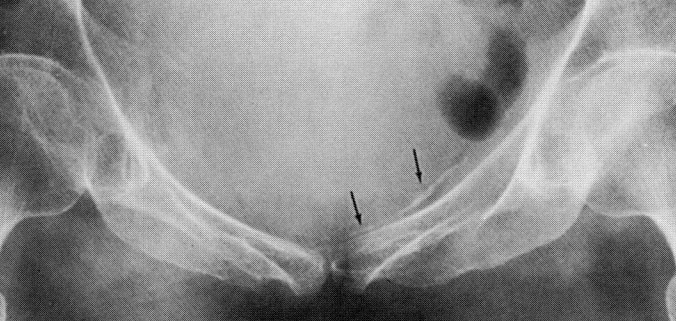

Figure 12–10. Fluid-filled loops of small bowel may simulate the "dog ear" sign of intraperitoneal fluid.

Figure 12–11. Examples of calcification in Cooper's ligament. This is seen in the elderly as an unusual form of physiologic calcification. (Ref: Steinfeld JR et al: Calcification in Cooper's ligament. *Am J Roentgenol* 121:107, 1974.)

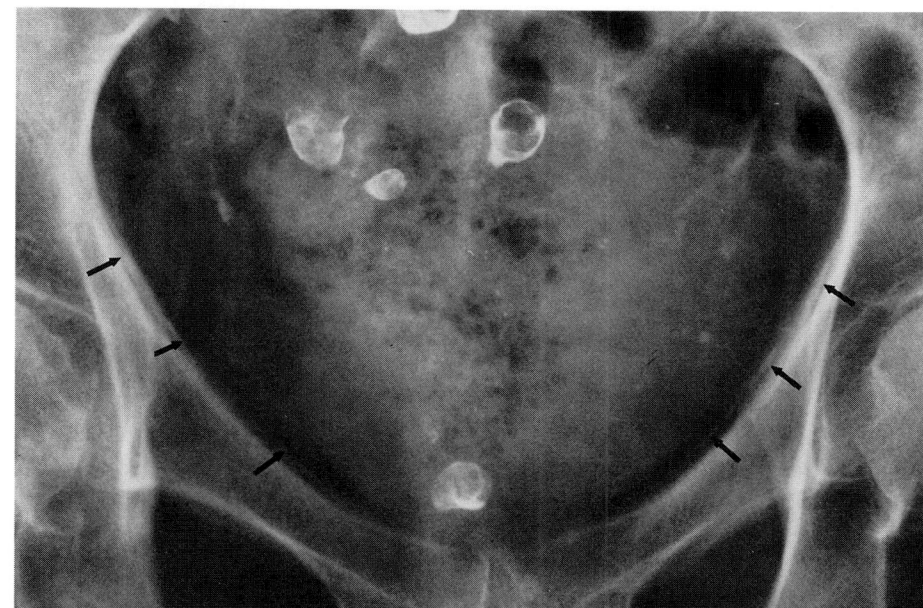

Figure 12–12. Unusually extensive calcification in Cooper's ligament.

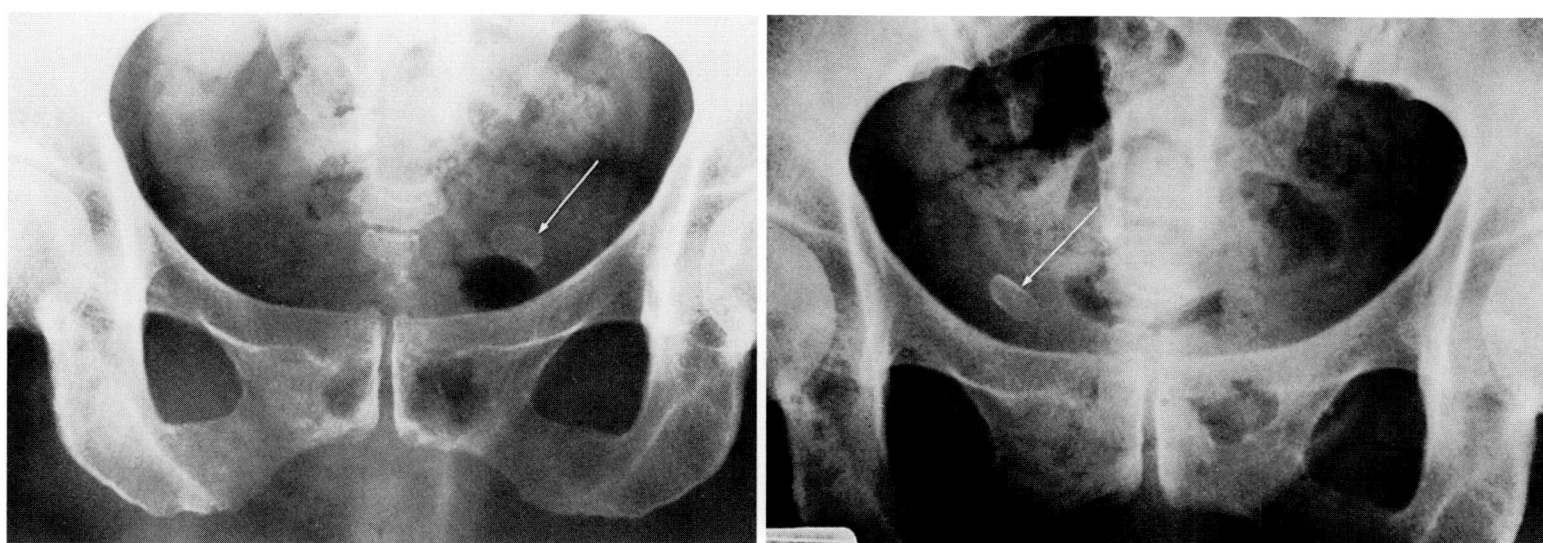

Figure 12–13. Calcified epiploic appendages that have fallen into the pelvis will shift from side to side, as illustrated in this patient. (Refs: Holt JF, MacIntyre RS: Calcified omental fat deposits: Their roentgenologic significance. *Am J Roentgenol* 60:612, 1984; Borg SA et al: A mobile calcified amputated appendix epiploica. *Am J Roentgenol* 127:349, 1976.)

Figure 12–14. Densities in the right side of the pelvis representing ingested bone meal. This appearance might be misinterpreted as psammomatous calcification of an ovarian malignancy. (Ref: Schabel S, Rogers CI: Opaque artifacts in a health faddist simulating ovarian neoplasm. *Am J Roentgenol* 130:789, 1978.)

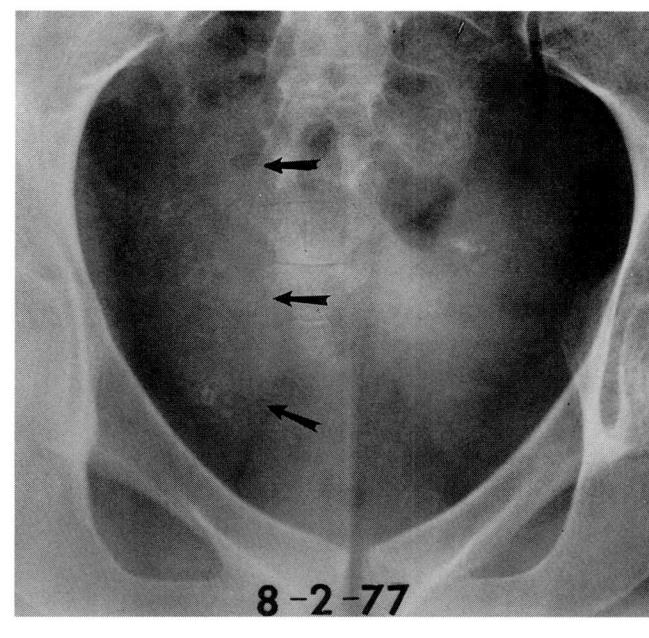

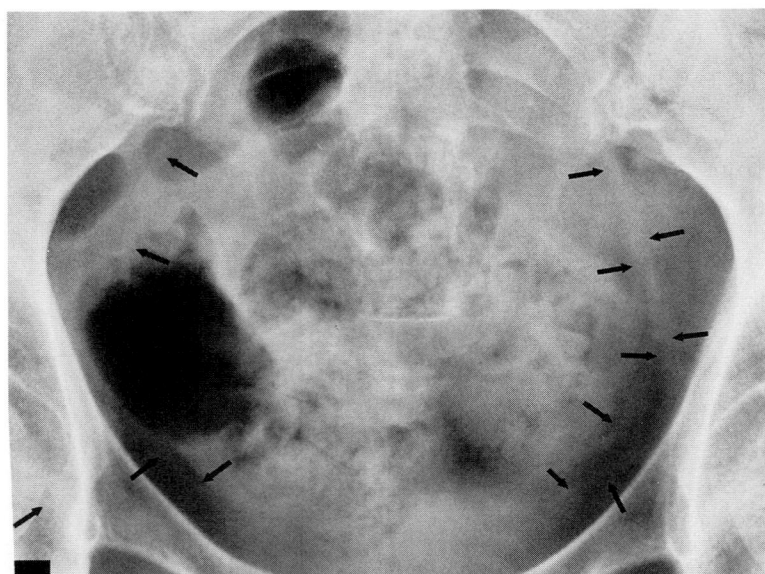

Figure 12–15. Visualization of the ureters without contrast by virtue of periureteral fat.

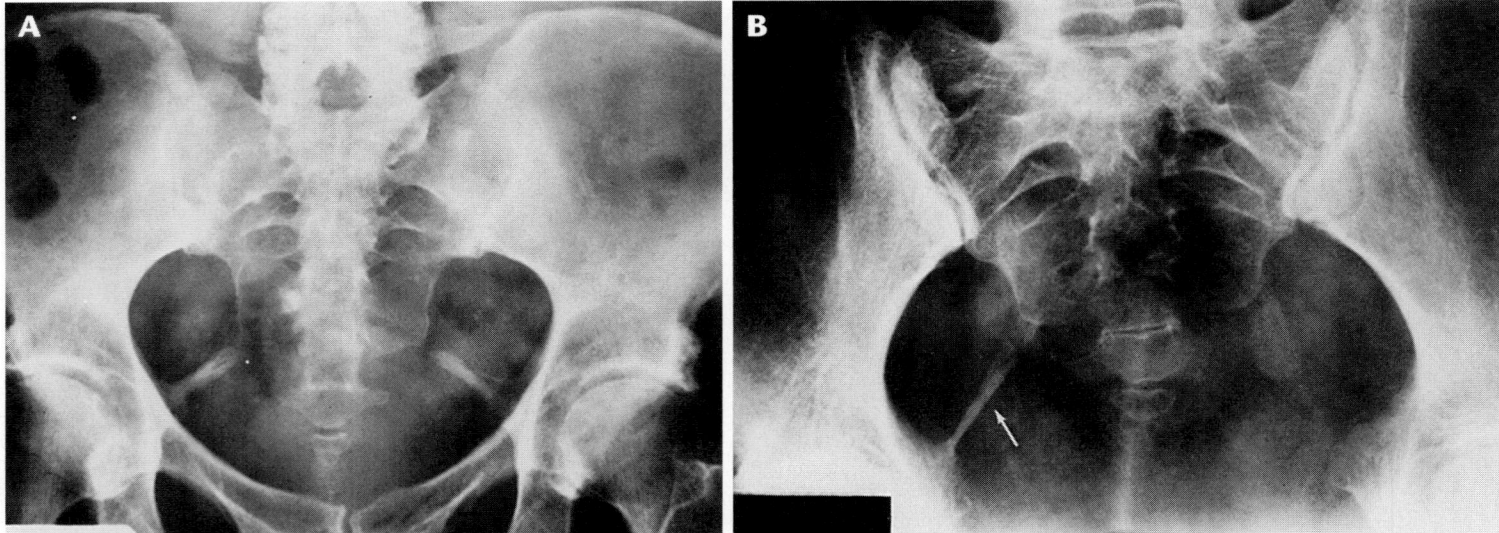

Figure 12–16. A and **B,** Examples of calcification of the sacrospinous ligaments.

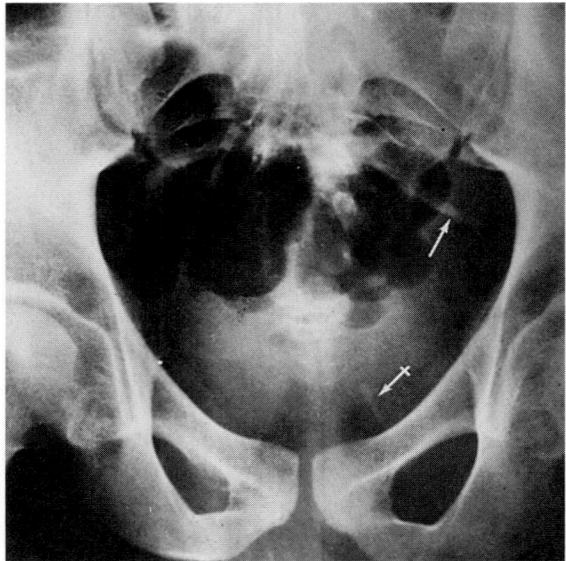

Figure 12–17. Calcification in the anterior sacral ligament (→) and in the sacrotuberous ligament (↦).

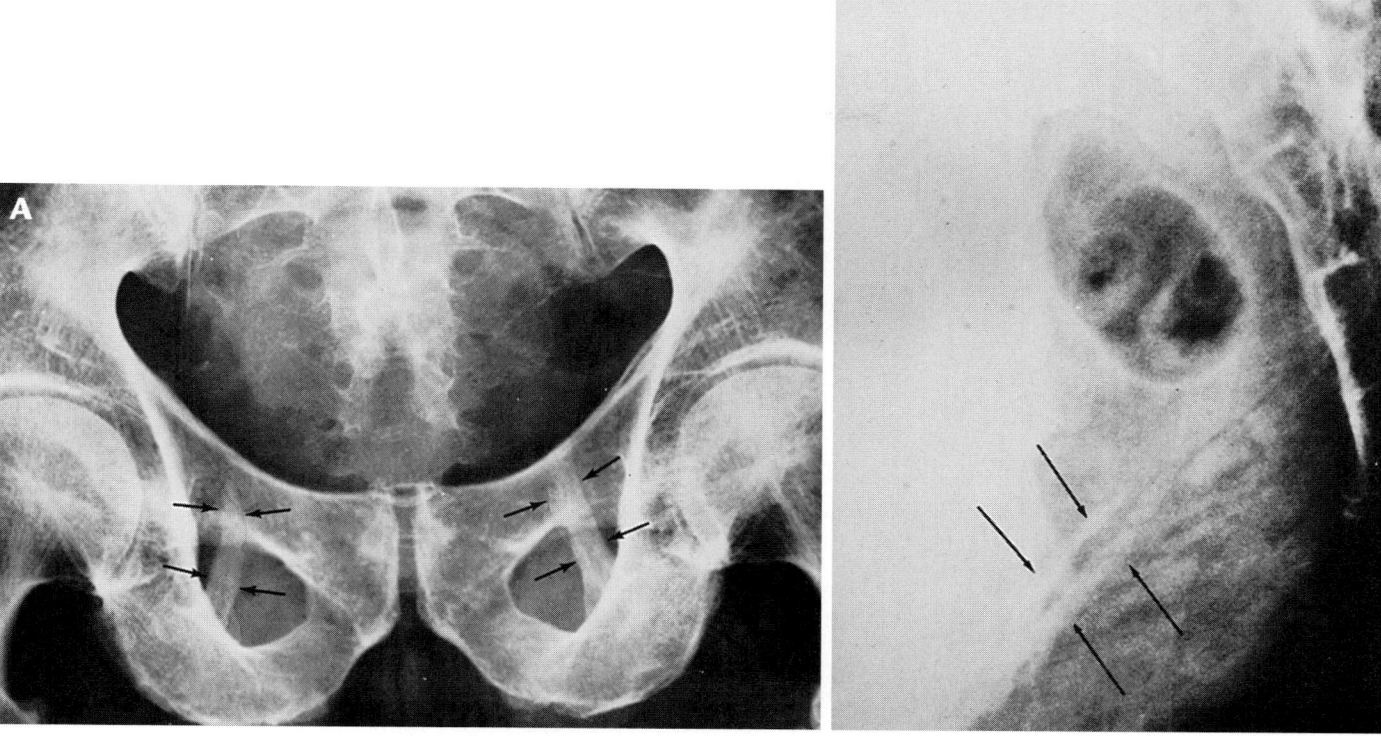

Figure 12–18. Calcification of the sacrotuberous ligaments. **A,** Frontal projection. **B,** Lateral projection.

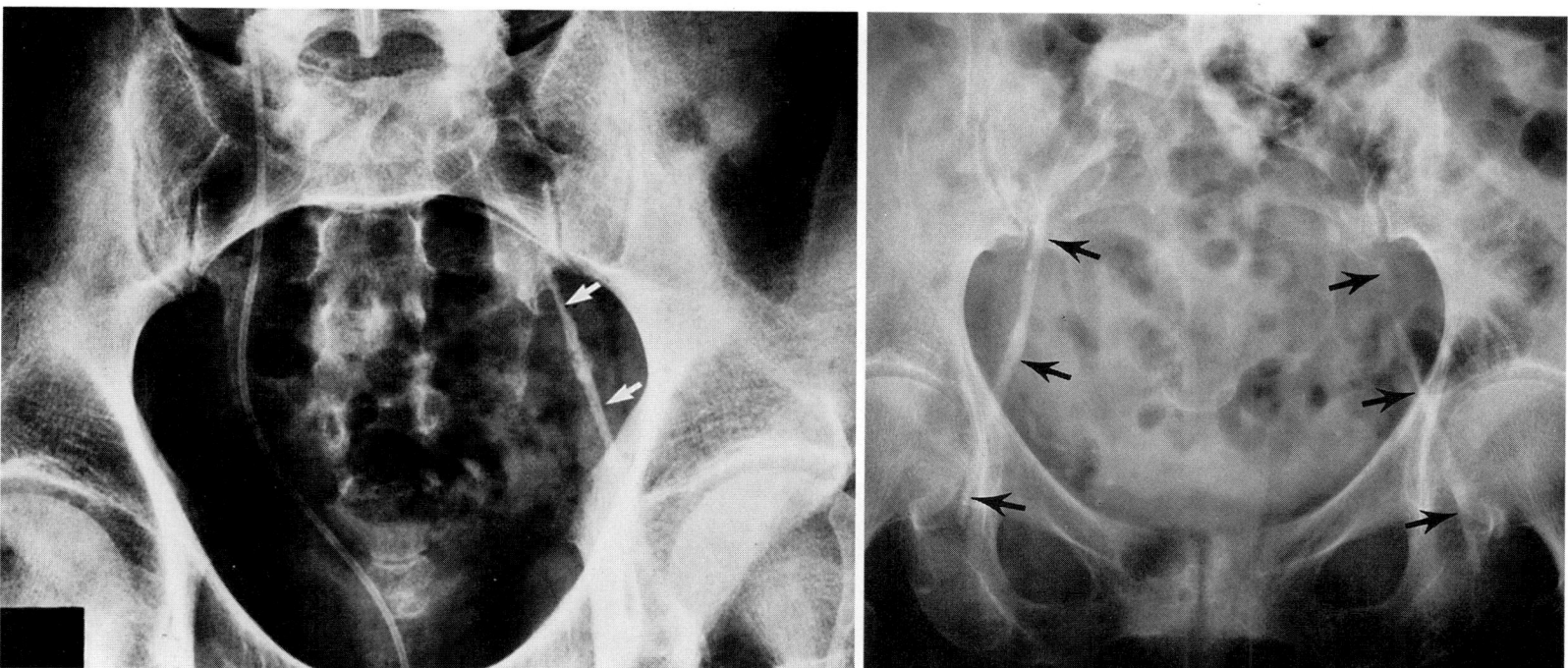

Figure 12–19. Long linear calcification of the sacrotuberous ligaments.

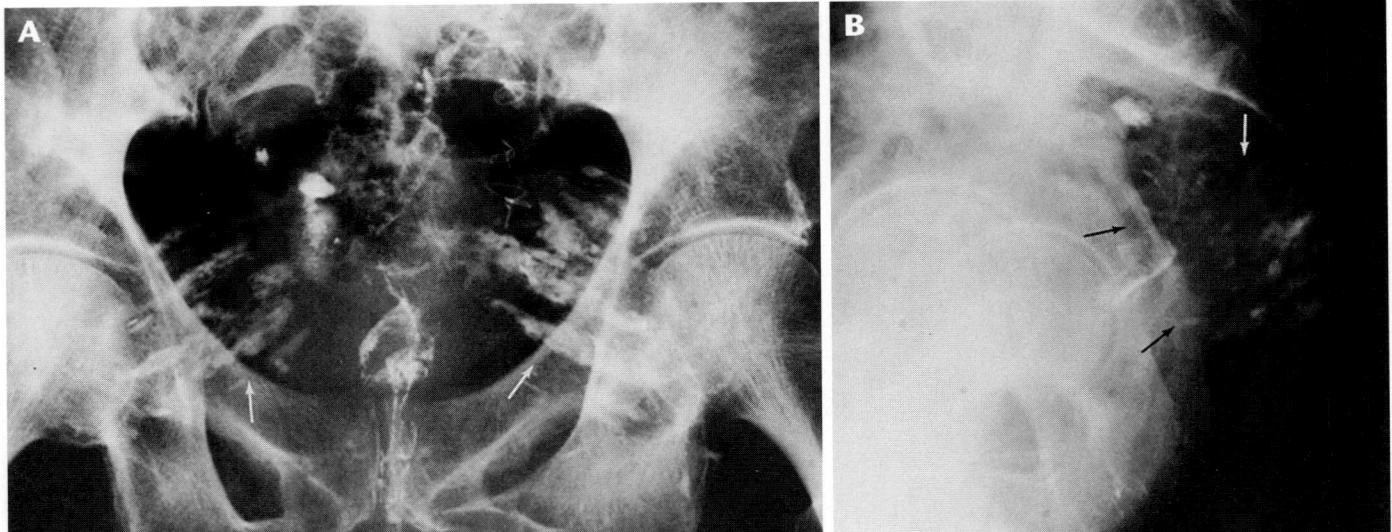

Figure 12–20. Calcification in the piriform muscles in an 82-year-old woman.

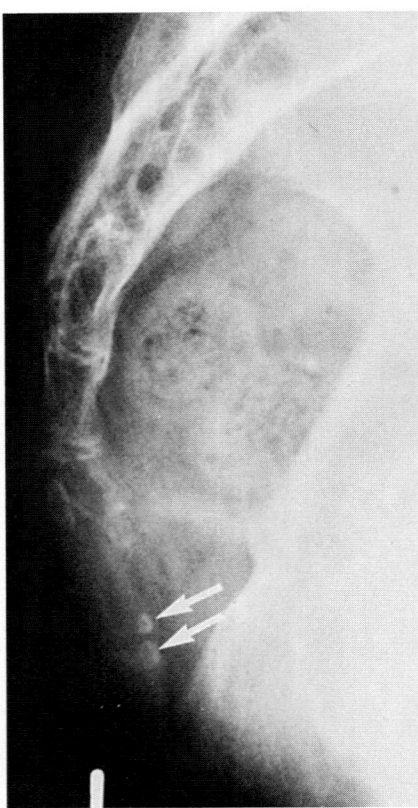

Figure 12–21. Calcification, probably within the coccygoanal ligament.

Figure 12–22. Calcification in the inferior pubic ligaments.

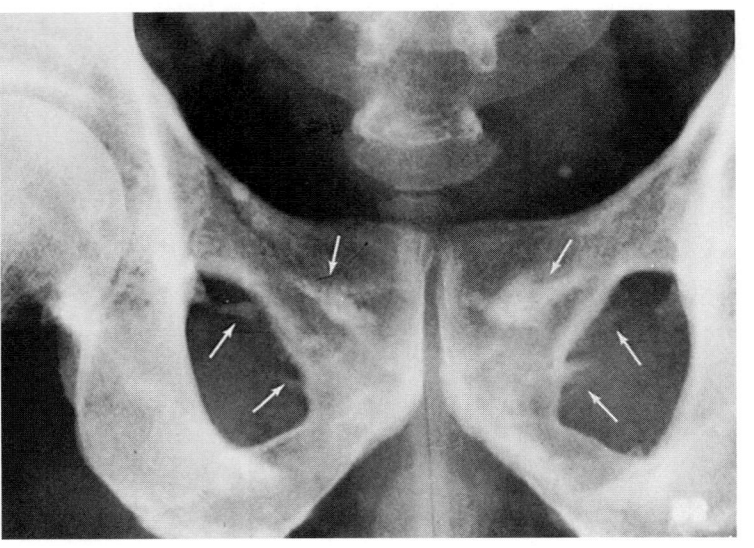

Figure 12–23. Ossification of the obturator foramen. (Ref: Birkner R, Consentius K: Ossification of the obturator foramen. *ROFO* 127:72, 1977.)

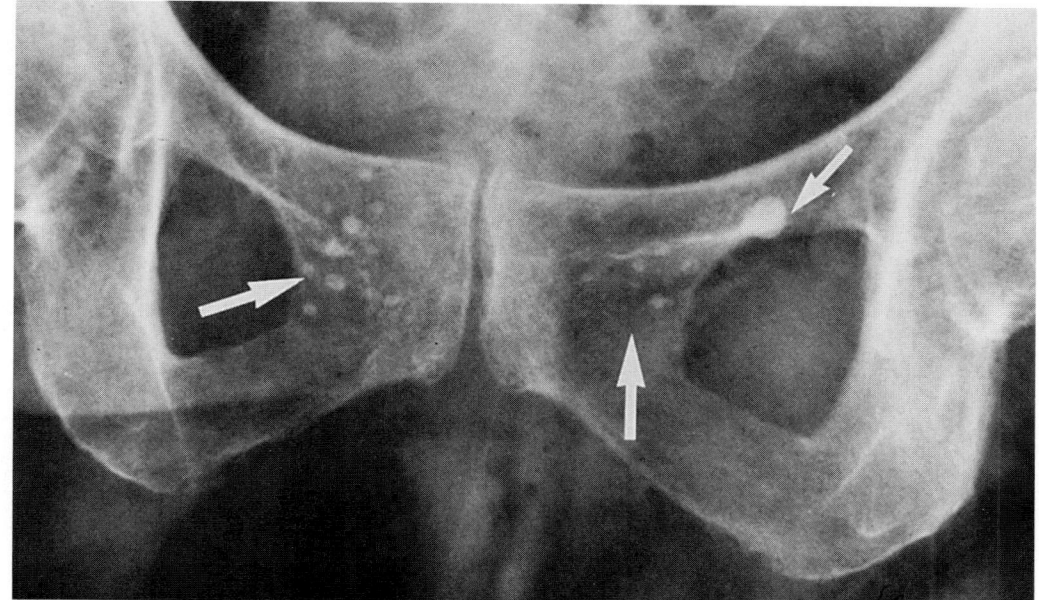

Figure 12–24. Multiple pelvic phleboliths of varying sizes.

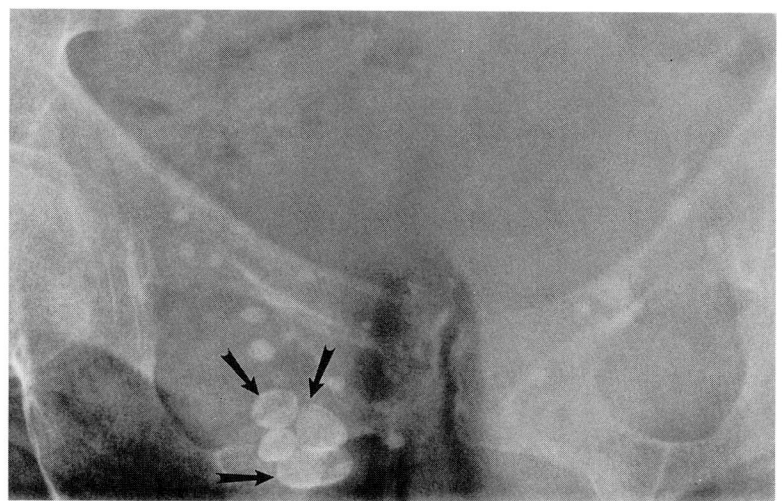

Figure 12–25. Huge phleboliths in a 94-year-old woman.

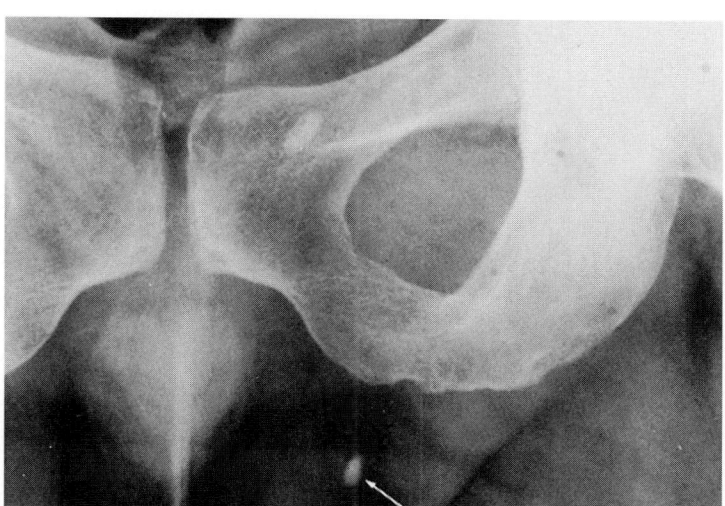

Figure 12–26. Phlebolith in the spermatic cord.

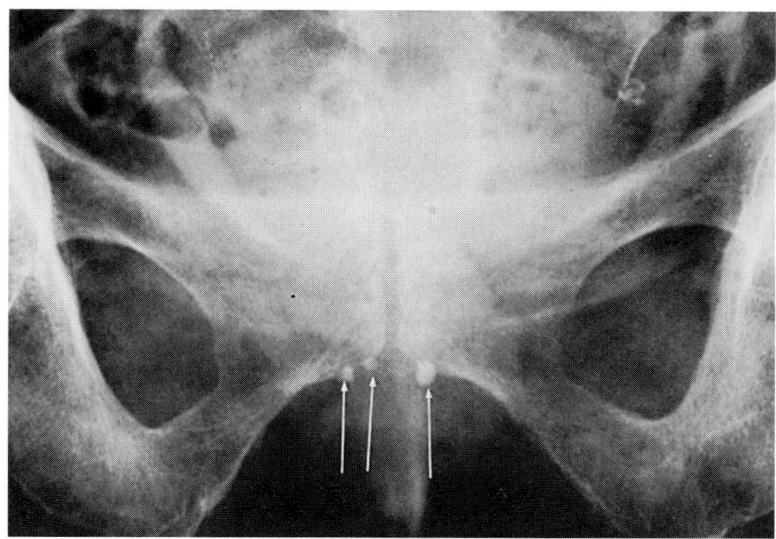

Figure 12–27. Vulvar phleboliths.

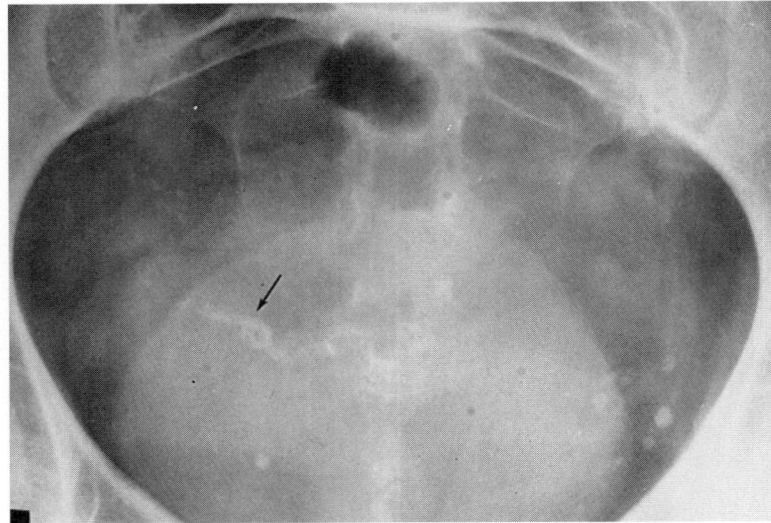

Figure 12–28. Calcification of the uterine arteries in an elderly woman.

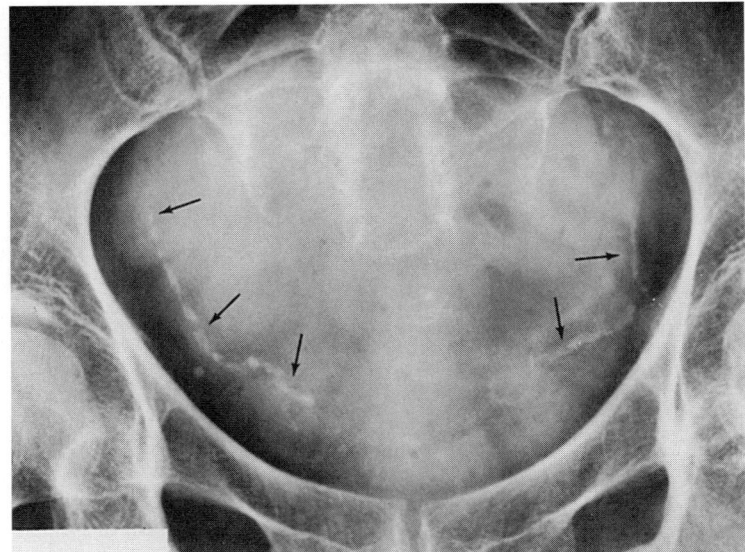

Figure 12–29. Calcification of the fallopian tubes in an elderly woman.

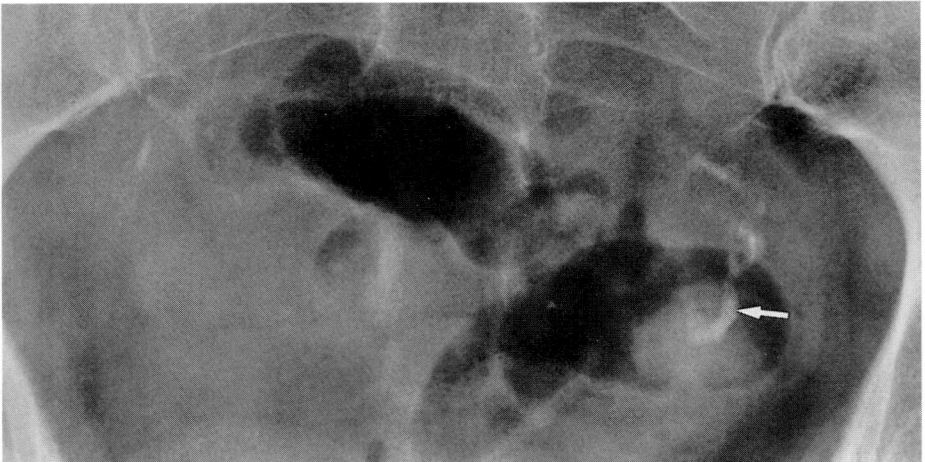

Figure 12–30. Unilateral calcification of the fallopian tube in an 80-year-old woman.

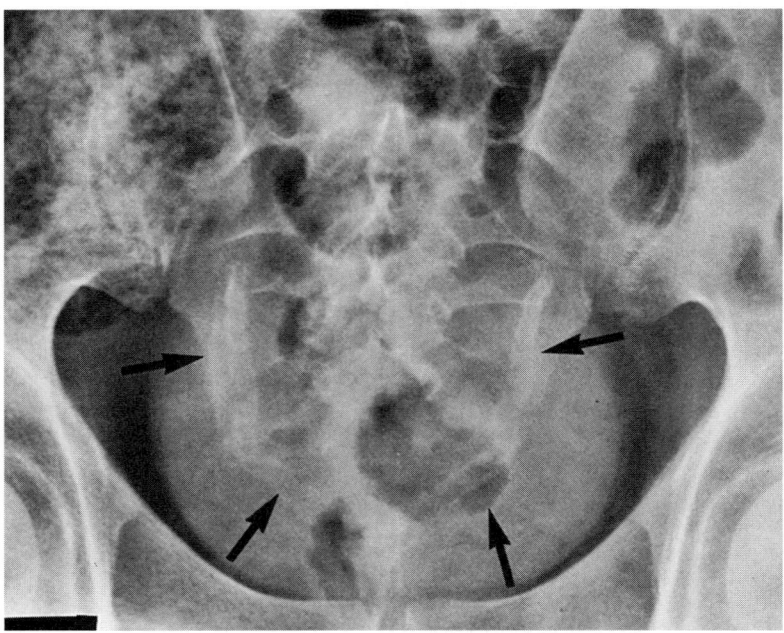

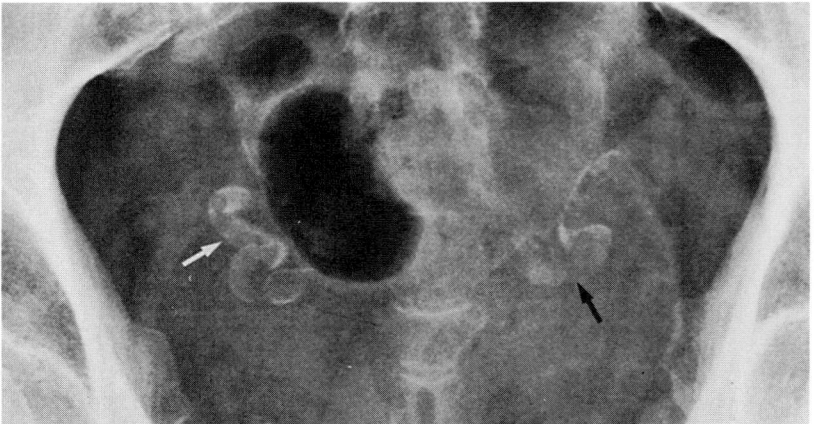

Figure 12–31. Two examples of calcified seminal vesicles. *Left,* 50-year-old man. *Right,* 71-year-old man.

CHAPTER 13

The Genitourinary Tract

The Kidneys

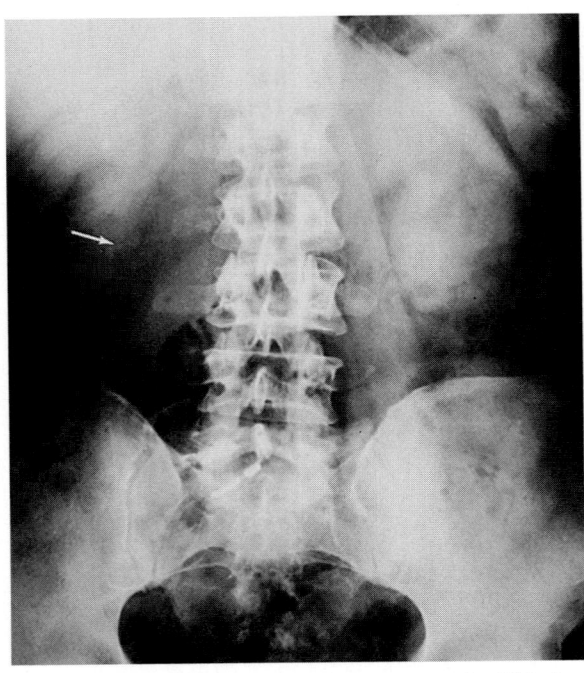

Figure 13–1. Apparent absence of one psoas muscle. This is seen in many normal individuals and is not necessarily of significance. (Ref: Elkin M, Cohen G: Diagnostic value of psoas shadow. *Clin Radiol* 13:210 1962.) Asymmetry of the psoas muscle is quite common and is usually of no clinical significance. (Ref: Goldfeld M, Loberant N: Unilateral "Vanishing Psoas": An anatomic variant. *Clin Imaging* 17:104, 1993.)

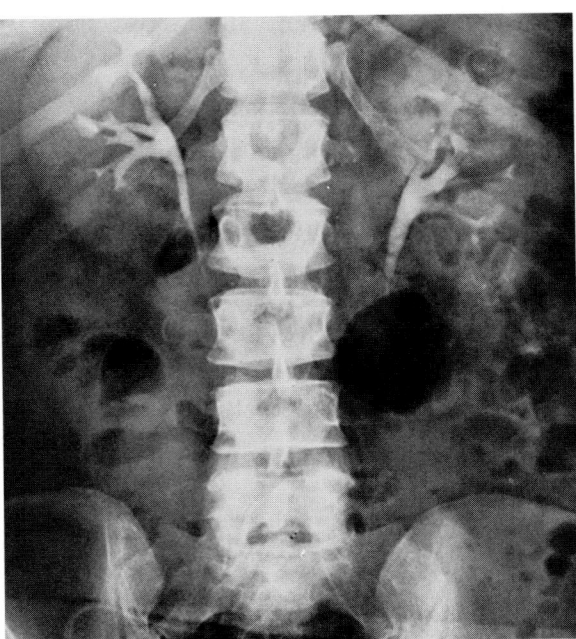

Figure 13–2. Low-lying left kidney. The left kidney lies at a level lower than the right in 5% of normal individuals. This finding is not therefore necessarily indicative of displacement. (Ref: McClelland RE: A low-lying left kidney. *J Urol* 75:198, 1956.)

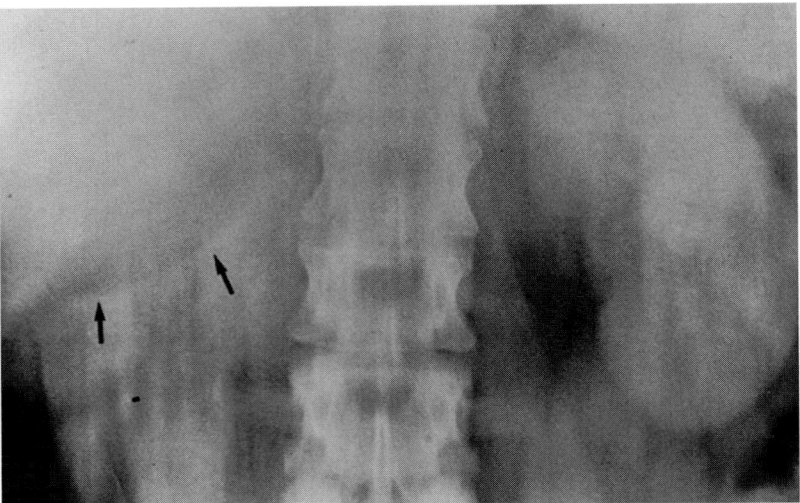

Figure 13–3. Costophrenic sulcus and the edge of the lung producing an unusual appearance in the nephrogram of the right kidney.

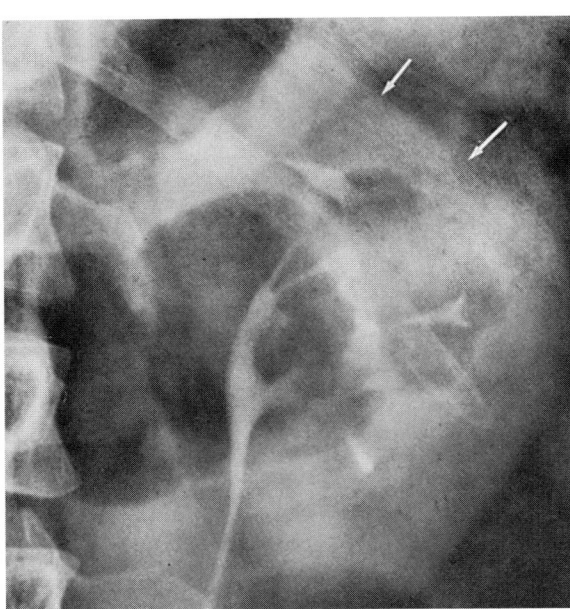

Figure 13–4. Splenic impression (←) on the left kidney that produces a "bump" in its midportion. (Ref: Olutola PO et al: Unusual renal distortion and displacement due to the spleen. *Pediatr Radiol* 12:185, 1982.)

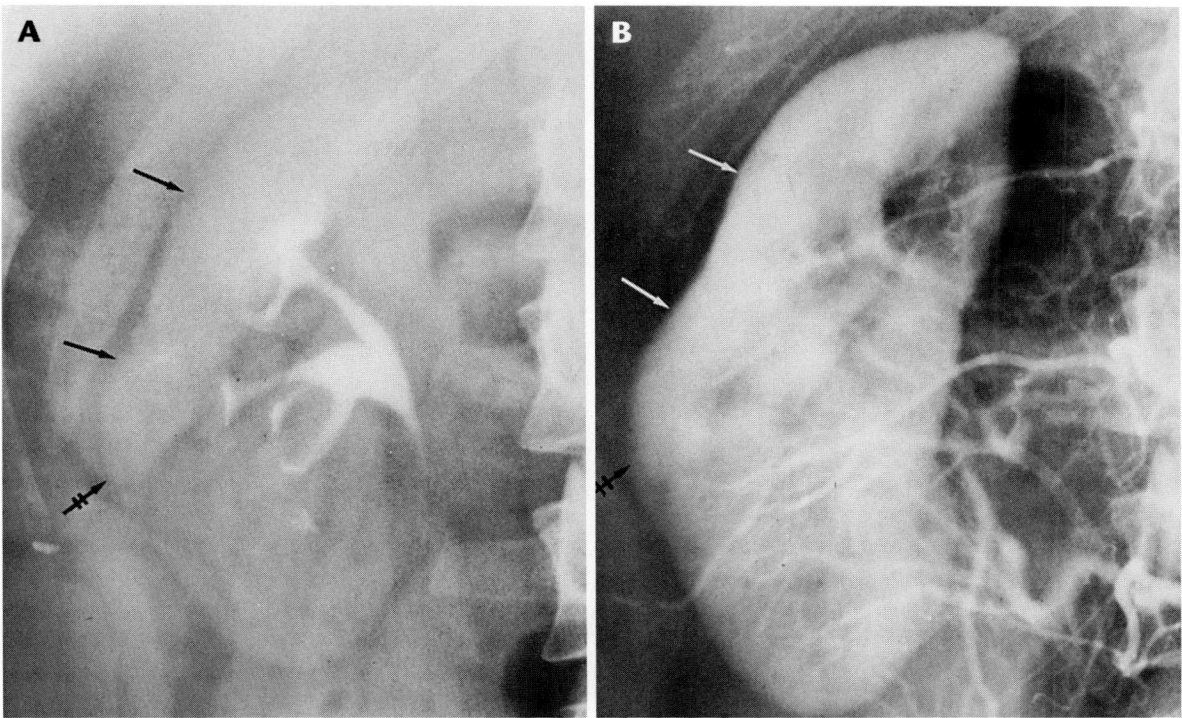

Figure 13–5. Hepatic impression (←) on the right kidney that produces a "bump" in its midportion (⊬). **A,** Urogram. **B,** Angiogram. (Ref: Doppman JL, Shapiro R: Some normal renal variants. *Am J Roentgenol* 92:1380, 1964.)

Figure 13–6. Fetal lobulation of the kidneys.

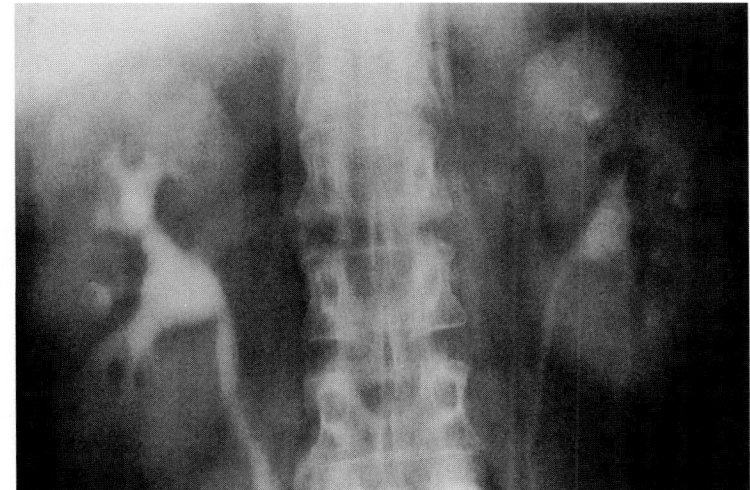

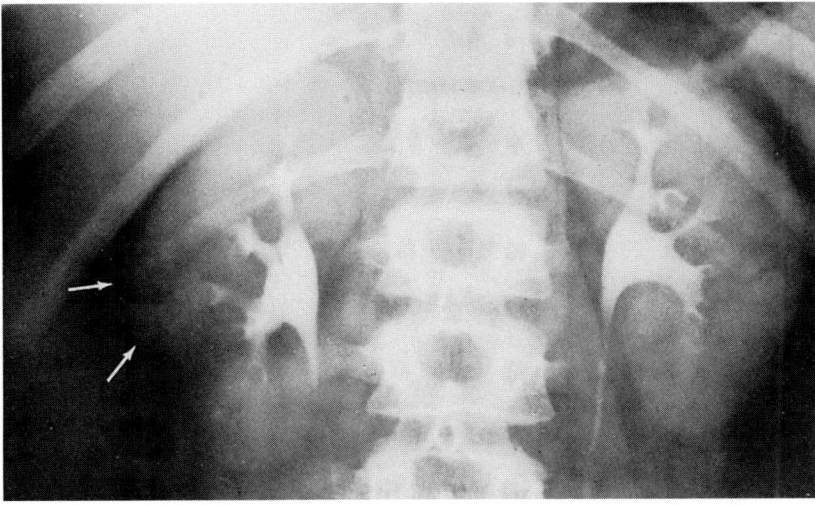

Figure 13–7. Nonsignificant variation in the outline of the right kidney.

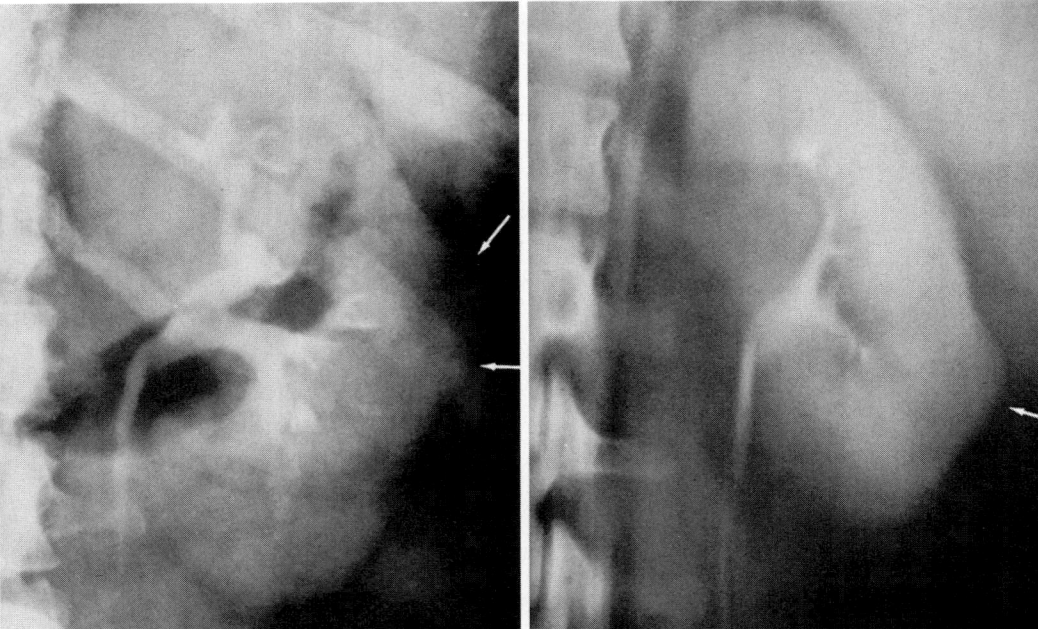

Figure 13–8. Two examples of the dromedary left kidney, an anatomic variation that simulates a mass lesion. (Ref: Harrow BP, Sloane JA: The dromedary left kidney. *Am J Roentgenol* 88:148, 1962.)

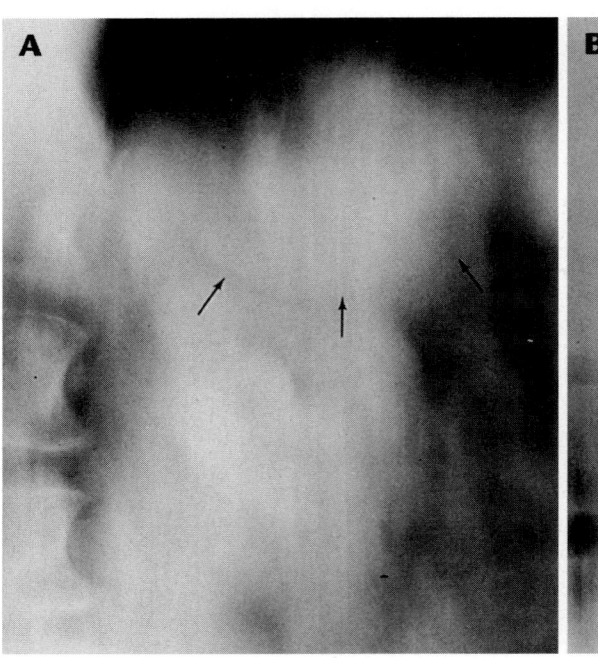
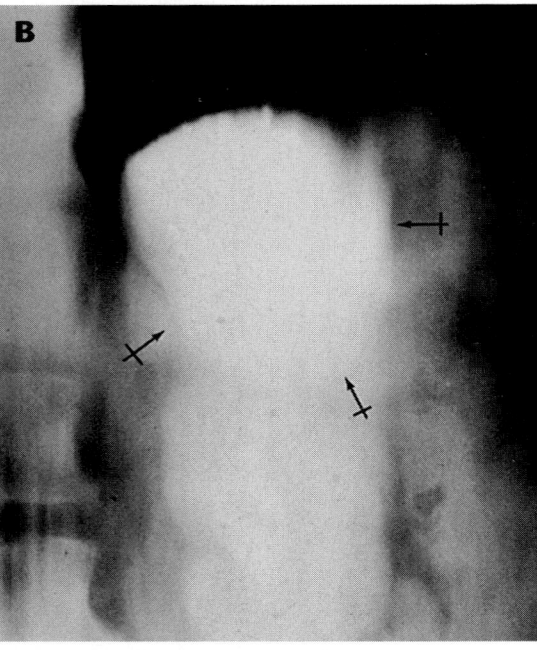

Figure 13–9. Gastric fundus simulating a suprarenal mass. **A,** Before ingestion of barium. **B,** After ingestion of barium. (Ref: Martire JR, Goldman SM: Left supra-renal pseudotumor. *Radiats Biol Radioecol* 17:12, 1977.) This pseudotumor may opacify on angiography and further obscure its proper identification. (Ref: Bjorn-Hansen RW, O'Brien DS: Aortographic opacification of the gastric fundus simulating neoplasm. *Am J Roentgenol* 100:408, 1967.)

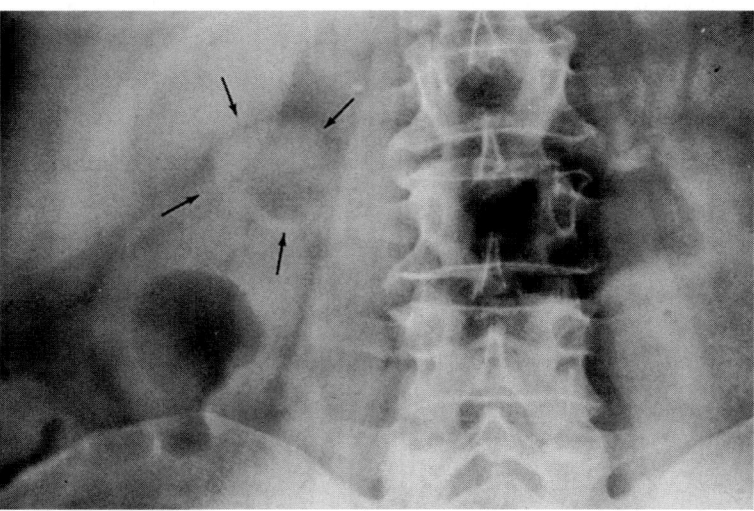
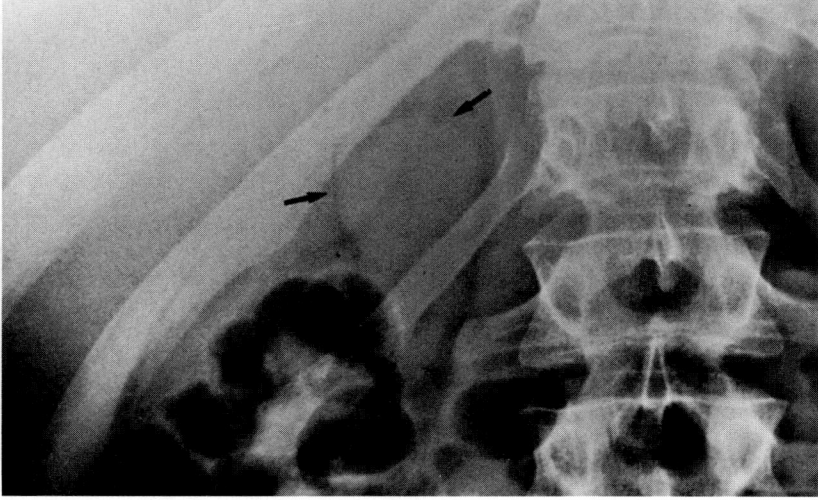

Figure 13–10. Two examples of spurious suprarenal masses produced by the duodenal bulb. *Left,* Fluid and air filled. *Right,* Fluid filled.

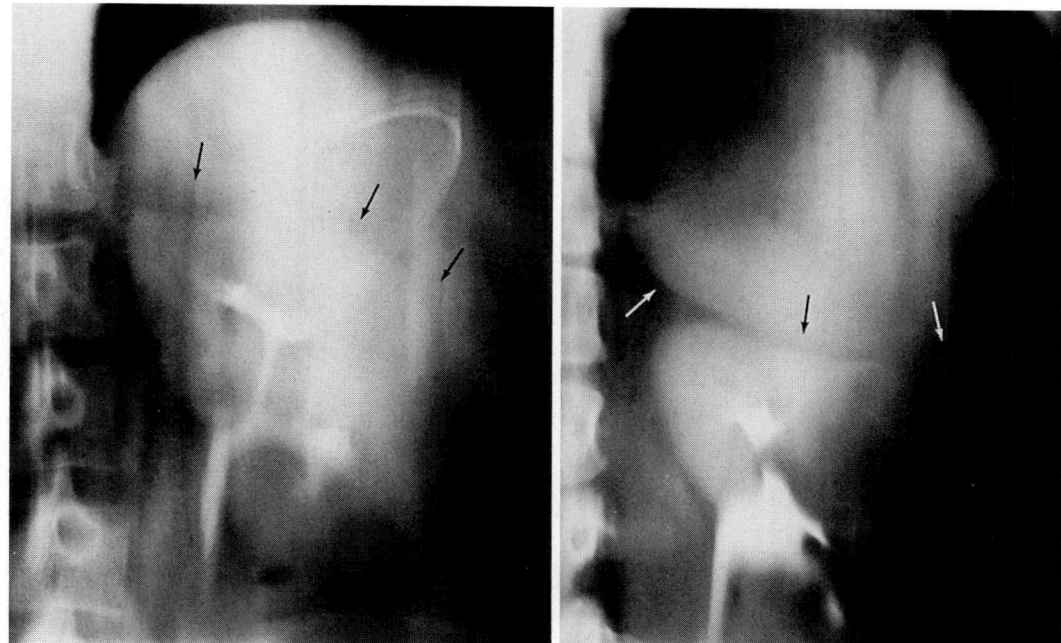

Figure 13–11. Two examples of renal pseudotumors produced by the spleen. (Ref: Madayag M et al: Renal and suprarenal pseudotumors caused by variations of the spleen. *Radiology* 105:43, 1972.)

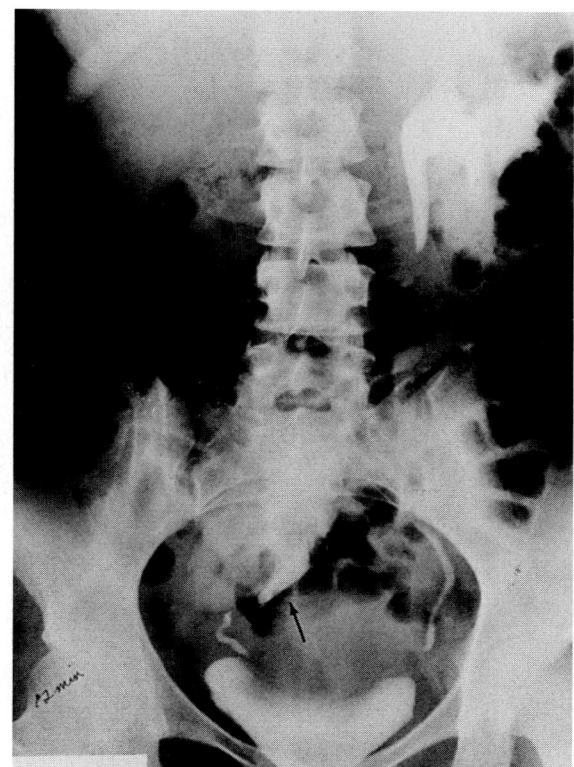

Figure 13–12. Pelvic kidney.

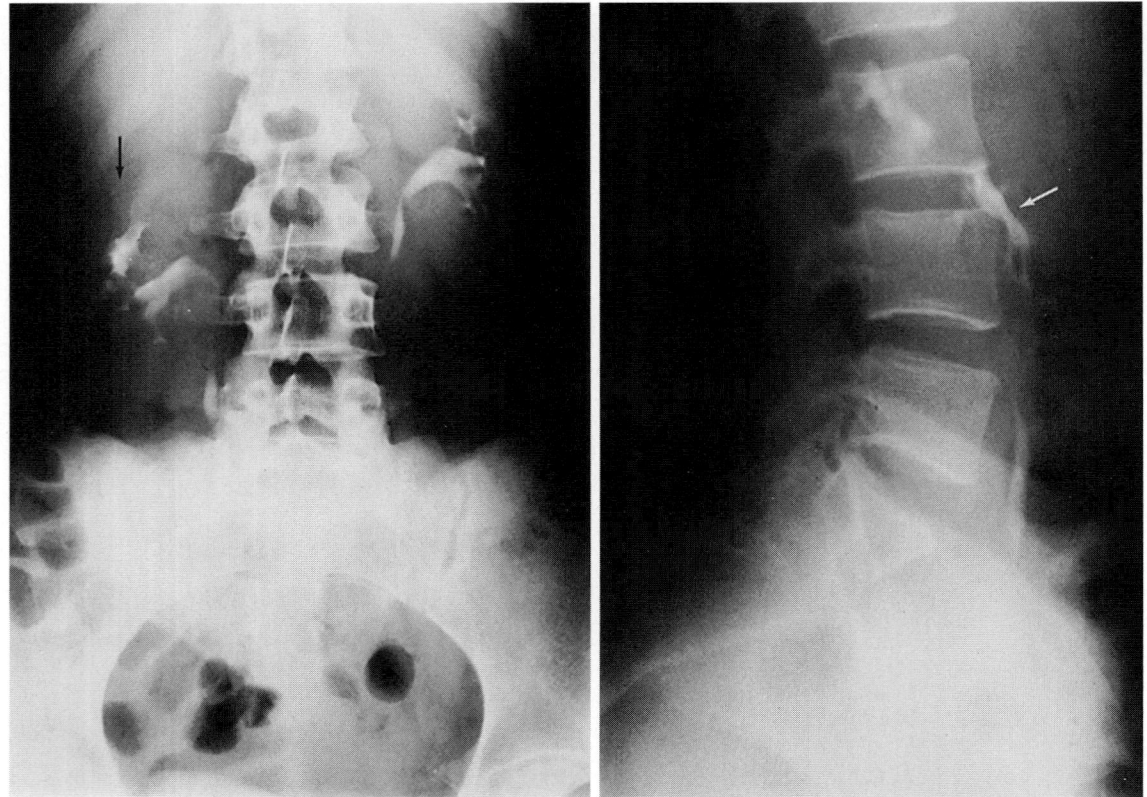

Figure 13–13. Ptotic right kidney. Note the configuration of its collecting system and its position in the lateral projection.

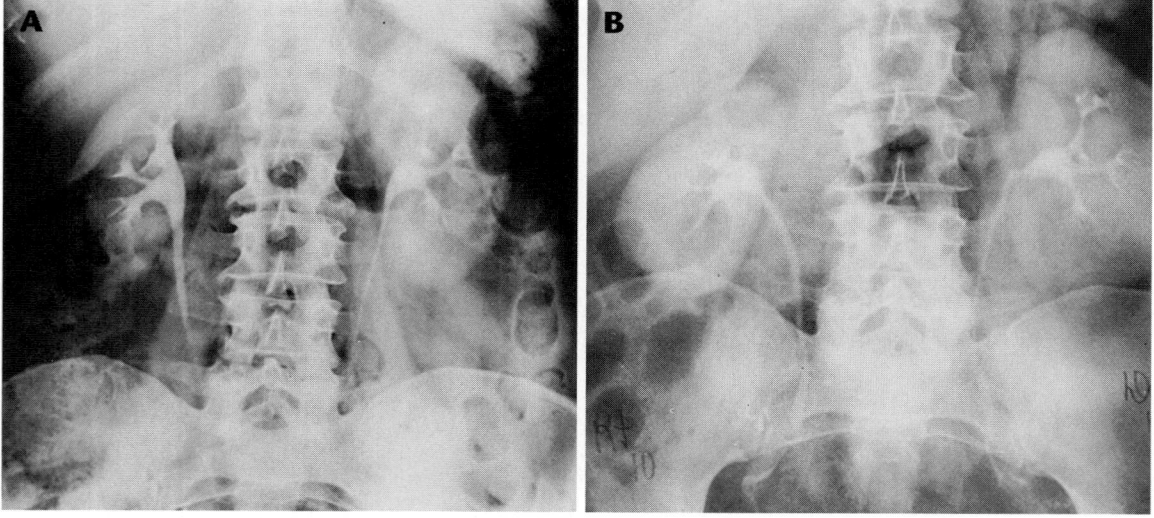

Figure 13–14. Variations in renal outline of the right kidney with respiration. **A,** Expiration. **B,** Inspiration.

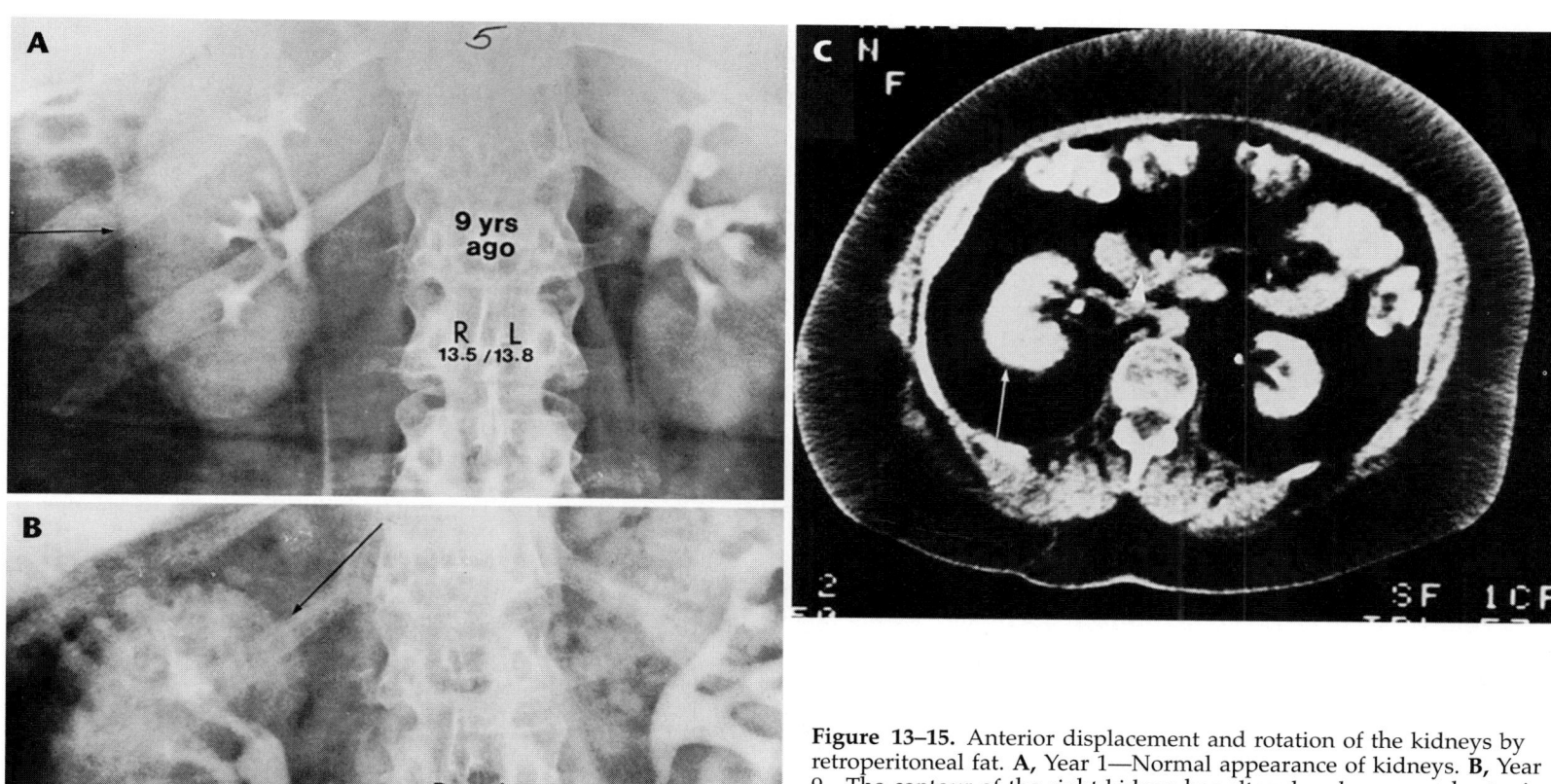

Figure 13–15. Anterior displacement and rotation of the kidneys by retroperitoneal fat. **A,** Year 1—Normal appearance of kidneys. **B,** Year 9—The contour of the right kidney has altered and appears shorter in its vertical dimensions. **C,** CT shows anterior displacement of the right kidney by fat. (Ref: Hooge WA et al: Anterior displacement of kidneys by fat. *J Can Assoc Radiol* 31:143, 1980.)

Figure 13–16. Duplication variant producing a discrepancy in renal size. The left kidney is duplex and is distinctly larger than the right. **A,** Plain film. **B,** Urogram.

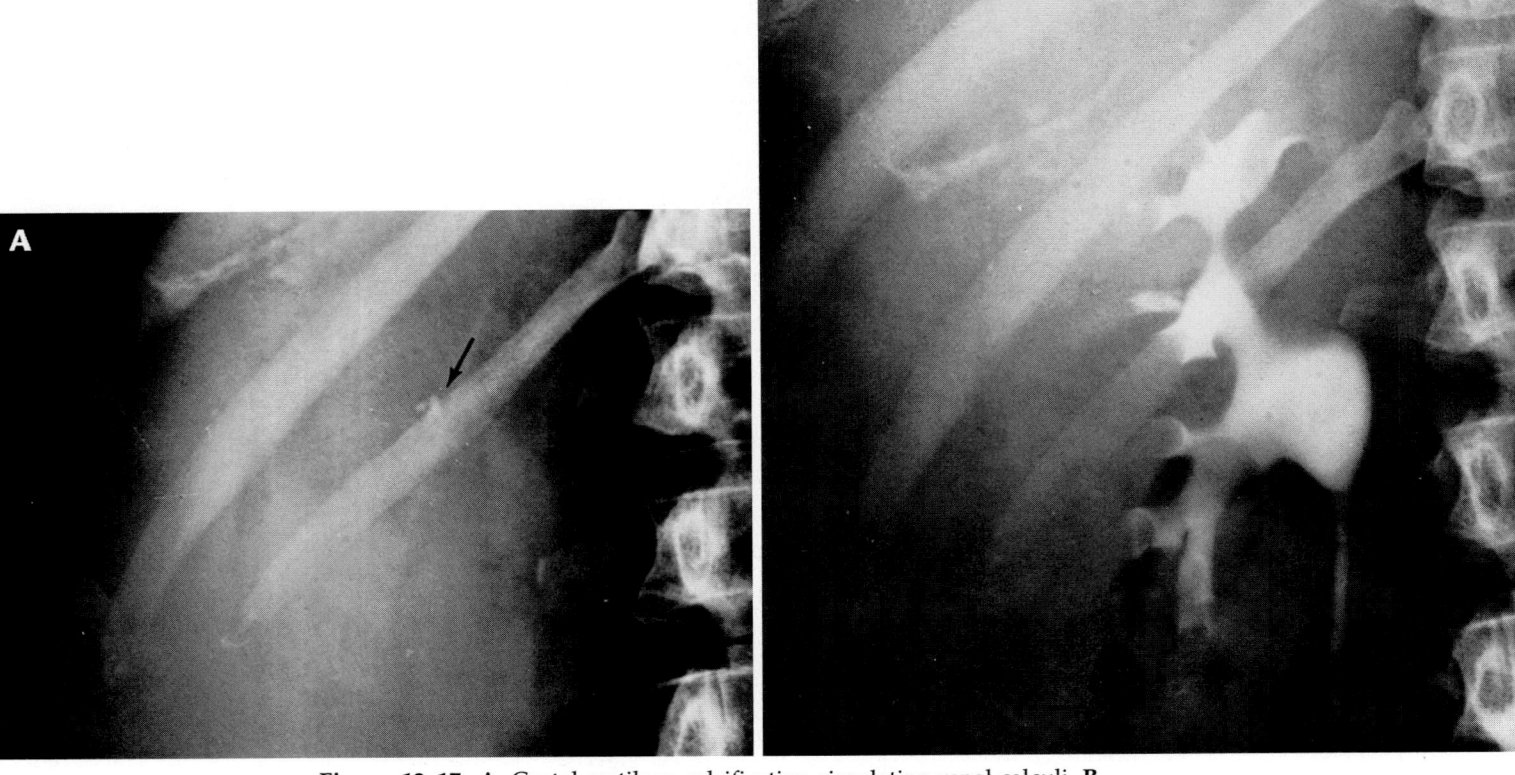

Figure 13–17. A, Costal cartilage calcification simulating renal calculi. **B,** Calcification is obscured by the contrast material in the urogram.

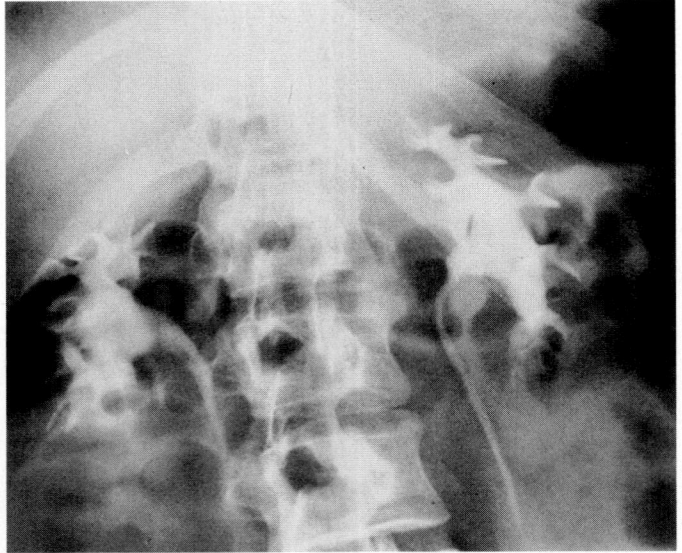

Figure 13–18. Multiplicity of calyces. This is an atavistic variant that may be mistaken for a pathologic state.

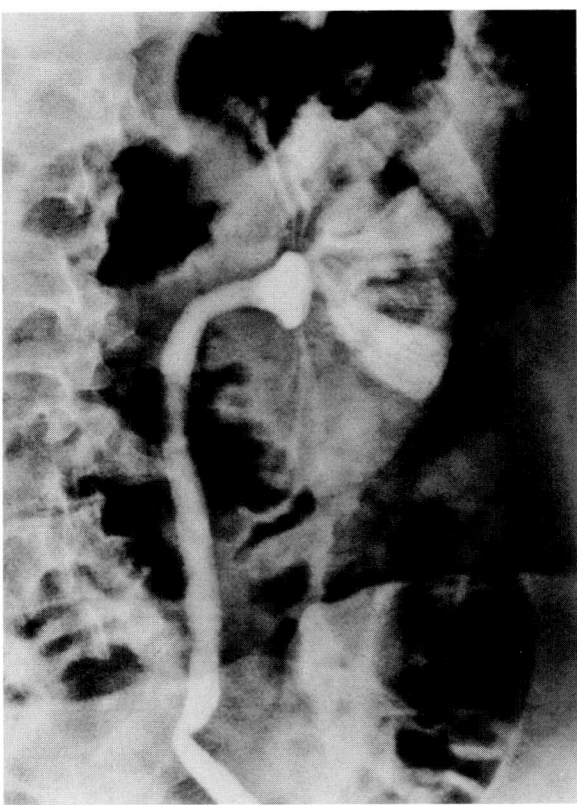

Figure 13–19. Unicalyx kidney. Another atavistic variant, representing the normal arrangement in monkeys, dogs, and rabbits. (Ref: Harrison RB et al: A solitary calyx in a human kidney. *Radiology* 121:310, 1976.)

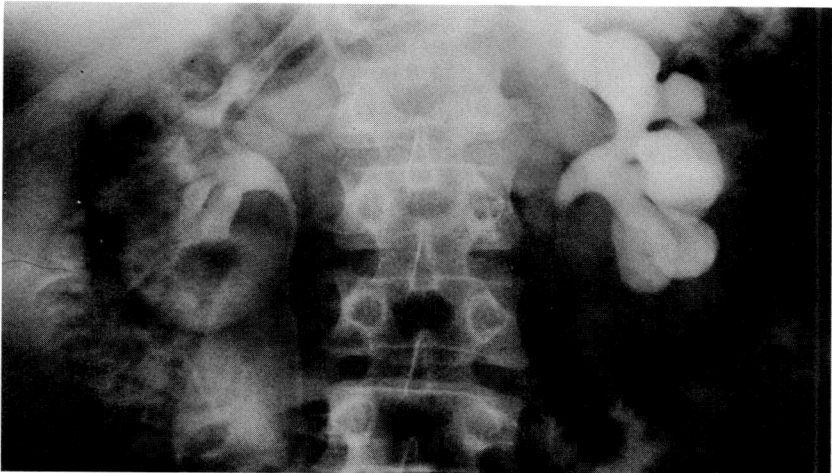

Figure 13–20. Megacalyces of the left kidney. This variant is often unilateral and represents a malformation of the renal papillae. The cortex is normal, but the medulla is hypoplastic. The dilated calyces and reduced parenchymal thickness resemble obstructive hydronephrosis or postobstructive atrophy. (Ref: Talner LB, Gittes RF: Megacalyces: Further observations and differentiation from obstructive renal disease. *Am J Roentgenol* 121:473, 1974.)

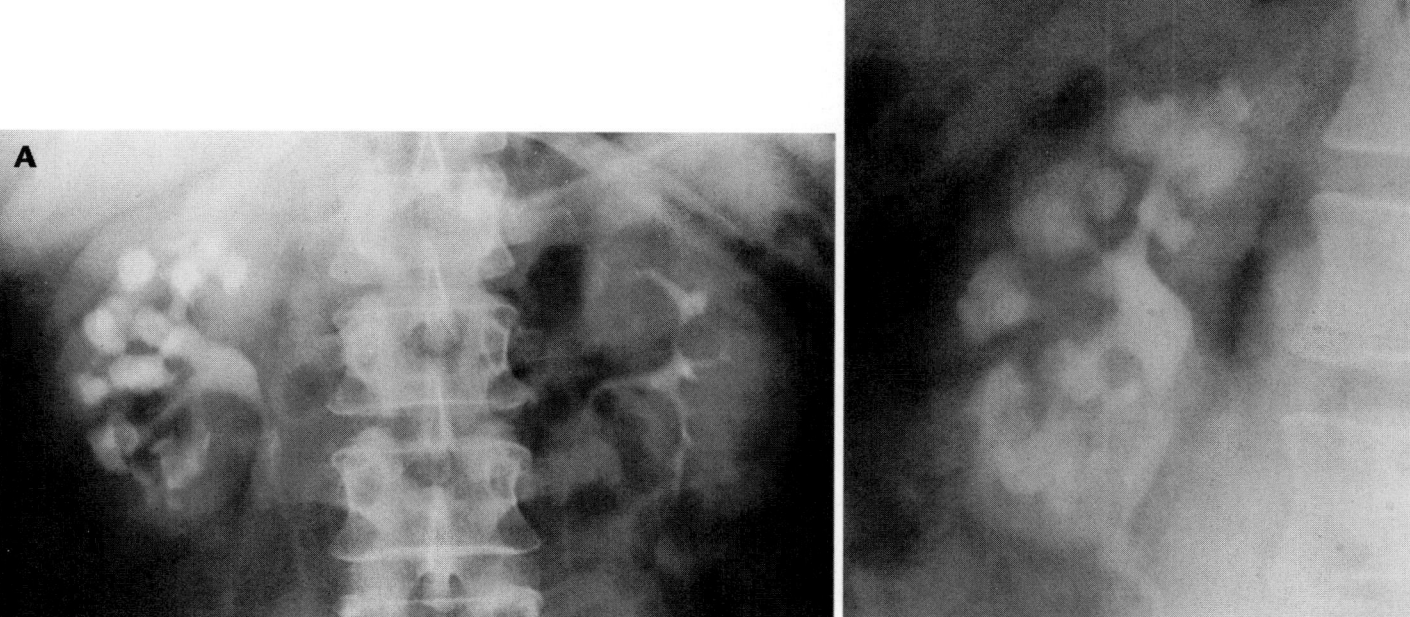

Figure 13–21. A, Megacalyces of the right kidney. **B,** Detailed view of the right kidney.

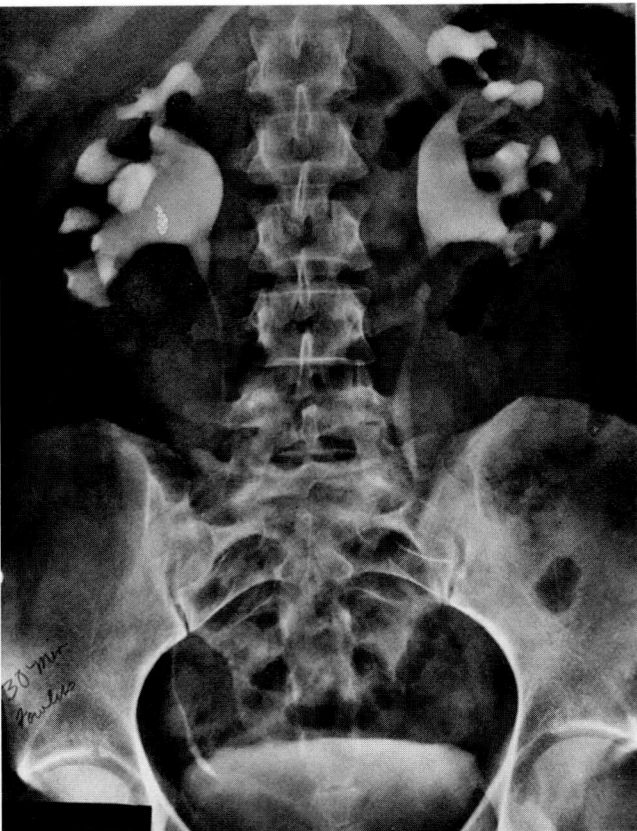

Figure 13–22. Bilateral megacalyces. This condition may be genetically transmitted. (Ref: Lam AH: Familial megacalyces with autosomal recessive inheritance. *Pediatr Radiol* 19:28, 1988.)

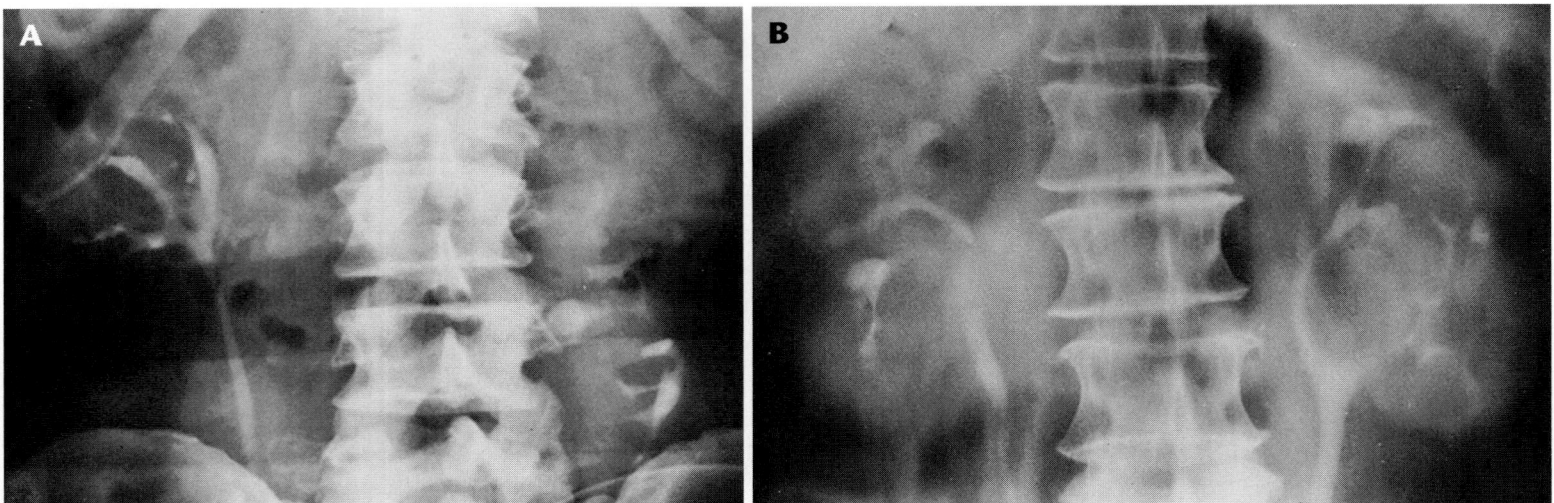

Figure 13–23. Two examples of extrarenal collecting systems. The clawlike configuration of the infundibula, best seen in the right kidney in **A,** is characteristic of this variation in development. Fifty percent of these individuals have associated renal disease. **B,** Bilateral extrarenal collecting systems. (Ref: Malament M et al: Extrarenal calyces: Their relationship to renal disease. *Am J Roentgenol* 86:823, 1961.)

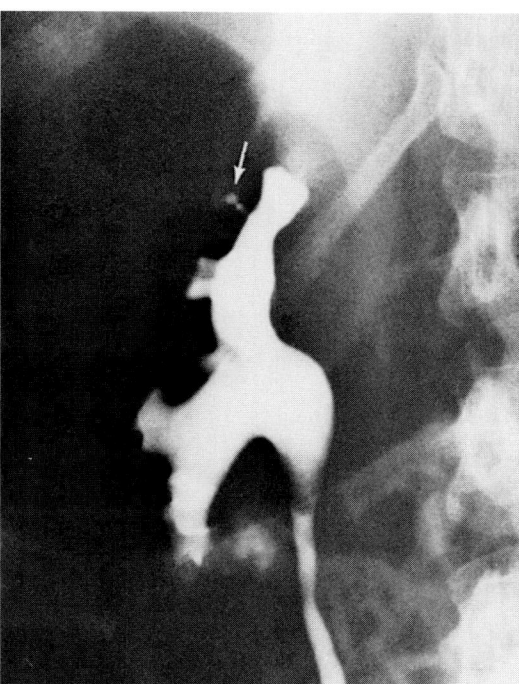

Figure 13–24. Miniature calyx. Tubular blush, produced by contrast material in the collecting tubules, is seen as a halo around this calyx. (Ref: Kunin M: The abortive calix: Variation in appearance and differential diagnosis. *Am J Roentgenol* 139:931, 1982.)

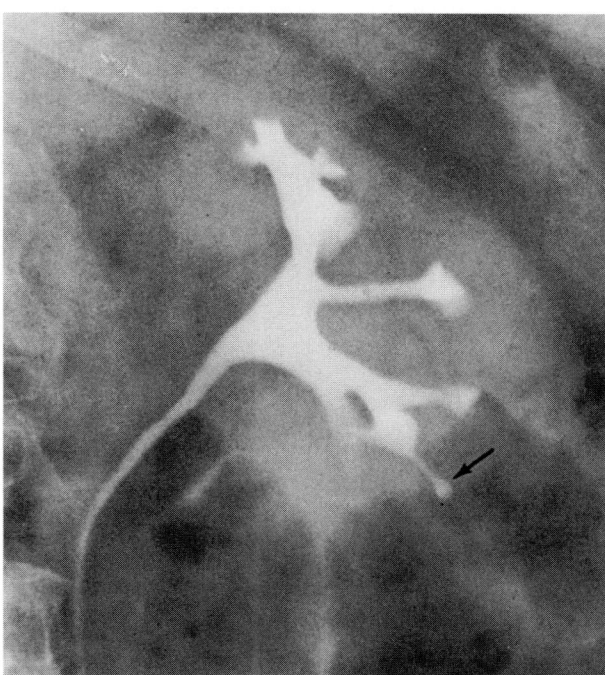

Figure 13–25. Accessory calyx arising from the lower calyceal group.

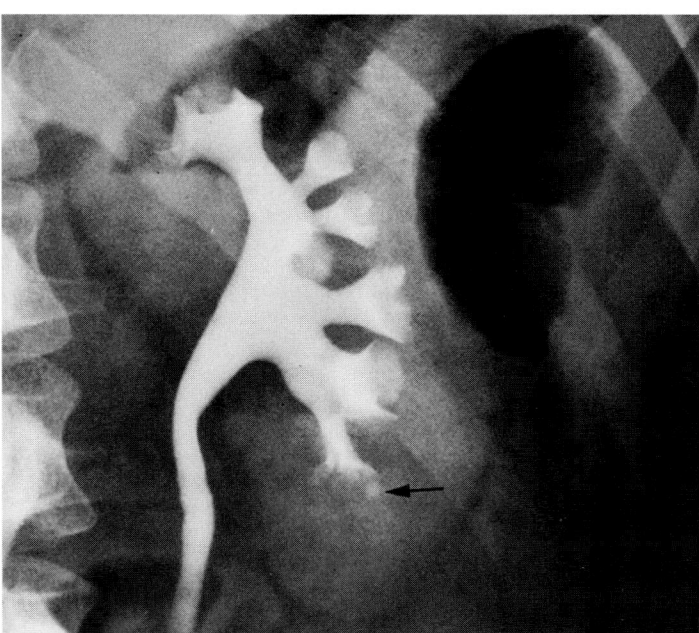

Figure 13–26. Small calyceal diverticulum.

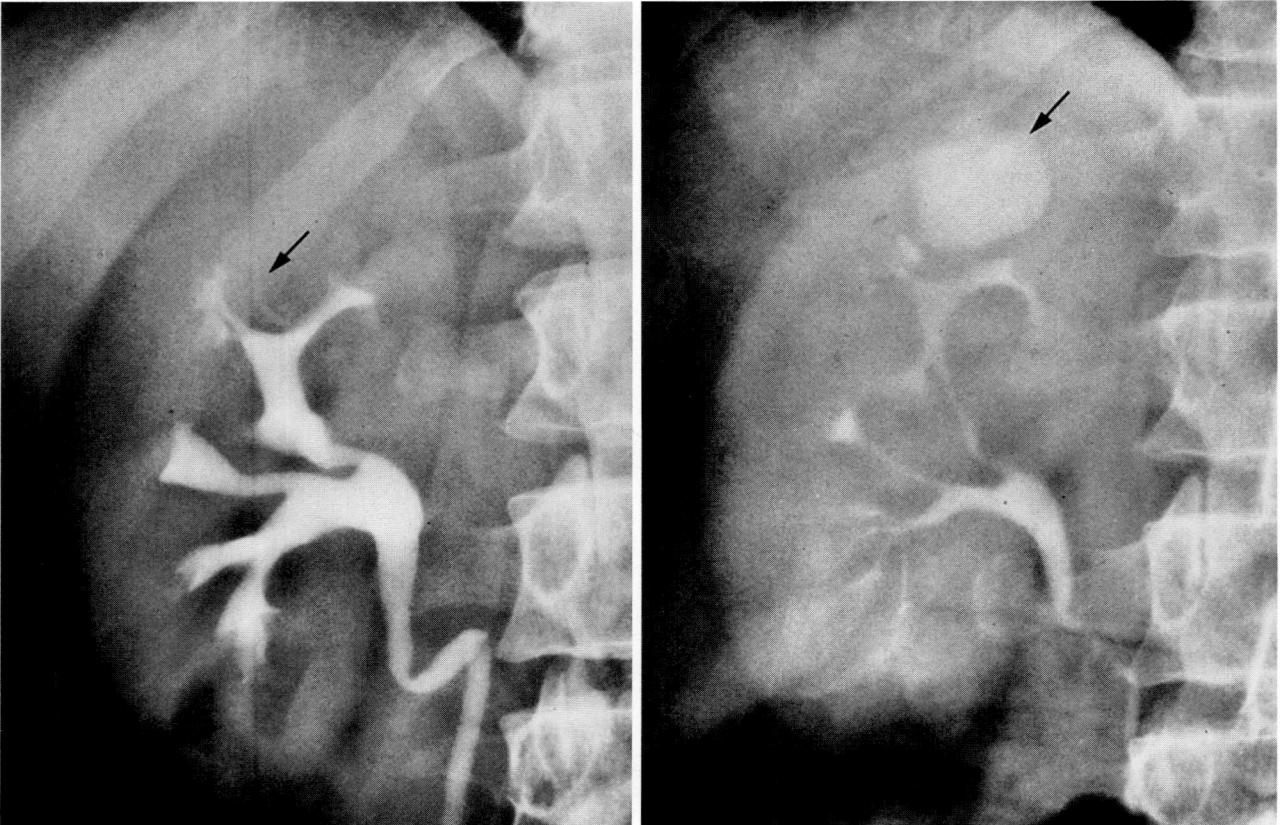

Figure 13–27. Calyceal diverticulum. *Left*, Early filling. *Right*, Late filling.

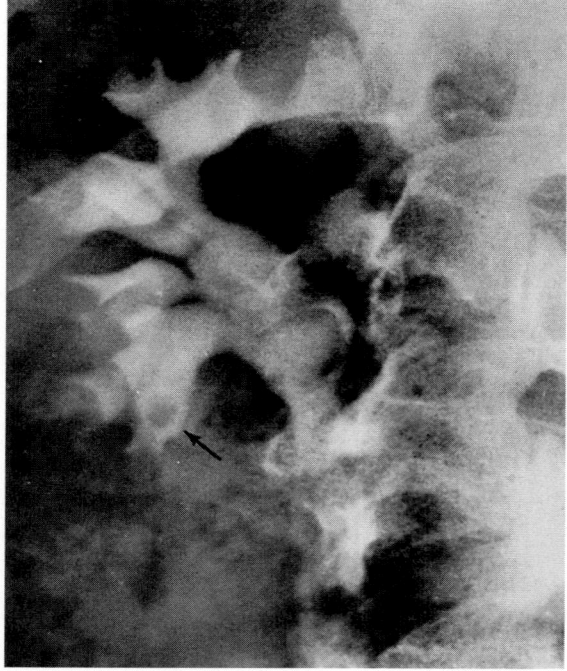

Figure 13–28. Calyx seen on end, simulating a filling defect.

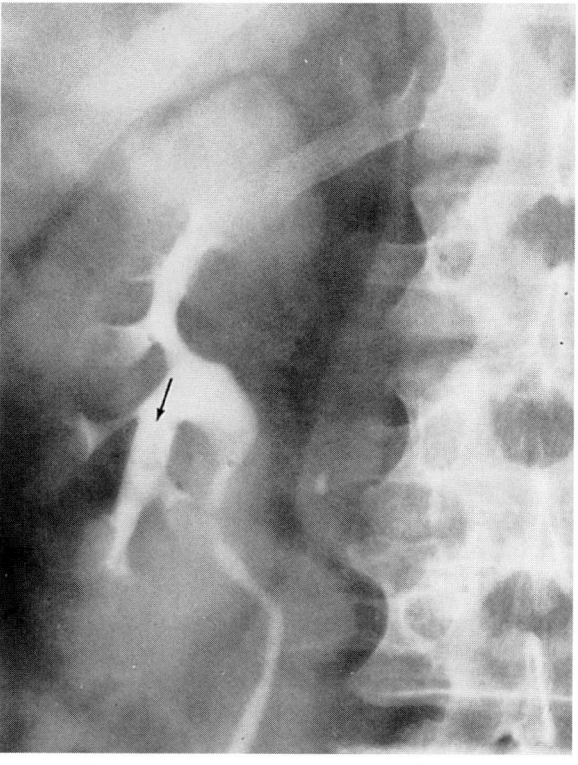

Figure 13–29. Aberrant renal papilla entering the infundibulum of the lower pole. (Ref: Binder R et al: Aberrant papillae and other filling defects of the renal pelvis. *Am J Roentgenol* 114:746, 1972.)

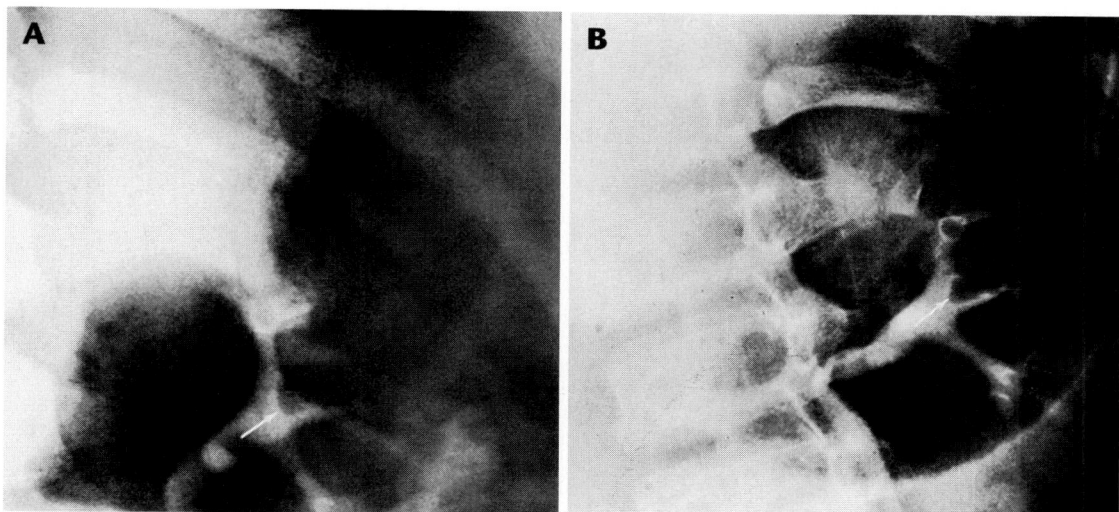

Figure 13–30. Aberrant renal papilla entering the renal pelvis. This variant may be associated with hematuria.

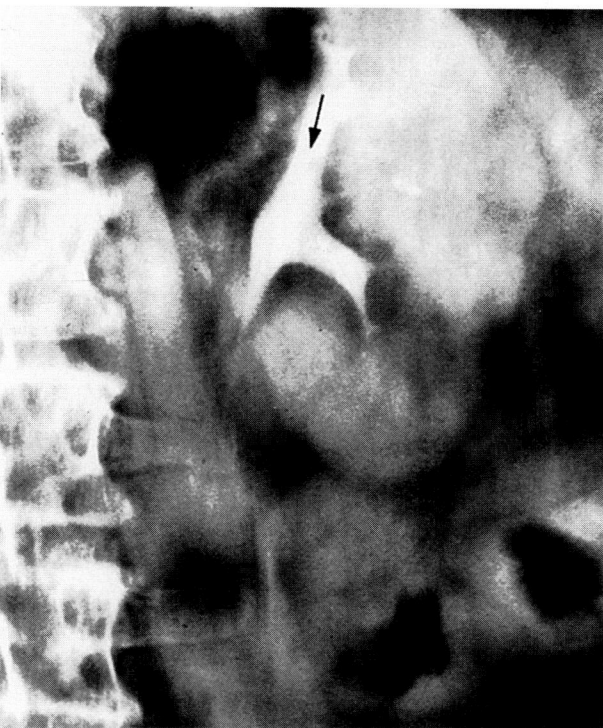

Figure 13–31. Another example of an aberrant renal papilla entering the renal pelvis.

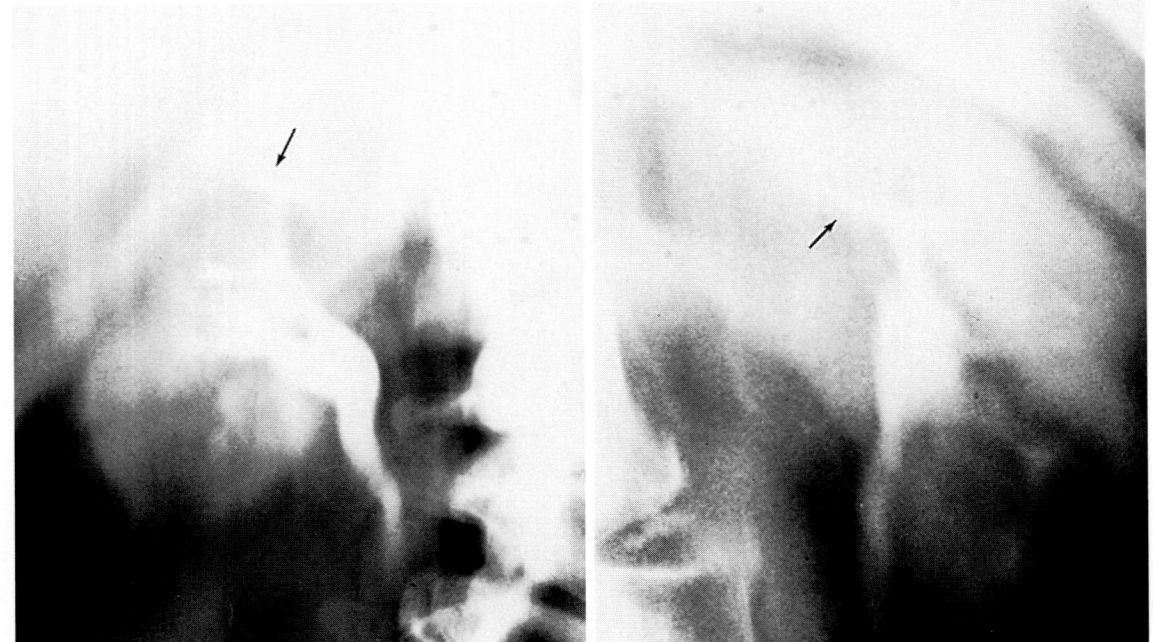

Figure 13–32. Flat upper pole calyceal groups that might be mistaken for distortion by an adjacent mass.

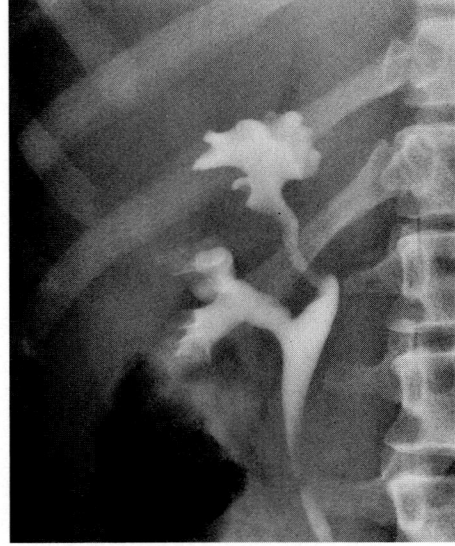

Figure 13–33. Composite upper pole calyces.

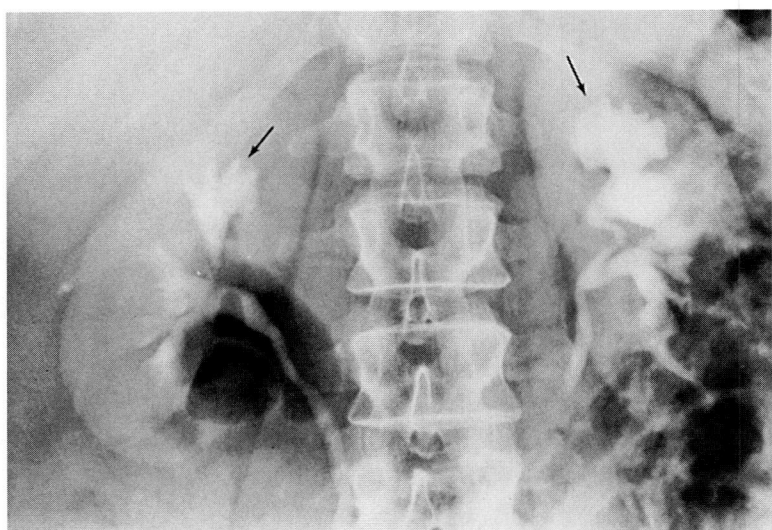

Figure 13–34. Large composite upper pole calyceal groups.

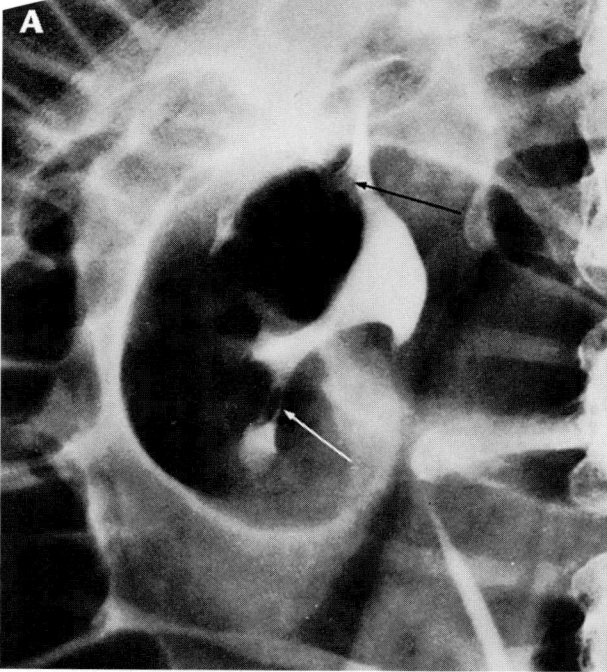

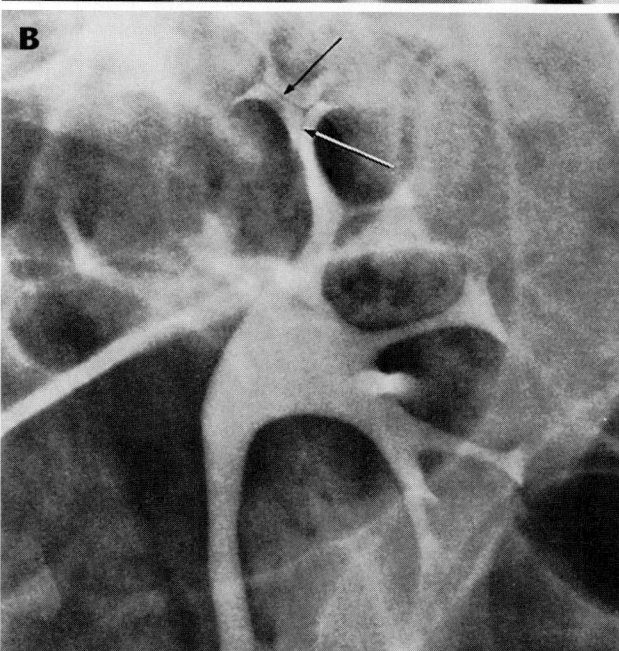

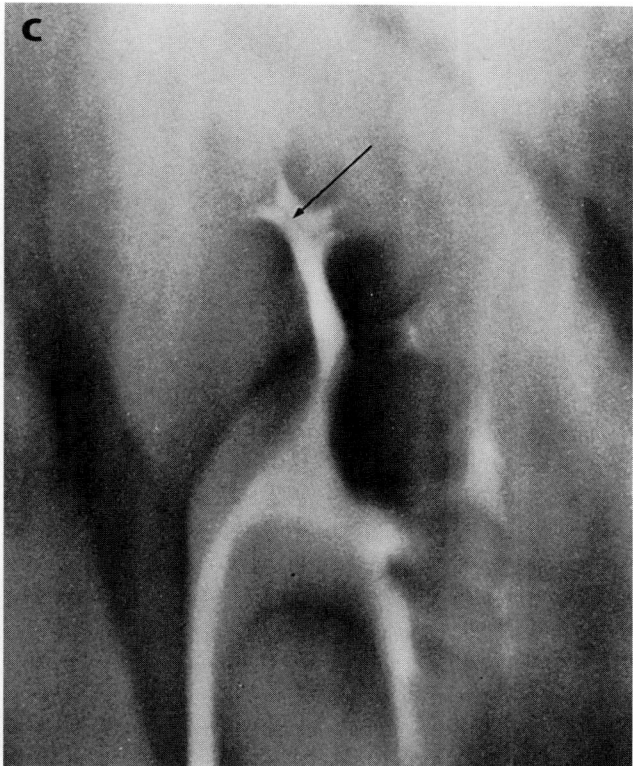

Figure 13–35. A and **B,** Mucosal folds seen within calyces and infundibula. **C,** Tomogram of left kidney shows the folds in the superior calyx. These folds do not indicate abnormality.

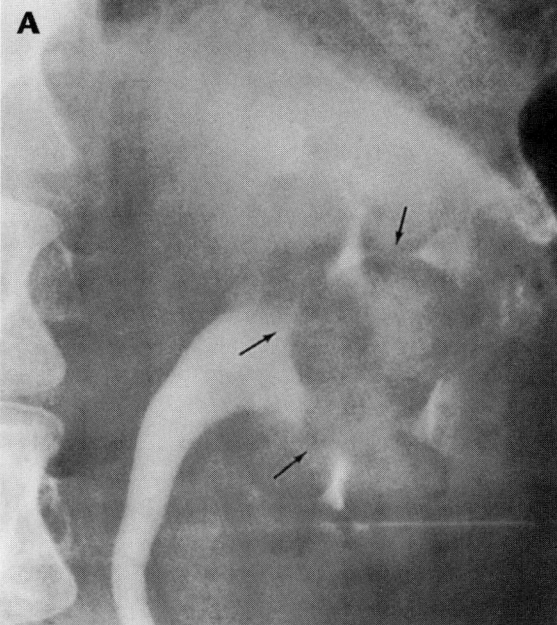

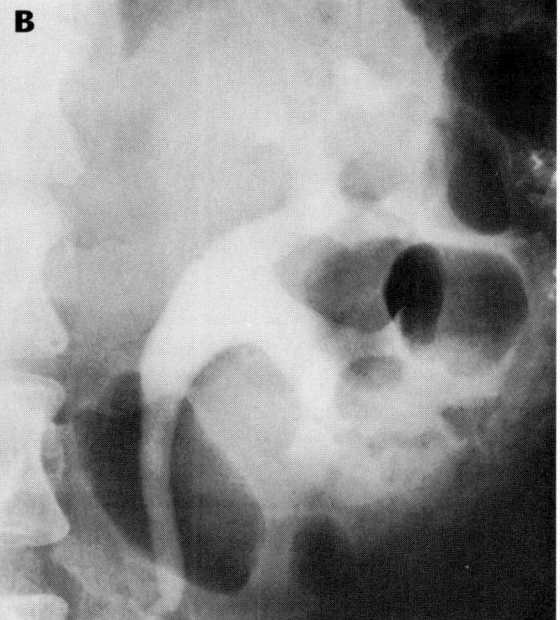

Figure 13–36. A, Incomplete filling of the calyces and infundibula may simulate a mass lesion. **B,** Mass effect is no longer seen with adequate filling.

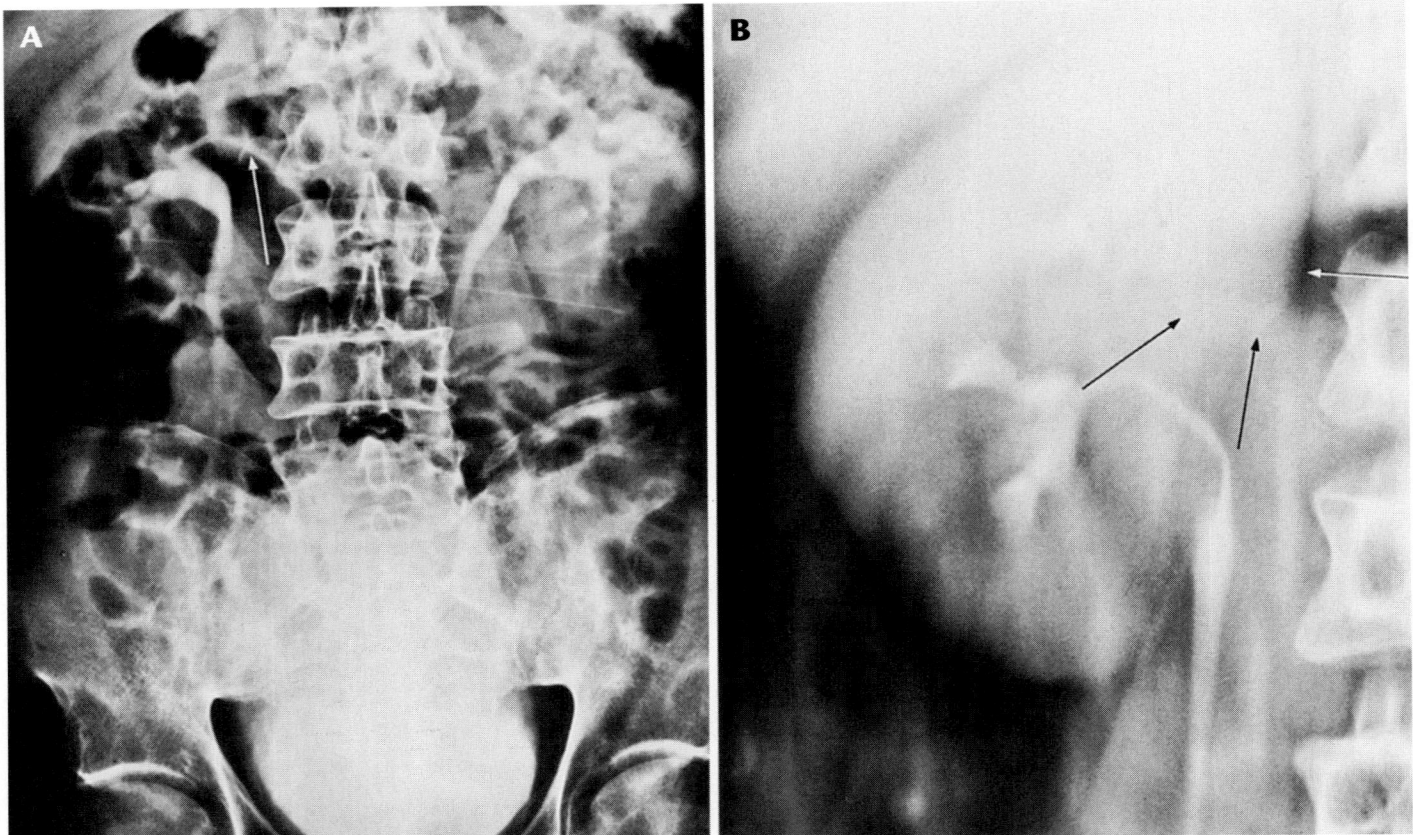

Figure 13–37. Bulge in the suprahilar region of the right kidney representing the hilar lip or renal uncus. **A,** Urogram. **B,** Nephrotomogram. (Ref: Feldman AE et al: Renal pseudotumors: An anatomic-radiologic classification. *J Urol* 120:133, 1978.)

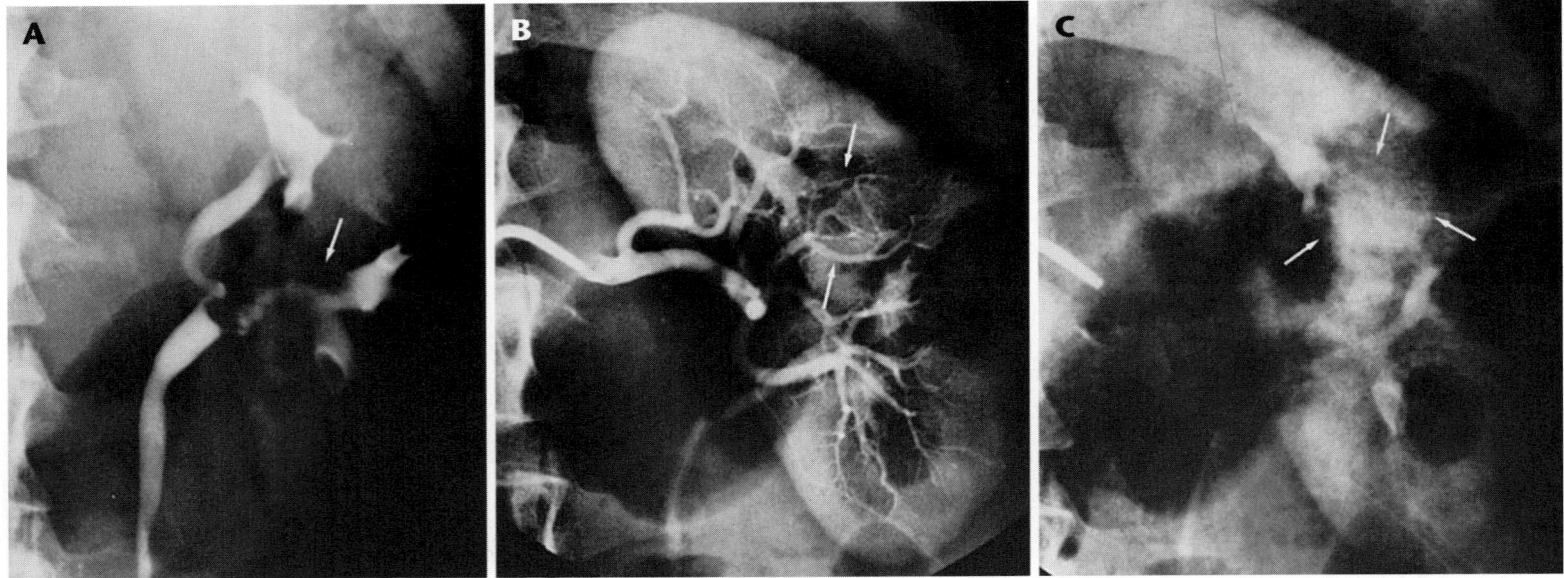

Figure 13–38. Deformity of the collecting system caused by excessive invagination of the cortical tissue in forming Bertin's columns. This entity is often found in cases with duplications of the collecting system and may simulate a neoplasm. **A,** Plain film. **B,** Arteriogram. **C,** Nephrogram. (Ref: Lopez FA: Renal pseudotumors. *Am J Roentgenol* 109:172, 1970.)

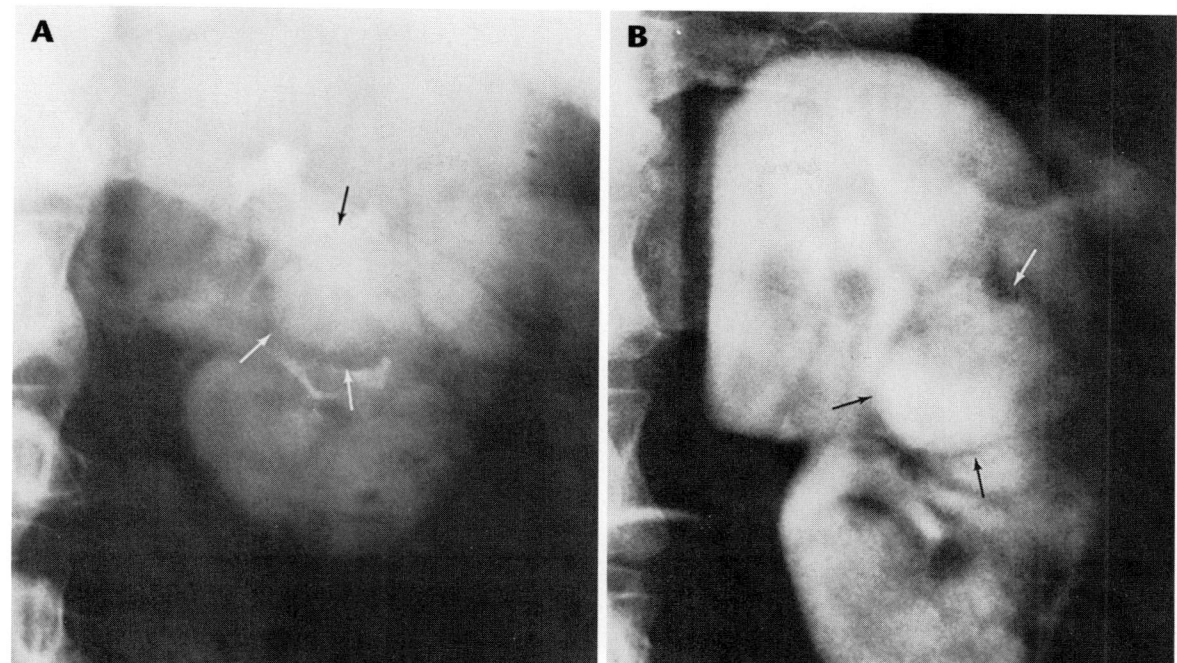

Figure 13–39. A, Additional example of the deformity of the collecting system caused by Bertin's columns. **B,** Nephrogram.

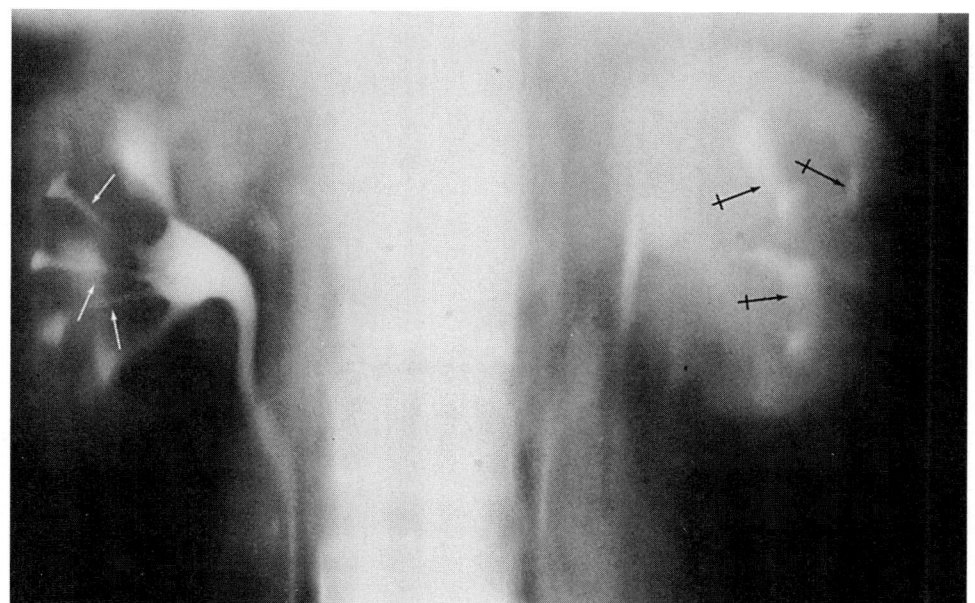

Figure 13–40. Renal pelvic lipomatosis. The deposition of large amounts of normal fat in the renal pelvis produces radiolucency, stretching, and elongation of the infundibula, best seen in the right kidney (←). On occasion it may resemble the changes of polycystic disease as seen in the left kidney (↔). (Ref: Ambos MA et al: Replacement lipomatosis of the kidney. *Am J Roentgenol* 130:1087, 1978.)

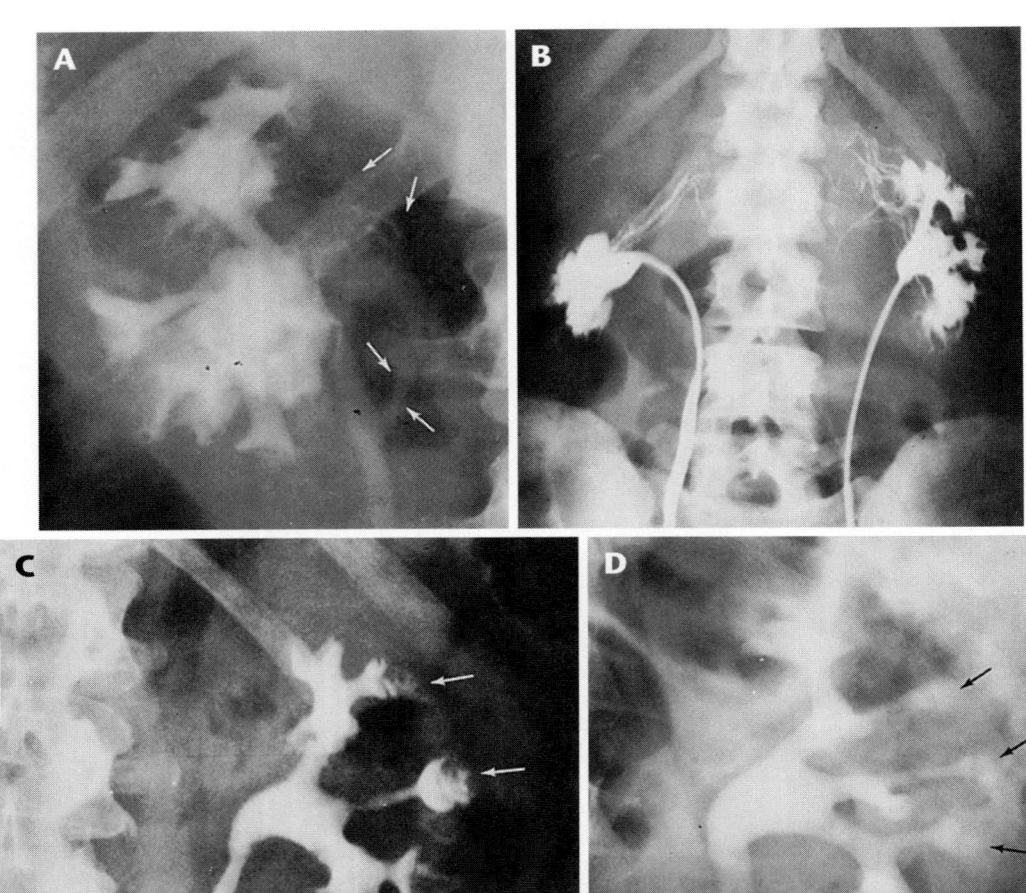

Figure 13–41. Backflow. **A,** Pyelovenous. **B,** Pyelolymphatic. **C,** Pyelotubular. **D,** Tubular blush produced by contrast material in the collecting tubules of the renal papillae. This should not be mistaken for the tubular ectasia of the medullary sponge kidney. (Ref: Ohlson L: Normal collecting ducts: Visualization at urography. *Radiology* 170:33, 1989.)

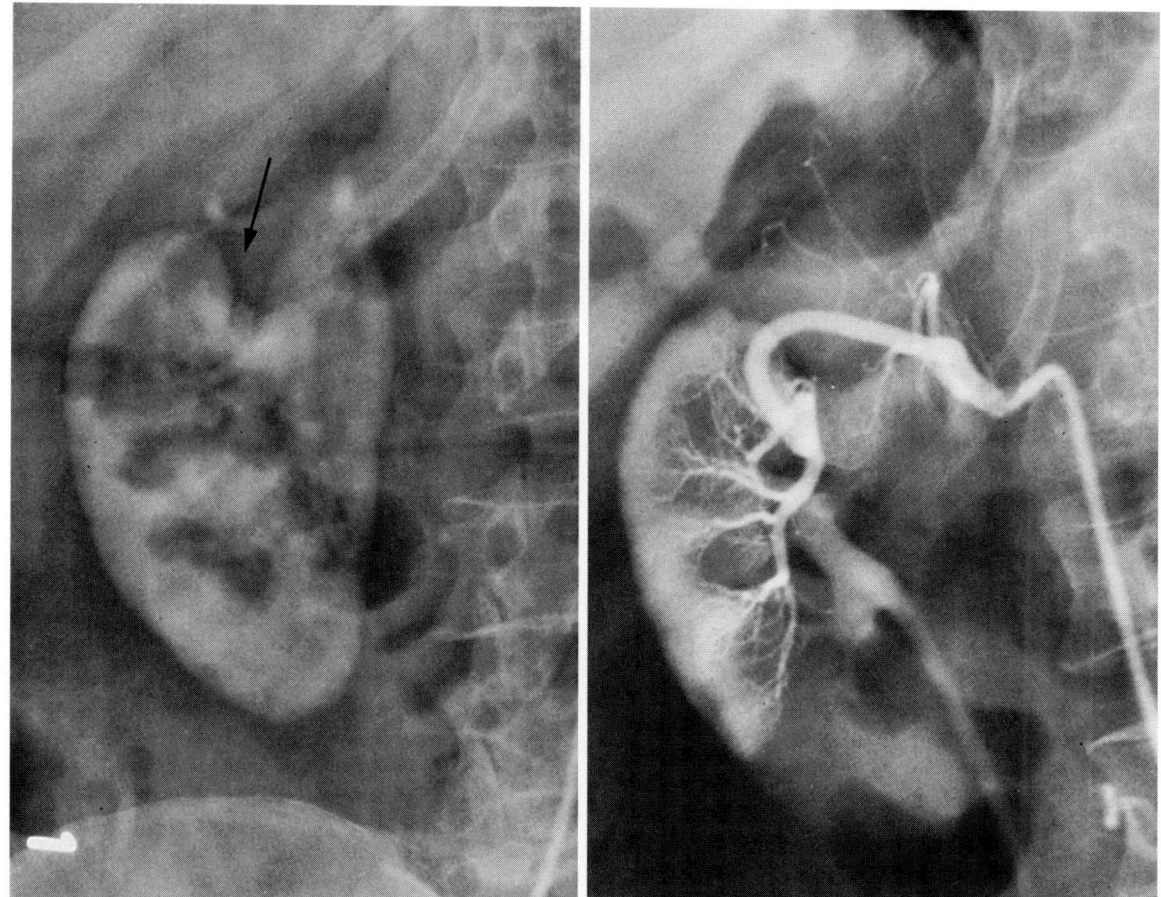

Figure 13–42. Accessory renal hilus. *Left,* Nephrogram shows a defect in the superior pole of the kidney *(arrow). Right,* Renal angiogram shows a renal artery entering the kidney at the area of the defect. A separate renal artery supplies the remainder of the kidney. Arteriography is usually necessary to distinguish the accessory renal hilus from a pathologic process. (Courtesy of Dr. Thomas F. Stephenson.)

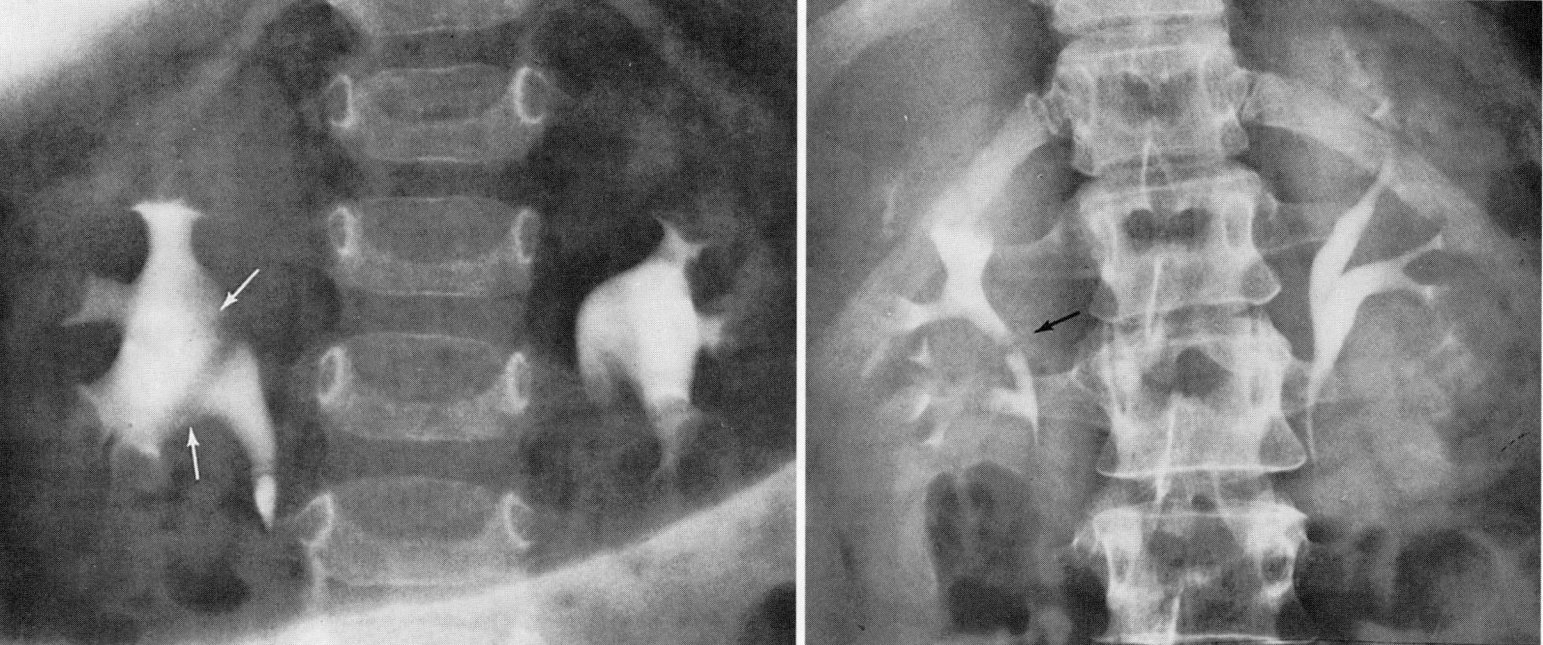

Figure 13–43. Two examples of vascular impressions on the renal pelvis. Most of these are not clinically important. (Ref: Baum S, Gillenwater JY: Renal artery impressions on renal pelvis. *J Urol* 95:139, 1966.)

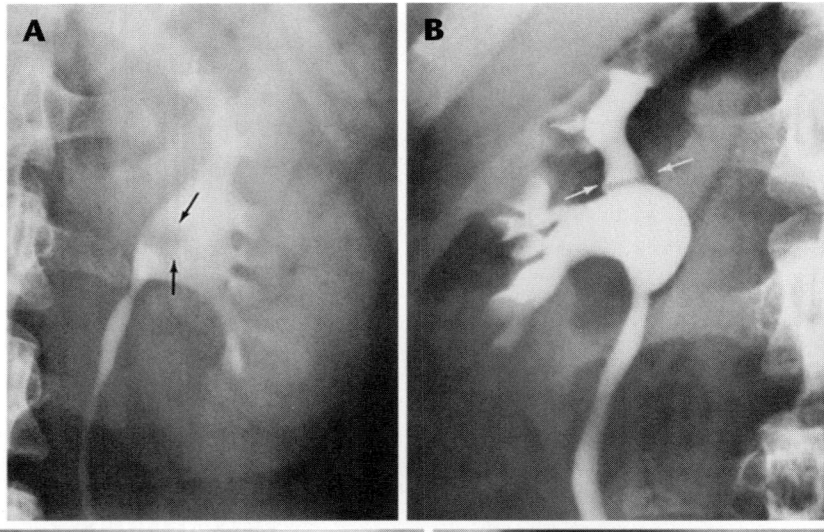

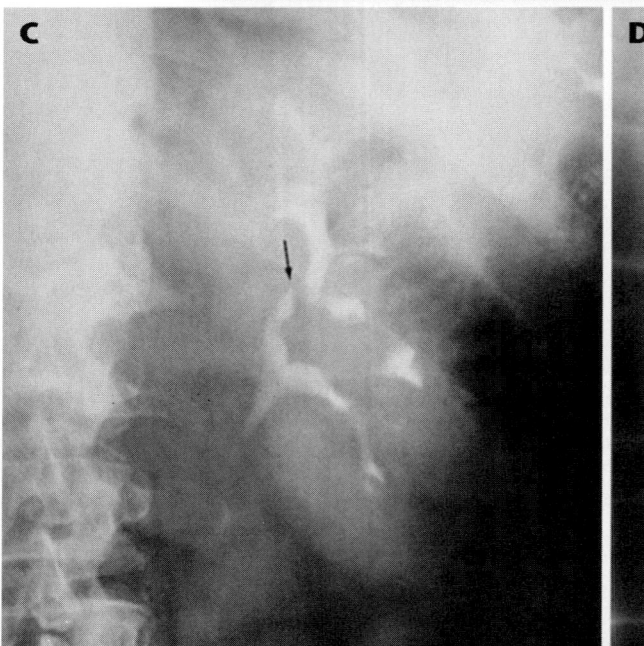

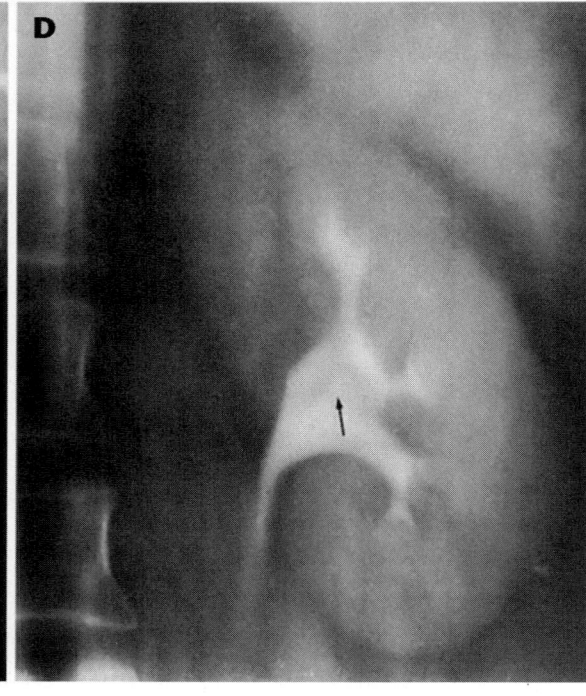

Figure 13–44. Four additional examples of vascular impressions on the collecting systems. (Ref: Nebesar RA et al: Renal vascular impression: Incidence and clinical significance. *Am J Roentgenol* 101:719, 1967.)

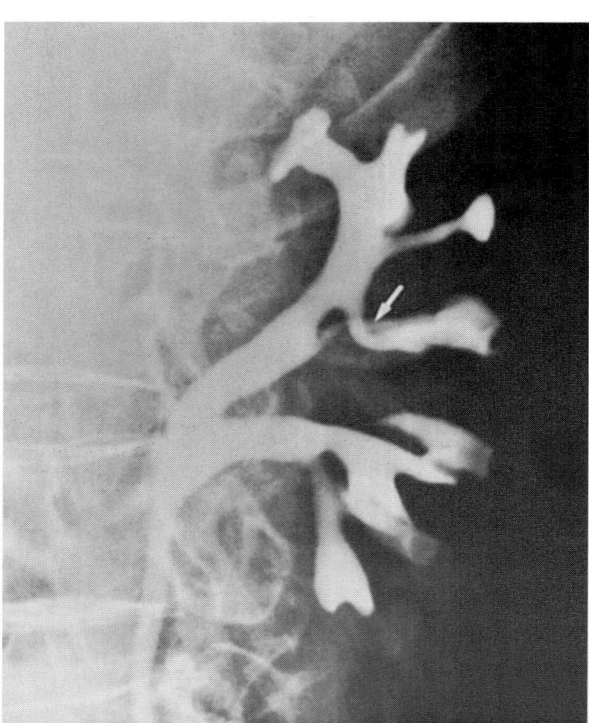

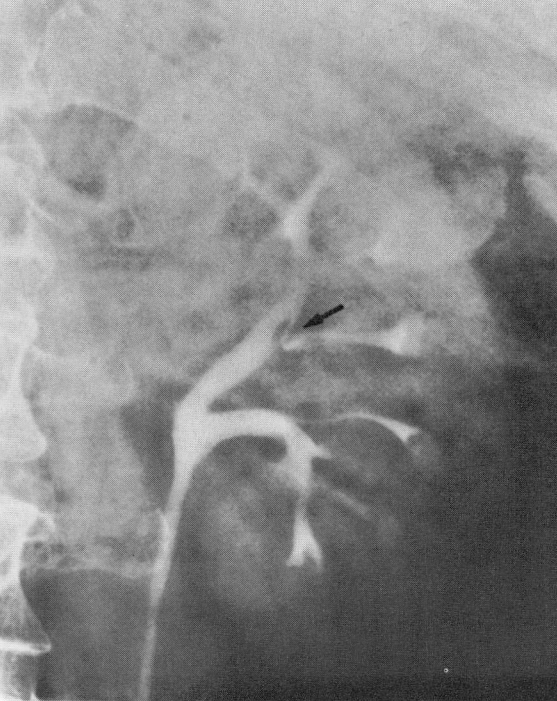

Figure 13–45. Tortuous infundibulum.

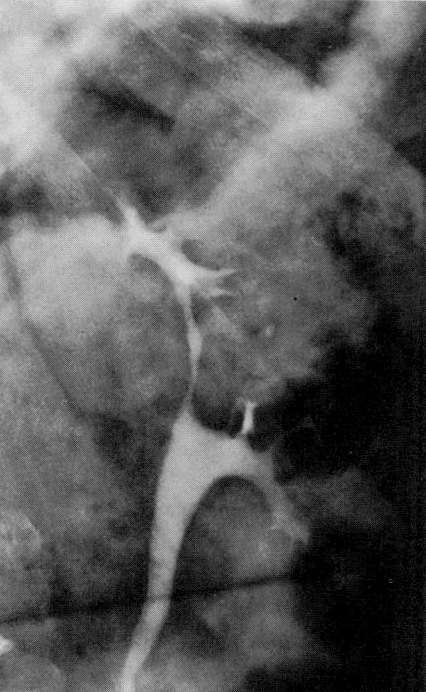

Figure 13–46. Unusual bifid collecting system.

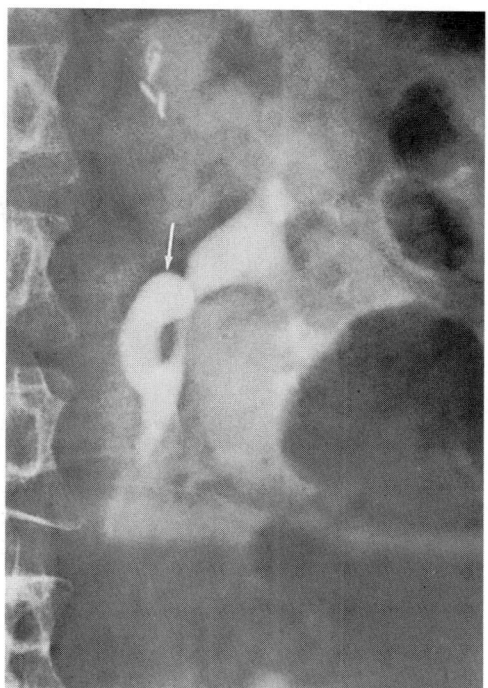

Figure 13–47. Abortive duplication of the renal pelvis.

Figure 13–48. Two examples of extrarenal pelves that simulate the changes of hydronephrosis. **A,** Bilateral extrarenal pelves. **B,** Duplicated extrarenal pelvis of the right kidney only.

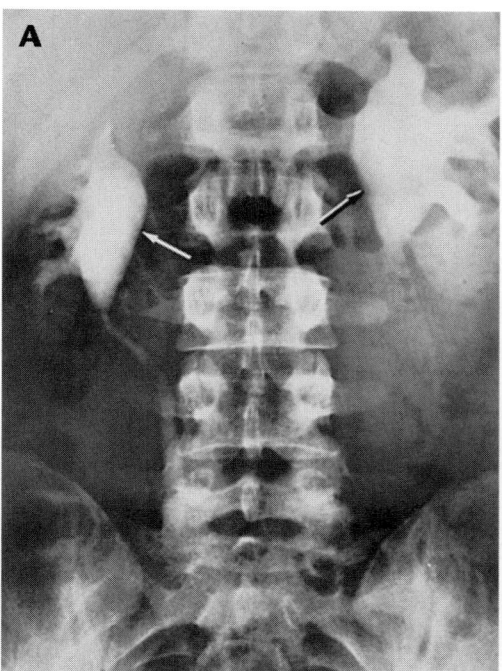
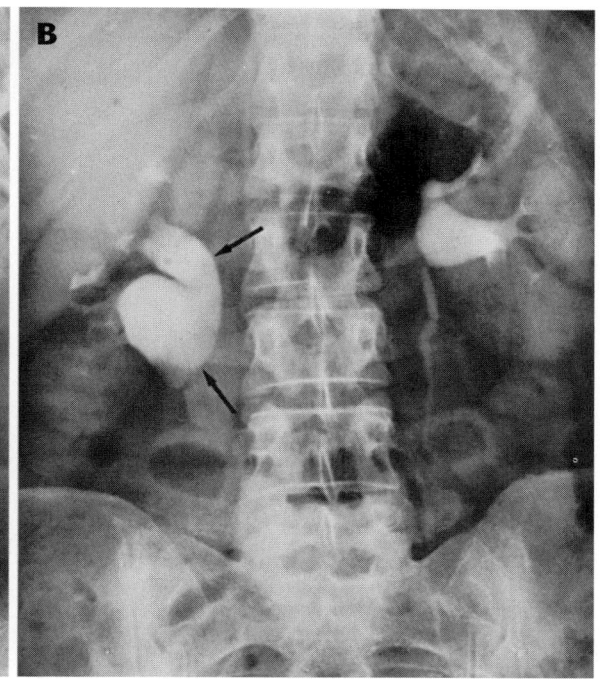

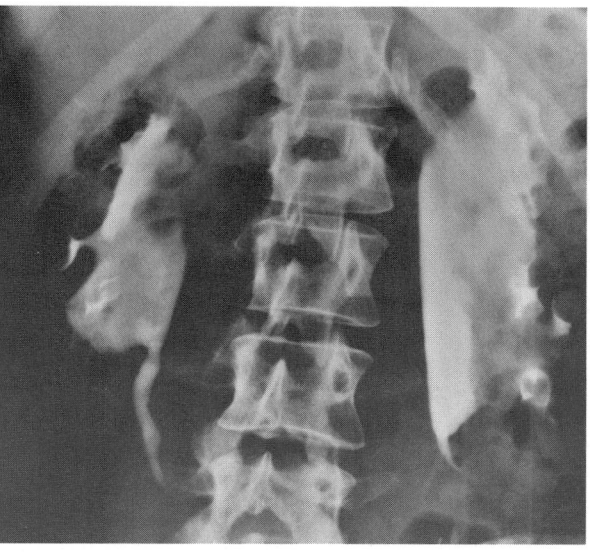

Figure 13–49. Very large extrarenal pelves.

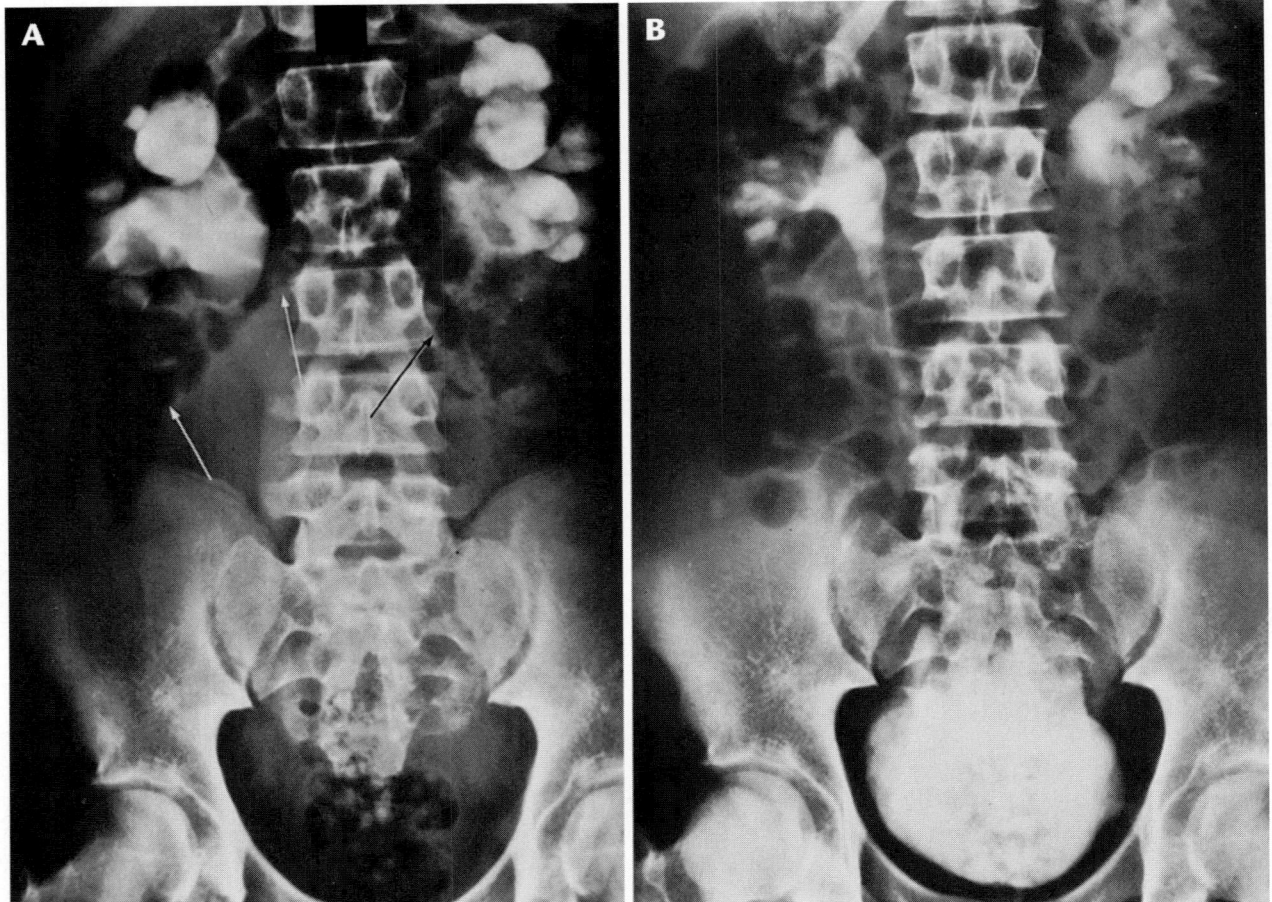

Figure 13–50. A, Simulated hydronephrosis produced by massive distention of the bladder *(arrows).* **B,** Appearance after bladder is emptied.

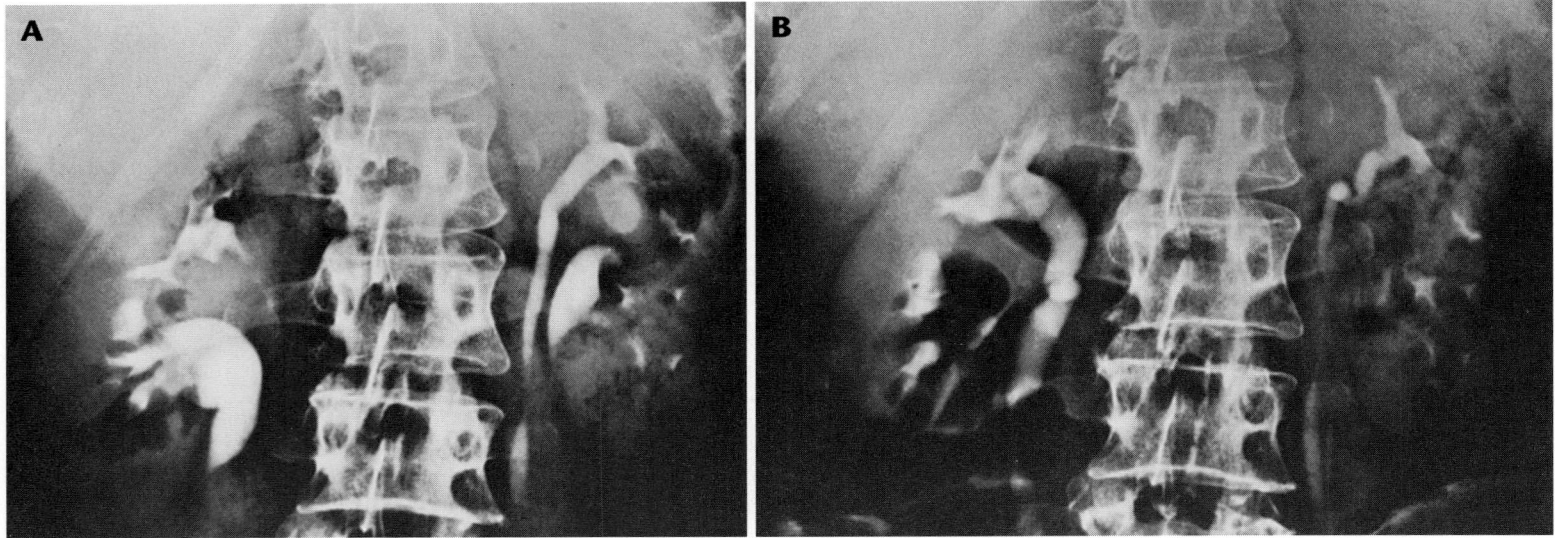

Figure 13–51. "Yo-yo" effect (saddle reflux) of pelvic emptying in duplex kidneys. **A,** Upper segment of the right kidney is emptying and the lower segment filling. **B,** Lower segment contracts and the upper segment fills by reflux. These are normal dynamics in duplex kidneys. The transient distention of the upper segment could be misinterpreted as pathologic dilatation. (Ref: Privett JRJ et al: The incidence and importance of renal duplication. *Clin Radiol* 27:521, 1976.)

The Ureters

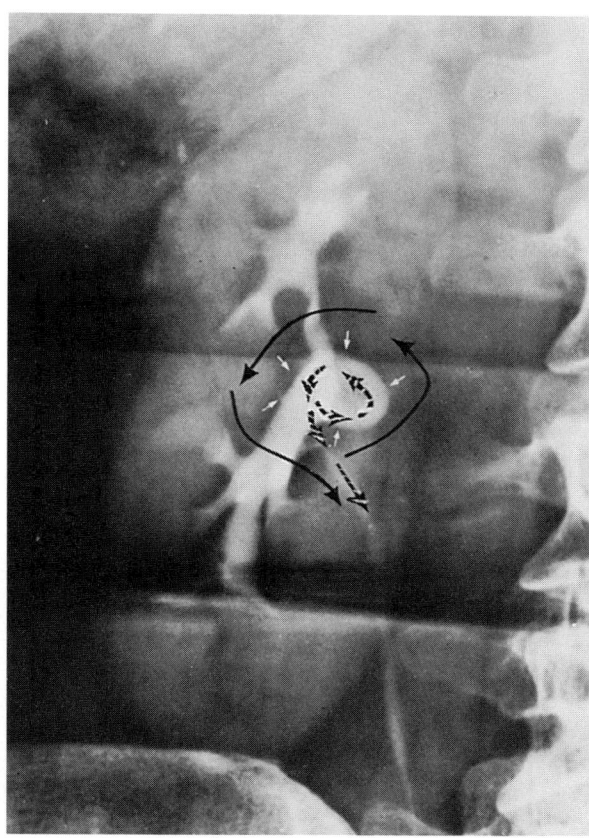

Figure 13–52. "Pigtail" renal pelvis showing an unusual course of the proximal portion of the ureter.

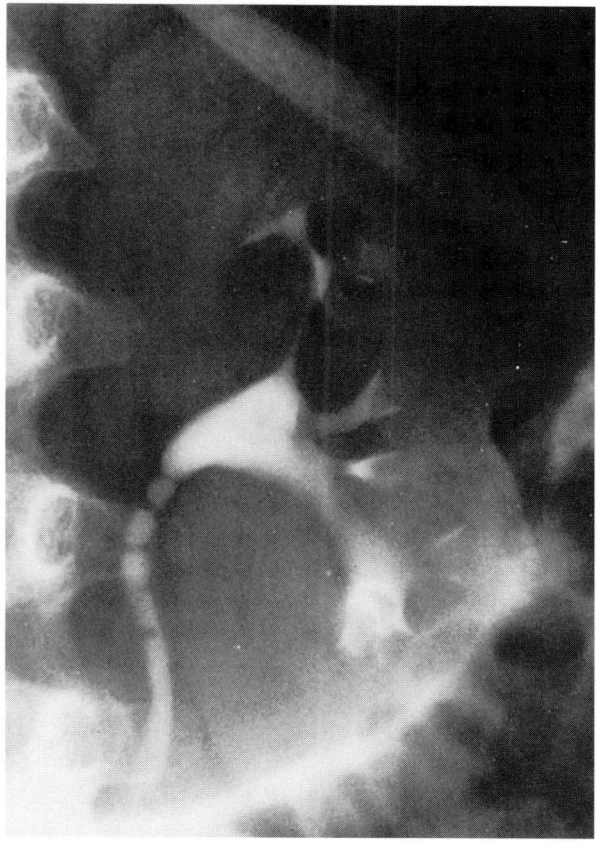

Figure 13–53. Transverse folds in the proximal ureter represent a normal variation in infants. They are believed to represent a persistence of normal fetal tortuosities. (From Kirks DR et al: Transverse folds in the proximal ureter: A normal variation in infants. *Am J Roentgenol* 130:463, 1978.) Similarly, longitudinal striations in adults are believed to be normal as well. (Ref: Parker MD, Clark RL: Urothelial striations revisited. *Radiology* 198:89, 1996.)

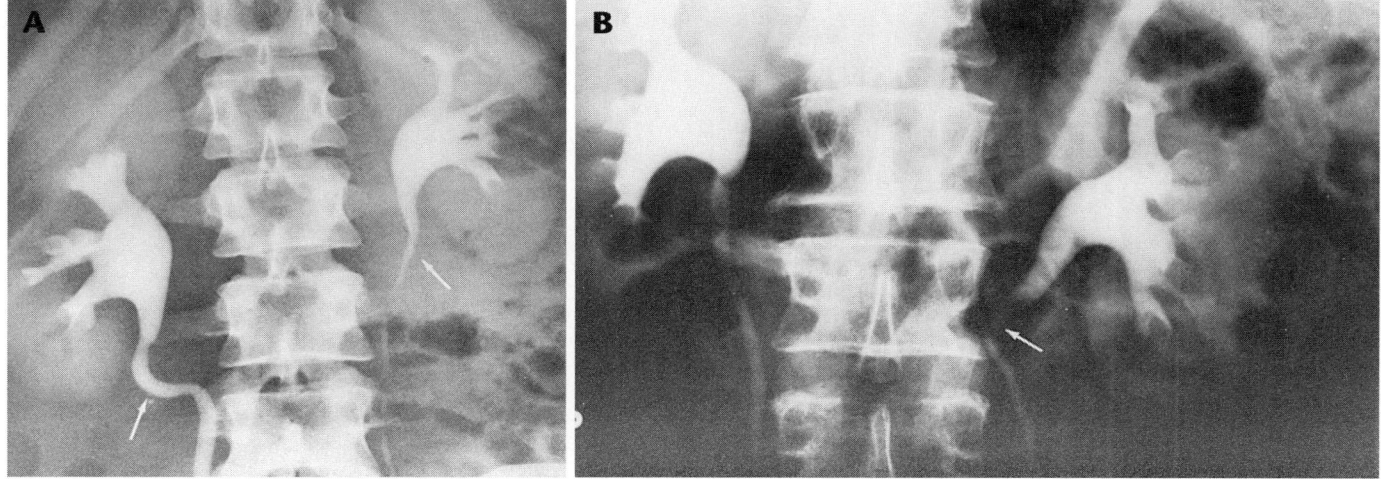

Figure 13–54. Normal deviations of the ureter, caused by the iliopsoas muscles. (Ref: Levine RB et al: Ureteral deviation due to iliopsoas hypertrophy. *Am J Roentgenol* 107:756, 1969.)

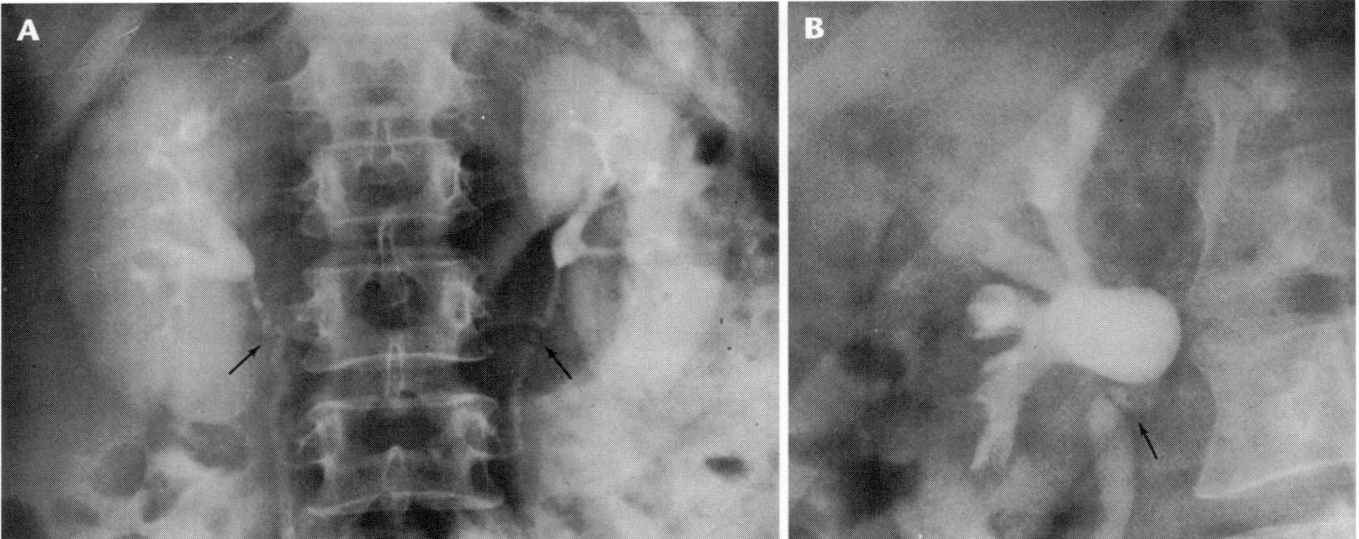

Figure 13–55. Peristalsis of the ureters should not be mistaken for pathologic changes.

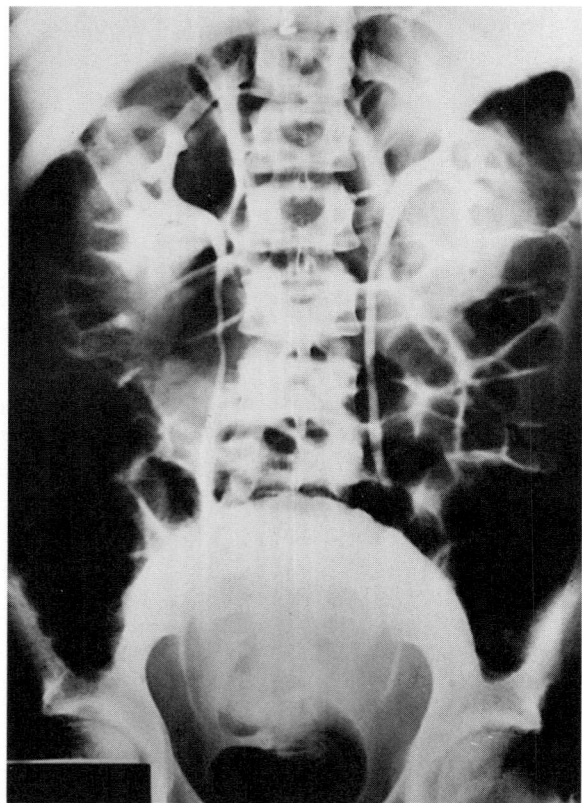

Figure 13–56. Full column filling of the ureters secondary to distention of the urinary bladder.

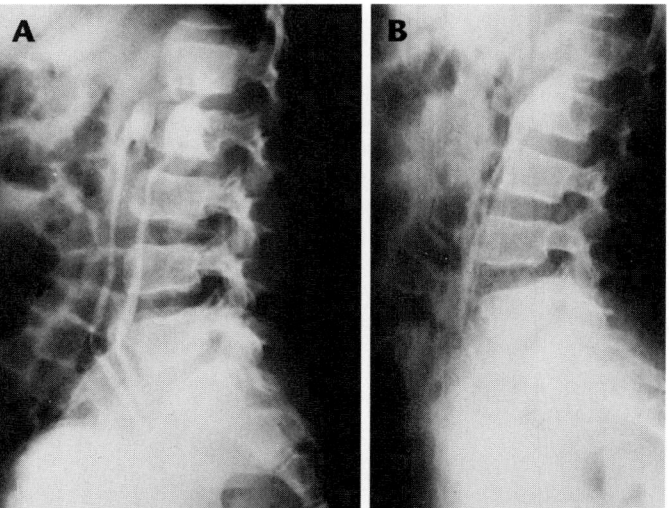

Figure 13–57. Variation in the position of the ureters with the technique of exposure. **A,** In the true lateral position, the upper kidney and ureter drop anteriorly. **B,** In the cross-table lateral view, the location of the ureters and kidneys can be compared more accurately. (Ref: Cook K et al: Determination of the normal position of the upper urinary tract on the lateral abdominal urogram. *Radiology* 99:499, 1971.)

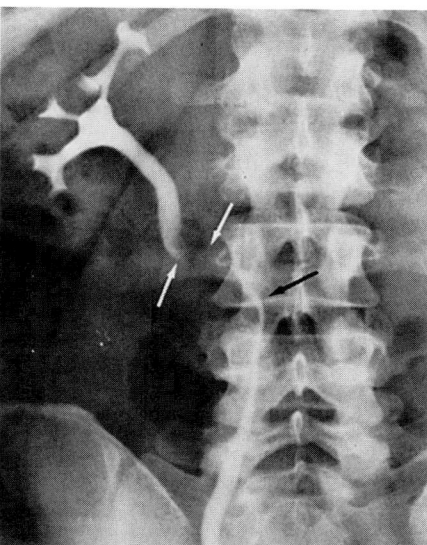

Figure 13–58. Retrocaval ureter coursing around the posterior aspect of the inferior vena cava. (Ref: Emmett JL, Witten DM: *Clinical urography,* 3rd ed. Philadelphia, WB Saunders, 1971, p. 1327.)

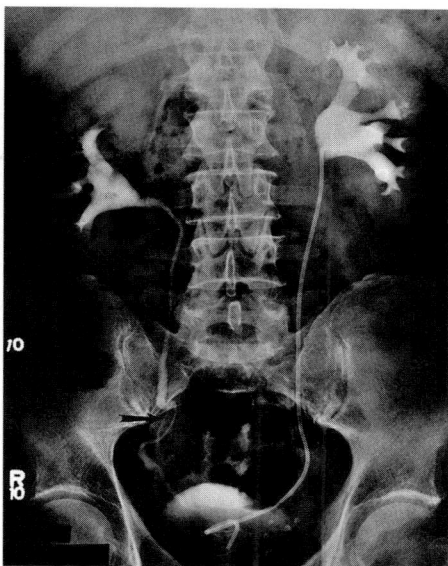

Figure 13–59. Retroiliac artery ureter, proved by angiography. (Ref: Hock E, Purkayastha A, Jay BD: Retroiliac ureter: A case report. *J Urology* 107:37, 1972.)

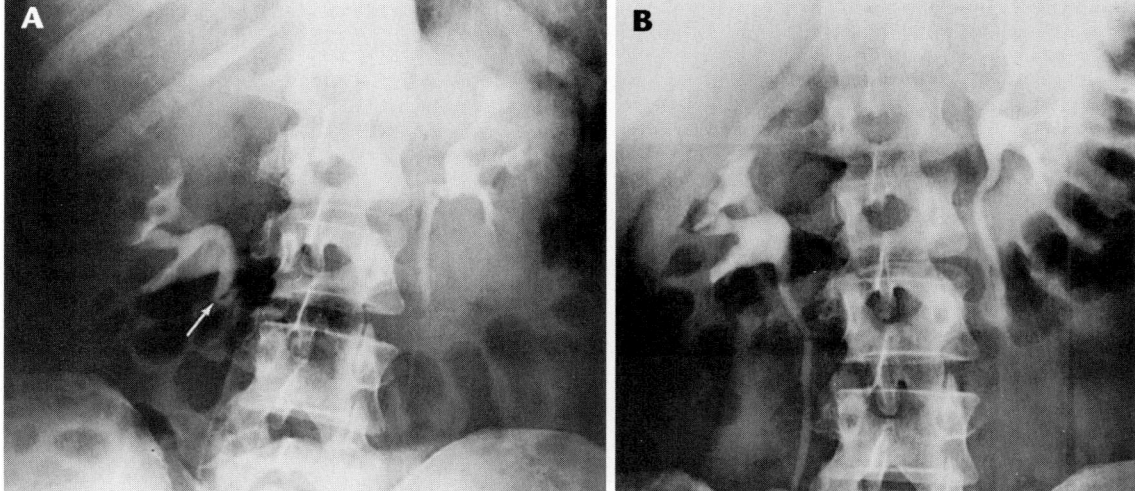

Figure 13–60. Effects of respiration on ureteral configuration. **A,** Inspiration. **B,** Expiration.

Figure 13–61. Visualization of the left ureter without a contrast agent, produced by periureteral fat.

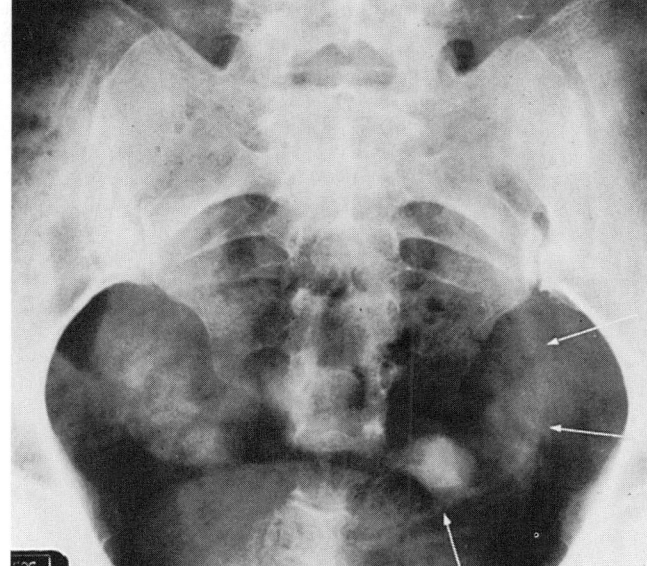

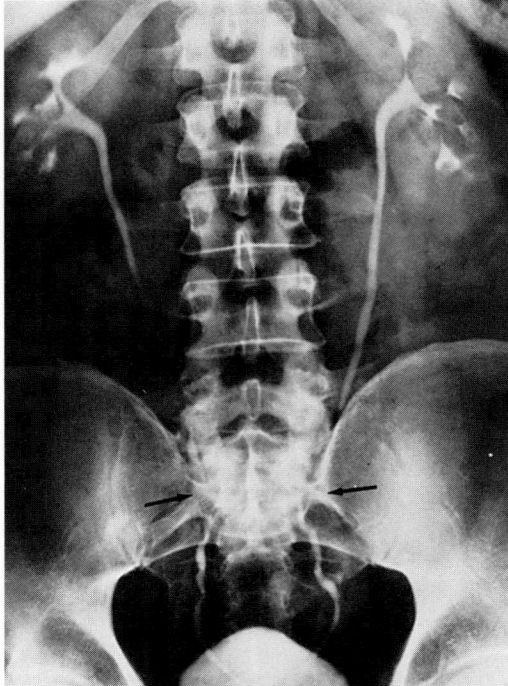

Figure 13–62. Medial deviation of the distal ureters as a normal variant caused by iliopsoas hypertrophy, and not secondary to retroperitoneal fibrosis. (Ref: Saldino RM, Palubinskas AJ: Medial placement of the ureters: A normal variant which may simulate retroperitoneal fibrosis. *J Urol* 107:582, 1972.)

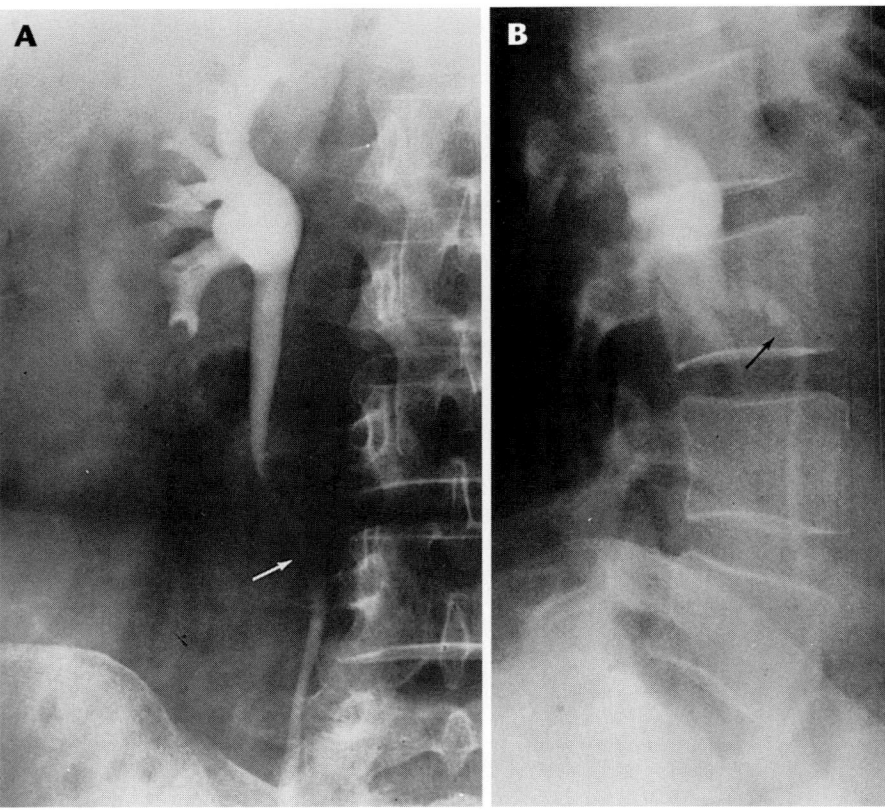

Figure 13–63. Ureteral displacement by hypertrophy of the iliopsoas muscles. This is a misleading finding, seen particularly in muscular young men, and may be unilateral. (Ref: Levine RB et al: Ureteral deviation due to iliopsoas hypertrophy. *Am J Roentgenol* 107:756, 1969.)

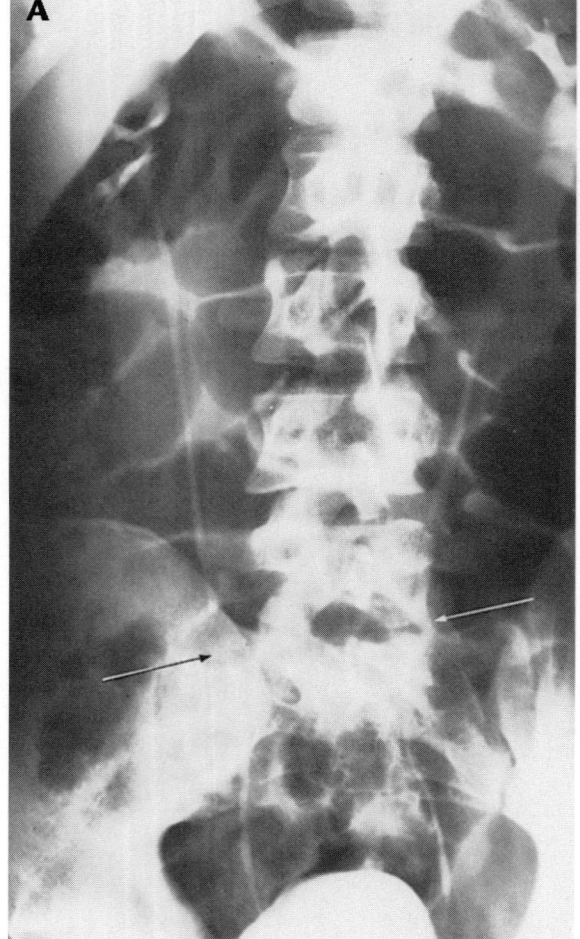

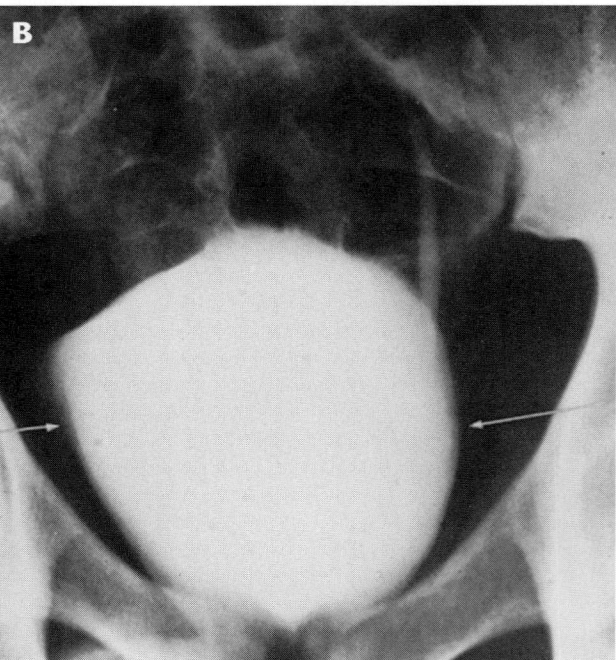

Figure 13–64. A, Medial deviation of the ureters by hypertrophied iliopsoas muscles. **B,** The muscles also produce medial displacement of the bladder. (Ref: Wechsler RJ, Brennan RE: Teardrop bladder: Additional considerations. *Radiology* 144:281, 1982.)

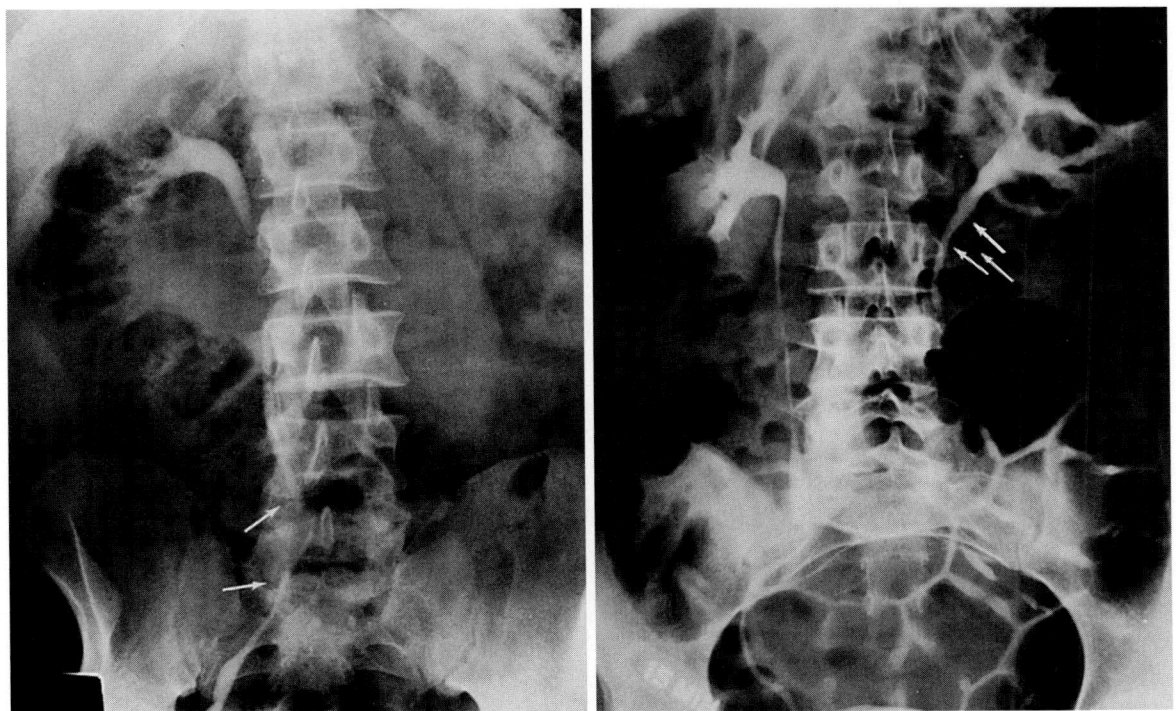

Figure 13–65. Two examples of unilateral deviation of the ureter caused by unilateral iliopsoas hypertrophy, both proved at laparotomy. (Ref: Ziter FMH: Unilateral ureteral deviation due to iliopsoas muscle hypertrophy. *J Can Assoc Radiol* 25:327, 1974.)

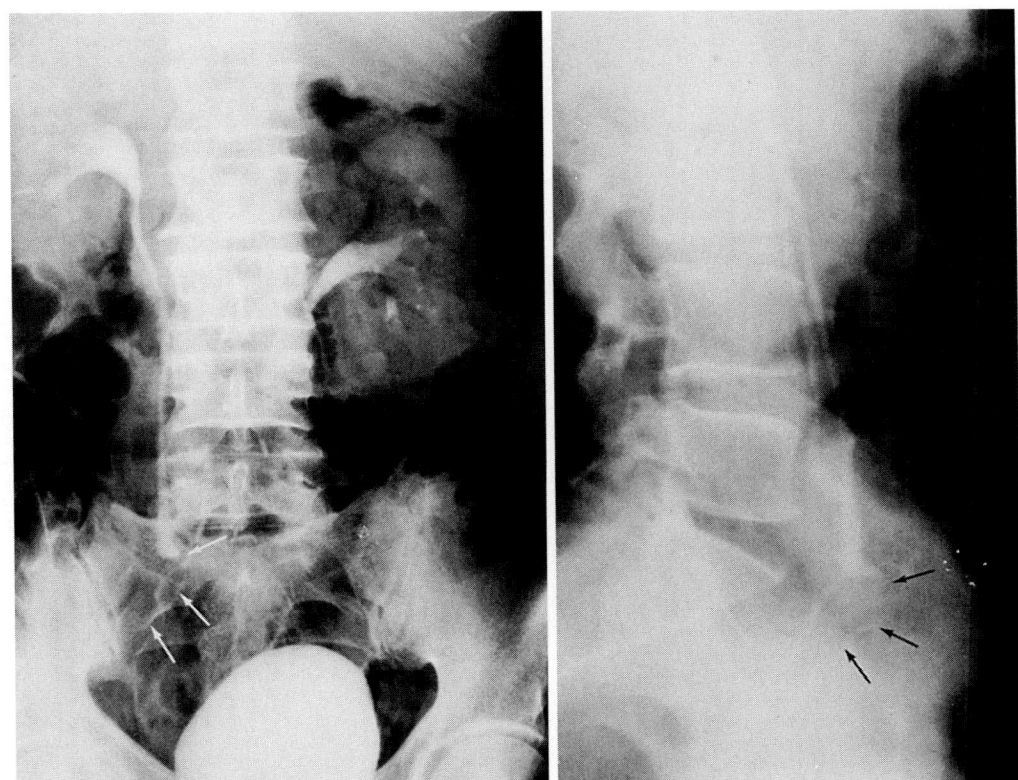

Figure 13–66. Deviation of the distal right ureter, produced by an ectatic iliac artery in an elderly man.

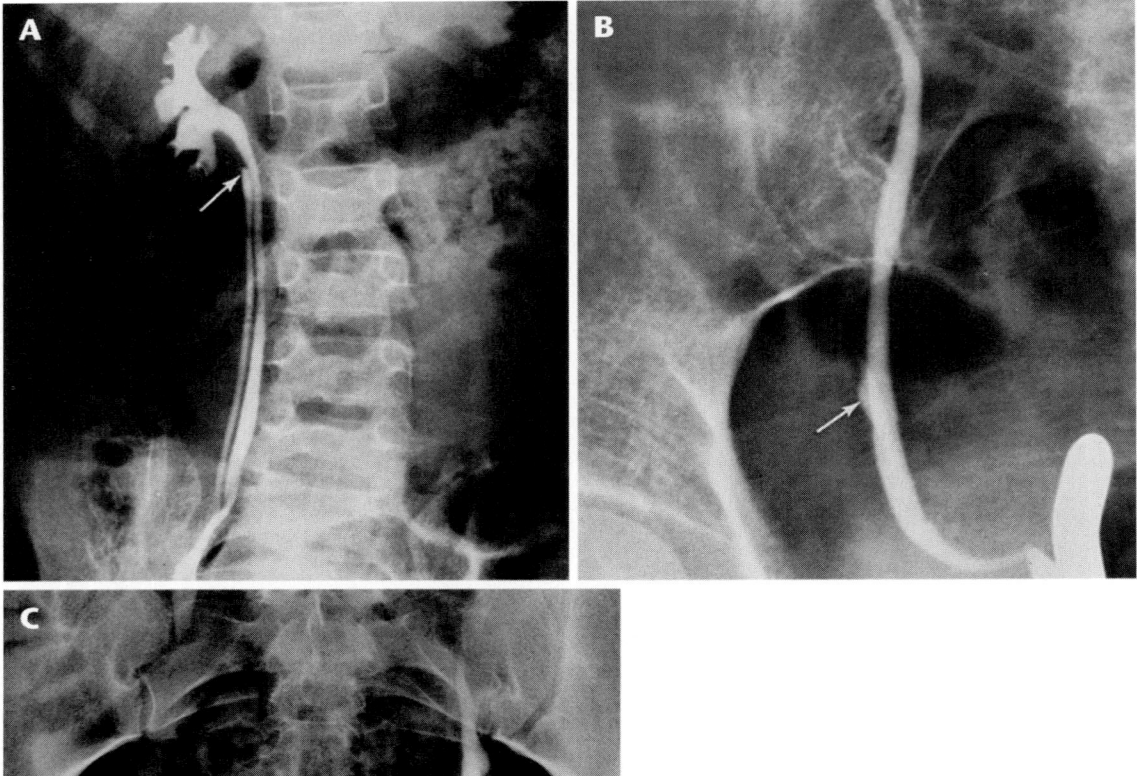

Figure 13–67. Three examples of blind duplication of the ureters. **A,** Termination at the renal pelvis. **B** and **C,** Termination in the pelvis. (Ref: Albers DD et al: Blind-ending branch of a bifid ureter: Report of three cases. *J Urol* 99:160, 1968.)

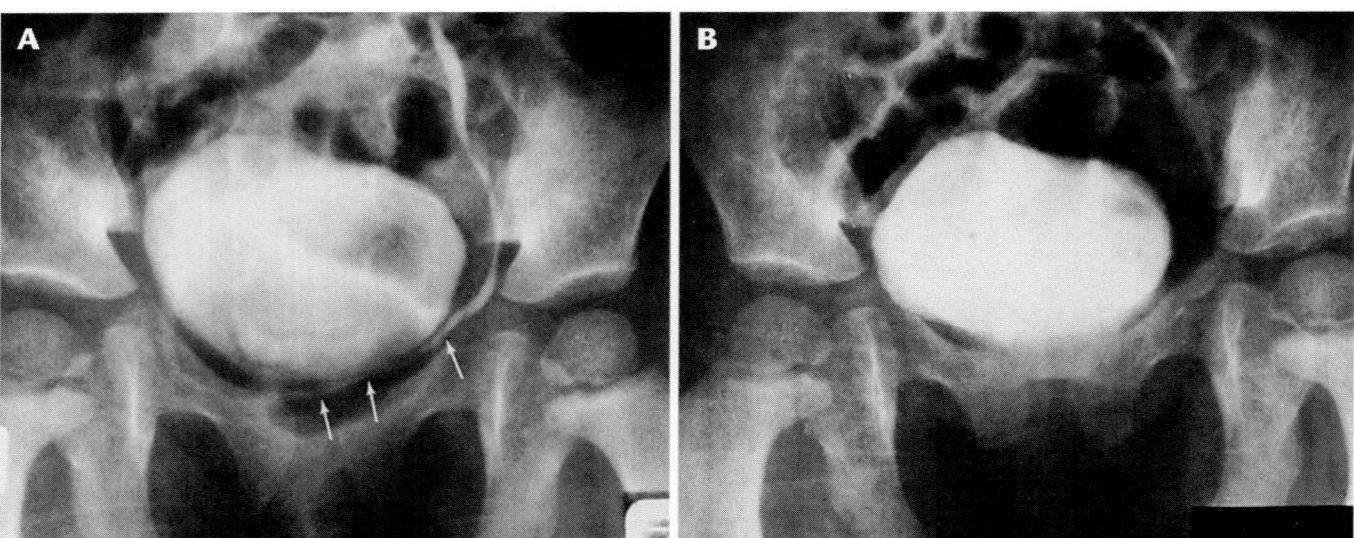

Figure 13–68. A, Pseudoectopic ureter seen in the prone position, in which the contrast material in the bladder gravitates toward the head into the dependent anterior dome and leaves the trigone area filled with nonopacified urine. The distal ureters appear to extend below the bladder. **B,** Supine film does not show the same effect seen in **A.** (Ref: Riggs W Jr, Seibert J: Pseudoectopic ureter on prone urogram. *Radiology* 106:391, 1973.)

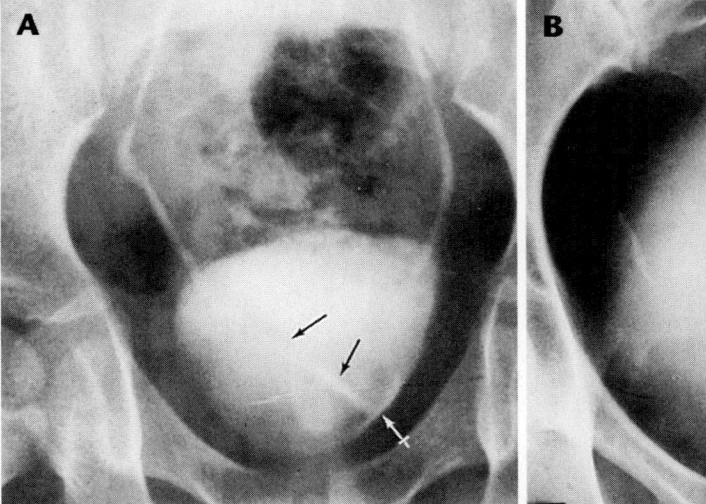
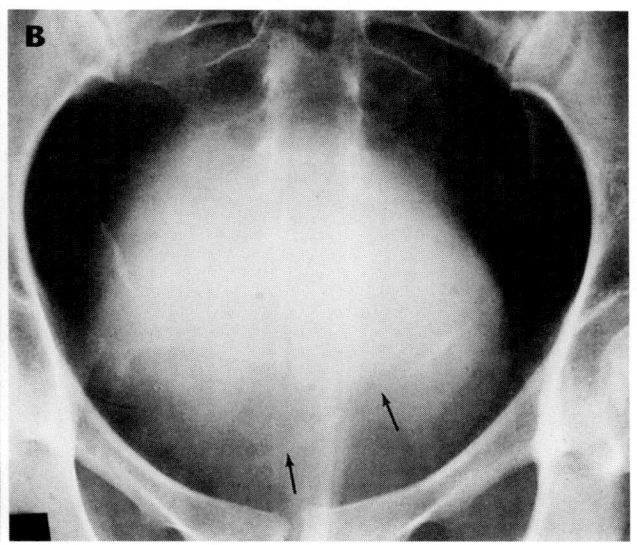

Figure 13–69. A, B, Two examples of the ureteral jet phenomenon. A stream of opaque medium leaving the ureter may simulate an anomalous configuration of the ureter. Note the impaction of the jet on the bladder wall in **A** (↔). (Ref: Kalmon EH et al: Ureteral jet phenomenon, stream of opaque medium simulating anomalous configuration of ureter. *Radiology* 65:933, 1955.)

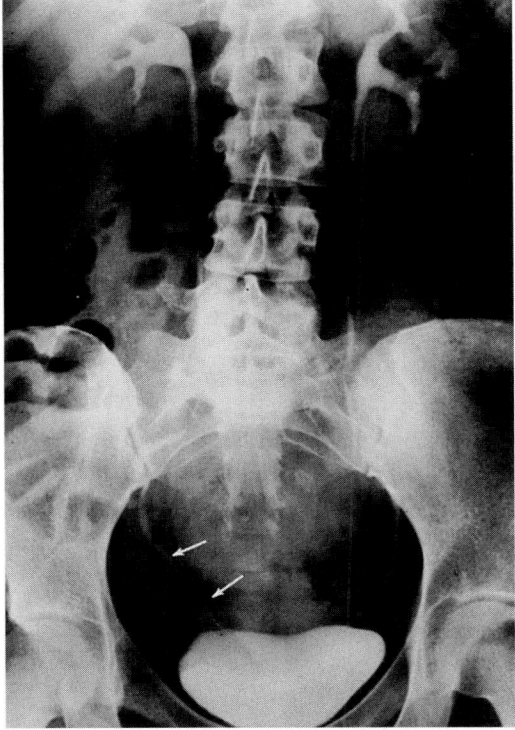

Figure 13–70. Asymmetry of the pelvic ureters in normal females, with medial deviation of the distal right ureter, is a normal variation. (Ref: Kabakian HA et al: Asymmetry of the pelvic ureters in normal females. *Am J Roentgenol* 127:723, 1976.)

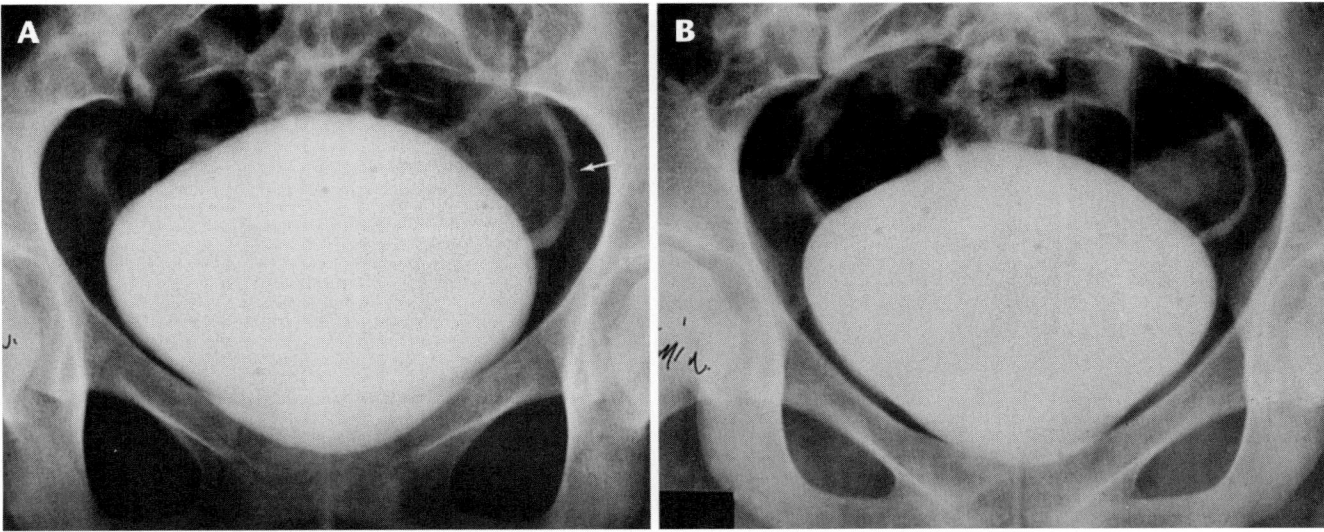

Figure 13–71. A, Apparent filling defect in the distal left ureter, resulting from peristalsis. **B,** After peristaltic wave has passed, the impression is no longer seen.

The Bladder

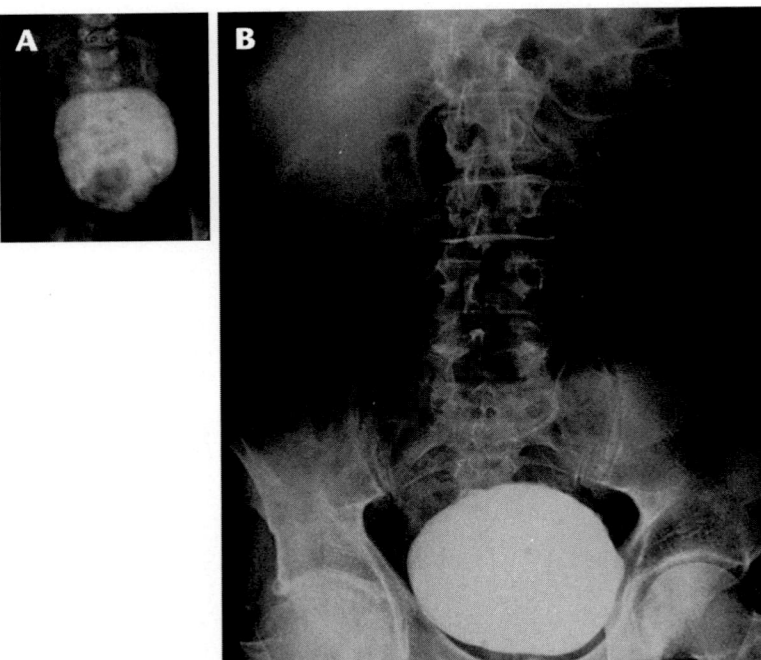

Figure 13–72. Proportional difference in size between the bladder and the total abdomen in the infant **(A)** and adult **(B)**. The bladder in the infant (as well as in the child) is capable of a much greater proportional degree of distention. (From Keats TE: Pediatric radiology: Some potentially misleading variations from the adult. *VA Med* 93:630, 1966.)

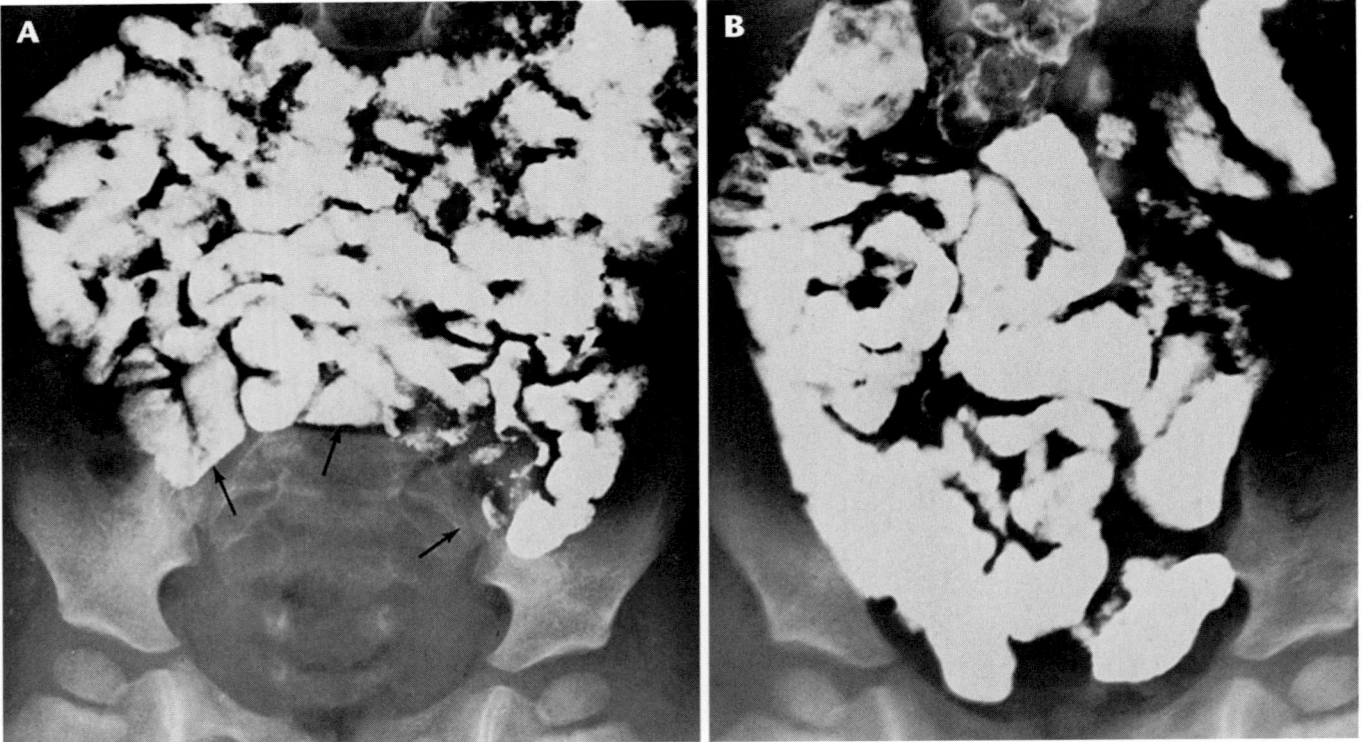

Figure 13–73. **A,** Normal distention of the bladder in a 2-year-old child, displacing the small bowel. **B,** After voiding.

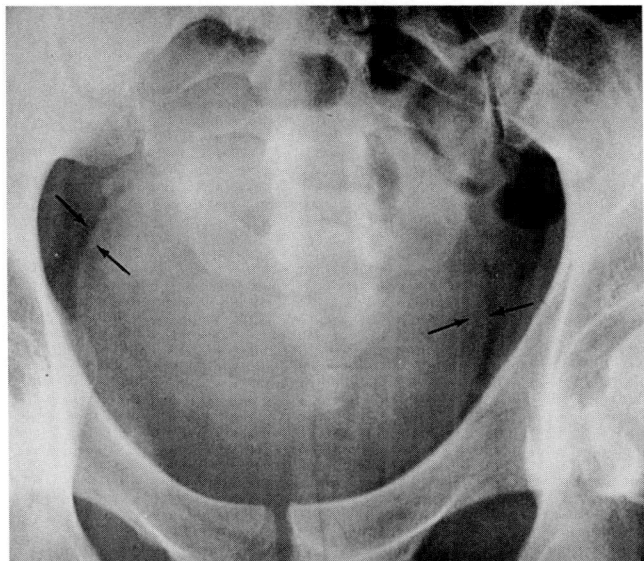

Figure 13–74. Visualization of the bladder wall as a result of the difference in radiographic density between muscle and urine and perivesical fat.

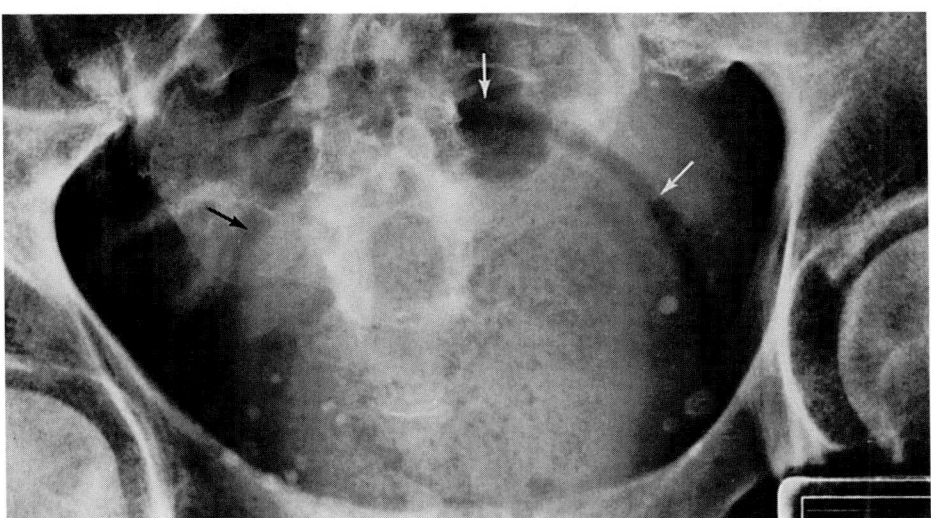

Figure 13–75. Perivesical fat producing an appearance simulating emphysematous cystitis.

Figure 13–76. "Bladder ears," a transitory extraperitoneal herniation of the bladder in infants. This is believed to represent a transient variation in normal development. (Ref: Allen RP, Condon VR: Transitory extraperitoneal hernia of the bladder in infants. *Radiology* 77:979, 1961.)

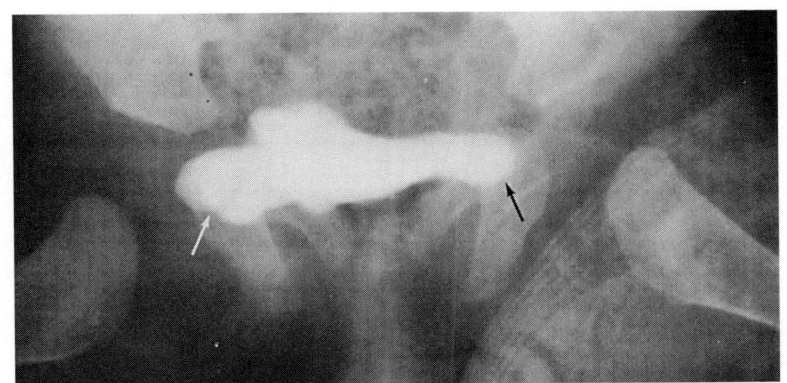

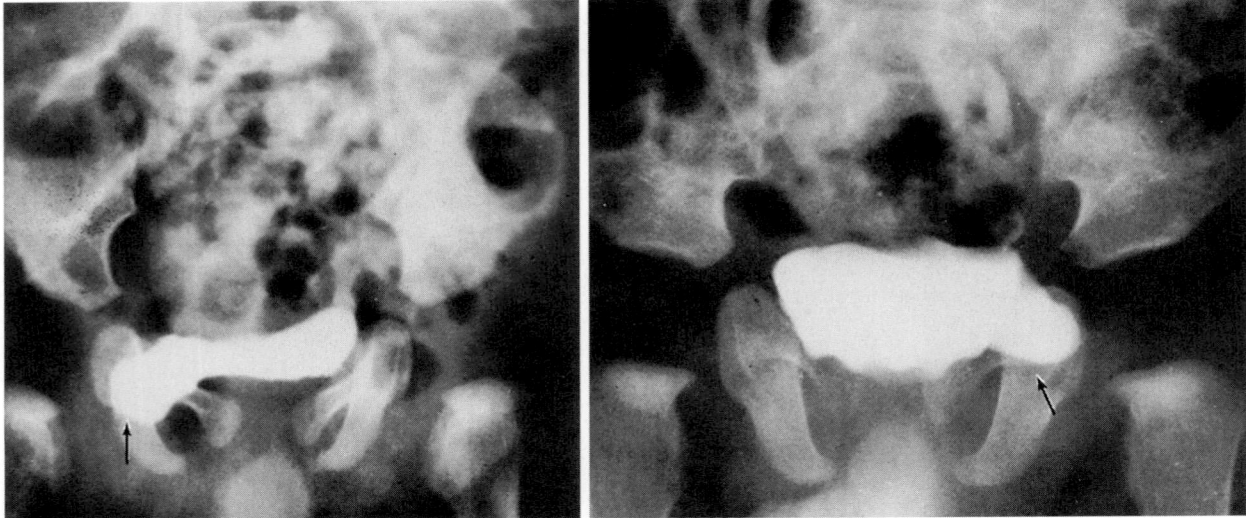

Figure 13–77. Examples of unilateral "bladder ears."

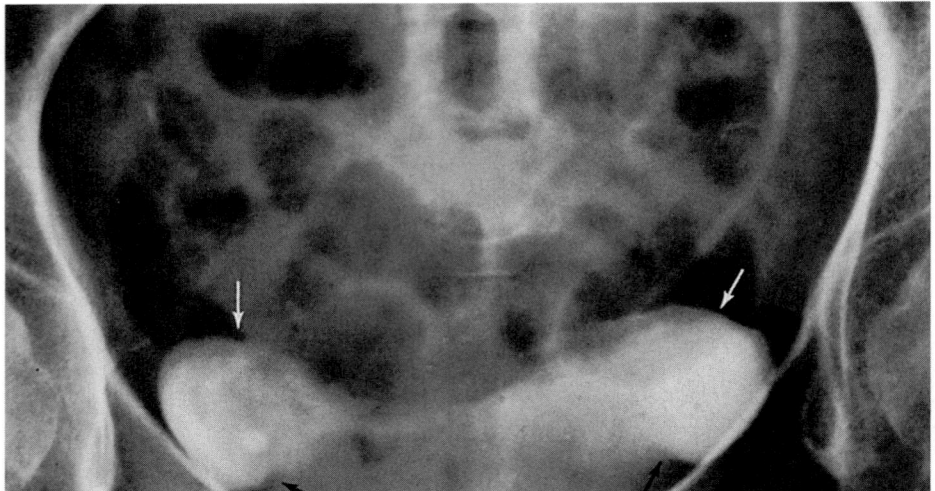

Figure 13–78. "Bladder ears" in a 53-year-old woman caused by laxity of the inguinal rings.

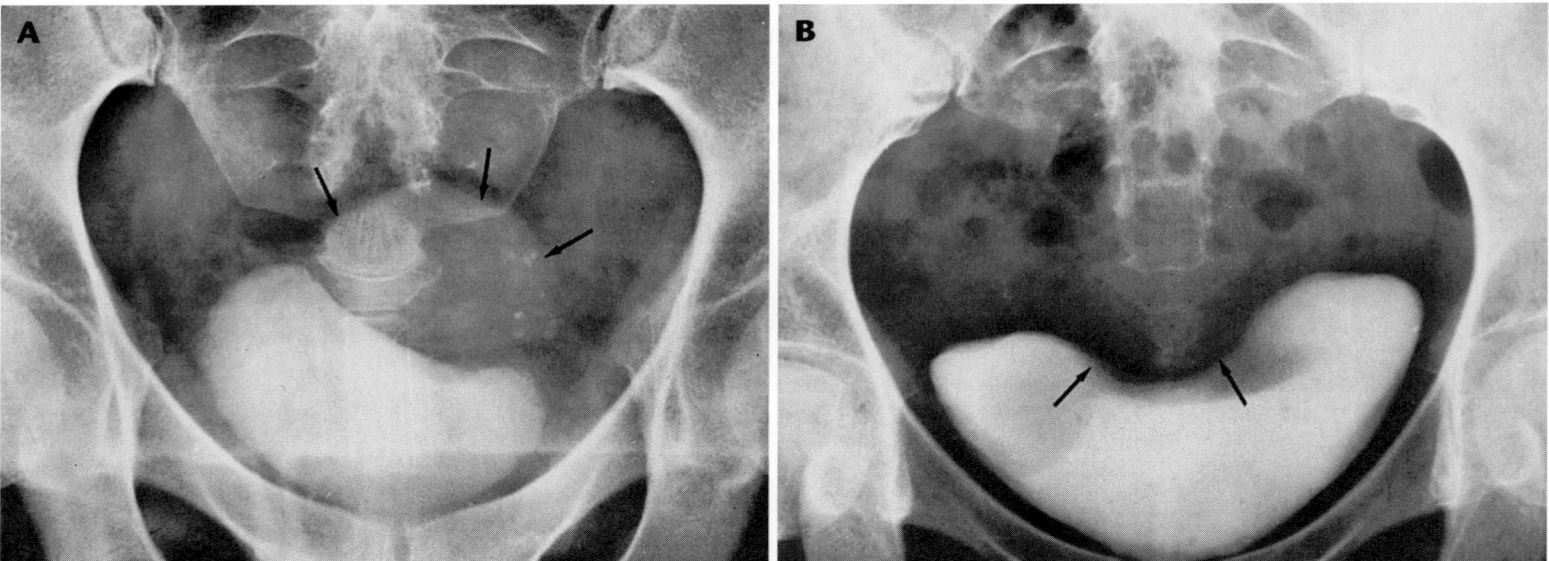

Figure 13–79. Two patients demonstrating uterine impression on the bladder. **A,** Shadow of the uterus is seen indenting the bladder. **B,** Shadow of the uterus is not seen above the impression on the bladder.

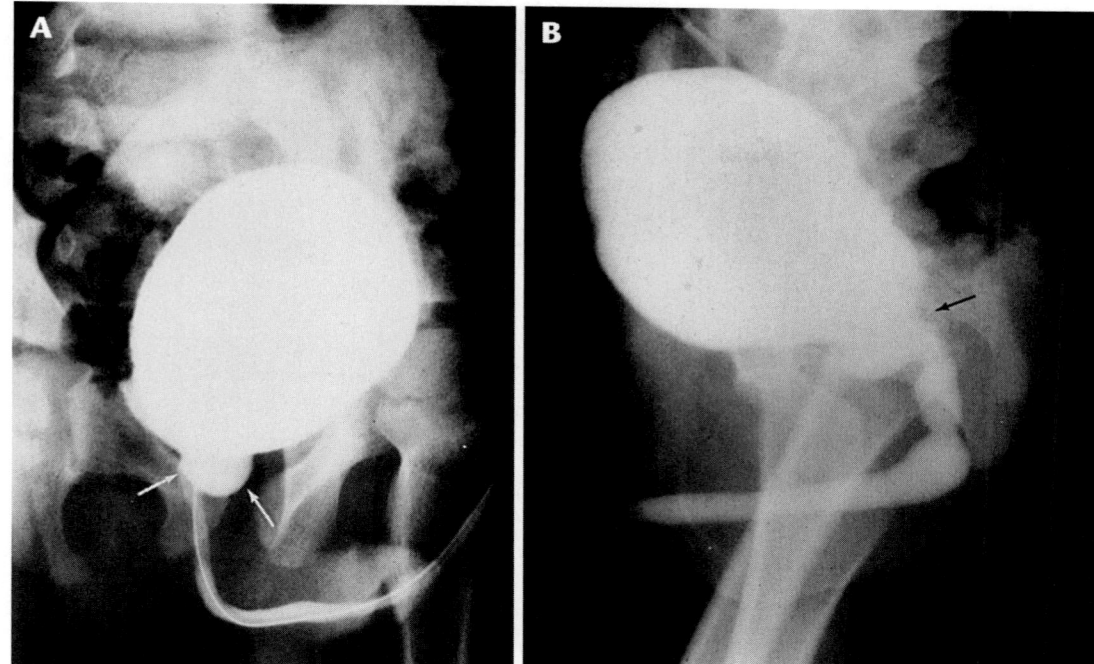

Figure 13–80. Normal physiologic variations in the contour of the base of the bladder during voiding. Note the asymmetric urethral distention in **A** (→) and the indentation produced posteriorly by the trigonal plate in **B** (→). (Ref: Shopfner CE, Hutch JA: The normal urethrogram. *Radiol Clin North Am* 6:165, 1968.)

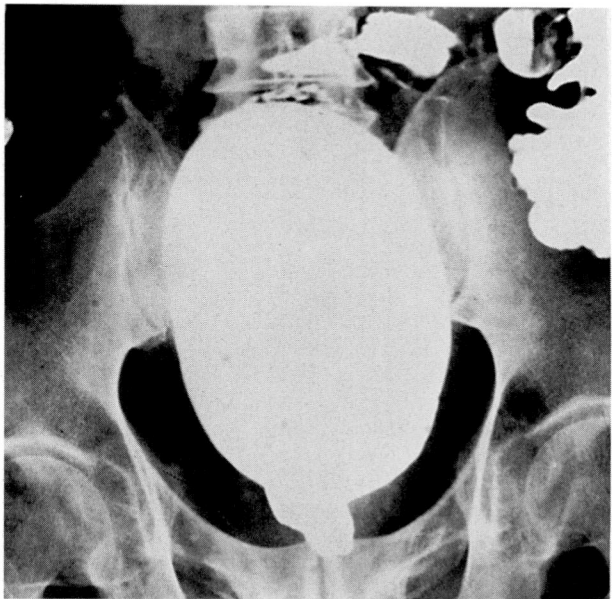

Figure 13–81. Elevation and elongation of the bladder, caused by accumulation of large amounts of fat in the pelvis. (Ref: Fogg LB, Smyth JW: Pelvic lipomatosis: A condition simulating pelvic neoplasm. *Radiology* 90:558, 1968.)

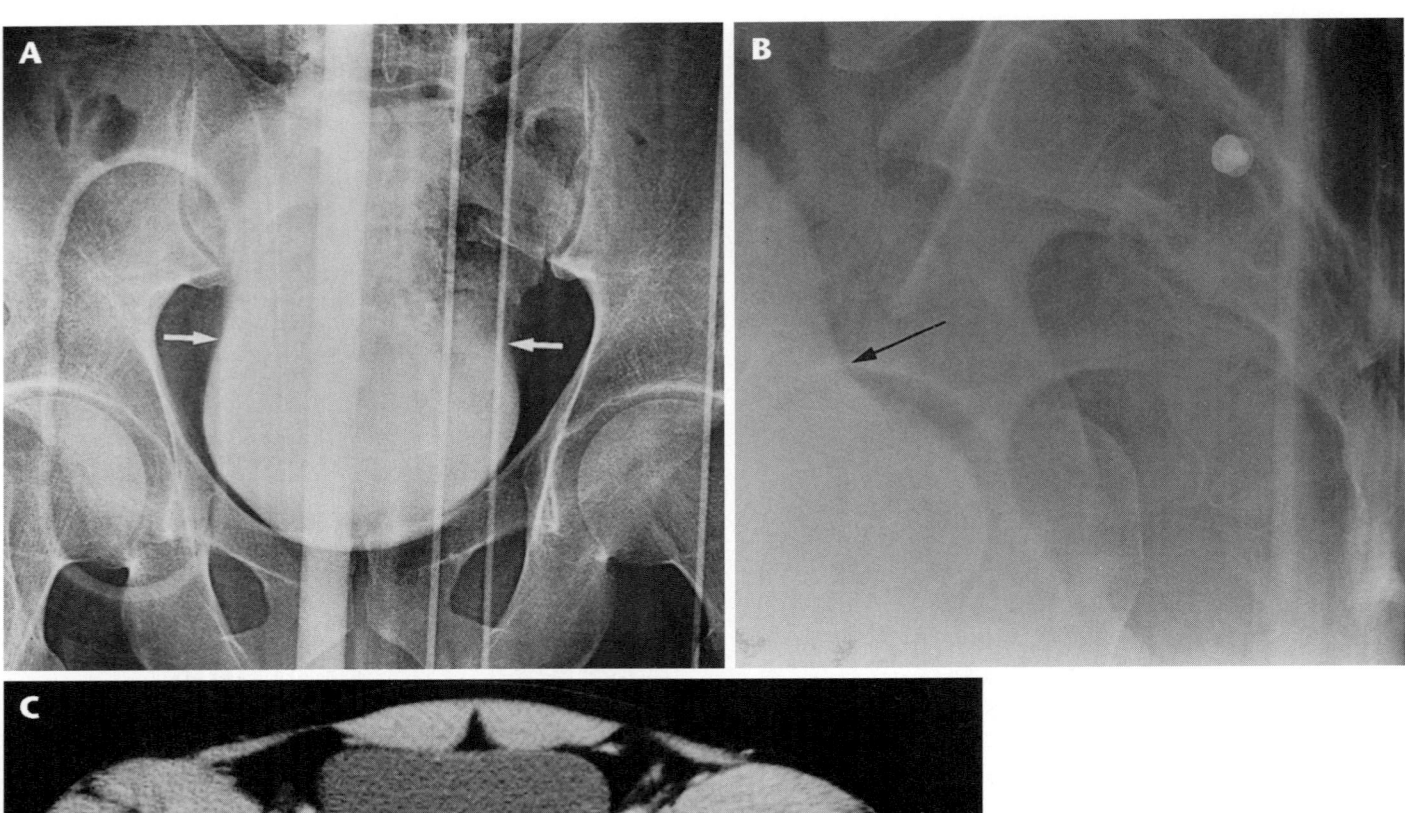

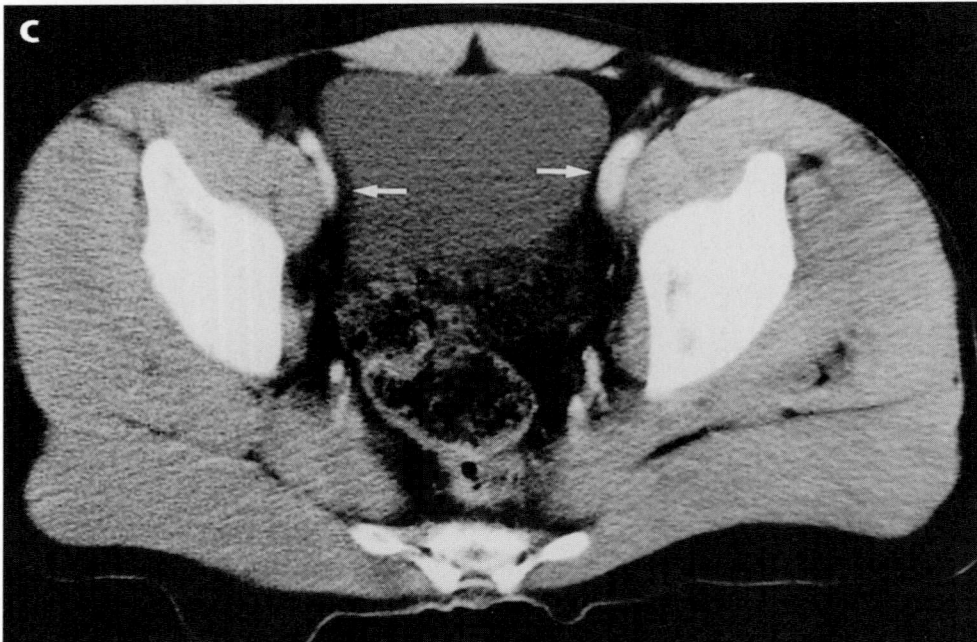

Figure 13–82. Unusual configuration of the bladder due to large psoas muscles. **A,** Frontal projection. **B,** Lateral projection. **C,** CT.

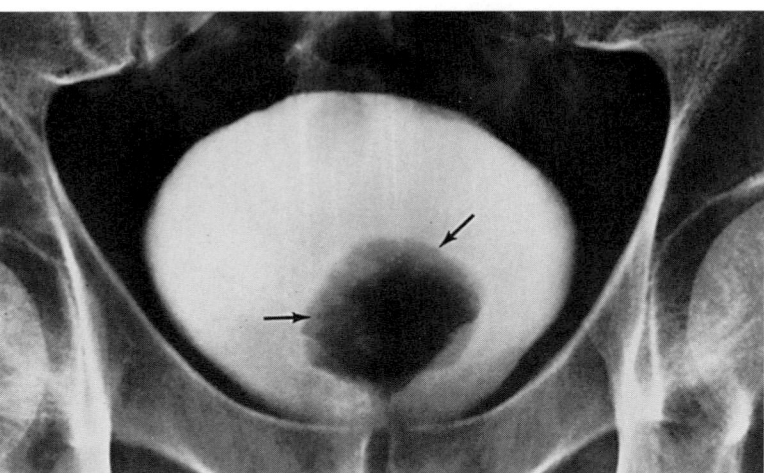

Figure 13–83. Gas in the rectum seen as a radiolucency within the contrast-filled bladder, simulating the filling defect of a bladder neoplasm.

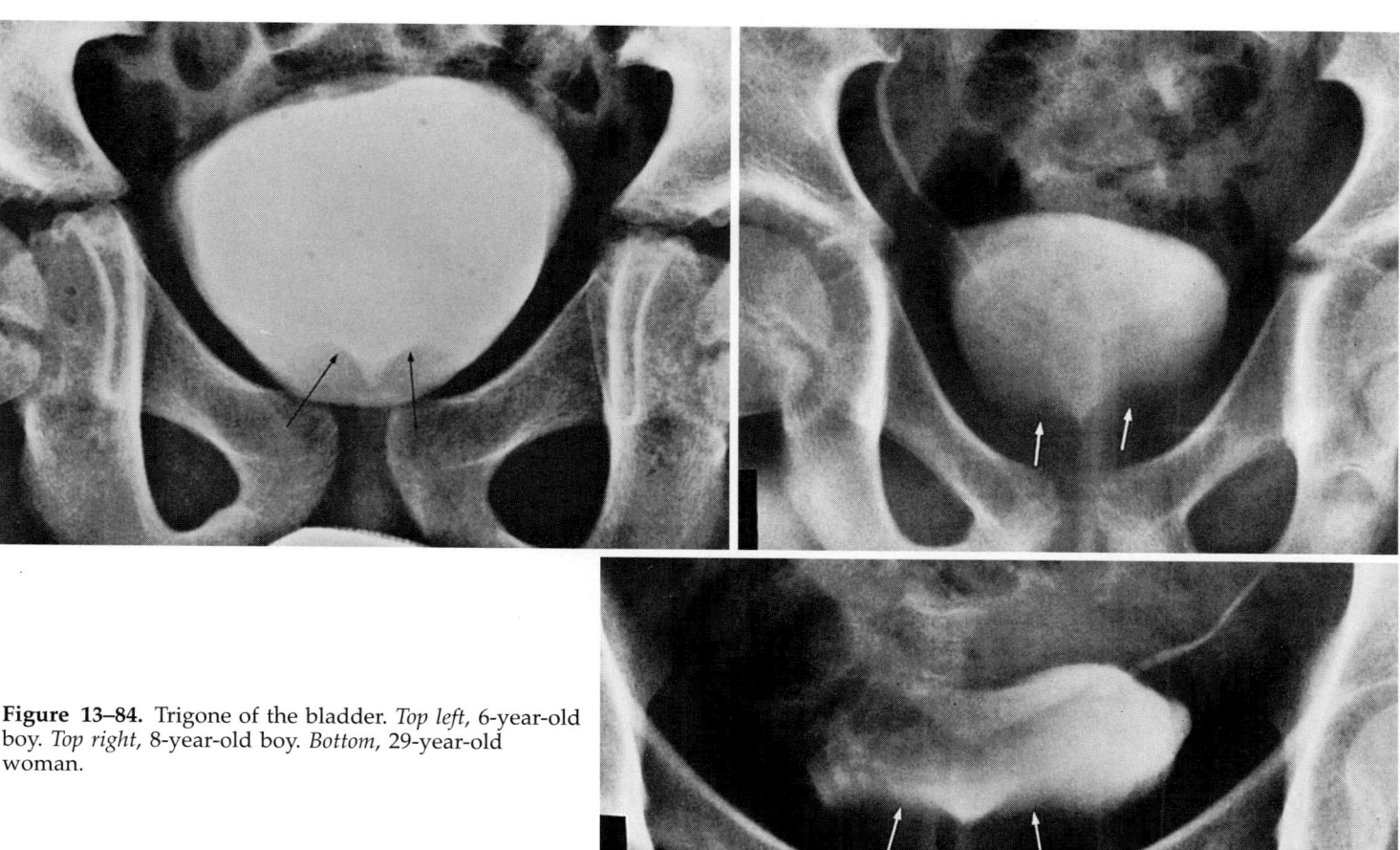

Figure 13–84. Trigone of the bladder. *Top left,* 6-year-old boy. *Top right,* 8-year-old boy. *Bottom,* 29-year-old woman.

Figure 13–85. The "female prostate," an indentation in the base of the bladder produced by asymmetry of the symphysis pubis. (Ref: Pope TL Jr et al: Bladder base impressions in women: "Female prostate." *Am J Roentgenol* 136:1105, 1981.)

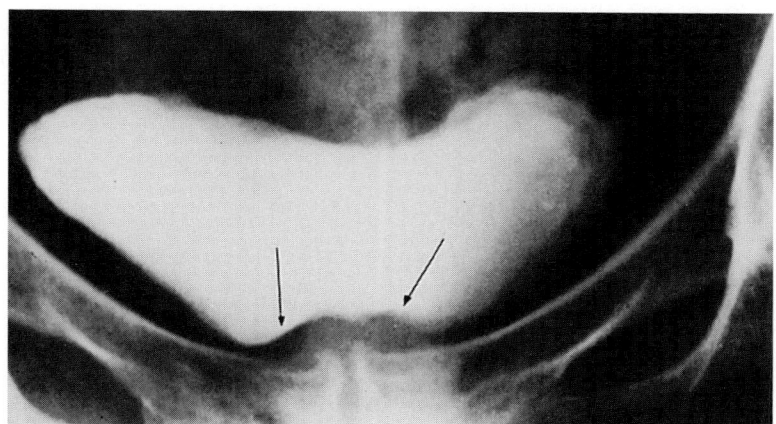

The Urethra

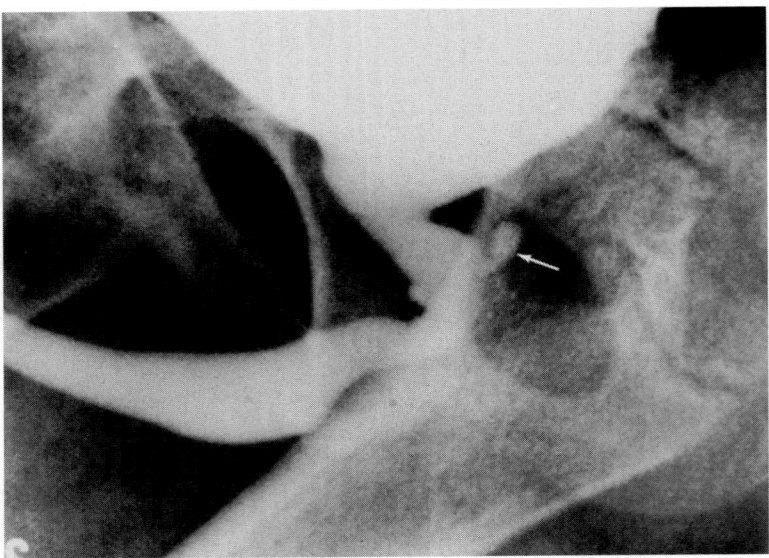

Figure 13–86. Prostatic utricle in an 8-year-old boy, not to be mistaken for a diverticulum.

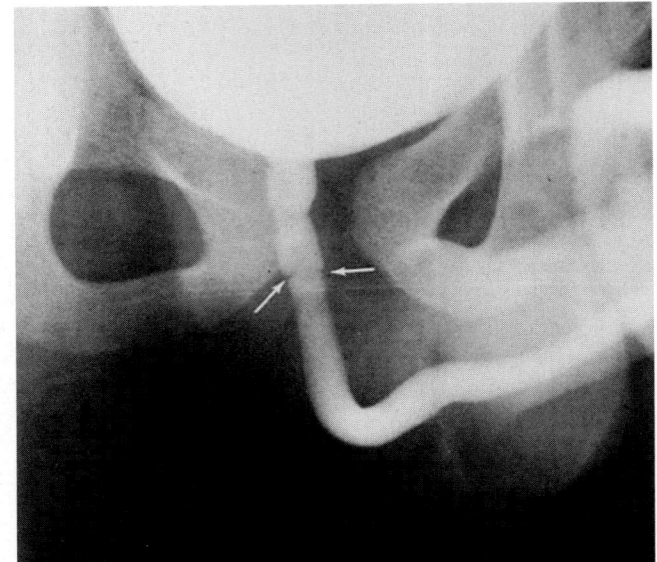

Figure 13–87. Plicae colliculi, not to be mistaken for valves.

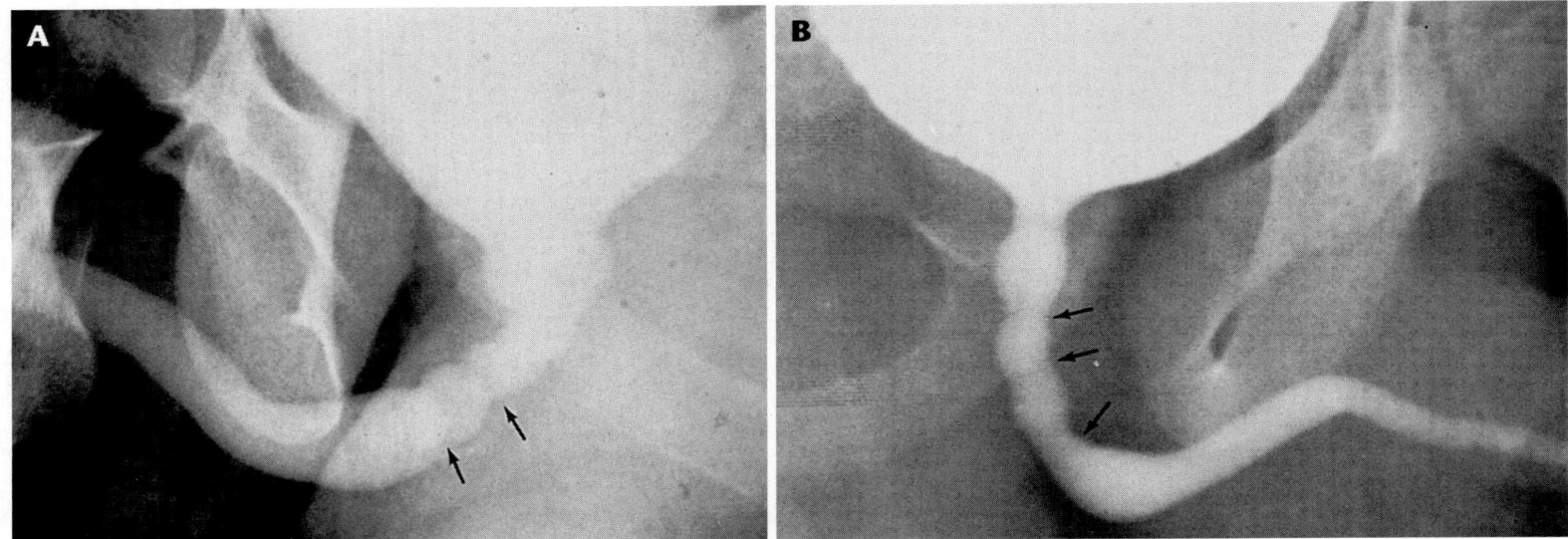

Figure 13–88. Two examples of normal intermuscular incisurae of the posterior urethra. **A,** 19-year-old man. **B,** 11-year-old boy. (Ref: Shopfner CE, Hutch JA: The normal urethrogram. *Radiol Clin North Am* 6:165, 1968.)

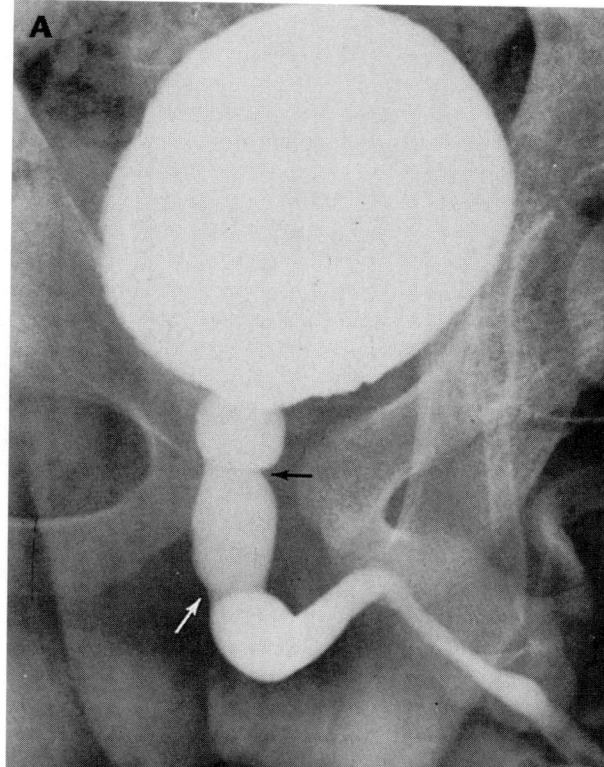

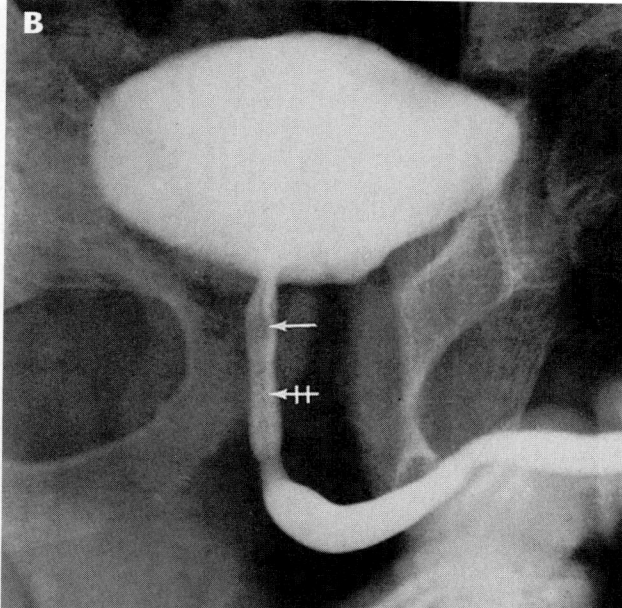

Figure 13–89. Another example of intermuscular incisurae of the posterior urethra in an 11-year-old boy. **A,** Urethra distended by retrograde injection. **B,** During voiding. Note the shadows of the verumontanum (←) and mucosal folds (←⊩).

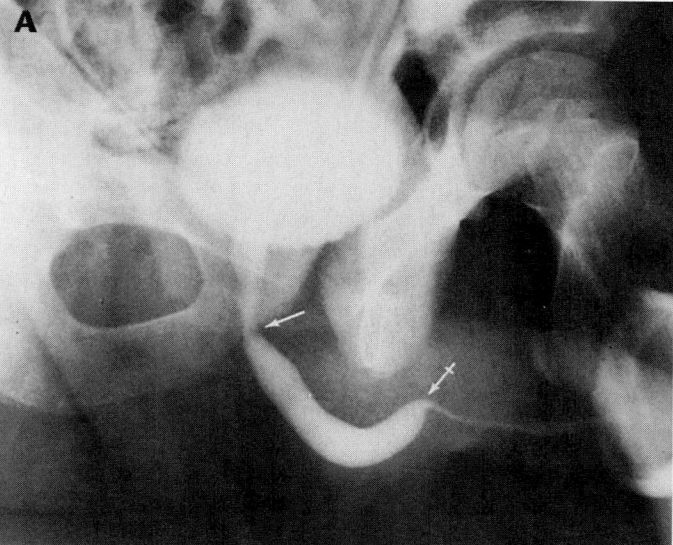

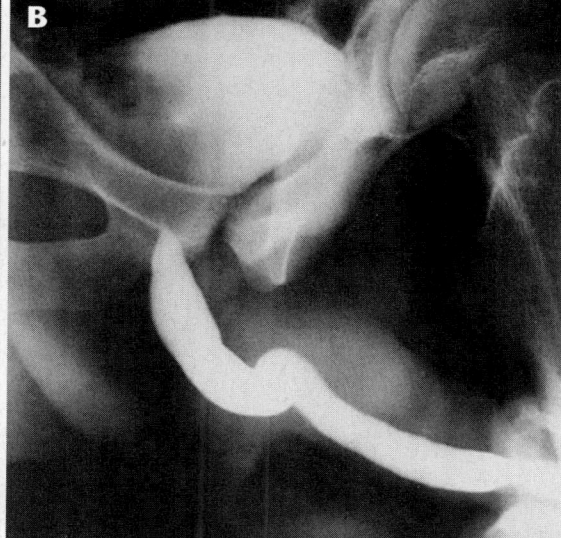

Figure 13–90. A, Voiding film. The external sphincter (→) and the insertion point of the suspensory ligament of the penis (↦) should not be mistaken for areas of organic narrowing. **B,** Retrograde examination.

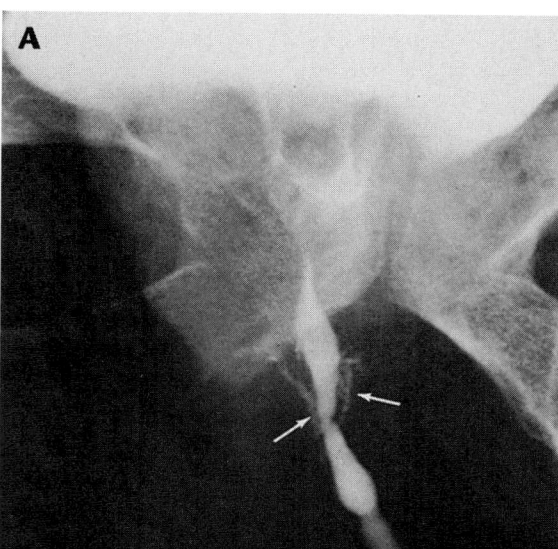

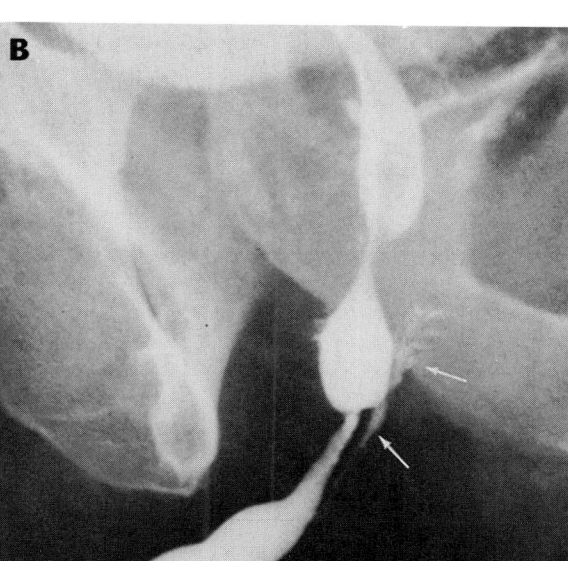

Figure 13–91. Cowper's glands, not to be mistaken for false passages.

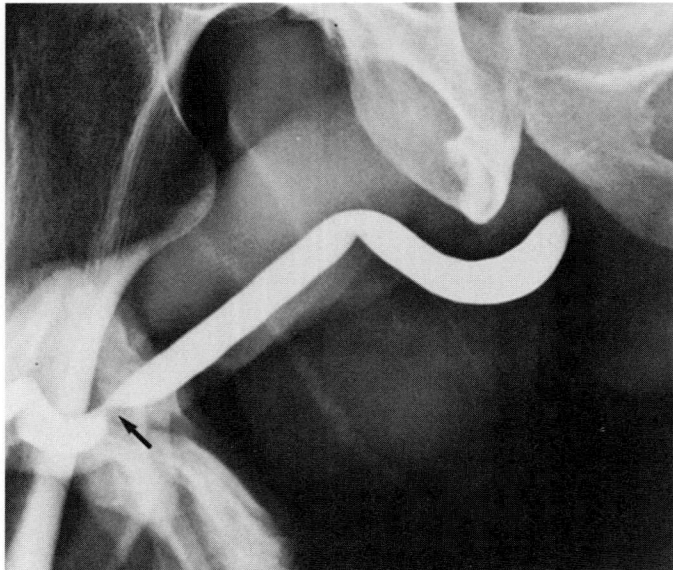

Figure 13–92. Finger pressure producing an apparent stricture of the urethra. A similar defect can be produced by pressure on the lip of the collecting receptacle. (Ref: Lebowitz RL: Pseudostricture of the urethra: Urinal artifact on urethrography. *Am J Roentgenol* 130:570, 1978.)

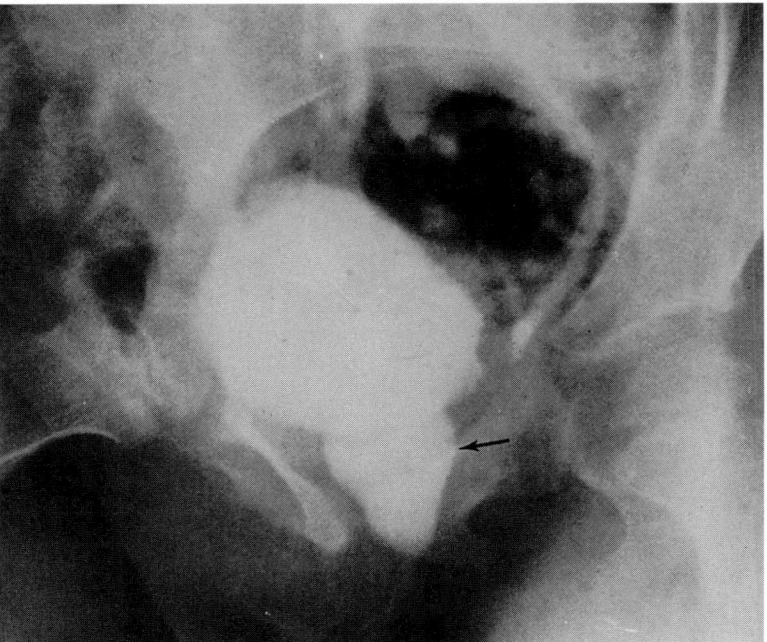

Figure 13–93. The "spinning top" urethra in a 6-year-old girl. This is believed to be a normal appearance seen in forceful voiding and is not the product of distal obstruction. (Ref: Whitaker J, Johnson GS: Correlation of urethral resistance and shape in girls. *Radiology* 91:757, 1968.) It has been stated that this configuration is the result of unstable contractions that are resisted by a voluntary increase in distal sphincter tension to prevent leakage of urine, and that it does not represent a normal variant. (Ref: Saxton HM et al: Spinning top urethra: Not a normal variant. *Radiology* 168:147, 1988.)

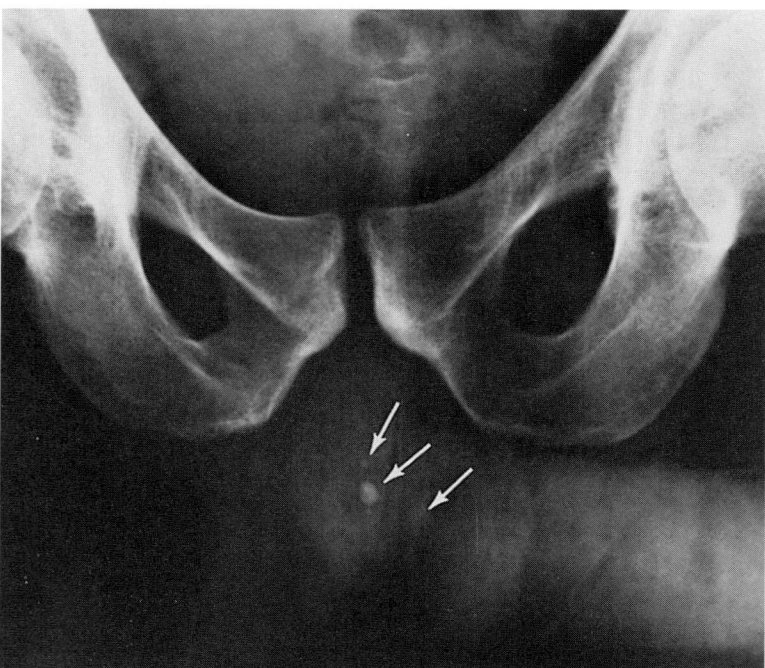

Figure 13–94. Phleboliths in the corpora cavernosa in a 40-year-old man, simulating urethral calculi.

The Genital Tract

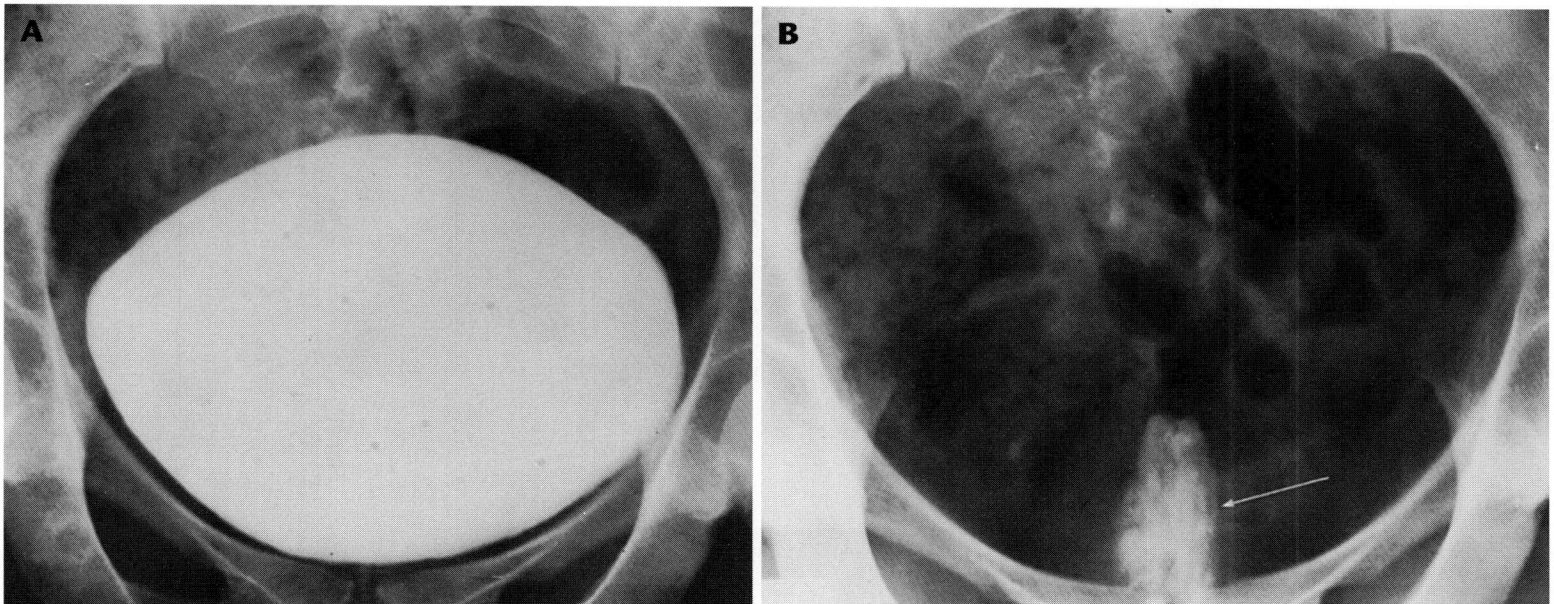

Figure 13–95. Intravaginal voiding. **A,** Cystogram. **B,** Vaginal residue.

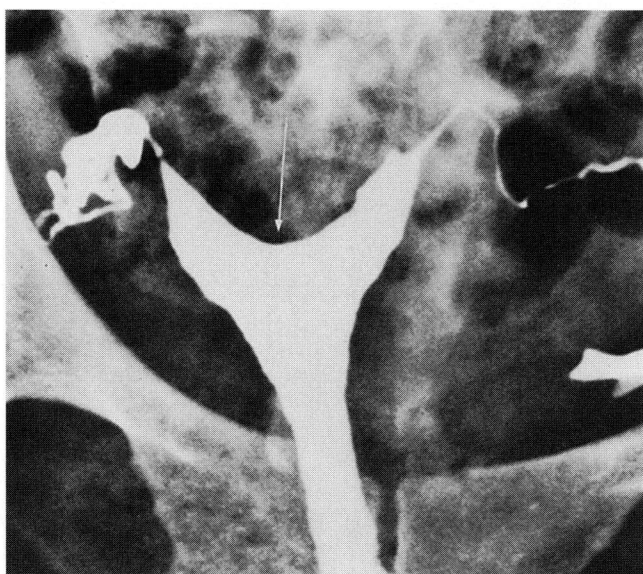

Figure 13–96. Arcuate uterus seen by hysterosalpingography. The impression in the fundus was misinterpreted as a myoma.

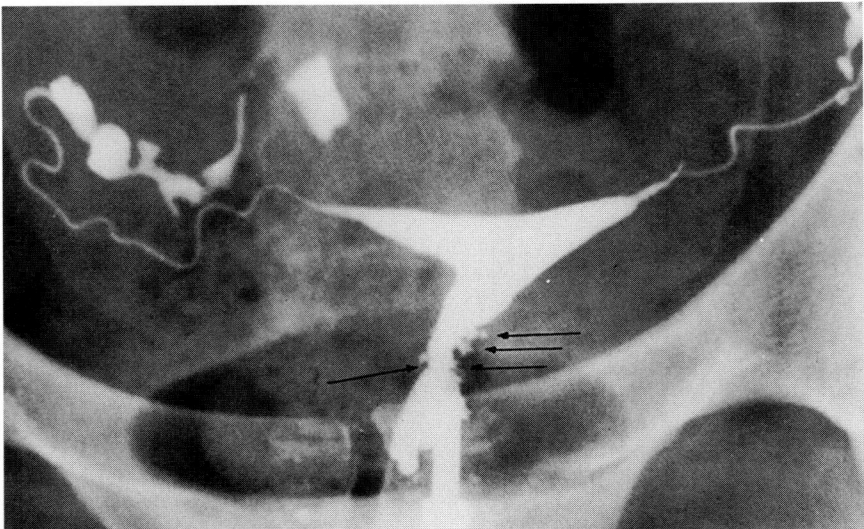

Figure 13–97. Normal filling of the endocervical glands on hysterosalpingography.

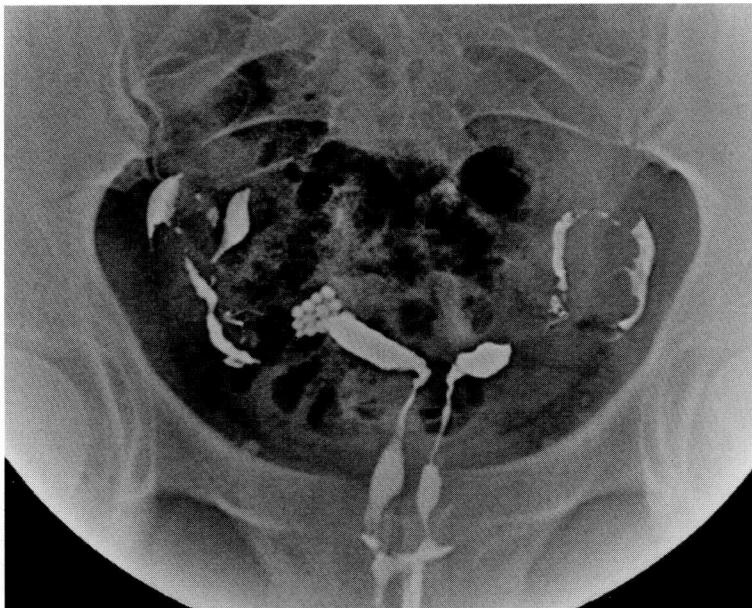

Figure 13–98. Uterus didelphys and complete vaginal septum constituting duplication of the vagina and uterus. (Ref: O'Neill MJ et al: Imaging evaluation and classification of developmental anomalies of the female reproductive system. *Am J Roentgenol* 173:407, 1999.)

Index